Burns' Pediatric Primary Care

Burns' Pediatric Primary Care

SEVENTH EDITION

Editors

Dawn Lee Garzon Maaks, PhD, CPNP-PC, PMHS, FAANP, FAAN

Clinical Professor
College of Nursing
Washington State University Vancouver
Vancouver, Washington

Nancy Barber Starr, MS, RN, CPNP

Pediatric Nurse Practitioner
Advanced Pediatric Associates
Centennial, Colorado

Margaret A. Brady, PhD, RN, CPNP-PC

Professor
School of Nursing
California State University Long Beach
Long Beach, California

Nan M. Gaylord PhD, RN, CPNP-PC, PMHS, FAANP, FAAN

Professor
College of Nursing
University of Tennessee
Knoxville, Tennessee

Martha Driessnack, PhD, PNP-BC

Associate Professor
School of Nursing
Oregon Health & Science University
Portland, Oregon

Karen G. Duderstadt, PhD, RN, CPNP, FAAN

Clinical Professor, Emerita
Department of Family Health Care Nursing
School of Nursing
University of California San Francisco
San Francisco, California

Associate Editor

Mary Dirks, DNP, RN, ARNP, CPNP-PC, FAANP

Clinical Professor and Assistant Dean for Graduate Practice
    Programs
College of Nursing
University of Iowa
Iowa City, Iowa

ELSEVIER

Elsevier
3251 Riverport Lane
St. Louis, Missouri 63043

Notice

Practitioners and researchers must always rely on their own experience and knowledge in evaluating and using any information, methods, compounds or experiments described herein. Because of rapid advances in the medical sciences, in particular, independent verification of diagnoses and drug dosages should be made. To the fullest extent of the law, no responsibility is assumed by Elsevier, authors, editors or contributors for any injury and/or damage to persons or property as a matter of products liability, negligence or otherwise, or from any use or operation of any methods, products, instructions, or ideas contained in the material herein.

Previous editions copyrighted 2017, 2013, 2009, 2004, 2000, and 1996.

Library of Congress Control Number: 2019939392

Senior Content Strategist: Sandy Clark
Senior Content Development Specialist: Laura Goodrich
Publishing Services Manager: Catherine Jacksoon
Senior Project Manager: Sharon Corell
Design Direction: Maggie Reid

Printed in Canada

Last digit is the print number: 9   8   7   6   5   4   3   2   1

Working together
to grow libraries in
developing countries

www.elsevier.com • www.bookaid.org

Contributors

Sandra Ann Banta-Wright, PhD, RN, NNP-BC
Assistant Clinical Professor
Pediatric Nurse Practitioner Program
Oregon Health & Science University
Portland, Oregon

Jennifer Bevacqua, RN, MS, CPNP-AC, CPNP-PC
Instructor, Pediatric Nurse Practitioner Program
Oregon Health & Science University
Portland, Oregon

Tami B. Bland, DNP, PNP-PC
Clinical Assistant Professor
College of Nursing
University of Tennessee, Knoxville
Knoxville, Tennessee

Catherine Blosser, MPA, HA, RN, PNP
Pediatric Nurse Practitioner, Retired
Multnomah County Health Department
Portland, Oregon

Cris Ann Bowman-Harvey, RN, MSN, CPNP-PC, CPNP-AC
Emergency Department
Children's Hospital Colorado
Aurora, Colorado
Faculty
Department of Pediatrics
University of Colorado
Denver, Colorado

Eliza Buyers, MD
Adolescent Gynecologist and Clinical Medical Director
Pediatric and Adolescent Gynecology
Children's Hospital Colorado
Senior Instructor
Department of Obstetrics and Gynecology
University of Colorado
Aurora, Colorado

Jennifer Chauvin, MA, BSN, RN-BC
DNP Candidate,
College of Nursing
Washington State University Vancouver
Vancouver, Washington

Donald L. Chi, DDS, PhD
Associate Professor
Oral Health Sciences
University of Washington
Seattle, Washington

Cynthia Marie Claytor, RN, MSN, PNP, FNP-C, CCRN
Graduate Nursing Faculty
Azusa Pacific University
Azusa, California

Daniel J. Crawford, DNP, RN, CPNP-PC, CNE
DNP Program Director
Clinical Assistant Professor
Edson College of Nursing and Health Innovation
Arizona State University
Phoenix, Arizona

Sandra Daack-Hirsch, PhD, RN, FAAN
Associate Professor
PhD Program Director
College of Nursing
The University of Iowa
Iowa City, Iowa

Renée Lynne Davis, DNP, APRN, CPNP-PC
Assistant Professor
School of Nursing
Saint Louis University
St. Louis, Missouri
Dr. Norman Pediatrics
Belleville, Illinois

Sara De Golier, BSN, MS, CPNP
Emergency Department
Children's Hospital Colorado
Aurora, Colorado

Ardys M. Dunn, PhD, RN, PNP
Associate Professor, Emeritus
School of Nursing
University of Portland
Portland, Oregon
Professor, Retired
School of Nursing
Samuel Merritt College
Oakland, California

Terea Giannetta, DNP, RN, CPNP, FAANP
Chief NP
Hematology
Valley Children's Hospital/Children's Hospital Central California
Madera, California
Professor, Emeritus
School of Nursing
California State University, Fresno
Fresno, California

Valerie Griffin, DNP, PPCNP-BC, FNP-BC, PMHS, FAANP
Assistant Clinical Professor
Director FNP Program
Southern Illinois University Edwardsville
Edwardsville, Illinois

Emily Gutierrez, DNP, C-PNP, PMHS, IFM-CP
Practice Owner
Neuronutrition Associates
Austin, Texas
Adjunct Faculty
School of Nursing
Johns Hopkins University
Baltimore, Texas

Susan Hines, RN, BSN, MSN, CPNP
Pediatric Pulmonary Medicine
Children's Hospital Colorado
Aurora, Colorado

Jennifer Michele Huson, MS, RN, CPNP, CNS
Nurse Practitioner
Pediatric Intensive Care
Children's Hospital Los Angeles
Los Angeles, California

Belinda James-Petersen, BS, MS, DNP, CPNP-PC
Pediatric Gastroenterology
Children's Hospital of The King's Daughters
Norfolk, Virginia

Rita Marie John, EdD, DNP, CPNP, PMHS, FAANP
Special Lecturer Consultant
Former PNP Program Director
Columbia University School of Nursing
Hillsborough, New Jersey

Victoria Keeton, MS, RN, CPNP, CNS
Clinical Professor
School of Nursing Department of Family Care Nursing
University of California San Francisco
Pediatric Nurse Practitioner
Children's Health Center
Zuckerberg San Francisco General Hospital and Trauma Center
San Francisco, California

Michelle McGarry, MSN, RN, CPNP, CUNP, FAANP
Certified Pediatric and Urology Nurse Practitioner/Program
  Director/President
Pediatric Effective Elimination Program Clinic and Counseling,
  PC
Highlands Ranch, Colorado

Jennifer Newcombe, MSN, PCNS-BC, CPNP-PC/AC
Nurse Practitioner
Pediatric Cardiothoracic Surgery
Loma Linda Children's Hospital
Assistant Professor
School of Nursing
Loma Linda University
Loma Linda, California

Sharon Norman, DNP, RN, CPNP, CNS, CCRN
School of Nursing
Oregon Health & Science University
Portland, Oregon
Randall Children's Hospital-Legacy Emanuel
Portland, Oregon

Catherine O'Keefe, DNP, CPNP-PC
Adjunct Associate Professor, Emerita
College of Nursing
Creighton University
Omaha, Nebraska

Sarah Obermeyer, PhD, CNM, WHNP, IBCLC
Assistant Professor
School of Nursing
Azusa Pacific University
Azusa, California

Adebloa M. Olarewaju, RN, MS, CPNP-PC
Pediatric Nurse Practitioner
Otolaryngology—Head and Neck Surgery
UC Davis Medical Center
Sacramento, California

Jaime Panton, DNP, MSN, BSN, CPNP-AC/PC
Assistant Professor
School of Nursing
Columbia University
New York, New York

Michele Polfuss, PhD, BSN, MSN, RN, CPNP-AC/PC
Associate Professor
College of Nursing
University of Wisconsin—Milwaukee
Joint Research Chair in the Nursing of Children
Nursing Research Department
Children's Hospital of Wisconsin
Milwaukee, Wisconsin

Sarah Elizabeth Romer, DNP, FNP
Assistant Professor
Adolescent Medicine, Pediatrics
University of Colorado Denver School of Medicine
Medical Director
BC4U Clinic
Children's Hospital Colorado
Aurora, Colorado

Ruth K. Rosenblum, DNP, RN, PNP-BC, CNS
Associate Professor
DNP Program Co-Coordinator
The Valley Foundation School of Nursing at San Jose State
  University
San Jose, California
American Nurses Association/California Board of
  Directory–Secretary

Susan K. Sanderson, DNP, MSN FNP, APRN
Professor
Outpatient Nurse Practitioner
Pediatric Infectious Diseases
University of Utah
Salt Lake City, Utah

Kathryn Schartz, BA, BSN, MSN
Pediatric Nurse Practitioner
General Academic Pediatrics
The Children's Mercy Hospital
Kansas City, Missouri

Alan T. Schultz, MSN, RN, CPNP-PC
Pediatric Nurse Practitioner
The Barton Center for Diabetic Education
Joslin Diabetes Center
Boston, Massachusetts

Isabelle Soulé, PhD, RN
Human Resources for Health Rwanda
University of Maryland
Baltimore, Maryland

Arlene Smaldone, PhD, CPNP-PC, CDE
Professor of Nursing
Dental Behavioral Sciences
Medical Center Assistant Dean for Scholarship and Research
School of Nursing
Columbia University Medical Center
New York, New York

Jessica L. Spruit, DNP, RN, CPNP-AC
Clinical Assistant Professor
College of Nursing
Wayne State University
Detroit, Michigan

Asma Ali Taha, PhD, RN, CPNP-PC/AC, PCNS-BC, CCRN
Associate Professor
Director
Pediatric Nurse Practitioner Program

School of Nursing
Oregon Health & Science University
Doernbecher Children's Hospital
Portland, Oregon

Helen N. Turner, DNP, APRN, PCNS-BC, AP-PMN, FAAN
Clinical Nurse Specialist
Anesthesiology and Perioperative Medicine
Oregon Health & Science University
Portland, Oregon

Amber Wetherington, MSN, CPNP-PC
University Pediatric Urology
East Tennessee Children's Hospital
Knoxville, Tennessee

Becky J. Whittemore, MN, MPH, BSN, RN, FNP-BC
Nurse Educator
Metabolic Clinic
Newborn Screening
Oregon Health & Science University
Doernbecher Children's Hospital
Institute on Development and Disbility
Portland, Oregon

Elizabeth E. Willer, RN, MSN, CPNP
Pediatric Nurse Practitioner, Retired
Department of Pediatrics
Kaiser Permanente
Walnut Creek, California

Teri Moser Woo, PhD, RN, ARNP, CPNP-PC, CNL, FAANP
Director of Nursing
St. Martin's University
Tacoma, Washington

Robert J. Yetman, MD
Professor of Pediatrics
Director of Division of Community and General Pediatrics
University of Texas—Houston Medical School
Houston, Texas

We would like to thank the previous edition contributors for their efforts in the Sixth Edition and whose work and ideas influenced this edition's content:

Michele E. Acker, MN, ARNP
Pediatric Nurse Practitioner
Seattle Children's Hospital
Seattle, Washington

Anita D. Berry, MSN, CNP, APN, PMHS
Director
Healthy Steps for Young Children Program
Advocate Children's Hospital
Downers Grove, Illinois

Cynthia Marie Claytor, MSN, PNP, FNP
Graduate Nursing Faculty
Azusa Pacific University
Azusa California

Joy S. Diamond, MS, CPNP
Pediatric Nurse Practitioner
Advanced Pediatric Associates
Children's Hospital Colorado
Aurora, Colorado

Mary Ann Draye, MPH, APRN
Assistant Professor, Emerita
DNP FNP Program
School of Nursing
University of Washington
Seattle, Washington

Susan Filkins, MS, RD
Nutrition Consultant
Oregon Center for Children and Youth with Special Health
Needs
Oregon Health & Sciences University
Portland, Oregon

Leah G. Fitch, MSN, RN, CPNP
Pediatric Nurse Practitioner
Providence Pediatrics, Carolinas HealthCare System
Charlotte, North Carolina

Lauren Bell Gaylord, MSN, CPNP-PC
Pediatric Nurse Practitioner
Etowah Pediatrics
Rainbow City, Alabama

Teral Gerlt, MS, RN, WHCNP-E, PNP-R
Instructor
School of Nursing
Oregon Health & Science University
Portland, Oregon

Denise A. Hall, BS, CMPE
Practice Administrator
Advanced Pediatrics Associates
Aurora, Colorado

Anna Marie Hefner, PhD, RN, CPNP
Associate Professor
Azusa Pacific University
Upland, California

Pamela J. Hellings, RN, PhD, CPNP-R
Professor, Emeritus
Oregon Health & Science University
Portland, Oregon

Susan Hines, RN, MSN, CPNP
Pediatric Nurse Practitioner
Sleep Medicine
Children's Hospital Colorado
Aurora, Colorado

Julie Martchenke, RN, MSN, CPNP
Pediatric Cardiology Nurse Practitioner
Oregon Health & Science University
Portland, Oregon

Michelle McGarry, MSN, RN, CPNP, CUNP
Certified Pediatric and Urology Nurse Practitioner/Program
Director/Owner
Pediatric Effective Elimination Program Clinic & Consulting,
PC
Highlands Ranch, Colorado

Peter M. Milgrom, DDS
Professor of Oral Health Sciences and Pediatric Dentistry
Adjunct Professor of Health Services
Director
Northwest Center to Reduce Oral Health Disparities
University of Washington
Seattle, Washington

Carole R. Myers, PhD, RN
Associate Professor
College of Nursing
University of Tennessee
Knoxville, Tennessee

Noelle Nurre, RN, MN, CPNP
Suspected Child Abuse and Neglect (SCAN) Nurse Practitioner
Oregon Health and Science University Doernbecher Children's
Hospital and CARES Northwest
Portland, Oregon

Catherine O'Keefe, DNP, CPNP-PC
Associate Professor/NP Curriculum Coordinator, Retired
College of Nursing
Creighton University
Omaha, Nebraska

Gabrielle M. Petersen, MSN, CPNP
Medical Examiner
Children's Center
Oregon City, Oregon

Ann M. Petersen-Smith, PhD, APRN, CPNP-PC, CPNP-AC
Assistant Professor
College of Nursing
University of Colorado Anschutz Medical Campus
Associate Clinical Professor
School of Medicine
University of Colorado Anschutz Medical Campus
Aurora, Colorado

Mary Rummell, MN, RN, CNS, CPNP, FAHA
Clinical Nurse Specialist
The Knight Cardiovascular Institute, Cardiac Services
Oregon Health & Science University
Portland, Oregon

Isabelle Soulé, PhD, RN
Human Resources for Health Rwanda
University of Maryland
Baltimore, Maryland

Robert D. Steiner, MD
Executive Director
Marshfield Clinic Research Foundation;
Professor of Pediatrics
University of Wisconsin
Marshfield, Wisconsin

Ohnmar K. Tut, BDS, MPhil
Adjunct Senior Research Fellow
Griffith University
Program Consultant Investigator
HRSA Oral Health Workforce Activities—FSM
Brisbane, Queensland, Australia
Affiliate Instructor
University of Washington
Seattle, Washington

Yvonne K. Yousey, RN, CPNP, PhD
Pediatric Nurse Practitioner
Kids First Health Care
Commerce City, Colorado

Reviewers

Brent Banasik, PhD
Scientist
Chemistry
Banasik Consulting Group
Seattle, Washington

Emily Souder, MD
Assistant Professor of Pediatrics
Drexel University College of Medicine
Attending Physician
Section of Infectious Diseases
St. Christopher's Hospital for Children,
Philadelphia, Pennsylvania

Preface

We are delighted to introduce the seventh edition and updated title of *Burns' Pediatric Primary Care*. With the retirement of three of the initial authors of this book, the team believed it was time to alter the title to call it what it is commonly referred to by those who love it and use it. Changes to this edition were made to ensure the contemporary relevance of topics and to support the educational needs of those in pediatric primary care. The editorial team consists of actively practicing pediatric nurse practitioners who understand the contemporary challenges and complexity of the primary care health care system. Each of the contributing authors of the chapters are experts in their fields. As always, every chapter has been thoroughly updated.

This book was initially developed more than 20 years ago as a resource for advanced practice nurses who were providing primary health care to infants, children, and adolescents. Currently, pediatric nurse practitioners (PNPs) and family nurse practitioners (FNPs) are the primary audience. However, physicians, physician assistants, and nurses who care for children in a variety of settings also find this book to be a valuable resource. This is the only nurse practitioner (NP) editorial team and NP-focused pediatric primary care text on the market.

*Burns' Pediatric Primary C*are emphasizes health promotion, disease prevention, and problem management from the primary care provider's point of view. Each chapter introduces key concepts, provides an evidence-based and theoretical care foundation, and includes a discussion of the identification and management of symptoms or conditions of specific disease entities. Experienced clinicians can simply jump to the topic or diagnosis in question while the novice can read the chapter for immersion into the topic. Additional resources for each chapter include websites to access organizations and printed materials that may be useful for clinicians and their patients and families.

Special Features of the Seventh Edition

Some features of the seventh edition about which we are particularly excited include the following:

- **NEW!** This edition includes a significant content reorganization. We made this change to reflect current understanding of the continuum of health and illness and to ensure that the flow and classification of information is intuitive to students and providers.
- **NEW!** Because of the evolving clarity of the primary care versus acute care roles, this edition now solely focuses on primary care management and the role of referral and consultation for acute care issues.
- **NEW!** Pediatric primary care providers see patients with a wide range of issues and health complexities. In order to reflect the depth and breadth of this role, nine new chapters were created. These include: a chapter on unique issues in pediatrics (Chapter 1), an overview of genetic and genomic concepts (Chapter 3), environmental issues that impact health (Chapter 4), children with special healthcare needs (Chapter 7), developmental management of newborns (Chapter 9), immunizations (Chapter 22), injury prevention and child maltreatment (Chapter 24), perinatal disorders (Chapter 19), and developmental, behavioral, and mental health promotion (Chapter 30).
- Unit 3 was redesigned to include typical developmental health issues and to emphasize health promotion and health protection. The first section includes developmental, behavioral, and mental health promotion. The second section covers the biophysical domains of nutrition, breastfeeding, elimination, physical activity and sports, sleep, and sexuality. The final section focuses on health protection in the areas of dental health, injury and child maltreatment prevention, and immunizations.
- Unit 4 was redesigned to include management of common diseases and disorders. This section no longer includes developmentally typical conditions and instead focuses on health restoration. Developmentally typical conditions and issues were relocated to Unit 3. The initial chapter in this unit details principles of pediatric disease management common to all ages.
- All other chapters have been updated and redesigned to reflect the highest level of contemporary evidence including *Healthy People 2020* (Healthy People, 2019) and the new edition of *Bright Futures* (Hagan et al., 2017).
- We expanded the use of algorithms to streamline the decision making for clinicians.

Organization of the Book

Children are a special population. Pediatric healthcare requires unique perspective grounded in a fundamental understandings of the complexities of child development, unique epidemiologic health influences, varied social determinants and environmental influences of health, and each child's unique genetic influences. These themes are carried throughout this book.

The book is organized into four major sections—Pediatric Primary Care Foundations, Management of Development, Pediatric Health Promotion and Protection, and Disease Management. Each chapter follows the same format. Standards and guidelines for care are highlighted, relevant child development is described, the physiologic and assessment parameters are discussed, management strategies are identified, and management of common problems is presented in a problem-oriented format. The scope of practice of the primary care provider is always emphasized with appropriate referral and consultation points identified.

It is our hope that this book continues in the tradition of the prior editions by supporting the primary care provider with the highest quality, evidence-based care strategies to foster improved health and wellness of children and their families.

Acknowledgments

A book of this size and complexity cannot be completed without considerable help—the work of the chapter authors who researched, wrote, and revised content; the consultation and review of experts in various specialties who critiqued drafts and provided important perspectives and guidance; and the essential technical support from those who managed the production of the manuscript and the final product. We are particularly grateful to Laura Goodrich, Sharon Corell, and Sandra Clark at Elsevier for their tireless support and advocacy during the development of this book.

Our Thanks to Family and Friends

- To my husband and greatest champion, Jeff, who always supports me and encourages me while giving me a safe place to recover and just be; to my amazing daughters, Rachel and Elizabeth, who give my life meaning; to the students, parents, and families who make me a better person; and to Amy DiMaggio, friends, and family for loving me and giving me wings. *Dawn Lee Garzon Maaks*
- Aloha and mahalo to my Jon, Jonah, and AnnaMei. I am ever grateful for the joy you bring to my life as well as your support of my time with "the book." Likewise, I am ever thankful for Denise and my APA colleagues who give me the flexibility and challenge to work hand in hand to provide model pediatric care. *Nancy Barber Starr*
- With deep appreciation for the circle of love and support from my dear family and friends who are always there surrounding me with warmth, laughter, and joy. *Margaret A. Brady*

- To my parents who first loved, supported, and encouraged me. To my husband, Mark, who loved me second and continues to love, support, and encourage me in all my professional endeavors. To my children, Curtis and Leah, who make life fun and will continue to do so with their own children. *Nan Gaylord*
- To my children and their children and their children who, along with children everywhere, are the living messages we send to a time we will not see. Here's hoping we have done well by them. *Martha Driessnack*
- The health of our nation's children is our most important resource. My hope is that this edition will contribute to that critical mission of improving the health and well-being of our children and families. Further, to my ever-patient husband who has sustained and bolstered me through the work on this edition! *Karen Duderstadt*
- With sincere gratitude and love to my amazing husband, Chuck, for his endless support and understanding during extended time dedicated toward my work on this edition. Thanks be to God for all my blessings, my parents for preparing me well for life's journey, and my children, Taylor and Jack, my pride and joy. *Mary Dirks*

References

Hagan JF, Shaw JS, Duncan PM: Bright Futures: guidelines for health supervision of infants, children, and adolescent, ed 4, Elk Grove Village, IL, 2017, American Academy of Pediatrics.

Healthy People 2020 (2019). Available at https://www.healthypeople.gov. Accessed March 30, 2019.

Contents

Burns' Pediatric Primary Care

1

Health Status of Children: Global and National Perspectives

KAREN G. DUDERSTADT

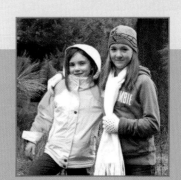

The health of all children is interconnected worldwide, and the health status of all children must be viewed with a global lens. Whether considering pandemic infectious diseases or global migration, incquitics in the health status of children globally and nationally are largely determined by common biosocial factors affecting health. Biosocial circumstances, or social determinants of child health, are shaped by economics, social policies, and politics in each region and country. There is a social gradient in health that runs from the top to bottom of the socioeconomic spectrum globally. Therefore the social gradient in health means that health inequities affect low-, middle-, and high-income countries (World Health Organization [WHO], 2018). Significant progress has been made in reducing childhood morbidity and mortality. However, a sustained effort is required globally and nationally to build better health systems to continue to positively impact child health outcomes. The framework of the United Nations Millennium Development Goals (United Nations Development Program [UNDP], 2015) and Healthy People 2020 (U.S. Department of Health and Human Services [HHS] Office of Disease Prevention and Health Promotion [ODPHP], 2018) goals set the mark for improving child health status.

This chapter presents an overview of the global health status of children, current health inequities, the progress achieved in the Millennium Development Goals and Healthy People 2020 targets, and the factors currently affecting the health of children in the United States, including food and housing insecurity. The chapter also discusses the important role pediatric healthcare providers have in advocating for polices that foster health equity and access to quality healthcare services for all children and families.

Global Health Status of Children

Thirty-one million children younger than 20 years old are part of the international migration of populations across continents (United Nations International Children's Emergency Fund [UNICEF], 2017). Among the world's refugees are an estimated 10 million children, who have been forcibly displaced from their home country, and 17 million more who have been displaced due to conflict

and violence (UNICEF, 2017). Immigrant children have increased health and educational needs that impact the health and well-being of communities; many of these communities have fragile healthcare systems. The United Nations Convention on the Rights of Children (UNCRC) charter was established 25 years ago and declares the minimum entitlements and freedoms for children globally, including the right to the best possible health (UNICEF, 2017a). The charter is founded on the principle of respect for the dignity and worth of each individual, regardless of race, color, gender, language, religion, opinions, origins, wealth, birth status, or ability. Immigrant children have the right to be protected under this charter (Box 1.1).

Health equity is the absence of unfair or remediable differences in health services and health outcomes among populations (WHO, 2016). Addressing health equity globally requires bold goals, political will with broad fiscal support, and a commitment within low-resource countries to prioritize the health of children and families as a primary goal.

Progress on the Millennium Development Goals

The United Nations (UN) Millennium Development Goals, adopted in 2000 with a deadline of 2015, produced the most successful movement in history by the UN to reduce child poverty globally (UNDP, 2015). The achievements are the result of the collaborations between governments, international communities, civil societies, and private corporations. Although the UNDP acknowledges shortfalls that remain, significant progress has been made globally in the 30 developing countries targeted. Although the rate of child mortality globally remains high, the global under-5 mortality rate declined by more than half, from 90 deaths per 1000 live births in 1990 to 43 deaths per 1000 births in 2015 (UNDP, 2015). The neonatal mortality rate fell to 19 per 1000 live births in 2016 from 37 per 1000 births in 1990. The highest rates of infant mortality occurred in two countries—39% of newborn deaths occurred in southern Asia and 38% in sub-Saharan Africa. Half of all newborn deaths occurred in just five

The UNICEF conventions include 42 articles that are summarized in the following list. They represent the worldwide standards for the rights of children. The conventions apply to *all* children younger than 18 years old. The best interests of children must be a top priority in all actions concerning children.
- Every child has the right to:
  - Life and best possible health
  - Time for relaxation, play, and opportunities for a variety of cultural and artistic activities
  - A legally registered name and nationality
  - Knowledge of and care by his or her parents, as far as possible, and prompt efforts to restore the child-parent relationship if they have been separated
  - Protection from dangerous work
  - Protection from use of dangerous drugs
  - Protection from sale and social abuse, exploitation, physical and sexual abuse, and neglect and special care to help them recover their health if they have experienced such toxic life events
  - No incarceration with adults and opportunities to maintain contact with parents
  - Care with respect for religion, culture, and language if not provided by the parents
  - A full and decent life in conditions that promote dignity, independence, and an active role in the community, even if disabled
  - Access to reliable information from mass media, television, radio, and newspapers, as well as protection from information that might harm them
- Governments must do all that they can to fulfill the rights of children as listed here.

[a]UNICEF stands for the full name United Nations International Children's Emergency Fund. In 1953, its name was shortened to the United Nations Children's Fund. However, the original acronym was retained.

countries: India, Pakistan, Nigeria, the Democratic Republic of the Congo, and Ethiopia (United Nations Inter-agency Group for Mortality Estimates [UN IGME], 2017).

Pneumonia, diarrhea, and malaria remain the leading causes of death globally in children younger than 5 years (UN IGME, 2017). The highest proportion of deaths due to these conditions are in children younger than 2 years old. *Rotavirus* is the most common cause of diarrhea globally, and *Streptococcus pneumoniae* is the leading cause of pneumonia—both are vaccine-preventable infectious diseases. Successful vaccination programs have markedly reduced the mortality caused by some infectious diseases, particularly measles and tetanus. Approximately 84% of children worldwide received at least one dose of a measles- containing vaccine in 2013, up from 73% in 2000 (UNDP, 2015). Other UNDP achievements include:
- More than 6.2 million malaria deaths have been averted between 2000 and 2015, primarily of children younger than 5 years in sub-Saharan Africa.
- More than 900 million insecticide-treated mosquito nets were delivered to malaria-endemic countries in sub-Saharan Africa between 2004 and 2014.
- The primary school net enrollment rate in the developing regions has reached 91% in 2015, up from 83% in 2000.
- More than 71% of births were assisted by skilled health personnel globally in 2014, an increase from 59% in 1990.

Undernutrition, low rates of breastfeeding, and zinc deficiency contribute significantly to the childhood mortality rates globally. As a micronutrient, zinc is essential for protein supplementation, cell growth, immune function, and intestinal transport of water and electrolytes, and it reduces the duration and severity of diarrhea and likelihood of reinfections (Khan and Sellen, 2015).

Sustainable Development Goals

Building on the successes of the UNDP, the Sustainable Development Goals (SDGs) came into effect in 2016 and will continue through 2030. The SDGs include 17 expanded goals, including climate change, economic inequality, innovation in industry and infrastructure, sustainable consumption, peace and justice, and a universal call to action to end poverty and to protect the planet and ensure that all people enjoy peace and prosperity (Fig 1.1) (UNDG, 2016). The UNDG initiatives include work in 170 countries and territories and provide support to governments to integrate the SDGs into their national development plans and policies. The plan focuses on key areas including poverty alleviation, democratic governance and peacebuilding, climate change and disaster risk, and economic inequality. Increased resources are needed to meet the data demand for the new development agenda. Global standards and an integrated information technology (IT) system are also needed for effective monitoring. If every country achieves the SDGs target by 2030, an additional 10 million lives of children younger than 5 years will be saved throughout the period 2017–30 (UNDG, 2016). Fig 1.2 illustrates 15 global challenges in countries collaborating to address the issue of health equity from a global perspective (The Millennium Project, 2014).

Health Status of Children in the United States

Child poverty rates in the United States remain higher than in other economically developed nations, and there are significant inequalities in race and ethnicity. In 2016, 19% of children—one in five children or 14.1 million—were living in poverty, with children comprising 32.6% of all people in poverty (Annie E. Casey Foundation, 2018). Mississippi and New Mexico have the highest rate of child poverty, at 30%. The rate of household poverty is 34% in African-American and Native American children and 28% in Latino children. In addition, 35% of children live in single-parent families, which often have fewer resources.

Despite having the highest health expenditure per capita in the world, infant mortality in the United States remains higher than other high-income countries; however, there has been a decline in infant mortality over the past decade largely due to a decline in sudden infant death syndrome (SIDS) from 50 per 100,000 in 2002 to 13 per 100,000 in 2015 (Khan et al., 2018). Inequality in infant mortality rates remain, and African-American infants have the highest mortality rate, at 1128 per 100,000 infants compared with 498/100,000 in non-Hispanic white infants and 466/100,000 in Latino infants (Khan et al., 2018). For children 1 to 19 years of age, mortality rates have declined over the past decade due to the decline in unintentional injury deaths. However, the rate of suicide mortality has increased slightly in children 10 to 19 years of age over the past decade, with the highest rate among non-Hispanic white youth in early and late adolescence. Rising suicide rates resulted in approximately 1400 additional deaths in 2015. Suicide by firearms increased in white youth 15 to 24 years of age, and intentional drug poisonings increased in African-American and Latino youth (Khan et al., 2018).

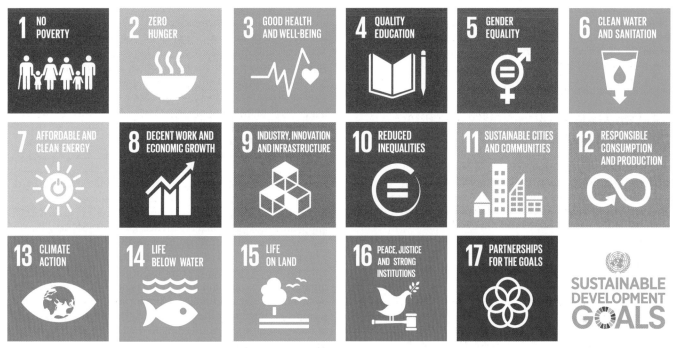

• **Fig 1.1** United Nations Development Program (UNDP) Sustainable Development Goals for 2030. (United Nations Development Program: the millennium development goals report 2015. UNDP. http://www.undp.org/content/undp/en/home/librarypage/mdg/the-millennium-development-goals-report-2015.html. Accessed September 10, 2018.)

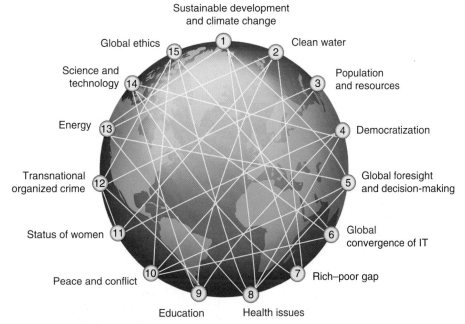

• **Fig 1.2** Fifteen Global Challenges Facing Humanity. *IT,* Information technology. (From http://107.22.164.43/millennium/challeng.html.)

Most concerning among the child health indicators is the percentage of overweight and obese children. Seventeen percent of children 2 to 19 years of age are *obese,* defined as a body mass index (BMI) greater than the 95th percentile for age on the BMI age- and gender-specific growth charts. The rate of obesity among adolescent males and females 12 to 19 years of age is currently 20.5% and has continued to rise over the past decade. Although rates of obesity among children and youth in the United States remain the highest among the high-income countries, surveillance studies show that the rate of overweight and obesity has stabilized among 2 to 5 year olds at 8.9% and the prevalence is less than the Healthy People 2020 goal of 9.4% in early childhood (Ogden et al., 2015). Obese and overweight children and youth are more at risk for developing adult health problems, including heart disease, type 2 diabetes, metabolic syndrome, stroke, and osteoarthritis. Of all the child health indicators, overweight and obesity significantly affect the cost of providing healthcare services in the United States.

Food and Housing Insecurity and Effect on Children's Health

Hunger and undernutrition are often associated with *food insecurity,* which exists when populations do not have physical and economic access to sufficient, safe, nutritious, and culturally acceptable food to meet nutritional needs. Food insecurity occurs in impoverished populations in developing countries and in industrialized nations, particularly among migrant populations. Children affected by migration and family separation are at risk for food insecurity and are vulnerable to further health consequences, including exposure to exploitation and child trafficking. Growing evidence about climate change indicates the dramatic effect on food crops that has led to food distribution issues globally, which is one of the primary contributors to the migration patterns and food insecurity (Fig 1.3). Globally, undernutrition is an important determinant of maternal and child health and accounts for 45% of all child deaths in children younger than 5 years of age (UN, 2015). Low rates of breastfeeding remain a problem in developed and developing nations. Children who are exclusively breastfed for the first 6 months of life are 14 times more likely to survive than nonbreastfed infants.

Despite many government food assistance programs in the United States, nearly one in five children in the United States lives in a food-insecure household. Children who are food insecure are more likely to have poorer general health, higher rates of hospitalization, and increased incidence of overweight, asthma, and anemia and to experience more behavioral problems. Factors other than income impact whether a household is food insecure. Maternal education, single-parent households, intimate partner violence, and parental substance abuse also contribute to food insecurity. Children living in households where the mother is moderately to severely depressed have a 50% to 80% increased risk of food insecurity (Gundersen and Ziliak, 2015).

Three-quarters of children spend some portion of the preschool years being cared for outside of the home. Depending on child care arrangements, the care can contribute to or ameliorate the effects of food insecurity for children. Young children who attend a preschool or child care center have lower food insecurity, whereas children cared for at home by an unrelated adult are at higher risk for food insecurity (Gundersen and Ziliak, 2015). The Supplemental Nutritional Assistance Program (SNAP), the Special Supplemental Nutrition Program for Women, Infants, and Children (WIC), and the School Breakfast Program (SBP) are federally funded programs with the purpose to combat childhood hunger. The average monthly WIC benefit for families is $43. Recent WIC data indicate the proportion of infant-prescribed formula declined over the past decade. This may reflect the trend of increased rates of breastfeeding in the United States reported in 2016 (Patlan and Mendelson, 2018).

Children living in poverty are also significantly affected by the affordable and adequate housing crisis in the United States, particularly immigrant children and families living in large metropolitan areas. Approximately 21% of persons experiencing homelessness in the United States are children (OHCHR, 2017). Although many children are reportedly experiencing sheltered homelessness, this lack of family financial stability, the

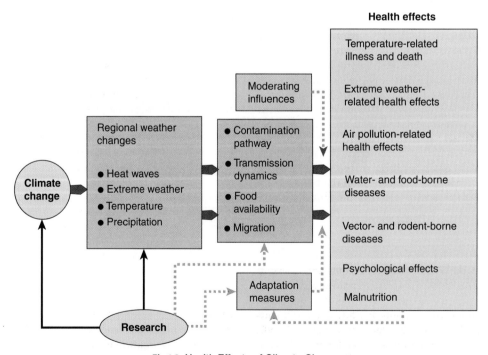

• **Fig 1.3** Health Effects of Climate Change.

limited housing supply in inner cities, and the high eviction rates negatively impact the education and physical and mental health of children.

Addressing Children's Health in the United States

Healthy People 2020

The Healthy People 2020 goals for children include foci specific to early and middle childhood and adolescents, social determinants of health in childhood, health-related quality of life for children, and specific disparities in child health to improve healthcare services and health outcomes. With increased proportions of children with developmental delays, Healthy People 2020 focuses on objectives to increase the percentage of children younger than 2 years old who receive early intervention services for developmental disabilities and to increase the proportion of children entering kindergarten with school readiness in all five domains of healthy development—physical health and well-being; social emotional development; approaches to learning; language development and communication; and cognitive development. The objectives set benchmarks to increase the percentage of young children who are screened for autism and other developmental delays at 18 and 24 months of age (National Center on Birth Defects and Developmental Disabilities, Centers for Disease Control and Prevention [CDC], 2015).

Reports indicate Healthy People 2020 objectives have been achieved in many areas. The United States surpassed the overall goal of a 10% reduction in infant and youth mortality in almost all age groups, averting 1200 child deaths in 2015 (Kahn et al., 2018). Infectious diseases among children in the United States—*Haemophilus influenzae* B, hepatitis B, group B streptococcal and pneumococcal infections, and meningococcal disease—declined, meeting or exceeding the Healthy People 2020 targets and indicating movement toward the 2020 objectives for completion of the vaccine series across age groups (National Center for Health Statistics [NCHS], 2016).

Healthy People 2020 objectives also address the need for increasing the proportion of practicing primary care providers, including nurse practitioners, to improve access to quality healthcare services. An integrated workforce can provide appropriate evidence-based clinical preventive services to reduce overall health care costs, as well as improve access and facilitate communication and continuity of care for children and families. Approaches to health care must be interprofessional and must consider the biosocial factors in the delivery of health care to achieve child health outcomes beyond those of the biomedical dynamics of disease (Holmes et al., 2014). The ODPHP advisory committee is building the Healthy People 2030 objectives on the foundational principles, mission, and overarching goals of the Healthy People 2020 framework.

Social Determinants of Health and Health Equity

The social determinants of health result in unequal and unavoidable differences in health status within communities and between communities. Individuals are affected by economic, social, and environmental factors in their communities. Social determinants of health recognize that home, school, workplace, neighborhoods, and access to health care are significant contributors to child health outcomes. Many of the Healthy People 2020 leading health indicators address social determinants of health. However, the targets often fall significantly below what is required to decrease the economic inequalities between communities and neighborhoods.

Some communities are addressing social determinants of health through connecting community safety and healthy child development and advocating for system, policy, and practice change (Prevention Institute, 2017). Exposure to neighborhood violence impacts children, and safer communities can promote social-emotional development for young children. Safe communities offer public places for children to play and community safety promotes economic development. Policies of community safety and early childhood development intersect and impact determinants of the sociocultural environment, physical/built environment, and educational/economic environment (Prevention Institute, 2017). Fig 1.4 illustrates a framework to help communities better understand and address the inequities that contribute to violence and how early experiences influence development over the life course.

Adverse Childhood Events and Impact on Child Health Outcomes

There is growing evidence about the disruptive impact of toxic stress on biologic mechanisms that impact childhood development. Early adverse stress is linked to later impairments in learning, behavior, and physical and mental well-being (American Academy of Pediatrics [AAP], 2014; Shonkoff et al, 2012). Toxic stress results from strong or frequent and prolonged activation of the body's stress response systems in the absence of the protection of a supportive, adult relationship (Shonkoff et al, 2012). The adversity can occur as single, acute, or chronic event in the child's environment, such as emotional or physical abuse or neglect, intimate partner violence, war, maternal depression, parental separation or divorce, and parental incarceration (Box 1.2). Adverse childhood events (ACEs) occur across all income groups, but 58% of children with ACEs live in homes with incomes less than 200% of the federal poverty level (FPL). African-American children are disproportionately affected by ACEs—6 out of 10 African-American children have experienced ACEs and represent 17.4% of all children in the United States with ACEs (Bethell et al., 2017). Emotional abuse is the most commonly reported ACE, followed by parental separation or divorce, and household substance abuse (Merrick et al., 2018).

Toxic stress in childhood has implications that carry over into adulthood. Evidence suggests that the results of the prolonged and altered biologic mechanisms lead to increased risk of chronic health conditions in adulthood, including obesity, heart disease, alcoholism, and substance abuse (Shonkoff et al., 2012). A child who has experienced ACEs is also more likely to engage in high-risk behavior, such as the initiation of early sexual activity and adolescent pregnancy. Limiting the impact of ACEs through effective interventions that strengthen communities and families and protect young children from the disruptive effects of toxic stress is critical to improve health outcomes throughout the life course for future generations (Merrick et al., 2018).

Child Health and Access to Care

Child heath is fundamental to overall child development, and children with health insurance are more likely to have a regular source of care and access to preventive healthcare services. Nationally, there has been significant progress over the past decade on

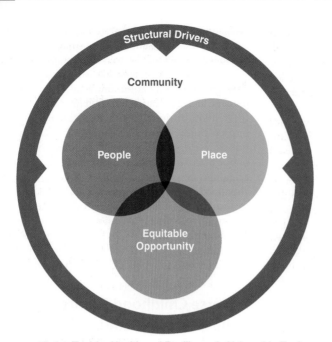

People
- Social networks & trust
- Participation & willingness to act for the common good
- Norms & culture

Place
- What's sold & how it is promoted
- Look, feel & safety
- Parks & open space
- Getting around
- Housing
- Air, water, soil
- Arts & cultural expression

Equitable Opportunity
- Education
- Living wages & local wealth

• **Fig 1.4** Tool for Health and Resilience in Vulnerable Environments (THRIVE) Clusters and Factors Impacting Early Child Development. (Prevention Institute & Center for Study of Social Policy; Cradle to community: a focus on community safety and health child development; 2017:1–47. http://preventioninstitute.org/sites/default/files/publications/PI_Cradle to Community_121317_0.pdf. Accessed October 12, 2018.)

• **BOX 1.2** **Adverse Childhood Events**

- Emotional abuse or neglect
- Physical abuse or neglect
- Sexual abuse
- Mother treated violently
- Household substance abuse
- Household mental illness
- Parental separation or divorce
- Incarcerated household member

---

expanding public insurance for children. In 2016, 4% of children lacked health insurance, which is half the uninsured rate in 2010 (Annie E. Casey Foundation, 2018). Alaska has the highest rate of uninsured children, at 5%, whereas just 1% of children in Massachusetts are uninsured. Inequalities remain among racial and ethnic populations as 7% of Latino and 12% of Native American children remain uninsured.

Thirty million children are currently covered by public insurance programs in the United States (Bettenhausen et al., 2018). The expansion of Medicaid and the Children's Health Insurance Program (CHIP) expanded healthcare access to primary care services for many low-and middle-income families and decreased avoidable hospitalizations and child mortality. States are dependent on federal financial support for Medicaid and CHIP, and the federal share of public costs exceeds 70% in some states (Bettenhausen et al., 2018). The public insurance eligibility rates vary across states, from 150% to 405% of the FPL income. A decrease in federal funding levels would limit access to public insurance enrollment and therefore access to preventive and acute care services. Hospitalizations represent the highest healthcare costs. Reductions in public insurance eligibility decreases access to

primary care and preventative services which shifts costs to hospitals and families. Sustained federal funding at current levels is needed to maintain access to vital healthcare services and improve child health outcomes.

Role of Primary Care Providers for Improving Child Health

Pediatric primary card providers (PCPs) have a key role in advocating for child health locally, nationally, and globally. Advanced Practice Registered Nurses (APRNs) provide continuity of care in the ambulatory care setting for underserved children with health conditions such as asthma, pneumonia, and vaccine-preventable conditions that might otherwise lead to greater use of costly emergency departments and hospitalizations. Increasing access to APRNs who deliver primary care services reduces healthcare costs, improves health outcomes, and produces health care savings—all steps that would allow the United States to lead rather than trail the other economically developed countries in child health indicators. In addition, APRNs are able to advocate for children and potentially influence economic and political decisions to ameliorate health disparities and increase health equality among populations and communities to build a healthier generation of adults.

Health Promotion and Evidence-Based Clinical Preventive Services

Many children are not receiving the recommended preventive services and developmental surveillance required for health promotion. There are many barriers to effective well-child care, including time constraints; low levels of reimbursement for preventive care and developmental screening services; lack of provider education in current strategies to identify child development, emotional, and behavioral problems; and lack of community referral sources to assist children, adolescents, and families. These issues have led to inconsistent quality of preventive healthcare services affecting children and families.

Much of the basis for primary care practice is not yet evidence based. Primary care would benefit from stronger scientific clinical research that could strengthen primary care principles and prevention. Lack of funding and infrastructure to support such primary care clinical research stands in sharp contrast to the organized commitment and emphasis on advancing knowledge in disease entities and treatment options. This gap provides an area of research open to pediatric nurse researchers and other pediatric healthcare providers trained in clinical research. Increased evidence in the primary healthcare domain would help to move the public dialogue toward a greater focus on primary prevention and away from a disease-focused healthcare system.

References

American Academy of Pediatrics (AAP). Adverse childhood experiences and the lifelong consequences of trauma (PDF online). 2014. www.aap.org/en-us/Documents/ttb_aces_consequences.pdf. Accessed September 12, 2018.

Annie E. Casey Foundation: The 2018 KIDS COUNT data book: an annual report on how children are faring in the United States, The Annie E. Casey Foundation (website). https://www.aecf.org/m/resourcedoc/aecf-2018kidscountdatabook-2018.pdf. Accessed September 12, 2018.

Bethell CD, Davis MB, Gombojav N, Stumbo S, Powers K. *Issue Brief: Adverse Childhood Experiences Among US Children, Child and Adolescent Health Measurement Initiative*. Johns Hopkins Bloomberg School of Public Health; October 2017. http://cahmi.org/projects/adverse-childhood-experiences-aces.

Bettenhausen JL, Hall M, Colvin JD, Puls HT, Chung PJ. The effect of lowering public insurance income limits on hospitalizations for low-income children. *Pediatrics*. 2018;142(2):1–8.

Gundersen C, Ziliak JP. The future of children: research report: childhood food insecurity in the U.S.: trends, causes, and policy options (PDF online). https://futureofchildren.princeton.edu/sites/futureofchildren/files/media/childhood_food_insecurity_researchreport-fall2014.pdf. Accessed October 30, 2018.

Holmes SM, Greene JA, Stonington SD. Locating global health in social medicine. *Global Public Health*. 2014;9(5):475–480.

Khan SQ, de Gonzalez AB, Best AF, Chen Y, Haozous EA, et al. Infant and youth mortality trends by race/ethnicity and cause of death in the U.S. *JAMA Pediatrics*. 2018;E1–E10.

Khan WU, Sellen DW. Zinc supplementation in the management of diarrhoea. World Health Organization (website). www.who.int/elena/titles/bbc/zinc_diarrhoea/en/. Accessed October 10, 2018.

Merrick MT, Ford DC, Posts KA, Guinn AS. Prevalence of adverse childhood experiences from 2011-2014 Behavioral Risk Factor Surveillance System in 23 states. *JAMA Pediatrics*. 2018:1038–1044.

Millennium Project. Global challenges for humanity. The Millennium Project (website). http://millennium-project.org/millennium/challenges.html. Accessed October 30, 2018.

National Center on Birth Defects and Developmental Disabilities. Centers for Disease Control and Prevention (CDC). Community report on autism. 2014 (PDF online). www.cdc.gov/ncbddd/autism/states/comm_report_autism_2014.pdf Accessed October 10, 2018.

National Center for Health Statistics (NCHS). *Chapter 23: Immunization and Infectious Diseases*. Hyattsville, MD: Healthy People 2020 Midcourse Review; 2016.

Office of United Nations High Commissioner for Human Rights (OHCHR): Statement on Visit to the USA, Philip Alston, UN Special Rapporteur on extreme poverty and human rights. 2017:1–13. https://www.ohchr.org/EN/NewsEvents/Pages/DisplayNews.aspx?NewsID=22533&LangID=E. Accessed on September 12, 2018.

Ogden CL, Carroll MD, Fryar CD, Flegal KM. *Prevalence of Obesity Among Adults and Youth: United States. 2011-2014. NCHS Data Brief*. no. 219. Hyattsville, MD; 2015.

Patlan KL, Mendelson M. *WIC Participant and Program Characteristics 2016: Food Package Report*. Prepared by Insight Policy Research Alexandria, VA: U.S. Department of Agriculture, Food and Nutrition Service, Project Officer: Anthony Panzera; 2018. Available online at: www.fns.usda.gov/research-and-analysis. Accessed on October 26, 2018.

Prevention Institute & Center for Study of Social Policy. Cradle to community. A focus on community safety and health child development. 2017:1–47. http://preventioninstitute.org/sites/default/files/publications/PI_Cradle to Community_121317_0.pdf. Accessed on October 12, 2018.

Shonkoff JP, Garner AS, Committee on Psychosocial Aspects of Child and Family Health, et al. The lifelong effects of early childhood adversity and toxic stress. *Pediatrics*. 2012;129(1):e232–e246.

UNICEF: Migration. Monitoring the situation of children and women. UNICEF 2017 (website). https://data.unicef.org/topic/child-migration-and-displacement/migration/. Accessed September 9, 2018.

UNICEF. Convention on the Rights of Children. UNICEF (website). https://www.unicef.org/crc/index_73549.html. Accessed September 9, 2018, 2017a.

United Nations Development Program. The millennium development goals report. UNDP (website). http://www.undp.org/content/undp/en/home/librarypage/mdg/the-millennium-development-goals-report-2015.html. Accessed September 10, 2018.

United Nations Inter-agency Group for Child Mortality (UN IGME) Estimation. *Levels & trends in child mortality: Report 2017, Estimates developed by the UN IGME*. New York: United Nations Children's Fund; 2017. http://childmortality.org/files_v21/download/IGME report 2017 child mortality final.pdf. Accessed September 10, 2018.

United Nations Development Group (UNDG). The sustainable development goals are coming to life. 2016. https://undg.org/wp-content/uploads/2016/12/SDGs-are-Coming-to-Life-UNDG-1.pdf. Accessed September 10, 2018.

U.S. Department of Health and Human Services (HHS) Office of Disease Prevention and Health Promotion. Healthy People 2020, HealthyPeople.gov. (website). www.healthypeople.gov/2020/default.aspx. Accessed September 10, 2018.

World Health Organization (WHO). Social determinants of health. WHO n.d.(website). http://www.who.int/social_determinants/sdh_definition/en/. Accessed September 10, 2018.

World Health Organization (WHO). Global health observatory (GHO) data: About the health equity monitor. WHO. 2016 (website). www.who.int/gho/health_equity/about/en/. Accessed September 26, 2018.

2

Unique Issues in Pediatrics

MARTHA DRIESSNACK

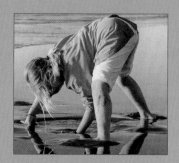

This chapter focuses on some of the unique issues that inform pediatric primary care, beginning with the inherent challenges of providing patient-centered care when the focus of care is a two-generation or dual patient. This introduction is followed by a brief discussion of contemporary contexts and theories that influence how we view children, as well as how the continued use of a developmental lens, although important, creates challenges. Also highlighted is the importance of early investment in lifelong health, with a particular focus on a child's first 1000 days, adverse childhood experiences (ACEs), and household and health literacy. The final section is a reminder that transitioning from a pediatric to an adult primary care system is critical for all children, but especially for adolescents and young adults with chronic physical and medical conditions.

Two-Generation or Dual Patient

One of the unique challenges in pediatrics is the two-generation or dual patient. Although the primary focus in pediatrics is the child, each child and/or adolescent comes with at least one parent or caregiver, if not three or four, and cannot be seen or cared for without this context. Taking time to understand and work with parents is paramount in pediatric primary care, but it is distinct from patient- and family-centered care (PFCC). In PFCC, providers acknowledge the patient's ultimate control over health-related decisions, while acknowledging that these decisions are contextualized within each patient's broader life experiences and family. The challenge of using a pure PFCC model in pediatric primary care is that there is not one patient, but two, and while the child is the focus, the parent is considered the authority in terms of decisions (Eichner, 2012).

For pediatric providers, one of the greatest challenges is how to access, acknowledge, and include the child's voice, which is often lost and/or overridden in healthcare. This tendency to lose track of and/or override children's voices is rooted in the long-standing tradition of seeing children using deficit-based or developmental lenses. Using these lenses there is a presumption of decisional incapacity in the patient and therefore deference to parental authority. This view is contrasted to how the patient is seen in adult healthcare, where there is a presumption of decisional capacity in the patient, with familial insight serving as adjunctive.

All health care providers are obligated to provide beneficial care to the patient. For adults this means the patient's needs and wishes take priority. In pediatrics, balancing the needs and wishes within the context of the dual patient continues to give rise to some of the most difficult and challenging care decisions,

especially as children's cognitive and executive function matures. Parents are clearly authorities and caregivers, but they are not surrogates. Pediatric providers need to seek out children's voices and encourage children's participation in care and health-related decisions over time.

Looking Through a Developmental Lens

How children are viewed influences how primary care providers (PCPs) interact with them. If children are seen only as works in progress using a deficit-based, developmental lens, they are regarded as human *becomings*, rather than as human *beings* (Driessnack, 2005). Children are not seen as agents in their own right, human beings who are capable of influencing their learning and others. Instead, our understanding of children and childhood is left to reports from adult surrogates. Although pediatric PCPs embrace the concept that every child is considered within the context of family, it does not mean that parents' perspectives are preferred or take precedence over the child's when health-related decision-making and plans of care are being considered.

Past dominance of deficit-based, stage theories as the lens through which children are primarily viewed is being challenged, replaced with a call for a more balanced understanding. This shift in understanding parallels the emerging emphasis on patient-centered care and shared decision-making. Although being patient-centered has some inherent challenges in pediatrics, it is a reminder to advocate for the voices of children, which too often are absent from health-related decision-making and plans of care. New tools and approaches are needed that access children's voices based on children's cognitive strengths and abilities. In the past, clinicians and researchers have relied on adult-developed and adult-centered tools and approaches, which have been *adapted* for use with children by adding pictures and/or simpler language. There is increasing realization that data from adapted, adult-centered tools have not adequately captured the voices and/or experiences of children, giving rise to national movements, such as *No More Hand-Me-Down Research* and *Nothing About Me Without Me*.

Understanding how children develop from conception through adolescence is foundational in pediatric primary care. Although a number of major theories have informed the study of child development over the past century, there are a few that have been resurrected, or borrowed from other disciplines, to examine the impact of modern societal contexts, rapid advances in science, and expanding worlds of media and technology (Table 2.1).

TABLE 2.1	Theories of Child Development	
Type of Theory	**Major Theorists**	**Focus**
Psychoanalytic	Freud Erikson	Personality formation through conflict resolution

Cognitive	Constructivist
	  Piaget
	  Vygotsky
	Information
	  processing
	  Siegler
		How children think

Learning	Pavlov Watson Skinner Bandura	How experience affects children's learning and behavior
Ethologic	Bowlby Lorenz	Biology and the role of early experiences during specific developmental periods
System	Bronfenbrenner Gottllieb Lerner Sameroff	How environmental and biologic systems interact and shape development

Among these theorists, Vygotsky and Siegler are highlighted here because they both provide pediatric primary care with a new understanding or alternative lens through which to view children and childhood.

Vygotsky's cognitive theory is not new. In fact, he was a contemporary of Piaget, whose stage theory of cognitive development remains a curriculum constant in many introductory psychology classes. Although contemporaries, they differed in how they viewed development. For Piaget, development precedes learning; for Vygotsky, learning precedes development. This is a subtle but important shift of focus. Piaget's cognitive theory, as with all other stage theories, uses a deficit-based lens, pointing out what children are not yet able to do at each stage, rather than what they can do. Vygotsky's theory, in contrast, uses a strength-based lens, looking at what children can do.

One group of theories that has emerged in this call for a more balanced understanding of development is information processing theory. This group of theorists (e.g., Siegler) has borrowed concepts from computer science, focusing on how information is received, processed, and stored, as well as how it then produces output. Like Vygotsky, information processing theory centers on the continuity of development; change occurs smoothly, gradually, and predictably over time. This view is in contrast to stage theories (e.g., Piaget), which center on discontinuity, the idea that development proceeds through a series of distinct stages over time with each stage qualitatively different from the last. The focus is less on whether children can solve a problem or complete a task correctly and more on how problems are solved or tasks approached.

Parents, Families, and Behavioral Economics

Parents clearly play an integral role as active agents on behalf of their children. Yet, in pediatrics, best practices are determined based on children's needs, not on the behaviors of their parents or the mental models, cultural influences, and worldviews that inform and guide parents in meeting those needs (Gennetian, Darling, and Aber, 2016). *Behavioral economics* is a relatively new field that combines insights from psychology, judgment, and decision-making with conventional economic theory to understand human behavior, especially in terms of individual influences on decision-making.

The introduction of behavioral economics represents a paradigm shift that is already making an impact, as policy makers embrace its approach to understanding a wide range of high-impact social issues, including obesity and poverty. Of particular interest in pediatric primary care is the role of cognitive load, which refers to an individual's current capacity to focus on and digest information. A parent's cognitive load can have far-reaching implications in pediatrics because any one individual can attend to only certain phenomena at any given point in time. Behavioral economics focuses on developing interventions that temporarily manipulate the salience of different cues, which can have large effects on decision-making. This shift to focus on salience created a new behavioral science term, *nudge,* and the teams examining such efforts are often called nudge units (Thaler, 2016; Thaler and Sunstein, 2009).

In this era of PFCC, pediatric PCPs can integrate the concept of nudging and nudge units, because there are many opportunities to nudge children's and parents' behaviors by making subtle changes to the context in which they make decisions. The shift in focus, drawing attention to the ways in which an individual's family, community, and cultural contexts affect people's real-world, in-the-moment decision-making, is at the heart of behavioral economics (Gennetian, Darling, and Aber, 2016). In addition to providing a new lens for considering individual and parent decision-making, behavioral economics and its focus on cognitive load and creating salience present an alternative lens for understanding larger social issues, such as poverty.

Early Investment in Lifelong Health

Early experiences shape the architecture of the developing brain and lay a foundation for long-term health. Health in the earliest years strengthens the systems that enable children to thrive and grow to be healthy adults. Ensuring that children have safe, secure environments, families, and communities in which to grow and learn creates a strong foundation for their futures and a thriving, prosperous society. New frameworks focus their attention not only on programs but also policies that support the foundations of children's health (Hoagwood et al., 2018). These new frameworks ask providers to work toward enhancing community efforts to change *social environments*, expanding their horizons beyond focusing their efforts solely on *people*.

Science shows that early exposure to adverse experiences can disrupt healthy development and have lifelong consequences. This new awareness is fueling a new way of looking at life, not as disconnected stages but as an integrated process across time—a *life course perspective* (Russ et al., 2014). At the forefront of this new perspective is the emergence of evidence surrounding adverse childhood experiences (ACEs) and their lifelong consequences. There are many other parallel bodies of evidence that all point to shifting attention upstream to early childhood, not only locally, but globally. Historically, early childhood interventions have focused on children of preschool age, but we currently know that interventions encompassing the period before conception through the first 2 years of life can greatly reduce adverse growth and health outcomes.

Clearly, what children experience in their earliest days and years of life shapes and defines their future. One of the best resources is Harvard's Center for the Developing Child. The World Health Organization (WHO), World Bank, and the United Nations International Children's Emergency Fund (UNICEF) have all drawn attention to the First 1000 Days of Life—from conception to birth (270 days), to a child's first birthday (+365 days), through to the second birthday (+365 days)—as a unique period where the foundations of health, growth, and neurodevelopment across the life span are established. All three global organizations contributed to and offered guidance to the pivotal series entitled Advancing Early Childhood Development: from Science to Scale (Lancet, 2016). Furthermore, a major focus of the United Nations' 2030 Sustainable Development Goals (SDGs) is on early childhood health and development to ensure that every child achieves her/his potential (United Nations, 2015). Accordingly, curricula offerings for parents and providers around the world have been developed (e.g., *ReachUpandLearn* and *Care for Child Development* [CCD]).

Equally intriguing is the science behind *Developmental Origins of Health and Disease* (DOHaD). This field examines models of causality and/or mechanisms that can trace the origin of many non-communicable conditions or chronic diseases (e.g., hypertension, metabolic syndrome) to environmental influences during early development. The link between early life environmental factors and later life diseases was originally called the Barker hypothesis, because Barker showed that poor nutrition during organ development could lead to increased risk for chronic disease later in life. His work highlighting the influences of adverse events that occur during early phases of human development on the pattern of an individual's health and disease throughout life provided the foundation for the more recent study of adverse childhood experiences.

ACEs are currently linked to risky health behaviors (e.g., smoking, alcoholism, drug use), chronic health conditions (e.g., obesity, diabetes, depression, heart disease, cancer stroke, COPD), low life potential (graduation rates, academic achievement, lost time from work), and early death (https://www.cdc.gov/violenceprevention/acestudy/index.html). Of note is that as the number of ACEs increases, so does the risk for these outcomes, which highlights the call for all pediatric PCPs to screen for and identify adverse events early in life. The research on ACEs continues to be tracked by the Centers for Disease Control and Prevention (CDC). The CDC and American Academy of Pediatrics (AAP) also provide toolkits and practice and provider resources. The AAP's resources and tools are housed within *The Resilience Project*.

Health Literacy

Health literacy is most often defined as the degree to which an individual is capable of obtaining, processing, and applying basic health information. In addition to general literacy and numeracy skills, health literacy requires knowledge of health topics. When individuals have limited health literacy, they lack knowledge or have misinformation about the body, the nature and causes of disease, disease risk, and the relationship between lifestyle factors, such as diet and exercise, and health outcomes. In pediatric primary care, parents' health literacy levels not only affect their children's but also affect their children's care. What parents learned about health or biology during their own education may currently be outdated or incomplete. According to the AAP, only 12% of adults have proficient levels of health literacy (Winkelman et al.,

2016). This is extremely important in pediatrics because health literacy is one of the strongest predictors of health. In pediatrics, PCPs need to assess parental health literacy levels up front, so that additional time may be added to encounters as needed. Furthermore, it is important for providers to remember that even parents with advanced literacy skills can be easily overwhelmed by health information, especially during stressful or hurried interactions.

Limited health literacy in adults has been linked to poor disease management skills, medication treatment errors, difficulties navigating the health care system, and poorer health care comes for themselves and their families (Orkan et al., 2018). In the past few years, attention has shifted upstream because the roots of health literacy are formed early in childhood as children are developing their health behaviors (Winkelman et al., 2016). Accordingly, childhood and schools are the newest population for targeted health literacy interventions. The *National Health Education Standards* (NHES) emphasize student comprehension of health promotion and disease prevention, offering unique opportunities for partnering with a growing number of school-based health centers (American Cancer Society, 2007).

Pediatric practices and PCPs are increasingly involved in these efforts as they support childhood literacy, the key precursor to learning. Office-based programs, such as *ReachOutAndRead*, ensure that children receive age-appropriate books and literacy-development instructions from their providers beginning with the first well-child visit. One of the simplest household literacy screening tools is the single-question query about the number of children's books in the home. The presence of 10 children's books is associated with adequate household literacy (Driessnack et al, 2014). The commitment to ensuring the presence of children's books in every child's home may well be one of the most impactful child health interventions undertaken in primary care. Enhancing both literacy and health literacy holds the potential to improve the health of children and to provide them with tools to be more informed and capable consumers in adulthood.

Transitioning to Adult Care

Transitioning from pediatrics to an adult primary care system is critical for all children but especially for adolescents and young adults with congenital and/or chronic physical and medical conditions (e.g., corrected congenital heart disease). Although advances in neonatal and pediatric medicine continue to improve the prognosis for children, care transition is increasingly identified as a critical process in health care management. Well-timed, -planned, and -executed transition plans enable all youth to maximize lifelong functioning and well-being and optimize their ability to assume adult roles and activities, regardless of their health care needs. Such transitions require interprofessional teams from both systems to work collaboratively with youth and their families, anticipating the unique medical, psychosocial, and educational needs as they move from child- to adult-centered care. Accordingly, the AAP and the National Center for Medical Home Implementation created a health care transition planning algorithm that specifies the protocol for managing the transition process (AAP, 2011). The guidelines highlight specific activities and decision points and provide a clear timeline suggesting transition plans begin by age 12. All PCPs are encouraged to adopt and adapt these materials for their practice.

References

AAP. *Adverse Childhood Experiences and the Lifelong Consequences of Trauma*; 2014. Available at: https://www.aap.org/en-us/Documents/ttb_aces_consequences.pdf.

AAP. Supporting the healthcare transition from adolescence to adulthood in the medical home. *Pediatrics*. 2011;128:182–200. https://doi.org/10.1542/peds.2011-0969.

American Cancer Society, Joint Committee on National Health Education Standards. *National Education Standards: Achieving Excellence*; 2007. Available at: https://sparkpe.org/wp-content/uploads/NHES_CD.pdf.

Care for Child Development (CCD). (https://www.unicef.org/earlychildhood/index_83036.html)

Driessnack M, Chung S, Perkhounkova E, Hein M. Using the newest vital sign to assess health literacy in children. *J Pediatr Health Care*. 2014;28(22):165–171. https://doi.org/10.1016/j.pedhc.2013.05.005.

Driessnack M. Children's drawings as facilitators of communication: a meta-analysis. *J Pediatr Nurs*. 2005;20(6):41–23. https://doi.org/10.1016/j.pedn.2005.03.011.

Eichner JM, Johnson BJ. *Patient- and family-centered care and the pediatrician's role*. AAP Policy Statement, 2012. https://doi.org/10.1542/peds.2011—3084.

Gennetian L, Darling M, Aber JA. Behavioral economics and developmental science: a new framework to support early childhood interventions. *J Appl Res Child*. 2016;7(2). Article 2. Available at: http://digitalcommons.library.tmc.edu/childrenatrisk/vol7/iss2/2/.

Harvard's Center for the Developing Child. (https://developingchild.harvard.edu/

Hoagwood KE, Rotheram-Borus MJ, McCaabe MA, et al. *The Interdependence of Families, Communities, and Children's Health: Public Investments that Strengthen Children's Healthy Development and Society Prosperity. NAM Perspectives*. Washington DC: Discussion paper, National Academy of Medicine; 2018.

Lancet. Advancing early childhood development: from science to scale. Available at: https://www.thelancet.com/series/ECD2016.

Orkan O, Lopes E, Bollweg TM, et al. General health literacy measurement instruments for children and adolescents: a systematic review of the literature. *BMC*. 2018;18:166. https://doi.org/10.1186/s12889-018-5054-0.

Reach Out and Read [ROAR]. (http://www.reachoutandread.org/)

ReachUpandLearn. (http://www.reachupandlearn.com/)

Russ SA, Larson K, Tullis E, Halfon N. A lifecourse approach to health development: implications for the maternal and child health research agenda. *Matern Child Health J*. 2014;18(2):497–510. https://doi.org/10.1007/s1099-013-1284-z.

Thaler RH. *Misbehaving: The Making of Behavioral Economics*. New York: W.W. Norton & Company, Inc; 2016.

Thaler RH, Sunstein CR. *Nudge: Improving Decisions about Health, Wealth, and Happiness*. New York: Penguin Books; 2009.

The Resilience Project. (aap.org/theresilienceproject)

United Nations. *Sustainable Development Goals: 17 Goals to Transform Our World*; 2015. Available at: https://www.un.org/sustainabledevelopment. Accessed June 9, 2018.

Winkelman TNA, Caldwell MT, Bertram B, Davis MM. Promoting health literacy for children and adolescents. *Pediatrics*. 2016;138(6):1–3.

3

Genetics and Genomics: The Basics for Child Health

SANDRA DAACK-HIRSCH AND MARTHA DRIESSNACK

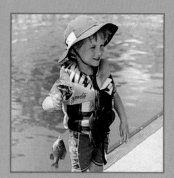

The future is not in front of us, but inside us.

Joanna Macy

Knowledge of the human genome continues to evolve, transforming not only the field of genetics, but also prior understanding of human embryology, physiology, and disease processes. In short, it is changing the way health care providers approach the diagnosis, treatment, and prevention of human diseases. The study of single genes and their role in inheritance has expanded to include the interaction of genes across the genome, as well as how these interactions are influenced by the environment, random events, and epigenetic factors and impact subsequent phenotypic changes. Very few diseases are entirely genetic and inherited, and health care providers should no longer characterize disorders as genetic or nongenetic. Rather, the astute clinician should consider to what extent genomics influences an individual's susceptibility to disease and, for that matter, an individual's potential/actual response to treatment (Fig 3.1).

At the same time, with the current emphasis on patient-centered care and patient engagement, children and families are becoming active participants in both their care and health care decisions. Of equal importance is the impact of the Internet, which delivers all forms of information in real time, accompanied by instant commentary and interpretation by anyone willing to weigh in. While healthcare is being transformed by the sheer volume of knowledge and technologies, it is also being transformed by its consumers. Today's children are right in the mix, growing up at the intersection of the genome era and information age (Driessnack, 2009).

A basic understanding of genomics is essential for all primary care providers (PCPs) to provide the best care. The medical home model of care identifies PCPs as holding a crucial role in the management of patients who have the potential for or have been diagnosed with an inherited or congenital disorder. Core competencies in genetics for nurses at all levels of practice have already been established, as communicated in *The Essentials of Baccalaureate Education for Professional Nursing Practice* (American Association of Colleges of Nursing [AACN], 2008), *The Essentials of Masters Education in Nursing* (2011), *The Essentials of Doctoral Education for Advanced Nursing Practice* (AACN, 2006), and the *Core Competencies in Genetics for Health Professionals* (National Coalition for Health Professional Education in Genetics [NCHPEG], 2007).

In addition, there are specific resources available for PCPs through the American Academy of Pediatrics (AAP) *Genetics in Primary Care* website (Table 3.1: American Academy of Pediatrics [AAP] Genetics in Primary Care).

This chapter provides a brief review of basic genetic and genomic concepts and terminology, genetic contribution to disorders, and patterns of inheritance, along with insights into obtaining a family history and conducting a pediatric assessment using a genetics lens. The concept of epigenetics, types of genomic testing, and some of the ethical challenges that can arise are introduced.

Basic Principles of Genetics

Each human is unique, established by the joining of one egg and one sperm, each of which provided a unique deoxyribonucleic acid (DNA) package. An individual's total DNA package is called a *genome*. Within each cell, genetic information flows from DNA to ribonucleic acid (RNA) to protein, with each gene coding for up to 20 different proteins. In other words, the information carried within the DNA dictates the end product (protein) that will be synthesized. This is known as the central dogma of biology (Fig 3.2). An individual's genome and the encoded protein products, in turn, interact with the individual's internal and external environment in very complex ways.

Deoxyribonucleic Acid

DNA is a molecule that contains genetic instructions for the structure and function of all living organisms. DNA is made up of a string of nucleotides, and each nucleotide consists of deoxyribose, a phosphate group, and one of four bases, called *adenine (A)*, *cytosine (C)*, *guanine (G)*, and *thymine (T)*. The two backbones of the DNA helix are formed by the deoxyribose and phosphate groups, whereas the rungs that hold them together are formed by complementary pairing (A-T and C-G) of the bases. The DNA helix is coiled tightly encircling histone proteins. Uncoiled, each DNA strand is approximately 6 feet long. Although each person has a unique DNA package that reflects one in several million possible combinations from the four grandparents' genetic material; the base sequences of any two human genomes are thought to be 99.9% identical. In short, people's DNA structure is more alike than different. Yet, the slightest alteration in an individual's DNA sequence can have devastating health consequences.

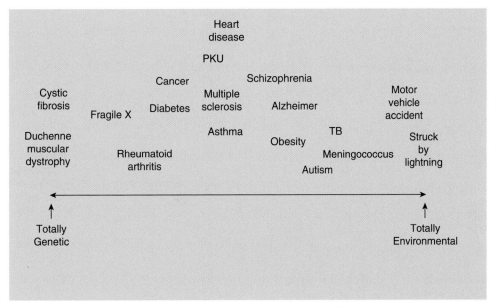

• **Fig 3.1 Spectrum of Disease Causation** *PKU,* Phenylketonuria; *TB,* tuberculosis. (From Health-Knowledge [website]; 2017. https://www.healthknowledge.org.uk/public-health-textbook/disease-causa-tion-diagnostic/2d-genetics. Accessed February 14, 2018.)

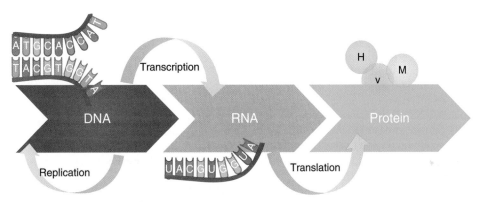

• **Fig 3.2** Central Dogma of Biology (From Genius [website]; 2018. https://genius.com/Biology-genius-the-central-dogma-annotated. Accessed February 14, 2018.)

For example, virtually every case of sickle cell anemia is caused by the smallest of genetic changes—a substitution of a single nucleo-tide (A→T). On the other hand, some DNA alterations have no known effect on an individual, whereas still others appear to pro-vide a benefit or protective action. The same single nucleotide alter-ation that is responsible for sickle cell anemia can confer a survival advantage to unaffected carriers challenged with the malaria patho-gen (Withrock, Anderson, Jefferson, McCormack, Mlynarczk et al., 2015). This is why sickle cell alterations, including both the trait and disease, persist in populations where malaria is endemic.

Chromosomes

Cytogenetics is the study of genetics at the chromosome level, where most of our genetic information is located. Each chromo-some is a strand of DNA. In the nucleus of all normal human cells, with the exception of gametes, are 46 chromosomes arranged in 23 pairs. Twenty-two of the pairs are called *autosomes*; they look the same in females and males. The remaining pair, the sex chromosomes, differs between females and males, with two X

chromosomes in females (XX) and one X and one Y chromosome (XY) in males. The 22 autosomes are numbered by size—from largest (1) to smallest (22). The picture of human chromosomes lined up in pairs is called a *karyotype* (Fig 3.3).

Human somatic cells are *diploid*, containing 23 paired chromo-somes. Diploid cells are replicated through the process of *mitosis*, which creates two identical daughter cells. In contrast, gametes, or germline cells (egg and sperm), are *haploid* cells, each containing only 23 chromosomes. Gametes are produced in the ovary or tes-ticle during *meiosis*, where there is an exchange of genetic material, through crossing over and recombination, resulting in a random assortment of maternally and paternally derived genetic material in the daughter cells. Fusion at fertilization restores the 46-chro-mosome (23-pair) complement, with one of each chromosome pair from each gamete, creating a unique human being.

A chromosome has a long arm (q) and a short arm (p). Geneti-cists often use a diagram, or *ideogram*, which shows a chromo-some's size and banding pattern. The bands are used to further describe the location of genes on each chromosome. For exam-ple, the cytogenetic location of the *CFTR* gene (cystic fibrosis) is

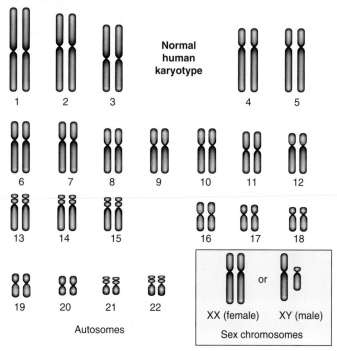

Normal
human
karyotype

1　2　3　　4　5

6　7　8　9　10　11　12

13　14　15　　16　17　18

19　20　21　22

XX (female)　or　XY (male)

Autosomes　　Sex chromosomes

• **Fig 3.3** Normal Human Karyotype (From Genetics Home Reference. Normal human karyotype. http://ghr.nlm.nih.gov/handbook/illustrations/normalkaryotype. Accessed November 16, 2015.)

7q31.2, which means the *CFTR* gene is located on the long arm (q) of chromosome 7, band 3, sub-band 1, and sub-sub-band 2. Other common symbols include *del,* for deletion; *dup,* for duplication; and + indicating an increased or − indicating a decrease in number. For example, 47, XY+21 indicates a male with three copies of chromosome 21 (Down syndrome), whereas 46, XX,8q− denotes a female with a deletion on the long arm of chromosome 8 (Genetics Home Reference, 2018).

At the ends of each chromosome are protective caps, or *telomeres.* Telomeres, specific repetitive sequences of noncoding DNA, contain and protect the genetic information on the chromosome. The telomeres shorten each time a cell divides, losing their protective function over time until cells can no longer replicate and divide, and therefore die. This shortening process is the focus of ongoing research related to aging and cancer. Emerging research now suggests that growing up in a stressful environment can also leave lasting marks on young chromosomes. In particular, children from poor and/or unstable homes have been shown to have shorter telomeres than their unaffected peers (Madhusoodanan, 2014). This line of research parallels the work of the adverse childhood experiences (ACE) study, whose findings suggest that as the number of stressors during childhood increase, the risk for adult health problems also increases in a strong and graded fashion (see Table 3.1: Centers for Disease Control and Prevention [CDC]a).

Genes

A gene is a specific *coding* sequence of DNA organized in small blocks of three letters (e.g., GGC, ATG), known as a *codon.* There are 64 different codons in the genetic code. To early geneticists, a gene was an abstract entity whose existence was only known through its reflected *phenotype,* or physical expression transmitted between generations. Later, genes on chromosomes were thought to be like beads on a string, each coding for one protein; however, it

TABLE 3.1	Online Resources
Resource	URL (Accessed February 21, 2018)
American College of Medical Genetics and Genomics (ACMG) ACT Sheets and Confirmatory Algorithms	http://www.ncbi.nlm.nih.gov/books/NBK55827
American Academy of Pediatrics (AAP) Genetics in Primary Care	https://www.aap.org/en-us/advocacy-and-policy/aap-health-initiatives/pages/Genetics-in-Primary-Care-Institute.aspx
Autism Speaks	https://www.autismspeaks.org/science/initiatives/autism-genome-project
Baby's First Test	http://www.babysfirsttest.org/
Centers for Disease Control and Prevention (CDCa)—ACE Study	https://www.cdc.gov/violenceprevention/acestudy/index.html
Clinical Pharmacogenomics Implementation Consortium (CPIC)	https://cpicpgx.org/
Centers for Disease Control and Prevention (CDCb)—Folic Acid	https://www.cdc.gov/ncbddd/folicacid/index.html
Genetic Testing Registry (GTR)	https://www.ncbi.nlm.nih.gov/gtr/
Genes In Life	http://www.genesinlife.org/
Genetic Alliance	http://www.geneticalliance.org/
MotherToBaby	https://mothertobaby.org/
NCHPEG National Coalition for Health Professional Education in Genetics Family History Collection and Risk Assessment	https://www.jax.org/education-and-learning/clinical-and-continuing-education/family-history
Online Mendelian Inheritance in Man, Neural tube defects, susceptibility to; NTD	http://omim.org/entry/182940
Positive Exposure	http://positiveexposure.org/
Recommended Uniform Screening Panel RUSP	https://www.hrsa.gov/advisory-committees/heritable-disorders/rusp/index.html

is now known that one gene codes for an average of three proteins. Today, genes are increasingly viewed through informational science and computational biology lenses, resulting in the infusion of information processing and systems language (e.g., upstream regulation). *Genotype* refers to an individual's collection of genes. The *phenotype* is the manifestation of the individual's genotype; however, more precisely, the phenotype is the result of gene expression, which is regulated by molecular mechanisms and modified by environmental factors. Phenotype includes an individual's physical and cognitive features, organ structure, and biochemical and physiologic nature.

Each human inherits two copies of each gene—one copy, or *allele,* from each parent. Alleles are forms of the same gene with differences in their DNA sequence. These differences contribute to each person's unique features. If the two alleles at any given location (locus) are similar, the individual is *homozygous*; if the alleles are different, the individual is *heterozygous*. For example, a child with cystic fibrosis may have identical CFTR gene sequences (e.g., mutation F508del) in both alleles, and as such would be called *homozygous* for that mutation, whereas this child's parents are heterozygous in their CFTR gene sequence, each with only one copy of the mutation allele and one copy of a normal allele.

In humans, genes can vary in size from 200 to more than 2 million DNA bases. Humans are thought to have between 20,000 and 25,000 different genes. Although every human cell contains every gene, not all genes are active at once; certain mechanisms activate them, turning them on or off at various developmental points or at various locations within the body. Each gene also has coding sequences (exons), separated by noncoding sequences (introns), and occupies a specific location (locus) on a chromosome. It was previously believed that differences in noncoding DNA sequences did not have relevance to human health and development. However, it is now known that some of these differences are associated with increased risk for common diseases, such as diabetes, heart disease, and cancer (Genetics Home Reference, 2018). In addition, a small number of genes are located in the mitochondria.

Mutations

An allele is typically regarded as a *mutation* when its genetic variation is found in less than 1% of the population or a *polymorphism* when it is found in greater than 1% of a population; however, the cutoff of at least 1% prevalence is somewhat arbitrary (Genetics Home Reference, 2018). The term *mutation* is usually used to mean a disease-causing variation, whereas a *polymorphism* is used to refer to a normal variation, or one that does not *directly* cause disease. But really the key difference between the classification of mutation and polymorphism is the frequency that each occurs.

One type of polymorphism is known as *single nucleotide polymorphisms*, or *SNP* (pronounced "snip"). SNPs are used to study the genetic contribution to multifactorial disorders, such as cleft lip and cleft palate, diabetes, heart disease, and cancer, as well as individual response to drugs (pharmacogenomics). A SNP is a single base pair alteration that is common in a given population. On average, SNPs are found every 300 to 2000 nucleotides in the human genome (Genetics Home Reference, 2018). Typically, SNPs are not directly disease-causing mutations; however, they are biologically relevant because they help identify individuals at increased risk for multifactorial disease. They also are used in pharmacogenomic testing to identify individuals at increased risk for adverse response to medications.

Mutations that directly cause disorders are further subclassified as *point mutations, nucleotide repeat expansions, copy number variants,* or *chromosome mutations*. It is important to remember that although these types of mutations can have a large effect on individual human health and development, human evolutionary changes are more likely to result from the accumulation over time of many mutations with small effects.

Point Mutations

Point mutations are single base pair changes (i.e., substitutions, deletions, or insertions), occurring at the level of the nucleotide, yet capable of changing the function of a gene or gene product. They are responsible for many single-gene disorders, including sickle cell anemia and cystic fibrosis. Point mutations should not be confused with SNPs. Although both are single nucleotide differences in a DNA sequence, a SNP, by definition, is present in at least 1% of the general population.

Deletions are mutations in which a section of DNA is lost or deleted. The number of base pairs deleted can range from one to thousands. Examples some syndromes cause by deletion mutations include 22q11.2 deletions syndrome, Duchenne muscular dystrophy, and neurofibromatosis type I.

Insertions are mutations in which extra base pairs are inserted into a new place in the DNA, making it longer than it should be. Like deletions, the number of base pairs involved ranges from one to thousands. Examples of some syndromes caused by an insertion include Duchenne muscular dystrophy and Charcot-Marie-Tooth Type 1A. Note that Duchenne muscular dystrophy was presented as an example for both insertion and deletion mutations. Many inherited and congenital syndromes are associated with more than one type of mutation; however, these different types of mutations involving the same gene result in the same syndrome.

Insertions and deletions are often collectively referred to as *INDELS*. Protein coding DNA is divided into codons. Insertions and deletions in the codons can totally change the gene message so that it cannot be coded or it cannot be coded correctly. This specific type of INDEL is called a *frameshift mutation*. Tay-Sachs, many types of cancers, and Crohn disease are some examples of disorders associated with frameshift mutations.

Nucleotide Repeat Expansions

A repeat expansion is a special type of insertion mutation that increases the number of times a short DNA sequence is normally repeated. When the number of repeats increases beyond the normally tolerated limit, the mutation (i.e., repeat expansion) results in a disorder that could be inherited. For example, almost all cases of fragile X syndrome are caused by an expansion of a trinucleotide (three-base-pair) repeat sequence (CGG) in the *FMR1* gene (Xq27.3) from a normal 5 to 40 times to over 200 times. The expansion makes the gene unstable, resulting in little or no protein output with an outcome of signs and symptoms of fragile X syndrome.

Copy Number Variations

A copy number variation (CNV) involves larger areas of chromosomes, beyond point mutations and repeat expansions. During egg and sperm production, unequal crossover events occur throughout the genome. When this happens, children may have lost (deletion) or gained (duplication) copies of genetic information that were present in either of their parents' chromosomes. Unlike other types of mutations that have been inherited for countless generations, geneticists now recognize that CNVs have a more recent origin. The study of CNVs has already enriched current understanding of autism and other neuropsychiatric diseases, such as mental retardation and schizophrenia (Yoo, 2015; see Table 3.1: Autism Speaks).

Chromosome Mutations

Chromosome mutations occur when even larger segments of a chromosome (involving many bands) are deleted, duplicated, rearranged, or translocated in such a way that there is a resulting alteration of the DNA sequence, a modification of the gene dosage, or a complete absence of a gene or several genes. For example, cri-du-chat syndrome (5p–) is caused by the deletion of the entire end of the short (p) arm of chromosome, whereas Down syndrome is caused by the addition of an entire chromosome. Chromosome mutations usually result in multiorgan, large effects, such as in Down syndrome, in which the individual can have neurologic, eye, ear, orthopedic, cardiac, and other abnormalities.

Genetics and Diseases

The term "genetic disorder" is in some ways an antiquated term. Nearly all diseases are now thought to have a genetic component, in that diseases are caused in whole, or in part, by changes in DNA sequence or gene expression (see Fig 3.1). Traditionally, disease and the respective genetic contribution are grouped under one of four categories: (1) single-gene disorders, (2) chromosome disorders, (3) multifactorial disorders, or (4) mitochondrial disorders. The genotype associated with a particular disease can be inherited, arise spontaneously, or be acquired over a lifetime. For example, some diseases are caused by inherited mutations; diseases can also be caused by spontaneous mutations that occur during the development of the gametes or in early human development (de novo), whereas most forms of cancers are the result of acquired mutations in a gene or group of genes that occur during a person's life. Mutations that are acquired during a person's life happen at the somatic level and occur either randomly or due to a random event or environmental exposure.

Single Gene Disorders

Single gene disorders (also referred to as *monogenetic disorders*) occur when the mutation affects one gene. The mutation may be present on one or both chromosomes, associated with one of three different *Mendelian* patterns of inheritance—dominant, recessive, or X-linked. Dominant disorders are caused by the presence of the gene mutation on just one of the two inherited parental alleles; recessive diseases require the presence of the gene mutation on both of the inherited alleles; X-linked diseases are monogenic disorders confined to the X chromosome. They can be dominant or recessive. Some examples of monogenic disorders that should be familiar to PCPs are sickle cell disease, thalassemia, neurofibromatosis, hemophilia, Duchene muscular dystrophy, cystic fibrosis, fragile X syndrome, polycystic kidney disease, Marfan syndrome, and Tay-Sachs disease.

Chromosome Disorders

Chromosome disorders occur with changes in the number or structure of an entire chromosome, or large segments of it. For example, Down syndrome (trisomy 21) is caused by an extra copy of chromosome 21, Prader-Willi syndrome is caused by the absence of a group of genes on chromosome 15, and chronic myeloid leukemia (CML) results from a translocation in which portions of chromosomes 9 and 22 are exchanged, resulting in a new, abnormal gene (Genetics Home Reference, 2018). Other examples of chromosomal disorders that should be familiar to providers in primary care are cri-du-chat syndrome (5p–), Williams syndrome, and DiGeorge syndrome, also referred to as *velocardiofacial* or *22q11 deletion syndrome.*

Chromosome disorders can also involve sex chromosomes, such as Klinefelter syndrome (XXY), which is caused by an extra X chromosome, and Turner syndrome (XO), which is caused by the absence of an X chromosome.

Another type of chromosomal disorder is called *mosaicism*, which occurs when an altered chromosomal arrangement occurs in some cells but not in others within the same individual. The clinical symptoms are usually milder, and the prognosis improves with fewer numbers of cells involved.

When taking a family history, PCPs should remember there is a high frequency of chromosomal disorders in spontaneous abortions and stillbirths. Further, the prevalence of chromosomal disorders due to nondisjunction increases with advancing maternal age.

Multifactorial Disorders

Multifactorial disorders result from a combination of genetic and environmental factors. Recurrence risks are based on empirical statistics—observations based on data collected from thousands of family histories transformed into probabilities. These disorders can cluster in families; the exact recurrence risk is difficult to predict because the individuals' or couples' precise genetic and environmental risks are usually not known. Therefore a population-based recurrence risk rather than a personal recurrence risk is given. One example of a multifactorial disorder includes neural tube defects (NTD), such as spina bifida or anencephaly. NTDs appear in females more often than in males, and once a child is born with an NTD, the chance for those parents to have another child with an NTD in a future pregnancy increases (see Table 3.1: Online Mendelian Inheritance in Man [OMIM]). The rate of NTDs decreases with sufficient maternal folic acid supplementation. Therefore the CDC recommends that all women of childbearing age consume 0.4 mg (400 µg) of folic acid daily (see Table 3.1: Centers for Disease Control and Prevention [CDC] b). In contrast, the rate of NTDs increases when mothers have uncontrolled diabetes or take certain medications (e.g., valproic acid). The specific combination of genetic factors or how they interact with each other or other environmental factors is unknown. Other examples of multifactorial disorders that should be familiar to PCPs are congenital heart defect, club foot, cleft lip/palate, pyloric stenosis, Hirschsprung disease, hip dysplasia, and asthma.

Teratogens

A *teratogen* is any agent that results in, or increases the incidence of, a congenital malformation. Although teratogens have traditionally been considered as environmental toxins altering critical embryonic and fetal development events, it appears that genomic factors can have significant modifying effects to the teratogen. The same teratogenic exposure can induce a severe malformation in one embryo, while failing to do so in another, even though the timing and dose of the exposure were similar (Wlodarczyk et al., 2011). A teratogen may also affect the embryo at one developmental point but not at a different one. The Organization of Teratology Information Specialists (OTIS) provides both health care providers and the public with evidence-based information about exposures during pregnancy and while breastfeeding (see Table 3.1: MotherToBaby). The world's most notorious teratogen is probably thalidomide; however, clinicians today are probably more familiar with fetal alcohol spectrum disorder (FASD), which results from prenatal exposure to alcohol. Teratogenic exposures can also include viruses, such as rubella, cytomegalovirus, and toxoplasmosis; medications, such as warfarin, lithium, tetracycline, and phenytoin; and maternal conditions such as type 2 diabetes and phenylketonuria (PKU).

Mitochondrial Disorders

Although the majority of an individual's DNA is found in chromosomes within the nucleus of a cell, a small amount of genetic material is found in the mitochondria located in the cytoplasm, outside the nucleus. This genetic material is known as *mitochondrial DNA (mtDNA)* and contains only 37 genes. Each cell contains hundreds to thousands of mitochondria, which also means there are more opportunities for mutations. Mitochondrial disorders are caused by mutations in mtDNA (i.e., nonchromosomal DNA) and are typically progressive disorders affecting the brain and muscles. Mitochondrial disorders are characterized by exclusively maternal (matrilinear) transmission. When many normal mitochondria are present, the effects from the aberrant mtDNA may be minimal. Some examples of mitochondrial disorders that should be familiar to PCPs are Leber hereditary optic neuropathy (LHON), Leigh syndrome, nonsyndromic deafness, mitochondrial encephalomyopathy, lactic acidosis, and stroke-like episodes (MELAS). Of note, mtDNA also provides individuals with genealogic information about their female ancestral line.

Patterns of Inheritance

Terminology

One of the important outcomes of taking a family history is the ability to recognize basic inheritance patterns; however, it is important to understand that there can be variable phenotypes, making some patterns of inheritance harder to detect. There are a few terms that clinicians need to understand, including penetrance, expressivity, pleiotropy, variable age of onset, and anticipation (Table 3.2).

Mendelian Inheritance Patterns

Disorders caused by mutations in a single gene are usually inherited in one of several patterns, commonly referred to as *Mendelian* (after Gregor Mendel, known as the father of genetics) patterns of inheritance. They include autosomal dominant (AD), autosomal recessive (AR), X-linked dominant, and X-linked recessive, as well as maternal or mitochondrial inheritance. In contrast, most chromosomal disorders are not passed from one generation to the next.

Autosomal Dominant

This type of single gene disorder is characterized by the inheritance of a single copy of a mutated gene located on one of the autosomal chromosomes (chromosome 1-22). The gene mutation is passed on from only one parent but results in an inherited disorder. The paired gene from the other parent is normal. The parent passing on the gene mutation typically has the disorder. For the offspring, the risk of inheriting the mutation from an affected parent is 50%, regardless of sex and independent of having an affected sibling (Fig 3.4). Children without the abnormal gene will neither develop the disorder nor pass it on. Examples of disorders with an AD inheritance pattern include Huntington disease, Noonan syndrome, and neurofibromatosis type 1.

The clinician reviewing a child's family history should consider AD inheritance when a specific phenotype appears in a family generation after generation, both sexes appear equally affected, and male-to-male transmission occurs. However, penetrance, expressivity, pleiotropy, variable age of onset, and anticipation can interfere with one's ability to recognize AD inheritance. Further, some AD disorders, such as achondroplasia, have a high rate of de novo (new) mutations, making it highly likely that a pedigree will not reveal additionally affected relatives.

Autosomal Recessive

This type of single gene disorder requires inheritance of two copies of a mutated gene (one from each parent) located on one of the autosomal chromosomes (chromosome 1-22). Offspring who inherit only one abnormal gene in the pair are considered *carriers*; they can pass that gene to their children but are typically unaffected.

TABLE 3.2	Definitions of Gene Expression Variables		
Term	**Definition**		**Examples**
Penetrance—complete or incomplete	Proportion (%) of individuals with a specific genotype that exhibit the corresponding disease phenotype. Complete: Everyone with a specific disease genotype (100%) manifests the corresponding phenotype Incomplete: Some (varying %) of the affected individuals manifest the phenotype		Complete: Huntington disease Incomplete: Breast cancer from BRCA1 or BRCA2 mutation
Expressivity (variable expressivity)	Degree to which a phenotype is expressed. Can vary by compilation and/or severity, even within families.		Van der Woude syndrome: Children can have a cleft lip, cleft palate, or both. Children can have pits near the center of the lower lip; mounds, and/or missing teeth.
Pleiotropy	One genotype results in multiple, seemingly unrelated phenotypes		Marfan syndrome: From joint hypermobility and limb elongation to aortic and heart disease, vision problems, caused by a dislocated lens in either one or both eyes, as well as varying severity, timing of onset, and rate of progression
Variable age of onset	Phenotypic expression does not emerge until later in life		Alzheimer or Parkinson disease
Anticipation	Some phenotypes become more severe and/or appear at an earlier age as a disorder is passed from one generation to the next		Myotonic dystrophy, fragile X syndrome, Huntington disease

For offspring of parents who both carry an AR mutation, there is a 25% chance of inheriting the mutation from both parents, thus developing the associated disorder, a 50% chance of inheriting one copy and becoming a carrier, and a 25% chance of not inheriting either mutation (Fig 3.5). Examples of AR disorders include cystic fibrosis, albinism, PKU, thalassemia, and sickle cell anemia.

The clinician reviewing a child's family history should consider AR inheritance when a specific phenotype affects multiple siblings and both sexes are affected. The phenotype is often not present in a family generation after generation. However, a family's geographic ancestry and ethnic background, as well as consanguinity, can influence the likelihood of AR disorders, making it more likely that the family will have affected family members in several generations. Examples of geographic ancestry increasing risk for AR disorders include (1) gene mutations associated with cystic fibrosis occur most frequently in populations of European descent and (2) gene mutations associated with sickle cell anemia occur more frequently throughout sub-Saharan Africa, the Middle East, and the Indian subcontinent (Williams and Weatherall, 2012).

X-Linked Inheritance

Although X-linked inheritance patterns have traditionally been separated into subcategories of X-linked dominant or recessive, there is a move toward collapsing these categories, considering X-linked inheritance patterns across a spectrum. However, for the purposes of this chapter, they will be presented separately.

X-Linked Dominant. When a disorder is classified as *X-linked dominant*, it means that a single abnormal gene on the X chromosome gives rise to the disease (Fig 3.6). If the father is affected (abnormal gene on his X chromosome) and the mother is not, all of his female offspring will inherit the disease-causing allele, but none of his male offspring, because daughters always inherit their father's X-chromosome, whereas sons inherit their father's Y-chromosome. If the mother is affected (one abnormal gene on an X chromosome)

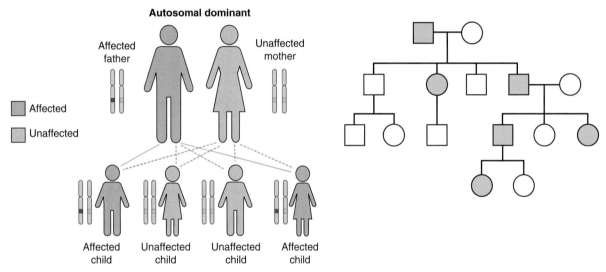

• **Fig 3.4** Autosomal Dominant Inheritance (From Genetics Home Reference. Autosomal dominant. http://ghr.nlm.nih.gov/handbook/illustrations/autodominant. Accessed November 16, 2015.)

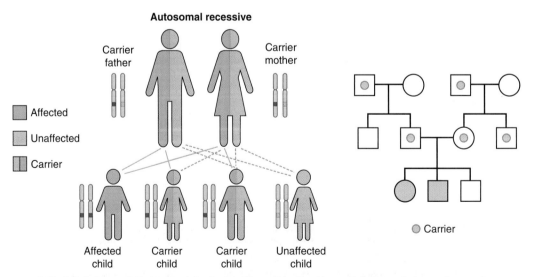

• **Fig 3.5** Autosomal Recessive Inheritance (From Genetics Home Reference. Autosomal recessive. http://ghr.nlm.nih.gov/handbook/illustrations/patterns?show=autorecessive. Accessed November 16, 2015.)

and the father is not, there is only a 50% chance that each daughter or son will inherit the disease-causing allele and manifest the disorder, because mothers have two X chromosomes to pass on.

The clinician reviewing a child's family history should consider X-linked dominant inheritance when a specific phenotype affects both sexes in each generation, with slightly more females

(X-linked dominant conditions are often lethal in males) and the absence of male-to-male transmission. Examples of disorders with X-linked dominant inheritance include Rett syndrome and vitamin D–resistant rickets.

X-Linked Recessive. When a disorder is classified as *X-linked recessive*, it usually occurs in males (Fig 3.7). This pattern is seen

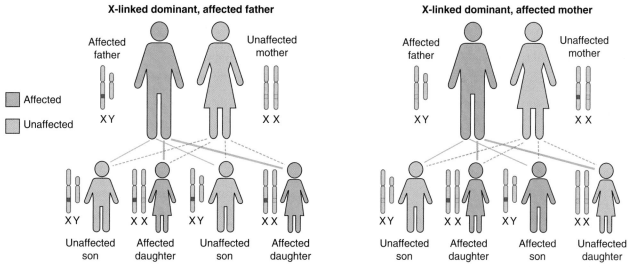

• **Fig 3.6** X-Linked Inheritance—Dominant (From Genetics Home Reference. Inheritance patterns. http://ghr.nlm.nih.gov/handbook/illustrations/patterns?show=xlinkdominantfather; and http://ghr.nlm.nih. gov/handbook/illustrations/patterns?show=xlinkdominantmother. Accessed November 16, 2015.)

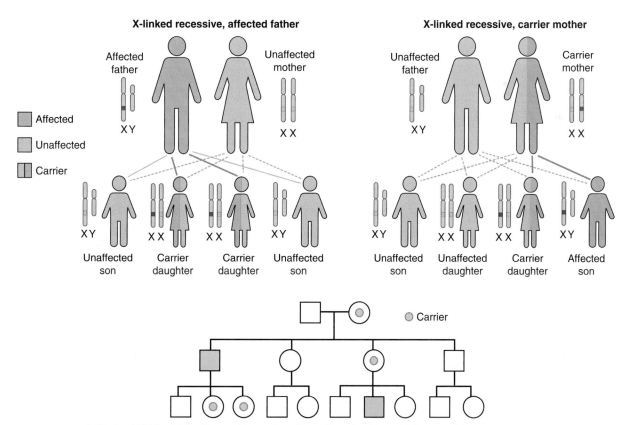

• **Fig 3.7** X-Linked Inheritance—Recessive (From Genetics Home Reference. Inheritance patterns. http://ghr.nlm.nih.gov/handbook/illustrations/patterns?show=xlinkrecessivefather; and http://ghr.nlm.nih. gov/handbook/illustrations/patterns?show=xlinkrecessivemother. Accessed November 16, 2015.)

because males have only one X chromosome, so a single, abnormal, recessive allele on that X chromosome is enough to cause the disease. When the father is affected, none of his sons will be affected, and all of his daughters will be *carriers*. If the mother is a carrier (one abnormal gene on one of her X chromosomes), there is a 50% chance that each son will be affected. Daughters have a 50% chance of being a carrier like their mothers. Although females can have an X-linked recessive disorder, it is rare.

When reviewing a child's family history, one should consider X-linked recessive inheritance when a specific phenotype is noted in males more often or more severely than females. Examples of X-linked recessive disorders include Fabry disease, hemophilia A and B, G6PD deficiency, and Duchene muscular dystrophy. As with AD inheritance, some disorders (e.g., Duchene muscular dystrophy) have high rates of de novo (new) mutations, thus rendering the past family history negative.

Nontraditional Inheritance Patterns

Mitochondrial Inheritance

Another inheritance pattern arises from the mtDNA, which accordingly is called *mitochondrial inheritance* (Fig 3.8). Mothers alone pass on mtDNA (i.e., matrilinear or maternal inheritance) because only egg cells contribute mitochondria to the developing embryo. Disorders that arise from mutations in mtDNA can appear in every generation, affecting both sexes. On average, males are more severely affected compared with females. Examples of disorders with maternal (mitochondrial) inheritance include LHON, myoclonic epilepsy with ragged red fibers (MERRF), and MELAS.

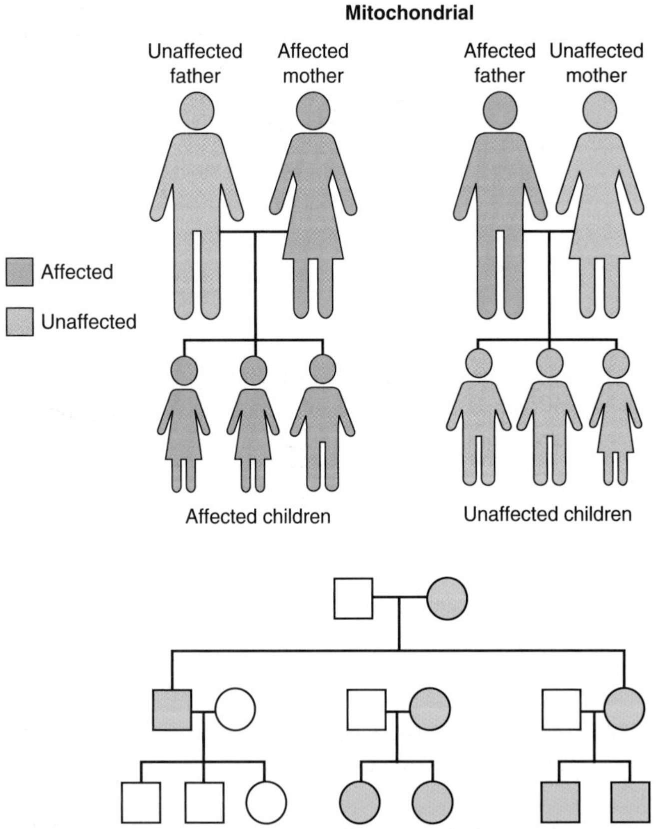

Mitochondrial

Unaffected father · Affected mother · Affected father · Unaffected mother

Affected / Unaffected

Affected children · Unaffected children

• **Fig 3.8** Mitochondrial Inheritance (From Genetics Home Reference. Inheritance patterns. http://ghr.nlm.nih.gov/handbook/illustrations/patterns?show=mitochondrial. Accessed November 16, 2015.)

Codominant Inheritance

A disorder is categorized as having a *codominant inheritance* when two different alleles for a gene can be expressed and different combinations result in slightly different proteins (Fig 3.9). There are a few genes with established codominant inheritance patterns; however, some disorders do not follow established patterns and are considered multifactorial in origin. Sometimes the specific gene(s) remain partially or fully unidentified. The best example of this type of inheritance is reflected in blood type (ABO blood group) determination.

Genomic Imprinting

Children typically inherit two copies of genes, one from their mother and one from their father, and both copies are active (i.e., turned on) in the cells together; however, in some cases only one copy needs to be expressed, and therefore the other copy is turned off or silenced during embryogenesis. The decision as to which gene remains working and which is silenced depends on the parent of origin. Only a small number of genes go through genomic imprinting, which occurs when the origin of the gene (maternal vs. paternal) is marked (imprinted) on the gene during the formation of egg or sperm cells through methylation. Imprinted genes tend to cluster together in the same regions of certain chromosomes (Genetics Home Reference, 2018). Improper imprinting can result in a child having two active copies or two inactive copies. Two major clusters of imprinted genes have been identified in humans, on chromosomes 11 and 15. Prader-Willi syndrome occurs when the paternally derived genes located in a specific chromosome 15 region are either improperly imprinted or deleted, whereas Angelman syndrome occurs when the maternally derived genes in the same area are either improperly imprinted or deleted. Thus the developing embryo does not detect a paternal or maternal copy of chromosome 15, producing one syndrome or the other. Beckwith-Wiedemann and Russell-Silver syndromes are other examples of disorders influenced by genomic imprinting.

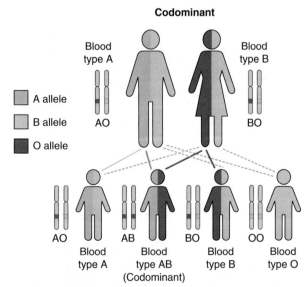

Codominant

Blood type A · Blood type B

A allele / B allele / O allele

AO · BO

AO · AB · BO · OO

Blood type A · Blood type AB (Codominant) · Blood type B · Blood type O

• **Fig 3.9** Codominant Inheritance (From Genetics Home Reference. Inheritance patterns. http://ghr.nlm.nih.gov/handbook/illustrations/patterns?show=codominant. Accessed November 16, 2015.)

Uniparental Disomy

When a child receives two copies of one chromosome, or a part of a chromosome, from one parent and none from the other parent, it results in uniparental disomy (UPD). The child will be homozygous for every gene located on that chromosome, which increases the possibility of inheriting an AR disorder. UPD can occur as a random event during the formation of egg or sperm cells, or may happen in early fetal development.

In many cases, UPD has no effect on a child's health or development, because most genes are not imprinted. Thus it does not matter if a child inherits both copies from one parent or one copy from each parent. However, in some cases, maternal or paternal inheritance of a specific gene is important. Examples of disorders that can arise from UPD include Prader-Willi and Angelman syndromes, which were also noted under genomic imprinting. Prader-Willi syndrome (caused by UPD) happens when the fetus inherits two maternal chromosome 15 (she or he is missing a paternally derived chromosome 15). Angelman syndrome (caused by UPD) happens when the fetus inherits two paternal chromosome 15 (she or he is missing a maternally derived chromosome 15).

Epigenetics

Epigenetics is the study of changes in gene expression that occur without a change in DNA sequence (Genetics Home Reference, 2018). Epigenetics regulates which genes get turned on and off. Its study is increasingly important in the identification and treatment of childhood diseases and developmental disorders. Unlike the genome, the epigenome is modifiable. The epigenome consists of molecular compounds that "mark" the genome and modify genetic expression by telling a gene or several genes what to do, when to do it, and where to do it. DNA methylation, histone modification, and/or microRNA (miRNA) are examples of three types of epigenetic modifications. *DNA methylation* involves the addition of a methyl (CH_3) group to the DNA, which modifies gene expression by turning the gene(s) off. *Histone modification* involves adding or subtracting molecules that in turn change how tightly coiled a segment of DNA is around its corresponding histone. DNA that is tightly coiled is closed to transcription, and therefore local genes cannot be expressed, whereas loosely coiled DNA is open to transcription and subsequent expression. *miRNA* regulate expression of target genes through posttranscription gene silencing. Different experiences or exposures may influence the epigenetic profile, including chemical exposures, diet, endocrine disruptive compounds, hypoxia, maternal physical state and age, placenta size, smoking, stress, and trauma. Many common adult disorders are now believed to be caused by epigenetic changes that occurred during that individual's embryonic development or in early childhood, such as obesity, heart disease, hypertension, diabetes, and obesity (Puumala and Hoyme, 2015).

Integration of Basic Genetics and Genomics into Pediatric Primary Care

Assessment

Family health history and the recognition of genetic red flags provide the foundation from which care evolves. Emphasis is on understanding genetic screening, working with children and families to understand the implications of a genetic workup and diagnosis, and coordinating care with genetic specialists. A complete head-to-toe physical and developmental assessment, combined with a comprehensive family health history, is important in identifying inherited and congenital disorders.

Family Health History and Pedigree

In primary care practice, taking the time to collect a child's family health history and pedigree can be just as important as information from a laboratory test, yet this is often underused or absent in today's increasingly time-constrained well child visits. Individual and family involvement in family health history got a boost in 2004, when the U.S. Surgeon General declared Thanksgiving as the ideal day to investigate and/or update one's family health history. An individual's family history should be updated annually.

Three-Generation Pedigree. The pedigree is a valuable visual record of genetic links and health-related information. It should include at least three generations and is much more helpful in visual form, rather than in lists or narrative formats. It is important to remember that most disorders have some genetic component, and the strength or pattern of traits or diseases may become apparent based on the number or pattern of individuals in a family who are affected. Table 3.3 suggests specific questions to use when conducting a comprehensive family health history. Insights about families are gained, not only because families share genes, but also because they also often share environments, behaviors, and culture—all of which contribute to shared health problems. See Figs 3.4 to 3.9 for the exemplars of pedigrees highlighting different patterns of inheritance.

All PCPs should be able to obtain, record, and interpret a three-generation pedigree, which is a construct that includes the health status of first-, second-, and third-degree relatives (three generations) of the individual's or child's family. Although the aim for clinical practice is a three-generation pedigree, asking about only two generations, or in some cases asking about four generations, may be more appropriate, depending on the trait or disorder and family size (see Table 3.4 for proportion of genetic material shared by family relationships).

There is a set of standardized pedigree symbols that have been adopted internationally (Bennett et al., 2008). An overview of the symbols, as well as how to connect them to illustrate various family relationships, is provided in Figs 3.10 and 3.11. There are also multiple Internet resources to assist children, families, and providers in obtaining and documenting family health histories, including Genetic Alliance's "Does It Run in the Family?" Toolkit (see Table 3.1: Genetic Alliance, NCHPEG Family History Collection and Risk Assessment, and Genes In Life).

The process of constructing a family pedigree should begin with the nuclear family, followed by added aunts and uncles, cousins, and grandparents. For all persons included in the pedigree, it is important to record their date of birth or age, relevant symptoms, traits, or disorders, as well as the ages of diagnosis, and the ages and causes of death. It is also important to record miscarriages, stillbirths, infertility, and any children relinquished for adoption. An additional query should be made about the presence or possibility of consanguinity or incest. When pieces of family history are missing, it is important to note the information as missing, because the absence of information does not mean the child has not acquired genetic risk.

Genetic Red Flags From the History. Genetic red flags indicate the potential for genetic risk. For some providers, it is easiest to remember the Rule of Too/Two. For some providers, it is easiest to remember simple rules (e.g., rule of too/two) or mnemonics (e.g., SCREEN, F-GENES) to remember the important components to look for or ask about when obtaining a family health history. (Table 3.5).

TABLE 3.3   General Screening for Genetic Conditions: The History

Question	Rationale/Comments
Does/has anyone in the family have/had a birth defect?	To identify conditions that affect others in the family. If answer is yes, try to get more information about the nature of the defect.
Has anyone in the family had a stillborn baby? A baby who died early? A baby who died unexpectedly?	To identify unrecognized syndrome. Babies who died very early may have inheritable metabolic disorders. Distinguish sudden unexplained infant death (SUID) and sudden infant death syndrome (SIDS).
Is there any chance that you and your partner are blood-related? Is this pregnancy a product of incest? Is there any history of consanguinity/incest in your extended family?	Consanguinity of partners closer than first cousins is a risk factor for autosomal recessive (AR) disorders. If yes, recommend genetics consultation.
Is there anyone in your family who routinely sees a health care provider for specific condition?	Significant if early onset, two or more close relatives affected. Remember to ask about hearing/vision, growth disorders. Genetic heart disease and genetic cancer risks are important. If yes, recommend genetic consultation and monitoring.
Have you or your partner, or any of your/your partners' parents/siblings had three or more miscarriages? How about infertility issues?	May indicate a chromosome translocation. If yes, order a karyotype of the mother or father (or both). Difficulties becoming/maintaining a pregnancy may indicate a genetic syndrome.
Does anyone in the family have learning problems, mental retardation/behavioral disorders, developmental delays?	Look for multiple members affected and associated with dysmorphic features. If yes, recommend genetic consultation.
What is your ethnic/geographic heritage background? Your partner's?	Discovering where an individual's ancestors come from can help identify certain ethnic and/or population risk factors.

TABLE 3.4   Degree of Relationship Between Individual Family Members and Shared Genetic Material

Relationship	Amount of Shared Genetic Material (%)	Example
First-degree relatives	50	Children, full siblings, biologic parents
Second-degree relatives	25	Grandparents, half siblings, aunts/uncles, nieces/nephews
Third-degree relatives	12.5	Cousins

In general, providers should pay attention if one or more of these genetic red flags emerge when taking a family health history: (1) multiple affected members with the same related disorder; (2) earlier age at onset than expected for the disorder; (3) a condition or disorder seen in the less-often affected sex; (4) the appearance of a disease in the absence of any known risk factors; (5) at-risk ethnicity or ancestral background; (6) unusual close relationships, such as consanguinity, by blood or through a common ancestor; (7) multifocal or bilateral occurrence in paired organs; (8) intellectual impairment with or without major or minor malformations; (9) women experiencing three or more miscarriages; and (10) individuals with two or more major malformations.

Physical Findings Indicating Inherited or Congenital Disorders

It is important not only to identify red flags in the history but also to identify physical findings that can point to the presence of a particular inherited or congenital condition(s). Findings that are particularly notable include physical abnormalities (e.g., multiple café au lait spots, growth problems, and congenital anomalies) and neurologic abnormalities (including hearing loss, vision loss, developmental delay, mental retardation, hypotonia, progressive muscle weakness, and hard-to-control seizure disorders). PCPs can hone their abilities by familiarizing themselves with advanced anthropomorphic measurement skills and by reviewing detailed descriptions and photographs of children and adults with various disorders (see Table 3.1: Positive Exposure).

Minor and Major Anomalies

Classification of features can appear somewhat arbitrary. A congenital anomaly or birth defect is an abnormality of structure or function that is present at birth. A physical finding is referred to as a *major* anomaly if it impairs normal body function (e.g., congenital heart disease, cleft palate), whereas a *minor* anomaly is more of a cosmetic variation, without impairing function (e.g., clinodactyly, small ear). This distinction is made because a genetic etiology is often considered when an individual has one major or more than two minor anomalies. Minor anomalies in the head, neck, and hand account for the majority of all minor anomalies (Table 3.6).

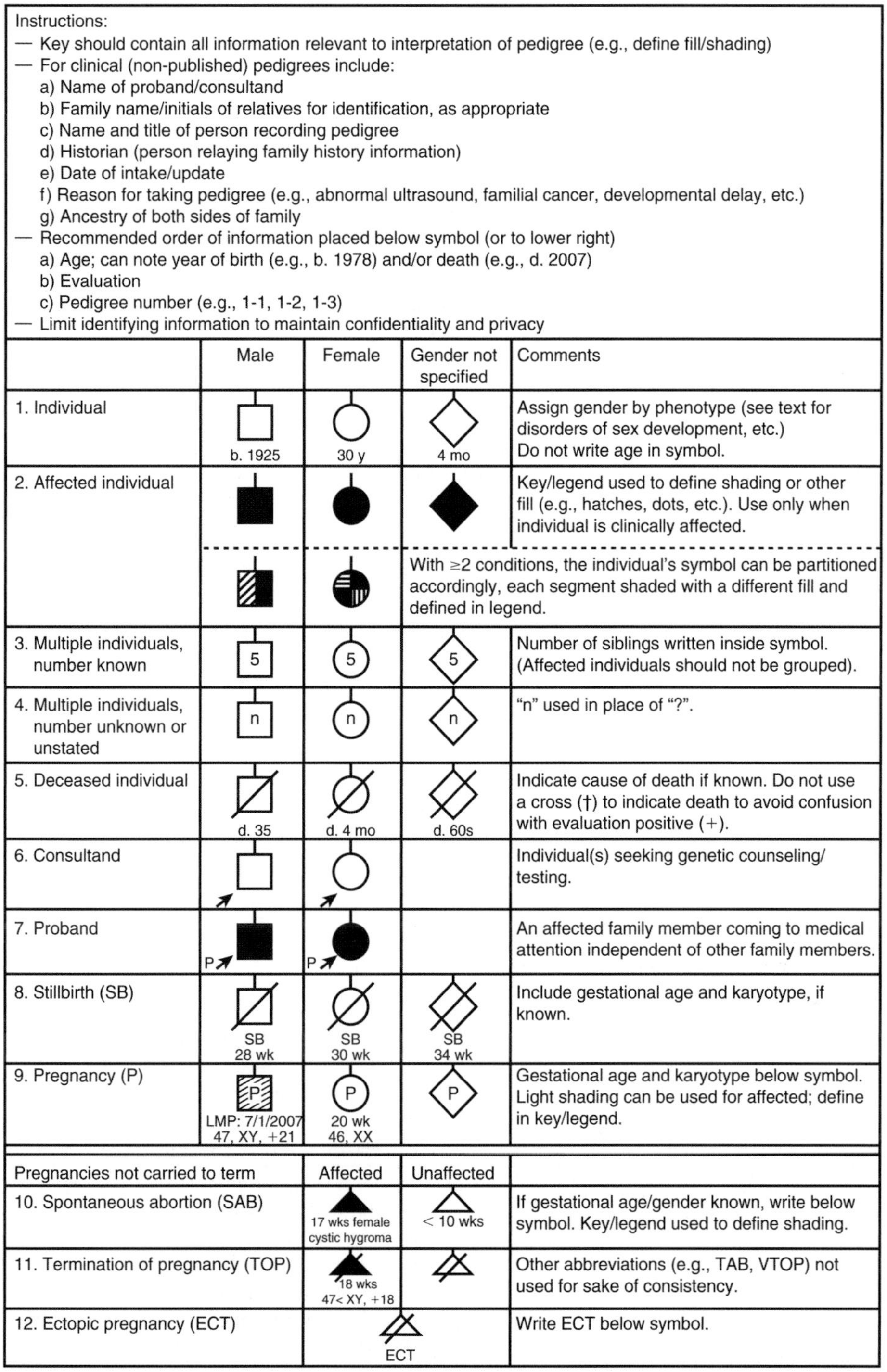

Instructions:
— Key should contain all information relevant to interpretation of pedigree (e.g., define fill/shading)
— For clinical (non-published) pedigrees include:
  a) Name of proband/consultand
  b) Family name/initials of relatives for identification, as appropriate
  c) Name and title of person recording pedigree
  d) Historian (person relaying family history information)
  e) Date of intake/update
  f) Reason for taking pedigree (e.g., abnormal ultrasound, familial cancer, developmental delay, etc.)
  g) Ancestry of both sides of family
— Recommended order of information placed below symbol (or to lower right)
  a) Age; can note year of birth (e.g., b. 1978) and/or death (e.g., d. 2007)
  b) Evaluation
  c) Pedigree number (e.g., 1-1, 1-2, 1-3)
— Limit identifying information to maintain confidentiality and privacy

	Male	Female	Gender not specified	Comments
1. Individual	□ b. 1925	○ 30 y	◇ 4 mo	Assign gender by phenotype (see text for disorders of sex development, etc.) Do not write age in symbol.
2. Affected individual	■	●	◆	Key/legend used to define shading or other fill (e.g., hatches, dots, etc.). Use only when individual is clinically affected.
	(partitioned/hatched)	(partitioned)		With ≥2 conditions, the individual's symbol can be partitioned accordingly, each segment shaded with a different fill and defined in legend.
3. Multiple individuals, number known	5	5	5	Number of siblings written inside symbol. (Affected individuals should not be grouped).
4. Multiple individuals, number unknown or unstated	n	n	n	"n" used in place of "?".
5. Deceased individual	⧄ d. 35	⦸ d. 4 mo	◇ d. 60s	Indicate cause of death if known. Do not use a cross (†) to indicate death to avoid confusion with evaluation positive (+).
6. Consultand	□↗	○↗		Individual(s) seeking genetic counseling/testing.
7. Proband	P↗ ■	P↗ ●		An affected family member coming to medical attention independent of other family members.
8. Stillbirth (SB)	⧄ SB 28 wk	⦸ SB 30 wk	◇ SB 34 wk	Include gestational age and karyotype, if known.
9. Pregnancy (P)	P LMP: 7/1/2007 47, XY, +21	P 20 wk 46, XX	P	Gestational age and karyotype below symbol. Light shading can be used for affected; define in key/legend.

Pregnancies not carried to term	Affected	Unaffected	
10. Spontaneous abortion (SAB)	▲ 17 wks female cystic hygroma	△ < 10 wks	If gestational age/gender known, write below symbol. Key/legend used to define shading.
11. Termination of pregnancy (TOP)	▲ 18 wks 47< XY, +18	△	Other abbreviations (e.g., TAB, VTOP) not used for sake of consistency.
12. Ectopic pregnancy (ECT)		△ ECT	Write ECT below symbol.

• **Fig 3.10** Pedigree Model Common pedigree symbols, definitions, and abbreviations. (Adapted from Bennett RL, French KS, Resta RG, et al. Standardized human pedigree nomenclature: update and assessment of the recommendations of the National Society of Genetic Counselors. *J Genet Couns.* 2008;17[5]:424–433.)

Malformations are birth defects that result from an intrinsic process, such as altered genetic or developmental processes. They typically result in a basic alteration in structure and occur early in gestation (e.g., cleft palate, anencephaly, limb agenesis). *Deformities* and *disruptions* are defects that result from an external process, resulting in an abnormal shape or positioning of a body part or organ. A deformity results from a distortion by a physical force, such as oligohydramnios or twins, on an otherwise normal structure (e.g., club foot), whereas a disruption refers to destruction of a tissue or structure that was previously normal (e.g., amniotic bands). In contrast, *dysplasia* is used to reflect abnormal cellular organization within tissues that results in a structural change (e.g., achondroplasia). When there is a set, recurrent pattern of features or malformations that often have a known genetic component,

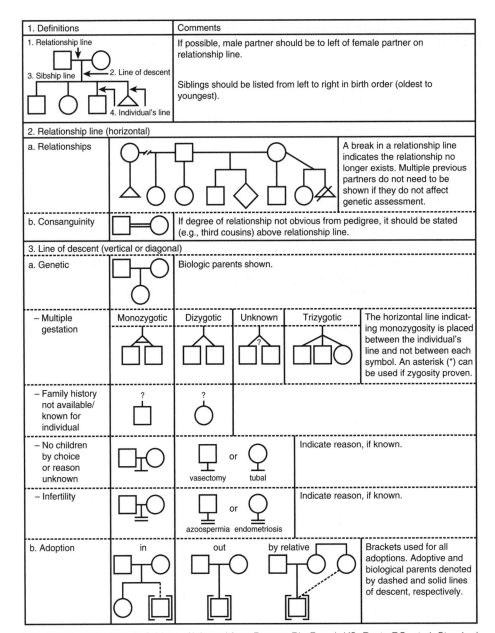

• **Fig 3.11** Pedigree Line Definitions (Adapted from Bennett RL, French KS, Resta RG, et al. Standardized human pedigree nomenclature: update and assessment of the recommendations of the National Society of Genetic Counselors. *J Genet Couns.* 2008;17[5]:424–433.)

it is called a *syndrome*. An *association*, on the other hand, is a group of anomalies that occur more frequently than would be expected by chance alone. Associations do not have a predictable pattern or a unified etiology (e.g., VACTERL association—V = vertebral, A = anal anomalies, C = cardiac, TE = trachea-esophageal fistula, R = radial and/or renal anomalies, L = limb anomalies). The numbers of malformation syndromes described are increasing daily. Health care providers need to think in terms of phenotypic analysis, which begins with a complete physical and developmental assessment.

Diagnostic Studies

No single genetic test can identify all disorders. Equally important, findings from genetic testing completed for one individual can impact other family members. The increased availability and use of genetic screening and testing in children led the AAP and the American College of Medical Genetics and Genomics (ACMG) to update their policy statements on newborn screening, diagnostic genetic testing, carrier testing, predictive genetic testing in children, and the disclosure of genetic test results (Hamid, 2013). In addition, they added a statement about direct-to-consumer genetic testing, strongly discouraging the use of this type of genetic testing in children. As highlighted in their policy statement, decisions about whether to offer genetic screening and/or testing should be informed by the best interest of the child (AAP Committee on Bioethics, Committee on Genetics and ACMG Social, Ethical, and Legal Issues Committee, 2013). The Genetic Testing Registry (GTR) is a robust resource for health care providers, and it provides current information about available genetic tests and where they can be done (see Table 3.1: Genetic Testing Registry [GTR]). Chapter 32 discusses managing primary care for children with congenital and inherited disorders.

TABLE 3.5	Mnemonics for Gathering and Interpreting the Genetic Health Data
Mnemonic	**Meaning**
Rule of Too/Two	**Too** many of something: individual is *too* tall, *too* short, *too* early, *too* young, *too* different, and so on *or* **Two** birth defects, *two* cancers, *two* in a family, or *two* generations involved
SCREEN	**S**ome **C**oncerns about traits or diseases that run in the family **R**eproductive problems History of **E**arly disease, death, or disability **E**thnicity of the patient **N**ongenetic risk factors or conditions that run in the family
F-GENES	**F**amily history: Multiple affected siblings in the same or individuals in multiple generations **G**roups (two or more) of congenital anomalies or anatomic variations **E**xtreme or exceptional presentation of a common condition(s), including early onset, recurrent miscarriage, bilateral disease **N**eurodevelopmental delay or degeneration (regression) **E**xtreme or exceptional pathology **S**urprising laboratory values

Adapted from Genetics in Primary Care Institute (GPCI): genetic red flags. https://www.aap.org/en-us/advocacy-and-policy/aap-health-initiatives/pages/Genetics-in-Primary-Care-Institute.aspx. Accessed May 21, 2018.

TABLE 3.6	Minor Malformations and/or Variations of Normal
General	Short/tall stature Body/limb disproportion Failure to thrive or obesity
Craniofacial features	Unusual head shape/circumference/fontanels Synophrys (fused eyebrows) Long eyelashes Hyper/hypotelorism Epicanthal folds Up/down slanting and/or short palpebral fissures Heterochromia, ptosis, cataract, glaucoma Low nasal bridge Abnormal ear position/shape/tags/pits Short, long, or flattened philtrum Malar flattening Prominent metopic ridge Bifid uvula, high arched/cleft palate Natal teeth/central incisor Micrognathia
Hands/feet	Abnormal creases Short/long digit(s) Prominent digital pads Clinodactyly (incurved fingers) Syndactyly (fused digits) Polydactyly Camptodactyly (bent/flexed) Dysplastic nails
Hair/skin	Abnormal hair line or color Increased numbers or anterior location of hair whorl Hirsutism Hypopigmented/hyperpigmented patches Pigmented nevi
Neck	Short, webbing
Chest	Widely spaced or supernumerary nipples Abnormal chest shape
Abdomen/genitalia	Redundant umbilicus Shawl scrotum

Screening

Screening is used in asymptomatic populations to identify individuals who need further evaluation and/or testing. Pediatric providers need to be familiar with newborn and prenatal screening. The family health history and specific tests that screen for disorders increasingly thought to have a genetic basis, such as autism, are also important screening tools.

Newborn Screening. Newborn screening is used to identify inherited and congenital disorders that can benefit from early diagnosis and treatment. Today, effective newborn screening involves a sophisticated network of coordinated efforts among public health agencies, PCPs, and specialists. It involves individual and family education, mass screening for a select subset of congenital or inherited conditions, and short- and long-term follow-up plans for newborns who screen positive. Each state determines the conditions included on their newborn screening panel; however, there is a national Recommended Universal Screening Panel (RUSP), which currently lists 34 core conditions and 26 secondary conditions, for which every baby should be screened. The RUSP is not a law, serving only as a guide for states. Clinicians should check the Advisory Committee on Heritable Disorders in Newborns and Children and Baby's First Test (see Table 3.1: RUSP; Baby's First Test), where the latest information on the conditions included in each state's newborn screening is continually updated.

Following up a positive newborn screen is stressful for both the clinician and the family. Being well prepared will make the initial contact with the family more effective. The ACMG developed action (ACT) sheets that provide clinicians with the steps to be taken after an initial positive screening result with an accompanying algorithm. Their website contains the latest versions of the ACT sheets, which are regularly revised based on new tests and information (see Table 3.1: ACMG ACT Sheets and Confirmatory Algorithms).

Prenatal Screening. Screening and diagnostic tests to detect inherited and congenital disorders have become standard prenatal care. Prenatal screening tests are typically offered to all women to screen for common syndromes (such as Down syndrome) and congenital anomalies (such as NTDs), or to select women who might be at higher risk based on age, ancestral or ethnic background, or a specific family history of the disorder. All forms of genetic testing for the specific purpose of diagnosing a fetus can be performed directly on the fetus by collecting fetal cells through a chorionic villus sample (CVS) or amniocentesis. In contrast, preimplantation testing is used to detect genetic changes in embryos created through assisted reproductive techniques before they are implanted to initiate pregnancy in the woman.

Diagnostic Genetic Testing

Diagnostic testing is used to confirm a diagnosis and is used in a symptomatic individual or in response to a positive screening test. Such tests are selected depending on the type or specific disease one is trying to confirm. Specific practice guidelines can help providers choose which test to order. For example, a chromosomal test would be used to confirm Down syndrome (trisomy 21) in a newborn, while a genetic test designed to identify missing or duplicated sections in the dystrophin (DMD) gene [Xp21.2] would be used to confirm Duchenne muscular dystrophy in a preschool male with delayed gross motor development and elevated CK/CPK levels. The test is designed to identify missing or duplicated sections in the dystrophin (DMD) gene [Xp21.2].

The main types of diagnostic genetic testing include karyotype, fluorescence in situ hybridization (FISH), biochemical testing, chromosomal microarray, molecular testing, and next-generation sequencing (Table 3.7). *Karyotype* is used to identify and evaluate the size, shape, and number of chromosomes. *FISH* is used to locate and detect a specific area of a particular chromosome, including subtle missing, additional, or rearranged chromosomal material by labeling a known chromosome sequence with fluorescent tags to see the location of genetic material. Unlike most other techniques used to study chromosomes, FISH does not have to be performed on cells that are actively dividing, making it more versatile. *Biochemical testing* is used to study the amount, activity level, or structure of proteins and enzymes that result from gene mutations. Many metabolic syndromes are screened for and diagnosed using biochemical testing. *Chromosomal microarray* is used to detect microdeletions or duplications (such as CNVs) in any of the chromosomes but not specific gene mutations. Microarray testing is noted to have a superior diagnostic yield over karyotyping for similar clinical features, including developmental disabilities (Ellison et al, 2012). *Molecular testing* is used to detect specific single gene mutations (e.g., deletions, insertions, and single base pair changes) known to cause single gene disorders. Molecular techniques are used to directly detect aberrant sequences changes in a targeted gene or short length of DNA or to indirectly detect aberrant changes in DNA structure by identifying size variations in fragments of DNA from the targeted locus or gene. *Next-generation sequencing* is used to detect a single mutation among many genes and can detect several sequence changes with one test.

Carrier Testing

Carrier testing is used to identify individuals who have one copy of a gene mutation that causes a known disorder when two copies are present (AR disorders). Individuals with one copy are often referred to as having the trait or being a carrier, rather than having the disease. Carrier testing is typically offered to individuals who are planning a family, focusing on information about the couple's risk of having a child with an AR or X-linked disorder. For example, parents can be tested to see if they are carriers of one of the mutations leading to cystic fibrosis or if they have sickle cell or thalassemia trait. Carrier testing is also done to identify nonmanifesting females of X-linked diseases. These women are referred to as "carriers" of X-linked diseases, such as Duchenne muscular dystrophy and hemophilia. Carrier testing in children is controversial. The AAP and ACMG do not recommend routine carrier testing in children, except when the carrier status has medical implications in childhood or for adolescents who are pregnant.

Other Testing

Predictive/presymptomatic tests are used when asymptomatic individuals are interested in learning if they have a gene mutation associated with a disorder and are typically offered when there is a family history of a single-gene disorder. This type of testing identifies mutations that increase an individual's *risk* of developing an inherited disorder (such as breast or colon cancer, Huntington disease, and hypertrophic cardiomyopathy), before they actually manifest signs or symptoms of the disease. The results help individuals and their providers make decisions about the need for increased screening, preventative measures, life planning, and reproductive planning. In general, these tests are not done in children because they are often associated with an adult onset. It is considered more ethical for children to make the decision about receiving this information when they are older and able to make such decisions as adults. However, there are single gene disorders that can and do manifest later in children, such as hypertrophic cardiomyopathy and certain forms of colon cancer. The use of predictive/presymptomatic testing should be guided by the child's best interests and should involve parental input (Hamid, 2013; Driessnack et al., 2013).

Pharmacologic testing (PGx testing) examines a person's genes to look at how drugs would move through the body, be broken down, or affect the body (Cheek, Bashore, and Brazeau, 2015). The primary purpose of PGx testing is to learn ahead of time what the best drug or best dose of a drug will be for a person, given their genotype. One of the biggest barriers to implementation of pharmacogenomic testing in primary care is the difficulty in translating genetic laboratory test results into actionable prescribing decisions. The Clinical Pharmacogenomics Implementation Consortium (CPIC) is an international consortium of professional volunteers and staff who facilitate the use of pharmacogenomic tests for patient care. CPIC's goal is to offset the translation barrier.

To facilitate clinical implementation of pharmacogenomic tests, CPIC created, curated, and made available peer-reviewed, evidence-based, updatable, and detailed gene/drug clinical practice guidelines. CPIC guidelines follow standardized formats and are published in a leading journal (in partnership with Clinical Pharmacology and Therapeutics), with simultaneous posting to their website. Entries are regularly updated (see Table 3.1: Clinical Pharmacogenomics Implementation Consortium [CPIC]).

Forensic testing is most often used in pediatric practice to establish biologic relationships between individuals, such as establishing paternity. Forensic testing can also be used to identify catastrophic victims and/or crime victims/suspects.

Ethical Issues

From the inception of the Human Genome Project, the National Human Genome Research Institute (NHGRI) had the foresight to anticipate the string of ethical, legal, and social issues that were to arise as part of advancing the science of genomic research. Housed within NHGRI is the Ethical, Legal, and Social Implications (ELSI) program. A few of the ethical issues include the rights to privacy and confidentiality, the rights to know, not know, the duty to warn, disclosure of incidental findings, and genetic discrimination.

The Genetic Information Nondiscrimination Act (GINA) was passed in 2008, with all aspects of the law in effect in November 2009. The intent of the legislation was to protect individuals from the misuse of genetic information in health insurance and employment and remove barriers to the use of genetic services. GINA does not affect healthcare. However, under GINA, *health insurers* cannot use an individual's genetic information to set eligibility requirements, establish insurance premiums, or request certain genetic tests. Further, *employers* cannot request, require, or purchase genetic information about an employee or family member, and they cannot use an individual's genetic information

	Karyotype	Fluorescence In Situ Hybridization (FISH)	Chromosomal Microarray	Molecular Testing[a]
Detects *large* deletions or duplications	X	X	X	
Detects deletions or duplication in *part* of a chromosome		X	X	
Detects *small* deletions or duplications			X	
Detects translocations	X			
Detects *very small* structure and sequence changes and single gene mutations				X

TABLE 3.7 **Diagnostic Genetic Testing**

[a]Including DNA sequencing.

in decisions about job hiring, firing, assignments, or promotions. Unfortunately, GINA does not provide protection when a condition is already diagnosed or manifest, even if that condition is genetic. Further, GINA does not apply to life, disability, or long-term insurers. The types of genetic information protected under GINA include family health history, carrier testing, prenatal genetic testing, predictive testing, and other assessments of genes, mutations, or chromosomal changes. There are a few groups exempt from GINA, which include members of the military, veterans receiving care through the Veteran's Administration, those using the Indian Health Service, and federal employees enrolled in the Federal Employees Health Benefits program. However, military, veterans, and federal employees have other protections that mirror GINA.

References

American Association of Colleges of Nursing (AACN). The essentials of doctoral education for advanced nursing practice, AACN (website). 2006. Available at: www.aacn.nche.edu/education-resources/essential-series.

American Association of Colleges of Nursing (AACN). The essentials of baccalaureate education for professional nursing practice, AACN (website). 2008. Available at: www.aacn.nche.edu/education-resources/essential-series.

Bennett RL, French KS, Resta RG, et al. Standardized human pedigree nomenclature: update and assessment of the recommendations of the National Society of Genetic Counselors. *J Genet Couns.* 2008;17(5):424–433.

Cheek DJ, Bashore L, Brazeau DA. Pharmacogenomics and implications for nursing practice. *J Nurs Scholarsh.* 2015;47:496–504.

Driessnack M. Growing up at the intersection of the genome era and information age. *J Pediatr Nurs.* 2009;24(3):189–193.

Driessnack M, Daack-Hirsch S, Downing N, et al. The disclosure of incidental genomic findings: an 'ethically important moment' in pediatric research and practice. *J Comm Genet.* 2013;4(4):435–444.

Ellison JW, Ravnan JB, Rosenfeld JA. Clinical utility of chromosomal microarray analysis. *Pediatrics.* 2012;130(5):e1085–e1092.

Genetics Home Reference. *Help me understand genetics.* U.S. National Library of Medicine, National Institutes of Health, Department of Health & Human Services. 2018. Available at http://ghr.nlm.nih.gov/.

Genetics in Primary Care Institute (GPCI): Genetic red flags. Available at: https://www.aap.org/en-us/advocacy-and-policy/aap-health-initiatives/pages/Genetics-in-Primary-Care-Institute.aspx. Accessed May 21, 2018.

Hamid R. New guidelines on genetic testing and screening in children. *AP Grand Rounds.* 2013;30:36.

Madhusoodanan J. Stress alters children's genomes: poverty and unstable family environments shorten chromosome-protecting telomeres in 9-year-olds, Nature (website). 2014. Available at: www.nature.com/news/stress-alters-children-s-genomes-1.14997.

National Coalition for Health Professional Education in Genetics (NCHPEG). Core competencies in genetics for health professionals (2007), The Jackson Laboratory (website). Available at: https://www.jax.org/education-and-learning/clinical-and-continuing-education/ccep-non-cancer-resources/core-competencies-for-health-care-professionals. Accessed February 21, 2018.

Puumala SE, Hoyme HE. Epigenetics in pediatrics. *Pediatr Rev.* 2015;36(1):14–21. https://doi.org/10.1542/pir.36-1-14.

Saul RA, ed. *Medical Genetics in Pediatric Practice.* Elk Grove Village: IL: American Academy of Pediatrics; 2013.

Williams TN, Weatherall DJ. World distribution, population genetics, and health burden of the hemoglobinopathies. *Cold Spring Harb Perspect Med.* 2012;2(9):a011692.

Withrock IC, Anderson SJ, Jefferson MA, McCormack GR, Mlynarczk, et al. Genetic diseases conferring resistance to infectious diseases. *Genes Dis.* 2015;2(3):247–254. https://doi.org/10.1016/j.gendis.2015.02.008.

Wlodarczyk BJ, Palacios AM, Chapa CJ. Genetic basis of susceptibility to teratogen induced birth defects. *Am J Med Genet C Semin Med Genet.* 2011;157C(3):215–226.

Yoo H. Genetics of autism spectrum disorder: current status and possible clinical applications. *Exp Neurobiol.* 2015;24(4):257–272. https://doi.org/10.5607/en.2015.24.4.257.

4

Environment and Child Health

JENNIFER BEVACQUA AND KAREN G. DUDERSTADT

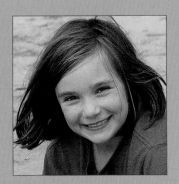

Introduction

The environment is a basic determinant of human health and illness. Although a direct cause-effect relationship between health and the environment is often difficult to determine, indoor and outdoor air pollution, second-hand smoke, unsafe water, lack of sanitation, and inadequate hygiene are responsible for one-third of the global burden of disease (World Health Organization [WHO], 2014). Children are particularly vulnerable to environmental factors due to their rapid growth and development in early childhood. Worldwide, one in four deaths of children younger than 5 years old can be attributed to unhealthy environments (WHO, 2017). Climate change, rising global temperatures, and increased levels of carbon dioxide have resulted in increased rates of asthma in children. Globally, it is estimated that 44% of asthma symptoms are related to environmental exposures, and the prevalence of children 5 years of age and older who report symptoms of asthma is 11% to 14% (WHO, 2017).

Principles for Understanding Children's Environmental Health

Children go through critical developmental periods or *windows of vulnerability* prenatally and during early childhood due to rapid brain development in the first 2 years of life. There are sensitive periods throughout childhood when rapid growth occurs and during which exposure to toxic or other harmful substances affects growth or damages organs or body systems. See Table 4.1 for environmental risk factors for children at different stages of development. Toxic substances are those chemicals in the environment capable of causing harm. *Toxicants* are environmental hazards from chemical pollutants, and *toxins* are environmental hazards from biologic sources. Toxicants that cross the placenta (e.g., drugs, carbon monoxide [CO], mercury, lead, and cotinine [from environmental tobacco smoke]) can contribute to low birth weight, spontaneous abortion, intrauterine growth retardation, and birth defects. The burden of disease and cost of environmental hazards stems primarily from exposure to toxic chemicals and air pollutants, and the related health conditions affecting children include lead poisoning, exposure to mercury pollution, childhood cancers, asthma, autism, intellectual and learning disabilities, and attention-deficit/hyperactivity disorder (Transande et al., 2015).

Children's rapidly developing and growing tissues more readily absorb environmental toxins; the lungs, skin, and gastrointestinal (GI) tract of newborns are highly permeable. At the same time, newborns' immature organ systems metabolize drugs more slowly and make it difficult for infants to detoxify and excrete harmful substances. Children consume more fresh fruit, water, milk, and juice per pound of body weight, and breathe more pollutants than adults, which increases exposure to pesticides or other chemicals (Axelrad et al., 2013). Children also engage in more outdoor activities and are physically closer to potentially harmful substances than adults. Running and rolling in grass are behaviors that increase exposure to pesticide poisoning and can trigger respiratory problems, including asthma exacerbations. For infants, crawling on floors and chewing on objects can result in lead poisoning. Children living in low-income communities are at higher risk than others due to poor nutrition, deteriorating housing with high levels of environmental lead contamination, and limited access to quality health screening and treatment. In addition to the immediate risk during childhood, children have a longer time span for exposure to environmental toxins (Landrigan, 2016). Adolescents are at increased risk if occupational hazards are present.

Epidemiologic Model of Environmental Health Hazards: Assessment of Risk

Using principles of epidemiologic relationships and toxicology, providers can better understand and explain to their patients and families the intersection between the environment and health.

A first step using an epidemiologic approach identifies the interactive factors in the environment, including *receptors* (hosts or living things that are susceptible or exposed to environmental agents); *toxins* or the agents (harmful substances that might cause damage); and the environmental *medium* or route (air, soil, water, or food) by which exposure could occur.

A second step of risk assessment using an epidemiologic model determines the possibility that harm could occur (National Research Council, 2003). A number of questions are asked when making this determination:

- *Hazard:* source of risk, a substance or action that can cause harm
  - How susceptible is the receptor to the agent (e.g., age, gender, genetics, diet, and general health)?

TABLE 4.1 Environmental Risk Factors for Children at Different Stages of Development

Developmental Stage	Developmental Characteristics	Exposure Pathways (Physical Environment)	Biologic Vulnerabilities	Appropriate Responses in the Social Environment
Preconception	Maternal and paternal health status	Maternal/paternal reproductive organs may be compromised. Maternal stores of toxicants in bones and fatty tissue can be mobilized during pregnancy	Problems with fertilization, implantation of ovum. Damage to ovum or sperm	Research and education regarding long-term effects of environmental contaminants on reproductive system and subsequent offspring
Prenatal	Fetal development dependent on maternal health status and environmental exposure	Maternal blood supply via placenta. Radiation. Noise. Heat	Tissue differentiation. Rapid cell division and growth. Organ development. Metabolic pathways incomplete	Prenatal education, programs, and regulations regarding: • Alcohol • Cigarettes • Drugs • Metals
Newborn (0-2 months old)	Nonambulatory. Restricted environment. High calorie, water intake. High air intake. Highly permeable skin. Alkaline gastric secretions (low gastric acidity to about 3 years old)	Food: Breast milk, infant formula. Dyes in clothing. Soaps and shampoos. Indoor air. Tap/well water in home	Brain: Cell migration, neuron myelination, creation of neural synapses. Lungs: Developing alveoli, rapid air exchange, narrow airways. Bones: Rapid growth and hardening. Other organs: Rapid growth. Poor enzyme detoxification	Newborn-sensitive programs and regulations regarding polychlorinated biphenyls. Lead in drinking water and dust particles. ETS. Educate parents and policy makers concerning environmental hazards
Infant/toddler (2 months to 2 years old)	Beginning to walk. Oral exploration (mouthing). Restricted environment and near floors. Increased time away from parents. Minimal variation in diet: High intake of fruits, vegetables, and milk products per body weight	Food: Baby food, food additives, milk and milk products. Air indoor layer effects: Air near floor contains more toxicants. Tap/well water in home and day care. Surfaces: Rugs, floors, lawns, playgrounds	Brain: Creation of synapses. Lungs: Developing alveoli, rapid air exchange, narrow airways	Child-sensitive programs and regulations regarding: • Radon in the home • Residential pesticide use • Lead abatement • ETS. Educate parents and policy makers concerning environmental hazards
School-age child (6-12 years old)	Beginning school. Playground activities. Increased involvement in group activities	Food at home and school. Air: School, outdoor. Water: School water fountains, tap/well water, swimming areas. Playgrounds: Wood preservatives, pesticides, and fertilizers. Other: Arts and crafts supplies, personal electronic equipment	Brain: Specific synapse formation, dendritic trimming. Lung: Volume expansion. Metabolic enzymes more active than in younger child	Child-sensitive programs and regulations regarding: • Asbestos abatement • Lead in school drinking water • Hazards in arts and crafts materials • ETS. Educate parents and policy makers concerning environmental hazards
Adolescent (12-18 years old)	Development of abstract thinking. Puberty. Growth spurt. Increased adherence to peer norms	Food. Air. Water. Personal electronic equipment. Other occupation. Self-determination: Smoking, inhalations	Brain: Continued synapse formation. Lung: Volume expansion. Gonad maturation: Ova and sperm maturation. Breast development. Bone growth and calcification. Muscle growth	Adolescent-sensitive programs and regulations regarding child labor and other issues, especially ETS. Educate parents and policy makers concerning environmental hazards

ETS, Environmental tobacco smoke.

Adapted from Gitterman BA, Bearer CF. A developmental approach to pediatric environmental health. *Pediatr Clin North Am.* 2001;48(5):1071–1083.

- *Exposure:* contact with a hazard where effective transmission of the agent may occur.
- *Dose-response relationship:* a change in amount or intensity to time of exposure is associated with increased risk.
  - At what quantity (i.e., dose) will the agent present a problem or cause a response in this receptor?
- *Risk:* likelihood (probability) and magnitude (severity) of an adverse event:
  - What is the concentration of the toxic agent? How much is there? How potent is it? What is the extent of contact of the toxic agent with the receptor?

A final step in this process compares the actual environmental condition with the applied action level, asking the following question:
- *Risk management:*
  - How long will it stay around? With the amount of exposure present, is the individual at risk for health problems?

Principles of Toxicology

Toxicology is the science dealing with detection, interpretation, and treatment of toxins or poisons. Toxicologic principles assess the exposure, absorption, distribution, metabolism, tissue sensitivity, and therapeutic or toxic effects related to the exposure to environmental toxins.

Exposure

Contact of a biologic, chemical, or physical agent with the skin, lungs, and GI tract constitutes exposure. The extent to which exposure creates a health problem depends on factors such as frequency and duration of exposure, concentration of the agent at the point of contact, and the susceptibility of the organism (e.g., an infant's skin burns much more easily than an adult's).

Absorption

Absorption is the process by which an agent is taken into the organism. It occurs in the skin, mucous membranes, lungs, or GI tract, and involves active or passive transport. Examples such as polychlorinated biphenyls (PCBs), which are lipid-soluble chemicals, are passively absorbed through the gut and stored in fat; lead is taken up through active transport in the GI tract and respiratory system and stored in bone *or other tissues* (Agency for Toxic Substances and Disease Registry [ATSDR], 2015).

Distribution

Toxic agents are distributed throughout the organism via the blood and lymph systems. The ability of an agent to cross the blood-brain barrier, the amount of blood flow to an organ, and the tissue uptake of a particular agent influence the degree to which a toxicant will be distributed throughout the body.

Metabolism

Metabolic enzymes in the body interact with toxic agents through oxidation, reduction, and hydrolysis of the agent or through conjugation and breakdown to promote elimination or excretion. Metabolism is influenced by the individual's age, gender, nutritional status, genetic makeup, presence of other drugs, and disease or illness.

Tissue Sensitivity

Susceptibility and reaction of tissue to a particular agent varies with increased tissue susceptibility during critical periods of gestation and early child development.

Toxic Effects

Toxic effects include a wide range of pathologic conditions. Prenatal exposures can result in sterility, infertility, miscarriage, stillbirth, congenital malformations, fetal growth retardation, prematurity, and chronic illnesses. Environmental toxins such as endocrine disruptors in small doses can have deleterious effects during pregnancy.

Children's Increased Risk for Environment-Related Illness

Clinical Findings

History

Assessment of environmental health hazards should be integrated into health visits of both well child visits and illness visits. Boxes 4.1 and 4.2 present questions to ask when screening children and families for environmental health history. Fig 4.1 presents environmental health history questions for pediatric asthma patients.

Physical Examination and Clinical Findings

The physical examination should cover all body systems. Evaluate agent-specific findings (e.g., burns caused by chemicals and neurotoxicity caused by mercury), but also look for subtle, nonspecific signs and symptoms (e.g., skin rashes, fatigue, headaches of unclear etiology). The effects of toxicants on the body are more commonly subclinical but may be readily noted. Moreover, effects can occur immediately or a period of time after the exposure. These factors may contribute to a provider missing physical manifestations of toxicant exposure if one does not have an index of suspicion.

• BOX 4.1   Screening Environmental History

The questions below are most often asked about the child's primary residence(s). One should always consider all places where the child spends time, such as day care centers, schools, and relatives' homes.
- Where does your child live and spend most of his/her time?
- What are the age, condition, and location of your home?
- Have you recently renovated or repaired your home, or do you have plans to do so?
- Does anyone in the family smoke?
- Do you have indoor pets?
- Do you have smoke detectors?
- Do you have a carbon monoxide detector?
- Have you had your home tested for radon?
- What type of heating/air system does your home have?
- Is your heating/air system inspected and maintained?
- What is the source of your drinking water?
  - Well water
  - City water
  - Bottled water
- What are the occupations of all adults in the household?
- Is your child protected from excessive exposure to the sun?
- Is your child exposed to any toxic chemicals of which you are aware?
- Does your child eat any odd items, such as paint chips, or chew on windowsills or other painted surfaces?
- Do you have any other questions or concerns about your child's home environment or symptoms that may be a result of his or her environment?

Data adapted from Agency for Toxic Substances and Disease Registry (ATSDR). *ATSDR Case Studies in Environmental Medicine. Taking a Pediatric Exposure History.* Atlanta: Centers for Disease Control and Prevention; 2013 and Etzel RA, Balk SJ. *Pediatric Environmental Health.* 3rd ed. Elk Grove Village, IL: American Academy of Pediatrics; 2012.

• BOX 4.2 Supplemental Environmental History

If a positive response is given to one or more of the questions in the Screening Environmental History, the primary care provider can ask the following questions:

General Housing Characteristics

- Do you own or rent your home?
- Was your home built before 1978? Before 1950?
- Has your child been tested for lead? If yes, what were the results?
- Is there a family member or playmate with an elevated blood lead level?
- Does your child spend significant time in a location other than your home?

Indoor Home Environment

- If a family member smokes, do they want to quit?
- Is your child exposed to smoke at school, day care, or a babysitter or relative's home?
- Do regular visitors to your home smoke?
- Does your home have carpet?
- Is the room where your child sleeps carpeted?
- Do you use a wood stove or fireplace?
- Have you had water damage, leaks, or a flood in your home?
- Do you see cockroaches or other pests in your home?
- Do you see rats and/or mice in your home?

Outdoor Environment/Air Pollution

- Is your home near an industrial site, hazardous waste site, or landfill?
- Is your home near major highways or other high traffic roads?
- Are you aware of Air Quality Alerts in your community?
- Do you change your child's activity when an Air Quality Alert is issued?
- Do you live on or near a farm where pesticides are used regularly?

Food and Water Contamination

- If you use well water, has it been tested? When? With what results?
- Have you tested your water for lead?
- Do you mix infant formula with tap water?
- What types of seafood do you and your child normally eat?
- How many times a week do you and your child eat: shark, swordfish, tilefish, king mackerel, albacore tuna, other?
- How often do you and your child eat organically grown fruits and vegetables?
- How often do you wash fruits and vegetables before giving them to your child?

Toxic Chemical Exposures

Consider this set of questions for patients with seizures, frequent headaches, or other unusual or chronic symptoms.

- How often are pesticides applied inside your home?
- How often are pesticides applied outside your home?
- Where do you store chemicals/pesticides?
- How often do you use solvents or other cleaning or disinfectant chemicals?
- Do you have a deck or play structure built of pressure-treated wood?
- Have you applied a sealant to that wood in the past year?
- What do you use to prevent mosquito bites to your children?
- How often do you apply that product?

Occupations and Hobbies

- What type of work does your child/teenager do?
- Do any adults who live with the child work around toxic chemicals?
- If so, do they shower and change clothes before returning to the home?
- Does the child or any family member have arts, crafts, ceramics, stained glass work, or similar hobbies?

Health-Related Questions

- Have you ever relocated due to concerns about an environmental exposure?
- Do symptoms seem to occur at the same time of day?
- Do symptoms seem to occur after being at the same place every day?
- Do symptoms seem to occur during a certain season?
- Are family members/neighbors/coworkers experiencing similar symptoms?
- Are there environmental concerns in your neighborhood, child's school, or day care?
- Has any family member had a diagnosis of any of the following: asthma, autism, cancer, and/or learning disability?
- Does your child suffer from any of the following recurrent symptoms: cough, headaches, fatigue, and/or unexplained pain (describe)?

Data adapted from Agency for Toxic Substances and Disease Registry (ATSDR). *ATSDR Case Studies in Environmental Medicine: Taking a Pediatric Exposure History.* Atlanta: Centers for Disease Control and Prevention; 2013 and Etzel RA, Balk SJ. *Pediatric Environmental Health.* 3rd ed. Elk Grove Village, IL: American Academy of Pediatrics; 2012.

Diagnostic Studies

Laboratory studies can be considered based on suspicion of exposure, overt signs and/or symptoms (Box 4.3). Regional Pediatric Environmental Health Specialty Units (PEHSU; www.pehsu.net) are a valuable resource, particularly in the event a patient needs evaluation for a less common substance.

Prior to ordering tests, the primary care provider (PCP) should understand that very few childhood exposures can be accurately identified, much less quantified and definitively linked to symptoms. Many agents have no defined reference or toxic ranges and have poorly defined toxic kinetics. How the offending agent is metabolized and potentially stored in the body (e.g., heavy metals in bone, persistent organic pollutants in adipose tissue) will affect the validity of serum testing. Also, many factors affect the outcome of exposure: dose, child's age, nutritional status, psychosocial and socioeconomic status, and developmental delay or genetic predisposition. These factors underscore how children may respond

• BOX 4.3 Laboratory Tests Available to Test for Environmental Toxins

- Plasma lead levels
- Gas-liquid chromatography (for polychlorinated biphenyls)
- Atomic absorption spectrometry (for mercury)
- Carboxyhemoglobin (for carbon monoxide poisoning)
- 24 hr urine (for heavy metals)
- Plasma cholinesterase levels (for pesticide metabolites, organophosphates)
- Urinary cotinine assays (for tobacco metabolites)

differently to the same exposure, further complicating exposures and their effects in children.

If the PCP has suspicion for an uncommon exposure, the regional PEHSU will provide expert advice on whether and how

Fig 4.1 Environmental History Form for Pediatric Asthma Patient.

Specify that questions related to the child's home also apply to other indoor environments where the child spends time, including school, daycare, car, school bus, work, and recreational facilities.

				Follow up/ Notes
Is your child's asthma worse at night?	❏ Yes	❏ No	❏ Not sure	
Is your child's asthma worse at specific locations? If so, where? _____	❏ Yes	❏ No	❏ Not sure	
Is your child's asthma worse during a particular season? If so, which one? _____	❏ Yes	❏ No	❏ Not sure	
Is your child's asthma worse with a particular change in climate? If so, which?_____	❏ Yes	❏ No	❏ Not sure	
Can you identify any specific trigger(s) that makes your child's asthma worse? If so, what? _____	❏ Yes	❏ No	❏ Not sure	
Have you noticed whether dust exposure makes your child's asthma worse?	❏ Yes	❏ No	❏ Not sure	
Does your child sleep with stuffed animals?	❏ Yes	❏ No	❏ Not sure	
Is there wall-to-wall carpet in your child's bedroom?	❏ Yes	❏ No	❏ Not sure	
Have you used any means for dust mite control? If so, which ones? _____	❏ Yes	❏ No	❏ Not sure	
Do you have any furry pets?	❏ Yes	❏ No	❏ Not sure	
Do you see evidence of rats or mice in your home weekly?	❏ Yes	❏ No	❏ Not sure	
Do you see cockroaches in your home daily?	❏ Yes	❏ No	❏ Not sure	
Do any family members, caregivers or friends smoke?	❏ Yes	❏ No	❏ Not sure	
Does this person(s) have an interest or desire to quit?	❏ Yes	❏ No	❏ Not sure	
Does your child/teenager smoke?	❏ Yes	❏ No	❏ Not sure	
Do you see or smell mold/mildew in your home?	❏ Yes	❏ No	❏ Not sure	
Is there evidence of water damage in your home?	❏ Yes	❏ No	❏ Not sure	
Do you use a humidifier or swamp cooler?	❏ Yes	❏ No	❏ Not sure	
Have you had new carpets, paint, floor refinishing, or other changes at your house in the past year?	❏ Yes	❏ No	❏ Not sure	
Does your child or another family member have a hobby that uses materials that are toxic or give off fumes?	❏ Yes	❏ No	❏ Not sure	
Has outdoor air pollution ever made your child's asthma worse?	❏ Yes	❏ No	❏ Not sure	
Does your child limit outdoor activities during a Code Orange or Code Red air quality alert for ozone or particle pollution?	❏ Yes	❏ No	❏ Not sure	
Do you use a wood burning fireplace or stove?	❏ Yes	❏ No	❏ Not sure	
Do you use unvented appliances such as a gas stove for heating your home?	❏ Yes	❏ No	❏ Not sure	
Does your child have contact with other irritants (e.g., perfumes, cleaning agents, or sprays)?	❏ Yes	❏ No	❏ Not sure	

What other concerns do you have regarding your child's asthma that have not yet been discussed?

(Used with permission of the National Environmental Education Foundation, Washington, DC. www. neefusa.org/resource/asthma-environmental-history-form. Accessed October 2, 2018.)

to test. Prior to ordering any tests, key questions for the PCP to consider include (American Academy of Pediatrics, 2012):

- Could the current health problem be related to an environmental exposure? What are the possible exposures in the child's environment?
- Did the potential exposure clearly occur prior to the onset of the health problem?
- Are laboratory tests available to document the exposure? Will the laboratory measurements accurately reflect toxicity if present? What is the cost of testing? What is the timeline from testing to receive results?
- Will the results change the treatment plan for the child and family? Will it inform care?

The diagnostic testing of hair is not recommended routinely, except for exposure to drugs in forensic examinations, but specimens must be sent to specialized, certified laboratories. Since toxins and toxicants are so ubiquitous in our environment (e.g., air pollution, personal care products, processed foods), hair is often contaminated with a multitude of chemicals, so hair levels may not accurately reflect serum levels of a toxicant or substance. Also, capillary finger sticks are not recommended due to the multitude of chemicals patients' hands come into contact with daily.

Approach to Management of Environmental Health Risks

In 2016, the Frank R. Lautenberg Chemical Safety for the 21st Century Act was passed in Congress, which modernized the Toxic Substances Control Act (TSCA) passed in 1976, the nation's primary chemicals management law. Provisions of the new law include (1) a mandatory requirement for the Environmental Protection Agency (EPA) to evaluate existing chemicals with clear and enforceable deadlines, (2) new risk-based safety standards, (3) increased public transparency for chemical information, and (4) a consistent source of funding for EPA to carry out the responsibilities under the new law. The EPA oversees management of approximately 85,000 chemicals in the United States, with a current pace of 2000 new substances annually. Only a small percentage of these chemicals have been tested for safety and risk to children and families due to the TSCA provision that "grandfathered in" many chemicals in existence prior to 1976. The new law has an improved process for monitoring safety of existing chemicals: prioritization, risk evaluation, and risk management (EPA, 2017). The law was enacted to minimize those populations most at risk for environmental hazards and to look more comprehensively at risk through enacting risk assessment of chemicals coming to market. The EPA has yet to execute a comprehensive framework in order to implement the law and has moved slowly to implement the rules.

The level of knowledge of the toxicology, human exposure, and interactions for numerous toxins and toxicants used in daily life is insufficient to permit definitive decision-making regarding protection of human health (American Academy of Pediatrics, 2012). Because of these uncertainties, the "precautionary principle" to controlling environmental health risks is favored by many leading U.S. health organizations, the European Union (EUR-Lex, 2016), and multiple international agreements also support this principle. The *precautionary principle* states that scientific uncertainty should not be used as a reason to postpone preventive measures. Invoking this principle allows action to be taken when there is valid concern that a chemical could be toxic. In effect, this principle moves the burden of proof of safety to the manufacturer when concern (meeting certain standards) has been raised, instead of recipients having to prove harm before action can be taken. Many scientists, organizations, and governments favor and have adopted the precautionary principle, yet the precautionary principle is not currently applied to chemical policy and has not been adopted by the United States.

Low-income populations are at higher risk for ill effects from environmental toxins and toxicants. The recent crisis in Flint, Michigan, highlights the dangers stemming from unacceptable levels of lead in the water system. The community water supply, previously drawn from Lake Erie, was changed by the State of Michigan and Flint administrators to the Flint River. This water supply changed the pH of the water, activating the lead in the pipe connectors in aging pipes connecting the city water supply to homes in Flint. Increased lead levels in the children in Flint doubled in the 2 years following the change in the water supply, and low rates of breastfeeding and also lead testing rates in the community compounded the risk to children and families. Significant activism by the pediatric community and environmental advocates over the course of 3 years, and a court decision was required to effect change in the community.

Entire communities can be threatened by aging infrastructure and resulting exposure to lead and other toxins. Providers should be aware of current inequities in their community and advocate for environmental justice issues. The environmental justice movement aims to rectify these inequities, and it includes the Office of Environmental Justice (OEJ), housed within the EPA (EPA, 2014), as well as numerous other non-governmental organizations.

Ambient Air Pollution

Outdoor Air

The Clean Air Act was revised and expanded in 1990, providing the EPA broader authority to implement and enforce public protections to reduce outdoor air pollutants. Since the implementation of the Clean Air Act, many gains have been made (e.g., six common air pollutants have decreased, automobiles have become cleaner over time, and ozone-depleting chemical production has decreased; EPA, 2017a).

However, despite these achievements, approximately 40% of the U.S. population lives in areas that still exceed safe levels for at least one of six air pollutants: CO, nitrogen dioxide, ground level ozone, lead, sulfur dioxide, and particulate matter (PM_{10}, complex mixtures of solid and liquid particles; EPA, 2017b). Coarse PM_{10}, such as dust and pollen, are 2.5 to 10 μm in diameter, whereas fine $PM_{2.5}$ such as combustion particles and organic compounds are less than 2.5 μm in diameter. Among the outdoor air pollutants, coarse, fine, and ultrafine particulate matter (from dust, dirt, soot, smoke, and liquid drops) have the greatest effects on human health (World Health Organization, 2017). Greenhouse gases (GHGs) (e.g., carbon dioxide, methane, nitrous oxide) are also now classified as pollutants, given their effects on the environment, thereby affecting human health.

The EPA has been charged with regulating emissions of 180 more pollutants (Table 4.2). Outdoor air pollution is responsible for 3.3 million premature deaths annually worldwide. This is in addition to the 3.5 million deaths per year caused by indoor air pollution (Lelieveld, 2015). Updated outdoor air quality information for anywhere in the United States is available at https://airnow.gov/.

Indoor Air

Indoor air quality can be affected by the same pollutants as outdoor air quality. In addition, indoor air exposures include tobacco smoke, cannabis (marijuana) smoke, carbon, asbestos, formaldehyde, volatile organic compounds (VOCs), radon, pesticides, and biological pollutants (National Institute on Drug Abuse, 2018). The EPA does not have regulatory power over indoor air quality. See Table 4.2 for more information on indoor air pollutants and their health effects.

Like most toxins/toxicants, effects can be acute, subacute, or chronic. The likelihood of acute effects to indoor air pollutants depends on age, preexisting medical conditions, individual susceptibility (based on genetics, nutrition, and other factors), and history of exposure (sensitization) to the pollutant compound(s). Certain pollutant exposures can mimic viral respiratory infections, asthma, pneumonitis, pulmonary hemorrhage, rhinitis, sinusitis, and recurrent hoarseness (AAP, 2012), causing difficulty in confirming the diagnosis. For this reason, it is important for the PCP to note the time and place where symptoms occur. If symptoms improve upon the patient leaving a certain area, then indoor air quality may be contributing to the problem. Long-term adverse effects from indoor air pollutants can erroneously be thought to be harmless, since they are not identifiable in the short-term. Radon is an example, as it causes no acute effects and is imperceptible in the air, yet long-term exposure to radon is the second leading cause of lung cancer in the United States. See Table 4.2 for strategies for limiting exposure to radon.

Management of Outdoor and Indoor Air Pollution

Over the last 50 years, air pollution has improved in the United States due to governmental protections and regulations by the EPA. Other large countries (e.g., China, India) without similar programs have not made these gains. Since air ignores political borders, it is important that we proceed with collective (societal), global action to control air pollution. Governmental protections and oversight of industry are necessary to ensure clean air for both children and adults. Thus, to improve our air quality for the 40% of Americans currently living in areas not meeting benchmarks, PCPs need to advocate for increasingly robust and modernized government and international protections.

For outdoor air pollution, protective measures include staying indoors when outdoor air pollution levels are high, utilizing portable or central air cleaning systems, limiting exercise (to reduce respiratory volumes), avoiding high air pollutant areas (e.g., traffic) when outside, and use of an M95 respirator mask (Laumbach, 2015). The efficacy of a respirator mask depends on the type of contaminant, type of filter, conditions of use, and fit. These masks are less likely to fit a child correctly. For indoor air pollution, source control (e.g., seal or enclose sources of asbestos), ventilation improvements (e.g., open windows and use fans while painting), and mitigation (e.g., install air cleaners) are options to improve air quality. CO detectors should be in every home and building. Homes or buildings with poorly vented heating appliances are most at risk for elevated CO levels.

Tobacco smoke has long been recognized as harmful to children's health. In addition, emerging research on cannabis smoke reveals harm to children's health (Herrmann, 2015). Smokers in the household should be educated and reminded that first-hand (direct smoking), second-hand (indirect smoking by being near active smokers), and third-hand (residual nicotine and other chemicals left on indoor surfaces) smoke are all harmful. It is imperative that the PCP educate and discuss the risks of smoking with adolescents, since 90% of smokers begin their habit by 18 years of age (CDC, 2017). See Table 4.2 for smoking cessation interventions.

Endocrine Disruptors

Endocrine disruptors are chemicals that mimic or disrupt naturally occurring hormones in the body, such as estrogens, androgens, and thyroid hormones. Endogenous hormones, and thus disruptors of these hormones, can affect the reproductive, neurological, and immune system of the developing fetus, infant, or child. Endocrine disruptors alter the function of endocrine hormones through a variety of mechanisms, including binding to hormone receptors to mimic natural hormones (potentially producing overstimulation), blocking/antagonizing hormone receptors, or altering the production or metabolism of endogenous hormones. Developing tissue is more vulnerable to endocrine disruption than mature tissues (Kabir et al., 2015). Further, endocrine disruptors can interfere with gene expression, changing developing tissues in permanent ways. There is also concern for latent effects of endocrine disruptor that are not apparent during the critical exposure period, but rather manifest in adulthood or during aging. Extremely low doses and extremely high doses may have significant effects; the toxicologic concepts of "dose-response" may not always apply to exposure to endocrine disruptors. Concentrations as low as one-tenth of a trillion of a gram (g) can alter the womb environment.

Endocrine disruptors are found extensively in the environment, including in food, water, soil, air, plastics, cosmetics, and drugs. They have a high degree of stability and do not degrade rapidly once discarded; thus they persist and continue to pollute the environment even in waste form. They are primarily ingested, but exposure can also occur topically, transplacentally, or perhaps in other unknown ways. The incidence of endocrine disruption is difficult, if not impossible, to quantify. Endocrine disruption generally does not result in acute illness for which the patient or caregiver would seek care, but rather is typically insidious. Specific chemicals or groups of chemicals, common exposure sources, health effects, and alternatives to their use are reviewed in Table 4.3. Reproductive system derangements caused by diethylstilbestrol (DES) is a high-profile, classic example of a severe endocrine disruptor. Millions of pregnant women were prescribed DES to prevent miscarriage, which was later proven ineffective, and their offspring had an unusually high incidence of genitourinary malformations, malignancy (clear cell adenocarcinoma of the vagina and/or cervix), pregnancy complications, and infertility. Bisphenol A (BPA) used in the current production of polycarbonate plastics and epoxy resins, DEHP Di (2-ethylhexl) phthalates used in the manufacture of consumer food packing, and polyvinyl chloride (PVC) medical devices are being studied in humans, as there is evidence for long-term effects of these chemicals in animal studies (PEHSU, n.d.). DES and other potential toxins under study highlight the danger and often latent effects endocrine disrupting agents can have on a developing human.

TABLE 4.2   Air Pollutants and Relationship to Disease

Substance	Source	Health Effects/Systems Affected	Signs and Symptoms	Prevention Strategies
Environmental tobacco smoke	First-, second-, or third-hand smoke from cigarettes, cigars, pipes Novel sources include e-cigarettes, snus, kreteks, bidis, hookahs, and dissolvable tobacco	Respiratory Cardiac Growth Neurologic	Bronchitis Bronchiolitis Pneumonia Asthma Otitis media Premature coronary artery disease Low birth weight Sudden infant death syndrome Cognitive delays	Adults and siblings in child's environment stop smoking or limit exposures as much as possible Enroll child in day care that is smoke-free Prevent child from starting smoking Recommend smoking cessation programs Health care provider recommendation of and support for decision to stop smoking
Radon	Air Water Generally concentrated in basements and underground	Respiratory	Lung cancer	Test air in basements and first floor of home for radon levels Avoid having children play in basements of homes with radon Consult mitigation company to reduce high levels Provide good ventilation in basement areas
Particulate matter	Outdoor: • Industrial pollution • Gasoline and diesel exhaust • Pollens • Natural phenomena (e.g., forest fires, volcanic activity) Indoor: • Wood stoves • Dust mites • Animal dander • Cockroach particles • Molds and more	Respiratory Cardiovascular	Bronchitis Pneumonia Wheezing Chronic cough Decreased lung function Asthma Lung cancer Cardiovascular conditions	When outdoor air pollution is high, keep children indoors Use high-efficiency particulate air filters for heating/air conditioning, vacuuming Check heating system to ensure it is clean Cover mattresses, wash bedding frequently, launder or discard stuffed animals
Molds	Damp areas (leaking roofs/walls/floors, wet basements, backed-up sewers) Humidifiers Steam from shower, bath, or cooking Wet clothes House plants Dry leaves	Respiratory Dermatologic Central nervous system	Cough Wheezing, dyspnea Sinus congestion Watery, itchy, light-sensitive eyes Sore throat Skin rash Headaches, memory loss, mood changes Myalgias, pain Fever	Maintain dry, clean environment Affected areas can be cleaned with hot water and detergent; may require deep scrubbing Bleach solutions are not routinely recommended; exceptional circumstances (i.e., the environment of immunocompromised patient) may require bleach solution to remove mold If unable to thoroughly clean, discard moldy materials to prevent spores from being released when materials dry Use dehumidifiers and air conditioners as necessary Fix leaks promptly Use exhaust fans in kitchens and bathrooms Ensure carpets do not stay damp
Asbestos	Construction materials: • Insulation • Ceiling and floor tiles • Shingles	Respiratory	Lung irritation Lung disease later in life with repeated exposure	Prevent exposure to asbestos products: If buildings that contain asbestos are in good repair, leave asbestos in place; if there is a question of possible exposure, contact a certified asbestos professional to check it Use asbestos abatement measures as appropriate when renovating If parents' workplace is a source of asbestos exposure, remove clothing and bathe before coming in contact with children

TABLE 4.3   Selected Endocrine Disruptors Including Pesticides

Chemical Group	Selected Sources	Known Toxic Effects[a]	Alternatives
BPA	• Hard, polycarbonate plastics (e.g., some water bottles) • Aluminum can linings • Thermal/carbonless receipts • Dental sealants • Plastic baby products (e.g., toys)	BPA acts as a weak estrogen. • Delayed onset of breast development in girls; adverse effect on oocytes and implantation • Externalizing behaviors (hyperactivity and aggression); abnormal neuronal circuit formation (those under thyroid hormone control) • Association with obesity and asthma, cardiovascular diagnoses, abnormal liver enzymes and diabetes	To reduce exposure to BPA and phthalates: • Buy low-fat dairy products; avoid high-fat foods (e.g., cream, whole milk, fatty meats) • Avoid canned and processed foods • When purchasing items, choose ones labeled phthalate-free and BPA-free • Minimize personal care product use, especially those with "fragrance" • Choose glass, stainless steel, ceramic, or wood instead of plastics for food storage • If using hard, polycarbonate plastics, do not use warm/hot liquids in them (BPA/Phthalates leach out of warmed plastics)
Phthalates	• Flexible, soft plastics and polyvinyl chloride products • Medical products: IV tubing, IV fluid bags, catheters, some medications (as excipient) • Food processing: plastics used in factory conveyor belts, jar lids, gloves, packaging, storage • Processed foods • High-fat dairy and meats	Phthalates are anti-androgenic. • Decreased anogenital distance (a marker of androgenization) • Altered sex hormone levels (e.g., luteinizing hormone, testosterone, sex hormone binding globulin) • Externalizing behaviors (hyperactivity and aggression) and declines in executive functioning • Abnormal sperm morphology in postpubescents	• Encourage frequent handwashing • Minimize handling of receipts • Take shoes off at home to avoid tracking in dust that may contain these chemicals • Keep carpets and windowsills clean to minimize chemical-containing dust • Avoid these plastics 3 PVC 6 PS 7 OTHER
Pesticides	• Residue on/in foods (often leaches into foods and cannot be "washed off") • Large-scale agricultural exposure (e.g., farm workers) • Small-scale garden and yard exposure • Contaminated drinking water • Pesticide-laden dust or residue that has settled on clothes, surfaces, floors, etc.	• Central nervous system dysfunction (neurologic and neurodevelopmental problems, polyneuropathy specifically) • Endocrine disruption (precocious puberty, thyroid dysfunction, hormone-mediated congenital defects [e.g., hypospadias] micropenis, poorly organized testis, abnormal ovarian morphology) • Cancer (specifically leukemias, lymphomas, neuroblastoma, Wilms and brain tumors) • Dermatologic problems • Respiratory problems including asthma exacerbations and pulmonary fibrosis	• Use Integrated Pest Management Principles (see text) indoors and outdoors • Consider tolerating low levels of non-harmful pests (e.g., ants, weeds) • Buy organic foods when possible; buy local when possible (increased travel time often necessitates pesticide use) • Keep children away from recently treated areas • Do not wear shoes or clothing that has been exposed to pesticides indoors • Store any pesticides out of reach of children
Perfluorinated compounds	• Industrial and consumer products that need surface protection (stain-, water- and oil-resistant coatings for cookware, sofas, carpets, mattresses, clothes [e.g., raincoats], shoes, food packaging, firefighting materials) and friction reduction (used in aerospace, automotive, construction and electronic industries). They are persistent pollutants (degrade very slowly). • Contaminated drinking water • Animal fats (e.g., certain types of fish)	• Anti-androgenic; decreased thyroid hormone levels • High cholesterol; elevated liver enzymes • Link to ulcerative colitis • Link to Cancer (kidney, testicular) • Preeclampsia • Adverse developmental outcomes	• Avoid stain-resistance treatments • Choose clothing that does not carry Teflon or Scotchgard tags • Use stainless steel cookware instead of nonstick cookware • Avoid greasy packaged foods (packages often contain grease-repellent coatings) (e.g., microwave popcorn bags, French fry boxes)

TABLE 4.3	Selected Endocrine Disruptors Including Pesticides—cont'd		
Chemical Group	Selected Sources	Known Toxic Effects[a]	Alternatives
PBDEs	• Flame retardants found in a wide range of products, including: electronics, plastics, paint, furniture, synthetic textiles • Animal fat (from bio-accumulating through the food chain) • Contaminated drinking water	• Associated with cryptorchidism; decrease thyroid hormone levels • Abnormal neuronal circuit formation (those under thyroid hormone control)	• Choose PBDE-free electronics and furniture[b] • Avoid contact with decaying or crumbling foam • Use a high-efficiency particulate air vacuum frequently • Use caution when replacing carpet (foam underneath often contains PBDEs) • Buy products made with natural fibers (cotton, wool) that are naturally fire resistant • Avoid high-fat meat and certain fish (generally the larger the fish, the more contaminated)
Polychlorinated biphenyls	• Industrial, lipophilic chemicals that have been banned for decades in most countries. Unfortunately, they are persistent pollutants (degrade very slowly) still found in the environment and in humans, including fetuses. • Animal fat (from bio-accumulating through the food chain) • Contaminated drinking water	• Lower sperm count, abnormal sperm morphology, reduced ability of sperm to penetrate oocyte; reduced anogenital distance; decrease thyroid levels (T4). Studies equivocal on pubertal timing alterations. • Abnormal neuronal circuit formation (those under thyroid hormone control)	• Children should avoid playing with old appliances, electrical equipment, or transformers • Avoid high-fat meat and certain fish (generally the larger the fish, the more contaminated)

[a]Not exhaustive lists. See Additional Resources for more information.

[b]Products made before 2005 may be the most hazardous. Seek out products made without flame retardants (this will be challenging).

BPA, Bisphenol A; *IV*, intravenous; *PBDE*, polybrominated diphenyl ethers.

Climate Change

Due to large-scale changes resulting from industrialization, the human population increased from approximately 1 billion worldwide in 1700 to over 7 billion today (Roser and Ortiz-Ospina, 2017). This dramatic increase in the number of humans on our planet—along with dramatic changes in the way we've come to live our lives—has led to an increase in GHGs in the atmosphere that block heat from escaping. Carbon dioxide, one of these gases, is released in natural processes, such as animal respiration and volcanic eruptions, but the amount has increased exponentially due to human activities, such as deforestation (fewer trees left to process carbon dioxide), land use changes, and the burning of fossil fuels (petroleum, coal, natural gas, and methane). Methane (from animal/agricultural sources), nitrous oxide, chlorofluorocarbons and water vapor alterations also play roles in warming our planet. Ninety-seven percent of climate scientists publishing peer-reviewed research (Cook, 2016) in leading scientific journals and organizations agree that unnatural climate change is occurring, and that the changes are caused by human activity (Climate Science Special Report [CSSR], 2017). The CSSR report and scientific evidence for climate change—the causes, effects, and solutions—can be accessed at https://science2017.globalchange.gov/.

Pediatric health consequences of climate change are exacerbated in communities with poor and disadvantaged children. These consequences include increases in
• Heat-related illnesses (e.g., heat stroke, fluid and electrolyte imbalances)
• Asthma and aeroallergy exacerbations due to more severe pollen seasons, increased particulate matter, ozone, heat, and indoor air pollutants
• GI illness due to contaminated water from altered precipitation events and increases in bacterial and algae growth
• Vector-borne disease (e.g., Lyme disease, malaria, La Crosse encephalitis)
• Food insecurity and malnutrition due to altered crop yields, crop destruction by weather disasters (e.g., floods, droughts), ocean warming and acidification, and decreased dietary diversity
• Negative mental health impacts due to weather events, displacement, potential political instability, and environmental degradation (Gamble et al., 2016; Sheffield and Landrigan, 2011; World Food Programme, 2017)

As PCPs, it is our aim to care for the health of children. Although our focus is often on individual treatment strategies and relief of symptoms, our patients and families are embedded in the larger social context, including the community and society at large. Advocating for a healthy environment for children is well within the providers scope of practice; however, climate change requires national and global governmental policy shifts to address urgent health issues and environmental impacts related to our changing climate and environment.

Additional Resources

Agency for Healthcare Research and Quality (AHRQ)
    www.ahrq.gov
Agency for Toxic Substances and Disease Registry (ATSDR)
    www.atsdr.cdc.gov
Centers for Disease Control and Prevention (CDC): National Center for Environmental Health
    www.cdc.gov/nceh
Children's Environmental Health Network
    www.cehn.org

Clean Water Action
www.cleanwateraction.org
Collaborative on Health and the Environment: CHE Toxicant and Disease Database
www.healthandenvironment.org/tddb
Environmental Health Perspectives
http://ehp.niehs.nih.gov/children
Environmental Working Group (EWG)
www.ewg.org
Green Guide for Health Care
www.gghc.org
Health Care Without Harm
www.noharm.org
Material Safety Data Sheets
www.ilpi.com/msds
National Environmental Education Foundation (NEEF)
www.neefusa.org
National Environmental Health Association (NEHA)
www.neha.org
National Institute of Environmental Health Sciences
www.niehs.nih.gov
National Safety Council
www.nsc.org
Pediatric Environmental Health Specialty Units (PEHSUs)
www.aoec.org/PEHSU.htm
TOXNET: Hazardous Substances Data Bank (HSDB)
www.toxnet.nlm.nih.gov/cgi-bin/sis/htmlgen?HSDB
TOXMAP: Environmental Health Maps
www.toxmap.nlm.nih.gov/toxmap/main/index.jsp
U.S. Environmental Protection Agency (EPA)
www.epa.gov

References

Agency for Toxic Substances and Disease Registry [ATSDR]. Toxic substances portal-Polychlorinated Biphenyls (PCBs). 2015. https://www.atsdr.cdc.gov/PHS/PHS.asp?id=139&tid=26. Accessed 10/30/2017.

American Academy of Pediatrics [AAP]. Council on Environmental Health. In: Etzel RA, ed. *Pediatric Environmental Health*. 3rd ed. Elk Grove Village, IL; 2012.

Axelrad D, Adams K, Chowdhury F, D'Amico L, Douglas E, et al. *America's Children and the Environment*. 3rd ed. Environmental Protection Agency [EPA]; 2013.

Centers for Disease Control & Prevention (CDC). *Youth and Tobacco Use*. 2017. https://www.cdc.gov/tobacco/data_statistics/fact_sheets/youth_data/tobacco_use/index.htm.

Climate Science Special Report [CSSR]. Fourth National Climate Assessment. Vol. 1. In: Wuebbles DJ, Fahey DW, Hibbard KA, et al., eds. Washington, DC; 2017. https://science2017.globalchange.gov/.

Cook J, Oreskes N, Doran PT, et al. Consensus on consensus: a synthesis of consensus estimates on human-caused global warming. *Environ Res Lett*. 2016;11(1-7).

EPA. *How the EPA Evaluates the Safety of Existing Chemicals*. 2017. https://www.epa.gov/assessing-and-managing-chemicals-under-tsca/how-epa-evaluates-safety-existing-chemicals.

EPA. *America's Children and the Environment*. 3rd ed. 2013a. https://www.epa.gov/sites/production/files/2015-06/documents/ace3_2013.pdf.

EPA. *Criteria Air Pollutants*. 2017b. https://www.epa.gov/criteria-air-pollutants.

EPA. *Environmental justice*. 2014. https://www.epa.gov/environmental-justice.

EPA. *Indoor Air Quality (IAQ)*. 2017c. https://www.epa.gov/indoor-air-quality-iaq.

EPA. *Progress Cleaning the Air and Improving People's Health*. 2017a. https://www.epa.gov/clean-air-act-overview/progress-cleaning-air-and-improving-peoples-health.

Etzel RA, Balk SJ. *Pediatric Environmental Health*. 3rd ed. Elk Grove Village, IL: American Academy of Pediatrics; 2012.

EUR-Lex. The precautionary principle. 2016. http://eur-lex.europa.eu/legal-content/EN/TXT/?uri=LEGISSUM%3Al32042.

Gamble JL, Balbus J, Berger M, et al. Ch. 9: Populations of Concern. *The Impacts of Climate Change on Human Health in the United States: A Scientific Assessment*. Washington, DC: U.S. Global Change Research Program; 2016.

Herrmann ES, Cone EJ, Mitchell JM, Bigelow GE, LoDico C, Flegel R, et al. Non-smoker exposure to secondhand cannabis smoke II: effect of room ventilation on the physiological, subjective, and behavioral/cognitive effects. *Drug Alcohol Depend*. 2015;151(1):194–202.

Kabir ER, Rahman MS, Rahman I. A review on endocrine disruptors and their possible impacts on human health. *Environ Toxicol Pharmacol*. 2015;40:241–258.

Landrigan PJ. Children's environmental health: a brief history. *Acad Pediatr*. 2016;16:1–9.

Laumbach R, Meng Q, Kipen H. What can individuals do to reduce personal health risks from air pollution? *J Thorac Dis*. 2015;7(1):96–107.

Lelieveld J, Evans JS, Fnais M, Giannadaki D, Pozzer A. The contribution of outdoor air pollution sources to premature mortality on a global scale. *Nature*. 2015;525:367–371.

National Institute on Drug Abuse. *Marijuana. What are the Effects of Secondhand Exposure to Marijuana Smoke?* 2017. https://www.drugabuse.gov/publications/marijuana/what-are-effects-secondhand-exposure-to-marijuana-smoke.

National Research Council. *Committee on Occupational Health and Safety in the Care and Use of Nonhuman Primates, Risk Assessment: Evaluating Risks to Human Health and Safety*. National Academy Press (U.S.); 2003. Available at: https://www.ncbi.nlm.nih.gov/books/NBK43454/. Accessed October 30, 2018.

Pediatric Environmental Health Specialty Unit (PEHSU). Healthcare Provider Guide: Phthalates and Bisphenol A (n.d.). https://www.pehsu.net/_Library/facts/bpahealthcareproviderfactsheet03-2014.pdf.

Roser M, Ortiz-Ospina E. *World Population Growth. Our World in Data* 2017. https://ourworldindata.org/world-population-growth/.

Sheffield PE, Landrigan PJ. Global Climate Change and Children's Health: threats and strategies for prevention. *Environ Health Perspect*. 2011;119(3):291–298.

Trasande L, Zoeller RT, Haas U, et al. Exposure to endocrine-disrupting chemicals in the European Union. *J Clin Endocrinol Metab*. 2015;100(4):1245–1255.

U.S. Chamber of Commerce. The precautionary principle. 2010. https://www.uschamber.com/precautionary-principle.

World Food Programme. *Climate Impacts on Food Security*. 2017. https://www.wfp.org/climate-change/climate-impacts.

World Health Organization [WHO]. Preventing disease through healthy environments. WHO (website). 2014. Available at: http://www.who.int/quantifying_ehimpacts/publications/preventing-disease/en/. Accessed September 3, 2018.

World Health Organization (WHO). The cost of a polluted environment: 1.7 million child deaths a year. WHO (website). 2017. Available at: http://www.who.int/news-room/detail/06-03-2017-the-cost-of-a-polluted-environment-1-7-million-child-deaths-a-year-says-who. Accessed June 4, 2018.

5

Child and Family Assessment

MARTHA DRIESSNACK AND DAWN LEE GARZON MAAKS

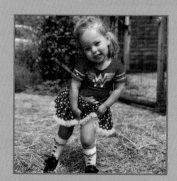

We are born out of relationships into relationships.

S. Bava

One of the unique challenges in pediatric primary care is that there is not one patient, but two. Pediatric primary care providers (PCPs) cannot care for children without also caring for their families. It is essential to move from child to family and back again during the assessment, although this process is complex. Ensuring children have safe, secure environments, families, and a community in which to grow and learn creates the foundation and building blocks, not only for their futures but also for a thriving, prosperous society.

The term "family-centered care" has slowly been replaced with the term "patient- and family-centered care" (PFCC) because it more readily captures the importance of engaging the family and patient, not only in a developmentally supportive manner but also as essential members of the healthcare team. This chapter provides assessment basics and foundational knowledge for the delivery of PFCC. In addition, evolving contexts and family composition, tools and approaches to assessment, and a brief overview of shared decision-making (SDM) in PFCC are discussed.

Child Assessment

Understanding how children develop from conception through adolescence is foundational to pediatric primary care, not only because it prioritizes *what* to assess at different ages, but it also informs *how* to approach children at different ages. Although the principles of examining children are very similar to adult examination, there are important differences in terms of approach, content, and patterns of disease. Of particular note is that in pediatrics, the history focus and physical examination changes over time as children develop. The following section highlights some of these important differences. These highlights focus on the unique issues of pediatric patients but are not intended to be as comprehensive as information found in a pediatric physical examination textbook.

Assessment Basics

Understanding the principles of growth, development, and maturation are key to assessing children over time. *Growth* refers to an increase in number and size of cells, as well as the increased size and weight of the whole or any of its parts. *Development* is a gradual change and expansion in capabilities, which represents advancement from lower to more advanced stages of complexity. *Maturation* represents an increase in competence and adaptability. A change in a structure's complexity is necessary for it to begin functioning or to function at a higher level. There are distinct pediatric growth and development patterns. For example, growth and development have a *cephalocaudal* (i.e., head-to-toe) and *proximodistal* (i.e., midline-to-periphery) progression. There is also a distinct pace/focus to growth, with the infant experiencing *rapid* growth (mostly head); toddler/preschooler experiencing *slow* growth (mostly trunk); school-age child experiencing *slow* growth (mostly limbs); and adolescents returning to *rapid* growth (mostly sexual maturation).

Each child progresses at her/his own pace. At the same time, growth and development occur on a spectrum. This knowledge means there are *ranges* of normal physical, social, emotional, and cognitive growth during infancy, childhood, and adolescence. One child gains weight quickly but is slower to speak, whereas another will acquire speech early but be slower to walk. Many children progress smoothly, whereas others do so in fits and starts. Remember to view deviations from the expected in the context of the whole child.

Measurement

A variety of measurements are obtained, recorded, and plotted to assist PCPs in assessing growth and pubertal development, including length/height, weight, body mass index, head circumference, and sexual maturity ratings. PCPs must know what to measure, how to measure, and what growth charts are best suited for each child. Growth charts are tools that contribute to forming an overall clinical impression of the child being measured; however, they are not intended to be used as a sole diagnostic instrument. Serial measurements are used to assess patterns and identify aberrations. The Centers for Disease Control and Prevention (CDC) recommends that providers use the World Health Organization (WHO) growth charts to monitor growth in infants and children from birth until 2 years of age and the CDC growth charts for children age 2 and older. Of note, the WHO growth charts are normed for *length* (*supine* measurement), whereas the CDC growth charts are for *height* (*standing* measurement). The occipital frontal (head) circumference (OFC) is normed for measurements on infants and children in an upright position. A complete set of these age- and sex-specific growth charts are located in the Appendix but can also be found, along with guidelines for use, at the CDC website (https://www.cdc.gov/growthcharts/index.htm).

Health Supervision, Surveillance, and Screening

Health supervision (routine well-child) visits are a core component of pediatric primary care because they provide ongoing opportunities to assess the health and function of the child and family. Each visit typically includes a health history, physical exam, screenings, and sharing of anticipatory guidance. Unlike ill-child encounters, during which the aim is to attend to the presenting malady, the health supervision visit is multifaceted, focusing on health promotion and anticipatory guidance, disease prevention, and disease detection. Each pediatric health supervision visit is guided by knowledge of growth patterns, developmental milestones, individual and age-related disease risk factors, and parent/family priorities and needs. Through ongoing assessment, the health and developmental trajectory for each child can be plotted and compared with normative data, much like length/height and weight, and any variation can be quickly attended to.

The timing and focus of health supervision visits are typically aligned with the American Academy of Pediatrics (AAP) Periodicity Schedule (https://www.aap.org/en-us/Documents/periodicity_schedule.pdf), which serves as a general guideline. Embedded in each visit is ongoing disease detection, which involves two techniques: surveillance and screening. *Surveillance* is the systematic collection, analysis, and interpretation of data for the purpose of prevention, because findings from health surveillance guide *primary* prevention measures. Surveillance is a continuous, long-term process, which may/may not include screenings. *Screenings* are targeted systematic actions at a single point in time that are designed to identify a preclinical condition or disease in individuals suspected of having or being at risk for the specific health impairment. Screening is recommended when the individual will benefit from early treatment or intervention and are part of *secondary* prevention measures. *Universal* screening is conducted on all children at defined time intervals or ages, whereas *selective* screening is conducted only on those children for whom a risk assessment suggests follow-up. Specific details about health supervision for each pediatric age group are included in Unit II.

History and Physical Exam

It is important to distinguish between the different types of primary care encounters, including the *routine well-child* encounter focused on screening for abnormalities of growth and/or development, the *ill-child* encounter focused on establishing the nature, cause, and extent of an acute or chronic illness/injury, and the *focused, single-purpose* encounter, such as to establish fitness for education or certain activities and the exam for signs of sexual abuse in child protection cases. However, there is not always a clear distinction between visit types. Single-purpose sports physicals can be completed within well-child encounters, problems with development, behavior, and growth may be noted during an ill-child visit, and recognition and documentation of child maltreatment can occur during any encounter and is an ever-present concern. What is important across all types of encounters is that all PCPs have a good working knowledge of growth, normal developmental milestones, age-related risk factors, and routine physical findings at different ages.

• BOX 5.1   Well-Child History (Comprehensive, Ongoing)

- Patient-identifying information/statement
  - Identify if this is a new or established patient/family
  - Child age, sex/gender
  - Accompanying adult(s)
- Reason for the visit
  - Highlight parental (and child) concerns/priorities
- Date of last visit
  - Interval history (with an established patient/family, seek an "update" of the comprehensive history on record)
- Past health/medical history
  - Prenatal/birth/neonatal history
  - Childhood illness/injury
  - Hospitalization/surgery/procedures
  - Allergies (food, medication, environment)
  - Immunizations
  - Medications (prescription, OTC, folk/herb, complementary/alternative therapies)
- Prior screening/results
- Review of systems—begin with global questions in each system; pursue areas of concern in further detail
- Current health
  - General habits/day-to-day functioning—nutrition, sleep, activity, elimination
  - Development/milestones—affective, cognitive, physical
  - Preventative health history—screenings, immunizations, health protection activities
- Family history
  - Family structure/function
  - Parenting
  - Family health history
  - Family ethnic/cultural beliefs/practices
  - Family health habits (e.g., literacy, smoking, seatbelts, helmets, guns)
- Household/environment
  - Family function—identify family members, role strain, or significant family changes.
  - Safety/risks—injury, exposure to violence, adverse childhood experiences, toxic exposures, social determinants of health, housing, and food security

---

History

A thorough, thoughtful health history is the first and often most critical step because it helps to focus the clinician's diagnostic reasoning and guides the physical exam. However, in pediatrics, it is important to remember that the history and physical examination often occur simultaneously. As children grow and develop the emphasis changes. Although each history needs to be individualized, be developmentally appropriate, and consider the child's family, health status, and physical/social environment, having a practical approach that encompasses key aspects of children's ongoing growth and developmental needs and progress is helpful. The typical elements of a *routine well-child* health history are presented in Box 5.1, and Box 5.2 presents the *ill-child* history. It is important to remember that ill-child encounters also provide an opportunity to assess a child's growth and development and ongoing needs, as well as to obtain scheduled surveillance and screening.

BOX 5.2   Ill-Child History (Episodic, Problem Focused)

- Patient-identifying information/statement
  - Identify if this is a new or established patient/family
  - Child age, sex/gender
  - Accompanying adult(s)
- Reason for the visit
  - Highlight parental (and child) concerns/priorities
- Date child was last well
- Interval/history of the present illness—chronologic description for each concern
  - Symptom analysis (onset, duration, course, symptom characteristics, aggravating/alleviating factors, exposure to illnesses/other causative factors, similar problems in close contacts, previous episodes of similar illnesses/symptoms, previous diagnostic measures, pertinent negative data, and the meaning of the concern for the family and child)
- Focused past health/medical history
  - Prenatal/birth/neonatal history
  - Illness/injury
  - Radiograph/lab tests/procedures
  - Hospitalization/surgery
  - Allergies (food, medication, environment)
  - Immunizations
  - Medications (prescription, OTC, folk/herb, complementary/alternative therapies)
- Review of systems
- Focused family history
  - Family health history
  - Family ethnic/cultural beliefs/practices
- Environment
  - Social determinants of health
  - Environmental aggravating/alleviating factors
  - Caregiver strain

Obtaining a history begins with the establishment of trust. Remember that, in any pediatric encounter, there are at least two historians in the room: the parent and child. Seek out and listen to both whenever possible.

Physical Exam

The easiest way to accomplish an accurate and complete physical exam is to secure the cooperation of the child; however, predictable, developmentally related fears or previous frightening experiences can impact a potentially positive encounter before it ever begins. Although the physical examination is traditionally conducted following the history, the reality of pediatric primary care often means moving back and forth from subjective data gathering to objective assessment techniques. Content of the physical exam varies depending on the child's age, cues from the history, and the various problems under consideration. This section focuses on unique issues of pediatric patients and is not intended to be as comprehensive as information found in pediatric physical examination textbooks. A list of principal findings that the provider are expected to identify is presented in Box 5.3, and Box 5.4 includes tips for developmental modification during physical exams. Additional discussion of physical examination techniques and findings are found in specific disease chapters.

Family Assessment

Rethinking Family—Changing Composition

The composition and context of a "typical" family unit have changed significantly. Fewer children are residing in homes with

both of their biologic parents and/or in homes with only one parent working. Currently, the typical family unit is hard to pinpoint because children nowadays can be part of a married, cohabitating, or kinship family; a single-parent, blended, or stepfamily; an intergenerational and/or grandparent-led household; a family with single-gender parents; or individual or sequential foster families, adoptive, or large, community-led families. It is not important what the family looks like, but how well it functions to meet the needs and support the growth and development of its members, especially children. Although the composition and context of families nowadays continue to expand in definition, it is important for PCPs to remember families are so integral to a child's well-being that unless the family is healthy, the child may be at risk. Little events or activities within families—the good, bad, and ugly—can have a dramatic impact on children and adults that stays with them for the rest of their lives.

Family Assessment—The Basics

Family assessment begins with the assumption that families are central to and inseparable from the health of children. The basic elements of family assessment include its: (1) anatomy or structure, (2) lifecycle or developmental stage, (3) functioning, and (4) presence of protective factors.

Assessing Family Composition/Structure

The current standard for assessing family composition or structure is to construct a three-generation pedigree, which provides a valuable visual record of family structure, genetic links, and health-related information. Insights about families are gained, not only because families share genes but also because they also often share environments, behaviors, and culture—all of which contribute to shared health problems. However, it is also important to note the pedigree includes genetically linked individuals and many families are composed of individuals who are not genetically linked. These individuals need to be included when documenting structure but are noted differently. Details about how to construct the three-generation pedigree are in Chapter 3.

Although both the three-generation pedigree and genogram include biologic or genetically linked relatives, a *genogram* expands the pedigree to include information about the sociocultural context of the family's relationships, much like the ecomap.

Assessing the Family Lifecycle

Just as children can be described in terms of their individual developmental stage, it is also possible to describe stages that occur throughout the life of a family unit. Special attention is given to families in several overlapping stages, as well as in transitions from/to different stages, because each has its unique focus, needs, and stressors. In any given family, each member is in a developmental stage, while the family is, as a unit, also going through various stages in the family life cycle. Sometimes, just acknowledging this is helpful.

Assessing Family "Functioning"

A number of tools are available to assess family functioning, including the family ecomap, Family APGAR, and SCREEM mnemonic. The *ecomap* is a graphic portrayal of the type, number, and quality of relationships or connections individuals have within their family and their community. It provides a snapshot of an individual's personal/social relationships, as well as how much energy the relationships use, by identifying each relationship as close/distant, strong/weak, mutual/one-sided, positive/negative,

• BOX 5.3   Essential Pediatric Physical Examination Data

- *General appearance:* Note the child's general state (e.g., Is the child alert? Active/interactive? Ill appearing?). Note general appearance (e.g., overall nutrition, color, respiratory effort, general body positions and movements). Does the child appear congruent with the stated age? What is the parent/child interaction? Are there any physical signs that may indicate the presence of a syndrome?
- *Head:* Assess size/shape (e.g., micro/macrocephaly, craniosynostosis, positional plagiocephaly), note size/appearance of fontanels, approximation/closure of suture lines.
- *Eyes:* PERRLA, EOMs, red reflex, cover/uncover, abnormal and/or asymmetric eye shape, movements, or color are standard elements. Vision screening begins early, beginning with whether or not the infant can fix/follow and respond to visual stimulation and later to formal vision screening beginning in early childhood.
- *Ears:* Shape/placement of the ear, response to auditory stimuli, and the presence of preauricular sinus/tags should be noted. Check that newborn hearing testing was done. Hearing screening also continues with assessment of an infant's response to voices/noises and language development. Formal audiometric evaluation begins in early childhood and continues through adolescence. Examination of the TM is one of the most common components of a pediatric exam.
- *Nose:* Newborns are obligate nose breathers. Assess for patency, septum position, and flaring. Note discharge. Infants/young children may explore/placing foreign bodies in nasal passages.
- *Mouth:* Assess for developmentally appropriate tooth eruption/shedding sequences, early/overt caries, abnormal mucosal color/lesions, uvula, intact palate, tonsil size/appearance, and tongue tie.
- *Neck:* Note ROM, noting any abnormalities (e.g., nuchal rigidity, webbed neck, torticollis) motion. Palpate thyroid. Note presence of thyroglossal/branchial cleft cysts/sinus.
- *Skin:* Note color/texture and nature/distribution of congenital/other lesions and/or rashes. Attend to lesions that might indicate the presence of disease or illness risk (e.g., hemangiomas, café au lait spots, acanthosis nigricans) or injury (e.g., color, shape, location of bruises) or are atypical for age (e.g., acne, secondary sexual characteristics).

- *Lymph nodes:* Note size, mobility, pain/tenderness, and warmth. Look for related cause.
- *Chest:* Assess for overall shape, congenital malformations (e.g., shield chest), and thoracic cage variations (e.g., pectus carinatum/excavatum). Note any dyspnea, retractions, and use of accessory muscles.
- *Breasts:* Note placement, discharge, and SMR.
- *Lungs:* Assess for symmetric expansion, air movement, and lung sounds.
- *Cardiovascular:* Assess heart sounds, noting abnormalities/presence murmurs. Note presence/nature of femoral pulses. Check peripheral perfusion/circumoral cyanosis.
- *Abdomen:* Assess for age-appropriate contour, distention/tenderness, organ position size, masses, umbilical hernia/erythema/leakage, inguinal bulging/hernia, and congenital malformations. Most umbilical hernias resolve by 2 years of age, whereas all inguinal hernias require surgical intervention.
- *Genitalia:* Note SMR. Assess for congenital/acquired variations, defects, or malformations (e.g., ambiguous genitalia, hypospadias, cryptorchidism, fused labia, vaginal discharge).
- *Anus:* Assess for patency/placement. Note abnormalities (e.g., bleeding, fissures, rectal prolapse).
- *Musculoskeletal:* Assess for full/symmetric ROM, presence of abnormal movements, joint laxity, abnormal/asymmetric tone/strength, extremity position/symmetry, gross/fine motor development, and presence of congenital/acquired abnormalities (e.g., tibial torsion, equinovarus, pes planus, metatarsus adductus, genu varum/valgum, femoral anteversion). Infants require ongoing hip evaluation (e.g., Barlow, Orotlani). Gait progression evaluation is standard. Careful attention to spine curvatures until growth is complete.
- *Neurologic:* Note presence/persistence of primitive reflexes. Assess overall alertness/interaction with others; cranial nerves, overall tone/abnormalities (e.g., spasticity, hypotonicity), tics, and seizure activity/abnormal movements. Assess for spinal dimple/lesion.

EOM, extraocular movement; PERRLA, pupils equal round reactive to light accommodation; SMR, sexual maturity rating.

• BOX 5.4   Physical Examination Approaches With Children

General: Infants/young children often dislike being placed on the examination table. Infants/toddlers can be easily examined on a parent's lap and/or knee to knee with the provider, creating a human "exam table." Young children are often easily distracted and/or enjoy simple playful interactions. Older children and adolescents can be modest/self-conscious and will do best if allowed to stay in street clothes with a drape if a more complete exam is needed.

Developmental considerations: Approach children at their eye level. Start examining peripherally (hands/feet) because this is often less threatening. Engage children, making the exam fun. A toy may help—either one that the child has brought or a penlight, or even an ear speculum rattling in a urine container can be a useful distraction. Make sure the child is comfortable and that hands and stethoscope/instruments are warm. Ask parents to assist with dressing/undressing young children. Be aware of sensitivities. Engage older children/teens throughout the process, make the exam informative, and allow child/teen to maintain control.

Deterring fears: Avoid predictable conflicts if possible (e.g., separating child/parent). Make parents your allies. Pay attention to your body language, voice, gaze, and touch. Maximize the child's cognitive ability (e.g., if a child has object permanence, you can play peek-a-boo or explaining each instrument and

having the child assist during the exam). Use what the child already enjoys/is doing as part of your exam. Avoid repetition of previous frightening experiences if possible or defer them to the end of the encounter.

Integrate play/books: Come prepared. Have age-appropriate and child-friendly toys, puppets, lights/gizmos, and books readily available. Be playful in the interaction when appropriate (e.g., pretending to blow out a light to initiate a deep breath). Enlist them as an assistant (e.g., holding the tongue depressor) or engage them in fun activities (e.g., see how long they can stand on one foot or if they can walk like a duck or penguin). Let them tell you a joke. Remember to smile.

Preparation: It is helpful to know what the parent understands, as well as what the parent has told the child will happen *before* you begin an exam or procedure. Clarify misconceptions. Have a trial run/role play with puppets or dolls. Encourage the child to ask questions before/during the process. Explain the exam or procedure step by step, focusing on what the child will experience (e.g., feel, taste, see, and/or smell) rather than solely on technical information. Pay attention to the child's comfort. Allow choices that are real (i.e., do not offer choices if there are not any).

nurturing/damaging, and/or secure/plagued by conflict. It is a valuable tool in determining a family's strengths, resources, needs, and deficits. The *Family APGAR* (Smilkstein, 1978) is used to assess a family's [A] adaptation, [P] partnership, [G] growth, [A] affection, and [R] resolve. It consists of five questions, which make it easy and quick to administer and a popular choice for evaluating family function in busy primary care settings (http://www.stritch.luc.edu/lumen/MedEd/family/apgar1.pdf). The *SCREEM* mnemonic is also used to identify a family's [S] social, [C] cultural, [R] religious, [E] economic, [E] education, and [M] medical resources, as well as their absence. For example, social interaction may be evident among family members or the family may be socially isolated.

Assessing for Protective Factors

Protective factors are conditions or attributes of individuals, families, communities, or the larger society that promote optimal child development, improve child resiliency, and reduce the likelihood of child abuse and neglect. Child health is particularly sensitive to family and community influences which may positively or negatively influence the child. Protective factors for child mental and physical health are grounded in a parent-child relationship that involves active, reciprocal, and nurturing interaction between parent and child; and parental developmentally appropriate teaching about social, emotional, and physical interactions with others. It includes loving opportunities to experience success and failure in ways that promote resiliency.

Adverse childhood experiences (ACEs) have profound impacts on mental and physical health (see Chapter 15). A number of evidence-based tools have been developed to assess the immediate

and long-term effects of adverse childhood experiences (ACEs), including the ACES Family Health History and Health Appraisal Questionnaire and the Parents' Assessment of Protective Factors (PAPF) (Kiplinger and Browne, 2014). The ACES *Family Health and Health Appraisal Questionnaires* are available from the CDC (https://www.cdc.gov/violenceprevention/acestudy/about.html) to collect information on child abuse and neglect, household challenges, and other sociobehavioral factors. There are female and male versions of each. The PAPF measures the presence, strength, and growth of five evidence-based protective factors: parental resilience, social connections, concrete support in times of need, children's social/emotional competence, and knowledge of parenting and child development.

Shared Decision-Making

Although the elements, principles, and positive health outcomes of SDM are well documented, there has been a lack of guidance for PCPs as to how to apply them in clinical practice. At its core, SDM is a process in which decisions are made in a collaborative way, trustworthy information is provided in accessible formats about a set of options, typically in situations where the concerns, personal circumstances, and contexts of patients/families play a major role in decisions (Elwyn et al., 2017). The very practical *three-talk model* of SDM (Fig 5.1) offers a clear pathway to application of SDM in practice (Elwyn et al., 2017). *Team talk* emphasizes the need to provide support to patients/families as they are made aware of choices, as well as eliciting their goals as a means of guiding decision-making processes. *Option talk* refers to the task of comparing alternatives, using risk-communication principles.

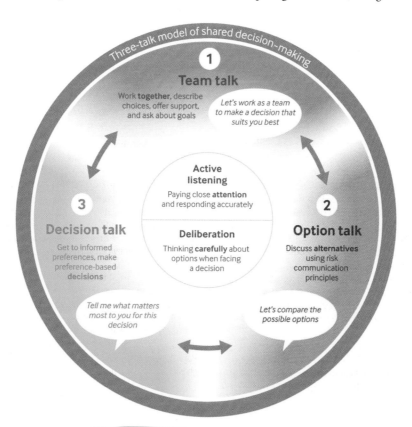

• **Fig 5.1** Three-Talk Model of Shared Decision-Making. (From Elwyn G, Durand MA, Song J, et al. A three-talk model for shared decision-making: multistage consultation process. *BMJ*. 2017;359:j4891. https://doi.org/10.1136/bmj.j4891.)

Decision talk refers to the task of arriving at decisions that reflect the informed preferences of patients/families, guided by the experience and expertise of the PCP. The three-talk model holds space open for collaboration and deliberation as the patient/family moves from *initial* to *informed* preferences to decision-making. The PCP role is one of active listening and decision support.

Additional Resources

Bright Futures

The AAP publishes *Bright Futures* (Hagan, Shaw, and Duncan, 2017), a national health promotion and prevention initiative focused on children and families, that provides age-specific guidelines, tools, and recommendations for health supervision visits (https://brightfutures.aap.org). Grounded in the life course framework, *Bright Futures* is built around the understanding that children and families are affected by a variety of biologic *(nature)* and ecologic *(nurture)* exposures, each of which can either promote healthy development or increase one's risk of disease or disability. The goal of *Bright Futures* is to support a child's life course in which strengths and protective factors outweigh risk factors.

Strengthening Families

Strengthening Families is a protective factors framework that summarizes best practices to achieve positive outcomes for all families. It is based on five protective factors: parental resilience, social connections, knowledge of parenting and child development, concrete support in times of need, and social and emotional competence for children. Each factor has been shown to protect against risk factors and poor outcomes for both children and families, as well as promote strong families and optimal development for children. *Strengthening Families* is one of the many resources offered through the Center for the Study of Social Policy (https://www.cssp.org/about), including *Cradle to Community*, which extends the focus beyond the family to advancing community approaches to safe communities and positive early child development.

References

Elwyn G, Durand MA, Song J, et al. A three-talk model for shared decision making: multistage consultation process. *BMJ*. 2017;359:j4891. https://doi.org/10.1136/bmj.j4891.

Hagan JF, Shaw JS, Duncan PM. *Bright Future: Guidelines for Health Supervision of Infants, Children, and Adolescents*. 4th ed. Elk Grove Village, IL: AAP; 2017.

Kiplinger VL, Browne CH. *Parents' Assessment of Protective Factors: User's Guide and Technical Report*. Washington, DC: Center for the Study of Social Policy; 2014.

Smilkstein G. The Family APGAR: a proposal for a family function test and its use by physicians. *J Fam Pract*. 1978;6:1231–1239.

6

Cultural Considerations for Pediatric Primary Care

ASMA ALI TAHA AND SHARON NORMAN

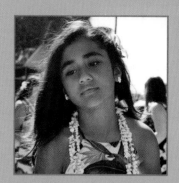

Recent political and economic crises have resulted in a marked increase in the migration of people across international borders, increasing contact among groups with widely varying backgrounds and worldviews. About 36% of the U.S. population belongs to a minority racial or ethnic group (United States Census, 2010); this is expected to reach more than 50% by 2050. Nearly 13% of U.S. residents are foreign-born and, depending on where they live, they range from 2% to 27% of their state's population (U.S. Census Bureau, 2013). Infants and children less than 5 years old who come from racial and ethnic minorities accounted for 50.3% of the U.S. population in 2015 (Cohn, 2016). Further, the fastest-growing population in the United States for the past 20 years comprises Latinos from Mexico, the Caribbean, and South and Central America. Over the past decade, the majority of refugees have immigrated from Africa and Asia, with the largest number coming from Burma and Iraq (Krogstadt and Radford, 2017). In 2016, Muslims accounted for 46% of the refugees and, for the first time, exceeded the number of Christian refugees (44%) (Krogstadt and Radford, 2017). This phenomenon of multiple religious and ethnic backgrounds has generated a greater awareness of the impact of dissimilar worldviews, values, and customs on the lived experiences of health and illness. Differences in values and customs often manifest themselves as health inequities and poor health status despite the best efforts of healthcare professionals. Achieving a goal of health equity where everyone has access to health care requires valuing everyone, using ongoing efforts to address preventable inequalities, and working to correct historical and contemporary injustices. This goal requires attention to population diversity and social determinants of health (see Chapter 1). Healthcare professionals are being called upon not only to increase their knowledge of other cultures but also to alter traditional ways of working with patients, families, and communities in response to that knowledge (Pernell-Arnold, Finley, Sands, Bourjolly, and Stanhope, 2012).

This chapter begins with a review of foundational concepts related to culture and the health care of children and families; it includes a cultural congruence model as a framework for providers, who can use it in caring for diverse groups. There is also a section on immigrant children, refugees, and international adoptees' unique health needs. For a comprehensive discussion of this topic we recommend the following books: *Immigrant Medicine* (Walker and Barnett, 2007) and *When People Come First: Critical Studies in Global Health* (Biehl and Petryna, 2013).

Culture

Culture is a complex, dynamic, learned pattern of behavior that is integral to the well-being of individuals and communities. No individual belongs to only one culture; each individual, family, and community represents a unique blend of overlapping and nested cultures that influence perception, attitudes, and behavior. Culture structures how we view the world; this includes our beliefs, attitudes, values, and expectations. Humans acquire culture both consciously and unconsciously throughout life. An individual's cultural reality is created within a specific context of experiences from parents, schools, community, and religious teachings. By 5 years of age, foundational aspects of culture have usually been internalized and further elaboration takes place during the teen years through peer socialization (Gilbert, Goode, and Dunne, 2007). Ethnicity, gender, age, sexual orientation, spiritual practices, geographic location, and social, educational, and economic status help shape one's cultural worldview. The degree to which we experience discrimination or persecution also influences our beliefs and behaviors.

Cultural Congruence Model

Although there are several cultural competence models, the cultural congruence model (Schim and Doorenbos, 2010) is based on Leininger's definition of culturally congruent care: it comprises those cognitively based assistive, supportive, facilitative, or enabling acts or decisions that are tailor made to fit with individual, group, or institutional cultural values, beliefs, and lifeways in order to provide or support meaningful, beneficial, and satisfying health care or well-being services. (Leininger, 1991, p. 49)

Based on Leininger's definition, Schim and colleagues developed a model for healthcare delivery to achieve cultural competence. It encompasses three levels: those of the client, provider, and system (Fig 6.1). The interconnectedness between levels at each encounter leads to a culturally congruent interaction. The model considers cultural competence a developmental process and learned behavior rather than an inherent attribute of the person, population, or agency. Congruence is defined as "the process of effective interaction between the provider and the client levels" (Schim and Doorenbos, 2010, p. 259). In contrast, cultural competence is an ever-evolving process.

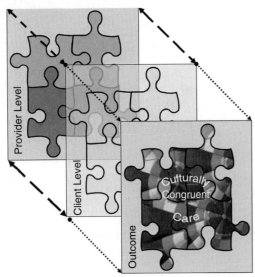

• **Fig 6.1** Three-dimensional Puzzle Model of Culturally Congruent Care. (From Schim SM, Doorenbos AZ. A three-dimensional model of cultural congruence: framework for intervention. *J Soc Work End Life Palliat Care*. 2010;6[3–4]:256–270. https://doi.org/10.1080/15524256.2010.529023.)

The Provider Level of the Model

Cultural Diversity. Diversity encompasses the differences and similarities between and within groups; however, it is commonly linked only to the phenotypic characteristics of individuals. Diversity goes beyond an individual's phenotypic characteristics to include communication, thought processes, and ways of living. Race, ethnicity, language, age, sex/gender, sexual orientation, socioeconomic status, education, religion, and individual experiences are also elements that contribute to the diversity construct. Communities are constantly changing in terms of their diversity. Providing culturally congruent care entails an ongoing assessment of the unique and evolving healthcare needs of the communities being served.

Cultural Awareness. Cultural awareness is a *cognitive* construct that allows us to appreciate the similarities and differences between people. Cultural awareness encompasses an understanding of oneself as a cultural being and one's conscious/unconscious biases toward others. Cultural awareness is developed through ongoing self-reflection and awareness of cultural traditions. Providers who are aware of their own beliefs and cognizant of a given cultural group's values and beliefs are able to develop a meaningful relationship with patients and families.

Cultural Sensitivity. Cultural sensitivity is an *affective* construct. Being open-minded to all cultures and attitudes is key to cultural sensitivity. Providers who are aware of their own cultural perspectives and who reflect on their beliefs and biases will demonstrate sensitivity and understanding when they are caring for individuals/families from different cultures. In addition, providers are socialized within their professions, and the organizational culture of practice settings influences the care domain.

Cultural Competence. Cultural competence is considered a *behavioral* construct. Competence is dependent on the actions taken in response to the demands of cultural diversity, awareness, and sensitivity. It is the provider's behavior that demonstrates the ability to bridge the cultural difference and to reduce barriers in each encounter. Schim and colleagues (2007) describe this process as dynamic and evolving over time as providers continue to expand their skills and knowledge and to develop new insight.

The Client Level of the Model

The client level of the model was also derived from Leininger's work. This level focuses on the client—patient, family, or community—while taking into account attitudes, beliefs, and behaviors regarding aspects of health and well-being. Several constructs may influence one's values and attitudes toward traditional western medicine. These constructs include family, home, nutrition and food patterns, education, decision making, values, beliefs and customs, personal space, and communication. Culturally congruent care occurs when there is harmony between the provider's plan of care and the client's unique cultural beliefs and practices (Schim and Doorenbos, 2010).

The System Level of the Model

The system level refers to the organizations that provide health or social services to individuals and families. For the system to provide congruent care, intentional strategies must be in place to serve the different populations for whom care is provided. Strategies to provide congruent care require organizational commitment and ongoing assessment of the communities' cultural needs, which entails establishing appropriate responses and mechanisms to support the community's service needs. Such strategies will minimize confounders of culturally congruent care, including racism, sexism, educational elitism, and homophobia.

Best Practices for Providing Culturally Congruent Care

Assessment Framework

In order to help providers offer culturally competent care, resources have been developed to guide their approach. The Office of Minority Health created the National Cultural and Linguistic Appropriate Standards (CLAS), which established a framework for organizations to improve health care quality, advance health equity, and help eliminate healthcare disparities. CLAS has four standards that are specific to communication and language assistance. These include offering language assistance to individuals with limited English proficiency (LEP), informing all individuals of the availability of language assistance verbally and in writing in their preferred language, ensuring the competence of individuals providing language assistance, and providing easy-to-understand printed and multimedia materials and signage in various languages in the service areas.

Providers can benefit from a structural framework in guiding family encounters. One culturally focused framework is the ETHNIC framework, which was developed by a group of physician faculty members at the Robert Wood Johnson School of Medicine and Dentistry of New Jersey in the Center for Healthy Families and Cultural Diversity. The framework includes a set of questions that providers can use in every encounter based on the mnemonic ETHNIC (Levin, Like, and Gottlieb, 2000) (Box 6.1).

Cowden and Kreisler (2016) identified two common pitfalls that providers may encounter when they are working with children of diverse cultural backgrounds: not knowing the child's culture and overestimating their own knowledge of the child's culture. Such pitfalls can lead to generalization and stereotyping, which in turn can lead to ineffective care.

• BOX 6.1 ETHNIC: A Framework for Culturally Competent Clinical Practice

E = Explanation	What do you think may be the reason you have these symptoms? What do friends, family, and others say about these symptoms? Do you know anyone else who has had or has this kind of problem? Have you heard about/read/seen it on TV/radio/newspaper? (If the patient cannot offer an explanation, ask what most concerns him or her about the problem.)
T = Treatment	What kinds of medicines, home remedies, or other treatments have you tried for this illness? Is there anything you eat, drink, or do (or avoid) on a regular basis to stay healthy? Tell me about it. What kind of treatment are you seeking from me?
H = Healers	Have you sought any advice from alternative/folk healers, friends or other people (nondoctors) for help with your problem? Tell me about it.
N = Negotiate	Negotiate options that will be mutually acceptable to you and your patient and that do not contradict but rather incorporate your patient's beliefs. Ask what your patient most hopes to achieve from this intervention.
I = Intervention	Decide on an intervention with your patient. This may include the incorporation of alternative treatments, spirituality, and healers as well as other cultural practices (e.g., foods eaten or avoided in general and when sick).
C = Collaboration	Collaborate with the patient, family members, other healthcare team members, healers and community resources.

Relationship-Based Communication

Strong, meaningful provider-patient relationships are essential in caring for culturally diverse patients and delivering high-quality care. The Relationship: Establishment, Development and Engagement (REDE) model provides a framework with strategies to enhance communication between the provider and patient. This model has three relationship phases: establishment, development, and engagement (Windover et al., 2014).

The establishment phase focuses on creating a safe and supportive atmosphere in order to make a personal connection, build trust, and collaborate with the child and/or family. The initial greeting between the patient and provider should convey value and respect. Additional key elements in this phase include reviewing the chart ahead of time, knocking and inquiring before entering the room, greeting everyone in the room while introducing yourself, positioning yourself at eye level, collaborating to set the agenda, introducing the computer if appropriate, and acknowledging any physical or emotional distress. Setting the agenda requires asking patients about their concerns using open-ended questions and avoiding interruptions. Ask the child and/or family "what else" until there are no further concerns. Encourage the child and/or family to prioritize their concerns, summarizing them in order of priority. If electronic health records are being used, explain the benefit and share computer information with the family while maintaining eye contact as much as possible. Empathy can be demonstrated using several tactics. The provider should recognize emotional cues, acknowledge the emotion, and respond immediately. The provider may need to clarify the emotion first or allow the child and/or family time and space without judgment.

The development phase of the relationship includes engaging in reflective listening, eliciting the patient's narrative, and exploring the patient's perspective. Engaging in reflective listening is accomplished with verbal and nonverbal actions. Examples of nonverbal actions include direct eye contact and nodding, whereas verbal actions include the use of phrases such as "go on" or "I see" and clarifying statements, such as "what I heard is . . ." The provider should avoid making judgments, becoming distracted, or redirecting the speaker. Open-ended questions are used to elicit the patient's narrative. The narrative is summarized to verify its accuracy. Exploring the patient's perspective involves asking about activities and the impact on the patient's ability to function, asking what the patient thinks is wrong, what the patient would like from the provider, and what worries her or him the most.

The engagement phase of the relationship includes sharing the diagnosis, collaboratively developing the plan, and ending with closure. Sharing the diagnosis involves orienting the patient to the education and planning components of the visit, presenting the diagnosis clearly, and framing the information with the patient's perspective in mind. Collaborative development of the plan involves describing treatment goals and options while being cognizant of the patient's preferences. Acknowledging the patient's contributions and scheduling any follow-up or consultation provides closure to the appointment.

Throughout the engagement phase it is important to achieve engagement with the patient by maintaining a dialogue. Open-ended questions provide information on the level of the patient's health literacy, understanding of the diagnosis, and personal preferences. The provider should present information in small chunks, include the use of visual aids, and assess the patient's emotional response to the information.

Immigrant Children, Refugees, and International Adoptees

Immigrant children are those who are foreign-born or born in the United States and living with a least one parent who is foreign-born (American Academy of Pediatrics Council on Community Pediatrics, 2015). Refugees are immigrants living outside their country of origin and cannot return owing to persecution or the fear of persecution due to their race, religion, or membership in a particular social or political group (Seery, Boswell, and Lara, 2015). Immigrants have unique challenges in maintaining health and well-being for reasons such as poverty, lack of health insurance, low educational attainment, and substandard housing as well as language barriers and medical conditions specific to their place of origin (Chilton et al., 2013).

In order to provide culturally competent care, resources have been developed to guide providers in their approach to care and establish standards of care for immigrant children. One resource for providers is the tool kit published by the American Academy of Pediatrics on the care of immigrant children (American Academy of Pediatrics Council on Community Pediatrics, 2015).

- Communicable diseases of public health significance
  - Active infectious tuberculosis
  - Active syphilis
  - Other sexually transmitted diseases (chancroid, gonorrhea, granuloma inguinale, lymphogranuloma venereum)
  - Hansen disease (leprosy)
- No documentation of vaccination against vaccine-preventable diseases (see Box 6.3)
- Physical or mental disorders with associated harmful behaviors
- Substance-related disorders (drug abuse or addiction)

Centers for Disease Control and Prevention. Technical Instructions for Panel Physicians and Civil Surgeons: Medical History and Physical Examination. 2016b. Retrieved from: https://www.cdc.gov/immigrantrefugeehealth/exams/ti/panel/technical-instructions/panel-physicians/medical-history-physical-exam.html.

Overseas Health Assessment

All immigrant children and international adoptees undergo health screening prior to being accepted for immigration into the United States. The screening is performed by Centers for Disease Control and Prevention (CDC) panel physicians and is intended to identify health-related conditions that prevent admission to the United States (Box 6.2). These conditions include communicable diseases considered to be a public health concern, vaccine-preventable diseases, physical or mental health disorders associated with harmful behavior, or a history of drug abuse or addiction (Centers for Disease Control and Prevention, 2016b). The screening includes a physical examination, evaluation for tuberculosis and for syphilis in those 15 years of age and older, and assessment of immunization status. Immunizations are required for vaccine-preventable diseases prior to immigration; although when vaccines are a series, only the first of the series is required for immigration eligibility (Box 6.3). For refugees, the U.S. Citizenship and Immigration Services (USCIS) has determined that immunization requirements are not mandatory at the time of their initial admission to the United States, although routine vaccines are strongly recommended and available through the vaccine programs (Centers for Disease Control and Prevention, 2016a). Refugees must meet the vaccination requirements when applying for an adjustment of status or permanent resident status in the United States (Centers for Disease Control and Prevention, 2016b). The vaccination requirements for immigration do not apply to adopted children 10 years of age or younger provided that prior to the child's immigration, the adoptive parent signs an affidavit stating that the parent is aware of U.S. vaccination requirements and will make sure that the child receives all required vaccinations within 30 days of arrival in the United States (CDC, 2017).

Domestic Health Assessment

Although the CDC and American Academy of Pediatrics (AAP) strongly recommend a health assessment for all foreign-born child immigrants, domestic health assessment for immigrants is not mandatory. The domestic health assessment is intended to identify acute and chronic conditions that need immediate treatment and/or follow-up as well as to initiate preventive services including immunizations (Box 6.4). The domestic health assessment should occur 30 to 90 days after arrival. The AAP recommends that

Under the immigration laws of the United States, a foreign national who applies for an immigrant visa abroad or who seeks to adjust status to a permanent resident while in the United States is required to receive vaccinations to prevent the following diseases:
- Mumps
- Measles
- Rubella
- Polio
- Tetanus and diphtheria
- Pertussis
- *Haemophilus influenzae* type B
- Hepatitis B
- Any other vaccine-preventable diseases recommended by the Advisory Committee for Immunization Practices (ACIP)

Each must be an age-appropriate vaccine as recommended by the ACIP for the general United States population and at least one of the following:
- The vaccine must protect against a disease that has the potential to cause an outbreak
- The vaccine must protect against a disease eliminated in the United States or that is in the process of being eliminated in the United States

From US Citizenship and Immigration Services (USCIS). Vaccination requirements, USCIS (website). www.uscis.gov/news/questions-and-answers/vaccination-requirements. Accessed October 9, 2017.

- Acute conditions: Infectious diseases (tuberculosis [TB], hepatitis B), dental caries, diseases of malnutrition
- Chronic conditions: Diabetes, malaria, parasites, others (e.g., thalassemia, sickle cell)
- Mental health conditions: Both acute and chronic and related to both circumstances of immigration and intrinsic variables (i.e., the condition would have manifested without immigration)
- Conditions related to the social circumstances of immigration:
  - Stress of transition, particularly a move from a rural to an urban environment
  - Posttraumatic stress disorders: Although children suffer psychologic trauma from war, dislocation, and violence, there are many factors (e.g., family attachment, peer support, and extended social networks) that serve to help the child cope and demonstrate resilience
  - Exposure to environmental and safety hazards in the new location (e.g., traffic and population density; farmworkers' occupational health)
  - Malnutrition secondary to poverty and lack of access to high-quality nutrients

international adoptees have a health assessment within 2 weeks of arrival in the United States. Culturally sensitive questions during the health assessment regarding the immigration experience, trauma experience, and family separation are required. When the experiences of immigrants are being assessed, cultural sensitivity and the creation of trust with the immigrant child and family are as important as assessing the health status of the immigrant during the initial visit.

The pediatric provider should be aware that screening and preventative care practices in the United States are foreign to immigrants, who need additional explanations in a culturally sensitive

---

• **BOX 6.5**   **Considerations for the Initial Screening of Immigrant Children**

- Birth country/ethnicity, country/countries of transit and length of time living in these countries, time in the United States
- Review all available records, including vaccine records (ask for overseas records)
- Past medical history including prenatal serology results of mother/health of mother, birth setting (home/medical facility), gestational age at birth, history of female genital cutting (FGC), other traditional cutting, transfusions, surgeries, tattoos
- Sexual history, including whether there is a history of sexual abuse
- Nutrition history, including foods available, to determine risk for specific micronutrient deficiencies
- Use of complementary and alternative medications
- Environmental hazard exposure history, including possible lead exposure risks
- Tobacco, alcohol, opium/heroin, betel nut, khat, other drug use
- Allergies
- Dental history
- Education: last year of school completed and literacy level of patient/parents as applicable, potential learning difficulty and/or need for special education
- Social history, including family structure, support in United States, school environment, individuals who live in the same home as the child, primary caretaker
- Complete history and physical examination, including vision, hearing, and dental evaluation
- Mental health evaluation using validated screening instrument (such as the Patient Health Questionnaire [PHQ-9], the Pediatric Symptom Checklist [PSC], or the Refugee Health Screener [RHS-15] for those over age 14) and specific screening for trauma
- Developmental screening (including use of an age-appropriate screening instrument)

From American Academy of Pediatrics. Immigrant Health Tool Kit; 2015. https://www.aap.org/en-us/about-the-aap/Committees-Councils-Sections/Council-on-Community-Pediatrics/Pages/Section-1-Clinical-Care.aspx#q3. Accessed March 20, 2019.

• **BOX 6.6**   **Physical Examination for Newly Arrived Immigrant Children**

- Growth evaluation (WHO for infants 0–2 years; CDC, NDSC >2 years)
- Skin evaluation
- Pubertal development
- Dental evaluation
- Blood pressure (evaluation ≥3 years or risk factors)
- Vision screen (≥3 years)
- Hearing screen (Newborn, ≥4 years)

From American Academy of Pediatrics. Immigrant Health Tool Kit; 2015. https://www.aap.org/en-us/about-the-aap/Committees-Councils-Sections/Council-on-Community-Pediatrics/Pages/Section-1-Clinical-Care.aspx#q3. Accessed March 19, 2019.

---

manner. The first primary care visit with a pediatric provider for immigrants, including refugees and international adoptees, should include a review of all medical records, a medical history, a developmental assessment, a psychosocial assessment, a complete physical exam and measurements, and tiered laboratory testing based on country of origin and risk factors (Box 6.5–6.7) (American Academy of Pediatrics Council on Community Pediatrics, 2015). Immunization status for vaccine-preventable diseases is reviewed and immunizations are immediately initiated based on the recommended schedule (Centers for Disease Control and Prevention,

2017). The CDC provides multiple resources that can assist in the decision to revaccinate or perform serologic testing for vaccine-preventable diseases; these resources can also serve to provide the names of vaccines that are given in other countries (Centers for Disease Control and Prevention, 2006).

Refugees and international adoptees often experience significant neglect and poor medical care prior to their arrival (Schwarzwald, Collins, Gillespie, and Spinks-Franklin, 2015; Seery et al., 2015). The refugee child has unique health care needs and is more likely than other immigrant children to have preexisting health problems. Infectious diseases are the most prevalent conditions among refugees. Parasites; tuberculosis; malaria; hepatitis A, B, and C; HIV; syphilis; gonorrhea; chlamydia; and Ebola are among the diseases seen in the immigrant population (Seery et al., 2015). Refugees at the highest risk of sexually transmitted diseases are those 15 to 24 years of age; also at risk are sexually active children and those with a history of sexual abuse (Seery et al., 2015).

Immigrant children may be malnourished, resulting in wasting and stunting. Intercountry adoptees and refugees often experience significant malnutrition and growth retardation (Schwarzwald et al., 2015; Seery et al., 2015. The most common nutritional issue is iron deficiency, although vitamin D deficiency is also common. Other potential nutritional deficiencies are micronutrients, including vitamin A, zinc, vitamin B12, iodine, vitamin B2, tryptophan, vitamin B1, and vitamin C (American Academy of Pediatrics Council on Community Pediatrics, 2015; Seery et al., 2015). Undiagnosed hemoglobinopathies, such as thalassemias or sickle cell disease, should be considered in those with anemia. Malnutrition most often includes undernutrition, but concerns are increasing for overweight and obese children immigrating from some African countries and Iraq (Centers for Disease Control and Prevention, 2013a). All refugees between 6 and 59 months of age should receive multivitamins with iron (Seery et al., 2015).

Immigrant children are often exposed to environmental toxins because of the impoverished living conditions in their country of origin. Elevated lead levels are seen more often in refugee children than native-born children (American Academy of Pediatrics Council on Community Pediatrics, 2015; Seery et al., 2015). A complete blood count, red blood cell (RBC) indices, and blood lead levels should be determined for all refugees on arrival to the United States (Seery et al., 2015). Children with elevated lead levels are required to have ongoing surveillance, especially since refugee children often continue to be exposed to lead after their arrival because of their poor living situations. All refugees aged 6 months to 6 years require ongoing lead-level surveillance regardless of the results of the initial lead level (Seery et al., 2015).

General health issues seen in immigrant children include pervasive dental problems, undiagnosed vision problems, and hearing deficits as well as developmental delay. Dental caries are seen in 60% to 90% of children worldwide (Seery, 2015); thus a thorough oral health assessment should be included in the comprehensive health care exam. Refugees are at high risk for developmental delay and behavioral issues (Seery, 2015). Developmental delays may be undiagnosed among immigrant children or detected at a later age (Martin-Herz, Kemper, Brownstein, and McLaughlin, 2012). The AAP recommends developmental surveillance and screening at regular intervals. Use of developmental screening tools will depend on the child's prior exposure/opportunity for acquisition of motor and language skills. An alternative option is to ask how the child is developing as compared with siblings or other children in the same culture.

• BOX 6.7 Medical Screening and Treatment Recommendations for Newly Arrived Immigrant Children

Tiered[a] laboratory screening/parasite treatment options for most immigrant children originating from resource-limited settings or from low socioeconomic circumstances

1. Tuberculosis testing: IGRA (TST if <5 years old)[b,1,9]
2. CBC/Differential[c]
3. Lead[d,6] in children 6 months–16 years
4. Hep B sAg[e,10,11]
5. Intestinal parasite evaluation (NB: for refugees, may omit if they received predeparture treatment per Centers for Disease Control [CDC] guidelines)
   - Stool O&P >24 h apart x 3[f] or presumptive treatment with albendazole
   - *Strongyloides* IgG[g] or presumptive treatment with ivermectin[g]
6. HIV[i]
7. Syphilis EIA, reflex RPR if positive[i,5]

Optional laboratory screening/presumptive treatment for children of specific ages, with specific exposures or risk factors
- Urine BHCG[j]
- Urine GC/*Chlamydia*[k]
- Hep C Ab[l]
- Newborn screen, per state guidelines[m]
- TSH[n]
- *Giardia* stool antigen[o]
- Hemoglobin electrophoresis[p]
- G6PD activity[q]
- Vitamin deficiency screening based on clinical presentation[r,8]
- Schistosoma IgG[s] or presumptive treatment for schistosomiasis[s]
- Praziquantel[s]
- Malaria thin and thick blood smears × 3[t] or malaria rapid diagnostic test[18] or presumptive treatment for *Plasmodium falciparum*[t]
- Atovoquone-proguanil[t] or artemether-lumafantrine[t]

[a]Consider laboratory tiering in this order when patients or healthcare facilities have no access to discounted financial coverage programs.
[b]Interferon gamma release assay (IGRA), tuberculin skin test (TST). Screen regardless of history of BCG vaccine.[1,9] If IGRA unavailable, may use TST at any age. Repeat TB screening in 6 months. NB: Repeat if there is chronic disease or malnutrition once medical issues have been managed, given that anergy may give a false negative result.
[c]Screen for anemia, eosinophilia (NB: absolute eosinophilia >400 warrants further workup).
[d]Repeat in 3 to 6 months in children 6 months to 6 years of age.[6]
[e]If never screened for infection, screen even if documentation of complete hepatitis B vaccine series. Vertical and horizontal transmission are possible.[10,11]

[f]Greater number increases sensitivity of test—most experts recommend two or three samples.
[g]Consider presumptive treatment with ivermectin without serology if greater than 15 kg, unless from loa loa–endemic countries.[30]
[h]If child is greater than 1 year old and has no history of seizures or other signs/symptoms of neurocysticercosis.*
[i]If prenatal lab results or recent maternal results available with negative screens and no risk for horizontal transmission, may omit.
[j]All pubertal girls (prior to vaccines or medication administration).
[k]All pubertal boys and girls or prepubertal boys and girls with history of sexual abuse.
[l]If history of HCV-positive mother, overseas surgery, transfusion, major dental work, IVDU, tattoos, sexual activity/abuse, FGC, other traditional cutting.[11]
[m]If no state-specific guidelines, infants <6 months old.
[n]All children 6 months to 3 years (screening for congenital hypothyroidism).
[o]If clinical suspicion based upon failure to thrive or gastrointestinal symptoms given low sensitivity of stool O&P and eosinophilia.
[p]To evaluate for SS, SC, S trait,[22] and thalassemias[29] in high-risk populations.
[q]For males from high-risk areas.[4,14]
[r]See CDC review of micronutrient deficiencies.[8]
[s]For immigrants from endemic regions of Africa[15] with no pre-departure treatment; May consider empiric treatment with praziquantel if greater than 4 years and if no history of known neurocysticercosis*).
[t]New immigrants from areas of sub-Saharan Africa (SSA) where Plasmodium falciparum is endemic[12] or with signs or symptoms of infection. For immigrants from SSA where P. falciparum is endemic,[12] if not pre-treated per CDC guidelines prior to departure and history of living in area with high malaria risk[12] consider treatment with atovoquone-proguanil or artemether-lumafantrine (if >5 kg), given that subclinical malaria infection is common and blood testing lacks sensitivity, particularly for specific refugee populations from areas that have greater than 40% endemicity (dark red on the endemicity map)[12] for malarial infection. For infants and pregnant teens with symptoms consistent with malaria, the CDC recommends blood PCR testing.
*Cysticercosis is a parasitic tissue infection caused by larval cysts of Taenia solium, also known as the pork tapeworm. These cysts can infect the brain (neurocysticercosis), which may present as seizures or neurologic deficits in children. It may also manifest as cysts in the muscles and other tissues. Presumptive treatment with praziquantel or albendazole in the setting of neurocysticercosis is contraindicated without concomitant antiepileptic and steroid pretreatment because these drugs may provoke significant brain inflammation and seizures. If child has history of seizures or neurologic deficits of unknown cause, do not treat with praziquantel or albendazole until the presence of neurocysticercosis has been eliminated through neuroimaging.
From the American Academy of Pediatrics. Immigrant Health Tool Kit; 2015. https://www.aap.org/en-us/Documents/3_AAP_MedicalScreening.pdf. Accessed October 9, 2017.
Numbered references in Box 6.7 may be accessed at the link provided.
FGC, Female genital cutting; G6PD, glucose-6-phosphate dehydrogenase; HCV, Hep C virus; IVDU, IV drug user; O&P, ova and parasite; PCR, polymerase chain reaction; S, sickle trait; SC, sickle cell; SS, homozygous trait.

Mental Health Assessment

Immigrant children may experience stressful situations prior to, during, or after immigration. It is not uncommon for immigrant children to be subjected to discrimination and to experience fear in the United States. Mental health conditions such as depression, posttraumatic stress disorder (PTSD), anxiety, somatization, sleep disturbances, and substance abuse are not uncommon among immigrant children. Mental health services should be recommended for the entire family when appropriate.

Approximately 11% of refugee children have been found to have PTSD (Fazel et al., 2012). Many refugees do not have a western perspective or vocabulary in terms of psychology so that questions have to be explained—with the assistance of an interpreter or bicultural worker—with specific examples or adapted to accommodate the refugees' frame of reference (Seery, 2015, p 332). Assessing the immigrant child, including refugees, involves screening for trauma, determining the influence of acculturation, consideration of changing social support structures, and resilience

(AAP Toolkit). It is essential to address mental health issues at the initial medical visit. The CDC provides a guideline for mental health screening during the first domestic assessment for newly arrived refugees (Centers for Disease Control and Prevention, 2013b).

Internationally Adopted Children

Internationally adopted children experience several stressors during their transition to a new country. They are removed from a familiar caregiver and place of residence, fly internationally, are exposed to a new language and culture, and are placed in a foreign environment with new caregivers. These children may experience grief from the loss of familiarity. They may be withdrawn, saddened, have reduced appetite, sleep excessively, and/or display aggressive behavior. Internationally adopted children have higher rates of emotional and behaviors disorders than other immigrants (Tan, 2016). The age at adoption influences long-term outcomes; children less than 6 months of age tend to have fewer developmental and behavioral disabilities compared with those 6 months old and older (Nalven, 2005). Children adopted after 24 months of age had more significant developmental and behavioral problems than those less than 24 months of age (Schwarzwald et al., 2015). International children adopted prior to 12 months of age are more likely to have typical English language development as compared with their native-born English-speaking peers. International children who are more than 1 year of age at adoption take 3 to 4 years to achieve parity in social language skills as compared with their native-born age-matched peers (Meacham, 2006).

Cultural Beliefs and Healing Practices

Immigrants often have health care beliefs and practices that are unfamiliar to the pediatric primary care provider. Pediatric primary care providers should be aware of the diverse cultures and healing practices in the communities they serve. Immigrants from Asia and the Middle East or populations, such as the Roma and Hispanics as well as other groups have unique beliefs and healing practices. Common healing practices for those from Asia include acupuncture, moxibustion, coin rubbing, and cupping. Acupuncture consists of inserting needles into specific energy points to stimulate energy in the body and mind and promote healing. Moxibustion is burning an herb above the skin to apply heat to acupuncture points, with the intent to promote healing and energy (Nguyen et al., 2016). Coin rubbing on the skin is used to scrape away the disease. Cupping involves placing a glass, plastic, or bamboo cup on the skin, creating suction next to the skin to improve Qi, or energy, as well as blood and lymph flow.

Traditional Chinese medicine is based on yin and yang, which are polar opposites (hot and cold, body and mind). The goal is harmony or balance between yin and yang through the use of herbs, acupuncture, and food to restore and maintain health. The herbs may be ingested as pills, powders, tinctures, or raw herbs or applied to the body as a balm. Traditional Vietnamese medicine focuses on nourishing the blood and vital energy. Illness is considered to be caused by "toxic wind" that enters the body from outside. Anxiety, PTSD, and other mental illnesses are considered disorders of the "wind" (Nguyen et al., 2016). Healing practices include herbal medicine, "wind scraping" (coin rubbing), "wind snatching" (fingers pinch and snap away the skin), acupressure, and bloodletting. The herbs may be teas or soups, pills, powders, or extracts.

The Hmong, an Asian ethnic population, believe that soul loss or soul separation is the source of the majority of illnesses (Lor, Xiong, Park, Schwei, and Jacobs, 2017). Healing practices include animistic folk healing and the healing power of traditional healers (shamans). Shamans communicate with the spirit world and correct the soul loss as well as treating physical injuries. The Hmong often use herbal medicine for natural causes and spiritual ceremonies for supernatural causes of illness (Lor et al., 2017). The Asian extended family is extremely influential and the oldest male in the family is often the decision maker and spokesperson.

Iraqi immigrants are predominately Arabs and usually practice their traditional medicine. Iraqis believe in preventative care for infant children; however, after infancy, visits to a primary care provider are made only for acute illnesses. A male will accompany a female to any appointment; typically males prefer male providers and females prefer female providers. It is not unusual for neighbors or relatives to bring a child along to the visit with the primary care provider. Prescriptions are needed only for "dangerous medicines" and in Iraq antibiotics are readily available from the pharmacy without a prescription (Regester, Parcells, and Levine, 2012). The Iraqi immigrant may expect to receive an antibiotic prescription with any illness. A significant stigma is associated with mental health conditions and it is believed that mental illness is incurable (Regester et al., 2012). The entire family is involved when major medical decisions are needed, although the Iraqi expects the physician to make treatment decisions and loses confidence in the provider if he or she does not recommend a treatment.

The Syrians, who are also Arabs, believe health is an absence of illness and a blessing from God (Wehbe-Alamah, 2014). To be free of illness a person must have a healthy body, mind, and soul, and it is believed that religious observance will strengthen health. Some Syrians look on illness as a physiologic or religious wake-up call (Wehbe-Alamah, 2014). The Syrians seek medical and professional treatment when ill. They believe in the "evil eye" (saybit ein/ain) and that this can be treated by mentioning god's name or reading certain chapters in the Qur'an or going to a sheikh (Muslim religious scholar/leader) who will typically read from the Qur'an. The majority of Syrians feel that caregiving is the responsibility of the family and community members. The Syrians believe in immunizations and make sure that their children are up to date with vaccinations. To prevent hernias and colic in newborns, a wide, thin cotton belt (zennar) is wrapped around the infant's abdomen.

Praying is considered a form of mental and physical exercise that strengthens the body and prevents harm and illnesses (Wehbe-Alamah, 2014). Drinking holy water (Mayet Zamzam) will maintain health, prevent illness, and cure diseases. Folk healing practices are utilized as a first-line treatment or in conjunction with professional treatment. Herbal teas are used for common colds, stomachaches, gas, and sore throats. Mint, chamomile, sage, anise, and cumin are among the herbs used to make tea, and each has a specific condition for which it is used. Antibiotics are commonly used at the first sign of a cold, as they are easily obtained. Ground coffee is used to treat minor bleeding by placing a large amount of coffee over the area of bleeding. Cupping is used by some Syrians to treat hypertension and diabetes. A Muslim sheikh is sought out to help cure or pray for someone who is ill, typically for chronic illnesses or states of mind believed to be caused by evil spirits (Wehbe-Alamah, 2014). A pharmacist may be asked to recommend a treatment if the Syrian cannot afford to pay a physician.

The Roma view ill health as normal and an inevitable consequence of adverse social experiences. They prefer to use their own cures, which include charms, talismans, and faith practices. The Roma also believe in luck, spirits, and ghosts. Instead of attributing diseases to bacteria and viruses, they believe that disease is caused by impurities and filthy places. They regard those who are not Roma as impure (Vivian and Dundes, 2004). The top half of the body, from the waist up, is clean and must be kept separate from the bottom half, which is considered marime (polluted) and to be regarded with shame (Vivian and Dundes, 2004). They believe that failure to keep the two areas separate can result in serious illness.

Healing practices used by Hispanics in treating children include massage and herbal remedies. Mothers may perform the massage or they may use a massage specialist (sobador). Herbal remedies are often teas or beverages such as manzanilla (chamomile), rice water, or yerba buena (mint tea) (Andrews, Ybarra, and Matthews, 2013; Hannan, 2015). Many Hispanics depend on powerful spiritual and folk healers (curanderos) to treat illnesses (Favazza Titus, 2014). Common folk illnesses include caida de mollera (sunken fontanel) in infants, *susto* (fright sickness), *empacho* (upset stomach), *mal ojo* (evil eye), and *envidia* (envy) (Hannan, 2015). Hispanic families believe in prayer and spiritual healing and may regard providers of western health care as unaware of the need for spiritual healing.

Barriers to Health Care Access

Inadequate health insurance, language and communication barriers, and the complexity of the health care system are barriers for immigrants seeking to access health care (Mirza et al., 2014). Lawful immigrant children are more than twice as likely to be uninsured (13%) as citizens (5%), whereas undocumented children are five times more likely to be uninsured (25%) (Artiga and Damico, 2017). The federal government permits states to require a 5-year waiting period prior to Medicaid or Children's Health Insurance Program (CHIP) eligibility for immigrant children. However, there are 31 states that do not require this 5-year waiting period (Brooks, Wagnerman, Artiga, Cornachione, and Ubri, 2017). Refugees are eligible for Medicaid and health insurance subsidies without the waiting period. Immigrant children may be eligible for Medicaid and Children's Health Insurance Program (CHIP), but some parents choose not to take advantage of it. Lack of enrollment in federal and state health insurance programs may be related to parental fear of accessing programs, concerns regarding the impact on their immigration status and sharing of information with immigration enforcement, as well as lack of knowledge regarding Medicaid or CHIP (Artiga and Damico, 2017).

Language Barriers

Lack of language support is one of the most common barriers to health care success for the resettled refugee (Mirza et al., 2014). In 2015, approximately 49% (21.2 million) of the 43 million immigrants ages 5 and older had Limited English Proficiency (LEP) (Jong and Batalova, 2017). The U.S. Census Bureau defines LEP as existing in any person age 5 and older who reports speaking English less than "very well." Language barriers can lead to lack of primary care, inadequate communication, confusion, dissatisfaction, and/or medical errors (Lee, Choi, and Lee, 2015). Limited health literacy impacts an individual's ability to communicate with physicians and care providers, implement self-management skills, understand medical conditions, and follow medical instructions (Lee, Choi, and Lee, 2015). Parents who have limited health literacy and LEP make more medication errors (Samuels-Kalow, Stack, and Porter, 2013). Clinically significant medical interpreter errors occur when an ad hoc interpreter is used rather than a professional medical interpreter (Flores, Abreu, Barone, Bachur, and Lin, 2012).

Professional interpreters should be used when health services are being provided to those with LEP. Interpreters who are familiar with the individual's culture and language are especially helpful because they are likely to be more sensitive to the nonverbal cues patients give. In some immigrant communities, especially those that are small, there may be few qualified interpreters. Also, as members of a small, closely knit community, both interpreter and client may find it awkward to discuss sensitive personal information in a clinical setting and then return to their culturally prescribed social roles in the community. In larger immigrant communities, several languages or dialects may be spoken; language barriers may arise even among people who speak the same language because communication patterns differ

among classes, subcultures, and regions in the country of origin. Also, there may be a wide range of literacy levels in all language groups. Contracting with a commercial technology-based company that provides telephone or video-remote interpreting may be a possibility in these instances. Telephone and video-based interpreters have been shown to be as effective as "in person" interpreters (Crossman, Wiener, Roosevelt, Bajaj, and Hampers, 2010; Nápoles, Santoyo-Olsson, Karliner, O'Brien, Gregorich, and Pérez-Stable, 2010).

Interpreters and providers may experience conflict related to control of the clinical situation. Providers may not be confident that the interpreter is accurately conveying their message or completely relaying the families' comments. Providers may see the interpreter as a tool to be used, not as a part of the team, whereas interpreters may take on a "codiagnostician" role, where they make decisions that can affect care without consulting the provider. Something as "minor" as neglecting to fully disclose what the client has said because the interpreter did not think it important, or the interpreter offering the client advice beyond that given by the provider, can compromise care. The provider must be sensitive to the relationship between the client and the interpreter. There must be a working relationship based on trust between the provider and interpreter as well as a clear understanding of the role of each; this must be actively negotiated (Brissett, Leanza, and Laforest, 2013; Hsieh, 2016; Steinberg, Valenzuela-Araujo, Zickafoose, Kieffer, and DeCamp, 2016).

The qualified interpreter stands or sits behind the provider so that he or she will not interfere with eye contact between the child, the parent, and the provider. If privacy is an issue, the interpreter can stand or sit behind a screen. If topics related to sexuality are to be discussed, clarify with the patient which gender he or she prefers the interpreter to be; generally, patients prefer interpreters of the same gender.

The interpreter should make an effort to translate the dialogue as closely and accurately as possible for both parties. This does not necessarily mean a "word-for-word" translation, especially since some English words have no equivalent in some other languages and vice versa. But when a provider's yes-or-no question results in a lengthy response, for example, the interpreter must ensure that the provider is apprised of what the whole statement means, including any seemingly unrelated data. It is especially difficult to convey emotion through verbal translation, and this component of communication may be lost or diminished when interpreters are used. This should not be perceived as lack of concern on the part of the child or family, and the provider should be alert for nonverbal cues. Such cues may have their own cultural connotation, however; therefore clarification should be sought (e.g., "You seem very upset; I noticed your face changed when we talked about _____. Are you worried about _____?"). Instructions for home management may have to be written by the interpreter in the family's language and reviewed before the family leaves.

Interpreters should work toward the following goals:
- Make the client's description and understanding of the problem clear to the provider.
- Communicate accurately the provider's interpretation and explanation of a health problem (e.g., pathophysiology) to the client.
- Facilitate the discussion to develop a management plan.
- Assess the child's and parents' level of knowledge and understanding of what is being said.

The provider should:
- Provide the interpreter a brief summary of the patient prior to any interpretive services
- Maintain eye contact with the patient/family
- Speak slowly and avoid jargon
- Avoid interrupting the interpreter
- Pay attention to body language and nonverbal cues (AAP Tool kit, p. 6).

Primary Care Management

Primary care providers face heightened challenges related to cultural barriers when they are working with immigrants. These cultural barriers may include differences in language, worldviews, cultural norms, and perceptions and interpretations of the meaning of health and illness. As a part of developing cultural humility and cultural competence, providers that care for immigrant populations need to develop a knowledge base including the following (Mishori, Aleinikoff, and Davis, 2017):

1. The political situation and experience of children and/or families in their country of origin.
2. Transition time experienced by the child and/or family: Were they in a refugee camp? Where? For how long? What were the conditions there?
3. Diseases common in the country of origin and in transition sites.
4. Effects on health that result from being a refugee (e.g., stress, malnutrition).
5. Legal context for refugees in the United States.
6. Effective management of trauma: physical, psychologic, and emotional.

The experience of inequality, marginalization, and stress can create lasting changes that lead to acute and chronic physical and mental health concerns (Morin and Schupbach, 2014). However, because of compromised coping, refugees may not use healthcare services, and following health care recommendations may be low on their list of survival needs. Immigrants use health services far less than do native-born U.S. residents (Yun, Fuentes-Afflick, Curry, Krumholz, and Desai, 2013); unauthorized immigrants in particular may make efforts to avoid public scrutiny and remain isolated from services and agencies. For a variety of reasons, the health status of immigrants deteriorates the longer they are in the United States (Akbulut-Yuksel and Kugler, 2016), and health care providers need to find ways to ensure that their health needs will be met. Communicating effectively on the initial health visit can set the stage. Clearly explaining the U.S. healthcare system to families is essential. The use of community-based participatory action to meet refugee health needs has been shown to be effective in situations where immigrant clients are involved in planning systems and primary care providers—including public health nurses, interpreters, social workers, and voluntary community agencies—have support from a larger system (Vaughn, Jacquez, Lindquist-Grantz, Parsons, and Melink, 2016).

Finally, providers must be alert to the fact that the care of second-, third-, and older-generation immigrants will differ from that of first-generation individuals or new arrivals. As they acculturate into the America lifestyle, immigrants begin to look and act more like others in their community; for example, adolescents take on the behaviors of their peer group and may seem like "typical" U.S. teenagers. But they do not have the same historical cultural context as their peers, and as a result, providers may make incorrect assumptions about adolescents or use cultural references in health education unfamiliar to them.

The provision of care to immigrant and diverse populations is a challenge to both health care providers and the health care system as a whole. High-quality care requires significant changes in beliefs, attitudes, and practices on the part of providers. It also requires changes in the way health care systems deliver care. By working sensitively with children and families, sharing ideas and information, learning from and about each other, and understanding differences and similarities, providers can become full participants in creating a new cultural context in the health care system and thus improve health care outcomes for immigrant populations.

Additional Resources

AAP (red book) immunization schedule. https://redbook.solutions.aap.org/redbook.aspx

Adoption intercountry. https://travel.state.gov/content/adoption-sabroad/en.html

American Refugee Committee International. www.arcrelief.org

American Translators Association. www.atanet.org

Bridging Refugee Youth and Children's Services. http://www.brycs.org/

Centers for Disease Control and Prevention Division of Global Migration and Quarantine. www.cdc.gov/ncezid/dgmq/

Centers for Disease Control and Prevention Recommendations of the Advisory Committee on Immunization Practices (ACIP). https://www.cdc.gov/mmwr/preview/mmwrhtml/rr5515a1.htm#tab1; https://www.cdc.gov/vaccines/schedules/easy-to-read/child.html

Centers for Disease Control and Prevention: Vaccine names in foreign countries. https://www.cdc.gov/immigrantrefugeehealth/guidelines/domestic/immunizations-guidelines.html

Centers for Disease Control and Prevention: Vaccine Program for US bound refuges. https://www.cdc.gov/immigrantrefugeehealth/guidelines/overseas/interventions/immunizations-schedules.html

Child Family Health International. www.cfhi.org

Cross Cultural Health Care Program. www.xculture.org

Curricula Enhancement Module Series. https://nccc.georgetown.edu/curricula/modules.html

Centers for Medicare and Medicaid Services: American Indian/Alaska Native. www.cms.gov/Outreach-and-Education/American-Indian-Alaska-Native/AIAN/

EthnoMED: Refugee Health Clinical Topics. https://ethnomed.org/clinical/refugee-health/refugee-health-clinical-topics

Health information in many languages, patient materials and provider information. https://healthreach.nlm.nih.gov/

Health insurance resources for refugees. https://www.acf.hhs.gov/orr/health

Health Resources and Services Administration (HRSA) and Office of Minority Health Resource Center. www.hrsa.gov/culturalcompetence; www.minorityhealth.hhs.gov/; www.minorityhealth.hhs.gov/omh/browse.aspx?lvl=2&lvlid=53

National Center for Cultural Competence. https://nccc.georgetown.edu/resources/title.php

National Network of Libraries of Medicine: Health Literacy and Cultural Competence. https://www.nlm.nih.gov/hsrinfo/health_literacy.html

National Network of Libraries of Medicine: Multicultural Resources for Health Information. https://sis.nlm.nih.gov/outreach/multicultural.html

Office of Minority Health (linguistics and culture). https://minorityhealth.hhs.gov/omh/browse.aspx?lvl=1&lvlid=6

Refugee Health Technical Assistance. http://refugeehealthta.org/physical-mental-health/mental-health/youth-and-mental-health/

Serologic vs revaccination approach. https://www.cdc.gov/mmwr/preview/mmwrhtml/rr5515a1.htm#tab12; https://www.cdc.gov/immigrantrefugeehealth/guidelines/domestic/immunizations-guidelines.html

The Kaiser Family Foundation: The Disparities Policy Project. https://www.kff.org/about-the-disparities-policy-project/

Think Cultural Health. www.thinkculturalhealth.org

U.S. Department of Health and Human Services, Administration for Children and Families, Office of Refugee Resettlement. www.acf.hhs.gov/programs/orr www.acf.hhs.gov/programs/orr/resource/voluntary-agencies

U.S. Department of State, Bureau of Population, Refugees, and Migration. www.state.gov/j/prm/

References

Akbulut-Yuksel M, Kugler AD. Intergenerational persistence of health: Do immigrants get healthier as they remain in the US for more generations? *Econ Hum Biol*. 2016;23:136–148. https://doi.org/10.1016/j.ehb.2016.08.004.

American Academy of Pediatrics. *Medical. Evaluation for Infectious Diseases for Internationally Adopted, Refugee, and Immigrant Children. Red Book: 2015 Report of the Committee on Infectious Diseases.* 30th ed. Elk Grove Village, IL: American Academy of Pediatrics; 2015:194–201.

American Academy of Pediatrics Council on Community Pediatrics. *Immigrant Child Health Toolkit.* Elk Grove village, IL: American Academy of Pediatrics; 2015. Retrieved from: https://www.aap.org/en-us/about-the-aap/Committees-Councils-Sections/Council-on-Community-Pediatrics/Pages/Immigrant-Child-Health-Toolkit.aspx. Accessed 8/15/2017.

Andrews TJ, Ybarra V, Matthews LL. For the sake of our children: Hispanic immigrant and migrant families' use of folk healing and biomedicine. *Med Anthropol Q*. 2013;27(3):385–413.

Artiga S, Damico A. *Health Coverage and Care for Immigrants.* The Henry J. Kaiser Family Foundation; 2017. Retrieved from: http://www.kff.org/disparities-policy/issue-brief/health-coverage-and-care-for-immigrants/.

Brisset C, Leanza Y, Laforest K. Working with interpreters in health care: a systematic review and meta-ethnography of qualitative studies. *Patient Educ Couns*. 2013;91(2):131–140. https://doi.org/10.1016/j.pec.2012.11.008.

Brooks T, Wagnerman K, Artiga S, Cornachione E, Ubri P. *Medicaid and CHIP Eligibility, Enrollment, Renewal, and Cost Sharing Policies as of January 2017: Findings from a 50-State Survey.* The Henry J. Kaiser Family Foundation; 2017. Retrieved from: http://www.kff.org/medicaid/report/medicaid-and-chip-eligibility-enrollment-renewal-and-cost-sharing-policies-as-of-january-2017-findings-from-a-50-state-survey/.

Centers for Disease Control and Prevention. *Recommendations of The Advisory Committee on Immunization Practices (Acip): Table 12 Approaches to the Evaluation and Vaccination of Internationally Adopted Children With no or Questionable Vaccination.* 2006. Retrieved from: https://www.cdc.gov/mmwr/preview/mmwrhtml/rr5515a1.htm#tab12.

Centers for Disease Control and Prevention. *Guidelines for Evaluation of the Nutritional Status and Growth in Refugee Children During the Domestic Medical Screening Examination.* 2013a. https://www.cdc.gov/immigrantrefugeehealth/guidelines/domestic/nutrition-growth.html. Accessed September 23, 2017.

Centers for Disease Control and Prevention. *Technical Instructions for Physical or Mental Disorders With Associated Harmful Behaviors and Substance-Related Disorders* 2013b. Retrieved from: https://www.cdc.gov/immigrantrefugeehealth/exams/ti/civil/mental-civil-technical-instructions.html.

Centers for Disease Control and Prevention. *Evaluating and Updating Immunizations during the Domestic Medical Examination for Newly Arrived Refugees.* 2016a. (May 2016 accessed September 23, 2017) Retrieved from: https://www.cdc.gov/immigrantrefugeehealth/guidelines/domestic/immunizations-guidelines.html.

Centers for Disease Control and Prevention. *Technical Instructions for Panel Physicians and Civil Surgeons: Medical History and Physical Examination.* 2016b. Retrieved from: https://www.cdc.gov/immigrantrefugeehealth/exams/ti/panel/technical-instructions/panel-physicians/medical-history-physical-exam.html.

Centers for Disease Control and Prevention. *Technical Instructions for Panel Physicians and Civil Surgeons: Epidemiology and Prevention of Vaccine-Preventable Diseases.* 2017. Retrieved from: https://www.cdc.gov/immigrantrefugeehealth/exams/ti/panel/vaccination-panel-technical-instructions.html. Accessed September 23, 2017.

Centers for Disease Control and Prevention. *Technical Instructions for Panel Physicians and Civil Surgeons: Epidemiology and Prevention of Vaccine-Preventable Diseases.* 2017. Retrieved from: https://www.cdc.gov/immigrantrefugeehealth/exams/ti/panel/vaccination-panel-technical-instructions.html#tbl1. Accessed September 23, 2017.

Chilton LA, Handal GA, Paz-Soldan GJ, Granado-Villar DC, Gitterman BA, Brown JM, et al. Providing care for immigrant, migrant, and border children. *Pediatrics*. 2013;131(6):e2028–e2034. https://doi.org/10.1542/peds.2013-1099.

Cohn D. *It's Official: Minorities Babies are the Majority Among the Nations' Infants, But Only Just.* Pew Research Center; 2016. Retrieved from: http://www.pewresearch.org/fact-tank/2016/06/23/its-official-minority-babies-are-the-majority-among-the-nations-infants-but-only-just/.

Cowden JD, Kreisler K. Development in children of immigrant families. *Pediatr Clin*. 2016;63(5):775–793. https://doi.org/10.1016/j.pcl.2016.06.005.

Crossman KL, Wiener E, Roosevelt G, Bajaj L, Hampers LC. Interpreters: telephonic, in-person interpretation and bilingual providers. *Pediatrics*. 2010;125(3):e631–e638. https://doi.org/0.1542/peds.2009-0769.

Favazza Titus SK. Seeking and utilizing a curandero in the United States: a literature review. *J Holist Nurs*. 2014;32(3):189–201.

Fazel M, Reed RV, Panter-Brick C, Stein A. Mental health of displaced and refugee children resettled in high-income countries: risk and protective factors. *Lancet*. 2012;379(9812):266–282. https://doi.org/10.1016/S0140-6736(11)60051-2.

Flores G, Abreu M, Barone CP, Bachur R, Lin H. Errors of medical interpretation and their potential clinical consequences: a comparison of professional versus ad hoc versus no interpreters. *Ann Emerg Med*. 2012;60(5):545–553. https://doi.org/10.1016/j.annemergmed.2012.01.025.

Gilbert J, Goode TD, Dunne C. *Cultural Awareness.* National Center for Cultural Competence; 2007. Retrieved from: https://nccc.georgetown.edu/curricula/awareness/index.html.

Hannan J. Minority mothers' healthcare beliefs, commonly used alternative healthcare practices, and potential complications for infants and children. *J Am Assoc Nurse Pract*. 2015;27(6):338–348.

Hsieh E. Emerging Trends and Corresponding Challenges in Bilingual Health Research. In: Hsieh E, ed. *Bilingual Health Communication: Working with Interpreters in Cross-Cultural Care.* New York: Taylor and Francis; 2016.

Jong J, Batalova J. *Frequently Requested Statistics on Immigrants and Immigration in the United States.* Migration Policy Institute; 2017. Retrieved from: http://www.migrationpolicy.org/print/15856#.Wce_XYprxmA.

Krogstad JM, Radford J. *Key facts about refugees to the U.S. Pew Research Center.* 2017. Retrieved from: http://www.pewresearch.org/fact-tank/2017/01/30/key-facts-about-refugees-to-the-u-s/.

Lee HY, Choi JK, Lee MH. Health literacy in an underserved immigrant population: new implications toward achieving health equity. *Asian Am J Psychol.* 2015;6(1):97. https://doi.org/10.1037/a0037425.

Leininger, MM. Culture care diversity and universality: a theory of nursing. New York: National League for Nursing; 1991.

Levin SJ, Like RC, Gottlieb JE. ETHNIC: a framework for culturally competent clinical practice. *Patient Care.* 2000;9(special issue):188.

Lor M, Xiong P, Park L, Schwei RJ, Jacobs EA. Western or traditional healers? Understanding decision making in the Hmong population. *West J Nurs Res.* 2017;39(3):400–415.

Martin-Herz SP, Kemper T, Brownstein M, McLaughlin JF. *Developmental Screening with Recent Immigrant and Refugee Children: A Preliminary Report.* 2012. Retrieved from: http://ethnomed.org/clinical/pediatrics/developmental-screening-with-recent-immigrant-and-refugee-children.

Meacham AN. Language learning and the internationally adopted child. *Early Childhood Educ J.* 2006;34(1):73–79. https://doi.org0.1007/s10643-006-0105-z.

Mirza M, Luna R, Mathews B, Hasnain R, Hebert E, Niebauer A, et al. Barriers to healthcare access among refugees with disabilities and chronic health conditions resettled in the US Midwest. *J Immigr Minor Health.* 2014;16(4):733–742. https://doi.org/10.1007/s10903-013-9906-5.

Mishori R, Aleinikoff S, Davis D. Primary care for refugees: challenges and opportunities. *Am Fam Physician.* 2017;96(2):112–120.

Morin P, Schupbach M. *Health in Sickness—Sickness in Health: Towards a New Process Oriented Medicine.* Portland, OR: Deep Democracy Exchange; 2014.

Nalven L. Strategies for addressing long-term issues after institutionalization. *Pediatr Clin North Am.* 2005;52(5):1421–1444. https://doi.org/10.1016/j.pcl.2005.06.010.

Nápoles AM, Santoyo-Olsson J, Karliner LS, O'Brien H, Gregorich SE, Pérez-Stable EJ. Clinician ratings of interpreter mediated visits in underserved primary care settings with ad hoc, in-person professional, and video conferencing modes. *J Health Care Poor Underserved.* 2010;21(1):301. https://doi.org/10.1353/hpu.0.0269.

Nguyen LT, Kaptchuk TJ, Davis RB, et al. The use of traditional Vietnamese medicine among Vietnamese immigrants attending an urban community health center in the United States. *J Altern Complement Med.* 2016;22(2):145–153.

Pernell-Arnold A, Finley L, Sands RG, Bourjolly J, Stanhope V. Training mental health providers in cultural competence: a transformative learning process. *Am J Psychiatr Rehabil.* 2012;15(4):334–356. https://doi.org/10.1080/15487768.2012.733287.

Regester K, Parcells A, Levine Y. *Iraqi Refugee Health Cultural Profile.* 2012. Retrieved from: https://ethnomed.org/culture/iraqi.

Schim SM, Doorenbos A, Benkert R, Miller J. Culturally congruent care: putting the puzzle together. *J Transcult Nurs.* 2007;18(2):103–110. https://doi.org/10.1177/1043659606298613.

Schim SM, Doorenbos AZ. A three-dimensional model of cultural congruence: framework for intervention. *J Soc Work End Life Palliat Care.* 2010;6(3-4):256–270. https://doi.org/10.1080/15524256.2010.529023.

Schwarzwald H, Collins EM, Gillespie S, Spinks-Franklin AA. Common issues faced by children and families in intercountry adoption. In: Schwarzwald H, Collins EM, Gillespie S, Spinks-Franklin AA, eds. *International Adoption and Clinical Practice.* 2015. Retrieved from: https://link.springer.com/book/10.1007%2F978-3-319-13491-8.

Seery T, Boswell H, Lara A. Caring for refugee children. *Pediatr Rev.* 2015;36(8):323–338. https://doi.org/10.1542/pir.36-8-323.

Steinberg EM, Valenzuela-Araujo D, Zickafoose JS, Kieffer E, DeCamp LR. The "battle" of managing language barriers in health care. *Clinical pediatrics.* 2016;55(14):1318–1327. https://doi.org/10.1177/0009922816629760.

Tan TX. Emotional and behavioral disorders in 1.5th generation, 2nd generation immigrant children, and foreign adoptees. *J Immigr Minor Health.* 2016;18(5):957–965. https://doi.org/10.1007/s10903-016-0388-0.

U.S. Department of Health and Human Services, Office of Minority Health. National Standards for Culturally and Linguistically Appropriate Services (CLAS) in Health and Health Care. https://www.thinkculturalhealth.hhs.gov/clas/standards. Accessed 8/15/2017

U.S. Census Bureau. How do we know? America's foreign born in the last 50 years. 2013. www.census.gov/library/infographics/foreign_born.html.

Vaughn LM, Jacquez F, Lindquist-Grantz R, Parsons A, Melink K. Immigrants as research partners: a review of immigrants in community-based participatory research (CBPR). *J Immigr Minor Health.* 2016:1–12. https://doi.org/10.1007/s10903-016-0474-3.

Vivian C, Dundes L. The crossroads of culture and health among the Roma (Gypsies). *J Nurs Scholarsh.* 2004;36(1):86–91. https://doi.org/10.1111/j.1547-5069.2004.04018.x.

Wehbe-Alamah H. Folk care beliefs and practices of traditional Lebanese and Syrian Muslims in the Midwestern United States. In: McFarland MR, Wehbe-Alamah HB, eds. *Leininger's Culture Care Diversity and Universality.* 3rd ed. MA: Jones and Bartlett Learning Burlington; 2014.

Windover AK, Boissy A, Rice TW, Gilligan T, Velez VJ, Merlino J. The REDE model of healthcare communication: optimizing relationship as a therapeutic agent. *J Patient Exp.* 2014;1(1):8–13. https://doi.org/10.1177/237437431400100103.

Yun K, Fuentes-Afflick E, Curry LA, Krumholz HM, Desai MM. Parental immigration status is associated with children's health care utilization: findings from the 2003 New Immigrant survey of US legal permanent residents. *Matern Child Health J.* 2013;17(10):1913–1921. https://doi.org/10.1007/s10995-012-1217-2.

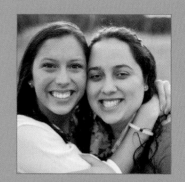

7

Children With Special Health Care Needs

KATHRYN SCHARTZ

Identifying the Population

The proportion of children with special health care needs (CSHCN) and complex medical conditions has increased over the past few decades, as these children live longer and premature and very low birth weight (VLBW) infants survive infancy. This emerging population has created new challenges for the health care system. Their conditions are chronic and often severe, requiring treatment and services over a lifetime. Their care spans inpatient, outpatient, and community-based settings and is often fragmented and poorly coordinated. Although they comprise a minority of the total pediatric population, their care exacts disproportionate costs, time, and social burdens (Berry, 2015). The impact of these conditions on children, families, providers, health professionals, and social/community agencies is immense.

This chapter provides a broad overview of the primary care issues for this population. Specific disorders and the unique care required for specific conditions are discussed in other chapters of this book (Unit 4). Primary care providers (PCPs) are uniquely suited to be care coordinators, an essential element in the care of CSHCN, and can be leaders in improving care for this most vulnerable population. The services necessary to care for CSHCN must be coordinated, as they occur across health care settings. PCPs must be well-versed in federal disability laws; current national, state, and local health care regulations; reimbursement and insurance issues; and the complexities of disease management.

The definition of CSHCN is broad and includes children with relatively minor, easily controlled conditions as well as those with multiple disorders causing life-threatening complications and devastating functional and/or developmental delays. According to the National Survey of Children with Special Health Care Needs (NS-CSHCN), the incidence of CSHCN in the United States in 2011 to 2012 was 19.8%, or 14.6 million children. This is an increase from 15.1% in 2009 to 2010 and 13.9% in 2005 to 2006 (U.S. Department of Health and Human Services [USDHHS], 2015). An early definition of CSHCN states "children with special health care needs are those who have or are at increased risk for a chronic physical, developmental, behavioral, or emotional condition and who also require health and related services beyond that required by children generally" (MCHB, 2018). This definition is broad and encompasses a wide range of disease and disability. For example, children with asthma or type 1 diabetes who require subspecialty and other health care services are included in

this population. Although they have more frequent hospitalizations and need lifestyle changes to thrive, they generally develop typically. Children who have global developmental delays, on the other hand, may need a myriad of subspecialty providers, multiple technologic devices and medications, have frequent hospitalizations as well as high rates of 30-day readmissions, and depend on a variety of community- and school-based services to meet their health care needs. The causes of special health care needs are many and are not easily defined; Table 7.1 lists some common conditions affecting such children.

It is vital to identify these children in order to individualize strategies for their care. The focus should be on decreasing unplanned hospital admissions and the use of emergency departments, facilitating health care access, reducing out-of-pocket expenses, and enhancing child and family satisfaction (Kuo and Houtrow, 2016). Specific medical diagnoses do not predict medical complexity. For example, some children with cerebral palsy develop typically and have minimal disability, whereas others have global developmental delays causing technology dependence for mobility, respiration, nutrition, and communication. Diagnostic codes predict individual health care needs and functional limitations inadequately, thus making them virtually meaningless for identifying CSHCN.

A subgroup of CSHCN—children with medical complexity (CMC)—have more complex and chronic health problems, significant functional limitations, neurologic impairment, high healthcare utilization, and an increased need for family support (Kuo and Houtrow, 2016). CMC are often identified as "medically fragile" or "special health care needs dependent" (Berry et al., 2015; Kuo et al., 2015).

Levels of Complex Care

PCPs must consider CSHCN encounter types and frequencies, the need for specialized therapies and equipment, functional ability limits, number and severity of chronic conditions, and community and home-care needs.

Primary Care

The role of the PCP in the care of CSHCN cannot be overstated. In spite of their many complex needs, these children require ongoing health maintenance, illness prevention, and developmental

TABLE 7.1	Common Diagnoses in Children With Special Health Care Needs
Mental health problems	• Attention deficit disorder • Mood disorders • Autism • Tic disorders
Atopic and rheumatic disorders	• Asthma • Juvenile rheumatoid arthritis • Systemic lupus erythematosus
Endocrine and metabolic diseases	• Growth disorders • Adrenal disorders • Disorders of sex development • Thyroid disorders • Inborn errors of metabolism • Diabetes mellitus • Posterior pituitary disorders
Congenital, genetic, or chromosomal defects	• Rare genetic diseases/syndrome • Sickle cell anemia • Septo-optic dysplasia • Mitochondrial disorders • Prader-Willi syndrome
Premature and/or very low birth weight infants	
Severe injuries or burns	
Static or progressive neuro-logic and neuromuscular disorders	• Cerebral palsy • Global developmental delays • Muscular dystrophy • Spina bifida • Seizure disorders
Respiratory disorders	• Cystic fibrosis
Cardiovascular disorders	• Cardiac defects • Long-term effects of acquired cardiovascular disease
Gastrointestinal disorders	• Inflammatory bowel disease
Childhood cancers	
Family psychosocial concerns	• Trauma/abuse • Homelessness • Undocumented immigration status • Overwhelming needs with limited resources

surveillance. Primary care is needed for routine vaccinations, common disease management, and family support and guidance. The PCP should be the gatekeeper and care coordinator as these children grow and develop. This becomes difficult, as PCPs often feel uncomfortable caring for these children for a variety of reasons. Many providers lack adequate information about specific and often rare health disorders. Care coordination requires collaboration among clinicians, case managers, family members, home care and school professionals, clinics, hospitals, and community-based services, and it is time consuming. Current billing and coding practices do not easily reimburse many of these activities. Although the Affordable Care Act (ACA) mandated changes to address this, current care models make care coordination cumbersome and difficult. Several care models have been proposed, with the patient-centered health home (PCHH) identified as the ideal model for managing complex health care needs.

Subspecialty Care

CSHNC may see up to 10 to 20 different healthcare professionals to manage their specific needs (Kuo et al., 2017). In many cases, the roles and responsibilities of each member of the health care team are not well defined, and care coordination is fragmented. It is important for PCPs to review subspecialty notes and recommendations, look for areas of duplication or contradictions, and help families understand recommendations and treatments. The sharing of health information across health care systems is challenging, making medication lists, up-to-date equipment needs, and care plans difficult to access. These problems lead to duplications, omissions, and errors in care.

For CSHCN who have clearly defined predictable conditions (e.g., spina bifida or cystic fibrosis), interdisciplinary specialty clinics be care coordinators and consultants for PCPs. The care coordination for children with less clearly defined conditions and with predictable health care needs is more difficult owing to use a myriad of subspecialists and services.

Tertiary Care

Children who rely on local PCPs for routine care may make several visits each year to subspecialists and require equipment and supply updates. Subspecialists often focus on their areas of expertise and not the whole child; they may not communicate with PCPs or other subspecialists, resulting in fragmented and poorly coordinated healthcare. PCPs are needed to integrate and manage subspecialty recommendations. Parents of CSHCN may become confused about which orders to follow and often become care coordinators by default. Emergency department providers, first responder personnel, and even primary care staff may not know what to do when equipment malfunctions or physiologic changes occur. PCPs can make sure that families have copies of their care plans and consultation notes. Parents need lists of health care provider contact information as well as providers of supplies and durable medical equipment (DME), medications, and therapies. Examples of these forms can be found via the American Academy of Pediatrics and the American College of Emergency Physicians (see the list of resources later in this chapter).

Home-Care/Community Services

Most care for CSHCN occurs outside the hospital setting. To care for their children at home, families need access to DME and supplies and may require in-home skilled nursing and therapy services. Unfortunately reimbursement for home health care is often difficult to obtain and may be limited to 8 hours a day. Children who require frequent care make heavy demands on caregivers' time and resources, so that such caregivers may not only find it difficult to work outside the home but also become vulnerable to exhaustion, isolation, and the feeling of being overwhelmed.

Components of Care

Technology Dependence and Medication

A significant proportion of CSHCN rely on technology for nutrition, oxygenation, neurologic function, and elimination. PCPs help coordinate care by ordering, improving access to these products and evaluating their use. Complex equipment (e.g., home ventilators, enteral feeding pumps, wheelchairs, hospital beds, and nerve stimulators) may be needed. Low-tech supplies may include such items as respiratory or feeding tubing, special formulas or diets, urinary catheters, and ostomy bags. Ongoing family education is essential to ensure the safe and effective use of all devices and to make sure that families know how to fix common complications (e.g., gastrostomy tubes falling out) without seeking urgent care.

CSHCN often require multiple medications. Polypharmacy leads to an increased risk of drug interactions and confusion about dosing and administration. Needed is ongoing review of medication necessity and limiting the use of medication to control drug side effects. PCPs can help families to find local compounding pharmacies, as many CSHCN cannot swallow pills or require medication not usually available in liquid form. Table 7.2 summarizes many of the complex care needs of CSHCN. Box 7.1 offers an example of a child with complex care needs.

Costs and Family Burden of Caring for Children With Special Health Care Needs

CSHCN comprise a small fraction of the pediatric population but have disproportionally high levels of medical costs, unmet health needs, substandard quality of care, and poor health outcomes. It is estimated that CSHCN make up 1% of the U.S. pediatric population but incur as much as one-third of pediatric health care spending (Kuo and Houtrow, 2016). CMC account for 55% of all hospital admissions and 80% to 85% of 30-day, unplanned readmissions (Berry et al., 2015). Most CSHCN health care costs come from hospitalization (Berry, 2015). Out-of-pocket costs and time spent caring for CSHCN can be significant and may lead to higher-level care when home-care needs are unmet. Almost three-quarters (73%) of CSHCN live in low- or middle-income families, and 22% are below the poverty line, thus adding to the impact of these social determinants of health (Kaiser Family

TABLE 7.2   Complex Care Needs

Surgery	• Congenital anomalies may result in life-saving and palliative surgeries within the first weeks of life; some children require a series of surgical repairs. • Orthopedic procedures to transfer tendons, lengthen muscles, or reduce joints to prevent contractures caused by spasticity, scoliosis, or joint subluxation and dislocation. • Insertion or removal of medical devices (baclofen pumps, vagal nerve stimulators, ventriculoperitoneal shunts, gastrostomy and jejunostomy tubes, colostomies, urostomies, and central venous ports). • Management of chronic illness comorbidities such as obstructive sleep apnea, gastroesophageal reflux disease, and severe dental caries.
Nutrition and gastrointestinal issues	• Poor absorption, failure to thrive, or overweight and obesity. • Difficulty sucking, chewing, and swallowing, which may contribute to aspiration and poor weight gain. Some children need assistive devices such as special nipples, whereas others require enteral feedings. • Changes in gastric smooth muscle tone that alter gastrointestinal motility and may cause reflux or severe chronic constipation. • Postsurgical impaired function for congenital conditions such as tracheoesophageal fistula, diaphragmatic hernia, anal atresia, Hirschsprung disease, and gastroschisis. • Children with enteral feedings require regular evaluation of gastrostomy or jejunostomy tubes, home care for tube maintenance, and access to durable medical equipment, supplies, and special formulas. • Consultation with dieticians to ensure adequate nutrition and with speech and occupational therapy to treat chewing and swallowing disorders. • Medications help with constipation, motility, absorption, and appetite. • Dietary supplements help ensure adequate vitamin and mineral intake.
Mobility/development/adaptive devices	• Physical, occupational, and speech therapy for the evaluation and treatment of mobility and/or developmental disorders. • Wheelchairs, walkers, braces, orthotic devices, and standers for mobility, ambulation assistance, and posture. • Eating utensils and other tools adapted to a child's ability and function to support independence. • Communication boards and other communication electronic devices. • Lack of mobility can interfere with uptake of calcium by bones, leading to osteoporosis.
Respiratory care	• CSHCN with muscle spasticity, scoliosis, contractures, and immobility may have mild to severe respiratory complications. • Children with gastroesophageal reflux disease or severe oropharyngeal dysphagia may have recurrent aspiration pneumonia. • Equipment including nebulizers, CPAP devices, suction, oxygen, tracheostomies, ventilators and cough assist devices. • Children with more severe respiratory conditions may require continuous skilled nursing care.
Neurologic	• Equipment including vagal nerve stimulators, baclofen pumps, ventriculoperitoneal pumps, cochlear implants, hearing aids, glasses. • Cognitive and developmental delays may require additional intervention.
Activities of daily living	• Assistance with elimination and toileting such as urinary catheterization and ostomy care. • Assistance with transfers or bathing ranging to complete dependence on caregivers for toileting, bathing, dressing, and mobility.

CPAP, Continuous positive airway pressure; *CSHCN,* children with special health care needs

• BOX 7.1   Example of a Child With Complex Care Needs

Alex

Alex, a 6-year-old child, is in foster care. He was born without complex health care needs but was abused by his caregiver in a shaken-baby incident and placed in foster care. His foster mother plans to adopt him. She has been caring for him since he was 9 months old. His history includes global developmental delays, quadriplegia with spasticity, severe cognitive impairment, cortical blindness, seizures, reactive airway disease, obstructive sleep apnea, recurrent ear infections, moderate, intermittent atopic dermatitis, bowel and bladder incontinence, severe gastrointestinal reflux with chronic aspiration, and chronic constipation. He has undergone four bilateral myringotomy tube placements, a tonsillectomy and adenoidectomy, a fundoplication with gastrostomy tube placement, and a baclofen pump implantation. He wears diapers, has an enteral feeding pump for continuous formula feedings. Alex uses continuous positive airway pressure (CPAP) at night; has a suction machine and nebulizer to use as needed; and is fitted for a wheelchair for transport to his special needs school, where he receives physical, occupational, and speech therapies. His foster mother is employed and performs his care in the evenings. At night, a home care licensed nurse provides care. Alex's medications include glycopyrrolate to minimize oral secretions, esomeprazole for reflux, divalproex and clonazepam for seizures, polyethylene glycol to manage constipation, albuterol and budesonide for respiratory problems, and topical barriers, steroid creams, and antibiotics to manage eczema flares and prevent or mitigate localized infections around his gastrostomy tube. He is seen in the baclofen clinic and is cared for by dermatology, orthopedics, neurology, gastroenterology, pulmonology, rehabilitation, and otolaryngology clinic subspecialists.

TABLE 7.3   Components of Medical Necessity Letters

Identifying information about child	• Name of the child • Parent/guardian name(s) • Insurance policy or Medicaid number • Date of birth of the child
Identifying information about provider	• Provider's name and credentials • Relationship to child (primary or subspecialty care) • Length of time caring for child
Date of last patient visit	• Date and reason for visit
Diagnoses	• Medical diagnoses (cerebral palsy, asthma) • Diagnoses "covered" by desired equipment or services (failure to thrive related to swallowing disorder) • Diagnoses must be specific (asthma) and not vague (wheezing)
Pertinent medical history	• Discussion of how problems progressed over time (swallowing dysfunction leading to chronic aspiration and poor weight gain)
Pertinent medical, developmental, or evaluative information	• Description of previously attempted treatments and how they worked or did not work • Discussion of inpatient hospital admissions or emergency department visits that occurred without the product or can be prevented by the product
Why product/treatment/evaluation is medically necessary	• Description of the product's use and how it affects the child's health status • Product's description, frequency of use, and relation to care goals (example: "The child requires tracheal suctioning up to 10 times every hour to clear the airway of tenacious secretions and improve oxygenation.")
Summary statement	• Emphasis on the reasons why the equipment or treatment is necessary • Restatement of product use

Foundation, 2017). CSHCN are at risk for fragmented care, with poor team communication, crisis-driven health care, and insufficient caregiver support.

Family-identified service needs change over time, as time devoted to the child's direct care, frequency of provider visits, care coordination needs, and the financial burdens all change. Financial stressors are particularly evident, as families balance their jobs, home care, and unreimbursed expenses.

Government Resources for Children With Special Health Care Needs

Medicaid and Supplemental Security Income

Approximately 44% of CSHCN use Medicaid, Children's Health Insurance Program (CHIP), or other public health insurance programs and more than a third (36%) of CSHCN rely on Medicaid as their sole health care coverage. The Supplemental Security Income (SSI) program provides financial help with care costs if the child has severe functional limitations caused by a physical and/or cognitive impairment likely to last longer than a year or to result in the child's death (Olson, 2017). Medicaid eligibility varies from state to state, so providers should familiarize themselves with the rules in their area. PCPs should encourage families to contact the Social Security Administration to begin the application process.

Durable Medical Equipment and Medicaid Reimbursement

PCPs must understand how to secure reimbursement for necessary services and supplies. In many cases, a Certificate of Medical Necessity (CMN) or DME Information Form (DIF) is needed for reimbursement authorization. For most health care plans,

obtaining DME requires a provider order and letter of medical necessity that must often be resubmitted annually. Unfortunately providers cannot bill for time spent completing this documentation. Links to sample letters are in the resource section at the end of the chapter. Table 7.3 identifies essential components of a letter of medical necessity.

Community and School-Based Services

Much of CSHCN routine care takes place outside of medical settings. Many providers lack knowledge of the nonmedical resources available to this population, including early intervention, public school services, financial assistance programs, respite care services, and support groups. Many developmental, educational, and psychosocial support services are provided in school settings by government and community. It is important for the PCP to be familiar with these services and the educational rights of children with disabilities. Because schools are mostly funded by local taxes, many smaller school districts lack the resources to provide these services.

Early Intervention and the Public School System

EI programs for children from birth to age 3 are managed by individual states and may include developmental, speech, physical, and occupational therapy; audiology; assistive medical technology; family training assistance; social work services; and service coordination. PCPs should refer any child with suspected disabilities or developmental delays to EI services for evaluation and therapy (Olson, 2017). Evaluation and service coordination are generally free, but other services may be billed to third-party payers or to families using a sliding scale, so referral to social work may be needed (Lipkin and Okamoto, 2015).

After age 3, CSHCN transition to services through the public school system. The Individuals With Disabilities Education Act (IDEA) and Section 504 of the Rehabilitation Act ensure free, appropriate education in the least restrictive environment possible for all children. Children with disabilities receive educational support in either general or special education classrooms; therapies including speech and occupational therapy; health care services needed during the school day; and emotional, behavioral, and psychologic services. PCPs should encourage families of children receiving EI services to contact their public school before the child's third birthday to begin the process of evaluation and educational planning. CSHCN may be eligible for an Individual Education Plan (IEP) or a 504 plan. Although not completed by PCPs, they can educate and encourage active participation by parents in this process.

Individual Education Plan and 504 Plan

An IEP outlines each child's educational goals as well as the types of scholastic supports and settings necessary to achieve them (Table 7.4).

Children who do not meet the criteria for an IEP may be eligible for a 504 plan if they can follow the curriculum without modification but require additional assistance in school settings such physical, sensory, or mental support.

Care Coordination

Navigating the increasingly complicated medical system is arduous. CSHCN require a wide range of physical, occupational, and speech therapies as well as home- and school-based nursing services to help manage their complex care. Families who live in rural and smaller urban settings who do not have ready access to a tertiary care center with pediatric subspecialists may have more fragmented community- and school-based services. This may mean that these children get some but not all of their needed therapies, thus compromising their full potential.

Parents often take on the role of care coordinators because of the complex care received across multiple settings. When PCPs act as care coordinators, this eases the burden on families, improves satisfaction, can help to improve health care outcomes and minimize health care expenditures. PCPs are ideal for this role because of their long-standing relationships with CHSCN and their ability to help families navigate the complicated and often intimidating health care system.

TABLE 7.4 Section 504 Plan and Individualized Educational Plan

Americans With Disabilities Act of 1990/Section 504 Plan	Individuals With Disabilities Education Act/Individualized Education Plan
Which Plan Fits the Child?	
For simple accommodations or minor changes	Needs a wide range of services or protections
Easier, faster, more flexible	More involved with mandated parental participation
Eligibility	
Based on identification of psychologic or physical disorder that "substantially limits" a "major life activity" (learning and/or behavior)	Must meet criteria of qualified disability (ADHD not included); often OHI; developmental delays, emotional disturbances, or SLD that seriously affect learning or behavior and "by reason thereof" needs special education and/or related services
Evaluation	
An evaluation (not formalized testing) compiled by the school from a variety of sources to confirm assumption	A complete evaluation compiled by a team of professionals including testing and information from a variety of sources
No money to cover evaluation or support/sustain accommodation	Federally funded
Can occur without parental knowledge or participation	Must have written consent to perform
Provisions	
A plan with individualized accommodations such as extra time to complete assignments, a copy of notes, providing a quiet place to take tests, or assistive technologies	An individualized IEP describes the child's learning problems, details services to be provided, sets annual goals, and defines how progress will be measured
No legal requirements for what is included in a 504, for parent involvement, or for mandated reevaluation	Changes made only in meeting and in collaboration with team
	Special provisions if suspended or expelled
	Reevaluation mandated every 3 years

ADHD, Attention-deficit/hyperactivity disorder; *IEP,* individualized education plan; *OHI,* other health impairments; *SLD,* specific learning disability.

Health Issues for Primary Care Providers

Many PCPs express discomfort in caring for these children because of a lack of knowledge of rare conditions or health care service requirements that may be beyond the scope of most PCPs. PCPs of CSHCN conduct comprehensive assessments, develop interdisciplinary care plans including subspecialty recommendations, review therapists' care, assist families in obtaining needed equipment and supplies, and help to coordinate care with schools. They also maintain an ongoing surveillance of the child's nutritional, mobility, and respiratory needs. The amount of time spent on the telephone, doing paperwork, reviewing medical records, and counseling parents is immense. Moreover, many of the activities of care coordination are not provided during face-to-face encounters or may require lengthy outpatient visits or telephone management; thus they are poorly reimbursed using standard fee-for-service models. In some cases, children are lost to primary care when they enter the world of tertiary and subspecialty care. Some families of CSHCN use PCPs only when local medical care is needed on short notice.

Strategies and Models to Improve Care for Children With Special Health Care Needs

Evidence suggests that CSHCN should have access to the following:
- Urgent care in an outpatient setting to treat acute health problems
- One or more ambulatory care providers who can comprehensively address acute problems, chronic medical needs, and functional and psychosocial issues
- Coordination of decision-making among all providers of care
- Proactive care planning to manage anticipated future problems and maximize well-being for the child and family (Kuo and Houtrow, 2016)

The Patient-Centered Healthcare Home

The patient-centered health care home (PCHH) is believed to be the ideal care model for CSHCN. The PCHH provides "accessible, continuous, comprehensive, coordinated, compassionate, culturally competent, and family-centered" care (American Academy of Pediatrics, 2004) and improves satisfaction and clinical and family outcomes for CSHCN. Table 7.5 lists the components of a PCHH. See the list of resources at the end of this chapter for additional information.

Shared Plan of Care

This is a comprehensive information compilation that, in partnership with the family, allows individualized care coordination. It is an especially useful tool for CSHCN with substantial care needs as it encompasses both clinical and nonclinical needs to achieve the shared goals of the patient, family, and caregivers (Wirth, 2016). There are four important elements of the care planning process: (1) identify the needs and strengths of the patient and family, (2) build essential partnerships, (3) create the plan of care, and (4) implement the plan of care (Table 7.6).

Supportive Care Needs for Children With Special Health Care Need

Respite Care

Because caring for children with complex care needs is unrelenting, families may need respite care to provide breaks from time to time. This can take place in homes or in institutional settings. Some states have access to federal funds to help support respite care services for families. Providers should be familiar with local services and help families to access them.

Support Groups and Services

Social support services are available through community-based services, parent training groups, and national organizations.

TABLE 7.5 Children With Special Health Care Needs Care in the Patient-Centered Healthcare Home

Plan of care	• Developed by PCP/designated care coordinator, child, and family • Collaboration with other providers, agencies, and organizations involved with the care of the patient
Central record or database (accessible to families and confidential)	• Pertinent medical information, including hospitalizations and specialty care • Updated medication list • Equipment, supplies, therapies with product information, suppliers, sizes
Care coordination	• Information-sharing among the child, family, and other providers • Referral to other health care professionals • Collaboration with agencies to obtain necessary services
Family support	• Support groups (online, national organizations) • Parent-to-parent groups • Social work • Mental health services
Communication	• Information sharing among specialists and other professionals • Families' understanding of recommendations and treatment options • Encouraging families to keep pertinent information and share this information with health care providers as needed

PCP, Primary care provider.

TABLE 7.6 Shared Plan of Care

Determine needs and strengths of child/family	• Consider each family's situation and abilities, strengths and needs, medical conditions, psychosocial factors, child/family development, environmental issues. • Financial strengths/needs.
Develop necessary partnerships	• Identify how providers, caregivers and children work together. • Shared agreement on goals. • Account for family preferences and best practices.
Develop a plan of care	• Identify roles and responsibilities of providers and families. • Include specific emergency care information. • Include fact sheets about rare conditions, legal documents about guardianship and/or health care decision-making.
Implement the plan of care	• Update the plan of care as needs change. • Evaluate and plan process at each encounter, assess progress toward goals and develop new goals as needed.

Families should be encouraged to seek out these services and to get involved in educational, advocacy, and other activities to alleviate stress and caregiver fatigue. Some conditions have national, state, and local organizations that parents can access online. For rare conditions, the National Organization for Rare Disorders website provides lists of disease-specific organizations and support groups.

Transition of Care

Of an estimated 4 to 5 million youth from 12 to 18 years of age with special health care needs, only around 40% will receive transitional care services (Zhou, Roberts, Dhaliwal, and Della, 2016). *Healthy People 2020* list initiatives for coordinating transition to adulthood for children with chronic conditions (U.S. Department of Health and Human Resources, 2010).

Unfortunately there are multiple barriers to effective transition. The diversity of clinical conditions makes standardization difficult. In many cases, there are no adult care providers qualified to treat what were once considered childhood diseases. Transitioning is a complex process requiring coordination and continuity of care across locations or levels of care. Six factors influence successful transition are as follows: (1) timing, (2) patient transition perceptions, (3) preparation for the transition, (4) posttransition patient outcomes, (5) barrier identification, and (6) transitions facilitating the identification of these factors (Zhou et al., 2016). CSHCN who can live independently must learn to perform self care activities, obtain vocational counseling, secure employment, and develop the skills needed for independent living.

Legal Issues

Parents of intellectually challenged CSHCN may face the problem of how to provide for their child's care when they become old or die. These children may become dependent on the state and face complex care decisions. PCPs should encourage parents to seek legal advice to set up a power of attorney and medical decision-making expertise to make sure that their wishes for their child are carried out, including the appointment of a guardian. They should legally determine palliative care options, health care decision authority, and other important considerations.

Additional Resources

Patient-Centered Medical Home

AAP Medical Home Resources. https://www.aap.org/en-us/professional-resources/practice-transformation/medicalhome/Pages/home.aspx

Emergency Information Form for Children With Special Health Care Needs. https://www.acep.org/by-medical-focus/pediatrics/medical-forms/emergency-information-form-for-children-with-special-health-care-needs/

Documents and Forms—Seattle Children's Hospital. https://cshcn.org/planning-record-keeping/documents/

Letters of Medical Necessity

Medical Home Portal. https://www.medicalhomeportal.org/issue/writing-letters-of-medical-necessity

Centers for Medicare and Medicaid Services. https://www.cms.gov/Medicare/CMS-Forms/CMS-Forms/CMS-Forms-List.html

National Survey Data. http://www.nschdata.org

Resources for Families

Support Groups

March of Dimes. https://www.marchofdimes.org

Our Kids. http://www.our-kids.org

Genetic and Rare Diseases Information Center. https://rarediseases.info.nih.gov/guides/pages/120/support-for-patients-and-families

Support for Families of Children With Disabilities. https://www.supportforfamilies.org

References

American Academy of Pediatrics. The medical home. *Pediatr.* 2004;113(5):1545–1547.

Berry JG. *What Children With Medical Complexity, Their Families, and Healthcare Providers Deserve From an Ideal Healthcare System.* Lucile Packard Foundation for Children's Health, Briefing Paper; 2015.

Berry JG, Hall M, Cohen E, et al. Ways to identify children with medical complexity and the importance of why. *J Pediatr.* 2015;167(2):229–237.

Kuo D, Houtrow A. Recognition and management of medical complexity. *Pediatrics.* 2016;138(6):e20163021.

Kuo DZ, McAllister JW, Rossignol L, et al. Care coordination for children with medical complexity: whose care is it, anyway? *Pediatrics.* 2017;141:S224.

Kuo D, Melguizo-Castro M, Goudie A, et al. Variation in child health care utilization by medical complexity. *Matern Child Health J.* 2015;19(1):40–48.

Lipkin PH, Okamoto J, Council on Children with Disabilities. The Individuals with Disabilities Education Act (IDEA) for children with special educational needs. *Pediatrics.* 2015;136:e1650–e1662.

Maternal & Child Health Bureau (MCHB). *Children with special health care needs.* 2018. Retrieved from: https://mchb.hrsa.gov/maternal-child-health-topics/children-and-youth-special-health-needs. Accessed April 5, 2018.

Olson K. After the visit: an overview of government and community programs supporting children with medical complexity. *Children.* 2017;4(5):35. https://doi.org/10.3390/children4050035.

U.S. Department of Health and Human Services, Health Resources and Services Administration, Maternal and Child Health Bureau. *Child Health USA 2014.* 2015. Retrieved from: https://mchb.hrsa.gov/chusa14/dl/population-characteristics.pdf. Accessed May 13, 2018.

U.S. Department of Health and Human Services. *Healthy People 2020: Understanding and Improving Health.* 3rd ed. Washington, DC; 2010.

Wirth B, Kuznetsov A. *Shared Plan of Care: a Tool to Support Children and Youth With Special Health Care Needs and Their Families.* National Center for Medical Home Implementation; 2016. Retrieved from: https://medicalhomeinfo.aap.org/tools-resources/Documents/Shared%20Plan%20of%20Care2.pdf. Accessed April 5, 2018.

Zhou H, Roberts P, Shaliwal S, Deilla P. Transitioning adolescent and young adults with chronic disease and/or disabilities from paediatric to adult care services – an integrative review. *J Clin Nurs.* 2016;25:3113–3130. https://doi.org/10.1111/jocn.13326.

8

Principles of Developmental Management of Children

DAWN LEE GARZON MAAKS

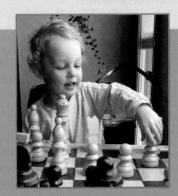

A critical part of the role of the pediatric primary care provider (PCP) is to provide developmental surveillance and anticipatory guidance to help parents and families adjust to their evolving roles as their child grows and develops. This requires a thorough understanding of child development, parental role development, and family function. This chapter presents an introduction to principles of development, developmental theories, methods of developmental assessment, and identification and management of developmental problems. Chapters 8 through 13 apply this content by age group, describe normal patterns of development, identify developmental "red flags," and recommend anticipatory guidance for families during infancy, early childhood, middle childhood, and adolescence.

Developmental Principles

Development is a lifelong, dynamic process. Milestone achievement in one phase sets the stage for the next phase. Development is a dynamic and reciprocal process influenced by the child's internal and external environments. Key principles provide a contextual understanding of developmental concepts. Exactly how these principles manifest in a particular child depends on the child's genetic background, personality or temperament, and intrauterine and extrauterine environments.

Principle 1. Growth and development are orderly and sequential. Although children differ in rates and timing of developmental changes, they generally follow certain predictable stages or phases. Specific examples include the rapid growth during the first year of life, progress toward independence throughout childhood, and the development of secondary sex characteristics during adolescence.

Principle 2. Growth and development pacing varies considerably between children. Some children demonstrate early skill in motor coordination, and others demonstrate early skill in language acquisition. These changes are unique to each child.

Principle 3. Development occurs in a cephalocaudal and proximodistal direction. An example of this principle is seen as infants develop increasing motor coordination, gaining head control before sitting and walking. Similarly, developmental progress occurs with controlled movements that first occur near the body's midline, such as rolling over, progress to distal coordination of the hands, such as mastery of the pincer grasp.

Principle 4. Growth and development increasingly integrates. Behavior that is taken for granted, such as self-feeding, occurs as a result of the acquisition of numerous small changes and skills. Simple skills and behaviors integrate into more complex behaviors as the child grows and develops.

Principle 5. Developmental abilities increasingly organize and differentiate. As a result of increasing maturation and experience, children's behaviors and responses to internal and external cues become more regulated, organized, and differentiated. The infant who cries and moves because of hunger is different from the hungry toddler who walks to the refrigerator and points.

Principle 6. The child's internal and external environments affect growth and development. Opportunities for play, societal norms, cultural values, family traditions, and family beliefs all influence child development. Similarly, children influence their environment to achieve desired experiences and opportunities.

Principle 7. Certain periods are critical to growth and development. Critical periods are points of time when developmental advances occur and are particularly susceptible to alterations due to internal and external influences. For example, fetal exposure to certain viruses during the first trimester of pregnancy increases the risk of congenital abnormalities.

Principle 8. Development is a continual process, often without smooth transitions. Developmental phases are marked by periods of change, growth, and stability plateaus.

Theories of Child Development

Developmental theories describe how children progress from infancy through adolescence and provide perspectives on childhood growth and development. PCPs need to stay abreast of changing ideas regarding child development and appreciate new pediatric developmental theories. Developmental theories are based on various cultures, personalities, environmental issues, philosophical beliefs, and investigative methods. When using a developmental perspective in practice, the provider should understand how the theory was developed and how it may relate to a particular family and child. Developmental theories provide guidelines for understanding the child's emerging behavior, personality, and physical abilities. It is usually necessary to combine several theories to holistically view the child.

Cognitive-Structural Theories: Language and Thought

Cognitive-structural theories examine the ways children think, reason, and use language. They are based on assumptions about central nervous system maturation and children's interactions with their environment. Individual differences are ascribed to genetic endowment and environmental influences.

Jean Piaget's observations, many of which were of his own children, provide an understanding of children's cognitive development and their perception and interaction with the world around them. Piaget (1969) described how children actively use their life experiences, incorporating them into their own mental and physical being over time. He emphasized how children modify themselves depending on their environmental experiences and their stage-related competency level. Piaget described four stages of cognitive development (Table 8.1).

Sensorimotor Stage (Birth to 2 Years)

At the sensorimotor stage, children learn about the world through their actions and sensory and motor movements. Key concepts during this period include object permanence, spatial relationships, causality, use of instruments, and combination of objects. The child's framework for learning is the self, and there is little cognitive connection to objects outside the self.

Preoperational Stage (2 to 7 Years)

Children next attempt to make sense of the world and reality. In this stage, they are egocentric and only able to reason when there are connections to concrete objects. They learn cause and effect, and their reasoning is often flawed. Children begin to use semiotic functioning, or the use of one thing to represent another. Intuitive reasoning emerges toward the end of this stage, but reasoning remains connected to the concrete reality of the here and now.

Concrete Operational Stage (7 to 12 Years)

Children use symbols to represent concrete objects and to perform mental tasks. This requires cognitive skill to organize experiences and classify increasingly complex information. Most schoolwork requires functioning at this level. This stage is characterized by flexibility of thought, declining egocentrism, logical reasoning, and greater social cognition.

Formal Operational Stage (13 Years Through Adulthood)

At this stage, adolescents begin abstract thinking, and imagining different solutions to problems. They develop increased awareness of health and illness and recognize how their behaviors impact health. Renewed egocentrism may be noted early in this stage as a result of a lack of differentiation between what others are thinking and one's own thoughts. This egocentric thinking eventually gives way to an appreciation of the differences in judgment between the adolescent and other individuals, societies, and cultures. This is the basis of an adolescent's ability to think about politics, law, and society in terms of abstract principles and benefits rather than focusing only on the punitive aspects of societal laws.

Information processing theory evolved from Piaget's work and holds that humans do not just respond to stimuli but process the information into scripts (similar to those used by computers) that guide behavior and social problem-solving (Huesmann, 1988). This model blends concepts of attention, perception, memory, social cues, and emotional states and how they influence the ability to encode and retrieve information.

Psychoanalytic Theories: Personality and Emotions

Psychodynamic theorists study factors that influence the individual's emotional and psychological behavior. Personality includes the characteristics of temperament and motivation, and concepts related to self-esteem and self-concept. Sigmund Freud (1938) was one of the most influential theorists in this area. Freud sought to link the conscious mind and the body through the unconscious mind (see Table 8.1). Some of his most significant contributions were his descriptions of the interactions of id, ego, and superego.

Anna Freud continued the work of her father, focusing particularly on children. Her studies developed the implications of psychoanalysis for raising normal children. She believed that psychoanalytic theory helps parents gain "insight into the potential harm done to young children during the critical years of their development by the manner in which their needs, drives, wishes, and emotional dependencies are met" (Freud, 1974).

Erikson (1964) expanded Freud's theories, describing the stages of the individual throughout the lifespan (see Table 8.1). Each stage presents problems that the individual seeks to master. Erikson believed that if problems were not resolved, they would be revisited again at future stages.

Sullivan (1964) emphasized the importance of self-concept and modulating environmental influences. He defined the parents and home as the most crucial cultural environment. Sullivan posited that progression toward mature relationships is based on communication skills and the integration of social experiences inhibited or enhanced by the parents' relationship between themselves.

Mahler and colleagues (1975) analyzed the development of an infant's evolving independence through study of the mother-infant dyad. Three phases of development were proposed: autism, symbiosis, and separation-individuation. They held that these phases account for the infant's gradually increasing awareness of self and others. In the autistic phase (3 to 5 weeks old), the infant has no concept of self but works, physiologically, to achieve extrauterine homeostasis. The second phase, symbiosis, refers to a period of undifferentiation or fusion with the mother in which infant and mother form a dual unity. Separation-individuation (from about 4 to 5 months old onward) is characterized by a steady increase in awareness of the separateness of the self and the other.

The context of separation and connectedness in infant attachment was explored by Stern (1985), Emde and Buchsbaum (1990), and Rogoff (1990). They propose that the quality and consistency of infant-caregiver relationships help the infant develop an affective, or emotional, sense of self. The early beginnings of the sense

TABLE 8.1   Comparison of Early Developmental Theorists

Age	Freud	KOHLBERG		PIAGET		ERIKSON	
		Stages		Stages/ Substages	Characteristics	Psychological Crisis	Themes
0–12 months	Oral stage	Stage 1 "premoral" preconventional level	1: Punishment avoidance and obedience	Sensorimotor stage: Reflexive stage: 0-1 month	Innate infant reflexes	Trust vs. mistrust	To get; to give in return
				Primary circular stage: 1-4 months	Repetitive responses		
				Secondary circular stage: 4-8 months	Outward-directed behaviors		
				Coordination of secondary circular stage: 8-12 months	Object permanence and goal-directed behaviors		
12-18 months				Tertiary circular reactions stage: 2-18 months	Causality and object permanence through several steps	Autonomy vs. shame	To hold on; to let go
18-36 months	Anal stage	Stages 1-2 preconventional level	2: Instrumental realistic orientation—recognizes needs in others as long as own needs are met	Mental combinations stage: 18-24 months	Memory used for problem-solving		
3–6 years	Oedipal stage	Stages 1-2 preconventional level		Preoperational stage: Preconceptual stage: 2-4 years Intuitive stage: 4-7 years	Increased use of symbols, especially language; representational thought, egocentrism, assimilation, and symbolic play Increased symbolic functioning, language, decreasing egocentricity, imitation of reality	Initiative vs. guilt	To make things; to play
6-11 years	Latency stage	Preconventional (stage 2): Up to 7 years Conventional (stages 3 and 4): 7-10 years Postconventional (stage 5): 10-11 years	3: Interpersonal acceptance of "nice" girl and "good" boy social concept—does not want relationships with others harmed 4: The "law and order" orientation—rules are not flexible or changeable 5: Social contract and utilitarian orientation—rules can change on social needs	Concrete operational stage	Flexible thought: Understands rules of reversibility and deconcentration, conservation, and identity Declining egocentrism: Ability to understand another's perspective Local reasoning: Understands concepts of relation, ordering, conservation; able to classify objects Social cognition: Improved sense of equality and justice	Industry vs. inferiority	To make things; to complete

Continued

(see Table 8.1)

TABLE 8.1	Comparison of Early Developmental Theorists—cont'd						
		KOHLBERG		PIAGET		ERIKSON	
Age	Freud	Stages		Stages/ Substages	Characteristics	Psychological Crisis	Themes
12-17 years	Adolescence (Oedipus complex)	Stages 5-6 post-conventional level	6: Universal ethical orientation principles are source of rules; inner conscience present	Formal operational stage	Development of logical thinking, able to work with abstract ideas; able to synthesize and integrate concepts into larger schemes	Identity vs. role confusion	To be oneself; to share being oneself or not being oneself
17-30 years	Young adult	Stages 5-6		Formal operational stage		Intimacy vs. isolation	To lose and find oneself in another

of self are based on three biologic principles: self-regulation, social fittedness, and affective monitoring (Emde, 1988). Infants with attachment security and a sense of connectedness are more likely to explore and be autonomous; they also have an internal working model to guide them in later attachments.

The concept of intersubjectivity, or mutual understanding of meaning and mutual engagement in social interactions, underlies attachment theory. Trevarthen and Aitken (2001) observed that even very young infants demonstrate an ability to interact with a sympathetic individual beyond an instinctive or reflexive manner. They concluded that the infant's capacity for self-regulation may be based in the operation of an intrinsic motive formation (IMF) developed in the parietotemporal region of the prenatal brain. Studies of the brain and infant behavior suggest that the IMF guides the newborn's ability to integrate sensory-motor coordination, orient to preferred stimuli (e.g., mother's voice), sustain mutual attention with an affectionate other, and anticipate what to expect in the environment. Successful development of the infant's "purposive consciousness" and the ability to cooperate with and learn from another depends on neurologic functioning and the presence of a supportive environment. Parents guide the infant to connect with others and experience shared affection. Major developmental influences of children include social interactions and engagement with their parents.

These theories help the provider assist parents to understand why, for example, infants who understand object permanence look over the side of the highchair for food or a toy that fell to the floor and smile and laugh when they spot it, because they knew it would be there. These same infants may call a parent to their room in the middle of the night; they now have "person permanence." They picture their parent in their mind and, perhaps experiencing normal separation anxiety, they want the parent to come to them. The PCP can use the concepts of attachment theory and intersubjectivity to explain that this behavior is normal for an infant trying to have his or her needs met. The behavior reflects healthy attachment and use of the parent as a secure base from which to explore the world.

The Role of Social Interaction in Cognitive Development

Kohlberg (1969) focused on theories of moral development and socialization, emphasizing the process by which children learn the expectations and norms of their society and culture (see Table

8.1). Kohlberg's work primarily involved male participants. Gilligan (1982) suggested that female thoughts and actions involve significantly different objectives and goals; specifically, that girls tend to think more in terms of caring and relationships, basing their moral judgments on complexities that they perceive in human interactions.

Fowler's (1981) theory described the spiritual dimension of human life, or the development of faith. This theory addressed the process of developing meaning in daily life. Faith is described as the structure that people use to build their lives. Fowler emphasized that achieving the stages is not due to intelligence but rather occurs through valuing, thinking, and interacting with others.

Vygotsky's (1978) theory of child learning states that as children interact with others, they develop as individuals within cultural contexts. They simultaneously develop memory, problem-solving skills, attention, and concept formation. Core to Vygotsky's theory is the "zone of proximal development," which is the difference between what a child can do on his or her own and what he or she can do with help from others.

Vygotsky believes that children learn by watching others, and that they learn best when their parents and caregivers provide them with opportunities in the child's zone of proximal development. This theory holds that cognitive development occurs in social, historical, and cultural contexts and that adults guide child learning. Development depends on the use of language, play, and extensive social interaction. One of Vygotsky's examples is the process of the child learning to point his or her finger. Initially, the infant points his or her finger without meaning; however, as people, and especially caregivers, respond to the finger pointing, the infant learns there is meaning to the movement. What starts as a muscle movement becomes a means of interpersonal connection between two people. This theory further holds that play and learning should be constructed to take into consideration the child's needs, inclination, and incentives. This theory supports the benefit of adult social learning opportunities via group interaction and observation.

Behavioral Theories: Human Actions and Interactions

Behaviorism, the study of the general laws of human behavior, focuses on the present and environmental influences of human behavior. Skinner's (1953) view of child development examined learning controlled through classic operant conditioning. Behavior modification therapy is largely based on Skinner's work. Bandura's (1962) social learning theory looks at imitation and modeling as a means of learning, emphasizing the social variables involved. Bijou and Baer (1965) responded to critics of behaviorism's view of the child as a passive object and argued that children's responses to environmental stimuli are dependent on their genetic structure and personal history.

Humanistic Theories

The humanists believe that individuals and those around them are responsible for the movement they make from one need plateau to another and include theorists like Maslow (1971), Buhler and Allen (1972), and Mahrer (1978). Maslow's hierarchy of needs included physiologic, safety, belongingness and love, esteem, and self-actualization. People must meet their basic needs for safety and physiologic needs before being able to work toward "higher" needs of belonging and self-actualization. Because of the developmental physical, emotional, and cognitive changes in childhood, pediatric patients have multiple critical stages where they require physiologic, safety, and emotional support in order to thrive and live happy, self-actualized lives.

Ecologic Theories

Human ecology theory (Bronfenbrenner, 1979) emphasizes the interdependence between environmental settings (roles, interpersonal relations, and activities) and the developing child. Development is described as the growing capacity to discover, sustain, or alter the self or the environment. Children are viewed as dynamic entities who increasingly restructure their environment. Environments, in turn, influence children, leading to mutual accommodation and reciprocity. Children's perceptions of the environment influence their behavior and development more than objective reality does.

Home and family, child care settings, schools, entertainment and recreational activities, their parents' work, and broad economic opportunities in society influence children. Role and setting changes, such as the birth of a sibling, have profound effects on the developing child. These can be mediated by family routines and rituals. Ecologic theory takes into consideration the whole child's environment and even delineates the strong influence that the quality of the parents' relationship with each other and each parent's individual development have on parent-child interaction. When parents successfully complete their own developmental tasks and they experience positive mutual feelings, the parent-child relationship is strengthened. Alternatively, when parents experience mutual antagonism or interference, the parent-child relationship may be impaired (Pridham et al., 2010). These theories are especially useful to assist PCPs to understand how interpersonal violence and unhealthy relationships impact child development.

Behavioral Economics

Behavioral economics is a relatively new theory of human behavior that comes from a blending of sociology, psychology, and economic theory. This theory holds that people make decisions based on three influences (World Bank Group, 2015; Gennetian et al., 2016). The first influence, automatic thinking, is mostly caused by limited human attention. This means that most people don't often think about their decisions but rather make them using "mental shortcuts" in an almost reflexive way. For example, when a school-aged child chooses a shirt from a full drawer of clothes, the natural tendency is to pull the first one they see or reach for their favorite

shirt without thinking if they are distracted or do not see the decision as important. This might result in grabbing an inappropriate shirt (short sleeved in the middle of winter). But when asked why, the response might be the familiar "I don't know" because there was no thought behind the decision. Situations that exacerbate automatic thinking are cognitive strain, having too many choices (the paradox of choice), or having decision fatigue.

The second tenant of this theory is that humans are inherently social and make decisions based upon cultural influences and norms, as well as an inborn desire to be altruistic, cooperative, and reciprocal. The result is that children have an intrinsic desire to please their parents and to be "good" children, but how they achieve this is largely defined by their social environment. Caregivers need to provide children social networks and their responses should tie to the child's behavioral cues. Sensitivity to children's cues involves responding within a few seconds with a response that meets the child's developmental stage and emotional needs and is directly related to the child's behavior (Gennetian et al., 2016).

The third influence, human decision-making, is rooted in social contexts and past experiences that provide behavior models. This is one of the reasons why anticipatory guidance usually includes parental modeling of good behavior. Children learn by watching others and using the observed behavior as a template. Positive reinforcement is another example of providing a child a behavioral mental model.

Behavioral economics not only helps describe how children behave and why they make the decisions they do, but it also serves as a model for how parents learn to parent. The role of the PCP is to help parents identify mental stressors that result in reactive instead of responsive parenting, establish a culture of appropriate parenting, and provide examples of strategies or "thought models" that can be used with their children.

Theories of Family and Parent Development

PCPs recognize that pediatric care occurs within the family context. Just as an infant is not born fully developed, families and parents grow and change over time. A wide variety of stimuli including sociocultural norms, changes in family members, learned behaviors from past experiences, and internalized individual expectations and desires influence parents and families. Family function and parental comfort and capability in their parenting role have profound impacts on child development and child well-being. Thus it is important for PCPs to be familiar with theories on how parents develop in their roles and how families develop as units.

Family Theories

Family systems theory provides a framework to help PCPs understand how family dynamics influence adult and child behaviors. Originally described by Bowen in the 1960s, this theory holds that an individual's emotional function has a profound impact on overall family health (Bowen, 1966). Differentiation of self and emotional fusion are key concepts in this theory. Differentiation of self refers to the individual's ability to recognize that he or she is a unique individual, with characteristics and traits different from those of other family members, who can function as a distinct person while developing and maintaining emotional connections to others. Emotional fusion reflects the ability to emotionally react to and communicate with others without conscious thought or speaking. Highly fused relationships can cause stress and anxiety because of fear of rejection and/or emotional distance. Anxious family

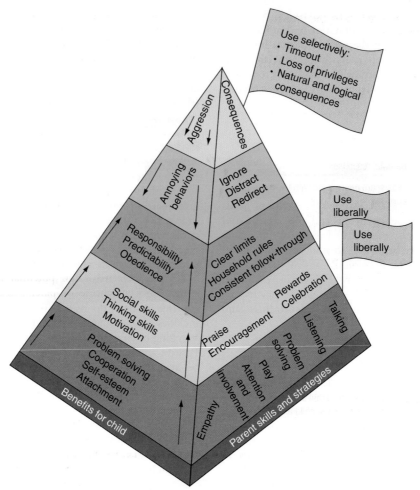

• **Fig 8.1 Parenting Pyramid.** (Modified from Webster-Stratton C. *The Incredible Years: A Trouble-Shooting Guide for Parents of Children Aged 2–8*. Seattle: Incredible Years Press; 2005.)

members, those with highly fused relationships, or those with poor self-differentiation, express their anxiety in ways that result in family dysfunction. This can cause parental discord, parent or child health or emotional problems, or triangulation, a process where anxiety and/or tension between two family members is passed on to a third family member (Lampis et al., 2017). This theory helps explain how parental relationship problems can result in child behavior difficulties or how an enmeshed parent-child relationship can result in inappropriate worries about child health and/or strain in the parents' relationship. PCPs help families to recognize triangulation and other signs of unhealthy self-differentiation and emotional fusion, modify unhealthy behaviors, and by referring to mental health specialists when significant concerns and dysfunctions occur.

Evolutionary life history theories explain how the family environment affects family conflict and child development (Hengartner, 2017). Core to these theories is the belief that families evolve over time and learned family behaviors have genetic influences; among them is the biologic imperative to reproduce. Family behaviors affect parenting practice and child development because children learn how to interact with others and develop social skills via interactions with family members. These theories hold that some parents focus on long-term pair bond (mating bond) outcomes and interpersonal relationships and are highly invested in their parenting role and their child's long-term success. Other parents focus more on short-term gains, forming pair bonds and less

on parenting. This can result in non-nurturing parent-child relationships, early onset sexual expression, and other externalizing behaviors, and inappropriate relationship expectations, especially in adolescent females.

Parent Development Theory

The parent development theory asserts that the parenting role begins in childhood, evolves over time, and is influenced by personal experience, social norms, the health of the parent-child relationship, family dynamics, and the child's own characteristics (Mowder, 2005; Sperling and Mowder, 2006). Fig 8.1 demonstrates factors that influence parental role development. Parent development theory defines the parent as the individual who assumes the responsibility of caring for and raising a child. Six characteristics of parenting are identified that vary in their importance based on the child's developmental needs (Table 8.2). These behaviors occur within a social context as part of the parent-child relationship and are dynamic. Parenting evolves as a child ages. For example, a parent of a toddler who is just learning to walk has a very different role from the parent of an adolescent who is a senior in high school and preparing to leave for college.

Expectations for parental behaviors are also shaped by societal norms and personal beliefs (Mowder, 2005). If parents view their role as primarily that of a disciplinarian, they may have very specific

TABLE 8.2	Parent Role Characteristics in the Parent Development Theory	
Role Characteristic	**Signs of Healthy Role Development**	
Bonding	Parents feel and express love and affection for the child. They positively regard the child.	
Discipline	Parents set limits for the child's behavior and make sure the rules are understood and followed. They give consistent parental responses.	
Education	Parents share information with their child to help them understand the world around them. They teach and guide their child, and they model good behaviors.	
General welfare and protection	Parents make sure their child is safe and has physical needs met. They provide a safe, healthy environment with adequate food, water, clothing, and shelter.	
Responsivity	Parents pay attention to their child and are responsive to cues from the child, addressing needs beyond those of general welfare and protection. They help, encourage, and support the child.	
Sensitivity	Parents listen to the verbal and nonverbal communication of the child and are able to accurately interpret the child's needs. They respect, empathize with and comfort the child, and give appropriate responses to the child's needs.	

Originally published by Pace University Press in Journal of Early Childhood and Infant Psychology, "Parent development theory: understanding parents, parenting perceptions and parenting behaviors," 1:45–64, 2005.

and defined ways they expect their child to behave, and many of the interactions they have with their child will focus on the child's behavior within the context of the parent's rules. On the other hand, parents who view their primary role as a nurturer and comforter may spend more time expressing love and affection for the child. There is no single approach to parenting, and parenting differs from family to family. Parenting roles are not fixed; parents may move from one role to another depending on the situational context.

It is important for PCPs to recognize that one parenting style does not "fit all." The PCP provides information and supports the knowledge and skills parents need for a healthy parent-child relationship. Concerns develop when there is a mismatch of parent role and child development or when strife in the parent-child relationship occurs.

Cultural Influences on Development

Cultural and ethnic traditions shape the development of infants, children, adolescents, parents, and families. PCPs should understand that cultural differences developmental milestones are normal until kindergarten (Hagan et al., 2017). Early milestones, such as eating solid food, weaning from the breast or bottle, sleeping through the night, and toilet training, may normally occur at different ages in different cultures. Parental responses to their children's needs also vary by culture. Accurate assessments of families

and children come from understanding the specific culture of a family and community. To understand family culture, additional assessment is needed beyond the traditional health history and physical examination. See Chapter 6 for more information.

Management Strategies in Child Development

Promoting Parent Development and Parent-Child Interaction: Anticipatory Guidance

Parents need clear information about expectations for child development, and providers must educate parents and families about normative development and best practices for managing development. The goal of anticipatory guidance is to help parents plan for and cope with anticipated changes and to increase parenting skills, confidence, and competence in problem-solving so that children can reach their maximum potential for health and wellness. Anticipatory guidance assists parents to adapt parenting styles and strategies to their child's temperament, growth, and development. Components include:

- Assess the child's development.
- Determine the parents' knowledge of child development.
- Determine the parents' knowledge of, and comfort and experience with, the parent role.
- Assess the parents' problem-solving and coping skills.
- Provide information about normative child development, including common developmental variations with age-appropriate written educational materials and referrals to additional sources (i.e., online resources, community and professional organizations, and support networks).
- Assist parents to develop realistic expectations of their child's development.
- Educate about parenting strategies and concepts.
- Conduct continuous process evaluation and reinforcement of healthy parental role development.

Promoting parent development through anticipatory guidance may be more challenging than providing physical care, especially when time is limited. The pediatric standard of care includes opportunities for providers to address parenting issues or concerns. Quick, pat answers to complex parenting issues do not facilitate parental growth. Creative strategies such as structured prenatal visits, hospital discharge rounds, early discharge newborn follow-up, breastfeeding consultations, well-child visits, and referrals can be used. Without an organized plan that connects the child's developmental needs, parents' concerns and educational needs, providers' abilities and resources, and community resources, it is easy to overlook, delay, or deny important parenting issues.

The interview and counseling conducted during anticipatory guidance should be based on a consistent framework such as Touchpoints (Brazelton and Sparrow, 2006), Bright Futures (Hagan et al, 2017), or Healthy Steps for Young Children (Minkovitz et al, 2007). No matter what framework is selected, anticipatory guidance should include information that helps reinforce positive health behaviors, minimizes or eliminates health risks, and facilitates optimal family functioning—all grounded in an understanding of the child's developmental stage and individual developmental needs.

There is a wealth of resources available to guide parents as they raise their children, and PCPs should be familiar with popular websites, parenting books, television shows, and parenting

TABLE 8.3 Comparison of Child-Centered and Family-Centered Care	
Child-Centered Care	**Family-Centered Care**
Goal: Focus on child's care.	*Goal:* Parental empowerment and child advocacy for the life of the child.
Child's needs are primary focus.	Family needs to assist the child are the focus.
Professionals decide on the plan of care.	Family and professionals decide on the plan of care.
Parents' opinions are not consistently requested or valued.	Parents' ideas are requested and valued.
Families are considered part of a particular group.	Families are all considered to be unique.
Parents participate as observers.	Parents are considered to be equal members at whatever level they are comfortable.
Parental differences are judged as not being in the best interest of the child.	Family culture, language, ethnicity, and structure are respected.
Test results of the child are the most important factor used to plan care.	Focus is on addressing parental concerns, issues, questions, and their need for assistance in problem-solving.
One-way communication is used—professional to parent.	Two-way communication is used with parents encouraged to have input into the child's care plan.

• BOX 8.1 Parenting Red Flags

Moderate Concern

Difficulty separating from child or prematurely hastening separation
Signs of feeling overwhelmed, apathic, or hostile
Fearful, dependent, apprehensive
Disinterested in or rejecting of infant or child
Overly critical, mocking, and censuring of child; undermines child's confidence
Inconsistent in discipline or control; erratic behavior
Highly restrictive or overly moralistic environment
Turning away from eye-to-eye contact

Extreme Concern

Extreme depression and withdrawal; rejection of child
Intense hostility, aggression toward child
Uncontrollable fears, anxieties, guilt
Complete inability to function in family role
Severe moralistic prohibition of child's independent strivings
Domestic abuse or violence in the home
Self-destructive behaviors—alcohol or drug abuse
Untreated mental health issues (e.g., parent with diagnosis of bipolar disorder, schizophrenia, or delusional disorder)

• BOX 8.2 Etiologies of Developmental Delays

- Central nervous system dysfunction
- Mental health problem
- Chronic disease affecting either functional abilities or activity tolerance (e.g., cardiovascular, visual, auditory)
- Child abuse and neglect
- Maternal or paternal stress
- Developmentally inappropriate animate or inanimate environment, or both
- Lack of parental knowledge of development
- Genetic syndromes
- Depression
- Attention-deficit hyperactivity disorder
- Autism spectrum
- Regulatory or sensory dysfunctions
- Unknown causes

"experts" so they can help parents better evaluate the parenting advice they contain. Giving parents positive feedback, being open to teaching, and listening to parents' concerns build parent confidence, create a trusting relationship, and establish comfort for bringing forth more difficult concerns when necessary.

Family-Centered Care

Children have the best healthcare outcomes when they receive individualized, developmentally grounded care. A partnership with the family is crucial for families to become comfortable and engaged in creating the plan of care for their child. Each family's cultural values, learning styles, and health beliefs and practices must be respected. The shift from child-centered to family-centered care is represented in Table 8.3.

Concerns about Delayed Development and Developmental Red Flags

Child development is exceptionally varied. A 2-year-old girl may use full complex sentences, whereas her 3-year-old neighbor relies on three-word directives (e.g., "Want milk, peeze.") to get what he desires. Both can be normal, but the differences may be striking, and parents may express concern that their child is "delayed." Prevalence estimates of developmental and behavioral disorders in the United States is approximately 15% (Bitsko et al., 2016). PCPs should keep in mind certain red flags for child development when seeing patients for well-child care or minor acute illnesses. Parenting red flags are listed in Box 8.1 and highlighted in each of the following chapters in this unit.

A standardized developmental screening is needed at every well visit and any time a concern is noted, with a follow-up developmental assessment, as appropriate. Children should be evaluated to determine if they are developing typically or if intervention is indicated. Information from the history, physical examination, developmental screening and assessment, hearing and vision screening, and other indicated tests are essential in making this decision.

It is also important to consider the cause of developmental delays (Box 8.2). Understanding possible causes helps the provider plan appropriate developmental care including parent counseling, educational programs, and referral choices (e.g., Which developmental specialist is best qualified to assess the child? Which treatment modality, such as speech or physical therapy, would be most effective?). The PCP should not assume that waiting will remedy a problem when parents express a concern or when developmental delays are noted. In addition, parents' stress and anxiety about their child can cause further problems. Some developmental problems can be fixed with home remedies (e.g., changing parenting or environmental factors), but sometimes developmental problems indicate serious systemic, particularly neurologic, dysfunctions.

Children with a confirmed developmental delay, those who fail to progress as expected, and those who lose developmental gains require immediate developmental assessment and diagnostic evaluation from developmental specialists and/or community early intervention programs, such as Early Head Start.

Talking With Parents About Developmental Delays

Talking with parents on a routine basis about their child's development usually makes it easier if developmental problems appear. It is essential for the PCP to listen and be sensitive to parental concerns. Typically, parents notice differences in the child first and seek reassurance or confirmation of problems from their health care provider. Parents report that they have expressed their concerns to their health care provider only to be reassured or told to "wait and see." Later on, as problems become more obvious and a referral is finally made, they are understandably frustrated that they were not listened to initially and that services to their child have been delayed.

When a problem is found, a strength-based approach can help soothe the experience of receiving "bad news." Each child has areas in which development is progressing, even if the progress is not consistent with typical development. Discussing these areas in addition to the parents' concerns is important. Focusing on strengths *first* provides parents with a framework for understanding their child's unique strengths along with any particular developmental challenges.

Parents may be overwhelmed with the news that their child has a developmental problem. To determine whether parents understand what they have been told, the provider can ask the parent how they are going to explain what has been discussed to others at home. To increase parents' follow-through, providers need to be very familiar with referral resources. They should walk the parent through the next steps in the process, and after allotting time for the family to complete the referral visit, follow up with a phone call or office or home visit with the family.

Above all, it is important to be honest, positive, and realistic. Most often, the long-term prognosis for developmental delays is unknown because of continuing brain development. Parents want to know what they can do and, specifically, how they can assist their child. They also need support and time to cope with their own feelings. Different families have different expectations for their children, so a child with mild delay may be more devastating to one family than a child with severe developmental delays may be to another.

Additional Resources

American Academy of Pediatrics (AAP), Section on Developmental and Behavioral Pediatrics (SODBP)
  https://www.aap.org/en-us/about-the-aap/Sections/Section-on-Developmental-and-Behavioral-Pediatrics/Pages/SODBP.aspx
Brazelton Touchpoints Center
  www.touchpoints.org
Bright Futures
  www.brightfutures.org
The Commonwealth Fund
  www.commonwealthfund.org
Hawaii Early Learning Program (HELP)
  www.vort.com
Healthy Steps for Young Children
  www.healthysteps.org
Parents as Teachers
  www.parentsasteachers.org
Zero to Three
  www.zerotothree.org

References

Bandura A. Social learning through imitation. In: Jones MR, ed. *Nebraska Symposium on Motivation.* Oxford: Oxford University Press; 1962:211–274.

Bijou S, Baer D. *Child Development II: Universal Stages of Infancy.* New York: Appleton-Century-Crofts; 1965.

Bitsko RH, Holbrook JR, Robinson LR, et al. Health care, family, and community factors associated with mental, behavioral, and developmental disorders in early childhood — United States, 2011–2012. *MMWR Morb Mortal Wkly Rep.* 2016;65:221–226. https://doi.org/10.15585/mmwr.mm6509a1.

Bowen M. The use of family theory in clinical practice. *Compr Psychiatry.* 1966;7(5):345–374.

Brazelton B, Sparrow JD. *Touchpoints: Birth to Three: Your Child's Emotional and Behavioral Development.* Cambridge, MA: DaCapo Press; 2006.

Bronfenbrenner U. *The Ecology of Human Development: Experiments by Nature and Design.* Cambridge, MA: Harvard University Press; 1979.

Buhler C, Allen M. *Introduction to Humanistic Psychology.* Monterey, CA: Brooks/Cole; 1972.

Emde RN. Development terminable and interminable. I. Innate and motivational factors from infancy. *Int J Psychoanal.* 1988;69:23–42.

Emde RN, Buchsbaum H. "Didn't you hear my mommy?" Autonomy with connectedness in moral self emergence. In: Cicchetti D, Beeghly M, eds. *The Self in Transition: Infancy to Childhood.* Chicago: University of Chicago Press; 1990:35–60.

Erikson E. *Insight and Responsibility.* New York: Norton; 1964.

Fowler J. *Stages of Faith: The Psychology of Human Development and the Quest for Meaning.* New York: Harper & Row; 1981.

Freud S. *An Outline of Psychoanalysis.* London: Hogarth; 1938.

Freud A. *The Writings of Anna Freud.* New York: International Universities Press; 1974. vol V.

Gennetian L, Darling M, Aber JL. Behavioral economics and developmental science: a new framework to support early childhood interventions. *J Applied Research Child: Informing Policy Child at Risk.* 2016;7(2). Available online at: http://digitalcommons.library.tmc.edu/cgi/viewcontent.cgi?article=1298&context=childrenatrisk Last.

Gilligan C. *A Different Voice: Psychological Theory and Women's Development.* Cambridge, MA: Harvard University Press; 1982.

Hagan JF, Shaw JS, Duncan PM. *Bright Futures: Guidelines for Health Supervision of Infants, Children, and Adolescent.* 4th ed. Elk Grove Village, IL: American Academy of Pediatrics; 2017.

Hengartner M. The evolutionary life history model of externalizing personality: bridging human and animal personality science to connect ultimate and proximate mechanisms underlying aggressive dominance, hostility, and impulsive sensation seeking. *Review Gen Psychol.* 2017;21(4):330–353.

Huesmann LR. An information processing model for the development of aggression. *Aggressive Behavior.* 1988;14:13–24.

Kohlberg L. Stage and sequence: the cognitive developmental approach to socialization. In: D. Goslin, ed. *Handbook of Socialization Theory and Research.* Chicago: Rand McNally; 1969:347–480.

Lampis J, Cataudella S, Busonera A, Skowron E. The role of differentiation of self and dyadic adjustment predicting codependency. *Contemp Family Therapy.* 2017;39(1):62–72.

Mahler M, Pine F, Bergman A. *The Psychological Birth of the Human Infant.* New York: Basic Books; 1975.

Mahrer A. *Experiencing: A Humanistic Theory of Psychology and Psychiatry.* New York: Brunner/Mazel; 1978.

Maslow A. *The Farther Reaches of Human Nature.* New York: Viking; 1971.

Minkovitz C, Strobino D, Mistry KB, et al. Healthy Steps for Young Children: sustained results at 5.5 years. *Pediatrics.* 2007;120(3):e658–e668.

Mowder BA. Parent development theory: understanding parents, parenting perceptions and parenting behaviors. *J Early Child Infant Psychol.* 2005;1:45–64.

Piaget J. *The Theory of Stages in Cognitive Development.* New York: McGraw-Hill; 1969.

Pridham KA, Lutz KF, Anderson LS, et al. Furthering the understanding of parent-child relationships: a nursing scholarship review series. Part 3: interaction and the parent-child relationship- assessment and intervention studies. *J Spec Pediatr Nurs.* 2010;15(1):33–61.

Rogoff B. *Apprenticeship in Thinking: Cognitive Development in Social Context.* New York: Oxford University Press; 1990.

Skinner BF. *Science and Human Behavior.* New York: Macmillan Free Press; 1953.

Sperling S, Mowder BA. Parenting perceptions: comparing parents of typical and special needs preschoolers. *Psychol Sch.* 2006;43(6): 695–700.

Stern D. *The Interpersonal World of the Infant: A View from Psychoanalysis and Developmental Psychology.* New York: Basic Books; 1985.

Sullivan H. *The Fusion of Psychiatry and Social Sciences.* New York: Norton; 1964.

Trevarthen C, Aitken KJ. Infant intersubjectivity: research, theory, and clinical applications. *J Child Psychol Psychiatry.* 2001;42(1):3–48.

Vygotsky LS. *Mind in Society.* 4th ed. Cambridge, MA: Harvard University Press; 1978.

World Bank Group. *World Development Report 2015: Mind, Society, and Behavior.* Washington, DC: International Bank for Reconstruction and Development/The World Bank; 2015. https://doi.org/10.1596/978-1-4648-0342-0.

9

Developmental Management of Newborns

NAN M. GAYLORD AND ROBERT J. YETMAN

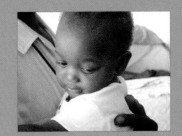

Standards of Care

The newborn, or neonatal, period includes the first 28 days of extrauterine life. The overall goals of the Healthy People 2020 objectives for this population are to improve maternal health and pregnancy outcomes, and to reduce disability rates in infants, thereby improving the health and well-being of women, newborns, children, and families in the United States (U.S. Department of Health and Human Services, 2018). A major focus of many public health efforts is improving the health of pregnant women and their newborns, reducing birth defect rates, decreasing newborn deaths, and addressing maternal and newborn death risk factors. This includes increasing breastfeeding rates, obtaining recommended universal screening panel (RUSP) for state-mandated diseases, reducing the proportion of children with a metabolic disorder who experience developmental delay which, in turn, requires special education services, and increasing the percentage of healthy full-term newborns who are placed to sleep on their backs.

The Guide to Clinical Preventive Services (U.S. Preventive Services Task Force, 2014) and/or the Advisory Committee on Heritable Disorders in Newborns and Children (Advisory Committee, 2017) recommend the following preventive services for neonates:

- Prenatal screening for Rh(D) incompatibility; human immunodeficiency virus (HIV); hepatitis B; syphilis; chlamydia and gonorrhea
- Promoting breastfeeding
- Screening neonates for sickle hemoglobinopathies to identify newborns who may benefit from antibiotic prophylaxis to prevent sepsis
- Screening for congenital hypothyroidism for all newborns within the first 4 days of life
- Screening for phenylketonuria (PKU) for all newborns before discharge from the nursery. Newborns who are tested before they are 24 hours old should receive a repeat screening test by 2 weeks old.
- Topical ocular prophylaxis of all newborns to prevent ophthalmia neonatorum
- Screening for developmental hip dysplasia

Bright Futures: Guidelines for Health Supervision of Infants, Children, and Adolescents (Hagan, Shaw, and Duncan, 2017) and the American Academy of Pediatrics (AAP) Committee on Practice and Ambulatory Medicine (AAP Task Force on Sudden Infant Death Syndrome, 2016) have detailed anticipatory guidelines for the newborn, first-week (2 to 5 day visit), and 1-month health supervision visits. *Guidelines for Perinatal Care* from the AAP and the American Congress of Obstetricians and Gynecologists (ACOG) is another thorough compendium of standards of caring for the newborn (Kilpatrick and Papile, 2017).

Anatomy and Physiology

The newborn's intra-to-extrauterine transition requires an extraordinary number of biochemical and physiologic changes. In utero, the placenta provides metabolic functions for the fetus. Oxygenated blood from the placenta arrives to the fetus through the umbilical vein. Because of high fetal pulmonary vascular pressure, this blood is shunted from the right to the left side of the fetus' heart through the foramen ovale or to the systemic circulation through the ductus arteriosus. At birth, the umbilical cord is clamped/severed and the newborn simultaneously begins to breathe and the high pulmonary vascular pressure drops, allowing blood to flow to the lungs for oxygenation. The foramen ovale and ductus arteriosus are no longer necessary and close. The newborn undergoes many other physiologic transformations, including the gastrointestinal tract absorbing nutrients and excreting waste, the renal system excreting wastes and maintaining chemical balance, the liver metabolizing and excreting toxins, and the immunologic system protecting against infection.

A predictable series of changes in vital signs, reactivity, and clinical appearance take place after the delivery in most newborns (Fig 9.1). The *first* period of reactivity includes sympathetic system changes, such as tachycardia, rapid respirations, transient rales, grunting, flaring and retractions, a falling body temperature, hypertonus, and alertness. Parasympathetic system changes during the first period of reactivity include the initiation of bowel sounds and the production of oral mucus. After an interval of sleep, the newborn enters the *second* period of reactivity. During this time, the oral mucus production again becomes evident, the heart rate becomes labile, the newborn becomes more responsive to endogenous and exogenous stimuli, and meconium is often passed.

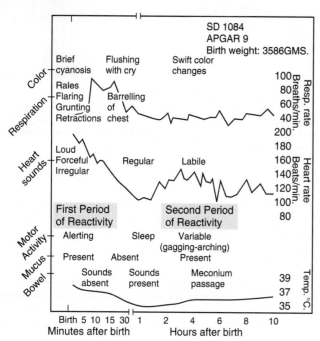

• **Fig 9.1** Summary of Normal Transition. *SD,* Standard deviation. (From Desmond MM, Rudolph AJ, Phitaksphraiwan P. The transitional care nursery. *Pediatr Clin North Am.* 1966;13:651–668.)

Pathophysiology

Assessment of the Neonate

History

• Past maternal health history
• Past obstetric history
  • Number of previous pregnancies; number of newborns born alive or stillborn
  • Number of elective or spontaneous abortions; number of preterm and term deliveries
  • Cesarean deliveries and indications for them
  • Health status of living children; if deceased, age and cause of death
• Family history
• Three-generation pedigree—focus on genetic conditions, congenital defects/diseases, intellectual disability, or other diseases/conditions, such as hypertension, hyperlipidemias, heart disease, or familial cancers
  • Age and health status of living relatives
  • Causes of death of family members
• Obstetric history
  • Current maternal health, including depression or other mental health conditions
  • Maternal age
  • Prenatal care—duration of
  • Medications used during pregnancy, including prescription, over-the-counter, and natural health products
  • Use of pregnancy-enhancing drugs or technology
  • Infections (including group B streptococcus [GBS] status and results of other screening tests) and illnesses during pregnancy
  • Alcohol, tobacco, or other drugs used during pregnancy
  • Environmental exposures to heavy metals (e.g., mercury, lead) or bacteria (e.g., *Listeria*)
  • Hypertension or glucose intolerance

  • Duration of labor, duration of ruptured membranes, analgesia, anesthesia, presentation and route of delivery, use of forceps or vacuum assist
  • Polyhydramnios (excessive fluid) or oligohydramnios (reduced fluid)
  • Stained meconium or foul-smelling amniotic fluid
  • Fever
• Social history
  • Emotional stressors during pregnancy, including homelessness or intimate-partner abuse
  • Unplanned or unwanted pregnancy
  • Financial and emotional support
  • Dietary considerations (e.g., strict vegan diet)
  • Educational background of parents
  • Partner's anticipated involvement in childrearing
  • Ages of other children in the home

Physical Examination

Immediately After Birth

Appearance, Pulse, Grimace, Activity, and Respiration (APGAR) Score. Immediate evaluation of the newborn at 1 and 5 minutes of age is a valuable routine (Table 9.1). The 1-minute score reflects the newborn's transition to extrauterine life.

• APGAR score: 8 to 10
  • Vigorous, pink, and crying
  • Requires only warming, drying, gentle stimulation
  • Occasionally requires oxygen for a short period
• APGAR score: 5 to 7
  • Cyanotic
  • Slow, irregular respirations
  • Good muscle tone and reflexes
  • Responds to bag-and-mask ventilation
• APGAR score: 4 or less
  • Limp, pale, or blue
  • Apneic, slow heart rate
  • Maximal resuscitative efforts with bag and mask, chest compressions, intravenous (IV) volume expansion, and drug therapy

TABLE 9.1 APGAR Scores

Sign	SCORE 0	SCORE 1	SCORE 2
ACTIVITY (muscle tone)	Limp	Some flexion of extremities	Well flexed
PULSE heart rate (bpm)	Absent	Slow (<100)	>100
GRIMACE—reflex irritability (response of skin stimulation to feet)	No response	Some motion	Cry
APPEARANCE—skin color	Blue; pale	Body pink; extremities blue	Completely pink
RESPIRATION—respiratory effort	Absent	Weak cry; hypoventilation	Good; strong cry

bpm, Beats per minute.

The 5-minute APGAR score is an indication of how well the resuscitation efforts have succeeded. Caution must be exercised when using the APGAR score to predict long-term mortality and developmental outcomes. The APGAR score is useful in determining long-term health outcomes only when combined with other factors, such as fetal status, umbilical cord or scalp blood pH, evidence of organ injury, or seizures (AAP, 2015). In actual practice, the decision to resuscitate (see Chapter 29) a newborn is based on a quick assessment (before 1 minute) of the heart rate, color, and respiratory rate, rather than the full 1-minute APGAR score, unless resuscitative decisions have been made prior to delivery when fetal anomalies are known.

Gestational Age. Maturational assessment of a newborn's gestational age is based on the physical examination (Fig 9.2). The assessment is done promptly (within 2 hours) after birth to confirm maternal estimated dates, and it is interpreted with information on the mother's menstrual history, obstetric milestones achieved during pregnancy, and prenatal ultrasonograms. A newborn's length, weight, and fronto-occipital circumference are measured and plotted on growth curves based on gestational age (Fig 9.3). Newborns whose weight falls above the 90th percentile for age are classified as large for gestational age (LGA); those whose measurements fall below the 10th percentile for age are classified as small for gestational age (SGA). Those whose measurements fall between the 10th and 90th percentiles are classified as appropriate for gestational age (AGA).

Temperature. Newborn body surface area relative to its weight is approximately three times that of an adult. Estimated heat loss rate in the newborn is four times that of an adult (Carlo, 2016). Body temperature falls precipitously in a cool and/or drafty environment unless adequate precautions are taken. Towel dry the newborn after birth to prevent evaporative heat loss and place skin-to-skin with the mother if the newborn is otherwise stable. Alternatively use a radiant warmer, wrap newborn in warm blankets, and cover the head to reduce heat loss when the baby is held by parents.

Lungs. During a vaginal delivery, the squeezing action on a newborn's chest as it passes through the pelvis and vagina assists in expulsion of amniotic fluid from the lungs. Further expulsion of amniotic fluid from the lungs and reversal of high pulmonary vascular resistance ensue with a newborn's first large breaths. Careful bulb suctioning assists in clearing the amniotic fluid from the naso/oropharynx. A newborn born by cesarean delivery does not experience the squeezing action of a vaginal birth and requires respiratory efforts and appropriate bulb suctioning to adequately clear the amniotic fluid. Auscultation of the newborn's lungs reveals bronchovesicular or bronchial breath sounds. Fine crackles can be present during the first few hours of life and is a normal variant.

Umbilical Cord. The normal umbilical cord contains two thick-walled arteries and a single thin-walled vein. Rarely, newborns have a single umbilical artery (SUA), which can be associated with congenital anomalies (e.g., cardiac, renal). There is increasing evidence to support delayed umbilical cord clamping for 30 to 60 seconds following birth has both maternal and newborn health benefits. This improves iron stores to prevent anemia in term and preterm newborns. In preterm newborns, this practice decreases the risk of intracerebral hemorrhage and necrotizing enterocolitis (American College of Obstetrics and Gynecology, 2017). It is important to note that delayed clamping decreases umbilical cord blood volume available for banking and families

that are considering umbilical cord blood banking should be educated about this.

After Stabilization

After a quick initial assessment in the delivery room to evaluate for obvious problems, a more complete physical examination is done (Table 9.2). When performing the physical examination, the newborn's gestational age, age in hours, and stage of transition must be considered.

Screening

All states in the United States require newborn screening for a variety of genetic and metabolic disorders, as well as selected congenital abnormalities, although the RUSP screening tests performed vary from state to state. Newborns should be screened based on state law. Typically, they are screened before discharge and if an initial screen was before 24 hours of life rescreening should be done by 14 days old. Although most newborns require no additional screening tests, some are at risk for predictable complications in the newborn period. Newborns born to mothers with poorly controlled diabetes and LGA or SGA newborns are at higher risk for hypoglycemia and usually require serum glucose level screening. Similarly, newborns with Coombs test positivity because of maternal-child blood incompatibility are screened for evidence of hemolysis. Some nurseries screen both mothers and newborns for syphilis; mothers should be screened for HIV and hepatitis B, unless it was done prenatally.

Universal hearing screening is recommended by 1 month old, and special attention is paid to any newborn at higher risk for hearing including those with low birth weight, rubella or other infection, malformation, trauma, asphyxia, prematurity, intensive care unit stay, or antibiotic use. Most hospitals and birthing centers complete the first screening using otoacoustic emissions (OAE) or auditory brainstem response (ABS) prior to discharge.

Two other screenings are typically completed prior to discharge: critical congenital heart disease (CCHD) using pulse oximetry; and bilirubin, transcutaneously or via serum analysis.

Management Strategies

Initial Care

Following birth, newborns require observation as they master the transition to the extrauterine environment. Components of care at this period include prophylaxis for ophthalmia neonatorum with antibiotic ointment and vitamin K injection (IM) for the prevention of classic and late onset hemorrhagic disease.

Establishing Feeding

The provider must ensure that the newborn and parents have well-established feeding patterns before discharge. Follow-up care is scheduled in 2 or 3 days to ensure adequate ongoing nutrition. See Chapter 17 for detailed information on breastfeeding and formulas.

Anticipatory Guidance Before Discharge
Physical Care

Umbilical Cord. *Bright Futures* guidelines for cord care includes leaving the cord to air dry and placing the diaper below the cord

MATURATIONAL ASSESSMENT OF GESTATIONAL AGE (New Ballard Score)

NAME _____ SEX _____

HOSPITAL NO. _____ BIRTH WEIGHT _____

RACE _____ LENGTH _____

DATE/TIME OF BIRTH _____ HEAD CIRC. _____

DATE/TIME OF EXAM _____ EXAMINER _____

AGE WHEN EXAMINED _____

APGAR SCORE: 1 MINUTE _____ 5 MINUTES _____ 10 MINUTES _____

NEUROMUSCULAR MATURITY

NEUROMUSCULAR MATURITY SIGN	SCORE							RECORD SCORE HERE
	-1	0	1	2	3	4	5	
POSTURE								
SQUARE WINDOW (Wrist)	>90°	90°	60°	45°	30°	0°		
ARM RECOIL		180°	140°-180°	110°-140°	90°-110°	<90°		
POPLITEAL ANGLE	180°	160°	140°	120°	100°	90°	<90°	
SCARF SIGN								
HEEL TO EAR								

TOTAL NEUROMUSCULAR MATURITY SCORE

SCORE

Neuromuscular _____

Physical _____

Total _____

MATURITY RATING

score	weeks
-10	20
-5	22
0	24
5	26
10	28
15	30
20	32
25	34
30	36
35	38
40	40
45	42
50	44

GESTATIONAL AGE (weeks)

By dates _____

By ultrasound _____

By exam _____

PHYSICAL MATURITY

PHYSICAL MATURITY SIGN	SCORE							RECORD SCORE HERE
	-1	0	1	2	3	4	5	
SKIN	sticky friable transparent	gelatinous red translucent	smooth pink visible veins	superficial peeling &/or rash, few veins	cracking pale areas rare veins	parchment deep cracking no vessels	leathery cracked wrinkled	
LANUGO	none	sparse	abundant	thinning	bald areas	mostly bald		
PLANTAR SURFACE	heel-toe 40-50 mm:-1 <40 mm:-2	>50 mm no crease	faint red marks	anterior transverse crease only	creases ant. 2/3	creases over entire sole		
BREAST	imperceptible	barely perceptible	flat areola no bud	stippled areola 1-2 mm bud	raised areola 3-4 mm bud	full areola 5-10 mm bud		
EYE/EAR	lids fused loosely: -1 tightly: -2	lids open pinna flat stays folded	sl. curved pinna; soft; slow recoil	well-curved pinna; soft but ready recoil	formed & firm instant recoil	thick cartilage ear stiff		
GENITALS (Male)	scrotum flat, smooth	scrotum empty faint rugae	testes in upper canal rare rugae	testes descending few rugae	testes down good rugae	testes pendulous deep rugae		
GENITALS (Female)	clitoris prominent & labia flat	prominent clitoris & small labia minora	prominent clitoris & enlarging minora	majora & minora equally prominent	majora large minora small	majora cover clitoris & minora		

Reference
Ballard JL, Khoury JC, Wedig K, et al: New Ballard Score, expanded to include extremely premature infants. *J Pediatr* 1991; 119:417-423. Reprinted by permission of Dr Ballard and Mosby- Year Book, Inc.

TOTAL PHYSICAL MATURITY SCORE

• **Fig 9.2** Classification of Newborns by Intrauterine Growth and Gestational Age. (From Ballard JL, Khoury JC, Wedig K, et al. New Ballard score, expanded to include extremely premature infants. *J Pediatric.* 1991;119:417–423.)

CLASSIFICATION OF NEWBORNS (BOTH SEXES)
BY INTRAUTERINE GROWTH AND GESTATIONAL AGE [1,2]

NAME_____   DATE OF EXAM _____   LENGTH_____

HOSPITAL NO. _____   SEX _____   HEAD CIRC. _____

RACE _____   BIRTH WEIGHT_____   GESTATIONAL AGE_____

DATE OF BIRTH_____

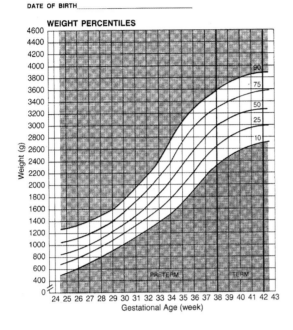

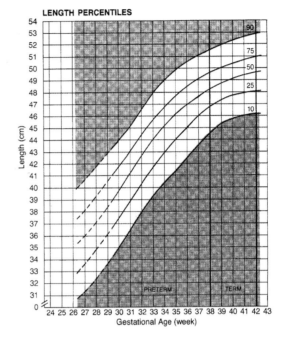

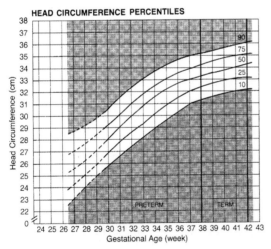

CLASSIFICATION OF INFANT*	Weight	Length	Head Circ.
Large for Gestational Age (LGA) (>90th percentile)			
Appropriate for Gestational Age (AGA) (10th to 90th percentile)			
Small for Gestational Age (SGA) (<10th percentile)			

*Place an "X" in the appropriate box (LGA, AGA or SGA) for weight, for length and for head circumference.

References
1. Battaglia FC, Lubchenco LO: A practical classification of newborn infants by weight and gestational age.
   J Pediatr 1967; 71:159-163.
2. Lubchenco LO, Hansman C, Boyd E: Intrauterine growth in length and head circumference as estimated
   from live births at gestational ages from 26 to 42 weeks. Pediatrics 1966; 37:403-408.

Reprinted by permission from Dr Battaglia, Dr Lubchenco, Journal of Pediatrics and Pediatrics.

A service of **SIMILAC® WITH IRON** Infant Formula

The Ross Hospital Formula System

A5860(0.05)/JULY 1993

ROSS ROSS PRODUCTS DIVISION
ABBOTT LABORATORIES
COLUMBUS, OHIO 43215-1724

LITHO IN USA

• **Fig 9.3** Newborn Maturity Rating and Classification. (From Ross Hospital Formula System. *Ross Products Division*. Columbus, OH: Abbott Laboratories; From Battaglia FC, Lubchenco LO. A practical classification of newborn infants by weight and gestational age. *J Pediatr.* 1967;71:159–163; Lubchenco LO, Hansman C, Boyd E. Intrauterine growth in length and head circumference as estimated from live births at gestational ages from 26 to 42 weeks. *Pediatrics.* 1966;37:403–408.)

TABLE 9.2 Newborn Physical Examination Findings

System	Findings
Measurements	• Vital signs—Check frequently in the first hours. Every 6-8 h when stable. • Evaluate temperature stability (97.7°F–99.3°F [36.5°C–37.4°C]) in open crib after birth. • Respiratory rate = 30 to 60 breaths/min. • Heart rate = 100-190 bpm. • Baseline weight, length, head circumference. Daily weight measurement with losses of up to 10% in the first 2-3 days are normal.
Skin	Normal dermatologic findings: Lanugo, vernix, dry and cracked skin.
Head	• Vaginally delivered newborns may have molding, overriding suture lines. • Fontanels: Anterior fontanel = about 2-3 cm in diameter; the posterior fontanelle = about 1 cm in diameter (Fig 9.4).
Face	• Facial structures and grimace should be symmetric. • Evaluate for dysmorphic features.

Eyes	• Check symmetry, size, and angle of palpebral fissures:
	  • Intermittent uncoordinated eye movements (disconjugate gaze) during the first weeks after birth are common, improving by 2-4 months old and resolving by 6 months old.
	  • Conjunctivae may be reddened due to the ocular prophylaxis agent.
	  • Note presence of red reflex bilaterally.

Ears	• Identify size, shape, position, skin tags or significant pits, and patency of the external auditory canal. • Universal screening for detection of hearing loss is recommended. Evaluate for low-set and/or posterior rotated ears.
Nose	• Nasal passage patency must be tested by obstructing one nostril at a time.
Mouth	• Evaluate size and symmetry of the lips, time spent with the mouth closed, appearance with movement.
Neck	• Assess for full range of motion.
Thorax	• Evaluate for shape and symmetry. Rounded appearance measuring about 2 cm less than the head circumference (approximately 33 cm) is normal. • Fullness and sometimes secretion of a white milky substance from nipples is normal and are secondary to maternal hormonal stimulation. • Supernumerary and inverted nipples are common.
Lungs	• Coughing, retractions, and an intermittently increased respiratory rate occur immediately after birth, transitioning by about 12 h of life to smooth and unlabored respirations at a rate of 30-60 breaths/min. • Rales or crackles are commonly heard immediately after birth as lung fluid is resorbed.
Heart	• Inspection: Observe for perfusion adequacy. • Palpation: Point of maximal impulse is at the fourth left intercostal space. • Auscultation: Heart rate is normally 100-190 bpm. Murmurs are common in the newborn period; many murmurs disappear after a few hours or days. Significant murmurs should be investigated. • Pulses: Brachial or radial pulses are compared with femoral or dorsalis pedis pulses for symmetry of impulse and strength. Measure oxygen saturation of the right hand and either foot. • Blood pressure: By Doppler device using a 2.5-4 cm wide and 5-9 cm long cuff, compare with normal for age and gestation. Systolic blood pressures greater than 96 mm Hg are considered significant hypertension in the newborn.
Abdomen	• Normal abdomen is slightly protuberant, is soft, moves smoothly with respirations, and has fine bowel sounds scattered throughout. • The liver is usually palpated 1-2 cm below the right costal margin; the spleen tip is often felt at the left costal margin; kidneys, deep within lateral aspects of the abdomen measuring 3-4 cm in size, may be palpated. • Umbilicus: Midline outpouching from the sternum to the umbilicus is seen with weak abdominal musculature (diastasis recti); a large and protuberant umbilicus occurs with an umbilical hernia. • First stool should pass in the first 24-48 h of life.

• Genitalia	• Male:
	  • The urethral opening should be at the tip of the penis. The foreskin should be completely developed. Testes not located in the scrotal sac or inguinal canal but retrievable to the scrotum are normal. Presence/absence of rugae.
	  • Hydrocele is identified by transilluminating scrotal fluid collection and is normal unless it is associated with inguinal hernia or it lasts more than 12 months.
	• Female:
	  • Labia majora are large and completely surround the labia minora.
	  • Labia and vagina should be patent, often with a white discharge.
	  • Blood-tinged fluid in small amounts by day 2-3 is normal.
	• Anus and rectum:
	  • Patency/placement of the anus should be noted.

TABLE 9.2	Newborn Physical Examination Findings—cont'd	

System	Findings
• Extremities, back, hip	• Intrauterine constraint and resultant molding cause mild curvatures of the feet and legs. • Fractures can occur anywhere as a result of the delivery process; note crepitus and range of motion in all extremities. Clavicles are particularly vulnerable. • Note dimples, hemangiomas, tufts of hair, or other lesions along the spine. • Perform Ortolani and Barlow maneuvers to assess for dislocated or dislocatable hips.
• Neurologic examination	• Observe tone, movement, and symmetry of the extremities while the newborn is awake. Elicit the following reflexes: rooting, suck/swallow, palmar grasp, Moro, ankle clonus (three or four beats is normal), stepping and placing response, truncal incurvation (Galant), asymmetric tonic neck.

bpm, Beats per minute.

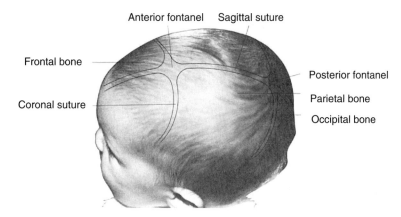

• **Fig 9.4 Fontanelles and Sutures.** (From Betz CL, Hunsberger M, Wright S. *Family-centered Nursing Care of Children.* 2nd ed. Philadelphia: Saunders; 1994:124.)

until it separates (Hagan et al., 2017). Alcohol application is no longer recommended. After cord separation, which usually occurs at 10 to 14 days old, a slight bloody discharge can be seen for 1 to 2 days. Bellybands or coins to cover the navel should be avoided because these increase the chance of infection. If a foul-smelling discharge or rapidly expanding erythema appears around the umbilicus, the newborn should be evaluated immediately for sepsis. If a granuloma appears after the cord falls off, an application of silver nitrate helps to heal it.

Circumcision. The decision to circumcise rests with the parents. In 2012, the AAP issued a policy statement on circumcision stating that there is no evidence for routine circumcision, but that the benefits of the procedure are greater than its risks. Additionally, this statement advocates for circumcision access for all families desiring the procedure (AAP Task Force on Circumcision, 2012). Providers can present both sides. Proponents of routine male circumcision claim that it keeps the glans penis cleaner; it lowers the chance for developing urinary tract infections (although the chance of urinary tract infections in uncircumcised males is only 1%); it reduces the incidence of penile cancer, phimosis, balanitis, adhesions, and occlusion of the urethral meatus; and it allows the boy to look more like his father/peers. The opponents of circumcision claim that it does not prevent sexually transmitted infection; that good hygiene prevents penile cancer; that circumcision leaves the glans open to the chance of cautery burns and meatal stenosis; and that because fewer boys are being circumcised, these boys will not be different from many of their peers.

Contraindications to circumcision include epi- or hypospadias, ambiguous genitalia, exstrophy of the bladder, familial bleeding disorders, and illness. Complications of circumcision are rare but include infections, bleeding, gangrene, scarring, meatal stenosis, cautery burns, urethral fistula, amputation or trauma to the glans, and pain. For newborns who undergo circumcision, procedural anesthesia is recommended. A variety of anesthesia techniques are available, including application of topical anesthetics (eutectic mixture of local anesthetics [EMLA] cream), dorsal penile nerve block, and subcutaneous ring block (Brady-Fryer et al., 2004; AAP Task Force on Circumcision, 2012). Helpful perioperative pain relief measures include sucrose on a pacifier, acetaminophen, soft music, and physiologic positioning of the newborn in a padded environment.

Care of the uncircumcised baby includes gentle cleaning around the genital area. The skin normally adheres to the penis and is not retractable at birth but loosens gradually as the baby grows. Counsel the parents not to force the foreskin back. If the baby is circumcised, the penis should be cleansed daily with cotton balls dipped in tap water followed by the application of a small amount of petroleum jelly to the tip of the penis for the first 2 or 3 days after the procedure with each diaper change to prevent discharge from the wound sticking to the diaper.

Bathing, Oils, and Powders. Newborns do not require daily baths. Tradition favors that the newborn not be immersed in a tub of water, but rather should be sponge bathed until the umbilical cord separates and the navel appears healed. Mild cleansing agents (such as Dove, Caress, Neutrogena, and Basis) are gentle enough for

• BOX **9.1** **Guidelines for Early Discharge of Normal, Healthy Newborns**

- No ongoing medical issues that require continued hospitalization
- Term newborn
- Stable vital signs for at least 12 h before discharge:
  - Rectal temperature of 97.7°F–99.3°F (36.5°C–37.4°C) in open crib
  - Heart rate 100-190 bpm
  - Respiratory rate less than 60 breaths/min
- Passage of urine and at least one stool
- Two successful feedings have been accomplished
- Normal physical examination
- Vitamin K received; no bleeding at circumcision site/umbilicus
- Baseline bilirubin—clinical significance of jaundice has been determined and appropriate follow-up plans made
- Evaluation and monitoring for sepsis based on maternal risk factors have been accomplished
- Newborn laboratory data, including maternal syphilis, maternal hepatitis B status, and human immunodeficiency virus (HIV), and newborn blood type and Coombs testing (as indicated) completed
- Appropriately timed neonatal genetic/metabolic, critical congenital heart disease (CCHD), and hearing screenings completed
- Hepatitis B #1 administered
- Mother has received (if needed) tetanus toxoid, reduced diphtheria toxoid, and acellular pertussis and influenza (CDC, 2016)
- Social support and continuing health care identified
- Social situation adequate: screen for drug abuse, previous child abuse, mental illness, lack of social support, lack of permanent home, history of domestic violence, communicable diseases in the household, teenage mother, inadequate transportation, or communication abilities
- Appropriate medical home identified with early follow-up care achievable, preferably within 48 h of discharge, but no later than 72 h in most cases
- Mother knowledgeable in the care of the newborn, including the following:
  - Feeding, with breastfeeding encouraged
  - Normal stool and urine frequency
  - Skin, genital, and cord care
  - Ability to identify illness (especially jaundice)
  - Proper safety (car seat, sleeping position, smoke-free environment, room sharing)
  - Smoke/carbon monoxide alarms in the home

From Benitz WE. Hospital stay for health term newborn infants. *Pediatrics.* 2015;135(5): 948–953.

• BOX **9.2** **Guidelines for 48- to 72-Hour Follow-Up Visit of the Normal, Healthy Newborn**

- Review delivery and discharge summary for any identified follow-up needs (e.g., hearing screening, specialty referrals)
- Assess the newborn's general health, weight, hydration, and jaundice; identify any new problems; review feeding, stooling, and urination; consider lactation consultation if needed
- Assess quality of bonding
- Reinforce maternal and family education
- Review outstanding laboratory data
- Perform/repeat neonatal screen or other tests (such as bilirubin), if indicated
- Develop plan for health care maintenance, including emergency care, preventive care, immunizations, and periodic screenings
- Evaluate mother for postpartum depression
- Refer to Women, Infants, and Children (WIC) program eligibility screening as appropriate.

From Benitz WE. Hospital stay for health term newborn infants. *Pediatrics.* 2015;135(5): 948–953.

newborns' skin. Oils and greasy substances are not recommended because they tend to clog the skin's pores and can cause acne or rashes. Powders should be avoided because inhaling the talc could lead to respiratory problems and increased cancer risk. For dry skin, a lotion (such as Keri, Eucerin, Aveeno, or Cetaphil) is recommended.

Diapers. Much controversy exists whether disposable or cloth diapers are the better choice for newborns. The need for frequent changing and proper cleansing is the important message to deliver.

Early Discharge and Follow-up

The Newborns' and Mothers' Health Protection Act of 1996, with final rules issued in 2008, prevents insurers from requiring hospital discharge before 48 hours for a vaginal delivery and 96 hours for a cesarean delivery (Department of the Treasury, Department of Labor, U.S. Department of Health and Human Services, 2008). Guidelines for early discharge of normal, healthy newborns are listed in Box 9.1 (Benitz,

2015). Prior to discharge, it is important to confirm plans for follow-up care within 48 to 72 hours, and plans for ongoing health maintenance (Box 9.2) (Benitz, 2015). Even newborns who are hospitalized longer may need follow-up care within the first few days of life. All parents leaving the hospital with a newborn should have a confirmed time and place for follow-up, in addition to contacts in case of an emergency or questions.

Common Neonatal Conditions

Skin Conditions

Table 9.3 lists newborn skin conditions.

Milia

Milia are multiple, firm, pearly, opalescent white papules scattered over the forehead, nose, and cheeks. Their intraoral counterparts are called *Epstein pearls.* Histologically, milia represent superficial epidermal inclusion cysts filled with keratinous material associated with the developing pilosebaceous follicle. No treatment is necessary because milia exfoliate spontaneously in most newborns over the first few weeks of life (Fig 9.5).

Sebaceous Hyperplasia

Sebaceous hyperplasia is characterized by prominent yellow-white papules at the opening of each pilosebaceous follicle, predominantly over the nose, forehead, upper lip, and cheeks. The overgrowth of sebaceous glands in response to the same androgenic stimulation that occurs in adolescence causes sebaceous hyperplasia. No treatment is required. These tiny papules diminish in size and disappear entirely within the first few weeks of life (Fig 9.6).

Erythema Toxicum

Firm, yellow-white 1- to 2-mm papules or pustules with a surrounding erythematous flare characterize erythema toxicum. Lesions are clustered in several sites. These lesions usually develop at 24 to 48 hours old. The cause is unknown, although examination of a Wright-stained smear of the lesion reveals numerous eosinophils. Up to 50% of newborns develop

TABLE 9.3 Comparison of Common Newborn Skin Conditions

Rash	Significant Maternal or Newborn History	Rash Description	Diagnostics	Management/Treatment
Milia	None	Firm, pearly, white papules over cheeks, nose, and forehead	None	Superficial inclusion cysts will spontaneously resolve
Sebaceous hyperplasia	None	Prominent, yellow-white papules over cheeks, nose, and forehead	None	Overgrowth of sebaceous glands will spontaneously resolve in first few weeks
Erythema toxicum	None Presents at 24–48 h	Yellow-white papules with an erythematous base over cheeks, nose, and forehead	Wright stain demonstrates large number of eosinophils Cultures are sterile	Clears within 2 weeks, completely gone in 4 months
Transient neonatal pustular melanosis	None More common in darker skinned newborns	Vesicopustules that rupture easily and leave a halo of white scales around a central macule of hyperpigmentation on trunk, limbs, palms, and soles	None	Spontaneous resolution in 2–3 days although hyperpigmentation can persist for up to 3 months
Sucking blisters	Results from vigorous sucking in utero on the affected part	Scattered superficial bullae on the upper arms and lips of newborns at birth	None	Will resolve without additional intervention
Cutis marmorata	Accentuated physiologic response to cold	Lacy, reticulated, red or blue vascular pattern	None	Transient and will resolve with warming
Harlequin color change	None	Half of the baby's coloring is red and the other pale	None	Transient and will resolve
Nevus sebaceous	None	Yellow, hairless smooth plaque on head or neck	None	Total excision prior to adolescence; refer to dermatologist
Herpes simplex virus (HSV) (See Chapter 31)	Mother may have active lesions or a history of disease	Grouped vesicles on erythematous base	DFA or ELISA detection of HSV antigens	Acyclovir

DFA, Direct fluorescent antibody; *ELISA,* enzyme-linked immunosorbent assay.

erythema toxicum, with a higher incidence in term than in premature newborns. Pyoderma, candidiasis, herpes simplex, transient neonatal pustular melanosis, and miliaria should be considered (see Table 9.3). No treatment is required; the course is brief and transient (Fig 9.7).

Transient Neonatal Pustular Melanosis

Transient neonatal pustular melanosis is characterized by superficial vesicopustules that rupture easily and leave a halo of white scales around a central pinhead-sized, hyperpigmented macule. Pustular melanosis is caused by increased melanization of the epidermal cells, with common sites being the trunk, limbs, palms, and soles. It is more common in darker-skinned newborns. Pyoderma and erythema toxicum are the differential diagnoses. No treatment is required. The pustular phase rarely lasts more than 2 to 3 days; hyperpigmented macules can persist for as long as 3 months (Fig 9.8).

Sucking Blisters

Sucking blisters are solitary or scattered superficial bullae on the upper limbs and lips of newborns at birth, commonly found on the radial aspect of the forearm, the thumb, and the index finger. These blisters result from vigorous sucking on the affected part

in utero. No treatment is required. These bullae resolve rapidly without sequelae.

Cutis Marmorata

Cutis marmorata is a lacy, reticulated, red or blue cutaneous vascular pattern appearing over most of the body surface. The vascular change is a response to exposure to low environmental temperatures. It represents an accentuated physiologic vasomotor response that disappears with increasing age. Persistent and pronounced cutis marmorata occurs in Down and trisomy 18 syndromes. Cutis marmorata usually resolves upon warming the newborn (Fig 9.9).

Harlequin Color Change

Harlequin color change is a division of the body skin coloring from forehead to pubis into red and pale halves. The cause is unknown. This occurs in up to 10% of newborns, usually between days 2 and 5 of life, but has been reported as late as 3 weeks following birth No treatment is indicated with this transient and benign condition (Valerio et al., 2015) (Fig 9.10).

Mongolian spots (congenital dermal melanocytosis), café au lait spots, salmon patch (nevus simplex), and port-wine stain (nevus flammeus, port-wine nevus)

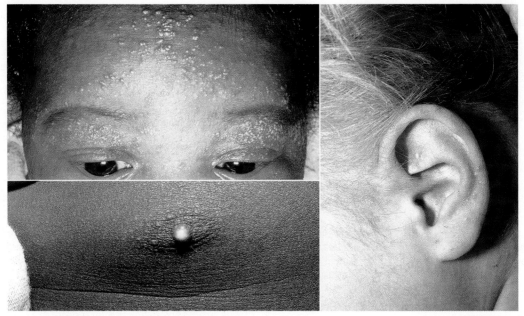

• **Fig 9.5** **Milia.** (From Cohen BA. *Pediatric Dermatology.* 4th ed. Philadelphia: Elsevier; 2013, Fig 2.18A.)

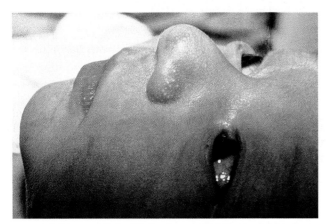

• **Fig 9.6** **Sebaceous Hyperplasia.** (From Paller AS, Mancini AJ. Cutaneous disorders of the newborn. *Hurwitz Clinical Pediatric Dermatology*. 5th ed. Philadelphia: Elsevier; 2016, Fig 2.10.)

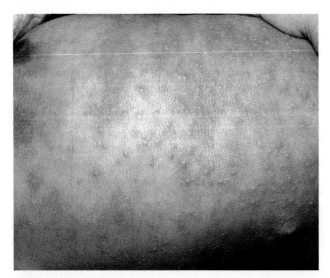

• **Fig 9.7** **Erythema Toxicum Neonatorum.** (From Paller AS, Mancini AJ. Cutaneous disorders of the newborn. *Hurwitz Clinical Pediatric Dermatology*. 5th ed. Philadelphia: Elsevier; 2016, Fig 2.13.)

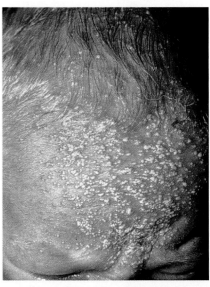

• **Fig 9.8** **Transient Neonatal Pustular Melanosis.** (From Paller AS, Mancini AJ. Cutaneous disorders of the newborn. *Hurwitz Clinical Pediatric Dermatology*. 5th ed. Philadelphia: Elsevier; 2016, Fig 2.17.)

See Chapter 34 for a discussion of these skin conditions.

Nevus Sebaceous

Nevus sebaceous is a yellowish, hairless, sharply demarcated smooth plaque usually on the head and neck. Histologically, these contain an abundance of sebaceous glands. With maturity, usually during adolescence, the lesions become verrucous with large rubbery nodules. During adulthood, the lesions are complicated by secondary malignancies, most commonly basal cell carcinoma. Total excision before the onset of adolescence is recommended. Referral to a pediatric dermatologist prior to adolescence is warranted (Fig 9.11).

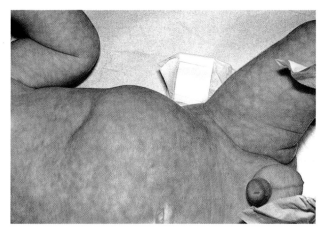

• **Fig 9.9 Cutis Marmorata.** (From Paller AS, Mancini AJ. Cutaneous disorders of the newborn. *Hurwitz Clinical Pediatric Dermatology.* 5th ed. Philadelphia: Elsevier; 2016, Fig 2.1.)

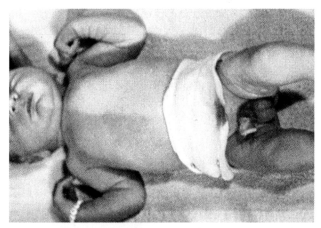

• **Fig 9.10 Harlequin Color Change.** (From Cohen BA. *Pediatric Dermatology.* 4th ed. Philadelphia: Elsevier; 2013, Fig 2.10.)

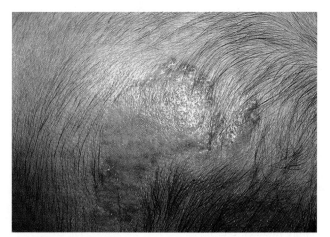

• **Fig 9.11 Nevus Sebaceous.** (From Cohen BA. *Pediatric Dermatology.* 4th ed. Philadelphia: Elsevier; 2013, Fig 2.82A.)

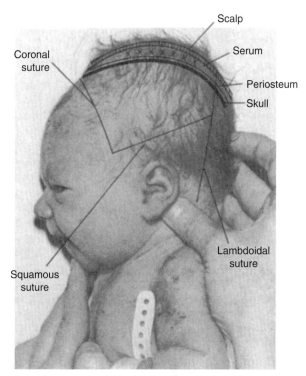

• **Fig 9.12 Caput Succedaneum.** (From Betz CL, Hunsberger M, Wright S. *Family-Centered Nursing Care of Children.* 2nd ed. Philadelphia: Saunders; 1994:124.)

Skin Dimpling

Deep skin dimples, pits, and creases can occur over bony prominences and in the sacral area. They can be normal variations or associated with underlying pathology and/or dysmorphologic syndromes. No treatment is indicated if isolated and not associated with other findings.

Preauricular Sinus Tracts and Pits

Sinus tracts and pits occur anterior to the pinna and can be unilateral or bilateral. They result from imperfect fusion of the tubercles of the first and second branchial arches during gestational development, are familial, more common in females and in African Americans, and occasionally are associated with ear and face anomalies and/or hearing loss. Excision rarely is required for chronic infections and drainage. Confirmation of normal newborn hearing evaluation is warranted.

Supernumerary Nipples

Solitary or multiple accessory nipples and sometimes areolae occur in unilateral or bilateral distribution along a line from the midaxilla to the inguinal area. The cause is unknown. Urinary tract anomalies very rarely occur in conjunction with the finding. Usually no treatment is necessary.

Head, Face, and Eye Conditions

Caput Succedaneum

Caput succedaneum is a diffuse, superficial swelling of the soft tissue of the scalp with possible underlying bruising; the swelling usually crosses the suture lines, but it can also be very localized (Fig 9.12). Caput succedaneum originates from trauma as the baby descends through the birth canal.

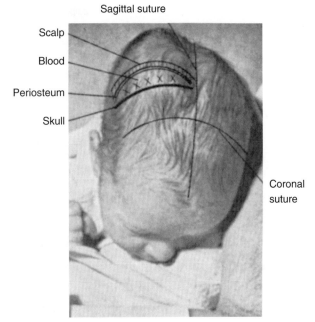

Sagittal suture

Scalp

Blood

Periosteum

Skull

Coronal suture

• **Fig 9.13** Cephalhematoma. (From Betz CL, Hunsberger M, Wright S. *Family-centered Nursing Care of Children.* 2nd ed. Philadelphia: Saunders; 1994:124.)

Clinical Findings

- Obvious swelling and bruising in the parietal regions of the scalp
- Superficial swelling that crosses suture lines
- Frequently associated with molding and/or traumatic delivery

Differential Diagnosis

Cephalohematoma and/or subgaleal hemorrhage are included in the differential diagnosis.

Management

No treatment is necessary because swelling resolves spontaneously over the first few days after birth. If there is associated bruising, observe the baby for the development of jaundice as the blood from bruising is reabsorbed.

Cephalohematoma

Cephalohematoma is a deep collection of blood in the subperiosteal area of the scalp that does not cross the suture lines. Frequently no noticeable surface bruising is seen (Fig 9.13). Cephalohematoma results from trauma possibly occurring during a difficult delivery. The swelling appears hours to days after delivery.

Clinical Findings.
- History may include primigravida and traumatic delivery
- Swelling in the parietal area that does not cross suture lines
- Rarely associated with a skull fracture, coagulopathy, or intracranial hemorrhage

Differential Diagnosis. Caput succedaneum, subgaleal hemorrhage, and cranial meningocele should be considered as differential diagnoses.

Management. No treatment is indicated because the condition resolves in a few weeks to months. Calcification of the hematoma can occur, which is felt as bony prominences on the cranium; resolution of a calcified hematoma may require months. It is important to monitor for hyperbilirubinemia.

Craniotabes

Craniotabes is thinning of the bone of the scalp. This is a normal variation of the parietal bone, usually near the sagittal suture line, most often seen in premature newborns.

Clinical Findings.
- A "ping-pong ball" effect when pressing on the parietal bone

Management. No treatment is necessary because craniotabes resolves spontaneously. If persistent, pathologic causes, such as rickets, should be investigated.

Jaundice. Jaundice, a clinically apparent accumulation of bilirubin in the skin, causes a yellow, orange, or sometimes green hue to the skin. Jaundice becomes apparent when serum bilirubin levels exceed 5 to 7 mg/dL and classically is described as advancing in a cephalocaudal pattern although the presentation is variable and serum levels cannot be estimated by clinical examination (Table 9.4). Physiologic jaundice is characterized by a rise in bilirubin from 1 to 3 mg/dL in cord blood to 5 to 6 mg/dL on the third day of life, declining to a normal adult level (<1.3 to 1.5 mg/dL) by 10 to 12 days in Caucasian and African American newborns. Newborns of Asian descent reach 8 to 12 mg/dL on day 4 to 5 and decline more slowly.

Early- and late-onset jaundice associated with breast-feeding are often included in the category of physiologic jaundice. Early-onset breast milk jaundice develops within 2 to 4 days of birth and occurs as a result of infrequent breastfeeding and insufficient intake leading to decreased intestinal motility. Late-onset breast milk jaundice develops 7 days after birth, peaks in the second or third week of life, and frequently persists unless breastfeeding is interrupted (see Chapter 16).

Nonphysiologic (pathologic) jaundice is typically considered to be jaundice that occurs too early, persists too long, and/or involves bilirubin levels that are too high. For example, jaundice that appears in the first 24 hours of life as well as jaundice lasting longer than 10 to 14 days are both considered pathologic, requiring attention. Kernicterus or bilirubin encephalopathy involves toxicity of the nervous system resulting from very high levels of bilirubin. The estimated minimal level of risk for kernicterus and thus consideration of exchange transfusion is 25 to 30 mg/dL in healthy term newborns without other risk factors (AAP, 2004; updated by https://www.ncbi.nlm.nih.gov/pubmed/?term=Maisels%20MJ%5BAuthor%5D&cauthor=true&cauthor_uid=19786452 Maisels et al., 2009).

Approximately 60% of term newborns are jaundiced in the first week of life (Ambalavanan and Carlo, 2016). Common causes include the following:
- Increased hemolysis: ABO, Rh, or other blood group isoimmunization; abnormal red blood cell shapes (spherocytosis, elliptocytosis, pyknocytosis, and stomatocytosis); red blood cell enzyme abnormalities (glucose-6-phosphate dehydrogenase deficiency, pyruvate kinase deficiency)
- Polycythemia: twin-twin transfusion, maternal-fetal transfusion, small for gestation age
- Delayed cord clamping
- Decreased rate of conjugation: immaturity of bilirubin conjugation (physiologic jaundice), congenital familial nonhemolytic jaundice (inborn errors of metabolism affecting glucuronyl transferase system and bilirubin transport), breast milk jaundice
- Abnormalities of excretion or absorption: delayed stooling (Hirschsprung disease, congenital hypothyroidism), sepsis, hepatitis (viral, parasitic, bacterial, toxic), metabolic abnormalities (galactosemia, glycogen storage disease, infant of diabetic mother [IDM], cystic fibrosis), biliary atresia, choledochal cyst, obstruction of ampulla of Vater (annular pancreas), drugs

TABLE 9.4 Diagnostic Features of the Various Types of Neonatal Jaundice

Diagnosis	Nature of Van Den Bergh Reaction	JAUNDICE		PEAK BILIRUBIN CONCENTRATION		Bilirubin Rate of Accumulation (mg/dL/day)	Remarks
		Appears	Disappears	mg/dL	Age (days)		
Physiologic jaundice							Usually relates to degree of maturity; newborn shows no signs of illness
Full-term	Indirect	2–3 days	4–5 days	10–12	2–3	<5	
Premature	Indirect	3–4 days	7–9 days	15	6–8	<5	
Hyperbiliru- binemia caused by metabolic factors							Metabolic factors: hypoxia, respiratory distress, lack of carbohydrates
Full-term	Indirect	2–3 days	Variable	>12	First week	<5	Hormonal influences: cretinism
Premature	Indirect	3–4 days	Variable	>15	First week	<5	Genetic factors: Crigler-Najjar syndrome, transient familial hyperbilirubinemia Drugs: Vitamin K, novobiocin
Hemolytic states and hema- toma	Indirect	May appear in first 24 h	Variable	Unlimited	Variable	Usually >5	Erythroblastosis: Rh or ABO incompatibility Congenital hemolytic states: Spherocytic, nonspherocytic Infantile pyknocytosis Enclosed hemorrhage—hema- toma Drugs: Vitamin K
Mixed hemolytic and hepa- totoxic factors	Indirect and direct	May appear in first 24 h	Variable	Unlimited	Variable	Usually >5	Infection: Bacterial sepsis, pyelonephritis, hepatitis, toxoplasmosis, cytomegalic inclusion disease, rubella Drugs: Vitamin K
Hepatocel- lular damage	Indirect and direct	Usually 2–3 days	Variable	Unlimited	Variable	Variable; can be >5	Biliary atresia; galactosemia; hepatitis, infection

From Brown AK. Diagnostic features of the various types of neonatal jaundice. *Pediatr Clin North Am.* 1962;9:589; as cited in Kliegman RM, Stanton BF, St Geme JW, et al., eds. *Nelson Textbook of Pediatrics.* 20th ed. Philadelphia: Elsevier; 2016.

Clinical Findings. The following are risk factors for the development of pathologic hyperbilirubinemia:
- Hemolytic disease, anemia
- Inborn errors of metabolism
- Prematurity (gestational age 35 to 36 weeks)
- Significant bruising or cephalohematoma
- Exclusive breastfeeding with significant weight loss or difficulty in feeding
- Jaundice that develops in the first 24 hours of life
- The total bilirubin increases more than 5 mg/dL/24 hours, is more than 12.5 mg/dL before 48 hours old, or the direct bilirubin exceeds 2 mg/dL
- Ethnic or geographic origin associated with hemolytic anemia (African or Mediterranean descent)
- Hepatobiliary disease
- Previous sibling required phototherapy

Physical Examination.
- Assess for jaundice within the first 24 hours and throughout the neonatal period. Usually, the face is affected first, followed by the shoulders, chest, and abdomen. Jaundice can be difficult to determine in dark-skinned newborns.
- The accuracy of estimating a newborn's true bilirubin level based on skin color alone is poor. However, a crude estimate of the level of jaundice can be based on the dermal zone in which the jaundice is noticed. This estimate should not be used to determine bilirubin levels or management; helps determine whether acquiring a total serum bilirubin (TSB) or a transcutaneous bilirubin (TcB) is warranted (Ambalavanan and Carlo, 2016).
  - Face—5 mg/dL
  - Mid-abdomen—15 mg/dL
  - Soles—20 mg/dL

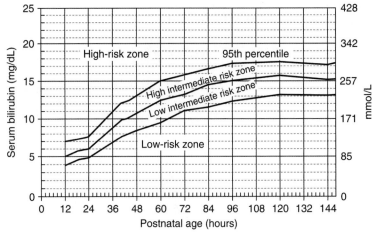

• **Fig 9.14** Nomogram for designation of risk in 2840 well newborns at 36 or more weeks' gestational age with birth weight of 2000 g or more or 35 or more weeks' gestational age and birth weight of 2500 g or more based on the hour-specific serum bilirubin values. (From the Academy of Pediatrics Subcommittee on Hyperbilirubinemia. Clinical practice guideline: management of hyperbilirubinemia in the newborn infant 35 or more weeks of gestation. *Pediatrics.* 2004;114:297–316.)

- Petechiae, bruising, hepatosplenomegaly, or signs of infection
- Lethargy, hypotonia, poor feeding, and loss of the Moro reflex are common initial signs of bilirubin toxicity to the brain (kernicterus). These symptoms are subtle and indistinguishable from those of sepsis, asphyxia, hypoglycemia, intracranial hemorrhage, and other acute illnesses in the neonate.
- Later signs of kernicterus include diminished tendon reflexes, respiratory distress, failure to suck, opisthotonos, bulging fontanelle, twitching of face or limbs, seizures, and a shrill, high-pitched cry.

Diagnostic Studies.
- TcB does not require a blood draw and is often used for the one-time mandatory screening prior to hospital discharge.
- A TSB level (indirect and direct) should be drawn on newborns who have: 1)a TcB more than 70% of the TSB recommended for phototherapy initiation, b) a TcB above the 75th percentile on the Bhutani nomogram, c) a TcB greater than 13 mg/dl at hospital follow-up, or d) are actively under phototherapy (Maisels, Bhutani, and Bogen, 2009).
- Additional blood can be drawn and held for further testing, eliminating a return visit, and/or unnecessary expense if all of the tests are not later indicated. Tests that may be indicated include:
  - venous ABO, Rh, blood type, isoimmune antibodies of mother (should be available at prenatal and delivering hospital), Coombs test on newborn (often done at delivery and held in the hospital's laboratory)
  - Hemoglobin, hematocrit, reticulocyte count

Conditions such as physiologic jaundice, breastfeeding jaundice, or congenital familial nonhemolytic jaundice cause elevated indirect (unconjugated) serum bilirubin with a normal reticulocyte count, hemoglobin and hematocrit, and negative Coombs test. Elevated indirect serum bilirubin with an increased reticulocyte count and low hemoglobin and hematocrit suggests increased hemolysis secondary to conditions such as isoimmunization (positive Coombs test, such as caused by ABO or Rh incompatibility), abnormal red blood cell shape, or red blood cell enzyme abnormalities. Elevated indirect and direct serum bilirubin with a negative Coombs test and a normal reticulocyte count indicate hepatitis, metabolic abnormalities, biliary atresia, choledochal cyst (in the bile duct), gastrointestinal or pancreatic obstruction, sepsis, or drugs.

Management and Prevention. Prevention of severe hyperbilirubinemia and bilirubin encephalopathy in newborns requires breastfeeding promotion and support, identification hyperbilirubinemia risk factors, early and focused follow-up based on the risk assessment, and treatment when indicated.

Management strategies for hyperbilirubinemia include:
- Promoting breastfeeding by advising mothers to put the baby to the breast 8 to 12 times/day for the first several days and discouraging the use of routine water or dextrose water supplementation.
- In the healthy full-term (>35 weeks) newborn, treatment course is determined by physical findings, bilirubin level according to age, and risk designation (Figs 9.14 to 9.16).
- Phototherapy treats elevated indirect hyperbilirubinemia. Home phototherapy can be used for those newborns without risk factors and with TSB levels 2 to 3 mg/dL less than those shown in Fig 9.15. Phototherapy is contraindicated with elevated direct bilirubin. During phototherapy, the newborn should be dressed only in a diaper, temperature monitored, fluid intake increased if possible, and oral drugs avoided due to decreased absorption. Three types of phototherapy are used:
  - Bililights are banks of overhead lights placed close to the newborn. This intervention requires eyepatches with removal at regular intervals, taking care to prevent corneal abrasions.
  - Biliblanket (fiberoptic pad) allows ongoing interaction between mother and newborn as the newborn is wrapped in a blanket with lights or with a pad placed under clothing.
  - Bilibed with lights under the baby and the baby lying on his/her back wrapped in material that light penetrates on the underside.
- It is important to continue breastfeeding during phototherapy. In breastfed newborns receiving phototherapy, supplementation with expressed breast milk or milk-based formula is only appropriate if the newborn's intake is inadequate, weight loss is excessive (>10% of birth weight), or the newborn seems dehydrated.

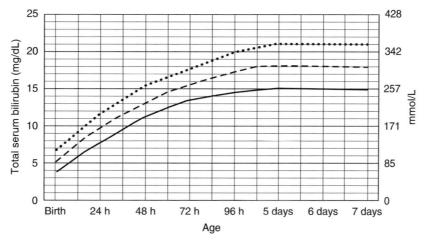

••• Infants at lower risk (≥38 weeks and well)
– – Infants at medium risk (≥38 weeks + risk factors or 35-37 ⁶/₇ weeks and well)
—— Infants at higher risk (35-37 ⁶/₇ weeks + risk factors)

• **Fig 9.15** **Guidelines for Phototherapy in Hospitalized Infants of 35 or More Weeks of Gestation.** (1) Use total bilirubin. Do not subtract direct-reacting or conjugated bilirubin. (2) The risk factors are isoimmune hemolytic disease, glucose-6-phosphate dehydrogenase deficiency, asphyxia, significant lethargy, temperature instability, sepsis, acidosis, or albumin <3 g/dL (if measured). (3) For well infants 35 to 37 ⁶/₇ weeks, total serum bilirubin (TSB) levels can be adjusted for intervention around the medium risk line. It is an option to intervene at lower TSB levels for infants closer to 35 weeks and at higher TSB levels for those closer to 37 ⁶/₇ weeks. (4) It is an option to provide conventional phototherapy in hospital or at home at TSB levels 2 to 3 mg/dL (35 to 50 mmol/L) below those shown but home phototherapy should not be used in any infant with risk factors. (From the Academy of Pediatrics Subcommittee on Hyperbilirubinemia. Clinical practice guideline: management of hyperbilirubinemia in the newborn infant 35 or more weeks of gestation. *Pediatrics.* 2004;114:297–316.)

• Rebound bilirubin testing (measurement of bilirubin after phototherapy is discontinued) is not required in full-term newborns with physiologic jaundice.
• Guidelines for exchange transfusion levels are available in the AAP practice parameter on the management of hyperbilirubinemia (AAP, 2004; updated by https://www.ncbi.nlm.nih.gov/pubmed/?term=Maisels%20MJ%5BAuthor%5D&cauthor=true&cauthor_uid=19786452 Maisels et al., 2009).

Sudden Unexpected Infant Death

The definition of sudden unexpected infant death (SUID) is the sudden death, explained or unexplained, of a child in infancy, especially those that occur during sleep. Included within SUIDS are explainable deaths such as unintentional suffocation or strangulation. Sudden infant death syndrome (SIDS) is a subcategory of SUID and includes a death that remains unexplained after a complete case investigation, including a complete autopsy, examination of the death scene, and review of the clinical history (Hunt and Hauck, 2016; AAP, 2016). Overall the number of deaths from SUID dropped from about 7000 infants/year before the initiation in 1992 of the "back to sleep" program to a persistent 3500/year currently. Non-Hispanic black and American Indian/Alaska Native infants have more than twice the risk of SUID than their white peers. Ninety percent of SIDS cases occur before about 6 months of age with a peak between 1 and 4 months of age (AAP Task Force on Sudden Infant Death Syndrome, 2016a; AAP Task Force on Sudden Infant Death Syndrome, 2016b). Brief, resolved unexplained events (now called "BRUE" and formerly called apparent life-threatening events [ALTE]) include events occurring in infants less than 1 year of age whereby there is a witnessed brief (<1 minute but usually <20 to 30 seconds) event where the child returns to baseline and has a normal history and physical examination (Tieder et al., 2016).

While the diagnosis of SIDS is one of exclusion because the specific cause remains unknown, explainable deaths associated with SUIDS are largely due to unintentional suffocations and strangulation. Thus the strategies to reduce SUIDS (including SIDS) are similar. SIDS cannot be predicted or prevented, although data show placing the newborn in a supine position decreases the incidence and is the recommended sleep position. The National Institutes of Health has monitored sleep position since 1992, and prone sleeping decreased from 70% to less than 15% today. At the same time, the SIDS death rate fell by about 67% in the United States (AAP, 2016a, 2016b). It is also recommended that newborns sleep in their parents' room, close to their bed but on a separate surface, for the first 6 months of life; data show that SIDS risk is reduced by as much as 50% with such sleeping arrangements.

Three main pathophysiologic mechanisms are considered to contribute to SIDS: decreased arousal, asphyxia and rebreathing, and thermal stress. Experts consider as possible causes respiratory obstruction, restrictive clothing, and hyperthermia. Factors associated with SIDS include precious BRUE, poverty, lack of prenatal care, low birth weight, SGA, preterm birth, young maternal age, high parity, maternal smoking and drug use, and co-sleeping.

Clinical Findings

History
• Maternal: Cigarette smoking, drug or alcohol use; no or limited prenatal care; bottle feeding; lower educational attainment;

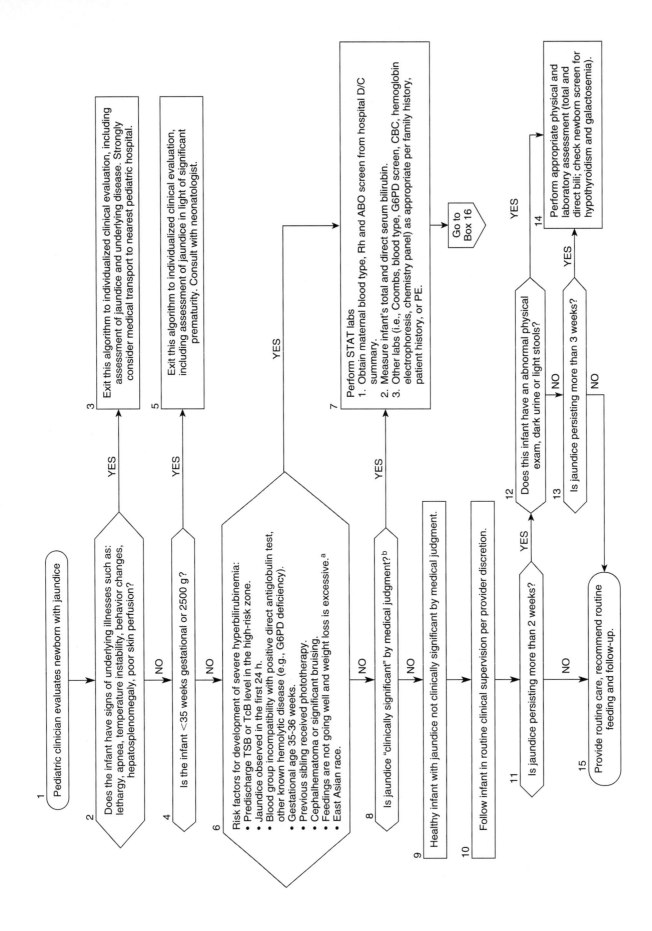

1
Pediatric clinician evaluates newborn with jaundice

2
Does the infant have signs of underlying illnesses such as: lethargy, apnea, temperature instability, behavior changes, hepatosplenomegaly, poor skin perfusion?

3
Exit this algorithm to individualized clinical evaluation, including assessment of jaundice and underlying disease. Strongly consider medical transport to nearest pediatric hospital.

4
Is the infant <35 weeks gestational or 2500 g?

5
Exit this algorithm to individualized clinical evaluation, including assessment of jaundice in light of significant prematurity. Consult with neonatologist.

6
Risk factors for development of severe hyperbilirubinemia:
• Predischarge TSB or TcB level in the high-risk zone.
• Jaundice observed in the first 24 h.
• Blood group incompatibility with positive direct antiglobulin test, other known hemolytic disease (e.g., G6PD deficiency).
• Gestational age 35-36 weeks.
• Previous sibling received phototherapy.
• Cephalhematoma or significant bruising.
• Feedings are not going well and weight loss is excessive.[a]
• East Asian race.

7
Perform STAT labs
1. Obtain maternal blood type, Rh and ABO screen from hospital D/C summary.
2. Measure infant's total and direct serum bilirubin.
3. Other labs (i.e., Coombs, blood type, G6PD screen, CBC, hemoglobin electrophoresis, chemistry panel) as appropriate per family history, patient history, or PE.

Go to Box 16

8
Is jaundice "clinically significant" by medical judgment?[b]

9
Healthy infant with jaundice not clinically significant by medical judgment.

10
Follow infant in routine clinical supervision per provider discretion.

11
Is jaundice persisting more than 2 weeks?

12
Does this infant have an abnormal physical exam, dark urine or light stools?

13
Is jaundice persisting more than 3 weeks?

14
Perform appropriate physical and laboratory assessment (total and direct bili; check newborn screen for hypothyroidism and galactosemia).

15
Provide routine care, recommend routine feeding and follow-up.

YES   NO

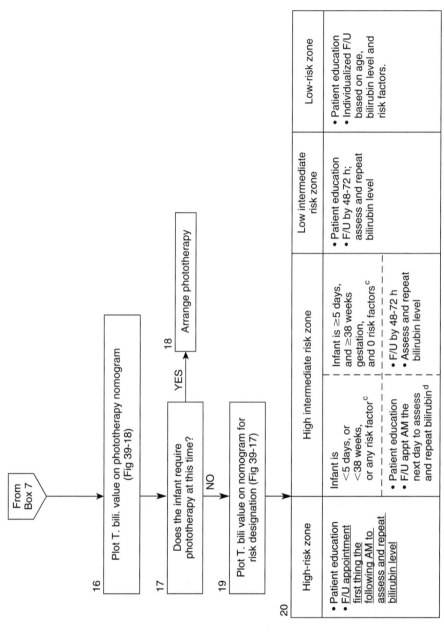

• **Fig 9.16** Algorithm for the Management of Neonatal Hyperbilirubinemia in the Outpatient Setting. *CBC,* Complete blood count; *D/C,* discharge; *ED,* emergency department; *F/U,* follow-up; *G6PD,* glucose-6-phosphate dehydrogenase; *PE,* physical examination; *Rh,* rhesus; *T. bili.,* total bilirubin; *TcB,* transcutaneous bilirubin; *TSB,* total serum bilirubin. (Modified and used with permission of the Multnomah County Health Department, Primary Care Division, Portland, OR.)

- Breastfeeding is recommended.
- Infants should be immunized (reduces risk by 50%).
- Place infants on their backs to sleep until at least 6 months old. The National Institutes of Health has a "Safe to Sleep" program with parent information, stickers, and video.
- Use a firm mattress. Do not use bumper pads, soft bedding, comforters, or have stuffed animals in bed. Infants should not sleep on a sofa or chair, on a waterbed, or in bed with an adult.
- Avoid overheating or too much sleepwear; room temperature should be 68°F–72°F (20°C–22.2°C).
- Avoid alcohol and drugs (including tobacco) while pregnant and breastfeeding, and while in bed.
- Do not allow cigarette smoking within the house or car.
- Avoid bed sharing and co-sleeping.
- Separate but proximate caregiver sleeping environments are recommended for the first 6 months to a year of life.
- Consider pacifier use at naptime and bedtime once breastfeeding established.

- Obtain a thorough history from the caretaker within a short period of time after the death. Do not accuse the family of any wrongdoing. Focus the questioning on the cause of death to better understand the circumstances.
- Reassure caretaker and family that it was not their fault and that in most instances death could not have been prevented.
- Offer support and counsel to families as soon as possible after death.
- Supply names of different support groups to help the family overcome grief.
- Provide follow-up for at least 1 year.
- Assist surviving siblings. Observe their reaction to the death and refer for counseling if necessary. Help them understand that it was not their fault and alleviate their feelings of guilt. Allow children to verbalize their feelings. Assist parents to deal with their other children; suggest that parents give extra love, attention, and reassurance to their other children.
- The use of home monitoring has not been shown to reduce the incidence of SIDS; their use is discouraged (AAP, 2016a). Box 9.3 lists measures that aid in the prevention of SUID.

unmarried; multiparity; maternal age younger than 20 years old; short intervals between pregnancies; anemia

- Newborn: Prematurity (<37 weeks' gestation); low birth weight (<2500 g) or SGA; twins or other multiple births; APGAR score less than 6 at 5 minutes; apnea; poor weight gain; anemia; intensive care unit stay; neonatal respiratory abnormality, bronchopulmonary dysplasia, previous BRUE; recent upper respiratory infection (URI) symptoms
- Socioeconomic, other: Low-income family; crowded living conditions; poor housing conditions; prior family SUID; prone sleeping position, soft bedding, overheating; co-sleeping, especially with parental tobacco, alcohol, or mind-altering drug use; race, ethnicity, culture (higher rates in African American, American Indian, and Alaska Native children)

Physical Examination

- No sign of injury (nonaccidental trauma must be ruled out)
- Frothy blood-tinged secretions in mouth and nares
- Intrathoracic petechiae on autopsy
- Retention of periadrenal brown fat on autopsy

Diagnostic Studies

Autopsy and death scene evaluation must be done. A skeletal bone survey may be done if a concern about abuse exists.

Differential Diagnosis

Aspiration; suffocation; newborn botulism or poisoning; cardiac or respiratory disease; hypoxemia; infection; metabolic disorders; child abuse, Munchausen syndrome, or shaken baby syndrome; and central nervous system (CNS) abnormalities should be ruled out. Bed sharing, especially if the parent is large, is associated with an increased likelihood of SUIDS-like deaths (AAP, 2016a, 2016b).

Management and Prevention

Management is aimed at assisting the family to cope with the loss of the child. The first response of the family is disbelief and shock.

Additional Resources

American SIDS Institute. http://sids.org/.
Canada's Agency for Drugs and Technologies in Health (CADTH): Newborn Screening. https://www.cadth.ca/newborn-screening-disorders-and-abnormalities-canada.
National Newborn Screening and Global Resource Center (NSGRC). http://genes-r-us.uthscsa.edu.
National Women's Health Information Center. www.healthywomen.org/.
SIDS: Safe to Sleep Campaign (National Institute of Child Health and Human Development). https://www.nichd.nih.gov/sts/Pages/default.aspx.
United Kingdom Newborn Screening. https://www.gov.uk/topic/population-screening-programmes/newborn-blood-spot.

References

Advisory Committee on Heritable Disorders in Newborns and Children. *Recommended uniform screening panel core conditions.* U.S. Department of Health and Human Services; 2017. Available at: www.hrsa.gov/advisorycommittees/mchbadvisory/heritabledisorders/index.html. Accessed April 16, 2018.
Ambalavanan N, Carlo WA. Jaundice and hyperbilirubinemia in the newborn. In: Kliegman RM, Stanton BF, St Geme JW, et al, eds. *Nelson Textbook of Pediatrics.* 20th ed. Philadelphia; 2016:871–875.
American Academy of Pediatrics (AAP). Clinical practice guideline: management of hyperbilirubinemia in the newborn infant 35 or more weeks of gestation. *Pediatrics.* 2004;114:297–316.
American Academy of Pediatrics (AAP). Task force on circumcision: circumcision policy statement. *Pediatrics.* 2012;130(3).
American Academy of Pediatrics (AAP). The Apgar score. *Pediatrics.* 2015;136(4):819–822.
American Academy of Pediatrics (AAP). Task force on Sudden Infant Death Syndrome, SIDS and other sleep-related infant deaths: updated 2016 recommendations for a safe infant sleeping environment. *Pediatrics.* 2016a;138(5): e20162938.
American Academy of Pediatrics (AAP). Task force on Sudden Infant Death Syndrome, Moon: SIDS and other sleep-related infant deaths: evidence base for 2016 updated recommendations for a safe infant sleeping environment. *Pediatrics.* 2016b;138(5): e20162940.
American College of Obstetricians and Gynecologists. Delayed umbilical cord clamping after birth. Committee Opinion No. 684. *Obstet Gynecol.* 2017;129. 35–10.

Ballard JL, Khoury JC, Wedig K, Wang L, Eilers-Walsman BL, Lipp R. New Ballard score, expanded to include extremely premature infants. *J Pediatric*. 1991;119:417–423.

Benitz WE. Hospital stay for healthy term newborn infants. *Pediatrics*. 2015;135(5):948–953.

Brady-Fryer B, Wiebe N, Lander JA. Pain relief for neonatal circumcision. *Cochrane Database Syst Rev*. 2004;4:CD004217.

Center for Disease Control (CDC). *Guidelines for vaccinating pregnant women*. https://www.cdc.gov/vaccines/pregnancy/hcp/guidelines.html. Accessed on March 10, 2018.

Department of the Treasury, Department of Labor, U.S. Department of Health and Human Services. Final rules for group health plans and health insurance issuers under the Newborns' and Mothers' Health Protection Act. *Fed Register*. 2008;73(203):62410–62429. https://www.gpo.gov/fdsys/pkg/FR-2008-10-20/pdf/E8-24666.pdf. Accessed on March 10, 2018.

Hagan JF, Shaw JS, Duncan PM, eds. *Bright Futures: Guidelines for Health Supervision of Infants, Children, and Adolescents*. 4th ed. Elk Grove Village, IL: American Academy of Pediatrics; 2017.

Hunt CE, Hauck FR. Sudden infant death syndrome. In: Kliegman RM, Stanton BF, St Geme JW, et al, eds. *Nelson Textbook of Pediatrics*. 20th ed. Philadelphia: Elsevier; 2016:1998–2006.

Kilpatrick SJ, Papile LA, eds. *Guidelines for Perinatal Care*. 8th ed. Elk Grove Village, IL: American Academy of Pediatrics and American College of Obstetricians and Gynecologists; 2017.

Maisels M, Bhutani V, Bogen D. Hyperbilirubinemia in the newborn infant >35 weeks' gestation: an update with clarifications. *Pediatrics*. 2009;124(4):1193–1198.

Stewart D, Benitz W. Umbilical cord care in the newborn infant. *Pediatrics*. 2016;138(3):e20162149.

Tieder JS, Bonkowsky JL, Etzel RA, Franklin WH, Gremse DA, Herman B, et al. American academy of pediatrics subcommittee on apparent life threatening events: clinical practice guideline: brief resolved unexplained events (formerly apparent life-threatening events) and evaluation of lower-risk infants. *Pediatrics*. 2016;137(5):e20160590.

U.S. Department of Health and Human Services. *Healthy People 2020 objectives*. HealthyPeople.gov *(website)*; 2018. Available at: www.healthypeople.gov/2020/topics-objectives. Accessed March 8, 2018.

U.S. Preventive Services Task Force. *Guide to clinical preventive services*. 2014, Agency for Healthcare Research and Quality (AHRQ) *(website)*; 2014. Available at: www.ahrq.gov/professionals/clinicians-providers/guidelines-recommendations/guide. Accessed March 8, 2018.

U.S. Preventive Services Task Force. *Ocular prophylaxis for gonococcal ophthalmia neonatorum—clinical summary of USPSTF recommendation*. U.S. Preventive Services Task Force *(website)*; 2011. Available at: www.uspreventiveservicestaskforce.org/uspstf/uspsgononew.htm. Accessed March 8, 2018.

Valerio E, Barlotta A, Lorenzon E, Antonazzo L, Cutrone M. Harlequin color change: neonatal case series and brief literature review. *AJP Rep*. 2015;5(1):e73–e76.

10

Developmental Management of Infants

SANDRA A. BANTA-WRIGHT

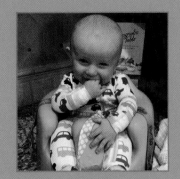

During infancy, there are phenomenal physical and developmental changes. All body systems mature while, simultaneously, developmental skills increase to allow the infant to respond and cope within the surrounding environment. The once solely dependent newborn awakens into the exploration of infancy.

Infant Mortality

Over the past decade, the overall infant mortality rate in the United States declined to 5.82 infant deaths per 1000 live births in 2014 from 6.86 in 2005 (Matthews and Driscoll, 2017). This is a 15% decline, but the declines are not equally distributed nor did they occur across all racial groups. Inequities between non-Hispanic blacks, Native Americans, and the non-Hispanic white population persist. Additionally, infant death rates decreased in all racial groups except American Indians and Alaska Natives. Infants born to non-Hispanic blacks have double the mortality rate of non-Hispanic white women. Another interesting trend is the rate of infant mortality related to maternal age. Mothers who are younger than 20 years (8.6) or older than 40 years (7.7) have a higher infant mortality rate than other age groups (Matthews, MacDorman, and Thoma, 2015).

The leading causes of infant mortality in 2016 were congenital malformations, low birth weight and prematurity, maternal delivery complications, sudden infant death syndrome, and unintentional injuries (Kochanek et al., 2017). Of these five leading causes, four declined, but deaths due to unintentional injuries increased by 11%.

Growth

It is important to realize that genetic, metabolic, environmental and nutritional aspects influence infant growth during the first year of life. Growth charts must be used to assess growth parameters. The World Health Organization (WHO) growth charts released in 2006 are still recommended as reference growth charts for children from birth to 24 months of age (Grummer-Strawn et al., 2010). The WHO used breastfed infants to establish the growth norm and provided a better description of physiological growth in infancy.

Weight

Typically, infants gain 150 to 210 g (approximately 5 to 7 ounces) weekly during the first 6 months of life. By 6 months, the infant's birth weight doubles. During the next 6 months, weight gain slows. By 1 year of age, the infant's weight triples from birth weight for an average of 9.75 kg or 21.5 pounds.

Height

Infant length increases an average of 2.5 cm (1 inch) a month during the first 6 months but slows during the next 6 months. While weight gain is steady and gradual, length increase occurs in sudden spurts. By 6 months of age, infants average 65 cm (25.5 inches) in length and increase to 72 cm or 29 inches by 12 months of age—almost a 50% increase from birth—due to truncal not leg increases.

Head Circumference

Like the rest of the growing infant, head circumference growth is rapid. During the first 6 months of life, head circumference increases approximately 1.5 cm (0.6 inches) per month. During the second 6 months of age, head circumference slows to only 0.5 cm (0.2 inches) per month. On average, the head circumference is 43 cm (17 inches) at 6 months and increases to 46 cm (18 inches) by 12 months, which represents a 33% increase from birth. During this time, the cranial sutures close. The posterior fontanel closes between 6 and 8 weeks of age while the anterior fontanel closes around 14 months, with a range between 12 and 18 months of age. During the first 12 months of life, the brain size increases by 2.5 times. Developmental milestone achievement illustrates brain growth and differentiation.

Chest Circumference

At birth the chest circumference is approximately 2 cm (0.7 inches) smaller than the head circumference but becomes approximately equal by age 12 months. During this time, the chest lateral diameter becomes larger than the anteroposterior diameter.

Vital Signs Maturation

Vital signs stabilize after the newborn period. The respiratory rate slows to 30 to 50 breaths/min. Infants use their diaphragms to breathe but abdominal respiratory movements are normal. The typical infant heart rate is 80 to 160 beats/min. Sinus arrhythmias are common, causing increased heart rates during inspiration and decreasing rates with expiration. During the first 3 months after birth, the diastolic pressure decreases as the right ventricle is no longer the main pump. Fluctuations in blood pressure can be observed during the various states of activity and emotions.

Body Systems Maturation

The dramatic changes of infancy are the most significant of any developmental phase. Infants have significant maturation of all body systems between 1 and 12 months of age. Neurologic and musculoskeletal maturation results in the development of purposive movements and initial speech. At birth, the newborn's total body fluid is 75% of weight, which decreases over the first year of life. They have a high percentage of extracellular fluid, predisposing them to fluid loss and dehydration. Renal system immaturity causes additional risk of dehydration and electrolyte imbalance.

The immunological system undergoes several changes during the first year of life. A full-term newborn receives a significant amount of maternal immunoglobulin G (IgG), which provides immunity for approximately 3 months postdelivery. Between 1 and 3 months, infants begin to synthesize IgG that reaches 40% of adult levels by 1 year of age. At birth, the newborn produces significant amounts of immunoglobulin M (IgM), which reaches adult levels by 9 months of age. Secretory IgA is absent at birth but is present in saliva and tears by 5 weeks. During infancy, the function and quality of T-lymphocytes, lymphokines, interferon-γ, interleukins, tumor necrosis factor and complement are reduced resulting in the infant's inability to optimally respond to infectious bacteria and viruses. The levels of IgA, IgD, and IgE are reduced and do not mature until after infancy.

At birth, the digestive system is immature with decreased enzymatic activity; saliva is present in minimal amounts but digestion does not fully function until 3 months of age. At this time, drooling becomes prominent due to the poor coordination of the swallow reflex. Gastric digestion is controlled by hydrochloric acid and rennin, an enzyme that acts on milk casein to cause curd formation, which facilitates milk retention and digestion. Pancreatic amylase, which is needed for the metabolism of complex carbohydrates, is deficient until approximately 4 to 6 months of age. In contrast, trypsin is present from birth in adequate amounts to catabolize proteins into polypeptides and amino acids. During infancy, the stomach enlarges to accommodate an increasing volume of food. By the end of the first year, the infant's stomach is able to tolerate three meals, two to three snacks, plus supplemental oral intake of either breastmilk or standard infant formula. During this time, parents notice a change in stool appearance from the soft yellow, cottage cheese consistency of a totally breastfed infant to the passage of incomplete solid food, such as corn and peas, in the stool. By the end of the first year, the infant's stools decrease to one to two a day instead of the more frequent movements that occur in the first few months. The liver begins gluconeogenesis, bilirubin conjugation, and bile secretion in the first few weeks after birth. In addition, intrahepatic and extrahepatic regulatory systems controlling ketone body metabolism are established during early postnatal life.

Infant Development

One Through Three Months Old

Physical Development

The infant experiences many physical and developmental changes during this time. These physical changes are discussed in detail in Table 10.1. Length increases by 1.4 inches (3.5 cm) and head circumference increases by 2 cm (0.8 inches) per month. The infant gains 14 to 28 g (0.5 to 1 ounce) per day and eats 8 to 10 times in a 24-hour period. Feedings vary in length from 20 to 30 minutes. Feedings that are outside this range need to be evaluated. At 6 to 8 weeks, the infant experiences a growth spurt and demands to eat more frequently (see section on "Crying" later in this chapter). During this time period, mothers of breastfed infants need encouragement that they are indeed making enough milk. Office weight checks can help parents understand their infant is gaining weight appropriately.

There is a change in infant's elimination pattern from stooling with each feeding to having one to two bowel movements a day or every other day. By 6 weeks of age, an infant may not have a bowel movement every day. The stools of breastfed infants tend to be more yellow than those infants fed standard commercial infant formula. In addition, the stools of breastfed infants tend to be seedier and pasty. Regardless of feeding type, the stool ranges from soft, loose, or even runny. Stools texture and frequency can identify a problem, such as a hard or dry bowel movement may reflect inadequate fluid intake. Wet diapers tend to occur after each feeding.

Sleep cycles become regular during this time, and infants this age sleep about 15 to 16 hours a day with well-defined patterns of sleep and awake. Infants with regular nap and nighttime routines are calmer. As sleep periods consolidate into more consistent nap routines, the infant may need more organized periods of play. Typically, infants have a fussy period in the late afternoon into the evening that should subside by 3 to 4 months of age. It is vital for the health care provider to discuss with parents plans to cope with the increased fussiness and crying before this time is upon them. "Shaken baby syndrome" should be discussed and the period of PURPLE crying introduced (see section on "Crying"). Parents need to know how to respond when they are feeling overwhelmed and frustrated by their infant's increased demands and should be encouraged to take a "parental time out" to allow the infant to cry in a safe environment. This may mean putting the infant in the crib and calling a support person when feeling overtired and stressed. All parents need a repertoire of coping skills during this time.

Gross and Fine Motor Skill Development

As primitive reflexes begin to fade, fine motor skills emerge. Infants attempt to grasp rattles, fingers, and clothing. There is visible head control. Body movements are symmetrical. By 3 months, the Landau reflex emerges when the infant is held horizontally in the air in the prone position. The strong grasp reflex begins to fade and hands are frequently open. When a rattle or similar object is offered, the infant will hold it but will not reach for it. They hold their own hands and pull at blankets and clothing.

Communication and Language Development

When the infant is in a quiet alert state, parents should be encouraged to look at their infant and observe how their infant looks back at them, and to observe how intently the infant looks at faces

TABLE 10.1 **Typical Growth and Development During Infancy**

Age	Physical	Gross Motor	Fine Motor	Language	Sensory	Socialization	Sleep
1 month	Gains 150-210 g (5-7 oz)/week (first 6 months); grows 2.5 cm (1 in)/month (first 6 months); primitive reflexes present; doll's eye and dance reflexes fading; obligate nose breathing	Turns head from side to side when prone; lifts head briefly when prone; marked head lag; asymmetric tonic neck test; sits with back rounded; when held standing, hips downward are limp	Hands mostly closed with non-directional hand swipes; strong grasp reflex; clenches on contact to rattle, necklaces, and hair	Shows anger, sadness, and joy; makes sounds while eating	Fixates eyes on an object 20-25 cm (8-10 inches) away; quiets to voices	Intently watches faces when talked to; fixes on colors; calms when spoken to	Sleeps 16-17 h/day; active sleep 50% of time
2 months	Posterior fontanel closes; crawling reflex disappears	Decreasing head lag when pulled to sit; lifts head and chest while prone; holds head upright but forward when sitting; symmetric tonic neck position	Hands frequently open; fading grasp reflex	Vocalizes more than crying; coos, vocalizes to familiar voice	Follows toy side to side when supine; searches for sounds; turns head to sounds	Has social smile; is more awake during the day	Sleeps more at night (8.5-10 h), and 6-7 h during the day; takes 3-4 naps
3 months	All primitive reflexes fading	Holds head erect when sitting, but bobs forward; minimal head lag when pulled to sit; body symmetric when prone; raises head and shoulders to a 45- to 90-degree angle when prone; begins to bear weight when standing; regards hand; Landau reflex emerges	Holds rattle, but will not reach for it; absent grasp reflex; hands kept loosely open; clutches own hand; pulls at blankets and clothes	Squeals to show pleasure; coos; begins babbling; vocalizes when smiling and when spoken to	Looks at mirrors, pictures of faces, shapes and colors; follows object 180 degrees; turns head to locate sound	Shows interest in surroundings; stops crying when parent(s) enter the room; recognizes familiar objects and faces; begins to be aware of strange stimuli or situations	Sleeps 15-16 h a day
4 months	Begins drooling; Moro and tonic neck reflexes disappeared	Minimal to no head lag when pulled to sit; balances head well in sitting position; sits upright if propped; raises head and chest 90 degrees off surface when prone; begins to roll prone to supine	Plays with own hands; pulls on clothing, blankets, hair, earrings, and eyeglasses; reaches for items; grasps with both hands; grasps rattle when placed in hand, but can't pick it up; mouths most objects	Vocalizations show mood; laughs out aloud; makes b, g, k, n, and p sounds	Focuses on objects 1.25 cm (0.5 inch) from face; begins eye–hand control	Enjoys interacting with others; fusses to demand attention; anticipates feedings when sees bottle or mother if breastfeeding (shows the beginning of memory); prefers certain toys	Develops regular sleep and wake pattern; self-soothes briefly; usually settles back to sleep; may sleep through the night without feeding; sleeps 12-15 h a day

TABLE 10.1   Typical Growth and Development During Infancy—cont'd

Age	Physical	Gross Motor	Fine Motor	Language	Sensory	Socialization	Sleep
5 months	Birth weight doubles by the end of this month	Rolls supine to prone; inserts toes in mouth when supine; keeps back straight without head lag when pulled to sit; holds erect when sitting; sits well with support	Uses palmar grasp to pull objects to mouth; holds one cube; plays with toes	Squeals in delight; begins to coo; vocalizes displeasure when objects taken away	Visually follows dropped object; localizes sound made below ear	Recognizes family members; smiles at mirror image; pats bottle or breast with hands; plays enthusiastically; may have rapid mood swings; discovers body parts	Sleeps for 10-11 h straight at night with 3 naps a day
6 months	Growth rate declines, gains 90-150 g (3-5 ounces)/week Height increases by 1.25 cm (0.5 inch)/month, chewing and biting begins	Rolls from supine to prone, lifts chest and upper abdomen and bears weight on hands when prone, sits in high chair with back straight; bears weight on legs when supported	Grasps, manipulates, and bangs small objects, releases one object when offered another; grasps feet and pulls to mouth; holds bottle if bottle feeding	Begins to imitate sounds, has one-syllable utterances, vocalizes to toys and mirror image; face brightens to own sounds	Adjusts posture to see an object; localizes sound made above ear	Recognizes parents; fears strangers; extends arms to be picked up; imitates sticking out tongue or coughing, definite likes and dislikes; searches briefly for dropped objects	Sleeps 13-14 h a day; uninterrupted night sleep with 2-3 naps
7 months		Lifts head off surface when supine; bears weight on hands when prone; sits erect momentarily then leans forward to tripod position; bounces when held standing	Grasps with one hand; holds two objects; bangs objects on table; transfers objects from one hand to the other; rakes at objects	Vocalizes four distinct vowels; combines vowel sounds with consonants to produce syllables (e.g., baba and dada) without meaning	Responds to own name; turns head to localize sound; has definite taste preferences; gaze fixates on very small objects	Imitates simple acts and noises; attracts attention by coughing or snorting; increasing stranger anxiety; worries when parent disappears from sight; plays peek-a-boo; refuses foods by keeping lips closed; bites in frustration	
8 months	Starts regular bladder and bowel patterns; parachute reflex emerges	Sits steadily unsupported for short periods of time; bears weight on legs when standing; may stand holding onto furniture; readily adjusts position to reach an object	Develops pincer grasp, releases objects at will ("the dropping game"); shakes rattle or bell; holds two cubes while eyeing a third; reaches for out of reach objects	Listens selectively to familiar words; consonant sounds include t and w; begins to have vocalizations with emphasis and emotion		Increased anxiety when parent is unseen; increased stranger anxiety; understands the word "no"; dislikes dressing or diaper changes	Can sleep through the night without a feeding; sleeps 11-12 h at night plus takes 2-3 naps daily

Continued

TABLE 10.1	Typical Growth and Development During Infancy—cont'd						
Age	Physical	Gross Motor	Fine Motor	Language	Sensory	Socialization	Sleep
9 months	Pincer grasp refines	Steadily sits on floor for up to 10 min; recovers if leans forward but may still fall over if leans sideways; pulls to stand when holds unto furniture; crawls	Hand dominance emerges; refines pincer grasp; compares cubes by bringing them together; grasps a third cube	Comprehends "no"; responds to simple verbal commands	Localizes sounds by turning head	Shows increased interest to please parent; fights having face washed by putting hands in front of face; fears of bedtime and being left alone begin	Sleeps 11-12 h each night plus 2 naps per day
10 months	Mature pincer grasp	Walks and begins to stand and walk holding on to furniture; changes from standing to sitting by falling down; begins to lift one foot as if taking a step; changes from prone to sitting position	Begins to grasp objects (e.g., chew toy, rattle) by handle	Says "mama" and "dada" with meaning; comprehends "bye-bye"; may say one-syllable words such as "hi" or "bye"		Develops object permanence; repeats actions that attract attention and cause laughter; plays interactively with others (e.g., as with pat-a-cake); stops behavior when told "no"; reacts to scolding or anger with crying; looks at and follows along with picture books; attempts to feed self; helps to dress by extending a leg or arm	Sleeps through the night for 11-12h without a feeding; takes 2 naps
11 months	Eruption of lower lateral incisor may begin	Pivots while sitting to reach toward back to pick up an object; walks while holding on to furniture or with both hands held	Has well-developed pincer grasp; explores objects more intently; offers objects to others and then intentionally drops object for them to be picked up ("the dropping game"); places one object into a container (sequential play); manipulates object to remove from a container	Continues to imitate speech sounds		When task is completed, experiences joy and delight; rolls ball forward when requested; anticipates body gestures in games and songs such as "this little piggy went to market"; plays games such as "peek-a-boo"; shakes head sideways for "no"	Sleeps 11-12 h at night without a feeding and takes 2 naps for a total of 2-2.5 h/day

TABLE 10.1	Typical Growth and Development During Infancy—cont'd						
Age	Physical	Gross Motor	Fine Motor	Language	Sensory	Socialization	Sleep
12 months	Triples birth weight; increased birth length by 50%; has equal head and chest circumference; anterior fontanel starts closing; Landau reflex fading; lordosis when walking	Walks holding one hand; attempts to stand without holding on to furniture; may take first steps; sits from standing position	Easily releases cubes into cup; builds two-cube towers; tries to release pellet into narrow-necked bottle; begins using spoon and cup; easily turns book pages	Says "mama" and "dada" and 3-5 other words; receptive language > expressive language; knows object names (e.g., ball, blanket); imitates animal noises; understands one-step commands	Follows rapidly moving objects; listens for sounds to return	Enjoys familiar settings of home and day care; begins to explore away from parent; shows joy and delight; gives affection by hugging or kissing when asked; gets angry when jealous; may cling to parent when unsure; may have a favorite object, such as a security blanket; searches for unseen objects (object permanence)	Sleeps 8-11 h at night with 1-2 naps

From Kliegman RM, Stanton B, St Geme J, et al, eds. *Nelson's Textbook of Pediatrics*. 20th ed. Philadelphia: Saunders; 2016 and Shelov SP, Altmann TR, eds. *Caring for Your Baby and Young Child: Birth to age 5*. 6th ed 2016. New York: Bantam Books; 2014.

when being talked to. This allows the infant and parents to connect if only for a few moments. Encourage parents to talk to their infant to begin language development. Infants start to coo and babble, which delights parents. Body movements continue to be a primary form of communication with snuggling, turning the head, and arching the back.

Social and Emotional Development

Infants becomes more social by imitating parental expressions and visually following the parent as well as attending to sounds by quieting body movements or demonstrating visual responses. By 3 months, the infant has a social smile, and smiles in response to their parent's voice. With the increase in activity, alertness and responsiveness, parents need to continue to observe for behavioral cues for the need to rest or decrease stimulation, rather than assuming the infant is ready for more stimulation.

Cognitive Development

Between 4 and 8 weeks of age, infants become more aware of their environment. They visually track faces and demonstrate various facial expressions, respond to sounds by turning their head, and attempt to imitate mouthing movements. By 3 months, infants enjoy toys and may wave their arms when a toy is brought into sight.

Four Through Five Months Old

Physical Development

At this age, infants have regular feeding, sleeping, and playing patterns. Many sleep through the night without a feeding. Between 4 and 6 months of age, they double their birth weight. Growth slows to a gain of 140 g (5 ounces) per week, length to 2 cm (0.8 inch) per month, and head circumference 1 cm (0.4 inch) per month and may be in spurts yet growth occurs in a steady upward curve. Weight gain is influenced by the amount of play and sleep.

Gross and Fine Motor Skills Development

As the Moro and asymmetric tonic next reflexes are integrated, they begin to roll from back to side first, then prone to supine. When prone, infants lift their head for increasing amounts of time. They first sit in a tripod position and progress to a straight back as they become stronger. When pulled to sit, there is no head lag. When held by their hands, they bear full weight and enjoy bouncing on the floor or parental lap. Floor and tummy time should be encouraged.

Fine motor skills are evident as infants play with their hands and reach clothing, earrings, hair, and eyeglasses. They grasp toys and attempt to hold or pat the breast or bottle. Eventually, they grasp objects with both hands and learn to mouth objects to feel, taste, and differentiate.

Communication and Language Development

The infant's vocalization increases with squeals of delight and they coo and add vowel and consonant sounds. The infant laughs (e.g., chuckles and deep belly laughs) to the delight of their parents. Infants this age look to locate rattles, bells, and other sounds.

Social and Emotional Development

At this stage, infants delight in social interaction while taking in more of their environment. Infants spontaneously smile and visually follow their parent by turning their head. They promptly look at and grab objects placed in front of them and vocalize displeasure when objects are taken away. Parents can use this interest in their surroundings to distract the infant by talking or playing.

Infants at this age discriminate between family members and strangers, demanding attention by becoming fussy. They enthusiastically want social, playful interaction and have rapid mood swings. This reciprocal recognition is an important aspect of attachment and parents need to recognize their child's unique, developing personality.

Cognitive Development

During this stage, infants seek out environmental objects like mirrors, their hands, and toys. They smile and mouth objects more. They have increasing eye-to-hand control.

Six Through Eight Months Old

Physical Development

With the addition of solids to their diets, infants decrease their intake of breastmilk or formula, beginning to chew and bite. Growth rate declines as the weight gain decreases to 90 to 150 g (3 to 5 ounces) per week for the next 6 months. In addition, height declines to 1.25 cm (0.5 inch) per month for the next 6 months. Some infants experience teething symptoms at 6 months as the central incisors emerge, and at 8 months with the lateral incisors.

Gross and Fine Motor Skills Development

Exploration of their environment is the infant's focus at this age. When prone, infants delight to lift chest and upper abdomen off surfaces, bear weight on hands, and begin to roll from back to abdomen. Instead of sitting in the tripod position, infants begin to sit erect momentarily and progress to sitting steady unsupported. The infant may begin to scoot while sitting, crawl, and rock in place when on the hands and knees. Some crawl while others push with their arms using frog-like leg movements while their stomachs remain on the floor. They eventually stand when supported and bounce when standing or holding on to furniture.

The infant now holds and drops objects to take another that is offered. They begin to transfer objects from hand to hand and to hold more than one object. They bang objects on surfaces and rake objects to grasp them. The pincer grasp (using the index, fourth and fifth fingers against the thumb) develops. It is entertaining to watch the infant release objects at will, play the "dropping game," and laugh in delight.

Communication and Language Development

Vocalizations continue to increase sound imitation, using pitch and tone with "raspberries" and coughing. Babbling includes one-syllable utterances such as "da," and "hi," and progresses to producing vowel sounds and chained syllables including "baba," "dada," and "kaka," without connecting meaning to them. By the end of 7 months, infant vocalizes four distinct vowel sounds and by 8 months adds consonant sounds. Infants delight in hearing their own sounds and "talk" with emphasis and emotion. They listen for familiar words from parents, and their receptive language increases as they listen and distinguish facial expressions and gestures. They may stop or become quiet when their parent says "no" or uses a different tone of voice.

This is a good time to read to infants using colorful simple board books with vivid drawings or pictures. Reading exposes the infant to "rare" words, which are particularly helpful in developing

vocabulary. The American Academy of Pediatrics (2016) recommends that infants not watch television or other forms of passive media such as videos prior to 18 months as this is an important time to expose the infant to language via human interaction.

Social and Emotional Development

Infants express frustration or reject being spoon fed, preferring to feed themselves. They point at objects, tug on clothing, vocalize loudly with varied pitch and tone and drop objects to get attention and communicate their needs. Issues of control begin to emerge. Parents should use the art of compromise, understand the infant's cues, engage the infant, and learn new parenting skills including how to deal with a determined, strong-willed child. Parents should understand that this new determination is a positive quality.

Cognitive Development

During this time, the infant is increasingly aware of their surroundings and expresses individual preferences more clearly. Toys teach the infant the concept of cause-and-effect when they pull on a string and a bell rings or a toy comes closer, and when releasing toys during the "dropping game." This causes a delightful smile and exclamation of joy. As the infant approaches 8 months, many begin to briefly search for an object or toy, a sign of object permanence. This continues to develop as the infant look for partially hidden toys and objects and plays "peek-a-boo."

Nine Through Twelve Months Old

Physical Development

Infants at this age have growth spurts and lags. Between 11 and 12 months of age, they gain about 0.5 kg (1 pound) per month. They usually eat three meals a day along with two snacks, one midmorning and one in the afternoon. Most infants transition to solid foods and demand to self-feed, not consistently eating the same amount during meals and developing food likes and dislikes. If the infant doesn't follow a normal growth pattern, estimate the caloric intake and address feeding issues in a timely manner.

The infant begins regular bowel and bladder elimination patterns, which may be incorrectly interpreted as toilet training readiness. Sleeping through the night becomes more consistent, but infants may fear being left alone, which may create struggles; having a favorite security toy or object may help.

Gross and Fine Motor Skills Development

By 9 to 10 months, infants easily crawl and some pull to stand or cruise by walking while holding onto furniture. They begin to take steps when their hands are held and, eventually, they take a few steps and progress from momentarily standing alone to taking cautious steps.

Fine motor skills entertain these infants. They delight in putting objects into containers and taking them out again. As they are read to, they easily turn the pages of a book either several pages at a time if paper or a single page if board.

Communication and Language Development

Receptive language growth includes the ability to understand simple commands, such as "put the block in the cup" or "give Mommy a kiss." They learn to mimic animal sounds like a dog or cat. Infants comprehend the question "what does a dog say?" and follow with the correct animal sound. They enjoy toys that make noise and participating in games such as "peek-a-boo" and "pat-a-cake." Overall, they comprehend more words than they verbalize, so their receptive language is greater than their expressive language. Their language includes around five words like "dada" and "mama" and they add simple syllable words such as "dog," but may not always be easily understood.

Social and Emotional Development

Infants demonstrate attachment to one person and exhibit less friendliness to others. They fear strangers, and may cry, turn away, and cling to their parent. They like to please parents and repeat actions that attract attention and cause laughter. They stop behavior and cry in response to a stern voice or a verbal command, such as "no-no." They love to interact with others and anticipate body gestures in games, such as "peek-a-boo" and songs such as "pat-a-cake" and "this little piggy went to market." Their delight becomes affection as they willingly "give Mommy a kiss." At the same time, they get angry and jealous and may adamantly shake their heads from side-to-side to say "no." Simultaneously, they delight in mastering new skills, such as helping to dress themselves by extending an arm or leg, and want others to notice their skills.

Cognitive Development

Infants complete more complicated tasks, such as attempting to stack blocks, but are not always successful. They start to do things on their own and see "cause and effect." They easily follow commands such as "put the toy in the box" and "take the toy out of the box." They master object permanence and enjoy active games such as "peek-a-boo" and "hide-and-seek." Their play is spontaneous and self-directed. They do not need lots of toys but enjoy simple objects such as pots and pans with an easily grip spoon to bang.

Developmental Assessment of Infants

Monitoring growth and development of infants is critical because of the rapid changes that occur. Delays or concerns need to be promptly evaluated, rather than using the "wait and see" approach. Referrals for interventions can make a tremendous difference in quality of life, learning, and later development. Sharing a concern about an infant's development with a parent is never easy, but it is important to ensure that the child receives the help they need. Having a consistent primary health care provider (PCP) enhances the ability to evaluate the infant and strengthens the provider–parent relationship to allow for providing anticipatory guidance, validating parental efforts, and reinforcing parental success.

Developmental Screening in Infants

As many as one in four children ages 0 to 5 years are at risk for developmental, behavioral or social delays or disability (Administration for Children and Families, 2017). Developmental screening is more in-depth than simple assessment and observation, and involves the use of an appropriate, validated developmental and behavioral screening tool. Universal developmental, behavioral, and social screening and surveillance of infants is recommended throughout infancy with formal norm-validated developmental screening at age 9 months (Hagan et al., 2018). Developmental surveillance includes acknowledging the parental concerns, obtaining a developmental and behavioral history, and completing a thorough examination of the infant's development. Routine well-child checks are recommended at 1, 2, 4, 6, 9, and 12 months, or whenever there are concerns. Table 10.2 includes evidence-based screening tools for use during infancy.

Further prompt evaluation is critical when screening identifies a potential developmental, behavioral, or social problem. A positive screen does not indicate a diagnosis. Early intervention programs are great community resources for infants with developmental delays.

Periodic Wellness Visits

The Prenatal Visit

The prenatal visit allows expectant parents to meet with a PCP to form a relationship between the PCP and the family. Topics to discuss include: what to expect after bringing the baby home, how they want to feed the baby, scheduled routine well-child visits, the importance of immunizations, family desires regarding circumcision, safe infant sleep, and car and firearm safety. There should be plenty of time for the expectant parents to ask questions. In addition, the PCP should explore parental expectations, observe the family dynamics, and explore social determinants of health such as living situations, cultural traditions, and family physical and mental health.

One Through Three Months Old

Regulation and Sleep-Awake Patterns

Infants sleep an average of 15 to 16 hours total, about 8.5 to 10 hours at night, and 6 to 7 hours during the day in 3 to 4 naps. Infants will develop an internal clock and sleep–awake patterns improve over time. By 3 months of age, infants' stomachs enlarge enough to allow them to feel fuller longer and sleep for extended periods of time.

- Structured feeding and nap times facilitate the infant's transition through the arousal states. Naptime and nighttime rituals help infants to develop a sleep routine.
- Discuss safe sleep. Remind parents to remove stuffed animals, comforters, and bumpers from cribs and bassinets. Review the dangers of co-sleeping.
- Place drowsy infants in the crib or bassinet to help them learn to self-soothe and go to sleep on their own.
- Help parents identify how family work routines, child care, breastfeeding patterns, and infant and parental temperament influence family sleep patterns and nighttime routines.

Strength and Motor Coordination

- Tummy time allows the infant to develop core strength and head, neck, and arm control. Parents can enhance this time with bright colored mats, baby-proof mirrors, and toys placed on the floor to entertain them while on their tummies.
- Encourage parents to show bright-colored pictures in board books, or smiling pictures of people in a magazine.
- Encourage parents to speak when their infant is supine to help get and keep the infant's attention.
- Encourage parents to offer easy-to-hold toys, such as rings or rattles. Regardless of prone or supine, encourage parents to provide frequent face-to-face time.

Nutrition

- Feedings become more consistent, and the infant has a strong need to suck, especially nonnutritive sucking on fingers, pacifiers, and toys.
- Feedings are important to meet nutritional and developmental needs. This is a time for close, affectionate communication between parent and baby.

TABLE 10.2   Standardized Screening Tools for Infants

Screening Tool/Ages	Purpose/Description	Number of Items	Time Frame	Website
Ages and Stages Questionnaires, edition 3 (ASQ-3) 1 month-5½ years	Developmental milestones Measures: communication, gross and fine motor, problem-solving, social, and overall development Written at the 4th- to 6th-grade level	30 items plus overall concerns	10-15 min to complete	www.brookespublishing.com
Bright Futures 2 days-21 years	Age appropriate child questionnaire that focuses on developmental milestones, nutrition, safety, and child and family's emotional well-being	14 items plus overall concerns		https://www.healthychildren.org
Child Development Inventories (CDI) 3-72 months	Measures gross and fine motor, language, social, and comprehension skills	60 yes/no questions	Less than 10 min	https://childdevrev.com/specialiststools/child-development-inventory
Parents' Evaluations of Developmental Status (PEDS) Birth-8 years	Screening/surveillance of development/social-emotional/behavior/mental health. Written at the 4th-5th grade level	10 items	2-10 min	www.pedstest.com
Survey of Wellbeing of Young Children (SWYC) 2-60 months	Age specific, based on the Pediatric Symptom Checklist (PSC). Every form contains sections on developmental milestones, behavioral/emotional development and family risk factors Written at 6th grade level	12-18 items with 1-3 subscales based upon age	<15 min	https://www.floatinghospital.org/The-Survey-of-Well-being-of-Young-Children/Overview.aspx

Screening Tool/Ages	Purpose/Description	Number of Items	Time Frame	Website
Battelle Developmental Inventory, edition 2 (BDI-2) Birth-8 years	Screening for early childhood developmental milestones Measures personal-social, adaptive, motor, communication, and cognitive ability	100 items	Takes 10-30 min; complete test in 1-2 h	www.riversidepublishing.com/products/bdi2/
Infant-Toddler and Family Instrument (ITFI) 6-36 months	Assesses infant, family, and home environment Includes gross and fine motor, social and emotional development, language, coping, and self-help		Parent interview: Takes two 45- to 60-min interviews	www.brookespublishing.com

Screening Tool/Ages	Purpose/Description	Number of Items	Time Frame	Website
Ages and Stages Questionnaire: Social-Emotional (ASQ:SE) 3-60 months	Screening of social-emotional development	34 items	10-20 min or less to administer	www.brookespublishing.com
Temperament and Atypical Behavior Scale (TABS) Birth-6 years	Screening for behavioral concerns Measures detached, hypersensitive and hyperactive, under-reactive, and dysregulated behaviors. Written at 3rd grade level	55 items	15-20 min to complete	www.brookespublishing.com

Screening Tool/Ages	Purpose/Description	Number of Items	Time Frame	Website
Short Sensory Profile (SSP) Birth-adult	Screens for sensory processing patterns Measures tactile sensitive, taste-smell sensitivity, movement, under-responsiveness, auditory filtering, low energy and weakness, visual and auditory processing	25 items	15-20 min	www.pearsonclinical.com

- They demonstrate cues for readiness to eat and satiation. For example, they may vocalize and increase their movements as they see the parents prepare for a feeding, and seal their lips, turn their head, or slow or stop sucking when they are satiated. Overfeeding occurs if parents do not recognize and respond to the infant's cues and stop feeding.
- Positive reinforcement for continued breastfeeding is essential and strategies for the mother who is returning to work are beneficial (see Chapter 16).
- Infants with little interest in feeding or not feeding enough to receive the necessary nutrition required for adequate growth need evaluation. If suspected, obtain a detailed feeding history including a minimum 3-day diet history and caloric analysis.
- Assess the infant's oral motor skills and general development because feeding difficulties may indicate other subtler developmental delays.
- Use a standard feeding assessment tool such as the NCAST Feeding Scale to assess the parent-child relationship and to develop individualized parent recommendations. If this cannot be done in the clinic, a referral to a comprehensive infant feeding disorders clinic, nutritionist, gastroenterology specialist, speech and language therapist, or psychologist should be considered.

Communication and Language

Parents should be encouraged to talk and sing to the infant during every day activities. The words do not necessarily matter, it is important for them to hear their parent's voice. Reading is another great way to encourage communication and language development.

Social and Emotional Growth

- Relationship development begins at birth and continues throughout childhood. Infants are social and desire to play with their caregivers. When they don't get the interaction they crave, this can result in a "fussy" baby.
- Infant temperament influences how the child approaches and reacts to the world. When parents understand their infant's temperament, they understand how their infant reacts and relates to the world around them. It is important to identify parent–child temperament mismatch (Chapter 15).
- Infants react to their parent's emotional states. Happy, healthy parents help make for happy, healthy babies. Parents need to develop strategies to have time together as a couple and do activities they find enjoyable. Providers identify criteria for child care resources and how to locate those resources.

Cognitive and Environmental Stimulation

- Encourage parents to provide a stimulating environment for their infants. Some parents may be stressed or have limited time to spend with their infants. Encourage them to use short, daily activities such as singing a nursery rhyme or song, dancing with the infant in their arms, blowing bubbles toward the infant, looking at pictures in the house and explaining who the people in the pictures are, or visiting the local public library to locate board books with brightly colored pictures to read each evening.

- Select toys that are safe and developmentally appropriate. Use caution with small toys that pose choking hazards (e.g., those with small pieces or that are smaller than the size of the infant's fist), and painted toys. Good choices include: high-contrast board books, toys that squeak or rattle, or an unbreakable mirror to look at themselves.

Four Through Five Months Old

Regulation and Sleep-Awake Patterns

At this age, infants can differentiate between day and night, and usually sleep 14 hours a day including 8 hours at night without a feeding. By 5 months, most infants sleep 10 to 11 hours straight. During the day, they nap from 4 to 5 hours usually spread out over 2 to 3 naps.
- Infants outgrow the bassinet and need to move to a crib.
- Bedtimes rituals are important to signal what is going to happen next, which builds a sense of security.
- Parents should modify routines to fit the infant's temperament.

Strength and Motor Coordination

- Increasing infant mobility means childproofing the home and the home of close relatives and friends. Measures include safety latches on drawers and cabinets, wrapping appliance cords, covering electrical outlets, and using gates for stairs or rooms. Avoid placing the crib near windows due to the presence of drapery and mini-blind cords.
- Floor time encourages motor strength and coordination. Parents can place a few bright toys just beyond their infant's reach to encourage rolling over to reach them. Time spent in playpens should be minimal.
- Even though movable walkers are no longer available in stores, they are readily available in second-hand stores and garage sales and should be avoided as they allow mobility beyond an infant's natural ability and faster than a parent's reaction time. Stationary activity centers are safer, but their use should be limited to avoid undue stress on the infant's developing hips.

Nutrition

- Drooling is common and can be due to teething but primarily occurs because of salivary gland maturation. The infant gradually develops the ability to swallow excessive saliva.
- Infants only need breastmilk or formula for the first 6 months of life though many parents desire to start solid foods earlier. Infants are ready for solids when they have good head control, can sit upright alone, and have a diminished tongue thrust reflex. All infants are different and develop at their own pace so parents must follow their child's cues.
- There is evidence that introducing allergenic foods by 6 months can decrease the risk of developing a food allergy. All infants should be evaluated for introduction to peanuts between 4 and 11 months of age (Fleisher et al., 2015).
- Spoon feeding helps the infant develop new oral-motor skills including tongue, lip, and cheek control. Infant cereal is typically one of the first solid foods offered and should be spoon fed, not mixed in a bottle or cup.

Communication and Language

Encourage parents to talk and to sing to their infant throughout the day as this encourages "back-and-forth talking" with their infant.

- Parents may notice infants start to babble using many of the characteristics of their native language. Although babbling may sound like nonsense, encourage parents to listen for changes in the infant's pitch.
- Promote daily reading time to develop the habits of quiet time, reading time, and parent–infant time together. Parents can explore colorful books with their infants describing the pictures, colors, and actions. The Imagination Library is a great resource for primary care as families can sign up to receive a new developmentally appropriate book for the child every month.

Social and Emotional Growth

- Nonnutritive sucking as a means of infant self-regulation. Sucking on fingers, toes and toys uses different oral-motor movements from those needed to suck on a pacifier.
- Information about infant development and strategies to deal with difficult behaviors is important. Parents should understand their child's behavior in terms of the infant's development. Encourage parents to change gears to change behavior. Because infants have very short attention spans, it is easy to distract them. For example, if the infant is determined to rip up the Sunday paper, encourage parents to offer a favorite toy to change his or her focus. Modeling desired behavior and redirecting behavior should be discussed before it is needed. Some parents may benefit from parenting classes or parent support groups that provide information on developmental milestones and anticipated changes. *Healthy Steps and Bright Futures* have one-page handouts that provide anticipatory guidance; this is available to download.
- Communication between parents about their roles, responsibilities, expectations, and differences is crucial, as is finding couple-time. Even though this may not seem vital, this time provides emotional well-being and allows them to better care for their infant.

Cognitive and Emotional Stimulation

- Infants this age are awake more and parents need strategies to provide more attention and play activities. Infants seek their parents' attention by cooing, babbling, smiling, or crying. Parents may need a list of activities such as providing the infant one or two toys then adding others when the focus wanes to stretch the activity out. Not all activities need to involve purchased toys, as infants enjoy common household objects such as pots, pans, plastic containers, and lids to stack, shake, or roll.
- Time spent outside can be an adventure. Explore other environments through walks to the park, the post office, the grocery store, and the neighborhood library.

Six Through Eight Months Old

Regulation and Sleep-Wake Patterns

- Encourage parents to have a sleep routine such as feeding, bath time, and story time to help the infant anticipate sleep. Put infants in their cribs when they are drowsy and awake, but not asleep.
- Allow infants who awaken at night to return to sleep on their own. If the infant does not return to sleep, encourage parents to intrude as little as possible, using only a soft voice, then gently touching, and finally holding the infant if other attempts fail.

Strength and Motor Coordination

- Floor time is essential at this stage as infants learn to scoot, crawl, and stand.
- Toys provide the infant with enticement to reach and to move with the end result of rolling, scooting, or crawling over to reach it.
- Parents must balance safety versus exploration. Childproofing needs to occur with the focus on the infant's point of view. Some parents find that getting down to the infant's level can identify hazards. Be aware of things that can be pulled down (e.g., electrical cords, table cloths, curtains, pot and pan handles), anything that can topple over (e.g., floor lamps), and electrical sockets. Padding sharp corners of coffee tables and mantles, removing small objects from the infant's reach, and keeping window covering cords out of reach are essential.
- Active supervision is the best way to prevent injuries as the infant becomes more mobile. This requires a parent or caregiver to be within reach and free of distractions while watching the infant. Infants should never be left unattended during baths.

Nutrition

- Many 6-month-old infants can go for 6 to 12 hours without a feeding. If the infant is still awaking for feedings at night, this is most likely a learned behavior. If not already started, solids should begin at 6 months. Breastfed infants need iron-fortified foods.
- The ideal high chair can make feedings more enjoyable for both the infant and parents, should be sturdy and stable, and stand up to heavy use, spills, and frequent cleaning.
- There is no evidence that waiting to introduce highly allergic foods, such as eggs, soy, peanuts or fish, prevents food allergy. All infants should be considered for peanut introduction between 4 and 11 months of age to prevent serious peanut allergy (Fleisher et al., 2015).
- Allow the infant to hold a spoon or cup to encourage self-feeding.
- It is important for infants to eat with their family at least once a day. The likelihood that infants will try new foods increases as they observe others eat. Distractions, such as toys and television, should be avoided. Mealtime conversation should be pleasant, helping all family members enjoy their time together.

Communication and Language

- Continue talking and singing to the infant using facial expressions and gesturing with arms. Name body parts while bathing the infant or changing a diaper.
- Read to the infant daily using a variety of brightly colored, age-appropriate books. Name family members in pictures around the home.

Social and Emotional Growth

- This is a time when many infants will develop a favorite toy or security blanket, which can ease the coming of separation anxiety.
- Infants begin to express feelings of discomfort, anxiety, pleasure, hunger, and being tired. In a new or different situation, infants seek comfort from parents or familiar caregivers and act anxious around unfamiliar people.

Cognitive and Environmental Stimulation

- Toys and objects that stack, involve a cause-and-effect reaction, and container play are ideal as are interactive games including "peek-a-boo" and "this little piggy went to market."
- Objects smaller than 2.25 inches (5.7 cm) long by 1.25 inches (3.2 cm) wide can cause choking hazards for children younger than 3 years old, and toys with small pieces that can break off should be avoided.

Nine Through Twelve Months Old

Regulation and Sleep-Wake Patterns

Predictability in the daily routine allows the infant to gain mastery over new situations. A daily schedule of mealtimes, snack times, and playtimes, a nighttime routine, and consistent caregivers increase the infant's sense of security during transitions. As infants enjoy the freedom that their increased mobility brings, they start to experience separation anxiety.

- Many infants latch on to a "comfort" object, such as a stuffed animal or blanket, which provides a sense of comfort and eases stressful situations. This love affair often lasts through toddlerhood or longer. A second, identical spare is vital in case the "favorite" gets lost; trade off the spare with the original so that both feel and smell the same.
- Infant temperament becomes more evident in activity and curiosity levels, and in adjustment to new situations. Help parents to identify strategies and creative solutions for temperament-based concerns.

Strength and Motor Coordination

- Infants refine old and achieve new motor skills. Parents should cheer the infant to further build upon cause-and-effect actions with positive reinforcement.
- Childproofing continues as the mobile and curious infant explores the surrounding environment. Medications and potentially hazardous items should not be stored in purses or other areas the infant can reach. Firearms should be in a locked cabinet and not just out of reach. Ammunition must be locked and stored separate from firearms. In addition, small objects, plastic grocery bags, and balloons must be kept away from the ever-curious infant. Making the home child-safe allows parents to spend more time playing and less time saying "No."
- Infants should not be left alone in the tub nor allowed to stand up to prevent a slippery fall into the water.

Nutrition

Food offered to infants at this age varies from pureed to blended foods, finger foods, and soft solids to a wide range of table foods. Regardless of the food type, self-feeding should be encouraged even though many parents struggle due to the "messiness" taking longer.

- Talk with parents about strategies to encourage self-feeding using fingers, spoons, and cups. Using hands and trying to use a spoon are important aspects of how an infant learns to self-feed and regulate his or her oral intake. Encourage parents to start out with one meal and snack for self-feeding with the goal to build up to full self-feeding.
- Hunger is inconsistent for infants. Three meals and two to three snacks a day are usually sufficient for infants this age. It is important to continue family meals and nondistracted eating.
- By 12 months, infants should be weaned from the bottle and pacifier, and transition to a cup.

Communication and Language

This is a fun time with infants as they are more interactive.

- Reinforce the infant's effort to communicate through gestures, pointing, and rather unclear vocalizations. Encourage the infant to "ask" for the item or the need. This provides groundwork for future speech development and socialization.
- While reading a book, parents can say "point to the cat" and "where is the red car?" imitating animal sounds while reading and allow infants to turn the page.
- While bathing, dressing, or diapering the infant, encourage naming body parts such as "this is your nose!" Name utensils during meals or when cooking, and describe food colors, smells, and taste, ("this is really sour"; "this is sweet.")

Social and Emotional Growth

- Degrees of independence and autonomy emerge in infants as they distinguish themselves from their parents.
- Discipline is a process to teach positive behaviors, rather than a punishment for negative behavior. It is easy to distract infants at this age by guiding their curiosity to other activities or objects.
- Parents may struggle to find the energy to deal with busy, on-the-go infants. Suggestions on how to cope with exhaustion and a busy infant may be needed (the parents having a simple dinner out together or letting the infant stay with someone for a few hours while the parents take a much-needed nap).
- Stranger anxiety can be difficult for parents to handle. Establishing a separation routine helps infants to understand that the parent is leaving but will return. Eventually, parents may feel sad or disappointed when their infant easily separates and enjoys time away from them.

Cognitive and Environmental Stimulation

Play is the work of infants. When parents participate in playing with their infant, the parent–child bond is strengthened while simultaneously stimulating cognitive development of the infant.

- Taking command during play fosters the infant's emerging independence and facilitates parents being able to model new activities and skills with interactive games such as a couch cushion obstacle course or singing "itsy, bitsy spider" and "wheels on the bus."
- A box or container of toys prevents toy boredom; encourage parents to rotate toys in and out of the box.
- A mixture of board books, blocks, stacking toys, and pull toys, and pretend toys, such a spoons and cups, help develop the infant's dexterity skills and promote self-feeding.
- "Messy" play provides further exploration and allows creativity (sandboxes and water tables, and gelatin).

Common Developmental Issues for Infants and Families

Parents' concerns during the infant's first year of life are often related to inexperience or lack of knowledge about infant growth and development. The majority of infants develop typically, but this includes a wide range of behaviors. Parents should have their questions and concerns acknowledged and be supplied with appropriate information about infant growth and development. When parents understand the complexity of normal infant growth and development, they are better able to parent and make healthy decisions for their family. Some of the more common developmental issues that trouble parents are discussed in this section.

Sleep

Infant sleep varies greatly from birth to 12 months of age. Initially, newborns sleep 16 to 17 hours. By 12 months of age, sleep decreases to 11 to 14 hours. However, if the infant is a poor sleeper and often disrupts parental sleep, discussions on ways to promote healthy sleep patterns needs to occur.

Nutrition

General guidelines for nutrition and breastfeeding are located in Chapters 16 and 17.

Crying

Crying infants cause parental concern that something is wrong with their infant. Strained parent–infant relationships can occur when parents cannot determine the cause of the irritability. It is normal for infants to cry up to 5 to 6 hours a day (Table 10.3). The developmental normal fussy period begins around 2 weeks old and can continue until about 3 to 5 months of age. Crying starts and stops for no apparent reason and is unrelated to anything that a parent does. Increased hard-to-soothe crying may not be the result of sickness or discomfort, but rather is a normal early behavioral development and is unrelated to parental skills. Labeling the crying as "colic" may or may not console stressed parents, and may result in reinforcing the parent's belief that something is wrong with their baby.

Colic is a controversial diagnosis and not one with a clear definition. It is often defined as excessive crying more than 3 hours a day in infants between 1 and 4 months old, for longer than 3 weeks. Instead of being medicalized, it should be recognized as a typical infant behavior. The Period of PURPLE Crying Initiative (www.purplecrying.info) is a resource for parents to assist them during the developmentally normal fussy period. The term PURPLE is an acronym that is used to describe specific characteristics of an infant's cry during this period and provides parents with knowledge that this is indeed normal and will pass in time (Fig 10.1).

When difficult-to-soothe crying occurs, a careful history and physical examination including a thorough gastrointestinal and neurological assessment should be performed. If the infant is gaining weight appropriately and has a normal physical examination, laboratory and radiographic studies are unnecessary. The main management is an acknowledgement by the provider of the tremendous difficulties the parents are dealing with and an inquiry about the well-being of the parents. There is no evidence to support changing formulas or using medications to manage crying. Herbal teas and supplements should be used with caution because of lack of standardization of strength and inadequate data to inform dosing.

The use of quiet "white noise"—noise that contains many frequencies with equal intensities—can help calm infants. Many parents realize their infants calm when the vacuum is running or a ceiling fan is on. Others notice a car ride provides a variety of noise from the engine, street, to calming music in the car. Discourage parents from putting the infant in a car seat on the dryer or using a blow dryer, in order to prevent falls and burns.

Postpartum Psychiatric Disorders

Maternal depression affects the cognitive development of infants and creates an environment of stress associated with attachment difficulties, developmental delay, behavior and mood disorders, abuse and neglect (Wouk et al., 2016). Postpartum depression affects approximately 11% of the population (Ko et al., 2017).

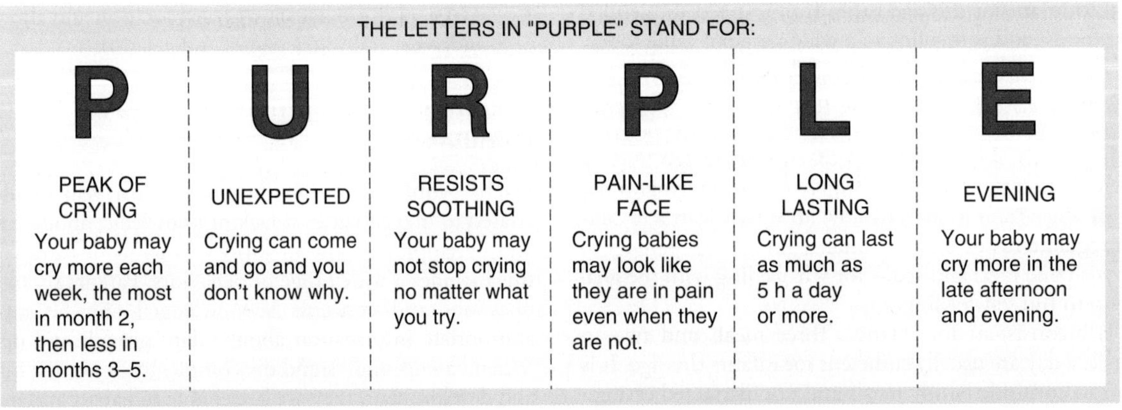

TABLE 10.3 Infant Cries	
Type of Cry	**Possible cause**
Vigorous and lusty	Healthy, full-term infant Healthy, premature infant

High-pitched, shrieking	Central nervous system, such as
	  Cornelia de Lange syndrome, like a
	  bleating sheep
	Cri-du-cat syndrome, like a cat meowing
	Cerebral irritability such as meningitis

Grunting	Sepsis Respiratory distress
Hoarseness	Hypothyroidism
Stridorous	Infection, such as croup or epiglottis Tracheal abnormalities Foreign bodies
Weak	Muscle weakness as in muscular dystrophy or myasthenia gravis

THE LETTERS IN "PURPLE" STAND FOR:

P	U	R	P	L	E
PEAK OF CRYING	**UNEXPECTED**	**RESISTS SOOTHING**	**PAIN-LIKE FACE**	**LONG LASTING**	**EVENING**
Your baby may cry more each week, the most in month 2, then less in months 3–5.	Crying can come and go and you don't know why.	Your baby may not stop crying no matter what you try.	Crying babies may look like they are in pain even when they are not.	Crying can last as much as 5 h a day or more.	Your baby may cry more in the late afternoon and evening.

• **Fig 10.1** The PURPLE Acronym for the Period (Meaning the Crying Has a Beginning and an End) of PURPLE Infant Crying. (Available online at: http://purplecrying.info/what-is-the-period-of-purple-crying.php.)

Between 50% and 80% of mothers experience "baby blues" or postpartum blues during the first 2 weeks after giving birth, which is characterized by crying, confusion, mood lability, anxiety, and a depressed mood (National Institute of Mental Health, n.d.). The symptoms appear during the first week postpartum, typically last a few hours to a few days, and have no negative sequelae. Mothers report feelings of inadequacy, unhappiness, and fatigue, which resolve.

Postpartum depression is a more serious problem than postpartum blues or "baby blues." Unlike baby blues, postpartum depression does not resolve by itself. It can appear days to months after the birth and can last for weeks to months. Postpartum depression makes getting through the day difficult due to periods of sadness, anxiety, and loss of interest in activities, and can affect maternal ability to care for the infant or herself. Postpartum depression is highest among new mothers who are:

- Less than 19 years of age and between 20 and 24 years of age
- American Native or Asian/Pacific Islander ethnicity
- Not a high school graduate
- Single
- Postpartum smokers
- Mothers with three or more stressful life events in the year prior to the baby's birth
- Mothers of a term, low-birthweight infant (<2500 g)
- Mothers of newborns admitted to a neonatal intensive care unit.

Mothers need to know that postpartum depression is treatable, and that treatment makes all the difference. Encourage the mother to seek treatment from a psychologist, psychiatrist, or other licensed mental health provider.

Postpartum psychosis is a severe psychotic disorder beginning within 4 weeks postpartum and includes delusions, hallucinations, and gross impairment of functioning. Maternal thoughts of harming herself and her newborn may occur. Postpartum psychosis is far less common than postpartum depression and postpartum blues. However, mothers with a history of bipolar disorder or schizo-affective disorder and those with a history or family history of postpartum psychosis are at an increased risk. The cognitive lapse that occurs with postpartum psychosis results in the mother's inability to care for herself, neglecting her infant's needs, and revealing unsafe practices.

In the first year after childbirth, suicide risk increases dramatically, becoming the leading cause of maternal death up to 1 year after delivery. Pediatric PCPs must inquire about maternal mental health. Each pediatric well-child check is an opportunity to screen mothers and families for factors that can affect infant growth and development. The 10 question Edinburgh Postnatal Depression Scale is an easy to administer screening tool, and a valuable and efficient way to identify mothers at risk for perinatal depression (Fig 10.2). Mothers who score 13 or more should be referred for further evaluation with an appropriate mental health professional. Intervention should be individualized.

Red Flags for Infant Development

Developmental delay in infants involves disorders that manifest as motor problems (e.g., cerebral palsy), communication problems (e.g., receptive or expressive communication), and/or cognitive problems (e.g., problem solving, mental retardation, specific deficits in processing information). Processing disorders include peripheral problems, such as deafness and blindness; central processing that results in motor, language, and perceptual dysfunction; and behavioral problems. Disorders may be degenerative (e.g., muscular dystrophy) or static (e.g., brachial plexus injury, cerebral palsy), and they may have clear signs in infancy or have delayed presentation. Signs and symptoms of developmental delay may also be a function of the disorder itself (e.g., progressive neurological loss) or secondary to the disorder (e.g., contractures with cerebral palsy).

All children develop at their own pace, so it is difficult to predict when they will learn a specific skill. Infant developmental problems can be difficult to identify, but the provider must be alert to "red flags" that place the infant at risk or indicate a potential problem. Parents may be the first to notice that their infant is lagging behind other infants of similar age and should be encouraged to discuss their concerns with their PCP. Pediatric providers need to listen carefully to parental concerns and be aware of the infant's history. The following are examples of specific risk factors for developmental delay disabilities:

- Maternal infections during pregnancy, such as cytomegalovirus infections
- Genetics, such as Angelman, fragile X, and Prader-Willi syndromes
- Maternal use of alcohol, tobacco, and drugs, both prescription and illicit
- Children who were low birth weight (<2500 g), premature (born prior to 37 weeks gestation), small for gestation (SGA), symmetrical intrauterine growth retardation (IUGR), or part of multiple gestations such as twins and triplets
- Children who have an older sibling with a developmental delay
- Children who were admitted to the neonatal intensive care unit and required long-term hospitalization
- Birth trauma

Potential problems need closer developmental surveillance and more frequent screening. They often require referral to developmental centers for more in-depth assessments and intervention. Table 10.4 outlines developmental findings that are indications for referral to a child development center, a state's early child development identification program, or a child development specialist. When indicators are present, referral should be made rather than waiting some months to validate observations. If a genetic condition is suspected, a referral to a pediatric genetic specialist may be indicated.

Edinburgh Postnatal Depression Scale (EPDS)

Name: _____ Address: _____

Your date of birth: _____

Baby's date of birth: _____ Phone: _____

As you are pregnant or have recently had a baby, we would like to know how you are feeling. Please check the answer that comes closest to how you have felt IN THE PAST 7 DAYS, not just how you feel today.

Here is an example, already completed.

I have felt happy:
- ○ Yes, all the time
- X Yes, most of the time
- ○ No, not very often
- ○ No, not at all

This would mean: "I have felt happy most of the time" during the past week.

Please complete the other questions in the same way.

In the past 7 days:

1. I have been able to laugh and see the funny side of things
- ○ As much as I always could
- ○ Not quite so much now
- ○ Definitely not so much now
- ○ Not at all

2. I have looked forward with enjoyment to things
- ○ As much as I ever did
- ○ Rather less than I used to
- ○ Definitely less than I used to
- ○ Hardly at all

*3. I have blamed myself unnecessarily when things went wrong
- ○ Yes, most of the time
- ○ Yes, some of the time
- ○ Not very often
- ○ No, never

4. I have been anxious or worried for no good reason
- ○ No, not at all
- ○ Hardly ever
- ○ Yes, sometimes
- ○ Yes, very often

*5. I have felt scared or panicky for no very good reason
- ○ Yes, quite a lot
- ○ Yes, sometimes
- ○ No, not much
- ○ No, not at all

*6. Things have been getting on top of me
- ○ Yes, most of the time I haven't been able to cope at all
- ○ Yes, sometimes I haven't been coping as well as usual
- ○ No, most of the time I have coped quite well
- ○ No, I have been coping as well as ever

*7. I have been so unhappy that I have had difficulty sleeping
- ○ Yes, most of the time
- ○ Yes, sometimes
- ○ Not very often
- ○ No, not at all

*8. I have felt sad or miserable
- ○ Yes, most of the time
- ○ Yes, quite often
- ○ Only occasionally
- ○ No, never

*9. I have been so unhappy that I have been crying
- ○ Yes, most of the time
- ○ Yes, quite often
- ○ Only occasionally
- ○ No, never

*10. The thought of harming myself has occurred to me
- ○ Yes, quite often
- ○ Sometimes
- ○ Hardly ever
- ○ Never

Administered/reviewed by_____ Date _____

SCORING

QUESTIONS 1, 2, and 4 (without an *) are scored 0, 1, 2 or 3 with top box scored as 0
QUESTIONS 3, 5, 6, 7, 8, 9, and 10 (marked with an *) are reverse scored, with the top box scored as a 3
- Maximum score: 30
- Possible depression: 10 or greater
- Always look at item 10 (suicidal thoughts)

Instructions for using the Edinburgh Postnatal Depression Scale:
1. The mother is asked to check the response that comes closest to how she has been feeling in the previous 7 days.
2. All the items must be completed.
3. Care should be taken to avoid the possibility of the mother discussing her answers with others. (Answers come from the mother or pregnant woman.)
4. The mother should complete the scale herself, unless she has limited English or has difficulty with reading.

Users may reproduce the scale without further permission providing they respect copyright by quoting the names of the authors, the title and the source of the paper in all reproduced copies.

• **Fig 10.2** Edinburgh Postnatal Depression Scale (EPDS). (From Cox JL, Holden JM, Sagovsky R. Detection of postnatal depression: development of the 10-item Edinburgh Postnatal Depression Scale. *Br J Psychiatry*. 1987;150:782–786; and Wisner KL, Parry BL, Piontek CM. Postpartum depression. *N Engl J Med*. 2002; 347[3]:194–199.)

TABLE 10.4	Developmental Red Flags: Newborns and Infants					
Age	Physical Development, Sleep and Temperament	Gross Motor, Strength and Coordination	Fine Motor, Feeding and Self-Care	Language and Hearing	Psychosocial and Emotional Growth	Cognition and Vision
3 months old	Weight gain <1 lb (0.5 kg)/month Head circumference not increasing or increasing >2 standard deviations on growth curve Problems with suck-swallow Difficulty with sleep-wake cycle Fussy baby	Asymmetrical movements Hypertonia or hypotonia No attempt to raise head when prone	Hands fisted with oppositional thumb No hand-to-mouth activity Feedings taking longer than 45 min Consistently waking hourly for feeding	Does not turn to voice, rattle, or bell No verbalizations, coos, squeals	Lacks social smile Withdrawn or flat affect Lack of consistent, safe child care Lack of eye contact	No visual tracking Doesn't fix on face or object
6 months old	Hasn't doubled birth weight Head circumference not increasing or too large Poor feeding or sleep regulation Poor self-calming	Persistent primitive reflexes Does not sit with support Head lag with pull to sit	Not reaching for objects Doesn't hold rattle Doesn't hold hands together Doesn't grasp at clothes	No babbling Does not respond to voice, bell, rattle, or loud noise Parent concern about hearing	No smiles No response to play Withdrawn or flat affect Lack of eye contact	Parental concerns about vision No reach for objects Doesn't look at caregiver
9 months old	Parent concerns about feeding or sleep Persistent night awakening Poor self-calming, self-regulation	Doesn't sit even in tripod position No lateral prop reflex Asymmetric crawl or other movements	No self-feeding No high chair sitting No solid foods Does not pick up toy with one hand	No single- or double-consonant sounds Doesn't respond to name or voice Lacks reciprocal vocalizations	Intense or absent stranger anxiety Does not seek comfort from caregiver Poor eye contact	Parent concern about vision No visual awareness Doesn't reach out for toys Doesn't explore toys visually or orally
12 months old	Hasn't tripled birth weight >2 standard deviation change on growth curve for weight, length, or head circumference Poor sleep-wake cycles Extreme separation anxiety	Not pulling self to stand Not exploring their environment	Persistently mouths objects Doesn't attempt to feed self or hold cup Cannot hold toy in each hand or transfer objects	Doesn't localize to sound Doesn't imitate speech sounds Doesn't use two or three words Doesn't point, or uses only gestures or pointing	No response to games, reading, or other interactive activities Withdrawn or flat affect Poor eye contact	Not visually following activities in the environment

Additional Resources

Brazelton TB, Sparrow JD. *Touchpoints—birth to three: your child's emotional and behavioral development.* Cambridge, MA: Perseus; 2006.

Bright Futures. www.brightfutures.org

Bright Futures Tool and Resource Kit. http://brightfutures.aap.org/tool_and_resource_kit.html

Fields D, Brown A. *Baby 411: clear answers and smart advice for your baby's first year.* 5th ed. Boulder, CO: Windsor Peak Press; 2011.

Hagan JF, Shaw JS, Duncan PM, eds. *Bright Futures: guidelines for health supervision of infants, children, and adolescents.* 4th ed. Elk Grove Village, IL: American Academy of Pediatrics; 2017.

Healthy Steps for Young Children: A National Initiative to Foster Healthy Growth and Development. www.healthysteps.org

Lancy DF. *The anthropology of childhood: cherubs, chattel, changelings.* 2nd ed. Cambridge, UK: Cambridge University Press; 2015.

National Capital Poison Center 1-800-222-1222. www.poison.org/actFast/1800.asp

National Center on Shaken Baby Syndrome/Period of PURPLE Crying. www.clickforbabies.org/

Nursing Child Assessment Satellite Training (NCAST). http://www.ncast.org/

Shelov SP, Altmann TR. *Caring for your baby and young child: birth to age 5*. 6th ed. Elk Grove Village, IL: American Academy of Pediatrics; 2014.

The Imagination Library. https://imaginationlibrary.com/

Zero to Three. www.zerotothree.org

References

Administration for Children & Families. *Birth to 5: Watch Me Thrive!* 2017. Retrieved from: https://www.acf.hhs.gov/ecd/child-health-development/watch-me-thrive.

American Academy of Pediatrics Council on Communications and Media. Media and young minds. *Pediatrics*. 138(5):1–6.

Eidelman AI, Schanler RJ, Section on Breastfeeding. Breastfeeding and the use of human milk. *Pediatrics*. 2012;129:e827–e841.

Fleisher DM, Sicherer S, Greenhawt M, et al. Consensus communication on early peanut introduction and the prevention of peanut allergy in high-risk individuals. *J Allergy Clin Immunol*. 2015;136(2):258–261.

Grummer-Strawn LM, Reinold C, Krebs NF, Centers for Disease Control and Prevention. Use of World Health Organization and CDC growth charts for children aged 0-59 months in the United States. *MMWR Recomm Rep*. 2010;59(RR-9):1–15.

Hagan JF, Shaw JS, Duncan B. *Bright Futures: Guidelines for Health Supervision of Infants, Children and Adolescents*. 4th ed. Elk Grove, IL: American Academy of Pediatrics; 2017.

Ko JY, Rockhill KM, Tong VT, et al. Trends in postpartum depressive symptoms— 27 states, 2004, 2008, and 2012. *MMWR*. 2017;66(6):153–158.

Kochanek KD, Murphy S, Xu J, Arias E. Mortality in the United States, 2016. *NCHS Data Brief*. 2017;(293):1–8.

Matthews TJ, Driscoll AK. *Trends in Infant Mortality in the United States, 2005-2014*. U.S. Department of Health and Human Services; 2017.

Matthews TJ, MacDorman MF, Thoma ME. Infant mortality statistics from the 2013 period linked birth/infant death data set. *Natl Vital Stat Rep*. 2015;64(9):1–30.

National Institute of Mental Health. (n.d.). Postpartum Depression Facts. Retrieved from: https://www.nimh.nih.gov/health/publications/postpartum-depression-facts/index.shtml.

Trachtenberg FL, Haas EA, Kinney HC, Stanley C, Krous HF. Risk factor changes for sudden infant death syndrome after initiation of Back-to-Sleep campaign. *Pediatrics*. 2012;129(4):630–638. https://doi.org/10.1542/peds.2011-1419.

11

Developmental Management of Early Childhood

VALERIE GRIFFIN

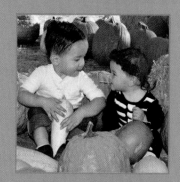

Developmental changes in the second through fifth years of life are subtler than those seen in the first year, yet they are highly significant. Children enter toddlerhood as babies, dependent on parents and caregivers for their survival, and leave this stage as accomplished children with skills, ready to enter the social world of school and community, and who have a sense of self that shapes the quality of their character for the rest of their lives. This chapter reviews many of the changes that occur in early childhood for toddlers (a child 12 to 24 months old) and preschoolers (a child 2 to 5 years old) and describes the role of primary health care provider (PCP) when working with these children and their families.

Development of Early Childhood

Physical Development

PCPs should use the World Health Organization (WHO) growth charts to monitor child growth from birth to 23 months, and the Centers for Disease Control and Prevention (CDC) growth charts to monitor growth in children 2 years of age and older. On average, a 2-year-old child weighs about 28 pounds (12.7 kg), is about 34 inches (86 cm) tall, and has a head circumference of about 18.5 inches (47 cm). The anterior fontanelle should completely close by 18 to 19 months. During the fourth and fifth years, skeletal growth continues as additional ossification centers appear in the wrist and ankle, and additional epiphyses develop in some of the long bones. Changes related to body systems are highlighted in Table 11.1.

Motor Skills Development

Developmental milestones include gross motor and fine motor skills. Gross motor skills involve the use of the large muscles. Fine motor skills include hand and finger development and oral-motor development (see Table 11.2 for a review of gross and fine motor milestones by age). Hand dominance usually develops between 2 and 4 years, but may not be emphasized until 4 to 6 years.

Communication and Language Development

During the first 3 years of age, speech and language skills develop rapidly. Language and communication development during early childhood is fundamental to social, cognitive, and academic growth (Hagan, Shaw, and Duncan, 2017). At 15 months, children speak few words but understand many; thus their receptive language is considerably greater than their expressive language. During Piaget's preoperational stage, children are likely to think symbolically and language becomes more mature. Beginning around 2 years of age, toddlers use words to convey their thoughts and feelings. They find joy in reciprocal communication. Rich reciprocal communication may be the most important speech development factor, especially for children under 3 years old (Head Zauche et al., 2017). Cognitive development is required for language development, because the child must decipher language rules independently, problem solve to understand the others' communication, and create symbols that reflect his or her ideas and emotions that can be understood by others. Literacy programs, including Reach Out and Read, and parental reading beginning in infancy foster language growth (Hagan et al., 2017).

Language development requires mastery of the following:
- Oral-motor ability to articulate sounds
- Auditory perception to distinguish words and sentences
- Cognitive ability to understand syntax, semantics, and pragmatics
- Psychosocial-cultural environment to motivate the child to engage in language use

Language milestones occur in two general categories—receptive and expressive language. Table 11.3 includes language development for infants and children younger than 5 years old.

Articulation

Young children practice articulation skills daily; and by age 2 years, speech sounds are 50% intelligible to a stranger. The intelligibility rate jumps to about 75% by 3 years of age. By 4 years, speech should be completely intelligible with the exception of particularly difficult consonants. By age 5 years, the tongue-contact sounds of "t," "d," "k," "g," "y," and "ng" are more intelligible.

TABLE 11.1	Physical Development of Toddlers and Preschool-Age Children
Body System	**Developmental Changes**
Dental	By 12 months, the child usually has 6-8 primary teeth By 3 years, the child has a complete set of 20 primary teeth, including second molars During the second year, calcification begins for the first and second premolars
Neurologic	Myelinization increases and cortical development occurs Both gross and fine motor skills are refined during early childhood Gross motor skills are smoother and more coordinated Fine motor movements are more detailed and sustained Visual acuity reaches 20/30 during the toddler years; hearing reaches maturity by age 4 years
Cardiovascular	Little change occurs in the second and third years By the fifth year, the heart size has quadrupled since birth By 5 years, the heart rate is 70-110 bpm Innocent murmurs and sinus arrhythmia are common The hematologic system should produce only adult hemoglobin by the fifth year The hemoglobin level approaches normal adult level
Pulmonary	As the diaphragm matures, abdominal respiration movement decreases By the end of the fifth year, respiratory movement is primary diaphragmatic Respiratory rate slows to about 20-30 breaths per minute
Gastrointestinal	By 2 years, the salivary glands reach adult size The stomach becomes more bowed and increases its capacity to about 500 mL Many children still require a nutritious snack between meals because of small stomach size During the second year, the liver matures and becomes more efficient in vitamin storage, glycogenesis, amino acid changes, and ketone body formation The lower edge of the liver may still be palpable By age 5 years, the gastrointestinal system is mature, allowing the child to eat a full range of foods Stools are more like those of adults
Renal	Kidneys are well developed and begin descending deeper into the pelvic area and grow in size Ureters remain short and relatively straight A 2-year-old child may excrete as much as 500-600 mL of urine a day A 4- to 5-year-old child excretes between 600 and 750 mL daily Urine characteristics are similar to adults
Endocrine	Quiescent time for sexual growth, with few hormonal changes Growth hormone stimulates body growth

Some sounds, such as the "zh," are not added until the child is 6 to 8 years old. Fig 11.1 identifies sounds articulated by children at specific ages.

During the second year, the child practices playful changes in pitch and loudness. Three- and 4-year-olds show normal hesitance in speech or stuttering. Stuttering may occur as a child is developing their language skills. They "stutter" by repeating words, especially those at the start of a sentence, or when excited, such as when they want to convey an important message (e.g., "Mommy, I… Mommy, I… Mommy, I want to tell you I hear the ice cream truck"). This normal speech variant does not include syllable repetition or cause undue stress for the child. While these disfluencies are usually temporary, they are considered abnormal if they cause significant stress for the child, last longer than 6 months, occur in children over 5 years old, or if they involve syllable instead of word repetition.

Children usually progress through a regular sequence of mispronunciations as they learn new articulation skills. At first, they omit the new sound and they try to substitute a more familiar sound for the new one (e.g., the "w" for "r" substitution, as in "wabbit" for "rabbit"). Distortion is followed by "addition" as the child adds an extra sound (e.g., "gulad" for "glad"). Knowing each of these steps allows the examiner to assure the parent whether the child is developing normally or needs additional monitoring.

Lexicon

Vocabulary, or lexicon, is the knowledge of the meaning and pronunciation of words. Vocabulary size is influenced by many factors, including environment, stimulation, intelligence, multilingualism, culture, and personality. Children usually understand more words than they are able to express, and addition of words to their expressive vocabulary comes with continued practice. Girls typically say their first word between 8 and 11 months, boys by about 14 months. Most 2-year-olds have more than 200 words in their vocabulary, and most 4- to 5-year-olds add approximately 50 words a month to their vocabulary. Five-year-olds should be able to define some words using other words (e.g., "cup" is "you drink with it," or "chair" is "to sit on").

Syntax

Syntax, or grammar, refers to the word structure in sentences or phrases. The ability to construct sentences that convey meaning

TABLE 11.2 Fine and Gross Motor Development Milestones for Early Childhood[a]

Age	Fine Motor	Gross Motor
12 months	Uses pincer grasp Points at objects Stacks two blocks Clasps hands together	Pulls self to stand Stands alone for 3-5 s Walks holding on to furniture Lowers self from standing to sitting without falling Rolls a ball
15 months	Puts blocks in a cup Drinks from a cup Holds utensils, some attempt to use Stacks two blocks	Stands alone well Walks forward and backward Stoops and recovers Climbs up stairs without alternating feet Pulls a pull toy
18 months	Builds tower of four cubes Scribbles spontaneously Puts blocks in large holes Drinks from cup with little spilling Removes socks Stacks 4-6 blocks	Throws while aiming Walks well independently Pushes and pulls toys Pulls toy while walking backward
24 months	Builds tower of seven cubes Circular scribbling Imitates folding paper once Turns doorknob Turns pages one at a time Unbuttons or unzips clothing Washes hands with assistance Uses a spoon	Throws overhand Runs well Climbs up on furniture Kicks ball Walks up and down stairs, may not alternate feet Walks with control Runs Jumps up Assists with dressing Able to pull pants down with assist
30 months	Builds tower of nine cubes Draws vertical and horizontal lines Imitates circle Buttons large buttons Holds fork in fist and attempts to use Dresses self with assistance	Jumps with both feet Climbs stairs alternating feet Stands on one foot for 1 s Walks on tiptoes
36 months	Builds tower of 9-10 cubes Imitates three-cube bridge Copies circle Uses scissors Brushes teeth but not well Puts on shoes Feeds self with utensils Plays with 1- to 3-piece puzzle Puts on shoes and socks Brushes hair Imitates drawing a cross Twists jar lids	Jumps with both feet Climbs ladders May pedal tricycle Balances on one foot 2-3 s Kicks ball with direction Catches a ball
48 months	Copies bridge from model Cuts curved line with scissors Dresses self independently Strings small beads Demonstrates hand preference Imitates a square Undresses self Buttons Strings beads Pours from small pitcher	Tries to skip using alternate feet Catches a bouncing ball Runs around corners lightly on toes and stops voluntarily Stands on one foot for 5 s Walks down stairs alternating feet Throws ball underhand

[a]Children develop at their own rate and often concentrate on one area of development and not necessarily on another. This chart provides general information and is not specific to any one child. To screen for developmental delays and concerns in early childhood a validated screening tool needs to be used.

Age of Customary
Consonant Production

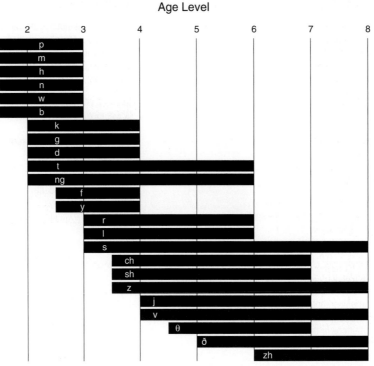

• **Fig 11.1 Average age estimates and upper age limits of customary consonant production. The solid bar corresponding to each sound starts at the median age of customary, articulation; it stops at an age level at which 90% of all children are customarily producing the sound (from Templin, 1957; Wellman et al., 1931). Source: Sander © 1972 American Speech-Language-Hearing Association.** Sander, E. K. (1972). When are speech sounds learned? *Journal of Speech and Hearing Disorders, 37*(1), 55–63. Templin, M. (1957). *Certain language skills in children: Their development and interrelationships.* Minneapolis, MN: University of Minnesota Press. Wellman, B., Case, I., Mengert, I., & Bradbury, D. (1931). Speech sounds of young children. *University of Iowa Study, Child Welfare, 5*(2), 1–82.

is a complex skill, proceeding through several stages in children including receptive, holophrastic, and telegraphic speech. Much of this skill is developed between 8 months and 42 months. By 8 months, children develop receptive language (i.e., they understand others who use a new word or structure before they are able to use it themselves). When asked "Where is the ball?" an 8-month-old searches for the ball. Between 12 and 18 months, children use holophrases, or single words, to express whole ideas. The child says "milk," perhaps to mean the whole sentence, "I want a glass of milk." A complex idea is expressed in one succinct word. Holophrastic sentences are denominative (labeling) or imperative (commanding).

Around 18 months, children begin using telegraphic speech, phrases that have many words omitted and sound like a telegram, to convey their message (e.g., "get milk," "go bye-bye"). At around 2 years old, children begin to expand their vocabulary and to form short sentences like "my big ball" and "the yummy cookie." This is the age when toddlers mimic phrases and gestures used by caregivers like "Oh, my goodness." Sentence structure becomes more complex as children move from active sentences, to questions, to passive and negative construction, and then add plurals (at 3 years old) and past tenses (at 4 years old) to their grammar. Three- or four-word sentences should be evident by 3 years; and by 5 years old, the child's syntax is close to adult style, including use of future tense and complete sentences of five or six words in length.

Semantics

Semantic development, the understanding that words have specific meaning and the child's use of words conveys specific meaning, is an ongoing process extending into adulthood. This development occurs in stages from global to more specific and requires interaction through conversation, listening, and reading. Words in any language have both denotative (the specific, concrete referent of the word) and connotative (a broader range of feelings aroused by the word) meanings. Even though children may be adept at using words correctly, they may have only a vague, diffuse connotative understanding of these words. For example, the 3-year-old child who drops a toy and uses an expletive that she heard when her father dropped a dish does not understand the connotative meaning of what she has said. As language progresses from simple to more complex, meaning and cognitive understanding evolve.

Each child develops speech at different rates. Hearing is vital to speech development. Table 11.3 lists common speech and language milestones.

Bilingualism

Raising children to be bilingual can help preserve the family culture and heritage, and studies suggest that fluent bilingual children have greater mental flexibility and enhanced employment

TABLE 11.3	Language Development of Toddlerhood	
Age	**Receptive Language**	**Expressive Language**
12-18 months	Follows one-step commands Each week understands new words Increased interest in naming pictures Differentiates environmental sounds Points to familiar objects and body parts when named Understands simple questions Begins to distinguish "you" from "me"	Uses all vowels, many consonants Increased use of real words Jargon is sentence-like Likes to use negatives (i.e., says "no" often) Names a few pictures By 18 months old, articulates 15-20 words and understands 50 Imitates non-speech sounds (e.g., cough, tongue click) Identifies body parts
18-24 months	Follows two-step commands without visual cues Vocabulary increases rapidly Enjoys simple stories and songs Recognizes pronouns	Imitates two-word combinations Dramatic increase in vocabulary, 200+ words Speech combines jargon and words Names self Answers some questions Begins to combine words Begins to use pronouns, such as my, me, and mine
24-30 months	Understands prepositions *in* and *on* Seems to understand most of what is said Understands more reasoning ("when you are finished, then …") Identifies object when given function (wear on feet, cook on)	Babbles less Two- to three-word sentences Repeats two numbers Increased use of pronouns Asks simple questions Joins in songs and nursery rhymes Can repeat simple phrases and sentences
30-36 months	Listens to adult conversations Understands preposition *under* Can categorize items by function Begins to recognize colors Begins to take turns Understands descriptive concepts, such as "big" and "little," "boy" and "girl"	Three- to four-word sentences Answers questions ("wear on feet," "to bed") Repeats three numbers Use of plurals Can help tell simple story
36-42 months	Understands *fast* Understands prepositions *behind* and *in front* Responds to simple three-part commands Increasing understanding of adjectives and plurals Understands "just one"	Understands and answers ("cold," "tired," "hungry") Mostly three- to four-word sentences Appropriate use of pronouns Gives full name when asked Begins rote counting Begins to relate events Lots of questions, some beginning prepositions (on, in)
42-48 months	Recognizes coins Begins to understand future and past tenses Understands number concepts—more than one	Uses prepositions Tells stories Can give function of objects Repeats longer than six-word sentences Repeats four numbers Gives age Good intelligibility Can explain what, who, where, and why
48-60 months	Responds to three-step commands	Asks "how" questions Answers verbally to questions, such as "How are you?" Uses past and future tenses Can use conjunctions to combine words and phrases

and lifestyle opportunities. Initially, normal toddlers from bilingual homes may show mild delays in initial spoken words and mixing of the words and phrases from the two languages.

Parents often ask primary care providers how to best introduce two languages to children. Often, they are told to use the one-parent-one-language approach. While this is often advised, the number of families who actually follow this advice has not been documented. Children who learn two languages at the same time may learn each at a slower rate than those children who are monolingual (Hoff and Core, 2015). Most children proficiently sort one language from the other, although they may "code switch" to the other language for clarity. They switch languages depending on the circumstances and the person with whom they speak. Some even translate for others, understanding that not everyone speaks or understands both languages. Ultimately, whether a second, third, or even more languages are learned simultaneously or sequentially, most children have one dominant language. Diagnosing language delays in bilingual children poses a challenge to providers but must be addressed.

Social and Emotional Development

Early childhood is marked by rapidly developing psychosocial skills. Emotions and cognition are interconnected so that assessment of any one area of development is somewhat arbitrary. Toddlers spend most of their time running about, verbalizing, and demanding to join in family activities. These are years of intense learning about and managing feelings (e.g., love, happiness, anger, frustration, aggression, and jealousy) and social skills (e.g., sharing, giving, and receiving affection). They learn the words that go with their feelings and, with guidance, the appropriate behaviors. A major developmental milestone for this age is the achievement of a sense of independence and autonomy. The road from depending on parents for everything to doing some things for themselves can be rocky and uneven.

During early childhood a child's ability to achieve independence is influenced, in part, by the strengths in his or her social environment. In particular, childhood adversity and the emotional/mental health of caregivers can significantly affect social-emotional development. Adverse childhood experiences (ACEs) and parental depression can cause toxic stress, which may affect the security of the infant–caregiver relationship leading to an increased risk of social-emotional problems later in life (Rock and Crow, 2017).

Toddlers need a great deal of love, warmth, and comfort, primarily from their parents and caregivers. Toddlers learn to give love and find satisfaction in pleasing their parents. They learn to respond to kisses, hugs, and cuddles that they receive by giving kisses, hugs, and cuddles in return. Toddlers who make these early attempts at giving love and are rejected or ignored soon stop trying and begin to find pleasure elsewhere. Toddlers with sensory issues learn to avoid some gestures unless they are in control and decide that they can handle the tactile or sensory feelings. Some toddlers find that thumb sucking, rhythmic body movements, and body manipulation are more pleasurable and reliable than person-to-person contacts.

Preschoolers develop more sophisticated ideas about feeling, giving, and sharing. Four- and 5-year-olds move away from the self-centered attitude of earlier toddlerhood and focus more on pleasing behaviors. At this stage, parents are the epitome of wisdom, power, integrity, and goodness. If early stages of the love relationship are not satisfied, preschoolers show more fears, inhibitions, explosive behavior, and demands for attention.

Toddlers and preschool-age children gradually increase their ability to follow commands consistently as they work to gain and maintain approval of adults and to behave the way "good" children are expected to. By the preschool years, children begin to show interest in table manners, being polite, saying "thank you" without a reminder, sharing, saying (and meaning) "I'm sorry," and taking turns. These social skills are learned through daily interactions at home, school, church, from parents, peers, relatives, and neighbors. Children learn to read others' social cues (e.g., the voice tone, facial expression, posture) and to correct their own behavior. Some children find these cues vague and difficult to learn, and parents can help by modeling, explaining, and discussing them.

During early childhood, children vacillate between being a big boy or big girl and mommy's or daddy's baby. They take great pride in doing as many things as possible for themselves, yet they need to feel totally secure in their parents' care. On some days, toddlers cling to their parents' side, not letting their parents out of sight; on other days, the child can play for short periods in the next room, trotting back every so often to see, touch, and hear the parent and be reassured by the parent's presence. The child who is securely attached uses the parent as a base from which to go out and safely explore the world. Gradually the periods of separation lengthen, and the child needs only to hear the parent's voice or to check occasionally for security. Separation anxiety occurs frequently during these years and can be traumatic for both parents and child.

Preschool children are much less dependent on their parents and frequently tolerate physical separation for several hours. As this sense of separateness increases, children are more aware that they are different from their surroundings, their families, and their friends. They begin to realize that other persons also have feelings, fears, and doubts. Peer dependence and learning about how to have and be friends becomes significant.

Toddlers like to have a choice in matters and quickly learn the power of the word "no." They can become extremely negative, practicing the power of "no" every day for months, even when their answer is actually "yes." As toddlers practice making choices, they are clumsy, awkward, and frequently wrong. This can be very frustrating for them, and their outraged responses can be equally annoying for their parents. Toddlers discover the delights of control over others and themselves. This not only increases their sense of power but also can lead to misunderstandings and hurt feelings if their parents do not read their moods properly. With time, they become more skilled, make better choices, have more successes, and feel more powerful. They no longer have to work so hard to show others their power, and the negative stage passes.

Preschool-age children are more verbal than toddlers and are able to perform many more self-care tasks (e.g., feed themselves using appropriate utensils, blow their own noses, and go to the bathroom unassisted). Interactions become easier and more enjoyable as the child learns to verbally express needs and feelings.

Peer Relationships

Toddlers may be fascinated by children their own age and demonstrate curiosity by physically examining the other child closely, poking, and probing. However, they generally do not engage with their peers in an interactive way. Parallel play is the norm. Preschoolers learn to interact with peers as their social world grows. As symbolic language develops, play becomes more interactive, cooperative, and shared. Play offers more than cherished memories of growing up; it allows children to develop creativity and imagination while developing physical, cognitive, and emotional strengths. Fantasy and make-believe are very important during these years. Imaginary play leads to "pretend play," role-playing, and creation of imaginary friends. Play is the major mechanism through which toddlers and preschoolers practice social roles, such as housekeeping, caring for baby dolls, "fixing" household items, going to work or school, cooking, and doing garden and yard work. Children need both structured and free play. Shared or cooperative play makes simple games of hide-and-seek and tag possible. Games with complicated rules can be frustrating to the preschooler, who prefers simple games with the option of making up the rules as the game proceeds. Cheating is common because the boundaries of acceptable play are not yet clear, and the earliest stages of moral behavior are only beginning to emerge.

Children today spend less time playing outside than previous generations, and they are more likely to play in their yard than any other location. Neighborhood environments play an important role in children's planned and incidental physical activity. Parents report that when they live closer to play areas, children are more active overall and more likely to engage in moderate-to-vigorous activity. When there are fewer connecting streets and more visually appealing play areas, children are more active in their neighborhood; also they are more likely to use public recreation spaces that are free from crime and have walk and cycle facilities. Creating safe and supportive neighborhoods may prevent overweight and obesity in children and adolescents (Borrell, Graham, and Joseph, 2016).

Morality

Morality, or the ability to know right from wrong, is based on external control during the toddler years and stems from their desire to please those they love. A child's success and failure at controlling the world influences their behaviors. Parents should focus more on helping the child to make safe decisions rather than moral ones. Toddlers cannot be expected to make correct choices if left alone in potentially dangerous situations because their internal sense of conscience is rudimentary and judgment is absent. Any room with electrical sockets, knobs for technical equipment, guns, open windows, unsecured television and furniture, or hot food represents a risk. As toddlers gain language skills, they begin to echo the parent's firm "no," but they do not understand the full meaning of the term. By 24 months, many toddlers show beginning internalization by saying "no" to themselves and stopping the act, or they may then continue with the act as they talk to themselves, still saying "no."

Preschoolers form a moral development foundation as they develop socioemotionally and cognitively. For the 4- to 5-year-old child, morality is more internally controlled. Instead of basing all decisions on the knowledge of the consequences of the act (e.g., "If I take a cookie, I will be sent to my room"), older children show an elementary understanding of what is right and wrong, fair or unfair. They recognize others' needs and may express a desire to help or comfort others. They begin to think ahead and are able to plan and control their urges, thus avoiding punishment. Four-year-olds can internalize some demands from their parents, and feelings of guilt can be elicited after some transgressions.

Body Image

Toddlers realize that they are separate persons and begin to take notice of their own bodies. They may become fascinated with gender differences and how their body's function. Bodily injury becomes a concern, and cuts and bruises elicit much discussion. Toward the end of the second year, children may notice the inner feelings of their bodies (e.g., the urge to move the bowels, the release and relaxation resulting from going to the bathroom, the discomfort of hunger, and the pleasure of eating). These are abstract feelings that toddlers cannot put into words but can show with actions.

Preschoolers are equally curious about their bodies but are more capable of understanding and expressing themselves. They reexamine themselves frequently, and worries over a lost tooth or a skinned knee are common. Curiosity about their bodies and those of others generates a wealth of innocent questions that generally require only a simple answer. Masturbation is considered a normal part of discovering parts of his or her body and the pleasurable feelings.

Cognitive Development

Cognitively, toddler thinking is highly concrete. According to Piaget, 18- to 24-month-old children use mental imagery and infer causality when they can see only the effect. For example, if they see a puddle of milk on the floor, they might say "uh-oh" because they recognize it was spilled by someone. By the end of the second year, children enter the preoperational stage with preconceptual and intuitive thinking. Primitive conceptualization processes begin with the development of symbolic thinking. A block becomes a car; words become symbols for ideas. The 3-year-old child continues to develop symbolic thinking, and this manifests through drawing and acting out elaborate play scenarios. However, children at this age generally are unable to take another's perspective but view the world egocentrically. Attending to one characteristic at a time is another feature of preschool thinking. For example, the child will try to fit a jigsaw puzzle piece using either color or shape, but not both.

Parents may have difficulty understanding preschool children's thoughts. On the surface, preoperational thinking has many characteristics that resemble adult thinking, and parents often believe that children are able to think as adults do. Preschool children, for example, are developing the use of language and the ability to symbolize concepts mentally. Some of their verbalizations appear quite precocious, as evidenced by the 3-year-old child who stares out the window and then states, "Look, Mommy, the trees are saying yes and no." Preschool children continue to be concrete and egocentric in their thinking, and their logic is the source of many communication problems between parents and children. Table 11.4 identifies major characteristics of preschool thinking and gives examples of each.

Language development through the toddler and preschool years remains one of the most sensitive indicators of cognitive development, and assessment tools plot language ability as a way of measuring cognitive levels. Social development and adaptive skills are also major indicators of cognitive abilities. Differentiation of the self from others, with increasing sensitivity not only to the rules and norms for social interaction but also to the perception of the perspectives and feelings of others, requires ever increasing cognitive capability. Finally, play quality is an indicator of cognitive development. Through play, children manipulate and learn to control their environment in safe, yet stimulating ways.

Developmental Assessment of Early Childhood

Developmental assessment is an essential part of each health supervision encounter and includes both ongoing surveillance and standardized developmental screening. Early identification of developmental and behavioral problems is key to providing early intervention. The process begins by establishing rapport with the parents/caregivers, reviewing parent report tools, and attending to their concerns. Data can be collected through parent interviews, standardized screening tools, observation of the interactions between the child and parents, physical examination, and laboratory or other diagnostic measures. If there are concerns about the child's development or if a child is identified through screening as having a potential problem, a thorough diagnostic assessment is required. Referral to an appropriate specialist should be made to determine the degree of developmental delay and to identify intervention strategies.

TABLE 11.4	Examples of Preschool Children's Thinking Using Piaget's Preoperational Stage
Characteristic	**Example**
Egocentrism	"It's snowing because I want to play in it"
Unable to see another's viewpoint	If John is holding a doll with its face toward Ann, Ann thinks John can also see the doll's face
Incomplete understanding of sequence of time	Knows names of time components (today, tomorrow, yesterday, minutes, days, weeks, and so on), but uses them inconsistently: "I'm not going to take a nap yesterday" Yesterday means any time before now; tomorrow means any time in the future Historical events are conceptualized in terms of the present: "Mommy, do you know George Washington?"
Developing sense of space and position: From experiencing them as a part of their activity, and to understanding them in detail and direction	Frequently used words: *in, on, up, down, at, under*
Evolving ability to categorize or order objects and phenomena	*Early preschooler:* No understanding of concept of class or groups; undisturbed to see a new Santa Claus on every corner *Cluster phenomena:* When asked to sort a series of blocks, the child may cluster a small, medium, and large block as a "baby," "mommy," and "daddy" block By 4-5 years, child is able to consistently use one or two categories to arrange objects in some order (color, number, form, or size)
Developing ability to establish causality (e.g., realism, animism, artificialism)	*Realism:* Intellectual (dreams are actually real) and nominal (a horse can only be called a horse, not a stallion or filly) *Animism:* 2- to 3-year-olds think objects possess innate person-like qualities that cause results: "The chair made me fall down" *Artificialism:* 3- to 4-year-olds think things are caused by some controlling force that controls the world
Transductive reasoning: from particular to particular	If the child does not like one particular vegetable, he or she will not like another particular fruit: "I can't eat my banana because my potatoes are burned"
Developing sense of conservation of quantity, weight, mass	Preschoolers are usually unable to conceptualize that change in shape does not affect quantity, weight, or mass of an object Generally, 50% of 5-year-olds have mastered conservation of quantity, and 50% of 6-year-olds have mastered conservation of weight or mass
Rigidity	Most children in the preoperational stage are very rigid in their thinking

Screening Strategies During Early Childhood

Toddlers and preschoolers require screening for gross and fine motor skills, communication and language, problem solving, and social, emotional, and cognitive development. This can be done at well-child visits and at visits for episodic illnesses. Validated screening tools provide a quick, inexpensive method of identifying potential delays or concerns. These tools are generally appropriate for all children, although culture and experience can affect outcomes. Parents can complete a screening tool in the waiting room, or providers can directly ask the parent questions. Providers should make sure they understand the parents' responses and clarify any concerns. Table 11.5 lists a variety of developmental screening tools. Tables 11.6 to 11.9 list questions that can be used to assess behavior and include the purpose or rationale for these questions.

Physical Development

Annually, toddlers and preschool children need anthropometric measurement, including blood pressure for children 3 and older and at-risk children. Hearing screening leads to early detection of hearing loss and should continue through the early childhood period. Age-appropriate visual acuity measurement is recommended starting at 3 years of age (Hagan et al., 2017). See Chapter 23 for information about dental health.

Motor Skills Development

Toddlers and preschoolers develop and refine their motor skills, driven by curiosity, desire for independence, and endless energy. Asking parents about the child's development is an important part of developmental surveillance. Gross and fine motor skills are best assessed using standardized, validated screening tools, such as the Ages and Stages Questionnaire-3 (ASQ-3).

Fine motor development is evaluated by assessing finger, hand, and oral movements. Gross motor skills are evaluated by assessing the child's large muscle skills, such as the ability to crawl, sit, walk, run, hop, skip, and climb. The quality of the child's movements during these activities is important to note as well.

Communication and Language Development

Communication is a vital part of being a happy, functioning human being, and language assessment is important during early childhood. A careful history of the child's abilities and pattern of learning (e.g., when did the child first articulate words?) provides much of the essential information. Listening to children and talking with their parents are essential, but the provider should also remember that parents may not be fully sensitive to speech problems because they are accustomed to hearing the child's speech. Physical examination helps to determine if physical structures

TABLE 11.5 Screening Tools for Toddler and Preschoolers

Screening Tool	Use	Website
Ages and Stages Questionnaires, ed 3 (ASQ-3) (2009)	Screening and surveillance of five key developmental areas: communication, gross motor, fine motor, problem solving, and personal-social For use with 1-month-olds to 5½-year-olds Parents report on 30 items plus overall concerns Written at the fourth- to sixth-grade level. Manual includes activity handouts for parents. Available in English, Spanish, and French	www.brookespublishing.com
Ages and Stages Questionnaire: Social-Emotional, ed 2 (ASQ:SE-2)	Screening and surveillance of social-emotional development: self-regulation, compliance, social-communication, adaptive functioning, autonomy, affect, and interaction with people Parents report on 32 items For use with 1- to 72-month-olds Takes 10-15 min or less to administer. Available in English and Spanish	www.brookespublishing.com
Battelle Developmental Inventory, ed 2 (BDI-2)	Screening for early childhood developmental milestones Measures personal-social, adaptive, motor, communication, and cognitive abilities Parents report on 100 items For use from birth to 8 years old Takes 10-30 min; complete test 1-2 h	www.riversidepublishing.com/products/bdi2/
Child Development Inventory (CDI)	Screening for motor, social skills, expressive language, language comprehension, self-help, letters, and numbers Parents report on 300 items For use with 15-month-olds to 6-year-olds Test takes 30-40 min to administer development milestones Measures fine motor, gross skills	www.childdevrev.com/index.html
Parents' Evaluation of Developmental Status (PEDS test)	Screening/surveillance of development, behavior, social-emotional, mental health, and autism Parents complete 10 questions For use from birth to 8 years old Test takes 2 min to administer Available in English, Spanish, Vietnamese, and many other languages	www.pedstest.com
Pediatric Symptom Checklist (PSC)	Psychosocial screen designed to recognize cognitive, emotional, and behavioral problems Parents complete 35 items For use with 4 to 11 years old Test takes 5-10 min to complete Available in English and dozens of other languages	www.massgeneral.org/psychiatry/services/psc_forms.aspx
Modified Checklist for Autism in Toddlers, Revised with Follow-Up (M-CHAT-R/F) (2013)	Screening for autism risk Parents complete 20 items. For use from 16 to 30 months Takes 5 min to complete Available in multiple languages	www.mchatscreen.com
The Survey of Wellbeing of Young Children (SWYC)	Screening for developmental milestones, behavioral/emotional development, and family risk factors For use from 2 to 60 months. Takes 15 min to complete	https://www.floatinghospital.org/The-Survey-of-Wellbeing-of-Young-Children/Overview.aspx

necessary for speech are intact (e.g., a cleft uvula may indicate an occult cleft palate that could interfere with the child's ability to shape words). See Table 11.10 for screening language assessment tools appropriate for use in primary care.

Language screening evaluates expressive and receptive language skills. Because language and cognitive skills are intricately interwoven, most intelligence tests have language sections that can be useful in assessing the total child. Expressive language screening places emphasis on articulation and vocabulary. Receptive language looks at comprehension, repetition, and follow-up of language heard (e.g., child's ability to follow directions).

Social and Emotional Development

Assessment of psychosocial and emotional development addresses the child's role in the family, success in making friends and working with peers, self-esteem, and feelings of contentment and security. This area of development should be assessed at each visit. The social emotional section of the ASQ assesses these behaviors but a more complete screening can be done by using the specific Ages and Stages Questionnaire: Social-Emotional-2 (ASQ: SE-2) for children 3 months to 5 years old. The Pediatric Symptom Checklist (PSC) is a validated screening tool that can be used beginning at 4 years old to screen for cognitive, emotional, and/or behavioral concerns (see Chapter 15).

TABLE 11.6 Surveillance of Physical Development and Motor Skills: Questions and Rationales

Question	Rationale for Question
Tell me about your child's health	Invites discussion of somatic issues and complaints
Do you have any concerns about your child's development?	Assesses parental concerns and allows to tailoring of assessment to identify them
Does your child appear to be developing similar to other children of the same age?	Assesses parent perceptions of physical development; developmental milestones
Has illness affected your child's daily activities?	Assesses possible chronic medical problem and effects on development
Tell me about your child's daily habits: elimination, toilet training, sleeping, eating	Assesses parent understanding of readiness, child's cues, changing behaviors, and current status
How does your child get from place to place?	Assesses gross motor skills (e.g., walks, climbs, runs, pedals tricycle), and activity level
How does your child feed himself or herself (e.g., cup, bottle, utensils)?	Assesses fine motor skills
Tell me about your child's play activities	Assesses gross and fine motor skills

TABLE 11.7 Surveillance of Communication and Speech Development: Questions and Rationales

Question	Rationale for Question
Do you have any concerns about your child's speech?	Assesses parental concerns and allows to tailoring of assessment to identify them
How does your child communicate needs and desires?	Assesses verbal and nonverbal communication strategies, vocabulary, and expressive language
How much do you think your child understands?	Evaluates cognitive level and receptive language
How does your child respond to one-step commands? To two- or three-step commands?	Evaluates receptive language; evaluates short-term memory and auditory sequencing
Does your child use plurals, pronouns, phrases, and sentences?	Indicates increased understanding of more complex structures
How well can you understand your child's speech? How well can others?	Indicates increased articulation ability

TABLE 11.8 Surveillance of Psychosocial and Emotional Development: Questions and Rationales

Question	Rationale for Question
Do you have any concerns about how your child gets along with others? Do you have any concerns about your child's emotions?	Allows tailoring of assessment to identify them
Is your child able to feed himself/herself, dress, and take care of his or her own toileting?	Assesses adaptive skills, comfort with own abilities
How does your child behave with family members he or she lives with? How does he or she behave with other family members?	Assesses child's development of roles within the family system; attachment should be evident
How do you guide or discipline your child without always saying "no"?	Evaluates adaptability, creativity, repertoire of parent's skills in response to child's behaviors
How does your child respond when you set limits?	Assesses child's understanding of limits of appropriate behavior, social rules, and self-control
How does your child react to strangers or new situations?	Evaluates child's ability to deal with increasingly complex social situations
Tell me about any tantrums your child has. What causes them? How does he or she behave? How do you respond?	Evaluates responses to stress, development of independence, and social control
What does your child do for play?	Indicates social and emotional well-being
How does your child behave around other children?	Considers social development with peers and development of appropriate play
What is your child's best friend's name? Does he or she have shared activities with peers?	Indicates child is developing a social circle and increasing opportunities for practicing new social skills
Does your child seem to understand the feelings of others?	Assesses empathy
Is your child afraid of anything in particular? How do you handle that fear?	Evaluates parent's responses to child's emotional stresses and understanding of child's view and feelings
Does your child have imaginary friends? Does she or he have a fantasy play time?	Allows child to explore emotions and developing roles in a safe way

Cognitive and Intellectual Development

After 2 years old, as thinking moves into the preconceptual stages, cognitive development is increasingly expressed through symbol systems and language. Toddlers begin to enjoy make-believe, and preschoolers love stories and become masters at games of pretend and fantasy.

Anticipatory Guidance for Early Childhood

Anticipatory guidance for toddlers and preschoolers helps parents and children transition from a highly dependent relationship to one in which the child has an established sense of autonomy with an evolving understanding of the self as a separate, creative, and powerful being. During the process, parents learn new communication

TABLE 11.9 Surveillance of Cognitive Development: Questions and Rationales	
Questions	**Rationale for Questions**
Questions Asked of 1- to 3-Year-Olds	
Tell me about a typical day. What sorts of things does your child do? With whom does she or he play? (Ask parent)	Assesses complexity of manipulation of objects, parallel and cooperative play, and role-playing
Can your child follow simple instructions? (Ask parent)	Assesses ability to retain and process instructions and respond to input
Does your child speak clearly? How much do you understand when your child speaks to you? Can your child understand what you say to him or her? (Ask parent)	Assesses progress in decoding, encoding, and using a language system effectively
How does your child behave with family members and other children? (Ask parent)	Indicates understanding of social systems and norms
What is your name? Are you a boy or girl? How old are you? (Ask child)	3-year-olds should know these facts
Questions Asked of 4- to 5-Year-Olds	
Ask child general information questions (e.g., colors, numbering, objects)	Assesses general fund of knowledge
Ask child what makes the sun come up	Illustrates child's belief about causality
Ask child about concepts of time (e.g., What time do you have lunch? What time do you go to bed?)	Assesses understanding of a relatively sophisticated concept
Ask child about spontaneous play (e.g., with puppets or dolls), imaginative use of play materials (e.g., clay, crayons, other toys)	Assesses imagination and magical thinking
Ask child to draw a person	50% of 4-year-olds draw a three-part person; by 5 years old, child can draw an eight-part person
How does the child behave in preschool or child care setting? (Ask parent)	Assesses language, social, and play development in relation to peers in a setting where expectations differ from those at home

and interaction skills with their children. Although the toddler and preschool years can be frustrating at times, the ultimate outcome of good communication and relationships that support the potential of both child and parent is worth the effort. According to the American Academy of Pediatrics recommendations for preventive pediatric health care and the *Bright Futures Guidelines,* providers should offer anticipatory guidance in all of the following areas: family support, child development, mental health, healthy weight, healthy nutrition, physical activity, oral health, healthy sexual development and sexuality, safety and injury prevention, and social determinants of health; they should also provide educational counseling and support services (Hagan et al., 2017).

Regulation and Sleep-Wake Patterns

- Discuss the need to assist toddlers and preschoolers to transition from one state to another. Consistent sleep and naptime schedules are essential. Use of a comfort object (e.g., teddy bear) and bedtime rituals help.
- Explain how children at this age process information and control themselves. They can be overwhelmed if they have too much stimulation.
- Explain that some children may have sensory integration issues that require structuring and modulation of their environment.
- Discuss how to help children identify and name their feelings. This ability will help them to more successfully organize and integrate the sensations they experience and respond appropriately.
- Encourage parents to provide opportunities for children to have some control and choice in daily activities (e.g., can select the story to be read at bedtime), while maintaining important rituals.
- Discuss sleep problems that may appear at this time, including sleep resistance, bruxism, nightmares, and somnambulism (see Chapter 20).
- Encourage parents to offer naps and opportunities for rest but not to force them on children. It is the parents' job to make sure the child has ample rest time.
- Encourage parents to form good sleep routines for the child, to provide positive reinforcement of healthy sleep behavior, and to use firm, loving, and consistent discipline when dealing with sleep refusal and other behavioral sleep problems.

Strength and Motor Coordination

- Encourage parents to provide a wide range of safe play opportunities that use both fine and gross motor skills.
- Urge parents to allow children to take the lead during play and to follow and expand on whatever the child is interested in.
- Encourage parents to provide their children with a variety of play activities that expose children to nature, such as the following:
  - Take children to a park or playground to run, throw balls, swing, and slide.
  - Encourage children to play with natural materials, water, sand, grass, and leaves.
- Provide children with age-appropriate play materials: stickers, pencils, crayons, paper, paints, utensils, blocks, cardboard boxes, and building toys.
- Explain how parents can incorporate motor skills practice as part of daily routines (e.g., have child help pour the milk, hold the cup, or squeeze the toothpaste; encourage child to do his/her own buttons, snaps, and zippers).
- Emphasize the need for constant adult supervision of children's activities.
- Discuss how parents can make the environment safer for their child: securing doors and using window guards; removing toxic substances and dangerous objects; providing toys that are developmentally appropriate and safely constructed.
- Reinforce teaching about car seat use and explain the need for larger car seats and booster seats as the child grows. Explain to parents the importance of modeling for the child by using their own seat restraint.
- Encourage bicycle helmet use with all riding toys and tricycles/bicycles.

TABLE 11.10 **Speech and Language Evaluation Tools**

Evaluation Tool	Age Assessed and Test Characteristics	Source
The Capute Scales: Cognitive Adaptive Test and Clinical Linguistic and Auditory Milestone Scale (CAT/CLAMS)	Use from birth to 36 months Interview Tests language and problem-solving skills to help clearly identify between the two	Paul H Brookes Publishing www.brookespublishing.com
Clinical Evaluation of Language Fundamentals—Preschool (CELF-P)	Use from 3 to 6 years Assesses receptive and expressive language	Pearson Assessment www.pearsonclinical.com/language/products/100000316/celf-preschool-2-celf-preschool-2.html
Early Language Milestone Scale (ELM Scale-2)	Use from birth to 36 months Tests visual and auditory receptive, and auditory expressive abilities. History, testing, and observation completed in 1-10 min	Pro-Ed www.proedinc.com
Goldman-Fristoe Test of Articulation	Use from 2 to 22 years old Assesses articulation skills	Pearson Assessments www.ags.pearsonassessments.com
Peabody Picture Vocabulary Test	Use from 2½ to 90+ years old Screens for receptive vocabulary	Pearson Assessments www.pearsonclinical.com
Receptive-Expressive Emergent Language Test, ed 3 (REEL 3)	Use from birth to 36 months Interview or direct observation of expressive and receptive language	Pearson Assessments www.linguisystems.com

Nutrition, Self-Care, and Safety

- Provide parents with information about healthy foods and nutritional needs of their child (see Chapter 17). Three meals and two nutritious snacks per day are encouraged.
- Discuss the parents' responsibility to provide children with healthy foods and to allow them to make choices from healthy food options; it is the parents' job to provide the child with nutritious foods, and it is the child's job to decide how much they will eat. Start with small portions of food will help the child choose a variety of foods. Discourage parents from making separate meals for their young children.
- Young children may go on "food jags," refusing some foods or requesting the same food day after day. Parents need to make sure the food eaten is nutritious.
- Explain how changes in toddlers' eating habits are caused by developmental changes (e.g., child has a decrease in appetite, is easily distracted, demonstrates more curiosity about what is going on around her than in eating, is more interested in using gross motor skills than in sitting still).
- Explain nonnutritive value of food and eating.
- Encourage self-feeding to help the child gain new skills (e.g., finger foods stimulate fine motor and cognitive development, in addition to fostering a child's sense of control and independence; eating together as a family can strengthen relationships and develop social skills).
- Encourage parents to structure family mealtimes that are pleasant and interactive; this may mean offering the toddler foods that can be eaten in short periods of sitting. Avoid making meals a power struggle.
- Discuss plans for weaning (if the child has not already weaned).
- Explain the importance of the child gaining mastery of self-care (e.g., toileting, bathing, dressing, eating) and the valuable role the parent plays as teacher in the process. Assist parents to cope with the frustration or tensions generated by toddlers and

preschoolers wanting to "do it myself." Ask the parents how they handle these situations.
- Ask if parents are concerned about the child becoming overweight.
- Remind parents that injury is a leading cause of early childhood morbidity and mortality so continued and updated child proofing the home is needed, and "choking foods" should be avoided (Chapter 24).
- Encourage young children to help with their self-care. They can brush their own teeth and hair and clean up in the bath, and the parents can go behind them to ensure that they did a sufficient job.

Communication and Language

Children learn and refine communication and language skills best through their interactions with others. When parents and caregivers listen to them, talk interactively with them, and read to them, children's language blossoms. Encourage parents to stimulate their child's language skills by doing the following:
- Read to children daily, using short, simple stories or picture books.
- Model appropriate language.
- Talk to the child, explaining in clear, simple language what is happening around the child; this helps increase vocabulary and the child's understanding of the world. Quality reciprocal speech is the best way to help children learn to express themselves (Head Zauche et al., 2017).
- Listen with care and respond actively to the child.
- Provide opportunities to interact verbally with other children and adults.
- Do not allow children younger than 2 years old to watch television, and limit television viewing, smartphone, tablet, and

videos to less than 1 hour of developmentally appropriate programs per day for older children. Remove televisions from children's bedrooms, watch programs with them, and talk about what is happening (Hagan et al., 2017).

Providers should give parents the following anticipatory guidance:

- Explain that children need constant reinforcement of their speech and language efforts, but remind them that nonverbal language, especially touch, remains crucial.
- Give parents an opportunity to explain their expectations for their child; discourage parental pressure on the child to perform (e.g., use of flash cards, requirement that child articulate sounds correctly), and point out that daily activities provide a wealth of opportunities to practice language skills.
- Reassure parents that language errors of young children usually disappear as children grow.
- Inform parents that children learn receptive language first, then expressive, and they may not understand meaning, especially connotative meaning, of what they hear or say (e.g., a 4-year-old child may innocently ask a stranger about his or her private body parts). Parents should explain clearly, simply, and unemotionally which words are appropriate and in which settings.

Social and Emotional Growth

The emotional development of toddlers is an area in which parents need anticipatory guidance and support. The balance between dependence and independence is constantly in flux for young children and their parents, and conflict can develop from inconsistent or extreme behavior. Toddlers and preschoolers master multiple social tasks during these years. They learn how to identify, control, and manage their feelings and emotions around anger, joy, love, and frustration. They learn about making and keeping friends, sharing, cooperative play, and living socially within a family. They learn to handle separation from parents, home, and neighborhood. To help families with this process, providers should:

- Reemphasize the role of parents as guides of their child's social and emotional growth. Parents must actively engage with their children, showing interest in their activities and giving them guidance on appropriate behavior.
- Encourage parents to give their children opportunities to expand social skills and form important attachments outside the immediate family by:
  - Providing toys that children can use creatively.
  - Allowing children to explore, guiding them to activities that are fun and stimulate their curiosity.
  - Structuring time for children to play in natural settings. "Nature play" enhances physical, mental, and emotional health of children (Seltenrich, 2015).
  - Allowing children to make choices when possible; do not give children a "choice" when there really is none (e.g., "Do you want to go to bed?"). Instead, use "toddler's choices" that allow the child to have a say and yet still get toward the final objective (e.g., "Do you want to put your pants on or your shirt on first? Do you want to take the bunny or the bear with you during your nap?").
  - Discussing differences among people openly and positively.
  - Helping children identify, name, and express feelings, both positive and negative.
  - Teaching children to manage anger and resolve conflicts without violence.
  - Limiting screen time and discussing television programs and movies to help children distinguish fantasy from reality.

- Taking children on trips to places of interest in the community.
- Arranging play times with other children; encourage cooperative play (e.g., tag, hide-and-seek).
- Reinforcing positive behavior ("catch the child being good").
- Making clear, consistent, and achievable expectations for the child.
- Differentiate discipline and teaching from punishment (see Chapter 15).
- Help parents to resolve different expectations for their children.
- Provide information to parents related to child development and what parents can expect their child to be able to do. The CDC has a number of free development handouts available online at https://www.cdc.gov/ncbddd/childdevelopment/index.html
- Recommend evidence-based parenting resources that provide information on developmental milestones, anticipated changes, and management strategies as children grow.
- Encourage parents to show affection in the family.
- Explain to parents that myths or fables can be important ways of teaching children abstract concepts, such as love, sharing, and giving.
- Inform parents of the need to provide children a feeling of safety and security. Parents can do the following:
  - Support use of comfort or transitional objects to allay fears (e.g., blanket).
  - Consider providing a nightlight.
  - Reassure if nightmares or fears occur and respond to the child's fears.
  - Explain about "good" and "bad" touch.
  - Reinforce that the child can always come to the parent for comfort.

Cognitive and Environmental Stimulation

- Explain to parents that toddlers and preschoolers are concrete and preoperational in their thinking. As a result, parents need to be ready to explain things over and over patiently, without expecting the child to understand the adult's interpretation clearly. Also, children may use words to convey thoughts and feelings, but many responses are repetitive, and trial-and-error problem solving is usually crude. They frequently attend to only one aspect of a problem, giving partial answers.
- Emphasize that parents should avoid putting their own meaning on the child's behavior or statements. For example, the child's statement, "What if you bought a new house and I had allergies to something in the house? I guess you'd have to get rid of me," should not be interpreted to mean the parents have somehow failed to show the child how much they love him or her. Rather the child can be exploring the concepts of place, ownership, belonging, size, or importance. In the child's mind, a house is much bigger than he or she is and may be more important. An appropriate response from the parent might be, "No, we'd probably have to get a new house or take out whatever is making you sick. Even if we just bought it, you are more important than any house, and we wouldn't want to lose you."
- Reassure parents that "Why?" will not continue to be the child's most frequent question. Toddlers and preschoolers are actively exploring meaning in their world and have learned that asking "Why?" brings them more information—and attention. As parents answer them, children begin to show threads of symbolic and more abstract thought.

Common Developmental Issues in Early Childhood

Sibling Rivalry

Interaction patterns between siblings vary and are affected by factors, such as gender, age, temperament, degree of attachment, nature of family interactions, types of discipline used in the family, and children's perceptions of how equally parents treat each child. Many toddlers or preschoolers regress when a new baby arrives, whereas older children may experience excitement, love, and enhanced self-esteem with a new sibling. Parents need to promptly limit any aggression expressed by the older child, provide love and attention, and talk about feelings. When older children fight, parents need to describe the situation and provide even-handed control. Blaming a child, except in a clear-cut instance of misbehavior, is usually unproductive. Promoting support, loyalty, and friendship is important for sibling interactions.

The birth or adoption of a sibling is a life-changing experience for the older sibling. Many parents voice concerns about the potential challenges with the older siblings, especially transient behavioral regressions that occur after a new infant is brought home. The developmental stage of the older sibling at the time of the new sibling's arrival is an important consideration in helping parents prepare their older child for the new sibling and in dealing with rivalry behaviors. For example, the 2-year-old child working on developing autonomy often feels highly vulnerable with the appearance of a new sibling.

Additionally, many school-age children experience feelings of sibling rivalry, which may continue in varying degrees as the children grow and develop. Sibling rivalry involves the realization by the child that he or she must share his or her parents' attention and affection. The child may feel threatened or displaced.

Assessment

To assess sibling rivalry after the arrival of a new infant, ask the parent whether the older child has:
- Manifested regressive behaviors since the new sibling arrived (e.g., bed-wetting, return to the bottle, temper tantrums, separation issues).
- Made negative comments about the new sibling or has demonstrated verbal or physical aggression toward the parents or new sibling.
- Voiced psychosomatic complaints.
  To assess sibling rivalry at any point, ask parents to:
- Describe sibling behaviors that concern them—fighting, verbal abuse, bickering.
- Identify any precipitating events or situations that seem to elicit negative behaviors between the siblings.
- Identify how rivalry behaviors between siblings were handled in the past and encourage the siblings to resolve the issues between them rather than the parents.
  The provider should also ask parents to describe how they reacted to the behaviors or verbal comments and if and how they have disciplined the child.

Management

The cornerstone of the management of sibling rivalry is anticipatory guidance and prevention. The provider needs to prepare parents before the arrival of the new sibling for the possibility of sibling rivalry and guide them in managing this situation. Before delivery or adoption:
- Explain to parents that at the time of the arrival of the new baby the other sibling(s) may exhibit regressive behaviors.

Do
- Allow children to vent negative feelings.
- Encourage children to develop solutions for problems with siblings.
- Anticipate problem situations.
- Foster individuality in each child.
- Spend time with children individually.
- Compliment children when they are playing together well.
- Tell children about the conflict you had with your siblings when you were a child.
- Define acceptable and unacceptable behaviors for sibling interactions.

Do Not
- Take sides.
- Serve as a referee.
- Foster rivalry by comparing siblings or their accomplishments.
- Use derogatory names.
- Permit physical or verbal abuse between siblings.

- Encourage parents to do the following:
  - Tell the child about the pregnancy or adoption of the new baby, using a time frame and language appropriate to the child's developmental stage.
  - Investigate the possibility of sibling preparation classes for older siblings.
  - Prepare the child for a change in daily routines and change in the amount of time he or she will have with the parents.
  - Give children realistic expectations of their interactions with the baby.
  - Include an older child in preparations for the new baby and in the excitement of the event (e.g., have the child visit the mother and baby in the hospital if possible).
  After the infant or child comes home:
- Encourage parents to consistently spend "alone time" each day with the older sibling.
- Have parents include the older sibling in the care of the new baby as appropriate (e.g., the toddler can help by bringing Mommy a diaper).
- Reinforce the older sibling's efforts to be a "big brother or sister"; praise the child for helping.
- Explain the need for tolerance when a child exhibits regressive behaviors, knowing the behaviors are not permanent.
- Educate parents about teaching children to distinguish between acceptable and unacceptable behaviors as well as accountability for negative behaviors.
  As siblings grow, parents should avoid intervening for minor squabbles; rather they should encourage child-centered articulation of more significant arguments, and intervene if physical or verbal abuse occurs. Box 11.1 has other strategies to help siblings develop healthy relationships.

Temper Tantrums

Parents struggle with how to handle temper tantrums, which are episodes in which the child is frustrated and angry and loses control of his or her feelings (see Chapter 15).

Toilet Training

Toilet training occurs in the toddler and preschool years and is usually complete by the time the child is 4 years old, with the majority

TABLE 11.11 Guidelines for Toilet Training Readiness Assessment

Skill Type	Description
Child's physical skills	Has voluntary sphincter control Stays dry for 2 h; may wake from naps still dry Is able to sit, walk, and squat Assists in dressing self
Child's cognitive skills	Recognizes urge to urinate or defecate Understands meaning of words used by family in toileting Understands what the toilet is for Understands connection between dry pants and toilet Is able to follow directions Is able to communicate needs
Child's interpersonal skills	Demonstrates desire to please parent Expresses curiosity about use of toilet Expresses desire to be dry and clean
Parental skills	Expresses desire to assist child with training Recognizes child's cues of readiness Has no compelling factor that will interfere with training (e.g., new job, move, newborn, and/or family loss or gain)

BOX 11.2 Management of Toilet Training

- Keep child as clean and dry as possible:
  - Change diapers frequently.
  - Use training pants or underwear when child stays dry for several hours during the day; use diaper at night.
- Talk to child about toilet training:
  - Praise child for asking to have diaper changed.
  - Explain connection between being clean and dry and using toilet.
  - Emphasize that the goal is to eliminate in the toilet, not to hold to stay clean and dry.
  - Provide opportunity for child to use toilet, especially before going out to play, going on a trip, before naps, and at bedtime; set an example with adult behavior.
  - Do not ask child if they need to go, rather set up a time schedule of every 1½ h for voiding, and state matter-of-factly it is time to go.
- Teach child how to use toilet:
  - Allow child to observe while parents or older siblings use toilet.
  - Demonstrate how to sit on toilet with feet supported and knees spread with forward pelvic tilt, use toilet paper, flush, and wash hands.
- Provide practice time for child:
  - Provide a potty chair or portable toilet seat.
  - Allow child to sit on potty chair with clothes or diaper on.
  - Encourage child to use potty chair while parent uses regular toilet.
  - Have child sit on potty chair without diapers for 5-10 min at a time.
  - Practice at times the child usually urinates or defecates.
- Provide a comfortable, safe-feeling environment:
  - Seat child facing backward on a regular toilet or provide a footstool to rest the feet on with knees wide and forward pelvic tilt.
  - Never flush the toilet when child is sitting on it. Use sticky notes to stop automatic flush on public toilets.
  - Stay with child for safety reasons.
- Give consistent, positive feedback:
  - Praise child for trying and for success.
  - Be understanding of child's refusal to use toilet.
  - Never demand performance.
  - Never make child sit on toilet if child resists.
  - Ignore or minimize undesired behavior.
  - Never scold or punish if a child wets or soils.
  - Use star chart or other reward for success or effort; consider having the reward the child is working toward in the bathroom so that the job and reward are clearly connected for the child.
- Do not praise excessively.

of children training between 2½ and 3½ years old. Successful toilet training requires sensitivity, understanding of development, good communication, hope, humor, and patience. In addition to becoming self-sufficient in their toileting, children should also learn that elimination is a natural and necessary process. As self-toileting is mastered, both parents and children should experience pride and satisfaction in having worked together to accomplish an important developmental task.

The healthcare provider plays an important role in providing anticipatory guidance to parents. Introduce the topic of toilet training at the 18-month visit; assess parents' expectations and plans, and provide ample opportunity for discussion and possible development of realistic toileting outcomes. It can also be useful to tell parents that age at toilet training is not related to or indicative of intelligence.

Parents perennially ask when is the best time to start toilet training. Providers should emphasize that every child is unique, and readiness cues should ultimately be used to decide when to begin training. Physiologic readiness develops by about 18 months. True voluntary sphincter control is a function of psychological and social development as well, so most children are not usually ready for independent toilet training until 24 months or older. Guidelines for assessing toilet-training readiness include physical, cognitive, interpersonal or psychological, and parental skills (Table 11.11). It is also essential that parents understand and can express to children that the goal is to use the toilet, not to hold in urine or stool. This is an important distinction, as holding of urine and/or stool can lead to bowel and bladder dysfunction (BBD).

As families from various cultural groups immigrate to the United States, health care providers need to understand family practices and be open to developing mutually agreed-upon approaches to toilet training. Many cultures start toilet training earlier or later than what is typically practiced in the United States, and toilet training strategies vary widely. As

such, it is critical to understanding parents' expectations for the process.

If begun too early, toilet training can be very stressful for both parents and children and can contribute to family dysfunction. Starting independent toilet training before 24 or after 30 months has also been found to be related to dysfunctional voiding and (in delayed training) constipation (Hodges et al., 2014).

Typically, children first learn nocturnal bowel control, and then daytime bowel control, daytime bladder control, and finally nocturnal bladder control. Average times for being fully trained are around 3 to 4 years old, with a normal age variation of up to 1 year for individual children.

There is little evidence regarding which, if any, toilet training strategy (e.g., child-oriented approach; operant conditioning) is most effective. When children and parents are ready to begin toilet training, several management techniques can be helpful (Box 11.2). If children resist training, the effort should be put on hold for a few weeks before trying again. It is important to stress to parents that none of these "holds" should be viewed as a failure for either parent or child. If toddlers seem to be toilet trained for a brief period and suddenly regress to wetting and soiling consistently, they should be placed back in diapers and the process begun again within a few weeks. It is extremely important that parents and children do not become engaged in a "battle for control" over toilet training. For example, providers should emphasize to parents that they should never ask the child, "Do you need to go potty, pee, and so on?" The answer will always be "No," and thus an immediate battle ensues that is not even about the actual toileting. Ultimately, it is the child's responsibility to control his or her bowel and urinary function, and toilet training is only one of the many tasks toddlers master on their way to independence. Parents have the responsibility to assist in the process by providing a positive environment and opportunities, teaching the techniques, and setting a positive example. It appears that a structured yet flexible approach that is responsive to the child's cues is likely to be most successful. Parents should be reassured that this needs to be individualized to each parent/child dyad and may be different for siblings.

Parents can become extremely frustrated if their expectations do not match the abilities and performance of their children, and child abuse related to toilet training may occur. PCPs play a crucial role in making the experience a positive one and preventing abuse by giving parents information about child development, techniques for managing the training process, and support and encouragement for their efforts. This includes proactively doing follow-up with families who express frustration or appear to be having difficulty with the toilet training process.

Child Care and Preschools

Child Care

Many parents return to work during the first year of their child's life and must make arrangements for child care. In 2016, 60% of children under 5 years old attended at least one weekly nonparenteral care arrangement (Corcoran and Steinley, 2017). In 2016, 65% of mothers with preschool-aged children (younger than 6 years old) were employed, and 75% of women with children between 6 and 17 years old were employed (Bureau of Labor Statistics, 2017). Child care issues affect millions of people and can be a source of significant parental concern. Parents are challenged with evaluating and selecting a qualified child care provider who provides a safe, nurturing, and developmentally appropriate setting. The individual needs of the child together with parental needs for work coverage and flexibility must be matched with the philosophy and constraints of the child care setting. The primary care provider is often called on to advise parents about how to select a suitable provider (Box 11.3).

Preschool

Entering preschool can be stressful for both the children attending the school and their families. Some children have difficulty adapting to the more structured school environment, whereas others are comfortable with limits and rules. Parents may find their child compared with other children, and a child with developmental delays (e.g., speech, motor, physical) may be singled out as different, not fitting in, or as having a behavior problem. Preschool and kindergarten were originally intended to help children learn separation, sharing, listening, paying attention, and simple social skills. Now, kindergarten students are often expected to show pre-academic skills, such as writing, counting, and letter and word recognition, in addition to the preschool social skills of paying attention and sitting still. In making their

> ## • BOX 11.3 A Five-Step Approach to Help Parents Select a Child Care Provider
>
> **Step 1**
>
> Begin searching for child care as early as possible. Deciding whether to use a child care center or an individual home is a very personal decision. It can take a while to find the right fit for your child and family.
>
> **Step 2**
>
> Familiarize yourself with local child care rules and regulations. Local and state child care licensing boards can provide lists of accredited child care facilities and information about the rules and regulations in your area. They also can provide information about formal child care complaints and violations.
>
> **Step 3**
>
> Visit potential child care sites. Drop in at different times and pay attention to the environment and how the staff responds to the children in their care.
> - Ask what the adult-to-child ratio is. Older children do not need the same level of attention as infants, so ratios tend to increase as the child ages. Make sure you know what the minimum state ratios are for your area.
> - Ask how many children are in each class/group. Think about your child's personality and needs and try to match the group size to what is best for your child. Large groups with multiple adults are very different from smaller groups with fewer adults.
> - Ask how child care providers are selected and what training and education they require. Caregivers with degrees in early child education (or who have special training) have skills that will foster your child's learning. It is important to know what kinds of continuing education caregivers receive.
> - Ask how often children change caregivers and ask about staff turnover. Children do best with consistent care and with regular caregivers. Just like they crave routine at home, children desire routines and consistent caregivers in child care.
> - Ask if the child care provider is accredited by a national organization. Accredited providers demonstrate they meet standards that are usually higher than state standards. National accreditation can be verified on the accrediting agency's website.
>
> **Step 4**
>
> When you make your decision about which child care provider to use, start by thinking about your child's and family's needs. Take into account all the information you received during your search.
>
> **Step 5**
>
> Stay involved with your child's child care. Talk to your child's caregivers. Don't be afraid to ask questions about your child's day and how he/she is doing during the day. Tell your child's caregiver about how your child is doing at home. For example, if your child is having trouble napping at home, asking about how naps are going at the child care can give you important information. Try to attend special events like field trips or holiday parties. You are your child's most important caregiver, and children do best when parents and child care caregivers work together as a team.
>
> Child Care Aware: Five steps to choosing care *(website)*. http://childcareaware.org/resources/printable-materials/. Accessed February 5, 2018.

preschool selection, parents should select a play-based learning curriculum, because this is the most comfortable way for young children to learn. Chapter 12 includes an in-depth discussion of school readiness.

When selecting a preschool, it is important to consider the following child characteristics:
- Social skills (e.g., ability to separate from parent for several hours)
- Language skills, both expressive and receptive

- Physical size
- Energy level (e.g., ability to actively participate)
- Neurologic maturation required for fine and gross motor activities (e.g., writing, cutting, coloring, climbing, running, walking)
- Neurologic maturation of sensory and cognitive function (e.g., visuospatial perception, tactile maturation, auditory processing, attending skills, memory)

Safety

Parents should safety-proof any environments their children spend time in but also need to know that safety-proofing is not enough; toddlers and preschool children need to have adult supervision at all times (see Chapter 24).

Developmental Red Flags in Early Childhood

Although there is a wide range of normal development, the provider needs to be alert to developmental red flags—signs of delayed or abnormal development. In addition to obvious abnormalities, minor problems that are left untreated can develop into major concerns; minor signs and symptoms that persist can indicate a more serious underlying problem, or a major problem can occur as a one-time event (e.g., a child who sets a fire). Some children and families are at high risk and need careful monitoring and guidance to detect problems at an early stage or to prevent their occurrence (e.g., very early premature infants, families with a history of violence, families with chronic medical or mental health problems, some single-parent families). The warning signs, or red flags, can be found in Table 11.12. Children who demonstrate these behaviors should be referred. Immediate referral is required for children who stop eating, demonstrate cruelty to animals or other people, are self-harmful, start fires, or talk of harming themselves, their peers, or others.

Physical Disorders

Children should be monitored for physical growth milestones. Further investigation, screening, and referral may be appropriate when children fall outside normal growth parameters or when children follow a normal growth pattern and begin to level off or fall below that range. If children have symptoms—they stop eating, complain of tiredness, are not as active as usual, or the parents state that the child has regressed—it is time to investigate.

Cognitive Disorders

Mental and cognitive delays are more difficult to recognize and categorize without the help of a screening tool or more in-depth assessment. These tools rank children based on a standardized score or against standardized criteria (e.g., word definition). Children with scores below 85 on intelligence scales, for example, predictably have more difficulty in school. Significant discrepancies between test scores taken over time also suggest problems. The causes of delay must be carefully assessed as well because some children may have a neurologic limitation, whereas others may be delayed because of material or environmental deprivation. Identifying the causes is necessary to plan effective interventions. In any case, when delays are suspected, prompt referral to developmental specialists or early childhood intervention programs for more detailed assessment is essential.

Language Disorders

Language delays or disorders are problems in learning communication systems and, when present, affect other areas of development, especially cognitive, social, and emotional development. Because language development is the best indicator of cognitive development, language delays may indicate serious issues that require developmental and educational intervention.

Children with language delays experience problems in either receptive or expressive language, or both. They may start talking late, talk very little as toddlers, or have prolonged stages of normal stuttering, distortion, and substitution.

Cognitive, familial, environmental, physical, psychological, or cultural factors can cause language delays. Language delays or disorders may occur if the child does not hear, is not immersed in a language-rich environment, or has a disorder, such as severe deprivation or autism. Speech disorders (i.e., problems producing sounds) are associated with physical problems (e.g., cleft lip, cleft palate, cerebral palsy, hearing impairments) or they can be idiopathic.

Language evaluation involves assessment of the child's physical, cognitive, social, emotional, and perceptual characteristics. Expressive and receptive language needs to be evaluated. The inability to use the symbols of language may be characterized by the following:

- Improper use of words and their meanings
- Inappropriate grammatical patterns
- Improper use of speech sounds

Speech disorders involve problems producing correct speech sounds and may be characterized by difficulty in the following:

- Producing speech sounds (articulation)
- Maintaining speech rhythm (fluent speech)
- Controlling vocal production (voice)

Management of children with language disorders requires a clear understanding of the nature of the problem. Referral to a specialist (e.g., pediatric speech pathologist) to make that determination is often the first step. Deficits identified in Table 11.10 are cause for referral for additional testing. Other criteria that warrant referral include the following:

- There are unusual connected speech confusion, reversals, or telescoping.
- There is a loss of previously acquired language skills.
- The child stops talking.
- The child reacts to his or her own speech with embarrassment or withdrawal.
- The child's voice is monotone, extremely loud, largely inaudible, or of poor quality.
- Pitch is not appropriate to the child's age and gender.
- Hypernasality or lack of nasal resonance occurs.

TABLE 11.12   Red Flags of Early Childhood Development

Age	Growth, Rhythmicity, Sleep, and Temperament	Psychosocial and Emotional Skills	Cognitive Abilities	Gross Motor, Language, and Hearing	Fine Motor, Feeding, and Self-Care	Strength and Coordination
12 months		No big smiles or joyful expressions		No babbling No recognizing name when called	Is not pointing or using sounds to get desired object; may just cry	No attempts at walking
15 months	No nighttime ritual Difficulty with transitions Parents express concern about temperament or control issues	Problems with attachment to caregiver	Lack of object permanence	No words Only single words by 16 months Lack of consonant production, uses mostly vowel sounds Consistent and frequent omission of initial consonants Does not imitate words No gestures or pointing	No self-feeding	
18 months	Poor sleep schedule Problems with control and behavior	Does not pull person to show something	Primary play: mouthing of toys No finger exploration of objects Lack of imitation Not using toys as they were intended	Unable to follow simple directions (e.g., "no," "jump") Excessive, indiscriminate, irrelevant verbalizing	Does not try to scribble spontaneously Unable to use spoon	Not yet walking or frequently falls when walking
24 months	Falling off growth curve Poor sleep schedule Awakens at night; unable to put self back to sleep	Absent symbolic play No evidence of parallel play Displays destructive behaviors Always clings to parent	No pretend play	No meaningful two-word phrases Use of noncommunicative speech (echolalia, rote phrases) Unable to identify five pictures Unable to name body parts No jargon History of greater than 10 episodes of otitis media	Unable to stack four or five blocks Still eating pureed foods Unable to imitate scribbles on paper Unable to dump pellet from bottle	Unable to walk downstairs holding a rail Persistent waddle walk Persistent toe walking
30 months	Resistance to regular bedtime Beginning behavior issues	Problems with biting, hitting playmates, parents Not able to play with others	Cannot follow two-step commands	Cannot name self Does not use pronouns	Unable to feed self Unable to build a tower of six blocks Unable to copy a circle shape Unable to imitate vertical stroke	Unable to jump in place Unable to kick ball on request

36 months	Problems with toilet training Unable to calm self	Not able to dress self Does not understand taking turns No expanded pretend play	Cannot name familiar colors Does not understand "same" and "different" Unable to recognize common objects Unable to recall parts of a story	Unable to give full name Unable to match two colors Does not use plurals Does not know 2 or 3 prepositions Unable to tell a story Unclear consonants Unintelligible speech Unable to speak in sentences	Unable to build a tower of 10 blocks Holds crayon with fist Unable to draw circle	Unable to balance on one foot for 1 s Toeing-in causes tripping with running
48 months	Lack of bedtime ritual Behavior concerns: Withdrawn or acting out Stool holding Problems with toilet training	Unable to play games, follow rules Unable to follow limits or rules at home (e.g., put toys away) Cruelty to animals, friends Interest in fires, fire starting Persistent fears or severe shyness Inability to separate from parent	Unable to count three objects Unable to recall 4 numbers Unable to identify what to do with danger, fire, and a stranger Consistently poor judgment	Difficulty understanding language Problems understanding prepositions Limited vocabulary Unclear speech	Lack of self-care skills—dressing feeding, Unable to button clothes Unable to copy square	Unable to balance on one foot for 4 s Unable to alternate steps when climbing stairs
60 months	Sleep problems Concerns with night terrors Hair pulling—scalp or eyelashes	Difficulty making and keeping friends; no friends Difficulty understanding sharing, school rules, organization of daily activities Cruelty to animals, friends Interest in fires, fire starting Bullying or being bullied Prolonged fighting, hitting, hurting Withdrawal, sadness, extreme rituals	Unable to count to 10 Unable to identify colors Unable to follow three-step commands	Speech pattern not 100% understandable Cannot identify a penny, nickel, or dime Abnormal rate or rhythm of speech	Unable to copy triangle Unable to draw a person with a body	Difficulty hopping, jumping

References

Borrell L, Graham L, Joseph S. Associations of neighborhood safety and neighborhood support with overweight and obesity in US children and adolescents. *Ethn Dis.* 2016;26(4):469–476.

Bureau of Labor Statistics. *News release, employment of characteristics of families summary.* Bureau of Labor Statistics (website); 2017. https://www.bls.gov/news.release/pdf/famee.pdf. Accessed February 5, 2018.

Child Care Aware. Five steps to choosing care *(website).* http://childcareaware.org/resources/printable-materials/. Accessed February 5, 2018.

Corcoran L, Steinley K. *Early Childhood Program Participation, From the National Household Education Surveys Program of 2016 (NCES 2017-101).* Washington, DC: National Center for Education Statistics, Institute of Education Sciences. U.S. Department of Education; 2017. Retrieved from: http://nces.ed.gov/pubsearch. Accessed April 4, 2018.

Hagan JF, Shaw JS, Duncan PM, eds. *Bright Futures: Guidelines for Health Supervision of Infants, Children, and Adolescents.* 4th ed. Elk Grove Village, IL: American Academy of Pediatrics; 2017.

Head Zauche L, Darcy Mahoney AE, Thui TA, et al. The power of language nutrition for children's brain development, health, and future academic achievement. *J Pediatr Healthcare.* 2017;31(4):493–503.

Hoff E, Core C. What clinicians need to know about bilingual development. *Semin Speech Lang.* 2015;36(2):89–99.

Rock L, Crow S. *Not Just "Soft Skills": How Young Children's Learning & Health Benefit from Strong Social-Emotional Development.* New York: Clinton Foundation; 2017.

Seltenrich N. Just what the doctor ordered: using parks to improve children's health. *Environ Health Perspect.* 2015;123(10).

12

Developmental Management of Middle Childhood

VICTORIA F. KEETON

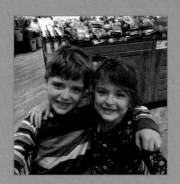

Children in middle childhood are busy, active, curious, and creative. With guidance and encouragement, they eagerly apply the skills they learned in early childhood as they move into structured school environments, home schooling, or community settings. The school-age years include middle childhood (6 to 9 years old) and late childhood (10 to 12 years old). Each school-age child is unique, and typical development patterns have broad parameters. Developmental goals of middle childhood include laying the groundwork for lifelong learning, creating a sense of self-worth, developing the ability to contribute to the world around them, and ultimately gaining satisfaction with life.

Primary health care providers (PCPs) must be familiar with theoretic models of physical, cognitive, and psychosocial development in order to provide holistic care for this age group (see Chapter 8). Providers can support children and their families to be successful in their achievements during these important years through appropriate anticipatory guidance and health promotion education.

Developmental Approach to Health Assessment and Health Promotion for Middle Childhood

This section discusses the developmental context for the elements of the preventive health visit in order to provide high-quality and comprehensive care for school-age children and their families.

Physical Development

The growth rate in middle and late childhood increases significantly from that of early childhood. Pre-pubertal children gain an average of 2 inches and 5 to 7 pounds/year (Duderstadt, 2018). Head circumference may increase slowly but is no longer routinely measured. Physical growth and neurologic maturation give children the ability to master many new skills. By middle childhood, the brain is about 90% of its adult size (Duderstadt, 2018). The cerebral cortex (responsible for intelligence) and the frontal lobe (responsible for problem-solving and decision-making) are the last to fully develop. Increasing brain maturation allows children

to complete increasingly complex motor and cognitive skills and to have greater control over their bodies. Visual development is generally complete by 6 years old (Duderstadt, 2018). Table 12.1 gives an overview of typical physical development for middle childhood.

School-age children may appear to be totally unaware of their bodies (e.g., the 9-year-old boy who does not change his shirt for 3 days). In fact, children at this age are extremely curious about changes happening to them as they grow and are sensitive to others around them. Highly literal in their thinking, they can be very frank with questions to people they trust (e.g., "Grandma, why are you growing a moustache?"). Their achievements and failures help them define who they are and are the basis for their evolving self-image. Social status among children is often based on physical competence; therefore the child's feelings about physical development can be as important as the physical growth itself. Their body images come from the experiences they have and feedback from family, peers, teachers, and others in the community. This feedback can help clarify their understandings and allow the child to gain self-confidence and feelings of worth.

Exploration of the sexual organs, including masturbation, is common in this period. Children in middle childhood will often compare their bodies with friends of the same sex. At the same time, they are learning the importance of social politeness (e.g., what is appropriate and how to behave in certain situations) and may be uncomfortable or shy about new or unusual situations. During puberty, children may have mixed feelings about physical changes occurring in the body, ranging from curiosity and excitement to anxiety and shame. These feelings may be amplified for children who are gender nonconforming, and the changes in their bodies may create discomfort or distress (see Chapter 21).

History

Begin with open-ended questions about any physical changes the child or caregiver notices and any concerns they have regarding growth or physical development. It is important to explore the child's feelings about body image and sexual maturation (as appropriate), as well as whether he or she has experienced bullying associated with body size or other physical characteristics. Investigate

TABLE 12.1	Physical Development in Middle Childhood
Body System	**Developmental Change**
Skin and lymph	At about 6 years old, tonsils and adenoids reach their largest size Prepubescence is characterized by more active sebaceous glands and vasomotor instability that can lead to uncontrolled blushing. Pubertal development can begin as early as 8-10 years old, including increased hair growth in axilla and genital regions
Head, eyes, ears, nose, and mouth	Head size becomes smaller in proportion to body size Undeveloped sinus cavities contribute to increased susceptibility to upper respiratory infections, sinus irritation, and sinus headaches By 6-7 years old, the retina is fully developed; visual acuity is 20/20 By middle childhood, the Eustachian tube becomes longer, narrower, and more slanted Primary teeth are intermittently shed and permanent teeth erupt
Pulmonary	Lungs gradually descend into the thoracic cavity By 8 years old, alveolar development is complete Tidal volume increases and normal adult respiratory rate is achieved (18-30 breaths/min) Increased maturation of the macrophagocytic activity of mucus and ciliary function in lungs makes the child more resistant to lower respiratory infections
Cardiovascular	By 5 years old, the heart is four times larger than at birth By 7 years old, the left ventricle thickens and is two to three times greater in size than the right; blood pressure increases to 90-108/60; cardiac volume increases; heart rate declines to 60-100 bpm; atherosclerosis begins
Gastrointestinal	Gastrointestinal tract size and function are adult-like
Genitourinary	By 6 years old, elimination patterns are established; greater than 90% of children are toilet trained Bladder capacity continues to expand Between 10 and 14 years old, puberty begins but can be normal in females after 8 years old or at 9 years old in males Delayed puberty is diagnosed if no secondary sex changes (e.g., breast budding; penis or testicle growth) are noted at 12 years old in girls and 14 years old in boys
Musculoskeletal	Long bones grow, leading to the taller, thinner school-age child Spine and legs become straighter Facial bones are actively changing as nasal accessory sinuses grow
Immune system	Rapid maturation of the immune system during middle childhood Allergic conditions may appear

statements suggestive of disordered eating or weight modification behaviors (see Chapter 30). A discussion about physical capabilities and endurance during peer play or sports can help elicit data about potential respiratory or cardiac problems, such as shortness of breath or fatigue with activity. Conduct a comprehensive subjective review of systems to obtain information about general physical function.

Physical Examination

A review of the child's objective growth measurements and trends is the most accurate way to assess for appropriate growth, including body mass index calculation to evaluate for healthy weight. Physical modesty is characteristic of middle and late childhood, so it is important to conduct the physical exam with consideration of the child's privacy (Hagan et al., 2017). The head to toe examination provides evidence of the development and function of each body system. Sexual maturity staging of the breasts and genitals should be included at every preventive health visit.

Anticipatory Guidance

Education and guidance for the child and caregiver includes a review of typical physical changes and average growth expected in the following year. It is important to remind them that physical growth and development follow individual trajectories and there is much variation among children during this period. This is also

an opportunity to discuss increasing independence in self-care and hygiene. Table 12.2 offers more detailed suggestions of anticipatory guidance in this area.

Gross and Fine Motor Development

School-age children gain strength and coordination, and become more physically capable, setting the stage for participation in sports and other physical activities. In middle childhood, gross motor skills are refined, allowing children to run, jump, climb, hop, skip, tandem walk, alternate their foot patterns, and use an overhand motion (Duderstadt, 2018). Activities that require balance and coordination (e.g., riding a bicycle, swimming, and roller skating) demonstrate children's expanding skills. In late childhood, gross motor skills become more controlled and purposeful, and are perfected with practice. A sense of competition is high as children try to outlast or outperform one another. Consequently, school-age children may enjoy participating in competitive activities such as sports.

Mastery of fine motor skills includes improved dexterity and better control of scissors and writing tools, such as crayons and pencils. Their drawings become more recognizable, showing details of eyes, ears, and other body parts. Digital technology is part of daily life in the classroom, and children progress in

TABLE 12.2	Developmental Anticipatory Guidance Topics in Middle Childhood
Physical	Promote nutrition and physical activity to support a healthy weight Explain relationship between good health and self-care In early middle childhood, supervise personal hygiene (e.g., brushing teeth, bathing, combing hair, and nail care) For older school child, supervision of hygiene is minimal; occasional reminders may be necessary Encourage shared decision-making and self-care during illnesses and for chronic disease management Teach about pubertal body changes and variations in timing of puberty
Motor	Encourage child's participation in daily exercise; limit screen time to <2 h/day Provide opportunities to be active that are fun, involve family or peers, and require cognitive or social skills Encourage healthful hobbies and activities fostering fitness and increased motor skills Encourage activities that require training, commitment, and effort, especially for an older child Avoid factors that decrease child's motivation to be active (e.g., overscheduling activities, or choosing activities that prioritize competition over enjoyment)
Communication	Read stories to child and listen to child read aloud Role model by reading and writing often Encourage child to make notes, keep a journal, and write letters to friends and family members Talk with and actively listen to child; play word games Enroll in extracurricular programs that offer child an opportunity to engage in active conversation with other children and adults Never punish by removing books or writing materials Limit screen time to 1-2 h/day; no television in bedroom
Cognitive	Stimulate younger child's thinking about comparisons and differences (e.g., changes in shape, volume, directions to and from school) to facilitate cognition at the concrete operations level Discuss variables in objects or situations as experienced, to help move thinking away from the earlier egocentric style Provide opportunities to gain knowledge through reading, outings, classes, and family discussions Engage experiences with other languages, music, and cultural groups; promote broader understanding of the world Establish regular homework time and environment that encourages focus and task completion with limits clearly defined Provide help early if school problems arise; seek school's assistance in securing resources and services to assist child at school (e.g., request an Individualized Education Plan) Recognize academic achievement to motivate further success Stay involved with school assignments and evaluate progress to support child's work Encourage problem-solving efforts Provide more complex opportunities at home (e.g., planning and cooking meals, planning family outings, and managing a budget)
Social	Encourage family to establish and recognize traditions or special family activities (e.g., birthday celebrations, Sunday afternoon walks, and videos and popcorn on Saturday night) Make clear home rules and expectations; apply consistently Teach respect for authority and help child learn to communicate well with other adults Play and work together as a family to teach child how to work together in a team (e.g., jobs or chores around the house) and to practice conflict resolution Provide opportunities for child to make and develop friendships with a variety of children, teaching how to initiate, sustain, and terminate relationships with friends; include child's friends in some family activities Teach how to read social cues and supervise experiences in which child can practice new skills successfully Discuss family values and rules; explain differences child may face when away from home Provide opportunities for appropriate behavior when values are challenged (e.g., "You can say, 'No, my mom won't let me do that,' and then walk away") Monitor communication activities on social networking sites; set and adhere to rules for Internet use and social networking sites both inside and outside the home
Emotional	Provide positive expressions of love, concern, and pride to promote self-esteem and a sense of family belonging Help child identify and appropriately express emotions, including feelings of aggression and anger Provide fantasy play opportunities to allow child to deal safely with emotions and concerns and to develop creativity Help child with decision-making and accepting consequences of actions Help child learn delayed gratification and increase frustration tolerance, while still remaining sympathetic Enhance goal setting and motivation with charts, calendars, and tally sheets. Let child set goals while caregivers monitor activities and point out options Provide opportunities to experiment with appropriate healthy behaviors that allow child to develop self-expression (e.g., school-age child can enjoy new hair styles or temporary tattoos) Provide opportunities to discuss emerging sexuality and sexual values in a safe and accepting manner

their mastery of keyboarding and touch screens. In early middle childhood, children become adept at dressing themselves, including being able to tie their shoelaces and manage buttons and zippers. Self-care skills (e.g., combing hair, brushing teeth) are improved. In late childhood, hand-eye coordination improves, and the child uses each hand independently with speed and smoothness. During this time, skill in playing musical instruments emerges.

TABLE 12.3	Progression of Communication Skills in Middle Childhood
6-7 years	Have basic syntactic abilities and can follow simple directions
	May not be accustomed to attending to total auditory stimuli (e.g., in the classroom environment)
	Still mastering connotative and semantic rules, such as understanding the concepts "before" and "after," relative clauses (e.g., "the cat was chased by the dog"), and the structures of sentences
	Difficult to follow complicated directions or cope with increased demands to recall information within a specific time frame
	Narrative skills can be poor; reading may be difficult
	Receptive language becomes strong; language decoding generally mastered; working on encoding information
	Organize previous knowledge and express it verbally or in writing; can solve word problems
	Articulation mastery of the "l" and "th" sounds may not be achieved until 7 or 8 years old
8-9 years	Significant syntactic growth with better use of pronouns and understanding of convoluted sentences
	Comparatives learned; able to distinguish qualities, such as more or less, near or far, and heavy or light
	Follow complex directions
	Begin to tell jokes because they understand different meanings of words
	Have better narrative and storytelling abilities, and summarization skills needed for activities such as explaining a task to other children
	Vocabulary grows with gradual improvements in grammar
10-12 years	Able to discuss ideas and understand inflections and metaphors
	Understand ambiguities of sentence structure, word meaning, and language; this contributes to their enjoyment of jokes and riddles
	Use concrete operational thinking to analyze and interpret language; more aware of the inconsistency in spoken languages
	Understand that words can mean more than their literal definition
	Able to answer questions involving sophisticated concepts
	Sentences should be grammatically correct; have more detail in their verbal skills
	Ability to verbally express emotion improves
	Language becomes a means of socializing with fewer gestures used

History

The history of gross and fine motor development in middle and late childhood centers on school performance, physical activity, and self-care. A review of participation in physical education or extracurricular physical activity may elicit concerns regarding gross motor abilities. Fine motor challenges may emerge in school as the child advances in writing tasks, and the caregiver may share concerns brought by the child's teacher. Competence in dressing, grooming and use of utensils during meals provide additional information about fine motor abilities.

If motor concerns were previously identified, there should be a school plan (such as an Individualized Education Plan [IEP] or 504 plan) that describes accommodations and services for the child, such as physical and/or occupational therapy (see Chapter 7). Copies of these plans can be uploaded into the child's medical record. These educational plans should be updated at least annually, so verify with the caregiver at each preventive visit if the child still requires support and whether the plan is up to date.

Physical Examination

Strength and coordination can be evaluated using a systematic musculoskeletal and neurologic examination. If the child participates in sports or other strenuous physical activity, a full 14-point preparticipation musculoskeletal examination should be included (see Chapter 19). Asking the child to write or draw during the visit is a simple way to evaluate fine motor abilities. Concerns about balance, coordination, strength, and mobility should be investigated depending on attention, school performance, and overall developmental function.

Anticipatory Guidance

Guidance for families surrounding motor skills includes the encouragement of physical activities and activities that promote dexterity, such as art or musical instruments. Children should be supported to consider various ways of being active that may not include team sports participation, such as dancing, riding a bicycle, swimming, or jumping rope. Explore ways children with physical limitations can participate in preferred activities and with their peers. Table 12.2 offers more detailed suggestions of anticipatory guidance in this area.

Communication and Language Development

The maturing brain is capable of increasingly complex receptive and expressive language skills. The child's language patterns provide insight into the status of the neurologic system. School-age children have a well-developed vocabulary and are able to retrieve words quickly; their expressive language should be fully intelligible (Hagan et al., 2017). Stuttering usually resolves by school age but may be seen if young children are overly eager to express themselves. Occasional or brief stuttering (repetition of sounds, syllables or short words) that does not cause the child distress is considered normal disfluency at this age (Perez and Stoeckle, 2016). Table 12.3 provides a more detailed summary of the progress of language development in this period.

Multilingualism is increasingly prevalent as societies become more and more diverse. Learning multiple languages has been shown to positively influence cognitive development (Barac, Bialystok, Castro, and Sanchez, 2014) and should be encouraged. Children who are learning English as a second language may need additional support as they try to juggle language learning with their other academic competencies. The assessment of communication skills in multilingual children should take into account their native language abilities; this also applies to children who are deaf or hearing impaired and use sign language for communication.

Communication disorders affect approximately 9% of children between the ages of 7 to 10 years of age (Black, 2015). Language delays and hearing impairment have been linked with motor coordination, behavior, and psychiatric comorbidities, such as attention-deficit and hyperactivity disorder (ADHD) (Stevenson, McCann, Watkin, Worsfold, and Kennedy, 2010). Although it is important that language delays be identified at a younger age, interventions and therapy for these conditions extend into school-age years. The perceptual difficulties experienced by these children require continued intervention to ensure learning success. Physical, occupational, and speech therapy are often necessary interventions through the school years (Muursepp, Aibast, Gapeyeva, and Paasuke, 2012).

History

School performance and reports from a child's teacher are good indicators of language skills. If language delays were identified and services rendered in the school system, a copy of the IEP or 504 plan should be requested and uploaded into the child's medical record. Each preventive visit provides an opportunity to verify with the caregiver if the child has received or requires support services. If the child presents with new concerns, these should be explored further, including a detailed history of hearing or related issues (such as frequent ear infections). Refer to school or other developmental specialists for formal diagnostic evaluation, if needed.

Physical Examination

Assessment of communication and language development is ongoing during the health care visit as the PCP talks directly with the child, probing for the child's level of understanding (e.g., Can the child follow directions? Does the child understand the PCP's explanations?). Pay attention throughout the visit to the child's articulation, vocabulary, sentence structure, and grammar. Note the child's ability to interact socially with the examiner, the caregiver, and others. If the provider does not speak the same language as the child, a certified interpreter should be used so that the child's command of his or her native language can be better appreciated.

Anticipatory Guidance

Mastering the ability to read, comprehend, and write is essential for the school-age child's academic success. Caregivers help advance vocabulary and grammar skills by engaging in conversation with and reading to their child. Emphasize the need to prioritize reading and writing activities over screen time and the use of electronic devices. Strong communication between the child's caregiver and teacher helps identify challenges early so that proper support can be provided (see Table 12.2).

Cognitive Development

In early childhood, children transition from preoperational thinking that uses intuitive problem-solving to early concrete operational thinking. Concrete operational abilities allow children to read, write, and communicate thoughts effectively. Magical thinking and egocentric logic fade, and concepts of conservation, transformation, reversibility, decentration, seriation, and classification emerge. Learning about the world, its people, and the views and values of others becomes possible. By late childhood, children should have well-developed concrete operational thinking. They are able to focus on more than one aspect of a problem and use logical thinking. New social skills appear with the ability to understand the viewpoints of others and the decline of egocentricity. Empathy, or the ability to share and understand another's

feelings, emerges—and with it, the capacity to make deep friendships (Hagan et al., 2017). School success fosters the development of a personal sense of competence. This is further facilitated by caregiver support.

Cognitively, school-age children face daunting challenges. They must master the intellectual skills of reading, writing, mathematics, science, and other academic work. Expectations for performance increase over the school years with examinations, graded papers, projects, and homework assignments. Many schools lack resources to maintain small class sizes or offer special programs for children with learning difficulties. Children with these issues are at risk for passing from grade to grade without remediation of their fundamental learning problems and with the stigma of failure. Unless struggling children are provided with social and remedial support, they may see school as an unpleasant burden, develop feelings of failure, and look for validation through nonacademic experiences. Social supports can help children cope with this stress, and interacting with healthy, interested, and caring adults is the strongest support children can have (Hagan et al., 2017).

History

Knowledge about the child's performance compared with that of their peers, the child's grades, and information from caregiver-teacher conferences provide data about cognitive abilities. Learning difficulties that arise should be explored further, including whether an evaluation and diagnosis has been made by a learning and developmental specialist. The use of school support services, such as tutoring, resource classes, or placement in a special education program, should be documented. If an IEP or 504 Plan is in place, it should be current from within the past year; a copy should be requested and placed in the child's medical record. For any new onset challenges, an assessment of vision and hearing concerns is important to determine whether impairment is a contributing factor.

Physical Examination

Assessment of cognitive development is difficult in school-age children. Generally, more detailed learning evaluations are more accurate than clinical judgments. Engaging the child in conversation throughout the visit and asking him or her to follow instructions with increasing complexity may provide initial data. If concerns arise in the history or physical exam, referral to an educational psychologist or other learning specialist is needed to obtain more definitive and objective information.

Anticipatory Guidance

Caregivers can support cognitive development by encouraging their child to engage with his or her environment and community in thoughtful ways. Conversations about everyday life and household tasks that promote age-appropriate advanced thinking related to problem-solving, empathy, and logic are helpful. Involvement in the child's schooling is important to know whether progress is being made and to evaluate the presence of quality and support received (see Table 12.2).

Social Development

The psychosocial development of school-age children puts to rest the notion that childhood is a "quiescent" period. During this time, they become skilled socially, separating from home and family, establishing friendships, negotiating with siblings and other family members, and working on developing a sound sense of who they are as unique members of the community (Hagan et al., 2017). The ability of children to form friendships depends on social cognitive development, a direct result of caregiver-child relationships during the developing years. As they move into the community, children maintain their role and feelings of belonging to a family, but also develop secondary attachments with other adults outside the home. Having positive relationships with adults outside the home is especially important when the family is not wholly functional or responsive to and supportive of the child (Hagan et al., 2017). It is also important in this age group to reinforce concepts around the recognition and avoidance of predatory adult behavior, both in person and through virtual media (Hagan et al., 2017).

It is important for school-age children to develop social interaction skills including how to understand social meaning and interpret others' social cues. They learn to form and engage in relationships through the initiation and termination of interactions with peers. Friends are generally chosen because of shared skills, interests, personality, and loyalty. Gaining social acceptance from one's peers depends on skills such as being socially responsive, understanding the group "rules," using the group jargon, being appropriately assertive, and being empathetic. Children who do not have those skills can experience a sense of failure when they are compared with their peers who do. Children often see themselves through the eyes of their friends. As early as 7 years old, some children are more concerned about a friend's opinion than about adults' opinions (Hagan et al., 2017). They develop "best friends" and dress and talk like their peers. A special-friend phase should occur at around 10 years old. With that friend, the child expands the self, learns altruism, shares feelings, and learns how others manage problems. Talking on the telephone, texting, emailing or using social media and sleepovers with friends become more common. These early friendships are the basis for later relationships. Family conflicts arise when peer activities and expectations conflict with family rules and values. Furthermore, the values of the family are challenged as the child learns that other families make decisions and have beliefs that differ from their own.

Relationships are crucial in normalizing biologic and behavioral systems in children exposed to adverse environments. Supportive, responsive relationships foster healthy child behavioral and biologic development (Thompson, 2014). Some children are given heavy responsibility at a young age. Many children care for themselves after school while their caregivers work, and may be alone, housebound, and unsupervised until adults return at the end of the day. Some also have responsibility for caring for younger siblings. Children with these responsibilities may need additional support to form or maintain social relationships with peers, as they do not often have opportunities to engage in social extracurricular activities (Rajalakshmi, 2015).

History

It is important to explore the child's success in making friends and working with peers, and his or her feelings of contentment and security. Asking the child to name one or more friends and probing into what the child does during school recesses or after school can provide helpful insight. The ability of a child to name a trusted adult aside from the caregiver is also important.

Physical Examination

Interaction between the child and examiner or others in the room can indicate social skills; however, it may be difficult to accurately assess this outside of a child's natural environment. Engaging the child in conversation throughout the visit and paying attention to the child's verbal and nonverbal behavior with the family and provider may be informative.

Anticipatory Guidance

During middle and late childhood, caregivers can support children by ensuring they have the social skills essential to succeed in school environments. The family environment is an ideal place to learn and practice these skills, and engaging in opportunities that facilitate collaboration, empathy, and conflict resolution with other family members is ideal. As the child begins to form relationships outside the home, it is important to remain aware of the nature and quality of these relationships and provide support and guidance for healthy interactions. Encouraging extracurricular activities may help to promote higher self-esteem, better school grades, and higher academic performance (see Table 12.2). After-school activity participation is associated with a reduction in withdrawal behaviors, depression, fighting, substance use, and engaging in other risky behaviors (Howie, Lukacs, Pastor, Reuben, and Mendola, 2010).

Emotional Development

Assessment of emotional development is an important aspect of the well child examination because 13% of children worldwide are affected by mental health disorders (Polanczyk et al., 2015). Anxiety is the most common mental health disorder of middle childhood, with most cases diagnosed before 12 years old. During the school-age period, children gain the ability to self-regulate, control impulse, and manage emotions (Hagan et al., 2017). By 7 years old, children should be competent functioning in a variety of settings (e.g., home, school, and playground). Emotional problems during these years often follow frustrations, losses, and situations in which the child's self-esteem is threatened or the child is faced with adversity.

Temperament affects the way that school-age children interact with peers, teachers, family, and others in their environment. As part of the process of developing relationships with others, they refine their ability to identify, label, and manage their feelings. However, their experiences are limited, and their cognitive abilities are still expanding. They need help labeling complex emotions, such as sadness, depression, worry, and envy. They also need help to consciously manage those and other feelings in acceptable ways. Children's coping abilities are significantly affected by the availability of social supports from caregivers (Thompson, 2014). A child's entry into school can be emotionally stressful for caregivers because they must adjust to a new social situation, routine, and a changing relationship with their child. Some caregivers feel that they have "lost" their child, watching him or her move from dependence on the family to participation in a new world of which the caregiver is not a part. Other caregivers anticipate the new opportunities facing the child and family and are ready to help their child cope with challenges that emerge in the school environment.

Impulse control is an important coping skill for school age children to continue to develop. Without impulse control, random behavior occurs; on the other hand, overly controlled children appear hostile, uncreative, or both. ADHD and disruptive behavioral disorders may emerge during this time. Behavioral challenges may impact a child's school performance, and disruptive behavior often leads to a negative pattern of disciplinary consequences that affect self-esteem and motivation.

TABLE 12.4   Developmental-Behavioral Screening Tools for Middle Childhood

Screening Tool	Target Population	Purpose
Caregiver's Evaluation of Developmental Status (CEDS)	Birth to 8 years old	Elicits caregiver concerns for their child's language, motor, self-help, language, behavioral and socioemotional abilities
Pediatric Symptom Checklist (PSC)	Children 4 through 16 years old (Y-PSC for youth 11 years old and over)	Generalized cognitive, emotional, and behavioral problems
Patient Health Questionnaire (PHQ-2, PHQ-9, PHQ-9 Adolescent)	12 years old and up	Depression and suicidality
Screen for Child Anxiety-Related Disorders (SCARED)	Children 8-18 years old	Childhood anxiety disorders
NICHQ Vanderbilt Assessment Scale	Children 6-12 years old	Caregiver and teacher evaluation of inattention, hyperactivity, conduct disorders, and anxiety or depression

By 7 years old, most children can name a site for their conscience (heart or brain), and school-age children tend to be rigid in their views of right and wrong, which is consistent with concrete thinking. They understand the relationships between responsibility and privileges and realize choices between right and wrong behaviors are within their control. Some children at this age act appropriately to get a direct reward, whereas others do their duty, viewing moral behavior as following the rules of higher authority. The ability to reason through difficult situations with a variety of influencing factors is heavily dependent on cognitive development; however, school-age children do not have the cognitive maturity to cope with all situations. The school environment, where rules and values may differ from those of the immediate family, must be confronted and negotiated daily. Social pressures may make it difficult to choose actions that the child believes are right. The pressures of gangs, drugs, and peers push many children to make decisions about their activities and behaviors before they are developmentally ready.

School-age children may face a variety of stressors in society, including violence, bullying, divorce, substance abuse in the family, early responsibilities, and lack of support in school. Adverse environments create stress in the lives of children that alter their development. Violence is a constant problem for many, not only in neighborhoods where children live and play but also within their families and schools. The biologic effects of stress undermine the child's ability to concentrate, remember things, and control and focus his or her own thinking (Thompson, 2014).

History

Psychosocial screening is an essential part of every preventive health visit. It is especially important to assess for life stress, anxiety, depression and suicidality, self-esteem issues, caregiver-child relationships, and a family history of mental and behavioral health disorders. Table 12.4 provides screening tools appropriate for the primary care setting with screening questions for emotional and behavioral concerns. In late childhood, it may be helpful to interview the child without the caregiver to assess for psychosocial concerns that he or she might not be comfortable discussing with the caregiver present. During the visit, the provider can role model the normality and acceptability of discussing emotional issues, which is especially important in families where there is strong stigma surrounding mental health disorders (see Chapter 15).

Physical Examination

An assessment of the child's affect is an essential component of the examination of health. Displays of sadness, worry and apathy are significant to note and explore. Caregiver and child interactions during the examination are also important to notice. During the skin assessment, the provider should observe for signs of self-harm or mutilation. Significant weight loss or gain should also be investigated further for both physical and emotional causes.

Anticipatory Guidance

The hallmark of successful school-age social and emotional growth is finding family and peer support while establishing individuality and independence. A nurturing home environment where children feel love and support from trusted adults is essential to their self-esteem development (Thompson, 2014). Caregivers can guide children by providing safe opportunities to identify and manage their emotions in a healthy manner. Role modeling coping skills and self-regulation of emotion provides additional support. Children should feel able to share emotional concerns without fear of judgment or stigma from caregivers (see Table 12.2).

Developmental Assessment of Middle Childhood

During middle and late childhood, caregivers should provide opportunities for children to adapt their needs and emerging skills to fit with family patterns of health maintenance such as nutrition, oral health, sleep, and safety. For school-age children, learning to take responsibility for their own health begins with simple goals and moves to more complex decision-making strategies. Table 12.5 provides a list of anticipatory guidance topics related to health maintenance in this period.

Nutrition

Careful attention to nutrition is important because 35% of school-age children are overweight or obese (Skinner et al., 2018). As children become more independent, their individual decisions around food choices and eating habits have significant impact on their nutritional health. Nutritional choices can be deficient in iron or vitamin C, and high-fat snack foods can become a habit. Consumption of sugar-sweetened beverages, high-calorie snacks,

TABLE 12.5	Anticipatory Guidance Topics for Health Maintenance in Middle Childhood
Nutrition	Ensure child has three nutritious meals and two nutritious snacks daily Establish an eating routine with at least one daily meal together as a family to preserve family time and share interests and experiences from the day's activities Monitor food choices and opportunities to determine best foods and beverages Teach about the importance of eating healthy foods and drinking water Encourage participation in meal planning, food shopping and selection, and meal preparation Discuss making nutritious choices for quick meals, school lunches, and when eating out Model healthy behaviors related to nutrition and other healthy self-care behaviors
Oral health	Encourage proper oral hygiene habits, including brushing and flossing Establish a dental home and schedule biannual visits Limit juice, soda, and candy consumption Ensure proper hygiene for orthodontic appliances Wear mouth guards during contact sports or other recommended protection against dental injury
Sleep	Set clear limits on expectations for healthy exercise, hours of sleep, and other health promotion behaviors Turn off screens at least 1 hour before bedtime Avoid exposure to violent or scary imagery in books or media, especially before bed Recognize "noncompliance" as a means of exerting independence; discussions about decision-making and healthy choices may be needed to resolve issues Model healthy behaviors related physical activity and sleep
Safety	Talk about safety and help child to think about safety aspects of activities Help learn "survival skills" (e.g., name, telephone number, address, use of 911, how to ask adults for help, and what to do if lost) Require protective gear when riding bicycles, skateboards, or scooters and as appropriate in sports activities Use booster seats or wear seatbelts as appropriate Use sunscreen (sun protection factor [SPF] 30 or higher) Teach to swim; supervise their activities near water Educate about hazards, both physical and social (e.g., pedestrian traffic on busy streets; stranger danger and unwanted touch; what to do if they find a weapon or syringe) Monitor all digital and social media use. Use security tools to prevent instant messages from strangers. Use parental controls to limit access on all electronic devices Provide opportunities to ask questions about sexuality, drugs, alcohol, and tobacco; encourage family discussion about these topics Educate that Internet and technology use is an opportunity—not a right Get rid of firearms or ensure they are unloaded and locked, with ammunition in a different location and the key is accessible only to caregiver Know child's whereabouts after school and know child's friends

and other high-calorie foods contribute to obesity in middle and late childhood, and monitoring and weight control programs are needed at earlier ages (see Chapter 17). Choosing nutritious foods while away from home and learning to eat new foods are areas for learning. School-age children can progress from simple (e.g., deciding to have a fruit or vegetable at each meal) to more complex engagement (e.g., helping plan some meals and participate in their preparation) in their nutrition. Providers should engage children and caregivers in discussions about their nutritional habits and provide guidance for healthy eating with a supportive and nonjudgmental approach.

Oral Health

During the school-age period, children begin shedding their primary teeth and their adult teeth emerge. Oral hygiene becomes increasingly important as the teeth grow closer together, making flossing an essential practice. Children in this age can be more independent in their brushing and flossing skills. Caregivers should remind them to engage in these practices twice daily and occasionally observe whether they are using the proper technique. Choosing water over sugar-sweetened beverages and limiting consumption of candy and sticky or gummy foods are healthy habits to encourage. In addition to examining the teeth for caries

or other problems, PCPs should assess whether the family has a dental home, and provide resources or referrals as needed. Chapter 23 provides more detailed information regarding oral health needs and management for school-age children.

Sleep

Sufficient sleep is essential to cognitive and metabolic health in children and contributes to academic performance and weight (Felso et al., 2017). Most school-age children sleep about 10 hours per night (range 8 to 14 hours) without naps, particularly during the school year (Hagan, 2017). Night terrors or sleepwalking may emerge (see Chapter 20). PCPs should assess amount and quality of sleep and explore problems related to falling or staying asleep. Caregivers can support healthful sleep habits by providing an environment conducive to uninterrupted sleep, encouraging calming bedtime routines, and limiting screen time before bed.

Safety

Unintentional injuries are common among school-age children. Often their growing bodies allow them to get into situations that they cannot get out of without help. They need guidance and direction to be safe and make safe choices. Child temperament plays a role in risk-taking behaviors, and boys are more likely to engage in risk behaviors than girls (Reniers et al., 2016). Increasingly, peers and influences outside the family during the school-age years impact children's decisions related to risk-taking behaviors (see Table 12.5).

With the widespread availability of social media, Internet safety is becoming a growing concern for school-age youth. Research suggests that the greatest risk factors for victimization that occurs via the Internet are family conflict, depression, conversing with unknown people about sex, and sending personal information to strangers (Livingstone and Smith, 2014). Victims of child maltreatment (physical, sexual abuse, or neglect) are at particular risk (Noll, Shenk, Barnes, and Haralson, 2013). Further information about safe use of social media is found in Chapter 13.

Common Developmental Issues for Middle Childhood

Developmental concerns, particularly those related to learning and the school environment, may emerge during the school-age period. The wide variation in the growth and development of children necessitates looking at these issues in the context of age, developmental competence, and peer and family functioning. Chronic conditions that impact children's development may have already been identified by the time they reach school age, or they may arise as new concerns during this time.

School Adjustment

School entrance is based on chronologic rather than developmental age, and generally begins with kindergarten enrollment at 5 years old. The process for determining children's readiness for school and preparing them for this transition takes place in early childhood. An estimated 30% of 5-year-olds are not ready for school, and this statistic increases to almost 50% for socioeconomically disadvantaged children (Isaacs, 2012). School participation requires skills to perform self-care, interact with a variety of new people, act with a sense of responsibility, and emotionally separate from the family and home base.

Children must learn to adapt many of their former behaviors as they adjust to life at school. Early wake times or the need to stay up late completing homework may lead to necessary adjustments in sleep schedules, and amount of sleep can impact learning, mood, and behavior. Children may either bring food or eat meals provided by the school, and thus experience increased independence over their dietary choices and eating habits. Elimination may be affected if a child is reluctant to use the school bathroom for defecation.

Self-regulation of attention, emotion, and behavior is essential to school success and is as important as intelligence in predicting academic achievement (Sawyer et al., 2015). Aggression or disruptive behaviors in early school years increase a child's risk for continued behavioral adjustment challenges with school staff and peers (Brennan, Shaw, Dishion, and Wilson, 2015). As they become adjusted to the rigor of an academic environment, children who lack necessary skills to meet school demands and expectations may be unsuccessful, and early school failure can result in significant negative consequences (Sawyer et al., 2015).

Caregivers may also need support as their children adjust to school. They may have difficulty adapting to their children's increasing independence, and worry about how to appropriately supervise and monitor them now that they spend more time outside the home. Some caregivers may have ambivalent attitudes toward their child's school and distrust the school's capacity to meet children's educational needs. Caregiver involvement is an important influence on children's academic and social development during the school-age years, and the primary care visit can be an optimal time to encourage relationship-building with the school. PCPs have a responsibility to work with caregivers and their communities to promote optimal development for children and their families during the transition and adjustment to school.

Clinical Findings

History. A child's adjustment to school is an evolving process, as every grade advancement and progression in development leads to new transitions and opportunities for adaptation. The PCP should consider the following areas:
- Ask the child about school, including likes and dislikes, examples of daily activities, and general level of comfort in the environment.
- Assess the caregivers' feelings about their child's school, including level of trust in administration and staff, sense of community with other families, and who they might go to for help if they had a concern related to their child's experience.
- Inquire about family activities, sibling school experiences, traumatic events, or separation of the child or caregivers, which may affect the child's adjustment in school.
- Investigate any stressors (e.g., chronic illness, economic issues, homelessness, and family disruption) that might compromise regular school attendance or school success.

Physical Examination. The child should have a complete physical examination with particular focus on the following areas to evaluate for any special needs that may require additional support at school:
- Neurologic function, including sensory, cognitive, and language abilities
- Affect and behavior, including symptoms of anxiety or depression

Assessment and Planning

Diagnostic Studies. Consider using a general psychosocial screening tool, such as the Pediatric Symptom Checklist (see Table 12.4), to elicit emotional or behavioral concerns related to school adjustment. Screening results should be evaluated in conjunction with history, observation, family situation, and previous experiences.

Management. Ensuring school adjustment involves sharing data between families, school staff, and PCPs—and offering the following anticipatory guidance:
- Encourage caregivers to visit the school, meet the teacher, and discuss their child's characteristics with the teacher. Encourage involvement in the classroom or school, if the caregiver is able, to become more familiar with the school environment.
- Urge children to share details of their daily school routines with caregivers, including any changes in eating and elimination habits.
- Help caregivers deal with their own stress of separation as their children progress in development and independence. Review their expectations for the child and identify what will be new and different with each school transition (e.g., new school year).
- Provide caregivers with available community and school resources to access to meet the developmental needs of their child.

- Be an advocate for caregivers and children with special needs to ensure the school adequately assesses both strengths and struggles of children, and develops a program of study (e.g., an IEP) that maximizes children's strengths.
- Reassure caregivers that difficulties in a child's adjustment to school may occur even with the best of caregiving.
- Monitor the child's progress throughout the year, advocating as necessary.

Learning Challenges

Learning challenges often present during the school-age years. The ability to manage school learning expectations requires growth in four cognitive areas: basic processing of information, memorization, increased attention span and recall of important events, and beginning problem-solving skills. Knowledge (the sum of what children know) rapidly expands during school-age as a result of schoolwork, experiences at home, and activities with friends. Knowledge organization improves as school-age children grow older and integrate existing concepts. Self-awareness, reflected by children's ability to predict performance, develops slowly and in areas in which children have the most knowledge. Children with learning challenges may have difficulties with basic thinking and processing, and/or have specific problems in language, attention, and organizational skills; higher cognitive functions, such as memory and sensory function; motor capacities; visuospatial analysis and neuro-motor function; and social awareness and behavior. Mental health and behavioral conditions may occur as a comorbidity with learning challenges and should also be considered (see Chapter 30).

Dysfunction in sensory integration (also referred to as sensory processing) may also interfere with learning. These children may require classroom modification and assistance to overcome their issues. Sensory integration can be particularly challenging for children with developmental or behavioral disorders such as autism or ADHD (see Chapters 15 and 30).

Early identification of learning challenges is important to ensure that children access resources that result in a positive school experience. The PCP must be alert to "red flags" that jeopardize children's school success and be ready to intervene with families and school professionals to obtain necessary evaluations and resources to address these problems (Table 12.6).

Clinical Findings

History. A complete history is needed to examine underlying or related etiologies for learning challenges. The history often provides the most information about how learning affects aspects of the child's life. It also identifies areas of strength on which the child and family can build strategies for managing the child's learning struggles. During the history, the provider should elicit the following information:

- Vision and hearing abilities, either reported by the caregivers or during routine school screenings
- Progress, interest, and success in school, including any sudden changes in school performance
- Changes or differences noted by caregivers or teachers in vocabulary or language, logical reasoning, or the ability to problem-solve
- Hyper- or hypo-sensitivity to sensory stimuli such as loud noises, bright lights, or specific textures; difficulty maintaining appropriate boundaries of physical space with others
- Reports of frequent fidgeting or inability to meet age-appropriate expectations for seated activities
- Concerns with peer interactions, particularly related to learning and progression of social skills
- Identification of learning problems by school or other outside professionals
- Request results of any educational testing done and school plans and placement based on needs and abilities.
- *Medical history:* Prenatal history, including in utero exposure to drugs, infection, toxins, and alcohol; neonatal history; recurrent or chronic medical conditions; allergies; medications; hospitalizations; syndromes; congenital, neurologic, metabolic, or endocrine conditions; current illnesses; vision and hearing problems; fetal alcohol spectrum disorder (FASD); history of accidents, concussions, or other brain injury
- *Developmental history:* Achievement or regression of developmental milestones, especially in language; experiences for achieving developmental skills at home or in preschool; daily routines and preferred play activities; temperament; behavioral concerns of caregivers; ability of the child to handle transitions and change; child's initiation of activities versus caregiver-guided activities; repetitive behaviors
- *Family medical history:* Family history of difficulties in school or school dropout, learning difficulties, ADHD, mental retardation, or genetic disorders; overall family members' functioning; substance abuse
- *Family social history:* Problem-solving and decision-making skills, use of community resources, financial resources, family stressors, substance abuse, homelessness, violence, criminal behavior

Physical Examination. The child should have a complete physical examination with particular focus on the following areas:

- General appearance, interaction with caregiver and examiner, and ability to follow commands
- The eye, including maneuvers to assess for nystagmus or strabismus
- Neuromuscular function, such as sensation, mobility, tone and strength in all extremities, and fine motor skills such as writing or drawing
- Mental status, including sensory, cognitive, and language abilities

Assessment and Planning

Diagnostic Screening. Screening in the primary care setting is focused on exploring physiologic etiologies for the child's learning differences, or any related comorbidities. Formal diagnosis of learning challenges is done outside of the primary care setting,

TABLE 12.6	Learning Challenges Seen in Middle Childhood
Fine motor	Dyspraxia Dysgraphia
Cognitive	Dyscalculia Auditory or visual processing disorder Intellectual disability
Communication	Dyslexia Dysphasia
Socio-emotional	Social communication disorder Autism spectrum disorders

and referrals to developmental, psychiatric or educational specialists may be helpful. Consider performing the following additional screening methods to assess for related health conditions, or to include in the referral to a specialist:

- Audiometry and visual acuity assessment
- Psychosocial screening for emotional or behavioral conditions (see Table 12.4)
- Additional testing may be recommended by specialist, such as genetic testing with chromosome studies, brain scans, or endocrine and metabolic testing

Management. The role of the PCP in the management of learning challenges is predominantly one of support, consultation, and resource provision for caregivers. Providers should encourage caregivers to pursue early diagnostic evaluation for their children. Chapter 7 includes information about the role of the PCP in early childhood intervention and educational supports, including IEPs and 504 plans.

School Refusal

School refusal is a term that was introduced in the 1970s to describe the heterogeneity of its causes. The prevalence ranges from 1% to 4% of all school-age children (Elliott and Place, 2017). Ninety percent of children who experience school refusal, commonly called *school phobia,* have a psychiatric diagnosis (Ek and Eriksson, 2013), such as separation anxiety disorder, simple and social phobias, or depression. Diagnostic criteria include the following: (1) severe difficulty attending school or refusal to attend school, (2) severe emotional upset when attempting to go to school, (3) absence of significant antisocial disorders, and (4) staying at home with the caregiver's knowledge. Children request to stay home from school with a variety of physical complaints, including stomachaches, headaches, dizziness, fatigue, or a combination of these. The symptoms gradually improve as the day progresses and often disappear on weekends. Unexcused school absences peak with the beginning of school entrance and again at 11 to 13 years old (Elliott and Place, 2017).

Clinical Findings

History. Because child, caregiver, family, and school environmental factors influence school refusal, an in-depth history exploring these areas is needed. Specific areas to emphasize during history-taking include:

- Patterns and characteristics of potentially somatic complaints (e.g., headache, abdominal or chest pain, or sleep difficulties)
- School environment and evidence of bullying, violence, mismatch with teacher, academic failure
- Socialization away from family: friends, involvement with peer group, participation in group activities
- Child self-concept and self-esteem; suicidal ideation or self-harm behaviors
- Patterns of isolation or withdrawn behavior; whether described as "shy" or "introvertive"
- Caregivers' feelings about child's attendance at school, evidence of overindulgence or overprotection
- Other symptoms of anxiety, such as pervasive worry or obsessive behavior
- Recent or anticipated loss or separation from caregiver or other family member, such as death or divorce
- History of traumatic event, including abuse or neglect
- Significant home responsibilities (e.g., caring for a chronically ill or substance abusing caregiver)

- Social determinants of health: housing status, food security, parent employment

Physical Examination. A complete physical examination and evaluation of mental status should be performed. PCPs should pay particular attention to the child's general emotional state, including interactions and engagement with the provider and caregiver.

Diagnostic Screening. The purpose of screening the child who is refusing school is to uncover underlying psychopathology or contributing physiologic conditions to provide appropriate referrals for diagnosis and treatment. See Chapter 30 for more in-depth information regarding the assessment and diagnosis of anxiety disorders. Laboratory analyses or diagnostic imaging are rarely necessary to differentiate somatic from organic complaints, and PCPs should be judicious and use evidence-based clinical judgment for the appropriate use of these resources. Table 12.4 describes validated tools that screen for psychosocial contributors most relevant to school refusal, for example:

- Pediatric Symptom Checklist (PSC), for general psychosocial screening
- Patient Health Questionnaire (PHQ), or Screen for Child Anxiety-Related Disorders (SCARED), for depression or anxiety

Management

Intervention is generally successful when behavioral measures are combined with supportive counseling of caregivers. In mild cases, school refusal can be managed in primary care through sufficient investigation of physical complaints. Evaluate somatic symptoms to rule out organic disease, without excessive medical attention or diagnostic testing. In addition, the provider should address environmental factors, such as bullying or home stressors, through communication with the school or community support services. Once there is a plan in place to evaluate the possibility of organic disease as well as address environmental contributors, children are encouraged to return to school. In many cases, once the above concerns are addressed, the symptoms resolve (Elliott and Place, 2017). Children with more severe presentations (those whose symptoms persist despite the above interventions, or those who screen positive for underlying psychopathology) should be referred to a mental health specialist and may benefit from interventions such as cognitive-behavioral therapy (CBT), or medications.

Key elements of primary care management of school refusal include the following:

- Support caregivers through a balance of validation of their concerns and encouragement to return the child to school as soon as possible.
- Collaborate with school personnel to intervene and address any factors in the school environment related to the child's reasons for refusal.
- Engage with social service agencies such as the local Department of Public Health, if needed, to assess the home situation and identify areas for social support.
- Provide referrals as needed for child or family counseling.
- Notify child protection services in the case of suspected abuse or neglect.
- Criteria for mental health referral include the following:
  - Symptoms are severe or do not improve within 2 weeks
  - Out of school for at least 2 months
  - Symptoms of depression, panic, or psychosis
  - Caregiver inability to cooperate with plan

- Transitions and progress in school and extracurricular activities
- Peer and family relationships
- Coping skills and problem-solving away from home
- Food choices, eating practices, and body image
- Oral hygiene
- Physical and sedentary activities
- Sleep patterns and hygiene
- Home and community safety
- Internet and social media practices
- Sexual development, gender identity, and sexuality

- Allergic rhinitis
- Asthma
- Constipation/encopresis
- Eczema
- Enuresis
- Obesity
- Scoliosis

Overview of the Preventive Health Visit in Middle Childhood

Middle childhood preventative health visits occur annually and are detailed in the following sections. Providers can best assist school-age children and families during these visits by reviewing the child's progress, validating caregiver efforts, and providing education and guidance.

History

The preventive health history includes a comprehensive summary of the child's physical, nutritional, neurodevelopmental, psychosocial, behavioral, and emotional status. The visit should begin by building rapport with the caregiver and the child. During middle and late childhood, direct questions first to the child, encouraging sharing aspects of daily routines, family experiences, school activities, and sensitive developmental concerns. Caregivers can then be invited to confirm or expand on data collected and to provide additional information. As with all children, family system assessment is crucial. For the school-age child, it is particularly important to evaluate how well the family is nurturing the child while supporting the child's efforts to become more independent and create a unique sense of self in the community. The provider should strive to integrate the preventive health history with anticipatory guidance, to elicit information about a topic and then provide education and advice within the same discussion. Box 12.1 provides a list of topics to address in the preventive health visit.

Physical Examination

Physical examination in the school-age preventive health visit includes a comprehensive assessment of all body systems, including growth and sexual maturity. It is also an opportunity for the PCP to elicit questions or concerns about body changes and to provide education and anticipatory guidance about physical development. Engaging the caregiver and child during the examination is important and can be done by providing a verbal summary of findings as the exam progresses. Findings that are atypical for the child's developmental and health status should be explored further. The PCP can assess for several developmental skills within the context of the examination and note any physical manifestations of delayed development. Box 12.2 contains information about common conditions that should be screened for during the physical examination in middle and late childhood.

Diagnostic Screening

Formal diagnostic screening in the preventive visit in middle childhood may include questionnaires, laboratory analysis, or other testing. Universal, annual assessment of development, overall psychosocial function, and body mass index is important. Selective screening may also be performed in children with specific risk factors or health concerns. Table 12.7 provides a summary of health screening recommendations for middle and late childhood.

Developmental surveillance (see Chapter 8) is an essential aspect of the visit history with the school-age child because preventive visits occur less frequently than in earlier childhood, and much can change from year to year. Developmental and psychosocial screening tools (see Table 12.4) may be used to allow the child, the caregiver, and the teachers to provide specific information about a child's development, behaviors, and emotional status. Caregiver reports of skills and concerns about language, fine motor, cognitive, and emotional-behavioral development are highly predictive of true problems (Woolfenden et al., 2014). Caregiver, teacher, and child perceptions about specific issues may differ, and a comprehensive assessment should include data from all involved.

Anticipatory Guidance

Anticipatory guidance for caregivers helps them understand, respond to, and guide various aspects of their child's behavior and development. Their support is essential to the child's adjustment and his or her ability to manage stressful life events. Caregivers typically welcome the suggestions and resources that health care providers give them. Because children assume more responsibility for self-care as they grow, age-appropriate anticipatory guidance should be discussed with them as well. Tables 12.2 and 12.5 include relevant anticipatory guidance topics. These lists are not intended to be exhaustive, but rather illustrated examples of how these concepts can be applied to everyday living.

Developmental Red Flags for Middle Childhood

The school-age child may present with more serious problems. Table 12.8 outlines "red flags" for children 6 to 12 years old. PCPs must be alert for indications that something more serious is occurring and, if needed, assess the child and family more thoroughly. PCPs can address risk factors with families to prevent further problems. In situations where the child has been referred, the PCP has a crucial role in working with other professionals to ensure that children and families receive timely and appropriate services.

TABLE 12.7 **Recommended Health Screening for Middle Childhood**

	Universal	Selective
Anemia	Identify dietary iron sources at every preventive health visit	Risk-based if poor nutrition or other medical indication
Blood pressure	Sphygmomanometry at every preventive health visit; if elevated, must perform manually twice and average two results	At any visit if previously elevated
Body mass index	Calculate from weight and height measurements and compare to Centers for Disease Control (CDC) growth charts at every preventive health visit	At any visit if overweight or obese
Development	Surveillance at every preventive health visit	At any visit if concerns from home or school
Dyslipidemia	Serum total cholesterol and high-density lipoprotein (HDL) at one preventive health visit between 9 and 11 years	Every 2 years if positive family history or other cardio-vascular risk factors
Lead toxicity	Serum lead level for new immigrants upon arrival	Risk-based if concerns for exposure
Oral health	Surveillance of brushing/flossing and fluoride at every preventive health visit	Risk-based if no dental home
Psychosocial/behavior	Surveillance of general socio-emotional concerns, caregiver depression, and social determinants at every preventive health visit	Standardized screening if concerns or risk-based for other mental health and substance abuse beginning at 11 years
Sexually transmitted infection	Surveillance of sexual abuse at every preventive health visit	Standardized screening if concerns or risk-based beginning at 11 years
Tuberculosis	Risk factor questionnaire at every preventive health visit	Tuberculin skin test or serum quantiferon level if concerns for exposure
Vision and hearing	Snellen chart and audiometry at 6, 8, 10, and 12 years	Risk-based if concerns from home or school

From Hagan JF, Shaw JS, Duncan PM, eds. *Bright Futures Guidelines for Health Supervision of Infants, Children, and Adolescents.* 4th ed. Elk Grove Village, IL: American Academy of Pediatrics; 2017.

TABLE 12.8 **Developmental Red Flags: Middle Childhood**

Motor skills	*Gross Motor:* Unable to catch a ball Unable to walk a straight line Poor coordination, endurance, strength Problems throwing or catching *Fine Motor:* Unable to print name Unable to tie shoes Difficulty holding pencil Illegible handwriting School failure related to handwriting skills
Cognition and perception	School failure related to attention or focus Unable to state age or days of the week Inability to perform basic addition or subtraction Lack of operational thinking: cause and effect, relationships of whole and parts, nonegocentric thinking Persistent difficulty understanding and completing school work Reports of double vision, blurred vision, or loss of vision or hearing
Communication and language	Unable to read and write simple words or phrases Unable to relate a simple story Inability to follow verbal instructions Problems with reading comprehension Speech not 100% intelligible
Social and emotional skills	Problems developing or maintaining peer relationships; unable to name a friend Lack of hobbies or interests Social isolation or withdrawal Persistently flat, depressed, or withdrawn affect Unable to sit still in class Cruelty to animals or people Illicit behavior such as fire setting, theft, vandalism Persistent defiance or deliberate disregard for rules Gang involvement Risk-taking behaviors: smoking, alcohol, sex

References

Barac R, Bialystok E, Castro DC, Sanchez M. The cognitive development of young dual language learners: a critical review. *Early Child Res Q*. 2014;29(4):699–714. https://doi.org/10.1016/j.ecresq.2014.02.003.

Black LI, Vahratian A, Hoffman HJ. *Communication Disorders and Use of Interventions Services Among Children Aged 3-17 Years: United States, 2012 (NCHS Data Brief No. 205)*. Retrieved from Hyattsville, MD: 2015.

Brennan LM, Shaw DS, Dishion TJ, Wilson MN. The predictive utility of early childhood disruptive behaviors for school-age social functioning. *J Abnorm Child Psychol*. 2015;43(6):1187–1199. https://doi.org/10.1007/s10802-014-9967-5.

Duderstadt KG. *Pediatric Physical Examination*. 3rd ed. St. Louis: Elsevier; 2018.

Ek H, Eriksson R. Psychological factors behind truancy, school phobia, and school refusal: a literature study. *Child Fam Behav Ther*. 2013;35(3):228–248. https://doi.org/10.1080/07317107.2013.818899.

Elliott JG, Place M. Practitioner review: school refusal: developments in conceptualisation and treatment since 2000. *J Child Psychol Psychiatry*. 2017. https://doi.org/10.1111/jcpp.12848.

Felso R, Lohner S, Hollody K, Erhardt E, Molnar D. Relationship between sleep duration and childhood obesity: systematic review including the potential underlying mechanisms. *Nutr Metab Cardiovasc Dis*. 2017;27(9):751–761. https://doi.org/10.1016/j.numecd.2017.07.008.

Hagan JF, Shaw JS, Duncan PM, eds. *Bright Futures Guidelines for Health Supervision of Infants, Children, and Adolescents*. 4th ed. Elk Grove Village, IL: American Academy of Pediatrics; 2017.

Howie LD, Lukacs SL, Pastor PN, Reuben CA, Mendola P. Participation in activities outside of school hours in relation to problem behavior and social skills in middle childhood. *J Sch Health*. 2010;80(3):119–125. https://doi.org/10.1111/j.1746-1561.2009.00475.x.

Isaacs JB. *Starting School at a Disadvantage: The School Readiness of Poor Children*. Retrieved from Washington, DC: 2012.

Livingstone S, Smith PK. Annual research review: harms experienced by child users of online and mobile technologies: the nature, prevalence and management of sexual and aggressive risks in the digital age. *J Child Psychol Psychiatry*. 2014;55(6):635–654. https://doi.org/10.1111/jcpp.12197.

Muursepp I, Aibast H, Gapeyeva H, Paasuke M. Motor skills, haptic perception and social abilities in children with mild speech disorders. *Brain Dev*. 2012;34(2):128–132. https://doi.org/10.1016/j.braindev.2011.02.002.

Noll JG, Shenk CE, Barnes JE, Haralson KJ. Association of maltreatment with high-risk internet behaviors and offline encounters. *Pediatrics*. 2013;131(2):e510–e517. https://doi.org/10.1542/peds.2012-1281.

Perez HR, Stoeckle JH. Stuttering: clinical and research update. *Can Fam Physician*. 2016;62(6):479–484.

Polanczyk GV, Salum GA, Sugaya LS, Caye A, Rohde LA. Annual research review: a meta-analysis of the worldwide prevalence of mental disorders in children and adolescents. *J Child Psychol Psychiatry*. 2015;56(3):345–365. https://doi.org/10.1111/jcpp.12381.

Rajalakshmi JTP. The effects and behaviors of home alone situation by latchkey children. *Am J Nurs Sci*. 2015;4(4):207–211.

Reniers RL, Murphy L, Lin A, Bartolome SP, Wood SJ. Risk perception and risk-taking behaviour during adolescence: the influence of personality and gender. *PLoS One*. 2016;11(4):e0153842. https://doi.org/10.1371/journal.pone.0153842.

Sawyer AC, Chittleborough CR, Mittinty MN, Miller-Lewis LR, Sawyer MG, Sullivan T, et al. Are trajectories of self-regulation abilities from ages 2-3 to 6-7 associated with academic achievement in the early school years? *Child Care Health Dev*. 2015;41(5):744–754. https://doi.org/10.1111/cch.12208.

Skinner AC, Ravanbakht SN, Skelton JA, Perrin EM, Armstrong SC. *Prevalence of Obesity and Severe Obesity in US Children, 1999-2016*. Pediatrics; 2018. https://doi.org/10.1542/peds.2017-3459.

Stevenson J, McCann D, Watkin P, Worsfold S, Kennedy C. The relationship between language development and behaviour problems in children with hearing loss. *J Child Psychol Psychiatry*. 2010;51(1):77–83. https://doi.org/10.1111/j.1469-7610.2009.02124.x.

Thompson RA. Stress and child development. *Future Child*. 2014;24(1):41–59.

Woolfenden S, Eapen V, Williams K, Hayen A, Spencer N, et al. A systematic review of the prevalence of parental concerns measured by the Parents' Evaluation of Developmental Status (PEDS) indicating developmental risk. *BMC Pediatr*. 2014;14:231. https://doi.org/10.1186/1471-2431-14-231.

13

Developmental Management of Adolescents and Young Adults

JAIME E. PANTON AND DAWN LEE GARZON MAAKS

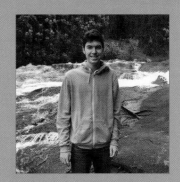

The changes a young person experiences during the transition from childhood to young adulthood are dramatic. The extent of physiologic growth and maturation during this time rivals that occurring during infancy. Social and psychological changes are also extreme and can create a tenuous sense of balance during this phase of development. The common question on the minds of most adolescents is "Am I normal?" Reassurance, information, and anticipatory guidance during well visits about what to expect as they grow are among the most valuable services a primary care provider (PCP) can offer the adolescent. This chapter focuses on the normal physical and psychosocial growth and development of adolescents and provides PCPs with a framework for structuring care of the adolescent and young adult client.

Adolescent and Young Adult Development

Puberty is defined as the development of secondary sexual characteristics and the biologic process that ultimately leads to fertility. The hormonal regulatory systems in the hypothalamus, pituitary, gonads, and adrenal glands undergo major changes between the prepubertal and adult states. Accompanying these changes are rapid growth in height and weight, development of secondary sex characteristics, and onset of fertility (Fig 13.1) (see Chapter 21). Normal development can be difficult to define and is, at best, an approximation rather than a precise parameter. However, even though the timing and progression of adolescent development varies, the sequence of events is orderly (Fig 13.2).

Adolescence refers to the psychosocial and emotional transition from childhood to adulthood and is influenced by social, genetic, and environmental aspects (Cabellero, 2016). The physical changes of puberty are accompanied by significant cognitive and psychosocial developmental changes that affect how adolescents view themselves and how the world views adolescents. Successful development in adolescence culminates in the achievement of goals that provide the basis for a healthy, productive adult life.

Physical Development

Sexual Maturity Rating

Pubertal growth and maturation can be divided into five stages, known as Sexual Maturity Rating (SMR) scales. These stages range from prepubertal (SMR 1) to adult (SMR 5) (Figs 13.3 to 13.5). Puberty is characterized by a period of rapid growth. Pubertal changes occur on a continuum, with individual differences in timing or tempo.

Female Stages. Females enter puberty earlier than males do, and their puberty usually progresses sequentially in the following pattern:

- Ovaries increase in size; no visible body changes occur.
- Breast budding (thelarche) begins as a result of estradiol secretion and traditionally occurs between 8 and 13 years old, with the average onset at 10.3 years (De Silva, 2018) (see Fig 13.3). Most girls (85%) experience the development of breast buds approximately 6 months before the appearance of pubic hair. African American girls, on average, reach thelarche at around 9.5 years and Caucasian females reach thelarche around 10.3 years (De Silva, 2018). The timing of the onset of breast development in females has no relationship to breast size at the completion of puberty.
- Rapid linear growth usually begins shortly after the onset of breast budding and reaches its peak about 1 year later. Most females reach peak height velocity (PHV) during SMR 2 and 3, at an average age of 11 or 12 years. Typically, by age 15, females have completed their linear growth (Klein et al., 2017). Early developers may experience a height spurt between 9 and 10 years old, whereas late developers may not experience a height spurt until between 13 and 14 years old. Final height is determined by the amount of bone growth at the epiphyses of the long bones. Growth stops when hormonal factors shut down the epiphyseal plates.
- Appearance of pubic hair (adrenarche or pubarche) commences at about 11.5 years old and is related to adrenal rather than gonadal development (i.e., thelarche) and is less valid than

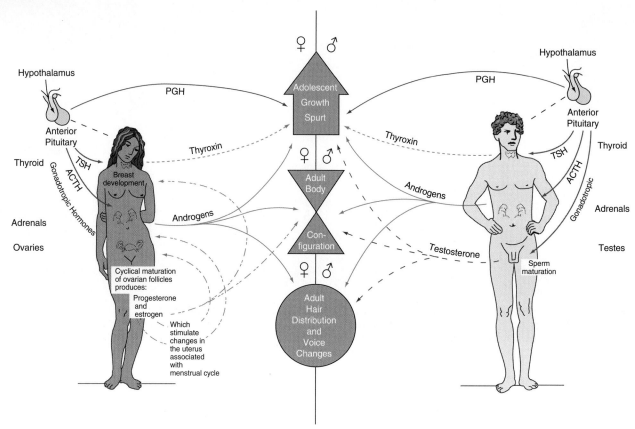

● **Fig 13.1** The Endocrine System at Puberty. *ACTH,* Adrenocorticotropic hormone; *PGH,* pituitary growth hormone; *TSH,* thyroid-stimulating hormone. (From Valadian I, Porter D. *Physical Growth and Development from Conception to Maturity.* Boston: Little, Brown; 1977.)

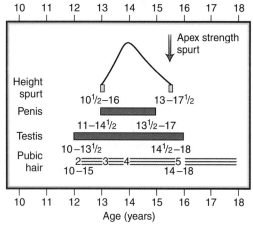

● **Fig 13.2** Sequence of Pubertal Events. Breast, genital, and pubic hair development indicate SMR stages 2 to 5. (From Marshall WA, Tanner JM Variations in the Pattern of Pubertal Changes in Boys. Archives of Disease in Childhood 1970;45:13–23.)

other secondary sex characteristics in assessing sexual maturation (see Fig 13.4).

• The first menstrual period (menarche) occurs, on average, at 12.5 years but age of onset ranges from 9 to 15 years. Menarche occurs approximately 2.5 years after thelarche (Klein et al., 2017). The mean age of menarche is highly dependent on ethnic, socioeconomic, and nutritional factors. It may be 18 to 24 months after

menarche before females establish regular ovulatory cycles. The American Academy of Pediatrics (AAP) and the American Congress of Obstetricians and Gynecologists (ACOG) recommend that PCPs recognize the menstrual cycle as a "vital sign" because of the need for education regarding normal timing and characteristics of menstruation and other pubertal signs (ACOG Committee on Adolescent Health Care, 2006; Hagan et al., 2017).

Changes in female body composition occur during puberty, and adolescent girls benefit from the PCP's reassurance that these changes are normal. Initial breast development usually begins as a unilateral disk-like subareolar swelling, and many adolescents and parents may initially present with concerns about breast tumors. Girls often have asymmetric breasts and need assurance that breasts become more or less the same size within a few years after the onset of breast budding. The female body shape changes as girls progress through puberty, with broadening of the shoulders, hips, and thighs. Girls experience a continuous increase in proportion of fat to total body mass during puberty. They enter puberty with approximately 80% lean body weight and 20% body fat. By the end of puberty, lean body mass drops to about 75%. Body fat is an important mediator for the onset of menstruation and regular ovulatory cycles. An average of 17% of body fat is needed for menarche, and about 22% is needed to initiate and maintain regular ovulatory cycles.

Pubertal changes in females occur at an earlier age than in past decades. Earlier sexual maturation is also influenced by race. Research suggests that nearly one-quarter of African American females, and 5% to 10% of Caucasian females between 7 and 8 years of age have signs of glandular breast tissue (Abreu and

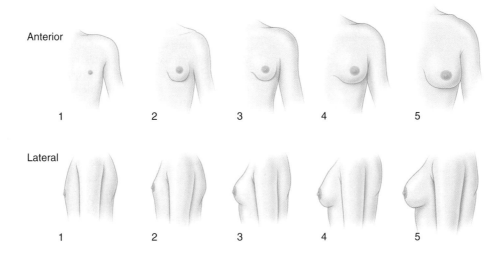

• **Fig 13.3** Normal Female Breast Development, SMR Stages 1 to 5. (From Duderstadt K. *Pediatric Physical Examination: An Illustrated Handbook.* 2nd ed. St. Louis: Elsevier/Mosby; 2014: 235. Original source Herring JA. *Tachdjian's Pediatric Orthopaedics.* 4th ed. Philadelphia: Saunders/Elsevier; 2008.)

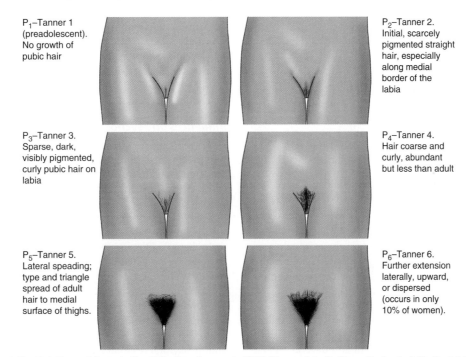

P_1–Tanner 1 (preadolescent). No growth of pubic hair

P_2–Tanner 2. Initial, scarcely pigmented straight hair, especially along medial border of the labia

P_3–Tanner 3. Sparse, dark, visibly pigmented, curly pubic hair on labia

P_4–Tanner 4. Hair coarse and curly, abundant but less than adult

P_5–Tanner 5. Lateral speading; type and triangle spread of adult hair to medial surface of thighs.

P_6–Tanner 6. Further extension laterally, upward, or dispersed (occurs in only 10% of women).

• **Fig 13.4** Normal Female Genitalia Development, SMR Stages 1 to 6. (From Duderstadt K. *Pediatric Physical Examination: An Illustrated Handbook.* 2nd ed. St. Louis: Elsevier/Mosby; 2014: 245.)

Kaiser, 2016; Klein et al., 2017). Females who develop secondary sex characteristics earlier than their peers are at increased risk for sexual assault, sexual abuse, dating violence, psychosocial issues, and depression (Chen, Rothman, and Jaffee, 2017; Mendle, Ryan, and McKone, 2017).

Male Stages. The physical changes of puberty generally occur sequentially in males as follows:
• The initial sign of male puberty is testicular enlargement and occurs on average at 11.5 years (Klein et al., 2017). Growth of the testes occurs approximately 6 months before the development of pubic hair in most males. If testicular enlargement does not precede other changes, the provider should consider whether the

adolescent is taking exogenous anabolic steroids. Once puberty begins, the left testis generally hangs lower than the right.
• Pubic hair development follows a pattern similar to that of girls (see Fig 13.5).
• The first release of spermatozoa (spermarche) generally occurs in midpuberty. However, it can occur at any stage of development from SMR 3 to 5 (Klein et al., 2017).
• Elongation and widening of the penis usually begin in SMR 3 and continue through SMR 5 (see Fig 13.5).
• Rapid growth in height occurs. The PHV occurs during SMR 3 to 4 and around age 13 to 14 years. Most males complete linear growth by age 17 (Klein et al., 2017). Boys generally lag

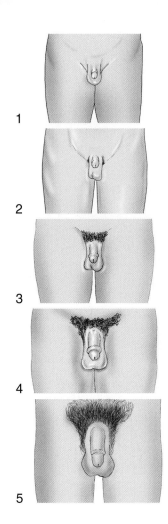

1

2

3

4

5

- **Fig 13.5** Normal Male Genitalia Development, SMR Stages 1 to 5. (From Duderstadt K. *Pediatric Physical Examination: An Illustrated Handbook*. 2nd ed. St. Louis: Elsevier/Mosby; 2014: 216.)

about 2 years behind girls, but 95% have their growth spurt between 12 and 16 years old. Males typically have a higher peak growth velocity than females. Males can continue to grow, although minimally, well beyond their teenage years.

- Change in the male voice coincides with the PHV.
- Development of axillary, facial, and body hair occurs. Axillary hair generally does not appear before SMR 4 pubic hair. Facial hair appears only after SMR 4 pubic hair and does so sequentially. It starts at the outer corners of the upper lip and moves inward, then appears on the upper parts of the cheeks and middle of the lower lip, and finally grows along the sides and lower border of the chin. The extent of body hair is determined to a large extent by genetic factors. Body hair develops gradually after facial hair. Body hair changes should not, however, be used to assess pubertal maturation related to changes in the endocrine system.
- The potential for reproduction occurs by the end of puberty in males.

As with girls, the body composition of adolescent males changes, sometimes causing great concern for the adolescent. The PCP can be an invaluable source of information and reassurance. In contrast to females, males generally increase muscle mass from approximately 80% to 90% and lose body fat during puberty.

Some changes associated with puberty may be unwelcome. Between 50% and 75% of males experience *gynecomastia,* a transient benign unilateral or bilateral enlargement of breast tissue, often occurring within a year of achieving PHV (Neinstein et al., 2016). Gynecomastia generally lasts 12 to 18 months and resolves completely by late puberty in nearly all cases. In a small percentage of males, however, some palpable breast tissue persists. Although generally benign, gynecomastia can occur secondary to anabolic steroid or illicit drug use. Additionally, acne may develop in early puberty. By midpuberty many males have moderate to severe acne, which can worsen throughout puberty. In cases of persistent gynecomastia or severe acne, the provider should ask if the adolescent is using alcohol, marijuana, or anabolic steroids, all of which can exacerbate these conditions.

Psychosocial, Emotional, and Cognitive Development

Adolescence is the time when the adolescent/young adult becomes independent and self-sufficient (Kilford et al., 2016). Adolescents transitioning from childhood to adulthood should achieve specific cognitive, emotional, and psychosocial developmental milestones that help them:

- Feel a sense of belonging in a valued group
- Acquire skills and master tasks that are important to the valued group
- Develop a sense of self-worth
- Develop at least one reliable relationship with another individual
- Demonstrate cognitive potential

Influences on Psychosocial, Emotional, and Cognitive Development

The adolescent's ability to achieve these milestones depends in part on brain functioning. Although full sized, the adolescent brain continues to develop functional ability. As with the infant brain, a process of pruning and reinforcement occurs, based on the stimuli, activities, and experiences of the teenager.

The brain is subject to chemical, hormonal, physical, and biologic changes. Dopaminergic and noradrenergic receptors become more active and neurotransmitter levels increase during adolescence. While there is an increase of dopamine in the prefrontal cortex (PFC), there is a decrease of dopamine in the accumbens, or "reward center" (Rees, Booth, and Jones, 2016). The PFC, which coordinates executive functions of abstract thinking, reasoning, judgment, self-discipline, ethical behavior, personality, and behavioral modification and emotions, experiences rapid growth. Emotional, social, and behavioral changes seen during adolescence are influenced by neural reactivity in the brain, particularly within the amygdala and PFC. Neuroimaging studies suggest the PFC also influences emotional regulation (Guyer, Silk, and Nelson, 2016). Current research indicates that gonadal hormones influence pubertal brain development and behavioral responses (Schulz and Sisk, 2016).

The hypothalamic-pituitary-adrenal axis, which is one of the body's principal stress response systems, changes significantly during adolescence. Additionally, the adolescent brain is particularly vulnerable to toxic stress from life events, abuse/maltreatment, mental illness, altered social interaction, and chronic illness. A stressful event may have a greater impact on neurodevelopment if the event occurs during adolescence compared to adulthood. Adolescents exposed to adverse experiences are at higher risk of

TABLE 13.1	Central Issues in Early, Middle, and Late Adolescence		
Variable	Early Adolescence	Middle Adolescence	Late Adolescence
Sexual maturity rating (SMR)	1-2	3-5	5
Somatic	Secondary sex characteristics Beginning of rapid growth Awkward appearance	Height growth peaks Body shape and composition change Acne and odor Menarche/spermarche	Physically mature Slower growth
Cognitive and moral	Concrete operations Unable to perceive long-term outcomes of current decision-making Conventional morality	Emergence of abstract thought (formal operations) May perceive future implications, but may not apply in decision-making Questioning social mores	Future-oriented with sense of perspective idealism; absolutism Able to think things through independently
Self-concept/identity formation	Preoccupied with changing body Self-conscious about appearance and attractiveness Fantasy and present-oriented	Concern with attractiveness Increasing introspection "Stereotypical adolescent"	More stable body image Attractiveness may still be of concern Emancipation complete Firmer identity
Family	Increased need for privacy Increased bid for independence	Conflicts over control and independence Struggle for acceptance of greater authority	Emotional and physical separation from family Increased autonomy
Peers	Seeks same-sex peer affiliation to counter instability	Intense peer group involvement Preoccupation with peer culture Peers provide behavioral example	Peer group and values recede in importance Intimacy/possible commitment takes precedence
Sexual	Increased interest in sexual anatomy Anxieties and questions about genital changes, size Limited dating and intimacy	Testing ability to attract partner Initiation of relationships and sexual activity May question sexual orientation	Consolidation of sexual identity Focus on intimacy and formation of stable relationships Planning for future and commitment
Relationship to society	Middle school adjustment	Gauging skills and opportunities	Career decisions (e.g., college, work)

From Kleigman RM, Stanton BF, St. Geme JW, et al.: *Nelson Textbook of Pediatrics*. Philadelphia: Elsevier; 2011, p 650.

anxiety, depression, and other mental health disorders (Tottenham and Galvan, 2016). See Chapters 15 and 30 for an in-depth discussion of mental health and illness.

Adolescents may be at risk of substance abuse disorders because of changes in the brain that occur during this time. The frontal lobe and limbic system are particularly susceptible to the effects of early alcohol and substance use. The limbic system impacts urges and cravings, and helps one control such urges. During adolescence, the area of the limbic system involved in urges and cravings is heightened, whereas the area involved in controlling urges is immature (Sharma and Morrow, 2016; Silveri, Dager, Cohen-Gilbert, and Sneider, 2016). Neuroimaging studies demonstrate decreased volume of the PFC, smaller temporal volumes, and decreased cortical thickness in adolescents with alcohol use and/or abuse (Silveri et al., 2016).

Drugs and alcohol have a significant negative effect on the adolescent brain by damaging the neural circuitry in the "reward" or motivation pathways and shutting down the body's ability to respond to stimuli that normally generate pleasurable feelings. In essence, the drug becomes the only thing that leads to pleasurable feelings; a craving for the drug is "etched" into the brain and thus the individual becomes addicted. In addition to contributing to addiction, brain changes resulting from exposure to alcohol, especially binge drinking, can lead to loss of memory and cognitive function. It is theorized that these changes occur because of

neurotoxicity and damage to the myelin sheath in the PFC (Coleman et al., 2014; Pascual et al., 2014). Genetic structures of individuals vary, however, and not all brains respond to drugs in this way, but the adolescent brain is highly vulnerable.

Principles of Behavior Changes

A wide variety of normal behavior characterizes the process of psychosocial, emotional, and cognitive development in adolescents (Table 13.1). Three general principles may be used to understand these changes:

- Transition is continual and generally smooth.
- Disruptive family conflict is not the norm.
- The quality of thinking changes from concrete to formal operational thinking.

Smooth Transition. The first principle of adolescent psychosocial development is that the transition from adolescence to adulthood is continuous and generally smooth. A commonly held myth is that adolescence is a period of "storm and stress." This view was originally described by G. Stanley Hall in 1908. Although his argument was not based on research, this myth continues to be widely believed. It is important to remember that adolescence is only one of many transitional phases in life, and although some experience significant challenges during these years, others pass through this critical time with relative ease.

Adolescent Survival Guide for Parents

- Start with clear rules and expectations before children are teenagers. Work on good communication with children early and continue through adolescence. State expectations and future consequences before trouble occurs (e.g., identify curfew expectations before the dance, not when the teen comes home late).
- Be firm and consistent with follow through.
- Be flexible and allow teenagers to negotiate nonsafety-related rules. Discussing principles and negotiating solutions are valuable life skills for the future. Do not negotiate rules that are nonnegotiable.
- Fighting and arguing are typical, often used by teens as they practice their developing reasoning skills. Often teens are engaged more recreationally than emotionally. Therefore, when the parent is tired, they should disengage and walk away. Try not to take what they say personally.
- Teenagers want parents to be involved, concerned, and ask questions. They just may not know it or know how to express their desire.
- Know who their friends are and call those parents from time to time. Compare household rules if possible.
- Be involved at their school as much as possible. Try to meet their teachers and stay in contact with them.
- Continue to involve teenagers in family activities, even when they no longer want to. Bringing friends along helps.
- Keep promises made to teens. This builds trust and respect and makes you a role model.
- Model good behavior. Adolescents recognize the hypocrisy of saying one thing and doing another.
- Don't forget that teenagers still need adult supervision at times.
- Keep communication lines open and don't be afraid to start conversations. Adolescents sometimes want to talk to adults but are nervous about speaking first.

Family Relationships Change. The second principle of adolescent psychosocial development is that the biologic, cognitive, and emotional changes experienced by adolescents require a reworking of family relationships. Some degree of adolescent-parent conflict is expected because of this, but disruptive family conflict is not the norm. Mundane, everyday issues (such as, which clothes to wear, hairstyles, household chores, curfew, and friends) are the usual sources of parent-adolescent conflict, and negotiation between parent and child is essential. Inexperienced in negotiation, adolescents will often argue a point to excess. It may help to remind parents that this verbal debate, or "arguing," is a normal behavior of teens that reflects their use of more abstract thinking skills. It is a way of practicing abstract thinking and engaging parents. However, the parent should not become too deeply engaged because the adolescent rarely is, and the "arguments" tend to blow over fairly quickly (Box 13.1).

Families should not experience one crisis after another. It is a cause for concern if family crises are the norm. When true turmoil exists, it usually represents psychopathology and will not be simply "outgrown." Careful assessment and treatment are required. Behavior that results in negative consequences is especially worrisome. For example, fights over hair color may not be worthwhile because hair color will grow out, but behavior that results in school and/or work difficulties should be addressed.

Cognitive Changes. The third principle of adolescent psychosocial development is about change in cognitive abilities. Adolescents develop what Piaget referred to as *formal operational thinking,*

characterized by the use of propositional thinking and abstract reasoning. The principal difference between concrete and formal operational thinking is the ability to reason using verbal manipulation rather than in terms of concrete objects. In early adolescence, thinking tends to be very concrete. The classic example is an adolescent who when asked, "Are you sexually active?" responds, "No, I just lie there," or when asked, "What brought you here to see me today?" answers, "The bus." Most teenagers acquire increasing sophistication in abstract thought after they are 14 years old. They learn to conceptualize about past and future events and to relate actions to consequences. During this process, adolescents begin to:

- Question values and often challenge familiar ones.
- Understand concepts of good and evil and understand human nature (e.g., not all authority figures are good people).
- Be aware of contradictions between what is said and what is done (e.g., adolescents are acutely aware when parents tell their children not to smoke or drink even though they do, or when they tell them to wear their seat belts although the parent does not).
- Understand the significance of their place within the construct of time (past, present, and future) and begin thinking about what they will be doing in the future (e.g., college, technical school, job, marriage, and family).

Although most teenagers develop the ability to translate experiences into abstract ideas and think about the consequences of actions, approximately one-third do not achieve more fully sophisticated thinking abilities, even as adults. Neurologic changes underlie the development of executive function, memory, social inhibition, intelligence, and cognition in adolescence. Emerging scientific evidence indicates that a combination of environmental influences (e.g., drugs, alcohol, and stress) and genetic susceptibility can have long-term effects on brain structure, cognitive ability, memory, and higher executive function (Conrod and Nikolaou, 2016).

Emotional Changes of Adolescence

Adolescence is often described as emotionally challenging and appropriately managing one's emotional responses is an important task during this time. The emotions of the adolescent may be exhibited more often and more intensely than the emotions of their adult counterparts (Guyer, Silk, and Nelson, 2016). Hormones present during puberty cause emotional and physical changes. As with physical growth and development, emotional changes appear differently in males than in females. Some males may experience an association between an increase in testosterone and sad or anxious feelings, acting out, aggressive behavior, or interest in sexual activity.

Some emotional changes that occur are not directly associated with hormonal changes. Research shows that boys with adultlike physiques are given more leadership roles, are more proficient in sports, are perceived as more attractive and smarter than their peers, and are more popular than others in their age group. In general, they demonstrate higher self-esteem in early adolescence. Late-maturing boys who are short and childlike in appearance until 15 years or older tend to show more personal and social maladjustment over the entire course of adolescence. They can be insecure, suggestible, vulnerable to peer pressure, and subjects of bullying or seen as weak, immature, and less competent than average. Males, as they progress through puberty, typically develop a more positive self-image and mood, whereas females may feel a diminished sense of attractiveness as their bodies mature. Boys tend to be more satisfied with their body image and, depending on their current size, may want to either gain or lose weight, whereas girls are more likely to express a desire to lose weight. Dieting and disordered eating usually develop in adolescence (see Chapter 30).

The emotional affect and behavior of pubescent females differ in other ways from those of males. Both early-maturing boys and girls demonstrate more risky behaviors than do adolescents who are late maturing, but girls are at greater risk as a result of romantic liaisons. Often these early bloomers get "bumped up" to an older group of peers and become the objects of sexual attention from older males. The developing body of early-maturing females may not match their chronologic age or emotional maturity. This difference can influence their behavior and place them at risk for early sexual activity, adolescent dating abuse, depressive symptoms, and antisocial behavior (Chen et al., 2017; Mendle et al., 2017).

Developmental Screening and Assessment

Principles and Approaches to Assessment

Throughout infancy, early childhood, and the school years, the focus of the health care visit is the parent or caregiver and the child as a unit. This dyad changes during adolescence. Adolescents must be evaluated independently of their parents, and developmental issues must be discussed privately with the adolescents. Nonetheless, parents remain concerned, and it is ideal that they be involved in their child's health care. Adolescents are part of the family system, and providers should work with adolescents to maximize communication with parents around health issues. Some providers believe that involving parents or other significant adults in the adolescent's care is essential. However, that decision is not always the provider's to make, and it may not always be in the best interest of the adolescent. Adolescents must be actively included in decisions about sharing information with others. For many sensitive health issues, providers need to help the teenager understand and evaluate the risks and benefits of involving family members. They must also provide guidance and support on how to best inform the family, if that is the final choice. This approach can help protect a teen from the parent who may be abusive or unsafe. It can also reduce the problem of parents who are upset if they feel they are denied information about the child they love and for whom they feel responsible.

Effective interviews with adolescent clients are based on the use of good general interviewing techniques: demonstrating respect for the client; establishing parameters of what can be accomplished during the visit; using appropriate body language, active listening, and communication techniques; and working with the client to develop a realistic, individualized treatment plan. The provider gives the message that the teenager and his or her concerns are important, that no judgments will be made, and that the provider and teenager are a team, working together to achieve the healthiest outcome possible.

Preserving confidentiality with the teenager is essential. Adolescents should be reassured that the provider will not share information with the child's parent or caregiver (general confidentiality) unless the adolescent agrees, or unless the health of the child or others may be compromised (e.g., threat of potential suicide, violence, evidence of an eating disorder). Providers must inform the teenager that there are limits to confidentiality (limited confidentiality). As "mandatory reporters," primary health care providers are required by law to report information that puts the child or others in danger (e.g., physical or sexual abuse; some states require reporting teen sexual activity, even if consensual, if an age

difference of 3 or more years exists between the couple). If adolescents perceive that their provider will maintain confidentiality, they are more likely to disclose more sensitive, relevant information and it has been found that even when providers tell adolescents that there are limits to their confidentiality, teens continue to disclose. However, the opposite is also true; adolescents who do not seek care because of privacy concerns are more likely to exhibit high-risk behavior (Gilbert et al., 2014). For teenagers who are hesitant to discuss sensitive issues, a questionnaire or checklist may be an effective way to collect information. Questionnaires used to identify adolescent strengths have been created by the Search Institute (see Chapter 15) and have been used by communities to enhance adolescent self-concept, whereas programs like the Rapid Assessment for Adolescent Preventative Services (RAAPS) can help PCPs identify risky adolescent behaviors (see Resources).

Assessment

Physical Development

Adolescents should have height, weight, body mass index (BMI), and blood pressure measured at each health maintenance visit. The growth trajectory should be evaluated, using growth grids to identify norms. The SMR should be recorded at each visit to evaluate progression of pubertal changes initiated by the endocrine system. Testicular growth can be directly assessed by palpation of the testes in the scrotum and comparison of their size with a standardized orchidometer. Self-assessment is generally reliable, and adolescent males can be asked to evaluate their own level of development if provided with standards against which to compare themselves. Varicocele, or enlarged veins palpable in the scrotum, may develop at sexual maturity and are not cause for alarm unless a discrepancy in testicular size is noted on examination. Gynecomastia in boys should be noted. Scoliosis may develop rapidly at this age, and assessment should be done annually. The thyroid gland should be palpated because goiter may appear in this age group. Additionally, the teen should be asked how he or she feels about their own physical growth and development. Dissatisfaction with body appearance might warrant further probing to elicit unhealthy behavior (e.g., bingeing and purging, steroid use) (see Chapter 30 for information about eating disorders).

Cognitive Development

Assessment should include questions about school attendance, school performance, and educational or career goals. School connectedness has been found to be a significant predictor of adolescent well-being; the extent to which a child connects to school depends on characteristics of both the child and the school (Bolland et al., 2016; Waters, Cross and Shaw, 2010). Children who are behind a grade have a much greater risk of dropping out of school, thus leading some to consider school failure as a form of adolescent failure to thrive. Chronic absenteeism, class skipping, and other types of school avoidance indicate a problem that may be related to cognitive ability and should be assessed in depth. Objective assessment of cognitive development, as with school-age children, requires formal psychological testing, which is best done, if needed, through schools.

Social and Emotional Development

Key areas to assess in social and emotional development include adolescents' emerging independence from family, relationships with peers, and goals for the future (an area that older teenagers should address more specifically than younger adolescents).

Adolescents should be interviewed about school, family, and peer relationships; safety (e.g., use of seat belts, driving, drowning); exposure to violence, abuse, or weapons; mental health issues, such as mood, depression, anger problems, or suicidal ideation; sexuality, sexual activity, and sexual orientation; and involvement in risk behaviors, such as tobacco, alcohol, prescription or street drug use, and eating disorders.

Parent Assessment

Parents also need advice, support, and encouragement. Normal adolescent mood swings can trigger strain on family relationships and result in arguments. Parents with balanced approaches that include unconditional love, clear boundaries, and consistent discipline are more likely to have adolescents with less depression, less risk-taking, and better academic success than authoritarian parents. It is important to assess parental concerns about their adolescent's health at each of the episodic wellness visits because these concerns can give insight into the teen's physical, socioemotional, and mental health, and they provide a glimpse into the family functioning and the health of the parent-child dyad. If problems exist in the parent's view, or a discrepancy and potential conflict emerge in the interviews, the provider should bring the teen and parent together to clarify the concern and offer counseling.

Anticipatory Guidance During Adolescence

Anticipatory guidance should be individualized to help the adolescent understand, respond to, and take responsibility for their own behavior and development (Table 13.2). Separate discussions need to be conducted with parents to help them understand and support their child's maturation and need for independence. In these discussions, the provider should clarify what values and expectations parents have for their child and how the teenager perceives those expectations. Some discussion points are outlined in each of the adolescent phases discussed later. They should be incorporated into the health supervision visit, but they are not all-inclusive, and they should not be covered exhaustively at each visit. Ideas for assessment and management of problems that emerge from these discussions can be found in subsequent chapters (e.g., sexuality issues are discussed in Chapter 21).

Phases of Adolescence

One simple way to understand adolescence is to divide it into three psychosocial developmental phases: (1) early, 11 to 14 years old or junior high school; (2) middle, 15 to 17 years old or high school; and (3) late, 18 to 21 years old or college, work, or vocational-technical school.

Each phase is characterized by certain behavior. Understanding such behavior assists in the evaluation of areas of concern to the adolescent or family. Within each developmental phase, adolescents deal with issues of autonomy, body image, identity development, and peer group involvement.

Early Adolescence (11 to 14 Years Old)

Early adolescence is the most difficult adjustment period for young people. Rapid changes occur simultaneously in all parts of the adolescent's life; cognitive skills may not keep pace with physical changes; emotional reactions may overwhelm the child's ability to understand and cope. Early adolescents are often confused, even frightened, by the changes they are experiencing. They can

be difficult people to be around, and the responses their behavior elicits from parents and other adults may be exactly the opposite of the support, caring, and understanding they desperately need.

Physical Development

Physical changes in early adolescence vary widely; some young people achieve SMR stage 3 or even 4, whereas others are still at SMR 2 by age 14 (see previous discussion of physical development).

Cognitive Development

As their thinking abilities develop, teenagers daydream frequently. Parents and teachers need to be reminded that daydreaming is cognitive work for adolescents and that they need time to participate in this activity. At the same time, early adolescents should be given the opportunity to use their growing reasoning skills to actively solve problems, explore values, and examine principles on which they make decisions. Early adolescents set idealistic goals that change frequently. One day they want to be an engineer and the next day a pilot or a parent who stays home to raise children. Some adolescents at this age experience a drop in academic performance in junior high school, which is related to motivation rather than ability.

Social and Emotional Development

Young adolescents begin to renegotiate relationships with parents and other significant adults and develop more intimate contacts with their peers. Because they lack experience and social skills, early adolescents may not yet be a part of an adolescent subculture and can be very lonely. At this stage, teenagers can appear to be anti-adult, preferring to spend more time with friends than with family, and suddenly finding their parents to be an embarrassment. This behavior is a normal and healthy step toward maturity and a first step toward independence. One way of demonstrating independence is to challenge parental authority. The early adolescent may become more argumentative and disobedient, refuse to do chores, and want to renegotiate rules (e.g., curfews, allowance, household responsibilities).

Wide mood swings—from euphoria to sadness—can occur within a matter of minutes. Normative mood fluctuations are linked to adolescent developmental processes and are characterized by their transient nature, commonly measured in hours or days. These emotional fluctuations can and should be distinguished from the unremitting, long-standing mood and behavior changes of serious depressive disorders.

During this period, adolescents become extremely body conscious as they adjust to the physical changes of puberty. They begin to spend more time in front of the mirror combing their hair, checking their skin, and putting on makeup. Clothes and appearance become more important for all teenagers, including those with a developmental delay or disability. The onset of secondary sex characteristics increases anxieties about menstruation, wet dreams, masturbation, and breast or penis size. This is an opportune time to dispel myths (e.g., masturbation causes blindness and acne) and to provide anticipatory guidance (e.g., a premenarcheal girl often has vaginal leukorrhea, a clear, mucoid discharge).

Early adolescents have a desire for greater privacy. They often spend more time in their room alone listening to music, using social media, texting, or talking on the phone. They magnify their problems and believe that no one could possibly understand what they are feeling. Much of the adolescents' time is used to develop new friendships as a greater number of opportunities become possible. Same-sex friendships occur, usually with one best friend.

TABLE 13.2	Adolescent Development and Related Anticipatory Guidance	
Area of Development	**Anticipatory Guidance**
Physical	
Experience growth from prepubescence to sexual maturity	Teach child about body functions (e.g., menstruation, nocturnal emissions) of both genders Teach about the timing and descriptions of primary and secondary sexual characteristics of both genders (e.g., changes in breasts, genitals, and hair) Discuss masturbation Discuss sexual orientation, sexual feelings
Reach adult parameters of height and physical growth by late adolescence	Provide counseling regarding substance abuse, safety, and unintentional injuries Teach and encourage correct and consistent use of helmets, seat belts, and proper sports equipment Emphasize safety and responsibility regarding access to and use of guns and other weapons
Become comfortable with one's body	Offer reassurance that physical findings are normal; explain what to expect; listen to adolescents' concerns; encourage exercise, sports participation, and body fitness; encourage healthy nutrition and sleep patterns
Cognitive	
Move from concrete thinking to ability to reason abstractly	Emphasize value of successful completion of school Discuss how meeting academic responsibilities is a priority and needs to be integrated with other activities Explain how changes in cognitive abilities may contribute to "overthinking" or a sense of confusion; encourage teen to do "reality checks" with a trusted adult Engage adolescent in conversation, explain procedures, and answer questions; listen
Develop personal value system and moral integrity	Encourage discussion of what the adolescent believes is important and what the adolescent finds valuable Help the adolescent develop skills in conflict resolution and prevention Discuss how learning to identify feelings is the first step in understanding how "feelings" influence mental and physical processes Discuss respect for rights, needs, and opinions of others; teach that maturation involves understanding and appreciating multicultural differences
Move from dependence on others to self for risk reduction	Provide information about how to resist peer pressure to engage in risky behavior Discuss injury prevention strategies at home, work, and school; emphasize dangers of weapons
Psychosocial	
Establish independence from parents	Explain to parents an adolescent's need for privacy and that not joining in all family activities is not a sign of rejection of the family; some privacy within the home should be expected
Develop sense of self-identity	Encourage adolescents to take responsibility for their own health care Encourage adolescents to take on new challenges; discuss plans for the future (e.g., school, work, and family) Help adolescents identify their own personal strengths and joys
Create new relationships with peers and other adults	Discuss importance of activities with peers; identify healthy ways to be part of a group Provide counseling on: • Avoiding gang involvement • Bullying, which may be physical, emotional, or sexual • Preventing the use of drugs, cigarettes, and alcohol • Stopping substance use for those who are using Discuss the notion that maturation includes increased independence *and* increased responsibility at home, school, and in the community Encourage the adolescent to participate in community activities Provide information and opportunity to discuss questions regarding sexuality, how to differentiate between "love" and "infatuation," how to be sexually responsible, and how to protect against pregnancy and STIs Discuss dating relationships; emphasize that healthy relationships are based on mutual respect. Discuss how to prevent date rape or other abusive relationships Advocate for safe social media usage

STI, Sexually transmitted infection.

These strong friendships may lead to fleeting same-sex experimentation as sexual feelings emerge and adolescents develop their sexual identity. Contact with the opposite sex is usually in groups (e.g., middle school dances with boys on one side of the gym and girls on the opposite side). Other sexual behavior of the early adolescent includes masturbating, telling dirty jokes, making lewd remarks to others, demonstrating interest in watching explicit sexual scenes in the media, or looking at images of nude individuals. Sexual experimentation may vary greatly, depending on the adolescent's subculture. For example, by this age, some teenagers have already experienced sexual intercourse or pregnancy, whereas others have not even held hands.

Early adolescents begin developing their own value system. They may try value systems other than the one that they learned from their family, often leaving family members befuddled or even threatened. Their peer group aids continued identity development.

Health Supervision

Annual health supervision visits are recommended. Critical components of the visit include developmental surveillance; assessing social and academic progress, including quality of interpersonal relationships and school performance; identifying emotional wellness (e.g., mood, mental health, sexuality); and risk reduction, including injury prevention, substance use prevention, and healthy sexuality. Immunizations for human papillomavirus (HPV), diphtheria and tetanus toxoids and acellular pertussis vaccine (DTaP), influenza, hepatitis A, and meningococcal meningitis are recommended. Serum lipoprotein analysis should be done if not done earlier in childhood.

Anticipatory Guidance

Anticipatory guidance for the early adolescent focuses on explaining the rapid changes that are occurring; helping the adolescent in the early process of developing self-concept, autonomy, and independence; and providing reassurance that he or she is "normal." The following should be specifically discussed:

- What physical changes to expect as puberty progresses.
- How the adolescent can best manage the rapid physical changes (e.g., engage in physical activity or sports; focus on injury prevention [e.g., bike helmets]; identify strategies to deal with beginning menstruation while at school; eat a well-balanced diet; get enough sleep).
- Nutritional needs: Increased iron and calcium intake is needed after menarche and during periods of rapid growth.
- What emotional and psychological changes are occurring, and what coping strategies do the child and family have to manage them.
- What it means to be sexually responsible, both physically and emotionally; include abstinence counseling.
- Transition to adult health care: Initial conversations regarding transitioning to adult health care should begin between 12 and 13 years of age. This consists of informing the teen and family about the practice's transition policies. Those with chronic health care needs should begin to learn about their condition and the management regime. By age 14 to 15, a transition plan should be developed with the adolescent and parent (AAP et al., 2011; Lestishock, Daley, and White, 2017).

Middle Adolescence (15 to 17 Years Old)

Middle adolescence is characterized by continued changes in physical, cognitive, and socioemotional development. Relationships evolve and peers can be highly influential during this time. The adolescent becomes increasingly aware of his or her appearance. Although middle adolescence often provides opportunities to develop the skills necessary for adulthood, it is also the time when the adolescent is at highest risk for developing mental health disorders. It is common for the middle adolescent to begin sexual and risky behavior experimentation (Hagan et al., 2017).

Physical Development

Physical development is nearing completion. Middle adolescents have less concern about body changes, but increased interest in making themselves more attractive. As body attractiveness increases in importance, teenagers spend more time with hairstyles, clothes,

and, for some, dieting or activities to build muscle mass. Middle adolescents defy the limits of their bodies, and many have periods of excessive physical activity followed by periods of lethargy.

Cognitive Development

Intellectual sophistication and creativity increase in middle adolescence. Practicing the skills of reasoning, logic, and decision-making strengthens the adolescent's ability to establish healthy adult patterns. School and extracurricular activities are often the focus of the middle adolescent's life. They demonstrate increased concern with neighborhood and societal issues, such as poverty, peace, and the environment.

Social and Emotional Development

Peer group involvement is intense and includes the establishment of a dress code, communication style, and code of conduct. Middle adolescents tend to be more non-adult than anti-adult, a characteristic of early adolescents. They spend twice the time with peers than adults. The need for peer contact is important for all middle adolescents, but it is especially important for teenagers with developmental disabilities, chronic handicaps, or both. However, peer involvement may be more limited for this group for any number of reasons (e.g., ostracism by the peer group, parental overprotectiveness, lack of social skills, and physical constraints).

Sexual drive emerges, and middle adolescents begin to explore their ability to attract a partner of the opposite gender, same gender, or both. Frequently, physical urges precede emotional maturity, and there is increased societal pressure to experiment with sex. Adolescents report that parents are the main influence on the adolescent's decision about sexual behaviors (Hagan et al., 2017). Further discussion about adolescent sexuality is found in Chapter 21.

Parental conflict peaks as middle adolescents argue and renegotiate issues, such as curfew, allowance, going to parties or movies, and dating. Rules and expectations must be clear by this stage.

Health Supervision

Annual health supervision visits are recommended, including annual influenza immunization; developmental surveillance; and assessment of social and academic progress, quality of interpersonal relationships, school performance, and emotional wellness (e.g., mood, mental health). Screening for sexually transmitted infections (STIs) is needed if the adolescent is sexually active. Papanicolaou (Pap) smears are no longer recommended until after age 21 years regardless of sexual activity. Tuberculosis and lipid screening is needed if risk factors are identified. If a plan for transition to adult health care is not already in place, one needs to be developed. These plans must be based on an assessment of the adolescent's ability to provide self-care, and the needs and desires of the teen and his or her family. Plans, once in place, should be reevaluated annually (AAP et al., 2011; Lestishock, Daley, and White, 2017).

Anticipatory Guidance

Anticipatory guidance for the middle adolescent focuses on the teen's expanding physical, cognitive, and socioemotional capabilities; consolidating self-concept; and identifying areas for continued growth and development. The provider should reinforce healthy behaviors and acknowledge and validate the adolescent's physical, intellectual, and social growth. Specifically discuss:

- Physical changes that allow for increasing skills; recommend regular, vigorous physical activity, fitness, and engagement in a wide range of activities.

- Dangers related to drug, nicotine, performance-enhancing drugs, caffeine, diet pills, and alcohol use.
- Injury and risky behavior prevention (e.g., use seat belts, bike helmets; safe driving; emphasize safe and responsible weapon use [e.g., for hunting], violence, technology use).
- Involvement in extracurricular activities (e.g., clubs, hobbies, volunteer work, and community activities).
- Nutrition and the relationship between good nutrition, health, and a positive body image. Emphasize healthy eating, limiting sugary and caffeinated beverages, and not skipping meals.
- Encourage healthy sleep habits (see Chapter 20).
- Importance of completing high school and making plans for the future.
- Sexuality. Emphasize:
  - Responsible sexual behaviors
  - Implications of sexual intercourse
  - Preventing date rape and other forms of intimate partner violence
  - Safe sexual practice for those who are sexually active
  - Prevention of STIs
  - Birth control, including emergency methods
  - Sexual orientation
  - Breast or testicular self-examination (Note: Although the U.S. Preventive Services Task Force [USPSTF] guidelines do not recommend self-examination [USPSTF 2011], this is common practice and is included in the *Bright Futures* recommendations); the USPSTF recommendations are challenged by many (Hendrick and Helvie, 2011; Thornton, 2016).
- Nature of peer relationships: based on mutual respect and caring? Gang involvement? Bullying?
- Nature of relationship with parents: reasonable limits set? Parents show interest and concern for teenager?
- Emotional maturity: how does adolescent resolve conflicts? Manage anger and/or frustration? Reduce stress?
- Potential for self-harm (e.g., cutting, bingeing, and purging).

Late Adolescence (18 to 21 Years Old)

Late adolescence is a time when the individual has a clearer self-concept, life choices are made, and decisions about how to contribute to society as a responsible adult are implemented. These are all examples of normal behavioral autonomy.

Physical Development

Physical development is typically complete, although the late adolescent's stature may continue to develop into his or her early 20s.

Cognitive Development

Late adolescents have adult reasoning skills. They are generally capable of understanding the consequences of their actions and behaviors, and can make complex and sophisticated judgments about human relationships. They no longer base their judgments about people on overt behavior, and have a good understanding of inner motivations, including multiple determinants of an action. Of course, neither teenagers nor adults consistently use this mature level of thinking, and some never reach this level of cognitive maturity.

Social and Emotional Development

By now, adolescents usually relate to the family as adults. Relationships with parents and family are gradually renegotiated to a more adult-adult basis. The role of the parent during late adolescence should be one of support. By the end of late adolescence, this parent's role optimally has progressed to autonomy for adolescents with continued strong family ties of affection. Once adolescence is complete, young adults often have a modified value system very similar to the one with which they grew up.

Much of the final identity shaping centers on late adolescents' perceptions of their future options as adults. Many are preparing for high school graduation or college entry. They work, enter the military, marry, or participate in a vocational or technical training program. In 2016, approximately 70% of high school graduates went on to study in colleges or universities, and 72% of those not attending postsecondary institutions were either working or looking for work (U.S. Bureau of Labor Statistics, 2016). In many significant ways, the years in college offer a "moratorium," or a prolonged adolescence, a time to further clarify one's self-image. College life offers both maximal autonomy and a structured, supportive environment in which to complete developmental tasks. Those who enter the workforce and leave home immediately out of high school have quite different tasks and experiences. Their identity may be formed earlier, because they do not have the added time and supportive structures of the college experience. They cannot delay facing the issues of earning a living, forming a family, and accepting other adult responsibilities. Adolescents who are unsuccessful in the educational system or the workplace (underemployed or unemployed) may establish an identity by joining gangs or becoming socially isolated. Some late adolescents opt to join the military, which may force them to take on adult responsibilities for which they may not be psychologically or emotionally prepared. Individuals affected by violence and other traumatic events can experience prolonged stress that jeopardizes their sense of self.

A substantial number of late adolescents have established their sexuality and entered into an intimate, committed partner relationship, including marriage. Partner selection is based more on individual preferences and less on the peer group's values.

Health Supervision

Annual health supervision visits are recommended, including an annual influenza immunization. Screening for STIs is needed if the adolescent is sexually active, and Pap smears should begin at age 21 regardless of sexual activity. Tuberculosis screening is needed if risk factors are identified. A fasting lipoprotein analysis is recommended once during late adolescence.

Providers should assist the adolescent in learning about health insurance, how to use the healthcare system, and to take responsibility for self-care. A plan for transition to adult care should be clearly developed by this time. Transition involves providing medical records and referring the adolescent to an adult health care provider. Many teens benefit from a pretransfer visit with an adult provider (AAP et al., 2011; Lestishock, Daley, and White, 2017).

Anticipatory Guidance

Anticipatory guidance for the late adolescent centers on the transition from being a teenager to taking on the responsibility and role of an adult. Specifically discuss:
- How physical exercise, good nutrition, sleep, and rest are incorporated into their lifestyle.
- Strategies to balance responsibilities of school, family, and job.
- Conflict resolution and stress management strategies.
- Choices made to achieve positive future goals and plan for the future—college, vocational training, military, and job or career.

- Ways the late adolescent clarifies values and beliefs; identifying talents and interests to be pursued, and taking on challenges that increase self-confidence.
- Relationships with family, parents, siblings, friends, significant others, and community.
- Injury prevention strategies.
- Sexuality. Emphasize:
  - Responsible sexual behaviors including safe sex for those who are sexually active.
  - Continued clarification of sexual orientation and the management of sexual feelings.
  - Prevention of STIs.
  - Prevention of date rape and other intimate partner abuse.
  - Birth control, including emergency methods. Childbearing may be a decision for some late adolescents.
  - Breast or testicular self-examination (see controversy discussed in middle adolescence).

Common Developmental Issues for Adolescents

Risk Behavior: General

Description

Risk behavior consists of actions that jeopardize adolescents' physical, psychological, or emotional health (Crandall et al., 2017). Risk behaviors include those related to drug, alcohol, nicotine use, and risky sexual behaviors. These behaviors are influenced by social factors, such as peer relationships, and developmental brain changes (Telzer et al., 2015). In the era of increased technological advances, risky behavior now includes the inappropriate use of social media (e.g., cyberbullying, "sexting") and the unsafe use of mobile devices (e.g., texting while driving). Although health-risk behaviors among adolescents have decreased in the past few years, they continue to be the major cause of morbidity and mortality for adolescents (CDC, 2016). It is a paradox of adolescence that developmental tasks (i.e., gaining independence, developing one's own values, becoming comfortable with one's body, and establishing meaningful relationships) may be achieved, albeit in negative ways, through risk-taking behavior. Adolescents needing peer affiliation and striving for increased autonomy are likely to explore, experiment, and otherwise push the limits of their personal experience—often in ways that put them at risk for health-compromising outcomes. Many adolescents engage in risk behaviors without apparent negative outcomes. Other behaviors may appear risky at first glance, but do not pose significant risk to the adolescent. It is also important to recognize that some teenagers who seem at high risk do not engage in risky behaviors. PCPs should recognize factors that are protective for and those that increase risk of risky behavior.

Factors That Contribute to Risk-taking. Although it is normal for behavioral experimentation to occur during this time, adolescents vary tremendously in their ability to think abstractly about the consequences of risky behavior. Their thinking is often characterized by the notion that "it can't happen to me." Although adolescents have increased abstract cognitive skills, thinking related to emotionally charged topics (e.g., substance use, sex, school performance, and peer pressure) is often less sophisticated. An adolescent who is drinking may be doing so in part to be accepted by friends or to feel a sense of independence and maturity. Because the behavior meets important developmental needs, it may be

difficult for the adolescent to look at it objectively and give it up. In addition, the effect of alcohol on brain function further limits the adolescent's reasoning ability.

Environmental factors, both social and physical, also influence adolescents' decisions to take risks. Factors that contribute to the adolescent risk behaviors include, but are not limited to, the following:

- Poor academic performance or low intellectual function
- Impulsivity or attention deficit-hyperactivity disorder
- Role models for deviant behavior (e.g., parents with mental health disorders or who abuse drugs or engage in criminal behavior)
- Lack of constructive support or encouragement from others in social environment
- Low self-esteem
- Sense of hopelessness or helplessness
- Child abuse or other types of adverse childhood experiences
- Depression or other mental-emotional disorders
- Illiteracy or lack of job skills
- Poverty
- Insufficient sleep

Protective Factors. Protective factors may help counter risk factors and help adolescents make healthier lifestyle choices. It is important for adolescents to have active parental influence during these critical years, and these relationships serve as strong protective factors for adolescents. Also, community support of positive adolescent behavior appears to minimize risk-taking. Examples of adolescent protective factors (Hagan et al., 2017) are:

- High self-esteem
- Family connectedness
- Sense of future
- Academic success
- Parental engagement
- Coping skills
- Relationships with caring adults
- Community involvement (e.g., school, religious institutions, volunteering)
- Access to recreation

Adolescents with multiple risk factors and few protective factors are more likely to engage in risk behavior, with potential health- and life-threatening results. These adolescents need prompt attention and assessment to determine the likelihood of negative outcomes. Conversely, resilient adolescents who are doing well, despite multiple risk factors, should be acknowledged and applauded.

Assessment

All adolescents should be assessed for their level of risk-taking behavior. The provider's approach to a discussion of sensitive issues should include ensuring confidentiality, providing privacy, using constructive communication strategies, and establishing rapport.

The HEEADSSS technique is a method of assessing risk behavior. Areas for assessment include **H**ome, **E**ducation and employment, **E**ating, **A**ctivities, **D**rugs, **S**exuality, **S**uicide/Depression, and **S**afety (Box 13.2) (Smith and McGuinness, 2017). Providers should also be alert for red flags at each developmental stage, because delays in development may contribute to negative behavior (Table 13.3).

The following are considered risky behaviors:

- Tobacco and other nicotine use (discussed later)
- Substance use or abuse, including alcohol
- Poor academic performance

• BOX 13.2 Questions for HEEADSSS Assessment

Questions focus on relationships with others, functioning at school and work, self-efficacy, resilience, and independent decision-making.

Home: Who lives with you? How are your relationships with the other people with whom you live? Have there been any changes at home? Do you feel safe at home?

Education/employment: What do you like/dislike about school? How is school going? How are your grades? Have you ever had trouble at school? Do you work? How many hours do you work? Where do you work? Do you have friends at school? At work?

Eating: Are you comfortable with your body? Are you interested in gaining/losing weight? How do you manage your weight? Tell me about how often you exercise. Tell me about what you normally eat every day.

Activities: What do you do for fun? What types of things do you like to do with your friends? What types of things do you like to do with your family? Do you play sports? Are you in clubs or other organizations? How much time do you watch TV? Use the computer? Text? Listen to music? What types of activities do you like to do online? On your phone?

Drugs: Do you, anyone in your family, or your friends use drugs/tobacco/drink alcohol? Have you ever used performance-enhancing drugs?

Sexuality: Do you date? Have you ever had a romantic relationship? What do you consider to be sex? Have you ever had sex? How many partners have you had? Are you interested in males/females or both? Have you ever had someone hurt or threaten you sexually? Do you use birth control/condoms? How often?

Suicide/depression: Do you ever feel like you are all alone or no one cares? Do you feel sad most of the time? Have you ever thought of actually hurting yourself? Do you ever need to use drugs (alcohol, tobacco, street drugs) to make you feel better? Have you lost interest in being with friends or doing things you previously liked to do?

Safety: Have you ever been hurt by or threatened by someone (who)? Have you ever been seriously injured? Do you use sports safety equipment? Do you use seat belts? Do you text/talk when you drive? Do you ever feel unsafe (where)? Have you ever been bullied? Have you ever met (or do you plan on meeting) someone you first met online?

- Risky sexual activity (including multiple partners, unprotected sexual intercourse)
- Drinking and driving
- Body dysmorphism or eating disorders (see Chapter 30)
- Behaviors that result in injury or violence
- Delinquency or involvement with gangs
- Violence-related behavior, such as carrying weapons or making threats of violence
- Mood disorders or signs of mental disorders
- Signs of physical, mental, sexual, or emotional abuse
- Poor nutrition and physical inactivity
- Inappropriate use of social media or technology devices

The consequences of such behavior can include addiction, school failure, pregnancy, STIs, injuries, conviction for driving under the influence, incarceration, or death. Half of all STI cases in the United States occur in 15- to 24-year-olds (CDC, 2017a). Engaging in chronic risk-taking behavior often arrests developmental progress toward adult emotional maturity.

Management

Interventions should be considered when the adolescent's behavior threatens the accomplishment of developmental tasks or the adolescent's health, safety, and well-being. Encourage adolescent behavior that supports the achievement of developmental tasks. Adolescents who pierce their noses, shave half of their hair, and spend evenings with friends, for example, may be irritating to parents, but their behavior can help them establish their autonomy, identity, and ability to relate to others. Historically, tattooing and body piercing were considered high-risk behaviors. However, recent literature does not consistently demonstrate that tattoos are associated with high-risk behaviors and normal body modification should be differentiated from nonsuicidal self-injury (Breuner and Levine, 2017).

The approach used for adolescent health care differs from that used with younger children. Early on, parents were central to the success of interventions. Although parents are still critical to successful intervention, PCPs must recognize that the teenager makes the decisions, and mediation between parent and teen may be necessary at times. The provider's role is to give the adolescent information and guidance to make the best-informed decisions possible.

Generally, high-risk teenagers require numerous services. PCPs need to know their state laws regarding adolescent health issues, how to access community resources, and how to use other professionals collaboratively. The following list identifies basic services that at-risk teenagers may need:

- Food resources for teenage parents and their children
- Temporary shelter
- Counseling and mental health services
- Foster care services for teenage parents and their children
- Local medical and social work services
- Local juvenile justice system and protective services
- Drug rehabilitation programs specifically designed for adolescents
- Alternative school and vocational education programs
- Sports, fitness, and community activities, including after-school programs
- Support programs such as Big Brothers or Big Sisters

Advocating for at-risk children and adolescents; involving their families, communities, and schools; and helping young people identify an individual who cares for them and trusts them are important actions all health care providers can take.

Risk Behavior: Tobacco Use

Description

Globally, the use of tobacco is the leading cause of preventable death. Most adults who smoke daily, began smoking before the age of 18. Despite decreases in traditional cigarette use, the rates of alternative tobacco product (ATP) use, such as hookahs and electronic cigarettes, have significantly increased in recent years. ATPs are marketed as a safer alternative to traditional cigarettes, yet evidence suggests these products are equally as harmful and potentially more harmful than cigarettes (Lee, Shearston, and Weitzman, 2016).

The National Youth Tobacco Survey reports in 2016, 20% of high school students and 7% of middle school students (nearly 4 million students) currently use tobacco products. Almost half of these students report using two or more tobacco products. In both groups, e-cigarettes were the most commonly used product (CDC, 2017b). In the past, regulation of ATPs has been minimal, but the Food and Drug Administration (2017) ruled that all products derived from tobacco will be regulated.

Many adolescents experiment with tobacco use but may stop after a short period before becoming addicted to nicotine. Tobacco dependence (addiction) varies from one individual to another and can appear at any time after initiating tobacco use, so prevention and early intervention are essential. As previously discussed, the

TABLE 13.3   Developmental Red Flags: Adolescent

Age	Physical and Sexual Development	Psychosocial Development	Cognitive Development
All phases of adolescence	*Physical development:* Poor vision close or distant Kyphosis or scoliosis Poor nutrition, poor oral health, caries, malocclusion Loss of appetite/underweight Chronic disease, such as heart disease, hypertension, dyslipidemia, diabetes, or a family member with a chronic or lifelong illness No physical activity; overweight Sleep disturbance	*Social habits:* Drug or alcohol abuse; blackouts Relationships: Permissive or authoritarian parental style No participation in home chores History of family violence School fights No close or "best" friend No identified peer group Friends or siblings in gangs Cruelty to animals Sexuality: Sexual orientation worries Mood: Pervasive sad mood, feelings of hopelessness, suicidal thoughts or gestures, history of previous suicide attempt Flattened affect without expressions of joy, sorrow, or excitement Excessive worrying or rumination Self-concept: Believes self to be "ugly" or "fat"; is dieting despite normal body size and shape Negative feelings of self-worth	Low IQ Behind in grade or failing classes Chronic absenteeism or class skipping Attention problems Lack of organizational skills for homework Disruptive behavior Lack of impulse control Unable to control own behavior (e.g., anger, impulsivity)
Early adolescence (11-14 years old)	Less than SMR stage 2 Female short stature or lack of height spurt Sexuality: Early sexual experimentation	*Sexuality:* Fears about emerging sexuality/sexual orientation Self-concept: Does not fantasize or dream about adult career	Unable to identify feelings
Middle adolescence (15-17 years old)	Kyphosis or scoliosis Less than SMR stage 4 Male short stature or lack of height spurt Male muscular growth without testicular maturation Male persistent gynecomastia and acne Female primary or secondary amenorrhea Risky sexual activity, including unprotected sexual intercourse and multiple sexual partners	*Social habits:* Drinking and driving Relationships: Excessively oppositional, defiant of all authority Abusive dating relationships Sexuality: Sexual orientation worries	Unable to differentiate emotional states from physical states Poor judgment
Late adolescence (18-21 years old)	Less than SMR stage 4 or 5 Risky sexual activity, including unprotected sexual intercourse and multiple sexual partners	No life goals Does not fantasize or dream about adult career Social habits: Drinking and driving Relationships: Lacks intimate relationships Abusive dating relationships Unable to separate from peer groups Unable to separate from parents Unable to keep a job Sexuality: Sexual orientation worries	High school dropout Persistent egocentrism Unable to reason or plan based on future and abstract concepts Poor judgment Chronic health care seeking for psychosomatic complaints

IQ, Intelligence quotient.

<table>
<thead>
<tr><th colspan="2">TABLE 13.4   Primary and Secondary Prevention and Tobacco Use Cessation Strategies for Adolescents</th></tr>
<tr><th>Primary Prevention</th><th>Secondary Prevention</th></tr>
</thead>
<tbody>
<tr>
<td>Provide multimedia, multisite health information, not limited to schools

Use social norms theory to encourage adolescent to forgo tobacco use

Emphasize skills to avoid peer pressure

Focus on adolescents' developmental need to belong to a social group</td>
<td>Ask at every visit whether adolescent or friends use tobacco

Inform adolescent of health risks of tobacco use and process by which one becomes addicted to nicotine; emphasize that it is easier to stop early

Develop mutual understanding of problem

Use brief motivational interviewing to spark interest in tobacco cessation

Determine realistic stop-use date

Help adolescent identify barriers to stopping and ways to overcome those barriers

Provide information about self-help and support groups; encourage adolescent to try to stop smoking with a friend

Provide nicotine patch pharmacologic cessation therapy where appropriate

Schedule follow-up visits to monitor progress; reinforce positive efforts

Assess parents' tobacco use patterns; provide information and support to stop use</td>
</tr>
</tbody>
</table>

adolescent brain is particularly susceptible to the influence of substances (like nicotine), and there is a resulting higher rate of dependence in teenagers than in adults.

Assessment

The Substance Abuse and Mental Health Services Administration and the AAP recommend clinicians screen for substance use, utilize a brief intervention, and if indicated, refer to treatment. Annual preventative visits serve as an opportunity to screen for substance use (Levy and Williams, 2016). Adolescents should be asked whether they or their friends smoke or use other forms of tobacco and ask about specific types of tobacco use (e-cigarettes, hookahs) during all visits. Utilizing a validated screening tool is the best approach. See Chapter 30 for a complete discussion on substance use.

Management

Adolescent tobacco management includes primary prevention, with a goal of keeping the child from starting to use, and secondary prevention with a goal of cessation (Table 13.4). Behavioral interventions in pediatric primary care for tobacco use are controversial and have been shown to be most effective for tobacco users with only mild nicotine dependence. The U.S. Public Health Service promotes the use of cognitive-behavioral strategies, motivational strategies, and examining the effects of social influence on smoking. Interventions should be tailored to the adolescent's readiness to change. Pharmacologic treatments can be offered for those with moderate to severe tobacco dependence, although these agents are only FDA approved for use in adults. Additionally, research on smoking cessation medications demonstrates nonadherence rates

and relapse after discontinuation of therapy to be barriers to use of pharmacologic agents (Siqueira, 2017).

Adolescents should be offered specific strategies and easily accessible support to assist with smoking cessation. One strategy is to provide the adolescent with a quit line referral number such as 1-800-QUIT-NOW and 1-800-44U-QUIT. These telephone-based interventions have been shown to help with tobacco cessation. Adolescents are also more likely to respond to provider education specific to how tobacco affects the adolescent's appearance, breath, and athletic performance. Education should specifically address the avoidance of ATPs as many adolescents view these products as safer than traditional cigarettes (AAP, 2015).

Another important source of tobacco exposure comes from parental tobacco use. Parental tobacco use increases the risk of their child using and becoming tobacco dependent. Anticipatory guidance should address effects of secondhand smoke on the adolescent's health. Evidence shows that even short messages can improve smoking cessation rates in families.

Risk Behavior: Self-Injurious Behaviors

Description

Nonsuicidal self-injury (NSSI) is a group of repetitive behaviors with the intent of purposefully causing physical harm to oneself but not with the intent of ending one's own life (Hornor, 2016). Symptoms must have occurred at least five times within the past year and be associated with at least two of the following:

- Previous negative emotions
- Preoccupation with and a repetitive desire to engage in the activity
- Feelings of relief from negative emotions or a sensation of positive feelings with activity
- Impaired interpersonal relationships (American Psychiatric Association [APA], 2013)

Excluded from this diagnosis are behaviors like piercings and tattoos, because these are seen as socially acceptable. NSSI behaviors vary widely and include cutting (the most common mechanism), scraping, hitting, burning or ripping of skin, subdermal tissue, or hair, hindering wound healing (does not include scab picking), and head banging (Hornor, 2016). The common factor among NSSI is that these behaviors are used as a coping strategy to relieve distress, anger, and stress and to create a sense of calm. Patients often report that the physical pain associated with these acts helps relieve emotional pain. These are not suicide attempts. However, individuals who engage in NSSI are more likely to attempt suicide, have an eating disorder, a history of abuse or trauma, a mood disorder, or psychological distress than those in the general population and should be assessed for suicide risk. NSSI is a component of borderline personality disorder but can be present in those without borderline personality disorder (Hornor, 2016).

NSSI typically begins in mid to late adolescence and declines in early adulthood, but at least 20% of those with NSSI behavior state the behaviors began prior to age 12 (APA, 2013; Lewis and Heath, 2015). Recent research indicates that the incidence of NSSI has increased by approximately 25% (Hornor, 2016). However, there are no historical data for comparison, and many studies do not differentiate NSSI from suicidal behavior. The incidence of NSSI that meets DSM V criteria in adolescents is 6.7% (Claes et al., 2015).

Although the behaviors associated with NSSI are not intended to result in suicide, research suggests as many as 70% of those with a history of NSSI have had at least one prior suicide attempt (Hornor, 2016). Characteristics of NSSI that are associated with increased risk of suicidality include more frequent NSSI behaviors, NSSI occurring over a longer period of time, multiple methods of NSSI, more severe methods used (such as burning), history of abuse, coexisting psychiatric disorders (borderline personality disorder, posttraumatic stress disorder) (Hornor, 2016).

Assessment

History should include focused questions about present and past experiences with self-injury, description of the frequency of these behaviors, and what emotional or mental responses the adolescent gets from self-injury. Given the association of NSSI with abuse, adolescents should be assessed for physical and emotional signs of abuse (see Chapter 24). Although self-injuries can decrease emotional pain, they often result in guilt. Therefore, adolescents who engage in NSSI often hide evidence of their activities, intentionally mask physical marks, and deny or will not disclose their NSSI behaviors, thus making diagnosis difficult. Suspicion should be raised if adolescents present with hoodies or heavy clothing on hot days, or when there is resistance to allow skin examination. The most common locations for NSSI injuries are the arms, legs, and front of the torso. There may be scratches or cuts in various stages of healing or that appear to be in patterns or that form words. Traction alopecia may be present. Adolescents should also be assessed for suicidality, because NSSI can be a predictive factor for future suicide attempts (see Chapter 15).

Management

Suicide and mental health assessment is needed when adolescents present with suspected NSSI. Self-injurers will often accept help during acute phases but lose motivation for help when symptoms are not as acute. The presence of any wounds should be recognized as a call for help. Appropriate therapeutic interventions include cognitive behavioral, dialectical, and family therapy. Therapeutic response is usually contingent on the self-injurer feeling recognized by the provider, and is achieved when positive emotional coping skills are learned. ● Prompt referral to a mental health professional is needed if symptoms of psychosis or suicide ideation are present (Hornor, 2016). However, not all adolescents who use NSSI need psychiatric referral. Those who have no other signs of mental illness and who are experimenting with self-injury, or who have engaged in NSSI because of peer pressure may not require immediate intervention but should have close follow-up.

Risk Behavior: Technology and Social Media Use

Description

Technology allows for increased connectivity and social interaction, and social media can be a positive influence when used appropriately. Social media allows adolescents to connect with friends, families, and classmates and gives them a platform to express their thoughts, feelings, and points of view to a broad audience. In 2015, adolescents reported using social media more than 1 hour every day (Uhis, Elison, and Subrahmanyam, 2017). More than 92% of people in the United States own a cellular phone, with the majority being smartphones (68%). On average, adolescents spend more than 2 hours daily on their smartphone.

Although there are benefits of social media and technology devices, such as developing friendships, increased self-esteem, and social support, there are also hazards to this increased access to social media and mobile devices (Atchley and Strayer, 2017; Uhis,

Elison, and Subrahmanyam, 2017). Nearly 10% of adolescents report experiencing cyberbullying; including having negative information reported about them, having personal information made public online; or receiving unwanted emails, messages, or texts. Peer cybervictimization, or "aggression communicated online intended to harm an individual of a similar age or social position" affects millions of U.S. adolescents and increases the risk of substance abuse, depression, and suicidality (Fisher, Gardella, and Teurbe-Tolon, 2016, p. 1727).

Assessment

Parents and PCPs should have open discussions with adolescents regarding their social media use. Risky social media usage includes:
• Cyberbullying and harassment
• Sexting: Sending nude or provocative photos, and/or sexual messages
• Depression and social withdrawal
• Signs of problematic technology use: Obsessing about social media use, avoiding interactions with others in order to engage online, getting in trouble because of social media use
• Meeting strangers through online profiles
• Unsafe use of mobile devices while driving

Management

It is important for PCPs to approach teens nonjudgmentally, because there is often a technology gap between adolescents who grew up with use of computers, tablets, and smartphones, and adults who begin technology use later in life. It is common for teens to state that adults don't understand how "everyone" uses social media and how not using technology can have a negative social impact. Providers should remind adolescents that electronic images and communications can be accessed and used by others even after being deleted. Therefore the teen needs to understand that any posting can, and possibly will be, shared with others and that digital footprints can be accessed years later and negatively impact their future (e.g., university admission and/or employment). Many adolescents do not realize that possession of nude or suggestive photos can be considered child pornography, although enforcement of this varies from state to state (O'Connor, Drouin, Yergens, and Newsham, 2017). Counsel teens not to post when they are emotionally upset (e.g., angry, sad, scared), because spur-of-the-moment expression can cause long-standing problems. Teach them that online profiles can be real but may also be complete fabrications that are designed to initiate a meeting with others under false pretenses.

An important part of managing social media usage involves parental education and supervision of online activity. Parents should have frequent, open conversations with adolescents about internet and social media use. The AAP has an online family media plan tool that helps families decide how to best set guidelines and limits on media use (available at www.healthychildren.org/English/media/Pages/default.aspx American Academy of Pediatrics, 2017).

Additionally, parents should address the issue of devices and distraction and the dangers of using mobile devices while driving. One study examining adolescents and motor vehicle crashes found that distractions (using a cell phone, looking for something in the vehicle, grooming, etc.) were a factor almost 60% of the time. Approximately one-quarter of all U.S. motor vehicle crashes are attributed to distractions by small screen devices according to the National Safety Council (Atchley and Strayer, 2017).

Finally, providers and parents should discuss the impact of media devices on sleep. Screen time is largely associated with negative sleep such as a delay in falling asleep and/or poor sleep (LeBourgeois et al., 2017). Parents are encouraged to remove media devices from the adolescent's bedroom and provide a central location outside of the bedroom to charge/store devices overnight. Parents and PCPs should talk with the adolescent about the benefits of adequate sleep, the potential consequences of poor sleep, and how to establish nighttime routines that promote healthy sleep including avoiding electronic media use before sleep.

Additional Resources

Adolescent Health Transition Project (AHTP). http://depts.washington.edu/healthtr

Alliance of Professional Tattooists, Inc.(APT). www.safe-tattoos.com

American Academy of Family Physicians www.aafp.org

American Academy of Pediatrics (AAP). www.aap.org

American Academy of Pediatrics (AAP): Talking to Kids About Social Media and Sexting. www.aap.org/en-us/about-the-aap/aap-press-room/news-features-and-safety-tips/Pages/Talking-to-Kids-and-Teens-About-Social-Media-and-Sexting.aspx

American Academy of Pediatrics Family Media Plan. https://www.healthychildren.org/English/media/Pages/default.aspx

Centers for Disease Control and Prevention (CDC). www.cdc.gov.

Family Acceptance Project. http://familyproject.sfsu.edu

Ginsburg K. *A Parent's Guide to Building Resilience in Children and Teens: Giving Your Child Roots and Wings.* Elk Grove Village, IL: American Academy of Pediatrics; 2006.

Got Transition: Resources for Health Providers. http://gottransition.org/providers/index.cfm

Menstrupedia. http://menstrupedia.com

National Runaway Safeline. www.1800runaway.org 1-800-RUNAWAY (786-2929)

Parenting Teens. www.parentingteens.com

Rapid Assessment for Adolescent Preventative Services (RAAPS). www.raaps.org

Rape, Abuse, and Incest National Network (RAINN). https://rainn.org/ 1-800-HOPE (4673)

Search Institute. www.search-institute.org

Sex, etc.—sex education for teens by teens. http://sexetc.org/

Society for Adolescent Health and Medicine (SAHM). www.adolescenthealth.org

References

Abreu AP, Kaiser UB. Pubertal development and regulation. *Lancet Diabetes Endocrinol.* 2016;4:254–264. https://doi.org/10.1016/@2213.8587(15)00418-0.

American Academy of Pediatrics (AAP). American Academy of Family Physicians, and American College of Physicians, transitions clinical report authoring group. clinical report: supporting the health care transition from adolescence to adulthood in the medical home. *Pediatrics.* 2011;128:182–200.

American Academy of Pediatrics. Clinical practice policy to protect children from tobacco, nicotine, and tobacco smoke. *Pediatrics.* 2015;136:1–10. https://doi.org/10.1542/peds.2015-3108.

American Congress of Obstetricians and Gynecologists (ACOG) Committee on Adolescent Health Care. Menstruation in girls and adolescents: using the menstrual cycle as a vital sign. *Obstet Gynecol.* 2006;108:1323–1328.

American Psychiatric Association (APA). *Diagnostic and Statistical Manual of Mental Disorders.* 5th ed. Arlington, VA: American Psychiatric Association; 2013.

Atchley P, Strayer DL. Small screen use and driving safety. *Pediatrics.* 2017;140(S2):S107–S111. https://doi.org/10.1542.peds.2016-1758M.

Bolland KA, Bolland AC, Bolland JM, et al. Trajectories of school and community connectedness in adolescence by gender and delinquent behavior. *J Community Psychol.* 2016;44:602–619.

Breuner CC, Levine D. Adolescent and young adult tattooing, piercing, and scarification. *Pediatrics.* 2017;140:1–17. https://doi.org/10.1542/peds.2017.1962.

Cabellero A, Granberg R, Tseng K. Mechanisms to contributing to prefrontal cortex maturation during adolescence. *Neurosci Biobehav Rev.* 2016;70:4–12. https://doi.org/10.1016/j.neubiorev.2016.05.013.

Centers for Disease Control and Prevention [CDC]. *STDs in adolescents and young adults*; 2017a. Retrieved from: https://www.cdc.gov/std/stats16/adolescents.htm.

Centers for Disease Control and Prevention [CDC]. *Tobacco use among middle and high school students-United States, 2011-2016*; 2017b. Retrieved from: https://www.cdc.gov/mmwr/volumes/65/wr/mm6514a1.htm. Accessed March 13, 2018.

Centers for Disease Control and Prevention [CDC]. *Youth Risk Behavior Surveillance-United States, 2015*; 2016. Retrieved from: https://www.cdc.gov/healthyyouth/data/yrbs/pdf/2015/ss6506_updated.pdf.

Chen FR, Rothman EF, Jaffee SR. Early puberty, friendship, group characteristics, and dating abuse in US girls. *Pediatrics.* 2017;139(6):1–9. https://doi.org.10.1542/peds.2016-2847.

Claes L, Luyckx K, Baetens I, Van de Ven M, Witterman C. Bullying and victimization, depressive mood, and non-suicidal self-injury in adolescents: the moderating role of parental support. *J Child Fam Stud.* 2015;24(11):3363–3373.

Coleman LG, Liu W, Oguz I, et al. Adolescent binge ethanol treatment alters adult regional brain volumes, cortical extracellular protein matrix protein and behavioral flexibility. *Pharmacol Biochem Behav.* 2014;116:142–151.

Conrod PJ, Nikolaou K. Annual research review: On the developmental neuropsychology of substance use disorders. *J Child Psychol Psychiatry.* 2016;57:371–394. https://doi.org/10.1111/jcpp.12516.

Crandall A, Magnusson BM, Lelinneth M, Novilla K, Dyer WJ. Family financial stress and adolescent sexual risk-taking: the role of self-regulation. *J Youth Adolesc.* 2017;46:45–62. https://doi.org/10.1007/s10964-016-0543-x.

De Silva NK. Breast development and disorders in the adolescent female. *Best Pract Res Clin Obstet Gynaecol.* 2018;48(4):40–50. https://doi.org/10.1016/j.bpobgyn.2017.08.009.

Fisher BW, Gardella JH, Teurbe-Tolon. Peer cybervictimization among adolescents and the associated internalizing and externalizing problems: a meta-analysis. *J Youth Adolesc.* 2016;45:1727–1743. https://doi.org/10.1007/s10964-016-0541-z.

Food and Drug Administration. *FDA's new Regulations for e-Cigarettes, Cigars, and all Other Tobacco Products*; 2017. Retrieved from: https://www.fda.gov/TobaccoProducts/Labeling/RulesRegulationsGuidance/ucm394909.htm#rule. Accessed March 13, 2018.

Gilbert AL, Rickert VI, Aalsma MC. Clinical conversations about health: the impact of confidentiality in preventative adolescent care. *J Adolesc Health.* 2014;55(5):672–677. 4-85.

Guyer AE, Silk JS, Nelson EE. The neurobiology of the emotional adolescent: from the inside out. *Neurosci Biobehav Rev.* 2016;70. https://doi.org/10.1016/j.neubiorev.2016.07.037.

Hagan JF, Shaw JS, Duncan PM, eds. *Bright Futures: Guidelines for Health Supervision of Infants, Children, and Adolescents.* 4th ed. Elk Grove Village, IL: American Academy of Pediatrics; 2017.

Hall GS. *Adolescence: its Psychology and its Relations to Physiology, Anthropology, Sociology, sex, Crime, Religion and Education.* Englewood Cliffs, NJ: Prentice-Hall; 1908.

Hendrick RE, Helvie MA. United States Preventive Services Task Force screening mammography recommendations: science ignored. *AJR Am J Roentgenol.* 2011;196(2):W112–W116.

Hornor G. Nonsuicidal self-injury. *J Pediatr Health Care.* 2016;30(3):261–267. https://doi.org/10.1016/j.pedhc.2015.06.012.

Kilford EJ, Garret E, Blakemore SJ. The development of social cognition in adolescence: an integrative perspective. *Neurosci Biobehav Rev.* 2016;70:106–120. https://doi.org/10.1016/j.neubiorev.2016.08.016.

Klein DA, Emerick JE, Sylvester JE, Vogt KS. Disorders of puberty: an approach to diagnosis and management. *Am Fam Physician.* 2017;96(9):590–599.

LeBourgeois MK, Hale L, Chang A, Akacem LD, Montgomery-Downs HE, Buxton OM. Digital media and sleep in childhood and adolescence. *Pediatrics.* 2017;140(s2):S92–S96. https://doi.org/10.1542.peds.2016-1758J.

Lee L, Shearston JA, Weitzman M. New alternative tobacco products–A threat to adolescent health. *Pediatric Rev.* 2016;37(7):310–312.

Lestishock L, Daley AM, White P. Pediatric nurse practitioners' perspectives on health care transition from pediatric to adult care. *J Pediatr Health Care.* 2017. https://doi.org/10.1016/j.pedhc.2017.11.005.

Lewis SP, Heath NL. Nonsuicidal self-injury among youth. *J Pediatr.* 2016;166:526–530. https://doi.org/10.1016/j.jpeds.2014.11.062.

Mendle J, Ryan R, McKone KM. Age at menarche, depression, and antisocial behavior in adulthood. *Pediatrics.* 2017;141:1–8. https://dio.org.10.1542/peds.2017-1703.

Neinstein LS, Katzman DK, Callahan T, Gordon CM, Joffe A, Rickert V. *Neinstein's Adolescent and Young Adult Health Care.* 6th ed. Philadelphia: Wolters Kluwer; 2016.

O'Connor K, Drouin M, Yergens N, Newsham G. Sexting legislation in the United States and abroad: a call for uniformity. *Int J Cyber Criminol.* 2017;11:218–245. https://doi.org/10.5281/zenodo.1037397.

Pascual M, Pla A, Miñarro J, et al. Neuroimmune activation and myelin changes in adolescent rats exposed to high-dose alcohol and associated cognitive dysfunction: a review with reference to human adolescent drinking. *Alcohol.* 2014;49(2):187–192.

Rees P, Booth R, Jones A. The emergence of neuroscientific evidence on brain plasticity: implications for educational practice. *Edu Child Psychol.* 2016;33(1):8–19.

Schulz KM, Sisk CL. The organizing actions of adolescent gonadal steroid hormones on brain and behavioral development. *Neurosci Biobehav Rev.* 2016;70:148–158. https://doi.org/10.1016/j.neubiorev.2016.07.036.

Sharma A, Morrow JD. Neurobiology of adolescent substance use disorders. *Child Adolesc Psychiatr Clin N Am.* 2016;25:367–375. https://doi.org/10.1016/j.chc.2016.02.001.

Silveri MM, Dager AD, Cohen-Gilbert JE, Sneider JR. Neurobiological signatures associated with alcohol and drug use in the human adolescent brain. *Neurosci Biobehav Rev.* 2016;70:244–259. https://doi.org/10.1016/j.neubiorev.2016.06.042.

Siqueira LM. Nicotine and tobacco as substances of abuse in children and adolescents. *Pediatrics.* 2017;139(1):e1–e13. https://doi.org/10.1542/peds.2016-3436.

Smith GL, McGuinness TM. Adolescent psychosocial assessment: the HEEADSSS. *J Psychosoc Nurs Ment Health Serv.* 2017;55:24–27. https://doi.org/10.3928/02793695-20170420-03.

Telzer EH, Fuligni AJ, Lieberman MD, Miernicki ME, Galvan A. The quality of adolescents' peer relationships modulates neural sensitivity to risk taking. *Soc Cogn Affect Neurosci.* 2015;10:389–398.

Thornton CP. Best practice in teaching male adolescents and young men to perform testicular self-examinations: a review. *J Pediatric Health Care.* 2016;30:518–527. https://doi.org/10.1016/j.oedhc.2015.11.009.

Tottenham N, Galvan A. Stress and the adolescent brain amygdala-prefrontal cortex circuitry and ventral striatum as developmental targets. *Neurosci Biobehav Rev.* 2016;70:217–227. https://doi.org/10.1016/j.neubiorev.2016.07.030.

U.S. Bureau of Labor Statistics. *Economic News Release: College Enrollment and Work Activity of 2016 High School Graduates (Website)*; 2016. Retrieved from: https://www.bls.gov/news.release/hsgec.nr0.htm. Accessed March 13, 2018.

U.S. Preventive Services Task Force (USPSTF). *Testicular Cancer: Screening*; 2011. Retrieved from: https://www.uspreventiveservicestaskforce.org/Page/Document/ClinicalSummaryFinal/testicular-cancer-screening. Accessed March 13, 2018.

Uhis YT, Ellison NB, Subrahmanyam K. Benefits and costs of social media in adolescence. *Pediatrics.* 2017;140I(S2):S67–S70. https://doi.org/10.1542/peds.2016-1758E.

Waters S, Cross D, Shaw T. Does the nature of schools matter? An exploration of selected school ecology factors on adolescent perceptions of school connectedness. *Br J Educ Psychol.* 2010;80(Pt 3):381–402.

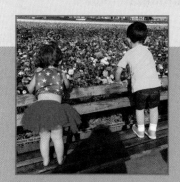

14

Introduction to Health Promotion and Health Protection

MARTHA DRIESSNACK

This chapter provides a brief introduction to the history and core concepts of pediatric primary care, including health promotion and protection, disease and/or disability prevention, and the pediatric medical home. The chapter also introduces *Bright Futures*, a national health promotion and preventive care initiative from the American Academy of Pediatrics (AAP). The chapter ends with a discussion of primary care versus primary prevention. Each subsequent chapter in this unit focuses on key health promotion and/or protection topics, including behavioral and mental health, nutrition, physical activity, immunizations, injury prevention, and child maltreatment.

There are a number of different pediatric primary care providers (PCPs), including pediatric and family nurse practitioners, pediatric and family physicians, and physician assistants. All are important and all are needed. In 2016, the Children's Health Fund shared that more than 20 million children (~28%) in the United States lacked sufficient access to essential health care. The fact that so many children are not getting the care they need to be healthy and to reach their potential represents an ongoing call to action to all pediatric PCPs:

> *Not only does failing to address health care access barriers threaten and undermine the health and wellbeing of children, but it also may have a direct impact on a child's ability to succeed academically and enter the workforce at their full potential. Loss of later productivity and the extraordinary costs of remediation will clearly have deleterious consequences for the future economic strength and vibrancy of the United States. The stakes could not be higher.*
> **[CHILDREN'S HEALTH FUND, 2016, p. 3]**

Pediatric Nurse Practitioners—Then and Now

In 1965, Dr. Loretta Ford and Dr. Henry Silver started the nation's first nurse practitioner (NP) program at the University of Colorado. As a result, Dr. Ford is often referred to as the mother of the NP movement and remains one of its greatest champions. One important piece of history is this first NP program was pediatric and focus was primary care. The emphasis in those early years was to expand public health nurses' roles, integrating the traditional role of the nurse with advanced training and authority in the delivery of primary care to children and families. This early focus on health promotion, protection, and disease prevention remains the mainstay of primary care pediatric nurse practitioner (PNP) programs across the country.

Today, the PNP role continues to evolve. The key difference between a primary care PNP and an acute care PNP is not the site where they practice, but the acuity of the patient for whom they are caring (ANA, 2015). Primary care PNPs, much like those in the early days with Dr. Ford, provide primary care, which includes well-child care and the prevention and/or management of both common pediatric acute illnesses and chronic conditions. In contrast, acute care PNPs provide care for acutely, critically, and chronically ill children who are unstable, experiencing life-threatening illness, are medically fragile and/or technologically dependent.

Pediatric Primary Care

Primary care represents one level of care within the larger health system. Subsequent levels of health care involve increased complexity, additional specialists, and specialized equipment. Accordingly, *primary* care is generalist care; *secondary* care requires specialized expertise; *tertiary* care requires both specialized expertise and equipment; and *quaternary* care requires highly specialized expertise and highly unusual or specialized equipment. Primary care is not site-specific; however, it is often incorrectly used synonymously with *out*-patient or ambulatory care, while subsequent levels of care are typically associated with *in*-patient or acute care.

Primary care is conceptualized as being more *person-* rather than *disease*-centered. It includes the provision of continuous, relationship-oriented care over time, rather than being a series

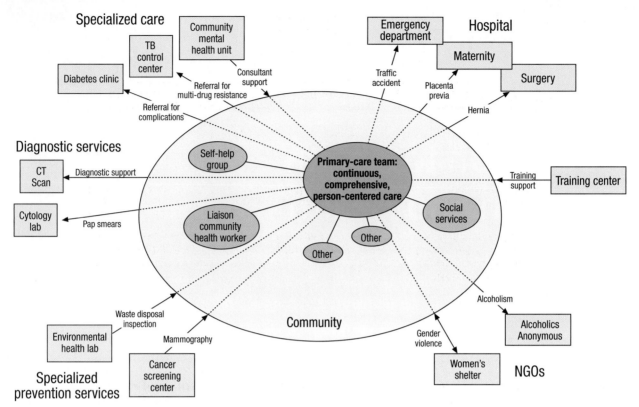

• **Fig 14.1** Primary Care as a Hub of Coordination: Networking Within the Community Served and With Outside Partners. (World Health Organization [WHO]. Primary health care: now more than ever; 2008:55. http://www.who.int/whr/2008/en/. Accessed June 1, 2018.)

of limited disease-based interactions. Pediatric primary care serves as the primary interface between the child/family and the health system, except in the case of serious emergencies. The emphasis is on health promotion and protection, and disease and/or disability prevention. It is designed to be a first contact point, not simply a point of entry into the health system. It is also designed to be the "hub" of coordination (Fig 14.1), providing continuity, as well as integrating subsequent care, regardless of where the care is delivered and who provides it. As comprehensive, continuous, and person-centered care, primary care is the ideal place for the establishment of the individual and family medical home.

The Pediatric Medical Home/Neighborhood

The pediatric *medical home* is a care model that delivers patient- and family-centered care, coordinated and tracked by a PCP within a community-based system, or *medical neighborhood*. A consensus statement on medical home principles was developed and jointly endorsed by the American College of Physicians (ACP), American Academy of Family Physicians (AAFP), American Osteopathic Association (AOA), and AAP in 2007. Understanding the unique needs of children, youth, and families, the AAP identified certain principles as critical for pediatric medical homes, the first of which was patient- and family-centered partnerships. They also identified *transitions*, in that the provision of high-quality, developmentally appropriate health care services must continue uninterrupted as the child moves along within systems from adolescence to adulthood (AAP, 2018).

Bright Futures—Health Promotion and Preventive Care Initiative

While there are many resources for primary care, *Bright Futures* is a national health promotion and preventive care initiative and a key resource for all pediatric PCPs (AAP, 2018). It provides theory-based and evidence-driven guidance for well-child care and preventive care screenings. The resource emphasizes the family as the child's primary source of strength and support and recognizes the importance of the child's and family's perspectives in clinical decision-making. This patient- and family-centered approach captures the importance of engaging both the family and the patient in a developmentally supportive manner as essential members of the primary health care team. Bright Futures is led by the AAP and supported by the Maternal and Child Health Bureau, Health Resources and Services Administration (HRSA).

Bright Futures identifies 12 key health promotion themes, including healthy development, family support, mental health and emotional well-being, nutritional health, physical activity, healthy weight, promoting lifelong health for families and communities, oral health, healthy adolescent development, safety and injury prevention, promoting the healthy and safe use of social media, and children and youth with special health needs. These themes align with the chapters that follow, providing a parallel resource for pediatric PCPs.

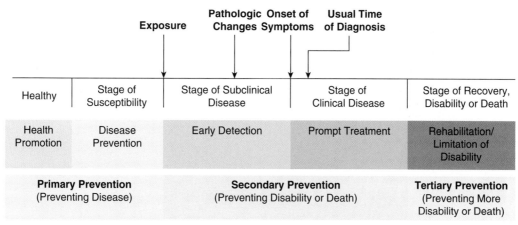

• **Fig 14.2** The Natural History of Disease Aligned With Levels of Prevention. (From Centers for Disease Control and Prevention [CDC]. *Principles of Epidemiology.* 2nd ed. Atlanta: U.S. Department of Health and Human Services; 1998. www.slideshare.net/nawanan/health-beyond-hospitals-lecture-for-ramathibodi-clinical-fellows.)

Primary Care Versus Primary Prevention

While primary care represents one of four levels of *care* within the larger health system, these levels are sometimes confused with levels of [disease] *prevention*. Disease prevention covers measures that not only prevent the occurrence of disease, but also arrest its progress and reduce its consequences once established. Preventive measures can be applied at any stage along the natural history of a disease, with the goal of preventing further progression of the condition. First described by Leavell and Clark (1965), primary, secondary, and tertiary *levels* of prevention are best understood in terms of the natural history of disease (Fig 14.2).

All healthcare providers aim to favorably influence the natural history of disease, but the anticipatory preventive actions they take are different based on the disease, disease stage, and the provider's role in the health system (CDC, 2017). Preventive care is an important task that is assigned principally to PCPs.

Primary prevention includes efforts that keep disease processes from becoming established by either eliminating the causes or increasing individual resistance to disease. Preventive actions are taken prior to the onset of disease to remove the possibility that a disease ever occurs. There are two subcategories in primary prevention: (1) health promotion and (2) specific protection. *Health promotion* involves health maintenance and education efforts, including lifestyle changes/choices, nutrition, and maintenance of safe environments. *Specific protection* involves actions targeted at specific diseases, such as immunizations, anti-malarial prophylaxis, and environmental modifications (such as fluoride). The term *primordial prevention* is sometimes inserted in front of (preceding) primary prevention to highlight efforts to prevent the emergence or development of risk factors in countries or populations in which they have not occurred.

Secondary prevention involves early diagnosis and prompt treatment, focusing on efforts that interrupt the disease process before it becomes symptomatic or halting the disease process at its incipient stage to prevent complications. The goal of secondary prevention efforts, including screening, early detection, and prompt treatment, is to cure the disease at the earliest stage, delay disease onset and/or duration, and reduce or reverse the transmission of disease.

Tertiary prevention efforts limit the physical and social consequences of symptomatic disease. The goal is to improve survival and/or quality of life. As with primary prevention, there are two subcategories: (1) disability limitation and (2) rehabilitation. *Disability limitation* focuses on early symptomatic disease and includes measures aimed at correcting the anatomic and/or physiologic components of disease, thus preventing or limiting the impairment or disability caused by the disease. *Rehabilitation* focuses on late symptomatic disease. The goal is to mitigate the ultimate effects of the disease by preventing total social and/or functional disability or by restoring the disabled persons to a useful and self-sufficient role in society through psychosocial, medical, and/or vocational services.

References

American Academy of Family Physicians (AAFP) American Academy of Pediatrics (AAP) American College of Physicians (ACP) American Osteopathic Association (AOA). *Joint Principles of the Patient-Centered Medical Home*; 2007. Available at: https://www.aafp.org/dam/AAFP/documents/practice_management/pcmh/initiatives/PCMHJoint.pdf. Accessed June 8, 2018.

American Academy of Pediatrics (AAP). *Building your medical home: an introduction to pediatric primary care transformation*; 2018. Available at: https://medicalhomes.aap.org/Pages/default.aspx.

American Academy of Pediatrics (AAP). *Bright futures.* Available at: https://medicalhomeinfo.aap.org/Pages/default.aspx. https://brightfutures.aap.org/Pages/default.aspx. Accessed June 8, 2018.

American Nurses Association (ANA). *Scope and standards of practice: pediatric nursing.* 2nd ed. Silver Spring, MD: American Nurses Association; 2015.

Centers for Disease Control and Prevention (CDC). *Introduction to public health.* In: *Public Health 101 Series.* Atlanta: U.S. Department of Health and Human Services; 2017. Available at: www.cdc.gov/publichealth101/public-health.html.

Children's Health Fund. *Unfinished business. 20 million children in U.S. still lack sufficient access to essential health care*; 2016. Available at: www.childrenshealthfund.org/advocacypublications/.

Leavell H, Clark AE. *Preventive medicine for doctors in the community.* New York: McGraw-Hill; 1965.

15

Behavioral and Mental Health Promotion

NANCY BARBER STARR AND DAWN LEE GARZON MAAKS

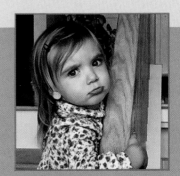

Fostering positive mental health and emotional well-being is a core task for children and those who raise them. The mental health status of children and adolescents has profound effects on a child's development, family functioning, and society as a whole. Positive mental health, also described as well-being, thriving, or flourishing, provides children with a strong foundation for the future. Educational achievement, economic productivity, responsible citizenship, lifelong health, and a thriving society depend on this foundation.

Mental health promotion begins with prenatal care that focuses on the mother's mental and physical health; becomes visible at birth with nurturing, responsive caregiving; and continues into the preschool years as young children learn to manage emotions. It is enhanced in school-age children and adolescents through friendships, peer relationships, and time spent in activities that shape the child's character and personality. Mental health is strengthened through healthy relationships and is maximized through the emotional and social skills of children and their caregivers. At all ages, responsive parenting, effective use of discipline, and a teaching-based style result in children who self-regulate their behavior, have a strong self-concept, and are socially competent. The ability to deal with stress and adversity is a critical component of mental health, and children develop that skill when they experience safe, secure, and nurturing relationships.

One of every five children experience a mental health issue, and 80% of mental health disorders begin in childhood (50% before 14 years old, 75% before 24 years old [Child Mind Institute, 2016]). Prevention, anticipatory guidance, early identification, and intervention have been proven to make a difference, and primary care providers (PCPs) with established therapeutic relationships with children and families are in the place to make a difference. They promote mental health and provide anticipatory guidance, understand normal child development and healthy parenting, have experience coordinating care with other health care specialists, and are familiar with chronic care principles and practice improvement. This chapter introduces the foundations of mental health promotion and provides assessment and management strategies to use with children and families, as well as strategies to deal with behavioral issues families may face as a child transitions from birth to adulthood. More significant mental health pathology in children is addressed in Chapter 30.

Mental Health Foundations

Emotional Well-Being: The Foundation for Health, Behavior, and Learning

Emotional well-being affects the ability to learn, concentrate, and be coherent, curious, and creative. It gives individuals a sense of self-confidence, self-worth, hope, and joy. Resulting from a dynamic developmental process that is hard-wired to attachment in infancy and is sensitive to social and emotional experiences, emotional well-being and mental health depend on social connections and a primary relationship that is stable, responsive, and recognizes children's needs. Positive mental health is correlated with solid social and emotional skills, and the ability to cope with stress and self-regulate emotions; it predicts physical health, happiness, school achievement, and success as an adult in the workplace (Moore et al., 2018).

Eight culturally sensitive, critical characteristics of well-being are identified in Table 15.1. In addition, three observable factors of well-being in children are (1) motivation (curious and interested in learning new things), (2) resilience (stays calm and in control when faced with a challenge), and (3) attention (follows through and finishes tasks) (Bethell, 2016).

Theories of Well-Being

Several theories of well-being exist including the Science of Thriving, Culture of Health, and Health Outcomes from Positive Experiences (HOPE), which are discussed here. Each contributes perspectives about the interrelationships among individual, family, and community factors to create opportunities for individuals, including children, to maximize their well-being rather than just survive. PCPs need to take a global approach to this area of health promotion for children and their families. These theories are broad and relevant to people of all ages but have particular salience to children, since they are learning and experiencing the world with fewer coping skills to deal with adversities. All these theories focus on the positive aspects of maturation—looking at building strengths in a supportive environment. That perspective is important for PCPs to bring to their work with children and families.

The *Science of Thriving* theory takes a holistic view of the central role of safe, stable, nurturing relationships (SSNR) related to

TABLE 15.1	Elements of Well-Being or Thriving	
Self-regulation[a]	Ability to recognize and control impulses, manage stress and emotions, and exert self-control
Attachment[a]	Positive relationship to, feelings of safety with, and trust in a parent or caregiver; co-regulation
Engagement/approaches to learning[a]	Cognitive, emotional, and behavioral engagement; interest, curiosity
Communication[a]	Ability to verbally and non-verbally express needs, preferences and emotions, and to listen and respond to the communication of others
Positive relationships with siblings and peers	Empathetic, open, warm, giving, and supportive interactions with other children
Executive functioning	Cognitive processes underline planning, goal-directed activity, and problem-solving, include attention, working memory, and inhibitory control
Positive self-concept and orientation to life	Compassion for self, optimism, meaning, and hope for life
Age-appropriate self-care	Ability and motivation to do things for self that are within own capacity

[a]Considered most critical.

From Kristin Anderson Moore et al. Flourishing From the Start: What Is It and How Can It Be Measured? 2017. Copyright Child Trends.

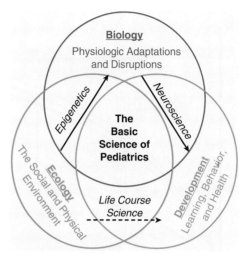

• **Fig 15.1** The Eco-Bio-Developmental Model of Human Health and Disease (From Garner A. Translating developmental science into healthy lives: realizing the potential. https://www.aap.org/en-us/advocacy-and-policy/aap-health-initiatives/EBCD/Documents/TranslatingSciencePPT.pdf. Accessed April 5, 2019.)

happiness and satisfaction and can apply abilities and talents in life. This approach has no "right way," but is based on recognizing that health is essential to every aspect of life and is the "bedrock of personal fulfillment and backbone of a strong, competitive nation," and requires collaboration between sectors (RWJF, 2018).

The *Health Outcomes from Positive Experiences (HOPE)* theory is based on not only actively promoting positive experiences that enhance healthy development, but also preventing and/or buffering the effects of adversity (Sege and Harper Browne, 2017). Four categories of essential interrelated experiences that maximize this process include (1) being in nurturing, supportive relationships; (2) living, developing, playing, and learning in safe, stable, protective, and equitable environments; (3) having opportunities for constructive social engagement and to develop a sense of connectedness; and (4) learning social and emotional competencies.

The Science of Early Childhood Development

Well-being is both an outcome of neurological development and an influencer of development. During a child's first 7 years, the brain rapidly develops, forming complex connections that are the foundation for strong physical health, cognitive functioning, and emotional relationships. Experiences in these earliest years are directly linked to the ability to succeed and thrive in life. More than 50 years of research and scientific debate in many fields clearly demonstrate that development results from an ongoing, reiterative dance between nature and nurture, or experience, biology, and behavior. Experiences can be protective and personal, or insecure and impersonal. Experiences interact with brain development (biology) to alter brain structure (epigenetics), and to create behaviors that are adaptive or maladaptive. See Fig 15.1.

All of these factors create feedback loops that move the person in a healthy or unhealthy direction. Currently the science of early childhood identifies three key concepts to explain how healthy development happens, what goes wrong, and what can be done to reestablish it (Center of the Developing Child at Harvard University, 2016).

healthy child development and flourishing. The theory embraces a proactive approach to promote healthy parenting, fosters positive mental health, prevents or mitigates the neurobiological and psychosocial impact of adverse childhood experiences (ACEs), and treats complex trauma through individual, family, and community endeavors (Bethell, 2016). This theory focuses on six key concepts: (1) the capacity for positive human development even in the face of adversity; (2) well-being as a learned ability; (3) of the interplay of human health and dynamics within the social, emotional, and environmental context we co-create; (4) a balance between conventional focus on negative development, risk factors, and pathology, with an explicit focus on strengths and what is already whole; (5) engagement of largely untapped capacities for self-led healing, resilience, and well-being at the individual, family, community, and societal levels; and (6) development of the social and emotional skills central to preventing interpersonal harm and poor self-care behaviors, and those that are essential to enhancing self-healing, resilience, and higher consciousness.

The *Culture of Health* theory is based in well-being as central to every aspect of our lives. This vision leads to individuals thriving and communities flourishing and supports children and families in building health, well-being, and equity for generations to come, based on diversity of beliefs, family customs, and community values. Well-being is defined as the extent to which people experience

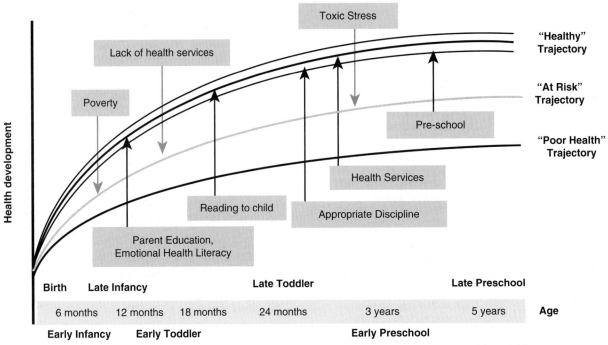

• **Fig 15.2** Life Course Perspective of Health Development (From Halfon N, Larson K, Lu M, et al. Life-course health development: past, present and future. *Matern Child Health J.* 2013;18[2]:344–365. https://doi.org/10.1007/s10995-013-1346-2.)

Concept 1: Responsive Relationships and Positive Experiences Build Strong Brain Architecture

As noted previously, positive relationships with responsive adults promote strong mental health in children. A number of principles underlie this concept.

Principle: the foundation of brain architecture is constructed early in life, but the brain continues to be built over time. Early childhood is the first window of opportunity where simple neural connections and circuits are being developed at a rate never to be repeated (both in cellular plasticity and in the number of connections developed), making these early years a sensitive period—a time of opportunity and vulnerability. With repetition, neural synapses become circuits that become pathways that lead to behaviors and skills that, in turn, influence the child's developmental trajectory and life course (Fig 15.2).

Repeated sensory input stabilizes synaptic connections; those synapses that are used are strengthened; those not used are pruned and eliminated. Skills that develop beget more skills, while deficits beget more deficits. Adolescence represents another sensitive period of both opportunity and vulnerability when the brain strengthens its most used connections, making them faster and more efficient, and prunes less-used ones. Though the foundation is set in the early years and cellular plasticity declines, the brain continues to adapt and change over a lifetime, being rewired in response to changes in the environment. However, as the brain ages, it takes more time, intensity, and repetition to reorganize.

Principle: epigenetic adaptation, or the interaction of genes and the experiences that a child has, shapes the circuitry of the developing brain. The interaction of early childhood ecology (the social and physical environment [epigenetics]) becomes biologically embedded (through physiologic adaptations and disruptions) and affects development (learning, behavior, and health). In other words,

gene expression can be altered (without altering DNA sequence) by positive and/or negative influences, with changes being either temporary or permanent. These changes influence adaptive behaviors, learning capacities, and lifelong physical and mental health. Positive experiences such as supportive environments and rich learning produce epigenetic changes that enhance development, while stressful experiences disrupt it. This is conceptualized in the Eco-Bio-Development Model of Human Health and Disease (see Fig 15.1).

Principle: children develop within an environment of relationships. This includes not only parents and family members, but others who play important roles in the child's life (e.g., caregivers, teachers, coaches, peers). Relationship interactions that are nurturing, reciprocal, and dynamic; occur in stimulating environments; and provide individualized attention that positively shapes a child's self-awareness and stimulates intellectual, social, emotional, physical, and behavioral development. This results in a child with self-confidence and sound mental health, and a motivation to learn and achieve. Children also develop the ability to control aggressive impulses, resolve conflict in nonviolent ways, and sustain friendships and relationships.

Principle: brains are built cumulatively, from the bottom up. Simple circuits lead to more complex circuits and adaptive skills. Inherent in this principle are sensitive or critical periods where the brain is unusually sensitive to the environment and experience. Different parts of the brain have sensitive periods at different times, requiring appropriate experiences for that stage. In early childhood, vision, hearing, and touch are critical, so sensory, social, and emotional experiences are key. Later on, creative play with opportunity for new experiences, active engagement, and learning from peers and adults is appropriate. After simple emotional and social capabilities develop, the groundwork is laid for prefrontal cortex development of executive skills and self-regulation.

Principle: the brain's many functions are mutually interactive with multiple systems throughout the body. Regulatory systems for the immune, neuroendocrine, metabolic, and cardiac systems are interconnected with brain circuitry in a way that affects learning and behavior. Especially important are the social, emotional, and language areas that are associated with the ability to experience and express different emotions and feelings. Cognitive development, including memory, learning, and executive function, involves multiple brain areas. When positively developed, emotions support executive function, leading to social competence, emotional well-being, and the ability to have successful relationships throughout life.

Concept 2: Adversity Disrupts the Foundations of Learning, Behavior, and Health

Principle: toxic stress responses can impair development and have lifelong consequences on learning, behavior, and health. Experiencing stress is a normal response to the challenges of life and is not necessarily a bad thing. The measure of stress is variable, depending on the individual's perception of (subjective) and reaction to (objective) the stress, and should be considered in terms of frequency, duration, and severity. The level of stress is key to the outcome (Table 15.2).

Stress reaches a toxic level in a dose-response relationship either by repetition of a stress or an accumulation of different stressors. Significant hardship or prolonged toxic stress can result in chronic or continuous activation of the fight-or-flight response; it can disrupt the development of the brain architecture and contribute to a hyperresponsive stress response and a lesser ability to calm and cope. Stress begins in the prenatal period but is especially impactful during the early childhood years as the brain foundations are being laid. Studies in the science behind the developmental origins of health and disease (DOHaD) and ACES (see Chapter 2) show a strong association between toxic stress, brain development disruption, functional learning differences, behavior and mental health, and immediate and long-term impacts on health and prosperity or one's life-course

trajectory. Though not an exclusive list, the most common ACEs can be categorized as (1) abuse (physical, emotional, or sexual); (2) neglect (physical or emotional); or (3) household dysfunction (e.g., mental illness, incarcerated relative, mother treated violently, substance abuse or divorce).

Concept 3: Protective Factors in Early Years Strengthen Resilience

Principle: providing the right ingredients from the start produces better outcomes than trying to fix problems later. It has been said that "it is easier to raise a healthy child than to fix a broken one." Although it is possible to change brain circuitry once established, it takes more effort from the individual and more resources from society to facilitate change later on in life.

Principle: positive early experiences, support from adults, and the early development of adaptive skills can counterbalance the lifelong consequences of adversity. Not all children who experience adverse events have negative sequelae later in life. Even one stable, responsive relationship provides support and scaffolding that not only prevents developmental disruption, but also builds key capabilities to protect against stress. This combination of positive experiences, supportive relationships, and adaptive skills is called *resilience*.

Principle: Both children and adults need core capabilities to respond to or avoid adversity, and these capabilities can be strengthened through coaching and practice.

From the brain development perspective, the following core life skills have been identified that help adults deal effectively with life, work, and parenting:

- Focus—Concentrating on what is most important at any given time
- Awareness—Noticing people and situations and how one fits in the picture
- Planning—Being able to make concrete plans, carry them out, and set and meet goals
- Flexibility—Adapting to changing situations
- Self-control—Controlling one's response to emotions and stressful situations

TABLE 15.2 Level of Stress, Response and Outcome

Level of Stress	Example	Response	Outcome
Positive stress = brief duration, mild to moderate severity, infrequent, normal and essential	Receiving an injection, beginning daycare or school, big test or project in middle or high school	Brief increase in heart rate with mild elevation in stress hormones. Socioemotional buffers (responding to nonverbal cues, consolation, reassurance, assistance in planning) allow a return to baseline stress response.	Quickly returns to normal. Builds resiliency and motivation.
Tolerable stress = sustained duration, moderate/severe severity, more frequently occurring	Car accident, death in family, natural disaster, frightening injury	Greater activation of stress response. Socioemotional buffers (above) allow a return to baseline stress response.	A single major, negative event does not mean long-lasting problems.
Toxic stress = severe intensity, frequent or prolonged duration	Physical, sexual, emotional abuse or neglect; caregiver substance abuse or mental illness; household or environmental dysfunction	Insufficient social-emotional buffers (deficient levels of emotion coaching, re-processing, reassurance and support) cause changes in baseline stress response.	Changes in brain architecture and function (hyperresponsive stress response with decreased calm/coping) that can affect learning and development and impact long-term health.

In youth these same capabilities are needed in order to manage school, outside interests, and social relationships successfully. Core capabilities require communication between the prefrontal cortex and other parts of the brain based in early childhood and adolescent brain development, but can be developed or coached through the entire life span. The interaction of these core capabilities allows the individual to focus on goals, resist distractions, and find alternate approaches (Fig 15.3).

Protective, Promotive, and Risk Factors

Children and their families experience both protective and health promotive factors as well as factors that put them at risk within their relationships. *Protective factors*, also called strengths or assets, are characteristics at the individual, family, neighborhood, or community level that moderate or buffer the negative effect on development. *Promotive factors*, often combined with protective, are those that aid healthy development. *Risk factors*, also called vulnerabilities or problems, are measurable characteristics that undermine healthy development. Protective factors and risk factors often interact in complicated ways, an example being a child's temperament, which can be either protective or a risk factor, depending on the situation and interactions that result. Protective factors for children are identified in Table 15.3; risk factors are identified in Table 15.4.

Relationships and Attachment

The ability to form relationships is a critical human trait that provides the glue for family, community, and society. Relationships range from transient and superficial to deep and enduring. Because the brain is designed to derive pleasure from interaction, early relationships provide attachment bonds that set a tone for all future relationships.

Safe, Stable, Nurturing Relationships

Interpersonal interactions create trust, respect, and connection with others. A competent, caring, positively attuned, engaged parent or caregiver addresses the child's physiologic and safety needs (protects), promotes healthy relationship and attachment (relates), and encourages foundational coping skills (nurtures). Parent and caregiver strategies that reflect a healthy parent-child relationship include using loving verbal and nonverbal communication, providing consistent routines, having frequent "fun" and play time, accurately reading child signals, and providing timely responses to the child's needs. Positive parenting is critical to children's ability to learn, self-regulate, and get along with others, and is a precursor to positive mental health.

Patterns of Attachment

Healthy attachment provides a child with attention, approval, and recognition of success that is critical to the development of healthy, happy, and self-confident children. Infants and young children with good attachments learn to cope and deal with adversity, develop the confidence to explore their world, and learn cognitive and social skills. The attachment between a parent and child is influenced by parent, child, and environmental factors, but can be categorized into patterns (Table 15.5). Observing the pattern, and helping families move toward secure attachment, builds the child's trust, comfort, and sense of self-worth.

Temperament

Temperament is inborn characteristics that describe an individual's emotional and behavioral response style across situations. It is

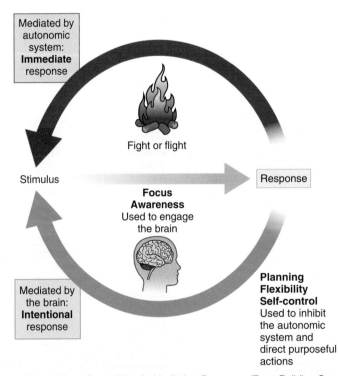

• **Fig 15.3** Interactions of Core Capabilities in Mediating Response (From Building Core Capabilities for Life, The Science Behind the Skills Adults Need to succeed in Parenting and the Workplace, 2016. http://www.ddcf.org/globalassets/child-well-being/16-0304-core-capabilities-for-life.pdf.)

TABLE 15.3 Protective/Promotive Factors for Child Well-Being

Relational/family	• Family support for children's executive functioning • Caregiver/adult responsiveness • Caregiver/adult warmth • Shared family activities • Parent/caregiver engagement with school and community • Safe and supportive home environment • Family routines • Stimulating home environment • Parenting skills and attributes (e.g., authoritative style) • Religious involvement • Enduring presence and positive support of caring adults and kin • Control over number and timing of children in the family
Contextual/community	• Relevant, high-quality, culturally appropriate available local services • Safe and healthy school environment • Safe and cohesive neighborhood, safe housing • Access to nutritious food • Access to jobs and transportation for the job • Access to medical care including wellness and behavioral health

From Kristin Anderson Moore et al. Child Well-Being: Constructs to Measure Child Well-Being and Risk and Protective Factors that Affect the Development of Young Children 2016. Copyright Child Trends.

TABLE 15.4 Risk Factors for Child Well-Being

Relational/family	• Economic downturns and material hardship • Parental depression/mental health problems • Parental substance abuse • Parental unemployment • Parental social isolation • Parental rigidity, harshness, or inconsistent discipline • Conflict/domestic violence • Parental history or maltreatment • Family stress • Family instability/turbulence • Toxic trauma, high level of adverse childhood experiences, accumulation of stresses • Younger child age at maltreatment, type of maltreatment • Removal from caregivers, placement with kin, placement stability • Inconsistent medical care
Community/contextual	• Exposure to violence/unsafe environment • Unavailable, inconsistent, poor-quality child care and other services • Negative peers • Unsupportive, negative child welfare service providers • Absence of foster care families • Lack of emergency housing • Inadequate recreational opportunities

From Kristin Anderson Moore et al. Child Well-Being: Constructs to Measure Child Well-Being and Risk and Protective Factors that Affect the Development of Young Children 2016. Copyright Child Trends.

different from personality, which reflects motivation, interest and drive. Although biologic in origin, temperament characteristics evolve and develop over time and are influenced and patterned by the social environment. Temperament is crucial to understanding how children interact with their environment, including their families (Box 15.1).

Characteristics of temperament are described in Box 15.1 and discussed later in this chapter. Temperament exerts an influence on children's psychosocial adjustment by affecting caretaker-child interactions. All nine traits are considered normal, even at extremes, but can predispose to behavioral, emotional, or functional difficulties by causing parental distress or when there is a poor fit with caregiver expectations and values. Temperament is sometimes described by types:
- "Difficult" child: intense, slow to adapt, withdrawing, negative mood, and irregular rhythmicity
- "Slow-to-warm-up": low activity level, low intensity, withdrawing, slow adaptability, negative mood
- "Easy": moderate-to-low intensity, fast adapting, approaching, positive in mood, regular or high rhythmicity

Goodness of fit refers to the congruence of a child's temperament with the expectations, demands, and opportunities of the social environment, including those of parents, family, and day care or school setting. Short- and long-term psychosocial adjustments are shaped by the goodness of fit between the individual's temperament and the social environment.

• BOX 15.1 Characteristics of Temperament

- Activity level
- Intensity of reaction
- Adaptability or flexibility tolerance
- Persistence and attention span
- Distractibility
- Rhythmicity
- Threshold of response
- Approach/withdrawal
- Mood

Family Assets

Relationships, interactions, opportunities, and values that provide SSNR and help families thrive have been identified by the Search Institute (Table 15.6). These assets are more commonly associated with young people's well-being than are family structure, income, education, immigrant status, community type, or other demographic factors, and they can be intentionally nurtured within a family.

Connectedness and Developmental Relationships

As a child matures, attachment leads to connection with others in schools, neighborhoods, and through religious or community activities that offer rich opportunities for the child. Relationships and experiences based on cultural identity, race, and ethnicity also help form identity and add to a sense of meaning and purpose.

TABLE 15.5	Attachment Patterns		
Pattern	**Parent**	**Child**	
Secure attachment	Is sensitive responsive, and available	Feels valued and worthwhile; has secure base; able to explore and master, knows parent is available; becomes autonomous. Engages with primary care provider, seeks and receives reassurance and comfort from parent.	
Insecure and avoidant attachment	Is insensitive to child's cues, avoids contact, and rejects	Feels no one is there for him, cannot rely on adults to get needs met, feels he will be rejected if needs for attachment and closeness are shown; asks for little to maintain connection and learns not to recognize his need for closeness and connectedness. May act fearful or angry with parent, may seek contact, then arch away and struggle, or may act extremely helpless or sad but not seek comfort or protection.	
Insecure attachment characterized by ambivalence and resistance	Shows inconsistent patterns of care, is unpredictable, may be excessively close or intrusive but then push away (seen frequently in depressed caregiver)	Feels he should keep the adult engaged because he never knows when he will get attention back; is anxious, dependent, and clingy.	

TABLE 15.6	Family Assets	
Types of Family Assets	**Description**	
Nurturing Relationships		
Healthy relationships begin and grow as we show each other we care about what each of us has to say, how we feel, and our unique and shared interests.	• Positive communication • Affection • Emotional openness • Support for sparks	
Establishing Routines		
Shared routine, traditions, and activities give a dependable rhythm to family life.	• Family meals • Shared activities • Meaningful traditions • Dependability	
Maintaining Expectations		
Expectations make it clear how each person participates in and contributes to family life.	• Openness about tough topics • Fair rules • Defined boundaries • Clear expectations • Contributions to family	
Adapting to Challenges		
Every family faces challenges, large and small. The ways families face and adapt to those changes together help them through the ups and downs of life.	• Management of daily commitments • Adaptability • Problem-solving • Democratic decision-making	
Connecting to the Community		
Community connections, relationships, and participation sustain, shape, and enrich how families live their lives together.	• Neighborhood cohesion • Relationship with others • Enriching activities • Supportive resources	

Used with permission from Search Institute, https://www.search-institute.org/wp-content/uploads/2018/02/Family_Assets_Framework.pdf.

Developmental relationships are close connections through which young people discover who they are, cultivate abilities, and learn how to engage with and contribute to the work around them (Search Institute, 2017). The Search Institute developmental framework focuses on relationships with an adult (teacher, coach), friend, sibling, or peer, in which each person is engaging and experiencing, contributing to, and benefitting from the interaction. Essential elements and associated actions are found in Table 15.7.

Social-Emotional and Spiritual Development

Social development enables children to contribute in positive ways to family, school, and community, leading to awareness of social values and expectations, building a sense of who they are and where they fit in society. *Emotional development* helps children understand what feelings and emotions are, gain emotional awareness of self and others, and learn how to manage emotions (Kids Matter, 2017). *Spiritual development*, different from religion, provides inner resource and identity, interconnectedness, purpose or meaning to life, and transcendence. Children with positive social-emotional skills can share feelings, manage themselves, relate and connect to others effectively (e.g., develop friendships), resolve conflict, and feel positive about themselves and the world. They serve as a buffer against toxic stress by turning off the physiologic stress response and lead to improved cognitive, linguistic, and self-regulation and executive functioning skills and improved moral outcomes (Weitzman and Wegner, 2016). Social-emotional skills are learned through modeling, nurturing, and practicing. Their mastery occurs as a result of a complex interplay within the developmental domains (emotional, social, cognitive, and physical). For example, character traits such as empathy and honesty (emotional domain) influence successful interaction with others (social domain) and contribute to a strong foundation for learning and problem-solving (cognitive domain). Whether these experiences develop depends on early experiences that influence the developing brain toward a strong or fragile foundation (physical domain) (Sege and Harper Browne, 2017).

TABLE 15.7 Developmental Relationships Framework

Element	Action
Express care—"Show me that you care."	Be dependable, listen, believe in me, be warm, encourage
Challenge growth—"Push me to keep getting better."	Expect my best, stretch my limits, hold me accountable, reflect on my failures
Provide support—"Help me complete tasks and achieve goals."	Navigate, empower, advocate, set boundaries
Share power—"Treat me with respect and give me a say."	Respect me, include me, collaborate, let me lead
Expand possibilities—"Connect me with people and places that broaden my world."	Inspire, broaden horizons, connect

Adapted from https://www.search-institute.org/wp-content/uploads/2018/05/Developmental-Relationships-Framework_English.pdf. Accessed June 15, 2018.

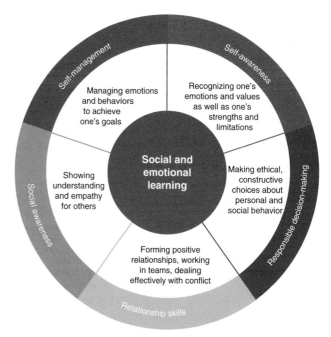

• **Fig 15.4** Social Emotional Learning Competencies (From KidsMatter www.kidsmatter.edu.au. Adapted from The Collaborative for Academics, Social, and Emotional Learning [CASEL]. *Sustainable Schoolwide Social and Emotional Learning [SEL]: Implementation Guide*. Chicago: Author; 2006.)

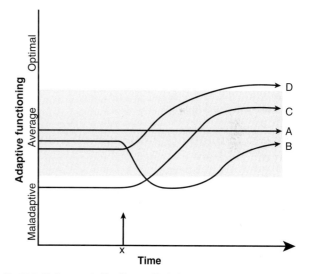

• **Fig 15.5** Pathways to Resilience Path A: relatively steady course even with acute trauma or chronic adversity. Path B: normal course with overwhelming adversity and eventual recovery. Path C: normalization, or a major shift in the quality of adaptation from poor functioning to good functioning over time. Path D: posttraumatic growth with improved adaptive function following trauma or adversity. (From Masten AS. Ordinary Magic: Resilience in Development. NY: Guilford Press; 2014.)

Bright Futures identifies key components of social-emotional development as (Hagan, Shaw Duncan, 2017):

- *Empathy.* Being able to understand how others feel leads to empathy, which is also expressed in generosity of action toward family and friends and volunteer activities.
- *Competence and mastery.* In a safe relationship and environment, children will explore, gaining skills and knowledge that result in a sense of competence and a feeling of mastery. Accomplishments in school, arts, athletics, and community service contribute to the child/adolescent's identity and self-concept.
- *Autonomy and independence.* As children grow, their interests and abilities expand and they are required to make more decisions. In this process, the parent role transitions to one of coach, giving guidance and helping children build life skills of self-advocacy and self-care, leading to independence and autonomy.

The Collaborative for Academic, Social and Emotional Learning (CASEL) identifies key competencies as self-awareness, social awareness, responsible decision-making, self-management, and relationship skills (Fig 15.4). Resilience and self-regulation are skills essential to mastering these developmental tasks.

Resilience and Self-Regulation

Resilience, which comes from the Latin verb meaning "to rebound," is broadly defined as the ability to overcome difficulty and succeed in life. It has been called "ordinary magic," as it arises from talents and resources everyone can access (Masten, 2014). Resilience can be learned, promoted, and supported through protective relationships, skills, and experiences. Children who are resilient have healthy social-emotional skills, specifically the intrapersonal skills of self-regulation, self-reflection, creating and nurturing a sense of self and confidence, as well as the interpersonal skills in which they can establish SSNRs.

Assessing resiliency in children requires looking at both the supportive elements in the child's life as well as the threats to child development and adaptation (i.e., the level of stress and degree to which stress is cumulative or allostatic). Four patterns or pathways of resilience are identified (Masten, 2014) in Fig 15.5.

Self-regulation involves a transition from reflexive responses in the newborn period to the ability to recognize and control one's thoughts and actions. Actions can either be automatic responses useful for threatening situations (fight or fight) or intentional responses that are conscious, proactive, and goal-directed. When the brain recognizes a situation that requires a response, the automatic self-regulation system initially responds. As conscious self-regulation develops, the individual is able to focus and prioritize action and modify or control the automatic self-regulation system (see Figure 15.3). The process of learning self-regulation is influenced by the individual child's abilities (e.g., attention, cognition, and impulsivity), temperament, genetics, and characteristics of their environment. Children best learn to self-regulate when they experience loving and nurturing parenting, and are provided consistent discipline, along with opportunities to learn without fear of negative outcomes if failure occurs.

Spiritual and Moral Development

Social-emotional development includes not only matters of the mind, but also of the spirit. As children mature and have personal experience with life events (e.g., birth of a sibling, death of a family member or friend), the foundation of their moral system is laid. Spiritual integrity is fundamentally a sense of meaning and purpose: one has a direction, control, and promise in a future. Morality is the quality of being that encompasses that which is right (justice or fairness) and that which is good (empathy or kindness). Faith is the basis for developing beliefs, values, and meaning, and is closely linked to spirituality. Empathy, a fundamental moral emotion, is an expression of the ability to understand the condition of another and to experience a visceral or emotional reaction to that condition—to quite literally take the perspective of another. Mature morality is constructed through social interactions in which individuals mutually "reverse" their thinking: each strives to understand and feel how the other is thinking and feeling, and as a result, each deepens his or her own understanding and emotions. Children's values and beliefs are reflected in different behaviors at different ages as they gain greater cognitive and social skills. As they develop moral integrity and spiritual values, healthy children achieve a positive sense of self, learn to value themselves and their contribution to the family and larger social system, and feel a sense of understanding and belonging.

Family and Community Influences on Mental Health of Children

Safe, stable, nurturing environments (at home, school, neighborhood, and community) are essential to children's well-being. Social determinants of health (SDoH), conditions in which people live, learn, work, play, worship, and age, affect a wide range of health, functioning, and quality-of-life outcomes and risks (CDC, 2018). Place (i.e., physical conditions of the child's environment), race, social-economic status (e.g., poverty), and other SDoH significantly impact the connectedness a child or family feels to the neighborhood in which they live and the community in which they participate. SDoH either support the development of well-being or add to the challenges faced by children and families. *Healthy People 2020* identifies improvements in economic stability (reducing poverty), social and community context, neighborhood, and environment as four overarching goals for the decade (Healthy People 2020, 2018).

Parent Well-Being and Parenting Style

Parents are a key element in responsive relationships and have the strongest effect in building positive experiences. Parental behavior may reflect efforts to "be like my parents were" or to "not do things wrong, like my parents did with me." Providers should acknowledge that parents are trying to do the best that they can and encourage them to relax and discover how to best

interact with their child. However, parents come with their own past experience, life stressors and changes, fund of knowledge (beliefs, education, strategies), temperament, experiences of being nurtured in childhood, perceptions (expectations, needs, and desires related to other people's reactions), and physical and emotional health. Research confirms the effect of the parents' personal history of being parented on the quality of parenting provided to children and the powerful influence on their perceptions of child behavior, beliefs about children and childrearing, and ultimately the parenting behaviors used in the home.

Describing the parenting styles can be useful in working with parents. In *authoritative* parenting, parents are present and set limits but still listen to the child and provide warmth and support, resulting in a child who is friendly, self-reliant, and self-controlled. *Authoritarian* parents establish strict rules and expect children to follow them "Because I said so," often punishing for not obeying, resulting in a child who may appear to follow the rules but stuffs anger inside, resulting in a lower social competence, self-regulation, and self-esteem. In *permissive* parenting, parents are warm, wanting to be their child's friend, but lax with rules, leading to children who have difficulty with self-regulation, tend to be aggressive and impulsive, and have more social issues. *Uninvolved* parents fulfill a child's basic needs, but demand little of the child and are not present nor responsive, resulting in children who lack self-control and have low self-esteem or confidence.

Newer descriptions of parenting models include the helicopter parent, the snowplow or lawnmower parent, and free-range parent. The *helicopter* parent is overly protective and thus controlling, wanting to protect the child from any danger and provide ultimate success. This parent micromanages everything about the child's life, wanting to be constantly aware of where the child is and intimately involved in every detail. The *snowplow* parent (also called the *lawnmower* parent) likewise desires the very best for their child and will go to any length to clear the path, removing any obstacle to future success. Though the motivation behind both of these is positive, the child emerges with a lack of confidence and feelings of inadequacy, often fearful themselves as they see life from the overly protective parenting style, and sometimes with feelings of negativity toward the parent. *Free-range* parenting believes that children are smart and capable, not in need of constant supervision. One of movement's mottos is "Fail! It is the new succeed! ", encouraging parents to let children get back out into the world, giving them independence, free time, and self-directed play.

Family Functioning and Dynamics

The foundation of mental health lies in safe stable, nurturing environments, but the initial groundwork is laid within families. The family is a dynamic social system that is usually the most powerful and constant influence shaping a child's development and socialization. The family provides emotional connections, behavioral constraints, and modeling that affect the child's development of self-regulation, emotional expression, and expectations regarding behaviors and relationships. The degree of satisfaction as parents is an important outcome measure of how well the family is functioning as a family unit. Common themes exist within all families, and six key dimensions (Box 15.2) have a significant effect on family functioning, contributing to cohesiveness, adaptability, and positive communication. To assist parents and children across the family life cycle and especially during times of stress, the provider must carefully assess these elements.

• BOX 15.2 Six Key Dimensions Affecting Family Functioning

Resources available to the family (e.g., social support network of extended family members, friends, and community), in addition to financial and other material assets. Families with limited resources or social support networks are more vulnerable to stressful life events than are families with resources and support systems in place.

Transitions and stresses (e.g., financial strains, illness, marital strain, family transitions, losses, and lack of effective coping strategies) necessitate change. Some are normal, some anticipated, and others unexpected; all can have a significant effect.

Childrearing styles (e.g., parenting behaviors, beliefs and actions) influence the environmental milieu in which the child learns about the world. Certain child-rearing styles (e.g., an uninvolved, permissive, or strict authoritarian parenting style) are ineffective and have dire consequences for the child's emotional health.

Values (e.g., spiritual, religious, cultural) provide a framework to find comfort, joy, and solace, and to guide, explain, and understand events being experienced.

Roles and structures vary from one family to another, within an individual family, and as family members grow and develop in response to external demands; shifts in the role of one family member affect other family members.

Coping style of the family speaks to the ways that demands are met, transitions handled, and concerns resolved. Positive or effective coping is characterized as a creative response to a change or stressor that results in a new behavior or attitude. Coping styles reflect habitual patterns of action. Over time, coping effort develops into a coping style.

Routines, Rituals, and Celebrations. *Routines* are activities that are done over and over in the same way and give a dependable rhythm to family life. By providing comfort and safety, they create a chance for trust and relationship and help children learn to deal with stress and transition by making everything appear normal. Routines help a child know what comes next and provide organization, giving children the confidence to try new things and gain competence. They can decrease anxiety, lower resistance to tedious tasks, and send messages about values. Common routines include bedtime and wake-up, mealtimes, "Stop and Drop," reading times, and playtime. *Rituals* are routines with a symbolic value and are often linked to cultural or spiritual belonging. Rituals help people learn to work together and provide social support. Family *celebrations* acknowledging even little milestones can provide positive time and family joy.

Communication. Communication is one of the most critical elements in a relationship. Healthy families are cohesive and adaptable with positive communication patterns. *Family cohesion* is an indication of the strength of the emotional bonding between family members. *Family adaptability* is the ability of a family system to appropriately change its power structure, role relationships, and relationship rules in response to situational and/or developmental stress. Communication patterns range from positive, respectful communication skills that convey messages (e.g., empathy, reflective listening, and supportive comments) to negative communication (e.g., double messages, double binds, criticism) that minimizes opportunities to share feelings. Family cohesion and adaptability are threatened and thwarted with negative communication patterns. The result of negative communication can be a chaotic household marked by high levels of family distress.

• BOX 15.3 Phases of Parenthood

Commander: In the first years, encourage a child's growth from discipline to self-discipline by explaining the reason for limits.

Coach: In the early and middle school years, teach growth from parent-direction to self-direction.

Counselor: In the teen years, encourage growth from dependence to independence.

Consultant: In the early adult years, let go, yet be available to help as requested.

From Hostetler B. The four phases of parenthood, Focus on the Family (website). 1998. www.focusonthefamily.com/parenting/parenting-roles/phases-of-parenthood. Accessed August 15, 2018.

Listening attentively, showing interest, and taking time is critical to helping children identify, handle, and express feelings by accepting and acknowledging what is said. Affection or warmth with emotional openness allows each family member to share their feelings. Maintaining a strength-based approach, looking for what a child does well but not being afraid to talk about disappointment, is key. Family communication when facing problems includes talking about what to do, working together to solve problems, knowing there are strengths to draw on, and staying hopeful even in difficult times. Approaches to communication may be facilitated by considering the four phases of parenthood (Box 15.3).

Growth Mind-Set. *Mind-set* is an important part of a child's well-being, not only in developing and stabilizing mental health, but also in repairing any damage. Families who encourage a *growth mind-set* teach a child that hard work is at the crux of success and that effort and practice are contributing factors that lead to continued (or expanded) growth. Praise for the process (i.e., effort, concentration, approach, or patience) allows them to focus on learning rather than performing, and an expandable mind-set provides resiliency in dealing with failure. Challenges are opportunities for growth, not fearful experiences of failure. In contrast, children who are approached with a *fixed mind-set* learn that success is due to a certain trait or talent, and when failure or challenge occurs, it must be due to lack of that trait or talent. These children often receive praise in the form of appreciation for a certain talent or trait (e.g., intelligence, musical or athletic ability), and their performance is their measure of worth. When they experience a perceived failure, they have nowhere to turn, believing the talent is all they have, so they expend their energy trying to bolster their own self-perception by looking for an excuse, blaming someone, or comparing themselves to someone who did not do as well as they did. Table 15.8 shows indicators of mind-set.

Assessment of Mental Health

Since mental health covers a broad range of dimensions, accurately identifying social, emotional, behavioral, and mental health status and the variables that influence that status is crucial. Mental health assessment focuses on the child's behavior (especially vis-à-vis the parent or caregiver) and on protective, promotive, and risk factors (see Tables 15.3 and 15.4). Correctly pinpointing these variables requires a more thorough history than does the diagnosis of many physical health problems. The comprehensive child and family assessment model found in Chapter 5 gives the PCP much information; however, screening tools assist in collecting information.

	TABLE 15.8 Indicators of Mind-Set		
Indicator	**Growth Mind-Set**	**Fixed Mind-Set**
What does the individual think it takes to succeed?	Effort, practice	Intelligence, talent
What does the individual think makes a genius?	Hard work	Innate ability
What is the individual's typical response to new challenges?	Yes, please	No, thank you
How does the individual respond to setbacks?	Looks for new approaches and strategies	Blames others, becomes defensive, or gives up
What might you see if the individual experiences failure?	Tries again with a new approach	Lies about performance, makes excuses
What might you expect if you know the test is very difficult?	Sustained effort at studying	Cheating, procrastination

The physical examination detects underlying physical conditions that may contribute to behavioral or emotional changes. During all health visits, the PCP should assess the quality of the verbal and nonverbal exchanges between infants, children, and adolescents and their parents and the PCP. Specific attention should be paid to the child's emotions and energy, and the presence or absence of interaction among those present in the examination room. An important question at every well and ill child visit is: *Do you have any concerns or worries about your child's mental/emotional health or his/her behaviors, or has there been a change in how he/she usually behaves at home or at school?* If a positive response is received, further symptoms analysis is warranted, including the degree of impairment, distress, severity of symptoms, frequency, intensity, duration, what is being done, and how helpful it is.

Principles of Conducting a Psychosocial Assessment

The manner in which the PCP conducts the history and physical examination is as important as the information obtained. Many caregivers and adolescents share their concerns only after a long period of trying to solve the problem themselves. They may be upset, worried, or frustrated. Many people are reluctant to discuss symptoms because of social stigmas against mental illness. Sufficient time should be scheduled for the history and physical. Providers are more likely to get a clearer picture of what is happening and gain the family's trust if they take the time to sit down and actively listen at length to both the caregiver's and child's concerns and perceptions. It is critical to avoid rapidly firing questions, restricting the history to only using a preprinted schedule of questions (even though validated screening tools provide critical information), searching the electronic health record, or taking notes that detract from giving full attention to the child and family. If a potentially significant but nonemergent problem is uncovered in the course of an episodic visit, a lengthier appointment should be

scheduled to avoid hurrying the assessment and potentially missing important data. It is essential to obtain information from the child's perspective and to use age-appropriate strategies.

To successfully assess mental health, the PCP should consider the following (King, 2016):
1. Remember the role trust can play in interaction with families and co-professionals.
2. Consider the role of time in unearthing clues when taking histories; set a return appointment to expand on concerns.
3. View family members as agents of change, for the patient, the parent and others around them.
4. Empower parents (and children) with whom you work—help them become active problem solvers, rather than simply providing them with specific answers.
5. Listen with curiosity, empathy, and support.
6. Associate or connect ideas that emerge as concerns with family history.
7. Record affect (nonverbal expressions of feelings) in responses, as well as specific answers.
8. Ask yourself who the real patient is; parents often think it is the child, but often it is parent or other family members.
9. Identify family secrets. When there is a problem in the child, it often stems from a family history of other issues (e.g., alcoholism, depression, mental illness, abuse).

Approaches to Behavioral Assessment of Children of Different Ages

Infants and Early Childhood

Observations of babies and toddlers with their caregivers offer valuable clues to the strengths and limitations of each partner. Structured and unstructured situations allow the observer to appreciate emotional exchanges and the quality of interactions between the infant and caregiver. For example, unstructured play with dolls and toys gives older toddlers and young preschoolers a way to spontaneously express their feelings and emotions; offers the PCP an opportunity to ask questions within a nonthreatening context; and can help evaluate the history provided by caregivers (e.g., if the concerning behaviors began shortly after the birth of a new sibling, playing with a baby doll, mother and father dolls, and a doll of the child's age and gender may help the child express his or her emotional state).

School-Age Children and Adolescents

Offer older preschoolers and young school-age children the opportunity to draw a picture of themselves and their family, asking them to tell a story about their picture. This allows the opportunity to evaluate the child's feelings and emotions and, if problems and concerns become apparent, clarify details from the child's perspective in a nonthreatening and familiar way. The school-age child and adolescent should be interviewed separately from their caregivers. Most children are comfortable talking about their feelings and experiences if they have a supportive listener. It is important to clarify issues related to confidentiality with both the adolescent and caregiver prior to initiating a mental health assessment. Tailor questions to the child's or adolescent's level of understanding, keeping questions simple and providing examples to younger children. Sample questions include:
1. "Tell me some of the things you do very well. What types of things do you have a hard time doing?" "If you could change one thing in your life, what would it be?"

2. "How are things going in your family?" "What do you like to do with your mom/dad?"
3. "How is school going?" "Do you ever feel scared?"
4. "You look very sad to me. Is there something that is making you sad?"
5. "Many children have things they worry about. What worries you most?"
6. "Everyone feels angry at times. What makes you angry? What do you do when you are angry?"
7. "Tell me what you think the problem is from your point of view."

History

In the collecting family health history, it is critical to check for any mental and developmental disorders in family members, including school failure, delinquency, substance abuse, learning disorders, reading problems, mood disorders, personality disorders, schizophrenia, attention-deficit/hyperactivity disorder (ADHD), autism, genetic syndromes, and birth defects. Though it should be routine, clarifying a child's achievement of developmental milestones, including social, emotional, and cognitive skills, is also crucial, as is identifying health supervision anticipatory guidance that has been provided. Beyond this initial data, the symptom analysis, family, and additional stress histories offer further insight.

Relationship as a Vital Sign, and PRN

The AAP suggests that assessment and support of early relationships be considered a *vital sign* to be assessed at every well-child visit. The acronym, PRN (protect, relate, and nurture), provides a focus for evaluating the relationship. Does the parent protect the child, relate to the child, and nurture the child during the visit? The vital sign concept emphasizes promotion, but also paves the way for secondary and tertiary interventions when needed.

The Symptom Analysis: Behavioral Manifestations

Parents are keen observers of their children, so it is wise to listen carefully to their observations and concerns. They may be troubled by behaviors that are developmentally normal, abnormal, or extremes of normal child behavior. By obtaining a clear idea of the concerns (Box 15.4), the PCP assesses the parent's knowledge level about child development and behavior, clarifies which behaviors are developmentally normal (but distressing to the caregiver), and/or confirms which behaviors fall outside the range of normal.

With this information, the PCP can develop a mutually agreeable plan of care with the parent(s). Eliciting information from teachers and other caregivers reinforces parent reports and provides a contextual understanding of child behavior. Underlying many behavioral concerns are the following issues:

- Lack of knowledge about normal development and behavior
- Unrealistic parental expectations for child behavior
- Parents' feelings hurt by the behavior or unable to empathize with how the child feels
- Unpredictable situational context that elicits or maintains problem behavior (setting, timing, who is present, triggers)
- Behavior that negatively affects relationships or child functioning
- Negative peer and/or teacher responses to and consequences of problem behavior
- Increasing frequency or severity of behavior

Family Stress History

All caregivers face stress and feelings of being overwhelmed from time to time. It is important to assist them to identify

---

> **• BOX 15.4** **The Symptom Analysis**
>
> - Describe your child's behavior.
> - What seems to make it better or worse?
> - How have you tried to help your child?
> - How does the behavior make you feel?
> - How do think your child feels?

situations in which they know the stress risk is greatest (Table 15.9). For example, certain developmental stages are commonly more taxing than others, and many young children have increasing behavioral problems in the late afternoon hours as fatigue increases and energy levels lag. Anticipatory guidance provides interventions to help caregivers predict and minimize these "at-risk" times. Those with mental illness have increased risk of role strain and parenting difficulties because of how their condition affects their perceptions and coping skills. It is helpful to specifically ask about family-related stressors because caregivers may not perceive these as sources of stress for their child. For example, a caregiver may welcome a job promotion that includes the need for travel and a significant pay increase. However, this same change may stress the child who is old enough to worry about how life will change with a traveling parent.

Social-Emotional Development and Behavioral Screening

Structured social-emotional, developmental and behavioral rating scales or checklists are valuable screening tools, especially those with established reliability and validity that provide norms as a basis for comparison. Key ages for assessment are 30 months, 4 years old, 8 years old, preadolescence, and adolescence. Chapters 10 through 12 describe age-appropriate developmental screens, but other social-emotional screening tools are available to PCPs (Table 15.10). When looking at behavioral concerns, a behavioral diary or log kept by caregivers, by the school-age child or adolescent, and by the teacher informs the PCP and family about the situational context for and severity of the behavior. This monitoring process itself often serves as an effective intervention. Even if children's scores do not reach a level of concern, attention must be paid to high scores, problem behavior witnessed over time, and attending circumstances. Suspicious or ambiguous findings may warrant a referral for a thorough developmental evaluation by a skilled psychologist or multidisciplinary developmental assessment team. Routine screening of mothers for symptoms of postpartum depression (PPD) is merited during health visits, especially in early infancy, as maternal PPD can negatively affect infant development (see Chapter 9).

Physical Examination and Diagnostic Studies

The PCP should complete a thorough physical examination with particular attention to physical anomalies, neurologic systems, and affect, cognition, and mental status. Part of a thorough exam includes documenting mental status, including the following components:

- Appearance (Dressed and groomed?)
- Attitude and interaction (Cooperative, guarded, or avoidant?)

TABLE 15.9   Additional Stress History

Topic	Sample Questions	Potential Stressors
Recent changes in the family, work, school, and other settings	What events or changes have occurred in your family in the past year?	Job promotion (more travel or time away) Move or parent deployment
Recent contextual changes in life circumstances, for better or worse, which provoke changes in the child's perception of self, family, or feelings of relationship security resulting in self-blame or a sense of betrayal	Who lives in your home? Have there been any recent changes at home or changes in family relationships? Any new health issues or deaths? Have parents separated or divorced or remarried? Has an older sibling moved away?	Changes in household composition (e.g., births, expansion to include elders) Risk of loss or loss of attachment figure(s) New role or responsibilities presenting a psychological challenge Child or sibling with special health care needs
Recurring experiences that a child may deal with	Tell me about the things you find difficult or stressful as a parent, especially in caring for this child. What is overwhelming? Who do you have to help you with child-rearing?	Parental overprotection, lack of supervision, restrictive or over permissive parenting Control struggles, ineffective limit-setting strategies, harsh discipline practices
Parents' personal history of being parented: it is important to have the caregivers share memories, good and bad, of their childhood and what they liked and disliked about the parenting they experienced	Tell me about your most favorite and least favorite memories of growing up. How is your parenting similar to and different from the parenting you received as a child? What are your expectations for your child?	Unhappy childhood, poor role models, unrealistic academic, athletic, or social expectations of the child, harsh discipline, poor family communication Reliance on the child by the parents for emotional comfort and support

- Activity level/behavior (Calm, active, restless? Psychomotor activity, abnormal movements, and/or tics?)
- Speech (Loud or quiet? Flat in tone or full of intonation? Slow or rushed? Does child understand and express appropriately?)
- Thought processes (Coherent, disorganized, flight of ideas, blocking [inability to fill in memory gaps], loosening associations [shifting of topics quickly though unrelated], echolalia, perseveration?)
- Thought content (Delusions, obsessions, perceptual disorders, phobias, hypochondriasis?)
- Impulse control (Aggressive, hostile, sexual?)
- Mood/affect (Depressed, anxious, flat, ambivalent, fearful, irritable, elated, euphoric?)

If physical findings are suggestive of health problems, pertinent laboratory tests (e.g., hemoglobin, thyroid test, antistreptolysin O [ASO] titer, blood lead level, serum electrolytes, drug tests for alcohol or illicit substances, or urinalysis) should be drawn. At times, the family history, developmental, and neurologic findings may warrant genetic studies or imaging of the central nervous system.

Mental Health Management Strategies

Management of mental health in children is two-pronged: promoting thriving as well as preventing and mitigating stress. In order to do this most effectively, prioritize the limited time PCPs have with families by doing the following (Clark and Garner, 2018): use the eco-bio-developmental framework to understand the life-course theory and developmental trajectories that affect child development; know biological threats to health and address environmental risks early; and proactively build wellness. As in all areas of pediatric primary care, the focus must be on both the child and his or her family. Parents need as much help as children, especially in the areas of mental health and behavioral management. Strategies discussed here are also relevant to many developmental problems of children and also to the management of neurodevelopmental and mental health problems, as discussed in Chapter 30.

Mental Health Promotion

Key components of mental health promotion include strengthening relationships, supporting family functioning and parenting, and providing strategies to facilitate social, emotional and cognitive growth. Chapter 2 describes the dual patient notion for pediatric primary care—the parent is a client as well as the child. Indeed, the family is a system made up of unique and independent parts—the family members who must interact to create a unified working whole, which benefits all within the constraints of individual strengths and weaknesses, and the environment in which the family unit exists. A key concept is that the child is most successful in achieving well-being if the parents are knowledgeable, healthy, and supported in their own lives. Further, parents must have their children's well-being as a core value they seek to develop and protect. Pediatric PCPs bolster parents and nudge them toward ever-changing parenting strategies in keeping with their children's needs. Promotion of good mental health in children requires a consistent focus on the parents.

Strategies to Build Relationships

Relationships are so key to child health and the future of the world that there are several national and international approaches recommended that can be incorporated in the PCPs daily routine. The following are some reliable options.

Essential Parenting. The CDC's parenting program identifies essential components of parenting, and provides tips, videos, and resources for each (CDC, 2018).

1. Communicate with your child by taking time to listen, let your child know when they have done something good, read with your child, make time to laugh, and avoid distractions.
2. Create structure and rules that provide consistency, predictability, and follow-through by providing choices, establishing routine, preventing temper tantrums.

TABLE 15.10 Screening Tools for Social-Emotional Development

Screening Tool	Age Group	Time/What Screens	Cost
Ages and Stages Social Emotional, ed 2. Available at: https://www.brookespublishing.com/product/asqse-2/.	1-72 months	10-15 min to complete; 1-3 min to score Social-emotional development	Cost; Brookes Publishing
Pediatric Symptom Checklist 17 and 35 item Available at: https://www.massgeneral.org/psychiatry/services/psc_home.aspx	4-16 years; Youth version; multiple languages	<5 min to complete; 2 min to score General psychosocial screening of externalizing, internalizing, and attention behaviors	Free
KYSS Assessment Questionnaire Available at: www.napnap.org/ProgramsAndInitiatives/MentalHealth/MentalHealthGuide/MentalHealthGuideHandouts.aspx	Older Infants and toddlers, preschool, school-age children and teens	<15 min to complete interpretive Mental health and psychosocial	Free; NAPNAP copyrighted
Survey of Wellness in Young Children Available at: www.floatinghospital.org/The-Survey-of-Wellbeing-of-Young-Children/Overview.aspx	Under 5 years old	15 min to complete Developmental milestones, behavioral/emotional development, family risk factors	Free; Tufts Medical Center
Strengths and Difficulties (SDQ) Available at: sdqinfo.org	Parent report 4-10 year and 11-17 years Youth report 11-17 years Teacher report 4-10 years and 11-17 years Baseline and follow-up	Five scales: Emotional symptoms, conduct problems, hyperactivity/inattention, peer relationship problems, prosocial behavior; and total difficulties score	Copyrighted, not in public domain
Child Behavior Checklist 2 (CBCL)	Preschool (18 months to 5 years) School age (6-18 years) for parent and teacher Youth (11-18 years)	Emotional and behavioral	Cost; requires training
Temperament Available at: www.preventiveoz.org	4 months to 6 years	Temperament questionnaire and profile Behavioral advice	Cost ($10 annual membership)
Temperament and Atypical Screening (TABS) www.brookespublishing.com	11 months to 71 months	15 question screener takes 5-10 55 question assessment takes 15-20 Detects detached, hypersensitive and hyperactive, reactive, and dysregulated behaviors	Cost; Brookes Publishing
Sensory Processing Disorder Checklist Available at: www.spdstar.org/basic/symptoms-checklist	Infant/toddler; preschool; school-aged; adolescent/adult	10-15 min to complete; interpretive	Free; Star Institute
Adverse Childhood Questionnaire (ASE-Q) Available at: https://centerforyouthwellness.org/cyw-aceq/	Child, teen and teen self-response	2-5 min to complete	Free; Center for Youth Wellness

3. Give directions: get your child's attention, give the direction, check compliance, and use discipline and consequences, by rewarding, praising, and paying attention to the positive or ignoring, distracting, natural and logical consequences, and time-out.

The First 1000 Days. The First 1000 Days initiative became an international movement focused on healthy nutrition to provide essential building blocks for brain development. The American Academy of Pediatrics (AAP) Early Brain and Child Development (EBCD) Initiative coupled nutrition with the development of SSNRs, incorporating the eco-bio-developmental model to provide optimal brain development. The action framework provides general principles for assessing and teaching at each well care visit during this time period based on *exploring* the socioemotional home environment, *building* relationships (reciprocity), *cultivating* development, and *developing* parent confidence and competence.

Other Strategies. There are multiple other strategies to build relationships, but two others that are widely used and easily adapted in PCP practice are Serve and Return and Circle of Security. Just as in many sports players serve the ball and it is returned, *Serve and Return* applies this concept to relationships to build healthier brains and social interaction. Harvard University's Center on the Developing Child identifies five steps to serve and return: (1) notice the serve and share the child's focus of attention; (2) return the serve by supporting and encouraging; (3) give it a name; (4) take turns and then wait, keeping the interaction going back and forth; and (5) practice endings and beginnings. A response that is sensitive, responsive, and attentive to the child's

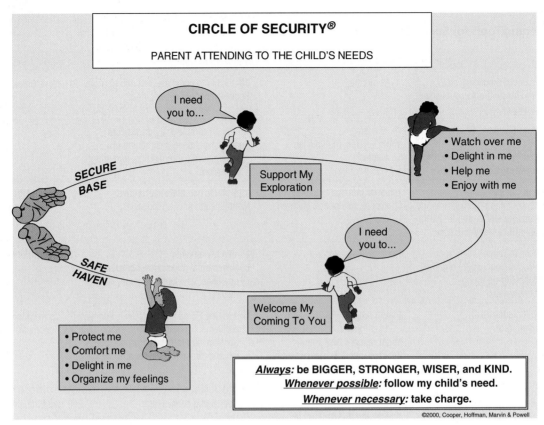

• **Fig 15.6** The Circle of Security (From Circle of Security Network. 2000. http://circleofsecuritynetwork.org/the_circle_of_security.html or https://www.circleofsecurityinternational.com/handouts. Accessed August 15, 2018.)

action provides a rich environment for continued interaction that becomes increasing complex as a child grows (https://developingchild.harvard.edu/resources/5-steps-for-brain-building-serve-and-return/).

The Circle of Security model (Fig 15.6) illustrates the ongoing process of attachment, co-regulation, and learning, where a child ventures out from a secure base to explore the world, growing in independence. Once things become difficult, the child returns to the safe haven for security and help in regulating their distress. The model applies to children of any age and is available in several languages and formats (www.circleofsecurityinternational.com).

Strategies to Promote Family Functioning and Parenting

By and large, parents want to do a good job of parenting and primarily need education, skills support, and help managing stress. These supports can easily be interwoven into anticipatory guidance that is provided routinely at well-child visits or can become brief intervention visits (discussed later). There are many different options to choose from when working with families, and selecting two or three favorites as mainstays works well for many PCPs. Routines, rituals, celebrations, family communication, and growth mind-set are discussed earlier in the chapter. Appropriate discipline and expectations of the child based on child age and development are discussed later. Some key parenting strategies are listed in Box 15.5. The Parenting Pyramid and Purposeful Parenting are two other frameworks widely used in pediatrics.

The Parenting Pyramid (see Fig 8.1), from the Incredible Years Parenting Program, illustrates the focus of positive parenting from both the parent side (skills and strategies) and child benefits. The base and foundation of the pyramid where the majority of time should be spent centers on connecting, teaching, and celebrating a child. From the base upward, clear and consistent limits, rules, and follow-through help direct the child's behaviors. The top layers of the pyramid address correcting behaviors which the child has already been taught but has not adhered to. If there is a problem at one layer of the pyramid, the solution is often in the layer below.

Purposeful Parenting, also called the 6 Ps, guides parents in helping their children learn, contribute, connect, and decrease stress (http://ohioaap.org/wp-content/uploads/2013/07/BPoM_PurposefulParenting.pdf).

The 6 Ps are *Protective*, meeting basic needs, feeling safe, but not being too overprotective; *Personal*, showing love and acceptance, being kind and gentle, and using positive teaching; *Progressive*, where discipline and parenting change depending on the child's stage; *Positive*, being loving, optimistic, and rewarding; *Playful*, being involved in and at times a follower in play; and *Purposeful*, keeping the end in mind and, at times when parenting is hard, looking for the purpose in child behaviors.

Two literacy-based programs are also effective in coaching parents. The *5 Rs of Early Literacy* include: (1) reading together every day; (2) rhyming, playing, and cuddling every day; (3) developing routines around meals, sleep, and family fun; (4) rewarding children with praise for successes to build self-esteem and promote positive behavior; and (5) developing relationships that are strong and nurturing. These activities are easy for parents to engage in while building skills and minimizing stress. The *Reach Out and Read* (www.reachoutandread.org) program provides parents of infants from 6 months to the start of school a book at clinic well visits as well as guidance to promote reading together.

• BOX 15.5 Positive Parenting Strategies

Attend to the Child Individually

- Respond to child's bids for attention with eye contact, smiles, and physical contact.
- Provide guaranteed child led special time daily: No interruptions, no directions, and no interrogations.
- Allow the child to make reasonable choices. Believe in the ability to learn, improve and grow.
- Comment on child's appropriate and desirable behavior frequently and positively throughout the day.
- Be available both physically and emotionally, to teach and model behavior.
- Do things with them, not just for them.
- Know your child's personality, temperament, dreams, and value your child's thoughts and opinions.
- Know your child's friends and encourage positive involvement with friends and activities.
- Prevent secondary gains for the child's minor transgressions by having no discussion, physical contact, perhaps even eye contact; be neutral and simply state the preferred behavior.
- Show up at their concerts, games, and events. Visit their schools.

Listen Actively

- Paraphrase or describe what the child is saying.
- Reflect the child's feelings.
- Share the child's affect by matching the child's body posture and tone of voice.
- Avoid giving commands, judging, or editorializing.
- Follow the child's lead in the interaction.
- Insist on family meals especially as a child get older.

Convey Positive Regard

- Communicate positive feelings (e.g., love) directly.
- Give directions positively, firmly, and specifically.
- Provide notice before requiring the child to change activities.
- Label the behavior, not the child.
- Strive for consistency.
- Praise competency and compliance; say thank you.
- Celebrate accomplishments.
- Apologize when appropriate.
- Avoid shaming or belittling the child.

Know Yourself as a Parent

- Understand and accept yourself, be aware of your own feelings.
- Acknowledge parental strengths and accept uniqueness.
- Take care of yourself and treat yourself with respect.

Discipline as a Parenting Strategy. Discipline is education that molds the behavior, mental capacities, or moral character of an individual. Punishment, on the other hand, is loss, pain, or suffering that is administered in response to behavior. Discipline is related to behavioral expectations of child and should be used to teach the child suitable behavior and to keep the child safe. Based in appropriate expectations, discipline modifies and structures behavior using positive behavior reinforcement (catching the child being good) more than negative reinforcement of undesirable behavior (time-out). Discipline reinforces social norms, helps a child fit into daily family and school routine, and makes child-rearing fun (Hagan, Shaw, Duncan, 2017). Parents' abilities to discipline appropriately are determined not only by their knowledge (or lack of) of appropriate ways to discipline, but also by their own responsibilities and stressors, their "fit" with the child, and past experiences.

The manner and intent of providing discipline are as important as the techniques used. Punishment should never include withdrawal of the parent's love or affection. When coming from a safe, secure relationship, the child learns to choose acceptable behaviors and develops self-control.

Expectations must be appropriate to the age, development, personality, temperament, strengths, and weaknesses of the child. If expectations are too high, children feel pressured and may feel failure even when they are doing their best. Expecting a child to do their "best" can be overly demanding because no one can consistently "do their best" all the time. Expectations that are too low diminish children's value and make them feel as if the parent has no faith in them. Although this is a sensitive issue, knowing where expectations begin (parent-driven or child-driven) and how they fit the child and family is important. Clearly stating expectations and identifying limits and consequences so that both the child and parent understand provide security for the child and prevent frustration, distrust, and further problems. Mistakes are accepted and expected, and resilience develops by helping the child learn to view failure or mistakes as chances to learn. A realistic assessment of the child's performance, emphasizing strengths and discussing strategies that lead to success, prepares children to approach future obstacles and disappointments constructively.

One of the easiest ways to provide discipline is by establishing structure (family routines), which really is just rules for how the family does things. Parents teach skills by modeling the desired behavior, but often, especially with younger children, by simply stating exactly what is desired followed by immediate reinforcement. As children grow, they should negotiate with their parents to help set the rules. Praise, with a specific description of what was accomplished, paired with the social values, is good reinforcement (e.g., "Great job sharing with your sister. It makes me proud that you know how to get along."). Gradually the child should move to ownership of behavior and being rewarded by the satisfaction of doing something well.

Consequences help children learn to socialize. Appropriate planned consequences are prompt, logically related to the behavior, appropriate to the child's age and developmental capabilities and the right size (i.e., smaller consequences allow the child to accept self-responsibility). Natural consequences (e.g., "You want to sleep in, but you are going to miss the bus, so I guess you wear your pajamas to school.") may be more accepted and remembered. As children grow, they should help determine the consequences for misbehavior. Time-out, being sent to the child's room, restricting a favorite activity, and turning off the television or video games are examples of successful consequences. Loss of privilege with a brief explanation teaches the child the why of the discipline (e.g., "You can't ride your bike tomorrow because you left it in the street.") Box 15.6 gives a few other basic principles of discipline.

Teaching problem-solving is also a part of discipline. Begin by providing opportunities to make choices and decisions. Teach the steps to problem-solving (stating the problem, expressing needs, considering alternatives, agreeing on a solution, and implementing and following through with the agreed-on solution). By taking time and letting the child work through the process, the child's confidence is built.

Managing Temperament. The provider can discuss with the parents how they view their child's temperament, how it fits with the parent's temperament or that of other family members, and what parent-child strategies can be used if conflicts emerge between the child's temperament and the caregivers' personal style. The intent is to alleviate guilt and frustration, to support the parenting role, and to assist parents to develop skills that enhance

• BOX 15.6   Additional Principles of Discipline

- Parents should talk with each other and agree on how to handle discipline and their child's misbehavior. They should distinguish between discipline and punishment.
- Interactions with children should focus on discipline or teaching, rather than punishment.
- Treat children with respect and empathy, even when being reprimanded for misbehavior.
- Misbehavior can often be prevented. When a child appears willful, bored, or out-of-sorts, distraction and active engagement with the parent (e.g., giving the child something to do; talking to, playing with, or dancing with the child) can stop misbehavior before it starts.
- Be alert to when children reach their limits (i.e., are nearing "meltdown" because they are tired, hungry, or overstimulated) and intervene to prevent problems from occurring. Children in a "meltdown" stage are not able to relate rationally to a parent's reasoned explanation or request; the underlying problem—hunger, lack of sleep, and so on—must be dealt with first.
- Parents may also need a "timeout" from the child to cool down and regain self-control and they should have a plan for help when they need respite.
- Use flexible limit setting, ("You have to wear a coat, but you may choose the blue or red one.").
- *Corporal punishment is unnecessary and has the potential to cause physical and/or psychologic damage.*

positive behaviors rather than exaggerate difficult temperamental characteristics. Supporting both the parents' and child's needs can prevent significant problems in the future. The PCP's understanding of the child's unique temperament helps parents and other caregivers better understand the child's behavior, especially when behaviors are perceived as confusing or problematic. As parents identify traits in their child's temperament, they gain a tool for understanding their child and managing responses to a variety of situations their child may face. In addition, parents benefit from understanding their own temperaments since "goodness of fit" between the child and parent is crucial (e.g., to a parent with a high activity level, a child with an average or low activity level might seem lazy or dull). No temperament characteristic is bad—just different (e.g., the persistent child may be "stubborn" when faced with discipline but may work for an extended period of time to understand a math problem or to master a technique for sports or musical performance).

Temperamental traits that parents find difficult to manage tend to engender parental criticism and irritability, power struggles, and restrictive parenting, and may be associated with behavior disorders, although temperament alone is not a risk factor for maladjustment. Critical mediators of the role of temperament in the development of behavioral disorders include parental psychological functioning, marital adjustment, childrearing attitudes and practices, and social support factors.

The goal of the PCP is to reframe temperament traits in such a way that they become more understandable and workable, enabling them to achieve "goodness of fit." Helpful strategies for parents, teachers, and other caregivers include (1) recognizing the child's innate behavioral qualities as temperament expressions, (2) understanding how temperament relates to behavior and that temperament is not amenable to change but can be worked with and reframed, and (3) encouraging caregivers to express their feelings and learn to develop strategies to work with the traits they find most challenging. Specific strategies for different temperament traits are found in Table 15.11.

TABLE 15.11   Strategies to Help Children With Different Temperaments

Temperament Characteristic	Strategy
Activity level—amount of child movement across different situations	Recognize activity level and plan high-energy activities (long walks, family outings). Plan activities to keep children busy in situations when quiet is required (such as during religious services).
Intensity of reaction—amount of reactive energy shown in response to both positive and negative events	Help children recognize their responses to positive and negative emotions. When an over-response occurs, teach children how to modify their behavioral response to their feelings.
Adaptability/frustration tolerance—how quickly the initial response pattern can be modified in desired direction	Provide reassurance when things don't go as planned. Teach how to deal with disappointment. Do not avoid situations in which frustrations may occur as part of developing emotional maturity is experiential.
Persistence and attention span—how long a child pursues activity especially in face of obstacles	Teach strategies to help stay on track. Help parents set realistic expectations of the child's attention span.
Distractibility—how easily external events or stimulation interfere or divert from ongoing activity	Take development and distractibility into consideration when doing tasks that require concentration (i.e., homework, quiet time).
Rhythmicity—regularity and predictability of sleep, feeding, and daily activity patterns	Keep normal sleep (including nap), wake, and feeding schedule in mind when planning activities and outings. Use normal elimination patterns as a guide during toilet training.
Threshold of response—sensitivity or amount of stimulation needed to evoke a discernible response	Recognize that not all children use the same strategies for calming and adapt to the child (i.e., use care not to over-respond to more mild situations such as when juice spills or things break).
Approach or withdrawal—response to anything new—food, people, places, toys, etc.	Recognize that new situations may be stressful. Teach skills and provide opportunities to deal with discomfort in a supporting and loving environment.
Mood—amount of pleasant, joyful, and friendly behavior typically shown in contrast to unpleasant, crying, and unfriendly behavior	Use positive reinforcement for good mood responses to situations. Ignore negative mood responses.

Social and Emotional Strategies

Helping children develop social-emotional skills comes easily to some parents, but others require direction and guidance. Some basic approaches are as follows:

- Infancy—help parents be attentive to their baby's likes and dislikes, sensitivities, and signals
- Older infants, toddlers, and preschoolers—allow the child to express and recognize the full spectrum of human emotion, from good to bad, as well as develop skills to cope with negative emotions
- Older children—support the child's self-esteem and help them explore a wide range of interests; ensure that overscheduling is avoided and there is plenty of "downtime" and relaxation
- Adolescence—provide clear expectations, sensitive support, pride in achievements, and positive affect toward the adolescent

Self-Regulation, Resilience, and Executive Function Skills. Three key skills that all children need to develop are self-regulation, resilience, and executive function. It can be helpful to remember that there are three stages of learning social-emotional skills. *Skill acquisition*, or show-and-tell, occurs as the child has the skill explained, then demonstrated, receives positive feedback with effort, and has the opportunity to practice. *Skill fluency*, or practice makes perfect, comes as the child practices the skill in various settings, links to similar situations, and is reminded of when to use the skill. *Skill maintenance and generalization,* "You've got it! ", comes as the child is reinforced in using the skill.

Self-regulation is the ability to manage emotions and behavior. Remaining calm in the face of changes, challenges, and frustrations is at the heart of self-regulation, sometimes also called self-control. Emotional dysregulation occurs when the child melts down and is unable to handle strong reactions. This reaction may be instantaneous, intense, and immediate, or it may build over time and lead to an outburst. The child's temperament and environment contribute to the ability to self-regulate. Self-regulation is taught by skill isolation and providing practice in a supportive environment (scaffolding) for the encouraged behavior. Practice runs, or breaking things into smaller steps to practice, are other effective techniques. Staying calm and taking time to evaluate what went wrong and why, and how it can be better next time, are other effective strategies for children to self-regulate (https://childmind.org/article/can-help-kids-self-regulation/; https://nurtureandthriveblog.com/how-to-teach-your-child-self-regulation/).

In order to build *resilience*, some stress is required. The PCP needs to assess what stresses the child has encountered and how the child is doing in the midst or aftermath of that stress. Promoting resilience can be as simple as attachment to a caring adult, giving a child choices, mastering a skill, assigning chores to give responsibility, learning to show appreciation, developing friendships, working as a team, learning to ask for help, and developing self-esteem and a sense of control.

Core life skills, which are developed and fine-tuned in adolescence, require self-regulation and *executive function* skills. The Center for the Developing Child (2018) identifies five ways to help build these skills: (1) practice with real-life situations (focus and flexibility), (2) spot and plan for triggers (awareness and self-control), (3) take another's view of stressors (awareness, flexibility, self-control), (4) focus on personally motivating goals (planning, flexibility), and (5) build on positive memories and small successes (focus, planning).

Promoting Strengths. Approaching any child from a strengths approach allows both the PCP and parent to focus on optimal outcomes. At times, parents may need help to identify strengths in their child, especially if parent-child fit is poor or parents are stressed themselves. One way that strengths can be classified are as *general* (e.g., independent, works well with others, creative, and curious), *social* (e.g., comforts others, follows routines, has a good sense of humor), *language* (e.g., expresses needs, participates in discussions, asks who, what, where), *literacy* (e.g., enjoys reading, tells stories, connects stories to life), and *math* (e.g., understands patterns in nature, thinks logically, remembers math facts). *Understood.org* has a list of specifics for each of these strengths (https://www.understood.org/en/friends-feelings/empowering-your-child/building-on-strengths/types-of-strengths-in-kids).

Developmental assets are another approach to identifying strengths in the child or family. Researched by the Search Institute, the 40 evidence-based assets relate skills, experiences, relationships, and behaviors evidenced as support, strengths, and noncognitive skills in self, family, school, and the community. These become building blocks that help children and adolescents grow into healthy, happy, and contributing members of society. Assets are applicable regardless of gender, culture, socioeconomic situation, or geographic location. The more assets a young person has, the more likely he or she is to make wise decisions and choose positive lifestyles while avoiding harmful or unhealthy choices. Developmental asset lists for adolescents (ages 12 to 18), middle childhood (ages 8 to 12), grades K to 3 (ages 5 to 9), and early childhood (ages 3 to 5) are available and have been translated into 14 different languages (www.search-institute.org).

Sparks, also identified by the Search Institute, are described as a key reason why some kids flourish instead of just getting by. Sparks are those interests, talents, and passions that motivate young people to grow, learn, and contribute and make positive choices about their activities and time, while leading them to express their unique personalities and contribute to the world. Kids who thrive have knowledge of their sparks and adults who support the development of these sparks. The 10 most common sparks identified by American teenagers are creative arts; athletics; learning (e.g., languages, science, history); reading; volunteering (e.g., helping, serving); spirituality or religion; nature, ecology, and environment; living a quality life (e.g., joy, tolerance, caring); animal welfare; and leading.

Prevent and Mitigate Effects of Stress

With an established, ongoing relationship, PCPs use their knowledge of brain development, the information they have about the family (protective and risk factors), and routine screening not only to promote mental health, but also to (1) help children figure out how to turn off their stress response (primary prevention requiring parent/child skills) and (2) intervene early if unable to turn off the stress response (secondary and tertiary prevention) (Garner, 2016). Identifying issues the family faces; preparing them for developmental challenges, temperament issues, predictable life events that impact children, such as moves or day care or school changes; and other common behavioral problems are often handled best at the PCP level. Teaching parents developmentally appropriate coping strategies for their children (e.g., symbolic play in preschoolers or developmentally appropriate books or movies with older children to help them express feelings and worries and gain control of their situation) are examples. However, initial interventions may not always be sufficient. Early detection and intervention and addressing unanticipated life events are the main components of secondary prevention. Social, emotional, or behavioral problems may emerge, even in the context of positive childrearing approaches. Early recognition of pediatric stress and mental illness is easier when care-givers have a realistic understanding of their child's development and PCPs actively screen for developmental red flags. Secondary prevention involves working collaboratively to identify and implement appropriate management strategies or to explain and reinforce the value of mental health recommendations. Tertiary prevention addresses major losses and trauma (e.g., victimization through sexual or physical abuse, parental marital problems, divorce, substance abuse, and parental psychopathologic conditions), in addition to any significant behavioral symptoms that impair daily functioning. Any child who experiences trauma should be referred to a mental health specialist for further assessment and intervention, even in the absence of behavioral manifestations of distress. In these cases, parents may not understand the need for referral, so it is helpful to frame the behavior problem as a "normal response" to stress and/or trauma, with the goal of referral being to maximize the child's growth and development. Many of these stressors are addressed later in this chapter or elsewhere in this book.

Violence Prevention

Violence is discussed in Chapter 24; this section focuses on the prevention of violence. The prevention of youth violence requires use of a public health model that addresses the complexity of causes and risk factors behind the problem. Some issues can be addressed in the primary care setting, whereas others require more active involvement in the community as a child and family advocate. Primary prevention of youth violence begins with strengthening relationships within families and helping parents be more effective. Start by identifying ways to prevent violence (e.g., discuss how the family can incorporate protective factors into their family life [Box 15.7] and minimize any risk factors [Box 15.8]). Strategies to achieve this include encouraging parents to be actively involved with their children, supervising youths and their activities, and monitoring the child's peer group (having friends who engage in conventional, nonviolent behaviors). Parents may need to be educated about the effect of violence on their children (media and technology), discussing ways to minimize exposure. Teaching about gun safety is always critical. Working to strengthen the developmental competencies of youth includes educating youths at an early age about violence and its prevention, teaching anger management and strategies for preventing a fight (role-playing), and promoting self-defense strategies, such as learning a martial art and discussing ways to manage difficult or potentially violent situations (Boxes 15.9 and 15.10).

Efforts should also be focused on helping improve the environment that youths are in, including supporting diversity training and bullying prevention programs in schools; supporting after-school programs for youth and work for community commitment to youth programs; working to make neighborhoods and schools safe places for youth; involving the community in a commitment to prevent violence; addressing the issues of media violence and of condoning violence as a way of life; enforcing current sale regulations and encouraging additional sale regulations of consciousness-altering substances (e.g., alcohol, marijuana) to youth; and supporting legislation to limit access to and carrying of guns.

Secondary prevention is focused on screening for potential problems, including assessing for violence risk factors at all health supervision and illness visits; screening for alcohol abuse problems; asking about weapons in the home (their presence, use, storage, and access); and caring for children exposed to or threatened by violence by addressing any physical or emotional problems resulting from violence in the primary care setting. Early intervention can prevent

---

• BOX 15.7 Protective Factors Against Youth Violence

Individual Protective Factors
- Intolerant attitude toward deviance
- High intelligence quotient
- High grade point average (as an indicator of high academic achievement)
- High educational aspirations
- Positive social orientation
- Popularity acknowledged by peers
- Highly developed social skills/competencies
- Highly developed skills for realistic planning
- Religiosity

Family Protective Factors
- Connectedness to family or adults outside the family
- Ability to discuss problems with parents
- Perceived parental expectations about school performance are high
- Frequent shared activities with parents
- Consistent presence of parent during at least one of the following: when awakening, when arriving home from school, at evening mealtime or going to bed
- Involvement in social activities
- Parental/family use of constructive strategies for coping with problems (provision of models of constructive coping)

Peer and Social Protective Factors
- Possession of affective relationships with those at school that are strong, close, and prosocially oriented
- Commitment to school (an investment in school and in doing well at school)
- Close relationships with nondeviant peers
- Membership in peer groups that do not condone antisocial behavior
- Involvement in prosocial activities
- Exposure to school climates that characterized by:
  - Intensive supervision
  - Clear behavior rules
  - Consistent negative reinforcement of aggression
  - Engagement of parents and teachers

Centers for Disease Control and Prevention, Injury Prevention & Control Division of Violence Prevention. Understanding and Preventing Violence: Summary of Research Activities Summer; CDC; 2013. https://www.cdc.gov/violenceprevention/youthviolence/riskprotectivefactors.html. Accessed August 11, 2018.

---

more serious problems later; referral may be necessary. Community programs that make home visits to mothers of new babies, especially those in low-income and teen-mother families; support groups for children who have suffered trauma or loss or witnessed violence (e.g., school counseling for traumatic experiences); and referral of families to community support programs, such as Big Brothers Big Sisters of America, are other effective interventions. Tertiary prevention is focused on treatment and rehabilitation programs for offenders and treatment for victims and their families. This can be difficult and costly and yield only mixed results.

In 2016, the CDC published a Comprehensive Technical Package for the Prevention of Youth Violence and Associated Risk Behaviors. This package identifies the following strategies to help communities focus on successful violence prevention. The six strategies are as follows: promote family environments that support healthy development; provide quality education early in life; strengthen youth's skills; connect youth to caring adults and activities; create protective community environments; and intervene to lessen harms and prevent future risk (David-Ferdon et al., 2016).

BOX 15.8 Risk Factors for Serious Youth Violence

Individual Risk Factors

- History of violent victimization
- Attention deficits, hyperactivity, or learning disorders
- Deficits in social cognitive or information-processing abilities
- Poor behavioral control
- History of early aggressive behavior
- Low intelligence quotient
- High emotional distress
- History of treatment for emotional problems
- Antisocial beliefs and attitudes
- Involvement with drugs, alcohol, or tobacco
- Exposure to violence and conflict in the family

Family Risk Factors

- Authoritarian childrearing attitudes
- Harsh, lax, or inconsistent disciplinary practices
- Low parental involvement
- Poor monitoring and supervision of children
- Low emotional attachment to parents or caregivers
- Poor family functioning
- Low parental education and income
- Parental substance abuse or criminality

Peer and Social Risk Factors

- Association with delinquent peers
- Involvement in gangs
- Social rejection by peers
- Lack of involvement in conventional activities
- Poor academic performance
- Low commitment to school and school failure

Community Risk Factors

- Diminished economic opportunities
- High concentrations of poor residents
- High level of transiency
- High level of family disruption
- Low levels of community participation
- Socially disorganized neighborhoods

Adapted from Centers for Disease Control and Prevention (CDC). Youth Violence: Risk and Protective Factors. CDC. www.cdc.gov/violenceprevention/youthviolence/riskprotectivefactors.html. Accessed August 18, 2018.

BOX 15.9 Tips for Talking With Teens About How to Keep Out of Trouble

- Do not carry a weapon; instead, "fight clean" (i.e., discuss the issue in conflict). Carrying weapons only makes one less safe; pulling out a weapon begins a cycle of retaliation.
- Do not go into harm's way. Avoid being around fights because the cycle of escalation and retaliation often involves innocent people.
- Avoid being caught alone; stay with friends.
- Do not be provoked into fighting. Words are said, and names are called, not because the names are true, but to provoke anger and a fight.
- If one becomes involved in a fight, try to end the incident on equal ground; that way anger is more likely to be diffused. The person who wins often takes on the aggressor role; the loser then becomes the scapegoat. Thus violence continues and becomes cyclic.
- Suggest discussions with friends about ways to handle potential situations in which a gun or knife might be brandished.
- Do not join gangs or associate with individuals who turn to violence as a way of settling differences.
- Report threats of school violence to adults.

BOX 15.10 Talking With Teens About Sexual Abuse/Assault

- Males as well as females can be victimized
- Alcohol intoxication or the use of drugs is a major factor in sexual assault. Prevention includes not placing oneself in harm's way by using such substances.
- Manipulative verbal threats and physically trapping the victim are common tactics used by perpetrators.
- Reluctance to report gang or date rape is common. However, keeping the rape a secret only leads to self-doubt and delays healing. The teen should report the rape immediately and seek professional counseling.

Counseling and Brief Evidence-Based Interventions

In addition to providing anticipatory guidance and assistance in developing healthy coping strategies, the PCP directly provides a variety of services that assist families in need of mental health services. Many PCPs work in collaboration with mental health providers through integrated care models. Community services such as home visits strengthen families and are often aimed at a risk population (premature babies, young mothers, low income). Art, music, or movement therapy allows a child self-expression, which improves well-being and confidence, and the opportunity to work with intense emotions, poor social skills, and low self-esteem. These therapies use physical activity and sensory integration to engage different parts of the brain, leading to relaxation and improved mood. The focus is on the process, not the product of these therapies with the parent or adult asking the child questions (without directing or judging) and talking about feelings that emerge.

The PCP can schedule *brief or very brief interventions* as billable office visits that can provide effective counseling strategies accomplished in 5 to 15 (max 30) minute time periods over one to multiple visits. These interventions serve as treatment or intervention while awaiting specialist care. A meta-analysis of 50 randomized, controlled trials of single-session interventions (SSI) showed improvement across all categories of mental health problems (Schleider and Weisz, 2017). The researchers also developed a 30-minute computer program to teach adolescents the growth mind-set, and they report the results were not only effective but lasting, even potentiating other therapies. Active monitoring (counseling and follow-up), behavioral approaches (e.g., checklists, reward charts, logical consequences, special times with parents [time-in] as well as time-out), and supportive counseling are effective. Additional strategies that can be used are discussed later.

Mindfulness

Mindfulness is defined as (1) paying attention, (2) on purpose, (3) in the present moment, and (4) nonjudgmentally. The goal of mindfulness is to take negative thoughts about one's past or fears of the future and listen to emotion and thoughts, recognizing that feelings rise and subside like the weather, and thoughts are just thoughts. This allows one to wait out the emotional overreactions (fight or flight) and come back to a calm state (intentional regulation). Among other benefits, mindfulness helps social and academic performance, improves sleep and self-confidence and immune function, changes maladaptive stress coping, and reduces anxiety and depression. It can be prescribed during health care visits (Rosenfeld, 2017) or taught to parents to help them cope (Hall, 2018) and in turn teach their children. Techniques as simple as "awareness walks" around the block, noticing sounds, sights, feelings, and smells; abdominal breathing; or focusing on a snow globe and watching the chaos of the snowflakes settle down can be helpful. Multiple initiatives, websites, classes, and apps (e.g., Calm, Breethe, Insight Timer) are available to help learn this technique.

Parent-Focused Interventions

Modifying a parent's perception of their child is considered evidence-based care for many mental health issues and can have a powerful effect on a child's well-being (Gleason, Goldson, Yogman, 2016). This approach reframes the parent's perception of the child, identifying their strengths and avoiding comparison with other children. Often based in child temperament traits, this can be used at any age and begins with the very first visit, identifying child and parent strengths as contributors to child skills development. For example, PCPs can take parents' negative perception of their child as destructive of everything in the house and change their focus to a positive by identifying the child as curious and investigative, like many inventors or scientists.

Collaborative Problem-Solving: The Nurtured Heart

The nurtured heart approach (Greene, 2018) looks at difficult behaviors as a child's red flag for *lagging skills* and inability to move forward in a struggle to meet parent or adult *expectations*. There are six Collaborative Problem-Solving (CPS) tenets: (1) emphasize problems (solving them) rather than behavior (modifying it); (2) work together (with the child), not unilaterally (imposed by parent); (3) use proactive not reactive problem-solving (timing is key); (4) understanding precedes helping (the child needs skill to meet expectations before behavior can be corrected); (5) children do well if they can, which is different from if they want to; and (6) children prefer doing well. Lives in the Balance (https://www.livesintheba lance.org) has a wealth of resources (e.g., Assessment of Lagging Skills, work sheets, FAQs, and a Bill of Rights) for this approach.

Motivational Interviewing

With an established partnership between PCP and family (shared decision-making) focused on a strength-based approach, MI establishes a solid base for counseling even in brief time slots. With open, respectful, encouraging communication, and nonjudgmental questions and reflective listening, MI provides information and then guides the child/family to identify beliefs, values, strengths, and readiness to change, and to plan self-guided behavioral change strategies. Taking a difficult situation, identifying strengths, and working with the child and/or family to problem solve not only helps in the moment, but also models problem-solving for other times. Stages of change are identified in Table 15.12. Tools for MI include agenda setting (client determines priorities), getting permission, open-ended questions to start, reflective listening, summarizing, eliciting self-motivational statement (change talk), willingness and importance (or confidence).

Common Factors Intervention (HELP)

Common factors are aspects that positively influence the patient-provider relationship's ability to change patient behavior. The factors are "common," as they are effective across mental health issues, settings and practitioners, across the life span, and can be used in brief interventions. The factors are alliance; empathy; shared goals; positive regard, affirmation, and optimism; genuineness; and a skilled, experienced clinician. The AAP Mental Health Task Force

TABLE 15.12	How People Change	
Stages of Change	**Intervention by Healthcare Provider**
Precontemplation—not considering change	Increase awareness
Contemplation—considering change, but ambivalent	Facilitate the resolution of ambivalence
Preparation—willing to accept direction, anxious about change	Help the client develop an action plan
Action—learning the new behavior	Solve problems related to new behavior
Maintenance—stable in new behavior	Review successes and reinforce healthy behavior
Relapse—reappearance of old behavior (a process, not an event)	Move into action once again

(Foy and Perrin, 2010) adopted the mnemonic HELP to assist PCPs in implementing this strategy: *H*ope (through strengths and assets), *E*mpathy (in communication), *L*anguage (using the family's words) and *L*oyalty (through support and commitment), *P*ermission (to go more in-depth), *P*artnership (working together to overcome), and *P*lan (incremental with follow-up).

Cognitive Behavioral Therapy Strategies

This is an interactive, short-term, problem-oriented therapy, focused on how one's thoughts, feelings, and behaviors interact. The goal is to modify unrealistic assumptions and change them by correcting cognitive distortions, reframing negative expectations, improving social skills and problem-solving. Steps in cognitive restructuring include:

1. Identify the situation—What made me upset?
2. Name the feeling—What was my response (usually fear and anxiety, sadness and depression, anger, or guilt and shame)?
3. Determine the thought—What am I thinking that is making me feel this way? How is this a thought problem (all-or-nothing, emotional reasoning, overgeneralizing, overestimation of risk, must/should/never, self-blame, catastrophizing)?
4. Challenge the thought—What evidence do I have for this thought? Is there an alternate way to look at the situation? What would someone else think?
5. Make a decision—Do things mostly support my thought or not?

Parent Training Models/Behavioral Therapies

Basic behavioral principles underlying parent training are (1) implement positive reinforcement to promote positive behaviors; (2) ignore low level provocative behaviors; and (3) respond in a clear, safe, consistent manner to unacceptable behaviors. Behavioral therapies are used in the classroom and in parenting and focus on the same principles. SAMHSA (https://www.samhsa.gov) has a national registry of evidence-based programs and practices based on behavioral therapies, limit setting, and problem-solving. Some of the best known of these methods are available in the Additional Resources.

TABLE 15.13 ABC Strategy for Assessing and Managing Behavioral Difficulties

	For Assessing Behavior	For Management
Antecedents	*What led up to this?* the events, actions or circumstances that happen immediately before the behavior (when, where, who, what)	Avoid or prepare for situations that are likely to cause behavior, and, as possible, give cues
Behavior	*What did the child do?* the observed behavior in detail, what need is not getting met	Interpret, ignore, teach or manage behavior—give it meaning and modify response
Consequences	*What did you do?* the action or response that immediately follows the behavior, including feelings	Remain calm, not reactive and consistent; model or show what to do, rather than tell what not to do

Referral and Follow-Up

While the PCP is ideally suited to work with families on promoting and developing mental health and helping families deal with concerns, referral is sometimes needed. The degree of impairment and the persistence of the problem are key concepts in determining if referral is indicated. Many of these issues are discussed in Chapter 30. *Bright Futures*, 4th edition, lists the following as situations that may be appropriate for referral: emotional dysfunction in more than one area (home, school, peers, activities, mood); acutely suicidal or signs of psychosis; diagnostic uncertainty; poor response to treatment; parents requesting referral; behavior creating discomfort for the PCP; and/or a previous difficult social relationship with the PCP (Hagan, Shaw, Duncan, 2017). Conveying the opportunity for referral in positive terms, including the ability to grow and improve oneself, rather than in negative terms, helps overcome barriers some people feel when approaching mental health intervention. Because specialized mental health services are in such shortage, the PCP must help the family find appropriate care and secure an appointment within a reasonable time frame.

An ongoing, supportive relationship between the PCP and child/family is necessary as they work to manage social and emotional issues. In addition to monitoring during regular well care, any issues that arise require follow-up, with the type and frequency dependent on the issue and the family. When referrals are made, follow-up is essential to make sure consultation or therapy has been arranged and families are comfortable with the provider.

Behavioral Issues

It is not uncommon for behaviors exhibited by children or adolescents to concern parents, relatives, teachers, or other adults. The issues of concern are often related to normal developmental or variations of normal for which the PCP provides education and reassurance, either in anticipatory guidance given during well-child checks or during brief intervention office visits. Newborn sleep, crying and colic, postpartum depression, toilet training, temper tantrums, breath holding, learning challenges, school refusal, risk behavior, tobacco, self-injury, and tech/social media are examples of these concerns that are addressed in Unit 2. Mental health issues (anxiety, depression, etc.) are discussed in Chapter 30.

Behavioral issues for children emerge from issues of nature— temperament and goodness of fit, neurodevelopmental and inherited vulnerabilities (autism spectrum disorder [ASD], ADHD, and mental health disorders), or medical conditions (brain injury, premature birth, auditory or visual disorders, side effects of medication, illness, etc.). Temperament and goodness of fit were discussed previously, and neurodevelopmental and inherited vulnerabilities are discussed in Chapter 30. Behaviors due to medical conditions are discussed with those conditions. Behavioral issues can also emerge from issues of nurture—parenting that is either too lenient or too controlling, disruptions in parent-child relationships (attachment)—affecting how the child views the world and how the child views self or serious life stressors (divorce, alcohol, adverse childhood events). This section organizes the more common behavioral concerns under the following framework: (1) difficulties in parental or interpersonal relationships, (2) social difficulties, (3) emotional difficulties, (4) bereavement, (5) difficulties with sensory perception, (6) recurrent physical symptoms, and (7) bullying.

When working with a family who has a behavioral concern, it is helpful to remember that all behavior has meaning and is often based on a need. The behavior may be indicative of stress that is greater than the child is able to cope with at that moment in time, or it may indicate a maladaptive response. The goal of the PCP is to understand the behavior not only from the perspective of the parent but also the child. The *Antecedent-Behavior-Consequence (ABC)* technique is helpful in analyzing and understanding the situation, but it can also be helpful in teaching the parents how to handle the behavior (Table 15.13). In following the assessment process detailed earlier, a picture of the child and family that is as complete as they will reveal can be established, which allows an assessment to be made and a plan to be formulated.

Utilizing a four-visit approach is often successful. The *first visit* is focused on reviewing the complete mental health assessment, identifying strengths, as well as using the ABC method to identify the problems or issues that need to be addressed. If extended time is available at the first visit, work can begin on deciding what strategies could be used. If not, the family should be asked to return within the week for a *second visit* in order to establish a clear approach. The family must be integrally involved in determining the issues and the management strategies, but the PCP bears the responsibility of guiding the discussion. The strategies, counseling techniques and brief interventions discussed in the previous section can be used as the PCP works with the family to determine an approach that the family can buy into. Within this first or second visit, the PCP can acknowledge the effort it requires to be a good parent, and the fact that children want to do well if they can (i.e., if they have the skills) (Greene, 2018). In addition, it is often helpful to provide intervention by reframing the situation or the child (e.g., he's not a brat, but curious and persistent), and/or pointing out skills that the child

Step 1: Provide practice of the appropriate behavior with feedback
Step 2: Praise and reinforce effort
Step 3: Model or point out others doing that skill
Step 4: Prompt the child to use the behavior when the situation arises

The behavior is
• Frequent
• Persistent over time
• Uncommon for child's age
• Maladaptive—causes serious changes in emotional maturation or social or cognitive functioning
• Turned inward (depression or self-destruction)
• Turned outward (complaints or aggression)
• Disruptive
• Distancing (withdrawal, denial, or somatization)

may be lacking that are contributing to the problem (e.g., it is not laziness; it is that she has not yet learned how to get dressed or throw a ball or plan out a school project). Providing a skills acquisition framework for "basic training" can give the parent a planned focus and the child an area in which to succeed (Box 15.11). These strategies can be used for a variety of behaviors, but work well in developing self-calming, social, and anger management skills. The *third visit* should be in a week or two in order to follow up on progress and troubleshoot when there are difficulties. Further visits can be scheduled as needed, but a fourth visit 6 to 8 weeks after the initial visit is important to ensure that progress has been made. If it has not, or there are other red flags (Box 15.12), referral should take place.

Difficulties in Relationship: Attachment and Parenting Style

Safe, secure, nurturing relationships are key to child well-being, and when these are missing, disrupted patterns of attachment (discussed earlier) emerge. Children may show unexplained withdrawal, fear, sadness, or irritability; a sad and listless appearance; no seeking of comfort or response to comfort; failure to smile; watching others closely but not engaging in social interaction; and failure to ask for support or assistance. It is critical to intervene as soon as possible, working with the parents as much as the children.

The relationship between parent and child is associated with parenting styles (discussed earlier). Impaired parenting occurs when there is a mismatch between caregiving behaviors and a child's developmental or situational needs result in inappropriate stimulation, inconsistent care, inappropriate supervision, developmentally inappropriate behavioral expectations, harsh words, child rejection, child abuse, or neglect. Caregivers face a tremendous challenge to adapt their parenting skills to the individual development and behavior of each child in their family. This may be evidenced by verbalization of dissatisfaction with their role, exacerbation of tensions between the parent and child, or inappropriate communication with the child. Child behaviors that may indicate impaired parenting include acting out, developmental regression, and other aberrant behaviors. Because of the unique characteristics of each child in a family, parenting strategies may be less successful with one child than with another, or the entire family unit may be dysfunctional due to parental problems.

Management

Difficulties in interpersonal relationships often present as parental complaints about some of the evidenced child behaviors. Using the relationship as a vital sign assessment at every visit and providing the strategies to build relationships and promote family functioning and parenting hopefully prevents problems and allows the PCP to get to know the family and be aware of the growing and developing relationships. Anywhere along the way if concerns are evident or expressed, a thorough mental health assessment often identifies some of the more specific issues. At this point, the

PCP may use counseling and brief interventions based in parent-focused training, or refer the parent and child to more intense programs and therapy.

Social Difficulties: The Shy Child, the Fearful Child, the Child with Lack of Moral Integrity

Children who struggle socially may lack social skills, may be shy or fearful, or may lack moral conscious or integrity. Some children by personality are outgoing and therefore more social, while others are quiet, reserved, deep thinkers and cautious. Some children may in reality only lack the skills that allow them to become more social. Helping parents know and understand their child, their strengths, and temperament type allows the parent to help the child learn the social skills they may be lacking. Social skills by age are discussed in Chapters 10 to 13.

Shyness is a common pattern of social inhibition with unfamiliar people, novel objects, or in unfamiliar situations caused by a temperamental disposition toward withdrawal that is linked to family factors. Children with social withdrawal rather than shyness have a lower rate of social interaction overall and do not warm up to social situations. Shy children are slower to approach peers or initiate play with an unfamiliar child and often spend more time observing the situation and other children before engaging. Infants show inborn bias in responding to unfamiliar events with anxiety, distress, or disorganization and withdrawal from social stimulation. During early childhood inhibition persists, evidenced by irritability, withdrawal, and clinging to the caregiver in new situations, but this diminishes normally by school age. School-age children who are shy continue to make fewer social approaches. Viewed by their peers as likable but shy, these children may be ignored or neglected by their peers. Behavioral inhibition in social situations may be adaptive if handled effectively by the caregiver and can indicate optimal self-regulation and conscience development. Although most shy children do not develop later internalizing disorders, extremely shy toddlers may be at risk for social withdrawal in later childhood and for developing an *adolescent* anxiety disorder.

Fears and phobias can also create social difficulties. Fear is the occurrence of various avoidance responses to particular stimuli; it is a state of apprehension in response to a threatening situation. In contrast, a phobia is a persistent, extreme, and irrational fear triggered by the presence or anticipation of the presence of a specific person, object, or situation. The onset of fears occurs normally during late infancy; they are a normal part of development and have a developmental function. Specific phobias occur in about 5% of the population and in 15% of children referred for anxiety-related problems. Phobias are determined by multiple factors, including genetic influences, temperament, parental mental health problems, and individual conditioning histories. Infants typically react fearfully to loss of physical support, heights, and unexpected stimuli. Toddlers experience separation anxiety and fear physical injury and strangers. Preschoolers fear imaginary creatures, animals, darkness, and being alone, and may demonstrate some persistent separation anxiety. Fear of animals and darkness extends into school age, but safety, natural events, and school- and health-related fears dominate. In preadolescence and adolescence, fears of bodily injury, economic and political catastrophes, and social fears are central. Fear and phobic reactions typically involve symptoms of autonomic arousal. The symptoms of autonomic arousal in those with phobias may evolve into panic attacks or phobic-avoidant reactions. Distinction must be made between normal developmental fears and phobias defined on the basis of persistence, magnitude, and maladaptiveness.

Although lack of moral integrity or conscious is not a clinically defined condition, some children demonstrate a lack of an age-appropriate capacity to respect others or the environment, to judge behavior as right or wrong, and to express empathy or remorse. They frequently engage in antisocial behaviors (see Chapter 30 for discussion of social aggression, conduct disorder, and oppositional defiant disorder). A multitude of factors contribute to poor moral reasoning and antisocial behaviors, including temperament, negative experiences in infancy and childhood (e.g., maternal depression, unresponsive parenting, and abuse), and environmental damage to neurologic systems. Many behaviors are typical of children, depending on age, developmental, and cognitive levels (e.g., lying, hitting, and refusing to share), but the child who lacks conscience expresses little or no remorse for negative behavior, demonstrating a callous demeanor (Viding et al, 2014); lacks internalization of a sense of justice, fairness, or right and wrong; fails to develop an ability to self-regulate behavior; and continues antisocial behaviors beyond the expected developmental age. Antisocial behavior and delinquency are behavioral disorders in which a lack of moral integrity is a key component.

Management

Parenting the shy child with warmth, sensitivity, and responsiveness fosters security in attachment and social competence. Social-emotional strategies discussed in the earlier section help build much-needed skills. Some of the most specific include focusing on strengths and building confidence, preparing the shy children for new situations by visiting new settings, identifying a sensitive adult to whom they may turn with requests or concerns, and negotiating for them to be allowed to watch and observe before engaging in play or other activities. Praise brave behavior and avoid overcomforting the child, as this reinforces the fear. For the school-aged child, playdates, practicing show-and-tell, and extracurricular activities help get past shyness. Insensitivity and a lack of responsiveness to the child foster a sense of insecurity and predict social withdrawal and associated internalizing disorders, including depression and anxiety.

Most fears are short-lived, are not serious, and do not predict adult mental health problems. Warmth, sensitivity, and responsiveness foster a sense of security for the fearful child. Strategies that are helpful acknowledge the child's fear as real while remaining calm without belittling the child; this gives perspective and helps the child learn to manage fear now and in the future. Point out that some fears are protective and reassure the child about measures that are in place to provide security.

Helping the child put the fear into words and rate the fear (up to my knees, my stomach, or my head) and using one-sentence self-statements, like "I can do this; it is not a big deal," helps the child develop coping skills. Letting the child know what to expect helps minimize fears. Teach children to monitor scary media and learn to walk away. Treatment of fears and phobias may focus on improving caregiver mental health, caregiver–child behavior management skills, and caregiver role satisfaction and self-efficacy. Parents must be cautioned against using fears as a form of behavioral control (e.g., threats of abandonment with toddlers or threatening a school-age child with an immunization) or as a discipline strategy (e.g., leaving a preschooler alone in a dark room). When the fear negatively affects the child's functioning, developmental progress, learning experiences, and level of comfort, referral is necessary. Various management strategies are available for treatment of phobias in children older than 5 years, including contingency management, cognitive-behavioral therapy (CBT), and family interventions.

Early and assertive intervention for the child with lack of moral integrity can help develop a healthier sense of moral self and decrease antisocial behaviors, especially if treatment emphasizes developing moral judgment and conscious. Storytelling, especially the personal narrative (the child's own story), can be used to explore moral and ethical issues. Interaction with older children who demonstrate higher levels of moral reasoning may be helpful. Discussing books or watching films, television, videos, and DVDs together allows for discussion of moral dilemmas and behaviors. Encourage parents to monitor, discuss, and limit the child's access to Internet and computer games. Assist the child or adolescent to clarify values (e.g., ask child or adolescent to talk about what is most important to them; or to describe what characteristics of other people [and themselves] they see as being the "best" or most desirable). However, if these strategies are unsuccessful, referral for psychiatric management may be necessary.

Emotional Difficulties: The Upset, Angry Child With Underdeveloped Coping Skills

Children who are upset often respond in anger to a perceived threat (e.g., fear, hurt, embarrassment). Small disappointments seem overwhelming (broken treasure, unfair discipline, scary bully), as they do not have context or developed coping skills. They may be frustrated and have difficulty expressing themselves, or they may be frustrated by a problem that is too big for them. Young children in particular may express themselves physically when they do not have the words to say what they want or how they are feeling—hitting, kicking, biting, throwing, yelling, or hot-headed outbursts over minor events. Ross Greene (2018) describes the explosive child with challenging behavior as one who is lacking skills in flexibility and adaptation, frustration tolerance, and problem-solving. Learning to understand and process emotions takes time and a positive, patient relationship. Children who are tired, hungry, out of sorts, overwhelmed, or anxious are more likely to have difficulty handling emotions. Lack of sleep not only makes one cranky; it impairs the ability to read facial expression (Dewar, 2016).

Management

Early intervention is essential for children who have difficulty coping or self-regulating. Teaching parents to use positive parenting strategies and supporting them in facilitating developmentally appropriate coping has been shown to be effective (Maaskant et al, 2017). The goal is for the child to learn to develop the skills that are lacking. It is helpful to have the family track patterns—place, time of day, people, and events, as well as the predictable behaviors that occur before the child loses control. Strategies in the Social-Emotional Strategies section are essential, as is the collaborative problem-solving approach, which provides many helpful tools. In general, encourage parents to:

1. Not to take the child's emotions personally, as they are usually not directed at the parent. Stay calm and be patient. Structure and routine give predictability and help the child remain calm.
2. Stay connected and maintain a positive relationship focused on what goes right, not on what goes wrong. Take time and avoid being hurried, especially during times of transition. Schedule times to be together to play and inject life with positive daily activities. Do not expect the worst; the self-fulfilling prophecy can prove true.
3. Be realistic in expectations of the child. Communicate clearly, and emphasize positive choices rather than prohibitions. Give the child tasks that can be accomplished, do not put them in situations that outstrip their ability, and remember the child needs practice and works at slower speeds than an adult.
4. De-escalate—Remove the child from an environment when escalating behavior is seen to allow the child to calm down and regroup in order to return to the activity less frustrated and aggressive. Eliminate trigger buttons (put away a favorite toy when friends come over).

The following strategies, liberally reinforced with praise for calm behaviors and any progress that is seen, help the child develop lacking skills.

1. Make a CALM plan. Determine activities (e.g., LEGOs, coloring) and teach strategies (e.g., deep breaths, blow bubbles, count to 10) that are calming. Create a safe spot for the child, but utilize "time-in" to help the child learn to regulate. Identify a cue word to communicate when calming is needed: "LEGOs."
2. Talk about emotions (all feelings are allowed) and work to figure out what was upsetting and how to handle it. With young children, start with mad, sad, happy, and scared. Create an anger thermometer: level 1 is happy, level 5 is angry feelings, and level 10 is ready to explode. Identify how the child's body is feeling at each of those levels.
3. Teach empathy and kindness through understanding the situation and seeing the other side. Ask the child how it would feel if that happened to him/her. Look at what is right in the situation instead of what is wrong. Foster cooperation and help settle arguments. Revise negative assumptions to be more flexible, optimistic, and relaxed toward others.
4. Brainstorm solutions to solve problems and negotiate conflicts. Practice what to say. Insist on making amends, which is not punishment; it is making things right.

If behaviors are severe or becoming more frequent or self-directed, causing injury to self or others, pets, or property, referral is needed.

Bereavement—Loss and Grief

Grief is a feeling of distress, sorrow, and loss, whereas *bereavement* is the process of dealing with loss. Many people use the terms *grief* and *bereavement* interchangeably. *Mourning* is the psychological process set in motion by loss of a loved one. The death of someone important to a child is one of the most stressful life events, and for children and adolescents, death of a parent or sibling is the most disturbing loss. However, children experience loss over many other events in life (birth of a sibling, death of an animal, loss of a friend, moving, parent separation, deployment or deportation, as well as crises [flood, fire, hurricane]). It is expected that most children and adolescents experience at least one significant loss before they reach adulthood, with an estimated 5% of children losing one or both parents to death before 15 years old.

The clinical picture of bereavement and grief depends in part on the concept of death. In infancy and toddlerhood, death is perceived as separation or abandonment, with no real cognitive understanding of death or ability to use the emotional resources to deal with loss. The central issue is the sense of loss or abandonment that can be due to temporary causes (e.g., caregiver travel, sibling hospitalization, natural disaster), long-term causes (e.g., caregiver separation, foster care placement), or permanent (e.g., death). Loss of a family member is particularly difficult because it results in the loss of the love and support from that person, significant effect on family functioning and resources, and changes in routines. In early childhood, children tend to perceive death as a continuation of life under different circumstances, with death personified and perceived as a punishment. School-age children grasp the irreversibility and finality of death, although they struggle with understanding the specific loss of the loved one. Adolescents are able to be more abstract and philosophical about death. At any given developmental stage, a child can resolve the effect of the death only at that developmental level. Thus bereavement resurfaces, and the significance of the loss needs to be reworked at each subsequent developmental stage.

In bereavement, infants and toddlers cry out or search for the absent caregiver, refuse the attempts of others to soothe them, withdraw emotionally, appear sad, and no longer engage in age-appropriate activities. Sleep and feeding are disturbed; they may display developmental regression and demonstrate extreme reactions to reminders of the missing caregiver through apathy, anger, or crying. For the older child, grief is a process that unfolds over time. Initially children may seem emotionally unmoved, but the initial shock and denial give way to depressive symptoms that can last for weeks or months. Depressive symptoms as a normal reaction to loss include sadness, feeling depressed, vomiting, bed-wetting, poor appetite, weight loss, insomnia, crying, internalizing symptoms (e.g., headache and stomachache), anxiety, guilt, and idealization of the person who died. Rage is a common reaction to the death of a parent, typically directed at the surviving parent and others in the immediate family. Angry behavior may also be directed at peers, compounding a sense of inferiority and alienation. Fears of dying, disease, and growing old are often stimulated. Identification with the deceased is common and needs to be assessed to determine whether this furthers or inhibits development. Similarly, a fantasy connection to a dead parent can develop and may be helpful. Guilt and responsibility are typical issues for children but are less problematic for adolescents. Adolescents often manifest a sudden "maturity," along with numbness, regrets, disorganization, and despair before closure and reorganization are achieved. It is not unusual for adolescents to develop stronger ties with friends and to distance from family while grieving.

In general, children at high risk for pathologic bereavement or depression have a previous history of individual and family problems. Symptoms of bereavement that should concern the provider and merit immediate referral to a mental health specialist include the following: long-term denial and avoidance of feelings; suicidal wishes and preoccupation with death; distressing guilt about actions taken or not taken; preoccupation with worthlessness; persistent anger; decline in school performance; social withdrawal; persistent sleep problems; or hallucinations beyond transitory experience of hearing the voice of, or seeing the image of, the deceased.

Management

Caregiver education facilitates effective bereavement management in children and adolescents. Communication is a must. It is critical for children to have an attachment to an adult who can be an effective source of support and involvement, as well as a focus for reactions to loss. There are several ways to support a child through bereavement.

1. Be honest. Children need to know what happened even if they don't ask. Considering their age, tell them as simply and honestly as you can. Do not use words like "asleep" or "lost," as children may understand that literally. Know that grief takes time.

2. Involve children in funerals or ceremonies. Children need to participate in the rituals around death as much as they choose. Such services and rituals provide even young children with an important way to grieve, especially if such involvement is supportive, appropriately explained, and congruent with the family's values.

3. Help children express their feelings. Children need to express and work through feelings and fantasies related to the loss. Be available to talk, answer questions, and share concerns. Find ways for them to express feelings (play, writing a letter, drawing or music). If they are old enough, it is helpful for them to know to expect a range of difficult feelings. Books about death, loss, and grieving for children and adolescents geared to various developmental levels may be helpful.

4. Share your feelings. Caregivers often need to be reassured that showing their own feelings (e.g., disbelief, guilt, sadness, and anger) is normal and helpful to children; it is also helpful to the child to let them know how the adult is coping with feelings. Sharing feelings about and memories of the family member who died is helpful as well.

5. Provide routine and support. Maintaining family routine as much a possible provides security. Extra time for closeness and comfort is essential. The child must be sensitively prepared for any changes occurring at the same time as the death, with the family advised to minimize these as much as possible.

6. Remember that grief resurfaces. Because bereavement resurfaces at subsequent developmental phases, counsel families proactively about the need to deal with grief at each developmental level. In addition, the PCP must assess symptoms over time as a possible manifestation of a new stage of bereavement.

7. Get extra help if needed. Any child who loses a parent before 5 years old warrants referral. Any child who is overly preoccupied with death, has persistent grief over months, persistent loss of performance, or feels like they would be better off dead also should be referred for further counseling.

Difficulties with Sensory Processing

Sensory input comes from not only vision, hearing, touch, taste, and smell, but also from position (proprioception) and movement (vestibular). Sensory modulation describes the child's ability to regulate and organize the intensity and nature of responses to sensory input in order to relate to the world around the child. The child who is *sensory overresponsive* responds too much, for too long, or to stimuli of weak intensity. The child who is *sensory under-responsive* responds too little or needs extremely strong stimulation to become aware of the stimulus. The *sensory seeking/craving* child responds with intense searching for more or stronger stimulation. Children with sensory difficulties often respond inappropriately to input, perceiving sensations that are pleasurable or positive in most individuals to be painful, irritating, and unpleasant, at times exhibiting extreme behaviors (e.g., tantrums or meltdowns in reaction to overwhelming physical sensations, or being overly aggressive in seeking stimulation). This inappropriate response affects the child's ability to adapt appropriate to daily life situations, learn, regulate attention and moods, and function in many social interactions.

Children with Sensory Processing Disorder (SPD) face many challenges in everyday life: they are sensitive to touch and pull away from hugs and cuddling; have trouble with transitions, family gatherings, parties, and vacations (things considered fun); do best with an environment that is predictable and routine; may have rigid control to try to manage sensory input; and can sometimes accomplish something if they put 100% effort into it but cannot always perform at 100%. Children who are overresponders have difficulties with clothing, physical contact, light, sound, and food. Children who are underresponders have little or no reaction to stimulation, pain, extreme hot or cold, and risk injuring themselves. Children who are sensory seekers are on perpetual overdrive and often in trouble with friends and family. Muscle and joint impairment (postural disorder) affect posture and motor skills (and can be described as floppy babies, a klutz, a spaz). Children with dyspraxia have difficulty recognizing and distinguishing shapes and textures, may have poor handwriting, or may have altered ability to do things like tying shoes, using buttons, or dressing themselves.

Infants may be colicky or fussy, have eating and sleeping difficulties, be fearful of movement, and resist being held or comforted. Preschoolers may not engage in purposeful interactive play; have delayed development; be defiant, irritable, and stubborn; resist transitions and certain activities; and have feeding, dressing, and sleep issues. The school-age child may have trouble with handwriting, figuring out steps in a game, organizing schoolwork; may be able to perform in school but may come home and fall apart; have difficulty handling transition; and be easily frustrated. Adolescents report trouble with social interactions, learning in the classroom, and physical skill development. They are at risk for inability to make friends, poor self-concept, academic failure, being labeled clumsy, uncooperative, disruptive, and out of control. Anxiety, depression, aggression, or other behavior problems are common.

The 5th edition of the Diagnostic and Statistical Manual of Mental Disorders (DSM-5) does not include a distinct diagnosis of sensory processing disorder, though it does acknowledge sensory over-responsiveness in a majority of children on the autism spectrum. Sensory processing issues can also occur with a wide range of emotional and behavioral disorders, but again, this is not exclusive to that diagnosis. Sensory issues can exist independently, comorbidly or as part of other diagnoses. Sensory issues are frequently found in premature children, gifted children, and those with neurodevelopmental disorders (e.g., autism and attention deficit disorder) and fragile X syndrome. In addition, sensory issues occur with environmental factors, such as institutionalization (overseas adoptees), severe physical or sexual abuse, poverty, lead poisoning, and alcohol and drug exposure. Research is ongoing for a neurobiologic and genetic basis for sensory processing difficulties (Conway, 2018). Advanced magnetic resonance imaging (MRI) differences in the white matter microstructure of the brain show decreased connectivity in areas of sensory perception and the auditory, visual, and tactile systems involved in sensory processing (Chang et al, 2014; Owen et al, 2013).

In spite of the disagreement about sensory processing disorder as a diagnosis, there is agreement that these children need early identification, psychoeducation, and referral for treatment. The PCP can screen, assess motor tone and planning, and determine if symptoms are part of another neurodevelopmental disorder. Red flags for sensory processing issues are found in Box 15.12. Screening tools can be found at www.sensorysmartparent.com or www.spdstar.org. If screening or assessment is concerning, evaluation and treatment is usually conducted by a specially trained occupational therapist (OT) using questionnaires, observational tools, and standardized tests.

Management

Early diagnosis and treatment for SPD increase positive child outcomes. The PCP can be actively involved in helping structure the environment and promote regulatory functioning. For the hyporesponsive child, active play (jumping on trampolines, swinging, swimming, and use of playground) is encouraged, and for the hyper-responsive child, calming activities (cozy corner with soft beanbag chair and decreased lighting and noise). Treatment by an OT trained in sensory integration is expensive and not always covered by insurance. The goal of therapy is to develop appropriate and automatic responses to sensations so that the child can function competently in play, at school, and in activities of daily living. Therapy includes the use of sensory stimuli in a sensory-rich environment, providing what is called *sensory nourishment* or a *sensory diet*. This fosters new neurologic connections, arousal and attention regulation, and social relationships. Counseling with families is essential, as they are often blamed or criticized for the child's behavior. Books and websites provide additional information. The OT in the school setting can often provide adaptations to help the child deal with their time at school.

Recurrent Physical Symptoms

Children may experience emotional stress as physical symptoms. The pain is often expressed developmentally—initially as stomachaches, in school-aged children as headaches, and in adolescence as trouble sleeping and fatigue. Focus on body sensation, heightened emotional response, poor coping skills, a sense of anger, and difficulty expressing emotional distress verbally can underlie the physical symptoms. Prior to adolescence, the incidence is equal in males and females, but after adolescence it is twice as frequent in females. History may reveal families that are overprotective or are experiencing stressors such as parental separation or divorce. Difficulties at school either academically or socially are often at the root of the complaints, especially in high-achieving families. At times there is a family member with similar symptoms, and maltreatment (emotional as well as physical and sexual) and other trauma must be considered.

The PCP must complete a thorough history and physical exam and lab studies as indicated, to ensure that there is no medical illness. At the same time, the parent and/or child can begin to keep a pain diary, recording the sensation, intensity, location, timing, and circumstances surrounding the pain. Approaching the medical and mental health piece simultaneously and explaining this approach as the most comprehensive is often most effective (Spratt, 2014). There are screening tools such as the Children's Somatization Inventory (CIS), with a child and parent version, and the Functional Disability Inventory (FDI), which assesses severity of symptoms that may be helpful in discerning what is going on.

Management

The PCP can begin working with the family to help them understand that physical symptoms are often a coping strategy for the child who has emotional discomfort that the child is not even aware of. The pain is real, and the goal is to help the child identify stress and learn how to cope in order to minimize the distress. Various counseling and evidence-based interventions can be used. Parents should be advised not to give attention to the pain but respond briefly and then help the child shift focus elsewhere. Strategies such as deep breaths, progressive relaxation, and use of distraction and guided imagery may be helpful. If the symptoms are disruptive of normal routine or are progressive or not improving, referral for mental health intervention is necessary. Cognitive-behavioral techniques and family therapeutic interventions to treat underlying stressors provide effective coping strategies and improve overall functioning. Referral is also necessary for children who have experienced maltreatment or trauma, or are at risk for somatic symptom disorders evidenced by intense worry about mild physical symptoms, acute anxiety, and interfering with school performance and relationships with family and friends.

Bullying

Bullying threatens well-being, and can cause physical injury and social and emotional problems. It affects the sense of safety of schools, neighborhoods, and society. Data collected in 2017 as part of the 12-month Youth Risk Behavior Study found that 19% of U.S. high school students reported being bullied on school property and 15% were bullied electronically (CDC, 2018). However, middle-school students reported the highest rates at 22%. *Bullying*, as defined by the CDC, is any unwanted aggressive behavior(s) by another youth or group of youths that involves power imbalance and is repeated or likely to be repeated multiple times. Bullying includes physical (hitting, tripping), verbal (name calling, teasing), or relational/social (e.g., spreading rumors or leaving one out of a group) aggression. Cyberbullying, another form of bullying over digital devices, includes sending, posting, or sharing harmful, false, or negative content about someone. Unfortunately, cyberbullying is available 24 hours a day, harder to detect, and more likely to become part of a permanent online profile. Youth rarely report bullying to an adult or care provider, often because the incidents typically occur when an adult is not present or has not witnessed any aggression. All states have legislation regarding bullying, but not all for cyberbullying.

Youth engaging in bullying behaviors can be described as a bully, a victim, or both—a category known as the bully/victim. Bullying behaviors cause harm or distress to the targeted youth, including physical injury, social and emotional distress, depression, anxiety, sleep difficulties, and lower academic achievement, and these youth are more likely to have depression, anxiety, eating disorders, health issues, and academic issues. Although most youth who are bullied do not consider suicide, the stress of bullying presents an increased risk of suicide in some young people. Youth who bully are at risk for substance abuse (tobacco and alcohol) and academic problems, and carry an increased risk for criminal activity and mental health disorders later in life. The bully/victim is at greatest risk for mental health disorders. Risk factors for youth violence have been identified by the CDC in the following categories: individual, family, peer and social risk, and community.

Management

Including violence prevention as part of routine well-child care is essential. However, bullying results in injury at many levels, and the PCP is likely to become involved when an injury has occurred, when there are mental health concerns, or during the psychosocial assessment during routine care. It is ideal to interview the youth separately from the parent; however, it is necessary to gather the history from both. Evaluate the youth's risk factors, family system, school performance, and the general presentation. Determine if the youth is considered the perpetrator, victim, or a bully/victim, and if any weapons were used or threatened (including the specific type). Obtain details of what occurred to the youth using open-ended questions, such as, "Tell me what happened," to elicit the story in the youth's own narrative. Assess for drug or alcohol use, and obtain details of any previous incidences. In addition, the PCP is responsible to report to both CPS and/or law enforcement when indicated.

The ideal goal is to stop bullying before it starts. There are many school-based bullying prevention programs, as well as community intervention programs (see Additional Resources). PCPs need to be familiar with the resources in the schools and community in which they practice and advocate for antibullying policies and bystander intervention trainings.

Parenting Challenges and Special Circumstances

Separation, Divorce, and Remarriage

Parental separation, divorce, and remarriage can all be emotionally stressful, complex events for families, and can lead to significant emotional disruption and disequilibrium for everyone. It is important to understand that separation and divorce are an ongoing processes, rather than one concrete event. Children may perceive the transition as a dramatic and painful time in their lives, and they experience grief because separation or divorce is a loss of family as the child knows it. Behavioral changes are an expected reaction as the child attempts to adjust to the changing family situation. Children (and parents) tend to more successfully adjust if there is a stable parenting foundation in the child's early years, if parents maintain a civil relationship with each other that focuses on what is best for the child, if they each provide warmth and praise for the child throughout the process, and if the child knows that both parents will remain involved in their lives. The goal of assessment of the family experiencing separation or divorce is to determine both the needs and strengths of the family in order to assist the family with healthy coping. Child-related factors to consider include the developmental stage of the children and common psychosocial reactions to divorce that typically occur at that stage. In addition, the psychosocial effect of the divorce on the parents and the economic consequences of divorce on the family unit must be determined (Box 15.13).

Remarriage creates a reorganized, often blended family through joining children from previous relationships after divorce or the death of spouses. The introduction of a stepparent and possibly stepsiblings may be beneficial for a child, or it can be a time of difficult adjustment. The majority of children within blended families gradually adjust well to their new family situations. Age and developmental stage affect the child's

• **BOX 15.13**   **Red Flags for a Sensory Processing Difficulties**

If more than a few of the symptoms fit the child, refer for evaluation.

Infants and Toddlers
- Problems eating or sleeping
- Refuses to go to anyone but a specific person
- Irritable when being dressed; uncomfortable in clothes
- Rarely plays with toys
- Resists cuddling, arches away when held
- Cannot calm self
- Floppy or stiff body, motor delays

Preschoolers
- Overly sensitive to touch, noises, smells, other people
- Difficulty making friends
- Difficulty dressing, eating, sleeping, and/or toilet training
- Clumsy; poor motor skills; weakness
- In constant motion; in everyone else's face and space
- Frequent or long temper tantrums

Grade Schoolers
- Overly sensitive to touch, noise, smells, other people
- Easily distracted, fidgety, craves movement; aggressive
- Easily overwhelmed
- Difficulty with handwriting or motor activities
- Difficulty making friends
- Unaware of pain and/or other people

Adolescents and Adults
- Overly sensitive to touch, noise, smells, and other people
- Poor self-esteem; afraid of failing at new tasks
- Lethargic and slow
- Always on the go; impulsive; distractible
- Leaves tasks uncompleted
- Clumsy, slow, poor motor skills or handwriting
- Difficulty staying focused at work and in meetings

response and ability to cope with changes associated with remarriage and new family relationships. Early adolescence is often a time of greatest difficulty in adjustment to remarriage, and a mother's subsequent pregnancy is a time of increased frequency and intensity of problems for young children. Some common issues occurring in newly blended families include complex relationships with new family members; altered relationships with established family members and possible feelings of betraying a biologic parent or being torn between parents; possible relocation and separation from family members and friends; continued or new tensions between parents and tensions between stepparents; rivalries between parents and stepparents; jealousy among stepsiblings; establishing new family traditions and values, while continuing to respect earlier family history, traditions, and loyalties that may be in conflict; unrealistic expectations by the child or stepparent (e.g., instant love, respect, and obedience from child); tensions within a blended-family household, creating anxiety and fear of another family breakup. The PCP's role includes assessing how the child is coping with these significant life changes and realignment of the family roles (see Box 15.10), and carefully considering any behavioral concerns. This information helps both the provider and the parents decide how to best focus their attention.

Common Reactions of Children by Developmental Stage to Divorce by Age Group

- 2-5 years: Regression, irritability, sleep disturbances, aggression
- 6-8 years: Open grieving and feelings of rejection or being replaced; whiny, immature behavior; sadness; fearfulness
- 9-12 years: Fear and intense anger at one or both parents
- >13 years: Worried about own future, depressed, or acting-out behaviors (e.g., truancy, sexual activity, alcohol or drug use, suicide attempts)

Economic Consequence of Divorce

- Devastating economic hardships and decline in living standards (especially for women due to nonpayment or delinquency in payment of child support)

Common Issues for Children of Divorcing Parents

- Continued tension, conflict, and fighting between parents
- Litigation over custody and visitation arrangements
- Abandonment by one parent or sporadic visitation (decreased availability) vs. denial of visitation
- Diminished parenting resulting from availability issues or emotional inaccessibility, distress, or instability
- Limited social support system outside nuclear family
- Feelings of loneliness or emotional abandonment, or both

Management

Anticipatory guidance given to parents who are in the process of separating and divorcing is outlined in Table 15.14. Custodial and visitation arrangements for children vary and may change as the child grows. Joint custody is an option that allows both parents the opportunity to participate in mutual decision-making about their child's life and welfare. Various living arrangements and visitation rights are possible with joint custody. In some instances, however, single custody is in the best interest of the child, and the noncustodial parent may have limited or no contact and involvement with the child. Custody disputes and exposure to parental conflict place additional stress on children and can increase their feelings of insecurity.

The goal of health education for children and parents experiencing these changes in the family unit is to help restore a sense of wholeness and integrity in children's lives. Providers must stress those factors that have been shown to significantly affect whether the child will experience a healthy adjustment to the divorce (Box 15.15). Successful efforts implemented during initial periods of disequilibrium and reorganization strengthen normal development and prevent future psychological trauma. A classic research study (Wallerstein, 1983) identified six psychological tasks that children of divorce must master, beginning at the time of parental separation and culminating in young adulthood (Box 15.16). If these psychological tasks are not achieved, the child's mastery of normal developmental tasks is negatively affected. Support can be provided with additional visits or telephone contacts with the family, and by focusing on the family's positive strengths and resilience.

The goal in remarriage is to foster positive parenting behaviors, protect child development, and enhance family functioning. Before remarriage, providers can counsel and guide parents regarding strategies for coping with transition in a blended family. Many children go on to develop strong and meaningful attachments to

their stepparents if the relationship is cultivated over time with careful sensitivity to the needs of the child, parent, and family. Some tips for families include:

- Discuss upcoming changes with your child before remarriage and address fears, feelings, and expectations.
- Keep the marriage strong by a nurturing husband-and-wife relationship.
- Blended-family parents need to agree on discipline issues, how to set limits, and type of discipline, remembering to be consistent.
- Start new family traditions, such as weekly family meetings.
- Be patient and as flexible as possible; do not expect your child(ren) to have an immediate positive relationship with the new stepparent.
- Spend quiet, alone time with your child as much as possible and preferably every day.
- Do not force your child to align with the new parent, and remember that a second parent does not replace the first; support and help maintain the relationship of your child with the other birth parent.

Deployment

In 2017, there were 1.3 million active duty military and more than 800,000 reserve forces (DoD, 2017), with 1.8 million children belonging to a military family—40% of them being under 5 years of age (Panton, 2018). A military family moves on average every 2 years. Deployments typically last 1 year, and parents may both be deployed at the same time. The average military child will change schools six to nine times, families often cannot keep their pets, and spouses face unemployment that is three times greater than the national average (Walters, 2016). These children face a multitude of stressors, and many families manage remarkably well. The Deployment Life Study (Meadows et al., 2017), a longitudinal study over a deployment cycle, assessed multiple outcomes, one of which was child and teen well-being assessed through emotional, behavioral, social, and academic functioning. Though there were exceptions, no significant effect of deployment was found on child and teen outcomes over the course of deployment, and changes that did occur were felt to reflect the passage of time and normal childhood development. However, an understanding of the stressors within each stage of the deployment cycle helps the PCP work with military families in mastering each stage (Panton, 2018). Predeployment is the time 3 to 6 months prior to departure, when the departing parent may have duties away from the family in preparation and the remaining parent makes arrangements to handle all family responsibilities. Parents and children may be overwhelmed and experience conflict, as well as stress and fear in anticipation of the separation. Deployment, lasting from 3 to 15 months, may be stable once a new routine has been established, or may be filled with ongoing changes and worry about the safety of the deployed parent. Postdeployment involves family reintegration and may be exciting and/or stressful as, once again, family routines and roles are readjusted.

Developmentally, the critical first 1000 days of an infant's life may be affected by parent absence or stress. In early childhood, there may be confusion with all the changes, and the level of parental stress may be the most critical factor in determining the child's reactions. School-aged children are at risk not only for stress related to deployed parents, but also for the multiple changes required of them through frequent moves. Adolescents who are dealing with their own unique issues often struggle as

TABLE 15.14 Anticipatory Guidance for Families Experiencing Separation or Divorce

Anticipatory Guidance	Discussion Points With Parents
Advise parents to prepare the child for the impending breakup.	• If possible, tell the child in advance of the breakup. Children who are appropriately prepared may cope better with the separation and change in family structure. • Discussions should focus on supporting the child's needs for reassurance and stability, not on blame, recriminations, or the parent's needs.
Explain to parents the need to discuss these key issues with their children.	• Discuss what arrangements have been made for the children to see departing parent unless visitation is not possible or problematic. Consider whether the children will be best served by continuing to see the departing parent when possible. • Explain what divorce means in language appropriate to the child's cognitive and developmental level; explain reasons for the divorce in the same terms. • Reassure children that they did not cause the divorce or separation, that they cannot correct their parents' unhappiness in the marriage, and that the divorce is the parents' decision. • Explain what the family structure will look like afterward and what changes will be necessary in the way the family functions. • Explain the visitation arrangements as soon as they are established. • Reassure children that they will be cared for, and they are not being abandoned by either parent, unless a parent disappeared or refuses involvement. • Tell children that feelings of sadness, anger, and disappointment are normal; encourage them not to "take sides," but love both parents. • Discuss how to handle special circumstances, such as when the "other parent" does not visit or simply leaves.
Discuss the need for consistency.	• Parents should strive to maintain consistent daily routines between the two households; encourage the use of security items that the child may depend on or carry familiar items between the homes during the transitional period. • Be consistent in disciplinary practices.
Suggest self-help measures.	• Children and parents may benefit from attending divorce recovery workshops, classes about families in transition, or peer support groups. • School counselors, religious groups, or community and social service agencies may be helpful resources.
Acknowledge grief.	• Providers should acknowledge the grief that both the parent and child are experiencing and provide support.
Discuss when referral for mental health counseling might be indicated.	• Children often demonstrate internalized or externalized psychosocial problems in response to divorce. Counseling may be indicated for the family members.

• BOX 15.15 Factors Affecting a Child's Ability to Achieve Healthy Adjustment to Separation and Divorce

• The opportunity for continued participation of the noncustodial or visiting parent in the child's life on a regular basis
• Custodial parent attempts to make visits with the other parent a routine event so that there is consistent contact (phone, visiting, email)
• The ability of the custodial parent to handle and successfully parent the child
• The ability of parents to separate their own feelings of anger and conflict and resolve their own hostility toward each other so that the child's need for a relationship with both parents is met
• The child does not become involved in parental conflict and does not feel rejected; the child should not be put in the middle
• The availability of a social support network
• The ability of parents to meet the child's developmental needs and to help the child master developmental tasks
• The child's overall personality, temperament, personal assets and deficits

• BOX 15.16 Six Psychological Tasks Children of Divorce Must Master

1. Acknowledge the reality of the marital breakup.
2. Disengage from parental conflict and distress and resume customary pursuits.
3. Resolve loss of familiar daily routine, traditions, and symbols and the physical presence of two parents.
4. Resolve anger and self-blame.
5. Accept the permanence of the divorce.
6. Achieve realistic hope regarding relationships—the capacity to love and be loved.

they are put in the position of carrying some of the responsibilities during deployment and then have to relinquish them postdeployment. A notable resilience factor for the adolescent with a deployed parent is support from other teens in the same situation (Meadows, et al., 2017).

Management

These children's needs are compelling and must be addressed. PCPs must recognize these military families, screen for potential stressors, be ready to provide coping strategies specific to their situation, and alert to need for mental health referral. Having a parent sent to an active combat zone with an undetermined return date may rank as one of the most stressful events of childhood. Children in such situations may be vulnerable, especially as the coping resources of the remaining parent (or guardian) may be compromised by his or her own distress and uncertainty. Children with a deployed parent have more emotional difficulties compared with their peers; older youth and girls of all ages report significantly more school-, family-, and peer-related difficulties if a parent was deployed (Panton, 2018). The longer the parental deployment and the poorer the nondeployed caregiver's mental health, the more likely the children will experience role-shifting and behavior problems during deployment and reintegration. Additional risk factors include history of rigid coping styles, family dysfunction, young families (especially first military separation), families recently moved to a new duty station, foreign-born spouse, families with young children, families without unit affiliation, pregnancy, and dual-career or single parents (Safran n.d.). Protective factors include resilience, family preparedness, active coping style, and positive psychological and mental health status of the at-home parent. Indications for referral include ineffective intervention after two visits, worsening symptoms or symptoms that continue for 3 months after redeployment, academic declines, situations where an at-home parent is having difficulty coping, or situations where the deployed parent is injured or fatally wounded (Panton, 2018).

Adolescent Parent(s)

Teen (ages 15 to 19) birth rates in the United States were 20.3/1000 in 2016, down from 61.8 per 1000 births in 1991 (HHS, 2018). However, the United States has significantly higher birth rates than other developed countries (CDC, 2017), and adolescent parents and their children are at high risk for medical, psychological, developmental, and social problems. Predictors of teen motherhood are listed in Box 15.17. Adolescents who become parents often face problems because they are not developmentally ready to assume the parenting role. Their developmental needs frequently conflict with the needs of their children, leading them to feel isolated, exhausted, and depressed. Children of adolescent mothers are more likely to have a low birth weight and ongoing child health problems, to grow up in homes without fathers, and to be raised in poverty or near poverty. There are teens who can successfully parent their infant if given support; however, preexisting family and individual factors that lead to teenage motherhood are relevant predictors of successful parenting. In order to better understand the environment in which a child will be raised, PCPs should ask about the adolescent parent's support system, their attitudes toward parenting, and sources of parenting advice. In addition, providers should determine the adolescent's school status, child care arrangements, financial situation, and plans for the future. Assessment of at-risk status varies, depending

---

• BOX 15.17 Predictors of Teen Motherhood

- Victim of sexual abuse as a child
- Adverse events in childhood
- Being a child of an addicted parent
- Family history of mental illness
- Lack of family involvement; an intolerable home situation as defined by the teen
- Poor academic achievement or school dropout
- Loss of a parent by death, separation, divorce, or foster placement
- Living in an impoverished social environment where adolescent pregnancy is commonplace and accepted
- Confusion about own sexual orientation

• BOX 15.18 Assessing Teen Parenting

When the teen is the parent of an infant:
- Parent-infant attachment: Is there evidence of healthy attachment or emotional or physical neglect?
- Confidence and ability of teen parent to care for her infant
- Conflicts between the teen's needs and those of her infant: Is the teen more interested in reestablishing an adolescent lifestyle or caring for the infant?
- Living arrangements: With whom and where are the teen and baby living?
- Degree of involvement of the social support network in the teen's and infant's life: Is the baby's other parent invested in the child? Support from extended family?
- Return to school or the workforce: What are the child care arrangements?
- Adequacy of financial resources
  When the teen is a parent of an older child:
- Parents knowledge level of child development and ability to cope with the variety of toddler behaviors
- How well the family unit is functioning
- Progress made by the teen toward reaching her life goals

---

on the stage of the teen (see Box 15.18). Addressing these issues on an ongoing basis contributes to more successful parenting and prevention of problems later in the child's or teen parent's life. The early childhood years are challenging, particularly for teens who themselves are survivors of abuse or neglectful parenting. As the child gets older, the teen mother transitions to the young mother role. Children of these mothers, especially those who are poor and living in urban settings, are more likely than their peers to have behavioral problems. In some cases, teen mothers may later become young grandparents, and the teen-pregnancy cycle repeats.

Management

Management strategies for the teen parent include:
- Maintain regular and frequent contact with the teen mother during the child's infancy and early childhood. Remember that the teen mother and the infant or child have their own separate needs for health supervision and guidance.
- Provide a supportive environment for the teen mother. Have a plan for follow-up so that teen mothers do not get lost in the system. Emphasize the strengths of the teen mother and praise her positive efforts. Involve other family members (e.g., grandparents, the father) in discussions about child-rearing issues, depending on the teen's wishes.

- Facilitate further education to minimize effects of poverty on child rearing.
- Refer to a community health nurse for home visits early in pregnancy and postpartum. This intervention is successful in delaying subsequent pregnancy and improving healthy parenting and family life.
- Provide referrals for resources and community agencies that can assist teen mothers (e.g., parenting classes or literature; support groups; special clinic programs that see both infants and teen mothers; Woman, Infants, and Children [WIC] program; early child intervention programs provided by school districts and Head Start).
- Intervene early when warning signs of potential neglect or abuse are evident and refer as necessary.

Premature or Multiple Birth

Premature infants present special issues for new parents. There may be an extended time between the child's birth and the time when parents are able to bring their infant home, with concerns about the child's physiologic vulnerability. Infant care costs and time commitments are increased. Parents may have the same concerns as parents of a full-term newborn, but their fears and anxieties about being responsible for a fragile newborn may be magnified.

A family faced with caring for newborn twins, triplets, or more, even while delighted, can be quickly overwhelmed by the responsibility and amount of work involved. Behavioral issues and the children's own unique relationships can be a challenge as multiples develop a special sibling relationship marked by loyalty and cooperative play, they function more independently, needing less parental attention, and develop their own language among themselves as young children.

Management

Assessing parents' attachment, fatigue levels, ability to seek and accept support, and plans for ongoing care is important. Similar to the situation of a multiple birth, exploring who is caring for the child and who is helping the parents is a priority. PCPs must assess for parental role difficulties at all visits to foster early identification and intervention for parental mental health and role difficulties.

Adoption

Adoption is the legal process that gives individuals who are not birth parents legal and permanent parental responsibility for children. Adoptions occur in a variety of different family types—married couples, single parents, gay and lesbian parents, grandparents, or other extended family members. Examples of types of adoptions include independent, identified, and international adoptions; surrogacy arrangements; intrafamily adoption; subsidized adoption of children with special health care needs; and open adoptions. Public and private agencies, independent adoption through attorneys, and foreign adoption services are potential avenues to assist in the placement of children.

Assessment of adopting families includes:
- Legal status, arrangements, and circumstances surrounding adoption process
- What, if any, contact will the birth parent or parents and birth family have with the child?
- Timing of finalization of the adoption and length of waiting period; how old was the child when the child was adopted?

- Decisions about how and when to tell the child about being adopted
- Support services available for the adoptive family
- Any known or suspected medical (including growth and development) child problems
- History of birth parent/family medical, genetic, or psychosocial concerns
- Information about the pregnancy, delivery, and neonatal period or subsequent medical problems

Management

Schedule a preadoption consultation, if possible, to review any issues or concerns. When considering adoption, parents often have many questions about the initial adoption period and the establishment of a family relationship. Issues that the provider should address include:
- Gradual disclosure of the adoption to the child done earlier rather than later, and children should always be told the truth about where they came from and why they were adopted.
- Discussion about adoption should be open, keeping in mind the child's developmental stage, cognitive abilities, and emotional needs, reassuring the child in words and actions that he or she is loved, and the adoptive parents will always be there.
- Addressing any myths, concerns, or fears that parents might have about adoption and their adopted child.
- A child's wish to know about or seek out the biologic parents is not a rejection of them.
- Adolescence can be difficult for adoptive children as they seek their own identity and deal with the fact that they are adopted.
- Adoption of an older child may present an extra challenge, especially if the child has been shuffled between homes or emotionally scarred by abuse or neglect. Telling parents about such challenges can help them better prepare to handle some of the difficulties that may lie ahead for their family and seek counseling early if needed.

Once adoption is finalized, close monitoring and support by the PCP during the initial adoption period are important. According to the AAP, all adopted children need a comprehensive medical evaluation immediately after their adoptive placement, and ongoing additional health supervision visits even when all appears to be going well. The medical evaluation should include age-appropriate vision, hearing, dental, and behavioral/developmental screenings. The presence of a social support network is important for adoptive families and often provides preventive resources, reassurance of competence, and encouragement. Families adopting older children and children with special needs may require extra assistance with family bonding and behavioral, mental health, and physical needs.

Foster Care

Children are usually placed in family foster care or a group home because of child maltreatment or because their biologic parents are unable to care for them. Some children are placed in foster care because they need specialized medical, psychiatric, or mental health care and developmental assistance beyond the ability of their biologic parents. Other children may need to be removed from a chaotic and unsafe family environment, or they may have been abandoned or orphaned. These children are at high risk for deep-seated feelings of insecurity, loss, and anger. The U.S. Department of Health and Human Services reported that 450,000 children were in foster care as of the end of September 2016. Half of all foster children live in foster homes with nonrelatives; about a third live with relatives, and the remainder are in group homes, institutions and other locations (USDHHS, 2018).

The PCP needs to conduct a complete assessment including exploring the reason for the child's placement in foster placement, physical or mental health issues that precipitated or resulted from separation from the birth parents, and evaluation of the foster parent. Information that is critical for the PCP to know about the foster child includes frequent history of chronic stress, hardship, and emotional trauma in their family; multiple placements and separation from siblings; involvement in family reunification programs and placement back with parents under the supervision of the child protective services; legal mandates in foster homes that mirror the children's ethnic, racial, and cultural identities as much as possible; health care has often been disjointed, and a disproportionate number of foster children have weight problems, medical issues, or developmental delays; and emancipation from the foster care system happens at 18 years old and is a major life change requiring preparation. A limited number of states extend foster care until age 21 years.

Management

Foster parents have a difficult role in society, wanting to be treated with respect and have their care and knowledge of their foster child acknowledged. They need assistance to provide the best care possible to the children in their care. Healthy Foster Care America (https://www.aap.org/en-us/advocacy-and-policy/aap-health-initiatives/healthy-foster-care-america/Pages/default.aspx), an AAP initiative to improve health and well-being, has multiple resources for the PCP. The Child Welfare League of America (https://www.cwla.org/) and the National Foster Parent Association (https://nfpaonline.org/) provide support and caregiving information for foster families.

Additional Resources

Bright Futures in Practice: Mental Health. http://www.brightfutures.org/mentalhealth
Center on the Developing Child. https://developingchild.harvard.edu/
Child Mind Institute. http://www.childmindorg
Committee on Psychosocial Aspects of Child and Family Health, American Academy of Pediatrics. https://www.aap.org/en-us/about-the-aap/Committees-Councils-Sections/Pages/Committee-on-Psychosocial-Aspects-of-Child-and-Family-Health.aspx
Community Resilience Initiative. https://resiliencetrumpsaces.org
Developmental Behavioral and Mental Health, National Association of Pediatric Nurse Practitioners. https://www.napnap.org/dbmh
Early Brain and Child Development, Initiative of American Academy of Pediatrics. https://www.aap.org/en-us/advocacy-and-policy/aap-health-initiatives/EBCD/Pages/default.aspx
Early Childhood Health Optimization, Florida State University Center for Prevention and Early Intervention. https://cpeip.fsu.edu/mma/pediatrician/pediatrician_resources.cfm
Essentials for Childhood. https://www.cdc.gov/violenceprevention/childabuseandneglect/essentials.html
Facts for Families, The American Academy of Child & Adolescent Psychiatry. https://www.aacap.org/AACAP/Families_and_Youth/Facts_for_Families/FFF-Guide/FFF-Guide-Home.aspx
Family Voices. http://www.familyvoices.org

Healthy Foster Care America. https://www.aap.org/en-us/advocacy-and-policy/aap-health-initiatives/healthy-foster-care-america/Pages/default.aspx
Lives in the Balance (collaborative & proactive solutions). https://www.livesinthebalance.org
National Alliance on Mental Illness (NAMI): Child and Adolescent Action Center. https://www.nami.org/Find-Support/Teens-and-Young-Adults
National Organization of Pediatric Nurse Practitioners: Mental Health Resources. https://www.nami.org/Find-Support/Teens-and-Young-Adults
Parent Child Interaction Therapy (PCIT). http://www.pcit.org
The Reach Institute. http://www.thereachinstitute.org
Reach Out and Read. http://www.reachoutandread.org/
Star Institute for Sensory Processing. http://www.spdfoundation.net
Sensory Processing Disorder (SPD) Resource Center. http://www.sensory-processing-disorder.com
Social and Emotional Development, Child Trends. https://www.childtrends.org/research-topic/social-and-emotional-development
Society for Developmental and Behavioral Pediatrics. http://www.sdbp.org
Strengthening Families: A Protective Factors Framework. https://www.cssp.org/young-children-their-families/strengtheningfamilies
Substance Abuse and Mental Health Services Administration (SAMHSA). http://www.samhsa.gov/children
The Community Resilience Initiative Resilience Trumps ACEs. https://resiliencetrumpsaces.org)
The Incredible Years. http://www.incredibleyears.com
The Resilience Project, Initiative of American Academy of Pediatrics. https://www.aap.org/en-us/advocacy-and-policy/aap-health-initiatives/resilience/Pages/Promoting-Resilience.aspx
Tools of the Mind. https://toolsofthemind.org
Triple P (Positive Parenting Practices). https://www.triplep.net/glo-en/home/

References

AAP Early Brain and Child Development. *Science.* Available at: www.aap.org/en-us/advocacy-and-policy/aap-health-initiatives/EBCD/Pages/The-Science.aspx. Accessed June 15, 2018.
American Psychiatric Association (APA). *Diagnostic and Statistical Manual of Mental Disorders (DSM-5).* 5th ed. Arlington, VA: American Psychiatric Association; 2013.
Bethell C. *The New Science of Thriving.* Available at: https://magazine.jhsph.edu/2016/spring/forum/rethinking-the-new-science-of-thriving/index.html Accessed September 15, 2018.
Center on the Developing Child. *Building the Core Skills Youth Need for Life.* Available at: https://developingchild.harvard.edu/resources/building-core-skills-youth/. Accessed September 15, 2018.
Center on the Developing Child at Harvard University. *From Best Practices to Breakthrough Impacts: a Science-Based Approach to Building a More Promising Future for Young Children and Families.* Available at: https://www.aap.org/en-us/advocacy-and-policy/aap-health-initiatives/EBCD/Documents/TranslatingSciencePPT.pdf.
Centers for Disease Control and Prevention (CDC). *Preventing Bullying.* Available at: https://www.cdc.gov/violenceprevention/pdf/bullying-factsheet.pdf; 2017.
Centers for Disease Control and Prevention (CDC). *Social Determinants of Health.* Available at: https://www.cdc.gov/socialdeterminants/ Accessed Sept 3, 2018.
Centers for Disease Control and Prevention (CDC). *About Teen Pregnancy.* 2017 Available at: www.cdc.gov/teenpregnancy/about/index.htm last. Accessed Sep 3, 2018.
Centers for Disease Control and Prevention (CDC). *Essentials for Parenting, 2018.* Available at: https://www.cdc.gov/features/parenting-essentials-index-html. Accessed April 21, 2019.
Chang Y-S, Owen JP, Desai SS, et al. Autism and sensory processing disorders: shared white matter disruption in sensory pathways but divergent connectivity in social-emotional pathways. *PLoS ONE.* 2014;9(7):e103038.

Child Mind Institute. *2016 Children's Mental Health Report*. Available at: https://childmind.org/report/2016-childrens-mental-health-report/. Accessed September 15, 2018.

Child Mind Institute. *The Debate Over Sensory Processing*. Available at: https://childmind.org/article/the-debate-over-sensory-processing/ Accessed September 15, 2018.

Child Trends. *Collaborative for Academic, Social and Emotional Learning (CASEL): what is SEL?*. Available at: https://casel.org/what-is-sel/ Accessed June 15, 2018.

Clark D, Garner A. *The first 1000 days: do you see what we see?* Available at: https://www.aap.org/en-us/advocacy-and-policy/aap-health-initiatives/EBCD/Documents/ALF-1000days.pdf Accessed August 15, 2018.

David-Ferdon C, Vivolo-Kantor AM, Dahlberg LL, et al. *A Comprehensive Technical Package for the Prevention of Youth Violence and Associated Risk Behaviors*. Atlanta: National Center for Injury Prevention and Control, Centers for Disease Control and Prevention; 2016. Available at: https://www.cdc.gov/violenceprevention/pdf/yv-technicalpackage.pdf. Accessed September 16, 2018.

Conway C. *The Unbearable Sensation of Being*. UCSF Magazine, Summer; 2018. Available at: https://www.ucsf.edu/news/2018/06/410786/living-with-sensory-processing-disorder.

Critz C, Blake K, Nogueira E. Sensory processing challenges in children. *J Nurse Practitioners*. 2015;11(7):710–716.

Department of Defense (DoD). Military Active-Duty Personnel, Civilians by State. Available at: http://www.governing.com/gov-data/public-workforce-salaries/military-civilian-active-duty-employee-workforce-numbers-by-state.html. Accessed September 15, 2018.

Dewar G. Taming aggression in children: *5 Crucial Strategies for Effective Parenting*. Available at: https://www.parentingscience.com/aggression-in-children.html; 2016.

Dickerson J. Sensory-related difficulties in children. *Pediatric News*. 2016.

Foy JM, Perrin J. American Academy of Pediatrics Task Force on Mental Health: enhancing pediatric mental health care. *Pediatrics*. 2010;125(suppl 3):S75–S108.

Garner A. *Translating Developmental Science into Healthy Lives: Realizing the Potential*. Available at: https://www.aap.org/en-us/advocacy-and-policy/aap-health-initiatives/EBCD/Documents/TranslatingSciencePPT.pdf.

Glascoe FP. Evidenced-based early detection of developmental-behavioral problems in primary care: what to expect and how to do it. *J Ped Health Care*. 2015;29(1):46–53.

Gleason MM, Goldson E, Yogman MW. *Addressing Early Childhood Emotional and Behavioral Problems*. Available at: http://pediatrics.aappublications.org/content/pediatrics/138/6/e20163025.full.pdf.

Greene R. *About the CPS Model*. Available at: https://www.livesinthebalance.org/about-cps Dewar.

Hagan JF, Shaw JS, Duncan PM, eds. *Bright Futures: Guidelines for Health Supervision of Infants, Children, and Adolescents*. 4th ed. Elk Grove Village, IL: American Academy of Pediatrics; 2017.

Hall AY. Mindfulness skill can help in parenting. *Pediatric News*. 2018;p18.

Health and Human Services. *The AFCARS Report No. 24*. Available at: https://www.acf.hhs.gov/sites/default/files/cb/afcarsreport24.pdf Accessed September 15, 2018.

Health and Human Services Office of Adolescent Health. *Trends in Teen Pregnancy and Childbearing*. Available at: https://www.hhs.gov/ash/oah/adolescent-development/reproductive-health-and-teen-pregnancy/teen-pregnancy-and-childbearing/trends/index.html.

Healthy People 2020. *Social Determinants of Health*. Available at: https://www.cdc.gov/socialdeterminants/faqs/#faq6.

Hostetler B. The four phases of parenthood, Focus on the Family (website); 1998. www.focusonthefamily.com/parenting/parenting-roles/phases-of-parenthood. Accessed August 15, 2018.

Kids Matter. *Social and Emotional Learning*. Available at: https://www.kidsmatter.edu.au/mental-health-matters/social-and-emotional-learning.

King H. *Learning to Care for Mental Health*. Available at: http://www.contemporarypediatrics.com/modern-medicine-feature-articles/learning-care-mental-health; 2016.

Martin JA, Hamilton BE, Osterman MJK, et al. Births: final data for 2016. *Nat Vital Statistic Rep*. 2018;67(1):1–55.

Maaskant AM, van Rooij FB, Overbeek GJ, et al. Effects of PMTO in foster families with children with behavior problems: a randomized controlled trial. *J Child Fam Stud*. 2017;26(2):523–530.

Masten AS. *Ordinary Magic*. NY: Guilford Press; 2014.

Meadows SO, Tanielian T, Karney B, et al. The Deployment Life Study: longitudinal analysis of military families across the deployment cycle. *Rand Health Q*. 2017;6(2):7. Available at: https://www.ncbi.nlm.nih.gov/pmc/articles/PMC5568161/#__sec6title. Accessed September 15, 2018.

Moore KA, Bethell CD, Murphy D, et al. *Flourishing from the start: what is it and how can it be measured*. Available at: https://www.childtrends.org/wp-content/uploads/2017/03/2017-16FlourishingFromTheStart-1.pdf. Accessed September 15, 2018.

National Institute for Children's Health Quality (NICHQ). *Promoting Young Children's Socioemotional Development in Primary Care*. 2016. Available at: https://www.nichq.org/sites/default/files/resource-file/Promoting%20Young%20Children%27s%20Socioemotional%20Development%20in%20Primary%20Care%20%282016%29.pdf; Accessed June 15, 2018.

Owen JP, Marco JP, Desai S, et al. Abnormal white matter microstructure in children with sensory processing disorders. *Neuroimage Clin*. 2013;2:844–853.

Panton J. Caring for military children: implications for nurse practitioners. *J Pediatr Healthcare*. 2018;32:435–444.

Perry B. *Six Core Strengths for Healthy Child Development*. Available at: http://www.cabrillo.edu/~ogarcia/Perry_Six_Core_Strengths.pdf Accessed July 2, 2018.

Reaching Children Initiative. *Cognitive Behavior Therapy for Children and Adolescents*; 2005.

Robert Wood Johnson Foundation (RWJF) and RAND Corporation. *Moving Forward Together: an update on building and measuring a culture of health*. Available at: https://www.rwjf.org/content/dam/COH/PDFs/MovingForwardTogetherFullReportFinal.pdf. Accessed June 15, 2018.

Rosenfeld AJ. Mindful kids, part1: origins and evidence. *Pediatric News*. 2017.

Schleider JL, Weisz JR. Little Treatments, promising effects? Meta-analysis of single-session interventions for youth psychiatric problems. *J Am Acad Child Adol Psychiatry*. 2017;56(2):107–115.

Schleider JL, Weisz JR. A single-session growth mind-set intervention for adolescent anxiety and depression: 9 month-outcomes for a randomized trial. *J Child Psychol Psychiatry*. 2018;59(2):160–170.

Sege RD, Harper Browne C. Responding to ACEs with HOPE: health outcomes from positive experiences. *Acad Pediatr*. 2017;17(&S):S79–S85.

Spratt EG. *Somatoform Disorder*. 2014. Available at: https://emedicine.medscape.com/article/918628-overview#a1. Accessed September 15, 2018.

USDHHS Children's Bureau. AFCARS Report #25, 2018. Available at: https://www.acf.hhs.gov/cb/resource/afcars-report-25. Accessed April 21, 2019.

UNICEF. The Adolescent Brain: a second window of opportunity. *A Compendium*. 2017. Available at: https://www.unicef-irc.org/adolescent-brain; 2017. Accessed June 1, 2018.

Viding E, Seara-Cardoso A, McCrory EJ. Antisocial and callous behavior in children. *Curr Top Behav Neurosci*. 2014;17:395–419.

Wallerstein JS. Children of divorce: the psychological tasks of the child. *Am J Orthopsychiatry*. 1983;53(2):230–243.

Walters JM. 12 *Things You Didn't Know About Military Families*. Available at: https://www.care.com/c/stories/4374/12-things-you-didnt-know-about-military-fami/. Accessed September 18, 2018.

Weitzman CM, Wegner L, Section of Developmental and Behavioral Pediatrics, et al. *Promoting Optimal Development: Screening for Behavioral and Emotional Problems*; 2016. Available at: http://pediatrics.aappublications.org/content/pediatrics/early/2015/01/20/peds.2014-3716.full.pdf. Accessed June 4, 2018.

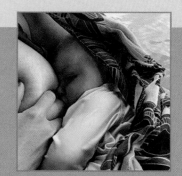

16

Breastfeeding

SARAH OBERMEYER

Human milk and breastfeeding are the optimal choice for newborn and infant nutrition and the normative method of feeding. Breast milk supports infant nutrition essential for optimal growth and development. In addition to healthy nutrients, breast milk contains many immune substances that protect the newborn against infections. Breastfeeding also offers parents and infants physical, psychological, and emotional benefits that last a lifetime. Breastfeeding should be promoted and supported whenever possible.

Promoting breastfeeding is the responsibility of all pediatric healthcare providers. They are called to engage in assessment, education, support, outreach, and advocacy as they promote breastfeeding. Breastfeeding is a learned skill for both the mother and the infant; providers must assess the mother's knowledge level and provide information and guidance to increase the skills of the mother-infant dyad as the breastfeeding experience develops. Providers need to educate mothers, fathers, and their families about the benefits of breast milk and how to recognize and prevent common breastfeeding problems. As a result, families can make educated choices about infant feeding practices and quickly seek professional advice and answers to their questions and concerns. Breastfeeding is supported when providers take the time to determine the cause of a breastfeeding problem, develop a plan to address the problem, and guide the family through difficulties; early assessment and intervention support a family in the decision to continue breastfeeding. Outreach and advocacy for breastfeeding are demonstrated when they contribute as members of hospital, clinic, and community committees, advisory boards, and task forces to develop policies that promote and support breastfeeding. Providers act as advocates for breastfeeding when they advise and educate colleagues about breastfeeding issues, teach breastfeeding content to students in the health professions, and serve as expert contacts for the media on issues related to breastfeeding. In all these activities, healthcare providers serve an important leadership duty in promoting and supporting breastfeeding.

Breastfeeding Recommendations

Major health professional organizations, including the National Association of Pediatric Nurse Practitioners (NAPNAP), the American Academy of Pediatrics (AAP), the American Academy of Family Physicians (AAFP), Association of Women's Health, Obstetric and Neonatal Nurses (AWHONN), and the American

Dietetic Association recommend breastfeeding exclusively for the first 6 months of life and then continued breastfeeding in combination with other nutrients for at least the first year (AAFP, 2014; AAP, 2012; AWHONN, 2015; Lessen and Kavenaugh, 2015; NAPNAP, 2013).

Breastfeeding goals for *Healthy People 2020* include the following targets:

- 81.9% of mothers will initiate breastfeeding in the neonatal period.
- 60.6% will be breastfeeding at 6 months old and 34.1% at 1 year old.
- 56.2% will be exclusively breastfeed through 3 months and 25.5% at 6 months.

There are also efforts to remove the barriers that mothers who are separated from their children (e.g., working mothers) encounter when attempting to breastfeed (U.S. Department of Health and Human Services [HHS], 2017). Although breastfeeding rates have increased in the United States, they continue to be well below the Healthy People 2020 goals (Centers for Disease Control and Prevention [CDC] Division of Nutrition, Physical Activity, and Obesity [DNPAO], 2014).

Much work remains to be done, and providers can make a major contribution to the success of efforts to support breastfeeding. One model that can be used to further these goals encourages providers to focus on interventions that (1) support the mother's self-efficacy to breastfeed, (2) provide lactation support to mother and family, and (3) increase lactation education for both mother and providers (Busch et al., 2014). Adequate education and support of the breastfeeding dyad by family members and providers is at the core of breastfeeding success.

Hospital-Based Support

Baby-Friendly Hospital Initiative

In 1991 the Baby-Friendly Hospital Initiative (BFHI) was developed by the World Health Organization (WHO) and the United Nations International Children's Emergency Fund (UNICEF) to recognize hospitals that provide optimal lactation support. This worldwide initiative trains providers and hospitals to promote breastfeeding internationally (UNICEF, 2009). The 10 criteria to meet a "baby-friendly hospital" standard are outlined in the original joint WHO/UNICEF statement (WHO/UNICEF, 1989) and are used to assess the quality of a lactation program.

Every facility that provides maternity services and cares for newborn infants should:

- Have a written breastfeeding policy that is routinely communicated to all health care staff.
- Train health care staff in skills necessary to implement this policy (18 hours of formal training are recommended).
- Inform pregnant women about the benefits and management of breastfeeding.
- Support initiation of breastfeeding within hour of birth.
- Show mothers how to breastfeed and maintain lactation even if they are separated from their infants.
- Give newborn infants no food or drink other than breast milk, unless medically indicated.
- Practice rooming in (i.e., allow mothers and infants to remain together) 24 hours a day.
- Encourage unrestricted breastfeeding.
- Give no artificial teats or pacifiers (also called *dummies* or *soothers*) to breastfeeding infants until breastfeeding is established, typically at 4 weeks of age.
- Foster the establishment of breastfeeding support groups; refer mothers to them on discharge from the hospital or clinic.

Currently, facilities in 152 countries have been designated "baby-friendly" internationally (WHO, 2018). As of March 2018, 489 hospitals and birthing centers in the United States (including the District of Columbia and the Commonwealth of Puerto Rico) held a "baby-friendly" designation, and, 23.72% of births in the United States were in "baby-friendly" facilities, greatly exceeding the Healthy People 2020 goal of 8.1%. (Baby-Friendly USA, 2018).

Benefits of Breastfeeding

With rare exception, breast milk is the ideal food for the human infant. Each mammalian species provides milk uniquely suited to its offspring, and milk from the human breast is no exception. It is a living fluid rich in vitamins, minerals, fat, proteins (including immunoglobulins and antibodies), and carbohydrates (especially lactose). It contains enzymes and cellular components, including macrophages and lymphocytes, in addition to many other constituents that offer ideal support for growth and maturation of the human infant. Amazingly, as the infant grows and develops, the properties of breast milk change. The sequence of colostrum, transitional milk, and mature milk meets the shifting nutritional needs of the newborn and infant. The milk of a mother of a newborn contains different concentrations of fat, protein, and carbohydrates and different physical properties, such as pH, when compared with the milk of the mother of a 1-month-old or 9-month-old infant. Premature infants in particular benefit when receiving colostrum from their own mothers or from a donor with an infant who matches the gestational age of the preemie because of the specific properties of preterm colostrum. In addition, some of the constituent properties in the milk are different from one time of the day to another. Breast milk has a higher composition of water in the morning when the milk has been in the breast for longer periods of time.

In addition to providing optimal nutrition for growth and development, breastfeeding confers many short- and long-term health benefits to infants. Initiation of breastfeeding at the time of birth allows the growth of protective bacteria necessary for a healthy microbiome. Continuation of breastfeeding promotes further growth of these bacteria, immunoglobulin A (IgA) secretion and decreased inflammation in the intestinal epithelial cells and underlying tissues. A protective barrier in the intestines is created

that prevents penetration of the intestine and may be able to inactivate some viral organisms. A review of studies examining the effect of breastfeeding on infant health revealed a lower risk of nonspecific bacterial infections, necrotizing enterocolitis, acute otitis media in early childhood, asthma, excessive weight gain, type 2 diabetes, and sudden infant death syndrome (SIDS) (Brenner-Jones et al., 2016; den Dekker et al., 2016; Al Mamum et al., 2015; Thompson et al., 2017). Many of the benefits of breastfeeding become more pronounced with a breastfeeding duration of at least 6 months.

There are also benefits for the mother that include establishment of the strong bond associated with successful nursing and decreased risk for breast and ovarian cancer (Ross-Cowerdy, 2017). In addition, breastfeeding is associated with short-term and long-term benefits that protect against cardiovascular risks associated with metabolic syndrome type, hypertension, and cardiovascular disease (Nguyen, 2017).

Breastfeeding also provides an economic incentive as a free and plentiful source of excellent infant nutrition. The cost of formula and other necessary supplies exceeds several thousand dollars each year for a family. It is estimated that suboptimal breastfeeding was related to 3342 deaths in 2014, as well as medical costs of $3.0 billion dollars and $1.3 billion dollars in nonmedical costs (Bartick et al., 2017). Investing in the establishment and support of extended breastfeeding may play a role in significant cost savings and preservation of health.

Contraindications to Breastfeeding

Although rare, contraindications to breastfeeding occur in some unique situations. Certain infections and many drugs or medications can be passed to the infant via breast milk. A small number of infant conditions also preclude breastfeeding. Contraindications to breastfeeding include the following (AAP, 2012):

- Infant with classic galactosemia
- Maternal diagnosis of human T-cell lymphotropic virus type I or II
- Maternal diagnosis of untreated brucellosis
- Maternal diagnosis of cancer and treatment
- Maternal human immunodeficiency virus (HIV) infection (except in some areas, see WHO recommendations [Box 16.1]; breastfeeding for HIV-infected mothers is not recommended in developed countries)
- Herpetic lesions on the mother's nipples, areolas, or breast (expressed breast milk can be fed to the infant)
- Maternal use of cocaine, phencyclidine (PCP), and cannabis

In certain situations where the mother and newborn must be separated because of illness, expressed breast milk may still be fed to the infant. The separation of mother and baby should occur if the mother is diagnosed with active, untreated tuberculosis (TB), active varicella developed 5 days prior or 2 days after delivery, or current H1N1 influenza virus with a fever (AAP, 2012).

Special Situations

Additional circumstances require special consideration regarding the advisability or management of breastfeeding. These circumstances include the following:

- Significant maternal or infant illness affecting the ability to feed
- Invasive breast surgery, in particular breast reduction in which the areola is removed and reattached

The primary goal is to balance the risk of human immunodeficiency virus (HIV) infection of the infant transmitted through breast milk with protection from other causes of child mortality that breast milk provides.

For HIV-positive mothers who live in countries where breastfeeding and antiretroviral treatments (ARTs) are promoted, the World Health Organization (WHO) recommends exclusive breastfeeding for the first 6 months and breastfeeding with nutritional supplements until 12 months.

National or subnational health authorities should decide whether HIV-infected mothers should either:

- Breastfeed and receive ARTs

or

- Avoid breastfeeding completely, implementing replacement feeding
- Replacement feeding should not be used unless it is:
  - Acceptable (socially welcome)
  - Feasible (facilities and help are available to prepare formula)
  - Affordable (formula can be purchased for 6 months)
  - Sustainable (feeding can be sustained for 6 months)
  - Safe (formula is prepared with safe water and in hygienic conditions)

From World Health Organization (WHO). Consolidated guidelines on the use of antiretroviral drugs for treating and preventing HIV infection: recommendations for a public health approach. WHO; 2013. www.who.int/hiv/pub/guidelines/arv2013/download/en/. Accessed April 5, 2018; WHO. Guidelines on HIV and infant feeding 2010: principles and recommendations for infant feeding in the context of HIV and a summary of evidence. WHO; 2010. www.who.int/maternal_child_adolescent/documents/9789241599535/en/. Accessed April 5, 2019.

- Documented history of milk supply problems
- Maternal smoking, which increases the risk of low milk supply and poor infant weight gain (AAP, 2012)
- If mothers cannot breastfeed their infants but want their baby to receive breast milk or if the infant requires breast milk to survive, a network of breast milk banks is available to families. Although it is expensive, the Human Milk Banking Association of North America (HMBANA) provides breast milk at three centers in Canada and 17 in the United States (see Additional Resources). Nursing mothers may also donate their milk to these banks. It is possible to buy breast milk online; however, this could be hazardous for the infant because many of these donors are unscreened and many samples purchased online have been found to be contaminated, unsuitable for consumption on arrival, or adulterated (Sriraman et al., 2018).

Induced Lactation and Relactation

Nongestational parents may wish to breastfeed an infant or toddler to provide an emotional bond and attachment. A lactation consultant can support the parent in establishing and maintaining breast milk supply, although there may be insufficient milk supply to solely support the infant's nutritional needs. Healthcare providers should closely follow the infant's weight gain and help the parents to determine the amount and type of supplementation based on the infant's age.

Lactation Consultants

Lactation consultants are trained to evaluate and support breastfeeding and intervene when necessary. The International Board of Lactation Consultant Examiners (IBLCE) licenses lactation consultants with specialized knowledge and clinical skills. These individuals are designated as International Board Certified Lactation Consultants (IBCLCs) and may practice in hospitals, public health or community agencies, or private practice. Consultation with a lactation consultant should be considered when the breastfeeding dyad needs assessment or intervention that is outside of the healthcare provider's skillset. Communication between the provider and lactation consultant is important in supporting the ongoing needs of the breastfeeding family.

Stages of Milk Production

Colostrum

Colostrum production begins at approximately 16 weeks of gestation. The pregnant woman may notice a small amount of yellow discharge on her nipple or clothing. After delivery of the baby, production of colostrum increases but is still of low quantity. This thick, rich, yellowish fluid has fewer calories than mature milk (67 vs. 75 kcal/100 mL) and is lower in fat (2% vs. 3.8%). It is rich in immunoglobulins, especially secretory immunoglobulin A (sIgA), and other antibodies. sIgA is important in the newborn because it coats the gut to protect against invasion of bacteria and decreases overall gut inflammation. In addition, colostrum is higher in sodium, potassium, chloride, protein, fat-soluble vitamins, and cholesterol than mature milk and facilitates the passage of meconium. Colostrum meets all nutritional needs of a healthy term newborn in the first few days of life. No supplementation is necessary.

Transitional Milk

Transitional milk appears between 32 and 96 hours after birth. The drop in placental hormones and increased prolactin levels triggers the transition of milk. Significant variability is seen in the constituent properties of transitional milk between mothers and within samples from the same mother. As a general rule, transitional milk has more lactose, calories, and fat and less total protein than colostrum.

Mature Milk

Mature milk gradually replaces transitional milk by the second week after birth and provides, on average, 20 kcal/oz. Ongoing milk production is supported by autocrine, endocrine, and metabolic controls.

Characteristics of Human Milk

The uniqueness of human milk to support the growth and development of the human infant cannot be overestimated. Scientists continue to find new components and to clarify the purposes of known components.

Water

Approximately 90% of human milk is water. Breast milk can meet the fluid needs of the infant without any water supplementation, even in tropical and desert climates.

Lipid (Fat) Content

Various lipids (fats) make up the second greatest percentage of the constituents of human milk. They are also the most variable component, with differences noted within a feeding, between feedings, in feedings over time, and between different mothers. On average, the fat content is approximately 3.8% and contributes 30% to 55% of the kilocalories in human milk. During feeding, the fluid content of the mammary gland becomes mixed with droplets of fat in increasing concentration. Thus the fat content is higher at the end of the feeding than it is at the beginning. The type and amount of fat in the maternal diet are thought to affect the type of lipid but not the total amount of fat found in the mother's breast milk.

The cholesterol content varies little in human milk and is approximately 240 mg/100 g of fat. Breastfed infants have higher plasma cholesterol levels than do formula-fed infants. Research on naturally occurring fatty acids found in breast milk, such as docosahexaenoic acid (DHA) and other long-chain polyunsaturated fatty acids (LC-PUFAs), indicates that they play an important role in brain and retinal development (Jackson and Harris, 2016). Maternal dietary changes to include greater amounts of omega-3 fatty acids can be beneficial in increasing the levels found in breast milk.

Protein

Approximately 0.9% of the content of human milk is protein. Protein levels are higher in colostrum than in mature milk. When milk is heated or exposed to enzymes as in digestion, a clot, or casein, is formed. The clear portion that remains is known as *whey*. In human milk, 60% to 70% of the protein is whey, which primarily consists of α-lactalbumin and lactoferrin, and 30% to 40% is casein. In contrast, cow's milk is 20% β-lactalbumin and 80% casein, with distinct chemical differences between the casein found in cow's milk and that found in human milk. The curds of human milk are more easily digested by the infant. Lactoferrin is an iron-binding protein, which is understood to reduce the available iron for iron-dependent pathogens and promotes growth of the intestinal epithelium. Other proteins include immunoglobulins, nonimmunoglobulins, and lysozyme—a nonspecific antibacterial factor (Walker, 2016).

Carbohydrates

The primary carbohydrate of human milk is lactose, which is synthesized by the mammary gland from glucose. Lactose is highly concentrated in human milk (6.8 vs. 4.9 g/100 mL in cow's milk) and appears to be essential for growth of the human infant. Lactose supports growth of pathogen-competing microflora in the intestines and enhances the absorption of calcium, a potentially important role because of the relatively low level of calcium in human milk.

Vitamins and Minerals

Human milk has more than adequate amounts of vitamins A, E, K, C, B_1, B_2, and B_6; however, the level of vitamin D in breast milk may not be adequate for breastfed infants. Further research is needed to determine exactly what supplemental dose of vitamin D is necessary for nursing mothers to ensure adequate concentrations in breast milk; however, the recommended 400 IU/day does not appear to be enough. It may need to be increased up to 16 times the currently recommended dose for mothers (Hollis et al., 2015). Direct, unprotected exposure to sunlight is a more effective way than diet for the body to get vitamin D and provides other

benefits to the infant; however, the AAP statement on prevention of vitamin D deficiency reports concern over direct sunlight without skin protection. In addition, sunscreen blocks vitamin D absorption. Therefore the AAP (2008) recommends a supplement of 400 IU/day, beginning shortly after birth for all infants, including those exclusively breastfed. Although low levels of iron are found in human milk, iron absorption from human milk is highly efficient, with 49% of the available iron absorbed in contrast to 4% from formula. A full-term infant who is exclusively breastfed for 4 to 6 months is not at risk for iron deficiency anemia with iron supplement (1 mg/kg/ day) beginning at age 4 months. Zinc is readily available in human milk and has an absorption rate of 41% versus 31% from cow's milk protein formulas and 14% from soy formulas.

Anatomy and Physiology

Pregnancy brings about the final stage of mammogenesis—growth and differentiation of the mammary gland and development of the structures to support breast milk production. Estrogen, progesterone, placental lactogen, and prolactin all play a role in mammogenesis. By approximately 20 weeks, the breast is capable of milk production. The actual production of breast milk is triggered by the fall in progesterone concentration after birth of the baby and delivery of the placenta. Placental retention inhibits milk production because of the influence of progesterone and other hormones.

Suckling by the infant is essential to establish and maintain lactation. The amount of milk production depends on stimulation of the breast, removal of milk from the breast, and release of hormones. The concept of "demand and supply" is an important one for providers and parents to understand. Suckling stimulates the hypothalamus to decrease prolactin-inhibiting factor and permits release of prolactin by the anterior pituitary, which leads to a rise in the level of prolactin. Prolactin levels are directly proportional to the level of suckling by the infant and are more important to the initiation than to the maintenance of lactation. The hypothalamus also stimulates the synthesis and release of oxytocin by the posterior pituitary (Fig 16.1). Oxytocin reacts with receptors in the myoepithelial cells of the milk ducts to initiate a contracting action that forces milk down the ducts. This action increases milk pressure called the *let-down reflex* or *milk ejection reflex*. Oxytocin also aids in maternal uterine involution, a mechanism protective of the new mother's life by reducing blood loss after birth.

Under the influence of the hormones mentioned previously, the mammary gland undergoes a dramatic change with an increase in size and rapid growth of the lobuloalveolar tissue. The alveoli are the site of milk production and combine in numbers of 10 to 100 to form lobuli. Twenty to 40 lobuli combine into lobes, and 15 to 25 lobes empty into a lactiferous duct. The ducts transport the milk to the nipple (Fig 16.2).

The nipple and surrounding areola serve as a visual and tactile target to assist with latch-on. The size and shape of the woman's breast and areola vary greatly. The size of the breast is not a predictor of breast milk volume or breastfeeding success. Women with small breasts can successfully breastfeed. However, the provider should be alert for the occasional presence of insufficient glandular tissue development, which is characterized by the absence of breast changes associated with pregnancy, a unilaterally underdeveloped breast, or conical-shaped breasts. The size, shape, and position of the nipple also vary among women. The nipple may be everted (protuberant from the breast), flat, or inverted.

Assessment of the Breastfeeding Dyad

Prenatal assessment focuses on maternal expectations for breastfeeding; knowledge about breastfeeding, especially techniques for getting off to a good start; and identification of any contraindications to breastfeeding. A nipple evaluation should be completed. All pregnant women should be assessed, regardless of past breastfeeding experience. In the early postpartum period, assessment focuses on the transition to breastfeeding and should include close observation of a feeding. In addition, signs of progress for successful breastfeeding should be reviewed, and the names and phone numbers of contact persons should be given to mothers for follow-up or questions.

Maternal History

Data should be collected about the following:
- Overall health, including documentation of any chronic illnesses or allergies
- Pregnancy history, especially any complications or need for medications
- Labor and delivery history, including medications, procedures, or complications
- Medications received in the early postpartum period
- Surgical interventions, especially to the breast or thoracic region
- Routine use of over-the-counter, prescribed, or recreational or street drugs, including tobacco, e-cigarettes, alcohol, and herbal preparations or supplements
- Nutritional status
- Previous breastfeeding experience
- Cultural expectations about breastfeeding
- Family and community support for breastfeeding

Infant History

Important infant data to gather include:
- Gestational age and age at the time of the assessment
- Overall health status
- Medications, other than routine protocol (e.g., vitamin K, eye drops), administered after birth
- Early responses to feeding attempts
- Congenital conditions, such as cardiac, respiratory, or orofacial conditions
- Trauma or complications during delivery
- Activities including circumcision, use of bilirubin lights, or use of bottle, cup, or tube feeding

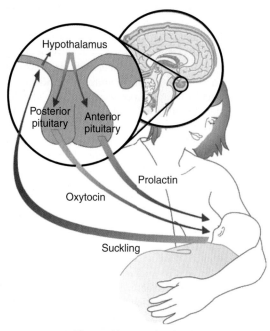

• **Fig 16.1** Neuroendocrine Loop.

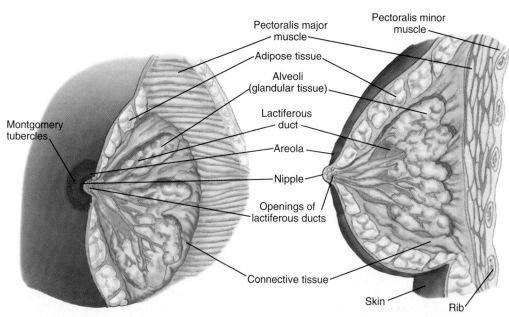

• **Fig 16.2** Anatomy of the Breast. (From Murray S, McKinney E, Holub KS, et al. *Foundations of Maternal-Newborn and Women's Health Nursing*. 7th ed. St. Louis: Elsevier; 2019.)

Maternal Examination

Examination of the mother should focus on an evaluation of the breast in the following areas:
- Presence of surgical scars on the breast or thoracic area
- Type of nipples—everted, flat, or inverted. It is not always possible to detect an inverted nipple by observation only. The "pinch test" may be needed to identify nipples that invert with tactile stimulation to the areola. To do the pinch test, place the thumb and forefinger on opposite sides of the areola approximately 1 to 1.5 inches back from the nipple-areolar junction. Gently compress as though bringing the two fingers together, causing the nipple to become more everted or inverted. This assessment should be conducted prenatally on every patient (Fig 16.3).
- Any nipple bruising or bleeding

The breast exam provides an opportunity for the healthcare provider to educate the mother on her breast anatomy and encourage breastfeeding preparation.

Infant Examination

Evaluation of the infant's oral-motor skills and structures is the basis for the examination. The examiner's finger should be inserted beyond the gum line nearly to the soft palate. The infant should be able to suck smoothly with upward motion of the tongue as the finger is drawn in for suckling. The hard and soft palate should be intact, without palpable clefts or submucosal clefts. The infant should be able to extend the tongue over the lower gum with no evidence of a tight frenulum. There are no standard objective criteria for diagnosis of what constitutes a frenulum that is *too* tight (i.e., ankyloglossia or "tongue-tie"). If frenulum tension is a concern, a trained practitioner and or a lactation consultant should examine the tension of the frenulum to determine its effects on the maternal and newborn breastfeeding dyad. Tongue tie release may be considered in some infants whose tongue does fully extend and who demonstrate consistent latch and suck problems, maternal

nipple damage, or insufficient breast milk transfer. Surgical release of a tight frenulum can significantly improve breastfeeding outcomes and transfer of breast milk (Ghaheri et al., 2017).

Positions for Breastfeeding

Getting off to a good start begins with positioning the baby at the breast in a way that is comfortable for both the mother and baby and that allows for good latch-on. The four most common positions are the cradle, cross-cradle, side-lying, and football-hold positions.

Principles of Correct Positioning

Several principles are common to all of the various positions for breastfeeding, including the following:
- Both the mother and the baby should be comfortable.
- The infant should be positioned "face on" at nipple height so that no head turning or tilting is required. The nipple should be directed toward the center of the infant's mouth.
- The infant should be lying belly to belly with the mother.
- The infant's body should be in good alignment, with a straight line from the ear to the shoulder to the hips.
- The infant's top and bottom lips should be flanged out (Fig 16.4).
- The infant's tongue should extend forward over the lower gum line and cup around the nipple and areola.
- Good latch-on results in quiet feedings. No "clicking" or "popping" sounds should be heard from the infant. After mother's milk is in, audible swallowing, such as a "glug" or air blowing out the baby's nose, should be heard.

Cradle Position and Cross Cradle Position

The cradle position (also called the *Madonna* or *cuddle position*) and its variation, the cross-cradle position, begin with the mother sitting upright with her feet on the floor or stool or her legs crossed in front of her. The infant is held or supported with pillows, with the mouth at nipple height, and the mother and infant are in a tummy-to-tummy arrangement. The mother uses her free hand to support the breast with her first finger and thumb forming a C shape, while keeping her fingers well back from the areola so that she does not interfere with latch (Fig 16.5). In the regular cradle

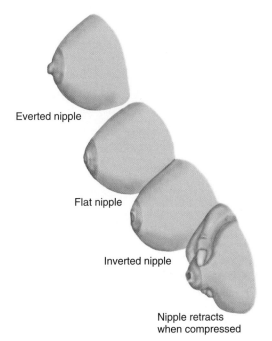

Everted nipple

Flat nipple

Inverted nipple

Nipple retracts when compressed

• **Fig 16.3** Nipple Shape and Pinch Test. (From Murray S, McKinney E, Holub KS, Jones R. *Foundations of Maternal-Newborn and Women's Health Nursing*. 7th ed. St. Louis: Elsevier; 2019.)

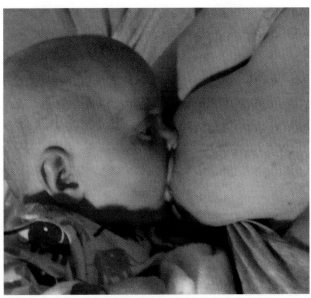

• **Fig 16.4** Lip Position.

position, the baby's head is supported in the crook of the elbow on the same side as the breast being suckled (Fig 16.6). In the cross-cradle position, the opposite hand supports the baby's head and shoulders. This position often works well for a premature infant because it provides extra head and trunk support and allows the mother to control the breast and nipple with her ipsilateral hand.

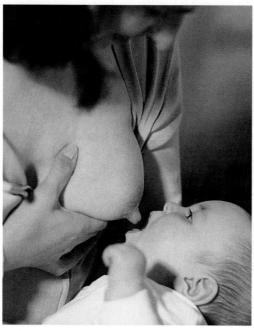

• **Fig 16.5** C-shape Hold on Breast. (© 2019 Medela.)

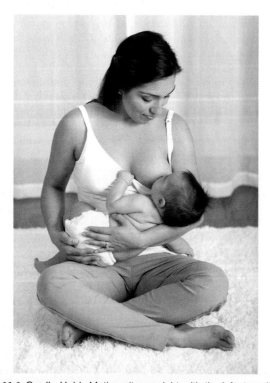

• **Fig 16.6** Cradle Hold. Mother sites upright with the infant positioned on her side and lays the baby's head and neck along her forearm. Baby's body is against her stomach (a tummy-to-mummy position). Pillows or a cushion can be placed behind mother for support or a breastfeeding pillow laid across her lap propping up the baby. The breastfeeding pillow should not lift the baby too high. Breasts should remain at their natural resting height to avoid sore nipples and a strained latch. (© 2019 Medela.)

After positioning the baby, the mother should draw the nipple from the infant's nose to chin to stimulate mouth opening. As the mouth opens and the infant extends his or her head upward, she should bring the baby close so that the lips come up and over the nipple and back onto the areolar tissue and the nipple rests on top of the baby's tongue. Once the baby appears latched on, the mother can check the lips for a flanged, open placement. At this point, the baby is very close to the breast, with the tip of the infant's nose touching it. Mothers often need to be shown that the baby is able to breathe without a need to press down on the breast tissue. If the baby appears to be pushed into the breast, the infant's buttocks should be brought closer into the tummy-to-tummy position. As the mother looks down at her baby, she should see a straight line from the baby's ear to the shoulders to the hips. Once the baby is suckling well, she can usually remove the hand that was supporting her breast and use it to cradle the baby in her arms.

Football Hold

In the football hold, the infant is supported off to the side of the mother. The football hold is often used to teach a newly breast-feeding mother the mechanisms of helping to support the baby's head while also controlling the position of the breast and nipple. This position is often used by a mother who had a cesarean delivery, because it does not require that the infant be positioned along her abdomen or by a mother of multiples when she would like to feed two babies at once. Finally, mothers with flat or inverted nipples are often able to achieve latch-on more easily with this position.

One or two firm pillows should be placed at the mother's side to help support the infant. The baby is in a side-lying position and flexed at the hips, with the buttocks back against the chair or couch. As in other positions, the mother may support her breast to assist with latch-on and remove her hand once the baby is suckling well (Fig 16.7).

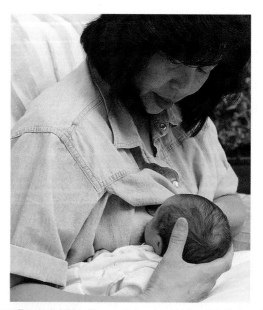

• **Fig 16.7** Football Hold. The mother supports the infant's head in her hand, with the infant's body resting on pillows alongside her hip. This method allows the mother to see the position of the infant's mouth on the breast, helps her control the infant's head, and is especially helpful for mothers with heavy breasts. This hold also prevents pressure against an abdominal incision. (From McKinney ES, James SR, Murray SS, et al. *Maternal-Child Nursing*. 4th ed. St. Louis: Elsevier/Saunders; 2013.)

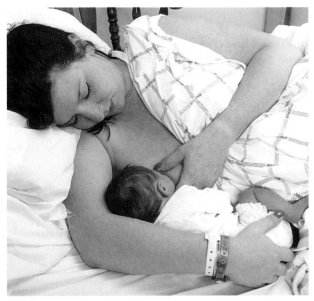

• **Fig 16.8** The side-lying position prevents pressure on episiotomy or abdominal incisions and allows the mother to rest while feeding. She lies on her side, with her lower arm supporting her head or placed around the infant. A pillow behind her back and between her legs provides comfort. Her upper hand and arm are used to position the infant on the side at nipple level and hold the breast. When the infant's mouth opens to nurse, the mother leans slightly forward or draws the infant to her to insert the nipple into the mouth. (From McKinney ES, James SR, Murray SS, et al. *Maternal-Child Nursing*. 4th ed. St. Louis: Elsevier/Saunders; 2013.)

Side-Lying Position

The side-lying or other lying-down variations are often helpful when the mother is uncomfortable sitting up or wishes to rest with her baby. When first learning to achieve latch-on, the side-lying position is not easy to use because the mother cannot see her breast and nipple quite as well and may need additional help to correctly position the newborn. With practice, the mother and infant can achieve latch-on without assistance.

In the side-lying position, the mother lies on her side, cradles her infant in her elbow, and supports the infant's back and neck. The mother or the nurse should arrange one to two pillows under the mother's head and shoulders and a rolled towel or blanket along the infant's back to keep the infant in a side-lying position. As in the cradle position, the mother may support her breast with her upper hand (Fig 16.8).

Physiologic Laid-back Position

The laid-back position is referred to as the physiologic or biologic nurturing position because it allows the mother to recline and allow gravity to bring the baby to the breast. In addition, the baby is in a position that is less likely to stimulate the startle (Moro) reflex and supports the innate feeding reflexes. In the laid-back position, the mother reclines in a position that supports her back and neck and brings her baby to her chest and allows the baby to rest its cheek against her breast. The baby is able to use the rooting and sucking reflexes to find the nipple, and the mother can support her breast to help guide the baby. When the baby has latched, gravity helps to maintain a deeper latch and the mother is able to relax and enjoy the breastfeeding session (Fig 16.9).

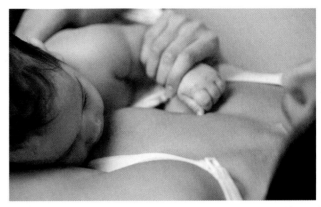

• **Fig 16.9** Laid-back Position. Also called biologic nurturing, this position allows the infant to rest against or beside the mother in a prone position. (© 2019 Medela.)

Ending a Feeding Session

When the feeding session has come to an end, the mother should attend to the way the baby releases the nipple. Suction on the nipple when the baby pulls back from the breast may result in nipple pain or trauma. The mother can insert her finger between the baby's lip and her breast to break the suction before bringing the baby away from the breast.

Dynamics of Breastfeeding

Early Feedings

The first breastfeeding should take place as soon after birth as possible. Full-term neonates often have an alert period for 30 to 60 minutes after delivery that is ideal for the first feeding practice. This first feeding should take place in the delivery area with encouragement by all in attendance. It will not delay, to any significant extent, any procedures required, such as weighing and measuring the infant, instilling ointment or drops in the infant's eyes, and giving a vitamin K injection. These procedures can be done while the baby remains on the mother's abdomen. The mother and infant should remain together as much as possible, with rooming-in preferable. The family's desire to promote close contact and initiate breastfeeding should be made clear to and supported by staff.

The infant usually goes into a deep sleep after the initial alertness and is difficult to wake for feeding. Parents should be instructed to watch for any awakening behavior, such as opening eyes or movement in the bed. Many newborns will not cry at this point, so parents need to be alert for these signs of feeding readiness. Full-term infants are born with stores of fluid and energy to carry them through this early transition to the nonuterine environment, a time of infrequent feeding and low volume of colostrum. The infant's stomach, liver, and kidneys are gearing up for the larger volumes of higher-fat food that will come in a few days. It is not necessary to provide any supplement, including water, to a healthy, full-term neonate.

During this transition time, assistance and support from an individual knowledgeable in breastfeeding can be helpful to the mother and infant as they practice latch-on and suckling. The infant should be encouraged to go to each breast for at least 10 to 15 minutes of active suckling, although some infants may spend even longer—up to 20 or 30 minutes. The infant's behavior is much more important during this time than the clock.

However, an infant who falls asleep in 5 minutes should be stimulated to continue active suckling. Rubbing the infant's back or foot or stroking the cheek or chin stimulates the infant to wake and begin sucking. Attention to proper positioning and technique becomes important as the frequency and duration of the suckling behavior increase. A mother is unlikely to get sore or cracked nipples when her infant is latched on correctly. These early feedings are excellent "practice" sessions both for the mother, who gains confidence in her breastfeeding ability, and for the infant, who gets first colostrum and then milk for the efforts at suckling.

The goal of discharge planning is to maintain successful breastfeeding and includes the following:

- Review proper positioning and signs of effective latch-on.
- Review signs of infant progress indicating adequate nutrition
- Arrange follow-up for 2 to 3 days after discharge.
- Provide a phone contact for questions and concerns.
- Encourage the mother to contact breastfeeding resources whenever she has questions.

Early efforts to provide contact and support during the transition to home will support the family and encourage them to maintain breastfeeding. Problems encountered during engorgement, sleep deprivation, and times of uncertainty or lack of confidence can be addressed quickly and directly rather than after a bottle is introduced or the mother's nipples are cracked and bleeding.

Frequency and Duration of Feedings

After the first 24 hours, the infant should be going to the breast 8 to 12 times (or every 2 to 3 hours) in 24 hours for approximately 20 to 45 minutes at each feeding. Frequent suckling stimulates milk production and establishes a regular routine. Exclusive feeding at the breast for the first 4 to 6 weeks should be encouraged to ensure the establishment of adequate milk supply and prevent any nipple preference. Parents need to be on alert if their infant sleeps more than 4 to 5 hours at a time or goes to sleep at the breast in 5 minutes. This infant must be actively wakened and stimulated for feeding.

If the mother and infant must be separated for one or more feedings or supplements are medically necessary, they may be given with a syringe, dropper, a cup, or a 5-Fr feeding tube placed at the breast. Proper instructions, close supervision, and follow-up are needed for each of these methods, and they should not be used routinely.

Hand Expression and Pumping

Routine pumping is unnecessary for mothers who are available for a feeding every 2 to 4 hours. If the mother and infant must be separated for more than one or two feedings, pumping should be part of the plan to assist with milk production. If the mother and infant are separated right after birth, pumping should begin as soon as possible, within the first 24 hours. The mother should pump six to eight times in 24 hours for 15 minutes if she is using a double-pump setup or 10 minutes per breast if she is using a single-pump setup. This routine mimics the desired feeding at the breast for the newborn. Instruct the mother to save even the smallest amounts of colostrum to give to her infant.

Hand expression and manual pumps work well for infrequent or short-duration pumping, and some women may choose to hand express exclusively. However, a hospital-grade, piston-style pump that permits pumping both breasts at the same time is ideal for a mother who has to pump for several weeks or months. No pump works as well as an infant in stimulating production, but frequent pumping does help in establishing a milk supply and provides the mother with a concrete, healthful contribution to her sick or preterm infant. As the volume of milk goes up over the first few days, the mother can see the success of her efforts. She should be counseled about the increase in breast milk production in contrast to the small volume of colostrum produced in the first few days.

Collection and Storage of Breast Milk

A mother should be reminded to wash her hands well before she begins pumping and to use clean containers for collection and storage. In addition, the pump parts should be thoroughly cleaned after each use. Many of the pump parts can go through a dishwasher; directions that come with the pump should be consulted for specific instructions on cleaning.

Milk collected from pumping should be stored in clean plastic bottles or disposable milk bags. It is preferable to store breast milk in small amounts so that only the amount that is needed is defrosted and used. The Academy of Breastfeeding Medicine recommends that saving breast milk from an unfinished bottle for use at another feeding be limited to 1 to 2 hours at room temperature. Milk that has been defrosted and not used within 24 hours should be discarded. Pumped breast milk should be refrigerated as soon after pumping as possible and can be stored there for up to 8 days. It can be stored with reusable cooler packs in a cooler for approximately 24 hours. If it is not going to be used during that time, it should be frozen. Breast milk can be stored for 3 months in a refrigerator freezer that maintains a steady temperature and can be stored for up to 12 months in a freezer in which 0°F is routinely maintained. Freezing breast milk has variable effects on its components. A reduction in calories, fat, protein, and lactoferrin is seen after 3 months of freezing, whereas other bioactive components such as sIgA, cytokines, and growth factors are consistent after 6 months of being frozen. The bottles or bags should be labeled with the date of collection and the oldest milk used first. If the milk must be transported to the hospital or day care facility, it should be placed in ice or on a blue ice unit to minimize the amount of warming or thawing (Academy of Breastfeeding Medicine Protocol Committee [ABM] et al., 2017a).

Growth Spurts

Just when parents begin to think that breastfeeding is well established, the first growth spurt occurs, and they may become concerned. The term *growth spurt* is used to describe those times during breastfeeding when the baby's growth demands exceed the breast milk supply at that moment. For 2 to 4 days, the infant seems to be "hungry all the time" and demands to be fed more frequently. During growth spurts, many babies cluster feed, needing to feed multiple times in a short period of time. The best response is to feed on demand and increase the number of feedings because increased stimulation of the breast increases milk production to the amount needed. However, an inexperienced parent may begin supplementation that can actually lead to a decrease in breast milk production. Once the level of milk production rises, the infant returns to the normal feeding pattern. Growth spurts tend to occur every 3 to 4 weeks, and parents seem to notice them less as time goes on. The behavior becomes an expected part of the breastfeeding experience.

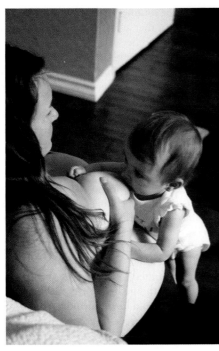

• **Fig 16.10** Breastfeeding Toddlers.

Breastfeeding Toddlers

Many mothers find breastfeeding an enjoyable experience and may continue into the child's second year of life. As the child grows, various changes in feeding position may support the breastfeeding dyad. Toddlers may try various positions of sitting and standing while feeding as they become curious about various ways of moving their bodies (Fig 16.10). In some cases, a second pregnancy occurs, and the mother chooses to breastfeed both the infant and toddler (tandem feeding). There are many benefits to breastfeeding toddlers who have a wide range of foods in their diet. Breastfeeding continues to provide immunity, strengthens the maternal-child bond, is a source of comfort to the child, and is readily available when the child needs quick nourishment and none other is available. Breastfeeding the toddler may reduce the prevalence of obesity in children (Hansstein, 2016).

Considerations for breastfeeding toddlers include:
- Breastfeed after the child has eaten a meal, not before
- Breastfeeding may not be on demand as with the infant; mothers can establish times and places when breastfeeding will occur
- If tandem feeding, always feed the infant first
- Have parent consult with the child's dentist regarding potential caries development with breastfeeding
- Have toddler brush teeth before bedtime but *after* breastfeeding

Weaning

The decision about the time for weaning is an individual one. Breastfeeding should be encouraged for at least 1 year, but individual circumstances may dictate a different choice for a family. Sometimes weaning is led by the mother and other times by the infant. Typically, a natural weaning process occurs as other foods become a part of the infant's diet and the infant begins to participate in self-feeding. When a family asks about the ideal time to begin weaning, counsel the parent(s) to consider a number of factors, including the desire of the mother, the developmental readiness of the infant, and any outside issues affecting the decision (social, environmental or family). Nutritional replacements for breast milk should be discussed when weaning is anticipated.

Whether weaning occurs as a planned or unplanned activity, it is best to implement it gradually. Some mothers use a plan over a week or so of having three feedings a day, then two, then one either in the morning or at bedtime. If necessary, the mother can use a breast pump to gradually decrease milk production and prevent breast engorgement, blocked ducts, and discomfort. An effective approach is to pump when uncomfortable and to pump only to comfort, not to empty. In situations where weaning was not an anticipated or planned event, the healthcare provider should help the mother to deal not only with the act of weaning but also with her feelings about it. Some mothers grieve the loss of the breastfeeding experience whether planned or unplanned.

In an effort to prevent premature weaning, providers should maintain close communication with families, especially those who are more likely to wean early. Early identification and support of these families may assist them to continue breastfeeding for a longer period. Factors associated with early weaning include postpartum depression (Dias and Figueredo, 2015), the perception of inefficient breast milk, and maternal dissatisfaction (Robert et al., 2014).

Clinical Indications of Successful Breastfeeding

Infant Weight Gain

Infant growth rates are dependent on a variety of factors, including genetics, type of feeding, and maternal nutrition and health during pregnancy. Normal newborn infants lose 5% to 10% of their birth weight in the first few days of life. It is helpful for parents to be aware of both the birth and discharge weights. Once the maternal milk volume increases, the infant begins to gain weight in the range of 0.5 to 1 oz/day or 4 to 7 oz/week. Many breastfed infants have regained their birth weight by 2 weeks, and others may take up to 3 to 4 weeks before return to birth weight is achieved (Paul et al., 2016). Breastfed infants usually double their birth weight by the time they are 4 to 6 months old and triple it by 1 year old.

The CDC recommends that providers in the United States use the WHO growth standards for children up to 24 months old. WHO standards are based on growth of an international population of healthy infants "predominately breastfed for at least 4 months and still breastfeeding at 12 months" (CDC, 2010). If growth charts other than WHO charts are used, breastfed infants show an apparent decline in growth from 6 to 9 months when compared with formula-fed infants, which may lead a provider to falsely conclude that the infant is not growing well. It is essential to assess developmental progress (see Chapter 5) and other measures of growth in all infants, as well as height, weight, and occipital frontal (OF) head circumference. Characteristics of a healthy breastfed infant include the following:
- Active and alert state
- Developmentally appropriate progress
- Age-appropriate height and OF head circumference
- Appropriate skin turgor and color
- Sufficient output of at least six wet diapers and several stools per day
- Contented and satisfied behavior after feeding

Urine Output Guidelines

In the first 2 days of life as the volume of breast milk is increasing, the infant may urinate only one to three times in 24 hours. By day 3, the infant should have three or more wet diapers in 24 hours; and by day 4, the infant should have four to six wet diapers per 24 hours. Over time, the infant should have a minimum of six to eight wet diapers in a 24-hour period. The urine should be light yellow with no strong odor. If parents are anxious or have a question about breastfeeding progress, a diary of wet diapers can aid the accurate assessment of progress. However, parents need to be alerted to the difficulty of doing accurate diaper counts with disposable diapers and may elect to insert a tissue liner into the diaper or to use cloth diapers for the first few weeks.

Stool Output Guidelines

In the first 24 hours after delivery, the baby should have at least one meconium stool followed by another on the second day of life. By the third day, stools are beginning to make the transition to the characteristic loose, yellow, seedy stools of breastfeeding, and the infant should begin having two to three stools in 24 hours. That number may continue to increase in the first few weeks of life. Some breastfed infants stool with every feeding. After the first month, the pattern may change again because some infants begin to stool less frequently and may go several days between stools. As long as the infant is healthy and gaining weight, there is no problem. However, infrequent stooling, especially in the first month, should stimulate a feeding history and possibly a weight check to make sure that the infant is getting enough breast milk.

Maternal Nutritional Needs During Breastfeeding

Maternal nutritional needs change during lactation. The characteristics of an appropriate diet in breastfeeding mothers are similar to that of a pregnant woman and include (Brown, 2016):
- Daily caloric intake of 300 extra calories over the prepregnancy recommendations based on weight and activity
- Water intake of 3.4 L/day
- Generous intake of fruits and vegetables, whole grain breads and cereals, calcium-rich dairy products, and protein-rich fish, meats, and legumes
- Rich sources of calcium, zinc, folate, magnesium, and vitamin B_6
- Supplementation with calcium if mother is avoiding dairy
- Supplementation of vitamin D if deficient

The mother should be encouraged to eat well for her own sake to keep herself healthy and to meet the energy demands of nursing. In addition, an adequate intake of fluid is necessary, but excessive use of fluids does not increase breast milk production. An easy guideline to remember for adequate fluid intake is maternal urine that is light yellow and has no strong odor. Eligible mothers and infants should be referred to the Women, Infants, and Children (WIC) special supplemental food program for nutritional counseling and for food supplements. Most WIC programs offer food supplements for the breastfeeding mother's diet because she does not need formula for the infant. Even with a diet that is adequate in nutrients and calories, a gradual maternal weight loss of 1 to 2 pounds per month usually occurs. In fact, breastfeeding is the ideal way to support a mother in returning to her prepregnancy weight.

No foods need to be routinely excluded from the maternal diet, unless there is evidence that a particular food bothers the infant. For infants with colic, mothers may wish to reduce or eliminate allergenic foods (e.g., cow's milk, eggs, peanuts, tree nuts, soy, fish, and wheat) in her diet; however, there is little evidence that elimination of foods is protective against colic symptoms. Certain foods, such as onions and garlic, may change the flavor and odor of the milk, but they do not negatively affect its quality. Infants begin to have exposure to the foods and flavors of their own culture through breast milk. The nutrient characteristics of breast milk are fairly stable.

The effects of alcohol intake on the breastfeeding infant occur in relation to the amount of alcohol the mother consumes and the timing of breastfeeding. Alcohol clears from breast milk in the same manner as it does from the mother's plasma and one drink may take 2 to 3 hours to be eliminated (Brown, 2016). Breastfeeding should occur when the mother is feeling neurologically normal (Hale, 2017).

Moderate intake of caffeine (1 to 2 cups of coffee per day) will not cause concerns for the infant. On the other hand, excessive caffeine consumption should be avoided until the infant is able to metabolize caffeine, which occurs at approximately 2 to 4 months of age (Brown, 2016).

Medications for Breastfeeding Mothers

Frequently, women question whether they can take certain medications while breastfeeding. Concerns relate primarily to two areas: (1) the effect of the drug on maternal milk supply and (2) the effect of the drug on the infant. General guidelines for providers related to maternal drug use include the following:
- Give drugs that are normally safe for infants or have been tested in infants.
- Avoid long-acting forms of a drug.
- Schedule feeding at times when the drug level is lowest. Often, breastfeeding immediately after taking the drug is the safest time.
- Observe the infant for changes in feeding pattern, fussiness, vomiting or diarrhea, or rash.
- Consider all appropriate options and select the drug with the lowest level in breast milk.
- Avoid drugs that inhibit prolactin release, such as estrogen, antihistamines, and ergot compounds.
- Be cautious about the use of herbal preparations.

Not all references available to providers offer adequate up-to-date information. Decisions about drug selection are difficult, especially when contraindicated drugs are being considered. The consequences of weaning and loss of breast milk for the infant must always be included in the deliberations. A comprehensive drug reference should be readily available for providers. Three excellent lactation-specific drug references are shown in Box 16.2.

Returning to Work

Women who return to work outside the home after initiating breastfeeding should be encouraged to continue breastfeeding and be supported in their decision with accurate information about how to manage both work and breastfeeding. Supporting the family in the mother's return to work includes education on how to best prepare for and make the adjustment back to the work environment (Box 16.3). The ideal work environment provides the following:

Hale TW, Rowe HE. *Medications and Mothers' Milk 2017*. 17th ed. Plano, TX: Hale Publishing; 2014. Updated and reprinted every other year.

U.S. National Library of Medicine, National Institutes of Health, Health & Human Services. LactMed: a TOXNET database, TOXNET. www.toxnet.nlm.nih.gov/newtoxnet/lactmed.htm. Accessed April 5, 2019. Updated weekly.

Woo TM, Wynne AL. *Pharmacotherapeutics for Advanced Practice Nurse Prescribers*. 4th ed. Philadelphia: FA Davis; 2015.

• BOX 16.3 Advice for Mothers on Returning to Work

Before Delivery

Discuss plans with employer before maternity leave and gain support of coworkers.

Provide employer with information to help in planning (see www.usbreastfeeding.org).

Discuss options with other employees who continued to breastfeed after returning to work.

Investigate pumps, including rental or purchase.

Identify a place to pump and to store breast milk at work.

During Maternity Leave

Practice method of breast milk expression that will be used at work (approximately 2-3 weeks).

Begin freezing milk. After the baby feeds at each breast, pump each breast and freeze in disposable milk bags. Although the amount will be small initially, the supply will increase with continued pumping.

Introduce bottle after breastfeeding is well established (usually approximately 3-4 weeks).

After Return to Work

If possible, arrange work hours to maximize times to nurse infant (e.g., arrive at work at 8:30 instead of 8:00).

Have a picture of your baby at the pump.

Plan on 15-30 minutes to complete pumping.

Wear clothes with easy access to breasts.

If possible, have caregiver bring baby for one feed each day.

Wash hands before and after pumping.

Rinse pump parts with cool water, then wash with dish detergent, and rinse well after each use.

Feeding Breast Milk

Warm or thaw milk in warm water. (Do not use microwave, because milk heats unevenly and presents a risk for burns.)

Refrigerate thawed milk for no more than 24 hours; do not refreeze.

Do not add milk to a bottle that has already been used.

- A location dedicated to pumping breast milk that is private, is convenient, and has access to a sink for washing up and a refrigerator for storage
- Breaks and lunchtime consisting of a reasonable amount of time in which the mother can pump or go to the infant: The average time needed to set up equipment, express milk, and clean up is between 20 and 30 minutes.
- Supportive colleagues and supervisors
- Maximum of 8 hours of work per day if possible

In addition to providing support and information to the mother, providers can advocate for community and corporate initiatives that promote these conditions in work settings. Women are more likely to continue breastfeeding if they have workplace support. Moreover, employers benefit from breastfeeding mothers, whose infants tend to be healthier; therefore the mother has fewer work absences and productivity increases (AAP, 2012). There are many resources available to employers to support lactation programs in their workplaces (see Additional Resources).

The National Conference of State Legislatures (NCSL) maintains a database on laws related to breastfeeding, including breastfeeding in public and breastfeeding in the workplace. Twenty-eight states, the District of Columbia, and Puerto Rico currently have laws specifically related to work and breastfeeding. Individual practitioners can access this website for an update on the laws in their location (www.ncsl.org/research/health/breastfeeding-state-laws.aspx) (NCSL, 2017).

Common Breastfeeding Problems

Flat or Inverted Nipples

A nipple can look as though it is inverted; however, a "pinch test" is necessary to determine what happens to the nipple during breastfeeding. If the nipple pulls in, it is inverted. If the nipple does not pull in, as happens most often, or everts with compression, it is considered to be flat.

Inverted nipples can make it more difficult for the infant to latch on in the early days because it is harder to pull the nipple into the mouth for suckling. As the baby continues to breastfeed, the nipple tissue elongates; with time, the problem usually becomes less severe, and successful breastfeeding is possible. Flat nipples do not generally change over time; rather, the infant develops a style to more easily latch on successfully. Adhesions cause retraction or inversion of the nipples. Flat nipples are often found in women with larger, pendulous breasts.

Differential Diagnosis

The differential diagnosis for flat or inverted nipples is dimpled, fissured, or unusually shaped nipples.

Management

Prenatal. If the patient is not at risk for preterm labor, breast shells can be used during the third trimester for inverted nipples. The obstetrician or nurse-midwife should be notified before their use. Shells are plastic, dome-shaped devices with small holes for ventilation. An opening in the portion that lies against the skin fits over the nipple, and gentle suction during use helps stretch the nipple tissue. The bra cup holds the shell comfortably in place, and the use of shells during the last trimester generally helps to stretch out adhesions in preparation for breastfeeding.

Postpartum. The provider should stay with the mother during early feeding attempts; give extra praise, reassurance, and support; and emphasize the need for extra patience and persistence. Encourage use of the football-hold position during feedings and have the mother lean slightly forward as she latches the baby on to her nipple.

Helpful suggestions for mothers:
- Wear breast shells between feedings.
- Manually pull or roll the nipple immediately before latch-on.
- Use a breast pump for 1 or 2 minutes before latch-on.
- Put a cold cloth or ice on the nipple for a few seconds before latch-on.
- Use a nipple shield to cover the nipple because it provides a rigid teat that may help the infant to latch.

- Avoid pacifiers and bottle nipples until the infant is 4 to 6 weeks old.
- If supplementation is medically indicated, use a syringe, dropper, feeding tube, or supplemental nutrition system.

Complications

Complications of flat or inverted nipples include frustration and loss of confidence; inadequate infant nutrition and its sequelae; severe maternal engorgement, plugged ducts, or mastitis related to milk stasis; and discontinued breastfeeding.

Sore Nipples

Nipple soreness is acute pain caused by irritation or trauma to the nipples and areola, often accompanied by a breakdown in skin integrity. Sore nipples have many causes, including:
- Improper latch-on and positioning at the breast
- Prolonged negative pressure
- Inappropriate suction release from the breast
- Use of or sensitivity to nipple creams and oils
- Incorrect use of breastfeeding supplies (e.g., pumps, shells, shields)
- Thrush (candidiasis)
- Leaking nipples that are not properly air-dried

Clinical Findings

The nipples, areolae, and breasts are tender, bruised, raw, cracked, bleeding, blistered, discolored, swollen, or traumatized.

Differential Diagnosis

The differential diagnoses for sore nipples include the following:
- Mild tenderness, which is sometimes described by new mothers as they are getting used to the infant's suckling
- Breast or nipple trauma from another cause
- Thrush (candidiasis)
- Mastitis/abscess
- Milk plugs at the nipple pores

Management

Prevention of sore nipples includes the early assessment of breastfeeding and latching, supporting the mother in various breastfeeding positions, and education about the use and maintenance of breastfeeding supplies.

The following measures can be taken to manage sore nipples:
- Assess breastfeeding at an early feeding. Prevent the problem by demonstrating and reinforcing the proper latch-on technique and positioning of the infant.
- Counsel mothers to seek help early for more than mild tenderness. Nipples can be damaged by constant high negative pressure and do not "toughen up" as breastfeeding progresses. Cracking and bleeding are not normal.
- Rub a few drops of colostrum or milk onto the nipple and areola after every feeding, and let it air-dry.
- Expose the nipples to air for short periods several times a day.
- Use breast shells to prevent the bra or clothing from rubbing against the nipple.
- Nurse from the least sore side first and use short, frequent feedings.
- Use a nipple shield during feedings to allow the nipple to heal.
- Pump the affected breast if pain is too severe to allow nursing.
- Use mild analgesics, as necessary.
- Refer to a lactation specialist as appropriate.

Severe Engorgement

Severe engorgement is characterized by bilateral intense fullness, soreness, and swelling of the breasts, beyond the normal fullness experienced as the milk transitions in volume. Engorgement is caused by milk stasis in the breast from inadequate emptying.

Clinical Findings

The following are seen in severe engorgement:
- Painful, hard, lumpy, swollen breasts
- Breasts usually warm to the touch
- Nipples flattened by the swelling

Differential Diagnosis

The differential diagnosis for severe engorgement is bilateral mastitis.

Management

The following are strategies to prevent severe engorgement:
- Nurse frequently, and make certain that latch-on and position are correct and audible swallowing is heard.
- Avoid long stretches between feedings in the early weeks as the milk supply is being established. Pump or express the breasts if a feeding will be missed.

If engorgement occurs, the following measures can be taken to manage engorgement:
- Take a hot shower, lean over the sink, and allow the water to run over the breasts, or wrap the breasts with warm, wet compresses for 5 to 10 minutes before nursing.
- Gently massage the entire breast or use an electric pump with intermittent suction on the minimal setting for several minutes after using wet heat to empty the excess milk in the breasts.
- Manually express milk before feeding to soften the areola and make it easier for the infant to latch on properly.

Mastitis

Lactational mastitis is an infection of the breast that can occur at any time during lactation, including pregnancy; *Staphylococcus aureus* is commonly reported as the causative agent.

Predisposing factors include:
- Stress, fatigue
- Cracked nipples, plugged ducts
- Constricting, improperly fitting bra
- Inadequate emptying of the breast
- Sudden weaning or a significant decrease in the number of feedings

Clinical Findings

The following are commonly noted in mastitis:
- Malaise
- Breast tenderness or pain
- A reddened, warm lump in any quadrant, sometimes associated with red streaking (Fig 16.11)
- Flulike symptoms, including fever, chills, and body aches. In general, flulike symptoms in a lactating woman are considered mastitis unless proven otherwise.

Differential Diagnosis

Differential diagnoses for mastitis include plugged ducts, severe engorgement, and breast abscess. Inflammatory breast cancer should be considered when appropriate treatment does not lead to resolution of symptoms.

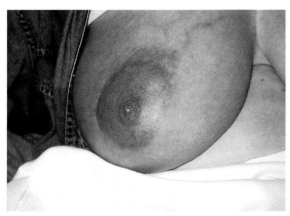

• Fig 16.11 Lactational Mastitis Characterized by Redness and Streaking Along the Duct. (From Goerke K, Junginger C. *Pflege konkret Gynäkologie Geburtshilfe: Lehrbuch für Pflegeberufe.* München: Elsevier; 2018.)

Management

Prevention of mastitis includes:
- Frequent breastfeeding
- Attending to cracked or sore nipples immediately
- Treatment of plugged ducts or blocked nipple pore with a warm compress, breast massage, and lecithin supplementation (reducing milk viscosity) (Lawrence and Lawrence, 2016)
- Oral *Lactobacillus salivarius* PS2 probiotics taken in late pregnancy appear to have a preventative effect on lactational mastitis (Fernández et al., 2016).

Recommendations for treatment of mastitis include the following:
- Empty the breast. Breast milk is not infected, and frequent breastfeeding should continue. If the breast is unable to be emptied through feeding at the breast, pump after the feeding has ended.
- Increase fluids, and use analgesics as necessary.
- Antibiotic use is considered when conservative management and supportive care are ineffective and symptoms persist beyond 12 to 24 hours. Treatment should be maintained for 10 to 14 days. Dicloxacillin, cephalexin, or clindamycin may be used for initial treatment of nonsevere mastitis in the absence of risk factors, such as methicillin-resistant *S. aureus* (MRSA) infection (Jahanfar et al., 2013). Mastitis that is not responsive to empiric antibiotic use should be evaluated for possible MRSA and treated appropriately (Amir, 2014).
- Rest (extremely important for healing).
- Take warm showers, or use warm wet compresses.
- Do not wean abruptly because of the possibility of mastitis progressing into an abscess.

Complications

Abscess and septicemia are potential complications of mastitis.

Nipple Preference

Nipple preference (also referred to as nipple confusion) occurs when an infant is accustomed to nursing from a bottle and is introduced to the breast. Different oral-motor skills are used in breastfeeding and bottle feeding, and infants who have been given a bottle or pacifier sometimes attempt to breastfeed using the same sucking pattern as with a bottle. This can make it difficult to obtain adequate nourishment and may contribute to maternal sore nipples. The infant may cry, fuss, or push away with their arms during attempts to nurse because they have become accustomed to feeding from a synthetic nipple and prefer the ease of sucking from it.

Clinical Findings

The following are seen in nipple preference: ineffective suckling at the breast; breast refusal; or sore, red, or bruised maternal nipples.

Differential Diagnosis

The differential diagnoses for nipple confusion are other causes of fussiness and refusal to feed (e.g., oral thrush, colic, gastroesophageal reflux disease).

Management

The following are recommended to manage nipple confusion:
- Avoid all rubber bottle nipples and pacifiers for the first 4 to 6 weeks or until the infant is breastfeeding successfully, unless absolutely necessary.
- Consult with a lactation specialist to retrain the infant to suck correctly at the breast by correct positioning, proper latch-on technique, suck training to repattern tongue movements, and supplementation via alternative methods if required.
- If supplements are medically indicated, give with an eyedropper, spoon, syringe, or cup or through a 5-Fr feeding tube (attached to a 20- or 30-mL syringe) taped to the areola or breast. The end of the tubing protrudes slightly past the end of the nipple so that the tube, nipple, and areola are in the infant's mouth.
- Using a thin silicone nipple shield may help the infant to successfully latch on. The shield may be used with the initial latch and then removed when the nipple has everted and the infant is sucking well. Cleansing and drying both the shields and breast after feeding are important to prevent skin breakdown and infection.

Complications

The following are complications of ongoing nipple preference: failure to thrive, hyperbilirubinemia, colic and crying, prolonged feedings, sore and cracked nipples, plugged ducts, mastitis, and frustration.

Breast Milk Jaundice

Breast milk physiologic jaundice is an elevated serum indirect bilirubin concentration, with the peak level occurring after the first week of life in an infant drinking an adequate amount of breast milk with no other signs of liver abnormality. The exact cause of breast milk jaundice is unknown; however, it is believed that an enzyme may be present in some mothers' milk that inhibits the action of glucuronyl transferase in the newborn, an enzyme which causes intestinal reabsorption of bilirubin. Breastfeeding jaundice (also called suboptimal intake jaundice) occurs in the first 2 to 7 days of life and is associated with low levels of intake, whereas breast milk jaundice may occur in infants with adequate transfer and consumption of breast milk (Academy of Breastfeeding Medicine Protocol Committee [ABM], 2017b).

Clinical Findings

Physical Examination. The following are seen with breast milk jaundice:
- Healthy and thriving infant
- Adequate stooling and voiding
- Appropriate weight gain
- Appearance of elevated bilirubin levels between day 7 and 10 of life
- Bilirubin peaks at approximately day 10 to 15
- Persistence up to the third month of life

Diagnostic Tests. The following tests are usually indicated: initial screening may use transcutaneous bilirubin (TcB) measurement; total serum bilirubin (TSB); and urine and other cultures, which are sometimes necessary to rule out infection.

Differential Diagnosis

The differential diagnosis for breast milk jaundice is pathologic jaundice.

Management

Encourage families to continue breastfeeding unless clinical signs of pathologic jaundice are observed. Rarely does breastfeeding need to be discontinued in an infant with breast milk jaundice. See Chapter 29.

Oral Candidiasis (Thrush)

When oral candidiasis is diagnosed in the infant or found on the nipple or areolae of the nursing mother, both members of the dyad should be treated. See Chapter 29.

Poor Weight Gain

Problems associated with poor weight gain occur at two different times and represent different challenges for management. During the newborn period, initiation of breastfeeding may not proceed normally, and the infant may actually continue to lose weight or, at best, gain very slowly. After the newborn period, infants may gain weight more slowly than expected given normal parameters for their age.

Poor weight gain has a number of contributing factors, including the following:

- Maternal: Infrequent or inadequate feeding because of poorly managed breastfeeding or environmental or social circumstances in the family system. In the first days after birth, this can occur because of the number of visitors the mother receives, making it difficult to breastfeed often enough to establish breast milk supply.
- Inadequate milk production
- Genetic predisposition, infection, organic disease
- Physical anomaly that prevents good suckling or swallowing

Clinical Findings

The following may be seen in poor weight gain:

Infant Factors
- Continued weight loss after 5 to 7 days old
- Failure to regain birth weight by 2 to 3 weeks old
- Failure to maintain an ongoing weight gain of 0.5 to 1 oz/day
- Weight below the third percentile for age (this finding can be a pattern over time or a sudden change)
- Lethargic, sleepy, inactive, unresponsive infant
- Newborn or young infant sleeping longer than 4 hours between feedings
- Dry mucous membranes, poor skin turgor

Technique Factors
- Ineffective latch-on or sucking
- Short time at the breast (the infant is removed before nursing is finished, thus reducing access to lipid dense milk and total consumption)
- Infant kept on a preset schedule despite cues for more feeding
- Infant given water between feedings to "get through" to the next feeding

- Infant encouraged or allowed to sleep through the night before 8 to 12 weeks old
- Fewer than eight feedings in 24 hours
- Infant fed in a distracting environment
- Infant in a day care setting that does not facilitate breastfeeding

Maternal Factors
- Does not initially respond to infant's cues for feeding or does not recognize that waking is needed to establish feeding
- Hectic schedule with limited time for breastfeeding
- Recent illness or significant weight loss
- Uses oral contraceptives or other hormones that decrease production of breast milk. Women wishing to use hormonal contraceptives that contain estrogen should wait until 6 months after birth when breast milk supply is well established and the infant is beginning to consume solids.

Differential Diagnosis

The differential diagnoses for poor weight gain are a pattern of slower but normal weight gain in healthy breastfed infants and failure to thrive.

Management

The following measures should be taken to manage poor weight gain:

- Complete a thorough history to elicit information regarding infant and maternal factors.
- Conduct a thorough assessment of breastfeeding techniques to accurately determine the extent to which mismanagement is a cause.
- Be alert for any infant who has lost too much weight and is unable to feed with vigor at the breast; such infants require an immediate infusion of calories for energy.
- Use a supplemental system at the breast if supplementation with expressed breast milk or formula is required.
- Provide instruction, encouragement, and reinforcement for correct breastfeeding techniques.
- Encourage and reassure the parents.
- Refer for treatment of physical or organic causes.

Complications

Complications of poor weight gain include developmental delay, poor bonding, and severe dehydration. In situations of early failure to establish breastfeeding, some infants may appear to be in a septic state and require hospitalization for rehydration and further evaluation.

Additional Resources

Ameda. www.ameda.com

Breast pumps and breastfeeding products. Australian Breastfeeding Association. https://www.breastfeeding.asn.au/

Human Milk Banking Association of North America. www.hmbana.org

Guidelines and information on human milk banking; a clearinghouse for member milk banks. International Board of Lactation Consultant Examiners (IBLCE). www.iblce.org

International board certification program for lactation consultants. International Lactation Consultant Association (ILCA). www.ilca.org

Annual conference with continuing education programs and peer-reviewed professional journal, *Journal of Human Lactation*

Kelly Mom Parenting and Breastfeeding. https://kellymom.com/

Evidence-based information on breastfeeding and parenting. Lactation Education Resources. www.lactationtraining.com/

Education materials and training course; parent handouts. La Leche League International. www.lalecheleague.org

Educational materials for breastfeeding families; annual workshops for lactation consultants and primary care providers. March of Dimes. www.marchofdimes.org/hbhb/

Healthy babies: Healthy business. Medela, Inc. www.medela.com

Breast pumps and breastfeeding products, referral hotline for consumers, and corporate lactation program. National Alliance for Breastfeeding Advocacy. United States Breastfeeding Committee (USBC). www.usbreastfeeding.org/

National group to promote and support breastfeeding. U.S. National Library of Medicine: TOXNET, Toxicology Data Network. www.toxnet.nlm.nih.gov

Up-to-date information on drugs and breastfeeding. WHO Global Data Bank on Infant and Young Child Feeding. www.who.int/nutrition/databases/infantfeeding/en/index.html

International information and links on infant, child, and maternal nutrition; links to WHO/UNICEF Baby-Friendly Hospital Initiative. Work and Pump. www.workandpump.com/

References

Academy of Breastfeeding Medicine Protocol Committee. ABM clinical protocol #8: human milk storage information for home use for full-term infants (original protocol March 2004; revision 2017). *Breastfeeding Med.* 2017a;12(5):390–395.

Academy of Breastfeeding Medicine Protocol Committee. ABM clinical protocol #22: guidelines for management of jaundice in the breastfeeding infant 35 weeks or more of gestation – Revised 2017. *Breastfeeding Med.* 2017b;12(7):250–257.

Al Mamun A, O'Callaghan M, Williams GM, Najman JM, Callaway L, McIntyre HD. Breastfeeding is protective to diabetes risk in young adults: a longitudinal study. *Acta Diabetologica.* 2015;52:837–844.

American Academy of Family Physicians (AAFP). *Breastfeeding, policy statement*; 2014. www.aafp.org/about/policies/all/breastfeeding-support.html. Accessed March 14, 2019.

American Academy of Pediatrics (AAP). Breastfeeding and the use of human milk. *Pediatrics.* 2012;129(3):827–841.

American Academy of Pediatrics (AAP). Prevention of rickets and vitamin d deficiency in infants, children and adolescents. *Pediatrics.* 2008;122(5):1142–1152.

Amir L. ABM Clinical protocol #4: mastitis. *Breastfeeding Med.* 2014;9(5):239–243.

Association of Women's Health, Obstetric and Neonatal Nurses (AWHONN). *Breastfeeding, position statement*; 2015. www.awhonn.org/?Breastfeeding. Accessed March 16, 2019.

Baby-Friendly USA. *Find Facilities*; 2018. https://www.babyfriendlyusa.org/find-facilities. Accessed March 14, 2019.

Bartick MC, Schwarz EB, Green BD, et al. Suboptimal breastfeeding in the United States: maternal and pediatric health outcomes and costs. *Matern Child Nutr.* 2017;13(1).

Brenner-Jones CG, Eikelboom RH, Jacques A, et al. Protective benefit of predominant breastfeeding against otitis media may be limited to early childhood: results from a prospective birth cohort study. *Clin Otolaryngol.* 2017;42:29–37.

Brown J. *Nutrition Through the Life Cycle*. 6th ed. Stamford, CT: Cengade Learning; 2016.

Busch DW, Logan K, Wilkinson A. Breastfeeding recommendations for primary care: applying a tri-core breastfeeding conceptual model. *J Ped Health Care.* 2014;8(6):486–496.

Centers for Disease Control and Prevention (CDC) Division of Nutrition. Physical Activity, and Obesity (DNPAO). *Breastfeeding report card*; 2014. www.cdc.gov/breastfeeding/pdf/2014breastfeedingreportcard.pdf. Accessed March 19, 2019.

Centers for Disease Control and Prevention (CDC). *WHO Growth Standards Are Recommended for Use in the U.S. For Infants and Children to 2 Years of Age*; 2010. https://www.cdc.gov/growthcharts/who_charts.htm. Accessed March 28, 2019.

den Dekker HT, Sonnenschien-van der Voort AMM, Jaddoe VWV, Reiss IK, de Jongste JC, Duijst L. Breastfeeding and asthma outcomes at the age of 6 years: the generation R study. *Pediatric Allergy Immunol.* 2016;27:486–492.

Fernández L, Cardenes N, Arroyo R, et al. Prevention of infections mastitis by oral administration of Lactobacillus salivarius PS2 during late pregnancy. *Clin Infec Dis.* 2016;62(5):568.

Ghaheri B, Cle M, Fausel S, Choup M, Mace J. Breastfeeding improvement following tongue-tie and lip-tie release: a prospective cohort study. *Laryngoscope.* 2017;127(5):1217–1223.

Hale T. *Medications and Mothers' Milk*. Springer Publishing; 2017.

Hansstein F. The impact of breastfeeding on early childhood obesity: evidence from the national survey of children's health. *Am J Health Promotion.* 2016;30(4):250–259.

Hollis B, Wagner C, Howard C, et al. Maternal versus infant vitamin D supplementation during lactation: a randomized controlled trial. *Pediatrics.* 2015;136(4):625–634.

Jackson K, Harris W. Should there be a target level of docosahexaenoic acid in breast milk? *Curr Opin Clin Nutr Metab Care.* 2016;19(2):92–96.

Jahanfar S, Ng CJ, Teng CL. Antibiotics for mastitis in breastfeeding women. *Cochrane Database Syst Rev.* 2013;2:CD005458.

Lawrence RA, Lawrence RM. *Breastfeeding: a Guide for the Medical Profession.* 8th ed. St. Louis: Elsevier/Mosby; 2016.

Lessen R, Kavenaugh K. Position of the academy of nutrition and dietetics: promoting and supporting breastfeeding. *J Acad Nutr Diet.* 2015;115(3).

National Association of Pediatric Nurse Practitioners. NAPNAP position statement on breastfeeding. *J Pediatr Health Care.* 2013;27(1):e13–e15.

National Conference of State Legislatures (NCSL). *Breastfeeding state laws*; 2017. www.ncsl.org/research/health/breastfeeding-state-laws.aspx. Accessed April 30, 2019.

Nguyen B, Jin K, Ding D. Breastfeeding and maternal cardiovascular risk factors and outcomes: a systematic review. *PLoS One.* 2017.

Paul IM, Schaefer EW, Miller JR, et al. Weight change nomograms for the first month after birth. *Pediatrics.* 2016;138(6).

Ross-Cowerdy M, Lewis CA, Papic M, Corbelli J, Schwarz EB. Counseling about the maternal health benefits of breastfeeding and mothers' intentions to breastfeed. *Matern Child Health J.* 2017;21:234–241.

Sriraman NK, Evans AE, Lawrence R, Noble L, and the Academy of Breastfeeding Medicine's Board of Directors Breastfeeding Medicine. Academy of Breastfeeding Medicine's 2017 position statement on informal breast milk sharing for the term healthy infant. *Breastfeeding Med.* 2018;13(1). https://doi.org/10.1089/bfm.2017.29064.nks. Mary Ann Liebert, Inc.

Thompson JMD, Tanabe K, Moon TY, et al. Duration of breastfeeding and risk of SIDS An individual participant data meta-analysis. *Child Maternal Health News.* 2017;140(5). https://childhealthnews.wordpress.com/2017/11/10/duration-of-breastfeeding-and-risk-of-sids-an-individual-participant-data-meta-analysis/. Accessed May 5, 2019.

United Nations International Children's Emergency Fund (UNICEF). *Baby-friendly hospital initiative training materials*; 2009. www.unicef.org/nutrition/index_24850.html?q=printme. Accessed March 16, 2019.

U.S. Department of Health and Human Services (HHS). *Maternal, infant and child health, morbidity and mortality: MICH-22: Increase the proportion of employers that have worksite lactation support programs*; 2014. www.healthypeople.gov/2020/topics-objectives/topic/maternal-infant-and-child-health/objectives?topicId=26. Accessed March 14, 2019.

Walker M. *Breastfeeding Management for the Clinician: Using the Evidence.* 4th ed. Burlington: Jones & Bartlett; 2016.

World Health Organization. *Baby friendly hospital initiative*; 2018. www.who.int/nutrition/topics/bfhi/en/. Accessed March 14, 2019.

World Health Organization/United. *Nations International Children's Emergency Fund (WHO/UNICEF). Protecting, promoting and supporting breastfeeding: the special role of maternity services: a joint WHO/UNICEF statement.* Geneva: World Health Organization; 1989.

17

Nutrition

ARDYS M. DUNN AND KAREN G. DUDERSTADT

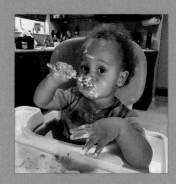

Optimal nutrition is the foundation for healthy physical and mental growth and development in infants, children, and adolescents. Children's ability to interact with their environment, to be curious, to explore and learn, and to have sufficient energy for exercise can be compromised without adequate nutrition. It is also essential for healing during acute conditions and successful management of chronic health conditions.

The goals of pediatric primary care providers (PCPs) are to assess if children are meeting their recommended daily dietary intake for age and weight/height ratio and to prevent any problems related to nutrition. To accomplish this, the PCPs must conduct thorough assessments, provide age-appropriate anticipatory guidance, develop clear and appropriate treatment plans, and refer the child and family to a pediatric nutritionist if needed. Dietary principles to guide PCPs include:

- Children's nutritional needs vary as they grow and are influenced by their state of health.
- A wide range of food choices and feeding behaviors are used to meet nutritional needs.
- Daily reference intakes (DRIs) are *guidelines* only.
- Parents and other caregivers are responsible for providing food choices that are nutritionally adequate and for establishing healthy eating patterns; to do so, they must be well informed.
- Family patterns of nutrition and eating are based on social, economic, cultural, and psychological dynamics.
- The PCP is a source of information regarding nutrition, feeding patterns, and healthy eating.
- The PCP works with a team of specialists including registered dietitians and nutritionists to manage children's nutrition status when providing care to children with nutritionally related challenges.

This chapter presents nutritional requirements of infants, children, and adolescents, as well as strategies providers can use regarding nutrition to help children be their healthiest. Nutritional standards are listed, followed by a review of the functions of specific nutrients in the body and the DRIs for these nutrients. These standards are recommendations—not requirements—and are often given as a range (e.g., 25% to 35% of energy intake in the form of fat), which reinforces the concept that there is latitude in healthy nutritional intake.

Pediatric Dietary Guidelines

The American Academy of Pediatrics (AAP) recommends exclusive breastfeeding until approximately 6 months old and continued breastfeeding, supplemented with appropriate foods for infants, for the first year or longer as mutually desired by mother and infant (AAP Section on Breastfeeding, 2012). The AAP also recommends 400 International units (IU) of vitamin D for all breastfed infants until they are 1 year old and for all children and adolescents during periods of rapid growth, particularly those with diets deficient in vitamin D (Kleinman and Greer, 2013). The National Committee for Quality Assurance (NCQA) recommends assessment of body mass index (BMI) for all children 3 to 17 years old (NCQA, 2018). The U.S. Preventive Services Task Force (USPSTF) recommends interventions to promote and support breastfeeding, that children ages 6 years and older be screened for obesity, and that children who are overweight or obese be given, or referred for, comprehensive intensive behavioral interventions to improve weight (USPSTF, 2017). The Institute of Medicine (IOM) has published ways to ensure that school food programs meet current dietary recommendations (IOM Committee on Nutrition Standards for National School Lunch and Breakfast Programs et al., 2010). *Bright Futures in Practice: Nutrition* (Holt and Wooldridge, 2011) presents nutritional guidelines, discusses issues and concerns related to pediatric nutrition, and outlines tools for providers to assess and manage nutrition in children.

The Food and Nutrition Board (FNB) of the National Academies of Science and the National Academy of Medicine list DRIs based on diets consumed in the United States and Canada. The DRIs include four categories of values (Box 17.1). DRIs identify parameters of nutrient intake that will meet body needs and prevent adverse effects of excessive intake. However, they do not set a standard basal requirement below which the diet is judged inadequate and can lead to pathology nor a standard that is sufficient for the body to maintain a healthy body reserve (normative requirement). The U.S. Department of Health and Human Services (HHS) and U.S. Department of Agriculture (USDA) publish Dietary Guidelines for Americans based on extensive analysis of scientific evidence on diet and nutrition and referencing the DRIs developed by the FNB. These guidelines address questions of nutritional adequacy, energy balance, weight management, and food safety and technology. They also make recommendations regarding intake of macronutrients, micronutrients, water, cholesterol, salt, and alcohol (HHS and USDA, 2015). These resources can assist families and providers to make healthful dietary decisions to meet the nutritional needs of individual children.

The authors acknowledge the work of Pamela Anain as an expert reviewer for the chapter.

Nutritional Requirements and Dietary Reference Intakes

The body requires energy, water, electrolytes, macronutrients, and micronutrients to survive. The nutritional requirements vary significantly by age, health status, and activity level.

Energy

Three body processes require energy, which is measured in kilocalories:

- Basal metabolism, primarily regulatory functions: respiration, digestion, temperature regulation, circulation, and so on. Most of the body's energy is used for this function, measured in basal metabolic rate (BMR) or resting energy expenditure (REE).
- Growth, which is greatest in infancy and adolescence.
- Activity, exercise, and other metabolic demands, including illness.

The body meets these energy demands, or estimated energy requirement (EER), by using stored energy sources or calories consumed on a daily basis. Macronutrients (protein, carbohydrates, and fats) and alcohol provide calories that supply energy. Caloric intake for children is recommended to be distributed among the three macronutrients, with each providing a certain percentage of total daily caloric intake. These recommendations are given as an acceptable macronutrient distribution range (AMDR) and are available at http://nationalacademies. org/hmd/~/media/Files/Activity Files/Nutrition/DRI-Tables/8_ Macronutrient Summary.pdf. They are based on age for children who are of average height, weight, and physical activity level. If more calories than those required for energy needs are consumed, they will be converted to fat and stored. The body requires essential nutrients and energy for growth and health. A diet high in calories (calorie dense) but low in nutrients (nutrient poor, consisting of what is often referred to as "empty calories") will result in excess weight gain, and the child will be undernourished. Data from the National Health and Nutrition Examination Survey (NHANES) show that 33% of American children's total energy intake came from empty calories as solid fat and added sugar (Poti et al., 2014).

Water

Water is the primary component of body tissue, and maintaining fluid balance is essential to good health. Because of the wide variation of healthful intake and output, there is no specific recommended daily requirement for water (Rush, 2013). Thirst is an adequate indicator of the need to take in more water. However, children do not always appreciate the feeling of thirst and may need to be offered water or foods that contain water. Infants present special concerns because they have a large skin surface per unit of body weight, their renal systems are not fully mature to process solutes, they have a high daily water turnover (up to 15% of body weight), and they are unable to express thirst. All of these factors make infants uniquely susceptible to rapid variations in water balance.

Water loss is increased by illness, activity, high altitude, high ambient temperature, and dry air. When more than 10% of body weight is lost without replacement, dehydration can become life threatening. If a child is vomiting and has diarrhea, water loss can be significant. Children who exercise strenuously, especially in a warm, dry environment, require additional water intake. However, after strenuous or prolonged exercise, high water intake without electrolyte replacement can lead to water intoxication See Chapter 19 for a discussion regarding dehydration and fluid intake after exercise.

Electrolytes

Sodium

Sodium functions primarily to regulate extracellular fluid volume. It also regulates osmolarity, acid-base balance, and the membrane potential of cells and is involved in the cell membrane transport pump, exchanging with potassium in intracellular fluid. Sodium loss occurs with vomiting, diarrhea, and perspiration. Sodium requirements vary with the rate of extracellular fluid expansion, which is most rapid in infants and very young children. It is not necessary to add sodium to the diet, even for children who exercise and perspire heavily. Most children on a typical American diet far exceed minimum requirements for sodium intake, with most sodium coming from salt added during food processing and manufacturing. For children 1 to 3 years old, 1000 mg/day is considered an adequate intake of sodium; for children 4 to 8 years old, the adequate intake is 1200 mg/day; and for children 9 to 18 years old, it is 1500 mg/day (FNB and IOM, 2005).

Potassium

Potassium helps to maintain intracellular homeostasis and contributes to muscle contractility and transmission of nerve impulses. Severe potassium deficit (hypokalemia) can lead to cardiac dysrhythmias and death. Excessive potassium (hyperkalemia) can cause cardiac arrest. The urinary and gastrointestinal systems regulate potassium levels, and extreme imbalances are generally due to disease processes or medication rather than dietary factors. Potassium requirements increase as lean body mass increases and are higher during the rapid growth of infancy and adolescence than during middle childhood. Fruits, vegetables, and fresh meat have high potassium content.

Chloride

Chloride functions with sodium to maintain fluid and electrolyte balance. Loss of chloride occurs through the same routes as sodium loss: vomiting, diarrhea, and perspiration. The major source of chloride is salt (NaCl or KCl) added to foods during processing. There is no recommended daily allowance for chloride, but adequate amounts are ingested with a normal diet.

Macronutrients

Protein

Protein is a fundamental component of all body cells. Dietary protein is broken down into amino acids, which are required for the synthesis of body cell protein and nitrogen-containing compounds, some enzyme and hormone activity, cell transport, and tissue growth and development. Ten "indispensable" or essential amino acids are not synthesized by the body and must be provided in the diet (phenylalanine, leucine, methionine, lysine, isoleucine, valine, threonine, tryptophan, histidine, and arginine [arginine is required in the diet for infants but not adults]). Depending on their age, children should receive 5% to 30% of daily calories from proteins.

Protein and amino acid deficiencies rarely appear alone but follow other dietary deficits (such as insufficient carbohydrate intake), although young children are vulnerable to protein deficiency when cow's milk is replaced with low protein beverages, such as plant-based milk (e.g., rice, almond) (Le Louer et al., 2014). Extreme stress and disease can deplete nitrogen, a process that contributes to tissue wasting and creates an increased demand for protein. Growth needs of the premature infant require higher levels of protein intake than those of infants born at term. The demand for protein is not increased with normal activity except with illness or to build additional muscle tissue during body conditioning.

Carbohydrates

Carbohydrates are the body's major dietary source of energy. More than half (45% to 65%) of children's body energy requirements should be supplied by carbohydrates (HHS and USDA, 2015). There are two forms of carbohydrates: simple sugars (the monosaccharides and disaccharides of sucrose, fructose, and lactose found in fruits, vegetables, milk, and prepared sweets) or complex carbohydrates (starches found in cereal grains, potatoes, legumes, and other vegetables). Most dietary carbohydrates should be in the complex form, and refined food products should be limited. Because carbohydrates are essential to facilitate protein synthesis, if carbohydrates are extremely limited or absent from the diet (e.g., as in a ketogenic diet used to manage intractable epileptic seizures [see Chapter 46]), the body uses stored triglycerides, oxidizes fatty acids, and breaks down dietary and tissue protein, leading to an accumulation of ketone bodies.

Fats

Lipids, fats, and fatty acids are used by the body to provide energy, to facilitate absorption of the fat-soluble vitamins (A, D, E, and K), and to maintain integrity of cell membranes and myelin. Two essential polyunsaturated fatty acids, linoleic acid (LA) and α-linolenic acid (ALA), are not produced by the body and must be included in the diet. These essential fatty acids are precursors of omega-6 and omega-3 fatty acids, respectively. LA is found in soy oil, corn oil, and sunflower, safflower, pumpkin, and sesame seeds. ALA is found in large quantities in flaxseed and flaxseed oil and in lower quantities in walnuts, canola oil, and wheat germ. Adequate amounts of omega-3 and omega-6 fatty acids are produced in the body if there is adequate intake of these two essential fatty acids and the vitamins and minerals (vitamins B_3, B_6, and C; zinc and magnesium) necessary to facilitate their conversion.

It is recommended that fat intake for children 1 to 3 years old be 30% to 40% of total caloric intake; children more than 3 years old should gradually adopt a diet of 25% to 35% of total calories from fats. Saturated fat intake should be minimal (<10% of total calories in the form of saturated fat), and trans fatty acids should be excluded from the diet (HHS and USDA, 2015). Numerous studies indicate that diets with high plant fibers, limited saturated fats, low cholesterol, and zero trans fats reduce serum cholesterol and low-density lipoprotein (LDL) levels without affecting normal growth and development (Oranta et al., 2013). When counseling parents, providers should emphasize that a diet with less than 20% of the total energy intake from fat can put the child at nutritional risk.

Micronutrients

Vitamins

Fat-Soluble Vitamins. Several characteristics of fat-soluble vitamins (A, D, E, and K) have implications for dietary assessment and management (Table 17.1). Fat-soluble vitamins can be stored for long periods of time in body tissues. Therefore temporary dietary deficiencies may not affect the body's growth and development. If stores are depleted and nutritional intake is inadequate over time, signs of vitamin deficiency appear. If intake of fat-soluble vitamins is excessive, which can occur when supplements are taken, toxic effects can appear. Fat-soluble vitamins are fairly stable when heated, as in cooking. Food preparation does not destroy fat-soluble vitamins as readily as water-soluble vitamins. They are absorbed in the intestines along with fats and lipids in foods. They require bile for absorption, and chronic conditions that compromise the hepatobiliary system put children at risk for decreased absorption of fat-soluble vitamins. Low-fat diets and increased intestinal motility or malabsorption syndromes put individuals at risk for fat-soluble vitamin deficiency. Fat-soluble vitamins do not contain nitrogen and do not act as coenzymes in cellular metabolism of nutrients.

Water-Soluble Vitamins. In contrast to fat-soluble vitamins, water-soluble vitamins (C and B vitamins) are stored in very small amounts in the body. If water-soluble vitamin intake is more than that needed by the body, absorption (primarily in the jejunum) decreases, and excess vitamins are excreted. As a result, daily intake of water-soluble vitamins is necessary, and there is little risk of toxicity from large doses. The B vitamins contain nitrogen and serve as essential coenzymes in the body's metabolism of nutrients. Niacin (vitamin B_3) plays a significant role in increasing high-density lipoproteins (HDLs).

Minerals and Elements

Three major minerals—calcium, magnesium, and phosphorus—are present in the body in amounts greater than 5 grams. DRIs have been set for boron, calcium, chromium, copper, fluoride, iodine, iron, magnesium, manganese, molybdenum, nickel, phosphorus, selenium, silicon, vanadium, and zinc. Recommended allowances for calcium, fluoride, iron, and zinc can also be found in the DRIs at https://www.nap.edu/catalog/11537/dietary-reference-intakes-the-essential-guide-to-nutrient-requirements.

Peak bone density is directly related to calcium intake during the years of bone mineralization, primarily before 20 years old. However, bone calcification continues for several years more, so to ensure maximum peak bone density, dietary calcium needs remain high until approximately 25 years old. Breastfed infants

TABLE 17.1   Vitamins: Function, Dietary Sources, Interactions, Deficiency, and Excess

Function	Dietary Sources	Interactions Affecting Absorption or Utilization	Signs of Deficit	Signs of Excess
Fat-Soluble Vitamins				
Vitamin A				
Vision, cellular differentiation and growth, reproductive and immune system function	Liver, fish liver oils, fortified milk, eggs, red and orange vegetables, dark green leafy vegetables	Facilitated by dietary fat, protein, and vitamin E Absorption of vitamin A is hindered by lack of protein, iron, or zinc	Anorexia, dry skin, keratinization of epithelial cells of respiratory tract, night blindness, corneal lesions, increased susceptibility to infections	Headache, vomiting, double vision, hair loss, dry mucous membranes, peeling skin, liver damage Toxic at 10 times the RDA Excessive intake of carotenoids (e.g., carrots) may cause hypercarotenosis, a benign condition of yellowing of the skin
Vitamin D				
Bone growth and development; regulates intestinal absorption of calcium and phosphorus	Sunlight, artificial ultraviolet light, fortified food products, especially milk, fish	Utilization compromised in patients with renal failure Increased exposure to sunlight increases synthesis Darker skin and aging skin inhibit synthesis	Inadequate bone mineralization, rickets or skeletal malformations, delayed dentition	Anorexia, nausea, vomiting, diarrhea, weakness, hypercalcemia, hypercalciuria, calcium deposits in soft tissue, permanent renal or cardiovascular damage
Vitamin E				
Antioxidant, traps free radicals, prevents oxidation of polyunsaturated fats	Vegetable oils, margarine, nuts, seeds, wheat germ, green leafy vegetables	Low serum levels have been associated with prematurity and congenital defects of the hepatobiliary system (e.g., cystic fibrosis, biliary atresia)	Macrocytic anemia and dermatitis in infants; neurologic defects in severe malabsorption	None known in dietary doses Supplements may cause hemorrhagic effects, especially if taken long term
Vitamin K				
Forms proteins that regulate blood clotting	Green leafy vegetables, milk, dairy products, liver	Inhibited by long-term antibiotic use, hyperalimentation, chronic biliary obstruction, or lipid malabsorption syndromes	Defective coagulation of blood, hemorrhages, liver injury	Vitamin K–responsive hemorrhagic condition, especially if patient is being treated with anticoagulants
Water-Soluble Vitamins				
Vitamin C				
Essential for collagen formation and function; promotes growth and tissue repair; enhances iron absorption; improves wound healing	Vegetables and fruits, especially citrus fruits, broccoli, collard greens, spinach, tomatoes, potatoes, strawberries, peppers	Vitamin C is easily lost in food storage and preparation with exposure to heat, oxygen, and water Exposure to cigarette smoke increases vitamin C requirement	Scurvy, cracked lips, bleeding gums, slow wound healing, easy bruising	Unknown; excess vitamin is excreted in urine
Thiamin (Vitamin B_1)				
Necessary for carbohydrate metabolism; promotes normal appetite and digestion	Whole grains, brewer's yeast, legumes, seeds and nuts, fortified grain products, organ meats, lean cuts of pork	Availability inhibited by presence of thiaminase (found in raw fish); alcohol contributes to thiamine deficiency Rarely, deficiency may follow gastric sleeve surgery for weight loss	Beriberi: muscle weakness, ataxia, confusion, anorexia, tachycardia, heart failure in infants	None by oral intake; excess excreted in urine
Riboflavin (Vitamin B_2)				
Necessary for oxidation-reduction reactions; essential for function of vitamin B_6 and niacin; helps to maintain integrity of skin, tongue, and lips	Dairy products, meat, poultry, fish; enriched or fortified grains, cereals, and breads; green vegetables, such as broccoli, spinach, asparagus, turnip greens	Positive nitrogen balance contributes to function of riboflavin	Oral-buccal cavity lesions, generalized seborrheic dermatitis, scrotal and vulva skin changes, normocytic anemia, dimness of vision	None known

TABLE 17.1   Vitamins: Function, Dietary Sources, Interactions, Deficiency, and Excess—cont'd

Function	Dietary Sources	Interactions Affecting Absorption or Utilization	Signs of Deficit	Signs of Excess
Niacin (Vitamin B$_3$)				
Essential for energy metabolism, glycolysis, fatty acids; maintains nervous system, integrity of skin, mouth, tongue	Meats, fortified grains, cereals, legumes. Milk, eggs, and meats contain tryptophan	Requires riboflavin for absorption and utilization. Grains treated with lime have more biologically available niacin. Dietary tryptophan converts to niacin	Pellagra: dermatitis, diarrhea, inflammation of mucous membranes, indigestion	No known toxicity with dietary doses; heat rush and flushing with excessive doses
Vitamin B$_6$ (Pyridoxine)				
Essential for metabolism of amino acids, lipids, nucleic acids, and glycogen	Chicken, fish, kidney, liver, pork, red meat, eggs, unrefined rice, soybeans, oats, whole wheat, peanuts, walnuts, fortified cereals	Riboflavin enhances function. Increased protein intake increases requirements for vitamin B$_6$	Seen in combination with other B-complex vitamin deficiencies; dermatitis, anemia, convulsions, neurologic symptoms, and abdominal distress in infants	Ataxia, sensory neuropathy when taken in gram quantities for months or years
Folate (Folic Acid, Vitamin B$_9$)				
Essential for amino acid metabolism and nucleic acid synthesis; red blood cell formation	Liver, fortified grain products, yeast, dark green leafy vegetables, green vegetables, legumes, orange juice, wheat germ	Only about 50% of folate in foods is directly bioavailable for absorption in intestine; more efficiently absorbed if serum levels are low	Megaloblastic anemia in severe cases; macrocytic anemia, glossitis, gastrointestinal disturbances; increased risk of neural tube defects and growth retardation in infants of folate-deficient mothers	None known in dietary doses; excessive folic acid supplementation may reduce serum levels of phenytoin, carbamazepine, and valproate and contribute to seizures in epilepsy controlled by these medications
Vitamin B$_{12}$				
Essential for neurologic function, adequate red blood cell formation, and DNA synthesis	Animal products: meat, eggs, and milk; shellfish; fortified foods	Absorbed in ileum; intrinsic factor mediated. In strict vegetarians, the vitamin excreted in the bile is reabsorbed	Megaloblastic anemia, neurologic symptoms, sore tongue, weakness	None known

DNA, Deoxyribonucleic acid; *RDA,* recommended dietary allowance.

or those who are fed an approved infant formula receive sufficient calcium and should not be given a supplement. Recommended daily requirement of essential minerals, their functions, dietary sources, and signs of deficit or excess can be found in Table 17.2. Iron (Fe) is the most common mineral deficiency in infancy and early childhood. Foods rich in iron are listed in Table 17.3.

Use of Vitamin and Mineral Supplements

National surveys reveal that many children in the United States have suboptimal nutrient intakes, particularly vitamins and minerals, due to a deficit of fruits and vegetables. School-age children are at high risk, and Project EAT (Eating Among Teens) data show that adolescents eat fewer fruits and vegetables as they get older (Nielsen et al., 2014).

Preterm or low-birth-weight babies and children with chronic illness may need supplements, and all pregnant teenagers should receive prenatal vitamins. The AAP recommends a vitamin D supplement (400 IUs) in breastfed infants, beginning at discharge from the hospital (which would be in the first days of life for infants delivered at home), and children and adolescents whose diet does not include an equivalent amount (Golden and Abrams, 2014). The Endocrine Society recommends vitamin D intakes of 400 to 600 IU/day for all children to maximize bone health (Pludowski et al., 2018). However, parents should be advised that, although supplements may be appropriate in some cases, they are not a substitute for a varied, nutrient-dense diet.

Assessment of Nutritional Status

Assessment of nutritional status is done to determine if there is deviation from normal growth and development, whether the child's diet is adequate, and variables that may be influencing the child's dietary intake. Much data can be collected in the

TABLE 17.2 Minerals and Trace Elements: Function, Dietary Sources, Interactions, Deficiency, and Excess

Mineral and Function	Dietary Sources	Interactions Affecting Absorption or Utilization	Signs of Deficit	Signs of Excess
Calcium				
Development of bone tissue; vital role in nerve conduction, membrane permeability, blood clotting, and muscle contraction	Milk and milk products, green leafy vegetables, broccoli, kale, and collards, soft bones of fish, sardines, foods processed or fortified with calcium	Absorption enhanced in the presence of vitamin D, adequate protein intake, during periods of rapid growth, and if dietary intake of calcium is low; inhibited by excess sodium or protein	Decreased bone strength, increased risk for fractures, paralysis	Constipation, increased risk for urinary stone formation; risk for decreased renal function
Phosphorus				
Essential for bone integrity and general metabolism; provides essential energy during the metabolic process	Almost all foods, especially meat, poultry, fish, milk, cereal grains; food additives in processed foods	Absorption inhibited by aluminum hydroxide in antacids and by excess iron	Bone loss, weakness, malaise, anorexia, and pain	None known
Magnesium				
Activates enzymes, facilitates cell metabolism, maintains electrical potential of cell membranes, enhances transmission of nerve impulses, assists to maintain adequate serum levels of calcium and potassium	Nuts, legumes, whole (unmilled) grains, green vegetables; bananas provide some magnesium	Absorption reduced with high-fiber diet, excess sodium, calcium, vitamin D, protein, and alcohol	Nausea, muscle weakness, irritability	None in healthy individual; with impaired renal function, excess may contribute to nausea, vomiting, hypotension, bradycardia, central nervous system depression
Iron				
Formation of the heme molecule; used in oxygen transport	Meat, eggs, vegetables, cereals, foods fortified with iron additives; Table 17.3 identifies a number of iron-rich foods	Absorption is enhanced if iron stores or daily intakes are low; presence of ascorbic acid increases absorption. Heme iron in meats is more bioavailable than nonheme iron from grains, fruits, and vegetables. Absorption inhibited if the iron-rich food is ingested with milk or caffeine or in presence of phytic acid, oxalic acid, or tannic acid	Anemia. Children are particularly susceptible to iron deficiency during periods of rapid growth combined with low dietary iron intake: from about 6 months to 4 years old and during early adolescence; menstruation puts adolescent girls at risk	Iron poisoning can be fatal; for a 2-year-old, a fatal dose is approximately 3 grams; for adolescents and adults, 200-250 mg/kg may be fatal
Zinc				
Cellular metabolism, growth, and repair	Meats, animal products, seafood (especially oysters), eggs	Absorption may be decreased if taken with high-fiber diet, excess iron, copper, folic acid, ascorbic acid	Anorexia, growth retardation, skin changes, immunologic abnormalities	Gastrointestinal disturbances, vomiting, acute toxicity, impaired immune response
Iodine				
Production of thyroid hormones	Water, seafood, airborne water from ocean mist, iodized salt, food processing related to milk and bread	None known	Thyroid dysfunction ranging from simple goiter to cretinism and mental retardation	Thyrotoxicosis; goiter, rare and not seen in children with intake up to 1 mg/day; toxic levels not known
Trace Elements				
Selenium				
Unknown	Seafood and organ meats; may be in grains grown in soil containing selenium	Intake linked to vitamin E intake; if vitamin E is adequate, selenium is likely to be also; may need to supplement in lactating women. TPN feedings contribute to deficiency	May be related to muscle weakness and pain, cardiomyopathy (Keshan disease) in young children	Nausea, abdominal pain, diarrhea, fatigue, nail and hair changes or loss; toxic levels not known

TPN, Total parenteral nutrition.

| TABLE 17.2 | Minerals and Trace Elements: Function, Dietary Sources, Interactions, Deficiency, and Excess—cont'd |

Mineral and Function	Dietary Sources	Interactions Affecting Absorption or Utilization	Signs of Deficit	Signs of Excess
Copper				
Normal growth	Organ meats, seafood, nuts, seeds; fetus stores copper in liver during gestation	TPN feedings contribute to deficiency; high vitamin C, molybdenum, or zinc intake may reduce retention or bioavailability	Bone loss, anemia, neutropenia, growth impairment	Liver disease, gastrointestinal symptoms, diarrhea, vomiting
Manganese				
Unknown, may be related to reproductive health, normal growth	Whole grains and cereals	Increased absorption during third trimester of pregnancy	Unknown; may be related to growth retardation	Unknown; may be related to learning disabilities, anemia
Fluoride				
Prevents dental caries, enhances bone health	Fluoridated water, tea, meat and bones of marine fish, potatoes, wheat germ	Processing foods in fluoridated water or cooking with Teflon increases content; cooking foods in aluminum reduces fluoride	Dental caries; may be related to poor bone health	Mottling of teeth, kidney disease, bone disease; may affect muscle and nerve function
Chromium				
Assists in glucose metabolism	Brewer's yeast, calves' liver, American cheese, wheat germ	TPN feedings can contribute to deficiency	May be related to impairment of glucose tolerance	Unknown; requires further study
Molybdenum				
Enzyme function	Milk, beans, breads, cereals	TPN feedings can contribute to deficiency	Unknown	Related to loss of copper; may lead to gout-like symptoms

TPN, Total parenteral nutrition.

intake interview or using a 3-day diet recall. Other tools available to assess diet include Bright Futures nutrition questionnaires for infants, children, and young adults www.brightfutures.aap.org/BrightFuturesDocuments/BFNutrition3rdEdition_tools.pdf (Holt and Wooldridge, 2011) and the Healthy Eating Index-2015 (www.cnpp.usda.gov/healthyeating index).

Dietary intake data should be combined with clinical, biochemical, and anthropometric information to provide a more complete picture of nutritional status. In addition, when doing nutritional assessment, it is important to remember that eating is a social, cultural, and economic activity. The nutritional value of foods is not the only variable in a child or family's decisions about what, how, and when to eat. In all cases the individual's true requirement and usual intake can only be approximated. Thus nutritional assessment is imprecise and must be interpreted in combination with other types of information about the individual.

History

Questions to elicit a history of nutritional status can be grouped into several categories:
- Nutritional status of mother during pregnancy
- Food and fluid intake of child and of family:
  - Type of feeding method used during infancy: If not exclusively breastfed, formula name and preparation. Any problems? When weaned? When solids started? Any allergies or intolerances noted?
  - Current nutritional intake of child, types and amounts of foods and fluids eaten (may use 24-hour recall, 3-day diet history, or length of time and frequency that child is at breast)
  - Additional intake (e.g., vitamin, fluoride, or iron supplements)
  - Is child's intake different from the rest of the family? How?
- Eating patterns or behaviors for both child and family:
  - Frequency of eating (nursing, meals, snacks)
  - Bottle feeding: Is bottle propped? Does child take bottle to bed at night or at naptime? Who feeds child?
  - Breastfeeding: On demand or scheduled? How flexible is mother to demands of infant? Is mother working? Is breast milk frozen and fed by someone other than the mother?
  - Describe mealtimes: Does family sit down together? Are meals prepared at home? Does child eat at school? How often are "fast foods" eaten? What amount of time is spent eating? How long does it take to feed child? Does the family view TV or other screen time during meals?
  - Does family eat out frequently? Fast food restaurants? How many times per week?
- Reactions to and attitudes about foods:
  - Any reaction to particular foods (e.g., vomiting, diarrhea, abdominal pain, rash)?
  - Food preferences or dislikes? How does child demonstrate likes and dislikes?
  - Cultural factors: What beliefs or attitudes does family have about how and what child should eat or how family should eat?
  - What is child's attitude about foods and eating?

TABLE 17.3	Iron-Rich Foods[a]		
Food	High Levels (5 mg/serving)	Moderate Levels (2-4 mg/serving)	Low Levels (<2 mg/serving)
Breads, grains, cereals, seeds[b]	Almonds (1 cup, whole, oil roasted) Cashews (1 cup, dry roasted) Pumpkin seed kernels (¼ cup, roasted) Fortified cereals Mixed nuts (1 cup, dry roasted with peanuts) Brown glutinous rice (1 cup, cooked) Sunflower seeds (1 cup, dry roasted) Watermelon kernels (1 cup, dried) Wheat germ (1 cup, toasted)	Bagel (1, egg or plain) Bread, Indian fry (1 piece) Breadstick (10, plain, without salt) Filberts (1 cup, dried) Gingerbread (1 piece) Muffin (1 wheat) Peanuts (1 cup, dried) White rice (1 cup, enriched, regular, cooked) Waffles (2 each) Walnuts (1 cup, dried)	Biscuits (1 each) Bread (1 slice, whole wheat) Egg noodles (1 cup, cooked) English muffin (1 each) Pancakes (1 each) Peanut butter (2 tbsp) Oatmeal (1 cup, cooked)
Fruits[b]	Apricot (1 cup, dried halves)	Avocado (1 whole) Currants (1 cup, dried Zante) Fig (10 each, dried) Pear (10 each, dried halves) Prune juice (1 cup) Raisins (½ cup)	Apple (1 medium, unpeeled) Apple juice (1 cup) Banana (1 medium) Dried mixed fruit (2 oz) Orange (1 medium) Orange juice (1 cup)
Vegetables[b]	Kidney beans (1 cup, cooked, fresh) Lentils (1 cup, cooked) Soybeans (1 cup, cooked) White beans (1 cup, cooked) Spinach (1 cup, cooked) Tofu (½ cup, cooked)	Black beans (1 cup, cooked) Garbanzo beans (1 cup, cooked) Refried beans (1 cup, canned) Beet greens (1 cup, cooked) Potatoes (1 medium, with skin, baked) Peas (1 cup, fresh, cooked) Snow peas with pods (1 cup, raw or cooked) Spinach (1 cup, raw) Molasses (2 tbsp, blackstrap) Spinach (1 cup, frozen, cooked)	Kidney beans (1 cup, canned) Green beans (1 cup, raw or cooked) Broccoli (1 cup) Carrots (1 cup) Corn (½ cup) Lettuce (1 cup) Potato (½ cup, baked, with skin) Sweet potatoes (1 cup, fresh, boiled, mashed) Tomatoes (1 cup fresh) Tomato juice (1 cup, canned) Turnip greens (1 cup, cooked)
Meats, poultry, fish, other protein sources[c]	Clams (3.5 oz, 5 each, or 1 cup = 22 mg iron) Oysters (3.5 oz) Beef heart meat (3.5 oz, cooked) Beef liver (3.5 oz, simmered) Veal liver (3 oz, simmered) Chicken liver (3.5 oz, cooked) Turkey liver (3.5 oz, cooked)	Ground beef (3 oz, cooked lean) Catfish (1 piece, floured, fried) Tuna (1 cup, canned, water packed) Lamb (3.5 oz, cooked)	Roast beef (3 oz, lean) Chicken (1 cup, dark or light meat) Egg (1, whole) Halibut (1 piece, baked or broiled) Ham (1 cup, roasted) Bacon (3 pieces, cooked) Pork (3 oz, lean shoulder roast)

[a]Cooking in cast iron pans increases iron intake, especially with high acid foods (e.g., tomatoes).
[b]Iron in plant foods is better absorbed when eaten with vitamin C or meat products.
[c]Iron in meat, poultry, and fish is more bioavailable than iron in other food sources.
Data Sourced from Hands ES: Nutrients in food, Philadelphia, 2000, Lippincott Williams & Wilkins.

- Feeding abilities of child: For example, does child choke, gag, vomit, have suck or swallow difficulties, or refuse certain foods, perhaps because of texture or smell?
- Any dietary restrictions in home or special diets? Vegan or vegetarian?
- Parents' and child's knowledge of foods and nutritional needs
- Management of foods in the family:
  - Who plans, purchases, and prepares food and meals for family?
  - What economic and environmental factors influence how food is managed? For example, are finances adequate to supply nutritious foods? Is there a refrigerator? Does family have transportation to carry larger amounts of food from store? Is there a full-service grocery store in the neighborhood? What is the socioeconomic status of family? Is food shopping budgeted? Are food stamps or other supplemental programs used?

- Health status affected by nutrition:
  - Special considerations for children or family related to food: Does child have special health care needs? Does child have a chronic condition that requires a special diet, formula, enzymes, or device for feeding?
  - Are any medications being taken that must be given with or without food?
  - Are any medications being taken that will affect the body's ability to digest or process foods?
  - Elimination patterns
  - Dental status and care of teeth
  - Patterns of wound healing, infections, colds, and mild illnesses
  - Any change in hair, nails, skin, or mucous membranes?
  - Tolerance for hot or cold weather?
  - Growth, activity, and exercise pattern: For example, has child been growing as parent expects? Has there been a

history of unusual weight gain or loss? Does child have energy to play? Is the child engaged in strenuous activity, competitive sports, or an athletic training program? an athletic training program?
- Family history: Hypertension, diabetes, hyperlipidemia, obesity, heart disease, allergies, eating disorders?

Physical Examination

A complete physical examination with vital signs should be done with a review of all systems. The AAP and Centers for Disease Control and Prevention (CDC) recommend measuring BMI in children 2 years old and older (CDC, 2018) and using World Health Organization (WHO) growth standards to determine weight to height ratio in children less than 2 years old (WHO, 2018). Plot all growth measures on appropriate growth charts (see Appendix).

Diagnostic Studies

Laboratory and diagnostic studies are performed as indicated:
- Hemoglobin or hematocrit
- Iron and ferritin levels, total iron-binding capacity, and transferrin saturation
- Serum levels for electrolytes
- Vitamin D levels on all children who are overweight or obese
- Bone radiographs for suspected iodine, vitamins C and D, or copper deficiency or to compare bone age with height age (age at which 50% of children reach the current height of the child)

Management Strategies for Optimal Nutrition

It is the parents' responsibility to provide healthful food that is adequate to meet the child's nutritional needs in an environment that makes eating enjoyable; it is the child's responsibility to decide what and how much of these healthful foods to eat (Satter, 1986). Critical to this interaction is a parent who knows which foods are healthful and which are not and who is aware of and responsive to the child's cues around feeding. Also essential is the parents' ability to provide healthful foods; this can be extremely difficult for some low-income families. Food insecurity is common, even in high-income countries (see Chapter 1) (Coleman-Jensen et al., 2014).

It is the providers' responsibility to counsel parents and children about making good decisions about nutrition and to facilitate families' access to healthful foods. PCPs may need to refer families to public health resources for assistance to find adequate food sources (e.g., Women, Infants, and Children [WIC] program; Supplemental Nutrition Assistance Program [SNAP]). and/or to pediatric dietitians for access to and management of special needs diets.

Developing Healthy Eating Habits

Healthy eating habits begin during gestation and continue throughout the life span. A healthy pregnancy most often leads to a healthy term newborn, ready to learn and master the skills of eating. The early childhood years are critical to establishing lifelong patterns of eating, and the responsibility of parents to provide healthful foods to their children cannot be overemphasized. Parents may rationalize giving their child empty calories rather than nutrient-rich food by stating, "That's all my child will eat,

and I know she needs the energy," but it is the parent—not the child—who decides if an 18-month-old's "treat" is French fries or fruit. Intervention by providers in the child's first year of life to teach parents which foods are healthy and encourage them to provide those foods helps establish healthy eating patterns in older children (Vitolo et al., 2012). Parents should be encouraged to provide the following:
- Positive examples of healthy intake:
  - Mostly plant-based foods (versus processed, edible food-products that contain additives, fats, and few nutrients) (Pollan, 2008)
  - Appropriate portions
  - Positive role models. Children learn eating behaviors by observation and instruction, and parents are the primary teachers in the process. Often that teaching is done without conscious reflection or planning on the part of parents but has lifelong ramifications. If children learn early that healthy, nutrient-filled foods are readily available and that their parents enjoy them, they are likely to enjoy them as well.
- Limits, but not prohibitions, on consumption of nonnutritious sugars and "sometimes" foods. Specifically, high-sugar, high-salt, and high-fat foods should make up a very small part of the diet; however, overly restricting them, especially in children, can contribute to unhealthy attitudes toward food.
- Food prepared in a form that stimulates children's appetites.

Parents are also responsible for a positive environment related to meals and should strive to provide the following:
- Regular, structured mealtimes when the family sits down to eat together; this may occur only once a day.
- Clear, developmentally appropriate expectations for children's behavior at mealtimes
- Developmentally appropriate access to and instruction in the use of utensils
- Appropriate supervision during mealtimes
- Developmentally appropriate opportunities to participate in planning, preparing, and serving meals
- Adequate exercise, sleep, and rest to stimulate appetites

Often parents will try to decide exactly how much their child should eat, rather than allow the child to choose from a variety of food. Appetite fluctuations and preferences are typical of children, and parents should be aware that children may appear to eat less than the parent thinks is sufficient or too much of one particular food to the neglect of others. If parents punish a child for not eating or force a child to eat, they have taken away the child's responsibility to choose. As a result, the child may develop an aversion to certain foods, overeat, or act out in other ways. Mealtimes can become contests of will between parents and children, creating feelings and patterns of interacting that extend far beyond the dinner table. Parents need to find out what healthy foods their children enjoy (e.g., it is perfectly all right to eat only carrots, peas, or broccoli as one's vegetable for several weeks in a row) and make those available. If provided a nutritious variety of foods they like, children tend to select those necessary for their healthy growth, in terms of both amount of calories and other nutrients. A general principle to keep in mind when considering portions is to serve one tablespoon of food per year of age. For children younger than 5 years old, one serving is approximately one-fourth to one-third of an adult serving; for older children, one serving is approximately one-fourth to one-half of an adult serving. However, children's appetites vary, and parents should be alert to cues that the child wants more or less of any particular food.

The range of nutrients available to the growing child will be greater with a wide variety of foods, but the introduction of new foods can create tension between parents and children. Parents should be informed that children may reject new foods, often because of taste or texture, as many as 15 to 20 times before they become accustomed to it and enjoy eating it. Parents should not be too concerned if a child refuses a particular food. Rather than force the child to try the new food or give in to the child's demands, the food should be removed without comment, then offered again at another meal. With a well-balanced diet, not eating a vegetable prepared at one meal, for example, will not compromise the child's health. However, parents should be encouraged to avoid becoming the child's "short-order cook," preparing a special dish if the child rejects what has been fixed for the family. If a child chooses not to eat much at a particular meal, he or she will be hungrier at the next. Between meals, children should be offered age-appropriate snacks, but snacks should not be a substitute for meals; "grazing" or eating whenever food is available tends to override the child's natural sense of satiety and encourage overeating.

Strategies that can be used to increase the chances of children accepting a new food include the following:
- Offer the food when children are hungry.
- Allow children to taste a little of the food rather than eating a full portion.
- Expose children to the food by preparing and serving the food without expecting them to eat it.
- Provide an example of parents eating and enjoying the food.
- Prepare the food the way children prefer: few spices, lukewarm, and recognizable.

Finally, remind parents that individuals do not need to eat all foods. The parent may not eat some foods because of a personal dislike (e.g., anchovies, sushi, or cilantro); children should be accorded the same courtesy if they have been offered the food numerous times and repeatedly demonstrate dislike. There are many food options for attaining the same nutrients. As children become older, parents can help them to master the social skill of politely trying new foods in new situations (e.g., visiting friends or dining in public places).

Nutrition Education

Nutrition education should include information about children's age and developmental abilities and characteristics; nutritional requirements; foods that meet children's nutritional needs; the relationship between diet and health conditions, including obesity and eating disorders; and strategies to facilitate the development of healthy eating behaviors. PCPs can also help parents to examine their own values and patterns related to eating, identify and reinforce those they would like to foster in their children, and eliminate those they see as negative.

MyPlate, MyPlate for Kids, and SuperTracker

MyPlate, MyPlate for Kids, and the SuperTracker are useful tools for educating families and children of all ages about a healthful diet (Fig 17.1). Based on current DRI guidelines, these tools can be used to calculate an individual's nutrient needs by age, gender, and activity level. They illustrate proportions of a healthy diet, emphasizing a foundation of grains, fruits, vegetables (particularly beans and peas), and lean meats, fish, and poultry. These tools provide in-depth information, resources, and a wide variety of nutrition-related activities to engage individuals in assessing and planning healthy nutrition. School nutrition is also addressed.

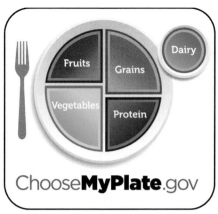

• **Fig 17.1** ChooseMyPlate (U.S. Department of Agriculture [USDA]. ChooseMyPlate [website]. choosemyplate.gov. Accessed October 10, 2018.)

Age-Specific Nutritional Considerations

Healthy eating habits are essential to good nutrition. Many eating problems, including obesity, are in part due to poor eating habits learned in infancy and early childhood that are then reinforced through the school-age and adolescent years. Special considerations related to developing healthy eating habits and specific nutritional needs are presented for each of the age groups in the sections that follow.

Newborns and Infants

Energy. Rapid infant growth requires high caloric intake. Adequate intake of breast milk or infant formula meets all energy needs for infants until they are 4 to 6 months old.

Fat. For proper myelination to occur, infants must have adequate fat intake. Children younger than 2 years old require more than 30% dietary fat for neural development. The lipids in breast milk and formulas meet these requirements. The AAP recommends transitioning to whole cow's milk at 12 months old and continuing for most children until 24 months old to promote healthy myelination of brain during this period of rapid brain growth. Fat is an important source of calories in infancy, and fat restriction is not encouraged, but appropriate fat content should be decided by parents and health care providers based on growth, appetite, intake of other foods, intake of other sources of fats, and potential risk for obesity and cardiovascular disease (National Heart, Blood, and Lung Institute [NHLBI]: Expert Panel on Integrated Guidelines for Cardiovascular Health and Risk Reduction in Children and Adolescents, 2011).

Vitamins. Vitamin D (400 IU daily) is recommended for all breastfed infants and infants who receive an unfortified formula from birth until they are 1 year old. Infants should have an adequate source of vitamin C after they are 4 to 6 months old. A multivitamin supplement is not recommended for healthy children receiving a well-balanced diet.

Iron. Iron deficiency is the leading cause of anemia in children, and iron supplements are necessary in some cases. Term infants who are breastfed usually have adequate iron supplies until they are 4 to 6 months old. Premature or low birth weight infants who are exclusively breastfed require iron supplementation for the first 12 months, and infants who are fed cow's milk before they are 12 months old are at high risk for iron-deficiency anemia. Iron-fortified cereals and iron-fortified formulas are excellent sources of dietary iron supplements for infants 6 to 12 months old.

TABLE 17.4 Specialized Infant Feeding Guidelines[a]: Formula Selection

Formula	Products	Indications	Contraindications	Main Features
Conventional cow's milk	Enfamil Infant Similac Advance Similac Sensitive	Healthy infants born >34 weeks gestational age	Cow's milk protein allergy	Protein: Intact cow's milk proteins (casein and whey)
Partially hydrolyzed	Enfamil Gentlease Good Start Gentle Good Start Soothe Similac Total Comfort	Note: marketed as intolerance formulas; not truly hypoallergenic Good Start Gentle: FDA approved for use in reducing risk of atopic dermatitis in high-risk infants	Cow's milk protein allergy	Protein: cow's milk proteins partially hydrolyzed into small peptides Note: Good Start and Similac: 100% whey
Extensive hydrolyzed	Alimentum, Nutramigen, Pregestimil	Hypoallergenic and used in cow's milk and soy protein allergy, protein maldigestion, or fat malabsorption	Severe cow's milk protein allergy	Protein: cow's milk proteins extensively hydrolyzed. Increased likelihood of tolerating whole cow's milk at age 1 year
Thickened	Enfamil A.R. Similac for Spit Up	Uncomplicated GERD Note: decreased efficacy when used with proton-pump inhibitor medications (e.g., Prilosec, Prevacid)	Premature infants <38 weeks GA Do not concentrate above 24 kcal/oz	Protein: intact cow's milk proteins Note: contains rice starch, which thickens upon contact with stomach acid Formulation maintains appropriate nutrient composition as opposed to adding cereal to formula
Soy	Enfamil Prosobee Good Start Soy Similac Soy Isomil	Vegan diet Family preference Galactosemia (Isomil and Prosobee powder only)	Prematurity Colic Constipation Cow's milk protein-induced enteropathy	Protein: soy protein isolates Note: all soy formulas are lactose free
Free amino acid	EleCare Infant (Abbott) Neocate Infant (Nutricia) PurAmino (Mead Johnson)	Cow's milk and soy protein allergy Multiple food protein allergies GERD Short bowel syndrome Malabsorption Eosinophilic esophagitis Galactosemia Note: limited availability and expensive		Protein: synthetic free amino acids Fat: EleCare and Neocate: 33% MCT oil Note: mixing ratios differ from standard formulas; refer to manufacturer's instructions
Low mineral	Breast milk Similac PM 60/40 (Abbott)	Impaired renal function Neonatal hypoglycemia		Protein: intact cow's milk proteins Note: breast milk's efficient absorption rate results in a naturally low mineral content Similac PM 60/40: Iron supplementation may be needed
Postdischarge premature	EnfaCare (Mead Johnson) Neosure (Abbott)	Birthweight >2000 g (4.5 lb.) and <34 weeks GA Can be used until 1-year corrected age Contraindications: full-term infants and FTT infants due to the risk of hypervitaminosis and hypercalcemia		Protein: intact cow's milk proteins Note: provides 22 kcal/oz at standard dilution

[a]These are general guidelines; not intended for use in the treatment of a specific clinical condition or without medical supervision.

FDA, U.S. Food and Drug Administration; *FTT,* failure to thrive; *GA,* gestational age; *GERD,* gastroesophageal reflux disease; *MCT,* medium-chain triglyceride.

From Oregon Academy of Nutrition and Dietetics. https://www.eatrightoregon.org/opnpg/page/pediatric-nutrition-resources. Accessed October 24, 2018.

Fluoride. The American Dental Association (ADA) recommends fluoride treatment starting at 6 months old in nonfluoridated communities (Casamassimo and Holt, 2014). Fluoridated water is the primary source of fluoride for children who live in communities with adequate fluoridation in local water supplies. Additional sources of dietary fluoride include foods cooked in fluoridated water, meats, potatoes, and wheat germ. The risk of excess fluoride in communities with fluoridated water is rare.

Infant Formulas. Breast milk is the ideal food for newborns and infants and should be promoted unless it is medically harmful to the infant. Most iron-fortified infant formulas provide adequate nutrition and, for some families, may be an appropriate alternative to breastfeeding. Table 17.4 outlines various types of commercial formulas available.

Occasionally infants demonstrate intolerance to formula, showing irritability, weight loss or slow gain, vomiting, diarrhea, constipation, other gastrointestinal problems, or atopic dermatitis. The PCP must work closely with parents to identify a formula tolerated by the infant, being careful to allow sufficient time for the baby to respond to a new formula as it is introduced. This can be a time- and energy-consuming process in which parents need support, reassurance, and encouragement. Referral to a registered pediatric dietitian may be indicated.

Gastroesophageal Reflux. All babies "spit up," especially directly after a feeding or when burped. A small regurgitation of undigested formula or breast milk is usually not of concern. Gastroesophageal reflux (GER) in infants can occur during, immediately after, or several hours after a feeding and can be exacerbated by increased intra-abdominal pressure (as with crying, coughing, defecation, or external pressure from movement or position). Children with insufficient lower esophageal sphincter tone are especially susceptible to GER. Reflux becomes symptomatic early in life, peaks at approximately 4 months old, and spontaneously resolves for most children by 12 to 24 months old.

Introduction of Solid Foods. Introduction of solid foods is recommended when the child is 6 months old. Development in a term infant makes this an appropriate time:

- Infants' sucking patterns have changed sufficiently to allow mastery of chewing and swallowing.
- Infants can sit with some support and are able to purposefully move their heads.
- Infants are able to grasp, pick up, and bring objects to their mouths.
- Iron stores present at birth are being depleted.
- Growth demands require nutrients other than those provided in milk alone.
- Developmental needs (cognitive, sensory, and motor) are stimulated by new foods, textures, smells, and tastes, and with the use of utensils.

Solid foods can be introduced in whatever sequence the family desires, often based on cultural or family customs. Cereals are convenient because they can be prepared in small volumes and mixed with formula or breast milk. In general, infants are able to pull the cereal from a spoon with their lips. Most infants are spoon-fed, but use of the process of "baby-led weaning" allows infants to feed themselves using their grasp, thus allowing the infant more control in the feeding process. To self-feed in this fashion, an infant must have the ability to sit with little or no support and to reach and grasp for objects. Although infants in many cultures are introduced to table foods as their first solid foods, further research is needed to determine the extent of benefits of "baby-led weaning" (e.g., protection from obesity, increased response to satiety cues, improved self-regulation, enhanced family eating patterns) (Brown et al., 2017). Whether fed by spoon or finger-fed, home-prepared foods, such as grains (e.g., oatmeal, bread, crackers, and rice), soft fruits, cooked vegetables, and pureed meats, can meet all the child's nutritional needs. Commercially packaged baby foods can provide adequate nutrition, but parents should examine labels to determine the amount of calories, fats, salt, sugar, and other additives. Box 17.2 lists some principles to keep in mind when beginning solid foods.

Eating Habits. Feeding on demand in early infancy is important, and neonates should not be allowed to sleep for long periods of time without feeding. Parents should be counseled to respond promptly to a child's feeding cues and to allow the child to initiate and guide the feeding interaction. However, feeding primarily to comfort a child should be discouraged, and parents are encouraged to recognize the different cries of an infant

---

> **• BOX 17.2 Principles for the Introduction of Solids into the Infant's Diet**
>
> - Introduce one food at a time to assess for adverse reaction.
> - If there is a family history of allergies or atopy, consider introducing iron-fortified rice and oatmeal cereals as the first food.
> - Introduce home-prepared or commercially prepared cereals, fruits, and vegetables in any sequence desired.
> - Prepare and provide a variety of foods appropriate to child's developmental abilities—strained, mashed, pureed, or finger foods.
> - Serving size approximately one tablespoon for initial serving for infant.
> - Include the child in family mealtimes.

---

during the hunger, sleep, and wake cycle. A child is not necessarily hungry every time he or she cries. Bottle-fed infants, whether formula or breast milk is given in the bottle, can easily be overfed. Parents or caregivers often urge the infant to take that extra half ounce just to empty the bottle even when the infant has indicated he or she wants to stop feeding. As a result, infants can learn to ignore feelings of satiety. Self-regulation of intake is evident in young infants, but by early childhood, children are influenced by social cues around feeding and can eat more than they need. Normal-weight term infants who are formula-fed and who rapidly gain weight in the first weeks of life appear to be at high risk for overweight (Feldman-Winter et al., 2018). All infants, whether breastfed or formula-fed, who are overweight at 6 months old are at risk for overweight as young children (van der Willik et al., 2015). Formula-fed infants introduced to solid foods before 4 months old are six times more likely to be obese at 3 years old than breastfed infants (Huh et al., 2011). Bottle feeding beyond 12 months old is also a risk factor for being overweight or obese.

A selection of varied, healthful foods gives the older infant a chance to explore textures, smells, colors, and taste. Feeding is also a time when older infants learn physical skills of fine motor control, cognitive skills of relationships between action and consequence, and skills of social exchange among family members.

Early Childhood

Energy and Protein. The growth rate in early childhood is slower than that of infants, resulting in decreased energy needs per unit of body weight. However, due to increased size and activity, these children require an increased number of total calories. Addition of muscle mass also demands a continued high protein intake.

Vitamin and Mineral Supplements. Vitamin D supplementation is recommended in early childhood for all children. Children who tolerate only *extremely* limited food choices or have inconsistent eating behavior may benefit from a multivitamin plus mineral supplement particularly for adequate daily intake of folate, vitamin A, and zinc.

Eating Habits. In early childhood, children learn how and what to eat by observing adults around them and by responding to the foods adults provide for them. They may show an initial aversion to new foods and may demonstrate "food jags," eating only a few kinds of food. With time, guidance, and patience, young children will learn to eat a wide variety of foods, become more skilled in managing eating, using utensils, enjoying family mealtimes, and demonstrating more distinctive food likes and dislikes. Parents should continue to be responsive to the child's cues for hunger and satiety, providing age-appropriate portions and not insisting on the "clean-plate" approach at mealtimes.

Middle Childhood

Energy and Protein. Energy and protein needs of school-age children vary depending on body size, growth patterns, and activity levels. Protein needs increase in older children as they gain more muscle mass. Active boys from 10 to 18 years old need between 2200 and 3200 calories a day, whereas active girls require approximately 1800 to 2400 calories daily.

Vitamin and Mineral Supplements. Poor eating habits and irregular meal schedules place school-age children at risk for deficiencies in iron, thiamin, vitamin A, and calcium. Nutrition education in school and at home can teach children in middle childhood about specific nutrient sources and encourage healthy eating habits. Vitamin D supplementation is recommended for all children, and supplementation with a daily multivitamin may be necessary for children who have an *extremely* limited diet and food choices. Vitamin B_{12} supplementation is required for children eating a vegan diet.

Eating Habits. Food likes and dislikes carry over from early childhood. There is great variation in appetite and intake as a result of uneven growth and activity levels. School-age children tend to skip some school lunch offerings and are more likely to snack with increased screen time. Families with hectic schedules or unstructured mealtimes often have an increased reliance on fast foods. Parents and children should identify healthy snacks and prepared foods that fit a busy family schedule. High-fat, high-calorie, low-nutrient snacks (e.g., chips, soda, and pizza) should be avoided on a daily basis and be a limited part of a child's diet.

Adolescents

Energy and Protein. The rapid growth rate of adolescents is remarkable. High levels of energy are needed to support this growth, and, if teens participate in sports or other exercise programs, additional caloric intake can be needed. Adequate protein intake is essential to produce muscle mass. The average intake of protein in the American diet is significantly greater than the DRI, so additional supplementation is usually not necessary.

Vitamin and Mineral Supplements. Thiamin, riboflavin, niacin, folate, iron, zinc, and calcium needs increase during adolescence. Adolescents with irregular eating habits or those who eat a diet with an extremely limited variety of foods are at risk for vitamin deficiencies, particularly vitamin A, vitamin C, and the vitamin B complex. Calcium intake is also limited in many adolescents and adolescent girls are particularly at risk for calcium and iron deficiency when menstruation begins. Adolescents who eat a vegan diet need vitamin B_{12} supplements. Vitamin D supplementation is recommended for all adolescents.

Eating Habits. Eating habits of adolescents are influenced by their increasing independence and social activity, perceptions of body image, and physical growth patterns. Adolescents often have erratic eating patterns; skip meals; eat high-fat, high-calorie, low-nutrient snack foods; and consume calories late in the day. Teens who participate in sports and adolescents who eat a vegetarian diet tend to have healthier eating habits than their non–sports-involved or meat-eating counterparts. Adopting a balanced vegetarian diet at a young age can establish lifelong healthy eating habits associated with lowered risk for obesity and chronic diseases (Segovia-Siapco et al., 2018).

Pregnancy in Adolescence. Nutrition for the pregnant teenager can be easily compromised and must be carefully monitored. Providers should carefully assess dietary intake and counsel the adolescent to eat a varied and healthful diet. The use of motivational interviewing by providers can help the teen to more actively engage in healthful prenatal care, increasing the chance of a successful pregnancy.

Pregnancy itself adds significant nutritional demands at the same time the teen is experiencing rapid growth, especially if she is less than 15 years old. In addition, many teens have irregular eating patterns and poor nutritional intake. As the fetus competes with the mother for nutrients, it is at high risk, and infants born to teenage mothers are more likely to be premature, have low birth weight, and experience chronic illness, disabilities, or death.

In addition to a healthful diet, the pregnant teen should take a prenatal vitamin and mineral supplement including iron, calcium, and folic acid. A daily intake of 1300 to 1500 mg of calcium (via food and supplement) is recommended. *All* girls capable of becoming pregnant should have a daily folic acid intake of 0.4 mg, increased to 0.6 mg with pregnancy.

Gestational weight gain in adolescents should be carefully monitored. Healthy adolescents who are still growing (i.e., they are <4 years after menarche) should gain the amount they would normally gain in 9 months if they were not pregnant plus a normal gestational weight gain. For teens who are 4 years past menarche, weight gain is similar to that of adult women. Adolescents who become pregnant when they are overweight or obese are at high risk for neonatal and perinatal morbidity (Todd et al., 2015); if they also have excessive weight gain during pregnancy, they are at risk for postpartum depressive symptoms (Cunningham et al., 2018). Gestational weight gains of 15 to 25 pounds in overweight and obese adult women and 15 pounds or less in morbidly obese women are associated with fewer adverse outcomes (Crane et al., 2009). There are no data on adolescents to match those of adult women, but weight gain should not be excessive.

Physical Activity

Physical activity is integral in relation to healthy nutrition. It is recommended that children and adolescents engage in 60 minutes of physical activity every day, most of which is moderate- or vigorous-intensity aerobic (exercise that makes them breathe hard); they should do vigorous activity at least 3 days a week and muscle- and bone-strengthening activity at least 3 days a week (HHS, 2018). Higher amounts of physical activity enhance bone health and reduce the risk of increased adiposity in children 3 to 6 years old (HHS, 2018). Increased activity creates a demand for more calories and nutrients and improves weight status; more sedentary behavior means that the body needs fewer calories, and sedentary lifestyles combined with poor eating habits can contribute to obesity.

Vegetarian and Vegan Diets

Vegetarian diets are increasingly common and offer striking health benefits. If children who eat a vegetarian diet continue to follow a plant-based diet into adulthood, they can expect to have lower levels of obesity, high blood pressure, heart disease, diabetes, and cancer. There are several different classifications of vegetarian diets:

- Vegans, or strict vegetarians, eat foods of only plant origin, including fruits, vegetables, grains, nuts, seeds, tofu, and legumes (e.g., beans, peas, lentils, and nuts).
- Lactovegetarians include milk and dairy products in their diet, in addition to all plant-based foods.
- Lacto-ovovegetarians consume eggs, dairy products, and all plant-based foods in their diet.

- Macrobiotic diets include whole grains, brown rice, vegetables, fruits, legumes, and seaweeds. Animal foods are limited to white meat or white fish and are consumed minimally, one to two times per week.
- Pescatarian diets are plant-based and include fish and shellfish but no other meat. Lacto-ovopescatarian diets add eggs and dairy products.
- "Flexitarians" have a diet that consists mostly of plant-based foods, but they occasionally eat fish, chicken, or some seafood, usually avoiding or severely limiting red meat.

Vegetarian and vegan diets can meet all nutritional needs of growing children, including athletes (Van Winckel et al., 2011). For children who are lacto vegetarians or lacto-ovovegetarians, or who from time to time eat fish or other meat, it is easy to achieve adequate nutrients needed for proper growth and development, and the diet of these children often meets Healthy People 2020 goals more often than do diets of their peers. However, vegetarian diets, especially vegan diets, may be deficient in some nutrients, specifically protein, vitamin B_{12}, iron, calcium, zinc, riboflavin, and (if exposure to the sun is limited) vitamin D. Attention must also be paid to ensure adequate intake of essential fatty acids (Table 17.5).

Clinical Findings

Nutritional assessment of the child with a vegetarian diet should include regular anthropometric measurements, diet recall and analysis, and laboratory assessment of vitamin B_{12}, zinc, iron, and vitamin D, especially if a previously healthy child presents with signs and symptoms of deficit of these nutrients (see Tables 17.1 and 17.2).

Management

Families and children who select vegetarian or vegan diets should be supported for their healthy dietary decisions, counseled about potential deficits, educated about alternative sources of nutrients that may be lacking in the diet, and assessed regularly to ensure adequate growth and development.

Consuming a variety of plants with different configurations of protein can meet the child's growth demands. This combination has often been called *complementary,* one plant providing the protein lacking in another. It is not necessary that these complementary proteins be eaten in the same meal; intake throughout the day is more important (Van Winckel et al., 2011). Examples of foods that provide adequate protein intake include combinations of legumes and grains, nuts, or seeds (e.g., peanut butter on wheat bread, beans and rice, lentils and rice, lentils and sunflower seeds, peas and rye or wheat, or tofu and almonds).

Vitamin B_{12}, in the form of a supplement or fortified foods, is required for the child who is a vegan because vitamin B_{12} is sufficiently bioavailable in animal-based foods only (Watanabe and Bito, 2018). Iron and zinc may also need to be supplemented in a child's vegetarian diet. Iron needs of vegetarians are calculated to be 1.8 times greater than nonvegetarians because the nonheme iron in plant-based foods is less bioavailable (phytates in grains and

TABLE 17.5	Vitamins, Minerals, and Nutrients at Risk for Deficit in Strict Vegetarian or Vegan Diets	
Vitamin, Minerals, and Nutrients at Risk for Deficit	Usual Sources	Alternative Sources in Vegan Diet
Vitamin D	Animal products: egg yolk, butter, liver, salmon, sardines, tuna; sunlight	Fortified cereals, milk, or margarine; sunlight (20-30 min/day, two or three times per week)
Vitamin B_{12}	Animal products only: meat, fish, eggs, dairy products	Fortified soy milk, fortified soy-based meat substitutes, nutritional yeast, fortified cereals, vitamin supplements
Riboflavin	Dairy products and meat are best sources; also eggs, dried yeast, grains, dark-green leafy vegetables, avocado, broccoli	Brewer's yeast, wheat germ, fortified cereal, beans, almonds, soybeans, tofu, dark-green leafy vegetables, avocado, broccoli, orange juice
Calcium	Dairy products are best source; also in some fruits, nuts, dark-green leafy vegetables	Fortified soy milk, dried fruits, almonds, sunflower seeds, filberts, whole sesame seeds, green leafy vegetables (at same meal, avoid eating spinach, Swiss chard, beet greens, whose oxalic acid hinders calcium absorption)
Iron	Iron in meat sources is more bioavailable than iron in plants; lentils, beans (cooked black, soy, garbanzo, lima) are good sources	All legumes, almonds, pecans, dates, prunes, raisins, fortified cereals, white or brown rice; absorption is enhanced by ascorbic acid–rich foods
Zinc	Meats, animal products, seafood (especially oysters), eggs; found in whole grains, brown rice, nuts, spinach; however, best plant sources also contain phytic acid, which inhibits zinc absorption	Whole grains, fortified cereal, brown rice, almonds, wheat germ, tofu, pecans, spinach
Omega-3 fatty acids	Fatty fish, eggs	Flax seed, chia seed, walnuts, soybeans
Protein	Animal products (meat, eggs, milk) that have all nine amino acids making them complete proteins	Plant-based foods are considered incomplete proteins because they do not contain all 9 amino acids. To remedy this, one can eat a variety of foods such as soy, legumes, nuts seeds, grains, cereals, potatoes, pasta.

legumes bind with iron to decrease its absorption). Iron absorption can be enhanced by combining intake with vitamin C found in fruits and some vegetables and by processing seeds and grains (e.g., soaking, sprouting, fermenting, or making into bread).

Phytates in grains and legumes also bind with zinc to inhibit its absorption. As with iron, eating zinc-rich foods (e.g., soy, nuts, cheese, legumes, and grains) with organic acids (e.g., citrus) and processing these foods by soaking, sprouting, or leavening with yeast increases zinc absorption.

Research indicates that children with a high fiber intake from a wide variety of plant-based foods grow well, have adequate energy intake, and experience a reduction in total serum and low-density cholesterol levels (Niinikoski and Routtinen, 2012). Like all children, those eating a vegetarian diet should emphasize a wide variety of nutrient-dense foods to achieve adequate intake.

It is important that PCPs offer advice, counseling, and support within the context of the child's and family's belief system. In the case of highly restrictive diets resulting in growth failure or vegetarianism as a form of eating disorder in the child, referral to a nutritionist and behavioral/mental health specialist is indicated ⬤.

Altered Patterns of Nutrition in Children

Nutritional needs of children can be altered for a variety of reasons, including illness, surgery, medications, chronic conditions, metabolic or endocrine dysfunction, and physical anomalies. The disease section of this text discusses specific conditions and the role of nutrition as part of the treatment plan for each. This section outlines more general considerations for conditions that require increased caloric intake, decreased caloric intake, supplemental or restricted diets, or physical alterations in diet management. This section also discusses childhood overweight and obesity.

In all altered patterns of nutrition, the family system must be an integral part of treatment; families of a child with special needs may face high stress and creating a positive feeding experience can facilitate a healthy parent-infant bond. PCPs can intervene by doing the following:

- Encourage parents to express their feelings.
- Listen without judging; acknowledge those feelings.
- Demonstrate techniques that increase feeding success.
- Explain the child's condition, treatments, and prognoses, both short and long term.
- Emphasize how the parent can be involved in the child's progress.
- Encourage parents to make decisions related to their child's care; provide suggestions and guidance as the child grows, as treatment is carried out, and as needs change.
- Give positive reinforcement for parents' success.

Disorders Requiring Increased Caloric Intake

Inadequate caloric intake should be suspected in any child with a weight-to-age ratio below the 10th percentile on standardized growth and BMI charts. For children who are genetically small or have a disabling condition that limits growth, a weight-to-length ratio or weight-to-height ratio below the 10th percentile indicates suboptimal nutrition. A number of conditions put children at risk for insufficient caloric intake, including the following:

- Conditions in which activity level is increased, either by purposeful or involuntary muscle work, such as athetoid cerebral palsy, attention-deficit/hyperactivity disorder, or chronic lung conditions

- A hypermetabolic state (sometimes complicated by secondary malabsorption), which may be present in the child who has acquired immunodeficiency syndrome (AIDS), cancer, burns, fever, or frequent infections or who has recently had surgery
- Chronic renal insufficiency
- Psychosocial factors, such as inadequate resources, poor feeding relationship with caregiver, and improper dilution of formula, which can lead to delayed growth and require increased calories for the child's catch-up growth
- Oral-motor impairment or chronic conditions, such as congenital heart disease, which can contribute to fatigue and poor feeding
- Low-birth-weight or premature infants
- Medical treatment (e.g., a child receiving corticosteroid treatment for Crohn disease)
- Conditions in which malabsorption occurs (e.g., cystic fibrosis)

When nutrition is inadequate, regardless of cause, the nutritional insult follows a predictable course. In the early stages, the child maintains or begins losing weight, then the child's linear growth slows or ceases. Finally, head circumference, indicating compromised brain development, levels off. Practical suggestions for increasing calories, protein, and nutrients needed for weight gain and growth are outlined in Box 17.3. A complete multivitamin and mineral supplement is also recommended.

For children who are underweight or growth retarded, it is not sufficient to simply increase intake to age-specific norms. These children require excess calories and protein for "catch-up" growth until growth is normalized. A method for calculating calories required for catch-up growth is presented in Box 17.4. Some chronic conditions may require more complex treatment, such as growth hormone therapy. Frequent monitoring of the child with inadequate caloric intake is necessary. Infants should be weighed at least weekly and length and head circumference measured once a month. Children more than 2 years old should be measured for height and weight at least once a month.

> **• BOX 17.3** **Strategies for Increasing Caloric Intake**

- Establish regular times for meals and snacks, 2 to 4 hours apart. Do not allow the child to nibble continually on small amounts of food.
- Keep mealtimes relaxed and pleasant. Avoid scolding, nagging, or forcing the child to eat.
- Allow the infant or child to provide cues regarding hunger and satiety.
- Use readily available, economic foods that are familiar to the child.
- Fortify milk by adding one cup of nonfat dry milk powder to one quart of whole milk. Drink or use to prepare cooked cereals, creamed soups, pancakes, pudding, milkshakes (do not use with children younger than 24 months old).
- Add additional butter or cheese to potatoes, vegetables, casseroles, rice, pasta, cooked cereals, etc.
- Encourage high-calorie snacks, such as dried fruits, nuts, bananas, cheese cubes, pudding or custard, cereal with whole milk, fruit yogurt (alone or as a dip for fruit), cheese or peanut butter on crackers, olives, or sliced or mashed avocado (as a dip for vegetables or crackers).
- Add instant breakfast mixes to whole milk.
- Use commercially prepared formula with high-calorie content (see Table 17.4).
- Use commercial liquid supplements, such as PediaSure, for children with lactose intolerance.

BOX 17.4 Estimating Catch-Up Growth Requirements[a]

Catch-up growth requirement (kcal/kg/day) = Calories required for weight age (kg/kg/day) × Ideal weight for age (kg) ÷ Actual weight (kg)
1. Plot the child's height and weight on the WHO or CDC growth charts.
2. Determine at what age the present weight would be at the 50th percentile (weight age).
3. Determine recommended calories for weight age (see Appendix, Estimated Energy Needs).
4. Determine the ideal weight (50th percentile) for the child's present age.
5. Multiply the value obtained in step 3 by the value obtained in step 4.
6. Divide the value obtained in step 5 by actual weight.

Disorders Requiring Decreased Caloric Intake

Health conditions that contribute to reduced energy output or decreased metabolic activity in children can require a decrease in caloric intake:
- Prader-Willi syndrome. Initially, the child with Prader-Willi syndrome is hypotonic and may demonstrate dysphagia and failure to thrive (FTT) as an infant. By 3 to 4 years old, the child becomes hyperphagic, lacking the internal regulation responsible for satiety.
- Down syndrome. Newborns with Down syndrome may have ≥10% weight loss and may be slow to regain their birth weight but are at risk for overweight as they grow.
- Myelomeningocele
- Hypothyroidism

The goal for children with medical conditions that reduce energy expenditure is to ensure that the child receives adequate nutrients without excessive caloric intake. Families should be referred to a registered dietitian to establish an appropriate caloric level and eating plan individualized to each child's growth needs. A complete multivitamin with mineral supplement is recommended as a restrictive diet can result in nutrient deficiencies. Children should be encouraged to engage in regular physical activity.

In some cases (e.g., children with brain dysfunction affecting hypothalamic control or Prader-Willi syndrome), access to food needs to be rigidly enforced and may include locks on refrigerators, cupboards, and garbage cans in the child's environment. Frequent monitoring is necessary to assess compliance and devise alternate strategies as indicated; weekly weight and monthly height measurements are recommended.

Disorders Requiring Restricted or Supplemental Diets

Nutritional status may be at risk if the hormones, enzymes, or cofactor activity necessary for body metabolism are either limited or produced in excess, or if absorption of nutrients is compromised. Under these conditions, nutritional intake must be adjusted by restricting diet or adding supplements (e.g., enzymes).
- Metabolic conditions or defects of absorption or transport (Table 17.6).
- Inflammatory bowel disease (Crohn disease or ulcerative colitis)
- Short bowel syndrome
- Celiac disease

TABLE 17.6 Metabolic Conditions Affecting Nutrition in Children

Organ Affected	Excessive Hormone/Enzyme Production	Deficient Hormone/Enzyme Production
Pancreas	Reactive hypoglycemia Organic or fasting hypoglycemia	Diabetes mellitus Cystic fibrosis
Thyroid	Hyperthyroidism Graves disease	Hypothyroidism
Parathyroid	Hyperparathyroidism	Hypoparathyroidism
Adrenal cortex	Cushing syndrome Corticosteroid therapy	Addison disease Congenital adrenal hyperplasia
Inborn errors of metabolism		PKU (deficiency of phenylalanine hydroxylase) Maple syrup urine disease Tyrosinemia Urea cycle disorders Organic acidemias Fatty acid oxidation disorders Galactosemia Glycogen or lysosomal storage disorders

- Cancer
- Infectious disease

The goals of nutritional intervention in these conditions are to provide for normal growth and development, maintain optimal health, prevent or delay complications related to progression of the disease (e.g., diarrhea, fistulas), and prevent or delay the need for more aggressive intervention (e.g., bowel resection). Referral to a registered dietitian is necessary, and the PCP should consult frequently with the dietitian.

Disorders Requiring Physical Alterations in Diet Management

Some physical conditions can create difficulty sucking, chewing, swallowing, or retaining food and liquids in the gastrointestinal tract and often require biomechanical or physical intervention:
- Cleft lip or palate
- Esophageal atresia
- Cerebral palsy
- GER disease
- Pyloric stenosis
- Stenoses, atresias, or fistulas secondary to surgery or environmental trauma, such as a chemical burn.

Treatment goals for these conditions include the following:
- Provide adequate nutrients for normal growth and development.
- Provide increased calories to add more weight if needed before surgical procedures.
- Strengthen child's resistance to infection.
- Prepare child to tolerate stress of surgical procedures.
- Facilitate healing processes postoperatively.

TABLE 17.7	Strategies for Feeding in Children With Cleft Lip or Palate	
Age	Problem Presented	Management Strategies
Infants	Poor suction when nursing	Individualize position used to feed infant; semiupright (60-90 degrees) position is often most effective.
	Nasal regurgitation	Breastfeed if possible; experiment with nipple position: position nipple toward side of mouth, do not put nipple into cleft.
	Swallows air	Use of longer, soft, or cross-cut nipples and squeezable bottles benefits infants with weak suck. Specialty nursing bottles require training of parents to ensure effectiveness. Use of prosthetic device may be helpful. Wean child by 12 months old. Tube or gavage feedings may be necessary in severe cleft. Burp frequently.
	Fatigue	Allow sufficient time for feeding; work toward providing adequate nutrients in 30 minutes.

- Ensure correct development and use of orofacial and oropharyngeal muscles and structures.
- Minimize disruption of family processes.
- Prevent development of feeding problems.

Table 17.7 lists strategies related to feeding children with cleft lip or palate.

Eating Disorders

An eating disorder is defined as eating (or not eating) in response to an external stimulus rather than in response to internal hunger cues. Although problems with feeding (e.g., colic, food refusal, picky eating) are common among children, anorexia nervosa, bulimia, and binge (or out of control) eating are the conditions most frequently identified as eating disorders in the pediatric population. These conditions are discussed in detail in Chapter 15.

Childhood Obesity and Overweight

BMI and weight-for-height ratios are used to define parameters of overweight and obesity in infants, children, and adolescents. Children 2 to 18 years old with a BMI greater than or equal to the 95th percentile for age and gender or those with a BMI greater than or equal to 30 (whichever is lower) are considered obese. Children with a BMI between the 85th and 95th percentiles for age and gender are overweight. For children younger than 2 years old, a weight-to-height ratio of greater than or equal to the 95th percentile is categorized as overweight.

As of 2014, 17% of children 2 to 19 years old in the United States were obese; 20.5% of adolescent males and females 12 to 19 years old were obese; this number has continued to rise over the past decade (Ogden et al., 2015). An additional 16.2% were overweight (Fryar et al., 2016). The prevalence of obesity among children 2 to 5 years old is 8.9%, which is approximately half

BOX 17.5   Risk Factors and Predictors of Overweight and Obesity in Children

- Maternal smoking during pregnancy
- Rapid weight gain in infancy, beginning at birth
- Bottle feeding
- Early introduction of solids
- Intake of high glycemic foods (e.g., sugars, soda, processed bakery goods) (contributes to disruption of normal balance of hormones and proteins, leading to hyperinsulinemia and insulin resistance)
- Limited intake of high-fiber foods (e.g., whole grains, fruits, vegetables) (contributes to disruption of normal balance of hormones and proteins, leading to hyperinsulinemia and insulin resistance)
- Use of food as a reward or a "comfort" during stress
- Sedentary lifestyle (e.g., watching television, screen time with technology, limited physical exercise)
- Television in the bedroom
- Overweight or obese parents
- Family stressors
- Significant differences in prevalence of overweight and obesity by race and ethnicity
- Middle or low socioeconomic status

that of children 6 to 11 years old (17.5%). There are significant differences in prevalence by race and ethnicity. The overall rate of obesity is highest among Hispanic youth (21.9%), followed by non-Hispanic black youth (19.5%) and non-Hispanic white youth (14.7%). Non-Hispanic Asian youth have the lowest rate of childhood obesity as measured by BMI at 8.6%; however, research suggests that Asian children and youth may have more fat at a lower BMI than non-Asian youth and may be at risk for associated health risks at a lower BMI (Fryar et al., 2016). The overall prevalence of childhood obesity remains greater than the Healthy People 2020 goal of 14.5%. However, for children 2 to 5 years old, the prevalence (8.9%) is slightly less than the Healthy People 2020 goal of 9.4% (Ogden et al., 2015).

Risk Factors and Predictors for Obesity

Obesity results from a complex relationship of genetics, environment, and the body's response to environmental factors, including neurohormonal regulation. Although studies show a variety of risk factors and predictors for obesity (Box 17.5), the specific moderators of excess weight gain vary and the relationship among variables is complex. Most obesity is a function of a genetic predisposition combined with environmental stimuli (Locke et al., 2015).

Biologic Mechanisms. Insulin and leptin are two major hormones that normally serve to control satiety and influence weight. Resistance to insulin and to leptin may contribute to the body's failure to register satiety. Chronic hyperinsulinemia may be the source of insulin and leptin resistance. Leptin normally stimulates the ventromedial hypothalamus (VMH), sending the message that the body has adequate energy stores. However, insulin and leptin share the same "signaling cascade" in the VMH, and if insulin levels are high, leptin is prevented from signaling its message of satiety (Lustig, 2008). Hyperinsulinemia thus prevents the message that the body is satiated from getting through, and overeating to satisfy a feeling of hunger can result. Hyperinsulinemia in children has three sources: genetics, epigenetics (small- and large-for-gestational-age infants experience hyperinsulinemia and insulin resistance), and environment. Environmental dynamics contributing to hyperinsulinemia are threefold:

- Increased stress leads to increased cortisol production, which can lead to insulin resistance.
- Decreased physical activity contributes to insulin resistance.
- Diet, especially high levels of fructose and decreased fiber, leads to excess insulin secretion.

"High glycemic" foods such as soda, sugar-sweetened beverages, juices, processed breads, pastries, and crackers are more quickly converted to serum glucose, and they stimulate a sharp rise in insulin production. With the high insulin level, glucose is moved quickly into cells, the extra insulin stays in the blood, and the resulting hypoglycemia stimulates hormone release that further increases appetite. The end result is overeating and increased fat storage (Lustig, 2008). High fructose consumption either as sucrose or high fructose corn syrup contributes to an increase in serum triglycerides and visceral fat that is associated with the recent increase in metabolic syndrome in children who are overweight or obese (Lustig et al., 2016).

Physical Activity and Screen Time. Decreased physical activity is a factor in the increased prevalence of childhood overweight and obesity. Children have increased time spent on sedentary activities including "screen time" with television, cell phones, tablets, and computers. Many schools have discontinued physical education classes (CDC, 2014), many children are driven to school rather than walking or riding bicycles, and many neighborhoods are unsafe for outdoor play.

A recent study found 96% of 13- to 24-year-olds watch free online video (on average, 11.3h/week), 71% view subscription online video (10.8 h/week), and 57% watch free online television (6.4 h/week) (DEFY Media, 2015). Excess screen time and having a TV in the bedroom are associated with increased risk of obesity (Wethington et al., 2013). Almost all children (96.6%) use mobile devices, and most start using them before they are 1 year old. At 2 years old, most children use a device daily and spend comparable screen time on television and mobile devices. Most 3- and 4-year-olds use devices without help, one-third are engaged in media multitasking, and three-fourths of children at 4 years old currently have their own mobile device (Kabali et al., 2015).

Increased screen time also exposes children to snack-food and sugar-sweetened beverage advertising that increases the likelihood that children will have these foods as part of their daily intake. This reinforces poor eating habits and is a primary contributor to childhood overweight and obesity.

Psychosocial and Environmental Factors. Numerous psychosocial and environmental factors put children at risk for being overweight (see Box 17.5). The low-cost availability of sugar-sweetened beverages in the environment contributes significantly to the added calories and sugar in the diets of U.S. children. Research links increased consumption of sugar-sweetened beverages and excess weight gain, dental caries, type 2 diabetes, and nonalcoholic fatty liver disease. Almost two-thirds of youth in the United States have at least one sugar-sweetened beverage daily (Rossinger et al., 2017).

In addition, food may be used to regulate emotions or cope with stress, or children may overeat in response to inappropriate body image perceptions or social pressure to be thin. Childhood depression and low self-esteem may contribute to overweight and obesity. Children who suffer neglect or abuse or have an overcontrolling parent may turn to food for comfort and overeat as a result. Research suggests that prenatal exposure to endocrine disruptors, such as bisphenol-A or estrogen, may predispose children to becoming overweight and obesity (Dhurandhar and Keith, 2014), and research is ongoing to assess the extent to which such exposure is associated with obesity or metabolic syndrome (Heindel et al., 2015).

Food Addiction. Addictive-like eating behaviors may play a role in obesity and overweight, although more research needs to be done to clarify the relationship (Mies et al., 2017). The Yale Food Addiction Scale for Children (YFAS-C) has been developed to facilitate this research (Gearhardt et al., 2013).

Clinical Findings

Assessing a child for overweight or obesity seems a simple matter: at the very least, calculate the ratio of height to weight and determine the child's placement on a standardized measure of BMI. However, both providers and parents often fail to conduct these measures and/or acknowledge the reality of the data. This failure represents a barrier to accurately define the problem of childhood overweight and obesity and support timely intervention. Many providers do not conduct thorough assessments or address the topic of weight in their routine well-child care. One study examining provider's perceptions found that 93.1% of physicians reported they had calculated BMI, but only 79% actually documented the data; and only 22% of the children found to be obese were documented as being so in the medical record (Chelvakumar et al., 2014). An earlier review of nearly 33,000 well-child visits for 2- to 18-year-olds found that providers diagnosed only 281 (0.78%) children with excess weight gain or obesity, despite the fact that approximately 15% of the population reportedly had BMIs equal to or greater than the 95th percentile (Cook et al., 2005).

In addition, most parents of overweight children perceive their child as normal weight or even underweight. A recent meta-analysis of studies worldwide found "the overall rate of parental underestimation of overweight/obese child's weight" to be 67.5% (corrected to 50.7% to allow for heterogeneity of study findings) (Lundahl et al., 2014). This analysis also found that one in seven parents underestimated their normal-weight child's weight; overweight parents were more likely to state that their normal-weight child was underweight. Another meta-analysis affirmed that 63% of parents of overweight children fail to recognize overweight of their child, and 86% of parents of overweight 2- to 6-year-olds fail to recognize it (Rietmeijer-Mentink et al., 2013). Difficult as it may be, PCPs and parents must acknowledge the problem of childhood overweight and obesity and intervene appropriately for change to occur.

History. The history should review patterns of eating and exercise for both the child and the family system. Also consider underlying factors and comorbid conditions, such as hypothyroidism, polycystic ovary disease, depression, diabetes, and cardiovascular disorders. The history should include the following:

- Dietary intake, including:
  - Total caloric intake and nutrient adequacy
  - Fat intake as percentage of total calories
  - Carbohydrate intake as percentage of total calories
  - Portion sizes
  - Amount of sugar-sweetened beverages, sodas, and 100% fruit juices consumed daily
- Eating patterns, including breakfast, frequency, and types of meals, snacking, fast food meals per week
- Exercise pattern and hours and type of sedentary activity
- Parental obesity
- Age at onset of excessive weight gain
- Family history of diabetes and cardiovascular disease (hypertension, congenital heart disease [CHD])

- Family or child history of hypothyroidism or other medical conditions that could contribute to being overweight
- Episodes of sleep apnea
- Social adjustment, peer group, friends
- Family and child readiness and ability to participate in a weight management treatment program based on healthy eating and activity
- Barriers to exercise and healthy eating (e.g., environmental constraints, physical disability)

Physical Examination. Perform a complete physical examination to determine child's level of fitness and anthropometric status:

- Blood pressure (measured with cuff that covers 80% of arm) and vital signs
- BMI for children older than 2 years and height-to-weight ratio for infants and children younger than 2 years old
- Skin (for acanthosis nigricans, skin tags over body, striae)
- Distribution of adiposity: central adiposity, adiposity in posterior neck
- Eyes (for arcus juvenilis)

Diagnostic Studies.

- HDL, cholesterol screening
- Random glucose test
- Thyroid screen: TSH, T_4
- AST, ALT
- HbA_{1c}
- Vitamin D level

Differential Diagnosis

Differential diagnoses include hypothyroidism and polycystic ovary disease, Down syndrome, and Prader-Willi Syndrome.

Management

For most children who are overweight or obese, the primary goal of weight management is to slow the rate of weight gain or maintain weight as the child grows, thereby allowing children to normalize their weight through their growth pattern. Weight reduction becomes the goal only if the child continues to gain weight rapidly or already weighs more than expected when fully grown.

Lifestyle Changes. Initially, lifestyle changes with active involvement of the entire family and regular monitoring by the PCP (anthropometric measures every 3 months) are recommended. When the entire family is involved, the overweight child has a much greater chance to normalize weight. PCPs can use motivational interviewing (described in Chapter 15) when working with children, adolescents, and their parents to make lifestyle changes for weight reduction. This approach allows the provider to:

- Educate parents about:
  - Strategies for developing healthy eating habits
  - Strategies to encourage physical activity in children
  - Children's growth patterns and nutritional needs
  - Children's communication around hunger and satiety
  - Risk factors for overweight and obesity
- Assist parents and children to clarify goals for weight
- Assist parents and children to identify barriers to weight loss and strategies to overcome them
- Assist parents to implement lifestyle changes consistent with the family's structure, abilities, and needs
- Provide ongoing support to families
- Identify, assess, and reward other parameters of progress with the child and family, such as improved dietary habits, increased physical activity, fitness, strength, and enhanced self-esteem.

• BOX 17.6 Parental Guidelines for Managing Childhood Weight Problems

- Do not put child on a diet (unless medically indicated and supervised). Instead, gradually modify *the entire family's* eating habits.
- Breastfeed infants if at all possible. If not breastfeeding and infant is at risk for overweight or obesity, consider providing lower protein formula (within the range of normal protein—the infant should *not* be given an inadequate protein intake). Higher protein content in infant formula has been found to be related to higher body mass index (BMI) and higher fat mass in infants and young children (Escribano et al., 2012; Weber et al., 2014).
- Respond to cues of satiety. Do not force infants to empty the bottle or children to clean their plates. They should eat only until they are full.
- Serve age-appropriate portions (e.g., one-quarter to one-third adult portion for young children).
- Schedule and maintain regular times for meals and snacks. Do not skip meals. Do not allow children to "graze" throughout the day.
- Have a family meal at least five or six times a week, eating, sharing, and enjoying food together.
- Reduce the number of meals eaten outside the home (e.g., in restaurants, fast-food chains).
- Serve low-calorie, low-glycemic, nutritious snacks, such as fresh fruit and vegetables, air-popped popcorn, pretzels, low-fat yogurt, frozen fruit juice bars, skim milk, and low-sugar cereals. Do not have high-calorie, high-glycemic snacks (e.g., chips, cookies, cakes, pies, ice cream, candy, soda pop, and doughnuts) in the home.
- Increase fiber intake. The Institute of Medicine's (IOM's) dietary reference intake (DRI) for dietary fiber is 14 g fiber/1000 kcal consumed or between 19 and 38 grams/day in children, depending on age (Kranz et al., 2012).
- Do not use food as a reward.
- Do not overly restrict a child's intake. This approach can actually lead to overeating and subsequent overweight.
- Promote physical activity. Start slowly, with low-weight–bearing exercise. Set reasonable goals and celebrate achieving them. Make daily exercise a priority. Encourage family participation, individual exercise, and team sports and structured activities with peers as appropriate. Strive for 1 h or more a day of vigorous activity.
- Limit "screen time" to 2 hours or less per day. Replace screen time with family activities, hobbies, or chores. Remove televisions from children's bedrooms (if present). Children who watch 4 or more hours of television per day are twice as likely as other children to become obese. Children are more sedentary when they watch television, and frequent food advertising is linked to increased snacking.
- Praise and reward children for the progress they make in reaching nutrition, activity, physical fitness, self-esteem, or weight goals.
- Emphasize the uniqueness of each child, pointing out special talents, abilities, and positive qualities.

If initial efforts at changing lifestyles are unsuccessful, referral to a nutritionist or registered dietician and a weight and exercise program for more rigorous management is indicated. Referral to a behavioral/mental health specialist may be indicated for some children and adolescents with low self-esteem or depression related to overweight and obesity. Box 17.6 outlines suggestions for counseling overweight children and their families. Medication or surgery may be appropriate for some children.

Medications. Medications should be used only after an intensive, formal trial of lifestyle change has proven ineffective and the child is excessively obese (>95th percentile) or overweight (>85th percentile) with comorbidities present (Boland et al., 2015); medication should always be used in conjunction with dietary changes and exercise. Providers should also inquire about whether the family or child is self-medicating and with what products. Several products are available over the counter (OTC) or as herbal or diet supplements.

Orlistat (decreases fat absorption) is approved by the U.S. Food and Drug Administration (FDA) for children 12 years and older and is available OTC and by prescription; OTC preparations are not recommended for children younger than 18 years old. Orlistat is contraindicated in individuals with gallbladder disease, malabsorption syndromes, pregnancy, and sensitivity to the drug. Major side effects of orlistat are fatty stool and gastrointestinal upset; fiber supplements (e.g., glucomannan) can be used to help control side effects.

Metformin does not have FDA approval for use in treatment of obesity and is not considered a weight-loss treatment, but it has been used off-label in monitored weight programs and has led to decreased BMIs (Styne et al., 2017). Metformin reduces hepatic glucose production, increases insulin sensitivity, and may reduce appetite. Although there are a number of amphetamine-like catecholaminergic and dopaminergic stimulants approved for use in obesity in adults, none are recommended for weight management in children and adolescents (Styne et al., 2017). The Pediatric Endocrine Society suggests that "clinicians should discontinue medication and reevaluate the patient if the patient does not have a greater than 4% BMI/BMI z score reduction after taking antiobesity medication for 12 weeks at the medication's full dosage" (Styne et al., 2017, p. 712).

Bariatric Surgery. The Pediatric Endocrine Society recommends bariatric surgery only for adolescents who meet the following criteria (Styne et al., 2017):
- Extreme obesity persists despite participation in a formal weight management program
- Have attained a Sexual Maturity Rating or Tanner 4 or 5 pubertal development and final or near-final adult height
- Have a BMI of greater than 40 kg/m^2 or a BMI greater than 35 kg/m^2 with significant comorbidities
- Have no underlying untreated psychiatric disorder
- Demonstrate ability to adhere to lifestyle changes such as healthy dietary and physical activity habits
- Have access to a Pediatric Bariatric Surgery Center that provides long-term follow-up

The American Society for Metabolic and Bariatric Surgery Pediatric Committee recommends that adolescents with class II (120% of the 95th percentile on CDC age and gender growth charts) and class III (140% of the 95th percentile) obesity be considered for metabolic and bariatric surgery (MBS) (Pratt et al, 2018). Furthermore, given the risks versus benefits of MBS, adolescents with severe comorbidities (e.g., depression, obstructive sleep apnea, type 2 diabetes, and fatty liver disease) should be considered for MBS to reduce the risk of persistent obesity and long-standing comorbidities (Pratt et al., 2018).

Community Changes. Individual and family interventions may not be sufficient to deal with the causes of obesity. For example, if children cannot safely play outside, it may be impossible for them to get the recommended 60 minutes of moderate-to-vigorous daily exercise they need. Community change is imperative to support individual and family efforts to lose weight. The CDC recommends community action in six different areas (see Additional Resources):
- Increasing access to affordable healthy foods
- Supporting healthy food choices
- Promoting breastfeeding
- Encouraging physical activity
- Providing safe communities in which to exercise
- Organizing at the grass roots to create and continue health-supportive change

PCPs can use the CDC Guidebook to advocate for their patients with community policy makers, giving them information about obesity as a public health problem and supporting public policy that creates positive change.

Complications

Children who are overweight or obese are at risk for hypertension, fatty liver disease, impaired glucose tolerance, diabetes, sleep apnea, orthopedic conditions (e.g., slipped capital femoral epiphysis), decreased energy and mobility, bullying, low self-esteem, depression, and suicide. They should be screened for conditions related to obesity at regular intervals and referred as indicated for further evaluation and treatment.

Adverse Food Reactions

A distinction is made between *food allergy*, a hypersensitivity to a food or food additive with a reproducible immediate or delayed immune system response (e.g., anaphylactic reaction to ingestion of nuts; atopic skin reaction), and *food intolerance*, a nonimmunologic inability to process or tolerate the food product (e.g., enzyme deficiencies [lactase] or PKU secondary to the body's inability to metabolize phenylalanine). Food can also be toxic (e.g., food poisoning or toxins from bacteria growing in the food) or create pharmacologic effects (e.g., headaches after eating ice cream). All are considered adverse reactions to food.

Although there has been an increase in reports of food allergies in the past two decades, their actual prevalence remains low. Parent reports suggest that 6.5% of children 0 to 17 years old have experienced a food allergy reaction in the past year (Black and Benson, 2018). However, based on serum immunoglobulin E (IgE), NHANES reported that an estimated 3.51% of the American population has food allergies to four foods (peanuts, cow's milk, eggs, and shrimp) (McGowan and Keet, 2013). As diagnostics become more sensitive and diverse, a more accurate measurement of food allergies will be possible (Sicherer and Sampson, 2018). Although few children are allergic to foods, food is the most common cause of anaphylaxis in children seen in an emergency department (Garbenhenrich et al., 2016). Factors contributing to adverse food allergies include the following:
- Heredity: Children with a history of food allergy in their family are more likely to have an allergy themselves. Children born with a metabolic disorder can have adverse reactions to specific foods.
- Infant diet: Breastfeeding may be protective against allergies, although the data about this are mixed. It also appears that solid foods should be introduced by 6 months of age, including foods that are considered allergenic (e.g., eggs, peanuts) (Sicherer and Sampson, 2018); later introduction may actually increase food sensitization (see Chapter 33).
- Immature gastrointestinal tract: Before 7 months old, the infant gastrointestinal tract is more permeable to large molecules, including most food proteins. Allergies to milk and eggs are more common in younger infants and are often outgrown with age and maturity.
- Compromised gastrointestinal tract: As a result of injury or illness, the gastrointestinal system can be more permeable to allergens, such as large proteins.
- Type of food: Some foods are more allergenic than others, and some individuals have greater sensitivity to certain foods. Only

a few foods—cow's milk, eggs, peanuts, soybeans, wheat, fish, crustaceans, and tree nuts (including almonds and cashews)—account for nearly 90% of IgE-mediated allergic reactions. Commercial baby foods that may appear to be only one fruit or vegetable can have eggs or milk added. Counsel parents on reading food labels.

- Allergic load or tolerance level: Conditions such as illness, stress, surgery, or trauma can place excessive metabolic demands on the body. An individual who is susceptible to food intolerance or allergy can have a reaction when these conditions are present. In addition, individuals may be allergic to more than one food and experience a reaction if more than one allergen is present.

Clinical Findings

The goals of a thorough clinical assessment are to determine whether an allergic reaction has occurred, whether it is related to food, to which food is it related, and how serious the problem is. This process is extremely challenging and can require referral to a registered dietitian or use of a team approach with primary provider, dietitian, and allergist for a more in-depth diagnostic work-up.

History. The history should assess the following:
- Age of child
- Suspected food
- Route of exposure: Ingested? Skin touched? Food dust inhaled?
- Amount of exposure
- Onset of symptoms relative to exposure
- Description of symptoms (gather data about change over the course of the reaction)
- Description of other factors that are present and may contribute to or aggravate an allergic response (e.g., stress, environment, exercise)
- Treatment given and child's response
- Does child have a previous history of symptoms following exposure to this food?
- What is the child's diet history? When and what types of foods were introduced into the diet?
- Does the child have a history of symptoms frequently seen in food allergies (e.g., respiratory distress, eczema, urticaria, rashes, colic, vomiting, diarrhea) unaccompanied by other signs of illness or history of exposure to infectious agents?
- Is there a family history of allergies, especially a history of reaction to certain foods?

Describe the child's usual intake. A food diary is an excellent mechanism for obtaining these data and includes the following:
- All foods and fluids ingested for at least 3 days
- How food is prepared (e.g., commercially, at home, fried, baked)
- How food is stored and fed to the child
- All medications, including herbs and dietary supplements
- Child's reactions to foods ingested (food-symptom diary). This can become a time-consuming, cumbersome task, especially if more than one food is involved; it requires real commitment on the part of parents.

Physical Examination. Signs and symptoms of adverse food reactions vary by type and severity, from a mild local reaction to life-threatening anaphylaxis, making it often difficult to diagnose the condition definitively. Table 17.8 lists possible clinical manifestations of food allergies or intolerances by body system. Height and weight should be monitored closely in children with food allergies because food elimination and use of alternative foods may compromise nutrition and affect growth. Chapter 33 reviews the

TABLE 17.8	Possible Clinical Manifestations of Food Allergies or Intolerances by Body System
System	**Symptoms**
Respiratory system	Chronic rhinitis Asthma Croup Cough Serous otitis media Bronchitis
Gastrointestinal system	Tingling and swelling of lips, mouth, throat Nausea, vomiting Diarrhea Colic Protein-losing enteropathy Bloating, flatulence Constipation Gastrointestinal blood loss Malabsorption
Integumentary system	Eczema Pruritus Atopic dermatitis Rashes Urticaria
Central nervous system	Headaches (sinus, migraine) Fatigue Drowsiness, listlessness Irritability Depression Excessive sweating
Circulatory system	Hypotension Cardiac dysrhythmias Anaphylaxis Pallor

clinical features of an allergic reaction in a child and relates it to the level of severity.

Diagnostic Studies. A double-blind, placebo-controlled food challenge is recognized as the "gold standard" for determining the presence of food allergy, but this is not usually practical for the clinical setting. Laboratory studies are used more commonly and include:

- Skin tests: The skin prick test (SPT) is very sensitive. However, cutaneous response may not correlate with a clinical systemic response. Antihistamine medications must be discontinued 3 to 20 days before the test, and the test should be avoided in children who have generalized skin lesions, dermographism, or a severe reaction to food following skin contact or inhalation.
- Serum IgE and eosinophil count (elevated serum IgE and eosinophilia >400/mm^3 are usually related to allergies). This test is done if the child cannot have an SPT done, but it can be expensive, especially if more than one food is suspected. Results must be interpreted carefully by an allergist because findings can reflect exposure to other allergens.
- Atopy patch tests: The atopy patch test looks for skin reaction to food but is not widely used in the clinical setting.
- Food elimination and challenge: When a food has been identified as a potential source of the problem, elimination and an oral food challenge can be used to confirm the diagnosis.

Medical supervision during the elimination and challenge is essential (to ensure prompt treatment in case of a severe reaction), and interpretation of responses should be done by an allergist or immunologist; overall the procedure has been found to be relatively safe (O'Keefe et al., 2014). The suspected foods are completely eliminated from the child's diet for at least 3 days and up to 4 weeks and then gradually reintroduced, one at a time. The initial reintroduction dose should be small and then increased until either a reaction recurs or the amount normally eaten is given. If exercise is thought to contribute to the initial allergic reaction, exercise must be part of the challenge. An allergy or intolerance is confirmed if symptoms cease when the food is eliminated and then reappear as it is reintroduced. If there is a possibility of a severe reaction to a food (e.g., anaphylaxis), the child should be hospitalized with emergency cardiovascular support available for the challenge part of this process.

Differential Diagnosis

The differential diagnoses for food allergy and food intolerance include:

- Reactions related to other environmental allergens
- Asthma as a result of other causes
- Immunodeficiency
- Psychological reactions to feeding
- Malabsorption syndromes (e.g., celiac disease), cystic fibrosis
- Lactose intolerance
- Chronic diarrhea
- Heiner syndrome, a milk-induced pulmonary disease with infiltrates, should be suspected in infants and young children who have persistent pulmonary disease without a clear cause.

Management

The goals of managing children with adverse food reactions are to maintain nutrition levels adequate for normal growth and development, prevent nutritional deficits, avoid exposure to offending food or foods, and respond promptly and appropriately to adverse reactions after exposure. Once a child has been assessed as to the cause and severity of the response, a treatment plan can be made. The National Institute of Allergy and Infectious Diseases (NIAID) has developed guidelines for managing food allergies (Burks et al., 2011). Prevention is always preferred, and early introduction of foods considered to be allergenic, especially peanut, is advised (Sicherer and Sampson, 2018).

Elimination Diet. The standard of practice is to avoid the offending food or foods. Efforts to eliminate the food from the diet raise challenging issues:

- The foods to which most individuals are allergic are very common and very nutritious. Extensive use of elimination diets can lead to malnourishment; these diets should be used for as short a time as possible.
- Sometimes the individual is allergic to the food in its raw form but can eat it in a cooked (heat-treated) form; completely eliminating it means unnecessary loss of a good source of nutrients.
- The food may contaminate other foods or be found in minute amounts in other foods (e.g., processed foods).
- Skin or inhalant contact may occur (e.g., breathing peanut dust) even if food is not eaten.
- Cross-reacting allergens may further limit diets.

Restricted foods need to be replaced with those of equivalent nutrient value in the context of a well-balanced diet. In addition, the physical problems caused by allergies (e.g., diarrhea, vomiting, dehydration, eczema) can create a need for extra nutrients to maintain health and foster growth. Consultation with a dietitian is recommended. For formula-fed infants allergic to cow's milk, hypoallergenic formula preparations are recommended (Lifschitz and Szajewska, 2015) (see Table 17.4). Extensively hydrolyzed cow's milk–based preparations may protect against allergy but can be expensive, and the infant may not accept the taste. Elemental formulas, synthesized free amino acids with vitamin and mineral supplements, can be used. Soy-based formulas are often a first-choice alternative for older infants, but many infants allergic to cow's milk are also sensitive to soy (see Chapter 33).

Oral Immunotherapy. Oral immunotherapy (OIT) has shown promise as an effective treatment for food allergy and may raise the threshold of reactivity in children with a range of IgE-mediated food allergies (Nurmatov et al., 2017). A recent study on preschool children with peanut allergy showed peanut-specific IgE allergy significantly declined in children treated with early OIT, although sensitization returned when the treatment was stopped. In the children in the study group, allergic side effects were mild to moderate (Vickery et al., 2017). However, allergic side effects are common and long-term follow-up is required to decrease reactivity. Immunotherapy for food allergies requires referral to a pediatric specialist, may require hospitalization for treatment, and should not be used routinely in clinical practice; safety is paramount and avoidance of the food allergen remains the standard of practice.

Revisiting the Food Challenge. The child's allergic status should be reevaluated at regular intervals. Food allergies and food intolerances are often outgrown; therefore the child may be challenged with most offending foods at intervals in the clinical setting. Cow's milk and egg allergies are often outgrown by 2 years old (Burks et al., 2012). Some foods appear to remain allergenic for longer periods (e.g., seafood, peanuts, and tree nuts) (Gupta et al., 2013). If the child's reaction has been serious or even life threatening, the parents may decide to continue to avoid the food. Many fatalities related to food allergies occur among older children, teenagers, and young adults.

Medication. Self-administered epinephrine is prescribed for children with moderate or severe allergies. Children, their parents, and other caregivers should be educated on intramuscular injection using a prepared epinephrine injection. Children at risk for food-related anaphylaxis should carry two doses of epinephrine. Antihistamines are prescribed for children with mild allergies, unless there is a history of a reaction to trace amounts of the allergen or the child has asthma from another cause; in these cases, epinephrine is appropriate. Children with food allergies should wear a medical-alert bracelet or necklace. School personnel should be informed of the child's allergy, and a medical plan should be implemented in the school.

Education. Education of families, children, and adults who are responsible for the child's well-being is critical. The provider can do outreach to teachers, schools, and day care centers with information about how to understand and safely manage the child's condition and be an ongoing source of suggestions, support, and advocacy for parents.

Complications

Complications of adverse food reactions include anaphylaxis, asthma, convulsive coughing (leading to aspiration and choking), malnutrition, gastrointestinal dysfunction, secondary skin infections, and disruption of family processes.

Toxic Exposures in Foods

Exposure to toxins and chemicals through the food chain contribute to many health problems in children. Chapter 44 examines the relationship between toxic exposure in foods and children's health.

Effect of Medications on Nutritional Status

Medications are designed to alter the body's biochemistry to promote healing. These biochemical changes can affect the individual's nutritional status in a number of ways. Some medications deplete essential nutrients from the body; others interfere with enzyme activity, absorption, distribution, and metabolism of nutrients. PCPs should consider nutritional implications of any medication and consult a pharmacologic resource for a full discussion of these dynamics.

Controversies in Pediatric Nutrition

Sugar Consumption

Diets high in sugar, particularly high fructose corn syrup and sucrose-fructose blends (e.g., sugar in soft drinks and juices) should be avoided in infants, children, and adolescents. Such diets tend to replace more nutrient-dense foods and contribute to overweight and obesity, dental caries, insulin resistance, metabolic syndrome, and other health problems. The American Heart Association (AHA) recommends that less than half of an individual's discretionary calories should come from added sugar (i.e., sugar not found naturally in fruits) (AHA, 2014). For the preschooler who consumes 1200 to 1400 calories/day, this equates to approximately four teaspoons of added sugar; for the 4- to 8-year-old child with a 1600 calorie intake, it is approximately three teaspoons; and for older children and adults who consume 2000 calories daily, it is approximately five to eight teaspoons each day. According to the Harvard School of Public Health, "the average can of sugar-sweetened soda or fruit punch provides the equivalent of 10 teaspoons of table sugar" (Harvard TH Chan School of Public Health, 2015).

Gluten-Free Diets

Gluten-free diets are the only known, effective treatment for celiac disease (see Chapter 40). Approximately 1% of the American population has a diagnosis of celiac disease, a statistic that has remained stable (University of Chicago, 2018). However, nearly 20% of individuals and families in the United States try to include gluten-free foods in their diet. A recent survey found that 53% of respondents who eat a gluten-free diet believe gluten-free foods are healthier and 27% believe that they will help them lose weight (Pauk, 2014). There is also an increasing number of self-diagnosed individuals with gluten sensitivity who state they have improved gastrointestinal symptoms on gluten-free products (Fryar et al., 2016). However, gluten-free grain products are often highly processed and not enriched with iron or folate. Sugar is often added to enhance the flavor of gluten-free products and can represent a health risk (Elliott, 2018). Gluten-free products may also be low in protein and are used for patients with metabolic diseases, such as PKU, who have a severely restricted protein allowance. Parents of children with gluten intolerance or sensitivity need to carefully assess gluten-free product labels.

Some individuals may be sensitive to wheat or other grains as in "nonceliac wheat sensitivity" and may have symptoms associated with wheat consumption, such as indigestion, abdominal pain, bloating, or fatigue. These symptoms may be due to dietary fermentable oligo-di-monosaccharides and polyols (FODMAPs) (e.g., fructose, lactose, fructans, galactans, polyols) and not exclusively wheat (Aziz and Sanders, 2014). The incidence of nonceliac gluten sensitivity is unknown.

Additional Resources

Academy of Nutrition and Dietetics. www.eatright.org
American Academy of Allergy Asthma and Immunology. www.aaaai.org
American Academy of Pediatrics Institute for Healthy Childhood Weight. https://ihcw.aap.org/Pages/default.aspx
American Diabetes Association. www.diabetes.org
American School Food Service Association. www.diet.com/g/american-school-food-service-association
Asthma and Allergy Foundation of America. www.aafa.org
BAM! Body and Mind. www.cdc.gov/bam/
Bright Futures Nutrition. http://brightfutures.aap.org/Nutrition_3rd_Edition.html
CDC Community Strategies to Prevent Obesity. www.cdc.gov/obesity/downloads/community_strategies_guide.pdf
CDC Division of Nutrition, Physical Activity, and Obesity. www.cdc.gov/nccdphp/dnpao
Food Allergy Research and Education. www.foodallergy.org
Gluten Intolerance Group. https://gluten.org/
Kids with Food Allergies. http://www.kidswithfoodallergies.org/
KidsHealth. www.kidshealth.org
National Academies Press (Daily Recommended Intakes). http://nationalacademies. org/hmd/~/media/Files/Activity Files/Nutrition/DRI-Tables/8_ Macronutrient Summary.pdf. https://www.nap.edu/catalog/11537/dietary-reference-intakes- the-essential-guide-to-nutrient-requirements.
National Agricultural Library/USDA. www.nutrition.gov
National Institute of Allergy and Infectious Diseases. https://www.niaid.nih.gov/
School Nutrition Association. https://schoolnutrition.org/
Shapedown: Weight Management for Children and Adolescents. www.shapedown.com
U.S. Department of Agriculture (USDA) ChooseMyPlate. www.choosemyplate.gov
U.S. Department of Agriculture (USDA) Healthy Eating Index. www.cnpp.usda.gov/healthyeatingindex
USDA Food Composition Databases. http://ndb.nal.usda.gov

References

American Academy of Pediatrics (AAP). Section on Breastfeeding: breastfeeding and the use of human milk. *Pediatrics.* 2012;129(3):e827–e841.
American Heart Association (AHA). *Sugar.101*; 2014. Available at: www.heart.org/HEARTORG/GettingHealthy/NutritionCenter/Healthy-Eating/Sugar-101_UCM_306024_Article.jsp. Accessed Oct 16, 2018.
Aziz I, Sanders DS. Patients who avoid wheat and gluten: is that health or lifestyle? *Dig Dis Sci.* 2014;59(6):1080–1082.
Black LI, Benson V. *Tables of summary health statistics for U.S. children: 2017 National Health Interview Survey*; 2018. Available at: www.cdc.gov/nchs/nhis/SHS/tables.htm. Accessed Dec 4, 2018.
Boland CL, Harris JB, Harris KB. Pharmacological management of obesity in pediatric patients. *Ann Pharmacother.* 2015;49(2):220–232.
Brown A, Jones SW, Rowan H. Baby-led weaning: the evidence to date. *Curr Nutr Rep.* 2017;6(2):148–156.
Burks AW, Jones SM, Boyce JA, et al. NIAID-sponsored 2010 guidelines for managing food allergy: applications in the pediatric population. *Pediatrics.* 2011;128(5):955–965.
Burks AW, Tang M, Sicherer S, et al. ICON: food allergy. *J Allergy Clin Immunol.* 2012;129(4):906–920.

Casamassimo P, Holt K, eds. *Bright Futures In Practice: Oral Health—Pocket Guide*. 2nd ed. Washington, DC: National Maternal and Child Oral Health Resource Center; 2014.

Centers for Disease Control and Prevention (CDC). *Bmi Percentile Calculator For Child And Teen*. Atlanta: CDC, U.S. Department of Health and Human Services; 2018.

Centers for Disease Control and Prevention (CDC). *Physical Education Profiles, 2012: Physical Education and Physical Activity Practices and Policies Among Secondary Schools at Select US Sites*. Atlanta: CDC, U.S. Department of Health and Human Services; 2014.

Chelvakumar G, Levin L, Polfuss M, et al. Perception and documentation of weight management practices in pediatric primary care. *WMJ*. 2014;113(4):149–153.

Coleman-Jensen A, Gregory C, Singh A. *Household Food Security in the United States in 2013, Err-173*. Washington DC: U.S. Department of Agriculture, Economic Research Service; 2014.

Cook S, Weitzman M, Auinger P, et al. Screening and counseling associated with obesity diagnosis in a national survey of ambulatory pediatric visits. *Pediatrics*. 2005;116(1):112–116.

Crane JM, White J, Murphy P, et al. The effect of gestational weight gain by body mass index on maternal and neonatal outcomes. *J Obstet Gynaecol Can*. 2009;31(1):28–35.

Cunningham SD, Mokshagundam S, Chai H, et al. Postpartum depressive symptoms: gestational weight gain as a risk factor for adolescents who are overweight or obese. *J Midwifery Womens Health*. 2018;63(2):178–184.

DEFY Media. *ACUMEN report: constant content. 3rd annual*; 2015 (PDF online) http://cdn.defymedia.com/wp-content/uploads/2015/10/Acumen-Report-Constant-Content.pdf. Accessed Oct 20, 2018.

Dhurandhar EJ, Keith SW. The etiology of obesity beyond eating more and exercising less. *Best Pract Res Clin Gastroenterol*. 2014;28(4):533–544.

Elliott C. The nutritional quality of gluten-free products for children. *Pediatrics*. 2018;132(2):1–8.

Escribano J, Luque V, Ferre N, et al. Effect of protein intake and weight gain velocity on body fat mass at 6 months of age: the EU Childhood Obesity Programme. *Int J Obes (Lond)*. 2012;36(4):548–553.

Feldman-Winter L, Burnham L, Grossman X, et al. Weight gain in the first week of life predicts overweight at 2 years: a prospective cohort study. *Matern Child Nutr*. 2018;14(1).

Food and Nutrition Board (FNB), Institute of Medicine (IOM). Dietary reference intakes for energy, carbohydrate, fiber, fat, fatty acids, cholesterol, protein, and amino acids. Washington, DC: National Academies Press; 2005.

Fryar CD, Carroll MD, Ogden CL. *Prevalence of overweight and obesity among children and adolescents aged 2-19 years: United States, 1963-1965 through 2013-2014*. National Center for Health Statistics (NCHS); 2016. Available at: https://www.cdc.gov/nchs/data/hestat/obesity_child_13_14/obesity_child_13_14.htm. Accessed Oct 28, 2018.

Garbenhenrich LB, Dolle S, Moneret-Vautrin A, et al. Anaphylaxis in children and adolescents: the European Anaphylaxis Registry. *J Allergy Clin Immun*. 2016;137(4):1128–1137.

Gearhardt AN, Roberto CA, Seamans MJ, et al. Preliminary validation of the Yale Food Addiction Scale for children. *Eat Behav*. 2013;14(4):508–512.

Gupta RS, Lau CH, Sita EE, et al. Factors associated with reported food allergy tolerance among US children. *Ann Allergy Asthma Immunol*. 2013;111(3):194–198.

Harvard TH Chan School of Public Health. *Added sugar in the diet*; 2015. Available at: www.hsph.harvard.edu/nutritionsource/carbohydrates/added-sugar-in-the-diet/. Accessed Oct 28, 2018.

Heindel JJ, Newbold R, Schug TT. Endocrine disruptors and obesity. *Nat Rev Endocrinol*. 2015;11(11):653–661.

Holt K, Wooldridge N, eds. *Bright Futures in Practice: Nutrition*. 3rd ed. Elk Grove Village, IL: American Academy of Pediatrics; 2011.

Huh SY, Rifas-Shiman SL, Taveras EM, et al. Timing of solid food introduction and risk of obesity in preschool-aged children. *Pediatrics*. 2011;127(3):e544–e551.

Institute of Medicine (IOM) Committee on Nutrition Standards for National School Lunch and Breakfast Programs, Stallings VA, West Suitor C, et al. In: *School Meals: Building Blocks For Healthy Children*. Washington, DC: National Academies Press; 2010.

Kabali HK, Irigoyen MM, Nunez-Davis R, et al. Exposure and use of mobile media devices by young children. *Pediatrics*. 2015;136(6):1–7.

Kleinman RE, Greer FR, eds. *Pediatric Nutrition*. 7th ed. Elk Grove Village, IL: American Academy of Pediatrics; 2013.

Kranz S, Brauchla M, Slavin JL, et al. What do we know about dietary fiber intake in children and health? The effects of fiber intake on constipation, obesity, and diabetes in children. *Adv Nutr*. 2012;3(1):47–53.

Le Louer B, Lemale J, Garcette K, et al. Severe nutritional deficiencies in young infants with inappropriate plant milk consumption [Article in French]. *Arch Pediatr*. 2014;21(5):483–488.

Lifschitz C, Szajewska H. Cow's milk allergy: evidence-based diagnosis and management for the practitioner. *Euro J Pediatri*. 2015;174:131–150.

Locke AE, Kahali B, Berndt SI, et al. Genetic studies of body mass index yield new insights for obesity biology. *Nature*. 2015;18(7538):197–206.

Lundahl A, Kidwell K, Nelson TD. Parental underestimates of child weight: a meta-analysis. *Pediatrics*. 2014;133(3):e689–e703.

Lustig RH. Which comes first? The obesity or the insulin? The behavior or the biochemistry? *J Pediatr*. 2008;152(5):601–602.

Lustig RH, Mulligan K, Noworolski SM, et al. Isocaloric fructose restriction and metabolic improvement in children with obesity and metabolic syndrome. *Obesity*. 2016;00(00):1–8.

McGowan EC, Keet CA. Prevalence of self-reported food allergy in the National Health and Nutrition Examination Survey (NHANES) 2007-2010. *J Allergy Clin Immunol*. 2013;132(5):1216–1219.

Mies GW, Treur JL, Larsen JK, et al. The prevalence of food addiction in a large sample of adolescents and its association with addictive substances. *Appetite*. 2017;118:97–105.

NHLBI. Expert Panel on Integrated Guidelines for Cardiovascular Health and Risk Reduction in Children and Adolescents: Summary report. *Pediatrics*. 2011;128(suppl 5):S213–S256.

National Committee for Quality Assurance (NCQA). *Weight assessment and counseling for nutrition and physical activity for children/adolescents (WCC)*; 2018. Available at: https://www.ncqa.org/hedis/measures/weight-assessment-and-counseling-for-nutrition-and-physical-activity-for-children-adolescents/. Accessed Oct 26, 2018.

Nielsen SJ, Rossen LM, Harris DM, et al. Fruit and vegetable consumption of U.S. youth, 2009-2010. *NCHS Data Brief*. 2014;156:1–8.

Niinikoski H, Ruottinen S. Is carbohydrate intake in the first years of life related to future risk of NCDs? *Nutr Metab Cardiovasc Dis*. 2012;22(10):770–774.

Nurmatov U, Dhami S, Arasi S, et al. Allergen immunotherapy for IgE-mediated food allergy: a systematic review and meta-analysis. *Allergy*. 2017;72(8):1133–1147.

Ogden CL, Carroll MD, Fryar CD, et al. *Prevalence of Obesity Among Adults and Youth: United States. 2011-2014*. Hyattsville, MD: NCHS data brief; 2015. No. 219.

O'Keefe AW, De Schryver S, Mill J, et al. Diagnosis and management of food allergies: new and emerging options: a systematic review. *J Asthma Allergy*. 2014;7:141–164.

Oranta O, Pahkala K, Ruottinen S, et al. Infancy-onset dietary counseling of low-saturated-fat diet improves insulin sensitivity in healthy adolescents 15-20 years of age: the Special Turku Coronary Risk Factor Intervention Project (STRIP) study. *Diabetes Care*. 2013;36(10):2952–2959.

Pauk S. The rise of gluten-free: trends in the US free-from market; 2014. Available at: www.chicagoift.org/members/presentations/Professional%20Dev_Presentation1_The%20Rise%20of%20Gluten%20Free.pdf. Accessed Oct 28, 2018.

Pludowski P, Holick MF, Grant WB, et al. Vitamin D supplementation guidelines. *J Steroid Biochemistry Mol Bio*. 2018;175:125–135.

Pollan M. *In Defense of Food*. New York: Penguin Press; 2008.

Poti JM, Slining MM, Popkin BM. Where are kids getting their empty calories? Stores, schools, and fast-food restaurants each played an important role in empty calorie intake among US children during 2009-2010. *J Acad Nutr Diet*. 2014;114(6):908–917.

Pratt JSA, Browne A, Browne NT, et al. ASMBS pediatric metabolic and bariatric surgery guidelines, 2018. *Surg Obes Relat Dis*. 2018;14(7):882–901.

Rietmeijer-Mentink M, Paulis WD, van Middelkoop M, et al. Difference between parental perception and actual weight status of children: a systematic review. *Matern Child Nutr*. 2013;9(1):3–22.

Rossinger A, Herrick K, Gahche J, Park S. *Sugar-Sweetened Beverage Consumption Among U.S. Youth, 2011-2014. NCHS Data Brief No. 217*. USDHHS; 2017.

Rush EC. Water: neglected, unappreciated and under researched. *Eur J Clin Nutr*. 2013;67(5):492–495.

Satter EM. The feeding relationship. *J Am Diet Assoc*. 1986;66(3):352–354.

Segovia-Siapco G, Jung S, Sabaté J. Vegetarian diets and pediatric obesity. In: Freemark M, ed. *Pediatric Obesity: Etiology, Pathogenesis and Treatment*. New York: Humana Press; 2018.

Sicherer SH, Sampson HA. Food allergy, a review and update on epidemiology, pathogenesis, diagnosis, prevention and management. *J Allergy Clin Immunol*. 2018;141(1):41–58.

Styne DM, Arllanian SA, Commor EL, et al. Pediatric obesity-Assessment, treatment, and prevention: an endocrine society clinical practice guideline. *J Clin Endocrinol Metab*. 2017;102(3):709–757.

U.S. Department of Health and Human Services (HHS). *U.S. Department of Agriculture (USDA). Dietary Guidelines for Americans, 2015-2020*. ed 8. Washington, DC: U.S. Government Printing Office; 2015. Available at: https://health.gov/dietaryguidelines/2015/resources/2015-2020_Dietary_Guidelines.pdf. Accessed Jan 20, 2019.

U.S. Department of Health and Human Services (HHS). *Physical activity guidelines for Americans*. 2nd ed. 2018. Available at: https://health.gov/paguidelines/second-edition/pdf/Physical_Activity_Guidelines_2nd_edition.pdf. Accessed Jan 20, 2019.

U.S. Preventive Services Task Force (USPSTF). *Obesity in children and adolescents: screening*; 2017. Available at: https://www.uspreventiveservicestaskforce.org/Page/Document/UpdateSummaryFinal/obesity-in-children-and-adolescents-screening1. Accessed Jan 20, 2019.

University of Chicago Medicine Celiac Disease Center. *Fact Sheet: overview of celiac disease*; 2018. Available at: www.cureceliacdisease.org/wp-content/uploads/FactSheet1_Overview-of-Celiac-Disease.pdf. Accessed Jan 20, 2019.

Van Winckel M, Vande Velde S, De Bruyne R, et al. Clinical practice: vegetarian infant and child nutrition. *Eur J Pediatr*. 2011;170(12):1489–1494.

van der Willik EM, Vrikotte TG, Altenburg TM, et al. Exclusively breast-fed overweight infants are at the same risk of childhood overweight as formula fed overweight infants. *Arch Dis Child*. 2015;100(10):932–937.

Vickery BP, Berglund JP, Burk CM, et al. Early oral immunotherapy in peanut-allergic preschool children is safe and highly effective. *J Allergy Clini Immunol*. 2017;139:173–181.

Vitolo MR, Bortolini GA, Campagnolo PD, et al. Maternal dietary counseling reduces consumption of energy-dense foods among infants: a randomized controlled trial. *J Nutr Educ Behav*. 2012;44(2):140–147.

Watanabe F, Bito T. Vitamin B12 sources and microbial interaction. *Exp Biol Med (Maywood)*. 2018;243(2):148–158.

Weber M, Grote V, Closa-Monasterolo R, et al. Lower protein content in infant formula reduces BMI and obesity risk at school age: follow-up of a randomized trial. *Am J Clin Nutr*. 2014;99(5):1041–1051.

Wethington H, Pan L, Sherry B. The association of screen time, television in the bedroom, and obesity among school-aged youth: 2007 National Survey of Children's Health. *J Sch Health*. 2013;83(8):573–581.

World Health Organization (WHO). *The WHO child growth standards*; 2018. Available at: www.who.int/childgrowth/standards/en/. Accessed Dec 3, 2018.

18
Elimination

ARDYS M. DUNN, MICHELLE MCGARRY, AND MARY DIRKS

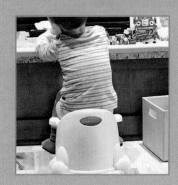

Metabolic by-products and wastes are eliminated from the body via the gastrointestinal (GI), renal, and integumentary systems. This chapter discusses normal bowel and bladder function and related normal developmental activities, such as toilet training. Problems that may require intervention (e.g., constipation, enuresis) or those related more directly to GI and genitourinary pathology are presented in Chapters 40 and 41. Dermatologic conditions are discussed in Chapter 34.

Healthy children demonstrate an extremely wide range of elimination patterns, and expectations about elimination vary with culture, social settings, and the parents' personal experience. As a result, parents may be unsure whether their child's pattern is problematic or not. Providers must offer assistance if a parent believes his or her child is experiencing a problem with elimination. The role of the primary care provider (PCP) is to conduct thorough and accurate assessments, provide anticipatory guidance for parents about what to expect as their child develops, and to help parents to recognize, understand, and facilitate healthy bowel and bladder function. Ineffective management of toilet training or lack of proper hydration may result in problems such as constipation, stool withholding, decreased appetite, vomiting, and urinary and fecal incontinence. Referral or intervention should be considered when an issue is complicated, out of normal developmental range, or causing distress to the parents and/or child.

Normal Patterns of Elimination: Bowel and Urinary

Elimination patterns are related to a child's age, intake of food and liquids, activity level, and health condition (e.g., fever can lead to dehydration and a subsequent decrease in urine output or transient constipation). Table 18.1 outlines specific differences in elimination patterns by age of child.

Assessment of Patterns

Assessment of elimination patterns begins with a thorough health history with questions asked of the parent or the child, depending on the child's age and ability. It is very important to get information from the child because parents may no longer be aware of habits, especially of older children. As variations of normal behavior become evident, relevant follow-up questions should be asked to clarify and complete the health picture.

Health History

Description of Current Status

The child's current elimination status can be assessed with the following questions:

- How often do you (asked of child) or does your child urinate? How many wet diapers does your baby have in a 24-hour period? Describe what the urine looks and smells like. How many times do you urinate at school (asked of school-age children)? What are the rules to get permission to go to the bathroom at school?
- How often do you (asked of child) or does your child have a bowel movement? Describe what the stools look, feel, and smell like. What is their size? How does your child act when having a bowel movement? Where does your child have bowel movements? Does your child use the toilet for both urine and stool? Does your child have aversions to having a bowel movement at school or in public restrooms?
- Is there anything unusual about your child's elimination habits? Does your child resist going to the bathroom, complain of pain, need to go often, or have a sense of urgency?
- Do you use any medications, including over-the-counter preparations or home remedies, to help your child with bowel movements?
- Describe your child's toileting habits. For example, at what time of day does your child have a bowel movement? Is this consistent?
- Ask parents of older infants: How do you think the process of toilet training will happen?
- Is your child toilet trained? When did training begin? Describe the process. How often do "accidents" happen? How do you (parent) feel toilet training is progressing? How stressed do you feel about the process and why?
- What names are used in your family for stool and urine, for body parts, and for the process of using the toilet? (Encourage use of accurate names).

Birth and Early Infancy History

Determine whether any problems with the child's urine or stool were present at birth and/or in the first month of life. Did the baby pass a meconium stool within 48 hours after birth? How soon after birth did the baby urinate? Was the baby breastfed? When were solids introduced and did that change stooling patterns or character?

TABLE 18.1   Normal Elimination Patterns by Age of Child

Age of Child	Bowel Function	Stool Characteristics	Urinary Function	Urine Characteristics	Signs of Adequate Function	Signs of Concern
Neonate	Meconium stool by 48 hrs old; then many small stools/day, typically 3-4 times daily	Breastfed infant stool is sticky, light yellow, curdy, with "sour" smell; formula-fed infant stool is darker, firmer, and smellier. Iron supplements can darken stool	Minimum of 6 times/day	Pale yellow or colorless	Moist mucous membranes; active; alert Grunting and straining are typical in infants as they pass stool; stool passes easily	Depressed fontanel; dry mucous membranes; fewer than 6 wet diapers a day; fewer than 1-2 stools/week; abdominal distention, vomiting; true constipation (see Rome IV criteria, Chapter 40) requires referral, especially in first month of life
Infant	Stooling typically decreases to one stool/day; breast-fed infant may go 8-14 days without stooling (AAP, 2012). Older infants begin to develop a pattern (e.g., first thing after waking in the morning)	Soft, semiformed, color depends on food intake; supplements	6-20 times a day	Pale yellow or colorless	See signs for neonate	
Toddler and preschooler	Patterns develop; usually 1 stool/day. Most children are toilet trained by 2.5-3.5 years old; bowel control typically precedes urine control	Soft, semiformed, color depends on food intake; supplements	Typically urinate 8-14 times a day; urge to urinate may be stimulated by cold, excitement, or stress	Pale yellow, no odor	Moist mucous membranes, active, alert Bedwetting is common until age 5 or 6. Stool passes easily	Fewer than 3-5 stools/week; illness or activity that increases need for fluids; vomiting, diarrhea
School-aged child	Adult function; 1-3 stools/day, 5-7 or more/week	Depends on food intake	Smaller bladder volume than adult; voids 6-8 times/day	Clear yellow; no odor	Increasing independence in toileting; may have poor hygiene	Dysfunctional voiding; daytime incontinence; nocturnal enuresis; encopresis may require referral (see Chapters 40 and 41)
Adolescent	Adult function	Depends on food intake; eating patterns	Adult function	Clear yellow; no odor		Sexual activity; eating disorders

Review of Systems

The review of systems should include the following questions:

- Has your child ever been constipated or had diarrhea? How do you define constipation and diarrhea? (See GI Chapter 40 for Bristol Scale of stool quality and the Rome IV criteria for functional constipation.) Is it persistent or only occasional? Did it start after a particular incident (e.g., illness, during toilet training, with a certain food or change in diet)? Providers need to remember that diarrhea can be a presenting symptom in constipation due to stool leaking around solid stool.

- Has your child ever had a urinary tract infection (UTI)? Describe the incident(s). How old was the child? Was there any fever, flank pain, or nausea and vomiting? Any work-up (e.g., ultrasonography [US], voiding cystourethrogram [VCUG])? What were the findings, treatment, and follow-up?

- Has your child had any illness, injury, or operation related to the bowel or bladder? Describe.

- Does your child have a physical condition or chronic illness that affects voiding or bowel movements?
- Is there a history of bed-wetting? At what age did it resolve?
- What medications, including over-the-counter preparations, herbs, or complementary medications, does your child take?

Family History

Determine whether any family members, including parents, have had problems with urination or bowel movements, and describe them (e.g., chronic constipation or diarrhea, bed-wetting; diagnosis of Hirschsprung disease). Has the child or family traveled or lived outside the United States? Does the family residence use well water?

Environmental and Psychosocial Issues

Environmental and psychosocial issues should be assessed, using questions such as:

- How do you, as a parent, feel about the issue of toileting?
- If appropriate, how often do you as a parent defecate/urinate?
- How do you interact with your child around toileting issues?
- How do you deal with toileting "accidents" (including bed-wetting)?
- What plans do you have for managing toilet training?
- Describe your child's typical diet.
- Tell me about the toileting facilities at your child's house, day care, and school. How do you think they affect your child's toileting habits?

Physical Examination

The physical examination includes external examination of the perineum, anus, and urinary meatus, including the base of the spine; and auscultation and palpation of the abdomen for bowel sounds, softness, masses, peristalsis, and tenderness. Perform an age-appropriate gross motor neurologic examination. A rectal digital exam is not warranted for healthy children.

Diagnostic Studies

Diagnostic studies may include:

- Urinalysis (with or without urine culture) as indicated based on symptoms
- Stool specimen for occult blood and ova and parasites, as indicated by history and symptoms
- Diagnostic imaging as indicated after initial laboratory work-up and assessment/management considerations (see Chapters 40 and 41)

Management Strategies for Normal Patterns

Toileting Skills

When to begin toilet training is a perennial question of parents. The AAP recommends that toilet training begins when the child and the parent are ready, which is not before 18 to 24 months old, although anticipatory guidance regarding toilet training readiness begins earlier (Wolraich, 2016).

PCPs should emphasize that every child is unique, and the child's development, readiness cues, parental expectations, and family circumstances should ultimately be used to decide when to begin toilet training. Learning to manage elimination for the child can be a stressful, messy project and, if begun too early, can actually take longer to complete than if begun when both the child and the family are ready. Starting too late can also be problematic because the initiation of toilet training after 36 months has been found to be related to constipation and dysfunctional voiding (Hodges et al., 2014). See Chapter 11, Developmental Management of Early Childhood, for a discussion of toilet training strategies.

Elimination Communication

Children around the world experience a wide variation in how elimination is managed; climate, environment, resources, family structure, and social dynamics all shape toileting practices of families and infants. In the United States, most infants are diapered until they master the art of self-toileting. Some families from various cultural groups who immigrated to the United States bring different expectations for toileting. For example, the process of *assisted toilet training* begins in the Vietnamese culture at approximately 3 months old, with most children trained by 24 months old (Duong et al., 2013). Currently, some U.S. families choose to use *elimination communication* (EC) or *natural infant hygiene* to manage their child's elimination (Bender and She, 2017). EC takes advantage of the regular elimination patterns of infants, especially older infants, and requires close communication between infant and caregiver. After the first few months and especially by the time they are 9 to 12 months old, infants generally have predictable elimination patterns; for example, they may have a bowel movement early in the morning or after feeding or stay dry for several hours and urinate immediately after waking from a nap. Infants may also give cues as to when they are urinating or defecating (e.g., grunting, straining, or becoming more still). Caregivers can use these patterns and cues to take the infant to the toilet. They can also introduce other elimination cues (e.g., the sound of running water, music, a swooshing sound in the infant's ear) when the infant is in position on the "potty," to encourage elimination. The infant is conditioned through practice and repetition to associate these cues with toileting, but the parent is being trained as well to be alert and responsive to the infant's signals.

Altered Patterns of Elimination: Bladder and Bowel Dysfunction

Bladder and bowel dysfunction (BBD) is any abnormal pattern in bladder and bowel function at an age when an individual is developmentally capable of control. A number of factors contribute to BBD, and the close relationship between bladder and bowel function, due to the function of the pelvic floor, is key to understanding this complex and varied condition; it is a set of conditions. Some children actively try to prevent bowel movements or urination (e.g., the school-aged child who has restricted access to bathroom facilities, the child who had a painful bowel movement and has decided that he or she does not want it to hurt, or the child who is "too busy" to stop and use the bathroom). The cause for each child is likely multifactorial, but in most cases, it is not necessary to know exactly why it happened. Parents can sometimes focus on the why, and, although having that information may help to prevent the problem from recurring, it is not necessary to treat and resolve the issue.

Urgency, frequency, and nocturnal and diurnal urinary incontinence are common in BBD. The child may have difficulty initiating urination or completely emptying the bladder. Persistent problems with incomplete emptying of the bladder can lead to UTI, vesicoureteral reflux (VUR), and (in severe or long-term situations) renal damage. Constipation can exacerbate bladder dysfunction by applying pressure to the bladder wall or restricting urinary flow. The child with BBD may experience stool incontinence (encopresis), either with or without constipation. Elimination problems also contribute to family difficulties, bullying, social isolation, emotional problems, and antisocial behaviors in families of children with fecal soiling (Koppen et al., 2016). Detailed discussions of these problems are presented in Chapters 40 and 41.

References

American Academy of Pediatrics (AAP). Breastfeeding and the use of human milk. *Pediatrics*. 2012;129(3):827–841.

Bender JM, She RC. Elimination communication: diaper-free in America. *Pediatrics*. 2017;140(1):e20170398. https://doi.org/10.1542/peds.2017-0398.

Duong TH, Jansson UB, Holmdahl G, et al. Urinary bladder control during the first 3 years of life of healthy children in Vietnam—a comparison study with Swedish children. *J Pediatr Urol*. 2013;9(6 Pt A):700–706.

Hodges SJ, Richards KA, Gorbachinsky I, et al. The association of age of toilet training and dysfunctional voiding. *Res Rep Urol*. 2014;6:127–130.

Koppen IJ, von Gontard A, Chase J, et al. Management of functional nonretentive fecal incontinence in children: recommendations from the International Children's Continence Society. *J Pediatr Urol*. 2016;12(1):56–64.

Wolraich ML, ed. *American Academy of Pediatrics Guide to Toilet Training*. 2nd ed. New York: Bantam Books; 2016.

19

Physical Activity and Sports for Children and Adolescents

MICHELE L. POLFUSS AND RENÉE L. DAVIS

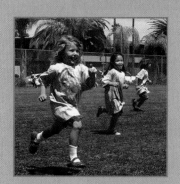

The importance of physical activity for all children and adolescents, including those with chronic health conditions and special health care needs, cannot be overstated. The benefits of children and adolescents engaging in regular physical activity are broad and include improving bone health, cardiorespiratory fitness, increasing lean mass and decreasing body fat, reducing symptoms of depression, and improving the individual's cognitive skills and ability to concentrate. Achieving a healthy lifestyle in childhood includes participating in physical activity in addition to optimizing nutrition and maintaining a healthy body weight. Physical activity is an essential component of overall health and the prevention of overweight, obesity, and the development of chronic health conditions (United States Department of Health and Human Services Office of Disease Prevention and Health Promotion, 2017).

Physical Activity: Overview

Physical activity is defined as "any bodily movement produced by skeletal muscles that requires energy expenditure" (World Health Organization, 2017a). While "exercise" is a subcategory of physical activity that is planned, structured, and repetitive, physical activity encompasses a broader definition (World Health Organization, 2017b). Physical activity in childhood and adolescence includes "free play, games, sports, transportation, chores, recreation, physical education, or planned exercise" and can occur in many contexts such as family, school, and the community (World Health Organization, 2017c).

Physical activity recommendations include children and adolescents participating in at least 60 minutes of moderate to vigorous physical activity daily and this timeframe can be divided into smaller sessions throughout the day. While most of the activity should be aerobic in nature, activities that strengthen muscles and bones should be performed at least three times a week (World Health Organization, 2017c). Currently, children and adolescents in the United States fail to meet the recommended national physical activity goals (Centers for Disease Control and Prevention, 2017a).

In the United States, the Centers for Disease Control and Prevention (CDC) biannual Youth Risk Behavior Surveillance

(YRBS) System monitors priority health risk behaviors of 9th-through 12th-grade students from public and private schools that contribute to leading causes of death, disability, and social problems. Important findings from the 2015 YRBS related to physical activity include (Centers for Disease Control and Prevention, 2017b):

- 48.6% of the students reported being physically active at least 60 min/day on five or more of the previous 7 days.
- 14.3% of the students did not participate in a minimum of 60 minutes of physical activity on any of the previous 7 days.
- 51.6% of the students attended a physical education class on 1 or more days in the average school week.
- Only 29.8% of the students attended physical education classes on all 5 days of the average school week.
- 57.6% (62% boys and 53% girls) played on at least one sports team related to their school or a community group during the 12 months before taking the survey.

When comparing each of the above statistics to the 2013 YRBS, no significant change occurred in any of the categories for children and adolescents in this age group.

In 2016, the National Physical Activity Plan Alliance released the United States Report Card on Physical Activity for Children and Youth. This document reported on 10 key indicators related to physical activity such as overall physical activity levels, active transportation, organized sport participation, active play, health-related fitness, and contexts such as family and peers, schools, and community including the built environment (Office of Disease Prevention and Health Promotion, 2017a). The two indicators that used the most recent data source of the 2015 YRBS resulted in a C– for Organized Sport Participation and a D+ for the School Environment based on the youth's attendance of physical education classes. The remainder of the grades for physical activity reported were poor (National Physical Activity Plan Alliance, 2016).

Physical activity has demonstrated a positive impact on cognitive function and brain structure and function, and psychological well-being may also be positively influenced by physical activity (Donnelly et al., 2016; Tandon et al., 2016). Physical activity is reported to have a positive impact on mental health, self-concept, and self-worth in children and adolescents (Liu, Wu, and Ming, 2015). In addition, physical activity can improve children's ability to control their symptoms of anxiety and depression and assist in their social development by providing opportunities for social interaction and building self-confidence (World Health Organization, 2017c).

The physical inactivity of youth is not only placing them at greater risk of developing chronic diseases such as cardiovascular disease, cancer, and diabetes, but it is dramatically increasing health care costs. If the decreased level of physical activity remains the same as it is currently, researchers estimate that more than eight million children or adolescents will be overweight or obese by 18 years of age. If 50% of youth would participate in 25 minutes of moderate to vigorous physical activity three times a week, they estimated that overweight and obesity prevalence would decrease by 4.2% and that direct medical costs would decrease by $8.1 billion annually (Lee et al., 2017).

In developing countries, increasing urbanization, poverty, high crime rates, structural barriers in the environment (e.g., lack of safe recreational areas, high traffic density, and overcrowding), and poor air quality contribute to inactivity in children and youth (World Health Organization, 2014). Globally, 3.2 million people die annually from risk factors related to physical inactivity.

Promoting Physical Activity: Guidelines and Standards

In the 2013-2020 Global Action Plan for the Prevention and Control of Noncommunicable Diseases, the World Health Organization (WHO) calls for a 10% increase in physical activity by 2025. The plan recommends 60 minutes a day of moderate to vigorous physical activity daily for children 5 to 17 years of age. They further state that activity beyond the recommended 60 minutes is beneficial and any activity is better than no activity. When promoting moderate to vigorous activity, it is important to understand that the intensity level of physical activity for one individual differs when compared to others based on their baseline level of fitness. General examples of moderate activity include brisk walking, dancing, or household chores. Examples of vigorous activities include running, fast cycling, swimming, or playing high-intensity sports such as soccer.

Guidelines and standards for physical activity were set in 2008 by the U.S. Department of Health and Human Services (DHHS) titled "Physical Activity Guidelines for Americans" and are broadly included in the goals of Healthy People 2020. Nutrition, Physical Activity, and Obesity is one of the 12 leading health indicators (Office of Disease Prevention and Health Promotion, 2017b). The guidelines provide specific clinical recommendations that address and promote physical activity for children from 6 years old through early adulthood. Children and adolescents should engage in a variety of physical activities that are age appropriate, enjoyable, and encourage sustained interest and participation. Recommendations include the following (Office of Disease Prevention and Health Promotion, 2015):

- Children and adolescents should strive for 60 minutes of physical activity daily; the minutes do not necessarily need to be contiguous.
- Physical activity should be of moderate to vigorous levels and include vigorous-intensity physical activity at least 3 days/week.

- Physical activity should include each of the following on 3 or more days per week: Aerobic activity for cardiovascular and respiratory fitness; resistance activities for muscle strengthening; weight loading for bone strengthening.

In 2017, DHHS Department of Public Health published a midcourse report that reviewed and highlighted the original guidelines and evidence in the literature to identify future recommendations and interventions that could increase physical activity in children in multiple environmental contexts (DHHS, 2017). The group focused on the following five settings: schools, preschool and childcare centers, community, family and home, and primary care settings. Their findings and recommendations include:

Schools should be a key player in increasing physical activity. Greater than 95% of children are enrolled in schools and spend an average of 6 to 7 h/day when school is in session. This provides an ideal venue to promote physical activity and reach a diverse and large audience of children. Suggestions for enhancing the physical education programs, providing classroom activity breaks, and before- and afterschool activity sessions and space were presented.

Preschool and childcare settings provide an opportunity to increase physical activity in children 3 to 5 years of age. Estimates of 60% of children not enrolled in kindergarten programs are enrolled in preschool centers. Recommendations included increasing the time children spend outside, providing equipment that promotes play such as balls and tricycles on common play spaces, and training staff on the delivery of structured physical activity sessions.

The community and/or built environment offered the opportunity to promote and increase activity for children and all members of the community through daily use. National, state, and local stakeholders are integral to this goal and the ability to increase physical activity and discussions surrounding transportation, urban planning, and public safety are key to meeting the physical activity guidelines. Increasing walkable and bikeable neighborhoods, reducing traffic and speed through speedbumps and traffic circles, and improving maintenance of community public spaces would encourage and support increased physical activity.

Health Benefits of Physical Activity

Physical activity plays an integral role and can provide a benefit for children with many chronic health conditions including:

- **Asthma:** Children with asthma may decrease participation in daily physical activity out of concern that the physical activity will trigger symptoms of their asthma, decreasing overall physical fitness. However, participation in aerobic activity has demonstrated an improvement to the individual's exercise capacity and reduction in their airway inflammation. Recent research found that asthma should not prevent children from participating in sports or physical activity (Gomes, 2015). Participation in sports requires their health care provider have the proper asthma plan in place, including medications and techniques for use of their inhalers prior to vigorous physical activity. Additional suggestions include to decreasing exercising in the cold or when needed, gradually increasing their fitness level, and performing proper warmup before participation in sports (American Academy of Pediatrics, 2015b).
- **Hypertension:** For hypertensive youth, regular to vigorous physical activity (30 minutes, 3 days/week) reduces blood pressure and improves physical fitness. Studies have shown direct relationship between activity level and reducing

systolic and diastolic blood pressure in children and adolescents (Durrani and Fatima, 2015; DuBose et al., 2015; Vale et al., 2015).

- **Metabolic syndrome and type 2 diabetes:** Physical inactivity increases the risk for metabolic syndrome, type 2 diabetes, and cardiovascular disease in adults and is related to increased levels of metabolic syndrome risk factors in children and adolescents. Once diagnosed, each of these diseases can be controlled or positively impacted through increased physical activity levels (Wu, Zhang, and Zhen, 2016). Engagement in aerobic exercise and resistance exercise can improve glycemic regulation (Bird and Hawley, 2016; Keshel and Coker, 2015). Aerobic exercise improves lipid profiles, specifically the HDL-C. LDL-C can improve when aerobic exercise is performed in combination with weight loss and mixed findings related to the impact of aerobic exercise on triglyceride levels were reported (Wang and Xu, 2017).
- **Obesity:** Children who engage in physical activity have lower body fat and improved health care outcomes. Children who participate in at least 55 min/day of moderate to vigorous physical activity were associated with lower odds of obesity independent of sedentary behavior (Katzmarzyk et al., 2015). Low-cost interventions in some school districts that involved simply increasing physical activity during the school day resulted in an increase in the level of physical fitness by 52% and helped combat obesity (Chin and Ludwig, 2013; Dobbins et al., 2013).

Physical Activity and Children With Special Health Care Needs

Children with intellectual or developmental disabilities have higher levels of obesity and participate in significantly less physical activity when compared to their peers without disabilities (Bandini et al., 2015). A recent study found children with intellectual disabilities were 40% less active than their peers and did not meet the daily recommendations for physical activity (Einarsson et al., 2015). General concerns with physical and motor limitations and challenges with social skills and communication can impede participation in physical activity (Must et al., 2014). Other contributing factors can include physical limitations related to the diagnosis, overprotective instincts of the caregivers, lack of opportunities in the school or community setting, lack of transportation, non-universal sports and playground equipment, or lack of understanding of how to integrate the child or understanding their skillset (Bandini et al., 2015). In a systematic review of the literature, nine of the 11 articles included reported significant positive improvements in physical activity when interventions were enacted (Frey et al., 2017).

Many children and adolescents with intellectual and developmental disabilities are capable of performing exercise or strenuous activities. Factors that facilitate participation in physical activity can be integrated within multiple environmental contexts starting within the home and family and extending to the medical home, school, and community. Similar to typically developing children, families should role-model and support participation in physical activity. The health care provider should assess body mass index regularly and provide guidance on physical activity and decreasing sedentary activity as needed with specific knowledge of opportunities to meet the needs of that individual child.

Schools should provide opportunities for physical activity and based on the Individuals with Disabilities Education Act, these opportunities should be inclusive of all children with disabilities (Must et al., 2014). When encouraging physical activity, age and developmental level of the child, physical limitations, and factors such as accessibility, socialization, and play should be integrated (Bandini et al., 2015).

Participation in sports for children with special needs has increased and the Special Olympics organization's enduring focus is to educate those with disabilities to make healthy lifestyle choices to improve their overall long-term health. The Special Olympics organization provides guidelines for healthy nutrition, lifestyle choices, and ways to increase one's level of physical fitness and holds sports health screening clinics. It also serves as a resource for community and health care professionals to learn about athletic participation and how to address health care disparities of children with special needs. Visit https://www.specialolympics.org/ for more information.

Special Consideration: Atlantoaxial or Atlanto-Occipital Instability

Children with Down syndrome are known to have low tone and looser ligaments that place them at greater risk of having a compression of the spinal cord causing nerve damage referred to as atlantoaxial instability (Bull, 2016). It is estimated that atlantoaxial instability affects 6.8% to 27% of individuals with Down syndrome (Myśliwiec et al., 2015). Diagnosis includes an x-ray obtained with the individual's neck in neutral position with forward flexion of the cervical spine (Myśliwiec et al., 2015). Individuals with atlantoaxial instability may exhibit changes in their ambulation, the ability to use upper extremities, complaints of neck pain, a new fixed head tilt, bowel or bladder dysfunction, or new unexplained weakness (Bull, 2016). Box 19.1 lists activities that should be avoided by those individuals with atlantoaxial and atlanto-occipital joint instabilities. They may, however, engage in most of the listed noncontact sports. Parents/guardians have the ability to decide if the athlete is permitted to perform in alternate activities.

• BOX 19.1   Sports Contraindicated for Youth With Down Syndrome and Conditions With Associated Atlantoaxial or Atlanto-Occipital Joint Instability

- Gymnastics
- Diving
- Butterfly stroke in swimming
- Diving start in swimming
- High jump
- Pentathlon
- Soccer
- Alpine skiing
- Equestrian
- Squat lift
- Judo
- Snowboarding
- Any warm-up exercises placing pressure on the head and neck muscles.

Data from Special Olympics. Article 2: Special Olympics Athletes; 2015. http://resources.specialolympics.org/Topics/General_Rules/Article_02.aspx.

During annual visits and preparticipation physicals, the provider should evaluate for signs of atlantoaxial instability and obtain an x-ray. Symptoms of possible spinal cord compression or atlantoaxial instability can include neck pain, localized neurologic pain, weakness, numbness, spasticity (unusual "tightness" of certain muscles) or change in muscle tone, gait difficulties, hyperreflexia, change in bowel or bladder function, or other signs or symptoms of injury to the spinal cord (Special Olympics, 2015). If abnormalities are present on x-ray, the child should be referred to a pediatric neurosurgeon or pediatric orthopedic surgeon for treatment. If there are symptoms suggestive of spinal cord compression and/or atlantoaxial instability, clearance for Special Olympics requires an additional thorough neurologic examination by a qualified physician. If the physician certifies that the athlete may participate in the activity and the athlete (or parent/guardian of a minor) signs a waiver provided by Special Olympics, the athlete may choose to participate in the sport of the athlete's choice (Special Olympics, 2015).

Strategies to Support Physical Activity for Children and Adolescents

Children and adolescents face a variety of barriers daily that influence their ability and choice to be physically active. Table 19.1 presents a socioecological model with different levels at which clinicians can promote physical activity. When promoting physical activity, it is critical to individualize the recommendations to include the effect of socioeconomics, race/ethnicity, gender, and the individual's community.

Health Care Providers' Influence on Lifestyle Behaviors

Health care providers have the unique opportunity to impact the individual's lifestyle through repetitive and sequential visits with the child and family during the child's transition from infancy through young adulthood. Acknowledging that physical activity is a behavior, the provider should be familiar with theories of change, motivation, and motivational interviewing to support behavioral change (see Chapter 15). If these techniques are used appropriately, the practitioner can support patient-centered care, educate the child and family, and increase motivation for the individual to competently manage his or her own health.

Counseling Families About Organized Sports for Their Children

Unstructured play from early childhood builds creativity and dexterity and should be encouraged; however, unstructured play has decreased in children's lives as parents, schools, and organizations recommend and offer more structured and goal-oriented activities. Society in the United States places a heavy emphasis on organized sport participation for youth as demonstrated by how schools are heavily involved in organized sports. Participating in organized sports has many benefits, including developing physical skills, creating friendships, learning to work as part of a team, following rules and fairness, and improving self-esteem.

The potential negative issues surrounding sport participation come when the context of the sport changes from fun to "win at all costs," which increases the level of stress and competition related to the sport. Behaviors and attitudes developed during sport participation, positive and/or negative, are engrained and carried into adulthood. While coaches are instrumental in development of these attitudes and behaviors, families play a key role in supporting the child by being actively involved and developing good sportsmanship. Specific examples include providing positive feedback and emotional support, having realistic expectations of their child's skills and abilities, keeping an open dialogue about the child's experiences with their coach and team, role modeling respectful behavior as a fan, and assisting the child to develop skills to handle losses and frustrations with the sport (American Academy of Child and Adolescent Psychiatry, 2013). Structured sports that promote developmentally age-appropriate participation support a child's physical, cognitive, and emotional health.

Early Specialization in Sports

Sports participation has increased in overall numbers and in the number of children ≤6 years of age who participate (Brenner and Council on Sports Medicine and Fitness, 2016). Recreational games and activities have decreased and been replaced by organized sports that are heavily influenced by coaches and parents. This shift often places an increased emphasis on winning and promotes year-round opportunities to play in one sport versus changing sport participation based on the season. The specialization in one sport is often prompted by the hope that the child's abilities and increased experience may lead to being noticed by a coach, media, an athletic scholarship, or professional play. In reality, only 1% will receive a scholarship and 0.03% to 0.5% will play professionally (Brenner and Council on Sports Medicine and Fitness, 2016).

While difficult to obtain accurate statistics, it is estimated that overuse injuries are responsible for 46% to 50% of all athletic injuries and that athletes who participate in a variety of sports have fewer injuries and play sports longer than their counterparts who specialized in one sport at an early age (Brenner and Council on Sports Medicine and Fitness, 2016). In addition to overuse injury, alternative consequences such as burnout, anxiety, depression, attrition, and social isolation from peers who are not active in the athlete's sport of choice may occur. If youth do decide to specialize in one sport, it is recommended they wait until after puberty to minimize injury risk and have the cognitive, physical, social, emotional, and motor skills to support their success with specialized training. Participation in multiple sports provides additional benefits for the athlete such as increasing agility, balance, coordination, and speed that can transfer from sport to sport. Box 19.2 provides guidance for the clinician on sports specialization in youth athletes.

Strength Training

Strength training or "resistance training" uses free weights, weight machines, resistance bands, or the individual's own body weight to allow the individual to build strength as they progressively exert force against the object of resistance (American Academy of Pediatrics, 2015e). Plyometric exercises, such as hops and jumps, use a combination of body weight and rapid movements to enhance power and "explosiveness." Strength training can be used for several reasons: to enhance performance in a particular sport, increase stamina, as a component of rehabilitation after some injuries, and, for some, to enhance muscle mass for appearance. Strength training is not meant to include power lifting or Olympic lifting (maximal lifting with

TABLE 19.1   Socioecological Model for Effective Promotion of Physical Activity by Health Care Providers

Level of Intervention	Examples
Individual Level	
Using the opportunity of the one-on-one interaction with the child and family members to understand their knowledge, attributions, and beliefs and to promote a positive outlook toward physical activity.	• Assess the child's baseline physical activity level at all patient visits. • Take interest in learning the interests of the child and family. • Discuss physical activity recommendations as part of healthy lifestyle. • Include recommendations on physical activity when providing obesity prevention, education, or obesity treatment. • Use motivational interviewing techniques to promote behavioral change for increasing physical activity. Base intervention on "stages of change" theory as a collaborative patient/provider model. • Role-model a healthy lifestyle.
Interpersonal Level	
Identify the child's relationships and who they interact with within their social networks, such as families, peer groups, and friendship-based social networks.	• Recommend social interactions when participating in physical activity as a mechanism to encourage accountability of the group and increase the enjoyment of the activity. • Initiate family goals to participate in physical activity regularly and together. • Role-model a healthy lifestyle and promote engagement in physical activities among clinic staff. • Be aware and provide suggestions for activities within the community that are oriented to youth and families.
Organizational Level	
Participate and be a leader on an institutional level by encouraging physical activity through policies and rules specific to assemblies of individuals. Common examples of assemblies include schools, religious or faith-based institutions, and the workplace.	Support activities that encourage organizational physical activity promotion, for example: • School programs, such as walk or bike to school days (e.g., International Walk to School Day that occurs yearly in October; see www.walkbiketoschool.org/). • Screen time awareness week. • Intramural programs. • Advise child care centers about ways to increase physical activity for children and staff. • Advise schools and parents about importance of recess and physical education (PE). • Encourage schools *not* to withhold recess as a punishment for misbehavior.
Community Level	
Communities include individuals who participate in interpersonal relationships within various local groups of institutions and organizations. Communities may be defined geographically, politically, culturally, or by other common characteristics.	Advocate for activities that help communities structure public space and promote physical activity: • Ensure safe and easily accessible park and playground space. • Promote affordable organized activities (e.g., scholarships to pay for team sports, after-school activities for low-income youth and local recreation department or YMCA offerings). • Advocate for bike lanes and walking trails in the community. • Advocate for vehicular speed control along major routes to schools to encourage walking/cycling safety. • Promote programs that teach bike safety and distribute low-cost helmets. • Advocate for keeping school buildings open after school for supervised physical activities. • Volunteer to sit on school boards or be a part of school parent teaching associations to advocate for physical activity within the realm of school.
Structure, Policy, and Systems Level	
Represents the local, state, and federal structures and systems that affect the built environment, surrounding communities, and individuals.	Advocate for changes in public policy: • Testify at hearings on importance of maintaining PE in schools. • Address zoning issues to maintain or increase green spaces, such as parks, bike trails, and walking trails. • Work with planners to ensure that communities are designed to promote family-friendly physical activity (e.g., adequate sidewalks/crosswalks, residential areas within walking distance to neighborhood schools, and adequate lighting at playfields and parks).

Some data from Centers for Disease Control and Prevention. (2017b). YRBSS Results. *Adolescent and School Health.* https://www.cdc.gov/healthyyouth/data/yrbs/results.htm.

ballistic movements) (American Academy of Pediatrics, 2015e). A strength training program should be supervised and designed to fit the needs, goals, and abilities of the child or adolescent. Supervision includes monitoring the use of low weight and high repetitions while taking ability to listen and to follow directions, existing motor skills and muscle strength, and technical proficiency in combination with biologic age and psychosocial maturity into consideration. Strength training programs, when done

• BOX 19.2 **Guidance for Clinicians on Sports Specialization**

- The primary focus of sports participation in youth is to have fun and foster lifelong physical activity skills. When specialization in one sport is decided, discuss what goals the youth has and confirm that these are his or her own goals and are safe and realistic.
- Recommending a total of ≥3 mo off over a year timeframe (in increments of 1 mo) from the specialized sport supports the youth's ability to recover physically and promote stability psychologically. Participation in other activities during this downtime is encouraged to remain active, meet guidelines, and to keep physically fit.
- During the specialized sport participation, recommending 1-2 days off per week decreases the athlete's risk of injury.

Data from: Brenner and Council on Sports Medicine and Fitness. Sports specialization and intensive training in youth athletes. Pediatrics. 2016;138(3):e1–e8.

• BOX 19.3 **Safe Practices for Strength Training for Youth Athletes**

- Preadolescents and adolescents should not engage in power lifting, body building, and maximal lifts until they reach physical and skeletal maturity.
- Integrating aerobic conditioning with resistance training can increase health benefits to the athlete.
- Include 10-15 min of warm-up and cool-down with each strength training session.
- Progression from no load or resistance to incrementally adding loads either through using body weight or other forms of resistance is recommended once the initial technique is achieved.
- Gradually increase weights by ≤10%/week.
- Recommend 2-3 sets of high repetitions (8-15) 2-3 times/week and for a minimum of 8 weeks in duration.
- The strength training program should focus on all major muscle groups including the core.
- Stop lifting if pain occurs. Any sign of illness or injury from the training program should be evaluated before returning to the program.
- Recommend young athletes use instructors or personal trainers who are certified or have special qualifications in pediatric strength training.
- Learn and use proper techniques when lifting.
- Adjust weight machines according to height.
- Advise athletes and families of the dangers of using performance-enhancing drugs.

Data from American Academy of Pediatrics. (2015f). Strength Training. Healthy Living. Retrieved from https://www.healthychildren.org/English/healthy-living/sports/Pages/Strength-Training.aspx.

properly, can increase strength by 30% to 50% over an 8-week period (American Academy of Pediatrics, 2015e). Box 19.3 lists general guidelines for youth strength training.

If a strength training program is supervised and individualized to the child/adolescent, the risk of injury is low. Potential injuries associated with include injury to the spine (e.g., injured growth plates and discs, disc herniation, spondylolysis), shoulder stress fractures, or muscle strains (American Academy of Pediatrics, 2015e). Additional concerns include the potential misuse of anabolic steroids or supplements to further increase muscle.

While potential for injury is present, the current consensus is that strength training is advantageous, even for young athletes, provided that it is done in a safe and supervised manner (Myers et al., 2017). Benefits of strength training include improved cardiovascular fitness, strength, flexibility, bone mineral density, blood lipid profile, and mental health (Lloyd et al., 2013). Furthermore, strength training is a beneficial tool in weight management as it improves body composition by increasing lean mass that can positively impact basal metabolic rate (Barbieri and Zaccagni, 2013). Strength training that is part of a well-rounded conditioning program has been shown to reduce blood pressure in hypertensive youth; when included in the preseason conditioning and training program for many sports, it correlates with a decrease in sports injuries (Lloyd et al., 2013).

Restrictions on who can safely do strength training include youth with severe or uncontrolled hypertension, seizure disorders, prior history of childhood cancers treated with chemotherapy, and children diagnosed with complex congenital heart disease (CHD). Individual cases should obtain clearance by the specialist involved with their care (e.g., neurologist, cardiologist) (American Academy of Pediatrics, 2015e).

Preseason Conditioning and Injury Prevention

A variety of strategies can be used to reduce the incidence and severity of injuries (see Chapter 24). Some of the more typical injury conditions that can be avoided with simple prevention strategies are included in Table 19.2. Readiness can be addressed from two perspectives—developmental readiness discussed previously and preseason conditioning readiness.

Preseason conditioning and strength training prepare the central nervous system (CNS) to react quickly to muscular stretching and shortening, which decreases overuse injuries (e.g., stress fractures, bursitis, and tendinopathies). Proper preseason conditioning should focus on enhancing strength, flexibility, and endurance, and improving natural sport-specific movements and agility. Conditioning helps to strengthen bone, facilitates weight control, improves balance and coordination, adds muscle mass, improves performance, and decreases amount of time needed for rehabilitation with injury. Players as young as 10 to 12 years old benefit from establishing overall motion patterns when they participate in warm-up programs. Coaches and fitness instructors should be certified and knowledgeable about age-specific training techniques and safety; adult training techniques should never be applied to children.

Intentional Weight Loss

Weight loss by adolescent athletes can be a dangerous practice. Weight loss through severe restriction of energy intake while participating in high levels of exercise is particularly harmful for young athletes who are still growing and can put the athlete at increased risk for injury during the season (Manore, 2015). Weight loss may originate from the desire to improve performance, for aesthetic purposes (i.e., figure skaters, gymnasts, or synchronized swimmers), or to meet mandatory weight requirements on the day of competition for certain sports (i.e., wrestlers, lightweight rowers, or jockeys). Use of extreme diets or unsafe weight-loss supplements should be identified and avoided. Nutritional counseling is essential with attention to the athlete's genetic makeup, determination if the goal weight is appropriate for the athlete's age and physical development, and evaluation of ability to sustain goal weight without unsafe practices, diets, or supplements (Manore, 2015).

TABLE 19.2   Common Injuries and Prevention Strategies

Medical Condition	Prevention Strategies	Comments
Muscle soreness	• Warm up body with a mix of static and dynamic stretching that prepares muscles for activity. Holding the stretch for a timeframe (i.e., toe touches and stretches) are static and activities that allow the body to continue to move are dynamic (i.e., jumping jacks). • Start with lighter weights and fewer repetitions when starting a new regimen.	• Soreness should be minor, resulting from microscopic muscle or connective tissue damage; it is a normal result of muscles that are adapting to a new exercise program. • Clinicians should explain this soreness ahead of time so that new exercisers do not use this condition as an excuse to stop their fitness regimen.
Strains and sprains	• Participate in a preseason conditioning program. • Tape site of previous injury. • Warm up body temperature before stretching. • Maintain playing surfaces. • Use proper footwear. • Limit practice time.	• Injuries are mostly related to pivoting sports, such as basketball, football, and volleyball. • Knee braces should not replace adequate conditioning specific to the sport. Use only after a formal diagnosis and management plan is in place following consultation with a provider or athletic trainer; braces should be only one aspect of acute or overuse injury treatment. Categories of knee braces include sleeves (help with swelling and support but infer no real stability; may have extra knee padding that helps with prevention in sports at high risk for blows to the knee); PTO brace or patellar strap/bands for added patellar stability; and hinged-knee braces (include prophylactic braces [protection of knee ligaments during contact sports]; and functional or rehabilitative [intended to prevent reinjury after torn knee ligaments or postoperatively]). Braces should not replace rehabilitation and surgery, if required.
Fractures	• Do strength-conditioning exercises. • Use proper techniques. • Take safety precautions. • Use protective gear that fits well, such as wrist guards.	• Most common fractures are of the elbow and femur. Depending on the age of the child, the growth plate may be open, which places the child at risk of injury to the growth plate and subsequent abnormal healing limitation to the future bone growth. Most fractures heal appropriately, with proper casting and observation, since the bone is still remodeling.
Stress fractures	• Use soft running and playing surfaces. • Use proper footgear. • Do strengthening exercises. • Stop activity when pain occurs.	• Stress fractures occur after repetitive force is placed on the musculoskeletal system without adequate time for healing to occur between activities. Children are at an increased risk because of weaker osteochondral junctions, decreased bone mineralization, thinner cortices, and variations in hormone levels.
Lacerations/contusions/abrasions (also see Chapter 24)	• Protective equipment is essential.	• Injuries are mostly related to baseball (contusion/abrasion), soccer, cycling, and ice hockey (lacerations).
Anterior leg pain syndrome or medial tibial stress syndrome (shin splints)	• Confirm proper body mechanics for the activity being performed. • Do not increase duration, frequency, or intensity of an activity too quickly. • Promote bone strength and density with including enough calcium and vitamin D in diet. • Use soft playing surface. • Use proper footwear (proper fit, impact-absorbing sole, insert for shoe). • When a shin splint is present, take adequate time to rest and heal or the athlete will risk progression to a stress fracture.	• Improper body mechanics can increase the risk for injury. • Do not increase duration, frequency, or intensity of activity too quickly. • During rest periods, the athlete can cross-train with nonimpact activities such as biking, swimming, and weights.
Plantar fasciitis	• Use proper footwear (cushioned with fitted heel counters or lifts). • Stretch calf and Achilles tendon. • Do ice massage after event. • Correct biomechanical errors. • Limit hills and speed work; increase soft-surface running.	• When plantar fasciitis is present, avoid activities such as running, jumping, or long periods of standing. • Roll a tennis ball in the arch of the foot to increase circulation and improve healing.

TABLE
19.2 **Common Injuries and Prevention Strategies—cont'd**

Medical Condition	Prevention Strategies	Comments
Blisters	• Wear socks. • Wear properly fitted shoes. • Use powder, petroleum jelly, an anti-friction product (highly recommended), or Second Skin on at-risk or reddened area(s).	
Head and neck injuries	• Have appropriate supervision and coaching that teaches proper skills, such as tackling. • Adhere to safety rules of the game. • Strengthen neck muscles. • Use appropriate equipment: helmets and face and mouth gear. • Follow concussion guidelines for RTP after injury (see Table 19.9).	• Greatest risks for these injuries are from cycling, diving, equestrian sports, football, gymnastics, ice hockey, wrestling, trampolines, football, rugby, and cheerleading. • Risks increase with age.
Eye trauma	• Although not required for most sport leagues, parents and coaches should mandate that children wear safety glasses or goggles when they play.	• Protective eyewear is made of ultra-strong polycarbonate that is 10 times more impact resistant and does not decrease the vision for the athlete.

PTO, Patellar tracking orthosis; *RTP,* return-to-play.

Data from: American Academy of Pediatrics, 2015c, 2015d; National Institute of Health National Eye Institute, N.D.; Orthopedic and Sports Medicine Center of Oregon, N.D.; Shelat and El-Khoury, 2016.

Considerations of Climate and Environment

Heat and Humidity

Core body temperature is a balance of heat generation and heat dissipation (see Chapter 28). A major contributor to core body temperature is the heat generated by muscle contractions. Exercising muscle generates 10 to 20 times the amount of heat of resting muscle, and sweating is the main mechanism that is used to rid the body of excess heat (Nichols, 2014). If the body is unable to rid itself of the excessive heat, body temperature will rise. Under ideal conditions, this can result in an increase of core body temperature of 1.8°F (1°C) in 5 minutes. When environmental heat or humidity excesses are added to the equation, the body must dissipate the heat at increased rates. Unless the usual heat dissipation mechanisms are properly working, heat stroke can result within 15 to 20 minutes. Heat is dissipated through evaporation (20% to 25%), convection (15%), and radiation (60%). It is dissipated only through evaporation when the environmental temperature exceeds body temperature and the humidity is 75% or less. There is no evaporation at 90% to 95% humidity. Thus the combination of high heat and high humidity greatly taxes the body's ability to effectively lower core temperature.

Previously, it had been thought that children were less effective at regulating their body temperature during episodes of exercising in the heat when compared to adults. More recent research indicates that children (9 to 12 years old) have sufficient cardiovascular capacity, effective thermoregulation, and exercise tolerance as long as they are sufficiently hydrated (Bergeron, 2016). With these new findings, there is now a greater focus placed on modifying internal and external risk factors related to heat illness. Internal factors that can be controlled include the athlete's fitness level, lack of heat acclimatization, and excess or inappropriate clothing including protective equipment. External factors include high heat stress; high humidity that reduces the efficacy of sweating in releasing body heat; lack of wind or air movement; individual exercise intensity (>75% VO_2 max) and duration (>1 hour); decreased planning or awareness of the risk of heat illness by the coach, parent, or athlete; delayed management of early heat illness; and decreased or lack of access to fluids and shade (Nichols, 2014).

Risk factors for heat illness include obesity, recent febrile illness, sickle cell trait (SCT), sweat gland dysfunction, uncontrolled diabetes mellitus (DM), hypertension, cardiovascular disease, diabetes insipidus, cystic fibrosis, recent concussions with residual CNS dysfunction, and history of malignant hyperthermia (Nichols, 2014). Medication use can predispose the athlete to heat illness. Examples include stimulants (amphetamines, ephedra, thyroid agonists, methylphenidate, alpha agonists), anticholinergics, antihistamines, benzodiazepines, alcohol, laxatives, tricyclic antidepressants, antipsychotics, illicit drugs (cocaine, heroin, lysergic acid diethylamino), and certain cardiovascular drugs (β blockers, calcium channel blockers, diuretics) (Nichols, 2014). Individuals with these predisposing risk factors need particular supervision because they might not recognize early warning signs of heat effects and may not hydrate adequately.

Dehydration

Dehydration is the imbalance of fluid between the intracellular and extracellular components. When the intra- and extracellular compartments are in balance the body maintains blood volume through regulation by the kidneys, hormones (antidiuretic hormone and aldosterone), and solutes such as sodium, potassium, proteins, and glucose (Adair, 2017). The intake of water and electrolytes maintain hydration and regulate the fluid shifts between the intracellular and extracellular compartments. As athletes exert energy, their active muscles generate heat, which raises their core temperature. The body responds by dissipating heat through circulation (warm blood sent to the skin; "flushed face"), evaporation (sweating), and hormonal adjustment (adjusting to the loss of electrolytes and water through sweat) (Adair, 2017). Hydration strategies are particularly important for children and adolescents as they get distracted and may forget about drinking fluids or they may be restricted due to logistics related to their activity (i.e., decreased breaks offered during their practice) (Castle, 2014).

Coaching staff should play a role in educating, monitoring, and supporting the athlete's ability to maintain hydration and should be proactive in providing drink breaks, having water bottles accessible, and reminding players to drink. Children 9 to 12 years old should replace lost fluids with 3 to 8 ounces every 20 minutes and 32 to 48 ounces every hour for adolescents (Castle, 2014). Fluid options may vary depending on the duration of exercise. For ≤1 hour of exercise, water is ideal. For ≥1 hour of exercise, a sports drink that contains some carbohydrates and replaces nutrients lost in sweat is useful (Castle, 2014). Drinking fluids with caffeine should be avoided because these beverages increase urine output, causing further dehydration. For monitoring hydration status, a sense of thirst is usually a late indicator of dehydration and should not be solely relied upon. On a scale of 1 to 9 with 1 being not thirsty and 9 being extremely thirsty, a score between 3 and 5 is related to 1% to 2% dehydration level. Urine color can be monitored with a goal of pale yellow indicating adequate hydration and any darker colors indicating dehydration. Urine color check charts can be ordered to post in locker rooms to assist athletes to prevent dehydration (www.hydrationcheck.com/about.php).

Sports Training Acclimatization for Prevention of Heat-Related Illnesses

Heat illness is recognized as a leading cause of death and disability in the United States for high school and college athletes. The National High School Sports-Related Injury Surveillance Study reported that heat illness is the third highest cause of sports fatalities in U.S. high school and college football players (Nichols, 2014). The month of August, typically when preseason conditioning and practices are held, accounts for 66.3% of exertional heat-related illness (Nichols, 2014). Heat-related illnesses are totally preventable. *Heat acclimatization* is the training process that gradually allows the athlete to physiologically adapt to exercising in high-temperature environmental conditions. This training typically occurs over 10 to 14 days with exercise sessions that last 60 to 90 minutes per day allowing the body to adapt by increasing plasma volume and sweat rates, adjusting kidney function by decreasing urinary sodium excretion, and increasing aldosterone production, sodium excretion, sweat threshold, sweat electrolyte content, and heart rate during workout (Nichols, 2014). For that reason, many sports associations at both the high school and collegiate levels require heat-acclimatization periods in their initial training schedules. Specific heat-acclimatization guidelines for athletic training are available at https://www.nata.org/press-release/032012/taskforce-guidelines-pre-season-heat-acclimatization-secondary-school-athletics.

Recreational Activities: Safety Issues

Recreational activities play a key role in maintaining and promoting physical activity and health. Activities that are recreational in nature can often be performed independently, may be performed as the youth's mode of transportation (i.e., cycling, skateboarding), or done for purely social reasons (i.e., pick-up game of basketball or playing at the park). Recreational activities are often relatively inexpensive when compared to organized sports. Although recreational in nature, these activities can still place the youth at risk for mild to serious injury (e.g., general body trauma, fractures, torn ligaments, or concussions) and should be reviewed with proper safety precautions identified. Table 19.3 identifies hazards linked to various recreational activities and related safety measures that providers can discuss with parents and children. Many recreational activities take place outdoors, encouraging children to engage actively with the environment and environmental health and safety concerns must be considered. The health care provider should discuss environmental safety including exposure to toxic compounds, use of protective equipment, traffic and pedestrian safety, and guidelines for lightning safety and sports that can be accessed at http://www.nsc.org/learn/safety-knowledge/Pages/news-and-resources-playground-safety.aspx.

Use of Helmets for Cycling and Winter Sports

In 2015 in the United States, there were more than 1000 deaths attributed to bicycle accidents, and greater than 450,000 bicycle-related injuries (Centers for Disease Control and Prevention, 2017a). States that have helmet laws have significantly lower mean unadjusted fatality rates in bicycle accidents in children younger than 16 years old (Meehan et al., 2013). Helmets are also recommended for winter activities such as skiing, snowmobiling, snowboarding, sledding, and ice skating (American Academy of Pediatrics, 2017c). See Box 19.4 for Proper Helmet Fitting Techniques.

Performance Enhancing Nutrition and Supplements

Proper nutrition is a critical component to optimize an athlete's growth and ability to perform. Prior to puberty, basic nutritional and energy requirements are comparable for boys and girls. Post puberty energy requirements vary depending on age, activity level, rate of growth, and physical maturation stage. If an imbalance exists in the form of an energy deficit, consequences such as short stature, delayed puberty, menstrual irregularity, loss of muscle mass, increased risk for injury, or decreased sports performance may occur. Excess energy can result in overweight or obesity, which also increases risk of injury or decreases the athlete's ability to perform.

Youth athletes should be able to meet 100% of their dietary needs from a balanced nutrition plan that includes a focus on the athlete's performance, hydration, and recovery. Supplements should only be used in selected medical conditions with known nutritional deficiencies, such as iron, calcium, or vitamin D (Thomas et al., 2016). Nutrition recommendations are summarized in Table 19.4. For additional information about certain metabolic requirements during exercise, see Chapter 17.

Macronutrients: Important for Sports Participation

Short-term, high-intensity activities (i.e., anaerobic activity, such as high jumping or diving) exclusively use carbohydrates (glucose) as a fuel source, whereas longer-duration activities (i.e., aerobic

TABLE 19.3 Recreational Activities: Their Hazards and Safety Recommendations

Activity and Hazards	Safety Measures
All-terrain vehicles (ATVs) • Loss of control	• No one <16 years old should drive or ride on ATVs. • Those ≥16 years old should take a hands-on training course offered by certified instructors. • Wear protective clothing (boots, goggles, helmet, long pants, and reflective outerwear). • Have flags, reflectors, and lights on ATVs. • Never carry passengers. • Never ride on public or paved roads or at night.
Motorcycles, motor scooters, mopeds, minibikes, minicycles, trail bikes • Collisions; inability to accelerate when mixing with other traffic; inadequate brakes	• Wear a helmet at all times. • Teenage motorcyclists should receive at least 30 h of professional instruction, including 10 h of driving in moderate to heavy traffic. • Discourage motorcycles for youth transportation. • Off-road vehicles (minibikes, minicycles, trail bikes) should not be used on the street.
Riding lawnmowers • Collisions or falling off when a passenger or operating; playing in vicinity of operating mower	• Be at least 16 years old and take an ATV course prior to operating riding mowers.
Snowmobiles • Collisions, rollovers (teenage boys and young males account for 75% of all collisions)	• The AAP recommends that no one under the age of 16 should operate, but the minimum age recommended by states varies as young as age of 10 or 12 after the youth obtains a state-certified safety certificate. • Adequate instruction/supervision by an adult is paramount. • Do not travel alone. • Wear protective clothing (boots, goggles, helmet, insulated outwear, and reflective clothing). • Travel only on designated trails, and avoid roads, railroads, waterways, and pedestrians.
Personal watercraft (jet skis/water scooters) • Collisions; turn-overs; ejections (some models can carry up to three passengers and reach speeds up to 60 mph)	• No one <16 years old should operate a personal watercraft (PWC). • Wear a U.S. Coast Guard–approved flotation device. • Do not jump waves. • Complete a safe boater course that includes instruction on personal watercraft (i.e., jet skis). • Do not operate a PWC if under the influence of alcohol. • Never operate in swimming areas or after sunset.
Golf carts • Collisions; loss of control; turn-overs	• Restrict drivers to those ≥16 years old. • Limit the number of riders. • Drive only at safe speeds; wear seat belts; use helmets. • Limit use to designated areas.
Community/school playgrounds • Falls, collisions	• Equipment and surfaces should be regularly inspected (includes sharp protrusions, detached matting, exposed concrete footings, tripping hazards) and maintained by schools and cities; all equipment should meet U.S. Consumer Product Safety Commission (USCPSC) guidelines. • Maintain good sight lines for supervision of child, based upon child's height. • Maintain barriers between playground and street. • Instruct children in proper use of equipment; monitor and enforce playground rules. • Surfaces should be constructed of shock-absorbing, single-unit materials (double-shredded bark mulch, shredded tires, or sand). Asphalt and concrete are unsuitable. • Separate areas for active and quieter play (e.g., swings from sandboxes) and by age. Have adequate entry and exit space around equipment so that children do not collide with each other or equipment. • Avoid metal or wood seats (best plastic or rubber); ensure equipment has no sharp edges and no openings that could entrap a child's head.
Roller sports (skateboards, scooters) • Falls, collisions (boys injured more than girls)	• Wear a helmet and other protective gear (e.g., wrist guards, elbow and knee pads). • Do not ride in or near traffic; utilize and promote skateboarding parks. • Check skating area for holes, bumps, and rocks; do not ride on uneven surfaces. • Limit skateboarding to daylight hours. • Children <5 years old should not use skateboards; 5- to 10-year-olds should be under an adult's supervision.
Swimming • Drowning (due to drain entrapment/entanglement; lack of swimming skills; inadequate supervision; lack of cardiopulmonary resuscitation [CPR] training by bystanders)	• Swimming pools should have drain covers, safety vacuum-release systems (SVRS), filter pumps with multiple drains, or other pressure-venting filters. Home pools should have pool alarms, fences, and covers. • All children should get swimming lessons and demonstrate proficiency. Non-swimmers require constant "arms-length" and "touch supervision." • Never swim alone or in the dark. • Face the waves vs. turning your back on them. • Wear protective footwear if surfaces are jagged. • If possible, swim where there are stationed lifeguards. • Parents, caregivers, and swim instructors should have CPR training.

Continued

TABLE
19.3 **Recreational Activities: Their Hazards and Safety Recommendations—cont'd**

Activity and Hazards	Safety Measures
Trampoline • Falls; doing acrobatic maneuvers (somersaults, flips); colliding with others using trampoline	The AAP does not recommend trampolines for home use. If there is a trampoline at home, general recommendations include: • Adult supervision at all times. • Extend padding to the frame, hooks, and springs. • Prohibit ladders; install netting and monitor the condition of the trampoline and parts frequently. • Prohibit somersaulting, multiple jumpers, and jumping onto trampoline from a higher surface. • Frequently inspect and replace protective elements; discard trampoline if parts are worn or damaged and replacement parts are unavailable. • Actively supervise children and enforce guidelines; adults should be ready to respond to medical emergencies. • Check homeowner insurance for coverage of trampoline-related injuries; if not covered, obtain a rider for trampoline-related injuries.
Winter sports (skiing, snowboarding) • Falls; collisions	• Dress warmly (insulated outerwear, hat, gloves, and slip-resistant snow boots); wear safety goggles when skiing, snowboarding, or snowmobiling. Wear sunscreen. • Wear special helmets made for skiers, snowboarders, and snowmobilers. When ice skating or sledding, wear a multi-sport or bicycle helmet if a ski helmet is unavailable. • Receive instruction from certified ski and snowboarding schools. • Use proper equipment; wear knee and elbow pads when ice skating and wrist guards when snowboarding. • Children <5 years old should only sled with an adult; children <7 years old should not snowboard; children <6 years old should not ride on snowmobiles without an adult. • Do not sled in or near streets or in areas with trees, fences, ponds, or light poles. Do not skate on river ice or ice that has thawed and refrozen. • Only one person should ride on a sled, unless child is riding with an adult. • Sit up and face forward; avoid sledding head first. • Steerable sleds are safer than snow disks or inner tubes. • Never ride a sled being pulled by a car, ATV, snowmobile, or other motorized vehicle. • Ice skate in designated skating areas.
Bicycle safety	• Always wear a bicycle helmet when riding a bicycle. • Wear fluorescent clothing that can increase the rider's visibility. • At night wear retro-reflective clothing to increase visibility. • Use lighting on the bike and/or the bicyclist including front white lights, rear red lights. • Follow rules of the road.

Data from American Academy of Pediatrics, 2015a, 2017a, 2017b, 2017c; Association of WI Snowmobile Clubs, 2017; Association, 2016; Centers for Disease Control and Prevention, 2017a; Foundation, 2015; National Safety Council, 2017; Nationwide Children's Hospital, N.D.-a, N.D.-c, N.D.-e; Pediatrics, 2015a, 2015b, 2017; University of Michigan, N.D.; University of Michigan Medicine, 2012.

• BOX 19.4 Proper Technique for Fitting a Bike Helmet

• Helmets should carry a U.S. Consumer Product Safety Commission (USCPSC) sticker. Additional certification labels to look for include ATSM, Snell, or ANSI. Adults should wear a helmet every time they ride to be a good role model for their child and others.
• Measure the child's head to have an indication of size. Using a soft tape measure or a string measure just above the eyebrows and ears while keeping the measure level.
• Bring the child along when purchasing the helmet and try on several sizes and models to find the best fit:
  • Position of the helmet should sit level and low on forehead with 1-2 finger widths above the eyebrow to the helmet.
  • The straps should create a "V" under and slightly in front of the ears.
  • The left buckle should be centered under the chin.
  • When buckled, the helmet should be snug with no more than 1-2 fingers fit under the strap and the chin.
  • Position the brim so that it is parallel to the ground when the head is upright: The child should be able to see the brim when looking up. This may require removing or installing inside pads to enable a snug fit, or it may require adjusting the sizing ring.
  • Securely fasten the chin strap to the point where the helmet will not shift over the eyes, rock side to side, or come off when the child shakes his or her head.

• Always replace a helmet after a crash, even if damage is not able to be visualized.
• Do not buy a helmet that you will grow into, it should fit at the time of purchase.
• Ensure the helmet is comfortable to increase the likelihood of wearing.

Centers for Disease Control and Prevention. (2017a). Bicycle Safety. Motor Vehicle Safety. Retrieved from https://www.cdc.gov/motorvehiclesafety/bicycle/index.html; National Highway Traffic Safety Administration. (2012). Fitting Your Bike Helmet. Retrieved from https://www.nhtsa.gov/sites/nhtsa.dot.gov/files/8019_fitting-a-helmet.pdf.

---

activity, such as running or cross-country skiing) use all three sources—carbohydrates, fats, and proteins. Complex carbohydrates (e.g., fruits, nuts, cereals, grains, pasta, and dried beans) are preferable to simple carbohydrates (such as bakery items, ice cream, and some crackers) because, although providing readily available energy, they do not cause the rapid spike in blood glucose levels with resultant insulin rebound that simple carbohydrates do. Hypoglycemia can result from insulin excess, which is counterproductive to the energy needed for sport participation. Each gram of carbohydrate contains approximately four kilocalories of energy. The glucose is stored as glycogen in muscles and liver. Carbohydrates should make up 45% to 65% of total calorie intake

TABLE 19.4	Nutrition Recommendations for Athletes	
Nutrient	**Recommendations**
Recommended daily caloric intake (from carbohydrates/ fat/protein)	• When participating in vigorous physical activity, may need 1650-3925 kcal (depending on gender and age) daily to maintain growth and development. • Allow appropriate vegetarian diets, work with a registered dietitian to ensure adequate micronutrients.
Vitamins and minerals: For energy production, hemoglobin synthesis, maintenance of bone health, immune function, and antioxidant protection	• Vitamins and minerals (with the exception of fluoride in unfluoridated regions) should be obtained from whole food vs. supplements. • Highest likelihood for deficiencies include iron and calcium (especially females after onset of menses). • Iron intake for boys and girls (9-13 years of age) is 18 mg daily and increases to 11 mg and 15 mg for boys and girls respectively ages 14-18 years old. • Iron-rich foods include meats, beans, and green leafy vegetables. Other sources include peanuts and iron-fortified cereals and dried fruits. • Calcium requirements of 1300 mg daily for boys and girls will optimize bone loading prior to skeletal maturation, which aids in osteoporosis prevention later in life. • Sources of calcium include milk, fortified orange juice, almonds, and broccoli. To absorb calcium, vitamin D needs to be present—many calcium sources are now fortified with vitamin D.
Carbohydrates: Help maintain blood glucose levels and replenish muscle glycogen stores	• 50% of the daily caloric intake for youth athletes should be from carbohydrate intake or between 3 and 8 g/kg body weight per day. • Use nutritious foods, such as fruits, vegetables, grains, and milk. • No specific guidelines for youth regarding ingesting carbohydrates during exercise exist. Suggestions to trial 30-60 g/h for exercise that lasts 60 min or longer and modify as needed. • Ingest 1-1.5 g/kg of body weight in carbohydrates in the 30 min post prolonged exercise.
Protein and/or amino acid supplements: Needed for normal cellular functioning and to facilitate muscle synthesis and repair	• 15%-20% of daily caloric intake should be from protein. No protein supplements needed; preference should be toward whole foods vs. supplements. • Depending on level of physical activity athletes may need more protein (1.4-1.7 g/kg/day) than their non-competing counterparts who need (0.8-1.2 g/kg/day). • Ingest 20 g of protein following exercise to maintain positive protein balance.
Fats: For energy and to aid vitamin absorption	• Fats are essential for the absorption of fat-soluble vitamins A, D, E, and K and aid in the synthesis of cholesterol and other hormones. • Limit intake of fats to 25%-30% of total caloric daily intake. • Low fat or diets with <15% of calories coming from fat have no documented health benefits and >30% can lead to excessive weight gain. • Fish oil (containing EPA and DHA) and conjugated linoleic acid (CLA) found in beef, lamb, and dairy products or in over-the-counter supplement form may benefit the athlete's performance. No research has documented ergogenic effects of EPA, DHA, or CLA or improvements in performance from taking these supplements.
Fluids with/without CHOs: For hydration, thermoregulation, may provide calories	• Plain water before, during, and after activity if physical exertion lasts no more than an hour. • Before exercise consume 5-7 mL/kg 4 h prior to exercise; during exercise continue hydration based on sweat loss (consider fluids with sodium to replace loss by sweat); after exercise consume 450-675 mL/0.5kg (consider fluids with added sodium to account for loss by sweating). • If exertion lasts more than an hour, fluids should contain CHOs; if exertion lasts more than several hours, fluids should also contain added sodium to maintain hydration and performance. • Avoid carbonated drinks because of delayed gastric emptying and intestinal absorption. • Avoid caffeine drinks as they increase diuresis.

CHO, Carbohydrate; *RDA,* recommended daily allowance.

Data from American College of Sports Medicine, 2013; Manore MM. Weight management for athletes and active individuals: a brief review. *Sports Med.* 2015;45(suppl 1):83–92; Smith, Holmes, and McAllister, 2015.

for youth 4 to 18 years of age. Approximately 3 to 4 g/kg body weight of carbohydrate-rich solid food, 3 to 4 hours prior to exercise are most effectively converted into needed energy. Ingesting fluid carbohydrates (1 g/kg of body weight) just before activities may improve performance (Thomas et al., 2016). After competition, carbohydrate intake is important in the first 30 minutes to 6 hours after exercise to improve the muscle glycogen resynthesis that occurs and assists the athlete for their next day's events (Rosenbloom, 2016).

Protein

Protein is not an initial source of energy but is useful for longer duration to maintain blood glucose through liver gluconeogenesis and assist in the building and repairing of muscle. Protein should equal approximately 10% to 30% of total caloric intake for youth 4 to 18 years of age. Adequate protein assists in preserving skeletal muscle integrity in the athlete who is physically active (Manore, 2015). In general, the athlete needs higher protein daily (1.4 to

1.7 g/protein/kg) as compared to those who are not physically active (0.8g/protein/kg) (Manore, 2015). Excessive protein may lead to an under consumption of adequate carbohydrates and fats, causing the excess protein to be stored as fat and increasing the risk of hypercalciuria with calcium loss and dehydration.

Fats

Dietary fats provide necessary essential fatty acids, absorb fat-soluble vitamins (A, D, E, K), protect organs, and provide a sense of satiety. Fats should equal 25% to 35% of the total daily calories for youth 4 to 18 years of age while limiting trans fats (Nemours Foundation, 2017).

Nutritional Supplements

Nutritional supplements are readily available to aspiring athletes who believe use of supplements will improve performance. Supplements generally are composed of one or more of the following: a vitamin, a mineral, an herb or other botanical, an amino acid, a dietary supplement that raises the total daily intake; a concentrate, metabolite, constituent, or extract; or a combination of the last four ingredients. Nutritional supplements are not well regulated, and advertisements tend to target young adults or adolescents. Often, there are inaccuracies in the labeling and amount of the ingredients included in the product, as well as contamination, and the inclusion of dangerous substances (Nationwide Children's Hospital, N.D.-d). Nutritional supplements in children and adolescents should be discouraged unless taken under the direction of a health care provider or registered dietician; vitamins and minerals are best gained through a healthy, well-balanced diet.

Sports Drinks Versus Energy Drinks

Sports drinks and energy drinks should not be confused with each other. Sports drinks provide benefits for athletes in certain circumstances such as prolonged duration of physical activity (see dehydration). Sports drinks are flavored beverages that often contain carbohydrates, minerals, electrolytes, and sometimes vitamins or other nutrients. However, sports drinks often contain sugar and, when consumed in place of water or low-fat milk, can lead to weight gain or tooth decay (Nationwide Children's Hospital, n.d.-b).

Energy Drinks

Energy drinks contain substances that are nonnutritive stimulants, such as caffeine, guarana, taurine, ginseng, or L-carnitine, as well as sugar, carbohydrates, minerals, and electrolytes (Centers for Disease Control and Prevention, 2016a). They are marketed to improve energy, weight loss, stamina, athletic performance, and concentration. Since energy drinks are not regulated by the FDA, the exact amount of caffeine is often unclear, but it can be 10 to 15 times the amount of caffeine in a can of soda (Nationwide Children's Hospital, N.D.).

The medical concerns regarding energy drinks are numerable, including the fact that the excess sugar found in these drinks can result in an increase in calories, obesity, and dental caries. Increased bone demineralization may occur based on either caffeine interfering with intestinal calcium absorption or less calcium being ingested if milk is being replaced by energy drinks. When consumed in combination with alcohol, the depressant effects of the alcohol can be masked by the stimulating effect of the energy

drink; users may feel wide awake and possibly underestimate their level of intoxication or impairment (Centers for Disease Control and Prevention, 2016a). When consumed in large amounts, the high caffeine content of energy drinks causes tachycardia, anxiety, and insomnia (Centers for Disease Control and Prevention, 2016a; Visram et al., 2016). If prolonged consumption occurs, additional symptoms can include agitation, tremors, and gastrointestinal distress.

Use of Ergogenic Drugs and Supplements

Ergogenic drugs refer to any legal and illicit substance used to enhance athletic performance, nutritional muscle-building, or sports supplements. Athletes use these substances as they are purported to increase energy (prolonging sports endurance), increase lean body mass, decrease adipose tissue, increase or decrease weight, improve cardiovascular function, and enhance overall sports performance. The steroid precursors, growth hormone, and ephedra substances have not been proven to enhance performance, and can have serious, long-term side effects of elevated blood pressure and cholesterol, blood-clotting and liver problems, mood swings, and reduced sperm production (Mayo Clinic, 2015a).

Many steroid precursors can be sold over the counter without stringent regulation by the U.S. Food and Drug Administration (FDA) (LaBotz and Griesemer, 2016). Dietary supplements are regulated differently than foods and drugs. Manufacturers are not required to prove that a product works or that it is safe before it is sold. Once on the market, if it can be proven to be unsafe, the FDA has the ability to remove it.

Young athletes can also be misled by advertising and messages from professional athletes and sports icons who use ergogenic drugs. Young athletes may use the performance-enhancing drugs as a mechanism to cope with their own insecurities related to their body image, peer pressure or pressure from others, or need to increase weight and/or muscles (Mayo Clinic, 2015b). Adolescents at higher risk of using performance-enhancing drugs include males who are involved in sports that demand strength, power, and speed, such as football, wrestling, gymnastics, baseball, basketball, and weight training.

All high school and collegiate sports associations have strongly worded policies prohibiting the use of performance-enhancing substances, actively enforce no-tolerance policies, and endorse the U.S. Anti-Doping Agency regulations and world anti-doping code. "Clean" team members can provide leadership by disavowing performance-enhancing drugs and emphasizing the integrity (fair play) of sports competition. Education of young athletes needs to include both benefits and risks.

Given the prevalence of these drugs, clinicians must be alert to youth who use them. Providers can note during their physical exam any potential signs or symptoms of ergogenic drug and supplement use such as rapid changes in body build; behavioral, emotional, or psychological changes; increased acne; or needle marks in the buttocks or thighs in females and males. Males may have enlarged breasts, male pattern baldness, and/or shrinking of testicles, and females may have smaller breasts, deepening of the voice, and excess body hair growth (Mayo Clinic, 2015a). Screening for substance use should be incorporated within the developmentally appropriate comprehensive history or the Preparticipation Physical Evaluation (PPE). Additional questions should be open-ended and specify different contexts (home, school, peer groups) before discussing the athlete's personal use. The AAP has guidelines for drug testing when there is high suspicion of use (LaBotz and Griesemer, 2016). Box 19.5 provides screening questions for performance-enhancing drug or supplement use and Box 19.6 has information for parents.

Anabolic-Androgenic Steroids

Anabolic-androgenic steroids (AASs) are equated with increasing muscle mass, speed, and agility (White and Noeun, 2017). The term *anabolic* refers to the drug's ability to stimulate protein synthesis; *androgenic* refers to the stimulation of male secondary

---

• BOX 19.5 Screening Youth for the Use of Body-Building and Other Performance-Enhancing Substances

1. Are you using any substances or supplements to improve your performance in your sports(s)?
2. Do you use any substance to improve your body's appearance, weight, or strength?
3. How do you feel you are doing at your sport? Is your performance where you would like it to be? Are you satisfied with how you are doing? If not, how are you planning to improve?
4. What are your goals with regard to your sport?
5. Are there people in your life (coaches, parents, self) who are pressuring you to improve your performance?
6. Do you know of any athletes or other peers who are using performance-enhancing substances?
7. What questions do you have about drugs or supplements or other things athletes might use to enhance performance?

Be sure to include questions about all drugs, body-building and other nutritional supplements, alcohol use, and needle use as per general adolescent health guidelines.

Adapted from (Holland-Hall, 2007).

• BOX 19.6 Guidance for Parents on Performance-Enhancing Drug or Supplement Use

- Be aware of the pressures that athletes are under through sport participation and overemphasis on winning.
- Be involved in your child's life and sport and do not hesitate to ask directly about drugs, alcohol, needles, bodybuilding or supplement use.
- Respect the coach and keep the coach informed of any pertinent issues that the athlete may be dealing with.
- If concern about drug or supplement use, communicate with the provider prior to the athlete's appointment so adequate attention to supplement use can be addressed during the appointment.
- Be aware of warning signs of drug or supplement use:
  - Perfectionism or low self-tolerance for not meeting standards or being perceived as "not good enough"
  - Worsening acne or abnormal hair growth
  - Complaints of chest pain or cardiac arrhythmia
  - Rapid weight loss or gain or changes in muscle mass
  - Acute and drastic mood swings
  - High blood pressure
  - Excessive exercise or time in the weight room
  - Secretive behavior
  - Voice changes (especially for females)

Information from LaBotz M, Griesemer B. Use of performance-enhancing substances. Pediatrics. 2016;138(1):e20161300.

---

sexual characteristics. AASs react with a variety of receptors in the body, including glucocorticoids, progestin, estrogen, and androgen. Endogenous anabolic steroid production starts in adolescence in the prepubertal male. The exogenous drug used by both sexes for performance enhancement or appearance is derived from testosterone and produces changes in the endocrine/reproductive, cardiovascular, hepatic, musculoskeletal, and neurologic systems. The AAS drugs are Class III controlled substances. AASs are available in oral, injectable, buccal, and transdermal forms and can be taken in "stacks" over 6- to 12-week cycles (LaBotz and Griesemer, 2016).

Clinical effects can be irreversible and extremely serious. Mild effects can include acne, weight gain, deepening voice, accelerated puberty, gynecomastia in males, or premature balding. With sustained use, some of the more serious side effects include cardiac failure, impotence, testicular atrophy, hepatic dysfunction suppression of the hypothalamic-pituitary-gonadal axis, neurologic changes (aggression and mania), premature closure of the epiphyseal plates of the long bones, and possible malignancy, and tendon or muscle injuries (due to disorganized collagen fibril alignment). In females, AAS use can cause irreversible menstrual irregularities and breast atrophy, virilization-enlargement of the clitoris, hirsutism, male pattern baldness, deepening of the voice with larynx changes, and amenorrhea. Mortality or life-threatening event statistics attributed to steroid use may be inaccurate as they can be masked by the diagnoses of cardiac arrest, liver, or kidney failure (Bird et al., 2015; LaBotz and Griesemer, 2016).

Androstenedione and Dehydroepiandrosterone

Androstenedione ("andro") and related dehydroepiandrosterone (DHEA) are prohormones that are converted to either testosterone or estrone. Androstenedione is a Class III controlled drug and DHEA may be purchased over the counter. These steroid precursors are used because of the mistaken belief that they will increase testosterone and produce the same effects on muscles and performance as seen with anabolic steroids. Studies, however, have not demonstrated any convincing measurable changes in athletic performance, strength, or muscle change (Nemours Foundation, 2015). Rather than show increases in testosterone levels, steroid precursors can significantly increase androstenedione and estradiol levels, causing the adverse changes seen with anabolic steroids. Changes include androgenizing effects in females, such as virilization; in males the side effects can include testicular cancer, infertility, stroke, and increased risk of heart disease. Similar to anabolic steroids, if used while the athlete is still growing, height can be stunted (Nemours Foundation, 2015).

Growth Hormone

Human growth hormone (HGH) is available in a biosynthetic, injectable form and is banned by sporting leagues. It is often used one or more times a month and youth use it to enhance athletic performance through anabolic mechanisms of increasing lean body mass and decreasing fat mass. However, it appears to worsen exercise capacity by increasing exercise-induced lactate levels. Potential negative effects related to high-dose HGH use include diabetes, cardiomyopathy, hepatitis, and renal failure. Athletes who take it report a "feel-good" sensation (probably caused by fluid shifts within tissues) and decreases in subcutaneous fat for a fit appearance.

Creatine and Other Supplements

Creatine is involved in the production of energy for muscular contraction and is found in fish, meat, milk, and other foods in small amounts. Creatine is made by the body naturally in the liver, kidneys, and pancreas. Synthetic creatine is an over-the-counter supplement used in the belief that it enhances athletic endurance by improving muscular contraction, strength, and performance. Studies performed in adults have reported mixed findings with some benefits for athletes who participate in intermittent high-intensity exercise with brief recovery breaks (i.e., sprinters or wrestlers); although no benefit was evident for one-third of the athletes studied (Nemours Foundation, 2015). In addition, no benefit in endurance or for aerobic performance has been demonstrated. Caution should be used in individuals who have kidney problems and the ACSM does not recommend that athletes under 18 years of age use creatine. Side effects include weight gain, diarrhea, cramps, and abdominal discomfort (Nemours Foundation, 2015).

Ephedra

Ephedra is a naturally occurring herb known as *ma huang*, and ephedrine is the main active ingredient. It has a chemical structure similar to amphetamine, enhances the release of norepinephrine, and stimulates the CNS. Ephedra was banned as an energy enhancer and diet aid in 2004 by the U.S. Food and Drug Administration (FDA), and in 2006, the retail sale of pseudoephedrine was regulated. Since the ban, ephedra has been replaced by other sympathomimetics that act similarly. Traditional Chinese herbal medicines, herbal teas, and medications that contain chemically synthesized ephedra are among the products not banned. Dietary supplements for bodybuilding and weight loss are readily available over the Internet and can include ephedra as a listed or unlisted ingredient. Many of these products also contain caffeine or caffeine sources such as yerba mate and guarana (Nemours Foundation, 2015).

Adverse reactions include insomnia, tachycardia, seizures, anxiety, dysrhythmias, dry mouth, headache, abdominal discomfort, tremors, or other life-threatening side effects (National Center for Complementary and Integrative Health, 2016). The active ingredients in ephedra are known to have serious interactions with amphetamines, antidepressants (tricyclics and monoamine oxidase inhibitors [MAOIs]), blood-thinning medications, blood pressure medication, caffeine, and narcotics.

The Preparticipation Sports Physical Examination for Sports

Almost 8 million youth participate in competitive high school athletics annually in the United States (National Federation of State High School Associations, 2017), and many more participate in recreational sports in school and community programs. The District of Colombia and all states except for Vermont require a PPE for high school sports (Caswell et al., 2015). There is not a standardized method or use of the PPE and the provider should check with their state for any special requirements. The AAP has classified the most common sports activities into three types: contact and collision, limited contact, and noncontact (Table 19.5). Table 19.6 provides recommendations and guidance on safe sports for various medical conditions and can be a useful reference for complex decision-making and making specific recommendations as to which sports are appropriate for youth with identified health problems.

The PPE historically served to detect cardiovascular risks for sudden death and inguinal hernias and provide liability protection and satisfy insurance regulations. Over the years, other objectives have been identified including:

- Evaluating health status (primary care prevention), including fitness level and preparticipation physical conditioning, grade-level eligibility, and emotional maturity level
- Detecting injuries, conditions, and illnesses from either inherited or acquired conditions that might limit competition and lead to significant injury, morbidity, or life-threatening medical emergencies
- Recommending alternative sports activities, as appropriate, or recommending exclusion of the child or youth from certain sports
- Providing anticipatory guidance about safety equipment for athletic participation
- Initiating further evaluation, referral, treatment, and follow-up of conditions impacting sports performance
- Promoting healthy choices while identifying lifestyle risk factors
- Recommending ways to improve athletic performance

For many adolescents, this requirement serves as an entry into the healthcare system and the PPE may be the only opportunity for pediatric health care providers to assess the health and health behaviors during the adolescent years. However, PPEs are not required for many recreational or club activities. To encounter these children, it has been recommended that *all* children (not just those in competitive or structured sports programs) be encouraged to have a PPE when they visit their primary care provider.

The completion of the PPE includes a prescreening health questionnaire targeting previous sports injuries; respiratory, neurologic, and cardiac health history; and the completion of standard PPE forms. The PPE monograph (Mirabelli et al., 2015) contains the recommended questionnaire, PPE, and clearance forms as well as guidelines for clinicians evaluating children with special needs (see Box 19.1) and the female athlete (see Boxes 19.12 and 19.13). Sports clearance forms can be accessed at https://www.rowpnra.org/wp-content/uploads/2015/05/Health-Form-PPE-4-forms.pdf.

Estimates vary but reports of 0.3% to 1.9% of athletes are disqualified from participation based on the findings of the PPE (Epocrates, 2016) and 3% to 13% require further evaluation (Sanders et al., 2013). The potential need for further evaluation prior to clearance is supported by the recommendation to have the athlete undergo the PPE 4 to 6 weeks prior to the start of the preseason training to allow additional evaluation to occur as needed (National Athletic Trainers' Association, 2014).

Mass PPE screenings are common in many school districts as an efficiency measure or because some youth may not have access to regular health care or difficulty making an appointment. However, mass screenings are a missed opportunity for building a trusted continuity patient-provider relationship and the ability to follow up on health care needs identified during the examination can be compromised. PCPs provide communication with parents, coaches, and trainers following the PPE, and can be involved in the care of the athlete if issues arise during participation.

TABLE 19.5 Classification of Sports According to Contact

Contact	Limited Contact	Noncontact
• Basketball[a,b]	• Adventure racing[c]	• Badminton
• Boxing[b,d]	• Baseball	• Bodybuilding[e]
• Cheerleading	• Bicycling	• Bowling
• Diving	• Canoeing or kayaking (whitewater)	• Canoeing or kayaking (flat water)
• Extreme sports[f]	• Fencing	• Crew or rowing
• Field hockey[b]	• Field events	• Curling
• Football, tackle[a,b]	• Floor hockey	• Dance
• Gymnastics	• Football, flag or touch	• Field events: Discus, javelin, shot-put
• Ice hockey[g]	• Handball	• Golf
• Lacrosse[b]	• High jump	• Orienteering[i]
• Martial arts[h]	• Horseback riding	• Powerlifting[e]
• Rodeo	• Martial arts[h]	• Race walking
• Rugby[b]	• Pole vault	• Riflery
• Skiing, downhill	• Racquetball	• Rope jumping
• Ski-jumping	• Skateboarding	• Running
• Snowboarding	• Skating: Ice, inline, roller	• Sailing
• Soccer[b]	• Skiing: Cross-country, water	• Scuba diving
• Team handball	• Softball	• Swimming
• Ultimate frisbee	• Squash	• Table tennis
• Water polo	• Volleyball	• Tennis
• Wrestling[a,b]	• Weight lifting	• Track
	• Windsurfing or surfing	

[a]Most hazardous for causing injuries (Kocher, 2015).

[b]Most frequent cause of concussions (Petteys and Nair, 2015).

[c]Adventure racing is defined as a combination of two or more disciplines, including orienteering and navigation, cross-country running, mountain biking, paddling, and climbing and rope skills.

[d]The American Academy of Pediatrics (AAP) opposes participation in boxing for children, adolescents, and young adults.

[e]The AAP recommends limiting bodybuilding and power lifting until the adolescent achieves sexual maturity rating 5 (Tanner stage V).

[f]Extreme sports with recent update.

[g]The AAP recommends limiting the amount of body checking allowed for hockey players 15 years old and younger to reduce injuries.

[h]Martial arts can be subclassified as judo, jujitsu, karate, kung fu, and tae kwon do; some forms are contact sports and others are limited-contact sports.

[i]Orienteering is a race (contest) in which competitors use a map and a compass to find their way through unfamiliar territory.

From Rice SG. Medical conditions affecting sports participation. *Pediatrics.* 2014;121(4):841–848. Used with permission.

TABLE 19.6 Medical Conditions and Sports Participation[a]

Condition		May Participate
Atlantoaxial Instability (Instability of the Joint Between C1 and C2)		
Explanation: Athlete (particularly if Down syndrome or juvenile rheumatoid arthritis with cervical involvement) needs evaluation; assess risk of spinal cord injury during sports especially with trampoline use.		Qualified yes
Bleeding Disorder		
Explanation: Athlete needs evaluation.		Qualified yes
Cardiovascular Disease		
• Carditis (inflammation of the heart)		No
Explanation: Carditis may result in sudden death with exertion.		
• Hypertension (high blood pressure) >13 years old		Qualified yes
• Elevated BP (120/<80 to 128/<80 mm Hg)	No limitations	
• *Stage 1 HTN (130/80-139/89 mm Hg)* with no end-organ damage, including left ventricular hypertrophy (LVH) or concomitant heart disease	No limitations or restrictions	
• *Stage 2 (≥140/90 mm Hg)* hypertension—no end-organ damage, including LVH or concomitant heart disease	Restrict from sports with high static or dynamic components until blood pressure is in the normal range.	
• Hypertensive with concomitant cardiovascular disease	Eligibility is usually based on the type and severity of the underlying cardiovascular disease.	
• Congenital heart disease		Qualified yes
Explanation: Consultation with cardiologist. Children with mild forms may participate fully in most cases; those with moderate or severe forms or who have undergone surgery need evaluation.		

Continued

TABLE 19.6   Medical Conditions and Sports Participation[a]—cont'd

Condition	May Participate
• Dysrhythmia (irregular heart rhythm) • Long QT syndrome • Malignant ventricular arrhythmias • Symptomatic Wolff-Parkinson-White syndrome • Advanced heart block • Family history of sudden death or previous sudden cardiac event • Implantation of a cardioverter-defibrillator *Explanation:* Consult with cardiologist. If symptoms (chest pain, syncope, near-syncope, dizziness, shortness of breath, or other symptoms of possible dysrhythmia) or evidence of mitral regurgitation on physical examination, refer for evaluation. All others may participate fully.	Qualified yes
• Heart murmur *Explanation:* If murmur is innocent, full participation is permitted. Otherwise, refer for evaluation (see structural/acquired heart disease, especially hypertrophic cardiomyopathy and mitral valve prolapse).	Qualified yes
• Structural/acquired heart disease	Qualified no
• Hypertrophic cardiomyopathy	Qualified no
• Coronary artery anomalies	Qualified no
• Arrhythmogenic right ventricular cardiomyopathy	Qualified no
• Acute rheumatic fever with carditis	Qualified no
• Ehlers-Danlos syndrome, vascular form	Qualified yes
• Marfan syndrome	Qualified yes
• Mitral valve prolapse	Qualified yes
• Anthracycline use *Explanation:* Consult with cardiologist because most of these conditions carry a significant risk of sudden cardiac death (SCD) associated with intense physical exercise.	Qualified yes
• Vasculitis/vascular disease • Kawasaki disease (coronary artery vasculitis) • Pulmonary hypertension *Explanation:* Consult with a cardiologist. Risk on the basis of disease activity, pathologic changes, and medical regimen.	Qualified yes
Cerebral Palsy	
Explanation: Evaluate to assess functional capacity to perform sports-specific activity.	Qualified yes
Diabetes Mellitus	
Explanation: All sports can be played with proper attention and appropriate adjustments to diet (particularly carbohydrate intake), blood glucose concentrations, hydration, and insulin therapy. Monitor before exercise, every 30 min during continuous exercise, 15 min after completion of exercise, and at bedtime.	Yes
Diarrhea, Infectious	
Explanation: Unless symptoms are mild and athlete is fully hydrated, no participation is permitted (risk of dehydration and heat illness) (see fever).	Qualified no
Eating Disorders	
Explanation: If eating disorder present, athlete needs medical and psychiatric assessment before participation.	Qualified yes
Eyes	
• Functionally one-eyed athlete • Loss of an eye • Detached retina or family history of retinal detachment at young age • High myopia • Connective tissue disorder, such as Marfan or Stickler syndrome • Previous intraocular eye surgery or serious eye injury *Explanation:* Boxing and full-contact martial arts are not recommended for functionally one-eyed athletes, because eye protection is impractical and/or not permitted. Some athletes who previously underwent intraocular surgery or had a serious eye injury may have increased risk of injury because of weakened eye tissue. Availability of eye guards approved by the American Society for Testing and Materials (ASTM) must be judged on an individual basis.	Qualified yes
• Conjunctivitis, infectious *Explanation:* If active infection, exclude from swimming.	Qualified no

Medical Conditions and Sports Participation^a—cont'd

TABLE 19.6

Condition	May Participate
Fever	
Explanation: Elevated core temperature may indicate pathologic medical condition (infection or disease).	No
Gastrointestinal	
• Malabsorption syndromes (celiac disease or cystic fibrosis) *Explanation:* Individual assessment for malnutrition or specific deficits; if treated adequately, may permit full activity.	Qualified yes
• Short-bowel syndrome or disorders requiring specialized nutritional support *Explanation:* Individual assessment for collision, contact, or limited-contact sports. Presence of central or peripheral, indwelling, venous catheter may require special considerations for activities and emergency preparedness for unexpected trauma to the device(s).	Qualified yes
Heat illness, History of	
Explanation: With likelihood of recurrence, needs assessment for presence of predisposing conditions; develop a prevention strategy for sufficient acclimatization, conditioning, hydration, and salt intake, as well as protective equipment and uniform configurations.	Qualified yes
Hepatitis, Infectious (Primarily Hepatitis C)	
Explanation: Ensure protection with hepatitis B vaccination before participation; cover skin lesions; use universal precautions.	Yes
Human Immunodeficiency Virus (HIV) Infection	
Explanation: As athlete's state of health allows (especially if viral load is undetectable or very low); cover skin lesions, use universal precautions; avoid sports likely to cause skin breaks/bleeding (e.g., wrestling and boxing). If viral load is detectable, avoid high-contact sports.	Yes
Kidney, Absence of One	
Explanation: Assess for contact, collision, and limited-contact sports; protective equipment may allow participation in most sports.	Qualified yes
Liver, Enlarged	
Explanation: Acutely enlarged liver: no participation because of risk of rupture; chronically enlarged or liver function compromised: individual assessment and sport dependent.	Qualified yes
Malignant Neoplasm	
Explanation: Individual assessment.	Qualified yes
Musculoskeletal Disorders	
Explanation: Individual assessment.	Qualified yes
Neurologic Disorders	
• History of serious head or spine trauma or abnormality *Explanation:* Individual assessment for collision, contact, or limited-contact sports.	Qualified yes
• History of simple concussion (mild traumatic brain injury), multiple simple concussions, and/or complex concussion *Explanation:* Individual assessment; no athletic participation while symptomatic and/or exhibiting deficits in judgment or cognition; graduated return to full activity.	Qualified yes
• Myopathies *Explanation:* Individual assessment.	Qualified yes
• Recurrent headaches *Explanation:* Individual assessment.	Yes
• Recurrent plexopathy (burner or stinger) and cervical cord neurapraxia with persistent defects *Explanation:* Individual assessment for collision, contact, or limited-contact sports; regaining normal strength is benchmark for return to play.	Qualified yes
• Seizure disorder, well controlled *Explanation:* Risk of seizure during participation is minimal.	Yes
• Seizure disorder, poorly controlled *Explanation:* Individual assessment for collision, contact, or limited-contact sports. Avoid archery, riflery, swimming, weightlifting, power lifting, strength training, and sports involving heights.	Qualified yes
Obesity	
Explanation: Increased risk of heat illness and cardiovascular strain; needs acclimatization, hydration, and potential activity and recovery modifications during competition and training.	Yes
Organ Transplant Recipient (and Those Taking Immunosuppressive Medications)	
Explanation: Individual assessment	Qualified yes

Continued

TABLE 19.6 Medical Conditions and Sports Participation[a]—cont'd

Condition	May Participate
Ovary, Absence of One	
Explanation: Risk is minimal.	Yes
Pregnancy/Postpartum	
Explanation: Individual assessment with modifications to usual exercise routines in later stages. Avoid fall risk activities and scuba diving. After birth, physiologic changes of pregnancy take 4-6 weeks to return to baseline.	Qualified yes
Respiratory Conditions	
• Pulmonary compromise, including cystic fibrosis *Explanation:* Individual assessment; sports may be played if oxygenation remains satisfactory during graded exercise test; need acclimatization and hydration with cystic fibrosis.	Qualified yes
• Asthma *Explanation:* If controlled and with education, only those with severe asthma need to modify their participation. If using inhalers, have written action plan and use peak flowmeter daily. Scuba diving is a high-risk activity.	Yes
• Acute upper respiratory infection *Explanation:* Individual assessment for all except mild disease (see fever).	Qualified yes
Rheumatologic Diseases	
• Juvenile rheumatoid arthritis *Explanation:* Individual assessment depends on involvement: cervical spine C1 and C2, risk of spinal cord injury; HLA-B27-associated arthritis; cardiovascular assessment for possible complications during exercise; if micrognathia, mouth guards; if uveitis, risk of eye damage from trauma.	Qualified yes
• Juvenile dermatomyositis, idiopathic myositis • Systemic lupus erythematosus • Raynaud phenomenon *Explanation:* If cardiac involvement, cardiology assessment required; if on systemic corticosteroid therapy, at higher risk of fractures and avascular necrosis; if on immunosuppressive medications, risk of serious infection; if myositis, active risk of rhabdomyolysis during intensive exercise with renal injury; photosensitivity with need for sun protection; if Raynaud phenomenon, risk to hands and feet with exposure to cold.	Qualified yes
Sickle Cell Disease	
Explanation: Individual assessment; as illness status permits, all sports may be played; avoid sport or activity that entails overexertion, overheating, dehydration, or chilling, or takes place at high altitude, especially when not acclimatized.	Qualified yes
Sickle Cell Trait	
Explanation: If sickle cell trait (SCT), generally no increased risk of sudden death or other medical problems; if high exertional activity, performed under extreme conditions of heat and humidity or increased altitude, complications can occur; need to progressively acclimatize.	Yes
Skin infections, including herpes simplex, molluscum contagiosum, verrucae (warts), staphylococcal and streptococcal infections (furuncles [boils], carbuncles, impetigo, methicillin-resistant *Staphylococcus aureus* [cellulitis and/or abscesses]), scabies, and tinea	
Explanation: During contagious periods, gymnastics or cheerleading with mats, martial arts, wrestling, or other collision, contact, or limited-contact sports not allowed.	Qualified yes
Spleen, Enlarged	
Explanation: If acutely enlarged spleen, participation avoided due to risk of rupture; if chronically enlarged, individual assessment needed.	Qualified yes
Testicle, Undescended or Absent	
Explanation: May require a protective cup depending upon sport.	Yes

[a]This table is designed for use by medical and nonmedical personnel. "Needs evaluation" means that the provider with appropriate knowledge and experience should assess the safety of a given sport for an athlete with the listed medical condition. Unless otherwise noted, this need for special consideration is because of variability in the severity of the disease, the risk of injury for the specific sports, or both.

Data primarily from Rice SG. Medical conditions affecting sports participation. *Pediatrics.* 2014;121(4):841–848. Used with permission. Hypertension data from Flynn JT, Daniels SR, Hayman LL, et al. Update: ambulatory blood pressure monitoring in children and adolescents: a scientific statement from the American Heart Association. *Hypertension.* 2014;63(5):1116–1135.

Medical Clearance and Liability Issues

The PPE, including all health history and physical examination findings, must be fully documented in the medical record. Recommendations based on the PPE include unconditional clearance; cleared with recommendation for follow-up; not cleared until further evaluation, treatment, or rehabilitation; or not cleared for any sport or level of participation in competitive sports. Counseling about more appropriate alternative sports should occur and be documented. In addition, the athlete and parents should be counseled that:

- Even though the examination appears "normal," data on the exact risks of a known sport are often limited and SCD is rare
- Safety and conditioning are imperative for prevention; injury is a more common cause of morbidity and mortality in sports than medical causes

Should the athlete, athlete's family, or guardian disagree with the provider's advice against participation in a certain chosen sport or activity, the provider needs to obtain the athlete's, parent's, or guardian's signed informed consent statement acknowledging understanding of the advice and potential dangers of participation and releasing the provider and organization from liability.

Components of the Preparticipation Physical Examination

Health History

The health history is the foundation of the participation physical exam and may reveal 88% of medical conditions and 67% of muscular skeletal problems (Mirabelli et al., 2015). See Box 19.7 for the routine recommended AAFP PPE health history information. When performing the history portion of the PPE, health care providers should also obtain the following history in order to better understand the scope of sports participation prior to clearance:

- The particular sports activity planned, the extent of participation, level of competition, and training schedule
- Coaching and supervision: What is the level of certification of the trainers and coaches?

• BOX 19.7 **Health History for Preparticipation Physical Examination**

The AAFP PPE history form is recommended and seeks information about the following:

- Thorough past medical history and family history
- Prior surgeries and any sequelae
- Previous trauma, especially musculoskeletal or central nervous system injuries (notably head injuries)
- Family history of cardiac risk factors, including unexplained drowning or unwitnessed car accidents (these can indicate an undiagnosed heart problem)
- Specific cardiovascular disease questions (see Box 19.8) including uncontrolled hypertension
- Prior heat-intolerance episodes
- Asthma, excessive dyspnea, fatigue associated with exercise, activity intolerance, or other allergic reactions
- Loss of function or absence of any paired organs (eyes, testes, kidneys)
- Seizure disorder or any other unexplained loss of consciousness
- Infectious mononucleosis (IM)
- Skin infection or recurrent skin infections, with a concern of MRSA
- Anatomic abnormalities, Down or Marfan syndrome, or history of Marfan syndrome in the family
- Obesity
- Medications, including supplement use, herbal remedies
- Immunization status
- Nutritional history—rapid weight changes, dieting, body perception
- History of sickle cell
- In females—menstrual history (see Box 19.12 regarding screening questions for the female athlete triad)

AAFP PPE, *American Academy of Family Physicians Preparticipation Physical Examination;* MRSA, *methicillin-resistant* Staphylococcus aureus.

- Hazardous playing and field conditions
- Injury prevention strategies, including level of preparticipation conditioning
- Nutritional changes needed for participation
- Risk behaviors present such as sexual history, use of drugs or performance-enhancing substances, smoking including e-cigarette use
- Family involvement, stress management during the competitive season, and how success will be measured
- Strategies to maintain schoolwork

Physical Examination

The PPE should be a comprehensive head-to-toe physical examination including vital signs (heart rate, blood pressure, height and weight) and vision and hearing screenings with particular focus on thorough cardiovascular, musculoskeletal, and neurologic exams. The 90-second musculoskeletal screening examination is recommended for all youth participating in sports (Fig 19.1). The examination focuses on musculoskeletal alignment, flexibility, and proprioception, which are effective measures of abnormalities and injury sequelae. Table 19.7 describes the components that should be included for examining different organ systems, including elements of the cardiovascular system. See Box 19.8 examination the cardiovascular screening examination for congenital and genetic cardiac disease. Additionally, the provider should include a genital examination in males. This examination provides information with regard to sexual maturity (Tanner stage or sexual maturity rating [SMR]; see Chapter 13) and provides an opportunity for counseling about general development, how to do a self-testicular examination, and the risk of testicular cancer, issues of reproductive health, and risks of sexually transmitted infections. The SMR level reflects muscle and spine maturity and is important in contact sports participation and weight and strength training. As the adolescent achieves greater sexual maturity, the risk of participation in high contact sports decreases although athletic injury remains a concern.

Diagnostic Studies

The use of echocardiographic screening has been proposed by cardiologists and others concerned about sickle cell disease the risk for youths who have a predisposition to this condition, and liability in sports participation. Despite the merits of augmenting the health history and physical examination with a screening electrocardiogram (ECG) and echocardiogram, their use as universal screening tools for youth participating in competitive sports remains controversial (Galas, 2014). In the United States, the ECG, echocardiogram, or exercise stress tests are not recommended as a requirement for all PPEs (Mirabelli et al., 2015).

Other diagnostic tests that may be indicated or mandated as part of the PPE health screening include hematocrit or hemoglobin recommended for adolescent females with heavy menstrual cycles, history of iron-deficiency anemia, or a history of iron supplementation or medications that could affect blood count; human immunodeficiency virus (HIV) testing for athletes with risk factors; sickle cell testing to confirm SCT in high-risk groups; lipid or cholesterol for overweight or obese athletes and those with a personal history of elevated lipid or cholesterol or positive cardiovascular risk factors. Urinalysis is not routinely recommended or supported by research. However, certain amateur recreational or professional organizations may require it as part of a drug screening policy.

- Appropriate for interscholastic, intramural, and extramural sports activities.

- A screening evaluation created to direct attention to problems but not evaluate the problems.

- Identifies the following conditions that might be adversely affected by athletic participation:

a. Congenital problems

b. Acquired problems

Questions such as the following are to be answered by the athlete and signed by BOTH the athlete and parent:
- Have you ever had an illness, condition, or injury that required you to go to the hospital, either as a patient overnight or in the emergency room or for x-rays; required an operation; caused you to see a doctor; caused you to miss a game or practice?

- Are you now or have you been under the care of a physician for any reason?

- Do you currently have any medical problems or injuries?

- Have you ever had a broken bone, joint sprain or ligament tear, muscle pull, head injury, neck injury or nerve pinch, dislocated joint, back trouble or problems?

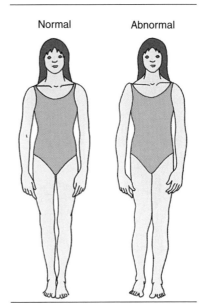

ACTIVITY 1

Normal   Abnormal

Instructions to patient:
  "Stand up straight and face me."

What is screened:
  Acromioclavicular joints, symmetry of extremities

ACTIVITY 2

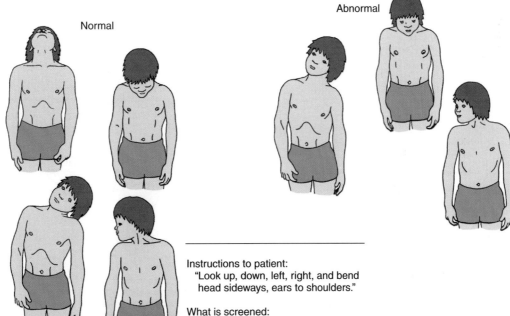

Normal

Abnormal

Instructions to patient:
  "Look up, down, left, right, and bend head sideways, ears to shoulders."

What is screened:
  Cervical spine range of motion

• **Fig 19.1** Illustration of the 90-second Sports musculoskeletal examination—cont'd.

ACTIVITY 3

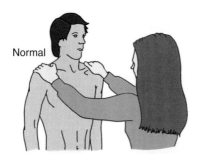

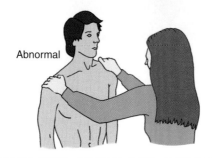

Instructions to patient:
"Shrug your shoulders." (Against resistance by examiner)

What is screened:
Trapezius strength

ACTIVITY 4

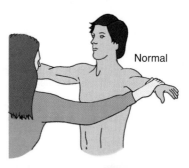

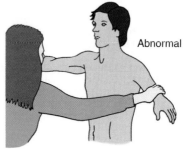

Instructions to patient:
"Hold arms outstretched from your sides and lift them." (Against resistance as examiner pushes down)

What is screened:
Shoulder range of motion

ACTIVITY 5

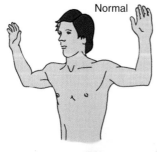

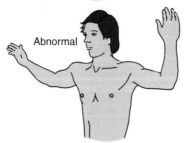

Instructions to patient:
"Raise your elbows at your sides 90 degrees. Rotate your hands backward."

What is screened:
Deltoid strength
Shoulder rotation

ACTIVITY 6

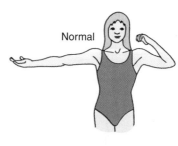

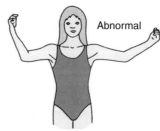

Instructions to patient:
"Hold arms straight out from sides, palms up. Flex and extend your elbows."

What is screened:
Elbow range of motion

• **Fig 19.1** Illustration of the 90-second Sports musculoskeletal examination—cont'd.

ACTIVITY 7

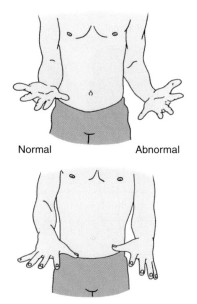

Normal   Abnormal

Instructions to patient:
   "Let your arms down again. Flex your elbows
   so that your hands reach straight out. Rotate
   your wrists, palms facing up, then down."

What is screened:
   Wrist range of motion (pronation/supination)

ACTIVITY 8

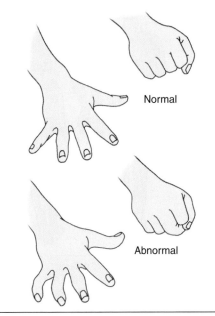

Normal

Abnormal

Instructions to patient:
   "Show me your hands. Spread your fingers
   out (examiner resists spreading). Make a fist
   and squeeze."

What is screened:
   Hand/finger range of motion and strength

ACTIVITY 9   Normal   Abnormal

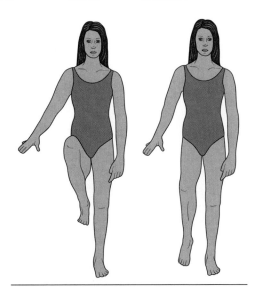

Instructions to patient:
   "Lift your right leg up, bent at the knee. Repeat
   using the other leg."

What is screened:
   Leg symmetry, knee or ankle effusion

Normal   **ACTIVITY 10**

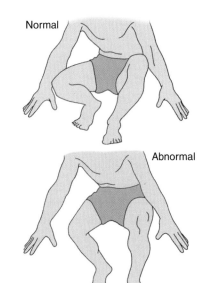

Abnormal

Instructions to patient:
   "Squat like a duck, and walk four steps
   away from me."

What is screened:
   Hip, knee, and ankle range of motion

• **Fig 19.1** Illustration of the 90-second Sports musculoskeletal examination—cont'd.

ACTIVITY 11

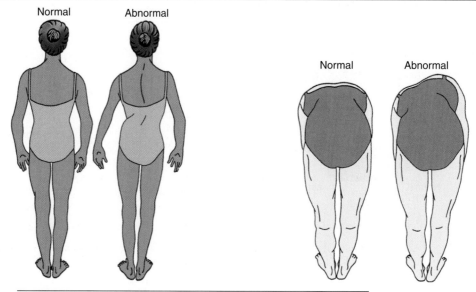

Instructions to patient:
  "Stand up straight. Keep your knees as straight as you can, and try to touch your toes. Straighten slowly."

What is screened:
  Shoulder symmetry, scoliosis, hip range of motion, hamstring tightness

ACTIVITY 12

Instructions to patient:
  "Stand up on your tiptoes."

What is screened:
  Calf symmetry, leg strength

• **Fig 19.1** Illustration of the 90-second sports musculoskeletal examination—cont'd. (Adapted from Ross Products Division, Abbott Laboratories, Columbus, OH, 43216. From For the practitioner: orthopaedic screening examination for participation sports. © 1981 Ross Products Division, Abbott Laboratories. Text adapted from Garrich JG. Sports medicine. *Pediatr Clin North Am.* 1977;24:737–747.)

TABLE 19.7	Components of Preparticipation Physical Examination

Examination Feature	Comments
Height and weight; BMI	Establish baseline and monitor for eating disorders, steroid abuse, and obesity.
Blood pressure, pulse	Assess in the context of participant's age, height, and sex.
General appearance	Excessive height and excessive long-bone growth (arachnodactyly, arm span greater than height, pectus excavatum) suggestive of Marfan syndrome.
Eyes	Important to detect vision defects; one of the eyes should have greater than 20/40 corrected vision. Lens subluxations, severe myopia, retinal detachments, and strabismus are associated with Marfan syndrome. Document anisometropia; absence of one eye can limit sport choices.
Cardiovascular (see Box 19.8)	Increased intensity and displacement at PMI suggests hypertrophy and CHF, respectively; murmur that intensifies with standing or Valsalva maneuver suggests hypertrophic cardiomyopathy; simultaneous delay between femoral and radial pulses or femoral pulse diminishment suggests aortic coarctation.
Respiratory	Observe for accessory muscle use or prolonged expiration and auscultate for wheezing. EIB requires exercise testing for diagnosis.
Abdominal	Assess for masses, tenderness, or organomegaly (especially liver, spleen, and kidneys). In females, assess for any pain, enlargement over hypogastric area or pelvis that might suggest pregnancy or gynecologic problem; proceed with further workup as indicated.
Genitourinary	Hernias and varicoceles do not usually preclude sports participation. Check for single, undescended testicle, and/or masses.
Musculoskeletal	Use the 90-s orthopedic examination (see Fig 19.1). Consider supplemental shoulder, knee, and ankle examinations as indicated specific to the chosen sport's injury prone areas.
Skin	Evidence of molluscum contagiosum, herpes simplex, impetigo, or lesions suggestive of MRSA, tinea corporis, or scabies would temporarily prohibit participation in sports where direct skin-to-skin competitor contact occurs (e.g., wrestling, martial arts).
Neurologic	Gross motor assessment with attention to equality of strength, especially with a history of recurrent stingers/burners, head injury. Usually sufficiently assessed during the 90-s musculoskeletal examination.

BMI, Body mass index; *CHF,* congestive heart failure; *EIB,* exercise-induced bronchospasm; *MRSA,* methicillin-resistant *Staphylococcus aureus; PMI,* point of maximal impulse.
Data from Hess, Mistry, and Herman, 2015; Mirabelli MH, Devine MJ, Singh J, et al. The preparticipation sports evaluation. *Am Fam Physician.* 2015;92(5):371–376.

• BOX 19.8 Cardiovascular Screening History and Examination Checklist for Congenital and Genetic Heart Disease

A thorough medical history with parental verification is recommended for high school and middle school athletes.

Personal History

1. Chest pain/discomfort/tightness/pressure related to exertion
2. Unexplained syncope/near-syncope (judged not to be of neurocardiogenic [vasovagal] origin; of particular concern when occurs during or after exertion)
3. Excessive exertional and unexplained dyspnea/fatigue or palpitations associated with exercise
4. Prior recognition of a heart murmur
5. Elevated systemic blood pressure
6. Prior restriction from participation in sports
7. Prior testing for the heart, ordered by a physician

Family History

8. Premature death (sudden and unexpected, or otherwise) before age 50 attributable to heart disease in one or more relatives
9. Disability from heart disease in a close relative <50 years of age
10. Hypertrophic or dilated cardiomyopathy, long QT syndrome, or other ion channelopathies, Marfan syndrome, or clinically significant arrhythmias; specific knowledge of certain cardiac conditions in family members

Physical Examination

11. Heart murmur (likely to be organic and unlikely to be innocent) auscultation should be with the patient in both supine and standing positions (or with Valsalva maneuver), specifically to identify murmurs of dynamic left ventricular outflow tract obstruction
12. Femoral pulses to exclude aortic coarctation
13. Physical stigmata of Marfan syndrome
14. Brachial artery blood pressure (sitting position); preferably taken from both arms

Data from (Maron et al., 2014).

Evaluation and Management of Sports Participation for Athletes With Chronic Health Conditions

Table 19.6 summarizes the AAP's recommendations regarding sports participation for youth with specific health conditions. Several high-risk conditions (chronic and acute) and diagnostic symptoms are discussed in the following sections in terms of their influence on decision-making and for the purposes of counseling and health management.

Asthma

Asthma is one of the most common respiratory conditions that impact children. Documentation of the child's history of symptoms, triggers, treatments, and interventions should be maintained and shared with the teacher and coach. As previously discussed, asthma or EIB should not prevent children from participating in physical activity. The one exception is scuba diving, which is not recommended for individuals with asthma or abnormal pulmonary function tests (Riner and Sellhorst, 2013). For other sports and general physical activity, the focus should be on the child's asthma control and having a plan that incorporates preventive measures and proper use of medications and inhalers (Gomes et al., 2015). Exercise can act as an additional trigger for bronchospasm in those with underlying reactive airway disease, or exercise may serve as the only trigger for bronchospasm. Comprehensive management of intermittent and persistent asthma and exercise-induced bronchospasm (EIB) is discussed in (see Chapters 33 and 37).

Cardiac Conditions

CHD encompasses a wide spectrum of cardiovascular problems or abnormalities from basic to complex. The ultimate goal for the health care provider performing the PPE is to recognize athletes who are at risk of significant morbidity or mortality from preexisting cardiac conditions that may or may not be diagnosed. The need for increased cardiac output and oxygen demands varies by sport and the child's ability to meet these demands will vary by the underlying condition, surgical repair work performed, and final anatomical structure. Regardless of the defect, participation in physical activity and athletics in some capacity is encouraged for most children and youth.

The American Heart Association (AHA) and American College of Cardiology (ACC) published a scientific statement on the eligibility and disqualification criteria for high school and college age athletes with cardiovascular abnormalities (Maron et al., 2015). The document provides recommendations that provide guidelines on the ability of the athlete to participate in competitive sports in middle school, high school, and college. The document is not meant to be used for basic recreational physical activity participation or as rigid mandates (Maron et al., 2015). A key takeaway is that the athlete's health and safety is the priority when determining eligibility to participate and personal motivation or interest in the sport on behalf of the athlete should not be a deciding factor (Maron et al., 2015). The ability to auscultate an organic murmur or detect warning signs (e.g., history of chest pain, excessive exertional dyspnea, or syncope) or history of sudden death due to unknown cause or family history of heart disease can raise suspicion and further testing is required to properly clear an athlete for participation. A 12-lead ECG or echocardiogram would be the initial recommended screening.

Cardiac Murmurs

Because cardiac murmurs are common in children, it is important to distinguish between benign and pathologic murmurs. For the PPE, evaluate heart sounds and listen for murmurs in each of four areas of the heart. A systolic murmur ≥grade 3, a murmur that disrupts normal heart sounds, radiation of the murmur, wide or fixed splitting of S_2, a murmur heard during diastole, or a murmur that

increases in intensity with the different positions or maneuvers should be further evaluated prior to clearance for sport participation (Conley et al., 2014). See Chapter 38 for a thorough discussion on the cardiac examination and interpretation of findings on physical exam.

Diabetes Mellitus

The goal for youth with both type 1 and type 2 DM is to support athletic participation and physical activity in a safe and supportive manner. Type 1 and type 2 DM are discussed in Chapter 45, including the management and monitoring issues for both type 1 and type 2 DM in terms of participation in sports. In general, youth with DM should follow the same physical activity recommendations of participating in 60 minutes of physical activity daily that is recommended for all youth. While full participation to the youth's capabilities and interest level is encouraged, acknowledging the risks of glucose variability that is possible with DM and the impact that physical activity can have on the individual's insulin needs is critical (Jaggers, Hynes, and Wintergerst, 2016). Each athlete should share their DM care plan with their coach and athletic trainer and confirm their comfort level in aspects of care associated with DM (Box 19.9). In addition, sharing the athlete's diagnosis with teammates and having them aware of general guidelines and treatment can increase the safety of the athlete and comfort with the necessary insulin checks and self-management performed by the athlete during practice and events. This is particularly important in children with type 1 DM, because athletic activity can increase short-term complications of hypoglycemia or significant hyperglycemia.

> **• BOX 19.9 Recommendations for the Care of the Athlete With Type 1 Diabetes Mellitus**
>
> 1. Provider may need to adjust blood testing schedule, insulin dosing, and general recommendations for safe participation in sport.
> 2. Athlete should frequently test and record blood sugars as recommended and as needed (often before, during, and after training or competition). Note conditions present during different training or competition sessions.
> 3. Follow insulin dosing schedule but be prepared for adjustments depending on level of physical activity. Avoid injecting insulin into the limb that is most active in the exercise performed (i.e., inject at a distant site) to avoid overly rapid insulin absorption.
> 4. Plan snacks appropriately. May need to increase snacks before, during, or after activity.
> 5. Pack extra testing supplies, pump supplies (if using pump), snacks, and water.
>   Wear medic alert bracelet.
>   Have emergency contact information readily available.
>   Have copy of diabetes management plan available.
> 6. Take control and put diabetes first, take breaks, or ask for help if needed. Do not exercise alone—use the "buddy system."
> 7. Tell coaches about diabetes diagnosis. Educate coaches and teammate of signs and symptoms of hypoglycemia-sweating, lightheadedness, shaking, weakness, anxiety, hunger, headaches, problems concentrating, and/or confusion. If severe, watch for fainting or seizures. Hyperglycemia symptoms include increased urination, dehydration, increased thirst, fatigue, weakness, and/or blurry vision.
>
> *Data from (American Diabetes Association, 2013; Kirk, 2015)*

Hypertension

Hypertension is the most common cardiovascular condition seen in competitive athletes. While physical activity is beneficial to cardiovascular health, further evaluation should be conducted before releasing an athlete to competitive, strenuous, intense training or activity. Recent AAP guidelines simplified hypertension classification categories for adolescents. Athletes should be allowed to participate in competitive sports once hypertensive and cardiovascular risk has been evaluated and/or if stage 2 hypertension with treatment has lowered blood pressure (Flynn et al., 2017). PCPs should also ask about the use of pharmacological agents that can be associated with elevated blood pressures including but not limited to (1) over-the-counter drugs such as decongestants, caffeine, and nonsteroidal anti-inflammatories; (2) prescription drugs such as stimulants, hormonal contraception, steroids, and tricyclic antidepressants; and (3) illicit drugs such as amphetamines or cocaine. See Chapter 38 for assessment, management, and treatment of hypertension.

Seizures

Children and adolescents with seizure disorders should be encouraged to participate in regular physical activity or sports (with a few exceptions) as physical activity has been associated with a positive quality of life and a possible reduction of seizure activity (Rauchenzauner et al., 2017). To date, studies do not demonstrate that exercise triggers seizures or that altered antiepileptic medication metabolism occurs during sports (Pimentel, Tojal, and Morgado, 2015).

Participation clearance for a specific sport should be based on the type and frequency of seizures, antiepileptic medication compliance, and presence of any comorbid conditions. The athlete, parents, coaches or trainers, and neurologist should be part of the discussion and plan for physical activity clearance and sport activities. In addition, consideration must be given to possible side effects (e.g., cognitive or behavioral changes, diplopia, dizziness, general fatigue, sedation, ataxia, tremors, hypohidrosis, dyskinesis, weight changes, decreased bone density) from anticonvulsant medication that could impair performance or put the individual at risk (Crutchfield, 2014; Rice, 2014).

If the seizures are well controlled, few restrictions are placed on sports participation including supervised contact sports, such as football, hockey, and wrestling. Youths participating in some cycling and those involving heights should weigh the risk and benefit of participating and follow recommendations given to them after considerable discussion about safety risks. Exclusion from sports or physical activities are based on risk of harm to self or others if a seizure occurred while participating. Activities such as water or water-based sports or high-altitude activities, such as scuba diving or skydiving, are generally prohibited competitively. If the seizures are poorly controlled, an individualized assessment, discussion, and medical decision are needed. The athlete with poorly controlled seizure activity should be excluded from contact, limited-contact, or collision category activities and/or dangerous activities until control has been achieved. Although contact sports have not been found to provoke seizures, head injury is always a risk (Knowles and Pleacher, 2012).

Sickle Cell Trait

SCT is generally benign and should not be a barrier to participation in sports, but in rare circumstances it can place the athlete at higher risk of an exertional sickle cell event or crisis that can be fatal (University of South Florida, 2017). These events are associated with intense exertion, severe heat, severe hypoxemia increased in high altitudes, acidosis, and red cell dehydration (Conley et al., 2014). These conditions can lead to the blockage of the small vessels that supply the vital organs leading to ischemia and muscle breakdown (rhabdomyolysis), the athlete collapses, and death can occur unless treatment is begun immediately. Persons with SCT appear to be at greatest risk when they are in a deconditioned state and perform short bursts of repetitive, high-intensity activity (e.g., sprints).

Athletes with SCT can participate in all sports, but they need to self-identify in order to ensure safety in training and in all aspects of participation. Precautions for the athlete include setting their own pace; performing gradual acclimatization to heat, humidity, and altitude; resting as needed; decreasing intense exertional activities to short bursts of less than 2 to 3 minutes; being aware and stopping activities if symptoms (e.g., fatigue, intense pain, swelling, muscle cramps, inability to catch breath) occur; not participating when ill; and staying well hydrated at all times (University of South Florida, 2017). Educating families about the risks of SCT and providing the option of SCT screening so that youths are aware of their SCT status are considered optimal practices. Working with the coach and athletic trainer on a proactive plan includes support for the athlete to moderate activity as needed, proper heat and humidity acclimation, adequate hydration, and understanding the conditions that increase the risk of a sickling crisis. If a sickle cell crisis occurs, it is a medical emergency that warrants calling 911. While waiting, the athlete should be cooled if overheated, receive oxygen, and respiratory and cardiac support should be performed as needed. Sickle cell disease and SCT is discussed in Chapter 39.

Acute Infectious Conditions

Infectious Mononucleosis

Infectious mononucleosis (IM) is a viral illness caused by the Epstein-Barr virus and more commonly affects adolescents and young adults. IM is covered in Chapter 31. Fever, pharyngitis, and lymphadenitis are common initial clinical manifestations, but splenomegaly (which occurs in about 50% of cases of IM) is the most concerning clinical issue for an athlete (Becker and Smith, 2014). There is a 0.1% to 0.5% risk of splenic rupture in those playing sports with this condition (Shephard, 2017). Splenic rupture can occur spontaneously (rare), but the risk of rupture increases when participating in a contact or collision sport or a sport in which there is an increase in intraabdominal pressure (e.g., rowing and weightlifting that require Valsalva maneuvers); the risk is at its highest within the first 3 weeks. Diagnosing splenomegaly can be a challenge as athletes often have well-defined and firm abdominal musculature making palpation of the spleen difficult and unreliable as a diagnostic tool. The only way to accurately diagnose splenomegaly is to get a baseline ultrasound and serial images over time. However, imaging is not recommended as a routine diagnostic measure or in return-to-play (RTP) decisions because there is great variance in normal spleen size along with the variance based on imaging (Shephard, 2017). Recommendations for RTP for the athlete with IM are as follows:

- Advise the athlete to avoid any form of exertion, including all sports during the first 2 to 3 weeks (minimum) after onset of symptoms when the spleen is more likely to enlarge.
- At 3 weeks after symptom onset, if afebrile and symptom-free, the athlete may return to light noncontact physical activities. No sport or activity is recommended if there is risk of chest or abdominal contact/trauma or if it involves increased intraabdominal pressure or Valsalva maneuvers.
- Full return to play should be made on a case-by-case basis based on clinical symptoms and physical exam as there is not a specific guideline or protocol. It is generally considered safe at 4 weeks after symptom onset, assuming the patient's physical stamina has returned and all clinical and physical symptoms have resolved. However, if the sport involved increases intraabdominal pressure, a longer recovery time may be suggested (Shephard, 2017).

Skin Infections

Communicable dermatologic conditions are a common concern in sports. Bacterial and tinea are the most common skin infections reported in high school athletes (89%) (Ashack et al., 2016). The potential of compromising skin integrity, injuries, close skin to skin contact, and sharing of equipment in sports increases the risk of infection with the highest incident in wrestling (73.6%) and football (17.9%) (Ashack et al., 2016). Utilizing this information reinforces the importance of prevention of infection. Athletes should be educated on proper personal hygiene, avoidance of sharing water bottles and towels, and thorough cleaning of equipment (Davies et al., 2017). Box 19.10 lists the most effective measures to prevent transmission of common skin infections among athletes through personal care and care of facilities. Table 19.8 outlines RTP recommendations for athletes with several of the more common communicable skin infections.

Human Immunodeficiency Virus and Other Blood-Borne Viral Pathogens

Physical activity and exercise should be encouraged for children and athletes with HIV, hepatitis B virus (HBV), and hepatitis C virus (HCV). When discussing sports participation clearance for those with an infectious blood-borne pathogen, the risk and benefits for the athlete participating and for those that could come into contact with the infected athlete should be discussed and considered. Coaches and trainers should be trained on universal precautions and transmission risk. Education for youth and adolescents in and out of sports should be on prevention of HBV through vaccinations, good personal hygiene tips such as not sharing razors or other personal items, as well as discussion about lifestyle behaviors and infection transmission routes that increase risk of infection. Mandatory screening for HIV or HBV is not recommended but should be decided on an individual basis based on risk factors.

To date, there has been no epidemiologic evidence of transmission of HIV infection through sports contact (Abalos and Petri, 2015). There is also no evidence that moderate intensity physical activity or the stresses of athletics are detrimental to the athlete with HIV. If the athlete is asymptomatic and without evidence of

• **BOX 19.10** Prevention of Transmission of Communicable Skin Infections Among Athletes

Prevention at an Individual Level

- Perform frequent hand washing using good technique (with soap or nonwater alcohol hand sanitizer with an ethanol content of at least 60%) by all athletes and trainers. Shower immediately after practice and game (preferably with antimicrobial soap, especially if doing a body contact sport such as wrestling, rugby, football); do not share soap or towels.
- Wash clothing, uniforms after each use (completely dry in a dryer).
- Regularly clean all personal equipment (e.g., helmets, body pads, knee/ankle sleeves, and braces).
- Wear protective clothing or gear designed to prevent skin abrasions or cuts.
- Keep cuts and abrasions covered with clean dry bandages or other dressings until healed. Do not use whirlpools or therapy pools that are not cleaned after each use until infections and wounds are healed.
- Do not share personal care items (e.g., bar soap, ointments from open containers, razors, towels, and/or cosmetics).
- Place a barrier (such as clothing or a towel) between skin and shared equipment such as weight-training equipment, saunas, and steam-room benches.

Institutional or Sports Organizational Preventive Measures

- Institutions and sports clubs must follow guidelines for cleaning and disinfecting all commonly used equipment. See "Cleaning and Disinfecting Athletic Facilities for MRSA" (www.cdc.gov/mrsa/community/environment/athletic-facilities.html) for information about cleaning common equipment.
- Coaches and training staff must be knowledgeable about communicable disease issues for their sport.
- Coaches should educate athletes about infectious disease guidelines including exclusion-from-play; RTP; hand washing and showering expectations; bagging up and uniform laundering expectations.
- Refer students to appropriate resources (e.g., team physician, athletic trainer, school nurse, or PCP) when infection is suspected.

CDC, *Centers for Disease Control and Prevention;* MRSA, *methicillin-resistant* Staphylococcus aureus; PCP, *primary care provider;* RTP, *return-to-play.*

Data from Centers for Disease Control and Prevention, 2016b, 2016c.

deficiencies in immunologic function, then the presence of HIV infection alone does not preclude participation. The highest risk for an athlete becoming positive for HIV occurs off the field.

HBV has a higher risk of transmission than HIV and HCV due to its ability to survive outside the body for longer periods of time and its resistance to many detergents, alcohol, drying, and temperature fluctuations. Nonetheless, the chance of transmission in sports is considered extremely low, and no exclusion for asymptomatic carriers is recommended. Sustained, close-physical-contact sports (e.g., wrestling) carry some risk, although minimal, of transmitting HBV. Some sports organizations (e.g., NCAA, International Olympic Committee) differ on their policies concerning athletes' HBV status or titers and current recommendations should be verified prior to exclusion. The NCAA states that it may be prudent to exclude athletes indefinitely with chronic HBV infections who are HBeAg positive or exclude those with an acute HBV infection until there is an absence of HBV e antigen (HBeAg) (National Collegiate Athletic Association, 2014). Athletes with acute hepatitis B may participate in sports once they are symptom-free and physically well.

TABLE 19.8	Recommendations for Return to Play for Athletes With Communicable Skin Conditions

Condition	Return-to-Play Guidelines
Tinea corporis	• Minimum 72 h on a topical fungicide • Extensive or active lesions lead to disqualification • Lesions must be covered with either bio-occlusive or gas-permeable dressing followed by underwrap and stretch tape
Tinea capitis	• Minimum 2 weeks systemic antifungal therapy
Herpes simplex virus (primary)	• Free of systemic symptoms of viral infection, fever, malaise, etc. • No new lesions for at least 72 h • No moist lesions; all lesions covered with a firm, adherent crust • Minimum 120 h on a systemic antiviral therapy, if prescribed (fully formed, ruptured, crusted-over lesions will not be affected by antiviral therapy) • Active lesions cannot be covered to allow participation
Herpes simplex (recurrent)	• No moist lesions; all lesions covered with a firm, dry, adherent crust • Minimum 120 h on a systemic antiviral therapy, if prescribed (fully formed, ruptured, crusted-over lesions will not be affected by antiviral therapy) • Active lesions cannot be covered to allow participation for practice or competition
Molluscum contagiosum	• Lesions must be curetted or removed • Localized or solitary lesions may be covered with a gas-permeable dressing followed by underwrap and stretch tape
Furuncles, carbuncles, folliculitis, impetigo, cellulitis, *Staphylococcus aureus* including MRSA	• No new lesions for at least 48 h • Minimum 72 h of antibiotic therapy (see also Chapter 34) • No moist, exudative, or draining lesions • Active lesions cannot be covered to allow participation
Scabies	• Negative microscopic skin prep before returning to practice or competition

MRSA, Methicillin-resistant *Staphylococcus aureus*.

Adapted from Davies HD, Jackson MA, Rice SG. Infectious diseases associated with organized sports and outbreak control. *Pediatrics*. 2017;140(4):e20172477.

HCV has the highest likelihood of being transmitted through blood or blood products, injecting drugs, or needle stick exposures. There have been no documented cases of sports-transmitted HCV infection (Abalos and Petri, 2015). Athletes with acute hepatitis C may participate in sports once they are symptom-free and physically well. Refer to Box 19.11 for a summary of standard blood-borne pathogen infection control measures for trainers and coaches.

Exercise-Induced Dyspnea

Exercise-induced dyspnea (EID) is one of the most common symptoms that can limit an athlete's performance or participation in physical activity both at a recreational and at a structured sports level. The similarity of subjective symptoms to asthma or EIB that are often reported during the history (i.e., coughing, cannot catch their breath or take a deep breath, or breathlessness) can easily lead to the unnecessary prescription of "asthma" medications (i.e., inhaled corticosteroids and pre-exercise β-agonists) (Depiazzi and Everard, 2016). During exercise, there is an increase in ventilation and cardiac output, so both systems need to be evaluated in order to reach a diagnosis. Cardiac conditions causing EID include pulmonary hypertension, exercise-induced arrhythmia, intracardiac shunting secondary a cardiac defect. Non-cardiac conditions (besides asthma and EIB) include dysfunctional breathing that may be functional (i.e., thoracic dysfunctional breathing secondary to pulmonary disease) or structural in nature (e.g., phrenic nerve palsy,

significant bronchomalacia, subglottic stenosis), gastric reflux, vocal cord dysfunction, physical deconditioning, anemia, subclinical pulmonary embolism, and hyperventilation syndrome. Acute illnesses that can present with EID include rhinitis, sinusitis, bronchitis, and pneumonia (Depiazzi and Everard, 2016). To assist the clinician with diagnosis, in addition to a thorough history and examination, spirometry and/or cardiopulmonary exercise testing can be useful tools.

High-Risk Conditions for Sports Participation

Sudden Cardiac Death in Young Athletes

The most frequent medical cause of sudden death in athletes is SCD with estimates ranging from 1 in 40,000 to 1 in 80,000 athletes annually (Wasfy et al., 2016). The incidence rate can vary depending on varied definitions for SCD. According to the National Collegiate Athletic Association there is an increased incidence in males, African American athletes as compared to Caucasian and Hispanic athletes, and the highest occurrences are in basketball followed by soccer and then football (Wasfy et al., 2016). The risk of SCD for African American male basketball players participating in Division 1 are estimated at 10 times higher than the overall athlete population (Wasfy et al., 2016).

Causes of SCD in youth athletes vary. In young athletes (<35 years of age), hypertrophic cardiomyopathy and anomalous origin of a coronary artery are the most common diagnoses that predispose the athlete to a ventricular arrhythmia. These conditions

• BOX 19.11 Recommendations for Trainers and Coaches to Prevent the Transmission of Blood-Borne Pathogens in the Sports Environment

- The health status of all athletes with regard to HIV and hepatitis should be held in confidence (as in all other health-related information).
- Individuals who care for injured or bleeding athletes should be trained in first aid and standard precautions.
- Standard precautions (blood, body fluids, secretions, and excretions regardless of whether visible blood is present) with the exception of sweat has replaced universal precautions (blood and body fluid).
- Have appropriate supplies and equipment that comply with standard precautions available (e.g., gloves, goggles, masks, bandages, appropriate waste containers, disinfectants). Any "sharps" or contaminated bandages, dressings, equipment, or clothing should be properly handled and disposed of consistent with facility guidelines.
- Athletes need to be instructed to report any bleeding wound obtained during an athletic event. If bleeding, the athlete should cease playing until the bleeding has stopped, and only return to play when the wound is covered with an activity-resistant covering. A contaminated uniform needs to be replaced before returning to play.
- If blood or body fluids were transferred to another individual with intact skin, the skin should be wiped first with an antimicrobial (*not* a chemical germicide for use on surfaces), then soap and water as soon as possible. Postexposure evaluation by a licensed health care professional should occur after any incident involving the athlete having non-intact skin, eye, mouth, mucous membrane, or parenteral (under the skin) contact with blood or other potentially infectious material.
- All athletes should be fully immunized against HBV.
- Educate about all the routes of transmission, particularly risky behaviors practiced when off the field of competition.

HBV, *Hepatitis B virus*; HIV, *human immunodeficiency virus*.

Data from National Collegiate Athletic Association (NCAA). 2014-2015 NCAA Sports Medicine Handbook. Indianapolis: National Collegiate Athletic Association Publishing; 2014.

can be asymptomatic, but a subset of athletes (approximately 30%) were reported with symptoms prior to the event (i.e., chest pain, shortness of breath, pre-syncope or syncope, palpitations, or decreased ability to perform at previous levels). Screening for family history risk factors, history of syncope, and history of cardiac disease or cardiac murmur in a child or adolescent are essential components of the PPE, yet these screening measures do not provide 100% assurance of determining SCD risk (Wasfy et al., 2016). The AHA and ACC advises against the use of the 12-lead ECG as a universal screening tool, although the European Society of Cardiology and International Olympic Committee do include a resting 12-lead ECG in addition to a focused history and physical examination (Wasfy et al., 2016). The use of ECG as a universal screening tool may increase the risk of false-positive or false-negative readings (5% to 20% of tests) depending on the ECG criteria and lead to over or under diagnosis of cardiac disease and exclusion from sports (Maron et al., 2015). If symptoms present in an athlete during activity, a full cardiac evaluation is needed that can include cardiac imaging, exercise testing, and electrophysiological evaluation (Wasfy et al., 2016). The ECG or other tests, such as echocardiograms, are indicated if the youth is at higher risk based on the 14-element questionnaire (see Box 19.8). See Chapter 38 for a discussion about the major underlying cardiac conditions that increase the risk for SCD. Other causes of SCD include:

- Anabolic steroids: Cardiac anomalies and possible myocardial damage remain under study (Statuta and Vaughan, 2015).
- Commotio cordis: A rare occurrence in which an athlete suffers a direct blow to the precordium by a projectile object, such as a baseball or softball, hockey puck, or lacrosse ball. If this happens at a vulnerable period of the cardiac cycle, it can trigger ventricular fibrillation. It is more common in children (mean age of 12 years old, perhaps due to an underdeveloped thorax) (Battle, Mistry, and Baggish, 2015).
- Exercise-induced bronchospasm (EIB): Although EIB may produce symptoms described as chest pain or chest discomfort, this can also be a sign of left ventricular outflow tract obstruction or coronary artery anomalies and should be further evaluated if the history and physical examination suggest a history of EIB.
- Premature coronary artery disease.

Although SCD often occurs without warning, secondary preventive measures are advocated in school districts and community settings. These measures include increasing awareness of the incidence of SCD in youth in competitive sports, recognition of early symptoms of SCD, athletic personnel trained to provide effective cardiopulmonary resuscitation (CPR), and access to an automated external defibrillator (AED) in school, sports fields, and community settings. When secondary prevention programs are implemented, the ability to successfully resuscitate youth increases for those previously diagnosed and undiagnosed with cardiac disorder (Galas, 2014).

Hernia

In male athletes, an examination for inguinal hernias is traditionally performed while the youth is standing. If an inguinal hernia is detected or suspicion is present, further evaluation is recommended (Conley et al., 2014). With inguinal or femoral hernias, athletes should be aware of potential complications including incarceration or strangulation. Depending on the type and size of hernia, individual recommendations will be made on the need for repair. The assessment and treatment of umbilical hernias can vary depending on the size of the hernia. If small, the athlete does not warrant being restricted from participation.

Absence of Paired Organs

When a youth has an impairment or absence of one of a paired organ and wishes to participate in a sport, the PCP should take several factors into consideration. These include the quality and function of the organ; probability of injury to that organ by participation in the sport; and what, if any, protective equipment is available and its effectiveness. Currently, there is no policy or consensus for sports clearance for those with one kidney. Athletes with a single kidney should be evaluated for functionality, likelihood of injury, and type of contact and counseled on the benefits and risks of physical activity (Mirabelli et al., 2015; Rice, 2014). A signed letter of understanding and waiver release by the student and parent or guardian for the athlete's record are indicated.

Sports that involve hard objects, sticks, racquets, or aggressive play (such as football or basketball) have greater risks for eye injuries. High school sports with the highest rate of eye injury or danger are baseball, followed by boys' basketball, girls' field hockey, and boys' wrestling. Serious eye injuries from hockey have dramatically decreased with the mandatory use of face masks (Boden et al., 2017). Approved eyewear is available for all sports except boxing, wrestling, and full-contact martial arts and studies have found a 90% decreased risk of eye injuries with protective eye wear (Protective eyewear for young athletes, 2015). All youth participating in organized sports should wear appropriate protective eyewear that is specified by the American Society for Testing and Materials (ASTM) or other organization with standards specific to football and lacrosse. Street-wear glasses and industrial education safety protective lenses are not appropriate substitutes. Contact lenses afford no protection.

The child who has one eye or best-corrected vision in one eye worse than 20/40 *and* a small face to fit should be required to wear molded polycarbonate sport frames (American National Standards Institute [ANSI] Z87.1 frames). It is better for the parent and child to choose a sport less likely to endanger the child's eye(s). For other functional one-eyed individuals, only participation in sports in which the use of eye protection is possible should be approved. For collision sports involving headgear (such as football, hockey, or lacrosse) the same safety ASTM-approved eyewear should be worn under the cage shield or mask with a chin strap on helmet. A history of detached retina is significant, and participation should be limited to non-strenuous sports until consultation with an ophthalmologist is complete (see also Table 19.6).

Young men with a single testicle can be adequately protected with the use of a hard-cup athletic supporter for contact and collision sports and those sports in which objects are projected at high speed. Young women with one ovary should not be restricted.

Musculoskeletal and Overuse or Traumatic Injuries

Overuse injuries are becoming more common in young athletes because of early sport specialization, year-round sports participation in multiple sports in the same season, and the increased demands put on young athletes by parents, coaches, and school settings. A common overuse injury unique to the skeletally immature athlete is apophysitis, which results from repetitive irritation, inflammation, and microtrauma at the growth plate. Overuse is associated with a significant proportion of musculoskeletal complaints in youth involved in competitive sports. An avulsion fracture can occur in youth with apophysitis as a result of a forceful muscle contraction displacing a small piece of bone from its origin. Apophysitis may present as a persistent or worsening pain symptom after a specific history of injury or with gradual onset of pain without specific injury. Persistent pain indicates the need for further diagnostics and referral.

Understanding the demands of a specific sport enables the PCP to more completely consider the various differential diagnoses, management, and an RTP plan. Successful RTP includes regaining strength and conditioning of the injured area. A program of gradual return to play with a trial of sports activities may be necessary before full RTP is accomplished. See Chapter 43 for further discussion on overuse injuries and trauma.

Overuse Injuries in Baseball/Softball. Young baseball/softball throwers and pitchers are at particular risk of overuse injury or apophysitis. There are specific guidelines that address this issue for pitchers (American Sports Medicine Institute [ASMI], 2013; Zaremski and Krabak, 2012):

- Do not pitch more than 100 innings in any calendar year
- Refrain from throwing overhead for 2 to 3 months/year (4 months is preferred); no competitive pitching for at least 4 months/year

- Watch and respond to signs of fatigue
- Do not play in both pitcher and catcher positions
- Follow daily and weekly pitch limits based on age; do not pitch on 3 consecutive days
- Do not use radar guns
- Pitchers should not pitch for more than one team at a time

Neck Injury

If there is a neck injury, the athlete should have a complete neck evaluation performed and demonstrate full range of motion and adequate strength in neck flexion and extension and symmetric strength during lateral flexion along with absence of neurological symptoms. If symptoms are present in the extremities, cervical radiographs that include flexion-extension views should be performed. If concern of cervical stenosis is present, further evaluation with radiographic studies is warranted (Conley et al., 2014).

Burners and Stingers

Burners and stingers (neuropraxia) are nerve root or brachial plexus compression or traction injuries and generally cause unilateral symptoms. This is a common injury in contact or collision sports, notably football and wrestling. Neuropraxia is derived from the sensation of a burn, stinging, electric, or "lightning bolt" sensation down an arm to the hand. The sensation can last seconds to minutes; up to 10% can last hours, days, or longer. Athletes can be cleared to return to their sport if they do not have any residual neck or radicular pain and demonstrate full range of motion and strength. If history of transient or recurrent quadriplegia has occurred, cervical radiographs are required prior to the athlete being cleared for participation. The athlete may require additional evaluation if the weakness lasts more than a few days, there are complaints of neck pain, the burners or stingers occur in both arms, or there is a prior history of burners or stingers.

Head Injury/Concussions

An estimated 3.8 million concussions occur each year in the United States as a result of sports and physical activity that involve head trauma (Broglio et al., 2014). It is estimated that 8.9% of all high school injuries in athletics are concussions. The sports posing the highest risk for head injuries are rugby, hockey, American football, volleyball, cheerleading, and baseball (Pfister et al., 2016). Helmets are required for many contact or high-risk sports such as skiing, baseball, and hockey (Bonfield, Shin, and Kanter, 2015). All 50 states have enacted concussion laws that cover education, assessment and emergency plans, athlete removal from play, and expert medical evaluation with RTP guidelines.

Less emphasis is now placed on loss of consciousness, post-traumatic amnesia, and retrograde amnesia as ways to diagnosis and classify the severity of concussion, as these only appear in a minority of injured athletes. Key points for sideline personnel and health care providers to remember in assessing young athletes for head injury (McCrory et al., 2017):

- Baseline (preseason) neurocognitive testing should be done on all athletes and used to compare any sideline assessments after an injury to avoid erroneous conclusions. In addition to the initial sideline assessment, serial assessments post injury are necessary.
- Recognize that a concussion may have occurred as most athletes show no obvious indications of concussion.

- Remove the player from play and do not allow the child to return to play on the day of injury.
- Sideline assessment is imperative for any athlete who receives a significant head blow or is not "acting themselves" no matter the degree of impact to the head.
- Concussion assessment and reassessment needs to be carried out by a certified trainer or health care provider who has been trained to evaluate and manage concussions. The Sport Concussion Assessment Tool 5 (SCAT5), the Concussion Recognition Tool version 5 (CRT5), and/or the Child SCAT5 is recommended by the 5th International Conference on Concussion in Sport as a sideline concussion assessment tool and is available at http://bjsm.bmj.com/content/bjsports/early/2017/04/26/bjsports-2017-097506SCAT5.full.pdf.

Both physical and cognitive rest is recommended after the diagnosis of a concussion. Cognitive recovery may lag behind physical symptom resolution, and cognitive recovery is a key factor in RTP decisions. Rest for 24 to 48 hours, then slowly and progressively, the athlete should become more active and begin progression through the Return to Sport (RTS) strategy steps. There should be at least 24 hours (or longer) for each step of the progression. If any symptoms worsen during exercise, the athlete should go back to the previous step. Resistance training should be added only in the later stages (stage 3 or 4 at the earliest) (Table 19.9). If symptoms are persistent (e.g., more than 10 to 14 days in adults or more than 1 month in children) or if the adolescent has 2 or 3 concussions without loss of consciousness or 1 to 2 concussions with loss of consciousness, referral to a specialist is indicated for further evaluation (McCrory et al., 2017). Chapter 46 discusses evaluation and management of traumatic brain injury and concussion.

Special Considerations for the Female Athlete

Injuries and the Female Athlete

With the rise in number of elite female athletes, the provider should be cognizant to injuries that are more prevalent in girls and female adolescents due to structural and growth differences, skeletal immaturity, hormonal changes, and nutrition (Stracciolini et al., 2017). Intensive sport training does not appear to delay the growth and sexual maturation of young female athletes. However, studies conclude that the differences in growth and maturation are more likely due to genetics and physique preselection rather than to extended, intensive training (Bergeron et al., 2015).

Knee injuries occur at higher rates in women in college noncontact sports and are related to mechanical injury (Agel et al., 2016) Sports with increased risk for females include basketball, field hockey, lacrosse, and soccer. It is theorized that the increased risk is due to several factors, including biomechanical, greater joint laxity in females, and hormonal effects on connective tissue. Anterior cruciate ligament (ACL) injuries occur at a 1.6 times more often in the female high school athlete compared to the male athlete (Gornitzky et al., 2016) ACL injury typically occurs during deceleration, landing, pivoting, or contact with another athlete. Many teams are utilizing some version of an ACL injury prevention training as part of their warm-ups in male and female sports, but these programs have shown mixed results in the reduction of injuries (Michaelidis and Koumantakis, 2014). Prevention programs with the best results included plyometric and strength training exercises with feedback on correct technique in addition to exercises specific to each sport (LaBella et al., 2014).

Other injuries common in the female athlete include those of the patellofemoral joint and shoulder (sustained during diving,

TABLE 19.9	Graduated Return-To-Sport Strategy After a Concussion	
Stage and Aim[a]	**Activity**	**Goal of Each Step**
1. Symptom limited activity	• Daily activities that do not provoke symptoms. • High school aged and younger youth should not return to sports until they have successfully returned to academics.	Gradual reintroduction of work/school activities
2. Light aerobic exercise	• Walking, or stationary cycling at slow to medium pace. No resistance training.	Increase HR
3. Sport-specific exercise	• Running or skating drills. • No head impact activities.	Add movement
4. Non-contact training drills	• Harder training drills (e.g., passing drills) May start progressive resistance training.	Exercise, coordination, and increased thinking
5. Full-contact practice	• Following medical clearance, participate in normal training activities.	Restore confidence and assess functional skills by coaching staff
6. Return to play	• Normal game play.	

[a]NOTE: An initial period of 24 to 48 hours of both relative physical rest and cognitive rest is recommended before beginning the RTS progression. There should be at least 24 hours (or longer) for each step of the progression. If any symptoms worsen during exercise, the athlete should go back to the previous step. Resistance training should be added only in the later stages (stage 3 or 4 at the earliest). If symptoms are persistent (e.g., more than 10 to 14 days in adults or more than 1 month in children), the athlete should be referred to a health care professional who is an expert in the management of concussion.

HR, Heart rate.

Data from McCrory P, Meeuwisse W, Dvorak J, et al. Consensus statement on concussion in sport-the 5(th) international conference on concussion in sport held in Berlin, October 2016. *Br J Sports Med.* 2017;51(11):838–847.

gymnastics, swimming, throwing, and volleyball) and stress fractures (Stracciolini et al., 2014). Stress fractures occur in 9.7% of female athletes and must be suspected in female athletes with low body weight and/or amenorrhea (Chen et al., 2013). Additional risk factors of stress fractures include menses that begin at a later age, greater than 8 hours of participation in sports per week, multiple years of running, a low dietary calcium intake, and positive maternal history of low bone mineral density or osteoporosis (Chen et al., 2013).

The Female Athlete Triad

The female athlete triad consists of three entities: (1) low energy availability with or without a disordered eating pattern, (2) menstrual dysfunction (amenorrhea or oligomenorrhea), and (3) low bone mineral density (osteopenia or osteoporosis) (Joy et al., 2014). The female athlete triad is associated with sports that emphasize a lean body mass, low weight maintenance, or retaining one's prepubertal physique. Disordered eating patterns can be due to either intentional caloric restriction (an eating disorder that may or may not encompass all the criteria for an anorexia or bulimia diagnosis) or an unintentional insufficient intake in calories that does not meet the athlete's metabolic demands of her body. Insufficient calories related to their activity and metabolic requirements causes low energy availability. The low energy negatively affects bone remodeling and mineralization and cause menstrual dysfunction (amenorrhea or oligomenorrhea). Inadequate bone mineralization during the critical adolescent years puts the teen at lifelong risk of osteoporosis, which increases the risk of stress fractures during adolescence and throughout life as well as skeletal problems at menopause.

There is also an increased risk for those with sports specialization at an early age and in abusive or unhealthy families (Weiss et al., 2016). Girls who participate in sports that emphasize leanness are at the greatest risk of the triad of disorders, including distance running, gymnastics, dance/dance team, figure skating, cheerleading, wrestling, light weight rowing, and pole vaulting (Weiss et al., 2016). It is estimated that the incidence of the female athlete triad with all 3 components in female high school athletes is 1.0% to 1.2% but could be as high as 16% in all female athletes (Weiss et al., 2016). The identification of the early existence of an eating disorder, weight loss, or menstrual irregularities from a PPE history and examination should alert the provider to take a more thorough history, provide testing, and initiate early treatment. The symptoms of the triad occur along a continuum rather than in unison and if one symptom is present, the athlete is at risk for developing additional components of the triad.

Screening questions utilizing the AAP's PPE health history and physical form can direct the provider to provide further screening or testing (Box 19.12). Box 19.13 lists recommendations for the clinician evaluating an individual identified as having the female triad. The initial goal of treatment is to increase energy intake and decrease energy expenditure. Therapy, participation, and return to play should be based on the risk categories and reassessed throughout treatment. Preventive counseling for all athletes should include nutritional energy needs for sports; importance of bone mineralization during child and adolescent years; bone health throughout life; importance of physical activity, calcium, vitamin D; and educating female athletes and families about this disorder.

• BOX 19.12   Screening Questions for Female Athlete Triad

Menstrual History
- Have you had a menstrual period?
- What was your age when you had your first period?
- When was your last period? How often do you have your periods?
- How many menstrual periods have you had in the past year?

Medications
- Are you taking hormones (estrogen, progesterone, birth control pills)?

Weight
- Are you concerned about your weight or body composition?
- Are you trying to or has anyone recommended that you lose or gain weight?
- Are you on a diet or do you avoid certain foods or food groups?
- Have you done anything to try to control your weight (purging, binging, fasting, diet pills or other botanicals)? Have you ever had an eating disorder?

Musculoskeletal
- Have you ever had a stress fracture?
- Have you been told that you have low bone density?

Data from Joy E, De Souza MJ, Nattiv A, et al. 2014 female athlete triad coalition consensus statement on treatment and return to play of the female athlete triad. Curr Sports Med Rep. 2014;13(4):219–232.

• BOX 19.13   The Female Athlete Triad: Recommendations for the Clinician

- Screen for all elements of the triad at the PPE and at annual physicals.
- If one component of the triad exists, screen for others.
- If an eating disorder is suspected, refer the athlete to a nutrition professional and a mental health professional for screening/treatment if indicated.
- Diagnosis of amenorrhea—screen for other causes (see Chapter 42). Functional hypothalamic amenorrhea is a diagnosis of exclusion.
- Screen for bone mineral density after a stress or low-impact fracture, 6 months of amenorrhea or oligomenorrhea, or as part of assessment for disordered eating pattern.

PPE, Preparticipation physical examination.

Data from Joy E, De Souza MJ, Nattiv A, et al. 2014 female athlete triad coalition consensus statement on treatment and return to play of the female athlete triad. Curr Sports Med Rep. 2014;13(4):219–232.

Additional Resources

2018 Physical Activity Guidelines for Americans. https://health.gov/paguidelines/second-edition/report/pdf/02_A_Executive_Summary.pdf

Academy of Nutrition and Dietetics: Sports, Cardiovascular, and Wellness Nutrition. https://www.scandpg.org/

American Academy of Family Physicians (AAFP). www.aafp.org/home.html

American Academy of Family Physicians (AAFP)—Sports Injury Prevention and Download PPE forms. www.aafp.org/patient-care/public-health/sports-medicine.html

American College of Sports Medicine (ACSM). www.acsm.org

American Orthopaedic Society for Sports Medicine (AOSSM). www.sportsmed.org

American Sports Medicine Institute (ASMI). www.asmi.org/research.php?page=research&section=positionStatement

BAM! Body and Mind (focused on Tweens). www.cdc.gov/bam

Centers for Disease Control and Prevention (CDC). www.cdc.gov

Centers for Disease Control and Prevention: Cleaning & Disinfecting Athletic Facilities for MRSA. www.cdc.gov/mrsa/community/enviroment/athletic-facilities.html

Health Equity Toolkit. https://www.cdc.gov/nccdphp/dnpao/state-local-programs/health-equity/index.html

Healthy People 2020. www.healthypeople.gov/2020/default.aspx

International Society of Sports Nutrition (ISSN). www.sportsnutrition-society.org

Lids on Kids: A Helmet—It's a Smart Idea. www.lidsonkids.org

Little League Pitching Rules. http://www.littleleague.org/learn/rules/pitch-count.htm

National Athletic Trainers' Association (NATA). www.nata.org

National Highway Traffic Safety Administration/Bicyclists. https://www.nhtsa.gov/road-safety/bicyclists

National Lightning Safety Institute. lightningsafety.com

Personal Watercraft Industry Association (rules and regulations listed by state). http://www.pwia.org/rules

Physical Activity Guidelines for Americans Youth Toolkit. www.cdc.gov/healthyschools/physicalactivity/guidelines.htm

President's Council on Fitness, Sports & Nutrition (PCFSN). www.hhs.gov/fitness/index.html

Safe Kids Worldwide. www.safekids.org

Special Olympics: Healthy Athletes. www.specialolympics.org/healthy_athletes.aspx

Sport Concussion Assessment Tool (SCAT5). http://bjsm.bmj.com/content/bjsports/early/2017/04/26/bjsports-2017-097506SCAT5.full.pdf

U.S. Anti-Doping Agency: True Sport Parent Handbook: A guidebook to developing young athletes and the role parents play. http://www.truesport.org/library/documents/resources/parent/parent_handbook.pdf

U.S. Youth Soccer Federation. www.usyouthsoccer.org

Walk & Bike to School. http://www.walkbiketoschool.org/

We Can! (Ways to Enhance Childhood Nutrition and Physical Activity). www.nhlbi.nih.gov/health/educational/wecan

World Health Organization (WHO) Global Strategy on Diet, Physical Activity and Health. www.who.int/dietphysicalactivity/en/

Youth Physical Activity Guidelines Toolkit. www.cdc.gov/healthyyouth/physicalactivity/guidelines.htm

References

Aaltonen S, Latvala A, Rose R, Kujala U, Kaprio J, Silventoinen K. Leisure-time physical activity and academic performance: cross-lagged associations from adolescence to young adulthood. *Sci Rep*. 2016;6:39215. https://doi.org/10.1038/srep39215. https://www.nature.com/articles/srep39215#supplementary-information.

Abalos K, Petri W. *Infectious Disease and Sports. DeLee & Drez's Orthopaedic Sports Medicine*. 4th ed. Philadelphia: Elsevier Saunders; 2015.

Adair D. *Hydration for Athletes. Sports Performance*; 2017. http://blog.nasm.org/nutrition/hydration-athletes/.

Agel J, Rockwood T, Klossner D. Collegiate ACL injury rates across 15 sports: National Collegiate Athletic Association injury surveillance system data update (2004-2005 Through 2012-2013). *Clin J Sport Med*. 2016;26(6):518–523. https://doi.org/10.1097/jsm.0000000000000290.

American Academy of Child & Adolescent Psychiatry. *Sports and Children. Facts for Families*; 2013. http://www.aacap.org/AACAP/Families_and_Youth/Facts_for_Families/FFF-Guide/Children-And-Sports-061.aspx.

American Academy of Pediatrics. *Bicycle Safety: Myths and Facts. Safety and Prevention*. 2015a. https://www.healthychildren.org/English/safety-prevention/at-play/Pages/Bicycle-Safety-Myths-And-Facts.aspx.

American Academy of Pediatrics. *Exercise and Asthma. Health Issues*; 2015b. https://www.healthychildren.org/English/health-issues/conditions/allergies-asthma/pages/Exercise-and-Asthma.aspx.

American Academy of Pediatrics. *Knee Pain: How to Choose the Right Knee Brace for Your Child*. 2015c. https://www.healthychildren.org/English/health-issues/injuries-emergencies/sports-injuries/Pages/Knee-Pain-and-braces.aspx.

American Academy of Pediatrics. *Shin Pain. Care of the YOuth Athlete Patient Education Handouts*. 2015d. https://www.healthychildren.org/English/health-issues/injuries-emergencies/sports-injuries/Pages/Shin-Pain.aspx.

American Academy of Pediatrics. *Strength Training. Healthy Living*; 2015e. https://www.healthychildren.org/English/healthy-living/sports/Pages/Strength-Training.aspx.

American Academy of Pediatrics. Strength Training. *Healthy Living*. 2015f. https://www.healthychildren.org/English/healthy-living/sports/Pages/Strength-Training.aspx.

American Academy of Pediatrics. *Summer Safety Tips from the American Academy of Pediatrics*. 2017a. https://www.aap.org/en-us/about-the-aap/aap-press-room/news-features-and-safety-tips/pages/summer-safety-tips.aspx.

American Academy of Pediatrics. *Trampolines: What You Need to Know*. 2017b. https://www.healthychildren.org/English/safety-prevention/at-play/Pages/Trampolines-What-You-Need-to-Know.aspx.

American Academy of Pediatrics. *Winter Safety Tips*. 2017c. https://www.aap.org/en-us/about-the-aap/aap-press-room/news-features-and-safety-tips/pages/Winter-Safety-Tips.aspx.

American College of Sports Medicine. Selected issues for nutrition and the athlete: a team physician consensus statement. *Medicine and Science in Sports and Exercise*. 2013;45(12):2378–2386. https://doi.org/10.1249/mss.0000000000000174.

Ashack KA, Burton KA, Johnson TR, Currie DW, Comstock RD, Dellavalle RP. Skin infections among US high school athletes: A national survey. *J Am Acad Dermato*. 2016;74(4):679–684. https://doi.org/10.1016/j.jaad.2015.10.042. e671.

Association of WI Snowmobile Clubs. *Snowmobile Safety/Classes*. 2017. https://www.awsc.org/Clubs/Resources-Links/Snowmobile-Safety.

Bae SK, Yatsuhashi H, Takahara I, et al. Sequential occurrence of acute hepatitis B among members of a high school Sumo wrestling club. *Hepatol Res*. 2014;44(10):E267–272. https://doi.org/10.1111/hepr.12237.

Bandini L, Danielson M, Esposito L, et al. Obesity in children with developmental and/or physical disabilities. *Disabil Health J*. 2015;8(3):309–316. https://doi.org/10.1016/j.dhjo.2015.04.005.

Barbieri and Zaccagni; 2013.

Battle R, Mistry D, Baggish A. Comprehensive cardiovascular care and evaluation of the elite athlete. In: Miller M, Thompson S, eds. *DeLee and Drez's Orthopaedic Sports Medicine: Principles and Practices*. vol. 1. Philadelphia: 2015;185–201.

Becker JA, Smith JA. Return to play after infectious mononucleosis. *Sports Health*. 2014;6(3):232–238. https://doi.org/10.1177/1941738114521984.

Becker PJ, Nieman Carney L, Corkins MR, et al. Consensus statement of the Academy of Nutrition and Dietetics/American Society for Parenteral and Enteral Nutrition: indicators recommended for the identification and documentation of pediatric malnutrition (undernutrition). *J Acad Nutr Diet*. 2014;114(12):1988–2000. https://doi.org/10.1016/j.jand.2014.08.026.

Bergeron M. *Hydration and Thermal Strain in Youth Sports: Responses and Recommendations to Minimize Clinical Risk and Optimize Performance in the Heat*; 2016. https://www.gssiweb.org/en/sports-science-exchange/Article/sse-158-hydration-and-thermal-strain-in-youth-sports-responses-and-recommendations-to-minimize-clinical-risk-and-optimize-performance-in-the-heat.

Bergeron MF, Mountjoy M, Armstrong N, et al. International Olympic Committee consensus statement on youth athletic development.

Br J Sports Med. 2015;49(13):843–851. https://doi.org/10.1136/bjsports-2015-094962.

Bird S, Goebel C, Burke L, Greaves R. Doping in sport and exercise: anabolic, ergogenic, health and clinical issues. *Ann Clin Biochem.* 2015;53(2):196–221. https://doi.org/10.1177/0004563215609952.

Bird S, Hawley J. Update on the effects of physical activity on insulin sensitivity in humans. *BMJ Open Sport Exerc Med.* 2016;2(1):e000143. https://doi.org/10.1136/bmjsem-2016-000143.

Boden BP, Pierpoint LA, Boden RG, Comstock RD, Kerr ZY. Eye Injuries in High School and Collegiate Athletes. *Sports Health.* 2017;9(5):444–449. https://doi.org/10.1177/1941738117712425.

Bonfield CM, Shin SS, Kanter AS. Helmets, head injury and concussion in sport. *Phys Sportsmed.* 2015;43(3):236–246. https://doi.org/10.1080/00913847.2015.1039922.

Brenner J. Council on Sports Medicine and Fitness. Sports specialization and intensive training in youth athletes. *Pediatrics.* 2016;138(3):e1–e8.

Broglio SP, Cantu RC, Gioia GA, et al. National Athletic Trainers' Association position statement: management of sport concussion. *J Athl Train.* 2014;49(2):245–265. https://doi.org/10.4085/1062-6050-49.1.07.

Bull M. *Atlantoaxial Instability in Children with Down Syndrome. Health Issues;* 2016. https://www.healthychildren.org/English/health-issues/conditions/developmental-disabilities/Pages/Atlantoaxial-Instability-in-Children-with-Down-Syndrome.aspx.

Castle J. *Defeating Dehydration;* 2014. http://www.nays.org/sklive/for-parents/defeating-dehydration/.

Caswell SV, Cortes N, Chabolla M, Ambegaonkar JP, Caswell AM, Brenner JS. State-specific differences in school sports preparticipation physical evaluation policies. *Pediatrics.* 2015;135(1):26–32. https://doi.org/10.1542/peds.2014-1451.

Centers for Disease Control and Prevention. *The Buzz on Energy Drinks.* School Nutrition; 2016a. https://www.cdc.gov/healthyschools/nutrition/energy.htm.

Centers for Disease Control and Prevention. *Methicillin-resistant Staphylococcus aureus (MRSA) infections: Cleaning and disinfecting athletic facilities for MRSA;* 2016b. www.cdc.gov/mrsa/community/enviroment/athletic-facilities.html.

Centers for Disease Control and Prevention. *Methicillin-resistant Staphylococcus aureus (MRSA) Infections: Prevention information and advice for athletes; what to do if you think you have MRSA;* 2016c.

Centers for Disease Control and Prevention. *Physical Activity Facts. Healthy Schools;* 2017a. https://www.cdc.gov/healthyschools/physicalactivity/facts.htm.

Centers for Disease Control and Prevention. *Bicycle Safety. Motor Vehicle Safety.* 2017a. https://www.cdc.gov/motorvehiclesafety/bicycle/index.html.

Centers for Disease Control and Prevention. *YRBSS Results. Adolescent and School Health;* 2017b. https://www.cdc.gov/healthyyouth/data/yrbs/results.htm.

Centers for Disease Control and Prevention. Bicycle Safety. *Motor Vehicle Safety.* 2017a. https://www.cdc.gov/motorvehiclesafety/bicycle/index.-.

Centers for Disease Control and Prevention. *Bicycle Safety. Motor Vehicle Safety;* 2017c. https://www.cdc.gov/motorvehiclesafety/bicycle/index.html.

Centers for Disease Control and Prevention. *When Thunder Roars, Go Indoors. Environmental Health;* 2017e. https://www.cdc.gov/features/lightning-safety/index.html.

Chen Y, Tenforde A, Fredericson M. Update on stress fractures in female athletes: epidemiology, treatment, and prevention. *Curr Rev Musculoskelet Med.* 2013;6(2):173–181. https://doi.org/10.1007/s12178-013-9167-x.

Chin JJ, Ludwig D. Increasing children's physical activity during school recess periods. *Am J Public Health.* 2013;103(7):1229–1234. https://doi.org/10.2105/ajph.2012.301132.

Conley KM, Bolin DJ, Carek PJ, Konin JG, Neal TL, Violette D. National Athletic Trainers' Association position statement: Preparticipation

physical examinations and disqualifying conditions. *J Athl Train.* 2014;49(1):102–120. https://doi.org/10.4085/1062-6050-48.6.05.

Crespo NC, Corder K, Marshall S, Norman GJ, Patrick K, Sallis JF, Elder JP. An examination of multilevel factors that may explain gender differences in children's physical activity. *J Phys Act Health.* 2013;10(7):982–992.

Crutchfield KE. Managing patients with neurologic disorders who participate in sports activities. *CONTINUUM: Lifelong Learning in Neurology.* 2014;20(6, Sports Neurology):1657–1666. https://doi.org/10.1212/01.CON.0000458968.40648.6f.

Davies HD, Jackson MA, Rice SG. Infectious diseases associated with organized sports and outbreak control. *Pediatrics.* 2017;140(4). https://doi.org/10.1542/peds.2017-2477.

Denny S. *Supplements and Ergogenic Aids for Athletes. EatRight;* 2014. http://www.eatright.org/resource/food/vitamins-and-supplements/dietary-supplements/supplements-and-ergogenic-aids-for-athletes.

DHHS Department of Public Health. *PAG Midcourse Report: Strategies to Increase Physical Activity Among Youth. Physical Activity Guidelines;* 2017. Available at: https://health.gov/paguidelines/midcourse/pag-mid-course-report-final.pdf.

Depiazzi J, Everard M. Dysfunctional breathing and reaching one's physiological limit as causes of exercise-induced dyspnoea. *Breathe.* 2016;12(2):120–129. https://doi.org/10.1183/20734735.007216.

Dobbins M, Husson H, DeCorby K, LaRocca RL. School-based physical activity programs for promoting physical activity and fitness in children and adolescents aged 6 to 18. *Cochrane Database Syst Rev.* 2013;(2):Cd007651. https://doi.org/10.1002/14651858.CD007651.pub2.

Donnelly JE, Hillman CH, Castelli D, et al. Physical activity, fitness, cognitive function, and academic achievement in children: a systematic review. *Med Sci Sports Exerc.* 2016;48(6):1197–1222. https://doi.org/10.1249/mss.0000000000000901.

DuBose K, McKune A, Brophy P, Geyer G, Hickner R. The relationship between physical activity and the metabolic syndrome score in children. *Pediatr Exerc Sci.* 2015;27(3):364–371. https://doi.org/10.1123/pes.2014-0134.

Durrani A, Fatima W. Effect of physical activity on blood pressure distribution among school children. *Advances in Public Health.* 2015;4. https://doi.org/10.1155/2015/379314.

Einarsson IO, Olafsson A, Hinriksdottir G, Johannsson E, Daly D, Arngrimsson SA. Differences in physical activity among youth with and without intellectual disability. *Med Sci Sports Exerc.* 2015;47(2):411–418. https://doi.org/10.1249/mss.0000000000000412.

epocrates. *Sports Preparticipation Physical;* 2016. https://online.epocrates.com/diseases/888/Athletic-preparticipation-physical.

Flynn JT, Daniels SR, Hayman LL, et al. Update: ambulatory blood pressure monitoring in children and adolescents: a scientific statement from the American Heart Association. *Hypertension.* 2014;63(5):1116–1135. https://doi.org/10.1161/hyp.0000000000000007.

Flynn JT, Kaelber DC, Baker-Smith CM, et al. Clinical practice guideline for screening and management of high blood Pressure in children and adolescents. *Pediatrics.* 2017. https://doi.org/10.1542/peds.2017-1904.

Frey G, Temple V, Stanish H. Interventions to promote physical activity for youth with intellectual disabilities. *Salud Publica de México.* 2017;59:437–445.

Galas JM. Sports participation during teenage years. *Pediatr Clin North Am.* 2014;61(1):91–109. https://doi.org/10.1016/j.pcl.2013.09.020.

Gomes E, Carvalho C, Peixoto-Souza F, et al. Active video game exercise training improves the clinical control of asthma in children: Randomized controlled trial. *PloS One.* 2015;10(8):e0135433. https://doi.org/10.1371/journal.pone.0135433.

Gornitzky AL, Lott A, Yellin JL, Fabricant PD, Lawrence JT, Ganley TJ. Sport-specific yearly risk and incidence of anterior cruciate ligament tears in high school athletes: a systematic review and meta-analysis. *Am J Sports Med.* 2016;44(10):2716–2723. https://doi.org/10.1177/0363546515617742.

Hess C, Mistry D, Herman D. Team Medical Coverage. In: 4 ed. Miller M, Thompson S, eds. *DeLee and Drez'z Orthopaedic Sports*

Medicine: Principles and Practice. Vol. 1. Philadelphia: Elsevier/Saunders; 2015:173–184.

Holland-Hall C. Performance-enhancing substances: is your adolescent patient using?. *Pediatric Clinics of North America.* 2007;54(4):651–662. https://doi.org/10.1016/j.pcl.2007.04.006. ix.

Jaggers J, Hynes K, Wintergerst K. Exercise and sport participation for individuals with type 1 diabetes: safety considerations and the unknown. *ACSMs Health Fit J.* 2016;20(6):40–44. https://doi.org/10.1249/fit.0000000000000249.

Joy E, De Souza MJ, Nattiv A, et al. 2014 female athlete triad coalition consensus statement on treatment and return to play of the female athlete triad. *Curr Sports Med Rep.* 2014;13(4):219–232. https://doi.org/10.1249/jsr.0000000000000077.

Katzmarzyk PT, Barreira TV, Broyles ST, et al. Physical activity, sedentary time, and obesity in an international sample of children. *Med Sci Sports Exerc.* 2015;47(10):2062–2069. https://doi.org/10.1249/mss.0000000000000649.

Keshel T, Coker R. Exercise training and insulin resistance: a current review. *J Obes Weight Loss Ther.* 2015;5(5):S5–003. https://doi.org/10.4172/2165-7904.S5-003.

Knowles BD, Pleacher MD. Athletes with seizure disorders. *Curr Sports Med Rep.* 2012;11(1):16–20. https://doi.org/10.1249/JSR.0b013e318240dc2e.

Kocher MS. Pediatric sports medicine: the young athlete. In: ed 4. Miller MD, Thompson SR, eds. *DeLee & Drez's orthopaedic sports medicine: principles and practice.* vol. II. Philadelphia: Elsevier/Saunders; 2015:1545–1554.

LaBella CR, Hennrikus W, Hewett TE. Anterior cruciate ligament injuries: diagnosis, treatment, and prevention. *Pediatrics.* 2014;133(5):e1437–1450. https://doi.org/10.1542/peds.2014-0623.

LaBotz M, Griesemer B. Use of performance-enhancing substances. *Pediatrics.* 2016;138(1). https://doi.org/10.1542/peds.2016-1300.

Lee B, Adams A, Zenkov E, et al. Modeling the economic and health impact of increasing children's physical activity In the United States. *Health Affair.* 2017;36(5):902–908. https://doi.org/10.1377/hlthaff.2016.1315.

Liu M, Wu L, Ming Q. How does physical activity intervention improve self-esteem and self-concept in children and adolescents? Evidence from a meta-analysis. *PloS One.* 2015;10(8):e0134804. https://doi.org/10.1371/journal.pone.0134804.

Lloyd RS, Avery DF, Stone MH, et al. Position statement on youth resistance training: the 2014 international consensus. *Br J Sports Med.* 2013;0:1–12.

Manore M. Weight management for athletes and active individuals: a brief review. *Sports Med.* 2015;45(suppl 1):83–92. https://doi.org/10.1007/s40279-015-0401-0.

Maron B, Friedman R, Kligfield P, Levine B, Viskin S, Chaitman B, Thompson P. Assessment of the 12-lead electrocardiogram as a screening test for detection of cardiovascular disease in healthy general populations of young people (12–25 Years of Age): A scientific statement from the American Heart Association and the American College of Cardiology. *Journal of the American College of Cardiology.* 2014;64(14):1479–1514. https://doi.org/10.1016/j.jacc.2014.05.006.

Maron BJ, Levine BD, Washington RL, Baggish AL, Kovacs RJ, Maron MS. Eligibility and disqualification recommendations for competitive athletes with cardiovascular abnormalities: Task Force 2: Preparticipation screening for cardiovascular disease in competitive athletes: A scientific statement from the American Heart Association and American College of Cardiology. *J Am Coll Cardiol.* 2015;66(21):2356–2361. https://doi.org/10.1016/j.jacc.2015.09.034.

Maron BJ, Zipes D, Kovacs RJ. Eligibility and disqualification recommendations for competitive athletes with cardiovascular abnormalities: Preamble, principles, and general considerations: A scientific statement from the American Heart Association and American College of Cardiology. *J Am Coll Cardiol.* 2015;66(21):2343–2349. https://doi.org/10.1016/j.jacc.2015.09.032.

Mayo Clinic. *Hazards of Performance-Enhancing Drugs. Healthy Lifestyle: Tween and Teen Health;* 2015a.

Mayo Clinic. *Tween and Teen Health. Healthy Lifestyle;* 2015b. https://www.mayoclinic.org/healthy-lifestyle/tween-and-teen-health/in-depth/performance-enhancing-drugs/art-20046620.

McCrory P, Meeuwisse W, Dvorak J, et al. Consensus statement on concussion in sport–the 5(th) international conference on concussion in sport held in Berlin, October 2016. *Br J Sports Med.* 2017;51(11):838–847. https://doi.org/10.1136/bjsports-2017-097699.

Meehan WP, Lee LK, Fischer CM, Mannix RC. Bicycle helmet laws are associated with a lower fatality rate from bicycle-motor vehicle collisions. *J Pediatr.* 2013;163(3):726–729. https://doi.org/10.1016/j.jpeds.2013.03.073.

Michaelidis M, Koumantakis GA. Effects of knee injury primary prevention programs on anterior cruciate ligament injury rates in female athletes in different sports: a systematic review. *Phys Ther Sport.* 2014;15(3):200–210. https://doi.org/10.1016/j.ptsp.2013.12.002.

Mirabelli MH, Devine MJ, Singh J, Mendoza M. The preparticipation sports evaluation. *Am Fam Physician.* 2015;92(5):371–376.

Must A, Curtin C, Hubbard K, Sikich L, Bedford J, Bandini L. Obesity prevention for children with developmental disabilities. *Curr Obes Rep.* 2014;3(2):156–170. https://doi.org/10.1007/s13679-014-0098-7.

Myers AM, Beam NW, Fakhoury JD. Resistance training for children and adolescents. *Transl Pediatr.* 2017;6(3):137–143. https://doi.org/10.21037/tp.2017.04.01.

Myśliwiec A, Posłuszny A, Saulicz E, et al. Atlanto-axial instability in people with Down's syndrome and its impact on the ability to perform sports activities – a review. *J Hum Kinet.* 2015;48:17–24. https://doi.org/10.1515/hukin-2015-0087.

National Center for Complementary and Integrative Health. *Ephedra;* 2016. https://nccih.nih.gov/health/ephedra.

National Highway Traffic Safety Administration. *Fitting Your Bike Helmet;* 2012. https://www.nhtsa.gov/sites/nhtsa.dot.gov/files/8019_fitting-a-helmet.pdf.

Nationwide Children's Hospital. (N.D.-a). *Golf Cart Safety.* http://www.nationwidechildrens.org/cirp-golf-cart-safety

Nationwide Children's Hospital. (N.D.-b). *New Guidelines: Sports and Energy Drinks. Sports Medicine.* http://www.nationwidechildrens.org/new-guidelines-for-sports-and-energy-drinks

Nationwide Children's Hospital. (N.D.-c). *Skateboarding Safety.* http://www.nationwidechildrens.org/cirp-skateboarding

Nationwide Children's Hospital. (N.D.-e). *Winter Sports Safety.* http://www.nationwidechildrens.org/cirp-winter-sports

National Collegiate Athletic Association (NCAA). *2014-2015 NCAA Sports Medicine Handbook.* Indianapolis: National Collegiate Athletic Association Publishing; 2014.

National Federation of State. *High School Associations.* High School Athletics Participation Survey; 2017:2016–2017. http://www.nfhs.org/ParticipationStatistics/PDF/2016-17_Participation_Survey_Results.pdf.

National Institute of Health National Eye Institute. (N.D.). *About Sports Eye Injury and Protective Eyewear. Sports and Your Eyes.* https://www.nei.nih.gov/sports

National Physical Activity Plan Alliance. *2016 United States Report Card on Physical Activity for Children and Youth;* 2016. http://www.physicalactivityplan.org/projects/reportcard.html.

National Safety Council. *Landing Lightly: Playgrounds Don't Have to Hurt.* 2017. http://www.nsc.org/learn/safety-knowledge/Pages/news-and-resources-playground-safety.aspx.

National Safety Council. *Landing Lightly: Playgrounds Don't Have to Hurt;* 2017. http://www.nsc.org/learn/safety-knowledge/Pages/news-and-resources-playground-safety.aspx.html.

Nationwide Children's Hospital. (N.D.-b). New Guidelines: Sports and Energy Drinks. *Sports Medicine.* http://www.nationwidechildrens.org/new-guidelines-for-sports-and-energy-drinks

Nationwide Children's Hospital. (N.D.-d). Supplements: To Use, Or Not To Use? *Sports Medicine*. http://www.nationwidechildrens.org/supplements-to-use-or-not-to-use.

Nationwide Children's Hospital. (N.D.). New Guidelines: Sports and Energy Drinks. *Sports Medicine*. http://www.nationwidechildrens.org/new-guidelines-for-sports-and-energy-drinks

Nemours Foundation. *Swimming. Kids Health*. 2015. https://kidshealth.org/en/kids/swim.html#.

Nemours Foundation. *Sports Supplements. Teen Health*. 2015. http://m.kidshealth.org/en/teens/sports-supplements.html.

Nemours Foundation. *A Guide to Eating for Sports. TeensHealth*. 2017. http://kidshealth.org/en/teens/eatnrun.html?WT.ac=ctg#.

Newsham K. Evaluating dyspnea in the athletic patient. *J Nurse Pract*. 2013;9(5):288–294. https://doi.org/10.1016/j.nurpra.2013.02.018.

Nichols A. Heat-related illness in sports and exercise. *Curr Rev Musculoskelet Med*. 2014;7(4):355–365. https://doi.org/10.1007/s12178-014-9240-0.

Office of Disease Prevention and Health Promotion. *Dietary Guidelines 2015-2020. Appendix 1. Physical Activity Guidelines for Americans*; 2015. https://health.gov/dietaryguidelines/2015/guidelines/appendix-1/.

Office of Disease Prevention and Health Promotion. *2016 United States Report Card on Physical Activity for Children and Youth Released*; 2017a. https://health.gov/news/blog-bayw/2016/11/2016-united-states-report-card-on-physical-activity-for-children-and-youth-released/.

Office of Disease Prevention and Health Promotion. *Leading Health Indicators*; 2017b. https://www.healthypeople.gov/2020/Leading-Health-Indicators.

Orthopedic and Sports Medicine Center of Oregon. (N.D.). *Trauma and Bone Fractures in Children*. http://orthosportsmed.com/trauma-and-bone-fractures-in-children/.

Pediatrics A, A. o. Lawn Mower Safety. *Safety and Prevention*. 2015a. https://www.healthychildren.org/English/safety-prevention/at-home/Pages/Lawnmower-Safety.aspx.

Pediatrics A, A. o. Life Jackets and Life Preservers. *Safety and Prevention*. 2015b. https://www.healthychildren.org/English/safety-prevention/at-play/Pages/Life-Jackets-and-Life-Preservers.aspx.

Pediatrics A, A. o. *ATVs are Dangerous to Children: Injuries Have Increased, Estimated ATV Deaths Up, but Data Is Incomplete*. 2017. https://www.aap.org/en-us/about-the-aap/aap-press-room/Pages/AAPCFAATVData.aspx.

Personal Watercraft Industry Association. *Rules and Regulations*. 2016. http://www.pwia.org/rules.

Petteys RJ, Nair NM. Head and spine diagnosis and decision making. In: *principles and practice*. ed 4. Miller MD, Thompson SR, eds. *DeLee & Drez's orthopaedic sports medicine*. Vol. II. Philadelphia: Elsevier/Saunders; 2015:1478–1483.

Pfister T, Pfister K, Hagel B, Ghali WA, Ronksley PE. The incidence of concussion in youth sports: a systematic review and meta-analysis. *Br J Sports Med*. 2016;50(5):292–297. https://doi.org/10.1136/bjsports-2015-094978.

Pimentel J, Tojal R, Morgado J. Epilepsy and physical exercise. *Seizure*. 2015;25:87–94. https://doi.org/10.1016/j.seizure.2014.09.015.

Protective eyewear for young athletes. (2004, reaffirmed 2015). *Ophthalmology*. 111(3):600-603. https://doi.org/10.1016/j.ophtha.2003.12.027.

Rauchenzauner M, Hagn C, Walch R, et al. Quality of life and fitness in children and adolescents with epilepsy (EpiFit). *Neuropediatrics*. 2017;48(3):161–165. https://doi.org/10.1055/s-0037-1599236.

Rice SG. Medical conditions affecting sports participation. *Pediatrics*. 2014;121(4):841–848. https://doi.org/10.1542/peds.2008-0080.

Riner W, Sellhorst S. Physical activity and exercise in children with chronic health conditions. *J Sport Health Sci*. 2013;2(1):12–20. https://doi.org/10.1016/j.jshs.2012.11.005.

Rosenbloom C. *Teen Nutrition for Fall Sports. Kids eat Right*. 2016. http://www.eatright.org/resource/fitness/sports-and-performance/fueling-your-workout/teen-nutrition-for-fall-sports.

Sanders B, Blackburn TA, Boucher B. Preparticipation screening – The sports physical therapy perspective. *Int J Sports Phys Ther*. 2013;8(2):180–193.

Shelat NH, El-Khoury GY. Pediatric stress fractures: a pictorial essay. *Iowa Orthop J*. 2016;36:138–146.

Shephard RJ. Exercise and the athlete with infectious mononucleosis. *Clin J Sport Med*. 2017;27(2):168–178. https://doi.org/10.1097/jsm.0000000000000330.

Smith J, Holmes M, McAllister M. Nutritional considerations for performance in young athletes. *J Sports Med*. 2015;2015:13. https://doi.org/10.1155/2015/734649.

Special Olympics. *Article 2: Special Olympics Athletes*; 2015. http://resources.specialolympics.org/Topics/General_Rules/Article_02.aspx.

Statuta S, Vaughan A. Doping and Ergogenic Aids: Sports Pharmacology. In: Miller M, Thompson S, eds. *DeLee and Drez's Orthopaedic Sports Medicine: Principles and Practice*. vol. 1. Philadelphia: Elsevier/Saunders; 2015:327–337.

Stracciolini A, Sugimoto D, Howell DR. Injury prevention in youth sports. *Pediatr Ann*. 2017;46(3):e99–e105. https://doi.org/10.3928/19382359-20170223-01.

Tandon P, Tovar A, Jayasuriya A, et al. The relationship between physical activity and diet and young children's cognitive development: A systematic review. *Prev Med Rep*. 2016;3(suppl C):379–390. https://doi.org/10.1016/j.pmedr.2016.04.003.

Thomas DT, Erdman KA, Burke LM. American College of Sports Medicine Joint Position Statement. Nutrition and Athletic Performance. *Med Sci Sports Exerc*. 2016;48(3):543–568. https://doi.org/10.1249/mss.0000000000000852.

University of Michigan. (N.D.). *Recreational Vehicle Safety*. http://www.med.umich.edu/yourchild/topics/rvssafe.htm.

University of Michigan Medicine. *Recreational Vehicle Safety. Your Child Development & Behavior Resources*. 2012. http://www.med.umich.edu/yourchild/topics/rvssafe.htm.

United States Department of Health and Human Services Office of Disease Prevention and Health Promotion. *Nutrition, Physical Activity and Obesity*; 2017. https://www.healthypeople.gov/2020/leading-health-indicators/2020-lhi-topics/nutrition-physical-activity-and-obesity.

University of South Florida. (2017, 6/01/17). For Athletes. *Educational Initiative on Sickle Cell Trait for the Athletic Population*. http://health.usf.edu/medicine/orthopaedic/sicklecell/athletes

Vale S, Trost SG, Rego C, Abreu S, Mota J. Physical activity, obesity status, and blood pressure in preschool children. *J Pediatr*. 2015;167(1):98–102. https://doi.org/10.1016/j.jpeds.2015.04.031.

Visram S, Cheetham M, Riby D, Crossley S, Lake A. Consumption of energy drinks by children and young people: a rapid review examining evidence of physical effects and consumer attitudes. *BMJ Open*. 2016;6(10). https://doi.org/10.1136/bmjopen-2015-010380.

Wang Y, Xu D. Effects of aerobic exercise on lipids and lipoproteins. *Lipids Health Dis*. 2017;16(1):132. https://doi.org/10.1186/s12944-017-0515-5.

Wasfy M, Hutter A, Weiner R. Sudden cardiac death in athletes. *Methodist Debakey Cardiovasc J*. 2016;12(2):76–80. https://doi.org/10.14797/mdcj-12-2-76.

Weiss Kelly AK, Hecht S. The Female Athlete Triad. *Pediatrics*. 2016. https://doi.org/10.1542/peds.2016-0922.

White N, Noeun J. Performance-enhancing drug use in adolescence. *Am J Lifestyle Med*. 2017.

World Health Organization. *Global Status Report on Noncommunicable Diseases*; 2014. http://apps.who.int/iris/bitstream/10665/148114/1/9789241564854_eng.pdf.

World Health Organization. *10 Facts on Physical Activity*; 2017a. http://www.who.int/features/factfiles/physical_activity/en/.

World Health Organization. *Physical Activity. Global Strategy on Diet, Physical Activity and Health*; 2017b. http://www.who.int/dietphysicalactivity/pa/en/.

World Health Organization. *Physical Activity and Young People Global Strategy on Diet, Physical Activity and Health*; 2017c. http://www.who.int/dietphysicalactivity/factsheet_young_people/en/.

Wu Y, Zhang C, Zhen Q. Metabolic syndrome in children (review). *Exp Ther Med*. 2016;12(4):2390–2394. https://doi.org/10.3892/etm.2016.3632.

Zaremski JL, Krabak BJ. Shoulder injuries in the skeletally immature baseball pitcher and recommendations for the prevention of injury. *PM R*. 2012;4(7):509–516.

20
Sleep

SUSAN HINES

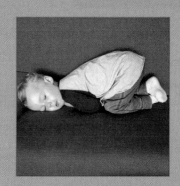

Adequate sleep is a necessary process for normal emotional, physiologic, and mental functioning in children. Sleep affects every aspect of a child's development and is considered a time of renewal for the mind and body. However, sleep is not simply a state of rest. The brain is more active during certain periods of sleep than it is in wakefulness, and researchers believe sleep is essential for brain development, which may be one reason that infants and young children spend the majority of their time asleep. Growth, healing, learning, processing of information, and many other functions are facilitated by the sleep state.

Sleep-Wake Cycle and Health

According to the American Academy of Sleep Medicine (AASM), sleeping the recommended number of hours (for the particular age of the child) on a regular basis is associated with better health outcomes, including improved attention, behavior, learning, memory, emotional regulation, quality of life, and mental and physical health. Furthermore, sleeping fewer than the number of recommended hours on a regular basis is associated with poor attention, behavior, learning problems, and depression (Paruthi et al., 2016a).

Evidence exists that inadequate sleep in adolescents can encourage high-risk behaviors such as substance abuse, suicide behaviors, and drowsiness while driving (Buxton et al., 2015). Insufficient sleep among school-aged children is associated with an increased risk of poor academic performance and depression (Yland et al., 2015). Insufficient sleep has been identified as a risk factor for obesity in all ages and can also increase the risk of obesity in adolescents regardless of physical activity.

Sleep difficulties are a common concern of all parents and experienced by approximately 25% to 30% of all children and adolescents regardless of age (Combs et al., 2016). Common sleep problems include behavioral insomnia, insufficient sleep, sleep disordered breathing (SDB), parasomnias, nightmares, periodic limb movements (PLMs), excessive sleepiness, and narcolepsy. Insomnia in children is defined as sleep onset delay more than 30 minutes (on average) per night, and/or frequent prolonged night waking with impaired daytime functioning (Tsai et al., 2016).

Electronic Devices and Sleep Problems

A shift toward poorer sleep in adolescents over the past decade has coincided with a sharp increase in the availability and use of electronic devices such as smartphones, video game consoles, computers, and tablets, along with television (Hysing et al., 2015). Current studies have found almost all American adolescents (97%) report having at least one electronic device in their bedroom (Yland et al., 2015). Along with entertainment, electronic devices play an ever-increasing part in the social lives of adolescents. Educational institutions also encourage electronic use for coursework. Therefore, parents may find it difficult to monitor whether their child is using their electronic devices for homework versus entertainment.

The timing of electronic use before bed is also significant because blue light emitted from screens suppresses the endogenous melatonin, and the suppression lasts throughout the night (American Academy of Pediatrics [AAP], 2017). A recent study examining technology-related behaviors found electronics (game playing) and online social media in the hour before bedtime were risk factors for shorter and poorer sleep, whereas time with family was protective of sleep duration (Harbard et al., 2015). Another recent study found cell phone use by adolescents late at night has been associated with poorer sleep quality, whereas physical activity can improve sleep quality and quantity (Arma et al., 2017). Making sure that children do not substitute electronic gaming for physical activity including outdoor play is vital.

The rise of electronic use is also affecting younger children. Screen time from computers and televisions is associated with reduced sleep duration among 9-year-olds (Yland et al., 2015). Even infants exposed to screen media in the evening hours show significantly shorter nighttime sleep duration than those with no evening screen exposure (AAP, 2016).

The 2014 National Sleep Foundation *Sleep in America* poll evaluated "Sleep in the Modern Family" to gather a contemporary picture of sleep in families with at least one school-aged child. The study found better age-appropriate sleep in households where well-established rules of sleep hygiene existed such as regular sleep-wake patterns and limited caffeine (Buxton et al., 2015). Sleep deficiency was more likely to be present when both parents and children had electronics devices on in the bedroom after bedtime (Buxton et al., 2015).

Parents play an important role in helping children and teens navigate media and should set expectations and boundaries to make sure the media experience is positive because negative media are very prevalent and accessible. According to the AAP, problems begin when physical activity, hands-on exploration, and face-to-face social interaction in the real world are displaced by media. Furthermore, too much screen time can also harm the amount and quality of sleep (AAP, 2017).

American Academy of Pediatrics Recommendations to Promote Adequate Sleep in Children

Electronic Device Recommendations

- Children younger than 18 months, avoid use of screen media other than video-chatting.
- Parents of children 18 to 24 months of age who want to introduce digital media should choose high-quality programming and watch it with their children to help them understand what they are seeing.
- Children ages 2 to 5 years, limit screen use to 1 h/day of high-quality programs. Parents should coview media with children to help them understand what they are seeing and apply it to the world around them.
- Children ages 6 and older, place consistent limits on the time spent using media and the types of media, and make sure media do not take the place of adequate sleep, physical activity, and other behaviors essential to health.

Further recommendations for media use and families include to: (1) designate media-free times together, such as dinner or driving, as well as media-free locations at home, such as bedrooms; (2) have ongoing communication about online citizenship and safety, including treating others with respect online and offline; (3) recommend that children not sleep with devices in their bedrooms, including TVs, computers, and smartphones; (4) avoid exposure to devices or screens for 1 hour before bedtime; and (5) discourage entertainment media while doing homework. The AAP developed a family media use tool that can help families to form a plan that is age appropriate for their children (https://www.healthychildren.org/English/media/Pages/default.aspx.).

Infant Recommendations

Although limited data exist about the best age at which to start behavioral strategies for sleep implementation, clinical experience suggests that between 3 and 4 months of age may be an ideal time. Behavioral interventions before 3 months of age are not recommended because infants still need to feed frequently. Placing infants into their crib drowsy but still awake allows them to initiate sleep independently in their own environment and enables them to return to sleep independently throughout the night. This strategy has been found to be the most important recommendation for parents in multiple studies (Kuhn, 2014). Nursing or bottle-feeding a baby to sleep after the newborn period is also not recommended, because the infant may learn to associate being fed with returning to sleep.

Adolescent Recommendations

"Chronic sleep loss in children and adolescents is one of the most common—and easily fixable—public health issues in the U.S. today," said pediatrician Judith Owens, MD, FAAP, lead author of the policy statement, "School Start Times for Adolescents," published in the September 2014 issue of Pediatrics. In 2014 the AAP released a statement recommending middle and high schools delay the start of class to 8:30 a.m. or later. Recommendations were based on biologic sleep rhythms of adolescents whose sleep-wake cycles begin to shift up to 2 hours later at the start of puberty. Furthermore, multiple studies have shown that adolescents who do not get adequate sleep are at risk of being overweight and suffering depression and that those who do get adequate sleep are less likely to be involved in automobile accidents and have better grades, higher standardized test scores, and an overall better quality of life (AAP, 2014). According to the AAP, napping, extending sleep on weekends, and caffeine consumption is common in sleep-deprived teens, but these measures do not restore optimal alertness and are not a substitute for regular, sufficient sleep. A study investigating the link between sleep and depression found that gradual sleep extension combined with sleep hygiene advice had a beneficial effect on depressive symptoms of adolescents with chronic sleep reduction (Lee et al., 2017).

Normal Sleep Stages and Cycles

Circadian Rhythm and Establishment of Normal Sleep Patterns

The circadian rhythm is an internal, endogenous clock that exists in all living organisms. This natural rhythm is synchronized to the 24-hour light-dark cycle and is genetically determined and typically lasts slightly longer than 24 hours. Circadian rhythms emerge at approximately 2 to 3 months of age and are affected by melatonin secretion from the hypothalamus. A special center in the hypothalamus, called the *suprachiasmatic nucleus (SCN),* releases melatonin in response to darkness, as perceived by a nerve pathway from the retina in the eye. This melatonin cycle is established between 4 and 6 months of age. The SCN initiates signals to other parts of the brain that control hormones, body temperature, and other functions that play a role in making us feel sleepy or wide awake (National Sleep Foundation, 2017).

Sleep Cycle

Normal sleep can be divided into two distinct phases: rapid eye movement (REM) sleep and nonrapid eye movement (NREM) sleep. NREM sleep can be further divided into three distinct stages as defined by changes in electroencephalographic (EEG) patterns. NREM sleep constitutes approximately 75% to 80% of total time spent in sleep, with the remaining 20% to 25% spent in REM sleep. These sleep stages make up sleep cycles, each lasting approximately 90 minutes, with about six of these cycles occurring per night.

Nonrapid Eye Movement Sleep

Stage 1 (NREM1 or N1)

NREM sleep is divided into three stages. N1 sleep is a state of drowsiness and occurs at the transition to sleep. Aside from newborns and children diagnosed with narcolepsy, the average child's sleep stage begins in N1 sleep. There may be eye-rolling movements, decreased body movements, and possibly opening and closing of the eyelids. Individuals may believe they are awake, but they cannot accurately report events that occurred during the time. N1 sleep typically accounts for 3% to 8% of the total sleep time.

Stage 2 (NREM1 or N2)

N2 sleep is somewhat deeper than N1, although a person can still be easily aroused. There is a slowing of eye movements, breathing, and heart rate during N2. Muscles weaken also, but a child can still reposition himself. N2 sleep accounts for approximately 45% to 55% of total sleep time.

Stage 3 (NREM3 or N3)

N3 sleep is also known as *deep, delta,* or *slow wave sleep (SWS).* During this stage of sleep, a child is even less responsive to the outside environment, and it can be very difficult to awaken a child during this stage. N3 sleep occurs in longer periods during the first half of the night, particularly during the first two sleep cycles, and represents approximately 15% to 20% of the total sleep time. Historically, NREM stage 4 (NREM4 or N4) was recognized, but, following the guidelines of the AASM, it is now included in the N3 sleep stage (American Academy of Sleep Medicine, 2014).

Rapid Eye Movement Sleep

REM sleep is characterized by increased EEG activity and bursts of REMs similar to a wake state. Individuals experience vivid dreams, with simultaneous muscle paralysis that is thought to protect the person from physically acting out the dream. REM sleep is considered a time for the brain to learn from the experiences of the day. The amount of REM sleep is highest at infancy, approximately 55%, and decreases to approximately 20% to 25% by 5 years old. The majority of REM sleep occurs during the latter portion of the night.

If children are deprived of REM or SWS, pressure to restore that particular phase of sleep mounts. A rebound pattern develops as the body shortens other stages of sleep to obtain the stage that it has been lacking. Furthermore, patients deprived of REM sleep become excitable and anxious, and those deprived of SWS often present with intense fatigue. It may be that REM is related to psychological recovery and NREM is related to musculoskeletal recovery.

The sleep cycle order is normally N1, N2, N3, and REM. There is a greater amount of deep sleep (stage N3) earlier in the night, whereas the proportion of REM sleep increases in the last two cycles just before natural awakening. Individuals often have brief arousals between sleep cycles, most are so brief that they cannot be recalled.

Sleep Patterns by Age Group

Sleep changes with age and in duration, cycling, and habits. The average duration is seen in Table 20.1. Differences in sleep are described in this section, although the trends vary from child to child. There are no clear differences in sleep patterns as children move from one age group to the next; changes occur gradually.

Newborns

Newborn sleep is different from the sleep of older infants and children. Infants younger than 6 months of age spend 50% of their sleep time in active REM sleep, compared with 20% to 25% in older children. REM sleep can be active in newborns with audible suckling. Newborns often enter REM sleep initially, unlike older children and adults who do not typically experience REM sleep until at least 90 minutes into the sleep cycle, and the sleep cycles are closer to 60 minutes. Active REM emerges more often during a sleep cycle in infants, resulting in shorter sleep cycles. By 6 months of age, the infant's sleep architecture closely resembles that of an adult's.

Newborns sleep a total of 10.5 to 18 h/day on an irregular schedule with periods of 1 to 3 hours spent awake (National Sleep Foundation, 2017). Sleep in newborns can last a few minutes to several hours, and they are often active during sleep with sucking, smiling, and twitching of arms and legs. Newborns need to feed frequently, and although not recommended, breastfeeding is often

TABLE 20.1 Average Sleep Duration by Age		
Age	Nighttime Sleep (Hours)	Daytime Sleep (Hours)
1 week old	8.25	8.25
1 month old	8.5	7
3 months old	10	5
6 months old	11	3.4
9 months old	11.2	2.8
12 months old	11.7	2.4
18 months old	11.6	1.8
2 years old	11.4	
3-5 years old	12.5	
5-11 years old	11	
12-17 year old	8-9	

Adapted from Dewar G. Baby sleep requirements: a guide for the science-minded. Parenting Science (website); 2008. www.parentingscience.com/baby-sleep-requirements.html. Accessed January 10, 2010; Dewar G. Newborn sleep patterns: a survival guide for the science-minded parent. Parenting Science (website); 2008. www.parentingscience.com/newborn-sleep.html. Accessed January 10, 2010; Jenni O, Molinari L, Caflisch J, et al. Sleep duration from ages 1 to 10 years: variability and stability in comparison with growth. *Pediatrics.* 2007;120(4):e769–e776; Rodriguez AJ. Pediatric sleep and epilepsy. *Curr Neurol Neurosci Rep.* 2007;7(4):342–347.

one of the most prominent reasons for bed sharing. Nighttime feeds are usually not necessary by 6 months of age, and many children will begin sleeping through the night; 70% to 80% will do so by 9 months of age (National Sleep Foundation, 2017).

Sudden Unexpected Infant Death

Sudden unexpected infant death (SUID) and sudden unexpected death in infancy (SUDI) are terms used to describe any sudden and unexpected death—explained or unexplained including sudden infant death syndrome (SIDS). SUDI describes infant death from suffocation, asphyxia, entrapment, infection, ingestions, metabolic diseases, and trauma (unintentional or nonaccidental).

SIDS is a subcategory of SUID defined as infant deaths that are unexplained after a thorough case investigation including autopsy, a scene investigation, and clinical history. The working model of SIDS pathogenesis is that death results from the interaction between a vulnerable infant and a potentially asphyxiating and/or overheating sleep environment (Moon, 2016). Deaths from SIDS drastically decreased since the AAP recommended that all infants sleep on their backs in the early 1990s. This was initially labeled the "Back to Sleep" campaign but is currently referred to as "Safe to Sleep" campaign. However, SIDS remains the leading cause of death in infants aged 1 month to 1 year (Zachritz et al., 2016). Currently, the occurrence of SIDS is greater than 1900 deaths/year, or 0.49 deaths/1000 live births (Moon, 2016). Ninety percent of SIDS cases occur before 6 months of age, with the peak between 1 and 4 months of age (Moon, 2016). The actual mechanisms for SIDS remain unclear; infants who die of SIDS are more likely to have been born premature and/or growth restricted, which suggests a suboptimal intrauterine environment (Moon, 2016).

In 2016 the AAP updated the SIDS prevention recommendations to include recent evidence that can help to prevent SIDS. These include the endorsement of room sharing without bed sharing; use of a pacifier; parental avoidance of illicit drugs, alcohol, and smoke; supine positioning on a firm sleep surface; avoiding bumper pads and the use of bedding; and avoiding overheating. Breastfeeding and routine immunization also remain in the recommendations as protective factors against SIDS.

Protective Factors for Infant Sleep

The APP currently recommends that infants sleep in the parents' room, close to the parents' bed but not in the same bed, ideally for the first year of life but at least the first 6 months (Moon, 2016). Infant cribs, bedside sleepers, play yard, portable cribs, and bassinets in the same room are all safe. The AAP has made this recommendation because this arrangement decreases the risk of SIDS by as much as 50% and is safer than bed sharing or solitary sleeping (infant sleeping in a separate room). In addition, room sharing lessens the chance of suffocation, strangulation, and entrapment that can be caused by cosleeping but allows for close proximity to the infant for feeding, comforting, and monitoring (Moon, 2016). Multiple studies have investigated the association of SIDS with prenatal and postnatal exposure to alcohol or illicit drug use, although substance abuse often involves more than one substance, and it can be difficult to separate other variables from smoking. However, sufficient evidence exists that bed sharing places the infant at particular risk for SIDS when there is parental alcohol and/or illicit drug use (Moon, 2016). Overheating is identified as a potential risk factor for SIDS but has not been proven. Multiple case-control studies report a protective effect of pacifiers on the incidence of SIDS, but the mechanism is not clear. However, pacifiers should not be hung around the infant's neck, nor should they be attached to the infant's clothes (Moon, 2016).

Health Professional Strategies to Reduce Sudden Infant Death Syndrome

Parental training on safe sleep education should be an integral part of hospital discharge for every newborn. All nursery staff, including nurses, doctors, social workers, nursing assistants, case managers and respiratory therapists, should receive safe sleep training. The most significant impact of the safe sleep environment education in reducing SIDS is the use of a flat sleeping surface and the avoidance of cosleeping (Zachritz et al., 2016).

Early Childhood

Toddlers need approximately 12 to 14 hours of sleep in a 24-hour period, and most toddlers transition to one nap at approximately 18 to 22 months of age (National Sleep Foundation, 2017). Sleep difficulties, such as resisting going to bed and nighttime awakenings, are common in this age group due to toddler's innate need for independence, as well as their increases in motor, social, and cognitive abilities. They are able to physically get out of bed, and this can become problematic. Separation anxiety, which is a normal developmental stage for children ages 6 months to 2 years, can also contribute to resistance at bedtime (AAP, 2015). Nighttime fears and nightmares are also common in this age group. Some families cosleep with their toddlers for cultural reasons, and other families cosleep when they are unsuccessful at getting children to sleep in their own beds.

3 to 5 Years of Age

Preschoolers typically sleep 11 to 13 hours each night, and most do not nap after they are 5 years of age. As with toddlers, difficulty falling asleep and waking up during the night are common. With further development of imagination, preschoolers commonly experience nighttime fears and nightmares. In addition, sleepwalking and night terrors (or sleep terrors) peak during preschool years. Regular daytime routines help to promote regular sleep patterns.

Middle Childhood 5 to 12 Years of Age

Children from 5 to 12 years of age need 10 to 11 hours of sleep. Some 5-year-olds still require a nap, but this need typically declines by first grade. If children still need naps in grade school, further evaluation is needed. Demands from school (homework), sports, and other extracurricular activities increase during this time. In addition, school-age children typically increase screen time and use of computers, smartphones, and TV. They also consume more caffeine products. All of these factors can lead to difficulty sleeping.

Adolescents

Most adolescents get less than the 8 to 9 hours of sleep as recommended by the Centers for Disease Control and Prevention (CDC) (Matthews et al., 2014). Adolescents have multiple reasons for not getting enough sleep, including:

- A natural shift in their sleep schedule: After puberty, a biologic shift of approximately 2 hours occurs in an adolescent's internal clock, making it difficult to fall asleep early.
- Early high school start times: In most school districts, the move to high school is accompanied by an earlier school start time, which can be as early as 7:00 a.m. Teens often have to wake up by 5:00 a.m. to get ready for school.
- Social and school obligations: Teens spend 30 to 35 h/week on average in class and an additional several hours per week doing homework. After-school activities, sports, and socializing often lead to late nights. As a result, most adolescents may be sleep deprived.

Parents of Asian children reported significantly more sleep problems than parents of Caucasians. Chinese parents reported the highest rates of perceived sleep problems in both younger children (0 to 3 years of age, 52%) and older children (3 to 6 years of age, 44%) (Mindell et al., 2013). Sleep habits in families differ; cosleeping practices, strategies for promoting sleep, and even what defines a sleep problem differ across cultures.

Assessment of Sleep

History

Chief Complaint

Evaluation of potential sleep problems involves a comprehensive history of the child's 24-hour routine, focusing on bedtime habits, sleep environment, and daytime behavior. The family medical history and the caregiver's attitudes and beliefs about what constitutes normal sleep are vital and can guide the investigation and treatment. See Box 20.1 for a review of family medical history. When sleep difficulties are noted, it is important to ask about the age when the problem began, precipitating events, presence of the symptoms on the weekends, holidays, and vacation, and if aggravating and alleviating factors are present. It is also necessary to ask about the effects on the child's daily living, as well as the impact on family members.

- Routines used for getting the child to sleep, sleep resistance, and parental response to objections.
- Sleep aids (such as pacifiers, blankets, and stuffed animals) and patting or rocking.
- Room environment, including cosleeping, room temperature, and electronics in the room.
- Nighttime behavior, such as prolonged awakening, night terrors, sleep walking, sleep eating, seizures, and head banging.
- Nighttime complaints of leg pain, restless sleep, and kicking which can be associated with periodic limb movements (PLMs).
- Sleep disordered breathing (SDB), such as snoring, gasping, apneas, cyanosis, headaches upon awakening, loud breathing, mouth breathing, neck hyperextension, and frequent position changes.
- Excessive secretions/drooling.
- Wake up times and daytime symptoms, such as difficulty waking up, falling asleep in class, hyperactivity, and overall emotional and cognitive functioning.
- Medications, caffeine intake (effects of caffeine can last up to 8 h), exercise, and diet.

Past Medical History and Review of Symptoms

Medical problems of the child are often associated with sleep difficulties. Pain and discomfort are important factors to consider. Assess the following:
- Obesity with sleep disordered breathing (SDB).
- Neurologic disorders (such as attention deficit hyperactivity disorder [ADHD], autism, cerebral palsy, and neuromuscular disorders) are associated with both behavioral sleep problems (BSPs) and SDB.
- Respiratory conditions, such as hypoxemia, asthma, laryngomalacia, and allergic rhinitis; obstructive sleep apnea (OSA) and asthma are prevalent respiratory disorders and are frequently comorbid conditions.
- Gastroesophageal reflux may contribute to OSA, especially in newborns and infants.
- Nocturnal enuresis, which can be associated with SDB.
- Dermatologic problems causing discomfort, such as itching with eczema.
- Pulmonary hypertension can be caused by untreated SDB and is important to assess.
- Failure to thrive secondary to increased caloric expenditure from increased work of breathing.
- Developmental delays, which can affect the child's ability to develop appropriate sleep behaviors.
- Epilepsy: Children with a seizure disorder are at increased risk for sleep disorders.
- Depression, anxiety, or other psychiatric problems can be significant in insomnia.

Family Assessment

Assess the following:
- Parental knowledge and expectations about infant and child sleep patterns.
- Parental ability and willingness to modify sleep hygiene.
- Family history of sleep disorders: SDB is often familial which is important information for clinicians.

- Recent divorces, separation, family or close friend death, or other family stressors.
- Recent changes in the living arrangements.

Physical Examination

A thorough physical examination should always be conducted, especially evaluating for signs of illness or pain in an individual presenting with a sleep issue. Vital signs should be obtained, including pulse oximetry, weight, body mass index (BMI), and blood pressure. Neurologic evaluation, including the child's muscle tone, needs to be completed because abnormal muscle tone can contribute to SDB. Special attention to obvious hyperactivity, anxiety, and/or depression is needed to fully evaluate the child. Physical findings that may indicate sleep apnea include swollen nasal turbinates, deviated septum, nasal polyps, open mouth posture, adenoid facies, large tonsils, narrow oropharynx, low-hanging palate, high-arched hard palate, micrognathia, or retrognathia.

Diagnostic Studies

A sleep-feeding-activity record for infants (Fig 20.1) or a 2-week sleep diary (Fig 20.2) can be useful for primary care providers and caregivers to identify patterns of awakenings and routines and is helpful when evaluating children with sleep disorder.

Sleep clinics may order an actigraphy study. *Actigraphy* measures light exposure and activity over a period of time (typically 1 week) in the home environment. A device is worn on the wrist that resembles a watch band. In general, there is a good correlation between the polysomnogram (PSG), a multiparametric test used in sleep medicine, and actigraphy-defined total sleep time, sleep latency, and sleep efficiency (percentage of time in bed spent sleeping) (Mullin et al., 2017). Actigraphy is also helpful for evaluating the effectiveness of insomnia treatments, because total sleep time is measured. Actigraphy is often used along with a personal sleep diary recorded by the child (if age appropriate) or the parent. Furthermore, actigraphy offers objectivity and can dispel sleep misperceptions, which are common in some pediatric populations. For example, some adolescents will report being awake most of the night when they are in fact sleeping a fair amount of time. Parents are not always able to monitor the amount of sleep of their child because they are sleeping as well.

Sleep in Children With Developmental and Neurologic Conditions

Children with neurologic disorders such as autism spectrum disorder (ASD) and ADHD have the highest rates of sleep problems of all children with mental challenges, and, like normally developing children, behavioral insomnia is the most common complaint.

Anxiety

Children with generalized anxiety disorder (GAD) also experience more insomnia when compared to their peers without anxiety. Youth with anxiety disorders who struggle to regulate high arousal negative emotions can be especially vulnerable to chronic sleep disturbances (Mullin et al., 2017). A study used both subjective

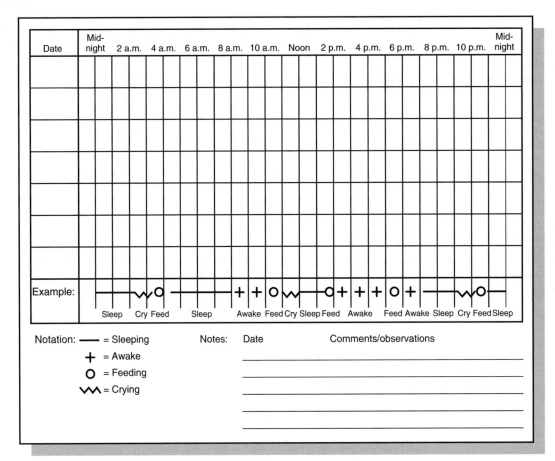

• Fig 20.1 Example of a Sleep-Activity-Feeding Record.

Two-week sleep diary	
Week 1:	Week 2:
Mon	Mon
Tue	Tue
Wed	Wed
Thu	Thu
Fri	Fri
Sat	Sat
Sun	Sun
Instructions: Describe your child's sleep each day. How long does your child sleep? What is the time it took to go to sleep? What are the hours of sleep? Describe issues during the night.	

• Fig 20.2 Two-Week Sleep Diary.

and objective methods to measure sleep in children with and without GAD; the objective measures were based on a combination of overnight sleep studies and actigraphy. These data estimate sleep and wake patterns as well as light exposure using established algorithms. The study found that decreases in nightly sleep duration were associated with increased morning anxiety but only among

children with GAD. This same study also found that relative to healthy controls, the GAD participants reported higher levels of bedtime fears/worries, restless legs, and overall insomnia symptoms, as well as greater daytime sleepiness (Mullin et al., 2017). These fluctuations in sleep duration may have contribute to daytime anxiety.

ADHD

Specific sleep disorders for children with ADHD include behavioral insomnia, SDB, and restless leg syndrome (RLS)/PLMs. SDB has been found in 25% to 57% of children with ADHD, causing further neurologic dysfunction (Tsai et al., 2016). Current recommendations for the initiation of pharmacotherapy in children with ADHD include assessment of sleep conditions before initiating the medications (Tsai et al., 2016). Interestingly, untreated sleep apnea, RLS/PLMs, and insufficient sleep in children without neurologic disorders can mimic symptoms of ADHD. Sleep difficulties among children with ADHD are thought to be related to shared neurobiologic pathways involving areas of the cortex responsible for regulation and arousal, the medication effects of stimulants used, and the presence of comorbid mental health disorders (Tsai et al., 2016). Methylphenidate, which is a first-line FDA-approved medication for ADHD, has been linked to insomnia in short- and long-term clinical trials (Tsai et al., 2016).

Autism

Approximately two-thirds of children with ASD have chronic insomnia. Currently, the strongest evidence on promoting sleep in children with ASD is sleep education including behavioral interventions, environmental changes, and exogenous melatonin (Souders et al., 2017). According to the revised International Classification of Sleep Disorders, behaviors associated with sleep problems in children with ASD include cosleeping, poor sleep efficiency, difficulty self-settling, frequent night waking, sleep onset latency, early waking, poor sleep hygiene (habits and practices before bed), irregular sleep-wake patterns, and daytime sleepiness (Cuomo et al., 2017). When assessing sleep difficulties in children with ASD, it is important to assess for SDB, PLMs, parasomnias, epilepsy, and narcolepsy. Medical problems such as parasomnias, PLMs, and SDB are common in children with ASD. Decreased muscle tone or hypotonia in children with ASD can cause or contribute to sleep apnea. This can occur during REM sleep when partial muscle paralysis occurs.

Strategies for Prevention and Management of Sleep Problems

Sleep Hygiene Promotion and Medications

Medications are not generally recommended as a first-line therapy for children with sleep problems. Behavioral therapy and establishing good sleep hygiene are the mainstays for any child with difficulties sleeping and need to be incorporated even if medication is used (Owens and Moore, 2017).

Early establishment of a dark, quiet, and slightly cool room for sleeping and a consistent sleep routine is helpful. Parents can use a variety of cues to set the sleep cycle, including daylight, darkness, meals, and activities. Making these cues clear to infants and children to help them establish healthy bedtime and sleep patterns is important. Exposure to light, even for brief periods of time, can prevent the secretion of melatonin, which is needed for sleep.

Melatonin has been shown to be beneficial for sleep disorders of different etiologies. Although melatonin is the most commonly prescribed medication for insomnia, wide variation exists in the dosing used and there are no clear guidelines for dosing in pediatrics. Antihistamines, such as diphenhydramine and hydroxyzine, are the most widely prescribed sedatives in the pediatric practice, but limited evidence exists to support their use (Bruni et al., 2017). Benadryl can be effective short term but should not be used in children who are prone to parasomnias. A review of pharmacologic treatment of insomnia in children found that zolpidem (Ambien) produced high levels of side effects and was not effective in increasing total sleep time or decreasing sleep latency (Barrett et al., 2013). Limited evidence exists to support the use of α-agonists such as clonidine to improve sleep onset latency, especially in children with ADHD (Bruni et al., 2017). Trazodone and mirtazapine, which are tricyclic antidepressants, are used for adults with insomnia and hold promise with children but require further studies (Bruni et al., 2017).

Recent studies have found that guanfacine (Intuniv), which is an α2-adrenergic agonist, can be helpful in treating hyperactivity, tics, or delayed sleep onset (Tsai et al., 2016). Atomoxetine (Strattera), once daily guanfacine extended release, and melatonin are all potential choices for children with ADHD who have severe sleep problems (Tsai et al., 2016).

A recent study revealed that classic conditioning helped to preserve the treatment effects of melatonin in children with sleep onset problems. Classic conditioning consisted of having children drink organic lemonade while taking melatonin and turning on a dim red-light lamp when children went to bed. Melatonin effectively advances dim-light melatonin onset and reduces sleep onset difficulties with a positive effect on health and behavior. The study found that children without comorbid conditions such as ASD and ADHD had some improvement with the red light classic conditioning even when melatonin was discontinued (Maanen et al., 2017).

Primary Care Interventions for Dyssomnias

When parents need further intervention strategies for sleep, several behavioral therapy techniques have been shown to be helpful. See Table 20.2.

Common Sleep Problems

Parasomnias

Parasomnias describe a group of sleep disorders that occur during NREM and REM sleep. NREM parasomnias include confusional arousals, somnambulism (sleep walking), night terrors, rhythmic movement disorders, benign neonatal sleep myoclonus, bruxism, and nocturnal enuresis. REM parasomnias include nightmares.

Precipitating factors for all NREM parasomnias include SDB, PLM, sleep deprivation, stress, fever, being overheated at night, a full bladder, and use of central nervous system depressant medications. These factors can interrupt sleep, and when this interruption occurs during deep sleep, it can cause a partial awakening resulting in a parasomnia (scary dream). Benadryl, which is a common sleep medication used in children, is known to precipitate parasomnias because it increases N3 sleep. Identification and treatment of primary sleep disorders such as PLMs and OSA often result in the resolution of parasomnia symptoms (Ifran et al., 2017).

TABLE 20.2	Primary Care Interventions for Dyssomnias
Unmodified extinction	Also known as *sleep training* or *systematic ignoring*, allows the child to cry it out. Parents implement a scheduled, presleep bedtime routine, placing children in bed and ignoring all subsequent sleep interfering behaviors until the morning. This method does not appeal to all families and relies on strict structure. Most families see results in approximately three nights.
Graduated extinction	Graduated extinction incorporates the same philosophy of establishing a bedtime routine but allows the parents to implement brief, planned checks on their child, assuring safety but with minimized parental attention (verbal and physical). The visits are systematically reduced until the child initiates and maintains sleep independently. This approach may take a few days to a few months.
Modified graduated extinction	An alternative form of graduated extinction allows the parent to sit with the drowsy child and then leave before the child falls asleep, promising to return. The parent may start by leaving for only several seconds but always returns, gradually extending the absences. The goal is for the child to fall asleep independently when the parent is out of the room. This approach can also take time but is beneficial for some families.
The bedtime pass	The bedtime pass targets bedtime resistance in children who are preschool to school age. The pass can be anything appreciated by the child; it is often helpful to have the child help make a ticket (laminating a favorite picture). The pass may be exchanged for one visit in the child's room after bedtime or one pass to come out from the room again that night. If the child uses the pass but then stays in his room until morning, the child receives a reward, such as a favorite breakfast. If the child does not use the pass at all, they get a "free reward" (e.g., 10 minutes of screen time or a sticker). Providing an immediate reward instead of later in the day is more effective.

Nonrapid Eye Movement Parasomnias

NREM parasomnias occur during N3 sleep and typically occur in the first third of the sleep cycle because that is when the majority of NREM sleep occurs. Furthermore, most NREM parasomnias occur at the end of the first sleep cycles, or approximately 90 minutes into sleep. Most children have memory of the events. Most episodes are brief, but they may last 30 to 40 minutes. Waking up the child during any parasomnia is not recommended because it can prolong the episodes. NREM parasomnias are often inherited. The movements exhibited during NREM parasomnias can be complex. Confusional arousals, night terrors, and sleep walking can all be normal for children; however, if they occur frequently, become prolonged, or pose a threat to safety (sleep walking), further evaluation is warranted.

Confusional Arousals

Confusional arousals occur when a child is awakened from a deep sleep during the first part of the night and is also known as excessive sleep inertia or sleep drunkenness (Ifran et al., 2017). Children will sit up in bed, appear dazed, and often react slowly to questions. Confusional arousals occur around 2 years of age and are typically benign but frightening for the parents. They generally diminish around 5 years of age.

Sleep Walking

Sleep walking or stalking typically begins as confusional arousals but can also begin with the child getting out of bed and running with complex movements. The child typically appears dazed with open eyes, and the speech is mumbled and slurred. Sleep walking is common, occurring in approximately 1% to 15% of children, and is usually benign. The parasomnias are common around 4 years of age and resolve around 8 years of age (Ekambaram and Maski, 2017). Of the parasomnias, sleep walking has the potential to be the most dangerous to the child (AASM, 2014).

Night Terrors

Night terrors are characterized by an extreme state of agitation when the child awakens from N3 sleep screaming. Dilated pupils, increased heart rate, and sweating are common. Like other arousals, they are typically short but can be prolonged with parental interference. Night terrors are reported in 1% to 6% of children, typically occurring after 18 months of age and resolved by 6 years of age (Ekambaram and Maski, 2017).

Rapid Eye Movement Parasomnias

Nightmares are frequently confused with night terrors, but they are distinctly different. Nightmares occur during REM sleep and are characterized by a sudden arousal from sleep to a fully awake state, whereas night terrors occur during N3 sleep and the child is, in reality, asleep during the event without recollection. Nightmares are typically recalled in detail even the next day. The average onset of nightmares is 36 to 72 months of age, affecting approximately 25% of all children 3 to 6 years of age (Ekambaram and Maski, 2017). Nightmares typically occur during the last portion of the night, whereas night terrors occur mostly in the first part of the night. Occasional nightmares are common in childhood, and reassurance is generally effective. However, recurrent nightmares can be associated with daytime stressors, and psychological evaluation may be needed.

Assessment of Parasomnias

History

The health history for parasomnias should include the following topics:
- Characteristics of the event, including timing in relation to sleep onset, frequency, and length
- Symptoms of SDB or PLMs
- Temperature of sleeping environment and sweating history of child despite the temperature
- Family history
- Medications
- Sleep patterns (how much sleep is obtained)
- Memory of the event

Treatment of Parasomnias

Parasomnias can be normal in all children, but if they are frequent, prolonged, or causing potential harm (such as a sleep walking episode where the child leaves the house), further evaluation is warranted. If SDB is present, evaluation with a sleep study and/or referral to a sleep provider, pediatric pulmonologist, or pediatric otolaryngologist is recommended. Normalizing sleep patterns and calmly guiding the child back to bed (if sleep walking) without attempting to awaken the child seem to be the most effective actions for parasomnias (Ekambaram and Maski, 2017). Placing a bell on the child's bedroom door to alert parents that the child is leaving the room and making sure the house is secure are needed for somnambulism.

Circadian Rhythm Disorders

Delayed Sleep Phase

The sleep cycle begins at a late hour and is followed by a late awakening. The child's internal clock for sleep and rest is not consistent with appropriate hours for sleep. Excessive naps or late morning waking may be related factors, especially for school-age children and adolescents. The differential diagnoses for delayed sleep phase are prolonged bedtime routine and oppositional disorder, which both involve active resistance to going to bed rather than the inability to fall asleep. Management approaches for delayed sleep phase may include:

1. Keep the nighttime routine in place, but awaken the child earlier each morning in 15-minute increments.
2. For the adolescent or older child who is off schedule by many hours (e.g., at the end of the summer when beginning the school year will require getting up earlier), it could take weeks to back up the cycle appropriately using 15-minute increments. In this case, it is better to go forward in time. In other words, have the child remain awake until the next evening and then go to bed at the desired hour, beginning the desired routine from that point.
3. Have the child or family keep a sleep log to document gradual change.

Advanced Sleep Phase

The sleep cycle begins too early with correlated early rising. Meals, naps, and bedtime should be delayed until the desired times. The early waking resolves itself.

Inappropriate or Unpredictable Schedules

Some people have a poorly organized sleep-wake cycle. This is described by some as a temperament problem of rhythmicity. The routines of eating, activities, and sleeping should be kept as regular as possible. The older child may need to learn to play quietly in bed until others awaken or until an alarm begins to play. At night, the child may need to learn to read or listen to music in bed when bedtime comes.

Chronic Health Conditions and Dyssomnias

Nocturnal Enuresis

Nocturnal enuresis is a common complaint in children. Primary enuresis occurs in children who have never attained dryness at night, whereas secondary enuresis occurs in children who have previously been potty trained. A strong family predisposition exists for primary enuresis. SDB has been associated with enuresis due to altered arousal response and sleep fragmentation. The pathophysiology of enuresis is seemingly linked to nocturnal obstructive events, causing increased intra-abdominal pressure and altered systemic blood pressure that induces natriuresis and polyuria by altering levels of antidiuretic hormone, and atrial and brain natriuretic peptides (Zaffanello et al., 2017). Resolution of secondary enuresis after medical or surgical treatment for obstructive sleep disordered breathing is common. Consequently, snoring, parasomnias, and restless sleep should be sought for all children with enuresis (Zaffanello et al., 2017). If enuresis persists after treatment of SDB, parasomnias, and restless sleep, a referral to a pediatric urologist is needed (see Chapter 41 for genitourinary disorders).

Restless Legs Syndrome and Periodic Limb Movements

RLS has long been identified as a parasomnia in adults. RLS is a sensory and motor disorder characterized by irritating sensations in the legs accompanied by an irresistible urge to move the legs, which typically helps. PLMs are repetitive jerks, typically in the legs, that are found by PSG to occur every 5 to 90 seconds. RLS and PLMs usually occur together, but PLMs may occur without RLS.

The prevalence of PLMs in school-age children has been estimated to be 1.9% to 3.6%; however, the presence is often unrecognized in younger children or those with delays secondary to communications deficits. The exact etiology still remains unclear, but genetic factors, dopaminergic dysfunction, and low iron storage status have been shown to play important roles (Munzer and Felt, 2017). Altered brain acquisition of iron has been identified as a major factor in RLS although blood iron levels may be normal (Munzer and Felt, 2017). Peripheral neuropathy and uremia are also causes of secondary RLS. Medications such as antidepressants, selective serotonin reuptake inhibitors (SSRIs), sedating antihistamines, and dopamine receptor antagonists may worsen or precipitate RLS. PLMs and nighttime arousals are increased with sertraline (Zoloft) treatment, so providers should pay attention to PLMs during SSRI treatment (Zang et al., 2013).

Clinical Findings and Treatment

Children will often complain of leg pain or itchy/crawly sensations. Affected children may complain to their parents that spiders or bugs are in their bed, and parents will find some improvement with massage. Sleep onset may be normal followed by arousal with the symptoms shortly thereafter. A recent study found the most striking single symptom of RLS or PLMs was awakening after 1 to 3 hours of sleep followed by screaming, crying, kicking, and slapping the legs or by verbally expressing that the legs hurt (Munzer and Felt, 2017). RLS and PLMs are associated with fragmented sleep, unrefreshed sleep, insomnia, daytime sleepiness, and hyperactivity. In general, the child has a normal physical and neurologic examination. Diagnosis of PLM/RLS is often based on the history and physical examination. If there are suspicions for SDB, a PSG is warranted; and if five or more PLMs per hour are experienced, PLMs are diagnosed. Growing pains, leg cramps, and Osgood-Schlatter disease are common differential diagnoses for RLS and PLM. Ferritin level is a measure of serum iron levels and can be a helpful laboratory test for PLMs. Ferritin levels less than 50 have been associated with RLS and PLMs in children and supplementation with ferrous sulfate (3 mg/kg/day) has been shown to drastically improve symptoms (Munzer and Felt, 2017). Clonazepam and gabapentin are sometimes used in treatment if ferritin levels are normal and other organic causes have been ruled out, but this should be initiated by a sleep specialist.

Head Banging and Bruxism

Rhythmic movement disorders involve head banging and body rocking and occur as the child is attempting to fall asleep and may repeat throughout the night when the child is trying to return to sleep. Head banging and body rocking are most commonly seen before 2 years of age. The disorder is typically transient and self-limited and rarely requires intervention (Gwyther et al., 2017).

Sleep bruxism, astereotypic grinding, or clenching of the teeth during sleep, seen in 8.2% of the population, frequently appears between 10 or 20 years of age, although there is a short-lived infant version. Bruxism may be associated with stress. A dental referral may be useful. Sleep bruxism is rarely associated with temporal lobe seizure activity in children.

Epilepsy and Sleep

In many cases a good clinical history can distinguish seizures from parasomnias. However, seizures arising from the frontal lobes often occur during sleep and, in many patients, are entirely restricted to sleep. Nocturnal frontal lobe epilepsy (NFLE) occurs as an inherited form (autosomal dominant NFLE) or sporadically, and the events can be more complex than typical seizures with vocalizations, complex automatisms, and ambulation. Routine EEG and magnetic resonance imaging (MRI) often show no abnormality, and the events can often mimic parasomnias. However, the patient often wakes up fully after the event, has recollection of the event, and typically has academic decline, which is not consistent with parasomnias where the patient has amnesia and sleeps through the event. The Frontal Lobe Epilepsy and Parasomnias (FLEP) scale, developed and validated by an expert panel, has been shown to delineate NFLE from parasomnias (Faludi et al., 2015). The FLEP scale contains specific questions about the age of onset, duration, timing, characteristics such as stereotypical movements and vocalizations, and recall.

Sleep Disordered Breathing

Children with SDB can manifest a continuum from simple snoring and upper airway resistance to OSA. OSA is characterized by upper airway obstruction, abnormal respiratory patterns, and fragmented sleep. The prevalence of OSA in children ages 2 to 6 is approximately 2% to 5%, but primary snoring estimates are as high as 17% (Roberts et al., 2016). Untreated OSA can result in various physical, mental, and cognitive problems. OSA has been shown to be a contributing factor to the pathogenesis of obesity by inducing leptin resistance and increasing ghrelin levels, which can potentiate cravings of high-calorie comfort foods. OSA generally causes insufficient sleep, compounding this metabolic insult (Falbe, et al., 2015).

A study (Hunter et al., 2016) performed on a large community-based sample of snoring and nonsnoring children aged 5 to 7 found that moderate to severe sleep apnea has a destructive impact on neurocognitive functioning. Even snoring alone had effects on neurocognitive functioning, leading to learning difficulties.

Clinical Findings

Signs of SDB can include snoring, gasping, apneas, increased work of breathing with paradoxic respirations, neck hyperextension, night sweating, tachycardia, restless sleep, and disrupted sleep. Persistent parasomnias can also be a sign of SDB secondary to arousals during SWS. Following arousals caused by SDB, the child will typically drift back to sleep, with the cycle repeating itself throughout the night, resulting in sleep fragmentation and nonrestorative sleep. Some children experience insomnia because of SDB either at sleep onset or awakenings after sleep onset. Symptoms may include behavioral problems, hypertension including pulmonary hypertension, failure to thrive, ADHD, and or daytime sleepiness. Risk factors include tonsillar or adenoid hypertrophy, obesity, craniofacial abnormalities, gastroesophageal reflux, neuromuscular disorders, and untreated allergic rhinitis. Children with neuromuscular disorders might not snore and should be evaluated with other criteria, specifically increased work of breathing, tachycardia, nocturnal sweating, and daytime symptoms.

Surgical and Medical Treatment of Sleep Disordered Breathing

Adenotonsillectomy (TA) is considered a first-line treatment for OSA (Roberts et al., 2016). The AASM and the AAP recommend a PSG to confirm and characterize obstructive sleep apnea syndrome (OSAS) before adenotonsillectomy (Rosen et al., 2015). However, the American Academy of Otolaryngology–Head and Neck Surgery recommends a PSG for children with certain complex medical conditions or when there is lack of agreement between tonsil size and reported severity of OSAS symptoms. The PSG allows the surgery team to understand the severity of the OSA so that perioperative and postoperative complications can be anticipated. This can also help surgeons to anticipate who needs a postoperative sleep study. Overnight pulse oximetry studies in the home are convenient, quicker to obtain, and less expensive than PSGs. However, home pulse oximetry studies can be inaccurate and yield erroneous data secondary to detachment from the patient, especially in young children and those with neurocognitive disorders.

TA is a relatively safe procedure because most children do not experience postoperative problems, especially after 3 years of age. The most common risk factors are pain and poor oral intake, with more severe complications including hemorrhage, dehydration, infection, and respiratory complications (Rosen et al., 2015).

Other surgical options include partial tonsillectomy, craniofacial surgery such as mandibular distraction for micrognathia, and tracheostomy for severe cases. The AASM recommends follow-up sleep studies on children at risk for residual SDB such as obesity, craniofacial abnormalities, and severe baseline SDB (Rosen et al., 2015). For some children, surgery is not an option, due to a lack of tonsillar or adenoid hypertrophy, young age, morbid obesity, family or surgeon preference, or other risk factors.

Nonsurgical options include positive airway pressure (PAP), nasal steroids, and leukotriene receptor antagonists (Montelukast), normal saline rinses, rapid maxillary expansion (RME), oral appliances, and weight loss (Rosen et al., 2015). Nasal steroids and Montelukast can be effective in mild to moderate OSA by reducing the lymphoid tissue, especially the adenoid. PAP therapy includes continuous positive airway pressure (CPAP), bilevel position airway pressure (BIPAP) bilevel support, and average volume assured pressure system (AVAPS) volume support. PAP therapy stents open the larynx to allow ventilation and is typically used without oxygen. CPAP is typically used to treat SDB, except in children with neuromuscular disorders or in those needing extra support with tidal volume or a back-up respiratory rate. PAP therapy delivers humidified air pressure via a nasal mask and ranges from 4 to 24 cm H_2O.

A PSG with a PAP titration is generally needed to determine the amount of pressure needed to normalize breathing and gas exchange. Auto CPAP machines can provide a range of pressure that can fluctuate to fit the patient's need and is frequently used in older pediatric patients. PAP therapy is typically managed by a sleep specialist instead of the PCP. Although PAP therapy is highly effective, it can be difficult to tolerate and parental involvement is necessary. Follow-up sleep studies are needed depending on the age and growth of the child.

Although adenotonsillectomy is considered the primary treatment for sleep apnea in children, RME has been shown to help prevent and treat SDB. RME is an orthodontic procedure used to expand a constricted maxillary or mandibular arch, correcting posterior crossbites and malocclusions. RME involves placing a temporary brace on the upper or lower maxilla that can be manipulated manually to widen the area for a specified time period (typically 8 months). Studies show that RME can also improve SDB by increasing the width of the nasal cavity, improving mouth breathing, and reducing airway resistance. The early detection of children with a high-arched palate and referral to a dentist for possible RME can also help to prevent SDB.

The Childhood Adenotonsillectomy (CHAT) study was designed to assist pediatricians, otolaryngologists, and families who are considering adenotonsillectomy to understand what adverse impact OSAS is having for the child and what the probability is that this adverse impact will be improved with surgery (Rosen et al., 2015). The study investigates whether baseline OSAS symptoms could predict postoperative changes in parent-perceived behavior, sleepiness, and quality of life regardless of PSG results. A parent sleep questionnaire (PSQ) containing 22 items that ask about snoring frequency, observed apneas, difficulty breathing during sleep, daytime sleepiness, inattentive or hyperactive behavior, and other pediatric OSAS features was used for the study. The PSQ takes approximately 5 minutes to complete and 1 minute to score. Higher scores indicated more OSAS-related symptoms.

The CHAT study found that results from the PSQ were clearly associated with baseline behavioral impairment, sleepiness, and reduced quality of life and predictive of their improvement after adenotonsillectomy (Rosen et al., 2015). The findings are important to clinicians because the PSQ may assist in their efforts to better identify candidates for adenotonsillectomy who are most likely to experience improvement in the key areas identified by the CHAT study to be responsive to the surgery (Rosen et al., 2015).

Central Sleep Apnea

Central sleep apnea (CSA) refers to absences of airflow that are related to failure of the ventilator control system to stimulate a breath (AASM, 2014). Unlike OSA, CSA is not associated with a snore or gasp and is common in children intermittently, especially following a sigh. When CSA occurs frequently or results in oxygen desaturations, it is considered pathologic. CSA is more common in premature infants or those with neurologic conditions, such as cerebral palsy, brainstem lesions, or Chiari malformations. CSA can also be induced by narcotic use.

A life-threatening condition called congenital central hypoventilation syndrome can present in newborns and should prompt immediate investigation and treatment. Premature infants typically outgrow CSA, and oxygen is often used to stimulate the ventilator control system. If hypoventilation is involved with CSA, bilevel ventilator support (BIPAP) with a backup rate is often used to restore normal gas exchange during sleep.

Narcolepsy

Narcolepsy is a disorder characterized by excessive daytime sleepiness, fragmented nocturnal sleep, and signs of REM intrusion, the most specific of which is cataplexy. Narcolepsy is an imbalance among wakefulness, REM, and SWS states that can range from mild to severe. Cataplexy is a brief sudden loss of skeletal muscle tone, which is typically brought on by laughter but can also be stimulated by other strong emotions. Neck, facial, and knee weakness are common cataplexy symptoms. Respiratory muscles are not affected. Individuals retain consciousness during cataplexy events, which can help to differentiate it from seizures. Not all people with narcolepsy have cataplexy. Excessive sleepiness, which is typically the first symptom to manifest, may present years before the cataplexy (AASM, 2014).

Other manifestations of narcolepsy include sleep-onset paralysis and hypnogogic hallucinations. Hypnogogic hallucinations are vivid dreamlike visual, tactile, or auditory hallucinations that occur as the patient is falling asleep. Children may complain of feeling someone whispering in their ear or breathing on their neck. Rarely can the patient decipher the whispering. Sleep paralysis is the total inability to move any muscles (except respiratory muscles) when falling asleep or waking up. Normal individuals may experience sleep paralysis due to sleep deprivation or even SDB and those conditions need to be ruled out before considering narcolepsy.

Narcolepsy with cataplexy is caused by a deficiency of hypothalamic hypocretin which is also named orexin and this can be measured in the cerebral spinal fluid. The HLA-DQB1*06:02 allele gene has been identified in most patients with narcolepsy. Narcolepsy with cataplexy occurs in 0.02% to 0.18% of the United States and western European populations. There is a low prevalence of familial cases. Narcolepsy typically occurs between 10 and 25 years of age; however, it is seen in children as young as 5 years of age. Diagnosing narcolepsy is complex, and a referral to a sleep specialist is warranted. Medication management is the core therapy for narcolepsy with cataplexy.

References

American Academy of Pediatrics (AAP). Adolescent Sleep Working Group: school start times for adolescents. *Pediatrics*. 2014;134(3):642–649.

American Academy of Pediatrics (AAP). *Separation Anxiety and Sleeping, Healthychildren.org (website)*. 2015. www.healthychildren.org/English/ages-stages/baby/Sleep/Pages/Separation-Anxiety-and-Sleeping.aspx.

American Academy of Pediatrics (AAP). Council on Communications Media: media use in school-aged children and adolescents. *Pediatrics*. 2017;138(5):3–6.

American Academy of Sleep Medicine. In: *International Classification of Sleep Disorders*. 3rd ed. Chicago: Am Acad Sleep Medicine; 2014. ICSD-3.

Amra B, Shahsavari A, Shayan-Moghadam R, et al. The association of sleep and late-night cell phone use among adolescents. *J Pediatr*. 2017;93(6):560–567. https://doi.org/10.1016/j.jped.2016.12.004.

Barrett JR, Tracy DK, Giaroli G. To sleep or not to sleep: a systematic review of the literature of pharmacology treatments of insomnia in children and adolescents with attention deficit/ hyperactivity disorder. *J Child Adoles Psychopharm*. 2013;23(10):640–647.

Bruni O, Angriman M, Calisti F, et al. Practitioner review: treatment of chronic insomnia in children and adolescents with neurodevelopmental disabilities. *J Child Psychol Psychiatry*. 2017;59(5):489–508. https://doi.org/10.1111/jcpp.12812.

Buxton OM, Chang AM, Spilsbury JC, et al. Sleep in the modern family: protective family routines for child and adolescent sleep. *Sleep Health*. 2015;1(1):15–27.

Combs D, Goodwin JL, Quan SF, et al. Insomnia, health-related quality of life and health outcomes in children: a seven-year longitudinal cohort. *Sci Rep*. 2016;68(5-6):165–177.

Cuomo BM, Vaz S, Lim Ai, Lee E, et al. Effectiveness of sleep-based interventions for children with autism spectrum disorder: a meta-synthesis. *Pharmacother J Hum Pharmacol Drug Ther*. 2017;37(5):555–578.

Ekambaram V, Maski K. Non-rapid eye movement arousal parasomnias in children. *Pediatric Ann*. 2017;46(9):e327–e331.

Falbe J, Davison KK, Franckle RL, et al. Sleep duration, restfulness, and screens in the sleep environment. *Pediatrics*. 2015;135(2):e367–e375.

Faludi B, Bone B, Komoly S, et al. Sleep disordered breathing and epilepsy: relationships and therapeutic considerations. *Ideoggyogy Sz*. 2015;68(11-12):374–382.

Gwyther ARM, Walters AS, Hill CM. Rhythmic movement disorder in childhood: an integrative review. *Sleep Med Rev*. 2017;10(35):62–75.

Harbard E, Allen NB, Trinder J, et al. What's keeping teenagers up? Prebedtime behaviors and actigraphy-assessed sleep over school and vacation. *J Adolescent Health*. 2016;58(4):426–432.

Hunter SJ, Gozal D, Smith DL, et al. Effect of sleep-disordered breathing severity on cognitive performance measures in a large community cohort of young school-aged children. *Sleep Neurol*. 2016;23(4):1035–1050.

Hysing M, Pallesen S, Stormark KM, et al. Sleep and use of electronic devices in adolescence: results from a large population-based study. *BMJ Open*. 2015;5(1):1–11.

Irfan M, Schenck CH, Howell MJ. Non-rapid eye movement sleep and overlap parasomnias. *Sleep Neurol*. 2017;23(4):1035–1050.

Kuhn BR. Practical strategies for managing behavioral sleep problems in young children. *Sleep Med Clin*. 2014;9:181–197.

Lee J, Na G, Joo EY, et al. Clinical and polysomnogram characteristics of excessive daytime sleepiness in children. *Sleep Breath*. 2017;21(4):967–974. https://doi.org/10.1007/s11325-017-1545-y.

Maanaen A, Meijer AM, Smits MG, Oort FJ. Classic conditioning for preserving the effects of short term melatonin treatment in children with delayed sleep: a pilot study. *Nat Sci Sleep*. 2017;3(9):67–79.

Matthews KA, Hall M, Dahl RE. Sleep in healthy black and white adolescents. *Pediatrics*. 2014;133(5):e1189–e1196.

Mindell JA, Bartle A, Ahn Y, et al. *Sleep in Young Children: A Cross-Cultural Perspective. Poster presented at 27th Congress of the International Pediatric Association*. Australia: Melbourne; 2013.

Moon RY. Task force on sudden infant death syndrome. SIDS and other sleep-related infant deaths: evidence base for 2016 updated recommendations for a safe infant sleeping environment. From the American Academy of Pediatrics Technical Report. *Pediatrics*. 2016;138(5):e1–e34.

Mullin BC, Pyle L, Haraden D, et al. A preliminary multimethod comparison of sleep among adolescents with and without generalized anxiety disorder. *J Clin Child Adolescent Psychol*. 2017;46(2):198–210.

Munzer T, Felt B. The role of iron in pediatric restless legs syndrome and pediatric limb movements in sleep. *Semin Neurol*. 2017;37(4):439–445.

National Sleep Foundation. *Sleep and The Circadian System (Website) Sleepfoundation.Org*. 2017. https://sleepfoundation.org/sleep-news/sleep-and-the-circadian-system.

Owens JA, Moore M. Insomnia in infants and young children. *Pediatric Ann*. 2017;46(9): E321–E320.

Paruthi S, Brooks LJ, D'Ambrosio C, et al. Recommended amount of sleep for pediatric populations: a consensus statement of the American Academy of Sleep Medicine. *J Clin Sleep Med*. 2016a;12(6):785–786.

Roberts SD, Kapadia H, Greenlee G, et al. Midfacail and dental changes associated with nasal positive airway pressure in children with obstructive sleep apnea and craniofacial conditions. *J Clin Sleep Med*. 2016;12(4):469–475.

Rosen CL, Wang R, Taylor HG, et al. Utility of symptoms to predict treatment outcomes in obstructive sleep apnea syndrome. *Pediatrics*. 2015;135(3):e662–e671.

Souders MC, Zavodny S, Eriksne W, et al. Sleep in children with autism spectrum disorder. *Curr Psychiatry Rep*. 2017;19(34):1–32.

Tsai M, Hsu J, Huan Y. Sleep problems in children with attention deficit/hyperactivity disorder: current status of knowledge and appropriate management. *Curr Psychiatry Rep*. 2016;18(76):1–9.

Yland J, Guan S, Emanuele E, et al. Interactive vs passive screen time and nighttime sleep duration among school-aged children. *Sleep Health*. 2015;1(13):191–196.

Zachritz W, Fulmer M, Chaney N. An evidence-based infant safe sleep program to reduce sudden unexplained infant deaths. *AJN*. 2016;116(11):48–55.

Zaffanello M, Piacentini G, Lippi G, et al. Obstructive sleep-disordered breathing, enuresis and combined disorders in children: chance or related association? *Swiss Med Wkly*. 2017;6(147):1–12.

Zang B, Hao Y, Jia F, et al. Sertraline and periodic limb movements during sleep: an 8-week open-label study in depressed patients with insomnia. *Sleep Med*. 2013;14(12):1405–1412.

21

Sexuality, Sex, and Gender Identity

MARY DIRKS AND TERAL GERLT

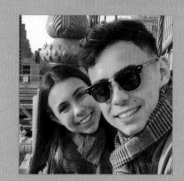

Sexuality and sex are not interchangeable concepts. Sexuality may be influenced by biological, ethical, spiritual, cultural, and moral issues, and includes an individual's beliefs, attitudes, values, and behaviors. Sex is what each individual is assigned at birth based on appearance of external genitalia, chromosomes, reproductive organs, and their functions. By assigning an individual a designation of male or female at birth, society has created a binary system that has traditionally ignored differences like intersex, also referred to as sexual differences. Achieving a sense of one's sexuality in its broadest sense begins with conception and continues throughout life. Despite what parents may want to think, their children will become sexual people. Knowledge of anatomy, physiology, and biochemistry of the sexual response system is important at various developmental stages and contributes to gender identity, sexual orientation, roles, relationships, and intimacy. The primary care provider (PCP) can play a crucial part in educating parents to anticipate, recognize, and guide their children through the stages of sexual development and gender identity. The primary care visit gives parents a chance to ask questions and solicit advice from the child's provider. Also, at age-appropriate times, the primary care visit provides children and adolescents with opportunities to explore questions they have about their sexuality. Current societal norms can create a challenging environment for children and adolescents who experience a same-sex attraction or who have questions about their developing bodies and feelings. This chapter focuses on sexual health promotion and gender identity, emphasizing that sexual development is a normal and healthy part of human growth.

Standards

Performing Preventive Services: A Bright Futures Handbook, developed by the American Academy of Pediatrics (Tanski et al., 2010); the U.S. Preventive Services Task Force (USPSTF) *Guide to Clinical Preventive Services 2014* (USPSTF, 2014); the still-used *Guidelines for Adolescent Preventive Services (GAPS),* developed by the American Medical Association (AMA, 1997); and the Sexuality Information and Education Council of the United States

(SIECUS) *PrEP Education for Youth-Serving Primary Care Providers Toolkit* (2016) offer the most comprehensive evidence- and consensus-based strategies concerning clinical preventive counseling and screening for adolescents. Together, these guidelines can inform providers of strategies that assist parents, children, and adolescents to promote healthy sexual development and prevent negative consequences of sexual behaviors. In addition, the National Coalition for Sexual Health's (NCSH's) *Sexual Health and Your Patients: A Provider's Guide* (Altarum Institute, 2016) and the Centers for Disease Control and Prevention's (CDC's) *Sexually Transmitted Diseases Treatment Guidelines, 2015,* recommend preventive and behavioral counseling for all sexually active teens at risk for sexually transmitted infections (STIs) and human immunodeficiency virus (HIV). Those individuals who initiate sex early, reside in detention facilities, attend STI clinics, or use injection drugs are particularly at risk, as are young men who have sex with men (Workowski et al., 2015). These strategies include the following:

- Ensuring a confidential environment in which the adolescent and health provider can freely exchange information
- Assessing and providing guidance toward the healthy accomplishment of physical, sexual, social, moral, cognitive, and emotional developmental tasks
- Supporting parental behaviors that promote healthy adolescent adjustment
- Providing health guidance that promotes wellness and healthy lifestyles, such as responsible sexual behaviors (e.g., abstinence, limiting the number of sex partners, and safer sex practices)
- Educating about the use of latex condoms to prevent STIs, including infection with HIV
- Educating about appropriate methods of birth control with instructions on how to use them effectively
- Interviewing annually about involvement in sexual and other "high risk" lifestyle behaviors (e.g., alcohol and drug use)
- Asking questions that explore the adolescent's sexual orientation, gender identity, number of sex partners in the previous 6 months, unintended pregnancy, and STI history
- Exploring whether or not the individual has exchanged sex for money or drugs
- Assessing sexual maturity stages for typical progression
- Screening sexually active adolescents for STIs (e.g., chlamydia and gonorrhea), and providing pregnancy and partner notification and referral for treatment

The contributions of Dr. Larry Newman were invaluable in completing this chapter, particularly the sections related to gender identity and sexuality of LGBTQ youth.

- Providing pregnancy testing and assisting with parent and partner notification
- Providing confidential HIV and syphilis screening of adolescents at risk for infection
- Initiating routine cervical cytology screening at 21 years old (American Congress of Obstetricians and Gynecologists [ACOG], 2017; American Cancer Society [Smith et al., 2018]; USPSTF, 2014) and annual interviews about any history of emotional, physical, and/or sexual abuse by caregivers, friends, or intimate partners
- Initiating the series of hepatitis B vaccinations for those 11 years and older if the series is not already completed
- Recommending routine human papillomavirus (HPV) vaccination for females and males age 11 or 12 years old, for females between 13 and 26 years and males between 13 and 21 years if not yet vaccinated, and through 26 years old for gay, bisexual, and other males who have sex with males, transgender, and immunocompromised persons (including those with HIV infection) not adequately vaccinated (CDC, 2016a). See Chapter 23 for a description of the three types of HPV vaccines and their indications for use.

Patterns of Sexuality

Historical and Cultural Context of Sexuality

The term *psychosexual development* is often used to describe the continuum of sexual development from infancy to adulthood. Historically, however, Freud first used this term as an integral concept in his theories of personality development—and eventually psychoanalysis. His concern was focused on the "sexual desires" that he believed were intrinsic formative drives, instincts, and appetites that led to one's behaviors and beliefs. The interplay between expressing these sexual desires and the perceived need to repress them led to his five psychosexual stages of typical sexual development: *oral*: 0 to 18 months old; *anal*: 18 to 36 months old; *phallic*: 3 to 6 years old; *latency*: 6 years old to puberty; and *genital*: puberty and beyond. The developmental characteristics and the ages at which he assigned the stages varied as Freud advanced his theory throughout his career.

Among others, Erikson furthered the discussion of sexual development by maintaining that children develop in predetermined stages. The stages were based on socialization and the effect this had on a child's personality, interactions with others, and self-esteem. Unsuccessfully fulfilling one stage prevented one from progressing to the next, until resolved. Successful completion of Erikson's stages related to the eventual healthy development of sexuality in terms of one's gender-role socialization, body image, social relationships, attitudes, values, and self-esteem.

In most Western cultures, gender has historically been considered absolute, based on sex assigned at birth, enduring for life, and defining the individual's personality and identity. Since the beginning of the 21st century, and with global Internet technology changing the way world views are disseminated, individuals have more opportunities to communicate their social realities regarding sexual values, norms, relationships, and behaviors. Some cultures are more accepting of those whose gender identity may not match the sex assigned at birth or whose sexual orientation does not fit within a heteronormative narrative. There are also cultures that have strict laws (cultural or religious) against the practice of anything other than heterosexuality. Providers must keep up with gender development concepts and standards of care of youth in this evolving environment (Ehrensaft, 2017).

Contemporary Definitions

Approaching sexuality as a paradigm of intersecting but distinctly separate factors between gender and sex helps providers appreciate the complexities of the child's developing sexuality. By understanding terminology and distinctions between seemingly similar constructs, PCPs can give more appropriate and effective patient care. The complexity of sexuality hinges on the key notion of gender. The following contemporary definitions explore this notion more fully:

- *Gender identity:* Gender identity is the internal perception of one's gender. Common identity labels include man, woman, gender queer, transgender, and more. Often confused with biological sex or sex assigned at birth, gender identity is self-determined. Numerous studies have begun to shed light on the complex interplay of cultural, environmental, and biologic factors that shape gender identity (Rosenthal, 2016). One's gender identity develops in stages according to age, stage, and cognitive development. Many theorists argue that gender identity is not fully established until a child has mastered the concept of gender permanency (5 to 7 years old). Others believe gender identity is achieved in the toddler and preschool years. Contemporary versions of gender development theory consider the transactional relationship among nature, nurture, and culture, known as the gender web, as neither fixed nor static at a certain age (Ehrensaft, 2017).
- *Gender expression:* The outward expression of maleness or femaleness, gender expression does not necessarily correlate with sex assigned at birth or gender identity. The expression of one's gender begins at preschool age and continues into adulthood. It is characterized by the emergence of behaviors, attitudes, and feelings that are labeled as male, female, or neutral. Previous research suggests that gender expression is dependent on testosterone and estradiol exposure. Testosterone levels, measured in amniotic fluid, appear to predict male-typical behavior in childhood.
- *Gender assignment or sex assigned at birth:* Gender assignment generally occurs at birth based on genital appearance and is the keystone in many societies for future gender socialization (i.e., gender identity). In most cases, genital appearance is determined from conception and is based on the 46XX and 46XY chromosome karyotypes and the appropriate masculinization effect of prenatal steroid exposure (testosterone and dihydrotestosterone). In approximately 1 in 4500 births, assigning gender may be difficult to do initially due to complex genital anomalies. In these cases, it is best to withhold a definitive assignment at birth. In the past, assigning gender to an intersex child was based on chromosomal analysis, and parents were often advised to have surgical "correction" performed—a procedure now seen as abusive. Studies have shown that gender of an intersex child is self-determined and that no medical or surgical intervention will change gender; it is best to allow children to self-identify gender as they develop (Fisher et al., 2016).
- *Sexual orientation* ("Whom do I love?"): This refers to an individual's feelings of sexual attraction and erotic potential. Rosenthal (2016) defines sexual orientation as to who an individual is attracted: a male, female, or someone else on the gender continuum. Sexual orientation is not dichotomous, and

individuals tend to fall along a continuum of sexual expression and desires rather than into exclusive categories. The phrase *sexual preference* implies choice and should not be used in reference to, or confused with, sexual orientation. Heterosexuality, homosexuality, and bisexuality are part of the normal spectrum of human sexuality and are equally valid and healthy developmental outcomes for youth (Bidwell, 2009). Possible genetic (neuroanatomic), hormonal (neurophysiologic), developmental, social, and cultural influences have been postulated as causing a particular sexual orientation, but none have been definitively identified. Adolescents may express different sexual behaviors, including short-term same-sex experiences. Teens may actually not be sexually active but label themselves as gay, lesbian, or bisexual because of whom they are physically or emotionally attracted to.

- *Sexual health* is defined as "a state of physical, emotional, mental, and social well-being in relation to sexuality. It requires a positive and respectful approach to sexuality and sexual relationships, as well as the possibility of having pleasurable and safe sexual experiences, free of coercion, discrimination, and violence" (World Health Organization [WHO], 2018). For sexual health to be attained and maintained, the sexual rights of all persons must be respected, protected, and fulfilled.
- *Sexual function* incorporates the biologic component of the human sexual response cycle and refers to the ability to give and receive sexual pleasure.
- *Sexual self-concept* is the psychological component of sexuality, the image one has of oneself, and the evaluation of one's adequacy in masculine and feminine roles.
- *Sexual relationships* refer to the social domain of sexuality and include the interpersonal relationships in which one's sexuality is shared with others.

Developmental Stages/Patterns of Sexuality

The PCP is in a unique position to incrementally educate parents about their child's sexual maturation starting in infancy, as well as to help parents distinguish between normal and problematic sexual behaviors. Anticipatory guidance not only enables parents to accurately understand their child's normal sexual development but also provides a structure for healthy parent-child sexual discussions in an ongoing open manner throughout the child's life. Table 21.1 discusses the components of development and behavior related to sexuality.

Infancy to 2 Years Old

Infants are reflexive beings, responding to their physical environment without hesitation or cognition. Sexual reflexes are present prenatally and are easily stimulated in the infant. It is not uncommon to observe a penile erection in prenatal ultrasounds or in the nursing child. Just as infants are fascinated by and explore their hands and feet, they explore their genitalia. Touching the genitalia—even masturbating—is pleasurable and soothing, is a natural part of exploring their environment, and begins as early as 3 to 5 months old. The provider should point out the spontaneity of this reflexive behavior so that a parent does not assign an adult sexuality interpretation to it.

Healthy parent-infant bonding requires physical contact and social interaction. Parents must hold, cuddle, stroke, talk to, look at, and respond to children if children are to develop a sense of trust on which intimacy and a positive self-image will be based in later years.

By the end of the first year, the child can differentiate between the sexes; some may even discriminate between sex-assigned toys. As society furthers its influence, children form their identities early and learn about their gender roles from the reinforcement of behaviors expected of males, females, or all individuals regardless of gender.

2 to 5 Years Old

Toddlers are able to recognize and pronounce themselves "I'm a girl" or "I'm a boy," but they can easily confuse gender in others and sometimes in themselves. Changing one's style of clothes, for example, can be perceived as a change in gender. Within the traditional model of gender development, children cannot integrate gender identity into their self-concept until they understand that gender is a permanent condition—an understanding that is thought to occur around 4 or 5 years old. Traditional theorists argue that gender identity is fully attained between 5 and 7 years old. Toddlers are extremely curious about their environment; they love to explore and experiment. Children in this age group have a cognitive awareness of the pleasure that self-pleasuring gives them and frequently masturbate, but, as with infants, they attribute no erotic or sexual meaning to their actions. They lack the concept of personal space and how their behavior may be misinterpreted as being sexual or improper. This is a good time for parents to discuss the notion of "private parts" and begin to teach the child that self-pleasuring is acceptable but should be done in private. Parental redirection is usually all that is required. The combination of curiosity and lack of self-consciousness characteristic of toddlers can contribute to embarrassing social incidents for their parents. They may be curious about what others look like under their clothes, touch other children's bodies, "play doctor," pretend to be Mommy and Daddy, and enjoy running around naked. By 4 years old, children may attach themselves more to the parent of the opposite sex.

Parents should be encouraged to use the appropriate names for body parts and bodily functions, even though they may also be using slang words. This enables children to better comprehend discussions with health providers, teachers, or health educators when the anatomical and physiologic terms are used.

Because preschool children at this age interpret statements literally and have "magical" thinking, their understandings of the physical self can be distorted, and lengthy explanations about body functions can be misunderstood. Parents should help children understand that their bodies come in different shapes, sizes, and colors; that all of these are equally important; that boys and girls also share many of the same parts, but different genital parts; and that sharing and respect are important aspects for developing friendships. It is appropriate for parents to introduce the notion of germs and hygiene, such as washing hands. This helps establish a framework for parents to advance the discussion to include STIs later in life. Situational factors can induce an increase in observed sexual behaviors in this age group, such as the birth of a new sibling, watching their mother breastfeed, and viewing another child's or adult's nudity.

5 to 9 Years Old

School-age children continue to have a high level of curiosity about sexuality, their bodies, and their environment. They are aware of the pleasure stimulation gives and continue to actively seek autoerotic arousal for enjoyment. Contact with other children may give them new ideas about sex, and exploration

	Typical Sexual Behaviors	Sexual Self-Concept	Sexual Role and Relationship
Infancy (birth through 1 year)	Orgasmic potential present Erectile function present May explore genital area during diaper changes	Gender identity reinforced	
Toddler	Genital pleasuring and exploration Sensual activity (e.g., hugging, stroking mother's breasts or other body parts)	Association of sexuality and good and bad Distinction between self and others	Sex role differences learned Discrimination between male and female role models Sexual vocabulary learned
Preschool	Sex play—exploration of own body and those of playmates; taking clothes off; showing genitals to other children or adults Self-pleasuring (masturbation) especially when tired	Gender identity understood as a permanent condition	Sex roles learned Parental attachment and identification
School age (5-11 years)	Masturbation (may occur more in public) Sex play between peers (playing "house" or "doctor"); exploration through looking at and touching genitals Asking questions and talking about sex Dressing up as the opposite sex as part of dramatic play	Curiosity about sex Sexual fears and fantasies Interest in aspects of sexual development Self-awareness as sexual being	Same-sex friends Off-color humor related to sexuality
Adolescence, pre-pubertal	Menarche (female) Seminal emissions (male)	Concerns about body image	Same-sex friends Sexual experiences as part of friendship
Adolescence, early	Awkwardness in first sexual encounter Masturbation, petting May or may not be sexually active May be aware of or question sexual orientation	Anxiety over inadequacy, lack of partner, virginity	Appropriate sex friendships Dating
Adolescence, late	May or may not be sexually active May be aware of or question sexual orientation	Responsibility for sexual activity	Intimacy in relationships learned
Young adult	Experimentation with sexual positions, expressions Exploration of techniques	Responsibility for sexual health (e.g., contraception, STI prevention) Development of adult sexual value system, tolerance for others	Giving and receiving pleasure learned Long-term commitment to relationship developed

STI, Sexually transmitted infection.

From Hillman JB, Spigarelli MG. Sexuality: its development and direction. In: Carey WB, Crocker AC, Coleman WL, et al., eds. *Developmental-Behavioral Pediatrics.* Philadelphia: Saunders; 2009.

games are typical (e.g., playing house or doctor) between same-age children, either of the same or opposite sex. This is normal behavior as long as a child is not emotionally distraught by the encounter or if it involves one child who is older than the other. Parents should avoid being overly alarmed if they witness this play. It is appropriate for parents to redirect the play to other activities. They should then discuss the situation later with their child to explore the experience, ascertain if the child was uncomfortable, and again emphasize the notion of privacy and respect for one's body. Box 21.1 discusses sexual actions beyond self-pleasuring and sexual play that can indicate possible sexual abuse.

By 5 to 7 years old, the use of sexual or "potty" language becomes evident—often to test parental reaction. Children at this age identify more with the same-sex parent; they tend to cluster into same-sex groups if given the opportunity. They are curious about where babies come from.

> ● **BOX 21.1   Signs That Sexual Play May Go Beyond Typical**
>
> - The behavior is not age-appropriate.
> - The behavior is prolonged.
> - The child looks anxious or guilty or becomes extremely aroused.
> - Child is being forced into sexual play through bribes, name-calling, and/or physical force.
> - Child knows more about sex/sexual acts than is appropriate for his or her age.

By the time children are about 8 years old, they begin to understand the significance of sexuality. They learn more about their body and body functions and "giggle" with children of their same sex when talking about sexuality, perhaps because they conceive that sex is a secretive topic. Unless parents actively communicate with their children, sexual lessons will be learned from peers, the media, jokes, and movies.

Parents and teachers are in key positions to teach children that their sexual curiosity and feelings are normal, to help boys and girls better understand how sexual development is an integral part of growing up, to use respectful language, and to reinforce that they are always available for questions (De Melker, 2015). Simple discussions about the body can introduce further discussions about hormones and reproductive systems. Establishing a good history of communication about sexuality and other subjects lays the groundwork for being accessible to update information as the child matures. This is also a good time for parents and others to reinforce the notion that there is diversity in families within which parents and adults love and care for children.

Some children may begin pubertal changes during this time and may be embarrassed by them. As their bodies change, they become curious and want to see others' bodies. Masturbation is still a way for them to explore their bodies. Sexual language is often used more to insult others or appear smart in front of their friends.

Preadolescence

Preadolescence is marked by the onset of pubertal changes. About this time, children understand sexuality as a normal part of life. Both males and females understand the changes that are occurring in each other's bodies and by 10 to 12 years old are ready to discuss sexual behavior and reproduction. Self-pleasuring as a result of sexual reflexes may now become connected to sexual fantasies, sexual behavior, and sexual relationships. It is still common for preadolescents to socialize and develop close relationships, mostly with members of the same sex. Both sexes often become uncomfortable or embarrassed about the changes in their bodies, particularly girls because breast development is more obvious to others. Privacy becomes more important.

Parents should discuss menstruation before it occurs so as not to cause undue alarm and have the child be caught "off guard." Being mindful of their values and beliefs, parents should discuss abstinence, STIs (including HIV), birth control, the HPV immunization for both sexes, consequences of early sexual activity (including teen pregnancy), and the influence of peer pressure. This is also a good time to discuss sexual orientation.

Adolescence

Adolescence is a period of rapid physical, emotional, and social change that presents a developmental challenge to both children and parents. In terms of sexuality, adolescents fit their sense of sexual being into their evolving self-image and personal identity; they learn about their bodies' (sometimes unexpected and embarrassing) sensual and sexual responses to stimulation, and they develop a sense of the moral significance of sexuality. The Guttmacher Institute (2017) reports that on average most adolescents will experience their first sexual intercourse by 17 years old, and that on average 66% of both sexes will have had sexual intercourse by the time they reach their 19th birthday. Activities such as group social functions, dating, participation in sports, and interactions at work and school provide opportunities to learn social and interpersonal skills of intimacy.

Learning how to communicate about sex, how to set limits, how to prevent misunderstandings, and how to say yes or no are important skills for adolescents. Equally important is the process of developing a set of sexual values. Whether the adolescent

practices abstinence, has a double standard for men's and women's sexual behavior, or is exploitative or nurturing in close personal relationships is a reflection of the adolescent's sexual values.

Sexuality in Individuals With Intellectual and Physical Developmental Disabilities

The sexual development of youth with intellectual and physical developmental disabilities (I/P/DD) is the same as those without such physical or cognitive limitations. The clinician needs to focus on the developmental level rather than chronological age when determining appropriateness of sexual behavior. For example, an individual with a cognitive level of a preschooler will normally exhibit sexual behaviors consistent with that developmental level.

The provider must also recognize that I/P/DD individuals have the same desires to make decisions and foster fulfilling relationships with others. Their abilities to develop healthy sexual identities and engage in sexual behaviors often largely hinge on society's comfort and proactive support concerning their right for healthy sexual expression, rather than on their disability itself. Individuals with I/P/DD may be viewed by society (including health providers, teachers, and parents) as being childlike, asexual, sexually inappropriate, having uncontrollable sexual urges, or being sexual deviants. Institutional isolation, overprotection, lack of awareness by others of their sexual needs, and pessimism about their potential often end up inhibiting the healthy sexual and psychosocial development of these individuals. As a consequence, many people with disabilities are vulnerable to sexual abuse and exploitation by those who house, employ, and take care of them. A person with a disability is three times more likely to be a victim of physical and sexual abuse; those with intellectual and mental disabilities are even more vulnerable. Sexual abuse victimization can lead to post-traumatic stress, low self-esteem, anxiety, depression, dissociation, eating disorders, sleep disorders, externalizing symptoms, adjustment disorders, and suicidal ideation (WHO, 2017).

People with I/P/DD largely acquire their sex education from formal educational programs and the media rather than from family or friends. Females may obtain such education in the form of abuse. These individuals are less likely to share their thoughts, feelings, and experiences with family and friends. Unless healthy sexuality is taught and supported, unhealthy and abusive sexuality can occur. Sex education can be effective for those with I/P/DD, and topics should include those listed in Box 21.2. The depth and length of discussion should vary depending on the type of disability (e.g., sex education taught to a child with autism would have a different focus than that taught to a child with Down syndrome). Excellent resources and books for parents, teachers, and clinicians can be accessed from Parent Advocacy Coalition for Educational Rights, SIECUS, and the Center for Parent Information and Resources (CPIR; see Additional Resources).

Factors That Can Alter Sexual Behaviors

Many factors can influence the frequency and number of different sexual behaviors exhibited by children. These include exposure to family nudity, co-bathing, limited privacy, exposure to pornographic materials, exposure to sexual acts (including in the media), extent of adult supervision, stressors (e.g., violence, parental absence, criminal activity, death, illness), sexual and physical abuse, neglect (can result in indiscriminate affection-seeking or

- Body parts
- Concepts of privacy and choice
- Masturbation
- Sexual abuse prevention
- Menstruation
- Homosexuality
- Marriage
- Sexual interaction
- Dating and intimacy
- Appropriate social behaviors
- Birth control, pregnancy
- Sexually transmitted infections
- Self-esteem
- Attitudes and values
- Sexual responsibility, privileges, and consent

interpersonal boundary problems), and psychiatric diagnoses (e.g., conduct disorder, attention-deficit/hyperactivity disorder [ADHD], oppositional defiant disorder) (Kellogg and Committee on Child Abuse and Neglect, AAP, 2009).

Assessment of Patterns of Sexual Development

Sexual development, questions, and concerns are present throughout childhood, although for many children, the onset of their first sexual intercourse is the cornerstone of their "sexuality." Assessment of sexuality and sexual maturation should be integrated into the health history, interview and discussion, and physical examination at *all* health maintenance visits. Creating a safe environment for discussion of sensitive topics when taking a sexual history is critical to establishing trust and open communication. Minimizing note-taking or charting during the visit and maintaining eye contact will also assist to build rapport. A useful tool for the clinician is the Child Sexual Behavior Inventory (CSBI; see Additional Resources). This tool is completed by parents and can help evaluate normal and age-appropriate sexual behaviors for those 1 to 12 years old. Developed to aid in evaluating whether a child has been or may have been sexually abused, the CSBI can provide assistance to the provider dealing with a parent who is concerned about their child's sexual behavior.

Confidentiality

Leading national healthcare associations endorse confidential health care for adolescents in accordance with state consent law regulations of minors (Guttmacher Institute, 2018). The provision of confidential care includes the adolescent spending time alone with the provider to discuss sexual and reproductive health issues. One-on-one time with teens is the standard of practice; it provides teens with regular opportunities to raise sexuality concerns and allows providers to give personalized information aimed at risk reduction (Breuner and Mattson, 2016). Despite these guidelines, many adolescents are not seeking health care due to concerns of confidentiality, especially from their parents. Studies have shown that the odds of avoiding medical

care due to confidentiality concerns increase in the presence of poor parental communication, high depressive symptoms, and suicidal ideation and/or attempt in the past year for both sexes (Copen et al., 2016; Fuentes et al., 2018). Females demonstrated a significant correlation between forgoing medical care due to confidentiality concerns when their histories included sexual intercourse, no birth control used with last sexual encounter, prior STI, or any alcohol use in the past year. With this information in mind, PCPs need to be clear about their policy of confidentiality with both the youth and parent before the need arises. This discussion needs to include confidentiality boundaries (i.e., severe mental health issues and safety) as well as billing statements that may be sent to parents.

History

The sexual history achieves several purposes. In addition to being a tool to collect information, the process itself gives permission to the child, adolescent, or parent to ask questions and receive reliable information regarding issues of sexual concern. It sets the stage to incorporate accurate, sexuality-specific education as a normal component of anticipatory guidance.

Types of Sexual Histories

The sexual history can be either comprehensive or problem-oriented. The comprehensive sexual history (Box 21.3) is detailed, encompassing all aspects of sexual information about individuals, their family of origin, siblings, and peer relationships. A comprehensive history is lengthy and may not be accomplished at the first visit or in a single interview; it can be anxiety-producing to have the client disclose such a level of detail during early visits, and clients can become fatigued by one lengthy interview.

In contrast, the problem-oriented sexual history (Box 21.4) usually focuses on the current complaint or assessment of specific behaviors, such as the risk of exposure to pregnancy or the acquisition of STIs. Problem-oriented sexual histories are shorter, more direct, and specific to the issue at hand.

Approach to Taking a Sexual History

The interviewer should do the following when taking a sexual history:
- Reassure the youth that asking sexual questions is a normal part of clinical practice: "I'm going to ask you a few personal questions about your life and well-being that I ask all my patients."
- Give appropriate, factual information; use medical-sexual terminology rather than slang, unless the client cannot relate to medical terms.
- Use language that validates the client's understanding of terms and concepts. For example, when talking with adolescents, the question "Are you sexually active?" seeks information regarding current activity on a planned and regular basis. The adolescent who has concrete cognitive abilities may respond negatively. However, the question "Have you ever had a romantic relationship with a boy or a girl?" allows for a more inclusive description of sexual activity. Define "sex" as oral, vaginal, or anal.
- Use open-ended questions. Questions that contain "why" can require a level of analysis beyond the capabilities of teens operating at a concrete level of cognition.
- Avoid assumptions of heteronormativity. Instead, ask questions such as "When you think of people to whom you are sexually attracted, are they males, females, both, neither, or are you not sure yet?" (SIECUS, 2016).

• BOX 21.3   Comprehensive Adolescent Sexual and Reproductive History

Background Data
Adolescent name, age (birth date), and sex
History of risky behaviors (e.g., drug history: onset, duration, and frequency of use of cigarettes, alcohol, and/or other illicit drugs)
Access to sexual social media (e.g., pornography), sexting
Parents':
    Ages
    Religions
    Educational levels
    Occupations
    Marital status
Child's feelings toward parent(s)

Childhood Sexuality
What were your parents' attitudes about sexuality when you were a child?
How did your parents handle nudity?
When do you first recall seeing a nude person of the same sex? Opposite sex?
Who taught you about sex, sex play, pregnancy, intercourse, masturbation, homosexuality, sexually transmitted infections (STIs), birth?
How often did you play doctor or nurse or have other sex play with another child?
Tell me about any other sexual activity (e.g., sexting) or experience that had a strong effect on you.

Adolescent Sexuality

Girls
Onset of breast development?
When did pubic hair appear?
Onset of menstruation (age, regularity of periods [initially, now])?
When was your last normal menstrual period (LNMP)?
What hygienic methods are used (pads, tampons)?
How were you prepared for menstruation? By whom?
What were your feelings about early periods? Later periods?
Have you had unusual bleeding or pains?

Boys
How were you prepared for adolescence? By whom?
Age of first orgasm (ejaculation)?
What were "wet dreams" like? How did they make you feel?
When did pubic hair appear?

Body Image
How do you feel about your body? Breasts? Genitals?
How much time do you spend nude in front of a mirror?
Have you ever texted a picture of yourself nude?

Masturbation
How old were you when you began?
What are others' reactions to your masturbation?
What methods do you use?
What are your feelings about it?

Necking and Petting
How old were you when you began? How often?
How many partners do you currently have?

Intercourse
How often have you had intercourse?
How many partners?

How often do you initiate sex?
How often do you currently have sex?
How often have you had oral sex?
Are your partners male, female, or both?
Type of intercourse: Penile-vaginal, orogenital, penile-anal, oral-anal

Contraceptive Use
What kinds of contraceptives have you used?
What are you using now?
Do you have any problems with contraceptives?
Do you use condoms?
How do you communicate about contraception with your partner?

Gender Identity
What does it mean to be transgender?
Do you think you might be transgender?
Have you known any transgender individuals?
How long have you identified as transgender?
What are your pronouns? (e.g., he, him, she, her, ze, hir)

Sexual Orientation
What does it mean to be lesbian, gay, or bisexual?
Do you think you might be lesbian, gay, or bisexual?
Have you known any lesbian, gay, or bisexual individuals?
How long have you known you are gay, lesbian, bisexual?
How often have you had sexual experiences? What kinds of experiences? What were the circumstances?

Seduction and Rape
When have you seduced someone sexually?
When has someone seduced you?
Have you participated in sexting?
Have you been raped?
Have you raped someone? How often have you forced someone to have sex?

Incest and Abuse
What kinds of touching did you receive in your home?
From your mother? Father? Brother(s)? Sister(s)? Other relatives? Others?

Prostitution
What feelings do you have about prostitution?
Have you ever accepted money for sex?
Have you ever had sex with a prostitute?

Sexually Transmitted Infections
How old were you when you learned about STIs?
Have you ever had an STI? Gonorrhea? Syphilis? Chlamydia?
Do you have any signs or symptoms of STIs now?

Pregnancy
Have you ever been pregnant? At what age?
How was it resolved—miscarriage, abortion, adoption, marriage, single parenthood?
Do you think there is a chance you are pregnant now?
Have you caused a pregnancy?

Abortion
What are your feelings about abortion?
Have you (or a partner) had an abortion? If yes, at what age? What were your feelings?
What about your feelings now? What about your feelings immediately afterward? What about your feelings after 1 year?

- Phrase questions that may be emotionally laden in a way that lets clients know that their experience may not be exceptional (e.g., "Many people have been sexually abused or molested as children; has this happened to you?").

When asking sensitive questions, phrasing the question in a way that normalizes it makes answering the question easier: "How often do you masturbate?" is better than "Do you masturbate?"

• BOX 21.4 **Problem-Oriented Adolescent Sexual History**

Describe the sexual concern, problem, issue, or difficulty that you have. Include the following history:

- Type of sex—oral, anal, and/or vaginal
- Condoms—consistency of use, for which sexual practices
- Previous sexually transmitted infections (STIs); medication allergies
- Most recent sexual encounter; number of partners in past 2 months
- Use of illegal drugs and alcohol by self and partner (include which drugs, frequency, route)
- Does patient and/or partner have sex with men, women, or both?
- Recent travel and location
- Any symptoms of dysuria, frequency, hematuria; adenopathy; fatigue; weight loss; night sweats; unexplained diarrhea; fever; rectal discharge, bleeding, constipation, pain?
- *Women only:* Additional symptoms of:
  - Vaginal discharge, bleeding, color of discharge; skin rashes, lesions, sores and location; pruritus (vulvar, anal, oral, other); pain (abdominal, vaginal, vulvar, anal, headache, joints)
  - Last normal menstrual period (LNMP), description, changes
  - Birth control method(s), consistency of use
- *Men only:* Symptoms of:
  - Penile discharge; lesions and/or pruritus (penis, scrotum, urethra, oral cavity); pain in testes
  - How do you feel about discussing this problem?
  - How long have you had it? When did this problem begin?
  - What do you think caused you to have this problem?
  - What might be contributing to this problem?
  - What kinds of things have you done to treat or solve this problem?
  - What health professionals have you seen?
  - What, if any, medication have you taken or are you taking?
  - Have you talked to anyone (e.g., friend, relative, provider)?
  - Have you read any books to solve this problem? What books?

Physical Examination

The physical examination serves to identify normal variations of sexual anatomy, the stage of sexual maturity rating (SMR), and any pathologic condition. The physical examination should include examination of the breasts, pattern of body hair growth, and external genitalia. In sexually active adolescents or when an abnormality is suspected, an oral, pelvic, and/or rectal examination may be indicated. Laboratory studies are performed only as indicated and can include cervical, urethral, rectal, and/or pharyngeal cultures; urine-based nucleic acid amplification test (NAAT); blood work for STIs (see Chapter 42); or genetic studies.

The physical examination should be performed with care and sensitivity. Very young children and toddlers make no distinction between examination of external genitalia and other body parts; young school-age children can be extremely modest, act embarrassed, and resist taking off their clothes for the examination. Older school-age children and adolescents can misinterpret the examination procedures and may feel violated or abused. The child needs to feel an element of control during the examination. By taking the time to provide clear explanations of procedures, using straightforward techniques, and involving the child in the examination (e.g., asking if the child wishes to have the parent or another adult present), the clinician can better achieve the fine balance necessary to perform a thorough, respectful examination.

Management Strategies

The health provider has two primary goals related to management of sexual development in children: first, to help children achieve a healthy sexual identity and function, and second, to provide support for parents to enable them to guide their children through the process. Counseling parents about children's sexual development can achieve both goals. Anticipatory guidance about sexual development and maturation that is age-appropriate should be provided to parents and their children. In particular, the provider must

- Assess the parent's level of understanding regarding typical physical and psychosocial sexual development in children.
- Provide or clarify information as needed.
- Provide strategies and support for teaching children about sexuality.
- Assist the parent to connect to community-based resources.

"Typical sexual behavior" is not always clear, and the range is especially wide in 2 to 6 year old children. Tables 21.1 and 21.2 provide information to help distinguish between the common, uncommon, and atypical displays of sexual behavior.

Setting the Stage

When working with children, the provider focuses on establishing and maintaining a positive relationship based on mutual trust and respect. The child needs to feel validated and comfortable revealing concerns and asking questions. In addition to using a constructive approach to taking a sexual history, a positive relationship can be achieved by

- Asking questions to give the message that the child is expected to be changing and is aware of and curious about those changes (e.g., "How are you feeling?" "How's your body?" "Do you notice that you're getting taller?" "Have you noticed your breasts getting any bigger?" "Boys' penises begin to get longer and wider as they become teenagers. Have you noticed any changes in yours?")
- Listening thoughtfully and carefully to the child's input
- Responding positively by answering the child's questions as fully as possible; being nonjudgmental, calm, friendly, and open; and having a sense of humor, yet taking the child seriously
- Using appropriate teachable moments during the health visit (e.g., when examining a 3-year-old child for inguinal hernia, the clinician can discuss appropriate and inappropriate touching with the child and his or her parent)
- Providing accurate information and referral resources as appropriate
- Respecting the child's need for privacy (e.g., knocking before entering the examination room, providing appropriate gowns, examining the child semiclothed)
- Maintaining confidentiality as appropriate, especially with an adolescent; however, children of any age may voice concerns about normal sexual development that need not be necessarily shared with the parent

Sexuality Education

For a child, developing healthy sexuality means gaining knowledge about physical changes; shaping a positive gender identity; clarifying one's sexual identity as straight, gay, or bisexual; establishing close, intimate relationships with others; and demonstrating

Age	Can Occur in All Children but Assess Child's Environment for Violence, Abuse, Neglect	Red Flags
TABLE 21.2	**Red Flags Related to Sexual Behavior of Children and Adolescents**	
12 years or younger	Asking peer/adult to engage in sexual act(s)[a] Simulating foreplay with dolls/peers (e.g., petting, French kissing) Inserting objects into genitalia[a] Imitating intercourse[a] Touching animal genitalia[a]	Preoccupied with sexual play Engaging in sexual play with children who are 4 or more years apart Attempting to expose others' genitals (e.g., pulling another's pants down) Precocious sexual knowledge Sexually explicit proposals or behaviors that induce fear/threats of force or that are physically aggressive (including written notes, graffiti) Compulsive masturbation; interrupts tasks to masturbate Chronic peeping, exposing self, using obscenities, exhibiting pornographic interests Simulating intercourse with dolls/peers/animals with clothing on or off Oral, vaginal, anal penetration of dolls, peers, animals Sexual behaviors that are persistent and cause anger in child if they are distracted
Older than 12 years	Pornographic interest Sexually aggressive themes/obscenities; may embarrass others with these Sexual preoccupation/anxiety interferes with daily activities Single occurrences of peeping, exposing self, simulating intercourse with clothes on	Chronic, public masturbation Degrading or humiliating self or others with sexual themes Grabbing or trying to expose others' genitals Chronic occupation with sexually aggressive pornography Sexually explicit talk or sexual behaviors with children 4 or more years younger (sexual abuse) Making sexually explicit threats (including written) Obscene phone calls, voyeurism, exhibitionism, sexual harassment Performing rape or bestiality Genital injury to others

[a]Uncommon but can occur in children 2 to 6 years.

From Hillman JB, Spigarelli MG. Sexuality: its development and direction. In: Carey WB, Crocker AC, Coleman WL, et al., eds. *Developmental-Behavioral Pediatrics.* Philadelphia: Saunders/Elsevier; 2009; and Kellogg ND. Committee on child abuse and neglect, AAP: clinical report—the evaluation of sexual behaviors in children. *Pediatrics.* 2009;124(3):992–998. Reaffirmed 2013.

the ability to make healthy judgments about sexuality and sexual activity. The questions a child asks and the behaviors displayed can embarrass some parents—who may respond in a manner that frightens, shames, or confuses the child. Parents who are engaged and comfortable talking about sexual health to their children result in adolescents who are more knowledgeable and proactive in seeking reproductive health care (Breuner and Mattson, 2016). Children are born as sexual beings, and parents, whether or not they are aware of it, are constantly providing lessons in sex education. The ways parents respond to a child's innate sexuality (innocent curiosity about sex, gender, and body parts and functions) and allow it to unfold are the core of a child's sex education.

Parents should be encouraged to take advantage of teaching opportunities in normal childhood sexual play and to answer questions simply and directly at the child's level of understanding (Box 21.5). Box 21.6 outlines what children should know about sexuality at different ages.

Research has shown clear evidence that comprehensive sexuality education leads to a reduction in the early onset of sexual intercourse and risky sexual behaviors (Breuner and Mattson, 2016). A comprehensive sexuality program should include information about sexual anatomy, reproduction, STIs, sexual orientation, gender identity, abstinence, contraception, and reproductive rights and responsibilities. This information should be provided to parents, religious and community groups, health care professionals, and school teachers, who, in turn, educate children. Sex education in the schools remains controversial and subject to federal, state, and local mandate as to content. With the passage of the Patient Protection and Affordable Care Act, signed into law

in March 2010, there are funds available for comprehensive sex education. States may apply for grants from the State Personal Responsibility Education Program (PrEP) but must use evidence-based elements in the curriculum (see Administration for Children and Families in Additional Resources). Box 21.7 lists criteria of effective curriculum-based comprehensive programs.

In 2008, the SIECUS partnered with Advocates for Youth, and Answer organizations to create the Future of Sex Education (FoSE) Initiative and published the National Sexuality Education Standards (FoSE, 2011). These standards are organized around seven key topics (anatomy and physiology, puberty and adolescent development, identity, pregnancy and reproduction, sexually transmitted diseases and HIV, healthy relationships and personal safety), and these concepts are discussed at four developmental levels (see Additional Resources).

Many professional nursing and medical organizations have policy statements or position papers that support comprehensive sex education in the schools and at home (ACOG, 2016; SAHM et al., 2014; SEICUS, 2018). They encourage abstinence as the adolescents' best choice to prevent pregnancy and STIs; they also encourage parental involvement. However, all statements agree that counseling and education on contraception, STIs, and HIV/acquired immune deficiency syndrome (AIDS) are essential.

Counseling of the Adolescent

Today's adolescents face multiple influences, including societal expectations that are at odds with the media's portrayal of sexuality; cultural norms, beliefs, and attitudes of the family of origin;

• BOX 21.5 Approaches to Teaching Your Child About Sex

- Find out what your child already knows. Understand the question before answering. Check to be sure your answer is understood. Make sure you answer the question that is asked, and give your child a chance to ask more questions.
- If your child asks a question about sexuality at an inconvenient time, set a time and place as soon as possible to answer the question.
- Discuss sex in a matter-of-fact way.
- Use correct terminology when talking about body parts; use dolls and books as guides.
- Keep the topics short and to the point. Keep the child's attention span in mind.
- Do not worry about telling children too much about sex. They tune out what they do not understand.
- Encourage questions. Never embarrass children or tell them they are too young to understand or that they will learn that when they grow up.
- Include values, emotions, feelings, and decision-making in your discussion. Do not focus only on biologic facts.

- Let your child know that people have different beliefs about sexuality.
- Bring up topics of STIs, including HIV/AIDS.
- Discuss anticipated changes of puberty before they occur. Do not wait until your child is a teenager. Discuss menstruation with both girls and boys.
- If you do not know the answer to your child's question, say so, and then look it up. Ask your pediatric PCP.
- If your child is masturbating in public or engaging in sex play, redirect him or her to other activities. At a later time, discuss where a more appropriate private place is for the child to masturbate.
- When your child uses obscene or derogatory words, calmly explain what they mean, why it is not appropriate to use them, and that use of certain words can be insulting (e.g., "gay"). Do not laugh or joke about your child's use of such words, because this can serve as encouragement.

AIDS, Acquired immune deficiency syndrome; *HIV*, human immunodeficiency virus; *PCP*, primary care provider; *STI*, sexually transmitted infection.

• BOX 21.6 Sexual Development: Content Children Should Know

By 5 Years Old:
- Use correct words for all sexual body parts.
- Be able to understand what it means to be male or female.
- Understand that their bodies belong to themselves, and they should say "no" to unwanted touch, but that having their private parts touched (for hygiene purposes by a parent) and during physical examinations by their health care provider when accompanied by a parent is normal.
- Know where babies come from; how they "get in" and "get out."
- Be able to talk about body parts without feeling "naughty."
- Be able to ask trusted adults questions about sexuality.
- Know that "sex talk" is for private times at home.

By 6-9 Years Old:
- Be aware that all creatures grow and reproduce.
- Be aware that sexuality is important at all ages, including at their parents' and grandparents' ages, and that it changes over time.
- Know and use proper words for body parts—their own and those of the opposite sex.
- Understand that there are many kinds of caring family types so that they do not see a single model of family as the only possible one.
- Be aware that sexual identity includes sexual orientation: lesbian, gay, heterosexual, bisexual, transgender.
- Understand the basic facts about how an individual acquires HIV/AIDS.
- Take an active role in managing their body's health and safety.

By 9-13 Years Old/Young Teens[a]:
- Be informed about human reproduction.
- Be aware of changes they can expect in their bodies before puberty (by 9-11 years old).
- Know how normal developmental changes begin, including normal differences and when those events occur for males and females.

- Know how male and female bodies grow and differ.
- Understand the general stages of the body's growth.
- Understand the facts about menstruation and wet dreams.
- Know that emotional changes are very common during this time.
- Understand that human sexuality is a natural part of life (by 12-13 years old).
- Be aware of how behavior can be seen as sexual and how to deal with sexual behavior (by 12-13 years old).
- Be aware that sexual feelings are normal and okay.
- Know how to recognize and protect themselves against potential sexual abuse and how to react to such dangers.
- Be able to recognize male and female prostitution and its dangers.
- Know how babies are made and what behaviors are likely to lead to pregnancy.
- Know that it is possible to plan parenthood.
- Understand that having a child is a long-term responsibility and that every child deserves mature, responsible, loving parents.
- Be aware that contraceptives (birth control methods) exist (and be able to name some).
- Know what abortion is.
- Know what STIs are.
- Understand how a person can get STIs.
- Be aware of how a person can protect himself or herself from STIs.
- Know how STIs are treated.

[a]Look for more detailed information and information about what older teens should know and understand about sexuality at www.plannedparenthood.org/parents/talking-to-kids-about-sex-and-sexuality.

AIDS, Acquired immune deficiency syndrome; *HIV*, human immunodeficiency virus; *STI*, sexually transmitted infection.

---

peer group pressure to conform; and the individual's own values and belief system. All these influences need to be considered and addressed when counseling the adolescent.

The PCP ideally uses the answers given by the adolescent in the sexual history to further guide the counseling and educational needs of that individual. It may take several visits for the trust relationship to grow before the adolescent is willing to divulge certain aspects of his or her sexual self. The provider's job is to assure the adolescent of the confidential nature of the relationship and provide opportunities for trust to develop.

• **BOX 21.7**   **Criteria of Effective Curriculum-Based Comprehensive Sexuality Education Program**

- Focus on clear health goals.
- Focus narrowly on specific types of behavior leading to the health goals.
- Address sexual psychosocial risk and protective factors that affect sexual behavior.
- Create a safe social environment.
- Include multiple activities to change each of the targeted risk and protective factors.
- Use instructionally sound teaching methods that actively involve participants, help them personalize information, and are designed to change the targeted risk and protective factors.
- Use activities, methods, and messages that are appropriate to the teens' culture, developmental age, and sexual experience.
- Cover topics in a logical sequence.
- Select educators with the ability to relate to young people and then train and support them.

Adolescents should be counseled that abstinence is the most effective strategy for the prevention of pregnancy, STIs, and HIV/AIDS. Further, they need to know that it is a choice to remain abstinent and a choice to become sexually active, not just something that happens; with each choice comes responsibilities. Open communication and respect for self and their partner will lead to choices that include protection from STIs and pregnancy.

When counseling adolescents, the provider's approach needs to be appropriate for the psychosocial developmental stage of the teen. Using Piaget's stages of development as the basis, counseling may be tailored accordingly. Early adolescents (12 to 14 years old) are concrete thinkers and cannot comprehend the abstract thought of "what if." Counseling language needs to be in simple concrete terms. Using pictures and direct questions and statements helps facilitate this. Middle adolescents (15 to 17 years old) are starting to understand abstract concepts but may often regress to concrete thinking in stressful situations. An adolescent at this age may demonstrate mature thought processes at one point in time yet revert to concrete thinking at another. The provider needs to adjust the approach to middle adolescents accordingly, help them identify the inconsistencies in their thought processes, and guide them through to the logical consequences. Late adolescents (18 to 21 years old) generally have abstract thought more firmly established and are future oriented. However, this ability varies, as with the general adult population.

Contraceptive and Safer Sex Counseling

It is important to use gender-neutral phrasing when discussing safer sex and contraception and not assume heterosexuality. Providers who provide contraceptive and safer sex counseling to adolescents should understand that the successful use of any method requires a complex process of knowledge, decision-making skills, and public behaviors. To use contraceptives and/or protective barriers successfully, an individual must master the following:

- *Knowledge.* For most adolescents, this means mastery of a barrier method (e.g., male or female condoms) to prevent an STI, in addition to a variety of hormonal methods for contraceptive purposes.

- *Ability to plan for the future.* Planning for the future requires self-admission that the adolescent will have sex in the future and the ability to take the steps necessary to use a method consistently and correctly.
- *Willingness to acquire needed contraceptive and/or barrier methods publicly.* The adolescent must be willing and able to be public with requests for contraceptive and/or protective devices (e.g., to purchase condoms at a local pharmacy or to seek services at the local clinic, school-based health facility, or private practice; see Chapter 42 for more in-depth information on contraceptive methods).
- *Communication skills.* Adolescents must have the ability to communicate with another person, such as their partner, health care provider, pharmacist or salesperson, about their individual contraceptive and/or protective barrier needs.

Special Counseling Needs

Children's sense of self; personality; relationship to others and to the physical world; cognitive, emotional, and spiritual abilities; perceptions; and expressions are all influenced by and, in turn, influence their sexual development. If children experience challenges with sexuality, all other aspects of development are affected. Issues of major concern include child sexual abuse (see Chapter 5) and adolescent pregnancy (see Chapter 42).

Lesbian, Gay, Bisexual, and Transgender Youth

The concept of sexual orientation includes at least three distinctive components: (1) sexual imagery (fantasies or attraction); (2) actual sexual behavior responsiveness; and (3) the person's self-identification as straight, lesbian, gay, or bisexual. Transgender is an umbrella term that describes individuals whose sex assigned at birth is incongruent with their gender identity. Sexual orientation is not related to gender identity.

Adolescent-specific data on sexual orientation are sparse due to difficulty in surveying, social stigma, and lack of personal awareness as to whom they are attracted. Approximately 8% of the population self-identify as non-heterosexual or bisexual (CDC, 2016b). These data suggest that today's adolescents are able to self-identify earlier than in the past and spend less time feeling unsure as to their sexual orientation (SAHM et al., 2014).

Management and Complications

The goal of the provider working with adolescents who are LGBT is the same as with any adolescent: promote healthy sexual development, assess social and emotional well-being, and encourage physical health through healthy lifestyle choices. It is important to support and validate the adolescent throughout the process of developing his or her awareness of and commitment to both a sexual orientation and gender identity and to provide a safe environment in which to access health care (SAHM et al., 2014). See Box 21.8 for LGBT terms and definitions.

The counseling needs of LGBT youth are much the same as with any adolescent. Specific interventions include the following: ensuring confidentiality, using correct gender pronouns and nonjudgmental language, displaying information that is important to LGBT youth, and providing information about available resources for support. Encourage abstinence, promote safer sex for those who are sexually active, and counsel about the association between substance abuse and unsafe sexual practices.

For many LGBT youth, adolescence unfolds without event, especially for those with family support, whereas others have a

• BOX 21.8 Glossary of LGBT Terms for Health Care Providers

Agender (adj.)—Describes a person who identifies as having no gender.

Ally (noun)—A person who supports and stands up for the rights of LGBT people.

Asexual (adj.)—Describes a person who experiences little or no sexual attraction to others. Asexuality is not the same as celibacy.

Assigned sex at birth (noun)—The sex (male or female) assigned to a child at birth, most often based on the child's external anatomy. Also referred to as birth sex, natal sex, biological sex, or sex.

Bigender (adj.)—Describes a person whose gender identity is a combination of two genders.

Biphobia (noun)—The fear of, discrimination against, or hatred of bisexual people or those who are perceived as such.

Bisexual (adj.)—Describes a person who is emotionally and sexually attracted to people of their own gender and people of other genders.

Bottom surgery (noun)—Colloquial way of describing gender-affirming genital surgery.

Cisgender (adj.)—Describes a person whose gender identity and assigned sex at birth correspond.

Cross-sex hormone therapy (noun)—The administration of hormones for those who wish to match their physical secondary sex characteristics to their gender identity.

Gay (adj.)—Describes those who are emotionally and sexually attracted to people of their own gender. It can be used regardless of gender identity, but is more commonly used to describe men.

Gender-affirming surgery (GAS) (noun)—Surgeries used to modify one's body to be more congruent with one's gender identity. Also referred to as sex reassignment surgery (SRS) or gender-confirming surgery (GCS).

Gender binary (noun)—The idea that there are only two genders, male and female, and that a person must strictly fit into one category or the other.

Gender dysphoria (noun)—Distress experienced by some individuals whose gender identity does not correspond with their assigned sex at birth.

Gender expression (noun)—The way a person acts, dresses, speaks, and behaves (i.e., feminine, masculine, androgynous).

Gender fluid (adj.)—Describes a person whose gender identity is not fixed and may feel more one gender some days, and another gender other days.

Gender identity (noun)—A person's internal sense of being a man/male, woman/female, both, neither, or another gender.

Gender nonconforming (adj.)—Describes a gender expression that differs from a given society's norms for males and females.

Genderqueer (adj.)—Describes a person whose gender identity falls outside the traditional gender binary. Other terms to describe people whose gender identity falls outside the traditional gender binary include gender variant, gender expansive, and so on.

Lesbian (adj., noun)—A woman who is emotionally and sexually attracted to other women.

Outing (verb)—Involuntary or unwanted disclosure of another person's sexual orientation or gender identity.

Pangender (adj.)—Describes a person whose gender identity is comprised of many genders.

Pansexual (adj.)—Describes a person who is emotionally and sexually attracted to people regardless of gender.

Queer (adj.)—An umbrella term used by some to describe people who think of their sexual orientation or gender identity as outside of societal norms; not embraced or used by all members of the LGBT community.

Questioning (adj.)—Describes individuals who are unsure about or are exploring their own sexual orientation and/or gender identity.

Top surgery (noun)—Colloquial way of describing gender-affirming surgery on the chest.

Trans man/transgender man/female-to-male (FTM) (noun)—Transgender persons whose gender identity is male may use these terms to describe themselves.

Trans woman/transgender woman/male-to-female (MTF) (noun)—Transgender persons whose gender identity is female may use these terms to describe themselves.

Transgender (adj.)—Describes a person whose gender identity and assigned sex at birth do not correspond. Also used as an umbrella term to include gender identities outside of male and female.

Transsexual (adj.)—Sometimes used in medical literature or by some transgender people to describe those who have transitioned through medical interventions.

Two-Spirit (adj.)—A contemporary term that connects today's experiences of LGBT Native American and American Indian people with the traditions from their cultures.

Outdated terms to avoid:
  Berdache
  Hermaphrodite
  Homosexual
  Sexual preference
  Sex change
  Transgendered/A transgender/Tranny

From National LGBT Health Education Center: A program of the Fenway Institute (SIECUS). Available from: www.lgbthealtheducation.org/wp-content/uploads/LGBT-Glossary_March2016.pdf. Accessed February 24, 2018.

---

rockier transition and engage in risky behaviors and experience complications. Family support and acceptance have been associated with increased levels of self-esteem, social support, and overall health. They have also been found to be protective against depression, suicidal ideation, and attempts, as well as substance abuse (McConnell et al., 2016). Maturity, access to accurate information, positive role models, and social support influence the LGBT youth's self-acceptance and success with intimate relationships (Roe, 2015).

Many sources report that LGBT youth engage in high-risk behaviors and face stress and victimization at a higher rate than their heterosexual peers (McConnell et al., 2016; Russell et al., 2014; SAHM et al., 2014), which may lead to poor health outcomes for these adolescents. Providers need to be aware of the increased risks surrounding LGBT youth and address these needs through education and counseling at every health visit. There are many great resources available.

Additional Resources

Administration, Administration for Children and Families, U.S. Department of Health and Human Services (HHS): State Personal Responsibility Education Program, Family and Youth Services Bureau (FYSB). www.acf.hhs.gov/programs/fysb/programs/adolescent-pregnancy-prevention/programs/state-prep

American Congress of Obstetricians and Gynecologists (ACOG), American Congress of Obstetricians and Gynecologists (ACOG). www.acog.org

Association of Reproductive Health, Association of Reproductive Health Professionals. www.arhp.org

Answer. www.answer.rutgers.edu/page/sexedstandards/

Center for Parent Information and Resources (CPIR), Center for Parent Information and Resources (CPIR). www.parentcenterhub.org

Child Sexual Behavior Inventory (CSBI). www.parinc.com/Products/Pkey/71

ETR Associates. www.etr.org

Family Equality Council. www.familyequality.org

Future of Sex Education (FoSE), Future of Sex Education (FoSE) Initiative. www.futureofsexed.org

Parent Advocacy Coalition for Educational Rights. www.pacer.org

Parents, Families, and Friends of Lesbians and Gays, Inc. (PFLAG). http://community.pflag.org

Planned Parenthood Federation of America. www.plannedparenthood.org

ReproLine. www.reprolineplus.org

Sexuality Information and Education Council of the United States (SIECUS), Sexuality Information and Education Council of the United States (SIECUS). www.siecus.org

Society for Adolescent Health and Medicine (SAHM), Society for Adolescent Health and Medicine (SAHM). www.adolescenthealth.org

References

Altarum Institute. *Sexual Health and your Patients: A Provider's Guide.* Washington, DC: Altarum Institute; 2016.

American Congress of Obstetricians and Gynecologists (ACOG). *Committee on Adolescent Health Care: Comprehensive sexuality education;* 2016. Available at: www.acog.org/Clinical-Guidance-and-Publications/Committee-Opinions/Committee-on-Adolescent-Health-Care/Comprehensive-Sexuality-Education.

American Congress of Obstetricians and Gynecologists (ACOG). Practice bulletin, screening for cervical cancer. *Obstet Gynecol.* 2017;120(5):1222–1238.

American Medical Association (AMA). *Guidelines for Adolescent Preventive Services (GAPS): Recommendations Monograph.* Chicago: American Medical Association; 1997.

Bidwell RJ. Gay, lesbian, and bisexual youth. In: McInerny TK, Adam HM, Campbell DE, et al., eds. *American Academy of Pediatrics Textbook Of Pediatric Care.* Elk Grove Village, IL: American Academy of Pediatrics; 2009:1358–1365.

Breuner CC, Mattson G, Committee on Adolescence, et al. Sexuality education for children and adolescents. *Pediatrics.* 2016;138(2):1–11.

Centers for Disease Control and Prevention (CDC). *HPV Vaccine Recommendations.* 2016a. Available at: www.cdc.gov/vaccines/vpd/hpv/hcp/recommendations.html.

Centers for Disease Control and Prevention (CDC). Sexual identity, sex of sexual contacts, and health-related behaviors among students in grades 9-12, United States and selected sites, 2015. *MMWR Surveill Summ.* 2016b;65(9):1–202.

Copen CE, Dittus PJ, Leichliter JS. Confidentiality concerns and sexual and reproductive health care among adolescents and young adults aged 15-25. *NCHS Data Brief.* 2016; (No. 266) :1–8.

De Melker S. The case for starting sex education in kindergarten. *PBS Newshour.* 2015. Available at: www.pbs.org/newshour/updates/spring-fever.

Ehrensaft D. Gender nonconforming youth: current perspectives. *Adolesc Health Med Ther.* 2017;8:57–67.

Fisher AD, Ristori J, Fanni E, et al. Gender, identity, gender assignment and reassignment individuals with disorders of sex development: a major of dilemma. *J Endocrinol Invest.* 2016;39(11):1207–1224.

Fuentes L, Ingerick M, Jones R, et al. Adolescents' and young adults' reports of barriers to confidential health care and receipt of contraceptive services. *J Adolesc Health.* 2018;62(1):36–43.

Future of Sex Education Initiative (FoSE). *National Sexuality Education Standards: Core Content and Skills, K-12;* 2011. Available at: http://www.futureofsexed.org/nationalstandards.html. Accessed August 10, 2018.

Guttmacher Institute. *Fact Sheet: Adolescent Sexual and Reproductive Health in the United States.* 2017. Available at: www.guttmacher.org/sites/default/files/factsheet/adolescent-sexual-and-reproductive-health-in-united-states.pdf. Accessed March 30, 2018.

Guttmacher Institute. *An Overview of Minor's Consent Law.* 2018. Available at: www.guttmacher.org/state-policy/explore/overview-minors-consent-law. Accessed March 30, 2018.

Kellogg ND. Committee on Child Abuse and Neglect, American Academy of Pediatrics (AAP). Clinical report—the evaluation of sexual behaviors in children. *Pediatrics.* 2009;124(3):992–998.

McConnell EA, Birkett M, Mustanski B. Families matter: social support and mental health trajectories among lesbian, gay, bisexual, and transgender youth. *J Adolesc Health.* 2016;59(6):674–680.

Roe SL. Examining the role of peer relationships in the lives of gay and bisexual adolescents. *Children & Schools.* 2015;37(2):117–124.

Rosenthal SM. Transgender youth: currents concepts. *Ann Pediatr Endocrinol Metab.* 2016;21(4):185–192.

Russell ST, Everett BG, Rosario M, et al. Indicators of victimization and sexual orientation among adolescents: analyses from Youth Risk Behavior Surveys. *Am J Public Health.* 2014;104(2):255–261.

Sexuality Information and Education Council of the United States (SIECUS). *PrEP Education for Youth-Serving Primary Care Providers Toolkit.* 2016. Available at: siecus.org/?s=PrEP+Education+for+Youth-Serving+Primary+Care+Providers+Toolkit+. Accessed February 24, 2018.

Smith RA, Andrews KS, Brooks D, et al. Cancer screening in the United States, 2018: a review of current American Cancer Society guidelines and current issues in cancer screening. *CA Cancer J Clin.* 2018. [epub ahead of print].

Society for Adolescent Health and Medicine (SAHM), Burke PJ, Coles MS, et al. Sexual and reproductive health care: a position paper of the Society for Adolescent Health and Medicine. *J Adolesc Health.* 2014;54(4):491–496.

Tanski S, Garfunkel LC, Duncan PM, et al. *Performing Preventive Services: a Bright Futures Handbook.* 3rd ed. Elk Grove Village, IL: American Academy of Pediatrics; 2010.

U.S. Preventive Services Task Force (USPSTF). Guide to clinical preventive services. *Recommendations of the U.S. Preventive Services Task Force.* 2014. Available at: www.uspreventiveservicestaskforce.org/Page/Name/tools-and-resources-for-better-preventive-care.

Workowski KA, Bolan GA, Centers for Disease Control and Prevention (CDC). Sexually transmitted diseases treatment guidelines, 2015. *MMWR Recomm Rep.* 2015;64(RR-03):1–137.

World Health Organization (WHO). *Responding to Children and Adolescents Who Have Been Sexually Abused. WHO Clinical Guidelines.* 2017. Available at: http://apps.who.int/iris/bitstream/handle/10665/259270/9789241550147-eng.pdf?sequence=1.

World Health Organization (WHO): Sexual Health 2018. Available at: http://www.who.int/topics/sexual_health/en/. Accessed August 10, 2018.

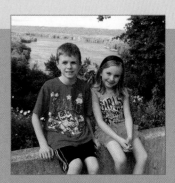

22

Immunizations

CATHERINE O'KEEFE

Vaccine Preventable Diseases

Childhood immunization is a mainstay of preventive disease control. It has reduced the burden of mortality and morbidity due to infectious diseases around the world and is extremely cost-effective.

Immunization is the process by which the body is artificially induced to mount a defense against certain foreign antigens; the immune system is primed to provide future protection with the next exposure to these same antigens. This is achieved by either (1) *active immunization* that involves introducing either a live attenuated vaccine or a toxoid (inactivated toxin) or (2) *passive immunization* that involves administering an exogenous antibody, such as an immunoglobulin.

All but five of the vaccines approved for general use in the United States are on the routine recommended vaccine schedule for all or specific populations of children and adolescents. Primary care providers (PCPs) may encounter children with vaccine preventable diseases due to under-immunization immunizations, barriers to immunization access, or personal belief exemptions. Many of these diseases rarely occur in the United States, but the high incidence of global travel leaves under-immunized populations vulnerable to reintroduction of preventable diseases from countries where the disease is endemic despite the availability of vaccines.

Every few years new vaccines become available, and vaccine schedules change almost annually. Thus the PCP needs to have updated knowledge annually on administration of vaccines across healthcare settings. Current vaccinology research (e.g., DNA vaccines and the nanoparticle approach) addresses new vaccine development, including *Shigella* conjugate vaccine for children, vaccines for herpes simplex virus (HSV) types 1 and 2, cytomegalovirus (CMV) to prevent congenital CMV, Marburg virus (a hemorrhagic fever disease), dengue fever, hantavirus, HIV, and others. Several cancer vaccines are under investigation. Other ongoing studies include development of a conjugate group B streptococcus vaccine for pregnant women to provide passive immunity to their fetuses, a vaccine to cover more serotypes of *H. influenzae,* and live and subunit parainfluenza type 3 vaccines. New vaccine delivery systems are being investigated that include skin-patch vaccines, edible vaccines, additional applications for nasal delivery, and needle-free injections. The Coalition for Epidemic Preparedness Innovations (www.cepi.net) was formed in response to recent worldwide life-threatening epidemics (e.g., Ebola) to advance the rapid development of vaccines against emerging pathogens (WHO, 2018a).

Barriers to Vaccination

Immunization of children requires many visits staggered over time to achieve and maintain adequate immunity from infancy through the teen years, a process that requires persistence and vigilance. Due to a variety of factors, PCPs frequently face barriers to full childhood immunization. These issues are very complex but can be grouped into family and community barriers, healthcare providers provider, and system barriers.

Family and Community Barriers

Parents fail to seek vaccinations for their children for many reasons. Specifically, parents express concerns that vaccines are not safe, may cause autism, overload or weaken the child's immune system, or are traumatic for children. Some parents feel the child is vulnerable to adverse reactions given a family history, the child's prematurity, or an underlying medical condition. Others had unsatisfactory past experiences with the healthcare system, distrust government agencies, live in a community supporting under-immunization, have personal religious beliefs against immunization, lack access to care, or have state policies that make it easy to exempt their child (Hough-Telford et al., 2016; Smith, 2017; Fadel et al., 2017; Spencer, Pawlowski, and Thomas, 2017). In addition, parents may perceive that there are other effective measures to avoid infection (e.g., handwashing/face masks) and that the potential risk of illness from preventable communicable diseases is overblown, or they may simply lack concern regarding the preventable illnesses (Fadel et al., 2017; Edwards and Hackell, 2016). Vaccines, though important to providers and public health agencies, may simply not rise to the level of importance above housing, food, and safety to motivate parents to seek out a source for immunization.

Lieu and colleagues (2015) identified geographic clusters of under-immunized communities in Northern California. Eighteen percent to 23% of children in these communities were under-immunized, compared with 11% in the general population. Whites, African Americans, and Hispanics have higher rates of under-immunization than Asians. Having higher education levels (i.e., graduate degrees) was associated with under-immunization. Full immunization was associated with having higher incomes, and living in poverty was associated with lower immunization rates. Social media platforms are used to identify those with antivaccine beliefs, with the intent of targeted education to those communities (Tomeny, Vargo, and El-Toukhy, 2017).

Healthcare Providers

Healthcare providers report confusion due to changing and complex immunization schedules, inadequate reimbursement, storage and stocking issues, documentation hassles, language barriers, counseling issues, unique immunization needs of special populations, and safety concerns as reasons for not offering vaccinations on-site.

System Barriers

System barriers, such as product recalls, new vaccines, shortages of vaccines, vaccine costs, program funding issues, and lack of a centralized vaccine registry, affect immunization rates (O'Leary et al., 2016; Giersing et al., 2017; Kempe et al., 2015; Farias et al., 2017).

Strategies to Improve Immunization Rates

Community Strategies

Successful community initiatives that raise immunization rates include partnerships between school-based immunization programs and primary care settings to reach large populations of under-immunized children (Perman et al., 2017; Lin et al., 2016; Nowalk et al., 2016).

Individual Provider Strategies

A healthcare provider's verbal cues can affect whether or not a parent chooses to vaccinate. Opel and colleagues (2015) found that providers who are presumptive (e.g., "these shots are due today") rather than participatory (e.g., "what shots do you want your child to receive today") in their discussion of childhood vaccines had fewer refusals by vaccine-hesitant parents, even within the context of initial vaccine resistance on the part of the parent (Opel et al., 2015; Hofstetter et al., 2017). Other important immunization discussion points for vaccine-hesitant parents include (Edwards et al., 2016; Holt et al., 2016):

- Acknowledge and respect the trusted relationship between provider and parent.
- Communicate a strong shared commitment with the parent to the health and well-being of their child.
- Listen to and query parents' reasons for refusing or delaying vaccines; not all vaccine-hesitant individuals have the same concerns.
- Be familiar with misconceptions and controversies regarding vaccines and be prepared to address them (e.g., thimerosal-free vaccines).
- Emphasize the safety of vaccines, the extensive testing before licensure, and the postlicensure safety surveillance programs. Explain the serious consequences of not vaccinating.
- Educate the family about the safety of multiple vaccines to be given at the same time. Mention that a healthy infant's/child's immune system capably fights off an estimated 2000 to 6000 germs (antigens) daily when playing, eating, and breathing. The number of antigens in any combination of vaccines on the current schedule is much lower than the daily exposure to many substances (150 antigens for the entire Advisory Committee on

Immunization Practices [ACIP] schedule) (American Academy of Pediatrics [AAP], 2018a).
- Emphasize the balance between risk and benefits of vaccination and that the risk associated with diseases is greater than the risk of a serious adverse vaccine reaction. Clarify that vaccines have the same effect on the immune system that the active disease does—without the morbidity and/or mortality seen in active disease.
- Provide a vaccine information statement (VIS) or other printed educational materials from the CDC VIS resources at https://www.cdc.gov/vaccines/hcp/vis/index.html.

If the parent refuses to vaccinate or delays vaccination, document discussion about risks, note that VIS was given, and have parent complete and sign a vaccine refusal form (see Additional Resources). If the parent is unwilling to sign the form, make a notation on the form, have it witnessed by clinic staff, and keep the refusal form in the medical record. Flag medical records of unimmunized or under-immunized children to alert provider(s) so that subsequent illness visits include those communicable diseases in the differential diagnoses; revisit the immunization discussion each subsequent visit. Providers are discouraged from dismissing families from their practice unless there is a substantial level of distrust, notable differences in the philosophy of care, or poor communication between provider and child/family. In such circumstances, advance notice in writing to parents must be given and medical care provided until a new provider is selected (AAP et al., 2018b). Providers should identify under-immunized sectors within their communities and be prepared to tailor their approach and interventions toward these areas, as well as work with public health officials to meet national vaccination benchmarks.

System Strategies

The Vaccines for Children (VFC) program enables PCPs to obtain ACIP-recommended vaccines without cost. These vaccines are provided free to children younger than 19 years old who are Medicaid-eligible, are uninsured, or who are Native American or Alaska Native. The VFC program pays for 50% of all vaccines administered to children in the United States younger than 6 years old (CDC, 2018a). In addition, children without immunization insurance coverage are eligible to receive vaccines at federally qualified health centers (FQHCs) and rural health clinics. The VFC program successfully reduces disparities in vaccination rates among low-income children (Srivastav et al., 2015; Walsh et al., 2016). All states receive a set level of federal VFC funds, but some augment that amount to cover more vaccines. Providers wishing to participate need only contact their local state Medicaid office to enroll; they need not be Medicaid-participating providers. Free vaccines plus their shipping costs and an administrative fee, which varies from state to state, are included in this incentive package; there is minimal provider paperwork.

The Affordable Care Act (ACA) stipulates that children younger than 19 years old who are enrolled in new group or individual private health plans with an in-network provider are immediately eligible to receive ACIP-recommended vaccines through the VFC program. Efforts to repeal the ACA and restructure Medicaid funding could jeopardize the success of such vaccine programs (Artiga and Petry, 2017; Buettgens, Kenney, and Pan, 2016). Advocacy for immunization funding as a public health priority ensures preventable disease coverage and promotes herd immunity.

Eliminating Vaccine Shortages

The Vaccine Management Business Improvement Project (VMBIP) addresses problems related to vaccine shortages, including vaccine procurement, ordering, distribution, and management. In addition, federal legislative proposals are ongoing to ensure federal-private sector partnerships to provide necessary incentives and protections to bring new vaccines to market (CDC, 2017). Information regarding vaccine shortages and expected procurement data are available through the CDC (CDC, 2018b). PCPs should develop a tracking system to recall patients whose vaccinations are delayed because of supply shortages and prioritize vaccinating high-risk children.

Understanding Vaccines

Live and Inactivated Vaccines

Inoculating a child with all or part of a modified product from a microorganism evokes an immune response–active immunity. Whole organisms (live, attenuated, or killed), modified proteins, and/or sugars are used to prepare certain vaccines and induce active immunity. Inactivated vaccines do not include a live organism in them. Live vaccines have an attenuated form of the virus, which induces immunity but does not produce disease. Anti-invasive, anti-adherence, antitoxin, neutralizing antibodies, or other protective responses begin soon after the vaccination is given. Live virus vaccines usually confer broader and longer-lived immunity than the inactivated types which require booster vaccines. Killed and inactivated vaccines provide systemic protection (immune globulin G [IgG] antibodies) but may fail to trigger local mucosal antibody (immune globulin A [IgA]) production, which can result in local colonization or infection that can be a problem during an epidemic. The active and inert vaccine ingredients differ among manufacturers and are listed on the manufacturer's vaccine information sheets. One must be aware of these components (such as antimicrobials) because of a patient's possible hypersensitivity.

Research is ongoing regarding the effect of environmental or inborne factors on the body's immune responses to vaccinations. Increased levels of prenatal and/or postnatal polychlorinated biphenyls (PCBs) are correlated with lower antibody response to tetanus and diphtheria vaccines in a birth cohort of children at 18 months and 7 years old (Grandjean et al., 2017a). This lower antibody response persisted in the birth cohort until adolescence (Grandjean et al., 2017b). Research is ongoing to identify genetic factors that account for the variation in immune response to the measles vaccine. This research can help inform future vaccine development and identify individuals with lower immune responses to vaccines (Haralembieva et al., 2017; Schald et al., 2017).

Safety of Childhood Vaccines

Adverse Reactions to Vaccines

After a comprehensive review of adverse events, the Institute of Medicine (IOM), now called National Academy of Medicine (NAM), determined there is no substantiated evidence of a causal relationship between thimerosal-containing vaccines or measles, mumps, rubella (MMR) vaccine and autism, attention-deficit/hyperactivity disorder (ADHD), speech/language delays, childhood-disintegrative disorder, Asperger syndrome, or Rett syndrome (IOM et al., 2012). The IOM also found no causal relationship when investigating the role of multiple vaccines and type 1 diabetes.

However, vaccines are not without adverse effects, and understanding such events is dependent upon learning more about the immune system, autoimmunity, and the effects of genetic variation on the immune response. The IOM (2012) found convincing evidence that

- The MMR, varicella zoster, influenza, hepatitis B, meningococcal, and tetanus–containing vaccines are linked to anaphylaxis.
- Vaccine injections can cause syncope, fainting, deltoid bursitis, shoulder pain, and loss of shoulder motion.

- After MMR, febrile seizures (benign and without sequelae) and measles inclusion body encephalitis (rare) in immunocompromised children can occur within a year of vaccination.
- Varicella zoster vaccine has a causal relationship to some adverse events (e.g., chickenpox rash; pneumonia, meningitis, hepatitis in children with immunodeficiencies; viral reactivation leading to meningitis or encephalitis).

The ACIP recommended vaccines are thimerosal-free or contain trace amounts with two exceptions: (1) multidose vials of inactivated flu vaccine and (2) multidose vials of one meningococcal vaccine that contains thimerosal. There are thimerosal-free alternatives available for each of these products (USDHHS—USFDA, 2018). Because of persistent concerns regarding the safety of the childhood vaccine schedule, the IOM is conducting a population study on vaccine schedule safety using data from the Vaccine Safety Datalink (CDC, 2018c; Glanz et al., 2016; McCarthy et al., 2017; McCarthy et al., 2016).

Vaccine Safety and Resources for Providers

The National Childhood Vaccine Injury Act (Public Law 99–660, amended by Public Law 101–239) requires standardized VIS consent forms for all vaccines, warning parents and caregivers about possible adverse events. VIS forms are available in 42 languages on the CDC website. The vaccine lot number, site of inoculation, and name of the person administering the vaccine must be included in the medical record. Healthcare providers are also required to report adverse events that occur after immunization so that unexpected patterns and safety concerns can be addressed. The vaccine lot number, site of inoculation, and name of the person administering the vaccine must be included in the electronic medical record. The suspected events should be reported to the Vaccine Adverse Event Reporting System (VAERS) using their standard confidential form. Information on which vaccine-associated injuries are reportable as well as official report forms can be downloaded from www.vaers.hhs.gov or from the U.S. Food and Drug Administration (FDA) website. Parents can also report adverse effects to VAERS.

Providers can also submit specific adverse event information on immunocompromised or targeted populations to the Clinical Immunization Safety Assessment (CISA) network for vaccine consultation and receive vaccine safety information about managing postvaccine adverse events.

Immunization Schedules in the United States

The ACIP of the CDC, the AAP, and the American Academy of Family Physicians (AAFP) annually approve a unified recommended childhood immunization schedule for the United States. Providers can download the most recent immunization schedules at the beginning of each calendar year from the CDC (https://www.cdc.gov/vaccines/schedules/index.html). There are three recommended immunization schedules: (1) for children 0 to 6 years old; (2) for children 7 to 18 years old; and (3) a catch-up schedule for children 4 months to 18 years old who start their vaccines late, who are delayed, or for whom an immunization history is unknown. Other countries may follow the WHO schedule or determine their own recommendations (see WHO http://www.who.int/immunization/policy/immunization_tables/en/).

Many factors influence the decisions about when vaccines should be administered. Maternal antibodies neutralize certain vaccines, so some are delayed until the child is 1 year old (e.g., measles). Infants vaccinated in the first year of life require more inoculations

TABLE 22.1	Tetanus Prophylaxis in Wound Management	
Previous Tetanus Immunization	**Clean, Minor Wounds**	**Other Wounds (Contaminated by Dirt, Feces, Soil, Saliva; Burns, Avulsions, Punctures due to Missiles, Crushing, Frostbite)**
Uncertain or fewer than three doses	Td or Tdap only[a]	Td or Tdap[a] and TIG[b] within 3 days
Three or more doses	Td or Tdap[a] *only* if last dose >10 years ago	Td or Tdap[a] if last dose >5 years ago

[a]In those 7 years old or older (including anyone in contact with infants >12 months old and healthcare workers), Tdap is preferred for prophylaxis as a booster dose if not given prior (applies if Td has been previously given; there is no minimum interval necessary between Td and Tdap); any subsequently needed prophylaxis or catch-up doses would be given as Td per catch-up schedule or every 10 years if caught up. In children younger than 7 years old, use DTaP (DT if pertussis is contraindicated).

[b]If TIG is not available, intravenous immunoglobulin (IVIG) can be substituted.

Td, Tetanus-diphtheria; *Tdap,* tetanus-diphtheria-acellular pertussis; *TIG,* tetanus immune globulin.

Data from American Academy of Pediatrics (AAP); Pickering LK, Baker CJ, Kimberlin DW, et al. Tetanus. *Red book: 2018* report *of the Committee on Infectious Diseases.* 31st ed. Elk Grove Village, IL: American Academy of Pediatrics; 2018.

than older children. Children who are not immunized in the first year of life should be vaccinated according to the most recent catch-up immunization schedule. Missed vaccinations should be given as soon as possible and do not require repeating doses.

Vaccines given outside the United States are acceptable as long as there is reliable written evidence of administration (including dates and number of doses), and the age and spacing are the same as the ACIP and CDC recommendations. It is reasonable to check antibody titers or reimmunize the child if in doubt. Diphtheria and tetanus toxoids with pertussis (DTP), diphtheria-tetanus-acellular pertussis (DTaP), *Haemophilus influenzae,* type B (Hib), bacille Calmette-Guérin (BCG), poliovirus, measles, mumps, rubella, and hepatitis B vaccines are routinely given globally, but *S. pneumoniae,* hepatitis A, and varicella vaccines are given less often. The ACIP offers general vaccination guidelines, including:

- If two live virus parenteral vaccines are given less than 28 days apart, the vaccine given second should be disregarded; repeat this second vaccine at least 4 weeks later.
- Do not aspirate the syringe before injection (unproven necessity); do not recap the needle after use.
- When multiple vaccines are given on the same extremity, the sites of injection should be at least 1 inch apart; the anterolateral aspect of the thigh is preferred.
- Use only written, dated records. Parent or guardian recollection of a child's immunization status may not be reliable.
- Reimmunization of an immune individual is not harmful.
- Reduced or divided doses of vaccines should not be given.
- In some circumstances (e.g., imminent travel, country epidemics, delayed immunizations) an accelerated schedule is available from the ACIP.

Techniques to decrease the pain of immunizations include applying pressure or rubbing near the injection site for about 10 seconds before vaccination; putting sucrose on the tongue or pacifier of an infant; having children blow a pinwheel or bubbles during the procedure; having the child sit upright on the caregiver's lap or hug the caregiver chest to chest. Pretreatment with acetaminophen and/or ibuprofen prior to immunizations is no longer recommended (AAP et al., 2018b).

The major vaccine contraindication is anaphylaxis with a prior dose or to a vaccine component. Those administering vaccines should know how to recognize and respond to syncope and severe allergic reactions, including anaphylaxis. Individuals with severe allergy to latex should not be administered vaccines that come from vials or syringes that contain latex (vial stoppers and syringe plungers can contain latex; see package insert). Personnel should

monitor and document storage requirements (temperature, safety precautions) daily. Failure to transport and store vaccines correctly can lead to vaccine failure (see the manufacturer' package inserts).

Inactivated Vaccines

Inactivated vaccines have killed antigen, including only the protein remnants that induce antibody responses. The inactivate vaccines include diphtheria-tetanus-pertussis, polio, Hib, hepatitis A, hepatitis B, human papilloma virus, meningococcus, and pneumococcus. Information about inactivated side effects, precautions, contraindications, and special case considerations of the attenuated or killed vaccines is available from the CDC, from the manufacturers' package inserts, or from a current AAP *Red Book.* Common side effects from the inactivated vaccines include mild to moderate fever and/or local swelling, pain, and erythema usually within the first 24 to 72 hours (e.g., to DTaP, tetanus-diphtheria [Td], or tetanus-diphtheria-acellular pertussis [Tdap], Hib conjugate, hepatitis B virus [HBV], pneumococcal conjugate [PCV-13]; AAP et al., 2015b). Side effects of meningococcal vaccine can also include headache and irritability. Sterile abscesses can occur due to a vaccine hypersensitivity response or hypersensitivity of a component of the vaccine such as aluminum (DTaP).

A history of anaphylaxis after any vaccine should be considered a contraindication to additional doses of the same vaccine until the child has undergone desensitization. Hypersensitivity reactions to components within vaccines may or may not preclude the administration of certain vaccines; allergy testing may be indicated. Vaccine package inserts should be consulted regarding hypersensitivities to ovalbumin, other egg white proteins, gelatin, yeast, and latex. Vaccine administration during pregnancy and following moderate to severe acute infections is also addressed in the vaccine package inserts.

Inactivated Vaccines in Current Use

Diphtheria-Tetanus-Acellular Pertussis Vaccine

DTaP vaccines are used for children younger than 7 years old; Tdap is given to those 7 years old or older. Acellular pertussis preparations have fewer side effects than the whole-cell vaccine (DTP), which is no longer available. Universal immunization with DTaP is the only effective control measure for these illnesses. Diphtheria and tetanus toxoids are highly effective vaccines. Tetanus prophylaxis as part of wound management (Table 22.1) is based on age, nature of the wound, type of prior Td toxoid vaccine, and vaccine reaction history.

The pertussis component is less effective. The duration of immunity after pertussis infection has not been established, but it is not lifelong. Recent pertussis outbreaks among fully vaccinated individuals have raised concerns about the durability of protection conferred by the current acellular pertussis vaccines (Klein et al., 2017). Young infants are the most vulnerable to the life-threatening complications of pertussis infection, while adolescents and adults are the predominant sources of infant disease. For this reason, adolescents should receive boosters with Tdap rather than with Td. In addition, the CDC and ACIP recommend antenatal vaccination at 27 to 36 weeks' gestation during each pregnancy to protect the mother and the developing fetus (Winter, Cherry, and Harriman, 2017; Gkentzi et al., 2017). Waning immunity, as well as changing antigenic and genotypic characteristics of the circulating *B. pertussis* strains, have prompted research and development of a new pertussis vaccine formulation as well as recommended booster doses of pertussis in adulthood (Kuchar et al., 2016).

Polio Vaccine

Only inactivated polio vaccine (IPV) is available for use in the United States; seroconversion to each of the three serotypes of polio ranges from 99% to 100% after three doses. The need for booster dosages of enhanced IPV has not been determined; immunity is believed to possibly be lifelong. The CDC provides guidelines for when polio vaccinations should be considered for those who are immunocompromised or at risk of imminent exposure from travel or outbreak, including adults. Oral polio vaccine (OPV) is currently used for global eradication, but the goal is to switch over to exclusive use of IPV once all global wild poliovirus has been eradicated (Orenstein et al., 2015).

Haemophilus Influenzae Type B Vaccine

Of the six serotypes, Hib is the most virulent, accounting for pneumonia, bacteremia, meningitis, epiglottitis, septic arthritis, cellulitis, otitis media, purulent pericarditis, and other less common infections, notably in those younger than 4 years of age. Hib was the most common cause of bacterial meningitis and epiglottitis in children in the United States and is now uncommon in children under 5 years old with herd immunity. Most new Hib infections in the United States occur in children who are under-immunized or in infants who have not completed their primary series (AAP et al., 2018b). Guidelines for chemoprophylaxis are available on the CDC website for exposed, unimmunized household contacts younger than 4 years old who are at risk of invasive Hib disease.

Hepatitis A Virus Vaccine

The primary HAV vaccine initiative focuses on children in order to prevent transmission to adults in whom the illness is likely to be serious. Current guidelines include universal vaccination for those 1 to 18 years old and for other subsets of the population. HAV is currently given as a two-dose series. The two inactivated HAV vaccines licensed in the United States have seroconversion rates of greater than 99% after the first booster is given. It appears that the long-term protective levels of these vaccines last for 14 to 20 years in children and at least 25 years in adults (CDC, 2018c). In some cases (e.g., areas where hepatitis A is endemic), a single dose may be adequate to provide protection (Stuurman et al., 2017).

HAV vaccine can be administered simultaneously with other childhood vaccines. The risk of vaccination to a pregnant woman is considered low to nonexistent. Seroconversion of immunocompromised patients (including those with HIV) may be suboptimal.

Either immunoglobulin or a single dose of HAV vaccine shows equal efficacy for preventing symptomatic disease if given within 14 days of exposure. Recommendations also target the following groups of individuals (CDC, 2018c; WHO, 2017):

- Those traveling to countries where HAV is endemic
- Those residing in and in contact with others from communities with a high HAV incidence or outbreak
- Children in diapers in day care centers with high rates of HAV
- Men who have sex with men
- Individuals with severe illness (e.g., chronic liver disease)
- Illicit-drug users (using injectable or noninjectable drugs)
- Those with blood-clotting disorders (e.g., hemophiliacs)
- Unvaccinated persons 1 year old or older who are household members and/or close contacts (including babysitters) of an international adoptee from a country of high or intermediate endemicity within 60 days after the adoptee's arrival.

Hepatitis B Virus Vaccine

Two recombinant HBV vaccines, composed of hepatitis B surface antigen (HBsAg) protein, are licensed in the United States. They are equally immunogenic and interchangeable when used according to the manufacturer's guidelines. The seroconversion rate is 90% to 95%, and immunogenicity appears to last 20 years or longer. Routine booster doses are not recommended, except for patients receiving hemodialysis or for other immunocompromised patients whose annual antibody to HBsAg level falls under 10 milli-international units/mL. This vaccine is safe during pregnancy and lactation. Test all pregnant women for HBsAg early in each pregnancy. The immunoprophylaxis management of newborns whose mothers are HBsAg positive is noted in Table 22.2.

Preterm infants weighing less than 2000 g should be immunized when they are 1 month old, while all newborns weighing 2000 g or more should be vaccinated prior to hospital discharge. In addition to young children and adolescents not previously vaccinated, there are other specific individuals who should be screened and/or, depending upon screening status, receive the HBV series (AAP et al, 2018b):

- Hemophiliac patients and other recipients of certain blood products
- Intravenous (IV) drug users
- Individuals with HIV, chronic liver disease, or on hemodialysis
- Heterosexual persons with a history of multiple sex partners in the previous 6 months or with recent sexually transmitted infections
- Men who have sex with men
- Household and sexual contacts of those who are HBsAg positive
- Foreign-born individuals (including adoptees) from countries with HBsAg prevalence
- Susceptible child who bit a person with chronic HBV infection
- Staff and residents of residential institutions for the developmentally disabled
- Staff and attendees of nonresidential day care and school programs for the developmentally delayed if an identified HBV carrier is known to attend or poses risk of infecting others
- Healthcare workers and others with occupational risk
- International travelers who travel to areas where endemicity for HBV is 2% or greater and who otherwise may be at risk
- Inmates in juvenile detention and other correctional facilities if unimmunized or under-immunized
- Individuals with diabetes mellitus between the ages of 19 and 59 years old

TABLE 22.2   Immunoglobulins Used in Children in the United States

Immunoglobulin	Reference Name	Indications for Use	Comments
Cytomegalovirus immune globulin intravenous	CMV-IGIV	For stem cell or organ transplants. Studies evaluating use for CMV transmission to newborns show no benefit over placebo.	Used in combination with IV ganciclovir to treat CMV pneumonia. In hematopoietic stem cell transplant recipients, CMV-IGIV and ganciclovir administered intravenously has been reported to be synergistic in treatment of CMV pneumonia.
Diphtheria antitoxin (from equine sera)		Life-threatening *Corynebacterium diphtheriae* disease.	Only available from CDC to treat life-threatening diphtheria; preferred route of administration is IV. Anaphylaxis and delayed serum sickness are possible adverse reactions and need to be weighed against risks of disease. Tests for reaction to animal sera should be performed.
Hepatitis B immune globulin	HBIG	Prophylaxis for those unvaccinated or under-vaccinated; who have discrete identifiable exposure to blood; exposed to body fluids that contain blood: • Newborns whose mothers are HBsAg positive. • Household contacts <12 months old who have received only one prior HBV vaccine and the second dose is not due. • Sexual contact or needle-sharing with known HBsAg-positive cases, including sexual assault or abuse victims. • Individuals with percutaneous or mucosal exposure to body secretions of known cases.	If mother's HBsAg status is unknown before delivery, infants should receive both HBV vaccine and HBIG within 12 h of birth or 24 h of blood exposure; vaccines administered after birth should be given at different injection sites. HBIG can be given within 7 days of delivery if mother tests positive for HBsAg postpartum but it is less effective. Sexual partners of known cases: give HBIG and HBV vaccine up to 14 days after last exposure; repeat vaccine at 1 and 6 months. Household contacts <12 months old: HBIG and three doses of HBV vaccine. If >12 months old, follow index case's antibody profile (if a carrier, vaccinate all household members). If children and adolescents have documented Hep B series and unknown seroconversion status, a booster dose is indicated. Hepatitis B vaccine can also be used for postexposure prophylaxis if given within 12-24 h after exposure.
Immune globulin	IG	Hepatitis A prophylaxis: • Household contacts and sexual partners of known cases. • Persons accidentally inoculated with a contaminated needle. • Newborn infants of infected, jaundiced mothers. • People with open lesions directly exposed to body secretions of known cases. • Children in schools where more than one case is reported. • All children and employees of child care centers where a case is reported. • Custodial care residents and staff in close contact with an active case. • Persons traveling to developing countries for less than 3 months. • HAV vaccine can be given concurrently with IG, if warranted, for those traveling internationally.	Is given within 2 weeks of exposure; can be used in children <2 years old; is thimerosal-free; >85% effective; dosage for those with continuous exposure to HAV differs from that given for short-term exposure. HAV vaccine can also be used for postexposure prophylaxis if given within 14 days of exposure.
		Measles prophylaxis: • To prevent or modify infection in unvaccinated children <1 year old and others at higher risk of complications who have been exposed to measles. • IGIV is recommended for pregnant women and the immunocompromised who are without immunity.	Not indicated in those who have had one dose of vaccine at ≥12 months old, unless immunocompromised. Given within 6 days after exposure; the dose for those immunocompromised differs according to the type and degree of immunodeficiency, whether IGIV has been given, and prior dosage amounts of immune globulin.

Continued

TABLE 22.2   Immunoglobulins Used in Children in the United States—cont'd

Immunoglobulin	Reference Name	Indications for Use	Comments

		Rubella prophylaxis:
		• Modifies or suppresses the clinical manifestations of the disease, urine shedding, and decreases the rate of viremia.
		• For use in:
		  • Early pregnancy after confirmed exposure and only if termination of pregnancy is not an option.
		  • Infants after maternal exposure.
		  • Older children not vaccinated with known exposure or at serious risk (immunocompromised).
			If pregnant woman is exposed to wild rubella or as a result of being accidentally vaccinated within 28 days of conception, fetus has theoretic risk of 1.3% of congenital rubella; Refer to OB-GYN.
			Administration of immune globulin and the absence of clinical manifestation of maternal rubella infection do not guarantee the infant will be born without congenital rubella syndrome. IgM antibody (not IgG) after immune globulin can be used to determine maternal infection after exposure.

Immune globulin intravenous	IGIV	FDA-approved for treating primary immunodeficiencies, chronic lymphocytic leukemia, bone marrow transplantation, HIV in children, ITP, Kawasaki disease; IGIV contains measles antibodies sufficient for measles prophylaxis (see Immune globulin).	Off-label use, including treatment for toxic shock syndrome, has created shortages.
Rabies immune globulin (human)	HRIG, RIG	For postexposure prophylaxis for rabies; used in conjunction with rabies vaccine. Administered once concurrently with human rabies vaccine.	Prior to use, consult with local health authorities.
Respiratory syncytial virus immune globulin	RSV-IGIV (Respi-Gam)	Reduces risk of RSV bronchiolitis or pneumonia in high-risk children. Provides additional protection against other respiratory viral illnesses; may be preferred over palivizumab in children with immune deficiencies or for premature infants prior to discharge in the RSV season for the first month of prophylaxis.	Palivizumab, a monoclonal antibody, is generally preferred over RSV-IGIV (see Chapter 37 Bronchiolitis).
Tetanus immune globulin	TIG	For individuals with tetanus-prone wounds who are under vaccinated (fewer than three tetanus toxoid vaccine doses) or whose vaccination status is unknown. For individuals with tetanus infection in combination with antibiotics (metronidazole or penicillin G). For immunodeficient patients, including those with HIV; they should be considered under-vaccinated regardless of actual tetanus toxoid status.	Tetanus-prone wounds include those contaminated with dirt (especially if around horses), feces, or saliva; puncture wounds; avulsions; wounds acquired as a consequence of missiles, burns, crushing, or frostbite. In infants <6 months old without the initial three-dose series, decision to use TIG depends on mother's tetanus toxoid immunization history at the time of delivery and if the wound is tetanus prone (e.g., out-of-hospital delivery and umbilical cord cut with non-sterile implement). TIG is given IM plus a dose of tetanus toxoid vaccine. If TIG not available, IGIV may be considered (not licensed for this use in the United States); equine TAT is another alternative to TIG (not available in the United States)—hypersensitivity testing required before use of TAT. Smaller dose is administered for tetanus neonatorum.

TABLE 22.2 Immunoglobulins Used in Children in the United States—cont'd			
Immunoglobulin	**Reference Name**	**Indications for Use**	**Comments**
Varicella immune globulin	VariZIG (varicella-zoster immune globulin)	Given to those exposed to varicella infection who are most susceptible to varicella and most likely to develop the disease and in whom complications of the infection would result: Household contacts. • Playmates with face-to-face contact (5 min to 1 h). Infant whose mother had varicella onset 5 days or less before delivery or within 48 h after delivery. • Immunocompromised children and adolescents without history of varicella, varicella immunization, or known to be susceptible. • Hospitalized preterm infants 28 weeks or more gestation whose mother lacks history of varicella or serologic evidence of protection. • Hospitalized preterm infants less than 28 weeks' gestation or less than 1000 g birth weight exposed in neonatal period regardless of mother's history or varicella-zoster virus serologic evidence.[a] • Other conditions: See CDC guidelines.	Available from FFF Enterprises 24 h/day (1-800-843-7477); strict adherence to forms and protocols required. Administered within 96 h after exposure; may be of benefit if given within 10 days (AAP, 2015b). Not indicated in infants whose mothers had zoster infection. In the absence of VariZIG, IGIV or acyclovir may be considered.[a]

[a]Consult with an expert in infectious disease or the CDC.

CDC, Centers for Disease Control and Prevention; *CMV*, cytomegalovirus; *FDA*, U.S. Food and Drug Administration; *HAV*, hepatitis A virus; *HBAT*, heptavalent equine antitoxin; *HBsAg*, hepatitis B surface antigen; *HBV*, hepatitis B virus; *HIV*, human immunodeficiency virus; *IG*, immune globulin; *IgG*, immunoglobulin G; *IgM*, immunoglobulin M; *IM*, intramuscular; *ITP*, idiopathic thrombocytopenia purpura; *IV*, intravenous; *IVIG*, intravenous immunoglobulin; *OB-GYN*, obstetrics and gynecology; *RSV*, respiratory syncytial virus; *TAT*, tetanus antitoxin.

Data from Goddard AF, Meissner HC. Passive immunization. In: Long SS, Prober CG, Fischer M, eds. *Principles and Practice of Pediatric Infectious Diseases*. 5th ed. New York: Elsevier; 2018:37–43; Pickering LK, Baker CJ, Kimberlin DW, et al., eds. *Red Book: 2018 Report of the Committee on Infectious Diseases*. 31st ed. Elk Grove Village, IL: American Academy of Pediatrics; 2018b.

The HBV vaccine series plus hepatitis immune globulin (HBIG) or an HBV booster dose (if previously immunized) are recommended for postexposure immunoprophylaxis for those with percutaneous or sexual exposure to an HBsAg-positive individual if given within 12 to 24 hours of exposure.

Human Papillomavirus Vaccine

Gardasil-9 (9vHPV) was licensed for use in 2014 and is recommended for males and females 9 through 26 years old. After 2016, the 9-valent vaccine was established as the only human papillomavirus vaccine (HPV) available in the United States (CDC, 2018d). The 9-valent HPV vaccine provides protection against the HPV types contained in the previous HPV4—6, 11, 16, 18—and an additional five HPV types—31, 33, 45, 50, and 58—that are responsible for the most common causes of cervical cancer worldwide (Huh et al., 2017). A 2-dose HPV schedule is approved for individuals who receive their first dose on or before 15 years of age, with a minimum of 5 months between the 2 doses (CDC, 2018d; D'Addario et al., 2017).

Pre- and postresearch studies show that HPV vaccines are safe with mild side effects (CDC, 2017d). Pregnant women should not receive the vaccine. Providers are encouraged to report any inadvertent exposure during pregnancy to HPV9 vaccine to the CDC, which is tracking such exposure on VAERS.

Influenza Vaccine

The influenza vaccine is formulated yearly based on epidemiologic forecasts. Usually one or two influenza A virus strains are changed based on the dominant influenza strain(s) projected to infect the population in the approaching flu season. Major changes in viral antigens generally occur at 10-year intervals with minor shifts occurring more frequently. These viral changes can prevent the body's immune system from recognizing the altered strain and mounting an immunologic response, thus requiring annual vaccination.

The ACIP recommends annual, universal vaccination for those 6 months old and older, unless contraindicated. Influenza disease rates are highest among children younger than 2 years old, in those 65 years old and older, and in those with high-risk medical conditions. Children serve as a major vector for influenza transmission because of their own high rates for contracting the virus; they also shed the virus at higher rates and for longer periods than adults. After even one influenza illness, people remain susceptible to other influenza strains; severe epidemics have occurred historically.

Two influenza vaccines are available. They either contain three virus strains (influenza A [H3N2 and seasonal H1N1] and one lineage of influenza B virus [trivalent]) or the two influenza A strains plus two lineages of influenza B viruses (quadrivalent). The inactivated influenza vaccine (IIV) is available as IIV3 or IIV4 in an intramuscular injection for those 6 months old or older. The quadrivalent *live*-attenuated inactivated vaccine (LAIV4) is no longer recommended (AAP Committee on Infectious Diseases, 2018b; Robison et al., 2017). Follow package inserts to determine the number of doses and dosage amounts for the age of the child.

The efficacy rate of the influenza vaccine ranges from 50% to 95% for IIV in healthy children older than 2 years (higher if the vaccine strain closely matches the circulating wild strain); the efficacy is lower in children younger than 24 months old. Immunity wanes up to 50% within 6 to 12 months after vaccination (AAP et al., 2018b). The vaccine should be given as soon as it becomes available before the onset of the yearly influenza season. It can be given any time until the anticipated end of the infective season to cover intermittent peaks (into May). It is acceptable to concurrently vaccinate with IIV and other inactivated or live vaccines.

Meningococcal Vaccine

Of the 13 serotypes of *Neisseria meningitidis*, serogroups B, C, Y, and W135 cause 90% of the meningococcal diseases in the United States. Most infections in children younger than 5 years old are attributed to serogroup B, whereas C, Y, and W135 cause three-fourths of infections in those 11 years old and older. Infections due to serogroup A are rare. Meningococcal disease is associated with high morbidity and mortality; fewer than 1000 infections are reported annually in the United States (CDC, 2018e). The vaccines that provide immunity to serogroups A, C, Y, and W-135 include three conjugate meningococcal vaccines (MenACWY-D and MenACWY-CRM; Menactra and Menveo) and a combination vaccine (HibMenCY/TT; MenHibrix) that contains the routine vaccines for Hib and *N. meningitidis* serotypes A and C and one meningococcal polysaccharide vaccine (MPSV4; Menomune [Cohn et al., 2013]). Ages, dosages, and schedules vary between the vaccines, and the provider needs to be familiar with the recommended regimens. Two vaccines for serogroups B, Trumenba and Bexsero, are currently licensed for individuals 10 to 25 years old and have been used to help stem the spread of disease during outbreaks caused by serogroup B in communities (notably college campuses). In 2015, the ACIP recommended use of serogroup B vaccines for those (10 to 23 years of age) who are at increased risk for serogroup B meningococcal disease (Patton et al., 2017). Consult the CDC/ACIP or manufacturer's package instructions regarding the current indications, precautions, timing of doses, need for boosters, and age restrictions for each of the vaccines. MenACWY-CRM is currently recommended as part of the routine ACIP immunization schedule for those 11 through 21 years old with a booster at age 16 years. The other vaccines are given to those at high risk for contracting meningococcal infection, including all adolescents; unvaccinated or partially vaccinated college freshmen living in dormitories; military recruits; those with HIV, functional or anatomic asplenia, or persistent complement deficiencies (including infants as young as 2 months old [see ACIP indications for use of MenHibrix in this instance]); travelers to hyperendemic or epidemic countries; or those exposed during a community outbreak attributable to a vaccine serogroup.

Pneumococcal Vaccines

There are 91 known serotypes of pneumococcus, and there has been a shift in the pneumococcal strains responsible for illness. Pneumococcal conjugate vaccine 13 (PCV13) covers 13 of those serotypes. PCV13 was licensed in 2010, succeeding PCV7, and is recommended for all children 2 through 59 months old; children 24 through 71 months old with uncompleted schedules

and underlying medical conditions (sickle cell disease, asplenia, chronic heart of lung disease, diabetes mellitus, cerebrospinal fluid leak, cochlear implant, or other immunocompromising disorders); and those 6 to 18 years old who have immunocompromised disorders, asplenia, cerebrospinal fluid leak, or a cochlear implant.

Children 2 years old through 18 years at high risk of pneumococcal disease should also receive two 23-valent pneumococcal polysaccharide vaccine (PPSV23) immunizations as part of their pneumococcal vaccine schedule. PPSV23 confers broader coverage against 23 pneumococcal serotypes rather than the 13 in PCV13. The number of doses varies according to the number of PCV13 vaccines given and the age of the child. No more than 2 PPSV23 doses should be given prior to 65 years old.

Live Virus Vaccines

Precautions Regarding Administration of Live Vaccines

It is important for providers to consult with infectious disease experts and authoritative reference resources when contemplating administering live virus vaccines (LAIV) to immunocompromised individuals. Recommendations differ according to the condition, degree of T-cell compromise, and anticipated length of illness (e.g., those with DiGeorge syndrome, HIV infection, cancer, immunosuppression, or other cellular immune problem). An individual with a low T-cell count or a cellular immunodeficiency can be seriously compromised if given an LAIV. Vaccine timing after reduction or cessation of chemotherapy or administration of an immune globulin varies; consult CDC/ACIP guidelines.

Measles-Mumps-Rubella and Measles-Mumps-Rubella-Varicella Vaccines

MMR is a trivalent vaccine; this combination is also offered as a quadrivalent vaccine with varicella (measles-mumps-rubella-varicella [MMRV]). Due to vaccine manufacturing and availability, it may be difficult to obtain measles, mumps, and rubella vaccines individually. The ACIP recommends that healthcare personnel demonstrate evidence of immunity to each of these diseases or receive the vaccine to protect themselves and their patients.

Measles Vaccine

A live attenuated measles vaccine using a chick embryo cell culture is licensed for use in the United States. Efficacy of the first dose at 12 months old is about 95%; after the second dose, seroconversion is about 98% (AAP et al., 2018b). Children who do not receive the second dose at 4 years of age should be revaccinated at the earliest possible time. Persons vaccinated with live vaccine and IgG, and those vaccinated before 12 months old, should be revaccinated with the recommended vaccine series. Palivizumab (Synagis) does not affect the MMR schedule.

The measles component is responsible for almost all the adverse reactions to the MMR vaccine. Transient rashes and fever of 103°F (39.4°C) can occur approximately 5 to 12 days after vaccination. Those with fever usually have no other symptoms, and the fever generally resolves within 1 to 2 (up to 5) days. Studies show that when the combination MMRV vaccine is given for the primary dose, the risk for febrile seizures increases twofold. When a separate varicella vaccine is given at the same time as MMR but in a different site in children between 12 and 23 months old, one additional seizure in 2300 to 2600 children can occur (AAP et al., 2018b). The AAP recommends that PCPs discuss this increased risk with parents and offer either the MMR and varicella separately as the primary dose for this age group or the combination

(MMRV). The MMRV given as the second dose at 4 years of age or older is not associated with the same increased risk for a febrile seizure (Ma et al., 2015).

The contraindications to measles vaccine include pregnancy or planning to become pregnant within the next 28 days; anaphylactic reaction to gelatin, egg, neomycin, or prior MMR vaccine; or a febrile illness. Planning is needed for those who need MMR and tuberculin skin testing simultaneously. There are selected recommendations for giving MMR to those with compromised immune systems and for those who have received immunoglobulins and blood products. Guidelines are available from manufacturer package inserts or from the CDC. Encephalopathy and encephalitis are rare complications of the vaccine, and they occur at a much lower rate than after the natural disease.

Measles Exposure or Epidemics

Recent measles outbreaks are largely due to unvaccinated individuals and importation of the disease from countries with endemic measles (CDC, 2018f; Hall et al., 2017). The measles vaccine provides some protection if given within 72 hours of measles exposure. Immunoglobulin used within 6 days of exposure to measles infection prevents or modifies the infection in susceptible individuals (e.g., contacts younger than 1 year old, children and adolescents with HIV infection and children born to HIV-infected women whose own HIV infection status is unknown). During measles outbreaks or anticipated travel, immunization can begin as early as 6 months of age but requires two additional vaccine doses at the routine recommended ages (AAP et al., 2018b).

Mumps Vaccine

The live-attenuated mumps vaccine is given in combination as MMR or MMRV. It is estimated to achieve an 80% seroconversion rate after one dose and 90% after two doses. Fever, parotitis, and orchitis have been rarely reported as side effects of the vaccine; causality has not been established for other effects, such as febrile seizures, rash, pruritus, nerve deafness, encephalopathy, encephalitis, purpura, or paralysis. These side effects occur at a much lower rate than they do after the natural disease. Contraindications are the same as for measles. Use of the MMR vaccine or immunoglobulin preparations are not effective as postexposure control measures for mumps; instead, infected individuals should be isolated for 5 days after the onset of parotitis (AAP et al., 2018b).

Rubella Vaccine

The live-attenuated rubella vaccine is given in combination with measles and mumps (MMR) or with added varicella (MMRV). The seroconversion rate is greater than 95% after one dose. Mild reactions to the vaccine include fever (5% to 15%), lymphadenopathy, rash (5%), joint pain (<1%) and arthralgia (usually seen more in unvaccinated postpubertal females; onset 7 to 21 days after vaccine), small peripheral joint pain, and paresthesias. Contraindications are the same as for the measles vaccine. If inadvertently given to a pregnant woman, there is no indication for pregnancy termination. However, the woman should be informed that the fetus is at a maximum theoretic risk of 0.2% of developing congenital rubella (AAP et al., 2018b). Refer to the AAP Red Book or the CDC for information regarding special vaccination precautions for children who are immunocompromised.

Females younger than 13 years old without documentation of rubella immunity (documented second dose of MMR or laboratory confirmation) should be the focus for vaccination. Routine prenatal screening for rubella susceptibility is warranted in postpubertal females, and they should be given the vaccine if indicated. Mothers found to be rubella-nonimmune during pregnancy should receive immediate postpartum vaccination.

Varicella Vaccine

This LAIV from the Oka strain of varicella-zoster virus (VZV) is well tolerated and immunogenic. The seroconversion rates range from 85% after one dose to 98% after the second dose. Two vaccines are licensed for use in the United States: (1) a single-antigen vaccine and (2) a quadrivalent vaccine with measles, mumps, and rubella (MMRV; Marin et al., 2016).

A small percentage of patients develop localized pain, erythema, and tenderness. Others may develop a mild, generalized maculopapular rash or a varicelliform eruption (generally nonvesicular) after vaccination. The varicelliform rash generally occurs within 2 weeks of vaccination, and wild-type VZV has been isolated from these lesions. A short period of fever may also occur 5 to 12 days after the vaccine. Given the low risk of secondary transmission, immunocompromised household contacts do not need to be isolated from recently vaccinated individuals. Those who contract varicella infection after being immunized usually have minimal fever, fewer than 50 lesions, and recover more rapidly than if they had not been vaccinated. These breakthrough varicella cases appear to be related to longer times since vaccination and severe cases are very uncommon (Leung et al., 2017).

When to Consider Postexposure Prophylaxis for Varicella Disease

Postexposure varicella-zoster immune globulin (VariZIG) is available to those for whom exposure poses significant risk (see Table 22.2) and should be provided within 10 days of exposure preferably within 96 hours (AAP et al., 2018b). As a substitute, nonspecific immunoglobulin G, acyclovir within 7 days, or varicella vaccine (given within 3 to 5 days after exposure) can be considered. However, there are limited data on acyclovir as a postexposure prophylaxis measure for immunocompromised children (Gershon, 2014). Guidelines for post varicella or herpes zoster exposure are published by the CDC and current *AAP Red Book*. Delay varicella vaccination by 5 months after VariZIG, unless varicella disease occurred despite VariZIG administration. Serologic testing to determine vaccine-induced antibody response may be unreliable and should not be used to determine susceptibility. The test is more reliable for diagnosing natural infection but not in those who are immunocompromised (AAP et al., 2018b).

Measles, Mumps, Rubella, and Varicella Vaccine

The combination MMR and varicella vaccine is as effective as when MMR and varicella vaccines are given separately, avoids potentially missing the administration of one of these vaccines, allows fewer vaccinations, and has excellent immunogenicity. See the earlier Measles Vaccine section regarding the increased risk of febrile seizures when the first immunization dose is given as the combined MMRV.

Rotavirus Vaccine

An estimated four out of five children are infected with rotavirus before 5 years of age. There are two rotavirus vaccines licensed in the United States: oral human-bovine reasserting pentavalent rotavirus (RV5) and oral human attenuated rotavirus (RV1). These have different dosing regimens, either a two- or three-dose oral series, for infants between 6 and 32 weeks old. An increased risk for intussusception follows both vaccines and usually occurs within 7 days following the first or second dose. In the United

States, this increased incidence means an estimated 1 in 20,000 to 1 in 100,000 might develop intussusception after either vaccine (CDC, 2018g). Both vaccines are effective and demonstrate similar safety and efficacy profiles. Ideally the same vaccine should be used for all doses, but this is not absolute if the prior vaccine name is not known or is unavailable. Infants in resource-poor countries do not appear to develop a robust response to either of the rotavirus vaccines. The reason for this may be related to maternal antibodies passed on to the infant either transplacentally or through breast milk (Sindhu et al., 2017). Contraindications to vaccination include a history of intussusception or severe combined immunodeficiency disease. Refer to the CDC website or AAP Red Book for information on further contraindications, warnings and precautions, and immunization of children with specific health conditions prior to administration.

Bacille Calmette-Guérin Vaccine

BCG live vaccine is not commonly used in the United States and was developed to prevent the spread of TB. The vaccines in use worldwide differ in composition and efficacy because of the differing attenuated substrains of *Mycobacterium bovis* from which they are derived. The vaccine is recommended at birth as a public health measure in more than 100 countries and provides suboptimal protection against primary pulmonary TB or reactivation of latent infection. The BCG efficacy in preventing disseminated and other potentially fatal effects from *Mycobacterium tuberculosis* disease (meningitis and miliary) in infants and children is approximately 80% (AAP et al., 2018b). For all populations worldwide, the efficacy of BCG is close to 50%; the variation is believed to be due to genetic differences in substrains, populations, concurrent infection with other diseases, or handling of the vaccine (WHO, 2018b). Countries have their own immunization schedules and generally a single dose of the vaccine is ideally given to non-HIV-infected infants at birth. New recombinant BCG and live attenuated TB vaccines are currently under development.

In the United States, BCG may be considered in infants and children with a negative tuberculin skin test (TST) who (1) live with persons with infectious pulmonary TB who are untreated or ineffectually treated, cannot be removed from those persons, and are without a source of long-term primary treatment; or (2) live with persons who have drug-resistant forms of TB (to isoniazid and rifampin) and cannot be separated from those persons. Before administering BCG in the United States, pediatric TB experts should be consulted. Healthcare workers in high-risk settings also may be candidates for BCG (AAP et al., 2018b). A complete guideline for the use of BCG is available from the WHO (see Additional Resources).

Smallpox Vaccine

The United States does not routinely use smallpox vaccine, which is reserved for pre-exposure or postexposure situations, such as bioterrorism. The vaccine contains a live vaccinia virus and protects against variola major and variola minor. In the case of a smallpox outbreak, high-risk individuals will be vaccinated per CDC guidelines issued at the time.

Passive Immunity

The Immunoglobulins

Passive immunization entails injecting an individual with a solution of preexisting antibodies to prevent or amend an infectious disease. These antibodies are derived from sera of pooled human immunoglobulin, illness-specific human immunoglobulin, antibodies formulated from animals, or monoclonal antibodies. Some common passive immunizations and their uses given to pediatric patients are listed in Table 22.2.

Passive immunization is reserved for individuals who suffer from immunodeficiencies in whom a live or attenuated vaccine could be dangerous or for those who have a problem making antibodies (Goddard and Meissner, 2018). An immunoglobulin is also indicated for unimmunized or under-immunized patients exposed to an infectious disease and whose incubation period is not long enough to allow complete active immunization. People at high risk for developing severe complications from an infectious disease should receive postexposure passive immunization. Some individuals who suffer from disease-produced toxins benefit from antitoxin passive immunization (e.g., a poisonous snakebite, tetanus, diphtheria, and botulism). All immunoglobulins manufactured in the United States are screened for HIV-1 and HIV-2; syphilis; human T-lymphotropic viruses (HTLV-1, HTLV-2); West Nile Virus; hepatitis B and C; most for *Trypanosoma cruzi* (Chagas disease); and selected ones for CMV. In addition, the United States requires manufacturers of IGIV and other preparations administered IV or IM to undergo procedures to inactivate or remove viruses (AAP et al., 2018b).

Immunoglobulins are given either IM or IV (IGIV). Most adverse reactions involve localized pain at the injection site but can also include flushing, headache, chills, sweating, and shock; children should not be given a product to which they have had a prior adverse reaction. Systemic reactions may occur, so administering personnel should be prepared to handle acute reactions and, in specific individuals, vasomotor or cardiac complications (e.g., elevated blood pressure, cardiac failure, or both). Off-label use is discouraged.

Some hyperimmune globulin preparations from human donors provide "super immunity" because of their high antibody levels to certain infectious diseases. These include those for hepatitis B (HBIG), rabies (RIG), tetanus (TIG), varicella-zoster (VariZIG), botulinum antitoxin (BIG), and cytomegalovirus (CMV-IGIV). Equine-derived antisera are available for botulism, tetanus, diphtheria, and rabies. These can produce more severe adverse reactions (including fatal anaphylaxis). They should be used with caution and only after hypersensitivity testing to animal sera is completed by a specialist.

Respiratory Syncytial Virus Prophylaxis

Palivizumab (Synagis) is the only product on the American market for use in infants at high risk for adverse outcomes from respiratory syncytial virus (RSV) infection. Palivizumab is a humanized mouse monoclonal antibody and is administered intramuscularly. It is given in five (maximum) monthly IM injections during RSV season (usually November through March or April, depending on the region) and is generally well tolerated. Palivizumab is safe and effective in reducing RSV hospitalizations in high-risk infants by 39% to 82%. Recurrent RSV infection can occur in the same child—even if he or she received palivizumab—due to more than one RSV virus circulating within any given community. It has a high cost-to-benefit ratio. Consider RSV prophylaxis for the following children (AAP et al., 2018b):

- Infants born before 29 weeks and 0 days of gestation during RSV season until they are 12 months old
- Children born prematurely at or before 32 weeks and 0 days of gestation who are younger than 2 years old with chronic lung disease (CLD) and who required treatment for their CLD within 6 months of the onset of RSV season (including oxygen

therapy); prophylaxis can be given to 2-year-old children with CLD of prematurity who continue to require medical support during the 6 months prior to the onset of RSV season
- Infants up to 12 months old with hemodynamically significant cyanotic or complicated congenital heart disease
- Infants up to 12 months old with neuromuscular disorder or congenital anomalies that compromise clearing of respiratory secretions

Consult the most current AAP Red Book or CDC for more specific recommendations, including the length of prophylaxis. Adverse reactions may include otitis media, rhinitis, upper respiratory tract infection, apnea, rash, and injection site reaction. Alanine amino transferase (ALT) and aspartate aminotransferase (AST) levels may increase and hemoglobin/hematocrit levels may fall. Once opened, a vial of palivizumab must be used within 6 hours (there is no preservative). It can be given concurrently with other vaccines.

References

American Academy of Pediatrics (AAP). *Vaccine Safety: Examine the Evidence, CDC* (website); 2018a. Available at: https://www.healthy-children.org/English/safety-prevention/immunizations/Pages/Vaccine-Studies-Examine-the-Evidence.aspx.

American Academy of Pediatrics (AAP) Committee on Infectious Diseases. In: Kimberlin DW, Brady MT, et al., eds. *Red Book: 2018 Report of the Committee on Infectious Diseases.* 31st ed. Elk Grove Village, IL: American Academy of Pediatrics; 2018b.

Artiga S, Petry U. Key issues in children's health coverage; 2017. Available at: http://files.kff.org/attachment/Issue-Brief-Key-Issues-in-Childrens-Health-Coverage.

Buettgens M, Kenney GM, Pan C. *Partial repeal of the ACA through reconciliation: coverage implications for parents and children*; 2016. Available at: https://www.urban.org/sites/default/files/publication/86706/coverage_implications_for_parents_and_children_1.pdf.

Centers for Disease Control and Prevention (CDC). Vaccine for children program, CDC (website); 2018a. Available at: https://www.cdc.gov/vaccines/programs/vfc/index.html.

Centers for Disease Control and Prevention (CDC). Vaccine Management Business Improvement Project (VMBIP) (website); 2017. Available at: https://www.cdc.gov/vaccines/programs/vtrcks/vmbip.html.

Centers for Disease Control and Prevention (CDC). Current vaccine shortages & delays (website); 2018b. Available at: https://www.cdc.gov/vaccines/hcp/clinical-resources/shortages.html.

Centers for Disease Control and Prevention (CDC). Vaccine safety datalink (VSD) (website); 2018c. Available at: https://www.cdc.gov/vaccinesafety/ensuringsafety/monitoring/vsd/index.html.

Centers for Disease Control and Prevention (CDC). Hepatitis A Questions and Answers for Health Professionals (website); 2018c. Available at: https://www.cdc.gov/hepatitis/hav/havfaq.htm.

Centers for Disease Control and Prevention (CDC). HPV Vaccine Information for Clinicians (website); 2018d. Available at: https://www.cdc.gov/hpv/hcp/need-to-know.pdf.

Centers for Disease Control and Prevention (CDC). Meningococcal Disease: Surveillance (website); 2018e. Available at: https://www.cdc.gov/meningococcal/surveillance/index.html.

Centers for Disease Control and Prevention (CDC). Measles cases and outbreaks (website); 2018f. Available at: https://www.cdc.gov/measles/cases-outbreaks.html.

Centers for Disease Control and Prevention (CDC). Routine vaccine recommendations: Rotavirus (website); 2018g. Available at: https://www.cdc.gov/vaccines/vpd/rotavirus/hcp/recommendations.htm.

Cohn AC, MacNeil JR, Clark TA, et al. Prevention and control of meningococcal disease –Recommendations of the Advisory Committee on Immunization Practices (ACIP). *MMWR.* 2013;82(2):1–32.

D'Addario M, Redmond S, Scott P, et al. Two-dose schedules for human papillomavirus vaccine: systematic review and meta-analysis. *Vaccine.* 2017;35:2892–2901.

Edwards K, Hackell J, AAP. The Committee on infectious diseases, the committee on practice and ambulatory medicine. Countering vaccine hesitancy. *Pediatrics.* 2016. https://doi.org/10.1542/peds.2016–2146.

Fadel CW, Colson ER, Corwin MJ, Rybin D, Heeren TC, Wang C, Moon RY. Study of Attitudes and Factors Effecting Infant Care (SAFE) study. Maternal attitudes and other factors associated with infant vaccination status in the United States, 2011-2014. *J Pediatr.* 2017;185:136–142.

Farias AF, et al. Association of physicians perceived barriers with human papillomavirus vaccine initiation. *Vaccine.* 2017;105:219–225.

Gershon AA. Varicella-zoster virus. In: Cherry JD, Demmler-Harrison GJ, Kaplan SL, et al., eds. *Feigin and Cherry's Textbook of Pediatric Infectious Diseases.* 7th ed. Philadelphia: Saunders/Elsevier; 2014:2021–2032.

Giersing BK, et al. Challenges of vaccine presentation and delivery: how can we design vaccines to have programmatic impact? *Vaccine.* 2017;35:6793–6797.

Gkentzi D, Katsakori P, Marangos M, et al. Maternal vaccination against pertussis: A systematic review of the recent literature. *Arch Dis Child Fetal Neonatal ED.* 2017;102:F456–F463.

Glanz JM, Newcomer SR, Jackson ML, et al. White Paper on studying the safety of the childhood immunization schedule in the Vaccine Safety Datalink. *Vaccine.* 2016;345:A1–A29.

Goddard AF, Meissner HC. Passive immunization. In: Long SS, Prober CG, Fischer M, eds. *Principles and Practice of Pediatric Infectious Diseases.* 5th ed. New York: Elsevier; 2018:37–43.

Grandjean P, Heilmann C, Weihe F, et al. Estimated exposures to perfluorinated compounds in infancy predict attenuated vaccine antibody concentrates at age 5 years. *J Immunotoxicol.* 2017a;14(1):188–195.

Grandjean P, Heilmann C, Weihe F, et al. Serum vaccine antibody concentrations in adolescents exposed to perfluorinated compounds. *Enviro Health Report.* 2017b;125(7).

Hall V, Banerjee E, Kenyon C, et al. Measles outbreak – Minnesota, April–May, 2017. *MMWR.* 2017;66(27):713–717.

Haralembieva IH, Ovsyamikova IG, Jennedy RB. Genome-wide associations of CD46 and IFI44L genetic variants with neutralizing antibody response to measles vaccine. *HumGenet.* 2017;136(14):421–435.

Hofstetter AM, Robinson JD, Lepere K, et al. Clinician-parent discussions about influenza vaccination of children and their association with vaccine acceptance. *Vaccine.* 2017;35:2709–2715.

Holt D, Bouder F, Elemuwa C, et al. The importance of the patient voice in vaccination and vaccine safety—are we listening? *Clin Microbiol Infect.* 2016;22:S146–S153.

Hough-Telford C, et al. Vaccine delays, refusals, and patient dismissals: a survey of pediatricians. *Pediatrics.* 2016;138(3):138–146.

Huh WK, Joura EA, Giuliano AR, et al. Final efficacy, immunogenicity, and safety analyses of a nine-valent human papillomavirus vaccine in women aged 16-26 years: a randomized, double-blind trial; 2017. www.thelancet.com (published online). Available at: https://doi.org/10.1016/S0140-6736(17)31821-4.

Institute of Medicine (IOM). Committee to review adverse effects of vaccines. In: Stratton K, Ford A, et al., eds. *Adverse Effects of Vaccines: Evidence and Causality.* Washington, DC: National Academies Press; 2012.

Kempe A, et al. Physician response to parental requests to spread out the recommended vaccine schedule. *Pediatrics.* 2015;35(4):666–677.

Klein NP, Bartlett J, Fireman B, et al. Waning protection following 5 doses of a 3-component diphtheria, tetanus, and acellular pertussis vaccine. *Vaccine.* 2017;35:3395–3400.

Kuchar E, Karlikowska-Skwamik, Han S Pertussis, history of the disease and current prevention failure. *Adv Exp Med Biol.* 2016. https://doi.org/10.1007/5584_2016_21.

Leung J, Broder KR, Marin M. Severe varicella in persons vaccinated with varicella vaccine (breakthrough varicella): a systematic review. *Expert Rev Vaccines.* 2017;16(4):391–400.

Lieu TA, Ray GT, Klein NP, et al. Geographic clusters in under-immunization and vaccine refusal. *Pediatrics*. 2015;135(2):280–289.

Lin CJ, et al. Reducing racial disparities in influenza vaccination among children with asthma. *J Pediatr Health Care*. 2016;30:208–215.

Ma SJ, Xiong YQ, Ziancy LN, Chen Q. Risk of febrile seizure of M-M-R-V vaccine: a systematic review and meta-analysis. *Vaccine*. 2015;33(31):3636–3649.

Marin MMM, Marti M, Kambhampati A, et al. Global varicella vaccine effectiveness: a meta-analysis. *Pediatrics*. 2016;137(3):e20153741.

McCarthy NL, Sukumaran NL, Newcomer S, et al. Patterns of childhood immunization and all-cause mortality. *Vaccine*. 2017;35:6643–6648.

McCarthy NL, Gee J, Sujumaran L, et al. Vaccination and 30-day mortality risk in children, adolescents and young adults. *Pediatrics*. 2016;137(3):1–10.

National Vaccine Injury Act

Nowalk M, et al. Maintenance of increased childhood influenza vaccination rates 1 year after an intervention in primary care practices. *Acad Pediatr*. 2016;16(1):57–63.

O'Leary SJ, Hurley LP, Kennedy ED, et al. Provider attitudes regarding vaccine tracking systems in private pediatric practices. *Acad Pediatr*. 2016;16:34–41.

Opel DJ, Mangione-Smith R, Robinson JD, et al. The influence of provider communication behaviors on parental vaccine acceptance and visit experience. *Am J Public Health*. 2015;105(10):1998–2004.

Orenstein WA, Seib KG. American Academy of Pediatrics committee on infectious diseases: eradicating polio; how the world's pediatricians can help stop this crippling illness forever. *Pediatrics*. 2015;135(1):196–202.

Patton ME, Stephens D, Moore K, MacNeil JR. Updated recommendations for use of Men B-FHbp serogroup B meningococcal vaccine – advisory committee on immunization practices (ACIP). *MMWR*. 2017;66(19):1–5.

Perman S, et al. School-based vaccination programmes: a systematic review of the evidence on organisation and delivery in high income countries. *BMC Public Health*. 2017;17:252–262.

Robison SG, Dunn AG, Richards DL, et al. Changes in influenza vaccination rates after withdrawal of live vaccine. *Pediatrics*. 2017;140(5):e20170516.

Schald DJ, Haralambiera IH, Larrrabee BR, et al. Heritability of vaccine-induced measles neutralizing antibody titers. *Vaccine*. 2017;35(10):1390–1394.

Sindhu KN, Cunliff N, Peak M, et al. Impact of maternal antibodies and infant gut microbiota on the immunogenicity of rotavirus vaccines in Africa, Indian and European infants: protocol for prospective cohort study. *BMJ Open*. 2017;7:e016577.

Smith T. Vaccine rejection and hesitancy: a review and call to action. *Open Forum Infect Dis*. 2017. https://doi.org/10.1093/ofid/ofx146.

Spencer J, Pawlowski R, Thomas S. Vaccine adverse events: separating myth from reality. *Am Fam Physician*. 2017;95(12):786–794.

Srivastav A, Zhai Y, Santibanez TA, et al. Influenza vaccination coverage of Vaccine for Children (VFC) –entitled versus privately insured children, United States, 2011-2013. *Vaccine*. 2015;33:3114–3121.

Stuurman AL, Marano C, Bunge EM, et al. Impact of universal mass vaccination with monovalent inactivated hepatitis A vaccines: a systematic review. *Hum Vacc Immuno*. 2017;13(3):724–736.

Tomeny T, Vargo C, El-Toukhy S. Geographic and demographic correlates of autism-related anti-vaccine beliefs on Twitter, 2009-2015. *Soc Sci Med*. 2017;191:168–175.

U.S. Department of Health and Human Services (USDHHS) –U.S. Food and Drug Administration (USFDA): Thimerosal and vaccines (website); 2018. Available at: https://www.fda.gov/BiologicsBloodVaccines/SafetyAvailability/VaccineSafety/UCM096228.

Walsh B, Doherty E, O'Neill C. Since the start of the Vaccines for Children program, uptake has increased, and most disparities have decreased. *Health Affairs*. 2016;35(2):356–364.

Winter K, Cherry JD, Harriman K. Effectiveness of prenatal tetanus, diphtheria, and acellular pertussis vaccination on pertussis severity in infants. *Clin Infect Dis*. 2017;64(1):9–14.

World Health Organization (WHO). Tracking the new vaccine pipeline (website); 2018a. Available at: http://www.who.int/immunization/research/clinicaltrials_newvaccinepipeline/en/.

World Health Organization (WHO). Hepatitis A: Fact sheet (website); 2017. Available at: http://www.who.int/mediacentre/factsheets/fs328/en/.

World Health Organization (WHO). WHO Report, BCG vaccine: WHO position paper, February 2018 –Recommendations. *Vaccine*. 2018b;36:3408–3410.

23

Dental Health and Oral Disorders

DONALD L. CHI

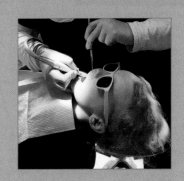

Oral health is increasingly recognized as a barometer of general health and well-being across the life span. Pediatric primary care providers (PCPs) are an essential part of the oral health team because they have early and ongoing contact with children and families, which provides opportunities for anticipatory guidance, specific prevention interventions, and early identification of oral disease. Accordingly, the American Academy of Pediatrics (AAP) Section on Oral Health provides education and training, including *SmilesForLife*, family resources, and practice tools, such as the *Oral Health Risk Assessment Tool, Oral Health Flip Chart*, and *Brush, Book, Bed* (https://www.aap.org/en-us/advocacy-and-policy/aap-health-initiatives/Oral-Health/Pages/Oral-Health.aspx).

This chapter offers information and practical answers for PCPs to ensure they have basic examination competencies; the ability to distinguish between normal and abnormal structures, pathology, and common oral diseases; provide oral health education; prescribe and apply preventive treatment (e.g., fluoride varnish); and recognize when to engage other members of the oral health team.

Dental Care Standards and Guidelines

Healthy People 2020 identified oral health as a priority, including 17 objectives that address the prevention and control of oral and craniofacial disease, conditions, injuries, and improvements in accessing preventive dental services and care. In 2010 the U.S. Department of Health and Human Services (HHS) launched a cross-agency initiative to improve oral health nationwide among children with Medicaid and the Children's Health Insurance Program (CHIP). Referred to as the *New Oral Health Initiative* (NOHI), it set both short- and long-term goals, calling for increasing accountability, expanding research and data collection, emphasizing disease prevention and oral health promotion, and reducing health disparities. They also introduced the concept of oral health care teams, including dentists, dental hygienists, dental therapists, and community dental health practitioners, as well as nondental professionals (e.g., PCPs). Their expanded view included a provision to reimburse PCPs for preventive dental services (e.g., oral examinations, risk assessment, fluoride varnish) (Institute of Medicine [IOM] and National Research Council [NRC], 2011).

The U.S. Preventive Services Task Force (USPSTF) subsequently issued two recommendations for preventing caries in children from birth to 5 years old: namely, PCPs should (1) prescribe oral fluoride supplementation starting at 6 months old if the water supply is fluoride deficient, and (2) fluoride varnish should be applied to the primary teeth of high-risk infants and children beginning at the onset of primary tooth eruption (Moyer and USPSTF, 2014).

The American Academy of Pediatric Dentistry (AAPD) recommends that pediatric PCPs encourage parents to establish a "dental home" for their children no later than 12 months old. Ideally, referral to a dentist should be considered as early as 6 months old or at the eruption of the first primary tooth (AAPD, 2017a). There are two additional factors that are important to optimize oral health for children: (1) regular exposure to fluoride, mainly through tooth brushing with fluoridated toothpaste and drinking optimally fluoridated water, and (2) minimizing sugary food and beverage intake. Sugar-sweetened beverages are particularly harmful to the teeth and U.S. children consume high volumes (Afeiche et al., 2018). Social factors, such as poverty, structural racism and implicit bias, and neighborhood features, can constrain whether a child or family is able to engage in optimal oral health behaviors (AAPD, 2017b).

Normal Growth and Development

Teeth

The structures of the mouth include the mucosa (buccal and gingival), palate, salivary glands, frenula, tongue, and teeth. Primary and permanent teeth have similar anatomy, differing primarily in the size and external shape of each tooth. Teeth are encased in mandibular and maxillary bone. A small opening at the root apex allows blood vessels and nerves to pass into the tooth. There are three layers: the outer enamel, dentin (softer than enamel), and pulp (inner most layer containing nerves and blood vessels).

Pattern of Tooth Eruption

The eruption of primary teeth typically begins with the lower central incisors and ends with the maxillary second molars (Fig 23.1). The sequence of eruption and the timing of eruption for each tooth are similar for boys and girls. Although there is some age variability in timing, the eruption sequence is important to document. In most children, the 20 primary teeth are fully erupted by age 2 years. Each primary tooth has a designated letter (A-T) (Fig 23.2). Tooth lettering begins at the second molar (tooth A) in the child's upper right quadrant, proceeds to the upper left quadrant (tooth J), continues down to the lower left quadrant (tooth K), and ends with the lower right mandibular second molar (tooth T).

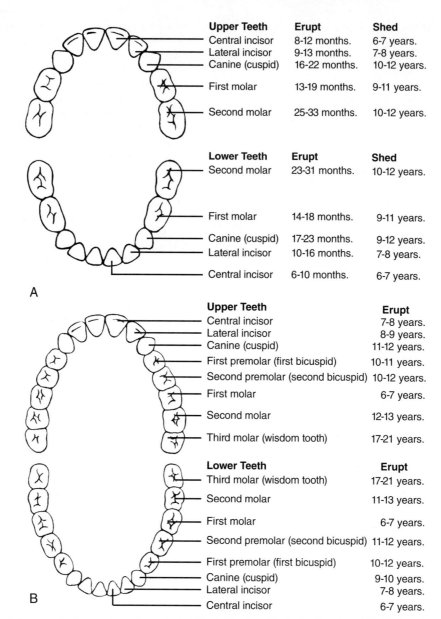

Upper Teeth	Erupt	Shed
Central incisor	8-12 months.	6-7 years.
Lateral incisor	9-13 months.	7-8 years.
Canine (cuspid)	16-22 months.	10-12 years.
First molar	13-19 months.	9-11 years.
Second molar	25-33 months.	10-12 years.

Lower Teeth	Erupt	Shed
Second molar	23-31 months.	10-12 years.
First molar	14-18 months.	9-11 years.
Canine (cuspid)	17-23 months.	9-12 years.
Lateral incisor	10-16 months.	7-8 years.
Central incisor	6-10 months.	6-7 years.

A

Upper Teeth	Erupt
Central incisor	7-8 years.
Lateral incisor	8-9 years.
Canine (cuspid)	11-12 years.
First premolar (first bicuspid)	10-11 years.
Second premolar (second bicuspid)	10-12 years.
First molar	6-7 years.
Second molar	12-13 years.
Third molar (wisdom tooth)	17-21 years.

Lower Teeth	Erupt
Third molar (wisdom tooth)	17-21 years.
Second molar	11-13 years.
First molar	6-7 years.
Second premolar (second bicuspid)	11-12 years.
First premolar (first bicuspid)	10-12 years.
Canine (cuspid)	9-10 years.
Lateral incisor	7-8 years.
Central incisor	6-7 years.

B

• **Fig 23.1** Eruption Sequence (A) Primary (Baby) Teeth Eruption Chart. (B) Permanent Teeth Eruption Chart. (©American Dental Association (2012). https://www.mouthhealthy.org/en/az-topics/e/eruption-charts. Accessed May 8, 2018.)

The permanent teeth begin erupting as children reach school age (~5 to 6 years old) and the jaw begins to grow. There is a total of 32 permanent teeth distributed among four tooth classes: 8 incisors, 4 canines, 8 premolars, and 12 molars. Permanent dentition eruption begins with the mandibular central incisors and ends with the maxillary third molars (a.k.a. *wisdom teeth*). The primary teeth shed as the permanent teeth erupt. The shedding and replacement of the primary molars by permanent premolars is usually complete by age 12 years. This period, when both primary and permanent teeth are present, is called *mixed dentition.*

Delayed tooth eruption (DTE) is when eruption of a tooth/multiple teeth is overdue, according to population norms based on chronologic age. Timely screening and recognition of DTE can minimize medical, developmental, functional, and esthetic problems resulting from untreated underlying local and systemic causes. Providers should also make note of children who have congenitally missing teeth (hypodontia) and extra teeth (hyperdontia).

Teething

Teeth typically erupt through the gums without causing any serious symptoms. However, it is important to note teething is not the cause of a report of *systemic* symptoms, such as diarrhea, high fever, vomiting, and cough, which should be addressed separately. Local gum irritation, irritability, and drooling are the most frequent symptoms of teething in infants and toddlers, peaking during the emergence of a child's primary incisors or front teeth (Massignan et al., 2016). A slight rise in body temperature is often reported but most often is not high enough to be considered a fever. This distinction is important. If a child develops a true fever, generally considered to be greater than 38°C (100.4°F), the inadvertent assumption that the cause is teething may lead parents and/or providers to miss an illness or infection that requires treatment. It is also important to remember other systemic symptoms, such as diarrhea, vomiting, and cough should not be attributed to teething.

The recommended treatment for teething discomfort is to offer a *chilled* rubber teething ring or a wet, *chilled* washcloth for

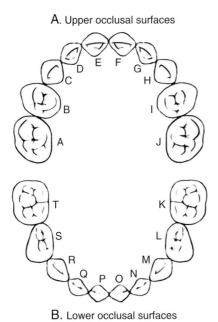

A. Upper occlusal surfaces

B. Lower occlusal surfaces

• **Fig 23.2** Lettering of Primary Teeth (A) Upper occlusal surfaces. (B) Lower occlusal surfaces. (Courtesy Jaemi Yoo, University of Washington School of Dentistry RIDE. Used with permission.)

gumming, massaging the gums, or allowing infants older than 6 months old to chew on a *chilled* hard food under supervision. Frozen objects (including those with a liquid component) should not be used because of the potential for trauma to the gums. A number of folk remedies are used, especially in communities with limited access to medical/dental care (Smitherman et al, 2005). For example, rubbing an alcoholic beverage (e.g., whiskey) on the gums, tying a penny on a string around the child's neck (creating a potential risk of strangulation), or using a honey-coated pacifier, which could cause tooth decay or introduce botulism, are discouraged. Topical application of salicylates (aspirin) can cause burns and should not be used. Topical anesthetic gels, especially those containing benzocaine, are not recommended because of the rare potential for methemoglobinemia (U.S. Food and Drug Administration [FDA], 2017). Silicone teething necklaces, worn by the adult, are becoming popular; however, the use of *amber* necklaces, in particular, and any necklace worn by the child is discouraged.

Performing the Oral Examination

Most important is that an oral examination should be systematic. Take the opportunity to note and point out normal development (e.g., erupted teeth, eruption patterns) and abnormalities (e.g., bloody or inflamed gums, tooth decay) to the parent(s). For an infant, have the parent immobilize the arms. With a tongue blade or toothbrush as a mouth prop, use a penlight and intraoral mirror for optimal visualization. Tip the head back to see the upper teeth. An alternative for examining a young child is for the provider and parent to sit across from each other knee to knee. The child faces the parent, and the child's head is then lowered into the provider's lap. The child's legs can be wrapped around the parent's waist if needed.

Clinical Findings

Oral Mucosa

The soft mucosal tissues are examined before the teeth. This exam should include an assessment of the tonsils for size and the presence

of inflammation or exudate. Start the examination with the inside of the lips and continue to the buccal mucosa, including the mucosal surfaces that connect and surround each tooth. Inspect the palate directly by tipping the child's head backward. Examine the dorsal and ventral mucosal surfaces of the tongue and floor of the mouth by retracting the tongue with a tongue blade or a dental mirror or by holding the tongue with cotton gauze. Note ulcerations, changes in color and surface texture, swelling, or fistulae of any of these tissues. When examining the gums, give special attention to any gingival swelling or recession. In racial or ethnic minority children, the gums may exhibit hyperpigmentation, which is normal. Note the presence and attachment of both frenula, noting the presence of "tongue tie" (a.k.a. ankyloglossia) and/or "lip tie." In infants, it is important to ask about difficulties latching onto the breast, because this may require surgical intervention. For older children, it is important to note the impact on speech. If speech is affected, a referral and/or surgical intervention is warranted.

Saliva

Note the quantity and quality of the saliva. Decreased salivary flow and changes in sensation around the facial nerve can result from infection or tumor in the parotid space or facial musculature or can be a side effect of dehydration or medications that cause xerostomia (dry mouth). Drooling commonly refers to *anterior* drooling, which peaks between 3 and 6 months of life. It should be distinguished from posterior drooling, which entails saliva spilling over the tongue through the facial isthmus. Drooling can be a significant and ongoing disability for a large number of pediatric patients with cerebral palsy and for a smaller number of patients with other types of neurologic or cognitive impairment.

Teeth

The number and types of teeth erupted, discoloration, irregularities, and asymmetries should be noted. Retract or lift the lips away so that the teeth can be examined systematically; beginning with tooth A and moving around to the left, ending with tooth J, examine the lingual surfaces of the upper teeth and the biting surfaces before repeating this examination on the lower teeth K through T. Teeth are best evaluated when dry. Variations in number, morphology, color, and surface structure should be noted, along with the presence of early caries, overt tooth decay, and/or the presence of previous dental work. Primary teeth may be malformed, incompletely formed, or chalky or have pitted enamel due to other systematic conditions, such as ectodermal dysplasia. In the case of traumatically previously injured teeth, the color and translucency of the injured tooth or teeth may be altered. Traumatized primary teeth that are discolored but asymptomatic and nonabscessed can be monitored. In addition, very low-birth-weight infants may present with enamel defects on primary teeth that increase dental caries risk (Nelson et al., 2013).

Aberrations in Primary Tooth Eruption and Gums

Natal and Neonatal Teeth

The prevalence of natal or neonatal teeth is estimated to be 1 out of 2000 to 3000 births and is equally common in boys and girls. The teeth usually erupt in pairs. Natal and neonatal teeth occur in approximately 50 different syndromes, of which approximately 10 are associated with chromosomal aberrations. More than 90% of these prematurely erupting teeth are mandibular central incisors with normal shape and color. Supernumerary teeth may be abnormal in shape and color and only loosely attached to the gingiva. Natal or neonatal teeth can lead to gingivitis, self-mutilation of the tongue, and trauma to the mother during breastfeeding; however, they should be extracted only if they are loose enough to involve risk of aspiration or sublingual ulceration or if feeding is severely disturbed. Most will develop normally with normal root structure (Khandelwal et al, 2013).

Atypical Tooth Eruption

Atypical tooth eruption can result from either *systemic* factors, such as prematurity, low birth weight, or genetic syndromes (e.g., Down, Turner), or *local* factors, such as a low-protein diet, adjacent supernumeraries, and dental tissue tumors. In general, children with chronic health conditions, who have delays in physical development, experience delayed but otherwise normal tooth eruption.

Preeruption Cysts

When a tooth starts erupting through the gingival tissue, a blood-filled cyst may precede it and alarmed parents may report a purple, reddish, black, or blue bump or bruise on their child's gums. If the enlargement is on the alveolar ridge, no treatment is indicated. The symptom will resolve as the tooth erupts.

Bohn Nodules

Bohn nodules are present at birth and appear as firm nonpainful nodules on the buccal surface of the alveolar ridge (Fig 23.3). They are remnants of dental lamina connecting the developing tooth bud to the epithelium of the oral cavity. No treatment is required because they will resolve spontaneously. If they appear in the midline of the palate, they are referred to as *Epstein pearls*.

Professional Dental Care

Fear of the Dentist

There is a significant relationship between parental and child dental fear, particularly in children 8 years old and younger (Themessi-Huber et al, 2010). Many parents of children with whom PCPs interact may have this fear and consequently avoid dental visits themselves. Approaching these parents using a calm, caring approach is imperative to help allay anxiety and fears. Early and

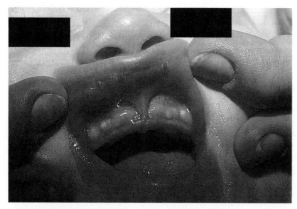

• **Fig 23.3** Bohn Nodules (From Eichenfield LF, Frieden IJ, Esterly NB. *Neonatal Dermatology.* 2nd ed. Philadelphia: Mosby/Elsevier; 2008.)

consistent primary prevention is the best way to avoid the development of fear and dental care avoidance. Allowing tooth decay to go untreated until a child needs extensive restorative intervention is not only costly, but it can also be traumatic.

Choosing a Dentist

The choice of a dentist and identification of a dental home is critical, especially for children who have had negative experiences with dentists. Many general dentists are highly skilled at working with children, so the absence of a pediatric dentist should not be a barrier to care; however, a dentist who is new to the child should be told about any prior dental experiences. Parents should be cautious about dentists with laser-based or other electronic diagnostic devices because these devices are often marketed as being capable of detecting "invisible" cavities and justify unnecessary fillings. The standard method of examination of the teeth is visual, using strong light and transillumination. Most tooth decay in permanent teeth in children occurs on the biting surface, and x-rays are of limited diagnostic value in such cases. When parents report excessive, new, or experimental dental treatments, PCPs can query the dental provider as a member of the oral health team.

First Dental Visit

The child's first dental visit should occur before the child's first birthday (12 months old) or within 6 months of the first tooth eruption. This first visit allows a dentist to begin to establish an ongoing relationship (dental home) for the child, provide education and anticipatory guidance, and deliver preventive care, such as topical fluoride if not performed by the PCP. Establishment of a dental home gives parents a familiar place to take their child for dental checkups and emergencies (e.g., dental/oral trauma, avulsion, dislodged filling). The first dental visit commonly involves a cleaning, dental examination, and topical fluoride treatment in the presence of the parent. For children younger than 3 years old, the parent may be asked to help position the child.

Dental Health Education

Dental health education is a crucial preventive strategy, and PCPs, with their ongoing and early contact with children and families, are ideally situated to introduce and reinforce proper oral hygiene/brushing techniques, emphasize the importance of fluoride, facilitate dental care access, and address nutrition intake, including the use of pacifiers, bottles, and no-spill cups. The PCP should review all materials for readability levels and inconsistencies. For example, the amount of toothpaste to use can be described as "pea-sized," but accompanying photos often show a long ribbon of toothpaste on the toothbrush. In addition, PCPs can address and dispel common oral health myths, such as tooth decay in baby teeth is not important because these teeth eventually fall out.

Well-child care is the ideal time to integrate dental health education and prevention. As noted earlier, the AAP has a number of educational resources and interventions. PCPs should introduce oral health-related education and anticipatory guidance, especially during early well-baby visits, to ensure that children have their first visit to the dentist by 12 months old. Earlier studies revealed that young children with a greater number of well-child visits between 1 and 3 years old were significantly more likely to have earlier first dental visits (Chi et al., 2013). Furthermore, Beil and Rozier (2010) found that children 2 to 5 years old who received a recommendation by a PCP to see a dentist were more likely to have a dental examination.

Bacterial Diseases of the Mouth

Tooth Decay

Tooth decay is a bacterial disease. The decay is caused by acid demineralization of the tooth's subsurface enamel. The acid is produced by bacteria (e.g., *Streptococcus mutans*) after metabolism of carbohydrates in the diet. Unless neutralized and buffered by saliva or remineralized with fluorides, the demineralization process leads to cavitation, or creation of holes. Although not involved in the initiation of cavities, lactobacilli are frequently found in cavities and contribute to their progression (Anil et al., 2017).

In infants, prolonged exposure to infant formula, sugary beverages such as juice, or breast milk is especially impactful when the infant is put to sleep with the nipple in the mouth or when allowed to "graze" on sweet fluids throughout the day. Frequent carbohydrate exposure, from continuous snacking, keeps the pH of mouth fluid near the tooth surface less than 5 and results in an acidic environment conducive to demineralization. The neutralization process does not have enough time to increase the mouth pH to a level that would allow remineralization. In children undergoing chemotherapy or radiation to the head and neck and/or who are immunocompromised, normal salivary flow and salivary buffering of acids can also be disrupted, putting them at risk for cavities.

The main risk factors in the development of cavities can be categorized as microbiologic, dietary, and environmental. Even though it is largely a preventable condition, tooth decay remains one of the most common childhood diseases. The major contributing factors for the high prevalence are improper feeding practices, familial socioeconomic background, lack of parental education, and lack of access to dental care, as well as the presence of tooth decay in other family members (Anil et al., 2017). Primary teeth are needed for proper nutrition and mastication, esthetics, phonetics, and maintaining space for permanent teeth.

Clinical Findings

- *Early* tooth decay: Early caries appear as white or brown horizontal lines or spots along the central gum line or gingival margin (Fig 23.4). When white lesions occur, the dentin is initially damaged. Then, as the lesion progresses, the hard enamel breaks, and a clinical cavity is evident.
- *Advanced* tooth decay: Advanced decay appears as cavitations in the teeth. Nearly all cavities in children's permanent teeth begin on the biting surface of the molars. The initial lesion appears as a pinhole surrounded by a white, opaque halo. As the lesion enlarges, greater damage to the enamel becomes apparent.
- Associated signs and symptoms:
  - Sensitivity: Cavities can be hot, cold, or sweet sensitive.
  - Localized dental or facial pain
  - Abscesses on the gums due to bacterial invasion of the pulpal tissue
  - Gingival inflammation
  - Possible lymphadenopathy or fever

PCPs should know that cavities may spontaneously arrest. This arrest is thought to occur when cavities are exposed to saliva high in fluoride or with changes in dietary and/or feeding practices. Arrested caries appear as open cavities that are black or dark brown. If the child has such open cavities in a primary tooth/teeth, is asymptomatic, and access to dental care is problematic, these teeth can be left alone and allowed to shed normally.

Management and Prevention Strategies

Active Decay. When tooth decay is present, decay can be arrested painlessly by topically treating the decayed surfaces with 38% diamine fluoride (NOTE: side effect is black staining of the lesion). This treatment was cleared by the FDA in mid-2014 (Horst et al., 2016). Even though cavities treated with silver diamine fluoride turn dark, parent acceptance is high (Crystal et al., 2017).

A decision to repair or remove teeth depends on the extent of damage and the length of time until the tooth would be normally exfoliated. Retention of primary molars is important because they hold space to allow the normal eruption of permanent successors. Larger cavities in primary teeth can be repaired atraumatically with plastic fillings or with steel or plastic crowns (Frencken, 2017; Innes et al., 2017). Teeth with deep cavities and draining abscesses are generally extracted. Young children may need to be sedated or receive treatment under a general anesthetic to meet extensive treatment needs, making tooth decay arrest with topical treatment and interim restorative care—at least until they get older to allow conventional dental treatment—a noteworthy option. In some cases, arresting decay will allow the space to be maintained and the tooth to be shed normally.

Cavities in permanent teeth are also repaired with either silver amalgam or tooth-colored composite resin (plastic) fillings. Approximately half of a silver amalgam filling is composed of liquid mercury, a binder for the other amalgam components (silver, copper, and other metals). Although mercury releases low levels of vapor, the FDA, based on scientific evidence, considers silver amalgams safe for children. The mercury levels from amalgams have been determined by the Environmental Protection Agency (EPA) and the Centers for Disease Control and Prevention (CDC) to be below the lowest levels associated with brain and kidney toxicity. They are also considered safe for use in pregnant and lactating women and children younger than 6 years old (FDA, 2014). However, amalgams are less commonly used currently, having been replaced by composite fillings. Severe cavities resulting in abscess formation in permanent teeth are treated with root canal therapy. Permanent molars either need to be capped after root canal therapy (e.g., crown) or treated with large amalgam fillings to avoid fracture.

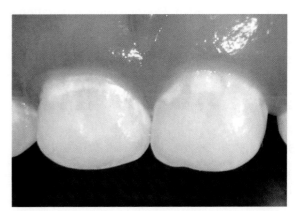

• **Fig 23.4** White Spots (From Cameron AC, Widmer RP, eds. *Handbook of Pediatric Dentistry*. 2nd ed. London: Mosby/Elsevier; 2003.)

Sealants. Pit and fissure (occlusal) plastic or glass-ionomer cement sealants are effective in preventing tooth decay in high-risk children (Mickenautsch and Yengopal, 2016). Poverty alone is not a good indicator of risk because at least half of poor children in the United States have no tooth decay. High-risk children are those who have experienced primary teeth decay and/or have ongoing exposure to diets with high amounts of refined carbohydrates and sugar-sweetened beverages. Sealants are polymerizing resin or glass ionomer coatings placed on the biting surfaces of primary molars at 2 to 3 years old and permanent molars at about 6 to 7 years old and 13 to 14 years old (Fig 23.5).

Fluoride Varnish. Early white spot lesions in primary and/or permanent teeth can be remineralized using topical fluoride varnish. Fluoride varnish is the agent of choice for young children. Fluoride gels are not recommended, because of the risk of acute toxicity. In many states, PCPs are permitted to apply fluoride varnish are reimbursed by insurance plans, including the Affordable Care Act (ACA), Medicaid, and CHIP programs. Twice-yearly applications have been shown to reduce tooth decay by approximately one-third. More frequent applications may be needed in high-risk children (every 3 to 6 months). The decision to place fluoride on a child's teeth should be based on the child's underlying risk for tooth decay (AAPD, 2017c). Plasma fluoride levels following applications of varnish are low and are not associated with toxicity or fluorosis.

To apply fluoride varnish:
1. Dispense approximately 0.25 mL of fluoride varnish into a small well. Prepackaged individual-dose systems come with their own well that is filled with varnish. To avoid risk of overexposure, use only the size package recommended for the age of the child.
2. Dry the teeth with air or gauze to remove excess moisture.
3. While keeping the teeth isolated from further moisture contamination, paint the varnish onto the teeth with a brush or applicator. Only a light coat is required. The varnish sets on contact with the slightly moist teeth.

PCPs are in a key position to have discussions with concerned parents about the safety of fluoride varnish, as well as other sources of topical fluoride (drinking water, toothpastes) important in cavity prevention (Chi, 2017).

Fluoride in Water, Infant Formulas, and Fluoride Supplementation. The most effective preventive measure against dental caries is optimizing community water fluoridation levels to no more than 0.7 milligrams of fluoride per liter of water (This recommended level updates and replaces the previously recommended range of 0.7 to 1.2 milligrams per liter). The fluoride level of public water supplies can be ascertained by calling the local health department. Children who consume fluoride-deficient water and who are at risk for caries will benefit from dietary fluoride supplementation (Moyer and USPSTF, 2014).

Providers should be aware of the status of fluoride in the community and routinely ask new families about fluoride in their water source. If the child is on a private water supply, the naturally occurring fluoride level should be tested before prescribing fluoride supplements. To prevent overdose, no prescription should be written for more than a total of 120 mg of fluoride. See Table 23.1 for adjusting the dose of fluoride supplements in relation to that found in the community/well water supply.

Current FDA regulations require that fluoride be listed on the bottled water or infant formula label only if fluoride is added during processing, but the concentration does not have to be stated.

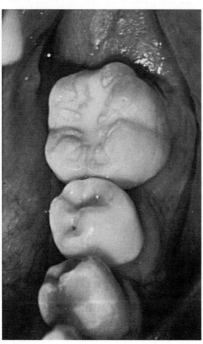

• **Fig 23.5** Sealant. (From Pinkham JR. *Pediatric Dentistry: Infancy Through Adolescence.* 4th ed. St. Louis: Saunders; 2005:537.)

TABLE 23.1	Recommended[a] Fluoride Supplementation Based on Drinking Water Fluoride Concentration		
	FLUORIDE ION LEVEL IN DRINKING WATER (PPM)[b]		
Age	**<0.3 ppm**	**0.3-0.6 ppm**	**>0.6 ppm**
Birth to 6 months old	None	None	None
6 months old to 3 years old	0.25 mg/day[c]	None	None
3-6 years old	0.50 mg/day	0.25 mg/day	None
6-16 years old	1 mg/day	0.50 mg/day	None

[a]Take all sources of fluoride into consideration—from water (including bottled) and amount and frequency of fluoridated toothpaste used in brushing.

[b]Optimal concentration of fluoride in water supply in mg/L or parts per million (ppm).

[c]2.2 mg sodium fluoride contains 1 mg fluoride ion.

From American Academy of Pediatric Dentistry (AAPD). Policy on the use of fluoride. *Pediatr Dent.* 2017;39(6):29–30.

A child who uses bottled water instead of fluoridated community water may need fluoride supplementation. On the other hand, powdered infant formulas reconstituted with fluoridated water may pose an increased risk of fluorosis because of the prolonged accumulative effect of fluoride on enamel development. The CDC maintains *My Water's Fluoride,* a website where people can find links to information on fluoride from their local water systems.

Fluorosis. Fluorosis is a complication of too much systemic fluoride exposure during the years of enamel development. With the increased availability of fluoride toothpaste, surveys showed there has been an increase in all levels of fluorosis (Beltrán-Aguilar et al., 2010). In mild cases, the fluorosis appears as lacey white streaks that are largely unnoticeable. Moderate fluorosis is similar in appearance but covers more of the tooth. In rare cases, severe fluorosis (Fig 23.6) appears as pitting and brown spots in the enamel. When the risk for caries is high, the benefit of fluoride outweighs the risk of mild or moderate fluorosis (AAPD, 2017c).

Toothbrushing. Parents should be taught to clean a child's teeth with a small toothbrush as soon as teeth erupt, using the "lift the lip" method. The technique involves having a parent lift the child's upper lip and use a soft toothbrush to cleanse each tooth surface. Parents should check regularly to see if dental problems are beginning, looking closely for the signs of demineralization. A demonstration by the PCP during a well-child visit is ideal. By making this an enjoyable routine, the child will become comfortable and any resistance should decrease (e.g., *Brush, Book, Bed*).

Toothpaste. Fluoridated toothpaste works by creating a reservoir of fluoride in the fluid layer of the plaque and saliva that are potentially being damaged by bacterial acids. Although fluoridated toothpastes sold in the United States have similar fluoride levels, the PCP also needs to know the fluoride content level in the community drinking water, other sources of fluoride the child might be consuming, and risk factors for tooth decay prior to recommending the use of fluoride toothpaste in all children (AAPD, 2017c).

Child-flavored toothpastes are easier to introduce. Toothpaste containing whitening or bleaching agents is contraindicated. A small amount of toothpaste should be used. Small is defined as a smear or "rice-sized" for children less than 3 years old and "pea-sized" for children 3 years old and older. The child should not rinse after brushing with fluoridated toothpaste. Swallowing these small amounts of toothpaste twice daily is not harmful; however,

the amount of toothpaste used should be controlled by an adult because young children swallow approximately 35% of what is brushed on. It is important to remember that added systemic intake of fluoride can lead to an increased risk of enamel fluorosis, which is particularly important prior to complete enamel maturation. In children at very high risk for tooth decay, parents should begin brushing teeth with fluoridated toothpaste with the eruption of the first tooth at 6 to 9 months old. Toothpastes and fluoride supplements should be stored out of reach of younger children. If a child ingests a large dose of fluoride, the caregiver should contact 911 immediately.

Diet. Sugar-sweetened beverages with energy-containing sweeteners, such as fruit juice concentrates, sucrose, or high-fructose corn syrup, are the primary source of sugars in Western diets. Fruit juice is not recommended for children younger than age 1 year. For children ages 1 to 3 years, juice should be limited to no more than 4 ounces per day and restricted to mealtimes. Because juices contain high concentrations of sugar, diluting juice with water will likely not prevent tooth decay. For children ages 4 to 6 years, juice intake should be limited to 4 to 6 ounces. For children ages 7 years and older, intake should be limited to 8 ounces.

Bottles should be used only for milk, infant formula, or water. Nursing mothers should not allow their infants to sleep attached to the nipple, and bottles should never be propped during naps or bedtime. Some Women, Infants, and Children (WIC) centers in the United States distribute no-spill training cups to promote appropriate eating behaviors and prevent tooth decay. However, personnel may not be aware of the potential danger of the cups themselves if sugar-sweetened beverages are available ad lib. It is ideal for parents to set established snack and meal times and avoid allowing their child to graze on foods and beverages all day. Use of vitamins containing table sugar (sucrose) and/or gummy vitamins that are sticky should be discouraged.

Topical Iodine. Polyvinylpyrrolidone (PVP) iodine (10% PVP-I or povidone-iodine [betadine solution]) can be painted on the teeth before the application of fluoride varnish for an additive effect to depress the tooth decay–causing bacteria in high-risk children (Tut and Milgrom, 2010). Application of topical iodine alone at 3-month intervals over 12 months has been shown to cause a significant reduction in the growth of flora (Simratvir et al., 2010). The teeth are dried with cotton gauze or air, and the povidone iodine is painted onto the teeth and gums with a cotton-tip applicator and then immediately wiped off with gauze or rinsed with air and water.

Abscesses. Abscesses may appear as swelling on the buccal or palatal gingival mucosa and frequently present with purulent drainage. A child with an abscessed tooth may not always report pain or sensitivity. Untreated abscesses require urgent dental referral because they may develop into life-threatening bony facial space infections, requiring surgical drainage and parenteral antibiotic treatment. If a dentist or oral surgeon is not immediately available for drainage and the abscess is uncomplicated, antibiotics and pain medication are appropriate interventions prior to further consult (Idzik and Krauss, 2013).

Periodontal Diseases

Gingivitis

Gingivitis is the presence of gingival inflammation without noticeable loss of alveolar bone or clinical attachment of structures that help to anchor the teeth. This condition is caused by plaque and is present in some degree in nearly all children and adolescents.

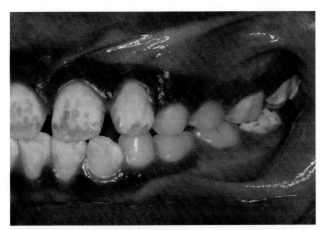

• **Fig 23.6** Severe Flurosis (From Neville BW, Damm DD, Allen CM, et al. Abnormalities of teeth. In: Neville BW, Damm DD, Allen CM, et al., eds. *Oral and Maxillofacial Pathology.* 4th ed. Philadelphia: Elsevier; 2016.)

Hormonal fluctuations inherent in puberty may be a determinant of altered inflammatory response to plaque in this age group (AAPD, 2017d). The gingiva will present with localized or generalized bleeding when brushed or flossed. The teeth will be covered in varying degrees of plaque and calculus secondary to poor or irregular hygiene. The teeth will not be loose. The treatment is brushing and flossing. It can take several days for the gingiva to respond to the improved hygiene. Gingivitis is reversible.

Aggressive Periodontitis

Aggressive periodontitis is a bacterial infection involving the gums and bone. It results in rapid loss of periodontal attachment and supporting bone around the primary or permanent teeth. The primary infection is by *Actinobacillus* and *Bacteroides* species in younger children and by *Treponema* species and other gram-negative rods in older children. Aggressive periodontitis is the most common type of periodontitis in children and adolescents. African-American children are at greater risk (AAPD, 2017d). The overall incidence is approximately 0.2% to 0.5% in children and adolescents, especially those 12 years old and older. For children with a familial history of periodontitis, frequent dental examinations and radiographs during the peripubertal period are essential.

The disease may be localized, involving the surrounding gums and bone around primary incisors and molars (localized), or generalized, involving all teeth. Teeth may become loose, but in the localized form there is generally no inflammatory response, suppuration, or fever. Children with suspected periodontitis should be referred to a dentist for local debridement (deep cleanings) and coordinated management with systemic antibiotics. The major complication of aggressive periodontitis is loss of bone and tooth attachment, resulting in the loss of teeth. Individuals should be counseled that tobacco products increase the risk periodontal disease and should be avoided.

Necrotizing Periodontal Disease

Necrotizing periodontal disease is an aggressive disease resulting in damage to the gum tissue between the teeth. Children typically have severe gingival pain and fever. The triangular area of gums between the teeth is ulcerated and necrotic and covered with a gray film. There may be a fetid mouth odor. The gum tissues harbor high levels of spirochetes, and invasion of the tissues has been demonstrated. Predisposing factors are viral infections (including human immunodeficiency virus [HIV] and other systemic diseases), malnutrition, emotional stress, and lack of sleep. Although the incidence in North America is less than 1% of children and adolescents, the prevalence is greater in individuals from Africa, Asia, and/or South America (Tinanoff, 2011a). Careful oral hygiene and a bland diet are recommended. As with all periodontal conditions, individuals should be referred to a dentist or periodontist.

Pyogenic Granuloma

Pyogenic granuloma is an inflammatory hyperplasia that is usually caused by low-grade localized infection, trauma, or hormonal factors. It is usually a small exophytic (i.e., outward growing) lesion that can be smooth, lobulated, and/or hemorrhagic. It typically occurs on the gingiva, lips, tongue, buccal mucosa, and hard plate. The surface color ranges from pink to red to deep purple, depending on how long the lesion has been present in the oral cavity. Pyogenic granulomas can occur after 4 years of age but are more common in pregnant women, including teens. Possible treatments include improved oral hygiene, 0.12% chlorhexidine gluconate

rinses, surgical excision, cryosurgery, or intralesional injections of corticosteroids. PCPs can begin with improved oral hygiene efforts and/or chlorhexidine; however, if it does not resolve, the individual should be referred to a dentist or periodontist.

Viral Diseases of the Mouth

Herpes Stomatitis

Herpes gingivostomatitis is a viral disease that results in oral and circumoral ulcers. It is usually caused by herpes simplex virus type 1 (HSV-1) (Fig 23.7) and most commonly affects children 6 months old to 5 years old. Antimicrobials are not appropriate because lesions heal without treatment in 7 to 14 days; however, supportive therapy, such as cold liquids and analgesics, is appropriate. Topical treatment with an equal mixture of diphenhydramine and Maalox may also provide symptomatic relief. It is recommended to remove the child from day care or school during the drooling phase of the illness. Encourage parents to clean the teeth with a soft toothbrush or cloth. Oral acyclovir can reduce the degree and length of symptoms if initiated within 3 days of the onset of the initial episode, while topical antiviral agents are ineffective (Prober, 2012).

Herpes stomatitis/labialis may be confused with aphthous ulcers (canker sores), ulcerative gingivitis, hand-foot-and-mouth disease, trauma, herpangina, or chemical burns. Rare conditions that may also cause similar lesions are neutrophil defects, systemic lupus erythematosus (SLE), Behçet syndrome, and Crohn disease. It is also important to remember that children with herpes are at increased risk for dehydration. Parents should be instructed to watch for signs and symptoms and seek medical care in such an event. Careful handwashing should be recommended to the child and the caregivers to prevent autoinoculation or transmission of infection to the eyes. An urgent referral to ophthalmology is needed if ocular spread is suspected.

Idiopathic Oral Conditions

Ankyloglossia (Tongue-Tie)

Ankyloglossia, or "tongue-tie," is caused by a short *lingual* frenulum that hinders tongue movement beyond the edge of the lips (Kotlow, 2013). The frenulum may lengthen as the child gets older and not require intervention. If the extent of the ankyloglossia is

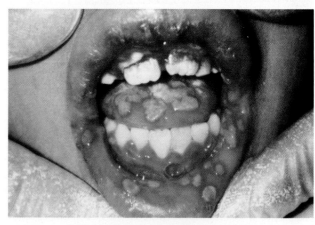

• **Fig 23.7** Herpes Stomatitis in an Infant.

severe, breastfeeding may be difficult and a minor surgical incision, called a frenotomy, may improve feeding (Cochrane, 2017). If speech is affected later in life, referral is also indicated. The evidence supporting frenotomy continues to vacillate about intervening for "tongue-tie," and for "lip-tie," caused by a short *labial* frenulum, when an infant is struggling to latch in breastfeeding (Maria et al., 2017).

Aphthous Ulcers (Canker sores)

The etiology of these recurrent, painful oral ulcers is not well understood. Infectious agents, such as *Helicobacter pylori,* HSV-1, and measles, have been implicated, as well as alterations of cell-mediated immunity. Emotional and physical stress, local trauma (e.g., orthodontic braces, toothbrush abrasion), hormonal factors, genetics, food hypersensitivity, and the presence of sodium lauryl sulfate (SLS) in toothpaste have also been implicated. Vitamin and mineral deficiencies contribute to recurrent oral aphthae, particularly deficiencies in several B vitamins (1, 2, 6, and 12), iron, folic acid, and zinc.

Lesions are present on alveolar or buccal mucosa, tongue, soft palate, or the floor of the mouth. The ulcers are shallow, surrounded with an erythematous halo, and covered by gray, yellow, or white plaques. There are three forms: minor (the most common), major, and herpetiform. *Minor* lesions are less than 10 mm in diameter, whereas *major* lesions (a.k.a. *Sutton disease*) are generally more than 1 cm in diameter and may take a month or more to heal and leave residual scarring. *Herpetiform* lesions are clusters of 1 to 2 mm lesions that may coalesce. Healing should be complete in approximately 7 to 10 days. Prodromal symptoms may occur, including localized tingling or burning. Aphthous lesions may be seen with inflammatory bowel disease, Behçet disease, gluten-sensitive enteropathy, HIV infection, and neutropenia.

The goal of treatment is to decrease the ulcers, relieve pain, and reduce frequency of occurrence. Maintaining good oral hygiene is essential. Minor lesions generally resolve spontaneously in 10 to 14 days and heal without treatment or scarring. A bland diet and oral analgesics may be appropriate. Vitamin or mineral replacement may prevent recurrence, if history suggests a deficiency. Over-the-counter treatments, such as triamcinolone hexacetonide in Orabase paste, fluocinonide gel covered by Orabase paste, or amlexanox 5% oral paste, may be applied 4 times per day for 3 to 4 days for pain relief and to promote healing. A mild mouthwash, such as sodium bicarbonate dissolved in warm water, may also provide comfort, and chlorhexidine gluconate mouthwash (0.12%) can reduce the severity of an episode. Thalidomide has been used in severe cases associated with HIV infection (Weiss et al., 2010). Consider additional diagnostic testing should symptoms and history suggest an infectious agent or gastrointestinal etiology.

Benign Migratory Glossitis (Geographic Tongue; Erythema Migrans)

Benign migratory glossitis (BMG) usually presents as asymptomatic, yellowish-white, circular, or serpentine-bordered lesions with atrophic red centers varying in intensity. The lesions appear on the anterior two-thirds of the dorsum of the tongue (Fig 23.8). The lesions may heal spontaneously and reappear on other areas of the tongue. The etiology is unknown. Occasionally BMG is associated with localized discomfort, especially when eating hot or spicy

foods. Proposed risk factors for BMG include immunologic factors, hormonal changes, use of oral contraceptives, diabetes mellitus, and stress. Patients can be reassured that the lesions are benign and do not generally require treatment.

Bruxism/Grinding

Bruxism is a condition of excessive grinding of the teeth that occurs when awake and/or during sleep. Children, 12 years old or younger, were more likely to report sleep-related bruxism, whereas those 13 years old or older experienced more wake-time tooth clenching. Underlying stressors may be a contributing factor. An increase in bruxism has also been found in children exposed to high or moderate amounts of second-hand smoke (Montaldo et al., 2012).

Primary teeth show marked wear; however, parents can be told that tooth grinding of primary teeth is not associated with damage to permanent dentition. Carra and colleagues (2011) found that both children with sleep-related bruxism and wake-time tooth clenching complained of jaw muscle fatigue. Those with wake-time tooth clenching had more headaches and loud breathing during sleep, whereas those with sleep-related bruxism reported more temporomandibular joint (TMJ) clicking and sleep and behavioral issues.

Evidence supporting the use of plastic night guards is anecdotal, as is support for behavioral methods, such as relaxation training (Lindemeyer, 2018). Elimination of gum chewing has been shown to be effective in helping to manage facial muscle pain and headache.

Dental Erosion

Dental erosion is a chemical process that leads to irreversible acid demineralization of tooth structure. Acids that cause dental erosion can be classified as intrinsic or extrinsic. *Intrinsic* acids include stomach acid introduced into the oral cavity by gastroesophageal reflux disorder (GERD), and/or vomiting. *Extrinsic* acids include acidic beverages, methamphetamines, citrus fruits (e.g., sucking on lemons), and medications (e.g., chewable vitamin C tablets). Factors that can aggravate dental erosion include xerostomia (a.k.a. "dry mouth") secondary to decreased salivary flow, medications that

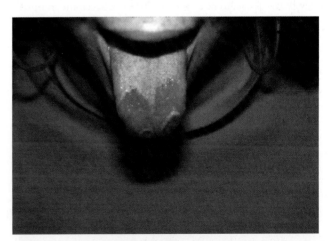

• **Fig 23.8** Benign Migratory Glossitis, or Geographic Tongue (From Morelli JG. Disorders of the mucous membranes. In: Kliegman RM, Stanton BF, St. Geme JW, et al., eds. *Nelson Textbook of Pediatrics.* 19th ed. Philadelphia: Saunders/Elsevier; 2011:2298, Fig 656.4.)

interfere with saliva composition or production (e.g., clonidine), dental attrition, and dental abrasion. Children and adolescents with bulimia nervosa frequently present with dental erosion. Children with asthma also have greater amounts of dental erosion, which may be due to increased gastroesophageal reflux in those with asthma, medications, or an increased consumption of erosive beverages taken to counteract the drying effect of inhalers.

Clinical manifestations of dental erosion include smooth, cupped-out teeth on chewing surfaces; fillings that are raised above the normal level of the tooth; overly shiny silver fillings; enamel cuffing along the gums; and tooth hypersensitivity. Mild to moderate dental erosion may be associated with complaints of tooth hypersensitivity. The differential diagnosis includes abrasion caused by gritty substances (coarse toothpaste or toothbrushes with hard bristles) and attrition caused by mechanical forces (tooth grinding [bruxism] or brushing too hard). Tooth decay should also be in the differential.

Early detection, diagnosis, and treatment of dental erosion are critical. Hot and cold sensitivity can be managed by using "sensitive teeth" fluoridated toothpastes, topical fluoride treatments, or silver diamine fluoride applied by the dentist. Unless the erosion is deep, fillings are not required. Typically, the problem can be managed by identifying and eliminating the etiologic agent. Over-the-counter products, such as soft toothbrushes, low-abrasive fluoridated toothpaste, and fluoride rinses, are helpful. Severe dental erosion can lead to dental nerve (pulp) exposures, which can necessitate root canal treatment.

Diastema

A space between any two neighboring teeth is referred to as a *diastema*. During the mixed dentition stage, when both primary and permanent teeth are present, a midline space between the upper front teeth is normal. There may also be diastemas present between other teeth. If the teeth are not otherwise crowded or misaligned, these spaces usually close by the time the permanent maxillary canines fully erupt, and referral is not needed. Diastemas caused by missing incisors or midline supernumerary teeth will persist in the permanent dentition stage and require early referral.

Another cause of a diastema is a prominent labial frenulum, which is the tissue connecting the upper lip to the area of the gums between the front upper teeth (Fig 23.9). Sometimes the frenulum is large and appears to be causing the space between the front teeth.

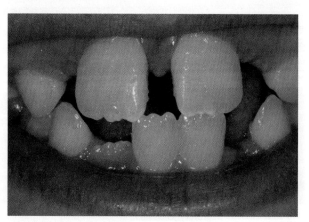

• **Fig 23.9** Diastema: Labial Frenum (Courtesy Donald L. Chi, DDS, PhD, Associate Professor, Department of Oral Health Sciences, University of Washington School of Dentistry.)

In general, the space closes as the jaws grow, and referral is not needed. Unnecessary or premature excision can result in scarring.

Gingival Hyperplasia

Gingival hyperplasia is a fibrous enlargement of gingival tissue around the teeth. The enlargement is typically caused by drugs (e.g., phenytoin, cyclosporine, nifedipine), hormones, chronic inflammation, or leukemia. It can also be idiopathic. The gingival tissue varies, appearing either normal, red-blue, or lighter than the surrounding tissue. It may be spongy or firm. In general, individuals are asymptomatic. Treatment consists of improved oral hygiene and 0.12% chlorhexidine gluconate mouth rinse. In cases in which the overgrowth interferes with chewing, gingivectomy is required.

Halitosis ("Bad Breath")

Halitosis is primarily associated with poor oral hygiene and/or tooth decay; however, its presence may signal systemic disease, sinusitis, sleep apnea, and/or airway related conditions. Halitosis is more common in individuals who are mouth breathers, who suffer from postnasal drip or dry mouth, or who use tobacco products. PCPs should encourage proper oral hygiene, including regular brushing (including the tongue), flossing, and dental visits, as well as avoiding sugar-containing breath mints and other candies that might cause tooth decay or erosion. Artificially sweetened gum or mints may be helpful. Individuals who have not had their teeth cleaned or an oral examination within the past 6 months should be referred to a dentist. For those with oral dryness, there are bioactive enzyme mouthwashes and lozenges available over the counter.

Malocclusion

Malocclusions have their basis in hereditary and/or environmental factors. Environmental factors include the premature loss of teeth due to trauma, caries, ectopic eruptions, and/or persistent use of a pacifier and/or thumbsucking beyond infancy. Southeast Asian populations have the greatest degree of severe malocclusion, and East Indian populations have the least (Hardy et al., 2012). In the United States, an estimated 57% to 59% of children younger than 18 years old require orthodontic treatment for malocclusion.

Malocclusions include anterior and posterior crossbites, as well as open bites. An *anterior* crossbite is due to crowding where one or more teeth are either behind or in front of the teeth in the opposing jaw while the others are in good alignment. With a *posterior* crossbite, one or more of the upper teeth is inside the opposing lower tooth. With an anterior *open* bite, the front teeth do not touch together when the back teeth are biting; these children may have a habit of passing their tongues through the space. They can also have problems speaking or chewing.

Malocclusion may have serious esthetic implications, affecting the self-esteem of the child or adolescent. Orthodontic treatment is not always available or affordable for many; however, whenever possible, PCPs should engage these dental health specialists earlier rather than later.

Mucocele

A mucocele is a salivary gland lesion caused by a blockage of a salivary gland duct. It is most common on the lower lip and has the appearance of a fluid-filled vesicle or a fluctuant nodule with the overlying mucosa normal in color. The most probable cause is trauma or a habit of lip biting. The individual should be referred to an oral surgeon for surgical excision (Fig 23.10).

Pericoronitis

Pericoronitis is due to a partially erupted lower wisdom tooth with a tissue flap covering part of the crown. A foreign body, such as a piece of food, is forced under the flap, causing a localized infection. In some cases, upper wisdom teeth will erupt with the crown rubbing against the buccal mucosa and cause pain. Partially erupted wisdom teeth can create an environment in which the distal surface of the second molar becomes decayed, because it cannot be cleaned. The gum tissue partially covering the tooth is inflamed and painful, and fever may be present. The tissue flap may show trauma from biting.

Not all wisdom teeth need to be removed. Most teeth that are fully covered in bone do not need to be removed and carry no significant risk. Similarly, if there is space for the erupting teeth, there is no reason to remove them. It is appropriate to wait for the teeth to fully erupt as much as they can because this maximizes the chance that they will not need to be removed and minimizes injuries associated with the surgery. Impacted teeth, unerupted teeth with cysts, and upper teeth that have erupted toward the buccal mucosa should be examined and assessed for surgical removal.

Removal of wisdom teeth always requires a risk-benefit calculation because there is significant morbidity associated with the surgery. Temporary or permanent nerve damage is possible, as is TMJ disorder (Huang et al., 2014). A common complication of wisdom tooth surgery is alveolar osteitis or dry socket. This painful condition is associated with the loss of the normal clot in the healing socket that exposes bone. Smoking and the use of oral contraceptives are risk factors. Pretreatment rinsing with 0.12% chlorhexidine gluconate mouth rinse reduces the risk of complications. Treatment at the time of surgery with a nonsteroidal antiinflammatory may reduce the extent of swelling postoperatively. Pain and foul taste in the mouth are the main symptoms, beginning 4 to 5 days after surgery. Referral to the dentist is imperative.

Ranula

A ranula is a cyst filled with mucin from a ruptured salivary gland. It most often appears as a large, soft, mucous-containing swelling in the floor of the mouth. The cyst should be excised by an oral surgeon (Fig 23.11).

Temporomandibular Joint Disorder (TMJ)

TMJ disorder includes chronic facial pain and mandibular dysfunction. It appears to be multifactorial in origin (Fillingim et al., 2011). Studies suggest that the onset of most TMJ disorders increases with age with greater occurrence during adolescence. Prevalence rates range from 4.2% to 25% in those 5 to 19 years old. Females have significantly higher rates (correlated to onset of puberty) than males (AAPD, 2017e). Third molar (i.e., wisdom teeth) removal can result in TMJ disorder (Huang et al., 2014).

Clinical symptoms may include self-reported facial (e.g., face, neck, temples, or jaw) pain once or more times per week associated with limitation in normal ability to open the mouth wide or with chewing; jaw locking; painful clicking, popping, or grating in jaw joint; and/or change in occlusion. On examination, the facial muscles are tender to palpation, often unilaterally, but there is usually no swelling or skin bruising. The individual will be afebrile. Tooth pain, if present, is nonspecific. There may be a deviation to the painful side when the mouth is opened. Pain, particularly in the chewing muscles and/or jaw joint, is the most common symptom.

The differential diagnoses include infection of the face, ear, or teeth; traumatic injury (e.g., fracture/dislocation of the jaw); myositis; sinusitis; headaches; neoplasm; arthritis; collagen diseases (e.g., SLE); congenital and developmental anomalies of the joint (rare); and capsulitis.

Conservative treatment should always be the first course of treatment because invasive, irreversible approaches have not proven effective (surgery, bite appliances, orthodontics, jaw implants, adjusting the bite) (National Institutes of Dental and Craniofacial Research [NIDCR], 2017 and National Institutes of Health [NIH], 2017). Recommendations include avoiding extreme jaw movements, soft diet, muscle relaxation and gentle stretching exercises, application of ice packs, analgesics, and antiinflammatory medication. A short-term, removable plastic splint (goes over the upper or lower teeth) may be fitted by a dentist to see if pain relief is achieved.

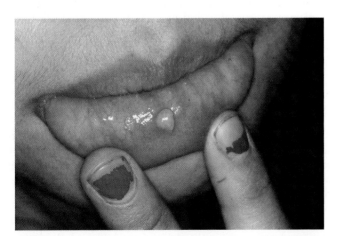

• **Fig 23.10** Mucocele (From Morelli JG. Disorders of the mucous membranes. In: Kliegman RM, Stanton BF, St. Geme JW, et al., eds. *Nelson Textbook of Pediatrics*. 19th ed. Philadelphia: Saunders/Elsevier; 2011:2298, Fig 656.2.)

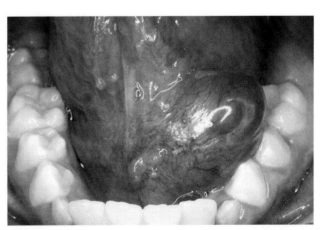

• **Fig 23.11** Ranula of the Floor of the Mouth (From Neville BW, Damm DD, Allen CM, et al., eds. *Oral and Maxillofacial Pathology*. 2nd ed. St. Louis: Saunders/Elsevier; 2002.)

Evidence does not support the supposition that chewing gum, bad bite, or orthodontic care causes TMJ disorder, but chewing gum may exacerbate it. Botox is currently being studied to see if it might be a useful treatment for chronic TMJ disorder. Individuals who do not respond to the basic recommendations need referral to specialized centers with expanded oral health teams that include dentists and psychologists, because adaptive behaviors to the discomfort or pain include being anxious, depressed, avoiding social interaction, developing other physical symptoms (e.g., migraines, tension headaches, back pain, ulcers, colitis), or seeking pharmacologic relief.

Traumatic Injuries to Oral Structures

Injuries to the face usually result in trauma to the soft tissues of the mouth, teeth, or jaws. Such trauma is one of the most common presentations of young children to dentists. Dental injuries occur secondary to falls, motor vehicle accidents, violence, abuse, contact with hard objects, and sporting activities. Although fewer traumas are seen from supervised, organized sports where children now wear mouth guards, a disproportionate amount of trauma results from unsupervised activities, such as skateboarding. Upper incisors are particularly vulnerable to dental injuries.

Age is a significant consideration in trauma to teeth. Most injuries cluster in three age groups: 1 to 3 years old (falls; physical abuse), 7 to 10 years old (bicycle; playground accidents), and 16 to 18 years old (sports injuries; fights; vehicular accidents) (Tinanoff, 2011b). It is important to rule out physical abuse because the orofacial region is commonly traumatized during such episodes. The PCP should be alert to the possibility of a closed head or neck injury if severe trauma is reported. If child abuse is suspected, call the child abuse hotline.

Clinical Findings

Because a dental injury may become the subject of litigation, a thorough history and examination is mandatory. When possible, an injury should be photographed.

History

- Circumstance—When and how did the trauma occur?
- Presence and/or history of other injuries?
- Safety—Is there any concern for the safety of the child and/or family?
- Family history—Is there a history of physical abuse or drug or alcohol use in the family?
- Impact—Are any problems/limitations occurring because of the trauma?
- Immunizations—Tetanus within the last 5 years? (This question is especially important with soil-contaminated wounds or with complete displacement of a tooth from its socket.)
- Recent dental work—For children presenting with trauma to the inside of the cheek, tongue, or lip, did the child recently receive local anesthetic for dental treatment?

Physical Examination. Blunt trauma tends to cause greater damage to soft tissues and supporting structures, whereas high-velocity or sharp injuries cause luxation (i.e., dislocation) and fractures of the teeth. Children with sports-related injuries can have teeth that are avulsed, fractured, or loosened, or displaced from their normal position.

The examination should include:

- Soft tissue: Palpate jaws/facial skeleton for potential fracture.
- Skin: Look for extraoral lacerations/facial wounds.
- Intraoral mucosa: Look for wounds, swelling, and bruising of the oral mucosa, gingiva, tongue, cheeks, and/or palate.

- Teeth: Look for:
  - Displaced, loose, missing, fractured teeth
  - Root fracture: Caused by injury to the tooth root
  - Bite problems: Check for abnormalities in occlusion
  - Pulp exposure: Bleeding from the broken stump of the tooth itself
  - Color change: Otherwise intact tooth turning dark from internal bleeding
  - Jaw movement: Deviation to one side; pain on opening; decreased range of motion (ROM)

Management and Complications. Most minor injuries to the oral soft tissues do not require suturing unless bleeding is a problem. Wound care should consist of irrigating the area with sterile saline and prescribing water-based 0.12% chlorhexidine gluconate mouth rinse for 2 to 3 minutes twice daily. Avoid alcohol-based rinses because use of these rinses may be painful. If it is determined that a child self-injured the inside of the cheek, tongue, or lip after receiving local anesthesia for dental treatment, the child should be referred to the dentist. Children with avulsed and fractured teeth, those unable to bite normally, and those with jaw injuries should also be referred to a dentist promptly to avoid tooth abscesses, dental pain, and problems with the eruption of permanent teeth.

Complications

Tooth avulsion: Avulsed primary teeth should not be replanted. If permanent teeth are knocked out, timing is important, and the following instructions can be provided over the phone. The child should be referred to a dentist at the same time:

Replant an avulsed permanent, clean tooth immediately. If the tooth is dirty, rinse it gently under cold running water (for <10 seconds), and then replant it (Andersson et al., 2012). Do not rub the root surface. If the tooth can be replanted, have the child bite gently on a handkerchief or clean cloth to keep the tooth in place. The dentist will be able to ensure that the tooth is in the right position and stabilized. If unable to immediately replant the tooth, place the tooth in transport media. *ViaSpan* or *Hanks' Balanced Salt Solution* is preferred. If those are not available, store the tooth in cold milk, physiologic saline, or saliva to prevent dehydration. The prognosis for successful replantation decreases with time. A tooth that is allowed to dehydrate will not be viable after 1 hour; however, it is still important to have a dentist evaluate as soon as possible because there are some interventions that can be taken for a tooth that has been out of its socket for longer than 60 minutes.

- Tooth fracture: If possible, have the child keep the pieces of permanent incisors and place them in saline or water to prevent drying. Sometimes the dentist can temporarily repair the tooth if the fragment is large enough. Tooth fractures with bleeding from the stump are emergencies. Simple fractures not involving the pulp or nerve tissue are not emergencies but still need attention/repair.

Patient/Family Education

Trauma compromises a previously healthy dentition and affects self-esteem and quality of life. In some cases the traumatized tooth may be asymptomatic and appear to be clinically normal. This tooth can subsequently become darker or can become spontaneously symptomatic, with the child reporting cold sensitivity, pain on chewing, or unprovoked pain.

It is important to identify and educate children who are at high risk for dental trauma–related injuries. Children and teenagers who participate in sports should be encouraged to wear mouth guards and helmets. Parents and coaches should also encourage youths to remove all intraoral piercings (e.g., tongue and lip rings or studs) while participating in sports. Parents, coaches, and physical education teachers should be alerted to the importance of including *ViaSpan* or *Hanks' Balanced Salt Solution* in first-aid kits to manage tooth avulsions.

Lifestyle Choices That Affect Dental Health

Oral/Intraoral Piercings and Tattoos

Adolescents may have piercings in the tongue and lower lip or tattoos on the buccal mucosa of the lips. Tissue around tongue studs may be infected, as evidenced by inflammation, swelling, and pain. The inflammation and pain may be an allergic response to the metals in the studs or piercings, particularly nickel. There also may be gum recession or fractures of the lower anterior teeth from metal studs, which can habitually click against the teeth. Tongues, especially after stud insertion, can become swollen.

Of note is that the mouth heals quickly and the inflammatory response should be resolved within 8 to 10 days without treatment. Swelling beyond this time period suggests infection or allergic response. Infection should be treated with 0.12% chlorhexidine gluconate mouthwash twice per day for at least 1 week and a broad-spectrum systemic antibiotic, such as penicillin or clindamycin. If mouth tissue is infected, the ornament should be removed, at least temporarily. If an allergic reaction to nickel is suspected, changing to gold or silver is advised. The PCP should ensure vaccinations are current, especially tetanus and hepatitis B. Deep neck infection, airway obstruction, bleeding, nerve damage, tooth fracture, systemic infections, and hepatitis have been noted. Adolescents contemplating or who have oral piercings should be counseled about:

- Potential for acquiring an infectious disease
- Using regulated practitioners
- Ensuring sterile equipment and noble metals are used
- Completing a hepatitis B vaccination series *before* seeking piercing
- Potential damage to the teeth and gums
- Need to remove studs and piercings during sports

Smokeless Tobacco and Betel Nut Use

Smokeless tobacco is a highly addictive substance. Because it is held in the oral cavity, it not only allows nicotine to enter the bloodstream, it is also detrimental to oral health. Fewer than 9% of all teenagers nationwide report using smokeless tobacco, and it is more prevalent among rural youth. Popular cultural events (e.g., baseball) and heroes/role models (e.g., rodeo riders; baseball players) can make the habit look "cool." Its popularity has also been attributed to intensive promotion and flavors, being viewed as a way to lose weight, and a way to get nicotine without having to frequent restricted smoking areas.

Betel nut (areca) may be crushed and chewed alone or combined with tobacco and held in the cheek like smokeless tobacco. It is the fourth most commonly used drug in the world; is carcinogenic; and is legal in the United States. Nearly 70% of adolescents in the Federated States of Micronesia use betel nut at least once per month, which is a growing concern for the mainland United States because of high rates of migration from the Pacific Islands (Milgrom et al., 2013).

PCPs should examine the posterior buccal vestibule of the lower jaw and the anterior buccal vestibule of the upper jaw. These are the areas where smokeless tobacco and betel nut are commonly held in the mouth. The intraoral findings include leukoplakia (matted white plaques on the soft tissues of the oral cavity), erythroplakia (matted red plaques), gingivitis and gum recession (particularly in the lower jaw), periodontitis, stained teeth, halitosis, and tooth decay (associated with tobacco products that have added sweeteners).

Individuals who use tobacco products and/or betel nut should be assessed for willingness to undergo tobacco cessation treatments. Active family involvement in the lives of children can help to prevent the start of smokeless tobacco use. If children have relatives who use tobacco products, PCPs may need to focus tobacco cessation efforts on these family members. Complications include lip and oral cancer, gingivitis, gum recession, periodontitis, and stained teeth. Studies on the oral effects of electronic cigarettes (e-cigarettes) are just beginning to emerge.

Tooth Whitening (Bleaching)

The desire for "whiter" smiles has resulted in increased demand for tooth whitening. Tooth whitening may be indicated for permanent teeth discolored or stained by trauma, fluorosis, tetracycline consumed during tooth development, or foods and beverages. Adolescents can be particularly self-conscious of discoloration. A pretreatment evaluation by a dentist is recommended prior to bleaching, to determine the etiology of the discoloration and any contraindications to the bleaching. The AAPD recommends judicious use of these products, particularly in a child with mixed primary and permanent teeth.

Tooth whitening can involve the use of over-the-counter kits, in-office treatment, or take-home bleaching trays that are customized by a dentist. The in-office tooth whitening process involves repeated short-term exposure of teeth to carbamide peroxide (typically in the range of 10%–38%) until desired results are achieved. Over-the-counter kits include lower concentration carbamide peroxide in trays or hydrogen peroxide in strips. Most products are used for 2-week periods. There are also numerous gels, rinses, gums, toothpastes, and paint-on films. Higher concentrations of hydrogen peroxide are more effective than lower concentrations. Up to 66% of those using bleaching agents can experience hypersensitive teeth and soft tissue/gum irritation, usually in the initial bleaching stages (AAPD, 2017f). Teeth will generally return to their normal sensation, gum status, and color if treatments are not repeated.

PCPs can educate parents that permanent teeth are naturally darker than primary teeth and in most cases do not need whitening. Unless there are major esthetic concerns that could affect a child's psychosocial development, tooth whitening should not be undertaken until all permanent teeth have fully erupted. This measure will also prevent shade mismatching that can occur when teeth are whitened during the mixed dentition stage.

Eating Disorders

PCPs and dentists may be the first provider to recognize an adolescent with an eating disorder. Purging by vomiting can result halitosis, dry mouth, tooth erosion, translucency, and sensitivity. Stomach acid damages the teeth, notably inside the upper front teeth.

Dental Care for Children With Special Health Care Needs

Children with chronic diseases or with congenital or acquired disabilities often require additional preventive strategies and individualized dental appointments based upon their particular needs and conditions. At-risk children include those with neuropsychological conditions (e.g., intellectual and developmental disability, autism spectrum disorder); sensory challenges (e.g., blindness, visual impairment, deafness, and hearing impairments); musculoskeletal or other structural difficulties (e.g., osteogenesis imperfecta, cerebral palsy, spina bifida, cleft lip/palate, paralysis); and chronic diseases (e.g., asthma, cardiovascular disorders, cystic fibrosis, chronic renal failure, diabetes mellitus, bleeding disorders, malignant disease, and epilepsy).

Low birth weight can be associated with structural tooth defects, which can lead to increased risk for tooth decay. Some individuals have a higher incidence of oral disease either because of a systemic problem or because of the secondary effects on tooth development, diet, medications, or the inability of caretakers to clean or maintain the teeth.

Risks include:

Diet: Children with special health care needs, including congenital heart disease, facial clefts, esophageal defects, generalized hypotonia, muscular dysfunction, or intellectual and developmental disability, often have feeding problems, nutritional alterations/needs, challenges, and forms. In addition, food is often retained in the mouth for a long time before it is swallowed.

Medications: Phenytoin commonly causes gingival hyperplasia. Box 23.1 lists classes of drugs that may reduce salivation and thereby increase susceptibility to caries.

Muscular function: Hypotonia may influence mouth breathing and salivation and cause drooling or chewing problems. Impaired manual dexterity may make it difficult for children to perform preventive oral hygiene routines. Hyperfunction may result in extensive tooth wear as a result of grinding of teeth. Children with feeding tubes face additional challenges because oral health may be overlooked. Preventive dental care for children with special health care needs varies with the complexity and difficulties presented by the child's condition and the family's ability to manage. PCPs are advised to ask about the status of dental visits and whether routine oral hygiene is being maintained. In addition, the following topics should be covered:

Diet: For children with reduced salivary secretion or impaired self-cleaning mechanisms of the oral cavity, parents or caretakers must be especially attentive to the child's diet. Restrictions in

---

• BOX 23.1 **Classes and Examples of Drugs Associated With Decreased Salivation and Xerostomia**

Analgesics: Nonsteroidal antiinflammatory drugs, narcotic analgesics
Antidepressants: Fluoxetine, amitriptyline
Antiemetics: Promethazine, metoclopramide
Antihistamines: Diphenhydramine, promethazine
Antihypertensives: β-Blockers, diuretics, angiotensin-converting enzyme inhibitors
Antipsychotics: Clozapine, chlorpromazine, risperidone

---

cavity-causing foods are necessary to prevent tooth decay. If sweetened medicinal syrups cannot be replaced by sugar-free alternatives, these medications should be taken at mealtime if permitted. Rinsing the mouth and teeth with water after a meal may help if brushing is not feasible. Water or artificially sweetened beverages should be recommended for drinks between meals.

Topical fluorides: A child with reduced salivary secretion, impaired muscular function, or with a cavity-causing diet may need an intense fluoride program in addition to careful oral hygiene. PCPs can apply 5% sodium fluoride topical varnish or prescribe a fluoride rinse, gel, or high-fluoride (1.1% sodium fluoride) toothpaste for home use. Carefully monitor the teeth of these patients and make prompt referrals when problems are noted.

Topical iodine: The teeth and gums can be painted with topical PVP-iodine once every 4 to 6 months. As previously discussed, there is evidence that topical 10% povidone-iodine suppresses tooth decay–causing flora without major changes in the overall flora (Tut and Milgrom, 2010). Children who have had major dental treatment because of extensive dental caries are obvious candidates for repeated iodine treatments. Iodine can be painted on the teeth at the same visit in which fluoride varnish is applied with the iodine wiped off with gauze before applying the varnish. PCPs can do this treatment if dental services are lacking.

References

Afeiche MC, Koyratty BNS, Wang D, et al. Intakes and sources of total and added sugars among 4 to 13-year-old children in China, Mexico and the United States. *Pediatr Obes.* 2018;13(4):204–212. https://doi.org/10.1111/ijpo.12234. Epub 2017 Sep 27.

American Academy of Pediatric Dentistry (AAPD). Policy on the dental home. *Pediatr Dent.* 2017a;39(6):29–30.

American Academy of Pediatric Dentistry (AAPD). Policy on social determinants of children's oral health and health disparities. *Pediatr Dent.* 2017b;39(6):23–26.

American Academy of Pediatric Dentistry (AAPD). Policy on the use of fluoride. *Pediatr Dent.* 2017c;39(6):29–30.

American Academy of Pediatric Dentistry (AAPD). American Academy of Periodontology (AAP)—Research, Science and Therapy Committee: periodontal diseases of children and adolescents. *Pediatr Dent.* 2017d;39(6):431–439.

American Academy of Pediatric Dentistry (AAPD). Best practices on acquired temporomandibular disorders in infants, children, and adolescents. *Pediatr Dent.* 2017e;39(6):354–361.

American Academy of Pediatric Dentistry (AAPD). Policy on the use of dental bleaching for child and adolescent patients. *Pediatr Dent.* 2017f;39(6):90–92.

Andersson L, Andreasen JO, Day P, et al. International Association of Dental Traumatology guidelines for the management of traumatic dental injuries: avulsion of permanent teeth. *Dent Traumatol.* 2012;28(2):88–96.

Anil, et al. Early childhood caries: Prevalence, risk factors, and prevention. *Frontiers in Pediatrics.* 2017. https://doi.org/10.3389/fped.2017.00157.

Beil HA, Rozier RG. Primary health care providers' advice for a dental checkup and dental use in children. *Pediatrics.* 2010;126(2):e435–e441.

Beltrán-Aguilar ED, Barker L, Dye BA. Prevalence and severity of dental fluorosis in the United States, 1999-2004. *NCHS Data Brief.* 2010;53:1–8.

Carra MC, Huynh N, Morton P, et al. Prevalence and risk factors of sleep bruxism and wake-time tooth clenching in a 7- to 17-yr-old population. *Eur J Oral Sci.* 2011;119(5):386–394.

Chi DL. Parent refusal of topical fluoride for their children: clinical strategies and future research priorities to improve evidence-based pediatric dental practice. *Dent Clin North Am.* 2017;61(3):607–617.

Chi DL, Momany ET, Jones MP, et al. Relationship between medical well baby visits and first dental examinations for young children in Medicaid. *Am J Public Health.* 2013;103(2):347–354.

Cochrane. Surgical release of tongue-tie for the treatment of tongue-tie in young babies; 2017. Downloaded from: http://www.cochrane.org/CD011065/NEONATAL_surgical-release-tongue-tie-treatment-tongue-tie-young-babies.

Crystal YO, Janal MN, Hamilton DS, et al. Parental perceptions and acceptance of silver diamine fluoride staining. *J Am Dent Assoc.* 2017;148(7):510–518.

Fillingim RB, Slade GD, Diatchenko L, et al. Summary of findings from the OPPERA baseline case-control study: implications and future directions. *J Pain.* 2011;12(11 suppl 3):T102–T107.

Frencken JE. Atraumatic restorative treatment and minimal intervention dentistry. *Br Dent J.* 2017;223(3):183–189.

Hardy DK, Cubas YP, Orellana MF. Prevalence of angle class III malocclusion: a systematic review and meta-analysis. *Open J Epi.* 2012;2:75–82.

Horst JA, Ellenikiotis H, Milgrom PL. UCSF protocol for caries arrest using silver diamine fluoride: rationale, indications and consent. *J Calif Dent Assoc.* 2016;44(1):16–28.

Huang GJ, Cunha-Cruz J, Rothen M, et al. A prospective study of clinical outcomes related to third molar removal or retention. *Am J Public Health.* 2014;104(4):728–734.

Idzik S, Krauss E. Evaluating and managing dental complaints in primary and urgent care. *JNP.* 2013;9(6):329–338.

Innes NP, Evans DJ, Bonifacio CC, et al. The Hall Technique 10 years on: questions and answers. *Br Dent J.* 2017;24(6):478–483. 222.

Institute of Medicine (IOM) and National Research Council (NRC). *Improving Access to Oral Health Care for Vulnerable and Underserved Populations.* Washington, DC: The National Academies Press; 2011.

Khandelwal V, Nayak UA, Nayak PA, et al. Management of an infant having natal teeth. *BMJ Case Rep.* 2013.

Kotlow LA. Diagnosing and understanding the maxillary lip-tie (superior labial, the maxillary labial frenum) as it relates to breastfeeding. *J Hum Lact.* 2013;29(4):458–464.

Lindemeyer RG. Treating bruxism in children. *Decisions in Dentistry.* 2018;4(2):53–56.

Maria CS, Aby JA, Truong MT, Thakur Y, Rea S, Messner A. The superior labial frenulum in newborns: what is normal? *Global Pediatric Health.* 2017;4:1–6. https://doi.org/10.1177/2333794X17718896. 2017.

Massignan C, Cardoso M, Porporatti AL, et al. Signs and symptoms of primary tooth eruption: a meta-analysis. *Pediatrics.* 2016;137(3):e20153501.

Mickenautsch S, Yengopal V. Caries-preventive effect of high-viscosity glass ionomer and resin-based fissure sealants on permanent teeth: a systematic review of clinical trials. *PLoS One.* 2016;11(1):e0146512.

Milgrom P, Tut OK, Gilmatam J, et al. Areca use among adolescents in Yap and Pohnpei, the Federated States of Micronesia. *Harm Reduct J.* 2013;10:26.

Montaldo L, Montaldo P, Caredda E, et al. Association between exposure to secondhand smoke and sleep bruxism in children: a randomized control study. *Tob Control.* 2012;21(4):392–395.

Moyer VA, US Preventive Services Task Force (USPSTF). Prevention of dental caries in children from birth through age 5 years: US Preventive Services task force recommendation statement. *Pediatrics.* 2014;133(6):1102–1111.

National Institutes of Dental and Craniofacial Research (NIDCR). National Institutes of Health (NIH): TMJ disorders, NIH (website); 2017. Available at: www.nidcr.nih.gov/oralhealth/topics/tmj/tmjdisorders.htm. Accessed November 1, 2017.

Nelson S, Albert JM, Geng C, et al. Increased enamel hypoplasia and very low birthweight infants. *J Dent Res.* 2013;92(9):788–794.

Prober CG. Herpes simplex virus Chapter 204. In: Long SS, Pickering LK, Prober CG, eds. *Principles and Practice of Pediatric Infectious Diseases.* 4th ed. Philadelphia: Elsevier; 2012.

Simratvir M, Singh SM, Chopra S, et al. Efficacy of 10% povidone iodine in children affected with early childhood caries: an in vivo study. *J Am Dent Assoc.* 2010;34(3):233–238.

Themessi-Huber M, Freeman R, Humphris G, et al. Empirical evidence of the relationship between parental and child dental fear: a structured review and meta-analysis. *Int J Paedr Dent.* 2010;20(2):83–101.

Tinanoff N. Periodontal diseases. In: Kliegman RM, Stanton BF, Schor NF, et al., eds. *Nelson Textbook of Pediatrics.* 19th ed. Philadelphia: Elsevier; 2011a.

Tinanoff N. Dental trauma. In: Kliegman RM, Stanton BF, Schor NF, et al., eds. *Nelson Textbook of Pediatrics.* 19th ed. Philadelphia: Elsevier; 2011b.

Tut OK, Milgrom PM. Topical iodine and fluoride varnish combined is more effective than fluoride varnish alone for protecting erupting first permanent molars: a retrospective cohort study. *J Public Health Dent.* 2010;70(3):249–252.

U.S. Department of health and human services (HHS). National Center for Health Statistics: Health, United States, 2013: trends and tables; 2014. Available at: www.cdc.gov/nchs/data/hus/hus13.pdf. Accessed May 5, 2018.

U.S. Food and Drug Administration (FDA). About dental amalgam fillings, FDA (website); 2014. updated 2017. Available at: www.fda.gov/medicaldevices/productsandmedicalprocedures/dentalproducts/dentalamalgam/ucm171094.htm. Accessed May 5, 2018.

U.S. Food and Drug Administration (FDA). FDA Drug Safety Communication: Reports of a rare, but Serious and Potentially Fatal Adverse Effect with the use of Over-the-Counter (OTC) Benzocaine Gels and Liquids Applied to the Gums or Mouth; Updated 8-4-2017. Available at: https://www.fda.gov/drugs/drugsafety/ucm250024.htm.

Weiss A, Nelson P, Dym H. Oral pathology for the primary-care clinician. *Clin Adv.* 2010;13(4):17–22.

24

Injury Prevention and Child Maltreatment

JAIME PANTON AND DAWN LEE GARZON MAAKS

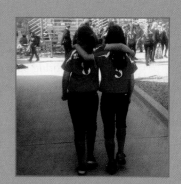

Injuries are the leading cause of death among children older than one year of age and adolescents, causing more death and disability than the other top causes combined. They are classified as unintentional or intentional. Unintentional injuries (UIs) are injuries that are unplanned and without intent to harm the child and include motor vehicle crashes, drowning, falls, fires, poisonings, and other causes. Conversely, intentional injuries result from purposeful inflicted harm, either by oneself or another and include suicide, homicide, or child maltreatment (physical abuse, sexual abuse, emotional abuse, or neglect).

Unintentional Injuries

Globally, over two million child deaths (ages 1 to 14 years) were documented in 2013, the largest proportion caused by motor vehicle crashes (Table 24.1) (Alonge, Khan, and Hyder, 2016). UIs are not simply accidents caused by a twist of fate but rather result from predictable and preventable occurrences, hence the change in terminology from accident to UI. The most common fatal UI in early childhood is drowning, while motor vehicle accidents (MVAs) cause more injury deaths in older children and adolescents (Centers for Disease Control and Prevention [CDC], 2016a). Known UI risks include child factors such as male gender, age (young children have the highest rates, adolescents have the highest fatality rate), child inattention, child oppositionality, child temperament, and risk-taking, and environmental factors include the presence of neighborhood hazards, presence of multiple children in the home, single parents, lower socioeconomic status, and lower family education levels. Young children depend on adults to prevent injury as most children under the age of 6 may be able to report safety rules but often do not actually follow them, and lack the ability to detect risk. Therefore, it is critical that parents have a realistic understanding of their child's development. Parents who overestimate their child's abilities (e.g., the 6-year-old who always knows to check for cars before he crosses the street) or underestimate their child's abilities (e.g., the parent who thinks their 15-month-old will not climb up stairs without a parent being there) may place their children at risk for injury because of inadequate parental supervision.

Principles of Injury Control

The most effective injury prevention education focuses on specific, usable information to decrease injury risk rather than broad, nonspecific recommendations. An injury control framework, such as the Haddon matrix, recognizes factors that contribute to injury in order to develop the most effective injury prevention programs (Table 24.2). Originally based on infection control theory, this theory identifies individual and environmental factors that occur in the pre-injury, injury, and post-events timeframes that affect whether injury occurs and the severities of those injuries.

Passive injury prevention is the most effective strategy for reducing injury and involves the implementation of safety measures that do not require caregivers to change their behavior to make the environment safer for their children. This strategy includes modification of everyday items in the child's environment. Examples include the use of child-resistant caps on medicines and cleaning products, and safety design in toys.

Another safety approach includes environmental modification, such as the use of smoke and carbon monoxide detectors, safe roadway design to reduce traffic volume and speed in residential neighborhoods, window locks, and firearm safety locks. Pediatric primary care providers (PCPs) can advocate for local and national prevention strategies and support programs, such as the Safe Kids USA campaign (www.safekids.org). They also play key roles by supporting injury prevention legislation, promoting initiatives to ensure consumer product safety, and implementing public health strategies to decrease injury. Public and consumer awareness is crucial for successful prevention programs and PCPs, as trusted advisors, are great sources of information about safe, developmentally appropriate toys and products.

Emergency preparedness is important for PCPs and parents. Although most children with serious injuries usually present in emergency departments or urgent care clinics, it is important for PCPs to remain current in basic life support techniques and to have injury management plans in place in case a severely injured child presents in primary care. Likewise, all parents and caregivers should be encouraged to enroll in a basic pediatric life support program, especially parents and caregivers of infants and children at risk for cardiopulmonary arrest.

Common Injury Mechanisms and Injury Control Methods

Unintentional injury control (previously referred to as injury prevention) involves the use of both passive and active strategies to impact individual, social, and physical environmental and vector/vehicle factors that contribute to this phenomenon. The most effective strategies are passive; for example, instituting graduated driving laws, requiring booster seats for older children, using safe road design, requiring minimal safety features for consumer products, and improving access to emergency services if injuries occur. Active approaches include strategies in which the individual takes part in the injury prevention plan such as a parent child-proofing cabinets and drawers containing medications and toxins.

There are three levels of injury control: primary, secondary, and tertiary. Primary interventions focus on how injuries can be prevented (e.g., anticipatory guidance). Secondary levels of prevention focus on decreasing injury severity and include strategies like seat belt and home smoke detector use. Tertiary prevention focuses on reducing morbidity and mortality once the injury occurs (e.g., on-scene management of injury).

Injury control requires a multidimensional approach that includes injury education about how to provide a safe environment and developmentally appropriate supervision, advocating for public health policies that influence injury outcomes, and advocating for safe design and consumer awareness. Effective injury control strategies are developmentally grounded and focus on modifying risk factors, and thus anticipatory guidance provided by PCPs at

TABLE 24.1   Common Causes of Unintentional Injury-Related Death by Age

Age	Mechanism of Injury Death	Anticipatory Guidance[a]
Infants	1. Accidental suffocation 2. Motor vehicle crashes 3. Drowning	• Back to sleep in parent's room but not in parent's bed • Review car seat safety guidelines, instruct parent/caregiver not to drive under the influence
Ages 1-4	1. Drowning 2. Falls 3. Motor vehicle crashes	• Constant supervision around water (pools, bathtubs, lakes, etc.) • Personal flotation devices (life jackets, not floaties) • Swim lessons beginning by age 4 years • Adequate fencing around pools • Do not leave child unattended near or inside of a vehicle
Ages 5-12	1. Motor vehicle crash 2. Drowning 3. Fires/burns	• Review car seat safety guidelines at every well visit • Consistent use of seatbelts • Swim lessons • Adult supervision around water • If on a boat or watercraft, wear Coast-Guard-approved life jacket • Functioning smoke alarms in the home
Ages 13-19	1. Motor vehicle crash 2. Poisoning 3. Drowning	• Prevent distracted driving • Consistent seatbelt use • Homes free of firearms • If a firearm is in the home, it must be stored unloaded and locked with ammunition stored separately

[a]Adapted from Bright Futures.
Hagan JF, Shawn JS, Duncan PM. *Bright Futures: Guidelines for Health Supervision of Infants, Children, and Adolescents.* 4th ed. Elk Grove Village, IL: American Academy of Pediatrics; 2017.

TABLE 24.2   Haddon Phase Factor Matrix for Understanding a Bicycle Injury in a 5-Year-Old Child

| Injury Phase | INJURY FACTORS | | | |
	Individual	Agent	Physical Environment	Social Environment
Pre-Event- Fall precursors	Inattention, bike riding skills, ability to respond to balance changes, sensory deficits	Speed, bald tires, worn brakes	Busy street, road hazards, steep grade on hill, visibility	Does not own bicycle helmet, parental supervision, residential street speed limits, beliefs about injury control
Event-What forces cause injury	Ability to control bicycle, distractions, clothing that protects skin from friction forces (road rash)	Head hits the road without a helmet, gravitational forces, child skids across the road, road surface type	Wet road, surface hardness, high curb on roadside, presence of vehicle on the road	Adult witnessing injury, understanding of injury severity, child injured in a location where he or she can be easily reached, bicycle helmet laws
Post-Event-Injury treatment and recovery	Child's health, ability of wrist fracture and skin to heal, extent of concussion	Did bicycle land on child?	Distance to emergent care, difficulty transporting child to care, quality of care	Ability to afford health care, ability to access follow-up care, family's ability to care for the injuries, social support

well-child visits should be geared to the developmental stage of the child. This includes assessing injury control techniques used within the home, reinforcing positive behaviors, and counseling about additional safety risks (Hagan et al., 2017). Written materials, audiovisual presentations, peer counseling, and one-to-one interaction with a health professional are all effective teaching and learning strategies. Use online resources like www.safekids.org and www.healthychildren.org to help parents find safety information at home. Provide safety information in moderate doses, with reinforcement or repetition at subsequent visits. Research suggests parents only retain a certain amount of information; therefore, only about four or five of the most developmentally appropriate teaching points should be discussed. Injury prevention education should be tailored to the risks of the provider's specific population. If firearm deaths are a leading cause of death in the area, anticipatory guidance should focus on safe storing of firearms in the home or removing firearms altogether from the home. Counseling should also be specific. For example, teaching parents how to purchase the appropriately sized bicycle helmet is more effective then general statements such as always wear a helmet.

Motor Vehicle–Related Injuries

MVAs are a leading cause of pediatric injury, death, and disability. Each year over 5000 children die as a result of MVAs, a number that represents 15% of the overall MVA deaths (Durbin et al., 2018). The greatest way to modify child MVA outcomes is through the use of child restraint systems. Teen driver distraction, substance use, risk-taking behaviors, and relative driving inexperience are known adolescent risk factors. All-terrain vehicles, snowmobiles, motorcycles, and other motorized vehicles also contribute to this phenomenon.

Passenger restraint systems, including infant seats, booster seats, and seatbelts effectively prevent significant injury. It is important to select and install car restraints according to the manufacturer's recommendations (Fig 24.1). Current child restraint guidelines (Durbin et al., 2018) call for the following:

- Infants and toddlers should be kept rear-facing as long as possible, at least until they outgrow the maximum height and weight for their car seat.
- Young children who have outgrown rear-facing seats should transition to a foreword facing restraint that includes a harness until they outgrow the height and weight maximums for their car seat.

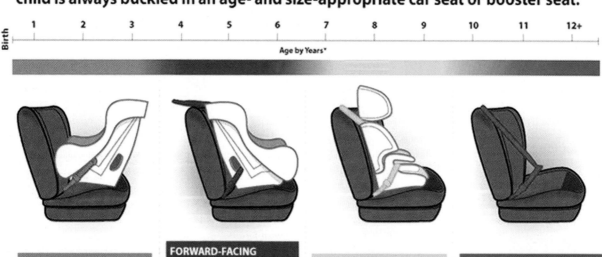

Using the correct car seat or booster seat can be a lifesafer: make sure your child is always buckled in an age- and size-appropriate car seat or booster seat.

REAR-FACING CAR SEAT

Birth until age 2-4

Buckle children in a rear-facing car seat until they reach the maximum weight or height limit of their car seat. Keep children rear-facing as long as possible.

FORWARD-FACING CAR SEAT

After outgrowing rear-facing seat until at least age 5

When children outgrow their rear-facing car seat, they should be buckled in a forward-facing car seat until they reach the maximum weight or height limit of their car seat.

BOOSTER SEAT

After outgrowing forward-facing seat and until seat belts fit properly

Once children outgrow their forward-facing seat, they should be buckled in a booster seat until seat belts fit properly. Proper seat belt fit usually occurs when children are 4 feet 9 inches tall and age 9-12.

SEAT BELT

Once seat belts fit properly without a booster seat

Children no longer need to use a booster seat once seat belts fit them properly. Seat belts fit properly when the lap belt lays across the upper thighs (not the stomach) and the shoulder belt lays across the chest (not the neck).

Keep children ages 12 and under properly buckled in the back seat. Never place a rear-facing car seat in front of an active air bag.

Recommended age ranges for each seat type vary to account for differences in child growth and height/weight limits of car seats and booster seats. Use the car seat or booster seat owner's manual to check installation and the seat height and weight limits, and proper seat use.

Child safety seat recommendations: American Academy of Pediatrics.
Graphic design: adapted from National Highway Traffic Safety Administration.
www.cdc.gov/motorvehiclesafety/cps

• **Fig 24.1** How to Select the Correct Car Seat (Courtesy CDC https://www.cdc.gov/features/passenger-safety/ingofraphic.html.)

- Once the harness car seat is outgrown, children should remain in booster seats until they are 4 foot 9 inches tall and are between 9 and 12 years old.
- Seat belts should not be used without a booster until: the shoulder belt fits across the mid chest, not the face or neck; the lap belt fits across the pelvis, not the lower abdomen; and the child can sit in the car with the legs bent without slouching for the entire length of the trip. Both chest and lap restraints should be used at all times.
- Children should not sit in the front seat until they are 13 years old.

Adolescent drivers require additional injury control strategies. These include (Hagan et al., 2017):
- Comprehensive graduated driving laws help decrease deaths and injuries caused by inexperience by controlling movement from the learner's permit to the independent license, limiting nighttime driving, limiting passengers for teen drivers, and by setting a minimum age at 18 for full licensure. These laws vary from state to state so PCPs should be aware of rules in their area.
- Parents should consider adding their own safety rules by creating a driving agreement. This covers restrictions, rules, and consequences for violations. An example can be found online at https://www.healthychildren.org/English/ages-stages/teen/safety/Pages/Teen-Driving-Agreement.aspx.
- Distraction is a leading reason for MVAs. Technology including phones and other electronic devices can be placed in "driving mode" so that they are not able to be used when moving. There are apps that prevent texting while driving. Other resources are available online at www.distraction.gov.
- Adults should model driving safety behaviors including seatbelt use, never driving when under the influence, avoiding aggressive driving, and never using technology while driving.

Falls

Falls are the leading cause of nonfatal injuries and the most common injury type. Every day in the United States, 8000 children require emergency room treatment for falls (CDC, 2016b). These occur with slips and falls, falls from a distance (stairs, windows, or balconies), during sports, secondary to infant walker use, from playsets, and in homes, schools, playgrounds, and child care settings.

The following points are important components of patient and parent fall control education:
- Always watch children on playground equipment. Ensure that there is sufficient padding from either wood chips or sand. Grass does not absorb fall energy well.
- Place skid pads underneath carpets and rugs and remove those that still slide even with skid pads.
- Place stair gates at the top and bottom of staircases. Consider using guard rails to prevent young children from getting access through spindles.
- Be cautious about leaving furniture and items that can be easily moved to allow a young child to reach areas by climbing.
- Use window guards for open windows above ground level.
- Always use bicycle helmets when using wheeled toys and bicycles. Recommend wrist guards and knee/elbow pads when skating.

Drowning

Drowning kills more young children between birth and 4 years old than anything other than congenital defects (CDC, 2016a). Supervision and environmental modification to decrease water access are leading drowning protective factors. Drownings commonly occur in bodies of water (lakes, rivers, oceans), swimming pools, bathtubs, and from falling head first into buckets, toilets, or other containers with liquids.

Drowning injury control occurs by teaching families to:
- Never leave young children unattended when they are around water. This includes bathtubs, kiddie pools, spas, above- and below-ground pools, and natural water features like creeks, ponds, etc. Do not assume that drowning children make noise.
- Parents should be careful of being distracted when watching children around water. This includes technology, conversations with others, and alcohol or other substance use.
- Everyone should learn basic water skills like how to float and basic swimming. Lessons can begin as early as age 1 year old, but the evidence for lessons prior to that age is lacking (AAP, 2018).
- Fence off pools with a latched gate.
- Use personal flotation devices whenever near or in bodies of water.
- Never leave unattended buckets of water or other liquids around young children. Five gallon and larger buckets are especially dangerous. A young child can drown in as little as one inch of standing water left in a bucket or container.

Fires/Burns

Burns are usually caused by scalding liquids in infancy and early childhood while flames cause most burns in older children. Young children's burns commonly occur when they splash themselves by pulling objects filled with hot liquids (e.g., grabbing pot handles from the stove, pulling tablecloths/table runners and causing hot food or liquids spill, bathing in water that is too hot) or playing with lit candles. Older children may mistakenly start fires or be burned with intentional fires. Residential fires can occur with the use of space heaters, smoking in bed, while cooking, and with electrical shorts.

The following points are important components of patient and parent education:
- Emphasize use of sunscreen protection (Chapter 34).
- Discuss home and environmental safety issues related to burn prevention at health maintenance visits. Key points to discuss with families include:
  - Install and maintain smoke alarms in the home on every floor and near rooms where people sleep.
  - Keep the hot water heater thermostat at 120°F or lower.
  - Turn pot handles away from the stove edge.
  - Never leave cooking food on the stove or hot food unattended.
  - Create and practice a family fire escape plan for the home.
  - Be careful about leaving hot mugs and bowls within reach of infants and young children.
  - Use table runners and tablecloths with caution as they can be used to pull hot items down on young children.
  - Place barriers in front of open fireplaces or heating stoves to limit access to young children.
  - Never leave space heaters within reach of young children, and never leave them unattended.
  - Use caution to ensue cords from hot items (irons, hair straighteners, curling irons) are left out of reach of young children.
  - Make sure ground-fault circuit interrupters (GFCIs) are functional and socket protectors and/or child-proof electrical outlets are in use in homes with young children.

- Reinforce injury prevention after a burn injury occurs (e.g., scald prevention, safekeeping of matches and cigarette lighters, safe use of electric cords and outlets).
- Teach burn first-aid measures (e.g., submerge minor burned area in tepid water; do not use butter, margarine, and oil-based creams and lotions; rinse chemical burns in cold water, and flush skin thoroughly for at least 20 minutes).

Poisoning

Poisoning is a major cause of pediatric injury. In the United States in 2016, more than 2.1 million poison exposure calls were made to the National Poison Control Center, almost half in children 5 years old or younger. In younger children, poison exposures are almost always unintentional (99%), but in adolescents 66% are intentional. In children 6 years of age and younger, the top causes of poisoning fatality include: fumes/gases/vapors, analgesics, unknown drugs, and batteries (National Poison Control Center, 2017). Disc/button battery(ies) or magnet(s) in any body cavity require emergent care because both can cause serious complications (e.g., corrosion of tissues, gastrointestinal perforation) and risk of death.

The American Association of Poison Control Centers (AAPCC) (2017) recommends the following to prevent childhood poisoning:
- Store the following up, away, out of the child's sight, in their original containers, and in cabinets with child-resistant locks:
  - All medications and pharmaceuticals, including OTC medications, vitamins, and supplements
  - Tobacco, e-cigarette products, marijuana (cannabis) products, and alcohol
  - Laundry and cleaning supplies
  - Pesticides and insect repellents
  - Button batteries
  - Any type of oil, lubricant, or other chemical
  - Personal care products, including cosmetics, contact lens cleaner, and hand sanitizers
  Other important strategies include:
- Never mix cleaning chemicals. Read and follow cleaning product label instructions.
- Apply insect repellent according to label instructions, not on hands, and wash off after returning indoors.
- Detect invisible threats (see Chapter 4) such as carbon monoxide, asbestos, radon.
- Do not share medicines with anyone else. Be cautious not to use more than one medication with the same active ingredient.
- Ensure proper medication disposal: visit http://disposemymeds.org, ask a pharmacist, or call the poison center (1-800-222-1222). Some communities host medicine take-back programs.
- Encourage smoking cessation for caregivers who use tobacco, nicotine, or cannabis.
- Avoid poisonous plants and mushrooms (varies by region).
- Store and prepare food safely. Visit https://www.foodsafety.gov for more information.
- Cosmetics and personal care products, cleaning substances, and analgesics are the top overall causes of pediatric exposures in children younger than 6 years old.
- PCPs should address poisoning and the increasing incidence of poisonings from laundry detergent packets/pods, analgesics (especially opioids), and marijuana (cannabis) products at opportune health care visits. The broad category of analgesics includes acetaminophen, ibuprofen, and aspirin in addition to opioids and other analgesics. The regional poison control center should be consulted in the case of any child ingestion or supratherapeutic doses (suspected or known; intentionally or unintentionally).
- Adolescents are more likely to intentionally abuse over-the-counter (OTC) medications, prescribed medications, or chemicals/illicit drugs for recreation. They are also at higher risk to attempt or complete suicide using poisons, OTC medications, or prescription medications.

Intentional Injuries

Intentional injuries, or child maltreatment, are a significant pediatric problem that must be recognized by PCPs. Child maltreatment is defined by the federal Child Abuse Prevention and Treatment Act (CAPTA) as "any recent act or failure to act on the part of a parent or caretaker which results in death, serious physical or emotional harm, sexual abuse or exploitation; or an act or failure to act which presents an imminent risk of serious harm" (Child Welfare Information Gateway, n.d.). These are considered minimal standards and serve as guidelines for states to define and manage child maltreatment. Child maltreatment is broken into four subcategories: neglect, psychological maltreatment, physical abuse, and sexual abuse. Some children only experience one type of abuse while others experience multiple abuse subcategories.

In 2016, there were over 4 million referrals made to child protective services (CPS) involving over 7 million children. Over 2 million of these referrals were responded to by CPS, and an estimated 676,000 children (9.1 per 1000) were found to be victims of abuse or neglect. When stratifying the data, the most common form of abuse was neglect (74.8%), followed by physical abuse (18.2%) and sexual abuse (8.5%). An estimated 1750 children in the United States were victims of fatal abuse (2.4 per 100,000) in 2016 (U.S. Department of Health and Human Services Children's Bureau, 2018).

There are a number of known child risk factors for maltreatment. Children fatally injured are more likely to be male and younger than 3 years of age. Children less than 1 year old have the highest victimization rate, with a rate of 24.8 per 1000, and most cases of abuse occur in children younger than 4 years. Females are more likely to experience maltreatment than males. Nearly one-half of all maltreatment victims are Caucasian (44%), 22% are Hispanic, and 20.7% are African American (U.S. Department of Health and Human Services, Children's Bureau, 2018; CDC, 2018). Children with behavioral and special health care needs, those with difficult temperaments, and those who are chronically ill are more at risk than their typically developing peers.

Family and environmental risk factors for maltreatment include poverty, children with special health care needs, parental substance abuse, and parental mental health disorders (Farrell et al., 2017; Maclean et al., 2017). Other important risk factors include the presence of a non-parental caregiver in the home (e.g., mom's male partner), parents with low education levels, families with large numbers of children, and parental history of being abused/neglected (CDC, 2018).

Research shows that adverse childhood experiences (ACEs), which include all forms of child abuse, significantly affect the physical and mental health of these adults (see Chapter 15). Child maltreatment is a significant contributor to poor health outcomes such as mental health disorders including depression, suicide, substance abuse, anxiety, as well as lung disease, heart disease, and early death (Hornor et al., 2017).

In 2012, Congress passed the Protect Our Kids Act, which led to the formation of the Commission to Eliminate Child Abuse and Neglect Fatalities (CECANF). Two years later, the CECANF began research on the causes of child maltreatment to make recommendations for prevention. The CECANF 2016 final report can be found online at https://www.acf.hhs.gov/sites/default/files/cb/cecanf_final_report.pdf.

General Assessment Guidelines

Healthcare workers only account for approximately 9% of CPS referrals (Hornor et al., 2017; U.S. Department of Health and Human Services, 2018). The importance of early identification and intervention cannot be overemphasized in order to minimize each child's ACEs risk. PCPs need to be alert to the possibility of child maltreatment. Thus, when an infant or child presents with certain injuries or behaviors, a careful and detailed history and physical examination must be conducted to identify all abusive injuries as well as to exclude all other possible etiologies. Box 24.1 lists behavioral signs that should alert the provider to the possibility of abuse that should be investigated further.

General Management Strategies

PCPs have two main goals when caring for children who are victims of maltreatment: help alleviate the negative effects of the ACEs, and in children presenting with behavioral concerns, provide more timely management of the child by considering ACEs as a potential underlying cause (Sege and Amaya-Jackson, 2017). The PCP should know when and how to refer families and victims for further assessment, treatment, and therapy when needed.

All states have mandatory reporting laws that require healthcare professionals to report *suspected or known* child maltreatment to the appropriate agencies. ⬤ If the history or physical examination is suspicious for child abuse, the provider should report to either CPS (also known as social services, department of human services, or department of family and youth services) or law enforcement. If the child is in imminent danger, a report should be made to both CPS and law enforcement. The burden to report minor injury or emotional maltreatment is just as great as the burden to report significant trauma resulting in grave bodily injury. Although the severity of injury is always an important consideration in treatment and disposition of the child, it does not determine, per se,

whether intervention by protective services or law enforcement will occur. Nonetheless, PCPs should know that only reasonable suspicion of abuse, not certainty, is required to make a report. All clinic personnel (including unlicensed staff) need to be aware of their role in reporting possible abuse as abuse may be observed in the waiting or examination rooms. Both civil and criminal immunity is ensured to mandated reporters who are acting within their professional role in making a required report. Because each state has its own reporting laws and procedures, PCPs should contact their state agency charged with protecting children for written guidelines about reporting laws and procedural policies related to child abuse. The telephone number for reporting suspicion of abuse should be readily available in each practice setting. If in doubt about the need to file a formal report regarding a particular situation, consult with staff at the local abuse reporting agency or with a child abuse specialist. The practice should have a list of child abuse resources in the community that can be accessed for guidance when needed.

Collaborating with child abuse teams and involving these providers in the child's care as soon as abuse is suspected can improve the assessment and management of abused children (Christian, 2015). A common error of those who provide medical care for children is to assume that two-parent families or families that present well could not be abusive. Therefore, it is important that providers be willing to assess their own biases when determining if a report to CPS is warranted.

Neglect

Neglect is defined as "failure of a parent or other person with responsibility for the child to provide needed food, clothing, shelter, medical care, or supervision to the degree that the child's health, safety, and well-being are threatened with harm" (Child Welfare Information Gateway, 2016, p. 2). Neglect by the parent or caregiver can be severe or subtle in its forms and effects, and occurs when children are not protected from danger, are placed in situations that threaten their health, or fail to receive adequate nurturance, supervision, clothing, shelter, food, education, and/or medical or dental care. Examples include the parent failing to respond to the child's physical, emotional, or education needs; lack of adequate supervision; or frequently missed medical appointments. A key factor in neglect is the extreme or persistent presence of these conditions in the child's environment. Risk factors for neglect are similar to the risk factors for other forms of abuse and include poverty, parental history of mental health disorders, substance abuse, paternal physical disability, and certain cultural practices.

Neglect is the most common form of child maltreatment and the consequences of neglect persist well into adulthood (U.S. Department of Health and Human Services, Children's Bureau, 2018).

Clinical Findings

The goal of assessment is to determine if neglect is occurring, whether the child's safety and welfare are threatened, and to identify other forms of abuse. General indicators of neglect are divided into child, home, and supervision factors (Box 24.2). PCPs can assess child factors in the primary care setting. Home and supervision factors are more difficult for the provider to assess from the clinical setting. Questions and discussion about the home situation should be included in the history (e.g., How are roles in the family divided? Who takes care of younger

---

> **• BOX 24.1   Behavioral Signs Associated With Child Maltreatment**

- Repeated injuries that are unexplainable or unusual
- Overly compliant or exhibits exaggerated fearfulness
- Clingy or indiscriminate attachment
- Extremes in behavior (aggressive or passive)
- Wary of physical contact with adults
- Frightened of a parent or another caregiver
- Exhibits drastic behavioral changes in and out of parental or caregiver presence
- Withdrawal from family or friends, poor school performance, depression or sadness, anxiety, aggressive or destructive behavior, or mistreating an animal or pet
- Suicidal (suicide attempts or plans) or engages in self-mutilation
- Displays sleep or eating disorders

children? Who prepares the meals? Does the family get Supplemental Nutrition Assistance Program (SNAP) or WIC? Does the child have unusual behaviors [e.g., hoarding food, stealing]?). If the child is attending Head Start, the provider can consult with Head Start staff who, in turn, can conduct a home assessment. However, if PCPs suspect neglect, a CPS report should be made. To determine the degree of adult supervision, factors such as the child's age and level of functioning, the length of time the parent is away, where the parent goes, whether the parent leaves a plan of supervision (e.g., relative or adult living next door or nearby who was readily available to the child), and how often the child is left alone are investigated. Most CPS hold parents to the standard of a "reasonable or prudent" parent. Economic factors are also considered when making judgments about parents' efforts to provide adequately for their children.

Differential Diagnosis

Differentiating willful neglect from neglect resulting from poverty, mental retardation, or mental illness is necessary. Willful neglect is a situation in which a parent knows how to seek resources for their family (such as, food stamps or rooming at a homeless shelter in severe weather conditions) but refuses to do so. Educational neglect (parent makes no provisions for the child to attend school) differs from truancy or elopement (i.e., when the child is sent to school but never arrives).

Management

Early recognition of child neglect is critical. The earlier neglect is experienced, the more likely the child will have negative consequences. Early intervention allows the provider to assess the parent's readiness to change and improve parental skills (Child Welfare Information Gateway, 2016). The CDC current recommendations include the use of behavioral parent training programs to help promote healthy parent-child relationships and reduce recurrence of abuse and neglect (CDC, 2016).

• BOX 24.2   General Indicators of Neglect: Child, Home, and Supervision Factors

Child
- Dirty, malnourished, poor hygiene, inadequately dressed for weather
- Inadequate medical and dental care (has multiple caries/decay)
- Always sleepy (chronic fatigue) or hungry
- Exhibits food insecurity behaviors (hiding, bingeing, stealing)

Home
- Fire hazards or other unsafe conditions
- Exposure to illegal substances
- No heating or plumbing
- Nutritional quality of the food inadequate
- Meals not prepared; food spoiled in refrigerator or cupboards

Supervision
- Child has history of repeated physical injuries or ingestion of harmful substances with evidence of poor supervision by adult caregiver
- Child cared for by another child
- Child left alone in the home, car, or anywhere without supervision (typically defined as a child younger than 12 years old who is left unsupervised during the daytime or a child <16-18 years old left unsupervised by an adult at night)

Psychological Maltreatment

There is not a universal definition for psychological maltreatment, but generally, definitions used include "injury to the psychological capacity or emotional stability of the child as evidenced by an observable or substantial change in behavior, emotional response, or cognition" and injury as evidenced by "anxiety, depression, withdrawal, or aggressive behavior" (Child Welfare Information Gateway, 2016, p. 3). It can take the form of acts of omission or commission, involve verbal or nonverbal communication, and can be done with or without intent to harm. Failure to adequately nurture children with support and affection is an example of emotional deprivation or an act of omission. Parents or caregivers who do not provide the normal experiences necessary for a child to feel loved, wanted, secure, or worthy are depriving their child of the emotional security that is critical for positive self-esteem. Parents or caregivers actively *commit* emotional abuse when they subject children to cruel statements and acts or reject, terrorize, ridicule, isolate, and corrupt the child. Torture, confinement, exposure to violence (witnessing interpersonal violence), and deprivation of food and water are extreme examples.

Parents or caregivers can ignore or reject their child for many reasons, including substance use, mental health disorders, personal problems, poor coping skills, poor parent role modeling, high stress levels or other preoccupying situations, or a personal history of emotional maltreatment. Psychological maltreatment should be differentiated from poor parenting skills. Risk factors for psychological maltreatment include multiple family stressors, family conflict, parental mental health disorders, or substance abuse. Children with chronic illness or those who are "different" from their siblings may become targets in the family system. Psychological maltreatment may contribute to failure to thrive (FTT), speech or sleep disorders, or a wide range of behavioral and emotional problems in children (e.g., withdrawal, aggressiveness, conduct and/or attachment disorders, depression).

Clinical Findings

There are generally no specific physical signs to indicate psychological maltreatment; therefore, PCPs must be aware of behavioral indicators suggestive of this type of maltreatment. Consistent or recurrent negative parental behaviors, willful cruelty, or unjustifiable emotional punishment are key indicators of psychological maltreatment, but the signs and symptoms can be subtler and may not indicate abuse. Therefore, a careful history is important. It is essential to interview parents, caregivers, and any child older than 3 years old.

The history can include the following:
- Past health history: Might be suggestive of neglect (e.g., little or no healthcare supervision, immunizations not up-to-date, earlier removal of a sibling for neglect)
- Interview with caregiver: Might reveal caregiver's negative feelings toward child, a state of feeling overwhelmed or depressed, plus feelings of being deprived or unloved; caregiver may be cognitively delayed
- Behavior problems with child in school or among peers (e.g., perpetrator or victim of bullying, withdrawal)
- Feeding and dietary history should be obtained, but may not be accurate; it can be helpful in distinguishing formula-preparation error from neglect
- Financial hardships: May be related to inability to provide for basic needs, especially food

Physical assessment of psychological maltreatment can be difficult. Nonorganic FTT can be related to physical and psychosocial factors, and both should be considered because they may be concurrent. Assessment of FTT is discussed in Chapter 40. Assessment for possible psychological maltreatment should include:

- *Child's behavior:* Extreme behavioral responses such as overly aggressive or unusually passive, seeks attachment from strangers, acts adult-like or infant-like, history of suicidality
- *Parent's behavior:* Presence of anger or dislike of child; may ignore, belittle, tease, or verbally abuse child; has lack of concern for child
- *Associated developmental delays:* Results from deficient psychosocial stimulation

Differential Diagnosis

Intentional mental injury should be distinguished from that caused by parental deficits, such as cognitive, psychological, and economic limitations. Psychopathology in the child resulting from other causes is also in the differential diagnosis.

Management

Because psychological maltreatment is generally difficult to prove, the provider must carefully document what was said in the interview and what behavioral indicators were found. Reporting concerns to the appropriate CPS agency is essential, as is close supervision of these families. Referral to a community health nurse for in-home assessment may be appropriate. Despite a lack of evidence about effective management strategies for victims of psychological maltreatment, referral to a mental health professional for evaluation should be considered to determine whether the behaviors or psychopathology, or both, in the child are due to parental emotional abuse or deprivation. Cognitive behavioral therapy and/or family therapy may be necessary, and parents may benefit from parental support groups and education, in addition to social service support to cope with demands on the family system (e.g., child care, nutritional education, access to economic resources, Early Head Start). The child may need to be placed out of the home. If a child has FTT, the condition must be treated clinically (see Chapter 40). Close and long-term healthcare supervision and follow-up plus psychosocial intervention and local case management by CPS are needed.

Patient and Family Education and Prevention

Prevention of emotional abuse generally involves the same prevention strategies as identified in the Physical Abuse section. Early recognition and intervention are the keys to preventing subsequent mental health problems. Frequent health visits to monitor the height and weight of infants who are falling behind are essential to prevent significant growth and development problems. Close follow-up is required for victims of all types of abuse and neglect.

Physical Abuse

Physical child abuse is defined as maltreatment involving "non-accidental physical injury to the child" (Child Welfare Information Gateway, 2016, p. 1). Certain states include acts that threaten harm and human trafficking as forms of physical abuse (Child Welfare Information Gateway, 2016). In some instances, the injury is a result of the parent or caregiver shaking, striking, or throwing the child in a moment of frustration or anger. Physical abuse can also be due to unreasonably severe corporal

or unjustifiable punishment, or caused by intentional, deliberate assault, such as burning, biting, cutting, poking, twisting limbs, or torturing.

Child physical abuse also occurs when a parent or caregiver falsifies the history or fabricates an illness in a child in order to receive attention from the medical community. This rarer form of abuse is known as *medical child abuse,* previously *Munchausen syndrome by proxy,* and has been defined as "a child receives unnecessary and harmful or potentially harmful medical care at the instigation of a caretaker" (Yates and Bass, 2017). Medical child abuse can lead to significant injury or harm to a child and is associated with high morbidity and mortality. Identifying medical child abuse can be difficult, and providers should be alert to some possible indicator, including a caregiver who frequently seeks another medical opinion when the child is not diagnosed with an illness, who does not accept reassurance that the child is healthy, or who does not accept normal results. Evaluation for medical child abuse often requires an extensive medical records review; therefore, concerns of medical child abuse should be referred to a child abuse specialist who can assist in the process.

Clinical Findings

Determining the presence of physical abuse can be difficult. Abused infants and children can present in various ways. A child or parent may disclose a history of an inflicted injury or a caregiver may bring the child in for treatment of an injury. Other than the perpetrator and victim, abusive events are rarely witnessed by others. Children may present with seemingly minor injuries or the injury may be life-threatening, in which case the patient must be stabilized before evaluation of abuse is conducted. Specific physical findings are often the key to a diagnosis of physical abuse. During routine exam, an undisclosed injury may be identified. In this situation, the parent/caregiver and/or child should be asked about the mechanism of injury and if treatment was sought for the injury. The PCP should have a high level of suspicion if there are discrepancies in the reported history of the injury and the child's age and developmental capabilities do not match or are unusual for either the type and/or severity of injury. For example, infants who are not yet independently mobile (e.g., cruising or crawling) should not have bruises.

Obtaining a meticulous and thorough history is important when evaluating the child with suspected abuse. Asking open-ended questions allows for the parent(s) or caregiver to provide history information without being influenced by the provider's interpretations. Then, if clarification is needed, the provider can ask specific questions. Important points to inquire about include details and timing of the event, what took place before the injury occurred, child's level of responsiveness, history of recent trauma, developmental level of child, and onset and progression of the symptoms. Additional information includes family history (bleeding disorders, orthopedic disorders), pregnancy history, forms of discipline used within the home, temperament of the child, history of previous abuse or abuse of other children in the home, history of CPS reports, substance abuse, and social/financial stressors (Christian, 2015). Red flags in the history include:
- Injury that is unusual for a specific age group.
- Injuries are unexplained or implausible (e.g., parent or caregiver cannot explain injury, is vague about how the injury occurred, gives discrepant accounts of what happened, or blames someone else); explanation does not match the type or mechanism of injury; or child is not developmentally capable of reported behavior.

- Parent or caregiver delays seeking care for the child, seeks inappropriate care (e.g., for something other than the true issue), or age of injury is inconsistent with the history (e.g., bruises are in late stages of resolution, yet parent states injury occurred a few hours earlier).
- Child, parent or caregiver, or both, hide injury (e.g., child wears excessive layers of clothing), or child is kept out of school (isolated).
- Presence of triggering behaviors, such as an inconsolable colicky infant, toilet-training accidents, or sleep or discipline problems that may have led to a violent response by a caregiver.
- Report of a crisis or stressful time for the family (e.g., financial difficulties) or intimate partner violence (IPV).
- Problem with substance abuse in the family.

Tables 24.3 and 24.4 describe common sites of injury and common characteristics of physical abuse by type of injury. Key considerations of abuse that should guide the physical examination include the following:

- Any injury in a perambulatory infant such as bruises, oral/dental injuries, fractures, intracranial bleeding, or abdominal injury
- Presence of multiple organ injuries
- Pattern of bruises, abrasions, lacerations (i.e., does it resemble a known object?)
- Presence of multiple injuries, particularly in different stages of healing
- Signs of other forms of abuse or neglect
- Severe injuries not otherwise explained
- "TEN 4" injuries: injuries occurring on torso, ear, neck and in children less than age 4 years and in ANY infant under 4 months old (Christian, 2015).

Behaviors are not definitive signs of physical abuse but are important areas to investigate for additional information including:

- Hypervigilance or difficulty regulating emotions
- Exaggerated emotional responses in the face of triggers such as a certain sight, smell, or sound

- Sleep disturbances
- Anger/irritability or withdrawal
- These behaviors may persist long after the maltreatment has ended (Sege and Amaya-Jackson, 2017).

Diagnostic Studies

The degree of diagnostic testing is based on factors such as severity of injury, age of child, and developmental level of the child. Consulting with child abuse specialists can help determine the most appropriate testing to order. Diagnostic tests to consider include:

- Blood coagulation studies: Platelet count, bleeding time, prothrombin time, partial thromboplastin time, von Willebrand panel, factor VIII level, factor IX level on any child who is severely bruised, has a history of "easy bruising" and suspicious bruises, or has intracranial bleeding
- Serum calcium, phosphorus, and alkaline phosphatase levels useful if bone disease is suspected; consider 25-hydroxyvitamin D and Parathyroid (PTH) levels
- Urinalysis, liver enzymes (aspartate aminotransferase [AST], alanine amino transferase [ALT]), amylase, and lipase to rule out abdominal trauma
- Review newborn screen and consider urine organic acids for suspected head trauma
- Radiographic studies:
  - Skeletal survey if physical abuse is suspected in any child under 12 months old and should be strongly considered in children 12 months to 3 years old. Table 24.5 gives details of which images are requested in a complete skeletal survey.
  - Local radiologic evaluation in an older child with limited range of motion or bony tenderness on examination.
  - Computed tomography (CT) scan and/or a magnetic resonance imaging (MRI) study whenever trauma to the face or head is suspected or on the basis of physical findings or symptoms. MRI is more sensitive for dating intracranial injuries, detecting subtle injuries, and identifying cervical spine injuries.
  - Abdominal CT with contrast when abdominal trauma is suspected, and if child is younger than 2 years old a skeletal survey should be obtained.

Other studies are ordered depending on physical findings.

Differential Diagnosis

Differential diagnoses are identified by type of injury:

- Normal bruising from accidental injuries that typically involve the knees, anterior tibia, and forehead
- Mongolian or melanin spots
- Cultural practices, such as coining (*cao gio*) or spoon rubbing (*quat sha*), sometimes practiced by Southeast Asian groups
- Burns, impetigo, bullous impetigo, or toxic epidermal necrolysis (scalded skin syndrome)
- Fractures: Osteogenesis imperfecta and rare bone diseases, such as rickets, scurvy, congenital syphilis, and neoplasms
- Head injuries: Metabolic disorders and accidental causes
- Bruising or bleeding (hematologic disorders, such as vitamin K deficiency, von Willebrand disease, hemophilia)

Management

Medical treatment of specific types of injuries is discussed in this text under the appropriate illness-related heading. If physical abuse is suspected, certain general management strategies should be followed. The provider must:

TABLE 24.3	Common Sites of Injury in Physical Abuse of Children
Location of Injury[a]	**Common Physical Finding**
Head area	Eyes—bilateral black eyes Earlobe—pinch and pull marks Cheek—slap marks, squeeze marks Upper lip and frenulum—lacerations or bruises Scalp—bare and broken hair, bruises
Neck	Choke marks
Trunk	Trunk—bite marks, fingertip encirclement marks, hand slap, pinch mark, belt mark Buttocks and lower back—paddling and strap marks
Anogenital	Pinch marks, penile wrapping with constrictive materials
Extremities	Upper arms—grab marks Ankles or wrists—tethering, friction burn marks Feet—pin or razor tattoo marks

[a]The shins, elbows, and knees are the most typical sites of accidental, non–child abuse injuries where bruises, cuts, and abrasions are most commonly seen.

TABLE 24.4 Common Characteristics of Physical Abuse by Type of Injury

Type of Injury	Key Considerations
Bruises, abrasions, and lacerations—surface and soft tissue	Pattern, shape, outline, or image of an object (e.g., handprint, cord, or buckle shapes) Location—sites other than over bony prominence (knees, shins, elbows, forehead) Number—more than one body surface or plane Multiple bruises
Burns—superficial or deep	Location: Burns on palms, soles, flexor surface of thighs or perineum; positive image of the shape of the object used to burn the child (e.g., curling irons, cigarette lighters, cigarettes, irons) Patterns, such as sharply demarcated or circumferential (e.g., sock, glove, zebra, branding, doughnut, or cigarette shape) Cigarette burns—7.5-10 mm round lesion, raised edges, and deep eschar
Human bite marks	Oval-shaped pattern, such as doughnut or double-horseshoe shape; can be on any part of the body; can have discrete tooth marks within the arcs or central ecchymosis between the arcs
Ligature marks	Typically, around neck or extremities; linear image at site where tool placed
Central nervous system/abusive head trauma	Radiographic findings (e.g., subdural hematomas, subarachnoid hemorrhages, skull fractures, suture spread), retinal hemorrhages; head trauma can have symptoms of irritability, lethargy, seizures, apnea, or coma Additional injuries may include posterior rib fractures and metaphyseal fractures
Internal organ trauma	Liver, bowel, spleen, pancreas, kidney damage consistent with blunt-force trauma May be no visible marks or bruises on abdomen May have symptoms of shock/sepsis Internal injury is second leading cause of death in child abuse
Skeletal fracture	Spiral fractures of long bones, avulsion of metaphyseal tips, multiple rib fractures in different stages of healing, subperiosteal proliferation reaction, unexplained fracture, especially in a young, nonambulatory child; fractures from birth injuries typically heal by 4 months
Poisoning or ingestion of medication	Deliberate poisoning or exposure to substance abuse via breast milk, passive inhalation of marijuana or other drugs
Medical child abuse (Munchausen syndrome by proxy)	Caregiver creates a fictitious illness or induces illness in child; signs and symptoms stop when perpetrator no longer has unsupervised contact with child

TABLE 24.5 Skeletal Survey

Area of Body	X-Ray View Requested
Skull	AP and lateral views
Spine	AP and lateral views
Chest/ribs	AP, lateral, and oblique views
Pelvis	AP views
Long bones	AP and lateral views
Hands	Oblique views
Feet	AP views

AP, Anterior-posterior.

- Report suspicions of physical abuse to CPS or law enforcement agencies, or both. The Health Insurance Portability and Accountability Act permits protected health information to be disclosed to CPS without the authorization of the legal guardian, but each state has their own laws regarding disclosure of health information to investigators (Christian, 2015).

- Carefully document findings and any statements made by parent or caregiver or child, or both.
- Secure photographic documentation of soft tissue injury or burn injury; this may be done by law enforcement personnel, CPS, or health care providers, as appropriate.
- Refer for appropriate medical treatment of injuries depending on type and severity of injury.
- The American Academy of Pediatrics recommends providers disclose to the parents that a CPS report has been made. This can be a challenging decision, but transparency can facilitate communication during and after the investigation (Christian, 2015).
- Refer to local Child Advocacy Center for specialized assessment and diagnosis if appropriate.
- Refer for mental health care. The need for long-term or intermittent therapy often depends on the individual child, the severity of the physical and emotional injuries, and other life events.

Patient and Family Education and Prevention

At-risk families have certain characteristics. A key to education and prevention is to identify families that have:
- A parental history of abuse during childhood or a history of exposure to interpersonal violence. Pursue affirmative responses with further questions as to what, if any, intervention(s) were taken.

- A family history of child maltreatment, including child death (categorized as extremely high risk), drug abuse, violent behavior, or serious mental illness.
- A mother or primary caregiver who does not show attachment to her infant, makes negative remarks about the child, or lacks basic parenting knowledge, skill, and motivation.
- Evidence of physical discipline of young infants.
- Family history of substance abuse and/or criminal activity.
- A lack of social support networks: Is the parent isolated?

The following interventions are recommended for at-risk children and families:

- Report immediately to CPS if abuse is suspected.
- Make early referrals for supportive services, including social service referrals, parenting classes, self-help groups (e.g., Parenting Support Programs or Alcoholics Anonymous plus battered women's services), respite care, public health nurse visits, or a combination of these.
- Provide close primary care supervision and ill-child follow-up visits.
- Use a multidisciplinary team approach to manage at-risk or high-risk families. A team approach gives objectivity to a situation.
- Use the services offered by community Child Advocacy Centers or child abuse prevention programs.

Sexual Abuse, Assault, and Human Trafficking

Sexual abuse is a complex form of child maltreatment and is often underreported. There were over 60,000 child victims of sexual abuse identified in 2015 and these victims only represent a percentage of children who were abused (Hornor, 2016). Child sex abuse definitions vary across disciplines, social systems, research efforts, and laws. Sex abuse can be defined to include acts of sexual assault or sexual exploitation of minors, or both. These acts can occur over an extended period of time or be a one-time incident; they may or may not involve force; they can involve threats of physical harm to a child or others in the family or emotional entrapment of the child; and the perpetrator often frames the incident as a secret between the victim and the perpetrator. In cases of child sexual abuse, multigenerational abuse is common. The perpetrator is usually known to the child and is often a "trusted" adult. For most policy makers and members of the public, child sexual abuse connotes sexual offenses at the hands of an adult. There is increasing evidence that juveniles perpetrate over half of the total estimate of sexual offenses, many of them peer acquaintances (Finkelhor et al., 2014).

Children normally explore their developing sexuality, but some children engage in sexual behaviors that go beyond harmless curiosity. Some, but not all, of these children have a history of being sexually abused themselves. Intervention is necessary when children demonstrate problem sexual behaviors that are inappropriate or harmful to themselves or others (Table 24.6). Abuse of children and adolescents involves a range of acts, including rape, rape by multiple perpetrators, incest, sodomy, lewd or lascivious acts on a child younger than 14 years old (e.g., fondling or touching of genital areas and breasts or inappropriate kissing), oral copulation, and penetration of genital or anal openings by a foreign object. Sexual exploitation includes activities such as pornography depicting minors and promoting prostitution by minors. Estimates of childhood sexual abuse range from 14% to 26%, with females having significantly higher incidence than males (Mooreland et al., 2018).

Human trafficking, also known as commercial exploitation of children, is a rapidly growing global issue. Many of these victims are children who have run away. National estimates show that one in seven endangered runaways who were reported to the National Center for Missing and Exploited Children (NCMEC) in 2017 was likely to be a sex trafficking victim. Eighty-eight percent of these children were in the care of social services or foster care when they ran (NCMEC, 2018). There is little research to date on these victims, however PCPs should know the risk factors for human trafficking and manifestations associated with child survivors. Factors include children and adolescent runaways, history of sexual assault/abuse, children and adolescents with substance abuse or living in a home with parental substance abuse, family dysfunction, and LGBTQ youth (Hornor and Sherfield, 2018; NCMEC, n.d.).

Clinical Findings

The pediatric PCP is likely to become involved in a child sexual abuse case in any of the following circumstances: if there is a spontaneous disclosure by the child; if a parent voices concerns about the possibility of abuse or reports a disclosure by the child; if there are suspicious physical or historical findings, or both; or if laboratory tests indicating sexually transmitted infections (STIs) or urine pregnancy test are positive. Child victims of sexual abuse do not often present with abnormal physical findings. On average, less than 10% of victims have an abnormal anogenital examination and less than 5% have a STI (Hornor, 2016).

The child or adolescent who has been sexually assaulted by a stranger usually discloses the abuse and comes to a provider for an immediate evaluation. This type of assessment is straightforward and involves the usual taking of a history and performing the medical examination (see Chapter 42) with collection of possible evidence if the incident occurred within 72 hours. These children are often seen in the emergency department of a local hospital or, ideally, at a special center that treats victims of child sexual abuse, such as a local designated child abuse center.

Child sex trafficking victims may present with certain red flags. Victims may be dishonest regarding their age and identity, have an overly controlling "boyfriend" present, have difficulty answering questions or rely on others to answer, or have tattooing or branding not easily explained. These children and adolescents do not often view themselves as victims, so PCPs must not rely on self-disclosure to identify them (NCMEC, n.d., 2017). Over half of children who are sexually abused do not disclose the abuse until adulthood. Some children were molested in the past but have only recently disclosed the abuse; in many instances, sexual abuse occurs over several years before the child discloses it. In other cases, the provider may suspect that a child is being or has been sexually abused. Assessment of these children should focus on three areas: behavioral indicators, physical indicators, and the interview of the child (see Table 24.6).

Ideally, an expert in the medical examination of children who have been or are suspected of being sexually abused should evaluate the child, so referral is essential. However, disclosure of sexual abuse may occur in the primary care setting, and the PCP must respond. When the parent first discusses concern of sexual abuse, the child should not participate in the discussion. The provider should gather information from the child and parent separately. When interviewing the child, the provider needs to be nonjudgmental, use language that the child understands, identify the words the child uses for the genital and rectal areas, have the child report what happened in his or her own words, and

TABLE 24.6 Behavioral and Physical Indicators of Sexual Abuse

Behavioral Indicators	Physical Indicators—Nonspecific	Physical Indicators—Specific	Lack of Significant Physical Findings
Loss of bowel and bladder control Regressive behaviors, such as newly manifested clinging and irritability in young children, thumb sucking, renewed need for a security object Sleep disturbances, inability to sleep alone, bed-wetting after having been dry at night Overeating or lack of appetite; compulsive behaviors or unusual fears and phobias Change in school performance; loss of concentration or easy distractibility Sexualized behavior or play inappropriate for developmental level (see Table 21.2) Depression or inactivity, poor peer relationships, poor self-esteem, acting-out, excessive anger Runaway, suicide attempts, prostitution or promiscuity, substance abuse, teen pregnancy, psychosomatic, gynecologic, and gastrointestinal complaints	Pain on urination; vaginal or penile discharge; vaginal, rectal, or penile bleeding Enuresis and encopresis Urethral or lymph gland inflammation; genital or perianal rashes; labial adhesions Pain in anal, gastrointestinal, pelvic, and urinary areas Genital injuries or signs, such as bruising, scratches, bites, grasp marks, or swelling of the genitalia that are unexplained or inconsistent with history	Blunt-force trauma (lacerations, bruising, abrasions, tears) to the genital or rectal areas, or both, that is inconsistent with the history or these same findings with a history of sexual contact or penetration Commonly encountered STIs: • Diagnostic of sexual abuse—gonorrhea (by culture) and syphilis if not perinatally acquired, nondelivery-related or nonpregnancy-related *Chlamydia* (culture is the only reliable diagnostic method), HIV, and herpes type 2 • Highly suspicious: *Trichomonas vaginalis* • Suspicious: Condyloma acuminatum (appearing after 3 years old and not perinatally acquired) • Possible: Herpes type 1 and nonvenereal warts (may be due to autoinoculation in the genital or anogenital area) • Uncertain: Bacterial vaginosis and *Mycoplasma* • Pregnancy, sperm, and semen are certain indicators of sexual abuse in young children	Lack of findings is often the result of delayed disclosure and the nature of the abuse. Most sexual abuse of young children does not involve penetrating trauma. "It's normal to have a normal examination." Even in cases in which a perpetrator was convicted for sexual abuse and perpetrators report penile-genital contact, a majority of victims had normal or nonspecific examinations.

HIV, Human immunodeficiency virus; *STI,* sexually transmitted infection.

Note: Most child victims of sexual abuse do not have any significant physical findings.

ask open-ended questions. Leading questions or coercive tactics should never be used. The provider must document what was said accurately and in words used by the child and/or parent.

After reporting the case to the local child abuse hotline, the PCP should work with CPS to ensure that a thorough assessment is conducted. This assessment includes a medical evaluation at a designated child abuse center with a complete physical examination and a forensic interview by a social worker, psychologist, or other trained professionals. The PCP must also assure the child and family of continued support, advocacy, and resources for them. Recanting a disclosure of sexual abuse is not uncommon because of fear of what disclosure can bring to the family or child, so reporting the case, referring to appropriate child abuse support services, and follow-up with the family are essential.

Diagnostic Studies

STIs are uncommon in sexually abused prepubertal children; less than 5% have an STI (Hornor, 2016). Routine screening and culture of all sites in asymptomatic prepubertal children is not recommended. However, STI testing should be considered if the child has disclosed genital-genital, anal-genital, oral-genital, or oral-anal contact; genital/anal discharge; or known exposure to an STI in the perpetrator or if a sibling has an STI. A positive STI test can be the first and sometimes only sign of sexual abuse (Hornor, 2016). Guidelines for STI diagnostic testing and management are found in Chapter 42.

When evaluating a child or teen who has experienced an acute sexual assault within the 72-hour time frame, it is important to assess the risk of possible human immunodeficiency virus (HIV) exposure. The current CDC recommendations state that each case should be discussed with a local HIV/infectious disease specialist to determine if postexposure HIV prophylaxis is needed. Each case is considered based on multiple factors, such as risk of exposure, single versus multiple perpetrators, and potential of complying with the recommended treatment protocol and follow-up with an HIV specialist. For further detailed information on medication regimes and follow-up, refer to the current CDC treatment guidelines for a child with acute sexual assault (https://www.cdc.gov/std/tg2015/sexual-assault.htm).

Differential Diagnosis

Differential diagnoses include straddle injury to the genitalia or rectal area, which produces labial ecchymosis, abrasions, or tears; penetrating vaginal trauma from accidental injury, such as jumping from dresser onto bedpost (needs careful investigation and should have an easily identifiable history); perinatally acquired STIs or STIs acquired through close contact but not sexual abuse; lichen sclerosus, poor hygiene, pinworm infestation that leads to vulvar skin irritation; and foreign body (frequently toilet paper in vaginal area) or other non-sexually transmitted bacteria causing vaginal discharge.

Management

An immediate forensic examination for a chain of evidence is required if trauma is present or the child gives a history that sexual abuse, including ejaculation, occurred within 72 hours. Colposcopy examination and specimen collection for semen, STI, pregnancy, and other evidence is done according to the local law-enforcement protocol for the evaluation of child sexual abuse or adolescent rape.

If the PCP is the first healthcare provider to see the child, he or she is likely to become involved in the following management issues:

- Careful documentation of the history and physical examination findings for medical-legal purposes
- Reporting of the case to law enforcement and social service agencies as required by law
- Referral for medical and psychosocial evaluation by experts in the field of child sexual abuse
- Referrals for crisis counseling of the child and other family members as needed
- Referrals for therapy in addition to support and encouragement for the child and family
- Treatment of STI: Follow-up STI cultures or blood work as indicated (e.g., HIV screening at the appropriate timelines). HIV is the only STI for which routine postexposure prophylaxis should be considered in children and adolescents. Current guidelines recommend against routine prophylaxis for chlamydia, gonorrhea, and trichomonas in prepubertal children.

Additionally, if STI treatment is indicated in prepubertal children, delay treatment until confirmative testing is performed. Prophylaxis is indicated for adolescents who are at higher risk of acquiring these infections if there has been genital-genital, anal-genital, or oral-genital contact within the past 72 hours (Hornor, 2016).

The child who demonstrates inappropriate sexualized behavior (i.e., beyond child behavior seen as a part of normal developmental curiosity—see Box 24.3) should be referred to a mental health specialist trained in child development and child mental health. Family therapy and education may also be necessary, because parents benefit from specific strategies (guided by the therapist), support, and counseling to cope with the situation and best help their child.

Patient and Family Education and Prevention

Prevention of later psychological problems related to child sexual abuse and revictimization is important. Prevention of sexual abuse involves instructing parents and caregivers about the need for early and consistent education of their children regarding:

- Good, bad, and secret touching of private parts
- How to say no or the use of self-defense techniques (e.g., yelling, kicking, or fighting back) if someone inappropriately touches them
- Telling a responsible adult
- Not to keep secrets

Parents should bring up the subject of sexual abuse as their child progresses through the various developmental stages. Young children who have been molested by a trusted adult often do not disclose for many years because they were threatened not to tell anyone or they interpreted the sexual activity (if it is not painful) as a sign of affection from the trusted adult and not as molestation. Later feelings of guilt, fear, and betrayal can emerge when children realize they were molested. Emphasize to parents that they must not place their child in high-risk situations (e.g., a parent who was abused by her father may have kept this a secret, blaming herself for what happened; she may erroneously believe that the perpetrator will not sexually abuse her child and may leave her daughter with him). Counsel that children are never safe around a pedophile.

During routine well visits, the PCP should:

- Provide families with information and educational reading materials about the topic of sexual abuse of children. Teaching should be tailored to the child's cognitive and learning abilities.
- Report promptly any suspicion of sexual abuse.
- Support efforts to target high-risk groups for intervention to prevent the continued spread of child abuse (e.g., children who have exhibited sexual curiosity beyond the bounds of normal or have experimented with but not yet victimized other children; hence they become a juvenile perpetrator acting out the sexual activity or violence done to them) (see Chapter 21 regarding normal sexual exploration and activities).
- Support public education efforts and community child sexual abuse prevention programs.
- Educate parents about the need to talk to their children about their daily activities, especially what their children did during the time they were not with the parents.

Violence

Violence is the outcome of aggressive behavior that becomes destructive and results in physical injury to people or damage to property. Characteristic features of violence are listed in Box 24.4. Violence is a major social and public health problem in the United States. A

• BOX 24.3 Sexual Problem Behaviors in Children

- Are clearly beyond the child's developmental stage (e.g., a 3-year-old attempting to kiss an adult's genitals)
- Involve threats, force, or aggression
- Involve inappropriate or harmful use of sexual body parts (e.g., inserting objects into the rectum or vagina)
- Involve children of widely different ages or abilities, such as a 12-year-old "playing doctor" with a 4-year-old
- Are associated with strong emotional reactions in a child, such as anger or anxiety
- Interfere with typical childhood interests and activities

National Child Traumatic Stress Network (NCTSN). Understanding and coping with sexual behavior problems in children—information for parents and caregivers. *http://nctsn.org/nctsn_assets/pdfs/caring/sexualbehaviorproblems.pdf. Accessed April 11, 2019*

• BOX 24.4 Key Features Characteristic of Violence

Continuity: Once it is used as a coping mechanism, violence becomes a habit that is hard to break.

Reciprocity: Violence generates violent behavior in others, increasing tension and eliciting negative responses.

Sameness: One form of violence becomes as acceptable as another. As its use becomes more common, violence permeates all of one's life.

Addiction: Violence gives a sense of power and control that, although temporary, is addictive.

Limitations of options or alternative actions: Reasoning is difficult in violent situations, and problem-solving abilities are not used.

Escalation: Violence begets more frequent and more intense violence, with potential for serious sequelae.

national survey on children's exposure to violence revealed that 37% of children and adolescents experienced physical assault in the previous year and 9% experienced an assault-related injury (Finkelhor et al., 2015). Although there are major differences in rates of violence-related injuries and death by ethnic groups, the majority of homicides involve people who know each other and are of the same race. Boys are more likely to perpetrate and be victims of physical violence, whereas girls are more frequently victims of sexual assault and interpersonal violence (Finklehor et al., 2015).

There is no one cause of violent behavior. Children from all socioeconomic backgrounds, genders, races, and communities experience violence directly or indirectly through news reports, social media, etc. Effective management of violence in families and communities depends on understanding major influences and key risk factors that contribute to or sustain violence.

Exposure to violence can lead to behavior problems and developmental issues, and can significantly affect physical and mental health. Homicide or serious injury can be the end result of violence. Data from the National Violent Death Reporting System show that in 2015, over 5400 children and youth under the age of 24 died as the result of violence (CDC, 2016a). The direct and indirect costs of violence in medical expenses, loss of productivity, and decreased quality of life are immense.

Clinical Findings

The assessment of youths who are victims of, witnesses to, or perpetrators of violent crime should focus on certain key pieces of historical information and the presence of risk factors to help determine the child's current safety and potential for future violence.

Youth who have experienced violence need a trauma-informed approach to determining the circumstances of their violent experiences. This means that children should be treated as children first and the goal of treatment is to not further victimize the child. The Substance Abuse and Mental Health Services Administration (SAHMSA) lists six principles of trauma-informed care including: safety; trustworthiness and transparency; peer support, collaboration, and mutuality; empowerment, voice, and choice; and cultural, historical, and gender issues. These and other PCP resources can be found online at www.integration.samhsa.gov/about-us/innovation-communities-2018/trauma-informed-approaches.

Management

The PCP is likely to become involved with the healthcare management of minor trauma resulting from assault, counseling after an incident of violence or threat of violence, and the prevention of youth violence.

In brief, the following are the key points in the management of minor assaults:
- Treat minor trauma or refer for necessary treatment
- Screen for alcohol and drugs
- Report the incident to law enforcement
- Refer to a social worker or mental health professional and to community programs as appropriate
- Work with parents and child to identify ways to prevent violence (e.g., discuss how the family can incorporate protective factors into their family life [Chapter 15]).

Youth Violence Prevention

See Chapter 15.

Intimate Partner Violence (Domestic Violence)

IPV is violence that occurs between individuals in a close relationship. IPV occurs in children, youths, and adults, and children who witness this violence are often significantly victimized. IPV includes physical violence, sexual violence, and/or emotional abuse and threats. It occurs in all socioeconomic, racial, gender, sexual-identity, and community groups. IPV can leave physical and emotional injuries. Children can also be physically injured during intimate partner disputes either by getting "caught in the crossfire" or in attempts to intervene. Children who witness violence between parents, family, and friends are almost always emotionally traumatized. Studies document that exposure to IPV can lead to poor academic and social outcomes. There appears to be a dose-response relationship between IPV and poor outcomes—the more severe or chronic the exposure, the poorer the outcomes.

Clinical Findings

Although most professional organizations recommend screening for IPV, the effectiveness of screening is unclear, and it is difficult to identify families where IPV occurs. Intimate partner abuse occurs in all strata of society and, when presented with screening questions, many victims are reluctant to disclose their victimization due to fear of the consequences.

Management

For the PCP, managing a child's exposure to IPV can be problematic. In most states, healthcare providers are mandated to report a child's exposure to IPV to CPS because it is considered a form of emotional child abuse. State agencies can then further assess the family functioning and can offer resources to help the perpetrator, the adult victim, and the children who are also being victimized. In all cases, care of families experiencing IPV requires a multidisciplinary, well-coordinated approach; referral and consultation with specialty treatment centers, social workers, and community health agencies are essential.

Patient Education and Prevention

The goal is to prevent IPV before it starts. Educating children about healthy behaviors and relationships can assist them in avoiding dating relationships that include violence. PCPs should review the negative effects of children witnessing conflict between adults, specifically parents. Little is known about preventing IPV in adults and further research is needed in this area.

References

Alonge O, Khan UR, Hyder AA. Our shrinking globe: implications for child unintentional injuries. *Pediatr Clin N Amer*. 2016;63. 267–181.

American Academy of Pediatrics. *Swim Safety Tips from the American Academy of Pediatrics* (website). 2018. https://www.aap.org/en-us/about-the-aap/aap-press-room/news-features-and-safety-tips/Pages/Swim-Safety-Tips.aspx.

Centers for Disease Control and Prevention, Centers for Disease Control and Prevention. *CDC Childhood injury report* (website). https://www.cdc.gov/safechild/pdf/cdc-childhoodinjury.pdf. Accessed April 11, 2019.

Centers for Disease Control and Prevention, Centers for Disease Control and Prevention. *Sexual Assault and Abuse and STDs* (website). https://www.cdc.gov/std/tg2015/sexual-assault.htm. Accessed April 11, 2017.

Centers for Disease Control and Prevention (CDC), Centers for Disease Control and Prevention (CDC). *Burn prevention.* (website). https://www.cdc.gov/safechild/burns/index.html. Accessed April 11, 2019.

Centers for Disease Control and Prevention (CDC), Centers for Disease Control and Prevention (CDC). *Injury Prevention & Control: Data & Statistics (WISQARS): Nonfatal and Fatal Injury Data* (website). https://www.cdc.gov/injury/wisqars/index.html. Accessed April 11, 2019.

Centers for Disease Control and Prevention, Centers for Disease Control and Prevention. *Child Safety and Injury Prevention: Fall Prevention* (website). https://www.cdc.gov/safechild/falls/. Accessed April 11, 2019.

Centers for Disease Control and Prevention, Centers for Disease Control and Prevention. *Preventing Child Abuse and Neglect: A Technical Package for Policy, Norm, and Programmatic Activities* (website). https://www.cdc.gov/violenceprevention/pdf/CAN-Prevention-Technical-Package.pdf. Accessed April 11, 2019.

Centers for Disease control and Prevention, Centers for Disease control and Prevention. *Child Abuse and Neglect: Risk and Protective Factors* (website). https://www.cdc.gov/violenceprevention/childabuseandneglect/riskprotectivefactors.html. Accessed April 11, 2019.

Child Information Welfare Gateway. *Definitions of Child Abuse and Neglect*. Washington, DC: U.S. Department of Health and Human Services: Children's Bureau; 2016. https://www.childwelfare.gov/pubPDFs/define.pdf.

Christian CW. The evaluation of suspected childhood physical abuse. *Pediatr.* 2015;135:e1337–e1354.

Durbin D, Hoffman BD. Council on injury. Violence and poison prevention: child passenger safety. *Pediatrics.* 2018;127(4):1–18.

Farrell CA, Fleegler EW, Monuteaux MC, et al. Community poverty and child abuse fatalities in the United States. *Pediatrics.* 2017;139. 2016–1616.

Finkelhor D, Shattuck A, Turner H. Hamby SL The lifetime prevalence of childhood sexual abuse and sexual assault assessed in late adolescence. *J Adolesc Health.* 2014;55:329–333.

Finklehor D, Turner HA, Shattuck A. Prevalence of childhood exposure, crime and abuse: results from the National Survey of Children's Exposure to Violence. *JAMA Pediatrics.* 2015;169(8):746–754.

Hagan JF, Shawn JS, Duncan PM. *Bright Futures: Guidelines for Health Supervision of Infants, Children, and Adolescents.* 4th ed. Elk Grove Village, IL: American Academy of Pediatrics; 2017.

Hornor G. Sexually transmitted infections and children: what the PNP should know. *J Pediatr Health Care.* 2016;31:222–229.

Hornor G, Bretl D, Chapman E, et al. Childhood maltreatment screening and anticipatory guidance: a description of pediatric nurse practitioner practice behaviors. *J Pediatr Health Care.* 2017;31:e36–e41.

Hornor G, Sherfield J. Commercial exploitation of children: health care use and case characteristics. *J Pediatr Health Care.* 2018;32:250–262.

Maclean MJ, Sims S, Bower C, et al. Maltreatment risk among children with disabilities. *Pediatrics.* 2017;139. 2016–1817.

Mooreland AD, Walsh K, Hartley C, et al. Investigating longitudinal association between sexual assault, substance use, and delinquency among female adolescents: results from a nationally representative sample. *J Adolesc Health.* 2018;63:320–326.

National Center for Missing and Exploited Children. *Child Sex Trafficking Identification Resource* (website). http://www.missingkids.com/content/dam/ncmec/en_us/documents/CST-Resource-blue-1.pdf. Accessed October 2, 2018.

National Center for Missing and Exploited Children. *Child Sex Trafficking in America: A Guide for Child Welfare Professionals* (website). http://www.missingkids.com/content/dam/ncmec/en_us/Child_Sex_Trafficking_in_America_Welfare_Prof.pdf. Accessed October 10, 2018

National Center for Missing and Exploited Children. *Key Facts* (website). http://www.missingkids.com/KeyFacts. Accessed October 10, 2018

National Poison Control Center. Poison Statistics. *National Data.* 2016. (website). https://www.poison.org/poison-statistics-national.

Sege RD, Amaya-Jackson L. Clinical considerations related to the behavioral manifestations of child maltreatment. *Pediatrics.* 2017;139: e1–e13.

U.S. Department of Health and Human Services Children's Bureau. *Child Maltreatment* (website). 2018. https://www.acf.hhs.gov/sites/default/files/cb/cm2016.pdf.

Yates G, Bass C. The perpetrators of medical child abuse (Munchausen Syndrome by Proxy)- A systematic review. *Child Abuse Neglect.* 2017;72:45–53.

25

Key Concepts, Assessment, and Management of Children With Acute or Chronic Disease

JENNIFER HUSON AND JENNIFER NEWCOMBE

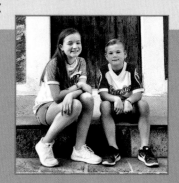

This chapter provides an overview of the care of the child with acute illness or chronic disease, and moves into a general discussion about the assessment, management, and educational approaches applicable to all disease processes. One of the major roles of the primary care provider (PCP) is to diagnose and manage patients consistent with national pediatric guidelines; this may involve telehealth measures in addition to providing care in the ambulatory or urgent care settings.

Key Concepts in Disease Management of Children

The PCP begins patient management by obtaining a presenting complaint and by taking a complete history. The PCP should be aware that the following factors are critical to establishing an accurate diagnosis and management plan:

1. Develop a trusting relationship with the child, adolescent, and caregivers.
2. Carefully observe the child and interactions with family members.
3. Pay attention to pertinent positive and negative historical and physical exam findings, avoid skewing questions toward a particular diagnosis.
4. Know age variant physiologic functions and developmental considerations.
5. Carefully consider differential diagnosis.
6. Tailor information and discussion to include the parent and/or patient in shared decision-making.
7. Take into account the patient and family's health literacy.
8. Obtain feedback from the family and child in order to ensure understanding and agreement about the diagnosis and management plan.

Shared Decision-Making as Part of Child- and Family-Centered Care

Families may face many decisions about medical treatment during the course of an acute illness or chronic disease management. Shared decision-making (SDM) is an interactive process in which the patient and family work together with the health care team to arrive at a mutually agreed upon treatment plan. Multiple definitions exist in the literature for SDM, but four characteristics are consistently described (Box 25.1). SDM is the basis for family-centered care with the ultimate goal of improved health and satisfaction (Adams and Levy, 2017).

As the SDM model increased in popularity, tools were designed to assist caregivers in making health care decisions. Decision aids for specific disorders provide education and discuss the risks and benefits of treatment options. These tools improve patients' knowledge of options and expectations of benefits and harms, and increase participation in SDM (Adams and Levy, 2017). Initially, healthcare providers were resistant to support SDM because of concerns related to efficiency in delivering patient care; however, a 2014 Cochrane review found that using decision aids did not significantly prolong the healthcare visit. The median time addition of their use to the patient encounter was only 2.5 minutes (Stacey et al., 2014).

SDM requires a collaborative approach; a provider neither assumes a paternalistic style, in which provider decisions are explained without choices left to the caregiver or child, nor a "hands-off" style, in which the provider offers options but gives no

• BOX 25.1　Characteristics of Shared Decision-Making

1. At least two parties must be involved
2. Information must be exchanged in both directions
3. All parties are aware of the treatment options
4. The knowledge and values of all those involved are considered equally

guidance regarding best choices. The SDM approach is somewhere in the middle; the provider, family, and child jointly decide the best course of action. In a life-threatening condition, where time is critical in providing care, an SDM approach may not be appropriate.

It is important for the clinician to document the details of the SDM conversation in the medical record, including (1) those present for the discussion, (2) issues addressed, (3) pertinent comments or concerns expressed, (4) perceived joint understanding, and (5) the current status of the plan. The ultimate goal of SDM is to collaborate to improve health and satisfaction (Adams and Levy, 2017).

Health Literacy

Health literacy impacts health outcomes and is an important consideration in pediatric health care (Keogh, 2014). Parents and children deserve the right to comprehensible healthcare information in order to make informed choices. The development of treatment plans in disease management requires special attention to the health literacy of clients. Written instructions and easy-to-read handouts with simple illustrations are useful. Simply giving oral or written instructions is not enough; the provider needs to make sure the receiver comprehends the information (Aslam, 2014). When designing handouts, use plain, conversational language, simple words, and short sentences without medical jargon to increase comprehension. It is important that written instructions are provided in the family's native language and are not designed for higher than a 5th grade reading level. Several tools assess the reading level and readability of the material (e.g., the Gunning Fog Index, the SMOG Readability Formula, and Flesch-Kincaid test). The U.S. Department of Health and Human Services (HHS) Office of Disease Prevention and Health Promotion (2010) recognizes the importance of health literacy, and has a National Action Plan to Improve Health Literacy. The goal of the plan is to deliver person-centered health services together with accurate and actionable information to promote lifelong learning and health.

Health Care Education

PCPs' effectiveness is enhanced by their ability to educate children and their families about the prevention of disease and management of common acute illnesses or exacerbations of chronic conditions such as asthma or atopic dermatitis. Parent-child education must be individualized and include unique child and family characteristics—age, education, health literacy, culture, family structure and function, economic status, stress, and access to community support and resources. Education can be immediate (e.g., discharge planning) or long-term (e.g., understanding, managing, and coping with chronic conditions).

Ninety percent of Americans routinely access the Internet (Center, 2017). Between 70% and 80% of adults have searched the Internet for health-related information, advice, or social support (Dol et al., 2017). Technology-focused education is becoming more advanced with interactive platforms. PCPs should develop a list of websites for parent/child education such as the American Academy of Pediatrics (AAP) health education information for parents in English and Spanish (www.healthychildren.org).

Following a healthcare visit, parents need information to make decisions related to that visit, especially in the case of an illness. Since most patients and families only remember about three main points from a discussion, written instructions are essential. It is important to consider where the patient and family are in the trajectory of the disease process. They may not need all the information about a specific condition during one visit and part of the plan should include what points are discussed at which visits. The key points to cover include diagnosis, management, possible complications, prevention, necessary follow-up, and barriers to care (Box 25.2).

• BOX 25.2　Health Care Education for Parents

Information on diagnosis includes:
- The cause, if known; epidemiology of infectious or noninfectious illnesses or medical conditions; communicability issues; and prevention guidelines, if applicable
- The rationale for procedures involved with diagnostic testing, including laboratory, radiographic, or imaging tests and the meaning of results
- Estimations of length of time before laboratory or imaging results are available, especially if long waiting periods (these are particularly frustrating for parents)
- Description of the disease, symptoms, course, and signs of improvement
- Recognition and discussion of cultural practices and beliefs about the illness or condition

Information on management includes:
- Return for any necessary follow-up or availability for a scheduled telephone conference
- Any special treatment or therapy, use of adaptive devices, and home monitoring tests
- Proper dosing of medication, the potential need to switch medications during treatment, and side effects of both prescription and OTC drugs
- Plan for administration of medications at school; completion of all appropriate forms, and instruction of school personnel on key issues related to pharmacologic therapy
- Any dietary needs or changes, hydration needs (i.e., electrolyte solutions or an increase in fluid intake), and changes in eating patterns that can be expected
- Potential benefit or harm from specific folk medicine or complementary and alternative medicine practices (including herbal, dietary supplements, or botanical preparations) if used alone or concurrently with prescribed or OTC medications
- Resources for sick care in the community that are accessible and affordable
- Safety and appropriateness of day care during the illness

Information on complications includes:
- Specific signs and symptoms that indicate worsening of the illness
- The need for immediate medical attention, or a return visit sooner than planned (e.g., a newborn with a fever of 100.4°F [38°C]; a child with severe lethargy, tender abdomen, labored breathing, stiff neck, bluish lips, purple "dots" on the skin, severe pain, inability to walk, or fever greater than 104°F [40°C])

Information should be given about prevention and barriers to care including:
- Possible recurrence and ways to prevent spread of illness
- Determining impediments preventing the parent or child from complying with the management plan (e.g., financial resources, inability to read, dysfunctional family, and/or transportation problems)
- Discussion about steps to correct these difficulties

OTC, Over-the-counter.

When discussing the management plan with parent(s) and/or child, sit down and make eye contact with them, if culturally appropriate. The parents' or caregivers' understanding of instructions should always be assessed by asking them to repeat what they have been told (teach-back method). By doing this, any misunderstandings can be addressed. The "Ask me three" plan (National Patient Safety Foundation, 2018) suggests obtaining feedback using these three questions: What is my child's main problem? What do we need to do? Why is it important for us to do this?

Chronic illness education should be directed to the caregivers and the child. The family's ability to understand the health plan needs to be considered when designing educational strategies. A clinician has a wide range of educational options during encounters including using strength-based counseling, audio and visual media aids, electronic communication, touch points, child-centered communications, and family-centered concepts. The illness severity and the child's age, maturity, and cognitive level are key factors that determine the child's degree of involvement in self-care activities. Children should be taught basic health promotion and disease prevention behaviors (e.g., hand washing) from early childhood. Likewise, they should be involved in the management of their illness to the fullest extent possible, considering their developmental capabilities and the complexity of their illness. The PCP may function as a liaison with school district personnel to effectively manage the illness while optimizing the child's educational and social experience at school.

Considerations for Care of Children With Illnesses

Parents as Observers of Illness

Most parents are alert to subtle changes in their children, so it is important to listen attentively when parents voice their concerns. A sick child who is considered high risk due to physical, mental health, or social problems merits closer observation and follow-up than does the average thriving child who becomes ill. If the child returns and is not significantly improved or is more symptomatic, the initial evaluation and diagnosis should be revisited by carefully analyzing the symptoms, investigating problems related to compliance or adherence, repeating the physical examination, reviewing likely differential diagnoses, and confirming the diagnosis before deciding on another management plan. Make sure to have the family's current contact information in case a telephone number is needed regarding the results of diagnostic tests or to monitor the course of the child's condition.

Parent Management of Illness

Parents should be encouraged to handle minor illnesses at home without calling for advice. Home instruction sheets designed for parents regarding common childhood illnesses or managing fevers (including medication dosage charts) are excellent resources. Additionally, parents should be given guidelines regarding when it is important for them to call (Box 25.3). During illness visits, parents should be told what to expect when their child is ill and should be given clear guidance about what situations require a return to clinic or a call for emergency medical services.

Working with Non–English-Speaking Families

With the diversity of dialects spoken in the United States, language can be a barrier in providing optimal health care. If a practice setting does not have access to an interpreter or native speaker, interpreter services can sometimes be obtained from local telephone services. It is important for the healthcare provider and the parent or caregiver to be able to communicate and understand each other.

Medication, Complementary Therapies, Pain, and Fever

Parents may need help to understand medication use and the importance of allowing time for the body's natural defense system to fight disease; such is often the case with viral illnesses in young children. Chapter 26 discusses prescribing principles in practice. Likewise, parents may seek complementary therapies as they offer other options or are felt to be safe; these are discussed in Chapter 27. Pain and fever can be very disturbing to parents who struggle to make their child comfortable or fear the worst. Management of these conditions is discussed in Chapter 28.

Urgent Care and Emergency Department Utilization

The emergency department (ED) is often used for primary care-related conditions (Grech et al., 2017). Parents bring their children to the ED instead of the PCP for convenience, perceived illness severity, or lack of access to a PCP (Schlichting, 2017). It is important for

---

> ### • BOX 25.3   Parent Guidelines for When to Contact the Primary Care Provider

Call immediately for an infant younger than 3 months old[a] with the following symptoms:
- Unusually sleepy
- Rectal temperature of 100.4°F (38°C) or higher
- Refuses to eat three or four times in a row
- Repeated bouts of diarrhea or vomiting
- Labored, wheezing, or grunting breathing pattern that lasts longer than half an hour
- Rash that looks like bleeding under the skin
- Yellow, jaundiced color or the baby develops pumpkin-colored skin
- Parent very nervous about baby's illness or general condition

Call immediately for an older child with the following symptoms:
- Seems unresponsive, does not make eye contact with you, or has cold and clammy skin that is not associated with vomiting
- Looks much sicker than usual with a routine illness
- Rash that looks like bleeding under the skin (purple blotches or spots)
- Any symptom that you believe to be unusual or frightening; this includes trouble breathing, stiff neck, severe headache, or very high fever

Call immediately after trauma or injury if:
- Child has struck his or her head and has either lost consciousness momentarily, has nausea or vomiting, or complains of severe headache; or if there is mental confusion, unbalanced walking, poor coordination, loss of memory, or a discharge coming from one or both ears
- There is continued swelling, tenderness, or a strange look to the injured part
- Child refuses to use an injured extremity for more than half an hour
- There is a deep puncture wound, a cut longer than 0.5 inch, or your child has not received a tetanus shot within the past 5-10 years
- There is injury to an eye that causes redness, pain, or tearing for more than 15 min
- Child has been bitten by an animal, and the bite has gone through the skin
- Child may have swallowed a toxic or poisonous substance

Call about symptoms:
- Concern about how your child looks
- Symptoms seem to be getting worse or last longer than expected
- Fever of more than 101°F (38.3°C) has lasted longer than 24 h
- Cough, cold, sore throat, or runny nose has lasted longer than 48-72 h
- Vomiting has lasted longer than 8 h, diarrhea longer than 24 h, or blood in the stool or vomit
- Child has severe stomach pains lasting longer than 4 h
- Symptom seems more severe than it has in the past
- Rash or other problem, and you are not sure what is causing it
- You are not certain whether the child needs to be seen by the healthcare provider

Call Emergency Medical Service (911) immediately and not your primary care provider:
- An infant younger than 3 months[a] who:
  - Is difficult to arouse
  - Has poor color, looks blue, difficulty breathing
  - Is limp and unresponsive

[a]Infants younger than 3 months, especially newborns, can quickly become acutely and gravely ill needing careful assessment by health providers.

---

the PCP to educate families on how and when to access care after hours as well as the appropriate use of urgent care and the ED in order to increase continuity of care for the child and minimize cost. Sturm et al., 2014 found a personalized handout with ways to obtain medical advice from the PCP leads to reduced non-urgent ED visits.

Primary Care for Chronically Ill Children

The critical issue in health promotion is to ensure an organized and coordinated approach to treatment of the child's specific disease or condition, and to ensure the child's primary health care

Common Issues or Concerns of Children and Families Related to Chronic Illness Care

- The high cost of treatment and the potential need for financial assistance
- Lack of, or barriers in, acquiring health care insurance
- Navigating the healthcare system and required paperwork
- The need for multiple healthcare providers and the frequent lack of coordination of services in providing continuity of care
- Family lifestyle alterations that may be required to care for the child
- Parents striving to normalize the child's condition and fitting into the family lifestyle
- The effect of stress on emotional and psychological well-being of all the members of the family
- The desire to be kept informed of their child's condition and progress
- The amount of parental education about disease process, pharmacology, and other therapeutic treatments required for the at-home care of the child
- How to best advocate for these children to access services through schools, state and community agencies, or special federally sponsored programs
- Treatments or procedures that may be embarrassing, painful, or time consuming
- Unpredictability of the child's condition and the potential for complications, frequent medical visits, hospitalizations, and death
- The developmental effect that chronic disease can have on a child, especially during adolescence and early adulthood (periods of increased vulnerability)
- Acceptance by peers
- Dealing with feelings (e.g., anger, sorrow) while attempting to cope with chronic illness
- Problems of non-compliance

• BOX 25.5 **Key Indicators That Affect Treatment Adherence in Children and Adolescents With Acute Illnesses or Chronic Diseases or Conditions**

Illness
- Severity of the illness and its predictability
- Length of illness and prognosis
- Effect of illness on functional and social activities of daily living

Management
- Complexity of treatment plan
- Length of time for each treatment, how often, and for what length of time treatments must continue
- Visibility of assistive equipment

Family
- Support network and size of family
- Financial resources; knowledge base and the understanding of illness or condition; overall cognitive skills; communication style
- Coping ability and skills; problem-solving skills
- Family's belief system and spiritual base

Child or Teen
- Age
- Cognitive, social, and emotional level of development; temperament
- Peer group; coping ability

Healthcare Provider and Environment
- Communication style of PCP with child, family, and other healthcare providers; belief in empowerment of parent and child/teen, as appropriate
- Organization of clinic or office setting to be child-, teen-, and family-friendly; need for adaptive modifications in their environment
- Number of healthcare providers involved in the child's care; team member collaboration and partnership among themselves and with the family
- Open and "blame-free" approach when adherence issues arise

needs are met. In doing so, the child can achieve their best potential. Healthcare management for children with a chronic illness includes: (1) assess their needs; (2) plan comprehensive health care for physical and psychosocial needs; (3) facilitate and coordinate services; (4) provide follow-up and monitoring of services; and (5) empower the child and family through education, counseling, and support. Although chronic illnesses are diverse in their severity and effect on the child, certain issues or concerns are common for children with chronic conditions and their families (Box 25.4).

The level or type of involvement in the treatment and management of a child with a specific chronic disease may vary depending on the situation of the child and family, and the healthcare provider's subspecialty. A holistic approach to care is important in order to address all aspects of care, including preventive care, health promotion, and child development. Strategies related to fostering the child's psychosocial development should also be addressed at each healthcare encounter.

Management of chronic pediatric illness should always include an assessment of quality of life. Child and/or caregiver perceptions about quality of life issues, such as physical and emotional pain and discomfort, may not be the same as those held by various healthcare providers. It is important to ask pertinent questions in gathering information about the goals of care from the child and/or caregivers. Healthcare management of children with chronic illness is about empowering them to live their lives to the fullest potential.

Family-centered care (FCC) is a collaborative approach to healthcare planning and decision-making that requires a partnership between the family and the PCP and takes place in a healthcare home model. By using a healthcare home model, members

of the healthcare team can communicate about a variety of issues. This model is discussed in Chapter 7. Communication with parents should be open and honest and they should be treated with respect and dignity. Parents of children with chronic conditions become experts in their child's care and should be viewed as partners in the management plan. The more complex the medical regimen, the greater the risk of non-adherence which can lead to serious medical complications, increased rates of hospitalization, greater length of hospital stay, and increased healthcare costs. Box 25.5 addresses key factors affecting adherence.

Assessment and Management of Children with Acute or Chronic Illnesses

History and Physical Examination

Chapter 5 discusses the complete history and physical examination of children from infancy through adolescence. In addition, each of the disease management chapters focuses on key questions to ask in history taking and highlights significant findings on physical examination. Careful attention must be given when analyzing the signs and symptoms of a child's illness, including the presentation of clinical findings, the course of the disease process, and its associated manifestations.

• BOX 25.6   **Indicators for Assessing Severity of Illness in Pediatric Patients**

1. Level of consciousness or quality of cry
   Strong cry with normal tone or content and not crying (NL)
   Whimpering or sobbing (MI)
   Weak or moaning or high-pitched cry (SI)
2. Hydration
   • Skin normal; eyes and mouth moist (NL)
   • Skin and eyes normal and mouth slightly dry (MI)
   • Skin doughy or tented and eyes may be sunken; dry eyes and mouth (SI)
3. Color
   • Pink (NL)
   • Pale hands, feet, or acrocyanosis (MI)
   • Pale or blue or ashen gray or mottled (SI)
4. Respiratory status
   • Normal (NL)
   • Nasal flaring, tachypnea, oxygen saturation of ≤95%, crackles (MI)
   • Grunting, tachypnea with more than 60 breaths/min, moderate or severe chest in-drawing (SI)
5. Reaction to stimulation by parent or healthcare provider—how a crying child reacts when held, patted on back, jiggled on lap, or carried
   • Strong cry and normal tone or content and not crying (NL)
   • Crying on and off (MI)
   • Cries continuously or minimal response (SI)
6. Sleep-to-awake or awake-to-sleep state
   • If awake then stays awake or, if asleep and stimulated, wakens quickly (NL)
   • Eyes close briefly then awakens or awakens but needs prolonged stimulation (MI)
   • Not able to arouse or falls to sleep (SI)
7. Response to social cues (being held, kissed, hugged, touched, quietly talked to, or comforted)—for infants 2 months old or younger use alert ratings
   • Smiles or alerts (NL)
   • Either briefly smiles or alerts to cue (MI)
   • No smile, face anxious, dull look, expressionless, or no alerting (SI)

MI, Moderately impaired; *NL,* normal; *SI,* severely impaired.

Data from McCarthy PL. Evaluation of the sick child in the office and clinic. In Kliegman RM, Behrman RE, Jenson HB, et al, eds. *Nelson Textbook of Pediatrics.* 18th ed. Philadelphia: Saunders; 2007; National Institute for Health and Clinical Excellence (NICE). Feverish illness in children under 5 years, 2013. Available from: www.nice.org.uk/guidance/CG160/chapter/1-Recommendations#/. Accessed April 3, 2019.

The physical examination is often a challenge when a young child is ill and uncooperative. Gathering as much data as possible by observation prior to examining the child and examining the child on the parent's lap can be helpful. The parts of the physical examination that are especially bothersome or frightening to a child should be performed last using a variety of distraction techniques from bubbles to smartphone applications. The child's ability to be comforted and overall appearance is important to accurately assess the severity of illness especially in infants and young children. If the child has a fever and looks ill, giving an antipyretic and reevaluating are key. Key indicators to evaluate during the history and the physical examination are listed in Box 25.6.

Considerations about Diagnostic Studies

Laboratory studies are used in secondary prevention to identify asymptomatic conditions (e.g., diabetes, high cholesterol, iron deficiency anemia, and lead poisoning), to diagnose conditions, and

to evaluate treatment response. Diagnostic studies and laboratory tests can be valuable, but keep in mind no diagnostic test or study is 100% accurate. False positives and false negatives occur; therefore these tests are only one part of formulating a differential diagnosis.

The Alliance for Radiation Safety in Pediatric Imaging launched the *Image Gently* campaign with the message to "child-size" the radiation used in children. Four tools were identified to accomplish this: (1) reduce the amount of radiation used, (2) scan only when necessary, (3) scan only the indicated region, and (4) scan once (not multiphase) (Image Gently, 2018). The Food and Drug Administration (FDA, 2017) promoted "shared responsibility" and identified "justified and optimized" as critical elements of the process. Shared responsibility includes manufacturers, providers, and caregivers taking a role. Justification means utilizing radiation only when needed to diagnose or answer a medical question, and when benefit outweighs risk. Optimization refers to the lowest radiation dose that still gives a quality reading as determined by age, size, and weight (Brooks, 2018). This puts the onus on the PCP to ensure there is clear benefit, order accurate tests that give the most information, are least invasive, establish a concrete diagnosis, and guide development of a treatment plan. The American College of Radiologists has information providers can use in ordering diagnostic studies based on the patient's symptoms. This website (http://acsearch.acr.org/list) provides a pediatric section with links to narrative and evidence-based information related to diagnostic studies. Useful points to remember about common imaging tests are detailed in Box 25.7.

Determining an Accurate Diagnosis

Following the history and physical examination, a diagnosis needs to be determined in order for a management plan to be formulated. Diagnostic errors are more common than realized and come from faulty data gathering or verification, as well as inadequate knowledge (Thammasitboon and Cutrer, 2013). Diagnostic errors remain a leading cause of malpractice claims (Nurses Service Organization, 2018). With increasing time constraints in clinical practice, difficulty in keeping track of patients in large group practices, and the development of the full clinical picture that may become evident only over time, it is important to use every available resource to elucidate difficult diagnoses. Four causes of error at the individual clinician level include: (1) availability heuristic—diagnosis biased by experience with past cases; (2) anchoring heuristic (premature closure)—relying on initial diagnostic impression despite subsequent information to the contrary; (3) framing effect—diagnostic decision-making unduly biased by subtle cues and collateral information; and (4) blind obedience—placing undue reliance on test results or "expert" opinion (AHQR, 2018). A more reflective thought process by the clinician can help avoid errors. Strategies to improve differential diagnostic skills fall into three major categories: (1) expanding clinical expertise, (2) avoiding cognitive processing errors, and (3) using cognitive aids in diagnostic decision-making. In order to expand clinical expertise, PCPs must be lifelong learners, increasing their expertise in both the science of diagnostic decision-making as well as closing the gaps in their knowledge about a variety of diseases. To avoid cognitive errors, the clinician must develop skills to avoid questions that are biased toward a particular diagnosis and understanding the importance of reflective practice. The use of evidence-based medicine and understanding the common errors of clinical practice improve the ability to make accurate diagnostic decisions. Several types of diagnostic aids, including using group

Conventional Radiographs

- Useful diagnostic tools if correctly ordered (e.g., the type of view[s] needed)
- Least expensive and readily available
- Involves radiation; for example, a single view chest radiograph effective radiation dose is up to 0.01 millisievert unit (AAP, 2018)

CT Imaging

- Costly
- Best for detecting calcifications and fresh blood; shows greater bone detail than MRI (Smith, 2011)
- Can be used with contrast material (taken by mouth, rectum, or injected via vein) for special evaluations, such as abnormalities affecting blood vessels; check for patient allergies to iodine, seafood, kidney disease, or prior reaction to contrast materials
- Images can be presented in frontal, transverse, or sagittal planes or obtained in three-dimensional imaging
- Breath-holding abilities must be considered; infants or young children may require sedation or general anesthesia
- Requires radiation exposure which increases the risk for developing cancer later in life (Darnell and Morrison, 2016). Therefore it is important CT examinations be performed only when absolutely necessary and scan only indicated areas. A head CT effective radiation dose is up to 2 millisievert unit (AAP, 2018).

MRI

- Ability to distinguish between mediastinal fat, blood vessels, and soft tissues (Thukral, 2015)
- MRI shows greater tissue detail than CT (Smith, 2011)
- Expensive and may require contrast
- Often requires sedation or anesthetic in infants and young children since immobilization is necessary (Thukral, 2015)
- Advanced MRIs include diffusion MRI, magnetization transfer MRI, fluid-attenuated inversion recovery, magnetic resonance angiography, magnetic resonance gated intracranial cerebrospinal fluid (liquor) dynamics, magnetic resonance spectroscopy, functional MRI, real-time MRI, and interventional MRI; usually ordered by specialists

Ultrasonography

- Gives two-dimensional images and measurements of internal organ systems; however, air-filled lungs and gas-filled bowel loops are impenetrable to ultrasound
- With Doppler ultrasound blood flow direction and velocity can be measured; a still picture of the image can be recorded as a permanent record, or sonography can be viewed as the image is being projected onto a video screen
- Highly dependent on operator skill and experience
- No sedation required, no radiation exposure; noninvasive; readily available

- Clearly identify whether this is a referral or a consult.
- State the child's name, age, tentative or actual diagnosis, and expectations of the consult/referral (e.g., "newly diagnosed type 2 diabetes mellitus; needs initial insulin control, and diet and physical activity recommendations").
- Discuss briefly the reason consultation or referral is requested.
- Give a synopsis of the history, clinical findings, prior management plan, and outcome of treatment if applicable.
- Identify pertinent past medical history, such as chronic illnesses or conditions.
- Provide pertinent family, educational, or social information, including insurance coverage if problematic.

an appropriate plan. Diagnostic decision support systems do not make a diagnosis but assist the clinician to form a list of differential diagnoses based on the patient's age, gender, geographic area, and symptoms. A tracking and follow-up system for diagnostic studies is critical in order for the provider to promptly note laboratory and diagnostic study results. Empowering patients by making sure they are engaged in the diagnostic process is also important (Thammasitboon et al., 2013b). Although a complete review of the numerous and various methods to reduce error is outside the scope of this chapter, an essential point to remember is that *reflective practice leads to improvement in diagnostic accuracy over time.*

Referral and Consultations

Pediatric PCPs may encounter clinical or behavioral problems that they are uncomfortable with or unprepared to treat and decide to consult or refer the patient. Although the two terms tend to be used interchangeably, there is a difference between a consult and a referral. *Referral* implies the patient will be assessed and managed by the provider referred to, whereas a *consult* implies the PCP wishes to continue to manage the patient's care but seeks consultation about particular aspects of the care. The goals of both processes are to enhance patient care and improve patient outcomes. Clear communication in an organized manner is essential for a successful referral or consult (Box 25.8). The PCP and the specialist must coordinate responsibilities for services (e.g., follow-up testing, monitoring, and treatments).

The PCP may ask a specialist to provide guidance through informal, "curbside" consults, but, due to malpractice concerns, many specialists are not receptive to this. It is difficult to provide all the needed information in this scenario. If an informal consultation is provided, the PCP should present information about the patient, as listed previously, and discuss potential management options. At the end of the informal consultation, the PCP should summarize in the patient's chart key areas that were discussed and agreed-upon recommendations.

Often overlooked sources of free consultation are state and local public health departments or agencies, health-related professional organizations, and some major medical centers that provide telephone consultation for providers in their community. Again, a notation should be placed in the chart if the case is discussed with a consulting agency. Connecting with colleagues on the Internet must be done securely; there are heavy fines for information transmitted without encryption over a secure server (see later discussion).

decision-making and seeking a second opinion on error-prone diseases, such as appendicitis, as well as the use of algorithms, diagnostic decision support, checklists, and point-of-care knowledge bases within EMRs or smartphones can improve the likelihood of a correct differential diagnosis. Consulting with or referring difficult patients to a more experienced healthcare provider and using computerized diagnostic decision support can help with a challenging pediatric situation and/or illness presentation. Data suggest computerized diagnostic systems give useful suggestions, provided all symptoms are entered correctly into the database. Internet-based decision support systems allow providers to consider a wider variety of differential diagnoses when formulating

The bond between the child, parent, and PCP is typically a strong relationship. When a patient is referred to another provider, the PCP must explain the reason for the referral to the child and parent, how the transfer of care will be managed, and when the patient will return to see the PCP. The information should be presented in a way that dispels fears of abandonment. If the PCP plans to seek a consultation, the child and parent should be informed by explaining the need for a second opinion or desire to collaborate with others. After the consultation, parents should be informed about the decision the consultant and PCP made in deciding the best course of action. Finally, the parent may seek consultation with an alternate healthcare provider. If so, treat this as the parent's need to collaborate in the child's care and listen carefully to the recommendation of the consultant. Be sure the consultant's reports are filed in the child's chart. It is helpful to maintain a list of specialty providers with their area of specialty or subspecialty, their fees for service (e.g., full fee or sliding scale), and which insurance plans reimburse their services. The child's insurance coverage is often a major factor in referral, and prior authorization from an insurance carrier may be needed.

National and Local Organizations and Resources

Parents and their children with specific disease entities or health conditions benefit from the educational materials, resources, and support national health organizations provide. Learning to live with a chronic disease or a disabling condition presents a challenge to families. Most national organizations provide written materials parents and children can easily understand about the cause, management, and treatment of the particular disease in question. These materials also help parents explain their child's condition to teachers and others. Many national organizations guide parents and children to support groups with families and children with similar diseases. These organizations assist parents to access unique services that benefit their children (e.g., enrolling in special camps and sports activities, learning about various legal rights of children with disabilities or handicapping conditions, and acquiring special adaptive equipment).

Many national and local health organizations also provide educational materials designed for health professionals and families about specific disease processes. An example is the National Organization for Rare Disorders (NORD) which assists providers and parents and offers information about various conditions or disease processes (www.raredisease.org). Healthcare providers should take advantage of the services these organizations offer and should have a listing of local community resources.

Documentation of Patient Visit

During a healthcare visit, PCPs should thoroughly document the patient's history, physical exam, diagnosis, and plan of care. Many malpractice claims against care providers are due to a lack of documentation. The old adage, "If it isn't in writing, then it wasn't done" has been used more than once to find providers liable and render a judgment in favor of the plaintiff. Good documentation practices are listed in Box 25.9.

Telehealth Management of Illnesses

Multiple communication technologies are available today to interact with patients and families. The use of brief electronic communication via email, text messaging, and social media are increasingly popular. Patients and families express considerable

---

• **BOX 25.9**   **Critical Components for Documentation**

- Be alert to a complaint or combination of complaints that are red flags for more serious illness (e.g., abdominal or chest pains, headache, syncope). Note pertinent positive and negative history and physical findings relative to these complaints.
- Identify differential diagnoses and rule out serious or life-threatening illness first. Be sure to gather enough data to either rule in or out the diagnosis based on history, physical findings, and diagnostic studies. "Rule outs" are no longer acceptable to insurance providers. Providers must use terms such as right lower quadrant pain rather than rule out appendicitis.
- Revisit an unresolved problem until it resolves. Reschedule a follow-up examination or use telephone or email contact with the family to determine if the complaint or illness resolved.
- Ensure there is a system in place to ensure that diagnostic studies were done, results received, and follow-up was done by the provider.
- Follow-up on referrals to other health care professionals or agencies and document the recommendations or treatments from these referral sources.
- Document missed clinic appointments through chart audits, which should be a regular part of practice quality improvement. Look for such information omissions, whether problems identified in earlier visits were addressed at subsequent visits until resolved, and compliance with routine health maintenance screenings.

---

interest in communicating with their providers using these methods. This section reviews telephone triage, text messages, email, and use of social media. It discusses possible problems associated with these modalities and what can be done to overcome the challenges.

Telephone Triage Systems

Telephone triage can also be called *telephone advice services, telephone consultations,* or *telenursing.* A major benefit of telephone triage is the ability to provide convenient access to healthcare professionals and healthcare advice. The major difficulty in providing telephone advice is the challenge of accurately assessing a situation without a physical exam. All PCPs should ensure their practice settings have a standardized approach to telephone triage. Nonemergent calls to a practice about a sick child during the day are usually routed through a receptionist, who can make an appointment, if appropriate, or transfer the call to a triage nurse or PCP. Many healthcare providers utilize standardized protocols for telephone triage. Triage protocols classify problems into one of several categories. These include life-threatening, emergent, urgent, non-urgent, recurrent, or mildly ill. Protocols vary slightly, but the major aim is to provide safe advice while avoiding unnecessary visits to an urgent care center or ED. Protocols may use a standardized algorithm to obtain a history and manage a specific health concern.

When using telephone protocols in a practice setting, training is essential and ensures consistency in the use of the system. Utilizing a management-by-telephone protocol should accomplish the following objectives: (1) allow the telephone triage provider to manage ill-child calls safely, (2) provide a standard of care and improve the quality of care, and (3) prevent omissions resulting from provider forgetfulness, interruption, or fatigue.

The individual doing the telephone triage must be receptive to the parent's concerns. Parents can be anxious and find it difficult to articulate the problem. The triage person needs to listen carefully to the caller; ask questions as dictated by protocol and by

• **BOX 25.10** Triage Questions

- Description: Tell me about the problem. What signs and symptoms are present?
- Duration: How long has the problem been present?
- Clinical changes: How has the child's behavior or activity level changed (e.g., eating, sleeping, playing, interaction with peers and family members)?
- Appetite: Has there been a change in the child's eating or drinking habits?
- Elimination: Have there been changes in bowel or bladder habits?
- Sleep pattern: Has there been a change in the child's sleeping habits?
- Environmental problems: Has there been any recent exposure, change, or stress in the child's environment?
- Cause: What does the parent believe may be contributing to or causing this condition?
- Management: What has the parent done for the condition, and what was the effect?
- Feelings: Does the parent feel anxious about the child's current condition?

judgment; process the information; determine the correct management protocol for the situation; give the necessary instructions to the parent; offer comfort and understanding to help the parent manage the illness; and document the encounter in a timely manner. The sequence of steps the triage provider must follow while using telephone protocols includes the following: collect data about the symptoms through open-ended and direct questioning, identify the problem or main symptom, develop a working assessment or differential diagnosis, decide on a triage category for the patient, select the correct protocol, and correctly advise the patient about the course of action. Questions should be asked in an effort to narrow the problem clinically from most to least severe. When using protocols, the provider needs to ensure each question is asked but can add additional questions when necessary. Screening questions that should be asked of parents are listed in Box 25.10.

Keep in mind protocols are a tool and should not override the provider's professional judgment. If the provider feels the patient needs to be seen despite what the telephone triage protocol states, then the patient should be seen.

One of the most important points to emphasize about the use of any telephone management system is the need to assess the comfort level of the parent with the advice provided. Parents should be asked at the end of the telephone contact whether they are comfortable with the plan of care. If the parent is not satisfied or is uneasy about the plan, PCP consultation should be an option. Finally, parents should be told to call back if their child's condition worsens or persists.

Call centers are another avenue pediatric practices use for handling sick calls after office hours. These centers may employ nurses and/or nurse practitioners who use telephone protocols to guide parents in the management of their child's illness until their regular healthcare provider is available. Call centers alleviate the burden of night call and are set up to use telephone protocols and a software program for documentation.

Documentation of sick calls and their disposition is an important element of a successful telephone triage system. All documentation should be part of the medical record. Written paperwork or electronic documentation must be scanned into the electronic medical record (EMR) so other providers have access, and are made aware of, the child's illness or medical condition. Important items to include in any documentation of a telephone communication

include: date and time; patient demographics—name, age, sex, and telephone number; patient history—chronic disease or condition; list of medications and their dosages; the chief complaint and a brief list of signs and symptoms, including their duration and frequency; documentation of sleeping pattern; activity level, appetite, and bowel and bladder elimination; diagnosis or working assessment; triage category (life-threatening, emergent, etc.); and instructions given about follow-up.

Texting and Email

Short message system (SMS) text messages have been increasing steadily since the emergence in smartphone technology. Although texting can be an efficient means of communication, there are potentially considerable privacy and security risks associated with this means of communication. HIPAA does not comment on text messaging because the law was created in 1996 before text messaging was available. However, effective September 2013, all providers must have the ability to have secure healthcare communications with an encryption protection platform as part of their mobile device assuring that if there is a loss of a mobile device, the user can be disconnected from the system to avoid a data breach. In addition, protected health information is not allowed to be stored on personal mobile devices if a personal mobile device is used on an open Wi-Fi network.

Most SMS communications are used to send appointment reminders, give educational messages, provide support to patients between visits, and track lab results. If text messaging is used by a provider evaluating a child's condition, it is important to ensure that the same information that would normally be asked in a telephone conversation is in the text message before giving any recommendations. Not all patients and families want to receive SMS; therefore patients and families must agree to the use of SMS messaging prior to sending out reminders or texts. Each practice needs to have a communication policy patients and families consent to using. Some practices have included requirements in their policy, such as encryption, passcode protection, registration of devices, or use of third-party secure messaging programs to avoid any breach of confidentiality.

As with SMS, emailing patients can be convenient, but has the same problems associated with SMS text messaging. Therefore it is important to limit this type of communication to encrypted networks in which the device can be turned off if lost. Again, there is a significant risk of data breach in emails, and there are no HIPAA secure devices for this purpose at this time.

Social Media

Many parents and youths spend more time on the Internet and social media than talking on the phone. If a provider is asked to connect on a social media platform there is the risk of disclosing personal patient information on these websites, leading to breaches in the patient-provider relationship. As a result, it is recommended clinicians avoid social media relationships with patients or their parents. The American Medical Association's policy statement addressing social media suggests (1) be careful to never post identifiable patient information, (2) monitor information to ensure its accuracy, (3) maintain appropriate professional boundaries, and (4) recognize posting can have a negative impact on one's own reputation and can result in reduced trust in the medical profession (Omaggio, Baker, and Conway, 2017).

Office Telephone and Electronic Messaging Policy

Practice settings should have an electronic messaging or telephone call policy that covers basic information about the office protocol for handling calls, requests for advice sent electronically about sick children, or other child-related concerns during office hours (e.g. well-child questions, prescription refills, after-hours calls, and weekend and holiday calls). Information should be provided to patients and families about who screens calls, when calls are returned, and after-hours coverage. There should also be a policy about answering electronic messages.

References

Adams RC, Levy SE. Shared decision-making and children with disabilities: pathways to consensus. *Pediatrics*. 2017;139(6).

Agency for Healthcare Research and Quality (AHQR). *Patient Safety Network: Diagnostic Errors*; 2017. Available at: https://psnet.ahrq.gov/primers/primer/12.

American Academy of Pediatrics. *What Every Pediatrician Should Know*. 2018. www.aap.org/en-us/about-the-aap/Committees-Councils-section-on-Radiology/Pages/What-Every-Pediatrician-Should-now.asp.

Aslam L. Patients safety and discharge teaching particularly in pediatrics, i-manager. *J Nurs*. 2014;4(3):20–24.

Brooks M. *Pediatric X-ray Imaging Safety a Shared Responsibility*; 2018. Available at: www.medscape.com/viewarticle/891170.

Center PR. *Internet/Broadband Fact Sheet*. 2017. http://www.pewinternet.org/fact-sheet/internet-broadband/.

Darnell K, Morrison GD. Minimizing the long-term effects of ionizing radiation in pediatric computed tomography examinations. *Radiol Technol*. 2016;87(5):495–501.

Dol S, Delahunty-Pike A, Sheren Siani, Campbell-Yeo M. *Ehealth Interventions for Parents in Neonatal Intensive Care Units: A Systematic Review*. Joanna Briggs Institute; 2017. https://doi.org/10.11124/JBISRIR-2017-003439.

Grech CK, Laux MA, Burrows HL, Macy ML, Pomeranz ES. Pediatric emergency department resource utilization among children with primary care clinic contact in the preceding 2 days: a cross sectional study. *J Pediatric*. 2017;188:245–251.

Keogh L. Health literacy and its importance for effective communication. *Part 2* 2014;26(4):32–36.

Image Gently. *Campaign Overview*; 2018. Available at: https://www.imagegently.org/About-Us/Campaign-Overview.

National Patient Safety Foundation (NPSF). *Ask Me Three*. NPSF (website); 2018. www.npsf.org/?page=askme3&terms="ask+and+three".

Nurses Service Organization (NSO). *Understanding nurse practitioner liability, CNA HealthPro Nurse Practitioner Claims Analysis 1998-2008, Risk Management Strategies and Highlights of the 2009 NSO Survey* (PDF online). 2018. http://international.aanp.org/Content/docs/UnderstandingNursePractitionerLiability.pdf.

Omaggio NF, Baker MJ, Conway LJ. Have you ever Googled a patient or been friended by a patient? Social media intersects the practice of *J Genet Couns*. 2018;27(2); 481–492.

Schlichting LE, Rogers ML, Gjelsvik A, et al. Pediatric emergency department utilization and reliance by insurance coverage in the United States. *Acad Emerg Med*. 2017;24(12). Available at: https://onlinelibrary.wiley.com/doi/abs/10.1111/acem.13281.

Stacey D, Légaré F, Col N, et al. Decision aids for people facing health treatment or screening decisions. *Cochrane Database Syst Rev*. 2014;1:CD001431.

Thukral BB. Problems and preferences in pediatric imaging. *Ind J Radiol Imag*. 2015;25(4).

Thammasitboon S, Cutrer WB. Diagnostic decision-making and strategies to improve diagnosis. *Curr Probl Pediatr Adolesc Health Care*. 2013;43(9):232–241.

Thammasitboon S, Thammasitboon S, Singhal G. System-related factors contributing to diagnostic error. *Curr Probl Pediatr Adolesc Health Care*. 2013b;43(9):242–247.

U.S. Department of Health and Human Services (HHS) Office of Disease Prevention and Health Promotion. Washington, DC: *National action plan to improve health literacy*; 2010.

26

Prescribing Medications in Pediatrics

CATHERINE G. BLOSSER AND JESSICA L. SPRUIT

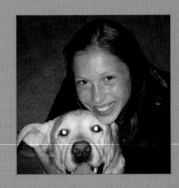

This chapter is designed to strengthen the health care provider's understanding about prescribing pharmaceuticals in pediatrics, including ways to enhance adherence. Providers should consult a comprehensive pediatric drug reference, the U.S. Food and Drug Administration (FDA), or pharmaceutical manufacturers regarding specific drugs, their classification, preparation, indications, dosing, side effects, interactions, and other considerations.

National Safety Goals Regarding Prescribing Medications

The Joint Commission has published National Patient Safety Goals (NPSG) that address several concerns regarding medication practices in ambulatory health care clinics. Since 2014, the goals have stressed the importance of reconciling medication information. The NPSG for ambulatory health care clinics, effective January 2018, direct health care providers to "maintain and communicate accurate patient medication information." To achieve this, health care providers determine the medications the patient is currently taking and the medications prescribed for that patient, and attempt to identify and resolve any discrepancies. Important information to be obtained from the patient and caregiver include the medication name, dose, route, frequency, and purpose. This information is also important when prescribing new medications, as potential interactions between medications must be considered. The Joint Commission directs healthcare providers to provide education about new prescriptions, including the name, dose, route, frequency, and purpose at the end of each care encounter. Additionally, providers should provide information about how to manage medications to patients and families during each interaction. Healthcare providers can support this management strategy by suggesting that the family maintain a medication list, update it as needed, and share it with their primary care provider (PCP) at each visit (The Joint Commission, 2018) (see Additional Resources).

Regulation and Safety of Pharmaceuticals

Less than 50% of drugs approved by the FDA in the United States have been specifically tested for use in some subset of the pediatric population (American Academy of Pediatrics [AAP], Committee on Drugs, 2014). This historical lack of drug testing in the pediatric population stems from several factors, which include economic disincentive (pediatric patients are a much smaller market than adult counterparts, especially because children are usually healthy); difficulty recruiting an adequate sample size; difficulty obtaining needed laboratory specimens from children in research studies; inability to obtain informed consent and questionable ethical use of placebo controls in children; possible discomfort, risks, and liability; additional ethical considerations when working with vulnerable population/minors; and difficulty in formulating acceptable medication delivery systems (e.g., tablets, liquids) for specific pediatric age groups (Edmunds and Mayhew, 2013; Institute of Medicine [IOM], 2012).

An internal review committee (Pediatric Advisory Committee [PAC]) at the FDA evaluates the post-market safety of all pediatric drugs, biologic products, and medical devices for children that have been granted patent exclusivity by the FDA. The PAC can request labeling modifications, areas where further investigation is efficacious, areas where further clinical trial data are necessary, and clinical trial design.

Under the Best Pharmaceuticals for Children Act (BPCA) and the Pediatric Research Equity Act (PREA) auspices, there have been over 500 pediatric labeling changes (e.g., ibuprofen labeling now includes doses for children 6 months to 2 years old and ranitidine labeling includes accurate dosing information for use in infants). Many medications, including anti-asthmatic and anticonvulsant medications, have been relabeled in response to these pediatric legislative initiatives, providing dosing information for a larger age range of patients. For updates on pediatric drug labeling changes, consult the FDA website (see Additional Resources).

Pharmaceutical labeling is required to provide drug information that is easily accessible and comprehensive for providers. The most important prescribing information about the benefits and risk of a drug, the date of initial product approval, and the phone number and website address to report adverse effects are now placed at the beginning of prescribing information and package inserts in a section called *Highlights*. Similar formatting must be included in electronic prescribing tools and other information resources.

The PAC recommends that pharmaceutical labels carry warnings about suicide, neonatal withdrawal/toxicity, and risks of off-label use for some drugs in pediatrics. Providers are responsible for reporting adverse effects and for monitoring the use of off-label drugs. All providers are encouraged to report adverse effects to the FDA MedWatch website (see Additional Resources). However, many clinical adverse effects of drugs in this age group may go unreported, and the true nature of a drug's safety may not be fully understood.

In the European Union, any company that applies to the European Medicines Agency (EMA) is required to include a pediatric investigation plan or obtain a waiver if a drug is not applicable for use in children. This provision, the Pediatric Regulation, also provides funding to study drugs no longer patent protected in children, with the results made available to the public.

Safety Issues With Pharmaceutical Manufacturers

Generic drugs account for 22% of prescribed drugs in the United States, but account for up to 88% of *filled* prescriptions. India is the largest exporter of these generics. China and India are the major exporters of low-value active pharmaceutical ingredients and excipients used in the production of finished drugs by other countries, including those manufactured in the United States (International Trade Administration, 2016). Concerns with counterfeiting, manufacturing safety lapses, substandard products, and falsified drug test results have led to an increase in FDA investigations, penalties, and enforcement measures within those countries. The availability of medications over the Internet at reduced prices further predisposes consumers to these risks. The National Association of Boards of Pharmacy created a verified pharmacy program on their website to help consumers buy safe medications (see Additional Resources). Chapter 27 also discusses safety and regulatory issues of imported herbs, botanicals, and dietary supplement products.

Issues With Pharmaceutical Testing

Increasingly, data on the effect of drugs are from clinical trials being conducted outside the United States; a limited study of late-phase trials of drug applications found that only 40% of studies were conducted entirely in North America. This practice raises many concerns including the applicability of data related to ethnic differences and genetic characteristics, challenges in overseeing such studies, and design and analysis of some questionable foreign trials (Khin et al., 2013). Global efforts are underway to address these issues by establishing standards for logistics, rigorous protocol development, review and protocol-driven clinical trials, internal auditing, and the use of established investigators at multicenter and multinational sites (Joseph et al., 2015).

Guidelines for Writing a Prescription

Prescriptions must be written in a manner that conveys accurate information to the pharmacist, the child, and/or parent or caregiver, and other clinicians accessing the child's chart. Among the most common errors in prescriptions are illegible handwriting, misplaced or ambiguous decimal points, omitted information, and inappropriate choice of medications (Lofholm and Katzung, 2018). Online resources are available to help reduce or document prescribing errors, including the Institute for Safe Medication Practices and National Coordinating Council for Medication Error Reporting and Prevention program (see Additional Resources). Electronic prescribing or e-prescribing (i.e., a computer-generated system) has greatly reduced prescribing errors (e.g., it allows the PCP to ensure legible script; cross-check the prescription against known allergies; calculate appropriate drug dosing based upon weight and/or body surface area; and note dosage limits, drug-drug interactions, and duplications) (Lofholm and Katzung, 2018; Porterfield et al., 2014). Prescribing accuracy can be enhanced by following the guidelines listed in Box 26.1.

• BOX 26.1 Guidelines for Accurately Writing a Prescription

- Limit each prescription to one medication.
- Prescriptions should be preprinted with names of prescribers in the practice setting; circle your name. (Pharmacist will know who to contact for questions/clarifications should the signature be illegible.)
- Eliminate drug abbreviations[a] (e.g., TCN could mean triamcinolone or tetracycline).
- Use computer-generated prescriptions whenever possible. If a handwritten prescription is needed, print out name of medication in block letters rather than write out the name in cursive.
- Provide concise dosage information[a]:
  - Use metric measures, such as milligrams or milliliters, rather than designating tablet, vial, teaspoon, tablespoon, or dropper. Most parents, including those who are non-English speakers or who have low literacy, can follow instructions on the use of metric measures (Lofholm and Katzung, 2018).
  - Write "unit" rather than a "U," which can be mistaken for a zero or a number.
  - Write "international unit" rather than IU, which can be mistaken for IV or the number 10.
  - Write "daily" rather than qd, which can be mistaken for qid.
  - Write "every other day" rather than qod, which can be mistaken for qid and qd.
  - Avoid a trailing or terminal zero (e.g., 9.0 mg), because the decimal point may be missed. Write 9 mg instead.
  - Lead with a zero before a decimal point (e.g., 0.15 mg) so that the decimal point is not missed.
  - Avoid using decimal points whenever possible (e.g., write 300 mg instead of 0.3 g).
- Do not use abbreviations for body parts[a] (e.g., o.d. [oculus dextra] for right eye).
- Avoid vague instructions that might cause confusion when patient is taking several drugs (e.g., avoid "take as directed" or "prn" without stipulating how often drug should be taken).
- Use generic, official, or trademarked name; avoid chemical names or coined names.
- Add the patient's age and weight to orient the pharmacist and help ensure age-appropriate prescription and dosage (e.g., tetracycline should not be prescribed to a 5-year-old child).
- Specify number of pills to be dispensed rather than stating a time duration. Adding refills for an acute treatment confuses duration of therapy and may preclude patient returning for a necessary recheck appointment.
- State indication or purpose of drug (alerts pharmacist and other physicians to appropriateness of medication and aids in counseling). This can be as simple as stating it is for a respiratory or skin condition (preprint the body system directly on the prescription for easy check-off).
- Add supplemental information (e.g., avoid sun exposure; do not take with grapefruit juice; take with food).
- Remain alert to lethal doses and compromising pathologic conditions (e.g., compromised renal or hepatic functions) that might affect drug levels.

[a]A complete list of abbreviations to avoid when writing prescriptions is available from www.ismp.org/tools/errorproneabbreviations.pdf.

IV, Intravenous; *qd, quaque die* (every day); *qid, quarter in die* (four times a day); *qod, quaquealtera die* (every other day).

Prescribing accuracy from Lofholm PW, Katzung BG. Rational prescribing & prescription writing. In: Katzung BG, ed. Basic and Clinical Pharmacology. 14th ed. New York: McGraw-Hill; 2014:chap 65; National Coordinating Council for Medication Error Reporting and Prevention. Recommendations to enhance accuracy of prescription/medication order writing; 2014. www.nccmerp.org/recommendations-enhance-accuracy-prescription-writing. Accessed January 10, 2018; Woo TM. Pediatric patients. In: Woo TM, Robinson MV, eds. Pharmacotherapeutics for Advanced Practice Nurse Prescribers. 4th ed. Philadelphia: FA Davis; 2016:1321–1335.

General Prescribing Guidelines

Pediatric patients pose unique considerations for medication management. Resist pressures from parents or other individuals to prescribe medications without a clear indication. A comprehensive understanding of over-the-counter (OTC) and prescription medication indications, contraindications, dosages, adverse reactions, and drug interactions, as well as knowledge of pharmacodynamics and pharmacokinetics of the drugs in the developing child, is essential for effective medication management. Some general points to keep in mind when prescribing drugs or recommending OTC medications in children include:

- Assess renal and hepatic systems for degree of maturation and function.
- Use clinical practice guidelines, if available.
- Be aware of the influence of advertising in prescribing practice. The newest agent may be more expensive, and there may be no evidence that its use leads to a better outcome.
- Use a decision-support system to investigate the possibility of drug interactions and side effects (e.g., an electronic medical record support system or an online application).
- Check for interactions between pharmacologic agents and any herbs, botanicals, or dietary supplements being taken concurrently.

Prescribing Medications for Children

In the past, the dosage for pediatric patients has typically been determined by extrapolating from the adult dose and proportionately reducing the dose based on the child's weight and drug side effect profiles. However, this approach does not take into account developmental changes in pediatric metabolism, the drug's pharmacokinetics, adverse effects (e.g., the connection between selective serotonin reuptake inhibitors [SSRIs] and potential suicide risk in adolescents), and medication delivery form. The fields of ethnopharmacology and pharmacogenetics/genomics provide health professionals with a better understanding of how genetics, age, developmental level of organs, the immune system, and metabolic rates influence the body's response to drugs. The phase I enzyme CYP2D6 (located on chromosome 22) for example, is responsible for variable metabolism and elimination of approximately 20% of drugs used clinically (Hibma and Giacomini, 2018). The maturing child is physiologically dynamic. Factors such as size, age, renal function, cardiac output, hepatic blood flow, concomitant drug use, disease, individual characteristics (including ethnicity and genetics), and maturation/development of body systems can lead to specific pharmacokinetic differences that affect any given drug effect and dosing decisions. Key fundamental principles to consider when prescribing medication for children are:

- Drug absorption: The absorption rate of medications administered through subcutaneous or intramuscular injection is affected by the blood flow to those tissues, where poor blood flow can result in delayed or reduced absorption. The immature gastrointestinal (GI) tract of neonates and young infants also influences the absorption of medications through decreased acid secretion, prolonged emptying, and irregular peristalsis. Finally, the thin stratum and large body surface of young children increase the concern for systemic absorption of topically applied medications (Woo, 2016). The younger the child, the more the absorption may vary.
- Drug distribution: The inherent physicochemical properties of a drug and the complex processes involved with growth and development in children affect drug distribution. Body weight (amount attributed to fat, protein, and intracellular water), bone and teeth maturation (e.g., tetracycline is deposited in growing teeth and can cause permanent staining), and pathologic factors that alter physiologic function must be taken into consideration. This is particularly important when prescribing for infants and young children (e.g., some drugs more easily cross the blood-brain barrier; a premature infant's blood-brain barrier is more permeable; and some conditions [e.g., meningitis, brain tumors, cranial trauma] can affect central nervous system permeability). Alterations in protein binding influence some drug distribution (e.g., increased free concentration of a medication such as diazepam and potential toxicity in preterm infants due to decreased protein binding) (Koren, 2018). The provider also needs to be aware of drugs contraindicated during breastfeeding (see Chapter 16 for suggested references).
- Drug metabolism: Most drugs are metabolized in the liver, requiring the provider to consider the maturation and function of the liver when prescribing medications. Although knowledge of drug metabolism is improving, little is known about the developmental pattern of phase I and phase II enzymes and activity in children (Woo, 2016). The decreased rate at which drugs are metabolized in neonates and young infants leads to slow clearance and prolonged elimination half-life. Later in childhood, however, the rates of metabolism through certain enzymes exceed adult levels, necessitating more frequent or higher doses. It is important that the provider is aware of the enzymatic activity required for drug metabolism and monitors drug levels as indicated (Koren, 2018).
- Drug elimination: The maturity of a child's renal excretion system has a significant effect on drug elimination. Glomerular filtration rate in neonates is approximately 30% to 40% of adults, however, the adult value is usually reached by 6 to 12 months of life. Common drugs cleared by the renal system (e.g., penicillin, gentamicin, digoxin) require dosage and dosing schedule changes and close monitoring in ill or immature infants (Koren, 2018).

Pharmaceuticals Used In Pediatrics: Off-Label Prescribing

Despite the lack of studies in the pediatric population and lack of pediatric labeling, an overwhelming number of drugs are prescribed for children. Such "off-label" use does not mean that the drug is being prescribed improperly or unethically for the condition or age. Evidence for the pharmaceutical use and safety in the pediatric age group may not have been submitted to the FDA, or the drug may not meet the "level of substantial evidence" needed for FDA approval. For example, many antibiotics, medications for asthma, dermatologics, ophthalmologic drops, and anti-psychotropic drugs are commonly prescribed off-label effectively.

Perils of Prescribing Off-Label

The practice of prescribing off-label is not without risk. Providers must balance patient safety against their judgment that the patient will derive the intended benefit. Some general guidelines when prescribing off-label include the following (AAP, Committee on Drugs, 2014):

- Consult the *Physician's Desk Reference,* Epocrates, or other reputable pharmacology application (app), or the package insert.
- Refer to published literature regarding a medication whenever possible. If publications are not available, use other scientific evidence and expert medical judgment.

- Check the FDA website for any warnings about the drug.
- Discuss recommendations for off-label treatment with the patient or family; document the decision-making process and the patient's/family's consent in the health record.
- Be mindful about the precautions that come with each drug, heeding warnings and contraindications.

Other Factors to Consider in Medication Management

Decisions about which drugs to use with children are not based simply on which one will be most effective in treating the child's clinical condition or which drugs are most typically prescribed. Ethical considerations must also be taken into account when prescribing, particularly where evidence of efficacy is weak or anecdotal and safety is a concern. Social and functional family issues must also be considered, as well as factors that influence adherence, such as taste, dosing regimen, and collaborative decision-making (Table 26.1). Parental education related to medication use is discussed in Chapter 25, and the reader is encouraged to review this discussion.

A child's developmental level and age affect the amount of influence parents have over the administration of, and adherence to, a medication regimen.

For *infants* it is important to take the following into consideration:
- The parent should be taught how to properly administer medications.
- Determine whether other caregivers will be administering the medication.
- Determine whether a simplified dosing schedule is necessary for a family (e.g., with children in day care).

Toddlers and *preschoolers* are beginning to exert their independence, and administering medication to this age group can be challenging. The keys to success with this age group are to:
- Choose a medication regimen with the fewest problems associated with administration (e.g., taste, frequency).
- Take into account palatability and doses per day.

School-age children developmentally are industrious, and they are often the most willing to take medications. Education should focus on:
- Both the parent who will supervise/administer the medication *and* the child who will be taking the medication.
- Letting the child choose the formulation if possible (liquid, chewable, or pills to swallow).
- Avoiding dosing during school hours if possible.

Adolescents often administer their own medication. The provider needs to closely collaborate with adolescent patients regarding their medication regimen by:
- Allowing them to have input about the dosing schedule and what will work best for them.
- Assisting the family with the transition from parental supervision to teen administration.

Medication Adherence

The 2015 survey data regarding ambulatory health care sponsored by the Centers for Disease Control and Prevention (CDC) found that 70.2% of pediatric healthcare visits resulted in a drug being provided or prescribed (CDC, 2018). Additionally, the number of chronically ill children and adolescents continues to increase as treatment modalities and survival rates improve, necessitating long-term medication use. Yet, 50% to 55% of pediatric patients do not consistently take their medication for chronic medical problems, with adherence rates declining more after the first six months of diagnosis (American Psychological Association [APA], Society of Pediatric Psychology, 2016). Failure to adhere to a medication regimen increases the use of healthcare services by children and adolescents with chronic medical conditions, such as asthma, epilepsy, human immunodeficiency virus (HIV), and inflammatory bowel disease (McGrady and Hommel, 2013). In addition, the lack of health insurance, the cost associated with obtaining medications, and the presence of learning disabilities contribute to poor adherence rates in those with chronic diseases (Capoccia et al., 2016; Dharmapuri et al., 2015).

The term *adherence* is currently used to describe whether or not a patient is taking the recommended pharmaceutical or following a recommended treatment regimen. Providers need to assess the child's and/or parent's barriers to medication adherence. Nonadherence needs to be proactively managed in order to improve clinical outcomes and cost effectiveness. Table 26.1 discusses general factors that contribute to lower adherence rates and suggests strategies to increase those rates. A myriad of research studies about adherence have led to the following conclusions:
- Adherence is not a steady state; therefore adherence needs to be assessed as part of each office visit.
- Open-ended questions that allow the patient/parent an opportunity to describe their adherence may provide more accurate information. Additionally, validated tools for assessing medication adherence are available and may be considered as an added measure of assessment (Capoccia et al., 2016). Some objective measurements can also be used to determine the level of adherence (e.g., laboratory measurements, dosage count, medication diaries, and refill rates).
- Adolescents are less likely to be adherent. Adherence rates in this age group can be increased by using technology such as personalized text message reminders and mobile health applications (Garofalo et al., 2016; Shellmer et al., 2016).
- Adherence is influenced by illness perceptions and medication beliefs. For example, if a family perceives asthma as an episodic illness, they are less likely to adhere to a daily medication regimen prescribed to control symptoms (Klok et al., 2015).
- Patients/families consider their trust in providers and the effectiveness and satisfaction of their communication when making decisions about medication adherence. Provider behaviors such as time spent with patients or communication skills and clinical systems that promote continuity and integration of care are necessary to enhance medication adherence (Conn et al., 2015).
- Adherence rates can improve by scheduling more follow-up visits and spending more time discussing the child's/parent's perception about the disease process, reasons for and benefits of the medication, and importance of adherence (Conn et al., 2015).
- A provider is more effective when practicing active listening, providing emotional support, using plain language, giving brief but complete instructions, and having the child and/or parent repeat instructions or "teach back," allowing adequate time for visits, using a wide range of teaching tools, and involving office staff in teaching activities.
- Health literacy has a significant impact on adherence. Strategies to overcome limited health literacy include providing verbal instructions and utilizing language that can be completely understood by patients (Miller, 2016).

TABLE 26.1 Factors That Influence Adherence to Taking Prescribed Pediatric Medications

Factors That Influence Adherence	Interventions That Improve Adherence
Length of treatment: Longer treatment contributes to poorer adherence.	*Shorten length of treatment if possible* (e.g., if multiple antibiotic regimens are equally as effective, select the one with the fewest days of therapy).
Medical condition: Adherence rates vary with chronic illnesses, frequency of medication changes, lack of physical symptoms, need of mastering techniques of medication administration, lack of immediate benefits of medication.	*Develop creative solutions to encourage adherence* (e.g., sticker charts; pill boxes; calendars; link dose to a personal daily habit, such as teeth brushing). Determine how drug regimen will fit into child's lifestyle and try to modify it to fit the child in order to increase adherence; repeat short educational instructions at every visit (include verbal and written instructions); assess for depression. Discuss barriers (e.g., does child have other priorities? Does treatment create a negative identity? Does child want to avoid unpleasantness?) and their underlying assumptions. Engage a family member or caregiver who will be assisting the child with their medications at home. Provide continuity of care.
Doses per day: The more medication doses that need to be administered per day, the poorer the adherence rate. This is particularly true with working parents and children in school who often miss midday doses.	*Simplify dosing regimen.* Prescribing medications that require once or twice daily dosing increases adherence (Woo, 2016). If possible, consider dispensing two bottles of a prescription medication so that some may be stored at home and some at school or day care. (This may be limited by insurance coverage and the ability to obtain two bottles.)
Palatability and ease of ingestion: Unpalatable medications are resisted by children, especially young children. Some children have difficulty swallowing some formulations (e.g., pills).	*Prescribe medications in a higher concentration when possible to reduce the volume required.* For example, when prescribing 250 mg of penicillin VK, select the suspension that includes 250 mg/5 mL rather than 125 mg/5 mL to reduce the amount of medication the child needs to swallow (Taketomo, 2017). *Choose the best-tasting medication, prescribe chewables or oral disintegrating tabs, or mask the taste.* If a medication has the same efficacy profile, the best-tasting (though that may not mean it tastes good) medication will be easier to administer to young children. Most pharmacies in the United States offer FLAVORx (for a small fee), which allows children or parents to custom choose how their liquid medicine will taste by masking or overriding the existing flavor (see Additional Resources). There is also the option of using flavoring syrups or crushing tablets, such as prednisone, and mixing with palatable semi-solid foods, such as chocolate syrup, jam, applesauce, or pudding. Before crushing any tablet or mixing a medication with syrup, the provider should check with a pharmacist to determine if the food is compatible with the medication. *Facilitate swallowing of pills and capsules.* Place pill in mouth and take a mouthful of water; turn head as far to the right as possible and swallow. Repeat on the left side and rotate sides, depending upon the number of pills in the treatment regimen.
Expense: Out-of-pocket costs may be difficult for some families to meet. Insurance coverage may not include medications.	*Choose the medication that has the lowest out-of-pocket expense for the family.* Prescribe generics when appropriate and offer information on insurance coverage and resources (e.g., discount cards, mail-order pharmacies, and medication assistance programs).
Belief systems: Religious and spiritual beliefs concerning medication containing ingredients of animal origin; concern with the safety profile and long-term effects of medications; seeing medication as a "crutch"; or if children or teens view themselves as "addicts" are all beliefs that can affect adherence.	*Counsel medication use issues with ethical and cultural sensitivity, especially in multi-faith communities.* Specifically address safety and side effects of drug regimen and elicit concerns. Use motivational interviewing techniques (see Chapter 15). Assess literacy and health literacy level.
Family/social factors: Issues such as working parents, poor transportation, homelessness, lack of social support, fatigue, family disruption, dysfunction, risky behavior (alcohol consumption and drug abuse), and level of literacy and health literacy can affect the ability to understand and adhere to a treatment regimen.	*Assess the family for issues that affect successful outcome.* If there is poor or less-than-expected outcome with a treatment regimen, the provider should determine if family issues are a barrier to adherence and address interventions to assist the family in identifying strategies that improve success. Assess literacy and health literacy levels.

- Incorporate all modes of teaching styles. The use of tools and emerging technologies are receiving more attention as a means to improve adherence rates. These tools include pictogram-based instruction sheets; telephone counseling; video or mobile games to improve knowledge, disease management adherence, and clinical outcomes; mobile phone apps; short, weekly text messages; pill boxes and organizers; and electronic monitoring devices that record inhaler use (see Additional Resources)

(Klok et al., 2015; Shellmer et al., 2016; Thakkar et al., 2016; Yin et al., 2017).
- Written instructions increase adherence rates. Consumer medication information (CMI) leaflets dispensed through retail pharmacies are intended to be short and comprehensive for consumers. They are written by third-party drug information companies and are not approved or regulated by the FDA. Patient package inserts (PPIs) are developed by the

pharmaceutical manufacturer and discuss risk information; they are lengthy, detailed, and intended for the use of medical providers.

- Ascertain who the child and family believe is the best support person (family member, outside friends, and so on) to work with to promote adherence to the medication regimen. Reinforcement techniques increase rates of adherence; have the child/adolescent and/or parents identify and use reinforcement strategies (e.g., stickers, special treats [a day at the zoo]). Establishing a provider/pharmacist collaborative management program for chronic treatment regimens increases adherence rates (Gums et al., 2014).
- Providers also need to self-critique any biases they have toward ethnically and socially diverse populations and overcome any cultural barriers.

Overprescribing Antibiotics: A Continuing Problem

Approximately 2 million illnesses and 23,000 deaths in the United States are attributed to drug-resistant bacteria each year (White House, 2015). In addition to the dangers associated with drug-resistant bacteria, other adverse events such as anaphylaxis are a growing problem (Fleming-Dutra et al., 2016). In response to this serious public health threat, a National Action Plan for Combating Antibiotic-Resistant Bacteria was developed in 2015. One of the goals outlined in this plan is to reduce inappropriate antibiotic use in outpatient settings by 50% (White House, 2015).

Approximately 12% to 28% of ambulatory care visits result in an antibiotic prescription. Upon evaluation, an estimated 30% of outpatient antibiotic prescriptions across all ages in the United States were deemed inappropriate (Fleming-Dutra et al., 2016). Antibiotics were often given without definitive bacterial confirmatory tests, or a broad-spectrum antibiotic was given without a clear indication (Gerber et al., 2014; Saleh et al., 2015). These data support the need for antimicrobial stewardship programs. Goals of pediatric antimicrobial stewardship programs include decreasing unnecessary use of antimicrobials, antimicrobial resistance, cost, and side effects of antimicrobials; and improving patient safety and outcomes (Goldman and Newland, 2015). Strategies to achieve these goals include increased training of prescribers and pharmacists, formulary limitations, and audits of prescribing practices with feedback (Goldman and Newland, 2015; Nichols et al., 2017). Antimicrobial stewardship programs have been proven to be effective, and the collaboration between the government, providers, health care facilities, and the community outlined in the National Action Plan has potential to continue to decrease the threat of antimicrobial resistance.

Advances in Pharmacologic Research: Maximizing Therapeutic Efficacy

As previously mentioned, genetic variations affect drug metabolism and an individual's response to a dosage. New research is also shedding light on "drug chronotherapy." This field of inquiry (chronobiology) demonstrates that the metabolism and tolerability of certain drugs depend upon the body's own biologic timing (circadian rhythm) of certain organs, tissues, and cells. Advances have been made to discern when certain pharmaceuticals should be taken to better align with these rhythms to produce better outcomes and allay side effects. The principles of chronopharmaceutics underlie the new regimens for treating certain cancers,

rheumatoid arthritis, and congenital adrenal hyperplasia. Additional studies are investigating the impact of circadian biology in diseases of the nervous system (e.g., attention-deficit/hyperactivity disorder [ADHD] and epilepsy), dermatologic conditions such as atopic dermatitis, and metabolic diseases (e.g., diabetes, obesity, and glucose metabolism disorders) (Manganaro et al., 2017; Selfridge et al., 2016; Vaughn et al., 2017).

Disposal of Pharmaceuticals

Most OTC and prescription drugs are not recommended to be disposed of at home (e.g., flushed down the drain or toilet). Trace amounts have been found in rivers, streams, and treated water, creating health concerns related to hormone disruption, antibiotic resistance, and synergistic effects. Community water treatment plants do not routinely filter out medicines. Providers should know which pharmacies in their area will take back unused or expired products or encourage patients to dispose of unused medications at hazardous recycling facilities or at a community-sponsored "take-back" program. The FDA website describes methods to dispose of unused medications, including disposal in household trash (sealed in a leak-proof container with used coffee grounds, cat litter, or other undesirable substance) (see Additional Resources). Additionally, the Drug Enforcement Agency has information regarding prescription take-back days and authorized collectors at their website (see Additional Resources). Also, before disposing of a medicine container, remove or scratch out all identifying information on the prescription label.

Additional Resources

Drug Enforcement Agency (DEA): Disposal of Pharmaceuticals. www.deadiversion.usdoj.gov/drug_disposal/index.html

European Medicines Agency. www.ema.europa.eu/ema/index.jsp?curl=pages/regulation/document_listing/document_listing_000068.jsp&mid=WC0b01ac0580925c45

Food and Drug Administration (FDA): New Pediatric Labeling Information Database. www.accessdata.fda.gov/scripts/sda/sdNavigation.cfm?sd=labelingdatabase

Food and Drug Administration (FDA): MedWatch: The FDA Safety Information and Adverse Event Reporting Program. www.fda.gov/Safety/MedWatch/default.htm

Food and Drug Administration (FDA): Disposal of Pharmaceuticals. www.fda.gov/Drugs/ResourcesForYou/Consumers/BuyingUsingMedicineSafely/EnsuringSafeUseofMedicine/SafeDisposalofMedicines/ucm186187.htm

FLAVORx. www.flavorx.com 1-800-884-5771

Institute for Safe Medication Practices. www.ismp.org

The Joint Commission (National Patient Safety Goals [NPSG], The Joint Commission (National Patient Safety Goals [NPSG]). www.jointcommission.org/standards_information/npsgs.aspx

National Association of Boards of Pharmacynabp.pharmacy

National Coordinating Council for Medication Error Reporting and Prevention. www.nccmerp.org/about-medication-errors

Mobile Phone Applications

The following apps provide treatment adherence and management programs for patients, family, and friends to alert when a medication is due or has not been taken. They can be downloaded free or at minimal cost from app stores for iOS or Android operating systems:

- Dosecast
- Mango Health
- MedCoach
- MediSafe
- Medi-Prompt

- MedMory
- MyMedSchedule
- MyMeds
- Pillboxie
- PillMonitor
- RxCase Minder
- RxmindMe.

Text Messaging

Memotext. www.memotext.com

Uses evidence-based screening tools to assess and personalize messaging for individuals and communicates with them about information based upon the individual's profile, condition, and desires for feedback.

Mosio Health Services. www.mosio.com/biz/solutions/health

Two-way text messaging web-based service that enables health care providers to proactively send and receive text messages to/from individuals or lists of individuals in a secure website.

Mobile Games: Available as Mobile Applications

HealthPrize Technologies. www.healthprize.com

Collects daily adherence data and rewards individuals with loyalty points, sweepstakes, and competitions; verifies refills.

References

American Academy of Pediatrics (AAP). Committee on Drugs. Policy statement: off-label use of drugs in children. *Pediatrics.* 2014;133(3):563–567.

American Psychological Association (APA). Society of Pediatric Psychology. *Fact Sheet: Adherence to Pediatric Medical Regimens for Chronic Disease.* 2016. Available at: www.societyofpediatricpsychology.org/medical_regimens.

Capoccia K, Odegard PS, Letassy N. Medication adherence with diabetes medication. *Diabetes Educ.* 2016;42(1):34–71.

Centers for Disease Control and Prevention (CDC). National ambulatory medical care survey: 2015 state and national summary tables. Available at: www.cdc.gov/nchs/data/ahcd/namcs_summary/2015_namcs_web_tables.pdf: Accessed February 24, 2018.

Conn VS, Ruppar TM, Enriquez M, et al. Healthcare provider targeted interventions to improve medication adherence: systematic review and meta-analysis. *Int J Clin Pract.* 2015;69(8):889–899.

Dharmapuri S, Best D, Kind T, et al. Health literacy and medication adherence in adolescents. *J Pediatr.* 2015;166(2):378–382.

Edmunds MW, Mayhew MS. Special populations: pediatrics. In: Edmunds MW, Mayhew MS, eds. *Pharmacology for the Primary Care Provider.* 4th ed. St. Louis: Elsevier/Mosby; 2013.

Fleming-Dutra KE, Hersh AL, Shapiro DJ, et al. Prevalence of inappropriate antibiotic prescriptions among US ambulatory care visits, 2010-2011. *JAMA.* 2016;315(17):1864–1873.

Garofalo R, Kuhns LM, Hotton A, et al. A randomized control trial of personalized text message reminders to promote medication adherence among HIV-positive adolescents and young adults. *AIDS Behav.* 2016;20(5):1049–1059.

Gerber JS, Prasad PA, Localio AR, et al. Variation in antibiotic prescribing across a pediatric primary care network. *J Pediatric Infect Dis Soc.* 2014;4(4):297–304.

Goldman JL, Newland JG. New horizons for pediatric antibiotic stewardship. *Infect Dis Clin North Am.* 2015;29(3):503–511.

Gums TH, Carter BL, Milavetz G, et al. Physician-pharmacist collaborative management of asthma in primary care. *Pharmacotherapy.* 2014;34(10):1033–1042.

Hibma JE, Giacomini KM. Pharmacogenomics. In: Katzung BG, ed. *Basic and clinical pharmacology.* 14th ed. New York: McGraw-Hill; 2018.

Institute of Medicine (IOM). *Safe and effective medicines for children: pediatric studies conducted under the Best Pharmaceuticals for Children Act and the Pediatric Research Equity Act.* 2012. Available at: www.nap.edu/catalog/13311/safe-and-effective-medicines-for-children-pediatric-studies-conducted-under.

International Trade Administration (ITA). Top markets report pharmaceuticals: overview and key findings. 2016. Available at: www.trade.gov/topmarkets/pdf/Pharmaceuticals_Executive_Summary.pdf.

Joseph PD, Craig JC, Caldwell P. Clinical trials in children. *Br J Pharmacol.* 2015;79(3):357–369.

The Joint Commission. Ambulatory health care national patient safety goals. 2018. Available at: www.jointcommission.org/assets/1/6/NPSG_Chapter_AHC_Jan2018.pdf.

Khin NA, Yang P, Hung HM, et al. Regulatory and scientific issues regarding the use of foreign data in support of new drug applications in the United States: an FDA perspective. *Clin Pharmacol Ther.* 2013;94(2):230–242.

Klok T, Kaptein AA, Brand PLP. Non-adherence in children with asthma reviewed: the need for improvement of asthma care and medication education. *Pediatr Allergy Immunol.* 2015;26(3):197–205.

Koren G. Special aspects of perinatal and pediatric pharmacology. In: Katzung BG, ed. *Basic and Clinical Pharmacology.* 14th ed. New York: McGraw-Hill; 2018.

Lofholm PW, Katzung BG. Rational prescribing and prescription writing. In: Katzung BG, ed. *Basic and clinical pharmacology.* 14th ed. New York: McGraw-Hill; 2018.

Manganaro S, Loddenkemper T, Rotenberg A. The need for antiepileptic drug chronotherapy to treat selected childhood epilepsy syndromes and avert the harmful consequences of drug resistance. *J Cent Nerv Sys Dis.* 2017. https://doi.org/10.1177/1179573516685883. eCollection.

McGrady ME, Hommel KA. Medication adherence and health care utilization in pediatric chronic illness: a systematic review. *Pediatrics.* 2013;132(4):730–740.

Miller TA. Health literacy and adherence to medical treatment in chronic and acute illness: a meta-analysis. *Patient Ed Couns.* 2016;99(7):1079–1086.

Nichols K, Stoffella S, Meyers R, et al. Pediatric antimicrobial stewardship programs. *J Pediatr Pharmacol Ther.* 2017;22(1):77–80.

Porterfield A, Engelbert K, Coustasse A. Electronic prescribing: improving the efficiency and accuracy of prescribing in the ambulatory care setting. *Perspect Health Inf Manag.* 2014;11(Spring):1g.

Saleh EA, Schroeder DR, Hanson AC, et al. Guideline-concordant antibiotic prescribing for pediatric outpatients with otitis media, community-acquired pneumonia, and skin and soft tissue infections in a large multispecialty healthcare system. *Clin Res Infect Dis.* 2015;2(1):1010.

Selfridge JM, Gotoh T, Schiffhauer S, et al. Chronotherapy: intuitive, sound, founded but not broadly applied. *Drugs.* 2016;76(16):1507–1521.

Shellmer DA, Dew MA, Mazariegos G, et al. Development and field testing of Teen Pocket PATH, a mobile health application to improve medication adherence in adolescent solid organ recipients. *Pediatr Transplant.* 2016;20(1):130–140.

Taketomo CK. *Pediatric & neonatal dosage handbook.* 24th ed. Hudson, OH: Lexi-Comp, Inc; 2017.

Thakkar J, Kurup R, Laba TL, et al. Mobile telephone text messaging for medication adherence in chronic disease. *JAMA Intern Med.* 2016;176(3):340–349.

Vaughn AR, Clark AK, Sivamani RK, et al. Circadian rhythm in atopic dermatitis – pathophysiology and implications for chronotherapy. *Pediatr Dermatol.* 2017;35(1):152–157.

White House. *National Action Plan for Combating Antibiotic Resistant Bacteria.* 2015. Available at: https://www.cdc.gov/drugresistance/pdf/national_action_plan_for_combating_antibotic-resistant_bacteria.pdf.

Woo TM. Pediatric patients. In: Woo TM, Robinson MV, eds. *Pharmacotherapeutics for Advanced Practice Nurse Prescribers.* 4th ed. Philadelphia: FA Davis Co; 2016.

Yin HS, Parker RM, Sanders LM, et al. Pictograms, units and dosing tools, and parent medication errors: a randomized study. *Pediatrics.* 2017;140(1):e20163237.

27

Complementary Medicine in Pediatric Primary Care With an Introduction to Functional Medicine

CATHERINE BLOSSER AND EMILY GUTIERREZ

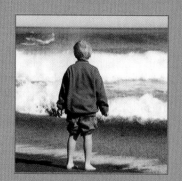

The clinical, academic, and philosophic foundations that drive conventional Western medicine are undergoing a paradigm shift. Boundaries of healthcare and health delivery systems that were once rigid and exclusionary continue to be challenged. This has resulted in therapies that were once regarded as unconventional or *alternative* to become accepted as an established part of the mainstream education and practices of nursing and medicine. Present-day terminology for the application of these therapies is *integrative* and/or *complementary* medicine; the term *alternative* medicine is no long used. The term *complementary* medicine is used throughout this chapter to describe *integrative* and/or *complementary* approaches. It is also notable that the National Institute of Health's (NIH's) National Center for Complementary and Alternative Medicine (NCCAM) is now known as the National Center for Complementary and Integrative Health (NCCIH).

In an integrative practice model, the primary care provider (PCP) is required to fully consider the complex interplay between biology, culture, psychosocial, environment, and lifestyle choices. The focus is on promoting health and healing and preventing future disease. The integrative model utilizes the most efficacious treatments from both allopathic and complementary therapies, being mindful of the scientific evidence behind both. In 2017, the American Academy of Pediatrics (AAP) published a consensus report on pediatric integrative medicine, saying, "In an integrative approach, evidence-based complementary therapies may be used as primary treatments or used in combination with conventional therapies" (McClafferty et al, 2017). This personalized approach is at the core of integrative medicine and also addresses 21st-century pediatric healthcare concerns and needs.

Functional medicine (FM) is a model of medicine that is associated with the application of complementary/integrative medical treatments. This model is also individualized and patient centered. It is based on a collaborative patient-practitioner partnership and focuses extensively on a biologic/metabolic pathway focusing on systems rather than on symptoms. In this way, it endeavors to determine the root cause of a disease, emphasizing the fact that

systems do not work in isolation but are interwoven in the presentation of chronic and complex disease. One condition might have many different causes and, similarly, one cause may result in many different conditions. Thus this model approaches assessment and management in a slightly different way from that of integrative or conventional medicine. This model is relatively new and research is active.

Integrative medicine gives the practitioner the ability to choose therapeutic tools outside of mainstream medicine. FM does the same but also goes a step further to stress prevention through nutrition, diet, and exercise; it emphasizes the use of different laboratory testing and other diagnostic techniques and then prescribes combinations of drugs and/or botanic medicines, supplements, therapeutic diets, detoxification programs, and stress-management techniques. An FM provider is a licensed health professional who has undergone specialty training and certification by the Institute for Functional Medicine or a similar academic institution (e.g., a physician, nurse practitioner [NP], naturopathic practitioner).

The underlying principles of each of these practice models are discussed in greater detail later in this chapter. Also covered are the foundations for understanding the use of complementary therapies in children, safety, and guidelines, clinical implementation strategies, and pharmaco-vigilance with dietary supplements. The choices of complementary therapies are expansive and diverse; some therapies are listed for a limited number of conditions. Some reliable references for treating an array of pediatric health conditions with complementary therapies are listed under Additional Resources, later in this chapter.

Standards and Guidelines

The Joint Commission's National Patient Safety Goals address medication reconciliation and require that all medications that a child or adolescent takes are accurately communicated (The Joint Commission, 2018). The name, dosage, frequency, and purpose of the complementary product(s) must be noted in the medical record so that the provider can ascertain if there are any contraindications to using the product at the same time as other medications. This helps to avoid negative outcomes and ensures access to this information for other healthcare providers.

The American Association of Colleges of Nursing (AACN) Quality Safety Education for Nurses graduate competencies include support of patient-centered care based on the individual's values, culture, ethnicity, and spiritual and social preferences—all reasons individuals choose complementary health practices. Providers should know their own boundaries in order to avoid adverse risk, use a positive organizational approach so that individuals feel free to discuss their use of complementary therapies, utilize teamwork between conventional and complementary health practitioners, research complementary health approaches, and monitor outcomes (AACN, 2012).

The AAP recognizes that the "best interest of the child" is always the guiding standard for providers, whether they are recommending a conventional or complementary medicine approach. Families should always be informed about the efficacy and safety of a particular treatment; they should also be told if there is a lack of information regarding a specific therapy. Providers are encouraged to keep an open mind, be nonjudgmental, be aware of cultural and ethnic practices of their patients, and educate patients about risks and benefits. The AAP offers the following standard (Adams et al, 2002, pp 662-663):

> If evidence supports both safety and efficacy, the physician should recommend the therapy but continue to monitor the patient conventionally. If evidence supports safety but is inconclusive about efficacy, the treatment should be cautiously tolerated and monitored for effectiveness. If evidence supports efficacy but is inconclusive about safety, the therapy still could be tolerated and must be monitored closely for safety. Finally, therapies for which evidence indicates either serious risk or inefficacy obviously should be avoided and patients actively should be discouraged from pursuing such a course of treatment.

In addition, any treatment must be viewed as hazardous if its use delays the provision of proven conventional care for a serious medical condition.

The NCCIH endorses strategies that emphasize safe and efficacious use of complementary medicine. These include better understanding of how and to what extent complementary medicine is used by the pediatric population and within demographic subpopulations (e.g., cultural groups); better understanding of the decision-making processes of patients who use or providers who recommend complementary medicine; studying the safety and risks of complementary medicine for the pediatric population; and developing and conducting research into specific complementary medicine interventions, practices, or disciplines that support healthy lifestyle behaviors (NIH, 2016).

The World Health Organization (WHO) issued the *WHO Traditional Medicine Strategy 2014–2023* to guide healthcare leaders of WHO Member States. This guide encourages Member States to formulate polices that recognize the potential contribution of traditional and complementary medicine (T&CM) to the overall health status and well-being of their populations; to promote safe, respectful, cost-efficient, and effective T&CM use by regulating and supervising products, practices, and providers of care; and to promote universal health coverage using integrative models in national health systems (WHO, 2013).

Use of Complementary Therapies by Children and Adolescents

The 2007 U.S. National Health Interview Survey (NHIS) provided the first comprehensive information regarding complementary medicine use by children in the United States (National Center for Health Statistics [NCHS], 2008). The last survey that included questions about this topic was conducted in 2012 with children 4 to 17 years of age (NCHS, 2013). Results revealed little change in the use of complementary treatments over time except for significant decreases in use among Hispanic children, in the use of a traditional healer, and in families with parents who had less than a high school education (Black et al, 2015). In 2012, approximately 12% of children used complementary medicine (excluding multivitamins and multiminerals). If specific vitamins and minerals were included, usage was approximately 55% of all children. A 2014 to 2015 study found over 60% of children used complementary medicine, most often vitamins, minerals, and massage (Kalaichandran et al, 2018). A large study in Canada revealed pediatric usage rates exceeding 75%, depending on the definition of complementary medicine. Concurrent use of complementary and conventional medicine was common (Adams et al, 2013).

Cultures that regard complementary medicine practices as mainstream rather than "alternative" may be using complementary medicine at higher rates. Specific subsets of children and their families in the United States tend to use complementary medicine therapies (Box 27.1).

The most commonly reported therapies used were *natural products*, frequently described as dietary supplements (e.g., echinacea, fish oil/omega-3, combination herb pills, or flaxseed oil/pills), chiropractic practices, deep breathing, yoga, homeopathic treatment, traditional healing, massage, meditation, diet-based therapies, and progressive relaxation (Black et al, 2015). Chiropractic/osteopathic manipulation was the most commonly used therapy that required a complementary medicine practitioner.

Complementary medicine therapies were used predominantly for head or chest colds, anxiety and stress, back and neck pain, other musculoskeletal conditions, attention deficit/hyperactivity disorder (ADHD), and insomnia. *Mind-body therapies* were most commonly used for anxiety and stress, insomnia, and nausea and vomiting; *biologically based therapies* were used for symptoms of fever, insomnia, reflux, and sinusitis; and *manipulation/bodywork* was used for abdominal pain, musculoskeletal conditions, and

---

• **BOX 27.1** **Characteristics of Children and Families Using Complementary Therapies**

- Child has a chronic illness, special needs, emotional, mental, and/or behavior issues
- Are non-Hispanic Caucasian
- Have a college-educated parent
- Family income above $65,000 per year
- Live outside of the southern United States
- Have taken prescription drugs within the past 3 months
- Have private medical insurance
- Have had more frequent visits to a conventional medical provider in the past 12 months
- Parent uses a complementary therapy (this is a key predictor)

From McClafferty H, Vohra S, Bailey M, et al. Pediatric integrative medicine. Pediatrics. 2017;140(3). https://doi.org/10.1542/peds.2017-1961

nausea and vomiting. Additional medical conditions or symptoms for which complementary medicine was used included allergies, asthma, dermatologic conditions, developmental disorders, gastrointestinal (GI) conditions, headaches, learning disabilities, overweight, and psychologic conditions (Black et al, 2015).

Little is known about the use of homeopathic product (HP) remedies in children. One study examined HP remedies that were administered to the same cohort of children at seven different times from birth to 8½ years of age (Thompson et al, 2010). Slightly less than 12% used HPs, with the most common age for administration around 7 years. Parents self-treated their children with HPs 46% of the time, whereas general practitioners prescribed HP 10% of the time. Chamomile for teething and colic and arnica for soft tissue bruising or cuts were the most commonly used products.

Specific practitioners who provide complementary therapies may include chiropractors, naturopaths, yoga instructors, herbalists, aromatherapists, homeopaths, acupuncturists, folk medicine practitioners (e.g., curanderos, shamans), and traditional Chinese medicine practitioners as well as others.

Scientific Studies of Complementary Medicine Therapies

Critics and advocates agree that whether the treatment is "mainstream" or "complementary," both conventional and nonconventional therapies need to be held to the standards of the scientific method. A landmark analysis in 2005 found that between one-third and one-half of the most acclaimed scientific medical research findings (across medical disciplines) were false, exaggerated, or riddled with conflicts of interest based on the evidence being later refuted (Ioannidis, 2005). Consequently, guidelines for all researchers to improve the credibility and efficiency of their studies are being actively promoted by the Meta-Research Innovation Center at Stanford University (Ioannidis, 2014). In this light, complementary medicine therapies are increasingly being subjected to the rigorous scientific study that meets Western criteria.

Randomized controlled trials (RCTs), meta-analyses, and systematic reviews have provided the strongest evidence for the efficacy and safety of various therapies. There has been a lack of these hypothesis-driven methodologies in the study of complementary treatments. In 2011, Snyder and Brown searched PubMed and found 111 research articles about complementary medicine therapies used in children. Of these, 81 studies examined the top five therapies. Studies that used RCTs, meta-analyses, or systematic reviews analyzed only the three most common therapies. Other methodologies included case-controlled or cohort/cross-sectional strategies. The majority of methodologies used did not provide solid empiric evidence for the use of most complementary therapies (Snyder and Brown, 2012). It is clear that more rigorous research is needed in this area; however, there are barriers to achieving this goal.

The nature of many complementary medicine therapies and the characteristics of those who use complementary medicine present a challenge to the use of hypothesis-driven research methods. Research in integrative medicine requires a shift from examining conventional research variables to looking at variables that focus on the unique characteristics of individuals in the context of their lives. This focus supports the "N of 1" approach, addressing the complexity of individual variability (Kravitz et al, 2014). The effectiveness of a complementary medicine treatment may also be influenced by the contextual or nonspecific effects of the relationship between the practitioner and the patient, a variable that is difficult to quantify. RCTs may not reflect the complexity of the symptom states or clinical responses most relevant to patients using complementary medicine therapies. For example, mind-body treatments affect a number of health domains and symptoms—all of which would have to be measured in a clinical trial.

Despite the difficulty of advancing a hypothesis-driven research agenda, much work is being done and more evidence being generated to support the use of complementary therapies. Advancements in technologies such as genomics, proteomics (study of proteins), metabolomics (study of chemical processes within living organisms), systems biology, and the analytic capacities of microprocessing and nanoprocessing has elicited new scientifically based insight into an individual's expression of health and illness. The NCCIH was established in response to the need for scientific studies into complementary medicine therapies. This organization has funded more than 2500 research projects nationally and internationally, and more than 3300 scientific articles have been published in peer-reviewed journals (NIH, 2017a). NCCIH does not specifically include children among its priority groups for federally funded research. However, the AAP Section on Integrative Medicine (SOIM) is making an effort to address this deficit by (1) working with the Pediatric Research in Office Settings (PROS) Network and NCCIH to do more targeted research among infants, children, and adolescents; (2) working with the U.S. Division on Health Care Finance and Practice Improvement to develop priorities, goals, and strategies for enhancing reimbursement for effective, appropriate complementary medicine therapies; and (3) highlighting effective pediatric integrative clinical care models for interested pediatricians.

The National Cancer Institute (NCI) and the Office of Cancer Complementary and Alternative Medicine (OCCAM) have also sponsored a number of clinical research trials and studies at medical centers to evaluate complementary medicine therapies for cancer. The Patient-Centered Outcomes Research Institute (PCORI)—a nonprofit, nongovernmental organization authorized by Congress in the Patient Protection and Affordable Care Act of 2010—funds clinical trials comparing the benefits and safety of at least two approaches known to be effective for a particular clinical disorder. These trials can include drugs, medical technologies, complementary medicine, behavioral interventions, and delivery systems (Selby, 2013). A number of academic centers in the United States have established centers for integrative medicine and are conducting ongoing research (e.g., the University of California-San Francisco, University of Maryland, Duke University, and Mayo Clinic).

The Pediatric Complementary and Alternative Medicine Research and Education Network (PedCAM) works to develop a pediatric complementary medicine research agenda through an international consensus-driven priority-building process. PedCAM disseminates a wide range of complementary medicine information and is building collaborative relationships among researchers, educators, clinicians, and policymakers, both nationally and internationally (see "Additional Resources," later in this chapter).

As a result of these efforts, studies of complementary medicine are increasingly found in the literature and in well-regarded Internet reference sites: PubMed, NCCIH, National Library of Medicine, and Cochrane Collaboration, to name a few. Some findings are clearly considered reliable and valid. Aetna Insurance Company, for example, recognizes that there is adequate evidence for the safety and effectiveness of acupuncture, biofeedback, chiropractic, and electrical stimulation for pain and covers these treatments in their policies (Aetna, 2018).

Integrating Complementary/Integrative and Functional Medicine into Pediatric Primary Care

Common Principles of an Integrative Care Practice Model

It is important for PCPs to understanding the basic principles common to integrative treatment modalities. These include the following:
- A focus on wellness that, in turn, prevents illness
- A belief in the body's ability to self-heal (external interventions that stimulate the body's internal healing processes are a focus of care)
- The understanding that health is a result of rebalancing the body's biologic systems
- An emphasis on using nutrition, plants, and other natural products to maintain or return to health
- Recognition and use of the individual's unique constitution and inner resources to achieve health; each individual has strengths that facilitate healing

Common Principles of a Functional Medicine Care Practice Model

The FM approach focuses on the underlying pathophysiology of biologic and metabolic systems and how they are interconnected and work together to contribute to disease. The intent is to arrive at a deeper understanding of the root causes of the illness. Seven core clinical imbalances are comprised by the contextual foundation for the individual's illness or illnesses. These include the following:
- *Assimilation*: How nutrients and fluids are broken down to provide energy and nutrition (through digestion, absorption, and microbiota of the GI tract as well as respiration)
- *Transport*: How nutrients are transported throughout the body (by the cardiovascular and lymphatic systems)
- *Structural integrity*: How the body holds up physically where there are disconnections (via subcellular membranes, arteries, veins, and tissues for musculoskeletal integrity)

- *Defense and repair*: How well the immune system is functioning to repair systems affected by inflammation and other insults (involving the immune system, inflammation, infection, and microbiota)
- *Communication*: How the body communicates within itself (the endocrine system, neurotransmitters, and immune messengers)
- *Energy*: Oxidation-reduction reactions that create adenosine triphosphate (ATP) (through energy regulation and mitochondrial function)
- *Biotransformation and detoxification*: The body's ability to interact with nutrients and convert them into inert waste products for elimination (involving toxicity and detoxification)

These seven underlying core biologic areas of focus are also connected to the psychologic, spiritual, and emotional state of the patient (i.e., cognitive function, perceptual patterns, emotions, regulation, grief, sadness, anger, meaning, purpose, and a relationship with a higher power). If these three are unbalanced, any of these seven core systems can be disturbed. See Fig 27.1 for an illustration of how the core imbalances interrelate and influence the disease process.

In the functional model the PCP looks for clues as to where the imbalance lies. The provider does this by following routine steps referred to as GOTOIT (Gather information, interview and physical examination); Organize information (establish a time line of symptom onset over a lifetime and plot it on the FM Matrix [Fig 27.2]); Tell the story back to the patient; Order and prioritize; Initiate treatment; and Track outcomes). The treatment plan often places a strong emphasis on nutrition as the key foundational piece for symptom and disease resolution. Other tools—such as dietary supplements, medications, and lifestyle modifications (including sleep, relaxation, exercise, and spiritual/emotional health)—may also be suggested. The time of onset of symptoms in a person's life is a key area of inquiry during the information-gathering stage. An example of a comprehensive pediatric FM intake form can be accessed from the Duke University Integrative Medicine website (see "Additional Resources," later in this chapter). Fig 27.2 illustrates the FM Matrix and how this tool can enhance the organization and analysis of an individual's health data as this information pertains to the seven areas of clinical imbalance.

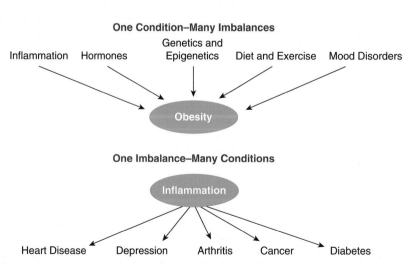

• **Fig 27.1** Functional medicine approach to a condition or specific symptom: core clinical imbalances—multiple influences. From Introduction to Functional Medicine, Jones and Quinn by The Institute For Functional Medicine.

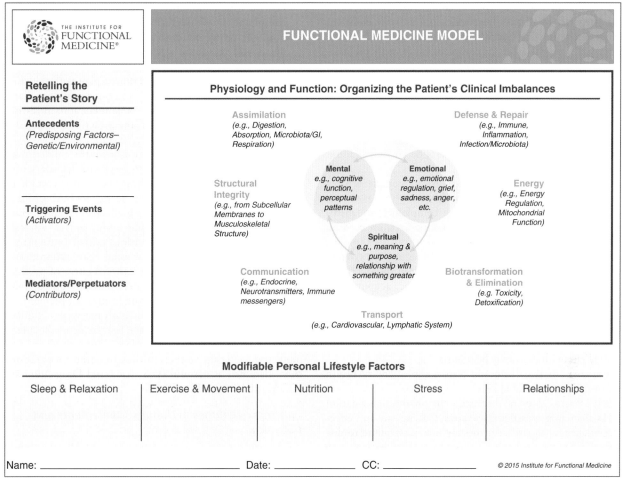

• **Fig 27.2** Function Medicine Model/Matrix. *GI*, gastrointestinal. From Jones D, Quinn S. Introduction to functional medicine, 2015. For the Institute of Functional Medicine. Available from: https://menoclinic.com/introduction-functional-medicine/. Accessed May 4, 2018.

Patient-Provider Communication Regarding the Use of Complementary Medicine

The topic of complementary medicine use must be broached nonjudgmentally to encourage disclosure, help the family clarify safety issues, and explore how complementary therapies might fit into a child's management plan. Parents may be reluctant to disclose their use of dietary supplements or complementary therapies to the PCP for fear of his or her judgment or disapproval, and providers do not routinely ask if parents are using them as a part of their care (Birdee et al, 2010). Some studies show that an estimated 40% to 60% of parents of pediatric patients disclose use of complementary and alternative medicine (CAM) to providers (Erlichman et al, 2010), but the number could be as low as 23% (Adams et al, 2013). Willingness to divulge the use of CAM can depend largely on the relationship the individual or family has with their provider (Adams et al, 2013). The provider-patient relationship and the trust that builds when they explore mutual goals form the foundation for ongoing dialogue. Such relationship-centered care is particularly important in dealing with children and adolescents with chronic illnesses that are not easily treated (Lin et al, 2018). The NIH addressed this issue by launching the "time to talk" campaign in 2009, providing tools and handouts to encourage better patient and provider communication and keep consumers better informed of complementary care issues

(NIH, 2017b, 2017c). Providers can facilitate this process by including the following in the child's health history:

- What complementary medicine *products* is the child taking, including "herbal" and "natural products," homeopathic and nutritional supplements?
- What complementary medicine *therapies* are being used (e.g., acupuncture, chiropractic, massage)?
- What other practitioners is the child seeing?
- What other kinds of activities are being used to address a particular problem?
- Has the complementary treatment helped the problem?
- What are the child's or family philosophy and self-care approaches to wellness and illness?

Safety, Legal, and Informed Consent Issues—Education in the Use of Addresses Complementary Medicine

Guidance is available for PCPs counseling families about complementary medicine that may involve medicolegal matters (McClafferty et al, 2017). Suggested considerations include these:

- Determine whether the parents intend to abandon accepted and effective conventional treatments if the child's illness is serious or life-threatening.

- Maintain knowledge about popular complementary practices, being prepared to discuss treatment options with children/families, including the benefits, possible limited evidence of efficacy, and side effects of the complementary medicine therapy; be respectful of the child's/family's values.
- Identify risks or possible deleterious effects, including diverting the child from an imminently necessary and effective conventional treatment.
- Educate families about evaluating information regarding complementary medicine treatments.
- Avoid communication of a negative bias or defensiveness about complementary medicine therapies.
- Offer to assist in monitoring and evaluating complementary medicine therapies chosen by the family.
- Evaluate the risk-benefit ratio of the complementary medicine therapy; base your judgment on support from medical literature.
- Understand the local and state statutes and regulations governing licensure of non-conventional providers and specific therapeutic modalities (e.g., naturopathic medicine, acupuncture, chiropractic, massage).
- Understand state statutes regarding child abuse and neglect—knowledge of complementary medicine being used as a substitute for conventional medical treatment of children with life-threatening illnesses may be reportable.
- Be familiar with the diagnostic tests complementary health practitioners use (see Table 27.1).

The PCP has a "duty of disclosure" to provide information about complementary medicine therapies that are safe and effective. As evidence for a particular therapy increases, failure to disclose information may become a liability issue (McClafferty et al, 2017). Blending the complementary and conventional treatment approaches requires thought and consideration.

For providers who incorporate complementary medicine therapies into their practices, informed consent for the therapy should be obtained and documentation made as for any conventional treatments that are discussed and/or refused. Providers should not refer children to complementary health providers without first having done a complete diagnostic evaluation, including the following:

- Determining the severity and acuteness of the illness and assessing curability, effective treatment, and adverse effects from using conventional medicine
- Studying the literature about the degree of invasiveness, safety, and efficacy of the chosen complementary medicine treatment for the particular malady
- Assessing the child's and/or parents' knowledge of and willingness to accept the risks and benefits of complementary therapy
- Reviewing any prescribed medications and drug interactions with complementary medicine botanicals

After the diagnostic evaluation of the child's complaint, the following steps should be taken to refer and/or assist those who wish to try complementary medicine therapy:

- Establish a "short list" of complementary/integrative/FM practitioners for referral purposes; be aware of the education, training, professional affiliations, and licensure status of any recommended complementary/integrative/FM practitioner if possible.
- Establish a collaborative relationship with complementary/integrative/FM practitioners on the "short list."
- Encourage the family to fill out a release of information form so both practitioners can share correspondence on patient care.

- Provide the child and family with questions to ask the complementary/integrative/FM practitioner during the first visit, including issues of cost, safety, efficacy of any treatment, and reasonable expectations of measurable improvement.
- Review the recommended treatment plan with the child/family; encourage the child/family to keep a symptom diary.
- Monitor the child's response to treatment at monthly intervals.
- Document concurrent use of any prescribed medications and assess drug/herb interactions.
- Document all clinical interactions with the child/family.

It is particularly important to ascertain the safety of certain treatment modalities by learning about any complementary products that the patient may be using, including side effects, possible interactions with other medications, and mechanisms of action. Mind-body techniques (e.g., prayer, guided imagery, spiritual healing, and relaxation) and acupuncture are not likely to interact with conventional medications. Providers should be aware of the possible harmful effect of products that are taken at high doses, such as herbal or phytomedicinal products, megadose combination nutritional supplements, colonics, or products taken in unconventional ways. Homeopathic remedies are highly diluted, have few adverse side effects, and are generally believed to be safe for infants, children, and pregnant and lactating women, although some preparations have been identified as harmful (U.S. Food and Drug Administration [FDA], 2018). See Box 27.3.

Pharmacovigilance of Dietary Supplements and Botanicals

A "dietary supplement" as defined in the Dietary Supplement Health and Education Act (DSHEA) of 1994 is a product taken by mouth that contains a "dietary ingredient" intended to supplement the diet (FDA, 2017). Supplements may include vitamins, minerals, herbs or other botanicals, amino acids, and substances such as enzymes, organ tissues, glandular extracts, and metabolites. Many supplements and/or their ingredients are imported (e.g., China and India are the primary exporters of low-value active pharmaceutical ingredients and excipients used internationally and in the United States in the manufacture of finished drugs [International Trade Administration, 2016]). Even though the FDA is charged with monitoring manufacturers supplying pharmaceutical drugs to the United States, oversight remains a large concern, and the FDA has added international inspectors owing to concerns about quality and safety. For supplements manufactured in the United States, the FDA publishes comprehensive regulations for Current Good Manufacturing Practices (GMP) that address the identity, purity, quality, strength, and composition of supplements, but it has no authority to approve or monitor them until there is a consumer complaint. Safety data, effectiveness, serving size, amount of nutrients, and other information are held by the manufacturers, who are under no legal obligation to disclose the information to the consumer or the FDA.

The majority of member states of the WHO regulate herbal products, although all face the same difficulty as the United States with products being made in countries other than those in which they are sold. There is an ongoing effort for further regional and international collaboration to regulate such products (WHO, 2013). The European Union (EU) is adopting uniform legislation to regulate herbal products that can be prescribed or recommended.

TABLE 27.1 Laboratory Tests in Integrative Medicine

Test	Explanation
Digestion/Nutrition	
Stool culture and analysis	Assesses digestion, absorption, metabolism, pancreatic function, inflammation, and fecal flora.
Intestinal permeability: double-sugar (lactulose and mannitol) challenge test	Measures the variable absorption of lactulose and mannitol.
Small bowel bacterial overgrowth: lactulose challenge test	Measures gas production (hydrogen and methane) over 2 h to determine the level of bacterial fermentation in the distal small intestine.
Lactose intolerance: challenge test	Measures gas production to determine whether lactose is digested properly.
Micronutrient testing	Assesses the level and function of specific nutrients in blood.
Essential Fatty Acids	
Plasma fatty acids	Reflects nutritional intake and intestinal absorption of EFAs. Rapid turnover is an indication of current fatty acid intake; allows assessment of triene-to-tetraene ratio (EFAs).
Red blood cell membrane fatty acids	Assesses fatty acid intake over past 2 to 4 months. Correlated with cardiovascular disease risk.
Environmental Testing	
Drinking water	Evaluates water for heavy metals, fluoride, and pH.
Environmental pollutants: 24-h urine	Tests urine for levels of common environmental pollutants such as xylene, styrene, paraben, and phthalates.
Heavy Metals	
Hair	Although of unknown value, hair tests for heavy metals have been used for the past 25 years by the U.S. Environmental Protection Agency to monitor environmental changes in toxic metals.
Urine • Random and timed urine tests • Postprovocation urine test	Used as a baseline evaluation before a chelating agent is given. A chelating agent, such as EDTA (to bind lead) and DMSA or sodium DMPS (to bind mercury) is given before a timed urine test. The amount of heavy metal excreted in the urine is an indication of total body burden before chelation. Test is useful to monitor treatment in an individual, but postprovocation reference ranges are not available.
Hormones	
Salivary/adrenal: hormone levels of DHEA and cortisol	Measure free hormone availability, which corresponds with adrenal function.
Salivary/female: hormone levels of progesterone, testosterone, and estradiol	Correlate with free hormone availability. Changes in salivary levels with hormone therapy make its use as a tool for monitoring treatment levels unclear.
Serum: hormone metabolites	2/16-hydroxyestrone ratio in blood predicts recurrence of breast cancer.
Urine: hormone metabolites	2/16-hydroxyestrone ratio in urine correlates with risk of breast cancer (low) and osteoporosis (high).
Immunology	
Immune function: flow cytometry	Assesses natural killer cell function as well as presence and activity of immune cells and cytokines.
Food allergies: serum immunoglobulins—IgE and IgG	Measures immunoglobulin activation in the presence of various food antigens. IgE, true allergic reaction to the food; IgG, intolerance.
Nutrigenomics	Broad-based term to represent genomic testing that highlights individual biochemical needs for particular macro- and micronutrients. Purely experimental at this point; no outcome studies have demonstrated clinical validity.
Oxidative Stress Markers	
Lipid peroxides, isoprostane, 8-hydroxydeoxyguanosine	Markers of oxidative end tissue damage to fats, proteins, and DNA.
Glutathione, TAC/TRAP superoxide dismutase	Markers of capacity to deal with oxidative stress.

DHEA, dehydroepiandrosterone; *DMPS,* dimercaptopropane sulfonate; *DMSA,* dimercaptosuccinic acid; *DNA,* deoxyribonucleic acid; *EDTA,* ethylenediaminetetraacetic acid; *EFA,* essential fatty acid; *TAC,* total antioxidant capacity; *TRAP,* total reactive antioxidant potential.

Adapted from Rakel D. Appendix: laboratory testing resources in integrative medicine. In: Rakel D, ed. *Integrative Medicine.* 3rd ed. Philadelphia: Elsevier; 2012:1004–1005.

Contamination and potency are of concern when patients use herbal (notably Ayurvedic herbal medicines) or folk remedies, as they can cause adverse reactions. Some traditional folk remedies or herbal preparations manufactured in third world countries contain heavy metals (e.g., lead, zinc, mercury, arsenic, aluminum, and tin), pesticides, and microorganisms. Other problems include content substitutions, adulterations, incorrect preparations, misleading advertising, improper labeling of contents, and failure to provide adequate amounts of the substance noted on the label. Prior nonproblematic use of a product by an individual may not be a predictor of a future drug reaction because of inconsistent potency; lack of standardization regarding which parts of a plant are used; variations in plant ripeness, storage, and regional growth conditions; and the unknown influence of fertilizers, pesticides, and herbicides used during cultivation.

Most herbal/natural health products (NHPs) consumed in the United States have been historically safe with few reports of adverse reactions (Karimi et al, 2015). A homeopathic teething compound has caused seizures and death in infants (Kaplan, 2017), but the most dangerous elements may be the pyrrolizidine alkaloids, which can cause liver complications or death. These compounds are found in comfrey, borage, coltsfoot, and species of *Crotalaria* and *Senecio*. These plants are often used in herbal teas, particularly in Jamaica, Africa, and South and Central America. Chaparral, germander, and a Chinese medicine called *jin bu huan* can also cause liver toxicity. See Boxes 27.2 and 27.3 for a summary list of herbs that are contraindicated in children and in pregnant and lactating women. In 1993, the FDA established *MedWatch*, a system for reporting adverse reactions to medical products and medications, including nutritionals and botanicals (see "Additional Resources" later in this chapter).

With 250,000 flowering plant species to consider, the burden of knowing what is safe to use or not becomes cumbersome. Although many herbs are harmless even in large amounts, others should be prescribed only by a knowledgeable herbalist or botanical professional. The Natural Medicines Therapy Research Center (TRC) has identified more than 1600 possible interactions between NHPs and conventional drugs (see "Additional Resources," later). Although some of these drug interactions are insignificant, others can be serious. The appropriate herb in the appropriate quantity—like pharmaceutical medicines—is necessary to obtain the intended benefits. The medicinal effect of an herb is thought to be the result of dozens of pharmacologically distinct actions. The herb may cause physiologic changes in numerous subtle ways, none of which alone would produce the desired response. This mechanism contrasts with conventional medicines, which generally act by one of a few mechanisms and use "physiologically more significant pharmacologic" dosing.

Standardized extracts are more likely to ensure that a specific amount of an active compound is present. Western herbalists often use *simples* (the compound is made from one herb), whereas Chinese and Indian (Ayurvedic) medicines often blend together more than one herb. See Table 27.2 for possible interactions between some pharmaceuticals and herbal preparations. Some useful guidelines for PCPs when they are either advocating or advising about herbal and dietary supplements include those listed in Box 27.4.

• BOX 27.2 Herbals, Botanicals, and Diet Supplements: Precautions for Use in Children

Do Not Use

- Borage *(Borago officinalis)*
- Chaparral *(Larrea divaricata)*
- Coltsfoot *(Tussilago farfara)* in herbal teas
- Comfrey *(Symphytum officinale)*
- Crotalaria species (rattle pods) in herbal teas
- Dietary weight loss supplements
- Dieter's teas containing senna, aloe, cascara, castor oil, rhubarb root, buckthorn, or other plant-derived stimulant laxative
- Ephedra (ma huang)
- Foxglove *(Digitalis purpurea)*
- Germander *(Teucrium chamaedrys)*
- Ginkgo seeds (these are toxic)
- Heliotropes
- Jin bu huan *(Lycopodium serratum)*
- Kava kava *(Piper methysticum)*

- Lobelia
- Monkshood/wolfsbane/aconite *(Aconitum napellus, A. columbianum)*
- Organ or glandular extracts
- Pennyroyal oil (*Mentha pulegium, Hedeoma* spp.)
- *Prunus* spp. (amygdalin, laetrile)
- Rattlebox (*Crotalaria* spp.)
- Sassafras
- *Senecio* (ragwort, groundsel, golden ragwort) in herbal teas
- St. Ignatius bean (contains strychnine and brucine)
- *Strychnos nux-vomica* tree seeds (contain strychnine)

Use With Restrictions

- *Echinacea:* Do not use in children younger than 2 years old
- Goldenseal/roots: Not for use in infants younger than 1 month old
- Pennyroyal: Do not prescribe for internal use
- Tea tree oil: Do not prescribe for internal use

From Fetrow CW, Avila JR. Professional's Handbook of Complementary and Alternative Medicines. 3rd ed. Philadelphia: Lippincott Williams & Wilkins; 2004; Kuhn MA, Winston D. Part II: herb monographs. In: Kuhn MA, Winston D, eds. Kuhn & Winston's Herbal Therapy and Supplements: A Scientific and Traditional Approach. Philadelphia: Lippincott Williams & Wilkins; 2008; Loo M. Integrative Medicine for Children. St. Louis: Elsevier; 2009, Chapter 7; U.S. Food and Drug Administration (FDA): FDA warning: consumers advised not to use Arrow Brand Medicated Oil &—Embrocation, Aceite Medicinal La Flecha, FDA (website). 2010: http:// www.fda.gov/NewsEvents/Newsroom/PressAnnouncements/ucm213596.htm. Accessed December 15, 2014; U.S. Food and Drug Administration (FDA). FDA warns consumers not to feed infants "Better than Formula Ultra Infant Immune Booster 117," 2004. FDA (website): http://www.fda.gov/NewsEvents/Newsroom PressAnnouncements/2004/ucm 108229.htm. Accessed December 15, 2014.

• BOX 27.3 Herbs and Botanicals Contraindicated in Pregnant and Lactating Women[a]

Avoid in Pregnancy[b]

Aloe	Thuga
Autumn crocus	Thyme
Barberry root	Uva ursi leaf
Black cohosh root	**Vervain**
Blessed thistle	White horehound
Blue cohosh	Wormwood
Buckthorn bark and berry	Yarrow
Burdock	Yohimbe
Calendula	**Avoid During Lactation[c]**
Cascara sagrada bark	Alfalfa
Chamomile (German and Roman)	Aloe
Chasteberry	Black cohosh
Cinchona bark	Bladderwrack
Cinnamon bark	Blue cohosh
Coltsfoot leaf	Borage
Comfrey herb, leaf, and root	Buckthorn bark
Dong quai	Buckthorn berry
Echinacea purpurea herb, injectable form	Bugleweed
Ephedra (Ma Huang)	Caraway oil
Evening primrose	Cascara sagrada bark
Fennel oil and seed	Chasteberry
Feverfew	Comfrey
Ginkgo biloba	Coltsfoot leaf
Ginseng (American and Korean)	Elecampane
Goldenseal	Ephedra
Hops	Fennel
Indian snakeroot	Fenugreek[d]
Juniper root	Garlic
Kava kava	Ginkgo biloba
Licorice root (>100 mg glycyrrhizin)	Ginseng
Mayapple root and resin	**Goat's Rue**
Motherwort	Indian snakeroot
Parsley herb and root	Joe-pye
Passion flower	Kava kava
Pau d'arco	Licorice
Pennyroyal	Mayapple root
Peppermint oil or leaf	Male fern
Petasites (butterbur) root	Peppermint oil
Red raspberry leaf	Petasites (butterbur) root
Rhubarb root	Rhubarb root
Rosemary	Rue
Sage leaf	Senna leaf
Saw palmetto	Stillingia
Senna leaf	St. John's wort
Shepherd's purse	Uva ursi
Slippery elm	Valerian
St. John's wort	Wormwood
Tea tree oil	Yarrow

[a]This table is not a complete list of all herbs that should be avoided during pregnancy; Chinese herbs with potent effects to regulate qi, move blood, or drain downward are contraindicated.

[b]As single herb or as an ingredient in a combination product; product is deemed unsafe, has insufficient evidence of safety, or is likely unsafe.

[c]Product is unsafe, has insufficient evidence of safety, or is likely unsafe.

[d]Used widely in some communities to increase production of milk in lactating mothers.

Data from Fetrow CW, Avila JR. Professional's Handbook of Complementary and Alternative Medicines. *Philadelphia: Lippincott Williams & Wilkins; 2004; Gardner Z, McGuffin M, eds.*

BOX 27.3 Cont'd

American Herbal Products Association's Botanical Safety Handbook. *2nd ed. New York: CRC Press; 2013; Kuhn MA, Winston D. Appendix A: herbs contraindicated during pregnancy and breast-feeding. In: Kuhn MA, Winston D, eds. Kuhn & Winston's Herbal Therapy and Supplements: A Scientific and Traditional Approach. Philadelphia: Lippincott Williams & Wilkins; 2008; Natural Medicines Comprehensive Database. Natural medicines used during pregnancy and lactation (website). 2014. http://naturaldatabase.therapeuticresearch.com/ce/ceCourse. aspx?s=ND&cs=&pc=11-102&cec=1&pm=5. Accessed December 12, 2014.*
From Petrie K. Section I: complementary and alternative medicine in maternity care. In: Ratcliffe SD, Baxtey EG, Cline MK, et al., eds. Family Medicine Obstetrics. 3rd ed. Philadelphia: Mosby; 2008.

• BOX 27.4 Key Guidelines for Use of Herbal and Dietary Supplements

- Use only single-herb supplements instead of combinations to prevent side effect confusion.
- Emphasize that "natural" does not mean "safe."
- Stop some herbal supplements at least 1 week before any scheduled surgical procedure to prevent any alterations in coagulation, blood pressure, or interactions with anesthesia; communicate cessation to the surgeon (Box 27.5).
- Exercise caution when purchasing herbal products over the internet.
- Avoid the use of herbs starting with the letter "G"—ginkgo, ginseng, garlic, ginger, or green tea if the patient is taking warfarin or a drug that is metabolized using the hepatic cytochrome P450 enzyme system. The "G" herbs can either potentiate or inhibit the drug, therefore altering the therapeutic effect or causing adverse effects.
- Research the NHP as thoroughly as possible and look for these labels:
- U.S. Pharmacopeia (USP) Dietary Supplement Verified seal: Product meets certain standards for contamination, adulteration, manufacturing processes, and pharmacologic properties.
- National Sanitation Foundation (NSF) International: Sets standards, tests, and certifies products and systems, including GMP for cleanliness, maintenance, and documented quality checks.
- Natural Products Association (NPA; formerly National Nutritional Food Association TruLabel program): Includes a GMP process and a Natural Seal certification process that ensures ingredient quality and purity.
- Consumer Lab (CL): Tests dietary supplements for composition, potency, purity, bioavailability, consistency of products.
- Generally Recognized as Safe (GRAS) in the United States: Recognized as generally safe for its intended purpose as part of the Federal Food, Drug, and Cosmetic Act.
- Herbal and NHPs manufactured and imported from Europe are generally regarded as safe because they have to comply with standards set by Commission E (Europe's equivalent of the FDA) (e.g., a label noting "original German formula" would be a good choice).
  - In England, an herbal product is licensed and meets standards of safety and quality if it has a Marketing Authorization (MA) or Traditional Herbal Registration (THR) Scheme number on the label.
  - Use websites, such as the American Botanical Council HerbClip Database, to determine if the product has been tested or reviewed. The Natural Medicines Comprehensive Database offers evidence-based information on safety, efficacy, interactions, and side effects for brand name conventional and NHPs. The NCCIH provides a list of herbal products that have been studied for specific conditions by that organization. The American Herbal Products Association (AHPA) evaluates herbal safety for all botanical ingredients sold in North America. Each herb is placed in one of three safety and interactions classes. There is also an internet application to help consumers learn about the safety and effectiveness of some popular herbs (see "Additional Resources," later).
- Reliable NHP labels for children include: Ortho Molecular, Master Supplements, Jarrow Formulas, Barleans, Designs for Health, Pure Encapsulations, Xymogen, Nordic Naturals, Thorne Research, Gaia Herbs, Klaire Labs, Metagenics, Quicksilver Scientific, Neurobiologix, Vital Nutrients, Pro Thera. Online provider-friendly dispensaries include FullScript and Emmerson Ecologics.

TABLE 27.2	Potential Interactions Between Some Pharmaceuticals and Botanical Products	
Drug Category	**Herbs**	**Effect of Herb on the Drug's Action**
Iron	Tannin-rich herbs (e.g., caffeine-containing herbs, cat's claw, tea, uva ursi)	Decreased drug effect (may be due to tannin binding with iron to decrease absorption).
Laxative, stimulant (e.g., bisacodyl)	Aloe, cascara sagrada, senna, yellow dock	May increase laxative effect.
Minerals	Fiber-containing herbs (flax, psyllium, acacia, slippery elm, marshmallow)	Decreased bioavailability, especially of Ca, Mg, Cu, Zn with psyllium.
NSAIDs	Gastric irritant herbs (e.g., caffeine, rue, uva ursi)	Increased side effects and may increase gastric erosion and bleeding.
	Nettles	Increased therapeutic effect—increased effect of antiinflammatory activity.
Oral contraceptives, combination	Licorice, St. John's wort	Both may increase blood pressure; St. John's wort may increase clearance and cause breakthrough bleeding.
Salicylates (e.g., aspirin)	Herbs that alkalinize urine (e.g., uva ursi)	Decreased plasma levels caused by increased urine secretion.
	Tamarind	Increased blood level of aspirin.
	Ginkgo, garlic	May cause prolonged bleeding by decreased platelet aggregation; eye hemorrhage.
Theophylline	St. John's wort	May inhibit drug's effectiveness.
Thyroid hormone	Horseradish	Decreased therapeutic effect by decreased thyroid function.
	Kelp	Increased therapeutic effect because kelp contains iodine, which may lead to hyperthyroidism.

This is not a complete list of potential drug-herb interactions; a comprehensive drug-herbal interaction checker (e.g., Natural Medicines Comprehensive Database website) should be utilized.

Ca, calcium; *Cu,* copper; *Mg,* magnesium, *NSAID,* nonsteroidal antiinflammatory drug; *Zn,* zinc.

Additional data from Danloff TA. Anesthesia and herbal supplements. *ASA Refresher Courses Anesthesiol.* 2012;40(1):7–17; and Laird J. Interactions between supplements and drugs: deciphering the evidence. *JAAPA.* 2011;24(12):44–46, 48–49.

Clinicians must be aware of conflict of interest and use discretion when they are prescribing supplements. Most supplement companies sell to clinicians at a 50% wholesale price, and selling a product to their patient at the manufacturer's suggested retail price gives providers a financial incentive to prescribe supplements. Although it is not illegal or malpractice to capture these financial incentives, it raises an ethical question; clinicians should prescribe only what is clinically necessary for optimal management.

Use of Aromatherapy

Aromatherapy (AT) has a long history of use as a complementary therapy in individuals of all ages. These plant extracts (essential oils) are either inhaled or delivered topically (mixed with a carrier oil or lotion [e.g., with vegetable-based fatty oils, such as grape seed or sweet almond oil]). AT is largely regarded as being a safe and gentle therapy for children. Its many uses include treating pain, nausea, stress, anxiety, insomnia, and abdominal pain, and other complaints. However, severe reactions to some essential oils can occur, as well as poisoning, allergic sensitivities (including cutaneous reactions), and worsening of symptoms of some disorders (e.g., use of essential oil of rosemary or sage may be contraindicated in those with high blood pressure or fennel in those with epilepsy). Essential oils used topically or in inhalation diffusers should be used only in small quantities in children (one to five drops). Before recommending any essential oil, it is important to review the specific safety information and recommended ages for the specific oil. The recommended dilution for infants and

> ● **BOX 27.5** **Botanicals to Discontinue Prior to Surgery**
>
> - Angelica
> - Anise
> - Arnica
> - Borage seed
> - Celery
> - Chamomile
> - Clove
> - Danshen
> - Dong quai
> - Echinacea
> - Ephedra
> - Fenugreek
> - Feverfew
> - Fish oil
> - Garlic
> - Ginger
> - Ginkgo
> - Ginseng
> - Goldenseal
> - Hawthorn
> - Horse chestnut
> - Kava
> - Licorice root
> - Onion
> - Papain
> - Parsley
> - Red clover
> - St. John's wort
> - Sweet clover turmeric
> - Willow bark
>
> *Not an all-inclusive list.*

children should be in the 0.5% to 1% range and not exceed 2% (see Additional Resources for a good reference on using essential oils and for figuring the safe dilution ratios for topical applications). All essential oils should be treated as medications and kept out of the reach of children; they should be purchased only if their bottles come with integrated drop dispensers, and all ingredients should be clearly labeled, including any added carrier oils.

Professional Oversight

Many states have licensing boards and professional organizations that set standards for nonconventional practitioners, including a requirement to carry malpractice insurance. The Federation of State Medical Boards has established policy and model guidelines for the use of complementary medicine therapies when a physician recommends the therapy or when comanaging the patient with a complementary medicine health provider. Licensing requirements are subject to change, and families should be encouraged to review the credentials of any practitioner they are considering using. Currently there is no national licensure for "complementary health providers" and state licensure requirements vary widely for different disciplines, like naturopathy (NIH, 2015). Before expanding their practice to incorporate complementary medicine modalities, NPs are advised to check the Advanced Nurse Practice Act of their state for the relevant standards of practice, educational requirements, and certification (if necessary), as well as the policies of their employer. Many courses about complementary medicine, functional and integrative medicine, and herbal medicines are offered by academic medical centers and affiliated institutions or by professional organizations in the United States. Integrative medicine conferences occur yearly in the United States, some of which are specific to pediatrics.

Common Complementary Therapies for Some Health Conditions

Complementary therapeutic interventions should be used at the discretion of the PCP, taking into account scientific evidence and the families' preferences for treatment. Ensure that the patient/parent/caregiver has given informed consent. Whereas the PCP may recommend a dietary supplement, the quality of the product should be discussed, as these products are available over the counter and accessible without a prescription. Although the studies on efficacy and safety of these supplements in children are significantly fewer than those in adults, the FDA has classified them as food products, and they are open to prudent use by the consumer. Dietary supplements are not required to come in childproof containers. Finally, providers should adequately and judiciously follow up on symptom resolution within a reasonable time period so that the plan of care can be revised as needed.

See the "Additional Resources" further on for references that can be recommended to providers wishing to learn more about or recommend complementary therapies for various pediatric health conditions.

The following topics cover some common diagnoses that have complementary medicine treatment applications (Table 27.3); the FM approach to each condition is discussed briefly as an example of the biologic-metabolic foundation of this model. Dosages are not included in Table 27.3 and must be determined by the clinician using appropriate references and/or original research studies in order to adhere to efficacy standards, age restrictions, and precautions and to avoid side effects (Kemper, 2016) (see "Additional Resources," later, which includes dosages for many of the complementary treatments listed). Each of these pathologies is also discussed in detail in respective disease chapters in this textbook (e.g., irritable bowel syndrome [IBS] is discussed in Chapter 40, Gastrointestinal Disorders).

Irritable Bowel Syndrome With Constipation and Diarrhea

The Institute for Functional Medicine has developed a program to restore gut health called the "5-R" approach to gut restoration

as part of the treatment for IBS. The goal of the 5-R program is to normalize digestion and absorption, achieve bacterial homeostasis, promote healing, and detoxify the body. The 5-Rs consist of the following:
1. Remove: Stressors and inflammatory triggers such as yeast, bacteria, or other food allergies or sensitivities.
2. Replace: Replace items needed for proper digestion, such as enzymes and hydrochloric or bile acids.
3. Reinoculate: Repopulate the microbiome with beneficial prebiotic, probiotic, and fibrous foods so that the beneficial microflora can flourish.
4. Repair: Consume reparative nutrients needed for gut barrier dysfunction such as zinc, fat-soluble vitamins, glutamine, essential fatty acids, and amino acids.
5. Rebalance: Address lifestyle factors such as adequate sleep and stress management.

From a FM standpoint, antecedents and triggers to IBS may include increased intestinal and epidermal permeability; iatrogenic causes such as antibiotics and nonsteroidal antiinflammatory drugs (NSAIDs); and environmental exposures such as allergens, pollution, a genetically modified organism (GMO), and pesticides. Genetic or epigenetic factors may also play a role (e.g., a predisposition to hypochlorhydria).

Attention-Deficit/Hyperactivity Disorder

FM approaches attention-deficit/hyperactivity disorder (ADHD) by addressing underlying pathophysiology contributing to the behaviors. Single nucleotide polymorphisms (SNPs) may be rate-limiting factors in how serotonin and dopamine are being processed. Botanical supplements and lifestyle factors can provide environmental epigenetic modulation of SNP function. It is also important to consider the child's gut, nutritional deficiencies (e.g., magnesium, zinc, iron, essential fats, and vitamin D may be lower) (Bener and Kamal, 2013), methylation, and broader processes such as thyroid or sleep disorders. Children with genetic mutations in their MTHFR 1298C and MTHFR 677T have a greater likelihood of impairment in transforming the synthetic form of folate into the methylated (and active) form that is needed for neurotransmission (Saha et al, 2014).

Headaches/Migraines

FM considers that frequent headaches and migraines can be due to an unhealthy decoupling of the acting potential of a resting neuron. Healthy neuronal mitochondria have lower resting potentials, lower oxidative stress, and higher resilience to environmental stimuli. In individuals with dysglycemia, anemia, inflammation, nutritional deficiencies (e.g., fatty acid, magnesium, B vitamins, calcium and vitamin D), and autoimmunity who lack exercise or experience environmental toxin stress, the neuronal membrane potential is closer to the action threshold that stimulates headaches and migraines. FM addresses such factors with exercise, liberal water intake (the daily goal would be at least half of the child's body weight in ounces), nutrition, and stress reduction to help achieve full headache remission.

Insomnia

Behavioral modifications around sleep and sleep routines are critical to teaching children how to get their best night sleep. Implementing healthy sleep hygiene habits is efficacious for improving

TABLE 27.3 **Complementary Treatments for Some Health Conditions**

System/Diagnosis	Benefits and Functional Considerations	Treatment	Possible Side Effects	Research Citations
Gastrointestinal • Irritable bowel syndrome (IBS)				
	Nutritional			
	Avoids foods that trigger immune response.	Follow Mediterranean diet; avoid processed foods (including fast foods), gluten, dairy, sugar, soy, shellfish, peanuts, eggs, beef, and pork.	None if adequate intake of calories, vitamins, and minerals.	Kemper, 2016
	May improve behavioral issues, especially in those with a neuropsychiatric disorder; some of those with nonceliac gluten sensitivity and/or IBS may also improve on a gluten-free diet.	Gluten-free diet.		Czaja-Bulsa, 2015; Makharia et al, 2015
	Prevents gut bacteria from using short-chain carbo-hydrates for fuel, thus ↓ hydrogen gas and other digestive symptoms.	Low fermentable oligo-, di-, mono-saccharides and polyols (FOD-MAP); ketogenic, low histamine, and specific carbohydrate diets may be tried.		Dolan et al, 2018
	If used in conjunction, selectively stimulates the growth and/or activity of intestinal bacteria and enhance probiotics to thrive.	Add fiber (soluble often helps better than insoluble, such as fruits, legumes, oat products); ↑ natural prebiotic foods (banana, onion, leeks, garlic, Jerusalem artichoke, raw asparagus).	None but can exacerbate IBS symptoms.	Curro et al, 2017; National Institute of Diabetes, Digestion and Kidney Diseases, 2017
	Dietary Supplements/ Botanicals			
	↓ Pain, flatulence, distention, bowel frequency.	Peppermint oil, enteric-coated only stated explicitly for enteric use.	Possible heartburn, rectal discomfort/burning.	Chumpitazi et al, 2018; Grund-mann and Yoon, 2014
		Iberogast (combination of nine herbal extracts; OTC).	↓ GI spasms; improves function and motility; relaxes stomach muscles; anti-inflam-matory and anti-bacterial; regulates stomach acid; ↓ gas and bloating.	Lapina and Trukhmanov, 2017
	Probiotics and Prebiotics			
	Improves quality of life; ↓ frequency and intensity of abdominal pain.	Mixture of *B. breve* M-16V, *B. longum* BB536, and *B. infantis* M-63; *L. rhamnosus*.	Do not use in those who are immunocompro-mised (can use kefir and yogurt) or in those with central lines.	Giannetti and, Staiano, 2016; Wegh et al, 2018

Continued

TABLE 27.3	Complementary Treatments for Some Health Conditions—cont'd			
System/Diagnosis	Benefits and Functional Considerations	Treatment	Possible Side Effects	Research Citations
	Bovine Immunoglobulins			
	Binds microbial components (e.g., yeast, dysbiotic bacteria, food antigens); ↑ GI homeostasis; improves nutrient/water absorption; ↓ diarrhea, gas, bloating.	Enteragam, a serum bovine immunoglobulin (SBI) is a packaged prescription medical food (10 g packets).	Should not be taken by those allergic to beef; shortness of breath has occurred.	SBI in EnteraGam has undergone RCT studies in adults with IBS-D, HIV-associated enteropathy, and IBD; has been used in children with ulcerative colitis (Soriano and Ramos-Soriano, 2017); RCT clinical study in children in progress at Louisiana State University Health Sciences Center in New Orleans
	Mind-Body/Other			
	Improves treatment outcomes; used with conventional treatments.	CBT, biofeedback, yoga, hypnosis, mindful meditation.	None.	Kemper, 2016
		AROMATHERAPY (for inhalation or massage only).	Not for ingestion.	
	Has antispasmodic and calming properties.	Roman chamomile, sweet fennel, peppermint, and ginger.		Purchon, et al 2014 (most studies done using peppermint oil)
Neurology				
• Attention deficit disorder (ADD) or attention-deficit/hyperactivity disorder (ADHD)				
	Nutritional			
	Certain foods and additives may cause neurotransmitter imbalances; possible fatty acid, vitamin, and mineral deficiencies; gut dysbiosis; or heavy metal toxicities; iron deficiency can interfere with behavior, memory, concentration.	See specific diet exclusions at the end of this table; correct any iron deficiency.	An elimination diet can put strain on family; best done in consultation with a nutritionist.	University of Maryland Medical Center, 2013
	Lowers ADHD scores in those adhering to this diet.	Mediterranean diet.	None.	Rios-Hernandez et al, 2017
	Dietary Supplements/ Botanicals			
	Regulates muscles and nerve function, help with irritability, attention span, mental confusion.	Magnesium.	Diarrhea, drowsiness, weakness, lethargy if overdose; drug interaction with antibiotics and antihypertensives.	Greenblatt and Gottlieb, 2017
	Regulates activity of brain chemicals, fatty acids, melatonin.	Zinc.	Higher doses can be dangerous.	Greenblatt & Gottlieb, 2017
	Decreases emotional lability and oppositional behavior.	Fish oil supplement of omega-3 (EPA) and omega-6 (DHA) in equal or higher EPA to DHA ratios.	Safe to try; ↑ EPA has anticoagulant effect.	Cooper et al, 2016

TABLE 27.3	Complementary Treatments for Some Health Conditions—cont'd

System/Diagnosis	Benefits and Functional Considerations	Treatment	Possible Side Effects	Research Citations
	Appears to increase levels of acetylcholine, norepineph-rine, serotonin, and dopa-mine; ↓ ADHD symptoms, especially if hyperactive/ impulsive, emotionally and behaviorally dysregulated.	Phosphatidylserine (PS) or Vayarin, a medical food (combo of 75 mg PS and omega-3).	Possible GI upset, head-ache, insomnia.	Hirayama et al, 2014
	Folate is a key precursor of serotonin and dopamine synthesis; folate deficiency due to generic mutation may produce ADHD symp-toms and lack ability to transform synthetic folate into active form needed for neurotransmission.	Folate (if patient has genetic mutations in MTHFR 1298C and MTHFR 677T).		Saha et al, 2014
	An antioxidant, pycnogenol ↓ inflammation to modulate oxidative stress by normal-izing catecholamine levels; ↓ hyperactivity; improves attention and visual/ motoric coordination and concentration.	Pycnogenol (Pinus pinaster, maritime pine bark, a mixture of polyphenols).	Possible irritability; do not take if pregnant or breastfeeding.	Schoonees et al, 2012; Trebatická and Ďuračková, 2015
	Mind-Body/Energy			
	For relaxation, anxiety, hyperactivity; discipline and conduct promotion; increase attention, con-centration and memory; decrease distractibility and behavioral problems.	Yoga, tai chi, gigong, exercise, music therapy (Hemi-Sync has music albums for ADHD), neurofeedback, Musiko with Pepe (a behavioral therapy–ori-ented group training for children), meditation.	None unless music is too high-pitched, fast, stimulating.	Culbert and Olness, 2010; Pel-ham et al, 2011; Rothmann et al, 2014; Sawni and Kemper, 2018;
• Headaches/ Migraines				
	Nutritional			
	↓ Headache severity and frequency.	Diet high in omega-3 (EPA) (cold-water fish, flax, chia, hemp, wild game, and enriched eggs); elimi-nate foods that typically cause headaches (see diet exclusions at the end of this table); ensure adequate hydration.	None unless allergic to fish.	Coeytaux and Mann, 2018
	Dietary Supplements/ Botanicals			
	↓ Migraine frequency and severity and ↑ quality of life.	Magnesium threonate, glycinate, or aspartate.	Diarrhea, gastric irrita-tion; hypermagnese-mia; use with caution in those with kidney or cardiac disorders.	Kovacevic et al, 2017
	↓ Number and duration of headaches but not frequency.	Riboflavin (B2).	None reported.	Talebian et al, 2018
	May have an effect on head-aches by platelet aggregation, ↓inflammatory promoters, and ↓vascular reactivity.	Feverfew (Tanacetum parthenium) (dried leaf standardized to a minimum of 0.2% parthenolide).	Mouth sores; abdominal pain; do not use in pregnancy or if any clotting issues.	Coeytaux and Mann, 2018

Continued

TABLE 27.3	Complementary Treatments for Some Health Conditions—cont'd			
System/Diagnosis	**Benefits and Functional Considerations**	**Treatment**	**Possible Side Effects**	**Research Citations**
	↓ Tension headaches.	Peppermint oil (10 g) in an ethanol solution (90%) (equals 10% peppermint product).	None unless sensitive to mint family.	Malone and Tsai, 2018
	↓ Migraine and tension headaches; abortive treatment for migraines; ↓ nausea/vomiting, phonophobia and/or photophobia.	Menthol, 6% to 10% topical oil (also found in Tiger balm).	None unless sensitive to menthol products.	Kemper, 2016; St Cyr et al, 2015 (used gel compounded with several botanicals)
	↓ Frequency of headaches.	CoQ 10.	Rare GI symptoms.	Coeytaux and Mann, 2018
	Mind-Body/Other			
	↓ Can all be used to reduce headaches.	Biofeedback, cognitive behavioral therapy, hypnosis, mindfulness meditation, spinal manipulation and acupuncture	None; can be used by people of different ages.	Coeytaux and Mann, 2018
		Aromatherapy.		
		Peppermint, lavender, and eucalyptus per inhalation diffuser or per massage in a carrier oil to back of neck or temple.	None unless allergic to essential oil used.	Purchon et al, 2014
• Insomnia				
	Nutrition			
		Avoid caffeine-containing products.		
	Dietary Supplements/Botanicals			
	Those with neurodevelopmental disorders and genetic single nucleotide polymorphisms in their CYP1A2 activity are more likely to have slower melatonin metabolism; advances circadian rhythms; ↑ sleep onset and sleep time.	Melatonin (fast-acting melatonin may help the onset of sleep, whereas extended release may help keep a child asleep for longer periods—anecdotal evidence).	Regarded as safe.	Bruni, 2015; Kemper, 2016; Naiman, 2018
	↓ Anxiety, stress, insomnia.	Lemon balm (*Melissa officinalis*) (look for combination of 80 mg lemon balm leaf extract and 160 mg valerian root extract); also used in aromatherapy, tincture, and topically in carrier oil.	None unless allergic to mint family.	Kemper, 2016; Naiman, 2018;
	Mild anxiolytic effects; promotes sleep.	Valerian root, crude herb, or standardized extract of 0.8%.	Rare GI irritation, headaches, dizziness, itching.	Kemper, 2016; Naiman, 2018
	Promotes sleep (especially in boys with ADHD).	L-theanine (Suntheanine).	Considered safe.	Lyon et al, 2011
	Aromatherapy			
	Improves sleep.	Lavender, roman chamomile, geranium, mandarin, and ylang ylang (*Cananga odorata*), jasmine have been used.	Review safety information.	Naiman, 2018; Purchon et al, 2014

TABLE
27.3
TABLE 27.3   Complementary Treatments for Some Health Conditions—cont'd

System/Diagnosis	Benefits and Functional Considerations	Treatment	Possible Side Effects	Research Citations
	Mind-Body			
	↑ Sleep quality.	Music therapy (can pair with muscle relaxation).	None.	Kligler et al, 2016; Street et al, 2014
		CBT, meditation, hypnosis, yoga, tai chi, acupuncture, light therapy.	None.	Kligler et al, 2016
MOOD DISORDERS				
• Mild to moderate anxiety/depression/ obsessive compulsive disorder				
	Nutritional			
	Boosts mood and vagal tone; modulate inflammatory responses to stressors; reduced odds of self-reported depression.	Mediterranean diet; also see ADHD diet at the end of this table; increase omega-3 fatty acids foods; ↑ tryptophan-containing foods (turkey, nuts, soybeans, cooked beans, peas); ↑ tyrosine-containing foods (eggs, aged cheese, tofu, seafood). Avoid SAD with processed foods.	Omega-3: rare interaction with anticoagulants.	Jacka et al, 2011; Kohlboeck et al, 2012; Quirk et al, 2013,
	DIETARY SUPPLEMENTS/ BOTANICALS			
	Acts as an intermediary in mood regulation by converting to serotonin to promote calmness, improve sleep and appetite.	5-Hydroxytryptophan (5-HTP).	Do not use if taking an SSRI, monoamine oxidase inhibitors (MAOIs), tricyclic antidepressants, alcohol, dextromethorphan, or are pregnant; may cause eosinophilia-myalgia syndrome. Possible GI upset.	U.S. Library of Medicine, 2017.
	↑ Alpha waves in the brain; promotes sense of calmness and relaxation; ↓ perception of stress; ↑ resilience; improve working memory, cognition, and attention.	Green tea (contains L-theanine, 25 mg per cup) or supplement with L-theanine (Suntheanine).	Considered safe.	Lyon et al, 2011 (study done in boys with ADHD); Mancini et al, 2017
	Altered folate metabolism may contribute to major depression and higher homocysteine; folate is used in monoamine neurotransmission.	L-methylfolate (vitamin B-9) or medical foods (e.g., Deplin). Found naturally in grains, fruits, vegetables, beans, and other foods.	Check for drug interactions if taking certain anticonvulsants. Regarded as safe.	Mech and Farah, 2016; Shelton et al, 2013
	Breaks down neurochemicals, such as dopamine, serotonin, and melatonin; thought to influence neuronal membrane fluidity.	S-Adenosylmethionine (SAMe).	GI upset.	Sharma et al, 2017 (studies done in adults)
	Inhibits reuptake of serotonin, norepinephrine, and dopamine, and appears to affect other neurochemicals such as glutamate and gamma-aminobutyric acid (GABA).	St John's wort *(Hypericum perforatum).*	Do not use if taking SSRI; occasional GI upset reported. Review Table 27.2.	Kemper, 2016

Continued

TABLE 27.3   Complementary Treatments for Some Health Conditions—cont'd

System/Diagnosis	Benefits and Functional Considerations	Treatment	Possible Side Effects	Research Citations
	Mind-Body/Other			
	Improves energy, mood, appetite, sleep, self-esteem.	Exercise (use as adjunct therapy).	Avoid if anorexic with compulsive overexercising.	Kemper, 2016; Kliger et al, 2016
	Enhance efficacy of other treatments; acupuncture alters neurotransmitter levels.	Yoga, meditation, hypnosis, imagery, tai chi, mindfulness-based CBT, music therapy, acupuncture.	None; rare with acupuncture.	Schneider and Wissink, 2018
	↓ Nonseasonal and seasonal affective disorder.	Phototherapy: Bright white (full-spectrum, 10,000-Lux light from special bulbs, lamps, light boxes).	None.	Perera et al, 2016
	Aromatherapy			
	↓ Irritability and anxiety; ↑ relaxation.	Bergamot, chamomile, lavender, rosemary, basil, peppermint, lemon grass, mandarin neroli, ylang ylang, jasmine, grapefruit, juniper, frankincense, clary sage, Douglas Fir essential oils.	None.	Purchon et al, 2014; Kemper, 2016; Sánchez-Vidaña et al, 2017
Respiratory • The allergic triad (allergies/atopic dermatitis/asthma)				
	Nutritional			
	Avoids foods that trigger an immune response.	Avoid processed foods (including fast foods), nitrates, nitrites, preservatives, artificial colors/dyes, preservatives, flavorings, hydrogenated and trans fats, including vegetable oils. Avoid gluten, dairy, sugar, soy, shellfish, peanuts, eggs, beef, and pork. Also see Specific Diet Exclusions at the end of this table. The Mediterranean diet is efficacious.		Mark, 2018
	Dietary Supplements/Botanicals			
	Inhibits histamines, leukotrienes and prostaglandins to ↓ inflammation; stabilizes mast cells.	Quercetin (occurs naturally in buckwheat, apples, onions, garlic, kale, tomatoes, broccoli, asparagus, berries, green tea). Available in coated tablets and novel food (Lertal); do not use the powdered form.	Occasional headaches and tingling of extremities; can cause kidney damage at high doses (>1 g/d). Do not take if pregnant or breastfeeding, if there is kidney damage, or taking certain steroids or aspirin.	Ariano, 2015; Mlcek et al, 2016. Presently in clinical trials with children 6-12 years with allergic rhino-conjunctivitis (U.S. Library of Medicine, 2017)
	↓ Inflammatory cytokines; improve airway responsiveness in those with asthma.	Omega-3 EPA (best as tuna, salmon, walnuts, flaxseed oil, and anchovies. rather than supplement); limit omega-6 fatty acids.	None.	Farjadian et al, 2016
	↓ Frequency of asthma attacks.	Vitamin D.	None.	Kemper, 2016

TABLE
27.3
Complementary Treatments for Some Health Conditions—cont'd

System/Diagnosis	Benefits and Functional Considerations	Treatment	Possible Side Effects	Research Citations
	Inhibits histamine release, promotes vasodilation; may ↓ EIB.	Vitamin C.	None at recommended doses.	Mark, 2018
	↓ Oxidative damage to lungs; ↑ asthma control.	Vitamin E (gamma-tocopherol may be more efficacious than alpha-tocopherol).	Do not exceed 400 IU a day.	Burbank et al, 2017; Cook-Mills and Avila, 2014
	Adequate levels necessary for lung function; improves asthma control.	Magnesium.	GI upset.	Mark, 2018
	Antioxidant; ↓ inflammation; levels found to be lower in asthmatics.	Selenium.	GI upset above 400 μg/day.	Mark, 2018
	An antioxidant and bioflavonoid that ↓ inflammation in allergic asthma.	Pycnogenol (*Pinus pinaster*, maritime pine bark, a mixture of polyphenols).	Occasional GI upset.	Lau et al, 2004; Mark, 2018
	↓ Atopic dermatitis in infants to 6 years; not found to decrease asthma.	Probiotics (*Lactobacillus rhamnosus* HN001 and Bifidobacteria tested; other strains under clinical study).	None; efficacious if given to pregnant women, breastfeeding mothers, and infants.	Forsberg et al, 2016; Slattery et al, 2016; Wickens et al, 2013;
	Improves eczema over mineral oil.	Coconut oil or sunflower seed oil topically.	None, unless sensitive to ingredients.	Evangelista et al, 2014; Goddard and Lio, 2015
• Otitis media				
	Nutrition			
	Determines cause of any rhinorrhea (e.g., due to allergies; poor immune resilience; ↑ susceptibility to infections; insufficient vitamin D, zinc, retinol, and/or EFAs).	Eliminate dairy, eggs, refined sugars; ↑ fruits and berries.	None; ensure adequate calcium intake.	Haywood, 2017; Tapiainen, 2014
	Dietary Supplements/ Botanicals			
	Regulates autoimmune processes; panaceal antibiotic; deficiencies associated with ↑ infections and influenza; ↓ viral loads; ↑ recovery time.	Vitamin D3.	None.	Becker, 2018
	Prevents *S. pneumoniae* from adhering to nasopharyngeal cells; ↓ occurrence of OM in healthy children enrolled in day care and possibly in healthy children with a URI or prone to AOM.	Xylitol (naturally found in plums, strawberries, raspberries, and rowan berries. Also in syrups, nasal spray, chewing gum and lozenges).	Rare gas and diarrhea when given in large doses (≥30 g/day).	Azarpazhooh et al, 2016
	Use as interim measure while waiting out probability OM will resolve naturally; ↓ pain.	Combination ear drops (available as Otikon) (garlic, mullein, St. John's wort, calendula, olive oil).		Kemper, 2016

TABLE 27.3   Complementary Treatments for Some Health Conditions—cont'd

System/Diagnosis	Benefits and Functional Considerations	Treatment	Possible Side Effects	Research Citations
	Probiotics			
	Antagonizes growth of *S. pyogenes* and *S. pneumoniae*; helps prevent streptococcal pharyngitis and OM.	*S. salivarius* K12 (BLIS K12) (Bactoblis).	None.	Di Pierro et al, 2016; La Mantia et al, 2017
	↓ Risk and recurrence of AOM.	*S. salivarius* 24SMB and *S. oralis* 89a nasal spray.	May not be commercially available yet.	La Mantia et al, 2017
	Mind-Body			
	Focuses on restoring normal neurological function through elimination of the subluxation complex, correcting chemical or lifestyle influences.	Osteopathic/chiropractic manipulation.	None reported but requires cooperation of child and skilled practitioner.	Becker, 2018 (studies mixed on efficacy)
• Common cold/upper respiratory infection/influenza (best prevention is the flu vaccine)				
	Nutritional			
	Inhibits neutrophil chemotaxis; ↓ mucous secretions; improves nasal airway resistance.	Chicken soup (use organic chicken and vegetables if possible); peppers (including cayenne), mustard, horseradish, salsa, other spicy foods.	None reported.	Barrett, 2018
	Mild antitussive effects.	Honey (locally sourced).	Do not use in children <2 years due to risk of *C. botulinum*.	Barrett, 2018
	Dietary Supplements/ Botanicals			
	↓ Duration and severity of common cold or possibly prevent it.	Vitamin C (natural sources: oranges, kiwi, bell peppers, strawberries, papaya, broccoli, Brussels sprouts, kale, guava).	Regarded as safe; can cause GI upset, diarrhea in high doses; do not exceed 10 g/day.	Rondanelli et al, 2018
	↑ Immune function; may ↓ incidence of influenza.	Vitamin D3 (natural sources include sunlight, fatty fish [tuna, mackerel, salmon], liver, cheese, and egg yolks; supplements may be necessary).	None at prescribed doses.	Kemper, 2016; Borella et al, 2014
	Maintains physical barriers; and mucosal membrane integrity exerts a direct antiviral effect on rhinovirus replication; ↑ recovery rate from URI.	Zinc lozenge supplement (and/or ↑ zinc-containing foods: lamb, pumpkin, beef, chickpeas, coca, cashews, kefir, mushrooms, spinach, chicken).	Toxicity with long-term use and high doses; do not use intranasal zinc.	Hemilä et al, 2017; Rondanelli et al, 2018

TABLE 27.3   Complementary Treatments for Some Health Conditions—cont'd

System/Diagnosis	Benefits and Functional Considerations	Treatment	Possible Side Effects	Research Citations
	Immunomodulatory effects on natural killer cell activation, stimulation of interferon B and release of nitric oxide and tumor necrosis factor α; ↓ severity and shortens duration of symptoms of acute bronchitis.	Umckaloabo (*Pelargonium sidoides*) (EPs 7630, Schwabe GmBh, or Gesellschaft mit beschrankter Haftung, meaning limited liability company in Germany).	May experience GI upset, including diarrhea; do not use if allergic to geranium family.	Kamin et al, 2018
	Illness prevention; ↓ symptoms and sick days.	*Echinacea purpurea* (do not use prophylactically).	Do not use in those with progressive and systemic disease. Risk of allergic reaction in children <12 years.	Karsch-Völk et al, 2015; Meincke et al, 2017 (mixed results for prevention or treatment of URI)
	Antiviral properties; expedites recovery from influenza; neutralizes hemagglutinins and enhances cytokine production; in vitro studies demonstrate effectiveness against human pathogenic bacteria as well as influenza viruses.	Elderberry Use Sambucol syrup or suspension by Natures Way only.	Source of this product is critically important as it is toxic in the wrong product.	Kemper, 2016; Krawitz et al, 2011
	Anti-inflammatory, antibacterial, antineoplastic, immunomodulatory; ↓ symptoms and duration of URI.	*Andrographis paniculata* (an Ayurveda herb) (use product containing 180-360 mg of andrographolide constituents).	Possible GI upset.	Hu, 2017; Natural Medicines Therapeutic Research Center, 2018
Probiotics				
	↓ Number and length of URI.	Studies done using *Lactobacillus acidophilus*, *Bifidobacterium lactis*, fructo-oligosaccharides, and *Lactobacillus rhamnosus* (LGG).	None.	Gerasimov et al, 2016; King et al, 2014; Laursen and Hojsak, 2018
Other Healing Techniques				
	Possible improvement in breathing and ↓ nasal secretions.	Saline nasal spray.	None.	Barrett, 2018

5-HTP, 5-hydroxytryptamine; *ADHD,* attention deficit/hyperactivity disorder; *AOM,* acute otitis media; *CBT,* cognitive behavioral therapy; *DHA,* docosahexaenoic acid; *EFA,* essential fatty acids; *EIB,* exercise-induced bronchospasms; *EPA,* eicosapentaenoic acid; *g,* gram; *GABA,* gamma-aminobutyric acid; *GI,* gastrointestinal; *HIV,* human immunodeficiency virus; *IBD,* irritable bowel disease; *IBS,* irritable bowel syndrome; *IBS-D,* irritable bowel syndrome with diarrhea; *IU,* international units; *mg,* milligrams; *OM,* otitis media; *OTC,* over the counter; *RCT,* randomized controlled trial; *SAD,* standardized American diet; *SSRI,* selective serotonin reuptake inhibitors; *URI,* upper respiratory infection; ↑, increase(d); ↓, decrease(d); >, greater than; <, less than

SPECIFIC DIET EXCLUSIONS:

Asthma: Eliminate dairy products, eggs, soy, wheat, peanuts, fish, yeast (breads, cheeses, and mushrooms); sulfites (dried fruits); pesticide residues (best to buy organic); food additives (e.g., tartrazine or yellow dye no. 5); citric acid; benzoates; aspartame.

Attention Deficit Disorder or Attention Deficit/Hyperactivity Disorder: Eliminate artificial colors (blue 1,2; green 3; orange 8; red 3, 40; yellow 5, 6), flavors, and preservatives (butylated hydroxyanisole [BHA], butylated hydroxytoluene [BHT—often in packaged cereals], tertiary butyl hydroquinone [TBHQ]), sweeteners (Truvia, Neotame, Alitame); naturally occurring salicylates (found in many fruits and vegetables); decrease refined foods and sugars; increase foods high in protein and complex carbohydrates; specific foods causing allergic reactions; buy organic foods; increase garlic, onions, eggs; increase foods high in calcium, magnesium, zinc, cold-water fish, walnuts, flax (omega-3). Can also try eliminating apples, oranges, benzoates (chewing gum, margarine, pickles, prunes, tea, raspberries, cinnamon, anise, and nutmeg), caffeine, corn, dairy, nitrates, propyl gallate, sulfites (dried fruits, mushrooms, potatoes, baked goods, canned fish, and relishes), peanuts, and tomatoes.

Headache: Avoid known dietary triggers (may need to try elimination diet [see Additional Resources]). Avoid aged cheeses, some nuts, onions, chocolate, aspartame, processed meats with nitrates (e.g., hot dogs/pepperoni), monosodium glutamate (MSG), refined sugar, processed carbohydrates; limit caffeine, avoid foods high in omega-6 fatty acids; ensure adequate hydration. Increase omega-3 fatty acids (wild salmon, herring, mackerel, cod, sardines; fish oil; flax and hemp seeds; walnuts; algae).

sleep (See Chapter 20). Despite developing these habits, some children continue to struggle to achieve optimal sleep. FM then focuses on the sources of dysbiosis. Yeast overgrowth, in particular, is targeted as it may cause hyperexcitability, agitation, irritability, and insomnia. Yeast overgrowth can be evaluated by serum measurements of *Candida* (IgG, IgA, and IgM) or by conducting urinary organic acids and look for *Candida* markers (such as arabinose, tartaric, carboxycitric, and tricarballyic acids). Treating yeast nutraceutically includes considering products such as grapefruit seed extract, caprylic acid, garlic, and oregano. Nystatin is a prescription consideration (see Chapter 34, treating candidiasis).

Depression/Anxiety/Obsessive Compulsive Disorder

The brain and gut (the enteric nervous system) are connected via the vagus nerve, and gut dysbiosis could be a root cause of a child's neuropsychiatric condition from a FM approach. Yeast and *Candida* overgrowth can be a contributing factor, especially with anxiety and poor sleep. Celiac disease and nonceliac gluten sensitivity can also manifest as psychiatric symptoms with few irritable bowel signs. High *(or low)* homocysteine can show poor methylation and poor detoxification. Infection titers (IgG, IgM), especially in children with an abrupt onset of symptoms, should be assessed for underlying infectious agents. Infections common with pediatric acute-onset neuropsychiatric syndrome (or PANs) (notably acute OCD onset) are *Streptococcus*, *Mycoplasma*, Lyme disease, herpes, and influenza. Clinicians should be aware of other physiologic contributors to cognitive imbalances such as hyper- or hypothyroidism. Lifestyle factors such as adverse childhood events (ACEs), must be assessed and addressed (see Chapter 30). It is also important that children meet their exercise needs several times a week to help with depression.

Common Cold/Upper Respiratory Infection and Influenza

Nutritional deficiencies can lead to poor infection resilience when a child is faced with an infectious trigger. Phytonutrient diversity is promoted by a diet rich in nutrients offered by the Mediterranean diet versus the standard American diet (SAD), which often includes fast foods. If a child is sick more than average, FM model advises the PCP to determine the child's levels of vitamin A, vitamin D, B12, folate, and zinc. Because the microbiome contains over 70% of the immune system's function, ensuring that the gut is balanced (by using the 5-R program) should also be a consideration.

Otitis Media

If otitis media (OM) is chronic, PCPs should look to the cause of the rhinorrhea and ask if there is a trigger that needs further evaluation and treatment. An FM clinician would consider whether the OM is a result of untreated environmental or food allergies or poor immune resilience leading to an increased susceptibility to contact infections. Is the child's nutritional status with vitamin D, zinc, retinol, and essential fatty acids adequate or are there some underlying deficiencies that need repletion?

The Allergic Triad (Allergies/Atopic Dermatitis/Asthma)

Prenatal and postnatal microbial exposure and diversity is critical for building the foundation of an infant's microbiome. Infants delivered by C-section or whose mothers had antibiotics do not benefit from an initial colonization of their systems. The interrelationship between a highly processed Western diet and gut microbiome receives much focus as a cause of allergic disease (Skypala and Vlieg-Boerstra, 2014). Ensuring optimal levels of vitamin D can help increase resilience to allergic disease. Genetic mutations in the vitamin D receptor gene can prevent optimal absorption, so a FM approach is to check serum levels of vitamin D if allergic disease is persistent.

References

Adams KE, Cohen MH, Eisenberg D, et al. Ethical considerations of complementary and alternative medical therapies in conventional medical settings. *Ann Intern Med*. 2002;137(8):660–664.

Adams D, Dagenais S, Clifford T, et al. Complementary and alternative medicine use by pediatric specialty outpatients. *Pediatrics*. 2013;113(2):225–232.

Aetna Health Insurance. *Complementary and alternative medicine*; 2018. Available at: http://www.aetna.com/cpb/medical/data/300_399/0388.html. Accessed: June 17, 2018.

American Association of Colleges of Nursing (AACN). *Graduate-level QSEN competencies: Knowledge, skills and attitudes*; 2012 Available at: http://www.aacnnursing.org/Portals/42/AcademicNursing/CurriculumGuidelines/Graduate-QSEN-Competencies.pdf. Accessed: June 16, 2018.

Ariano R. Efficacy of a novel food supplement in the relief of the signs and symptoms of season allergic rhinitis and in the reduction of the consumption of anti-allergic drugs. *Acta Biomed*. 2015;86(1):53–58.

Azarpazhooh A, Lawrence H, Shah P. Xylitol for preventing acute otitis media in children up to 12 years of age. *Cochrane Database Syst Rev*. 2016;3(8):CD007095. https://doi.org/10.1002/14651858.CD007095.pub3.

Barrett, 2018 B: Viral upper respiratory infection. In: Rakel D, ed. *Integrative Medicine*. 4th ed. Philadelphia: Elsevier/Saunders; 2018. Ch 18.

Becker D. Otitis media. In: Rakel D, ed. *Integrative Medicine*. 4th ed. Philadelphia: Elsevier; 2018. Ch 16.

Bener A, Kamal M. Predict attention deficit hyperactivity disorder? Evidence-based medicine. *Glob J Health Sci*. 2013;6(2):47–57.

Birdee GS, Phillips RS, Davis RB, et al. Factors associated with pediatric use of complementary and alternative medicine. *Pediatrics*. 2010;125(2):249–256.

Black LI, Clarke TC, Barnes PM, et al. Use of complementary health approaches among children aged 4-17 years in the United States: National Health Interview Survey, 2007-2012. *Natl Health Stat Rep*. 2015;(78):1–19.

Borella E, Nesher G, Israeli E, et al. Vitamin D: a new anti-infective agent? *Ann NY Acad Sci*. 2014;1317(1):76–86.

Bruni O, Alonso-Alconada D, Besag F, et al. Current role of melatonin in pediatric neurology: clinical recommendations. *Eur J Paediatr Neurol*. 2015;19(2):122–133.

Burbank A, Duran C, Pan Y, et al. Gamma tocopherol-enriched supplement reduces sputum eosinophilia and endotoxin-induced sputum neutrophilia in volunteers with asthma. *J Allergy Clin Imm*. 2017;141(4):1231–1238. https://doi.org/10.1016/j.jaci.2017.06.029. Epub 2017 Jul 20.

Chumpitazi BP, Kearns Gl, Shulman RJ. Review article: the physiological effects and safety of peppermint oil and its efficacy in irritable bowel syndrome and other functional disorders. *Aliment Pharmacol Ther*. 2018;47(6):738–752.

Coeytaux R, Mann J. Headaches. In: Rakel D, ed. *Integrative Medicine*. 4th ed. Philadelphia: Elsevier; 2018. Ch 12.

Cook-Mills M, Avila P. Vitamin E and D regulation of allergic asthma immunopathogenesis. *Int Immunopharmacol*. 2014;23(1):364–372. Published online 2014 Aug 29. https://doi.org/10.1016/j.intimp.2014.08.007.

Cooper RE, Tye C, Kuntsi J, et al. The effect of omega-3 polyunsaturated fatty acid supplementation on emotional dysregulation, oppositional behavior and conduct problems in ADHD: a systematic review and meta-analysis. *J Affect Disord.* 2016;190:474–482.

Culbert TP, Olness K. *Integrative Pediatrics.* New York: Oxford University Press; 2010.

Curro D, Ianiro G, Pecere S, et al. Probiotics, fibre and herbal medicine products for functional and inflammatory bowel disorders. *Br J Pharmacol.* 2017;174(11):1426–1449.

Czaja-Bulsa G. Non coeliac gluten sensitivity - a new disease with gluten intolerance. *Clin Nutr.* 2015;34(2):189–194.

Di Pierro F, Colombo M, Biuliani MG, et al. Effect of administration of Streptococcus salivarius K12 on the occurrence of streptococcal pharyngo-tonsillitis, scarlet fever, and acute otitis media in 3 year old children. *Eur Rev Med Pharmacol Sci.* 2016;20(21):4601–4606.

Dolan R, Chey W, Eswaran S. The role of diet in the management of irritable bowel syndrome: a focus on FODMAPs. *Expert Rev Gastroenterol Hepatol.* 2018;12(6):607–615. https://doi.org/10.1080/17474124.2018.1476138. Epub 2018 May 18.

Erlichman J, Salam A, Haber BA. Use of complementary and alternative medicine in pediatric chronic viral hepatitis. *J Pediatr Gastroenterol Nutr.* 2010;50(4):417–421.

Evangelista MT, Abad-Casintahan F, Lopez-Villafuerte L. The effect of topical virgin coconut oil on SCORAD index, transepidermal water loss, and skin capacitance in mild to moderate pediatric atopic dermatitis: a randomized, double-blind, clinical trial. *Int J Dermatol.* 2014;53(1):100–108.

Farjadian S, Moghtaderi M, Kalani M, et al. Effects of omega-3 fatty acids on serum levels of T-helper cytokines in children with asthma. *Cytokine.* 2016;85:61–66.

Forsberg A, West CE, Prescott SL, et al. Pre- and probiotics for allergy prevention: time to revisit recommendations? *Clin Exp Allergy.* 2016;46(12):1506–1521.

Gerasimov SV, Ivantsiv VA, Bobryk LM, et al. Role of short-term use of L. acidophilus DDS-1 and B. lactis UABLA-12 in acute respiratory infections in children: a randomized controlled trial. *Eur J Clin Nutr.* 2016;70:463–469.

Giannetti E, Staiano A. Probiotics for irritable bowel syndrome: clinical data in children. *J Pediatr Gastroenterol Nutr.* 2016;(63 suppl 1):S25–S26. 2016. https://doi.org/10.1097/MPG.0000000000001220.

Goddard A, Lio P. Alternative, complementary, and forgotten remedies for atopic dermatitis. *Evid Based Complement Alternat Med.* 2015:676897, 2015. Published online 2015 Jul 15. https://doi.org/10.1155/2015/676897.

Greenblatt J, Gottlieb B. *Finally Focused: The Breakthrough Natural Treatment Plan for ADHD that Restores Attention, Minimizes Hyperactivity, and Helps Eliminate Drug Side Effects.* N.Y: Harmony Books; 2017.

Grundmann O, Yoon SL. Complementary and alternative medicines in irritable bowel syndrome: An integrative view. *World Journal of Gastroenterology.* 2014;20(2):346–362.

Haywood M, Alade A, Vijendren A, et al. Late presentation of egg white and milk protein allergy as rhinitis and otitis media. *Br J Hosp Med (Lond).* 2017;78(2):112–113.

Hemilä H, Fitzgerald JT, Petrus EJ, et al. Zinc acetate lozenges may improve the recovery rate of common cold patients: an individual patient data meta-analysis. *Open Forum Infect Dis.* 2017;4(2).

Hirayama S, Tersawa K, Rabeler R, et al. The effect of phosphatidylserine administration on memory and symptoms of attention-deficit hyperactivity disorder: a randomised, double-blind, placebo-controlled clinical trial. *J Hum Nutr Diet.* 2014;27(s2):284–291.

Hu X, Wu R, Logue M, et al. Andrographis paniculata (Chuān Xīn Lián) for symptomatic relief of acute respiratory tract infections in adults and children: a systematic review and meta-analysis. *PLoS One.* 2017;12(8):e0181780.

Ioannidis JP. Why most published research findings are false. *PLoS Med.* 2005;2(8):3124.

Ioannidis JP. How to make more published research true. *PLoS Med.* 2014;11(10):31001747.

Institute of Medicine (IOM). Committee on the Use of Complementary and Alternative Medicine by the American Public, Board on Health Promotion and Disease. *Complementary and Alternative Medicine in the United States.* Washington DC: National Academies Press; 2005.

International Trade Administration (ITA). *2016 Top Markets Report Pharmaceuticals: overview and Key Findings.* Available from https://www.trade.gov/topmarkets/pdf/Pharmaceuticals_Executive_Summary.pdf. Accessed May 1, 2018.

Jacka F, Kremer P, Berk M, et al. A prospective study of diet quality and mental health in adolescents. *PLoS One.* 2011;6(9):e24805. https://doi.org/10.1371/journal.pone.0024805.

Kalaichandran A, Barrowman N, Chan I, et al. Use and perceived effectiveness of complementary health approaches in children. *Paediatr Child Health.* 2018;23(1).

Kamin W, Funk P, Seifert G, et al. EPs 7630 is effective and safe in children under 6 years with acute respiratory tract infections: clinical studies revisited. *Curr Med Res Opin.* 2018;34(3):475–485.

Kaplan S. Hundreds of babies harmed by homeopathic remedies, families say. *STAT Scientific American.* 2017.

Karimi A, Majlesi M, Rafieian-Kopaei M. Herbal versus synthetic drugs; beliefs and facts. *J Nephropharmacol.* 2015;4(1):27–30.

Karsch-Völk M, Barrett B, Linde K. Echinacea for preventing and treating the common cold. *JAMA.* 2015;313(6):618–619.

Kemper K. *The Holistic Pediatrician Twentieth Anniversary Revised Edition: A Pediatrician's Comprehensive Guide to Safe and Effective Therapies for the 25 most Common Ailments of Infants, Children, and Adolescents.* NY: Harpers Paperbacks; 2016.

King S, Glanville J, Sanders ME, et al. Effectiveness of probiotics on the duration of illness in healthy children and adults who develop common acute respiratory infectious conditions: a systematic review and meta-analysis. *Brit J Nutr.* 2014;112(1):41–54.

Kligler B, Teets R, Quick M. Complementary/integrative therapies that work: a review of the evidence. *Am Fam Physician.* 2016;94(5):369–374.

Kohlboeck G, Sausenthaler S, Standl M, et al. Food intake, diet quality and behavioural problems in children: results from the GINI-plus/LISA-plus studies. *Ann Nutr Metab.* 2012;60(4):247–256.

Kovacevic G, Stevanovic D, Bogicevic D, et al. A 6-month follow-up of disability, quality of life, and depressive and anxiety symptoms in pediatric migraine with magnesium prophylaxis. *Magnes Res.* 2017;30(4):133–141.

Kravitz RL, Duan N. *DEcIDE Methods Center N-of-1 Guidance Panel. Design and Implementation of N-of-1 Trials: A User's Guide.* Rockville, MD: Agency for Healthcare Research and Quality; 2014. Available at: https://effectivehealthcare.ahrq.gov/topics/n-1-trials/research-2014-5. Accessed: June 16, 2018.

Krawitz C, Mraheil M, Stein M, et al. Inhibitory activity of a standardized elderberry liquid extract against clinically-relevant human respiratory bacterial pathogens and influenza A and B viruses. *BMC Complement Altern Med.* 2011;11:16. Published online 2011 Feb 25. https://doi.org/10.1186/1472-6882-11-16.

La Mantia I, Varricchio A, Ciprandi G. Bacteriotherapy with Streptococcus salivarius 24SMB and Streptococcus oralis 89a nasal spray for preventing recurrent acute otitis media in children: a real-life clinical experience. *Int J Gen Med.* 2017;10:171–175.

Lapina T, Trukhmanov A. Herbal preparation STW 5 for functional gastrointestinal disorders: clinical experience in everyday practice. *Dig Dis.* 2017;35(suppl 1):30–35. https://doi.org/10.1159/000485411. Epub 2018 Feb 8.

Lau B, Riesen S, Truong K, et al. Pycnogenol as an adjunct in the management of childhood asthma. *J Asthma.* 2004;41(8):825–832.

Laursen R, Hojsak I. Probiotics for respiratory tract infections in children attending day care centers-a systematic review. *Eur J Pediatr.* 2018. https://doi.org/10.1007/s00431-018-3167-1. [Epub ahead of print].

Lin JL, Cohen E, Sanders LM. Shared decision making among children with medical complexity: results from a population-based survey. *J Pediatr*. 2018;192:216–222.

Lyon M, Kapoor M, Juneja L. The effects of L-theanine (Suntheanine) on objective sleep quality in boys with attention deficit hyperactivity disorder (ADHD): a randomized, double-blind, placebo-controlled clinical trial. *Altern Med Rev*. 2011;16(4):348–354. 2011.

Makharia A, Catassi C, Makharia GK. The overlap between irritable bowel syndrome and non-celiac gluten sensitivity: a clinical dilemma. *Nutrients*. 2015;7(12):10417–10426. https://doi.org/10.3390/nu7125541.

Malone M, Tsai G. The evidence for herbal and botanical remedies. *Clinican Rev*. 2018;28(5):22–28.

Mancini E, Beglinger C, Drewe J, et al. Green tea effects on cognition, mood and human brain function: a systematic review. *Phytomed*. 2017;34:26–37.

Mark JD. Asthma. In: Rakel D, ed. *Integrative Medicine*. 4th ed. Philadelphia: Elsevier/Saunders; 2018. Ch 29.

McClafferty H, Vohra S, Bailey M, et al. Section on Integrative Medicine: pediatric integrative medicine. *Pediatrics*. 2017;140(3). https://doi.org/10.1542/peds.20171961.

Mech AW, Farah A. Correlation of clinical response with homocysteine reduction during therapy with reduced B vitamins in patients with MDD who are positive for MTHFR C677T or A1298C polymorphism: a randomized, double-blind, placebo-controlled study. *J Clin Psychiatry*. 2016;77(5):668–671.

Meincke R, Pokladnikova J, Straznicka J, et al. Allergy-like immediate reactions with herbal medicines in children: a retrospective study using data from VigiBase. *Pediatr Allergy Immunol*. 2017;28(7):668–674.

Mlcek J, Jurikova T, Skrovankova S, et al. Quercetin and its anti-allergic immune response. *Molecules*. 2016;21(5):623.

Naiman R. Insomnia. In: Rakel D, ed. *Integrative Medicine*. 4th ed. Philadelphia: Elsevier; 2018. Ch 9.

National Institute of Diabetes and Digestion and Kidney Diseases. *Eating, diet, & nutrition for irritable bowel syndrome*; 2017. Available at https://www.niddk.nih.gov/health-information/digestive-diseases/irritable-bowel-syndrome/eating-diet-nutrition. Accessed November 12, 2018.

National Institute of Health (NIH), National Center for Complementary and Integrative Health (NCCIH). *Credentialing, Licensing, and Education*; 2015. Available at: https://nccih.nih.gov/sites/nccam.nih.gov/files/Credentialing_08-11-2015.pdf. Accessed: June 17, 2018.

National Institute of Health (NIH), National Center for Complementary and Integrative Medicine (NCCIM). *2016 Strategic Plan*. Available at https://nccih.nih.gov/about/strategic-plans/2016/Objective-3-Foster-Health-Promotion-Disease-Prevention. Accessed May 4, 2018.

National Institute of Health (NIH), National Center for Complementary and Integrative Health (NCCIH). *Research*; 2017a. Available at: https://nccih.nih.gov/research. Accessed: June 19, 2018.

National Institute of Health (NIH), National Center for Complementary and Integrative Health (NCCIH). *Be an Informed Consumer*; 2017b. Available at: https://nccih.nih.gov/health/decisions. Accessed: June 17, 2018.

National Institute of Health (NIH), National Center for Complementary and Integrative Health (NCCIH). *Safe use of Complementary Health Products and Practices*; 2017c. Available at: https://nccih.nih.gov/health/safety. Accessed: June 17, 2018.

Natural Medicines Therapeutic Research Center (TRC). *Andrographis [Monograph]*; 2018. Available at: https://naturalmedicines.therapeuticresearch.com/databases/food,-herbs-supplements/professional.aspx?productid=973#mechanismOfAction. Accessed: January 20, 2018.

Pelham Jr WE, Waschbusch DA, Hoza B, et al. Music and video as distractors for boys with ADHD in the classroom: comparison with controls, individual differences, and medication effects. *J Abnorm Child Psychol*. 2011;39(8):1085–1098.

Perera S, Eisen R, Bhatt M, et al. Light therapy for non-seasonal depression: systematic review and meta-analysis. *BJ Psych Open*. 2011;2(2):116–126. 2016. https://doi.org/10.1192/bjpo.bp.115.001610.

Purchon N, Cantele L. *The Complete Aromatherapy & Essential Oils Handbook for Everyday Wellness*. Toronto, Canada: Robert Rose; 2014.

Quirk S, Wiliams L, O'Neil A, et al. The association between diet quality, dietary patterns and depression in adults: a systematic review. *BMC Psychiatr*. 2013;13:175. https://doi.org/10.1186/1471-244X-13-175.

Ríos-Hernández A, Alda JA, Farran-Codina A, et al. The Mediterranean diet and ADHD in children and adolescents. *Pediatrics*. 2017;139(2):e20162027.

Rondanelli M, Miccono A, Lamburghini S, et al. Self-care for common colds: the pivotal role of vitamin D, vitamin C, zinc, and *Echinacea* in three main immune interactive clusters (physical barriers, innate and adaptive immunity) involved during an episode of common colds—practical advice on dosages and on the time to take these nutrients/botanicals in order to prevent or treat the common cold. *Evid Based Complement Alternat Med*. 2018. https://doi.org/10.1155/2018/58213095.

Rothmann K, Hillmer JM, Hosser D. Evaluation of the musical concentration training with Pepe (MusiKo mit Pepe) for children with attention deficits [in German]. *Z Kinder Jugendpsychiatr Psychother*. 2014;42(5):325–335.

Saha T, Dutta D, Rajamma U, et al. A pilot study on the contribution of folate gene variants in the cognitive function of ADHD probands. *Neurochem Res*. 2014;39(11):2058–2067.

Sánchez-Vidaña D, Pui-Ching Ngai S, He W. The effectiveness of aromatherapy for depressive symptoms: a systematic review. *Evid Based Complement Alternat Med*. 2017;2017:5869315. Published online 2017 Jan 4. https://doi.org/10.1155/2017/5869315.

Sawni A, Kemper K. Attention deficit disorder. In: Rakel D, ed. *Integrative Medicine*. 4th ed. Philadelphia: Elsevier; 2018. Ch 7.

Schneider C, Wissink T. Depression. In: Rakel D, ed. *Integrative Medicine*. 4th ed. Philadelphia: Elsevier/Saunders; 2018. Ch 5.

Schoonees A, Visser J, Musekiwa A, et al. Pycnogenol (extract of French maritime pine bark) for the treatment of chronic disorders. *Cochrane Database Syst Rev*. 2012;4. https://doi.org/10.1002/14651858.CD008294.pub4.CD008294].

Selby JV. The patient-centered outcomes research institute: a 2013 agenda for "research done differently." *Popul Health Manag*. 2013;16(2):69–70.

Sharma A, Gerbarg P, Bottiglieri T, et al. S-Adenosylmethionine (SAMe) for neuropsychiatric disorders: a clinician-oriented review of research. *J Clin Psychiatry*. 2017;78(6):e656–e667. https://doi.org/10.4088/JCP.16r11113.

Shelton R, Manning J, Barrentine L, et al. Assessing effects of l-methylfolate in depression management: results of a real-world patient experience trial. *Prim Care Companion CNS Disord*. 2013;15(4):PCC.13m01520. Published online 2013 Aug 29. https://doi.org/10.4088/PCC.13m01520.

Skypala I, Vlieg-Boerstra B. Food intolerance and allergy: increased incidence or contemporary inadequate diets? *Curr Opin Clin Nutr Metab Care*. 2014;17(5):442–447.

Slattery J, MacFabe D, Frye R. The significance of the enteric microbiome on the development of childhood disease: a review of prebiotic and probiotic therapies in disorders of childhood. *Clin Med Insights Pediatr*. 2016;10:91–107. Published online 2016 Oct 9. https://doi.org/10.4137/CMPed.S38338.

Snyder J, Brown P. Complementary and alternative medicine in children: an analysis of the recent literature. *Curr Opin Pediatr*. 2012;24(4):539–546.

Soriano R, Ramos-Soriano A. Clinical and pathologic remission of pediatric ulcerative colitis with serum-derived bovine immunoglobulin added to the standard treatment regimen. *Case Rep Gastroenterol*. 2017;11(2):335–343. https://doi.org/10.1159/000475923.

St Cyr A, Chen A, Bradley K, et al. Efficacy and tolerability of STOPAIN for a migraine attack. *Front Neurol*. 2015;6:11. Published online 2015 Feb 4. https://doi.org/10.3389/fneur.2015.00011.

Street W, Weed D, Spurlock A. Use of music in the treatment of insomnia: a pilot study. *Holist Nurs Pract*. 2014;28(1):38–42.

Talebian A, Soltani B, Banafshe HR, et al. Prophylactic effect of riboflavin on pediatric migraine: a randomized, double-blind, placebo-controlled trial. *Electron Physician*. 2018;10(2):6279–6285.

Tapiainen T, Paalanne N, Arkkola T, et al. Diet as a risk factor for pneumococcal carriage and otitis media: a cross-sectional study among children in day care centers. *PLoS One*. 2014;9(3):e90585.

The Joint Commission. *National Patient Safety Goals*; 2018. Available at: https://www.jointcommission.org/2018_national_patient_safety_goals_presentation/. Accessed: June 17, 2018.

Thompson EA, Bishop JL, Northstone K. The use of homeopathic products in childhood: data generated over 8.5 years from the Avon Longitudinal Study of Parents and Children (ALSPAC). *J Altern Complement Med.* 2010;16(1):69–79.

Trebatická J, Ďuračková Z. Psychiatric disorders and polyphenols: can they be helpful in therapy? *Oxid Med Cell Longev.* 2015;2015:248529. Published online 2015 Jun 9. https://doi.org/10.1155/2015/248529.

U.S. Food and Drug Administration (FDA). *FDA 101: Dietary supplements*; 2017. Available at: https://www.fda.gov/forconsumers/consumerupdates/ucm050803.htm. Accessed: June 17, 2018.

U.S. Food and Drug Administration (FDA). *Homeopathic products: is the FDA concerned about the safety of homeopathic products?* 2018. Available at: https://www.fda.gov/Drugs/DrugSafety/InformationbyDrugClass/ucm589282.htm. Accessed: June 17, 2018.

U.S. Library of Medicine. *Efficacy and safety of Lertal® as an add-on to standard therapy for allergic rhinoconjunctivitis in pediatrics*; 2017. Available at https://clinicaltrials.gov/ct2/show/NCT03365648. Accessed September 3, 2018.

University of Maryland Medical Center. *Attention Deficit Hyperactivity Disorder. UMMC (Website)*; 2013. https://www.scribd.com/document/283151788/Http-Umm-Edu-Health-Medical-Altmed-Condition-Attention-Deficit-hyperactivity-disorder-1. Accessed August 31,2018.

Wegh C, Benninga M, Tabbers M. Effectiveness of probiotics in children with functional abdominal pain disorders and functional constipation: a systematic review. *J Clin Gastroenterol.* 2018. https://doi.org/10.1097/MCG.0000000000001054. [Epub ahead of print].

World Health Organization (WHO). *Traditional medicine strategy 2014-2023.* Geneva: WHO; 2013. Available at: http://www.searo.who.int/entity/health_situation_trends/who_trm_strategy_2014-2023.pdf?ua=1. Accessed: June 17, 2018.

Additional Resources

General Information:
Academic Consortium for Integrative Medicine & Health.
https://www.imconsortium.org/
Institute for Functional Medicine.
www.ifm.org/functional-medicine/
Linus Pauling Institute Oregon State University.
http://lpi.oregonstate.edu/
MedWatch.
https://www.fda.gov/safety/medwatch/
Pediatric Complementary and Alternative Medicine Research and Education Network (PedCAM).
http://www.pedcam.ca/
U.S. Food and Drug Administration.
https://www.fda.gov/
Comprehensive Pediatric Functional Medicine Intake Form
Duke University Integrative Medicine.
https://www.dukeintegrativemedicine.org/wp-content/uploads/2018/01/Pediatric-Medical-Intake-71225-1.pdf

Elimination Diet,
University of Wisconsin Integrative Medicine Department.
http://projects.hsl.wisc.edu/SERVICE/courses/whole-health-for-pain-and-suffering/Clinician-Guide-Nutrition-Elimination-Diet.pdf

Essential Oils/Aromatherapy

Tisserand R, Young R. *Essential Oil Safety: A Guide for Health Care Professionals.* 2nd ed. Philadelphia: Churchill, Livingstone, Elsevier; 2014.
Functional/Integrative Lab Resources:
Doctor's Data.
https://www.doctorsdata.com/
Genova Diagnostics.
https://www.gdx.net/
Great Plains Laboratories.
https://www.greatplainslaboratory.com/
Alleless Medical.
https://foodallergy.com/
Precision Analytical.
https://dutchtest.com/
Genomix Nutrition.
https://www.gxsciences.com/
Igenex.
https://igenex.com/
Herbal/Botanical Safety,
American Botanical Council HerbClip Database.
http://cms.herbalgram.org/herbclip/index.html
American Herbal Products Association.
http://www.ahpa.org/
National Center for Complementary and Integrative Health online app: HerbList (available free from the Apple App store and Google Play store).
Natural Medicine Comprehensive Database. *Natural Product/Drug Interaction Checker*; 2018. http://naturaldatabase.therapeuticresearch.com/nd/Search.aspx?s=ND&cs=&pt=7&rli=1&sh=.
Natural Medicines Therapy Research Center (TRC) (Subscription required to access).
http://trchealthcare.com/solutions/natural-medicines
References for Complementary Therapies used in Pediatrics
Culbert T, Olness K: *Integrative pediatrics*, New York, 2010, Oxford University Press.
GreenMedInfo—The World's Natural Health Resource, *http://www.greenmedinfo.com/* (professional membership fee required).
Kemper K. *The Holistic Pediatrician Twentieth Anniversary Revised Edition: A Pediatrician's Comprehensive Guide to Safe and Effective Therapies for the 25 most Common Ailments of Infants, Children, and Adolescents.* New York: Harpers Paperbacks; 2016.
Loo M. *Integrative Medicine for Children.* Philadelphia: Elsevier; 2009.
McClafferty H. *Integrative Pediatrics: Art, Science, and Clinical Applications.* New York: Routledge; 2017.
Misra S, Verissimo A. *A Guide to Integrative Pediatrics for the Healthcare Professional (Springer briefs in public health).* New York: Springer International Publishing; 2014.
Natural Medicine Comprehensive Database. *http://naturaldatabase.therapeuticresearch.com/home.aspx?cs=&s=ND* (professional membership fee required).
Rakel D, ed. *Integrative Medicine.* 4th ed. Philadelphia: Elsevier; 2018.

28

Pediatric Pain and Fever Management

HELEN N. TURNER AND CRIS ANN BOWMAN-HARVEY

Pediatric Pain Management

Our knowledge of pain and its management advanced exponentially in the last 50 years and resulted in dramatic changes in pain management for infants, children, and adolescents. Prior to the mid-1980s, it was thought infants did not feel or remember pain so there was no need to treat it. Coinciding with this was concern that many pain medications were not safe for pediatric patients. Today, we recognize the critical need to minimize pain related to medical care and have the necessary resources to do so safely and effectively.

Overview of Pain

Pain has an evolutionary purpose—the painless interval post injury allows the fight or flight response to occur and then incites injury awareness which provokes withdrawal from the painful stimuli. Early painful experiences are significant events and can produce long-term consequences for the child. Preterm infants are particularly vulnerable and undergo numerous painful procedures. Studies document early and under treated pain have long-term negative physiologic and psychological consequences such as increased pain sensitivity, decreased effectiveness of analgesia during subsequent procedures, persistent pain, increased stress responses, and behavior and learning difficulties (Anand, 2017).

Standards for pediatric care necessitate incorporating pain management and prevention in every treatment plan, from minor painful procedures to more serious illness or injury and persistent pain. Understanding nociception, types, mechanisms, and sources of pain is critical to developing a successful treatment regimen. Nociception is the neural process of encoding the noxious stimuli which results in pain perception. This is a four-part process (transduction, transmission, perception, modulation) when sensory nerve endings (nociceptors) are activated by chemical, mechanical, thermal, or mixed stimuli (Fig 28.1). Pain assessment, diagnosis, and treatment are determined by the type of pain (Box 28.1) and the mechanism or etiology of the pain (Box 28.2). The neural foundations and pathways necessary for nociception develop early in fetal life. At approximately 32 weeks of gestation, myelinization of the brain stem and thalamic tract is complete and the beginning of the neuronal pain inhibiting mechanism appears. This continues developing until well after the newborn period. Because of neural plasticity, newborns subjected to repetitive acute pain may develop central neural changes that predispose them to pain vulnerability, cognitive effects, and opioid tolerance (Committee on Fetus and Newborn and Section on Anesthesiology and Pain Medicine, 2016).

Pain is "an unpleasant sensory and emotional experience associated with actual or potential tissue damage or described in terms of such damage" (International Association for the Study of Pain [IASP], 2017). Persistent pain is pain that lasts 3 to 6 months or longer or lasts longer than the expected healing time for an injury. Approximately 30% of children experience persistent pain, with the most commonly reported being headaches, abdominal pain, and musculoskeletal pain (Huguet et al., 2016). Children and adolescents with persistent pain are at greater risk for anxiety, depression, and sleep disturbances, and they may experience more emotional and functional problems than their peers. The prevalence of the co-occurrence of persistent pain and mental health disorders is about 25% (Tegethoff et al., 2015). Persistent pain affects children's school attendance, participation in hobbies, appetite, and quality of life, and results in increased health services. Because it is not always feasible to eliminate pain, effective management with minimal side effects and return of function are the primary goals of treatment.

Factors Influencing Pediatric Pain Management

Physiological

- Genetics and age influence levels of neurotransmitters or medication responses.
- Established pain is more difficult to control, making pain prevention and timely pain management critical goals.
- Persistent pain is rarely associated with sympathetic nervous system arousal; therefore, children with persistent pain may not appear to be in pain. This lack of outward expression of symptoms may impede pain evaluation and treatment.

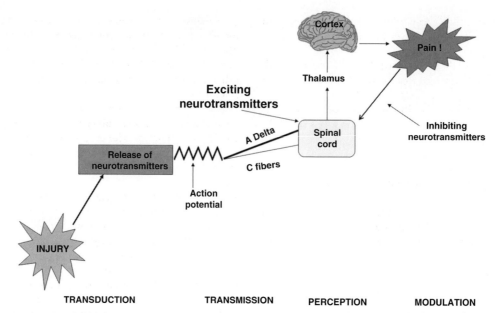

• **Fig 28.1** Nociception *Transduction:* Painful or noxious stimuli are translated into electrical signals at sensory nerve endings and forwarded to the spinal cord via A-delta fibers and C fibers. A-delta fibers are large, myelinated, fast, and when activated result in sharp, stinging sensations. In contrast, C fibers are small, unmyelinated, slow, and their activation results in dull, aching, burning, and diffuse sensations. *Transmission:* Electrical impulses are forwarded through the sensory nervous system through both the peripheral and central nervous systems. *Perception:* The emotional and physical experience of pain. *Modulation:* Alteration of information by endogenous mechanisms results in lessening or amplification of the pain signal. (Adapted from Curtiss, personal communication, 2017. Czarnecki ML, Turner HN, eds. *Core Curriculum for Pain Management Nursing.* 3rd ed. St. Louis: Elsevier; 2018.)

• BOX 28.1 Types of Pain

- *Procedural (incidental):* Short-term acute pain caused by medical investigations and treatment.
- *Acute:* Sudden onset, usually associated with trauma, injury, or medical case and resolves in a predictable and expected timeframe.
- *Persistent:* Pain that continues beyond the expected healing time. Persistent pain no longer has a purpose. Factors not necessarily related to the initial cause of pain may perpetuate it.
- *Recurrent:* Returning or occurring again following a pain-free period.
- *Mixed:* Acute pain in the setting of persistent pain.

• BOX 28.2 Mechanisms of Pain

- Nociceptive pain: occurs when nociceptors (mechanical, chemical, thermal) are stimulated
  Somatic: from bones, joints, muscles, and skin; may be superficial or deep
  Visceral: from viscera or pleura
- Neuropathic pain
  Central: disease or injury of central nervous system (CNS)
  Peripheral: disease or injury of peripheral nervous system (PNS)
  Mixed: combined dysfunction of CNS and PNS
- Inflammatory pain
  Inflammatory process itself alters nociceptors such that threshold to response is lowered
  Nerve recruitment occurs
  Wind up (dysregulation of amplification and modulation) occurs
- Psychogenic pain
  Not a diagnostic term
  Psychological factors play significant role
  Report of pain may not match symptoms
  Pain is real!

Psychosocial

- Individual physiologic and psychologic states influence pain perception and response.
- Developmental stages (e.g., cognitive, emotional, and physical), age, and temperament significantly affect pain interpretation, expression, and control. Therefore, pain management must be tailored to the individual child.
- Cognitive factors influencing pain perception include the child's memory, level of understanding, sense of control, attachment of meaning to a painful situation, and expectations regarding pain.
- Emotional factors affecting a child's pain perception include anxiety, fear, frustration, anger, and depression.
- Consider biopsychosocial and spiritual manifestations of persistent pain when treating pediatric persistent pain.
- Involve pediatric patients and families in the pain management plan including assessment, management, and

education. Educate parents about their role in engaging and providing distraction and comfort to their child during and after painful procedures (e.g., vaccinations, ear examinations, and incision and drainage procedures). Educate the parents of children with persistent pain to effectively manage pain and support the child in developing strategies to effectively cope with pain.
- Consider culture, family learning patterns, and language barriers (e.g., pain beliefs, folk remedies, and how pain is expressed).

- Others' reactions to a child's pain influences the treatment plan and should be included in the plan. Family harmony or conflict are pediatric pain influencers.
- Socioeconomic status and other social determinants of health impact access to medications, treatments, and pediatric pain specialists.
- Children with pain experience disparities related to race, ethnicity, and culture.

Barriers to Effective Pain Management

Barriers to effective pain management tend to fall into three areas: the patient and family, the primary care provider (PCP), and healthcare systems. These barriers in isolation or combination result in inadequate pain control. PCPs must be cognizant of these barriers and the negative effect they have on pain management strategies.

Patient and Family

- Fear of the possible treatment (e.g., getting an injection, addiction) or of not believing they have pain
- Difficulty conceptualizing, quantifying, and communicating a pain experience
- Fear of worsening or progression of disease
- Cultural differences about the significance of pain, and pain expression and treatment

Healthcare Providers

- Outdated knowledge (e.g., belief in the myth that infants and children do not feel pain, or if they do, there is no consequence)
- Lack of current knowledge regarding assessment, treatment options, and pain physiology
- Inaccurate assumption that pediatric pain management takes too much time and effort
- Fear of adverse effects of analgesic medications, including respiratory depression and addiction
- Personal values and beliefs about the meaning and value of pain

Healthcare Systems

- Restrictions on certain analgesic medications related to diagnosis, age, or off-label use
- Limited insurance coverage for nonpharmacologic modalities
- Legislative barriers to PCP access to opioids
- Failure to hold providers accountable for pain care
- Lack of developmentally appropriate assessment tools

Pain Assessment

A systematic approach to pediatric pain assessment begins by obtaining a pain history from the child and the parent. Ask the child and parent what words they use for pain (e.g., "owie," "boo-boo," "ouchie," "hurt"), and use these words. Behavioral observations and physiologic findings provide additional information necessary for a comprehensive pain assessment. Pain evaluation in children needs to be multidimensional. Collect data about what children say related to their pain, assess for physiologic and emotional manifestations of pain, and investigate other pertinent contributors to the child's pain.

Pediatric pain assessment can be challenging given developmental and cultural considerations that influence pain expression. These include whether distressed behaviors manifested by either verbal or nonverbal children of various ages indicate pain or if other causative factors (e.g., anxiety, fear, stress, or hunger) are responsible.

Self-report is the gold standard for assessment but is dependent on the child's cognitive ability to understand pain severity on a continuum (Hauer and Jones, 2018). Children as young as 3 years old may be capable of quantifying their pain and translating it to a visual representation. Factors that influence self-report of pain include:
- Situational influences (e.g., setting, person asking, or what the child expects to happen as a result of their answer).
- Children may underreport pain if they lack knowledge that pain can be treated, if they fear their pain may upset their parents, or they are concerned the treatment may be worse than the pain (e.g., injection).
- Some children overstate their pain to receive increased attention. This tends to be an unconscientious, learned behavior.
- Various factors and perceptions affect a child's report of pain, including nausea, anxiety or fear of talking to a health care provider, disappointing or bothering others, receiving an unpleasant medication, or the need to be re-hospitalized. Younger children may confuse fear with pain. Adolescents may not want to miss an athletic event or disappoint their teammates, so they may underreport their pain or deny being in pain.
- Children with developmental delays may have difficulty reporting pain, be less precise in their reports, or be unable to communicate their pain. However, self-report is always preferred over observational tools when possible. These children are no less sensitive to painful stimuli than children with typical development.

Developmental factors must be considered in pain assessment. Infant and toddler assessment relies on pain-related behaviors, typically nonverbal responses (e.g., facial expression, limb movements, and crying). Many toddlers use their own words to indicate pain and report its general location but cannot describe pain severity. Preschoolers say they have "none," "a little," or "a lot" of pain and some may be able to use pain scales such as the Faces scale. During middle childhood, they describe location, intensity, and quality of their pain, while adolescents provide more descriptive information.

Reliable, valid, sensitive, and easily understood instruments specific to acute or persistent pain should be used but should not be the sole determinant for evaluation or treatment. Self-report tools, pain journals, and other objective pain measures help to quantify pain before treatment and serve to evaluate the treatment effectiveness. Multiple web-based tools are available. For children unable to self-report, observational pain scales are available. A child's pain assessment is not complete until the provider considers self-report data as well as individual and contextual factors related to the child's clinical history, child and family preferences, and responses to previous treatments (Twycross et al., 2015). Commonly used pediatric pain scales are summarized in Table 28.1.

Pain History

A systematic interval history and examination are needed when pain does not abate as expected or there is a change in quality, intensity, duration, or location. The following information should

TABLE 28.1	Commonly Used Pediatric Pain Scales	
Scale	**Population**	**Comments**
Observational		
PIPP	Premature infants	
N-PASS	Premature infants and neonates	Some evidence for use with older infants; quantifies both pain and sedation
NIPS	Premature and term infants	
COMFORT Behavior Scale	Non-communicating children with cognitive impairment	
CRIES	Infants up to 6 months	
FLACC	2 months–4 years Non-communicating children with cognitive impairment	
rFLACC	Non-communicating children with cognitive impairment	Allows for addition of child-specific behaviors
INRS	Non-communicating children with cognitive impairment	Pain cues based on parent/caregiver input
Self-Report		
Wong-Baker Faces	4 years and older	End anchors may lead to under reporting of pain
FPS-R	4 years and older	
VAS	4 years and older	
Oucher	4 years and older	Multiple ethnic versions available
Poker Chip	4 years and older	
Eland Color Tool	4 years and older	
Numeric	8 years and older	Child must be able to understand seriation or rank and order

CRIES, Crying, Requires oxygen, Increased vital signs, Expression, Sleeplessness; *FLACC,* Faces, Legs, Activity, Cry, Consolability; *FPS-R,* Faces Pain Scale Revised; *INRS,* Individualized Numeric Rating Scale; *NIPS,* Neonatal Infant Pain Scale; *N-PASS,* Neonatal Pain, Agitation, and Sedation Scale; *PIPP,* Premature Infant Pain Profile; *rFLACC,* Revised FLACC; *VAS,* Visual Analog Scale.

be obtained during the history (refer to Box 28.3 for helpful mnemonics):

- Intensity (mild, moderate, severe, or overwhelming)
- Location (including areas of radiation and referral)
- Quality—how pain is described by child or parent (e.g., stinging, burning, throbbing, or squeezing feeling or "big ouchie") and any pain behaviors noted
- Aggravating or alleviating factors

• BOX 28.3 Pain History Mnemonics

- **QUESTT** is a classic strategy for *how* to evaluate a child's pain (Baker and Wong, 1987):
  Question
  Use pain rating scales
  Evaluate behavior
  Secure parents' involvement
  Take cause of pain into account
  Take action and evaluate
- **PAINED** identifies the specific elements (*what*) of an assessment (Lynch, 2001):
  Place: Location(s) of pain; keep in mind the possibility of radiating or referred pain; using a body diagram can be helpful
  Amount of pain: Pain intensity score, duration of pain, pattern of onset (e.g., continuous or intermittent)
  Intensifiers: What makes the pain worse (e.g., position, movement, or time of day)?
  Nullifiers: What makes the pain better (e.g., position, heat or cold, or medications)?
  Effects: Consequences of pain medication (e.g., relief or side effects) and effects of pain on activities of daily living and quality of life
  Description: Quality of pain (e.g., dull, sharp, aching, stabbing, or cramping)

- Timing and duration (e.g., when it started, was there an identifiable cause, is it present all the time or does it come and go, is it worse in the morning or evening)
- Impact on function and daily activities
- Other associated symptoms, such as nausea, anxiety, tachycardia, or diaphoresis
- Past pain experience, including the child's memory of a painful experience and the treatment
- Cultural beliefs about pain and treatment

Physical Exam Focus Points

Note the child's appearance, posture, and gait. Carefully inspect for any signs of trauma and palpate for areas of hypersensitivity and tender points in muscles or tendon insertion sites.

Behavioral Indicators

Nonverbal cues are important indicators of pain (Box 28.4) and may be the only sign of pain in preverbal or nonverbal children. Infants in pain tend to sleep less, are irritable and agitated, do not feed well or refuse to feed, and have increased muscle tone. Older children may sleep to cope with pain so sleep is not necessarily an indication of a comfortable child. It is important to remember behaviors in cognitively impaired children are very individualized and may differ from those typically associated with pain.

Physiologic Indicators

Physiologic parameters (e.g., heart rate, oxygen saturation, respiratory rate and pattern, and blood pressure), diaphoresis, palmar sweating, and pallor are neither sensitive nor specific indicators of pain, particularly in children with persistent pain. Pulse-oximetry readings may decrease due to increased oxygen consumption or breath-holding. Other physiologic responses to pain include

• BOX 28.4 **Examples of Behavioral Indicators of Pain**

- Vocalizations
  - Crying
  - Whimpering
  - Whining
- Facial expressions
  - Grimacing
  - Tightly closed eyelids
  - Grinding or clenching teeth
- Breath holding
- Body positioning
- Changes in sleep patterns (more or less)
- Actions
  - Rubbing or touching the painful site,
  - Avoiding the painful site, or
  - Guarding the affected area
  - Withdrawal from touch
  - Protecting an injured limb
- Social withdrawal
- Vigilance
- Anger

changes in metabolic functioning (e.g., hypermetabolism, hyperglycemia, or lipolysis), decreased gut motility, sodium and water retention, and cytokine production.

Laboratory and Imaging Studies

Diagnostic testing is not usually needed. Consider checking a vitamin D level as there is some evidence to suggest hypovitaminosis D may contribute to pain and increased inflammatory cytokines (de Oliveira, Hirotsu, Tufik, and Anderson, 2017).

Management of Pediatric Pain

The goal of pediatric pain management is to safely and effectively reduce pain, limit side effects and minimize medication use. Positive outcomes of effective pain management include improved function (ability to perform daily activities), increased satisfaction for the child and parents, an enhanced recovery process, and a positive script learned by the child related to pain and its management for future use. In some situations (e.g., after surgical procedures, severe burns, or persistent pain), complete "freedom" from pain may not be possible. However, much can be done to alleviate pain in these situations through the multimodal, developmentally appropriate, nonpharmacologic and pharmacologic interventions. Multimodal therapy is more effective than high-dose single medications and reduces the risk of toxicity and adverse side effects (Lundeberg, 2015). Refer to Table 28.2 for examples and strategies for common painful acute conditions.

Pharmacologic Considerations

There may be interactions between nutraceutical (or natural) preparations and medications used to manage pain. It is imperative to know all the substances (pharmaceutical or other) a child uses to provide appropriate counseling regarding potential undesirable or dangerous interactions. Opioids have common side effects (Table 28.3) and a plan to prevent or mitigate them is essential.

TABLE 28.2 Common Acute Painful Pediatric Conditions and Pain Relief Strategies

Condition	Pain Relief Strategies
Otalgia	Acetaminophen or NSAIDs Warmed compresses pressed against the ear
Pharyngitis	Acetaminophen or NSAIDs Antibiotics if GABHS Saltwater gargles Anesthetic lozenges for older child
Stomatitis	NSAIDs Bland diet Saline mouth rinses for older children Diphenhydramine-calcium carbonate (in a 1:1 preparation) to coat the mucous membranes Sucralfate
Musculoskeletal injury	**RICE**—**R**est, **I**ce, **C**ompression, and **E**levation Immobilization of affected area Cold for the initial 48-72 h NSAIDs
Fractures and sprains	NSAIDs Opioid analgesics if severe fracture or sprain Topical NSAIDs give relief in soft tissue trauma, strains, and sprains
Laceration	LET procedure: Use on open wounds that are simple lacerations of head, neck, extremities, or trunk that are <5 cm in length; use 3 mL max; place LET mixed with cellulose on open wound and cover with occlusive dressing, or place two cotton balls soaked with LET in the wound Contraindications: Allergy to amide anesthetics, gross contamination of wound; do not use on mucous membranes, digits, genitalia, ear, or nose

GABHS, Group A β-hemolytic streptococcal infection; *LET,* lidocaine (4%), epinephrine (0.1%), and tetracaine (0.5%); *NSAID,* nonsteroidal anti-inflammatory drug.

TABLE 28.3 Management of Common Opioid Side Effects

Side Effect	Considerations	Medications
Nausea	Exclude other processes, such as bowel obstruction. Consider switching to different opioid. Use antiemetics.	Metoclopramide Ondansetron
Pruritus	Exclude other causes, such as drug allergy. Consider switching to different opioid. Use antipruritics.	Diphenhydramine Hydroxyzine
Constipation	Encourage water, fruit, and vegetables, and high-fiber diet if appropriate. Regular use of stimulant and stool softener laxatives.	Docusate Bisacodyl Polyethylene glycol

From Ku LC, Smith PB. Dosing in neonates: special consideration in physiology and trial design. Pediatr Res. 2015;77:2–9; and Lu H, Rosenbaum S. Developmental pharmacokinetics in pediatric populations. J Pediatr Pharmacol Ther. 2014;19:262–276.

• BOX 28.5 **Factors Producing Age-Related Differences in Analgesia Responses**

- Infants (until approximately 6 months of age) have delayed hepatic enzyme maturation resulting in altered drug metabolic inactivation. Analgesics metabolized in the liver, such as opioids, have a prolonged elimination half-life in newborns and young infants.
- Glomerular filtration is reduced in the first few weeks of life, which results in slower elimination of opioids and their active metabolites.
- Toddlers' and preschool children's renal clearance of analgesics is greater than adults.
- Neonates and young infants have decreased plasma protein binding for many drugs, resulting in greater concentrations of pharmacologically active unbound medication.

• BOX 28.6 **Examples of Common Pediatric Painful Procedures**

Circumcision
Heel stick, capillary sampling
Tape removal
IM/SQ injection
Urinary catheterization
Dressing change
Wound care
Suture placement/removal
Occupational or physical therapy consultations
Cast application
Nasopharyngeal swabs or scraping
Lumbar puncture
Venous or arterial sampling or catheterization

IM, Intramuscular; SQ, subcutaneous.

A consideration in administering analgesics is whether there is a need to maintain serum concentration levels. While medicating around-the-clock (i.e., regardless of pain intensity at the time of administration) is a long-held practice in some situations, a Cochrane review by Hobson, Wiffen, and Conlon (2015) concludes there is limited evidence to recommend around-the-clock administration over as needed (PRN) therapy. Consider the child's response to previous pain medications and doses and adjust accordingly. Refer to Box 28.5 for factors producing age-related differences in analgesia responses.

Procedural Pain Management

- Multimodal (physical, psychological, and pharmacologic) approach to pain management before, during, and after procedures that may cause pain or anxiety for the child and family is essential. Emergent procedures do not negate use of some combination of pain and anxiety relief; many interventions may be employed without time delay.
- Family members (any person[s] who plays a significant role in child's life) are critical in alleviation of child's pain and anxiety as they are a primary source of strength and support.
- Administer intramuscular (IM) injections using a rapid injection technique without aspiration.
- Avoid placing child supine during painful procedures. Holding a baby or young child in a bear hug and placing an older child in a sitting position is preferable.
- Pre-procedural dosing with acetaminophen and an appropriate nonsteroidal antiinflammatory drug (NSAID) mitigate postprocedural pain.
- Refer to Box 28.6 for examples of common pediatric painful procedures. Proper planning and preparation for any procedure will make it easier for the clinician, less distressing for the family, and provide the opportunity for a child to demonstrate mastery of appropriate coping techniques.

Prior to Procedure

- Establish a mutually agreed upon developmentally appropriate comfort plan for use during the procedure. Table 28.4 describes developmentally based procedural pain management techniques used in primary care settings for relief of pain associated with common procedures.

- Educate about the procedure and comfort management options; tailor information to meet the patient and family needs.
- Use a procedure room, if available.

During the Procedure

- If pain and/or anxiety are not well controlled during the procedure, stop the procedure and provide additional comfort measures.
- One person should provide verbal coaching and leadership in a calm manner.
- Ensure the environment remains safe and relaxed for the patient and family.

After the Procedure

- Discuss and evaluate the procedure with the patient and family.
- Document procedure, patient's experience, and recommendations for future procedures.
- Develop and implement a comfort plan for post-procedure pain as needed.
- Circumcision: Neonatal male circumcision, when properly performed, prevents phimosis, paraphimosis, and balanoposthitis and is associated with decreased incidence of penile cancer and decreased urinary tract infections (UTIs) in neonates (American Urological Association [AUA], 2017). Consider medical benefits and risks, and ethnic, cultural, religious, and personal preferences during the informed consent process. See Box 28.7.

Acute Pain Management

Refer to a current pediatric dosing reference for specific dosing and time intervals.

Mild pain. Acetaminophen and a NSAID are effective and safe for managing mild acute pain in children, however NSAIDs should be used with caution in infants less than 6 months old.

Moderate to severe pain. For this pain, use of an oral opioid (e.g., oxycodone, hydrocodone, or morphine) may be considered although use of acetaminophen and/or NSAIDs reduces opioid consumption by 30% to 40% (Walker, 2015). Because of concerns of respiratory depression, the US Food and Drug Administration (US FDA, 2017) announced contraindications for the use of codeine and tramadol in children.

TABLE 28.4 Developmentally Based Procedural Pain Management Techniques

Age	Recommended for Use Before Pharmacologic Measures		Onset
	Physical/Psychological Interventions	Pharmacologic Interventions	
Preterm neonate	• Developmental positioning • Swaddling • Breastfeeding *(before, during, after procedure)* • Skin-to-skin contact • Non-nutritive sucking • Oral sucrose • Music *(as appropriate)*	• Acetaminophen if appropriate • Topical anesthetic cream (for infants >28 weeks gestation; *maximum application duration 1 h)*[ab]	• 30 min • 30 min
Newborn— (≥37 weeks gestation) 3 months	• Procedure room[c] • Swaddling • Breastfeeding (before, during, after procedure) • Skin-to-skin contact • Non-nutritive sucking • Oral sucrose • Music	• Topical anesthetic cream (maximum application duration 1 h)[ab] • Acetaminophen if appropriate • Urojet (sterile) lidocaine jelly for urinary catheterization • For patients >6 weeks old: Atomized/ intranasal midazolam for sedation during procedures	• 30 min • 30 min • 1-2 min • 5 min; Max effect: 10 min
3-6 months	• Procedure room[c] • Swaddling • Non-nutritive sucking • Oral sucrose • Breastfeeding (before, during, after procedure) • Skin-to-skin contact • Non-nutritive sucking • Music • Approved pet therapy	• Topical anesthetic cream[ab] • LET procedure[d] • Acetaminophen if appropriate • Urojet (sterile) lidocaine jelly for urinary catheterization • Viscous lidocaine for nasogastric tube (NGT) insertion • Atomized/intranasal midazolam for sedation during procedures	• 30-60 min • 1-2 min • 30 min • 1-2 min • Use to lubricate tip of tube • 5 min; Max effect: 10 min
7-12 months	• Procedure room[c] • Non-nutritive sucking • Oral sucrose to encourage sucking • Breastfeeding (before, during, after procedure) • Singing/music • Distraction • Positioning for comfort[a] • Approved pet therapy • Ice/cold pack application	• Topical anesthetic cream[ab] *or* • 1% lidocaine via J-Tip device *or* • 1% lidocaine intradermal injection • LET procedure[d] • Acetaminophen or NSAID if appropriate • Urojet (sterile) lidocaine jelly for urinary catheterization • Viscous lidocaine for NGT insertion • Atomized/intranasal midazolam for anxiety	• 30-60 min • 30-60 s • 30-60 s • 1-2 min • 30 min • 1-2 min • Use to lubricate tip of tube • 5 min; Max effect: 10 min
1-2 years	• Procedure room[c] • Non-nutritive sucking • Singing/music • Distraction • Positioning for comfort[a] • Hand holding • Reading/telling stories • Medical play • Television/games • Approved pet therapy • Ice/cold pack application	• Topical anesthetic cream[ab] *or* • 1% lidocaine via J-Tip device *or* • 1% lidocaine intradermal injection *or* • Vapocoolant (ethyl chloride) *or* • Bacteriostatic saline injection • LET procedure[d] • Nitrous oxide gas for anxiolysis • Acetaminophen or NSAID if appropriate • Urojet (sterile) lidocaine jelly for urinary catheterization • Atomized/intranasal lidocaine for NGT insertion • Intranasal midazolam for anxiety	• 30-60 min • 30-60 s • 30-60 s • Immediate • 30-60 s • 1-2 min • 2-3 min • 30 min • 1-2 min • Use to lubricate tip of tube • Immediate • 5 min; Max effect: 10 min
Toddler/pre- school 2-5 years	• Procedure room[c] • Singing/music • Distraction • Positioning for comfort[a] • Hand holding • Reading/telling stories • Medical play • Television/games • Guided imagery (≥3 years) • Blowing bubbles/deep breathing techniques (≥3 years) • Tactile stimulation prior to injection (≥4 years) • BuzzyBee • Approved pet therapy • Ice/cold pack application	• Topical anesthetic cream[ab] *or* • 1% lidocaine via J-Tip device *or* • 1% lidocaine intradermal injection *or* • Vapocoolant (ethyl chloride) *or* • Bacteriostatic saline injection • LET procedure[d] • Nitrous oxide gas for anxiolysis • Acetaminophen or NSAID if appropriate • Urojet (sterile) lidocaine jelly for urinary catheterization • Cetacaine spray for NGT placement • Viscous lidocaine for NGT insertion • Atomized/intranasal lidocaine for NGT insertion • Atomized/intranasal midazolam for anxiety	• 30-60 min • 30-60 s • 30-60 s • Immediate • 30-60 s • 1-2 min • 2-3 min • 30 min • 1-2 min • Immediate • Immediate • Immediate • 5 min; Max effect: 10 min

Continued

TABLE 28.4	Developmentally Based Procedural Pain Management Techniques—cont'd		
	Recommended for Use Before Pharmacologic Measures		
Age	**Physical/Psychological Interventions**	**Pharmacologic Interventions**	**Onset**
School-aged 6 years and older	• Procedure room[c] • Positioning for comfort[a] • Reading/telling stories • Blowing bubbles/deep breathing techniques • Medical play • Hand holding • Television/games • Guided imagery • Music • Tactile stimulation prior to injection • BuzzyBee • Approved pet therapy • Ice/cold pack application	• Topical anesthetic cream[ab] *or* • 1% lidocaine via J-Tip device *or* • 1% lidocaine intradermal injection *or* • Vapocoolant (ethyl chloride) *or* • Bacteriostatic saline injection • LET procedure[d] • Nitrous oxide gas for anxiolysis • Acetaminophen or NSAID if appropriate • Urojet (sterile) lidocaine jelly for urinary catheterization • Cetacaine spray for NGT placement • Viscous lidocaine for NGT insertion • Atomized/intranasal lidocaine for NGT insertion • Atomized/intranasal midazolam for anxiety	• 30-60 min • 30-60 s • 30-60 s • Immediate • 30-60 s • 1-2 min • 1-2 min • 30 min • 1-2 min • Immediate • Use to lubricate tip of tube • Immediate • 5 min; Max effect: 10 min

[a]EMLA is contraindicated in patients with congenital or idiopathic methemoglobinemia or in infants less than 12 months old who are being treated with sulfas, acetaminophen, benzocaine, chloroquine, dapsone, nitrofurantoin, phenobarbital, phenytoin, or quinine.

[b]Topical anesthetic cream refers to eutectic mixture of local anesthetics (e.g., EMLA) and liposomal 4% lidocaine cream (e.g., L.M.X.4).

[c]L.M.X.4 contraindicated with allergy to amide anesthetics.

[d]Lidocaine (4%), epinephrine (0.1%), and tetracaine (0.5%) (LET) procedure: use on simple lacerations of head, neck, extremities, or trunk that are <5 cm in length; use 3 mL max; place LET mixed with cellulose on open wound and cover with occlusive dressing, or place two cotton balls soaked with LET in the wound. Contraindicated with allergy to amide anesthetics, gross contamination of wound; do not use on mucous membranes, digits, genitalia, ear, or nose.

NSAID, Nonsteroidal antiinflammatory drug. Compiled by Alles K, Bateman A, Turner HN.

• BOX 28.7 Pain Management Plan for Circumcision

Prior to Procedure
• Acetaminophen 15 mg/kg 1 h prior to procedure
• Topical anesthetic cream
• Hold and comfort infant (breast feed if possible) while supplies are gathered
• Position infant in semi-recumbent position on a padded surface with arms swaddled
• Maintain thermoregulation of the environment to prevent cold stress

During Procedure
• Analgesic/comfort techniques: in addition to at least one anesthetic
• Administer 24% sucrose or breast milk orally 2 min before penile manipulation
• Injectable anesthetic options (injection techniques should use slow injection speed, small-gauge needle, warmed solution)[a]:
  • Subcutaneous block (circumferential at midshaft or at the level of the corona at 10- and 2-o'clock positions) OR
  • Dorsal penile nerve block
• Pacifier for non-nutritive sucking, if sucrose or breast milk contraindicated

Following Procedure
• Remove infant from restraint immediately, soothe, and return to parent
• Continue oral acetaminophen (15 mg/kg) around the clock every 4-6 h for at least 24 h
• Instruct family on administration of acetaminophen and circumcision care

AAP Committee on Fetus and Newborn and Section on Anesthesiology and Pain Medicine. Prevention and Management of Procedural Pain in the Neonate: An Update. *Pediatrics*. 2016;137(2):e20154271.

• Tramadol and codeine should not be used in children under 12 years old.
• Tramadol should not be used in children under 18 years old for T&A pain.
• Tramadol and codeine should not be used in children between 12 and 18 years who are obese or have conditions such as obstructive sleep apnea (OSA) or severe lung disease.

Persistent Pain Management

Persistent pain is most successfully treated by a coordinated, planned, interprofessional approach including disciplines like medicine, psychology, physical therapy, occupational therapy, and nursing. It is essential all team members are communicating a consistent message as an integrated team. Evidence supports the use of psychological interventions (e.g., relaxation, parent interventions, and cognitive strategies) as key management components to reduce persistent pediatric pain. These strategies reduce pain symptoms and disability post treatment and should be emphasized (Fisher et al., 2014).

The PCP must be diligent in assessing for the presence or development of sleep disturbances, adverse childhood experiences (ACEs), depression, anxiety disorders (e.g., situational, separation, social), posttraumatic stress disorder, panic disorder, and obsessive-compulsive disorders as these comorbidities impact pain experience and coping. PCPs collaborate and coordinate interprofessional treatment plans and work in partnership with the child and parent. The goal of managing persistent pain is development of a comprehensive multimodal treatment plan that improves quality of life and all domains of daily functioning.

Pharmacologic measures. NSAIDs and acetaminophen are commonly used to treat persistent pain. Gabapentin is frequently used to treat neuropathic pain. Due to few adverse side effects, it is considered a first-line therapy. Assess the efficacy of pharmacologic therapy by having the child or parent use a pain intensity rating scale and keep a diary of the child's activities and pain. On follow-up visits, question whether symptoms have improved, side effects are present, and function has improved.

If a child's pain is not controlled, referral to pain management specialists is indicated. The following therapies may be considered:

- Antidepressants (e.g., selective serotonin reuptake inhibitors [SSRIs], serotonin–norepinephrine reuptake inhibitors [SNRIs], tricyclics [TCAs] and atypicals), opioids, anticonvulsants, muscle relaxants, and other selected medications may also be used, however, these patients require close monitoring for worsening of depression, suicidality, and unusual behavior, especially during the first few weeks of therapy. Educate family members to closely observe the patient and communicate changes in the patient's condition.
- Botulinum products may be used for certain pain conditions in children such as seventh cranial nerve disorders, dynamic muscle contractures associated with cerebral palsy, and migraine headaches. Pain specialists work with children and their families during the administration of this drug, but the PCP should be familiar with adverse and life-threatening reactions associated with this drug.
- Invasive techniques, such as neuroablative procedures and spinal cord stimulation are occasionally used as a last resort.

Nonpharmacologic measures. Physical therapy, relaxation, massage, guided imagery, biofeedback, hypnosis, heat and cold, distraction, transcutaneous electrical nerve stimulation (TENS), music therapy, craniosacral therapy, acupuncture, and psychological therapy are part of the multimodal management of persistent pain.

Additional measures. There are parental strategies that encourage optimal coping with persistent pain issues (Fisher et al., 2014). These include the following:

- Not giving excessive attention, special privileges, or rewards when the child reports pain.
- Encouraging normal activities, within reason, during pain episodes (e.g., going to school, doing chores).
- Spending time during the day doing quiet, low-key activities when the child cannot go to school or participate in other events. Activities, such as playing games and excessive screen time, may reinforce for the child not wanting to participate in "well" activities.
- Lessening the focus on pain by not repeatedly asking the child about his or her pain.
- Reinforcing the child's role in self-management through the use of nonpharmacologic strategies based on developmental appropriateness. When the child reports pain, ask, "What do you think you can do to help lessen your pain?" followed by encouragement of nonpharmacologic strategies.

The PCP should be aware of clinical practice guidelines found online addressing pain management related to common pediatric conditions like sickle cell anemia (https://www.nhlbi.nih.gov/health-topics/sickle-cell-disease) and arthritis (http://www.kidsgetarthritistoo.org/).

Partnership in Care

Several critical elements related to pain management and administration of pain medications must be emphasized to parents and children. They include:

- Only take pain medication as prescribed.

- Store pain medications under lock and key and properly dispose when no longer needed.
- Myths related to addiction and the use of opioids should be discussed, if applicable.
- Use multimodal pain management. Medication alone is not sufficient to manage persistent pain and cognitive-behavioral therapies are helpful in acute pain situations.
- Counsel about drinking alcohol with opioids, using opioids for conditions other than for which they were prescribed, and the importance of not sharing medications.
- The PCP needs to be informed of all prescribed, over-the-counter (OTC), and natural therapies used.
- Pain medication used for more than 10 to 14 days may need to be tapered and not abruptly stopped.
- Pain medication works most effectively when taken before the onset of severe pain.
- Common side effects such as constipation, dizziness, nausea, drowsiness, sweating, and flushing may occur with pain medications. The PCP should be aware of these problems so appropriate interventions can be provided.
- Assess for improvement in daily function and decrease of pain and related symptoms.
- Follow-up assessment by phone or appointment determines whether optimal pain control is achieved, evaluates whether pharmacologic side effects are minimized or effectively managed, and ensures the causative factor of the pain was correctly identified.

Overview of Pediatric Fever

Fever is an abnormal elevation of body temperature that occurs as part of a specific biologic response mediated and controlled by the central nervous system (CNS). It is one of the most common reasons that parents seek health care advice. The pathophysiology of fever is a result of an alteration in the thermoregulatory center of the preoptic nuclei of the anterior hypothalamus. Exogenous pyrogens, such as bacteria, and endotoxins generate release of endogenous pyrogens (such as cytokines), regulate inflammatory cell (C-reactive protein [CRP], haptoglobin ceruloplasmin, amyloid A, and fibrinogen) release of prostaglandin E, and raise the thermoregulatory set point (Lye and Densmore, 2018). Heat production is caused by increased cellular metabolism, involuntary shivering, and autonomic responses such as vasoconstriction and behavioral responses such as covering oneself.

Normal body temperature is considered to be 37°C (98.6°F); most pediatric literature defines fever as 38°C (100.4°F) in infants under 2 months and 38.3°C (101°F) over 2 months. Fever in a child can be infectious and or noninfectious and be beneficial and harmful. Although viral infections are responsible for most children's fever, the differential for fever includes bacterial infection, reaction to immunizations, autoimmune and inflammatory disease, cancer (leukemia and lymphoma in particular), medication (antibiotic and seizure medication), tissue damage, and other disease states. The normal physiologic hypothalamic body temperature set-point is altered by many different agents. Febrile illnesses in neonates are usually the result of congenital infections or infections acquired at delivery (e.g., late-onset group B streptococcal infection), in the nursery (especially in premature infants), at home (e.g., pneumococcal or meningococcal infection), and those acquired as a result of anatomic or physiologic dysfunction (e.g., renal). Temperatures higher than 105.8°F (41°C) are rarely of infectious origin but are due to CNS dysfunction (e.g., malignant hyperthermia, drug fever, heat stroke).

TABLE 28.5	Types of Thermometers and Measurement Sites
Type of Thermometer	**Measurement Site**
Contact electronic	Axilla, oral, rectal
Non-contact infrared forehead	Forehead; naval if forehead is not available
Infrared tympanic membrane	Ear

Factors Influencing Pediatric Fever Management

Parents are often concerned about fever and its possible harmful effect on their children. Some people fear all fevers are dangerous and believe any fever over a certain point is "too high" or has a serious cause. They may relate concern about brain damage and seizures. Many families believe all fevers should be treated, and if not treated, the fever will continue to rise. They also think once medication is given, the fever should resolve completely. Unfortunately, there are times when PCPs also are susceptible to some of these beliefs.

Fever Assessment

Several noninvasive methods measure the core temperature of the body. Table 28.5 lists types of thermometers and measurement sites. The most invasive measurement of fever is rectal thermometry. Although it is considered the most accurate for assessing core body temperature, its use in outpatient health care settings is only recommended for children less than 12 months of age who are at risk for serious infections or trauma. It is contraindicated in cases of suspected neutropenia. Oral thermometry is a more comfortable method generally used in children old enough to cooperate (over 5 years of age). It is more accurate than axillary measurement though the results can be swayed by mouth breathing, tachypnea, exercise, hot or cold drinks, and thermometer position. Axillary thermometry is used in cases of neutropenia, though the result will always be lower than rectal thermometry. Infrared thermometry is measured in the tympanic membrane or on the forehead and temporal artery. The tympanic membrane has additional sources of blood supply to the tympanic membrane, so the reading can be affected by poor positioning, cerumen, and otitis media. When the thermometer tip is not securely fitted in the canal, the reading measures the temperature of the ear canal, skin, or cerumen. Infrared contact and no contact forehead thermometers measure the amount of heat produced by temporal arteries at the surface of the skin on the forehead. The infrared thermometers can be affected by sweating or vascular changes. Both tympanic and temporal thermometers are well tolerated and easy to use; however, rectal temperature remains the gold standard for children 3 years of age or younger unless it is contraindicated for a medical reason.

History and Physical Exam

In addition to the actual temperature assessment, a careful history and physical examination are critical. The following should be included:
- Duration and degree of fever

- Associated symptoms: Vomiting, diarrhea, respiratory symptoms, rash (particularly petechiae or purpura), feeding pattern, irritability, inconsolability, change in play activities, lethargy (level of consciousness characterized by poor or absent eye contact, failure to recognize parents, or lack of interaction with persons or objects in the environment)
- Review of known exposures (family illness, contacts with other ill children, day care contacts); recent travel history
- Past medical history of chronic illness, malignancy, splenectomy, shunt, indwelling catheter, immunologic disorders, recurrent or serious bacterial infection (SBI)
- Neonatal history of complications, prior antibiotics, prior surgeries, or hyperbilirubinemia
- Current medications, including antipyretics, antibiotics, herbs, and dietary supplements
- Immunization history, particularly with Hib conjugate and pneumococcal conjugate vaccines

All patients should have a complete physical exam and be fully undressed. In a febrile pediatric patient, the overall clinical appearance of the child with fever should be considered prior to concentrating on the fever itself. A toxic (ill appearing) appearing child is considered at risk until proven otherwise and needs a thoughtful workup. The appearance of a child who has a benign illness and a high fever is usually very different (i.e., does not appear as ill) than a child with a serious infection who still appears ill even after fever reduction. Important considerations include:
- Is the neonate lethargic, fussy, irritable, inconsolable, or exhibit a decrease in activity?
- Is there airway, breathing, and circulation (ABC's) compromise?
- Are there symptoms suggestive of serious bacterial illness (e.g., fever, bulging anterior fontanel, respiratory system changes, lethargy and other CNS symptoms, evidence of skin infection or rashes, skin perfusion, and turgor)?

Management of Pediatric Fever

Fever as a Friend

Fever is a known host defense that exerts beneficial effects against a variety of invading microorganisms by impairing survival and reproduction via phagocytosis or decrease in required nutrients such as free iron (Lye and Densmore, 2018). Fever can also be curative and maximize antimicrobial treatment. It is often self-limited. Fever phobia is common among parents who have little knowledge about the beneficial role it may play, therefore educating parents about fever can be helpful in lowering their anxiety. Consider the following topics: fever is a symptom and a normal response to fighting an infection; fever in itself is not dangerous; brain damage does not occur at temperatures under 107.6°F (Varnell, 2018). How sick the child looks is much more important than what the temperature is; fever makes a child feel worse and medication is primarily given to make a child more comfortable.

Non-Pharmacologic Measures

Strategies for fever control include:
- Adequate hydration
- Reassurance to parents and advice that not all fevers need to be treated
- Appropriate clothing; do not bundle in additional clothing or coverings

TABLE 28.6	Antipyretics: Infants and Children (12 Years Old and Younger)	
Drug	Dosage	Comments
Acetaminophen	10-15 mg/kg every 4-6 h PO (not to exceed five doses/24 h) *or* 10-20 mg/kg every 4-6 h per rectal suppository as needed (not to exceed five doses in 24 h)	Drug of choice. Temperature reduced by 1.8-3.6°F (1-2°C) within 2 h; 15 mg/kg/dose as effective as ibuprofen at 10 mg/kg/dose.
Ibuprofen	For temperatures <102.5°F (39°C): 5°mg/kg/dose every 6-8 h as needed For temperatures ≥102.5°F (39°C): 10 mg/kg/dose every 6-8 h as needed	Use in children 6 months old to 12 years old; maximum daily dose of 40 mg/kg; temperature stays lower for a longer period of time with ibuprofen vs. acetaminophen. Use with caution if decreased liver function, asthma, or coagulation disorder.

PO, Per os (by mouth, orally).

- Ambient environment temperatures of around 72°F (22°C)
- Tepid water baths for temperatures greater than 104°F (40°C); sponging should be stopped if the child starts to shiver; ice-water baths and alcohol sponging should not be done

Pharmacologic Measures

- Antipyretic agents acetaminophen and ibuprofen work in the same manner by inhibiting prostaglandin synthesis without affecting the baseline body temperature (Taketomo et al., 2014). Alternating these antipyretics carries with it an increased risk of medication errors and possible toxicity. Therefore, before using this regimen, careful consideration of the risk versus the benefits must be weighed taking into consideration parental abilities. Table 28.6 lists dosages.
- Naproxen sodium is marketed as a "fever reducer," however, it has not been well studied as an antipyretic in children and should not be used for this purpose.
- Aspirin should never be used in pediatric patients due to possibility of Reyes syndrome, bleeding, and other harmful side effects unless prescribed by a specialist for other significant benefit that outweighs risk.

Fever Without Focus in Infants and Young Children

When approaching a child with fever, an objective diagnosis can be reached by completing a careful history and physical examination and following diagnostic, assessment, and management guidelines based on age, symptoms, estimated risks, associated diseases, and immunization status. *Fever without focus, also called fever without source,* is an acute febrile illness in a child under 24 months of age in which the fever etiology

is not apparent after careful history and physical examination. Approximately a third of all febrile children in this age range do not have localizing signs of infection. The younger the infant, the greater the concern about the possibility of an SBI or invasive bacterial illness (IBI) due to decreased immunologic competence, therefore, the greater the need to rule out this possibility. Although the cause of the majority of these fevers is viral infection (enterovirus, influenza, respiratory syncytial virus [RSV], rotavirus, adenovirus, herpes virus-6, or parechovirus) (Barbi et al., 2017; Pelton, 2018), a workup for bacterial disease is still necessary. In the past all infants under 90 days of age received a complete sepsis workup, but due to the advent of the *Haemophilus influenza* type b and *Streptococcus pneumonia* vaccines, the incidence of SBI is greatly reduced. Currently, most common SBIs that cause fever in children with no clinical symptoms are UTI, pneumonia, and bacteremia. Children between birth and 24 months old are at greatest risk for unsuspected occult bacteremia with *Escherichia coli* as the most common cause. *E. coli* is also the leading cause of UTI and meningitis in this group with *Group B Strep* the next most common. Another factor that has changed the evaluation of febrile children is the introduction of rapid antigen testing for bacteria and viruses as well as CRP and procalcitonin (PCT) biomarkers.

The workup and management of infants and children less than 24 months of age with fever without localizing signs is based on age: neonate (birth to 28 days), young infant (29 days to 90 days), and older infant or toddler. Four criteria (Boston, Rochester, Philadelphia, and Milwaukee) developed in the 1990s serve as the framework for much current evaluation of fever in these children. Newer models (e.g., 5 Stage Decision Tree, Yale Observation Scale, Pneumonia Rule, and Meningitis Rule) have been developed in an attempt to increase diagnostic predictions. In spite of the variety of tools, no consensus has been reached on any one protocol, and overall the trend seems to be moving toward individualizing the approach to each infant (decreasing use of lumbar punctures [LPs] and in-hospital care for well-appearing infants (Gomez et al., 2016)).

Clinical Findings

Complete history and physical exam are indicated as discussed earlier in the chapter. For the neonate with a rectal fever of 38°C (100.4°F) or more, questions should focus on presenting illness, prenatal history and care, birth history including intra-partum fever and maternal *Streptococcus group B* status, and postnatal care. In the young infant who has begun to develop a more complex immune system, consideration of vaccine status and recent immunizations are pertinent.

Clinical assessment of appearance is key and can give an accurate impression of the child's status as well as severity of illness. This is accomplished by taking the time to stop before touching and look at the infant's general appearance or level of interaction, work of breathing, and circulation to skin (also called Hands-off or Pediatric Assessment Triangle.) In addition to this key initial assessment, a provider's feeling that something is not right is often very accurate (Barbi, 2017). Evaluation of red flags is also critical to assessment (Box 28.8).

Diagnostic studies based on age and symptoms can include:
- Urinalysis with urine culture by catheterization or needle aspiration

- Complete blood count (CBC) with differential, absolute neutrophil count (ANC), and blood culture
- Procalcitonin (PCT) and C-reactive protein (CRP)
- Alanine aminotransferase (ALT) and aspartate aminotransferase (AST) if herpes suspected
- Cerebrospinal fluid (CSF) studies and culture (bacterial and viral); consider herpes simplex virus (HSV) polymerase chain reaction (PCR)
- Chest x-ray if respiratory symptoms not indicative of bronchiolitis (cough, tachypnea, grunting)
- Stool culture if diarrhea with blood or mucus in stool
- RSV or influenza PCR if in season

Management

Management decisions are based on age, results, and patient presentation. Neonates under 28 days of age with fever should be hospitalized and receive a full septic workup including but not limited to a CBC with differential, blood cultures, catheterized urinalysis with urine culture, a lumbar puncture to examine the CSF for infection and HSV. A chest radiograph and stool cultures may be done as indicated. After workup, antibiotics (Table 28.7) and possibly acyclovir are started empirically until results of all cultures are known and a clearer picture of the illness is identified.

The young infant (29 to 60 days) if ill appearing, should be admitted with complete workup and followed clinically as described in the neonatal section above. However, if the infant appears to be healthy with no chronic problems and was full term with an uncomplicated nursery course, a full septic workup may not be indicated, and management is based on exam and data collected. Fig 28.2 details the approach to this group of infants. After initial evaluation, the infant who meets low-risk criteria (see Box 28.9) can be sent home with strict follow-up including reevaluation in 12 to 24 hours, access to emergency care if condition worsens, and daily follow-up of culture results with immediate return if cultures become positive. Parents need to receive instruction on signs and symptoms that indicate worsening of illness (see Box 28.8). If there is any uncertainty about the family's ability to follow-up or provide care, the infant should be admitted. If low risk criteria are not met, admission and further workup is necessary.

The infant from 60 to 90 days, if well appearing, should have a urinalysis and urine culture done, and possibly a CBC with

TABLE 28.7	**Empiric Antimicrobial Regimens for Febrile Infants Under 90 Days of Age Without Focus of Infection**
Age	**Antibiotic Regimen[a]**
Neonate under 28 days	• Ampicillin AND cefotaxime (if meningitis concern) or gentamicin • Add acyclovir if HSV concern[b] and workup performed • Add vancomycin if meningitis concern
Infant (29-60 days)	• Ceftriaxone or cefotaxime • Add acyclovir if HSV concern[a] and workup performed • Add vancomycin if concern for meningitis • Add gentamicin for broader Gram-negative coverage
Infant (61-90 days)	• Ceftriaxone or cefotaxime • Add vancomycin if indicated

[a]All cultures should be obtained prior to antibiotic administration.

[b]Ill appearing, hypothermia, abnormal neurologic status or seizures, vesicular rash, exposure to HSV, hepatosplenomegaly.

HSV, Herpes simplex virus.

differential, blood culture, and PCT. An exception could be the infant who received immunizations within the past 24 hours and has a temperature that is below 38.6°C (101.5°F). Otherwise management proceeds as for the 28- to 60-day-old infant.

Any child under 2 years of age with fever without focus warrants a urinalysis and urine culture, and any of the following positive findings can constitute a preliminary diagnosis of UTI: urine leukocyte esterase, nitrite, leukocyte count, or Gram stain.

Fever of Unknown Origin

The definition of *fever of unknown origin (FUO)* in children is a temperature greater than 38°C (101°F) or greater on several occasions, of more than 3 weeks duration, and with failure to reach a diagnosis despite 1 week of intense investigation (Gompf, 2017). The PCP must first rethink and reevaluate historical, clinical, and laboratory data, with an infectious disease consultation often recommended. Many FUOs are atypical presentations of common disorders, notably infections (accounting for more than one-third of cases) or rheumatologic and connective tissue diseases (e.g., juvenile rheumatoid arthritis, systemic lupus erythematosus [SLE]) (Cho et al., 2017). In children younger than 6 years old, the most common causes of FUO are UTI/pyelonephritis, respiratory illness, localized infection (abscess, osteomyelitis), juvenile arthritis, and, rarely, leukemia. In adolescents, the most common causes include TB, inflammatory bowel disease, autoimmune disorders, abscesses, chlamydia, lymphoma, as well the causes listed for children under 6 years. In the United States, infectious diseases associated with most diagnoses of FUO include Epstein-Barr virus (EBV), cat-scratch disease *(Bartonella henselae),* complicated UTIs, Lyme disease, and osteomyelitis. Neoplastic conditions and AIDS generally have symptoms other than just fever (see Box 28.9).

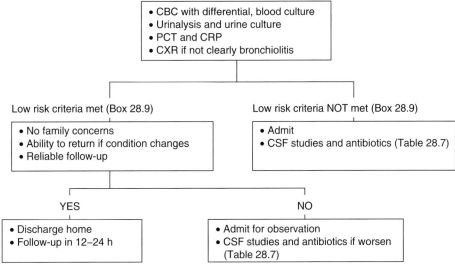

- **Fig 28.2** Approach to healthy-appearing febrile infants 29 to 60 days of age. *CBC*, Complete blood count; *CRP*, C-reactive protein; *CSF*, cerebrospinal fluid; *CXR*, chest x-ray; *PCT*, procalcitonin.

• BOX 28.9   Low Risk Criteria for Young Infant with Fever of Unknown Origin

- Well appearing, easily consolable
- Previously healthy infant with uncomplicated nursery stay, no chronic problems
- Full term (>37 weeks)
- No focal bacterial infection
- No systemic antibiotics within 72 h
- Negative urinalysis (WBC <5-10/hpf; neg leukocyte esterase and nitrate, neg Gm stain)
- WBC >5000 and <15,000 mm^3
- ANC ≤1500 bands/mL
- Procalcitonin >0.3 ng/mL
- No discrete infiltrates on CXR if done
- Stool smear negative if done

ANC, Absolute neutrophil count, CXR, chest x-ray; WBC, white blood cells.

Clinical Findings

History

A careful detailed history helps distinguish between recurrent fever episodes and those that need further evaluation. Recurrent fevers that resolve with well periods between suggest an etiology of multiple self-limiting infections. The history should include:

- A careful analysis of symptoms or signs, a meticulous review of systems, history of the fever pattern, and patient's age
- Note of past medical history of recurrent infections, surgery, transfusions, and contact with ill individuals
- Medication use, including over-the-counter and herbal/natural/dietary supplements
- Family medical history, including autoimmune disease or inflammatory bowel disorder; genetic background (inherited periodic fever syndromes [e.g., familial Mediterranean fever, hyperimmunoglobulinemia D with periodic fever syndrome], tumor receptor–associated periodic syndrome)
- Family pets including reptiles, pet immunization history, or exposure to wild or other domestic animals
- Unusual dietary habits (eating squirrel, rabbit, or other unusual animal meat)
- History of pica; history of travel (location; travel immunizations; water/food ingested; if returned home with travel souvenirs containing dirt, rocks, or earth-contaminated artifacts)

Physical Examination

The physical exam should begin with general assessment of patient appearance, activity, vital signs, and growth parameters. Special attention needs to be paid to:

- Skin: Presence of rashes, lesions, nail fold capillary abnormalities; presence or absence of sweating
- Mouth: Note a smooth tongue with absence of fungiform papillae; presence of candidiasis, ulcers, dental abscess, or abnormal dentition
- Throat: Exudate, erythema
- Local or generalized lymphadenopathy or hepatosplenomegaly
- Palpation/percussion of sinus and mastoid areas for tenderness; tap upper teeth
- Eye examination noting exudate, erythema, palpebral or bulbar conjunctivitis, conjunctival hemorrhages, papillary reaction; a complete ophthalmologic examination is indicated to fully evaluate for uveitis, chorioretinitis, proptosis
- Deep tendon reflexes and joint examination, and palpation of bones for tenderness or swelling
- Pelvic exam may be indicated in adolescent females and testicular exam in males; genital ulcers may be noted in females or males
- Rectal examination and guaiac test

Diagnostic Studies

Laboratory studies are dependent on a history and physical examination. Studies may include:

- CBC with differential and smear, erythrocyte sedimentation rate (ESR), CRP, PCT, and liver chemistries
- Serologic tests for specific diseases as suggested by history and examination
- Aerobic blood cultures (may require serial specimens to rule out endocarditis, osteomyelitis, or deep abscesses)
- Urinalysis plus urine cultures
- Mantoux skin test or interferon gamma release assay (IGRA)

- Chest, sinus, mastoid, and GI tract radiographs may be indicated
- Heterophil antibody and antinuclear antibody titer in older children
- Echocardiogram if subacute endocarditis is suspected; radionuclide scans, total body CT, MRI, ultrasounds, or biopsies; if bone marrow biopsy, cultures for bacteria, acid-fast bacillus (AFB), and fungus

Management

Children with FUO often have treatable or self-limiting diagnoses. Infectious disease consultation may be advised with consideration of hospitalizing the child if there is evidence of systemic illness or failure to thrive, the child is very young, the parent(s) anxiety is extreme, or an extensive workup is planned. Otherwise, the child should be followed with frequent visits, documented fever pattern, and other specialized tests if screening tests indicate the need, or if other physical findings develop. Treatment is based on the underlying diagnosis, and empiric use of antibiotics should be avoided.

References

AAP Committee on Fetus and Newborn and Section on Anesthesiology and Pain Medicine: Prevention and management of procedural pain in the neonate: an update. *Pediatrics*. 2016;137:(2): e20154271.

American Urological Association. *Policy Statement: Circumcision*. 2017. Retrieved from: http://www.auanet.org/guidelines/circumcision.

Anand KJS. *Prevention and Treatment of Neonatal Pain*. 2017. Retrieved from: https://www.uptodate.com/contents/prevention-and-treatment-of-neonatal-pain?search=neonatal%20pain&source=search_result&selectedTitle=1~19&usage_type=default&display_rank=1.

Baker CM, Wong DL. Q.U.E.S.T. T.: a process of pain assessment in children. *Orthopedic Nurs*. 1987;6(1):11–21.

Barbi E, Marzuillo P, Neri E, et al. Fever in children: pearls and pitfalls. *Children*. 2017;4:81.

Cho CY, Lai CC, Lee ML. Clinical Analysis of fever of unknown origin in children: a 10-year experience in a northern Taiwan medical center. *J Microbiol Immunol Infect*. 2017;50(1):40–45.

Committee on Fetus and Newborn and Section on Anesthesiology and Pain Medicine. Prevention and management of procedural pain in the neonate: an update. *Pediatrics*. 2016;137(2):1–13.

de Oliveira DL, Hirotsu C, Tufik S, Anderson ML. The interfaces between vitamin D, sleep and pain. *J Endocrinol*. 2017;234:R23–R36.

Fisher E, Heathcote L, Palermo TM, de C Williams AC, Lau J, Eccleston C. Systematic review and meta-analysis of psychological therapies for children with chronic pain. *J Pediatr Psychol*. 2014;39:763–782.

Gomez B, Mintegi S, Bressan S, et al. Validation of the "Step-by-Step" approach in the management of young febrile infants. *Pediatrics*. 2016;138(2):e20154381.

Gompf S. *Fever of Unknown Origin (Fuo): Practice Essentials, Background, and Etiology*. Available at: https://emedicine.medscape.com/article/217675-overview.

Hauer J, Jones BL. *Evaluation and Management of Pain in Children*. 2018. Retrieved from: https://www.uptodate.com/contents/evaluation-and-management-of-pain-in-children?search=pediatric%20pain&source=search_result&selectedTitle=1~150&usage_type=default&display_rank=1.

Hobson A, Wiffen PJ, Conlon JA. As required versus fixed schedule analgesic administration for postoperative pain in children. *Cochrane Database Syst Rev*. 2015. https://doi.org/10.1002/14651858.CD011404.pub2.

Huguet A, Olthuis J, McGrath PJ, et al. Systematic review of childhood and adolescent risk and prognostic factors for persistent abdominal pain. *ACTA Paediatrica*. 2016;106:545–553.

International Association for the Study of Pain (IASP). *IASP Taxonomy*. 2017. https://www.iasp-pain.org/Taxonomy.

Ku LC, Smith PB. Dosing in neonates: special consideration in physiology and trial design. *Pediatr Res*. 2015;77:2–9.

Lu H, Rosenbaum S. Developmental pharmacokinetics in pediatric populations. *J Pediatr Pharmacol Ther*. 2014;19:262–276.

Lundeberg S. Pain in children—are we accomplishing the optimal pain treatment? *Pediatr Anesthesia*. 2015;25(1):83–92.

Lye PS, Densmore EM. Fever. In: Kliegman RM, Lye PS, Bordini BJ, Toth H, Basel D, eds. *Nelson Pediatric Symptom-Based Diagnosis*. Philadelphia: Elsevier; 2018:701.

Lynch M. Pain as the fifth vital sign. *J Intravenous Nurs*. 2001;24(2):85–94.

O'Conner-Von S, Turner HN. American Society for Pain Management Nursing (ASPMN) position statement: male infant circumcision pain management. *Pain Manag Nurs*. 2013;14:379–382.

Pelton SI. Evaluating fever in the first 90 days of life. 2018. Available at: https://www.mdedge.com/chestphysician/article/162390/neonatal-medicine/evaluating-fever-first-90-days-life. Accessed April 12, 2019.

Tegethoff M, Belardi A, Stalujanis E, Meinlschmidt G. Comorbidity of mental disorders and chronic pain: chronology on onset in adolescents of a national representative cohort. *J Pain*. 2015;16(10):1054–1064.

Twycross A, Voepel-Lewis T, Vincent C, Franck L, von Baeyer CL. A debate on the proposition that self-report is the gold standard in assessment of pediatric pain intensity. *Clin J Pain*. 2015;31(8):707–712.

U.S. Food and Drug Administration (US FDA). *US FDA Drug Safety Communications. Fda Restricts Use of Prescription Codeine Pain and Cough Medicines and Tramadol Pain Medicines in Children; Recommends Against Use in Breastfeeding Women*. 2017. https://www.fda.gov/downloads/Drugs/DrugSafety/UCM553814.pdf.

Varnell H. *Fever, When You Should Worry and When You Can Reassure*. Children's Hospital Colorado 10 Minute Talk; 2018.

Walker SM. Pain after surgery in children: clinical recommendations. *Curr Opin Anaesthesiol*. 2015;28(5):570–576.

29

Perinatal Conditions

ROBERT J. YETMAN AND NAN M. GAYLORD

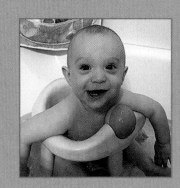

The neonatal period is remarkable for the vast array of biophysiologic changes that must occur as the neonate transitions from intrauterine to extrauterine life, including cardiopulmonary, thermo-metabolic regulation, nutrition, elimination, and acquiring immunity. It is not surprising that, in the United States approximately two-thirds of all deaths in the first year of life occur during the newborn period (birth to 28 days) with the highest risks in the first hour, followed by the first 24 hours of life (Mathews and Driscoll, 2017). The most common challenges are referred to as the neonatal energy triangle: hypoxia, hypothermia, and hypoglycemia. However, there are also many psychosocial transitions that need to occur for the newborn and family. An understanding of fetal development, needs, risks, and pertinent psychosocial and biophysical findings is necessary for primary care providers (PCPs), not only to assist the neonate's transition to extrauterine life, but also to provide family education. This chapter focuses on common perinatal and neonatal issues, diseases, injuries, and conditions, building on the newborn content found in Chapter 9.

Pathophysiology

High-Risk Pregnancy

Many newborn problems are due to poor and/or incomplete transition to extrauterine life, which can be secondary to premature birth, congenital anomalies, and/or adverse effects of delivery (e.g., birth asphyxia) (see Chapter 9; Fig 9.1). High-risk pregnancies are those with factors that increase the chances of spontaneous abortion, fetal demise, premature rupture of membranes and delivery, intrauterine growth retardation (IUGR), and selected fetal/maternal diseases or disorders. Identification of high-risk pregnancies is a key step toward anticipating or preventing neonatal problems (Box 29.1). Obtaining a three-generation pedigree can also be helpful in highlighting risks (see Chapter 3).

Acquired Health Problems

In utero exposure to poor nutrition, alcohol, drugs, infection, and maternal conditions (e.g., hypertension and diabetes) can result in prematurity and fetal abnormalities. The risk for many neonatal problems increases with a maternal age younger than 20 years old and older than 40 years old (see Box 29.1).

Perinatal Complications and Injuries

The term *birth injury* includes mechanical and anoxic trauma incurred by the newborn during labor and delivery. Predisposing risk factors for birth injury include macrosomia, prematurity, cephalopelvic disproportion, dystocia, prolonged labor, and breech presentation. Birth injuries include caput succedaneum, cephalohematoma, subgaleal hemorrhage, skull fractures, subconjunctival and retinal hemorrhages, intracranial hemorrhage, nerve palsies (brachial, phrenic, facial), fractured clavicle or humerus, ruptured liver or spleen, and hypoxic-ischemic insults. Infants with injuries need treatment immediately after birth. PCPs who attend births or care for newborns need to be familiar with perinatal conditions that subject the newborn to a higher risk and to be prepared to intervene quickly using the most up-to-date Newborn Resuscitation Program (NRP) guidelines.

Immediately After Birth

The first minute of life is referred to as the golden minute. NRP guidelines walk those in attendance through the needed assessment beginning with three items: (1) term gestation, (2) adequate breathing/crying, and (3) good muscle tone. When these are present, routine care begins along with ongoing standardized assessments. Resuscitation efforts may be necessary if the newborn does not meet an adequate threshold in these areas. At the end of the first minute is when the first Apgar score is universally recognized and routinely used for assessment. The 1-minute Apgar score assesses how well the newborn tolerated the birthing process, and the 5-minute Apgar score assesses how well the newborn is adapting to her/his new environment. The Apgar score is not used to determine the need for resuscitation (see Chapter 9; Table 9.1). The need for newborn resuscitation is based on a standardized algorithm of assessment and decision points provided by NRP guidelines (AAP, 2016) (see Figure 29.1).

Premature/Special Needs Newborns

Premature and special needs newborns (e.g., congenital anomalies, disease states, social situations) require early and ongoing assessment, newborn/family intervention, and referral before discharge (Box 29.2) to ensure that adequate family support/education and newborn follow-up are in place (AAP, 2017).

Common Neonatal Conditions

Skin & HEENT

Amniotic Band/Constriction Syndrome

In utero fibrous strands that encircle fetal parts can cause permanent depression and deformity of the entrapped tissue. Found in otherwise normal infants, these bands are thought to result from

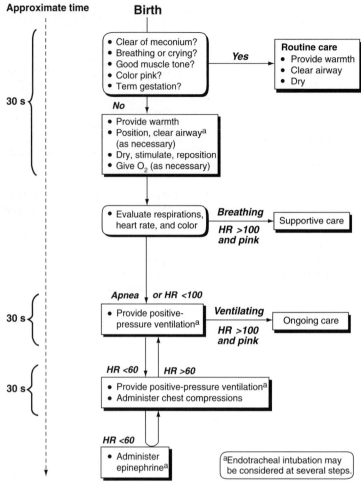

• **Fig 29.1** Resuscitation in the Delivery Room. *HR,* Heart rate. (From Niermeyer S, Kattwinkel J, Van Reempts P. International guidelines for neonatal resuscitation: an excerpt from the Guidelines 2000 for Cardiopulmonary Resuscitation and Emergency Cardiovascular Care: International Consensus on Science. *Pediatrics.* 2000;106[3]:29 and consistent with AAP NRP 7th Edition Guidelines, 2016.)

intrauterine rupture of the amnion with formation of fibrous strands. Sometimes there are associated abnormalities, including craniofacial anomalies and thoracic or abdominal wall defects. Treatment depends on the severity of the deformities. Constriction bands on the limbs are often managed in consultation with plastic surgery.

Branchial Cleft and Thyroglossal Cysts and Sinuses

Branchial cleft cysts and sinuses can be unilateral or bilateral, open onto the cutaneous surface, or drain into the pharynx. They are located along the anterior border of the sternocleidomastoid muscle and form as a result of improper closure during embryonic life. Thyroglossal cysts and sinuses are defects located in or near the midline of the neck, extending up to the base of the tongue. Thyroglossal cysts occasionally contain aberrant thyroid tissue and mucinous material. Both anomalies appear to have familial clusters, but also occur spontaneously. Once these anomalies are discovered, surgical consultation is required.

Cleft Lip and Palate

Clefts of the lip and/or palate (CLP) are immediately recognizable disruptions of normal facial structure. They represent embryonic failures in development that can occur in isolation or as part of a broad range of chromosomal, mendelian, or teratogenic syndromes.

A genetics consultation is recommended. Collectively CLP has a major clinical impact requiring surgical, dental, orthodontic, speech, hearing, and psychological treatments or therapies throughout childhood. They are among the most common birth defects worldwide, occurring more often in males than females.

Clinical Findings

- Varying degrees of cleft, from a small notch to a complete separation
- Unilateral or bilateral
- Involvement of the soft and/or hard palate
- A bifid uvula may indicate a submucosal cleft palate

Management and Complications

Referral to an ear, nose, and throat (ENT) specialist is required as surgical repair is indicated, the timing of which is individualized. Special feeding techniques are used until surgery can be performed. Breastfeeding and bottle feeding may be successful, depending on the severity of the cleft. Interprofessional team management is now standard, both in the short and long term, as speech, hearing, dental/orthodontic, and ENT care will be ongoing, along with patient/family psychosocial education and support. Middle ear, nasopharyngeal, and sinus infections, as well as associated hearing loss can occur.

• BOX 29.1 Factors Associated With High-Risk Pregnancies

Demographic Social Factors

Maternal age <20 years old or >40 years old
African American race
Developmentally delayed mother or low educational status
Illicit drug, alcohol, cigarette use
Poverty, unemployed, homelessness
Unmarried or lack of support
Emotional or physical stress, including depression and other mental health problems
Poor access to or use of prenatal care, underinsured, or uninsured

Medical History

Diabetes mellitus
Hypertension, maternal hypercoagulable state, sickle cell disease, congenital heart disease
Autoimmune disease, including rheumatologic illness (SLE)
Chronic medication
Sexually transmitted infections (colonization: herpes simplex, GBS, syphilis, HIV)

Prior Pregnancy

Intrauterine fetal demise or neonatal death
Previous infertility
Prematurity or low birthweight infant
Intrauterine growth retardation
Congenital malformation
Incompetent cervix
Blood group sensitization, neonatal jaundice
Neonatal thrombocytopenia
Hydrops
Inborn errors of metabolism

Present Pregnancy

Uterine bleeding (abruptio placentae, placenta previa)

Infection

Inception by reproductive technology
Poor weight gain or abnormal fetal growth
Multiple gestation, parity more than 5
Preeclampsia or eclampsia
Premature rupture of membranes
Short interpregnancy time
Polyhydramnios or oligohydramnios
High or low maternal serum alpha-fetoprotein

Labor and Delivery

Premature labor (<37 weeks) or prolonged labor
Postdates (>42 weeks) or prolonged gestation
Fetal distress
Immature L/S ratio: Absent phosphatidylglycerol
Breech presentation
Meconium-stained fluid
Nuchal cord
Forceps or cesarean delivery
Apgar score <4 at 1 min

Neonate

Birth weight <2500 g or >4000 g
Birth before 37 or after 42 weeks of gestation

Male Sex

SGA or LGA
Hypoglycemia
Tachypnea, cyanosis
Congenital malformation
Pallor, plethora, petechiae

GBS, *Group B streptococcus;* HIV, *human immunodeficiency virus;* LGA, *large for gestational age;* L/S, *lecithin-sphingomyelin ratio;* SGA, *small for gestational age;* SLE, *systemic lupus erythematosus.*

HEENT

Congenital Cataracts, Glaucoma, and Retinopathy of Prematurity (Chapter 35)

Cardiac Conditions (Chapter 38)

Transient Tachypnea of the Newborn

Transient tachypnea of the newborn (TTN) results from incomplete evacuation of fetal lung fluid in full-term infants, leading to decreased pulmonary compliance and tidal volume, and increased dead space. It is more common in cesarean deliveries. The two most common differential diagnoses are RDS and pneumonia (see Table 29.1).

Respiratory Conditions

Neonatal Respiratory Distress Syndrome

Neonatal respiratory distress syndrome (NRDS), formerly known as *hyaline membrane disease,* results from surfactant deficiency, resulting in alveolar atelectasis (Table 29.1). It is increasingly referred to as surfactant deficiency disorder (SDD). Most cases of NRDS occur in newborns born before 37 to 39 weeks. The more premature the baby is, the higher the chance of respiratory distress syndrome (RDS) after birth. NRDS can also be due to genetic problems with lung development. Antenatal steroids, postnatal surfactant, and newer ventilation techniques have reduced mortality from RDS to approximately 10% (Carlo and Ambalavanan, 2016a).

History and Clinical Findings

- Sibling who had RDS
- Maternal diabetes
- Cesarean delivery or induction of labor before the baby is full-term
- Problems with delivery that reduce blood flow to fetus/newborn (e.g., asphyxia, cold stress)
- Multiple pregnancy (twins or more)
- Preterm, precipitous or cesarean delivery

Physical Examination

- Tachypnea, grunting, intercostal retractions, nasal flaring, duskiness, and/or cyanosis
- Breath sounds may be normal but often are diminished with harsh tubular quality
- Fine rales on deep inspiration

Diagnostic Studies

A radiograph of the chest shows a fine reticular granularity of the parenchyma and air bronchograms. Blood gas results indicate hypoxemia, hypercarbia, and mixed metabolic/respiratory acidosis.

Management, Prognosis, and Prevention

Supportive care and mechanical ventilation are used as indicated. The administration of synthetic corticosteroids to women expected to deliver prematurely is indicated to reduce the severity

• BOX 29.2 Guidelines for Discharge and Follow-up of the High-Risk Neonate

Discharge Planning

- Demonstrate adequate weight gain, temperature control in open crib for 24 h, competent feeding without cardiorespiratory compromise, and mature and stable cardiorespiratory function for 5 to 7 days without caffeine.
- Ensure adequacy of immunizations based on infant's chronologic age and appropriate metabolic screenings are completed.
- Screen for anemia and nutritional risks; begin therapy, if indicated.
- Conduct fundoscopic evaluation if necessary.
- Ensure appropriate hearing screen has been completed.
- Identify all active medical or social problems through a review of the medical record and physical examination of infant; ensure home readiness has been evaluated, especially for the technologically dependent child.
- Complete car seat evaluation. Limit long car rides for 6 months and have another adult in the back when possible.
- Review with a family member the medications, feeding schedules, well-child care, signs of illness, change in health status, safety instruction, and appropriate response and follow-up for infants with active medical conditions.
- Identify family and community resources if infant is to be discharged on home oxygen therapy.
- Ensure adequate training of at least two appropriate family members in cardiopulmonary resuscitation (CPR) and, if applicable, home apnea monitor or other equipment use.
- Consider the need for: a home visit to assess environment, a visiting nurse, social services, respite care, support groups, early intervention services, referral to the Women, Infants, and Children (WIC) program, and/or a lactation consultant if breastfeeding.
- Ensure that follow-up care is arranged to include a primary care provider, neurodevelopmental follow-up, and surgical or other subspecialty providers, if indicated.

Follow-up Planning

- Schedule follow-up hearing screen (if necessary) for infants with craniofacial abnormalities, in utero infections, birthweight less than 1500 g, meningitis, exchange transfusion for hyperbilirubinemia, ototoxic medications exposure, Apgar score of ≤4 at 1 min or ≤6 at 5 min, ≥5 days of mechanical ventilation, diagnosis of a syndrome associated with hearing loss, failed initial screening, or family history of deafness.
- Ensure that by about 4 to 6 weeks of chronologic age a dilated binocular indirect ophthalmoscopic examination has occurred for neonates with a birthweight of 1500 g or less or with a gestational age of <32 weeks, a birthweight between 1500 and 2000 g, or gestational age of more than 32 weeks with an unstable clinical course. Additional examinations may be recommended based on the results of this first evaluation.
- Primary care follow-up visits every 1 to 2 weeks, especially if infant is on oxygen therapy and/or a cardiorespiratory monitor.
- Of prime interest at each routine primary care outpatient visit should be growth and development, preventative care, guidance, parental education with referral for additional evaluations if any concerns are identified. Ensure that the referral to Early Intervention program is complete.

TABLE 29.1 Clinical Comparison of Transient Tachypnea of the Newborn and Respiratory Distress Syndrome	
Transient Tachypnea of the Newborn	**Respiratory Distress Syndrome**
Seen in infants delivered at or near term, often in infants born by cesarean section	Found almost always in premature infants, with the greatest incidence in infants weighing <1500 g
Increased respiratory rate is present; grunting and intercostal retractions are not always present	Usually, respiratory rate is increased, infants grunt at expiration, nasal flaring is noted, and sternal and intercostal retractions are common
Cyanosis is not a prominent feature	Cyanosis in room air is a prominent feature
Air exchange is good; rales and rhonchi are usually absent	Auscultation reveals diminished air entry
Begins at birth, usually resolving in the first 24-48 h of life	Progressive respiratory distress in the first hours of life
Chest radiograph shows central perihilar streaking with slightly enlarged heart and fluid in the fissure	Chest radiograph demonstrates reticulogranular, ground-glass appearance, and air bronchograms
Typical course involves gradual decrease in respiratory rate with resolution in about 72 h	Course variable depending on infant's gestational weight and age; usually, respiratory distress syndrome improves after 5 days of life
No specific therapy other than maintaining oxygenation is usually necessary	Artificial surfactant and antenatal administration of steroids to the mother can reduce the severity of this disease; mechanical ventilation is common

and mortality due to RDS as well as reducing the incidence of severe intraventricular hemorrhage (IVH), necrotizing enterocolitis (NCE), and neurodevelopmental impairment. After delivery, the immediate introduction of exogenous surfactant to the newborn has been found to reduce mortality rates and to improve short-term respiratory status in preterm infants. The overall prognosis depends on the severity of the disease and the birthweight of the infant. The only fully effective preventive measure is the elimination of prematurity (Carlo and Ambalavanan, 2016a).

History and Clinical Findings

- Tachypnea, expiratory grunting, intercostal retractions
- No adventitious auscultation findings
- Occasionally requires minimal oxygen
- Usually disappears within 24 to 48 hours

Diagnostic Studies

A chest radiograph shows prominent pulmonary vascular markings, fluid lines along fissures, over aeration, flat diaphragms, and occasionally pleural fluid.

Management and Prognosis

If the infant is not in significant respiratory distress, close observation, and transcutaneous oxygen saturation monitoring is sufficient until the absorption of fetal lung fluid is complete and tachypnea resolves. The need for supplemental oxygen therapy should be based on close oxygen monitoring. The use of mechanical ventilation in TTN is rare. Infants usually recover rapidly within 24 to 48 hours without intervention.

Meconium Aspiration Syndrome

Meconium aspiration syndrome occurs in term or postterm infants. This syndrome is a serious pulmonary disorder characterized by small airway obstruction, chemical pneumonitis, and secondary respiratory distress. In utero fetal distress and anoxia increase intestinal peristalsis and relax the anal sphincter, resulting in the release of meconium into the amniotic fluid. Thick meconium is aspirated either in utero or with the first breath. Approximately 10% to 15% of all newborns are meconium stained, but only 5% of these infants develop respiratory problems (Ambalavanan and Carlos, 2016).

Clinical Findings

- Meconium in the amniotic fluid and below the vocal cords on resuscitation
- Tachypnea, intercostal retractions, grunting, and cyanosis within hours of delivery

Diagnostic Studies

A chest radiograph shows patchy infiltrates, coarse streaking of both lung fields, and flattening of the diaphragm.

Management, Prognosis, and Prevention

An infant born with meconium in the amniotic fluid but who is vigorous (strong respiratory effort, good muscle tone, and a heart rate of higher than 100 beats per minute [bpm]) does not need intubation and suctioning as had been previously recommended. Rather, ongoing treatment of the vigorous infant includes supportive care and standard management of respiratory distress. The intubating and suctioning of meconium-stained infants are no longer recommended for the depressed infant. Rather, resuscitation should be performed if the depressed infant follows the same recommendations as for an infant with clear fluid (ACOG Committee Opinion, 2017). Severe meconium aspiration cases may require extracorporeal membrane oxygenation (ECMO). The mortality rate is increased in infants born with meconium staining. Meconium aspiration syndrome accounts for a significant proportion of neonatal deaths. Residual lung problems are possible, and central nervous system (CNS) injury from asphyxia can occur.

Gastrointestinal and Abdominal Conditions

Esophageal Atresia and Tracheoesophageal Fistula

In esophageal atresia (EA), a blind pouch occurs in the esophagus with or without an associated fistula. Most infants (87%) have a proximal pouch, with the associated fistula connecting the distal esophagus and the trachea (Fig 29.2). This defect occurs in 1 in 2000 to 4000 births. Affected infants born prematurely and those that have associated cardiac anomalies have the highest risk for mortality. About 50% of infants with EA have a syndrome, most commonly VACTERL syndrome (consisting of **V**ertebral dysgenesis, **A**nal atresia [imperforate anus], **C**ardiac anomalies, **T**racheo-**E**sophageal fistula, **R**enal anomalies, and **L**imb anomalies). An evaluation for associated findings, especially cardiac and vertebral, is warranted (Khan and Orenstein, 2016).

History and Clinical Findings. The history *includes* maternal polyhydramnios and inability to pass a nasogastric tube into the stomach during resuscitation at birth or afterward in the nursery, especially in a child with respiratory distress or vomiting. The diagnosis may be suspected prenatally with polyhydramnios and when a small stomach sac and blind pouch is found on prenatal

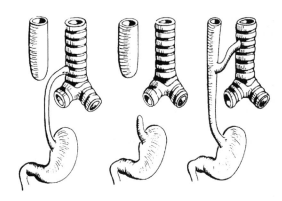

• **Fig 29.2** The Three Most Common Types of Esophageal Atresia and Tracheoesophageal Fistula (From Bruch SW, Kunisaki SM, Coran AG. Congenital malformations of the esophagus. In Wyllie R, Hyams JS, Kay M, eds. *Pediatric Gastrointestinal and Liver Disease*. 5th ed. Philadelphia: Saunders/Elsevier; 2016.)

ultrasonography but is difficult to diagnose (Garabedian, Verpillat and Czerkiewicz, 2014) and may need additional evaluation.

Physical Examination
- Excessive oral secretions that require frequent suctioning
- Choking, coughing, and cyanosis, particularly during feedings
- Spitting or vomiting

Diagnostic Studies. Chest and abdominal radiographs show the nasogastric tube coiled in the pouch in the thoracic region confirms EA, and air in the stomach suggests an associated tracheoesophageal fistula (TEF). Carefully performed water-soluble x-ray evaluation of the upper esophagus demonstrates the anatomy of the atresia and identifies the presence, if any, of an associated TEF.

Differential Diagnosis. RDS, meconium aspiration, and congenital heart disease should be considered.

Management, Complications, and Prognosis. This is a surgical emergency requiring immediate intervention. A nasogastric tube is inserted into the blind pouch to prevent aspiration until surgical repair can be accomplished. Preoperatively the infant should be placed in a prone position and suctioned frequently. Pneumonia, atelectasis, aspiration, postoperative strictures, and repeated surgery are possible complications. The survival rate postoperatively approaches 100% unless other congenital anomalies are present. Approximately 50% of affected infants have other congenital anomalies (Khan and Orenstein, 2016).

Duodenal Atresia

Duodenal atresia (DA) is a complete obstruction of the duodenum, ending blindly just distal to the ampulla of Vater. DA occurs in about 1 in 10,000 births. It is associated with prematurity in 50% of cases, and other congenital anomalies are common, including congenital heart disease, malrotation, and annual pancreas. About half of the patients with DA have chromosome abnormalities with Down syndrome seen in about one-third of such patients (Bales and Liacourus, 2016).

History and Clinical Findings. The history includes maternal polyhydramnios and is more common in prematurity and in infants with chromosomal abnormalities, especially Down syndrome. The infant presents with bilious vomitus, absence of abdominal distention, and jaundice.

Diagnostic Studies. Abdominal radiographs show a "double-bubble" pattern in the upright position secondary to air in the stomach and a distended duodenum.

Differential Diagnosis. Malrotation, duodenal obstruction for other reasons, and annular pancreas should be considered.

Management, Complications, and Prognosis. Surgical intervention is indicated once the diagnosis of DA has been made. Feedings should be discontinued and gastric suctioning applied. The prognosis depends on early identification and treatment and other associated anomalies. Aspiration of gastric contents can occur as a complication of this condition. Evaluation for associated anomalies, such as heart disease, skeletal anomalies, and renal abnormalities, is warranted

Malrotation With Volvulus

Malrotation with volvulus in the newborn period is the twisting of a loop of bowel, causing intermittent or acute pain and obstruction with vomiting. It occurs in 1 in 500 live births, half of whom present with symptoms in the first month of life (Kennedy and Liacourus, 2016).

Clinical Findings. Physical findings include abdominal distention and bilious vomiting.

Diagnostic Studies. Intestinal obstruction is demonstrated on plain abdominal radiograph. Contrast studies demonstrate a "bird's-beak" obstruction in the proximal duodenum and a spiral (corkscrew) configuration of the duodenum.

Differential Diagnosis. Duodenal obstruction or atresia and annular pancreas are in the differential diagnosis.

Management, Complications, and Prognosis. In the symptomatic infant, fluid replacement and surgical repair are indicated. The prognosis depends on early identification of the volvulus and rapid surgical repair. Perforation, necrosis of the bowel, sepsis, and peritonitis are possible complications.

Pyloric Stenosis

Pyloric stenosis is caused by a hypertrophied pyloric muscle, resulting in a narrowing of the pyloric sphincter. Pyloric stenosis occurs in 1 to 3/1000 live births, with a four- to sixfold increase in males compared with females (Hunter and Liacourus, 2016). It tends to be familial and is seen more commonly in Caucasian first-born males.

History and Clinical Findings
- Regurgitation and nonprojectile vomiting typically after the first week of life that progresses to nonbilious, progressive projectile vomiting around 2 to 3 weeks old
- Insatiable appetite with weight loss, dehydration, and constipation
- There is an association of pyloric stenosis with the administration of oral erythromycin in the first 2 weeks of life
- Weight loss
- A distinct "olive" mass might be palpated in the epigastrium to the right of midline
- Reverse peristalsis visualized across the abdomen is frequently reported in the literature but is rarely seen in practice

Diagnostic Studies. Most common is ultrasound with measurement of the pyloric muscle thickness. If ultrasound is unavailable or inconclusive, an upper gastrointestinal series demonstrates a "string sign," indicating a fine, elongated pyloric canal.

Management and Prognosis. Surgical intervention (pyloromyotomy) is corrective. Vomiting and fluid and electrolyte imbalance need to be corrected, although they are less common postoperatively. Feedings should be introduced gradually. The prognosis is excellent.

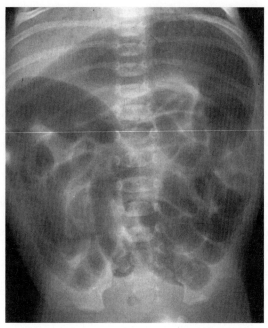

• **Fig 29.3** Dramatic Dilation of Bowel Consistent With Hirschsprung Disease (Photo courtesy of Lawrence H. Robinson, professor of Radiology and Pediatrics, University of Texas Medical School, Houston, TX.)

Hirschsprung Disease (Congenital Aganglionic Megacolon)

Hirschsprung disease is an absence of ganglion cells in the bowel wall, most often in the rectosigmoid region, resulting in a portion of the colon having no motility. This disorder occurs in 1 in 5000 births. It is the most common cause of neonatal colon obstruction and accounts for approximately 33% of all neonatal obstructions. The disease is familial, affects males four times more commonly than females, and is common in children with trisomy 21 as well as a variety of other syndromes. Thus a careful examination is performed to identify additional anomalies that are sometimes present (Fiorino and Liacourus, 2016).

History and Clinical Findings
- Failure to pass meconium within the first 48 hours of life
- Distended abdomen with bilious vomiting
- Failure to thrive, poor feeding
- Chronic constipation, vomiting, abdominal obstruction
- Diarrhea, explosive bowel movements, or flatus
- Down syndrome

Diagnostic Studies. Radiographs (plain or with contrast) indicate dilated bowel loops (Fig 29.3). A rectal suction biopsy showing the absence of ganglion cells is diagnostic.

Differential Diagnosis. The differential diagnosis includes ileal atresia with microcolon, small left colon syndrome, and meconium plug/ileus syndrome (often associated with cystic fibrosis [CF]). In the older child, the differential diagnosis includes acquired functional megacolon, colonic inertia, chronic idiopathic constipation, lower spine malformations, and constipation.

Management. Surgical resection of the affected bowel is indicated, with or without a colostomy.

Imperforate Anus

Imperforate anus is the lack of a rectal opening. This condition occurs in about 1 in 3000 births, many of which are associated with another anomaly, often VACTERL syndrome. Congenital heart disease, EA, intestinal atresia, annular pancreas, intestinal malrotation or duplication, bilateral absence of the musculus rectus abdominis, trisomy 21, finger and hand anomalies, omphalocele, bladder exstrophy, and exstrophy of the ileocecal area are among the associated conditions (Akay and Klein, 2016).

History and Clinical Findings. The history includes failure to pass meconium or the passage of meconium from an unexpected location. Findings may include no obvious opening in the rectal area. In girls, stool passage may occur through a rectovaginal fistula, and in boys a fistula in the median raphe or to the bladder can be identified. The diagnostic studies to evaluate this condition vary depending on clinical findings including plain films, ultrasound, and urinalysis.

Management. Immediate surgical consultation and repair with or without performing a colostomy is indicated. Long-term management related to bowel functioning is often needed as some children will have challenges with bowel emptying or incontinence.

Omphalocele and Gastroschisis

An omphalocele is a protrusion of the sac of intestines into the base of the umbilical cord where the intestines are covered by the peritoneum without overlying skin. Occurrence is 1 in 5000 to 10,000 births. Gastroschisis is similar in appearance with intestinal contents protruding through the abdomen with no protective peritoneal covering. Gastroschisis occurs in about 1 in 10,000 to 20,000 live births. With omphalocele, serious associated conditions occur in 50% of newborns including chromosomal abnormalities (trisomy 13 and 18), congenital diaphragmatic hernia (CDH), and a variety of cardiac problems. Concomitant hypoglycemia and macroglossia suggest Beckwith syndrome. Associated congenital anomalies are rare with gastroschisis (Carlo and Ambalavanan, 2016b).

Clinical Findings. Examination reveals a saclike protrusion covered by the peritoneum without overlying skin at the mid abdomen.

Management and Complications. Maintain body temperature. Apply protective gauze and wrap the lesion with Mersilene mesh to prevent heat and fluid loss, and infection. When the infant is stable, surgical repair is indicated. Ileus is a common complication.

Necrotizing Enterocolitis

NEC is characterized by varying degrees of mucosal or transmural intestinal necrosis. The usual onset is in the first 2 weeks of life, but it can be later in very low birthweight infants. The cause is unknown, but the condition is less common in infants who are breastfed and have minimal feeds before bolus feeds are initiated. Infants that have immature colons that have become necrosed from trauma or injury are at an increased risk of developing this condition. NEC occurs in 1% to 5% of neonates in the neonatal intensive care unit, with the vast majority of these cases occurring in very low birthweight premature infants. While NEC is most common in preterm infants, the condition is also seen in full-term infants; particularly those with a history of birth asphyxia, congenital heart disease, and after rotavirus infections (Maheshwari and Carlo, 2016b).

History and Clinical Findings
- Prematurity, small for gestation (SGA), asphyxia, polycythemia
- Maternal hemorrhage, preeclampsia, cocaine exposure in utero
- Exchange transfusions, umbilical catheters

- Congenital heart disease
- Abdominal distention, vomiting, bloody stools (25%)
- Apnea, lethargy
- Evidence of disseminated intravascular coagulation (DIC), rapid progression of shock

Diagnostic Studies
- Sepsis work-up should be done.
- An abdominal radiograph shows pneumatosis intestinalis, a specific air pattern.

Differential Diagnosis. The differential diagnosis includes sepsis, intestinal obstruction, volvulus, Hirschsprung disease, anal fissures, and neonatal appendicitis.

Management, Complications, and Prognosis
- Prescribe systemic antibiotics following sepsis work-up.
- Stop feedings, initiate gastric suctioning, maintain electrolyte balance, give oxygen as needed, and initiate surgical consultation.
- Obtain serial abdominal radiographs to follow the course of disease.

The mortality rate is 10% to 30%. Ileus and perforation are early complications. Sequelae to NEC include feeding intolerance, stricture formation, and short-bowel syndrome, especially after intestinal resection (Maheshwari and Carlo, 2016b).

Meconium Ileus

Meconium ileus is intestinal obstruction caused by meconium bowel impaction. Meconium ileus is associated with CF and maternal polyhydramnios. About 80% to 90% of patients have CF; about 10% to 15% of patients with CF have meconium ileus (Bales and Liacouras, 2016).

History and Clinical Findings
- Failure to pass meconium within 48 hours of life.
- Abdominal distention and persistent bilious vomiting.

Diagnostic Studies. A radiograph shows bowel loops of varying width, often with a grainy appearance due to trapped gas bubbles at the points of heaviest meconium concentration.

Management and Prognosis. Treatment is individualized including high enemas (with water-soluble contrast material) or laparotomy. The survival rate is good. Underlying disorder identification should be considered. Referral to a gastrointestinal specialist may be necessary, and to a CF team if CF is confirmed.

Diaphragmatic Hernia

In diaphragmatic hernia, abdominal contents herniate into the thoracic cavity. A diaphragmatic hernia is caused by failure of the pleuroperitoneal canal to close completely during embryologic development. It occurs on the left side 80% to 90% of the time with a frequency of about 1 in 2000 to 5000 live births, and is more common in females. While most cases of congenital diaphragmatic hernia (CDH) are sporadic, up to 30% have associated anomalies including CNS, EA, omphalocele, and cardiac lesions (Maheshwari and Carlo, 2016a).

History and Clinical Findings. These lesions are often diagnosed on prenatal ultrasound. After birth, immediate respiratory failure occurs secondary to pulmonary hypertension or pulmonary hypoplasia. The degree of respiratory distress is related to the amount of functional lung capacity. Any newborn with respiratory distress should be evaluated for diaphragmatic hernia.
- Respiratory distress with tachypnea, cyanosis, absence of breath sounds
- Scaphoid abdomen, bowel sounds heard in the chest (rare)
- Heart tones best heard in the contralateral chest

Diagnostic Studies. A chest radiograph shows fluid and air-filled loops of intestine in the chest. The mediastinum is displaced toward the unaffected side, usually to the right.

Management and Prognosis

- As soon as the diagnosis is suspected, the infant should be positioned with the head and chest higher than the abdomen.
- Intensive respiratory support, which often includes ECMO.
- Surgery, with intensive respiratory and metabolic support.

The mortality rate is about 30%, depending on the degree of lung hypoplasia (Maheshwari and Carlo, 2016a).

Umbilical Hernia

Umbilical hernia is a weakness or imperfect closure of the umbilical ring.

Clinical Findings. Findings include a reducible soft swelling in the umbilical area often associated with diastasis recti.

Management, Prognosis, and Education. Surgery is not required unless the hernia persists beyond about 5 years of age, strangulates, becomes nonreducible, or dramatically enlarges in size. Most umbilical hernias resolve spontaneously by 1 year old, but some can take up to 4 to 5 years to resolve. Lesions with fascial defects greater than 1.5 cm in diameter have a lower rate of spontaneous closure. Incarceration is extremely rare. Counsel parents to avoid taping coins or placing bellybands over the umbilicus; these efforts do not help, can contribute to infection and are a choking risk if swallowed.

Genitourinary and Renal Conditions

Hydrocele and Inguinal Hernia

See Chapter 41.

Acute Renal Failure

Newborns normally produce 1 to 3 mL/kg/h of urine and urinate within the first 48 hours of life—almost all within the first 24 hours of life. A stressed neonate may develop decreased renal function. Urine output less than 0.5 mL/kg/h indicates acute renal failure. Multiple causes of renal failure include stress during the prenatal period, dehydration, sepsis, anoxia, shock, administration of nephrotoxic drugs, renal dysgenesis, obstructive uropathy, congenital heart disease, hemorrhage, and renal vein thrombosis.

History and Clinical Findings

- Decreased or no urinary output; maternal oligohydramnios
- Pallor, edema, lethargy, vomiting, seizures, coma
- High or low blood pressure
- Pulmonary edema, congestive heart failure or arrhythmias
- Abdominal mass, myelomeningocele or prune-belly syndrome

Diagnostic Studies. Order the following, as indicated:

- Catheterization or bladder tap to confirm adequacy of urinary output
- Urinalysis to identify hematuria or pyuria
- Urine osmolarity, sodium, and potassium values to measure kidney filtration
- Serum blood urea nitrogen, creatinine, sodium, and potassium values to measure kidney filtration (although in the first days of life these may reflect maternal renal function)
- Complete blood count (CBC) including differential and platelets for evidence of thrombocytopenia, sepsis, or renal vein thrombosis

Management and Prognosis

- Replace fluid loss (approximately 30 mL/kg every 24 hours), then restrict fluid and diet.

- Maintain strict intake, output, and fluid and electrolyte balance.
- Monitor blood pressure.
- Dialysis is sometimes indicated.
- The prognosis depends on the cause and the degree of renal failure.

Hydronephrosis

Hydronephrosis is a significant dilation of one or both kidneys caused by an obstruction of the ureteropelvic junction, posterior urethral valves, ectopic ureterocele, prune-belly syndrome, or ureteral or ureterovesical obstructions. Obstructive uropathy is slightly more common in males.

History and Clinical Findings

- Findings on prenatal ultrasonogram
- Asymptomatic in early stages
- Decreased urinary output or abdominal mass

Management and Prognosis. Surgical repair may be necessary depending on the cause of the hydronephrosis and if spontaneous resolution does not occur by 6 to 12 months of age. The longer the obstruction lasts, the less likely renal function will return to normal.

Cystic Kidney Disease

The presence of multiple kidney cysts of various sizes and shapes is a genetic disease. The autosomal dominant form usually appears in the fourth or fifth decade of life and is associated with hepatic cysts or cerebral aneurysms. The adult form (autosomal dominant) occurs in 1/400 to 1000 individuals; the juvenile form (autosomal recessive) is diagnosed most commonly during the prenatal or neonatal periods due to abdominal masses, and occurs in 1/10,000 to 40,000 live births (Porter and Avner, 2016).

History and Clinical Findings

- Maternal oligohydramnios due to decreased fetal kidney function resulting in pulmonary hypoplasia
- Evidence of Potter syndrome (low-set ears, micrognathia, flat nose, arthrogryposis, and IUGR)
- Abdominal lobular mass
- Hematuria
- Hypertension

Differential Diagnosis. A renal ultrasonogram is done to document the disorder. Multicystic dysplastic kidney, hydronephrosis, von Hippel-Lindau disease, Wilms tumor, and renal vein thrombosis are included in the differential diagnosis.

Management and Prognosis. The infant presenting with the juvenile form of the disease typically has respiratory failure and requires aggressive ventilator support. Both forms require careful monitoring of kidney function, renal ultrasound for the enlargement of cysts, and observation for signs and symptoms of infection. Hypertension may be difficult to control. Nephrectomy may be necessary if cysts do not regress in size or a significant complication develops. Dialysis or transplantation is sometimes considered for those infants with profound renal failure. With severe involvement of the juvenile form, the neonate is at risk for death from pulmonary or renal insufficiency.

Renal Artery or Vein Thrombosis

Injury to the kidney occurs when there is decreased blood flow to the kidney due to thrombus formation.

History and Clinical Findings. This condition is associated with asphyxia, dehydration, shock, sepsis, hypercoagulable states, and maternal diabetes. Sudden onset of gross hematuria may be noted. Findings include a firm flank mass. Ultrasonography shows marked enlargement of the kidney; Doppler flow studies show reduced flow to affected kidney(s). The hematocrit is low, and the urine contains protein and often blood.

Differential Diagnosis. Other causes of hematuria (e.g., hydronephrosis, cystic disease, Wilms tumor, hemolytic-uremic syndrome, and renal abscess) are included in the differential diagnosis.

Management
- Maintain fluid and electrolyte balance.
- Monitor blood pressure.
- Nephrectomy is not necessary unless chronic infection or uncontrollable hypertension occurs.

Neuroblastoma

A neuroblastoma is a solid tumor of unknown cause that originates from neural crest tissue along the craniospinal axis. The majority of neuroblastomas develop in the abdomen, usually in the adrenal gland. About 600 new cases of neuroblastoma are diagnosed each year; it is the most commonly diagnosed neoplasm in neonates (Zage and Ater, 2016).

Clinical Findings
- An unexplained fever, mass, and symptoms related to the site of the tumor
- Ascites and/or firm, irregular, nontender mass in abdomen
- Pallor, hypotension, irritability
- Possible external tumors in newborn, such as skin lesions similar to those of congenital rubella syndrome

Diagnostic Studies. The following help to assess and stage the disease:
- CBC, basic chemistry panel
- Renal radiographs to detect calcifications
- Ultrasound, computed tomography (CT) or magnetic resonance imaging (MRI) of abdomen
- Radiograph or CT scan of chest
- Skeletal survey or bone scan
- Urine catecholamines, homovanillic acid (HVA) and vanillylmandelic acid (VMA)
- Bone marrow aspirate and biopsy

Differential Diagnosis. Wilms tumor, hydronephrosis, renal vein thrombosis, and lymphoma are included in the differential diagnosis.

Management and Prognosis. Although some neuroblastomas regress without therapy (usually only those in children younger than 1 year old), treatment generally involves surgical removal followed by radiation therapy or chemotherapy. The prognosis depends on the age of the patient and the stage of the tumor.

Renal Agenesis

Renal agenesis is failure of the kidney to form normally. Bilateral agenesis is incompatible with life, and occurs in 1 in 3000 births (Elder, 2016).

History and Clinical Findings. Maternal oligohydramnios is noted in bilateral agenesis. Unilateral renal agenesis usually is detected on prenatal ultrasound or when the child is evaluated for other congenital anomalies or for urinary tract infection.
- Single umbilical artery associated with unilateral agenesis
- Associated anomalies involving the gastrointestinal or urinary tract and skeleton, especially with Potter syndrome (bilateral agenesis)
- Low-set ears, senile appearance, broad nose, and receding chin consistent with Potter syndrome

Management and Prognosis. Monitor for proteinuria and hypertension. Infants with bilateral disease often die shortly after birth due to pulmonary insufficiency.

Endocrine Conditions

Congenital Hypothyroidism and Congenital Adrenal Hyperplasia

See Chapter 45.

Metabolic Conditions

Hypoglycemia

In the term infant, serum glucose levels rarely fall below 35 mg/dL in the first 3 hours of life, below 40 mg/dL between 3 and 24 hours of life, or below 45 mg/dL thereafter. Infants at higher risk of developing hypoglycemia include late preterm infants exposed to maternal steroids, SGA infants, and those born to diabetic mothers, asphyxia at birth, sepsis, erythroblastosis fetalis, glycogen storage disease, or galactosemia (Table 29.2).

Management and Prognosis. Infants with symptomatic hypoglycemia, particularly low birthweight infants and infants of diabetic mothers, are at risk for poor intellectual development compared with asymptomatic infants. Prognosis for normal intellectual function is guarded in infants with prolonged and severe hypoglycemia.

Infant of a Diabetic Mother

An infant of a diabetic mother (IDM) is born to a mother whose pregnancy is complicated by poorly controlled gestational or insulin-dependent diabetes mellitus. Maternal hyperglycemia causes fetal hyperglycemia and hyperinsulinemia, leading to increased hepatic glucose uptake and glycogen synthesis, accelerated lipogenesis, and augmented protein synthesis (Carlo, 2016) (see Table 29.2).

Management, Complications, and Prevention. Cardiomegaly is common (30%), and heart failure occurs in 5% to 10% of infants. Congenital anomalies are increased threefold; cardiac malformations (15 times greater) and lumbosacral agenesis are most common (Carlo, 2016). Symptomatic neonatal hypoglycemia, which can occur upon cutting of the umbilical cord, increases the risk of impaired intellectual development. Strict management of blood glucose levels in mothers with diabetes decreases the risk of severe problems in the infant.

Hematologic Conditions

Polycythemia

Polycythemia is characterized by a central hematocrit of 65% or higher. Polycythemia occurs with a variety of conditions, including IDM, cyanotic congenital heart disease, and infants with IUGR and chronic fetal hypoxia resulting in stimulated erythropoietin production and increased red blood cell production. Polycythemia occurs in 1% to 2% of term appropriate-for-gestational-age births, depending on the etiology (see Table 29.2).

History and Clinical Findings. Born to a diabetic mother (infants may also have hypoglycemia), recipient of a twin–twin transfusion, delayed clamping of umbilical cord, trisomy conditions, and maternal hypertension.
- Cyanosis (persistent fetal circulation), tachypnea, respiratory distress irritability, lethargy, feeding disturbances, early jaundice
- In severe cases, stroke, seizures, renal vein thrombosis

Management and Prognosis. Most asymptomatic infants are normal, but long-term problems may include speech deficits, abnormal fine motor control, reduced intelligence quotient (IQ), and other neurologic abnormalities.

TABLE 29.2 Identification and Management of Hypoglycemia, Infant of Diabetic Mother and Polycythemia in the Newborn

Condition	Clinical Finding	Workup	Management
Hypoglycemia	Blood glucose <30 mg/dL; infant with history of SGA; mother with poorly controlled diabetes (IDM); at risk for sepsis, asphyxia, erythroblastosis fetalis, lethargy, poor feeding, regurgitation, apnea, jitteriness, pallor, sweating, cool extremities and seizures	Serum glucose—measure within 1 h of birth, every 2 h until 6-8 h of life, then every 4-6 h until 24 h of life	Give normoglycemic high-risk infants oral or gavage feedings with breast milk or formula at 1-3 h of life and continue every 2-3 h for 24-48 h; IV glucose at 8 mg/kg/min if serum glucose less than 30 to 35 mg/dL and oral feedings poorly tolerated.
Infant of diabetic mother (IDM)	IDM: Large, plump infant; puffy facies; plethora; hyperactivity first 3 days; ± hypotonicity, lethargy, poor suck; ± cardiomegaly and murmur	Intensive observation and care Serum glucose—measure within 1 h of birth, then frequently for the next 6-8 h, especially for macrosomia or growth restriction	If clinically well and normoglycemic, start oral or gavage feedings with infant formula or breast milk within 2-3 h old and continue at 3-h intervals. If infant is unable to tolerate oral feeding, discontinue feeding and give 10% glucose by peripheral IV infusion at a rate of 4-8 mg/kg/min. Treat hypoglycemia, even in asymptomatic infants, with IV infusions of glucose.
Polycythemia	Cyanosis, tachypnea, respiratory distress; hyperbilirubinemia; infant with history of diabetic mother; IUGR, postmaturity, SGA exposed to chronic hypoxia; recipient of twin–twin transfusion; delayed clamping of umbilical cord; plethora; and feeding disturbance	Hematocrit ≥65%	Phlebotomy and replacement with saline or albumin or partial exchange transfusion to reduce hematocrit to 50%.

From Hughes HK, Kahl LK. *The Harriet Lane Handbook.* 21st ed. Philadelphia: Elsevier; 2018.
IUGR, Intrauterine growth restriction; *IV,* intravenous; *SGA,* small for gestational age.

Hemorrhagic Disease in the Newborn

Severe transient vitamin K-dependent clotting factor deficiencies lead to Vitamin K dependent bleeding (VKDB). Hemorrhagic disease is caused by vitamin K deficiency is caused by a lack of free vitamin K in the mother and absence of bacterial intestinal flora normally responsible for the synthesis of vitamin K in the infant. Vitamin K–dependent clotting factors (II, VII, IX, and X) are normal at birth, but decrease within 2 to 3 days, increasing the incidence of early-onset bleeding in all newborns. Breast milk is a poor source of vitamin K; late-onset bleeding (occurring 1 to 3 months after birth) is rare but may be seen in exclusively breastfed infants. A particularly severe form of deficiency of vitamin K–dependent coagulation factors occurs in the first day of life in women receiving the anticonvulsants phenytoin and/or phenobarbital.

History and Clinical Findings
- Anticonvulsant (phenytoin or phenobarbital) use by the mother
- Prematurity
- Exclusive breastfeeding without vitamin K supplementation
- Failure to administer parenteral vitamin K at birth
- Neonatal hepatitis or biliary atresia
- Gastrointestinal, nasal, subgaleal, or intracranial bleeding or bleeding at the site of an injection or circumcision

Diagnostic Studies. Prothrombin time, blood coagulation time, and partial thromboplastin time are prolonged.

Differential Diagnosis. This disorder may result from DIC or congenital bleeding disorders unrelated to vitamin K.

Management, Prognosis, and Prevention

- In the child with evidence of hemorrhagic disease, intravenous (IV) infusion of 1 to 5 mg of vitamin K is needed. Improvement of coagulation defects and cessation of bleeding should occur within a few hours.
- If a newborn is delivered at home, confirm that vitamin K was given.
- Prevention of early- and late-onset bleeding is achieved by routinely giving 1 mg of natural oil-soluble vitamin K intramuscularly within 1 hour of birth.
- Prognosis of a child sustaining a hemorrhagic event depends on the site and extent of bleeding.
- Some parents object to parenteral vitamin K. Oral formulations are available but are unlicensed and ineffective against early onset of disease as the peak efficacy of oral vitamin K is 24 hours with continued dosages required over the first 3 to 4 months of life. Full efficacy of parental vitamin K is obtained 4 to 6 hours after injection and the infant is fully protected against VKDB (CDC, 2017).

Anemia

Anemia is characterized by less than the normal range of hemoglobin for birthweight and postnatal age. Anemia is caused by factors before, during, or immediately after birth and occurs secondary to acute blood loss before or during delivery.

History and Clinical Findings
- Congenital aplastic or hypoplastic anemia
- Twin–twin transfusion

- Unexpected tearing or delayed clamping of umbilical cord resulting in neonatal blood loss
- Internal hemorrhage (fracture, cephalhematoma, internal organ trauma, gastrointestinal, pulmonary, or other injured organ)
- Umbilical stump or circumcision bleeding
- Hemolysis
- Pallor, congestive heart failure, and shock are possible

Management and Prognosis. Treatment depends on the cause and symptoms. An asymptomatic full-term infant with a hemoglobin level of 10 g/dL might be observed, whereas a symptomatic neonate born after abruptio placentae or with severe hemolytic disease of the newborn requires transfusion. Treatment with blood should be balanced by concern about transfusion-acquired infection with cytomegalovirus (CMV), HIV, and hepatitis B and C viruses. Prognosis depends on the cause and severity of the anemia.

Blood in Vomitus or Stool

Bright red or dark red blood in the vomitus or stool can be seen without clinical evidence of blood loss. This problem often is caused by maternal blood ingestion during delivery.

Clinical Findings. Visible bright red or dark red blood in vomitus or stool.

Diagnostic Studies. Blood of maternal origin can be differentiated from infant blood by testing for fetal hemoglobin using the alkali denaturation test (APT).

Differential Diagnosis. The differential diagnosis includes infant gastrointestinal bleeding caused by trauma, bowel duplication, intussusception, volvulus, bowel hemangioma or telangiectasia, rectal prolapse, vitamin K deficiency, or anal fissure.

Management. No treatment is necessary if blood is of maternal origin, although breakdown of maternal blood may exaggerate neonatal jaundice.

Orthopedic Conditions

Fractured Clavicle and Brachial Palsy

See Chapter 43.

Polydactyly and Syndactyly

Polydactyly is a condition that varies from a skin tag to a fully formed finger or toe with a nail; they most commonly extend from the postaxial side. Postaxial polydactyly is an inherited condition in the African American population. In the Asian and white population preaxial duplication is more common. In contrast, syndactyly can be identified by finding fingers or toes fused by skin and sometimes bone. Syndactyly and polydactyly occur in isolation or as part of a variety of syndromes (Carrigan, 2016; Winell and Davidson, 2016).

History and Clinical Findings. A positive family history is found in 30% of cases (Carrigan, 2016; Winell and Davidson, 2016). In polydactyly, a floppy digit is seen on the foot or hand. It varies in degree of formation. Syndactyly is webbing of two digits, partially or to the tip of the digit.

Management. For polydactyly, surgical removal of the floppy extra digit is indicated. If the digit is stabilized by bone, surgical removal is deferred until the patient is older, when function can be assessed. Surgical separation of syndactyly is recommended by at least 2 to 3 years of age. Close physical examination for other congenital anomalies is recommended.

Central Nervous System Conditions

Congenital Hydrocephalus

Congenital hydrocephalus is an over accumulation of cerebrospinal fluid (CSF) in the brain's ventricles at birth (Kinsman and Johnson, 2016). Malformations, infections, IVH, and disorders in brain development can lead to congenital hydrocephalus. The incidence varies depending on which of these conditions is causative. Cranial ultrasonography shows dilated ventricles. Often an MRI is obtained to further define the anatomy.

History and Clinical Findings
- Head circumference enlarging or rapidly increasing in size
- Cranial sutures separated by large, tense fontanelles

Management. Medications that decrease CSF production (e.g., acetazolamide), a ventriculoperitoneal shunt, or both are used. Referral to a pediatric neurosurgeon should be prompt. Refer to Chapter 46 for ongoing management of hydrocephalus.

Intraventricular Hemorrhage

IVH occurs within the ventricles of the brain, usually within the first 72 hours of life. Risk factors include prematurity, RDS, hypoxic-ischemic or hypotensive injury, increased or decreased cerebral blood flow, hypertension, hypervolemia, and reduced vascular integrity. The incidence of IVH decreases with increasing gestational age. Infants weighing less than 1000 g are particularly prone to severe IVH (Carlo and Ambalavanan, 2016c).

History and Clinical Findings
- Risk factors (as listed in previous paragraph above)
- Majority of cases are asymptomatic
- Diminished or absent Moro reflex, apnea
- Poor muscle tone, lethargy, somnolence
- Periods of pallor or cyanosis
- Inadequate suck
- High-pitched, shrill cry; seizures
- Bulging fontanel or sudden increase in head circumference

Diagnostic Studies. Ultrasonography is used to classify IVH into grades I to IV based on the presence and quantity of blood in the ventricles or brain tissue. Screening cranial ultrasounds are routinely performed on all premature infants. The initial screening typically is done between 7 and 14 postnatal days, and follow-up studies are done based on the infant's clinical course and initial findings (AAP, 2017).

Management and Prognosis. Prevention and treatment may include the following:
- Prevention
  - Glucocorticoid given antenatally at 24 to 34 weeks of gestational age for pregnancies at risk for pre-term delivery to reduce the severity of RDS and associated hypoxia
  - Supportive care including meticulous fluid and electrolyte management and avoidance of wide swings in blood pressure
  - Careful respiratory care to avoid hypocarbia and hypoxia
  - Minimal stimulation
  - Indomethacin in the very low birthweight infants reduces the incidence of severe IVH
- Treatment
  - Acetazolamide decreases CSF production
  - Repeated lumbar punctures
  - Ventriculoperitoneal shunt or external ventriculostomy

Outcome is related to white matter involvement, with grade IV lesions being associated with the most adverse outcome.

TABLE 29.3	Hypoxic-Ischemic Encephalopathy in Term Infants		
Signs	Stage 1	Stage 2	Stage 3
Level of consciousness	Hyper alert	Lethargic	Stuporous, coma
Muscle tone	Normal	Hypotonic	Flaccid
Posture	Normal	Flexion	Decerebrate
Tendon reflexes/clonus	Hyperactive	Hyperactive	Absent
Myoclonus	Present	Present	Absent
Moro reflex	Strong	Weak	Absent
Pupils	Mydriasis	Miosis	Unequal, poor light reflex
Seizures	None	Common	Decerebration
Electroencephalogram	Normal	Low-voltage changing to seizure activity	Burst suppression to isoelectric
Duration	<24 h if progresses, otherwise may remain normal	24 h-24 days	Days to weeks
Outcome	Good	Variable	Death, severe deficits

Adapted from Sarnat H, Sarnat M. Neonatal encephalopathy following fetal distress: a clinical and electroencephalopathic study. *Arch Neurol.* 1976;33:696; cited in Kliegman RM, Stanton BF, St Geme JW, et al., eds. *Nelson Textbook of Pediatrics.* 20th ed. Philadelphia: Saunders/Elsevier; 2016.

Hypoxic-Ischemic Insults

There are three stages of newborn hypoxic-ischemic insult (stages I, II, and III, or mild, moderate, and severe) (Table 29.3). Brain damage results from fetal hypoxia or ischemia over an extended period followed by metabolic and respiratory acidosis. Compensatory mechanisms, such as shunting blood through the ductus to maintain brain, heart, adrenal, kidney, liver, and intestine perfusion ultimately fails if the insult is severe enough. Depending on the organ(s) most damaged, a variety of signs and symptoms can be seen; 20% to 30% of infants with hypoxic-ischemic encephalopathy die in the neonatal period, and up to 30% to 50% develop permanent neurodevelopmental disabilities. Causes of the initial hypoxic or ischemic insult include abruptio placentae, hemorrhage, cord compression, mechanical injury, severe maternal hypertension or diabetes, and inadequate resuscitation of the infant (Carlo and Ambalavanan, 2016c).

Clinical Findings. Infants can have apnea, pallor, cyanosis, and bradycardia unresponsiveness to stimulation. Seizure activity can be a consequence of a hypoxic-ischemic event.

Management and Prognosis. Management consists of whole body or selective cerebral hypothermia, seizure control, and end-organ damage management. The prognosis depends on the effectiveness of managing the underlying symptoms. Severe complications (hypoxia, hypoglycemia, shock) and encephalopathy characterized by flaccid coma, apnea, and seizures are

associated with a poorer prognosis (Carlo and Ambalavanan, 2016c). An infant who remains neurologically abnormal after the initial recovery phase (2 weeks) is more likely to have suffered permanent neurologic impairment. A low Apgar score at 20 minutes, absence of spontaneous respirations, and persistence of abnormal neurologic signs at 2 weeks of age predict death or severe cognitive and motor deficits; Apgar scores done at 1 and 5 minutes are far less predictive of outcome (AAP, 2015).

Myelomeningocele

A myelomeningocele is the result of failure to close the posterior neural tube and the vertebral column. This is the most severe form of neural tube defect occurring in 1/4000 live births (Kinsman and Johnston, 2016). Genetic and environmental factors play a causative role (see Chapter 46 for more information).

History and Clinical Findings
- History of poor prenatal intake of folic acid and exposure to hyperthermia or valproic acid
- Sac-like cyst containing meninges and spinal fluid covered by thin layer of partially epithelialized skin; 75% found in the lumbosacral area
- Flaccid paralysis of lower extremities
- Absence of deep tendon reflexes
- Lack of response in lower extremities to touch and pain
- Constant urinary dribbling

Management, Prognosis, and Prevention. Surgical repair, sometimes in utero in advanced centers, and multidisciplinary supportive management are indicated. The mortality rate is 10% to 15% in aggressively treated children with most deaths occurring before 4 years old. At least 70% have normal intelligence, but seizure disorders, hydrocephalus, learning disabilities, and neurogenic bowel and bladder are more common than in the general population (Kinsman and Johnston, 2016). Prenatal folic acid supplementation (400 mcg/day) with a daily multivitamin helps prevent neural tube defects and should be taken by all females of childbearing age. Prenatal vitamins have at least 400 mcg of folic acid/vitamin; however, additional folic acid supplementation (4000 mcg) is recommended for those women who have a previous child with a neural tube defect (AAP, 2017).

Infections of the Newborn

Four mechanisms for acquiring neonatal infections exist:
- Transplacental, when the mother acquires an organism that invades her bloodstream and passes through the placenta
- Vertical, when organisms in the vagina invade the uterine amniotic fluid
- Exposure during the birth process
- Horizontal, when the newborn is exposed to environmental agents after birth

Syphilis is transplacentally acquired; herpes, gonorrhea, group B streptococcus (GBS), *Listeria, Escherichia coli,* and *Chlamydia trachomatis* are typically vertically acquired (Martin and Fanaroff, 2015). Staphylococcal infection is the most common horizontal infection. The most common means for horizontal transmission is unwashed hands.

Risk factors for newborn sepsis include early rupture of amniotic membranes, preterm labor, prolonged rupture of membranes, maternal fever, maternal diagnosis of chorioamnionitis, maternal tachycardia, fetal tachycardia, and malodorous amniotic fluid. The neonate with sepsis can be asymptomatic or, due to delayed immune response to local infection, display nonspecific

• BOX 29.3 Neonatal Sepsis

History

"Not doing well"
Temperature instability (often hypothermia)
Jitteriness
Poor feeding, vomiting
Irritability or lethargy
Apnea or respiratory distress
Seizures

Physical Examination

Jaundice
Pallor
Petechiae or purpura
Rash
Hepatosplenomegaly
Poor tone and perfusion
Tachycardia or bradycardia
Tachypnea
Cyanosis, grunting, flaring, retractions

Laboratory Evaluation

Blood for CBC with differential, platelet count, and culture (evaluating for anemia; increase or decrease in WBC count with left shift; thrombocytopenia); serum ammonia for urea cycle defects
Urine for analysis and culture typically not done in the first 72 h of life because of low yield
CSF often obtained for protein, glucose, cell count, and culture (evaluating for elevated protein and WBC count; depressed glucose)

Management

Combination broad-spectrum antibiotic coverage for gram-positive cocci, gram-negative bacilli, and *Listeria* is recommended. Consider adding coverage for herpes infection when suspected. *Listeria* is treated with ampicillin; *GBS* can be treated with the penicillins and the cephalosporins; gram-negative organisms are well covered by aminoglycosides and some cephalosporins.

CBC, Complete blood count; CSF, cerebrospinal fluid; GBS, group B streptococcus; WBC, white blood cell.

infection symptoms, such as poor feeding or temperature instability (Martin and Fanaroff, 2015). Organisms quickly invade the systemic circulation, and significant deterioration occurs before it can be clinically recognized. Because of the serious nature of neonatal sepsis, a newborn with significant risk factors or a clinically unstable neonate without perinatal risk factors warrants investigation and initiation of appropriate antibiotics (Box 29.3).

Toxoplasmosis

Toxoplasmosis is caused by *Toxoplasma gondii,* an obligate intracellular protozoan. *T. gondii* infects most species of warm-blooded animals, particularly cats. Cats excrete oocysts in their stools; intermediate hosts include cattle, pigs, and sheep. Humans become infected by consumption of poorly cooked meat or by accidental ingestion of oocysts from soil or in contaminated food. Depending on the timing of the infection, 17% to 65% of untreated women who acquire toxoplasmosis during gestation transmit the parasite to their fetuses (McLeod, Van Tubbergen and Boyer, 2016).

History and Clinical Findings

* Prematurity and low Apgar scores
* Infants with congenital infection may be asymptomatic at birth (AAP, 2018)

* Jaundice, anemia, hepatosplenomegaly
* Chorioretinitis, microcephaly

Diagnostic Studies. CT of the brain shows calcifications or hydrocephalus. The CSF shows high protein, low glucose, and evidence of *T. gondii.* Serum-specific immunoglobulin G (IgG), IgM, and IgA antibodies against toxoplasmosis are elevated.

Differential Diagnosis. Sepsis, syphilis, and hemolytic disease are considered in the differential diagnosis.

Management, Prognosis, and Prevention. Pyrimethamine plus sulfadiazine (with folic acid supplementation) for up to 1 year is often recommended. Treatment usually eliminates the manifestations of toxoplasmosis, such as active chorioretinitis, meningitis, encephalitis, hepatitis, splenomegaly, and thrombocytopenia. However, infants with extensive involvement at birth often have mild to severe impairment of vision, hearing, cognitive function, and other neurologic functions. No protective vaccine is available. Pregnant women should be informed not to handle raw meat or contaminated cat litter, to wash fruits and vegetables before consumption, to cook meat and eggs well, and to drink pasteurized milk.

Congenital Rubella

Rubella is a ribonucleic acid (RNA) virus. It is transmitted by person-to-person contact; the virus infects the placenta and is transmitted to the fetus. It occurs more frequently in the winter and spring.

History and Clinical Findings

* Maternal infection before 16 weeks of gestation results in highest rate congenital defects
* Negative maternal rubella titers at beginning of pregnancy
* As many as 50% of infected women are asymptomatic (AAP, 2018)
* May be asymptomatic in the newborn period
* Cataract or glaucoma and microphthalmia, hearing loss
* "Blueberry muffin" skin lesions, congenital heart disease
* Intellectual disability

Diagnostic Studies. The diagnosis of rubella typically is made through the measurement of serum immunoglobulins. Alternatively, the rubella virus can be isolated from nasopharyngeal secretions, conjunctiva, urine, stool, and CSF.

Management and Prevention. No specific drug therapy is available. Monitoring and intervention for developmental, auditory, visual, and medical needs improve the quality of life for these children. Congenital rubella is now a rare occurrence because of widespread administration of an effective vaccine (AAP, 2018). All women of childbearing age should have rubella serology titers, and vaccine should be given to IgG-seronegative, nonpregnant women.

Cytomegalovirus

CMV, a member of the herpesvirus family, is transmitted via intimate and household contact with virus-containing secretions and blood products. When CMV is introduced into a household, it is common that all members will acquire the infection. CMV transmission to the infant occurs via the placenta, passage through an infected maternal genital tract, or postnatally by ingestion of CMV-positive human milk. Infections occur worldwide and most humans are infected by the time they reach adulthood. About 0.5% to 1% of all live-born infants are infected in utero and excrete CMV at birth. As many as 90% of infected newborns are asymptomatic. Fetal damage is worse following an infection in the first half of the pregnancy. Infection can be primary (new exposure in a previously CMV negative mother) or nonprimary (acquisition of different strain or reactivation of existing strain) (AAP, 2018; Martin and Fanaroff, 2015).

History and Clinical Findings
- Maternal infection (although many women are asymptomatic)
- SGA and/or IUGR
- Jaundice, hepatosplenomegaly
- Petechial rash, chorioretinitis
- Cerebral calcifications, microcephaly

Diagnostic Studies. CMV is isolated in urine, saliva, or other body fluid cultures; recovery of the virus from a target organ is strong evidence of its pathology. Detection of viral deoxyribonucleic acid (DNA) by immunofluorescence antibody (IFA) are available. Proof of congenital infection requires obtaining specimens within 2 to 4 weeks of birth. Viral isolation or a strongly positive test for serum IgM anti-CMV antibody, especially with a fourfold rise in titers, is considered diagnostic.

Management, Prognosis, and Prevention. Treatment of symptomatic infants with oral valganciclovir for 6 months results in improved audiologic and neurodevelopmental outcomes at 2 years of age (AAP, 2018). The prognosis of symptomatic congenital CMV infection is poor; a 3% to 10% mortality rate is seen, and up to 50% of children have isolated sensorineural hearing loss. Between these two extremes, psychomotor retardation, microcephaly, seizures, chorioretinitis, optic atrophy, intellectual disability, and learning disabilities are seen. Susceptible pregnant women exposed to the urine and saliva of CMV-infected children who attend day care centers are at high risk for acquiring the infection (AAP, 2018). Reinforce hand washing and simple hygienic measures in this population.

Group B Streptococcus

GBS, a gram-positive diplococcus, is a leading cause of sepsis in infants from birth to 3 months old, resulting in significant perinatal morbidity and mortality rates. Early-onset disease usually occurs within the first 24 hours of life but can occur in the first 7 days of life; late-onset disease occurs during the second week of life through 3 months of age.

The organism colonizes the maternal genitourinary and gastrointestinal tracts. Pregnant women are usually asymptomatic, but they can manifest chorioamnionitis, endometritis, or urinary tract infection. Infants born of women who are highly colonized are more likely to become infected. GBS is acquired by newborns following vertical transmission (e.g., ascending infection through ruptured amniotic membranes or contamination following passage through the colonized birth canal). As many as 50% of infants with early-onset disease are symptomatic at birth. The highest attack rate of early-onset GBS is in high-risk deliveries, premature SGA infants, very low birthweight infants, or those with prolonged ruptured membranes. Full-term infants account for 50% of cases. Colonization of pregnant women and newborns ranges from 15% to 35%. The incidence of early-onset GBS disease declined from 1 to 4 cases per 1000 live births to 0.24 cases per 1000 live births due to widespread chemoprophylaxis (AAP, 2018).

History and Clinical Findings
- Infants born before 37 weeks of gestation
- Rupture of membranes 18 hours or longer
- Maternal fever during labor above 100.4°F (40°C) oral
- Previous delivery of a sibling with invasive GBS disease
- Maternal chorioamnionitis including rupture of membranes and maternal fever with at least two of the following:

- Maternal tachycardia (heart rate greater than 90 bpm)
- Fetal tachycardia (heart rate greater than 170 bpm)
- Maternal leukocytosis (white blood cell count greater than 15,000/mm^3)
- Uterine tenderness
- Foul-smelling amniotic fluid
- Poor feeding, temperature instability
- Cyanosis, apnea, tachypnea, grunting, flaring, and retracting
- Seizures, lethargy, bulging fontanelle
- Rapid onset and deterioration

Diagnostic Studies. Cultures of blood, CSF, or both are definitive; Gram stain of body fluids typically sterile is presumptive evidence of infection.

Differential Diagnosis. RDS, amniotic fluid aspiration syndrome, persistent fetal circulation, infection or sepsis from other organisms, and metabolic problems are included in the differential diagnosis.

Management, Prognosis, and Prevention. Initiate antibiotic therapy with a penicillin (usually ampicillin) and an aminoglycoside, often gentamicin, until GBS has been differentiated from *E. coli* or *Listeria* sepsis or other organisms (AAP, 2018). Duration of therapy is 10 (bacteremia without focus) to 14 days (uncomplicated meningitis) minimum. Consultation with pediatric infectious disease specialists is recommended.

Screening of all pregnant women for GBS at 35 to 37 weeks of gestation is recommended. Antepartum treatment of asymptomatic mothers carrying GBS is not recommended. The mortality rate of early-onset disease is as high as 20%; mortality rate is highest in very low birthweight infants and in those with low neutrophil count (<1500/mm^3), low Apgar scores, hypotension, apnea, and a delay in antimicrobial therapy initiation. Chemoprophylaxis of high-risk, colonized, pregnant women is effective for preventing early-onset GBS infection. The American Academy of Pediatrics (AAP, 2018) developed consensus guidelines that outline screening and risk-based GBS prevention. Treatment consists of IV penicillin or ampicillin given to high-risk women at the onset of labor, repeated every 4 hours until the infant is born.

Listeriosis

Listeria monocytogenes is a small gram-positive rod isolated from soil, streams, sewage, certain foods, silage, dust, and slaughterhouses. Food-borne disease transmission is related to soft-ripened cheese, whole and 2% milk, uncooked hot dogs, undercooked chicken, raw vegetables, and shellfish. The newborn infant acquires the organism transplacentally, by aspiration or ingestion at the time of delivery. Late-onset disease (typically at 8 to 30 days) is also possible, usually presenting with meningitis and a fatality rate of approximately 25%.

History and Clinical Findings
- Brown-stained amniotic fluid
- Generalized symptoms of sepsis
- Whitish posterior pharyngeal and cutaneous granulomas
- Disseminated erythematous papules on skin

Diagnostic Studies. Culture blood, CSF, meconium, and urine. The CSF shows elevated protein, depressed glucose, and a high leukocyte count. Cultures of the placenta and amniotic fluid also may be helpful.

Management and Prognosis
- Administer IV ampicillin and an aminoglycoside (gentamicin) as initial therapy for severe infections.
- The duration of therapy is 14 days for infections without meningitis and at least 21 days for infections with meningitis (AAP, 2018).

Transplacentally acquired listeriosis often results in spontaneous abortion. The death rate of premature infants with *Listeria* pneumonia noted within 12 hours of birth approaches 100%. The mortality rate varies from 14% to 56% if the disease develops within the first week of life, and it is especially high in premature infants. Intellectual disability, paralysis, and hydrocephalus occur in survivors of *Listeria* meningitis (Martin and Fanaroff, 2015).

Congenital Varicella

Varicella-zoster virus (VZV) is a herpesvirus. Humans are the only infection source for this highly contagious virus. The infectivity rate for congenital varicella syndrome is 2% when exposure occurs between 7 and 20 weeks of gestation (LaRussa and Marin, 2016).

History and Clinical Findings
- History of maternal chickenpox infection
- Limb atrophy
- Scarring of the skin in a dermatomal distribution
- Microcephaly
- Eye manifestations

Diagnostic Studies. Diagnosis of congenital VZV is made by a history of maternal infection, and viral DNA identification by polymerase chain reaction in tissue samples.

Management, Prognosis, and Prevention. Experts recommend acyclovir for pregnant women with varicella, especially in the second or third trimester (AAP, 2018). Varicella-zoster immune globulin (VariZIG) is recommended for the term newborn infant whose mother had chickenpox onset within 5 days before delivery or within 48 hours after delivery. All exposed premature infants younger than 28 weeks of gestation or 1000 g or less birthweight should receive VariZIG; exposed premature infants 28 weeks of gestation and older whose mothers lack serologic evidence of disease or a reliable history of disease also require VariZIG (AAP, 2018). Despite having received VariZIG, about 50% of infants may still develop a mild varicella infection. If VariZIG is not available, then immunoglobulin intravenous (IGIV) is recommended. VariZIG is not indicated if the mother has varicella-zoster (shingles) only. Airborne and contact precautions are recommended for neonates born to mothers with varicella for 21 days from last exposure or 28 days if they received VariZIG.

Target prevention efforts to potential mothers. Varicella vaccination is recommended for nonpregnant women of childbearing age who have no history of varicella infection (AAP, 2018) (see Chapter 31).

Sexually Transmitted Infections

Gonorrhea

Neisseria gonorrhoeae is a gram-negative diplococcus that occurs only in humans. The organism lives in exudate and secretions of infected mucous membranes, and is transmitted primarily through sexual contact and birth. Gonococcal infections in the newborn are acquired primarily during delivery.

History and Clinical Findings. There is a history of maternal gonococcal infection. Findings include conjunctivitis, and rarely septicemia, pneumonia, or joint infection.

Diagnostic Studies. Culture of eye and body fluids (blood, joint fluid, abscess) are positive for *N. gonorrhoeae*.

Management and Prevention. Administer a single dose of intramuscular ceftriaxone 25 to 50 mg/kg (not to exceed 125 mg) for the prophylaxis of infants born to mothers with active gonorrhea. Because gonorrheal conjunctivitis can rapidly lead to blindness, all infants are given eye prophylaxis at birth with erythromycin 0.5% ophthalmic ointment (AAP, 2018).

Chlamydia

Chlamydial infection is caused by an obligate intracellular parasite, *C. trachomatis,* and is the most common sexually transmitted infection in the United States. Acquisition occurs in approximately 50% of infants born vaginally to infected mothers and in some infants delivered by cesarean section with intact membranes. The risk of developing conjunctivitis is 25% to 50% in infants who have acquired *C. trachomatis;* the risk with pneumonia is 5% to 30% (AAP, 2018).

History and Clinical Findings
- History of maternal chlamydial infection
- Conjunctivitis a few days to several weeks after birth
- Infant commonly afebrile with normal activity level
- Pneumonia 2 to 19 weeks after birth

Diagnostic Studies
- Although not approved by the U.S. Food and Drug Administration, nucleic acid amplification tests (NAATs) have published sensitives and specificities as high as those for culture.
- Routine bacterial cultures are not helpful.
- When NAATs are not available, Gram stain and culture of discharge from the eye (must include epithelial cells from the palpebral conjunctival sac because chlamydia is an obligate parasite) are necessary for diagnosis.

Management and Prevention. Oral erythromycin or azithromycin will be given for both conjunctivitis and pneumonia (AAP, 2018; Workowski and Bolan, 2015). Appropriate treatment of the pregnant woman before delivery prevents disease in the newborn. Prophylaxis with oral erythromycin of the asymptomatic infant born to an untreated but *Chlamydia*-positive woman generally is contraindicated because of the increased risk of developing hypertrophic pyloric stenosis.

Syphilis

Syphilis is caused by the spirochete *Treponema pallidum,* which crosses the placenta in an infected mother. Routine maternal serologic testing is legally required during prenatal care in all U.S. states.

History and Clinical Findings
- Maternal infection and positive serologic testing
- The majority of neonates are asymptomatic at birth
- Failure to thrive, restlessness, fever, persistent rhinorrhea
- Maculopapular or bullous dermal lesions, hepatosplenomegaly

Diagnostic Studies. Individualize evaluation depending on the adequacy of maternal syphilis treatment and follow-up. Consultation with infectious disease may be indicated. CSF evaluation shows high protein, low glucose, high white blood cell count, and positivity on Venereal Disease Research Laboratory (VDRL) test. Serum liver enzymes are elevated with liver involvement and serum rapid plasma reagin (RPR) test is positive.

Management and Prognosis. For proven or highly probable congenital syphilis, the CDC recommends 10 consecutive days of crystalline penicillin G 100,000 to 150,000 units/kg/day (Red Book, 2018-2021). For infants with less certain evidence of syphilis, alternative regimens are available; reference to the latest CDC guidelines or the AAP Red Book is recommended. Untreated congenital syphilis can lead to severe multiorgan involvement. Infants who are appropriately treated have a good prognosis.

Herpes Simplex Virus

Three clinically distinguishable categories of herpes simplex virus (HSV) (Fig 29.4) infection exist: (1) disseminated disease; (2)

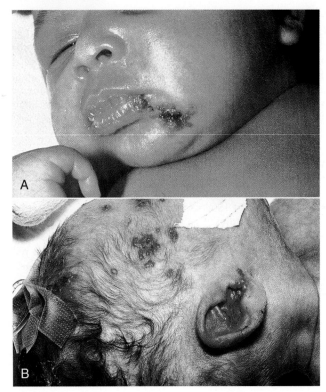

• **Fig 29.4** Herpes Simplex Virus (From Cohen BA. *Pediatric Dermatology*. 4th ed. Philadelphia: Elsevier; 2013, Fig 2-45A and B.)

CNS disease; and (3) disease restricted to the skin, eyes, and mouth (AAP, 2018). HSV is transmitted by direct contact with infected maternal genitalia during the birth process. Transplacental transmission occurs but has been reported in only a few cases. The risk of neonatal infection is highest with primary genital infection (see Chapter 31 for further discussion).

History and Clinical Findings. The mother may have active lesions and deliver vaginally. Vesicles in the skin, eye, and mouth are found. Signs or symptoms of encephalitis, pneumonia, or sepsis also can be present.

Diagnostic Studies. The virus is isolated in tissue cultures obtained from vesicles, nasopharyngeal or conjunctival swabs, urine, stool, and tracheal secretions; alternatively, vesicle scrapings can be evaluated for antigens with rapid diagnostic tests.

Management, Prognosis, and Prevention. Acyclovir is given for 14 days (skin, eyes, and mouth infection), up to 21 days (disseminated or involving the CNS) for HSV (AAP, 2018). Additionally, treatment with ophthalmic drugs (1% trifluridine, 0.1% iododeoxyuridine, or 0.15% ganciclovir) is used for infants with ocular involvement (AAP, 2018). Despite effective antiviral therapy, disseminated neonatal HSV infections and localized encephalitis are associated with considerable morbidity and mortality. Some obstetricians provide antiviral therapy in the final weeks of life for women with a history of HSV. The risk of acquiring this serious infection is lowered by performing cesarean delivery before rupture of membranes in any pregnancy in which signs or symptoms of HSV infection occur.

Human Immunodeficiency Virus

The human immunodeficiency virus (HIV), a retrovirus, is transmitted to the newborn via the placenta or at birth secondary to exposure to maternal blood (see Chapter 31).

Drug Exposure

Neonatal Abstinence Syndrome

Although the incidence varies by location, maternal drug abuse affects about 5.8/1000 births (Ko et al., 2016; Patrick et al., 2015). Complications of maternal drug abuse include higher risk of infection including syphilis, gonorrhea, hepatitis, and HIV; psychiatric, nervous, and emotional disorders; and abruptio placentae. Elimination of in utero drug exposure can occur only if high-risk mothers are identified and referral to a substance abuse prevention program occurs.

The use of "street drugs" and prescription medications place the infant at risk for poor neurologic outcomes and withdrawal symptoms at birth. Drugs of abuse generally can be divided into opioids, CNS stimulants, CNS depressants, and hallucinogens. The onset of neonatal symptoms begins at birth or up to about 14 days after birth; with symptoms lasting from a few days to 18 months. Symptomatic neonates need both pharmacologic and nonpharmacologic intervention for withdrawal symptoms; asymptomatic neonates need nonpharmacologic interventions as identified later (Hudak and Tan, 2012/2016). The use of an objective scoring tool helps guide therapy. The Neonatal Drug-Withdrawal Scoring System (Lipsitz, 1975) (Table 29.4) is a relatively simple numeric system using a value of 4 as an indication of significant withdrawal signs. A more comprehensive scoring system (21 symptoms and different assigned score for each) is the Modified Finnegan's Neonatal Abstinence Scoring Tool (Finnegan, 1990), which can be found at www.lkpz.nl/docs/lkpz_pdf_1310485469.pdf.

Cocaine (Crack) Exposure

Cocaine is a local anesthetic and CNS stimulant that some believe to be a teratogen that crosses the placenta.

Clinical Findings. Includes maternal exposure to cocaine or crack, and positive maternal and/or infant urine drug screen. Premature labor, abruptio placentae, intrauterine growth restriction, and fetal asphyxia with meconium staining are possible. Many infants show no adverse effects from maternal cocaine use and no clinically documented neonatal withdrawal syndrome for cocaine has been identified (Carlo, 2016a).

Management, Complications, and Prevention
• Do not breastfeed because cocaine is detectable in breast milk.
• Close neurodevelopmental follow-up and testing are necessary through the first several years of age.
• Involvement of the Department of Child and Family Services is essential.

Heroin and Methadone Exposure

Heroin and methadone are narcotics that cross the placenta.
History and Clinical Findings
• Maternal exposure to heroin or methadone
• Urine drug screen positive for opiates in mother and/or infant
• Increased incidence of stillbirths and SGA infants, but not congenital anomalies
• Tremors and hyperirritability often coarser than those with hypoglycemia
• Limbs rigid and hyperreflexic, fist sucking
• Skin abrasions secondary to hyperactivity
• Tachypnea, poor feeding, high-pitched cry
• Vomiting, diarrhea
• Low birthweight or SGA in 50% (Carlo, 2016a)

TABLE 29.4 Neonatal Drug-Withdrawal Scoring System

SIGNS	SCORE			
	0	1	2	3
Tremors (muscle activity of limbs)	Normal	Minimally increased when hungry or disturbed	Moderate or marked increase when undisturbed; subside when fed or held snugly	Marked increase or continuous even when undisturbed, going on to seizure-like movements
Irritability (excessive crying)	None	Slightly increased	Moderate to severe when disturbed or hungry	Marked even when undisturbed
Reflexes	Normal	Increased	Markedly increased	
Stools	Normal	Explosive, but normal frequency	Explosive, more than 8 days	
Muscle tone	Normal	Increased	Rigidity	
Skin abrasions	No	Redness of knees and elbows	Breaking of the skin	
Respiratory rate/minute	<55	55-75	76-95	
Repetitive sneezing	No	Yes		
Repetitive yawning	No	Yes		
Vomiting	No	Yes		
Fever	No	Yes		

Reprinted with permission from Lipsitz PJ. A proposed narcotic withdrawal score for use with newborn infants: a pragmatic evaluation of its efficacy. *Clin Pediatr.* 1975;14(6):592–594.

Heroin withdrawal symptoms occur in the first 48 hours of life in 75% of affected newborns, depending on the daily maternal dose, duration of addiction, and most recent maternal dose. Symptoms of methadone withdrawal occur in up to 90% of affected newborns. A higher incidence of symptomatology is seen if the last dose was taken within 24 hours of birth. Overall the withdrawal syndrome is more severe and more prolonged with methadone than with heroin (Carlo, 2016a).

Differential Diagnosis. The differential diagnosis includes hypoglycemia and hypocalcemia.

Management and Prevention. Supportive management, such as swaddling, frequent feedings, and protection from external stimuli is needed. Education regarding sudden infant death syndrome is imperative because these infants are at increased risk. Child protective services must be involved before discharge. Medications (e.g., morphine, clonidine, buprenorphine, phenobarbital, and methadone) can be used if symptoms—such as severe irritability, vomiting and diarrhea, seizures, temperature instability, or severe tachypnea—are noted. Pregnant women who are addicted to heroin should be encouraged to enter a treatment program.

Fetal Alcohol Syndrome
See Chapters 3 and 32.

Additional Resources

Birth Defect Research for Children, Inc. www.birthdefects.org
Centers for Disease Control and Prevention (CDC): Birth Defects. www.cdc.gov/ncbddd/birthdefects/index.html
Centers for Disease Control and Prevention (CDC): Infectious Disease Information. www.cdc.gov/DiseasesConditions/
Cleft Palate Foundation. www.cleftline.org
Compassionate Friends. www.compassionatefriends.org
Group B Strep Association. www.groupbstrep.org
Infant Loss Resources. http://infantlossresources.org/
March of Dimes (Local chapters found online). www.marchofdimes.com
National Perinatal Association. www.nationalperinatal.org

References

Akay B, Klein MD. Surgical conditions of the anus and rectum. In: Kliegman RM, Stanton BF, St Geme JW, et al., eds. *Nelson Textbook of Pediatrics.* 20th ed. Philadelphia: Elsevier; 2016:1894–1897.

Ambalavanan N, Carlo WA. Meconium aspiration. In: Kliegman RM, Stanton BF, St Geme JW, et al., eds. *Nelson Textbook of Pediatrics.* 20th ed. Philadelphia: Elsevier; 2016:859–860.

American Academy of Pediatrics [AAP]. Clinical Report. Hospital Discharge of the High-Risk Neonate. *Pediatrics.* 2008;122(5):1119–1126. Reaffirmed May 2011.

American Academy of Pediatrics (AAP), Kimberlin DW, Brady MT, Jackson MA, Long SS, eds. *Red Book: 2018 Report of the Committee on Infectious Diseases.* 31st ed. Elk Grove Village, IL: American Academy of Pediatrics; 2018.

American Academy of Pediatrics (AAP). The Apgar score. *Pediatrics.* 2015;136(4):819–822.

American Academy of Pediatrics (AAP). Folic acid for the prevention of neural tube defects. *Pediatrics.* 1999;104(2):325–327. Reaffirmed 2017.

American Academy of Pediatrics (AAP) and American Heart Association. Eds. Weiner GM, Zaichkin J, Kattwinkel J. *Textbook of Neonatal Resuscitation.* 7th ed. Elk Grove Village, IL: American Academy of Pediatrics. Accessed at: https://www.aap.org/en-us/continuing-medical-education/life-support/NRP/Pages/NRP.aspx. September 4, 2018, 2016.

AAP Committee on Fetus and Newborn and ACOG Committee on Obstetric Practice; Kilpatrick SJ, Papile LA, eds. & associate eds. Macones, GA, Watterberg, KL. *Guidelines for Perinatal Care.* 8th ed. AAP and ACOG Publishers; 2017.

American Academy of Pediatrics and American College of Obstetricians and Gynecologists Committee on Obstetric Practice, Kilpatrick SJ, Papile LA, eds. & associate eds. Macones, GA, Watterberg, KL. Brain injury: hemorrhagic and periventricular white matter brain injury. In: *Guidelines for perinatal care.* 8th ed. AAP and ACOG Publishers; 2017:411–412.

American College of Obstetricians and Gynecologists (ACOG) Committee Opinion no. 689: delivery of a newborn with meconium-stained amniotic fluid. *Obstet Gynecol.* 2017;129:e33–e34.

Bales C, Liacourus CA. Intestinal atresia, stenosis, and malrotation. In: Kliegman RM, Stanton BF, St Geme JW, et al., eds. *Nelson Textbook of Pediatrics.* 20th ed. Philadelphia: Elsevier; 2016:1800–1804.

Carlo WA. Metabolic disturbances. In: Kliegman RM, Stanton BF, St Geme JW, et al., eds. *Nelson Textbook of Pediatrics.* 20th ed. Philadelphia: Elsevier; 2016:897–899.

Carlo WA, Ambalavanan N. Respiratory tract disorders. In: Kliegman RM, Stanton BF, St Geme JW, et al., eds. *Nelson Textbook of Pediatrics.* 20th ed. Philadelphia: Elsevier; 2016a:848–867.

Carlo WA, Ambalavanan N. The umbilicus. In: Kliegman RM, Stanton BF, St Geme JW, et al., eds. *Nelson Textbook of Pediatrics.* 20th ed. Philadelphia: Elsevier; 2016b:890–891.

Carlo WA, Ambalavanan N. Nervous system disorders. In: Kliegman RM, Stanton BF, St Geme JW, et al., eds. *Nelson Textbook of Pediatrics.* 20th ed. Philadelphia: Elsevier; 2016c:834–844.

Carrigan RB. The upper limb. In: Kliegman RM, Stanton BF, St Geme JW, et al., eds. *Nelson Textbook of Pediatrics.* 20th ed. Philadelphia: Saunders/Elsevier; 2016:3302–3309.

Centers for Disease Control and Prevention (CDC). Prevention of perinatal group B streptococcal disease—revised guidelines from CDC, 2010. *MMWR Recomm Rep.* 2010;59(RR–10):1–36.

Centers for Disease Control and Prevention (CDC). *Facts about Vitamin K Deficiency Bleeding*; 2017. Accessed at: https://www.cdc.gov/ncbddd/vitamink/facts.html. September 4, 2018.

Elder J. Congenital anomalies and dysgenesis of the kidneys. In: Kliegman RM, Stanton BF, St Geme JW, et al., eds. *Nelson textbook of pediatrics.* 20th ed. Philadelphia: Saunders/Elsevier; 2016:2554–2556.

Finnegan LP. Neonatal abstinence syndrome: assessment and pharmacotherapy. In: Nelson N, ed. *Current Therapy in Neonatal-Perinatal Medicine.* 2nd ed. Ontario: BC Decker; 1990.

Fiorino KN, Liacouras CA. congenital aganglionic megacolon (Hirschsprung disease). In: Kliegman RM, Stanton BF, St Geme JW, et al., eds. *Nelson Textbook of Pediatrics.* 20th ed. Philadelphia: Elsevier; 2016:1809–1811.

Garabedian C, Verpillat P, Czerkiewicz I, et al. Does a combination of ultrasound, MRI, and biochemical amniotic fluid analysis improve prenatal diagnosis of esophageal atresia? *Prenatal Diagnosis.* 2014;34(9):839–842.

Hudak ML, Tan RC, American Academy of Pediatrics (AAP) Committee on Drugs and Committee on Fetus and Newborn. Neonatal drug withdrawal. *Pediatrics.* 2012;129(2):540–560. Reaffirmed 2016.

Hughes HK, Kahl LK. *The Harriet Lane Handbook.* 21st ed. Philadelphia: Elsevier; 2018.

Hunter AK, Liacourus CA. Pyloric stenosis and other congenital anomalies of the stomach. In: Kliegman RM, Stanton BF, St Geme JW, et al., eds. *Nelson Textbook of Pediatrics.* 20th ed. Philadelphia: Elsevier; 2016:797–1799.

Kennedy M, Liacourus CA. Malrotation. In: Kliegman RM, Stanton BF, St Geme JW, et al., eds. *Nelson Textbook of Pediatrics.* 20th ed. Philadelphia: Elsevier; 2017:1803–1804.

Khan S, Orenstein S. Esophageal atresia and tracheoesophageal fistula. In: Kliegman RM, Stanton BF, St Geme JW, et al., eds. *Nelson Textbook of Pediatrics.* 20th ed. Philadelphia: Elsevier; 2016:1783–1784.

Kilpatrick SJ, Papile LA, eds. *Guidelines for Perinatal Care.* 8th ed. Elk Grove Village, IL: American Academy of Pediatrics and American College of Obstetricians and Gynecologists; 2017.

Kinsman S, Johnston MV. Congenital anomalies of the central nervous system. In: Kliegman RM, Stanton BF, St Geme JW, et al., eds. *Nelson Textbook of Pediatrics.* 20th ed. Philadelphia: Elsevier; 2016:2802–2819.

Ko JY, Patrick SW, Tong VT, Patel R, Lind JN, Barfield WD. Incidence of neonatal abstinence syndrome–28 states, 1999-2013. *MMWR Morb Mortal Wkly Rep.* 2016;65:799–802.

LaRussa PS, Marin M. Varicella-zoster virus infections. In: Kliegman RM, Stanton BF, St Geme JW, et al., eds. *Nelson Textbook of Pediatrics.* 20th ed. Philadelphia: Elsevier; 2016:1579–1586.

Lipsitz PJ. A proposed narcotic withdrawal score for use with newborn infants: a pragmatic evaluation of its efficacy. *Clin Pediatr.* 1975;14(6):592–594.

Mathews TJ, Driscoll AK. *NCHS Data Brief: Trends in Infant Mortality in the United States, 2005-2014*; 2017. Available at: https://www.cdc.gov/nchs/data/databriefs/db279.pdf.

Maheshwari A, Carlo WA. Diaphragmatic hernia. In: Kliegman RM, Stanton BF, St Geme JW, et al., eds. *Nelson Textbook of Pediatrics.* 20th ed. Philadelphia: Elsevier; 2016a:862–864.

Maheshwari A, Carlo WA. Necrotizing enterocolitis. In: Kliegman RM, Stanton BF, St Geme JW, et al., eds. *Nelson Textbook of Pediatrics.* 20th ed. Philadelphia: Elsevier; 2016b:869–871.

Martin RJ, Fanaroff AA, Walsh MC. *Fanaroff & Martin's Neonatal-Perinatal Medicine: Diseases of the Fetus and Infant.* 10th ed. Philadelphia: Elsevier/Saunders; 2015.

McLeod R, VanTubbergen C, Boyer KM. Toxoplasmosis (Toxoplasma gondii). In: Kliegman RM, Stanton BF, St Geme JW, et al., eds. *Nelson Textbook of Pediatrics.* 20th ed. Philadelphia: Elsevier; 2016:1723–1733.

Patrick SW, Davis MM, Lehmann CU, Cooper WO. Increasing incidence and geographic distribution of neonatal abstinence syndrome: United States 2009 to 2012. *J Perinatol.* 2015;35(8):650–655.

Porter CD, Avner ED. Anatomic abnormalities associated with hematuria. In: Kliegman RM, Stanton BF, St Geme JW, et al., eds. *Nelson Textbook of Pediatrics.* 20th ed. Philadelphia: Elsevier; 2016:2512–2517.

Tinanoff N. Cleft lip and palate. In: Kliegman RM, Stanton BF, St Geme JW, et al., eds. *Nelson Textbook of Pediatrics.* 20th ed. Philadelphia: Elsevier; 2016:1771–1772.

Workowski KA, Bolan GA, Centers for Disease Control and Prevention (CDC). Sexually transmitted diseases treatment guidelines, 2015. *MMWR Recomm Rep.* 2015;64(3):1–140. Available at: http://www.cdc.gov/std/tg2015/tg-2015-print.pdf.

Winell JJ, Davidson RS. Toe deformities. In: Kliegman RM, Stanton BF, St Geme JW, et al., eds. *Nelson Textbook of Pediatrics.* 20th ed. Philadelphia: Elsevier; 2016:3254–3256.

Zage PE, Ater JL. Neuroblastoma. In: Kliegman RM, Stanton BF, St Geme JW, et al., eds. *Nelson Textbook of Pediatrics.* 20th ed. Philadelphia: Elsevier; 2016:2461–2464.

30

Neurodevelopmental, Behavioral, and Mental Health Disorders

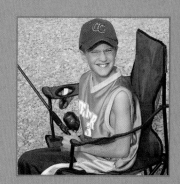

DAWN LEE GARZON, NANCY BARBER STARR, AND JENNIFER CHAUVIN

The term *mental health disorder* describes conditions that affect behavioral, emotional, and neurologic development; and neurologic development: stress, altered coping from difficult life circumstances, and psychiatric illness. *Neurodevelopmental disorders* are conditions recognized early in development, characterized by delays, deficits, or impairments in personal, social, academic, or occupational performance, or functioning. More specifically, the challenges affect emotions, behaviors, attention, memory, learning ability, and the ability to socialize, self-regulate, and maintain self-control. Neurodevelopmental disorders as defined in the DSM-5 include autism spectrum disorder (ASD), attention deficit/hyperactivity disorder (ADHD), specific learning disorder, intellectual development disorder, communication disorders, and motor disorders. The term *behavioral health disorder* includes emotional health issues, substance use and abuse, and neurodevelopmental and mental health disorders. It is a broader and more preferred term to mental health. There are many reasons for pediatric behavioral health issues, including exposure to environmental toxins, such as lead and mercury, genetic inheritance, chronic toxic stress, lack of opportunities to develop coping and resiliency, and adverse childhood experiences (ACEs). Anxiety and depression arise from a genetic predisposition, neurohormonal influences, and/or stresses of modern family life. Epigenetics, or the role of nongenetic influences of gene expression, may be a significant contributor to behavioral health disorders. Known epigenetic influences include trauma, ACEs, and toxic stress, including child maltreatment, parenting style, nutrition, hormones, environmental toxins, social support, drugs, and family interactions (Tost, Champagne & Meyer-Lindenberg, 2015). Common childhood stressors that can negatively impact child behavioral health include parental divorce or separation, domestic violence, child abuse or neglect, death of a parent or sibling, natural disasters, familial mental illness, exposure to media reports of traumatic events, school problems, interpersonal conflict, and/or prolonged separation (e.g., incarceration or military deployment) from a loved one.

The 2015 America's Children: Key National Indicators of Well-Being showed that 5% of responding parents identified their 4- to 17-year-old children as having severe emotional difficulties, impaired concentration, challenging behavior, or inability to get along well with others (Wallman, 2015). Significant problems were identified for 6% of males and 4% of females. Children living in families with incomes at the federal poverty level were twice as likely to have significant issues than those whose family incomes were at least twice the federal poverty level. Children living with only their mother (8%) were more likely to have significant problems compared with children living in two-parent families (4%). Lastly, 43% of parents reported seeking help from a general physician, whereas 55% consulted a behavioral health specialist for their child's treatment.

Children and adolescents in the United States are not getting the behavioral health care that they need. National estimates indicate that 21% to 23% of children have a mental health or substance use disorder (SUD), and that those with a psychiatric diagnosis represent the most severely impaired; those with mild symptoms often go unrecognized (Chun et al., 2016). Only half of the children and adolescents who meet diagnostic criteria for a behavioral health disorder visited a healthcare provider for treatment of their condition in the past year, and fewer than 20% receive the treatment that they need (Wallman, 2015). There is a particular shortage of pediatric behavioral health providers and child psychiatrists, especially in rural areas and for children and teens from lower socioeconomic backgrounds. This is the rationale for the development of the pediatric primary care mental health specialist (PMHS) certification, thus allowing for recognition of advanced expertise of pediatric nurse practitioners with demonstrated expertise in primary care mental health. Primary care providers (PCPs) must take active roles in the identification of and early intervention for children and adolescents with mental health disorders. *Bright Futures* call for assessment of family psychosocial functioning at all routine health supervision visits and routine screening for mental health issues using validated instruments for older school-age children and adolescents (Hagan et al., 2017).

Early behavioral health influences include the child's genetic composition and the intrauterine effects on the developing fetus. Known maternal factors that influence child behavioral health include maternal nutrition, especially vitamin B_{12}, folate and folic acid intake, and maternal stress including her own behavioral health, experiencing a natural disaster or chronic toxic stress, and maternal sustained psychosocial stress (Stevens, Rucklidge & Kennedy, 2018; Van den Bergh et al., 2017). Severe prenatal macro- and micronutrient deficiency is associated with the development of depression, autism, schizophrenia later in life as well as congenital central nervous system abnormalities (Stevens et al., 2018). There are known genetic links for conduct disorder (CD), bipolar disorder, depression, schizophrenia, attention-deficit hyperactivty disorder (ADHD), substance abuse, antisocial behavior, generalized anxiety disorder (GAD), and obsessive-compulsive disorder (OCD) among others.

From infancy through early adulthood, changes in the limbic system, specifically the amygdala and hippocampus, influence emotional development and the emergence of affective disorders, substance abuse, and high-risk behaviors. However, none of these brain differences alone appear to be necessary or sufficient for psychopathology to occur. Rather, environmental strengths and vulnerabilities and cumulative life experiences more strongly influence the number and severity of symptoms and the adaptive competencies that the child displays at any age. Activation of the hypothalamic-pituitary-adrenal (HPA) axis triggers release of cortisol, and elevated serum cortisol levels are toxic to central nervous system neurons, inhibiting the growth of dendrites and neurons and causing the death of neurons. There are profound effects of chronic stress during the final phase of brain growth when the brain prunes away unused neurons and dendritic connections. Children who experience chronic posttraumatic stress disorder (PTSD) following maltreatment have decreased hippocampal, prefrontal cortex, and amygdalar volumes (Morey, Haswell, Hooper, et al., 2016).

Neurodiversity is a concept that explains neurodevelopmental issues as differences or variations in brain structure or wiring rather than abnormalities. The framework allows children and families to approach challenges as differences rather than deficits, and it offers the perspective that the goal is to provide support to those who are neurodiverse in order to enable them to fully participate. This perspective is especially useful in removing barriers and advocating for a variety of teaching strategies with learning and attention issues. However, in order to receive support and services, a disability needs to be identified.

Caputo's triangle is a way to conceptualize neurodevelopmental disorders that represents them as a triangle with three main developmental streams representing brain function: motor, cognition, and social behavior (Voight, 2011). These streams have an associated *spectrum* and *continuum*: the spectrum identifies each stream as ranging from mild to severe, and the continuum represents the associated deficits or comorbidities in one or both of the other streams. The motor stream consists of gross motor, fine motor, and oral motor (speech, chewing, and swallowing) skills (on the mild end, the clumsy child or dysgraphia). The cognitive stream includes intellectual ability, language and communication, and nonverbal skills (on the mild end, a slower learner or letter identity and position difficulties). The social-behavior stream includes social abilities, attention, and impulse/hyperactive dimensions (on the mild end, a shy, inattentive, or hyperactive child).

Assessment and Management of Behavioral Health Disorders

A behavioral health disorder is a sustained behavior change that results in functional impairment. Because these problems cover a broad range of behavioral, emotional, and psychological disorders, many of which include genetic influences, the accurate identification of emotional, social, behavioral, and mental health status requires a thorough history and a physical examination. A targeted history should focus on child behavior and functional impairment

(Table 15.9 and Box 15.3). The physical examination detects underlying physical conditions that can result in behavioral or emotional changes. PCPs must recognize that common illness symptoms, such as fever, can change a child's behavior because of malaise, arthralgias, pain, or other physical symptoms. Chapter 15 includes details about the history, physical examination, and diagnostic evaluation of pediatric patients with behavioral health concerns.

Making Mental Health and Behavioral Diagnoses

Making behavioral health diagnoses is often difficult. PCPs must decide whether behaviors are within normal limits for age, temperament, family, health, and other factors. Comorbidities are common. In practice, several things may need to be addressed: the behavior, the family effects, nutrition, sleep, and other interrelated issues. In many cases, a behavioral health specialist such as a clinical psychologist or psychiatrist may be required to assist in diagnostic decision-making.

Management Strategies

After the diagnosis, the PCP must decide how to manage and/or co-manage problems with other pediatric specialists. Pediatric PCPs manage more behavioral health problems than ever before, largely because of the scarcity of behavioral health services or inadequate insurance coverage that makes behavioral health care out of reach for many families. However, many PCPs lack adequate education to manage complex problems. In addition, it is financially difficult for many busy primary care practices to offer the extended appointments needed for high-quality behavioral health care, and reimbursement for these services is different than that provided for medical care.

Evidence demonstrates the best outcomes occur when behavioral health and primary care are integrated; however, this model is not standard and PCPs must plan for how to manage children and youth with behavioral health issues. This includes, but is not limited to, determining referral sources to therapists and other behavioral health providers, identifying appropriate screening tools, and educating themselves about behavioral health. There are very good education programs available through organizations like The Reach Institute (www.thereachinstitute.org), Project Teach (www.projectteachny.org), and the National Association of Pediatric Nurse Practitioners (NAPNAP) (www.napnap.org). Almost half of the states in the United States have free phone consultation with a psychiatrist or other behavioral health provider to help PCPs identify and manage affected youth. A list of participating states and contact information is available online at http://web.jhu.edu/pedmentalhealth/nncpap_members.html.

As a rule, if the cause of the problem is a life event with acute, short-term consequences (such as the death of a pet or a friend moving away) or a common developmentally normal but troublesome behavior (e.g., temper tantrums or sibling rivalry), it can be managed in the primary care setting. More enduring problems, such as loss of a parent or major depression, may require collaboration or consultation with or referral to a pediatric behavioral health specialist.

Appropriate care of pediatric behavioral disorders always requires an interprofessional approach. Pharmacotherapy alone is never appropriate, nor should it be used without a thorough evaluation. Clinical practice guidelines further emphasize the need for treatments to be evidence-based and inclusive of short- and long-term follow-up plans. All ethical issues regarding consent and assent are especially important in mental health care. Caregivers and patients should be aware of treatment risks, benefits, and alternative options.

PCPs can find information from the Developmental Behavioral and Mental Health special interest group of the NAPNAP which has a comprehensive website for providers at www.dbmhresource.org/. Additionally, the American Academy of Pediatrics provides information about evidence-based psychosocial interventions online at www.aap.org/en-us/Documents/CRPsychosocialInterventions.pdf. This resource is updated multiple times a year. This webpage includes a wealth of information about the evidence-based diagnosis and management of pediatric behavioral health disorders, training resources, and links to practice guidelines and screening resources.

Common Behavioral Health Disorders

Anxieties

Anxiety

Anxiety causes apprehension and is differentiated from fear in that the stimuli is unknown or nonspecific. It is a normal developmental phenomenon that is experienced by every person at some point and may actually serve to heighten the senses and help in stressful situations. Anxious responses include somatic symptoms mediated by the autonomic system and include tachycardia, tachypnea, hypertension, gastrointestinal distress, tremor, sweating, and enhanced vigilance and reactivity. Anxiety that persists at high levels and causes maladaptive behavior warrants diagnosis and treatment. Anxiety disorders include conditions associated with childhood such as separation anxiety disorder (SAD), GAD, social anxiety disorder, OCD, agoraphobia, and PTSD. SAD, GAD, and social anxiety are often referred to as the pediatric anxiety disorder triad as they often happen in the same individual and have similar life courses and treatments. Anxiety disorders are some of the most common child and adolescent psychiatric conditions and are estimated to affect 15% to 20% of youth (Wehry et al., 2015). Children diagnosed with anxiety disorders tend to have multiple problems, have social functioning impairments, and are more likely to live with parents who experience symptoms of anxiety or mood disorders than their nonaffected peers. Anxiety disorders typically emerge in the preschool years although they are often not diagnosed until middle childhood. Children with early onset of these disorders generally have greater impairment of social and personal development, and thus have a much greater likelihood of poor subjective views of their personal mental and physical health, social relationships, career satisfaction, and home and family relationships in adolescence and adulthood.

Risk factors include (1) genetics (familial heritance and specific gene loci), (2) temperamental disposition for behavioral inhibition and/or shyness, and (3) social environment or life circumstances (e.g., parental distress, dysfunction, or trauma). Youngsters with anxiety disorders are at high risk for comorbid mood disorders and adolescent substance abuse.

Separation Anxiety Disorder

The essential feature of SAD is an abnormal reaction to real, impending, or imagined separation from major attachment figures, home, or familiar surroundings. Separation anxiety is a normal developmental phenomenon from about 7 months old through the preschool years. Some infants and toddlers experience excessive levels of distress with separation from their major caregiver and they cry, cannot be comforted, or refuse to be cared for

and comforted by a competent, substitute caregiver. Alternatively, older infants, toddlers, and preschoolers may act aggressively toward the substitute caregiver or intentionally injure themselves.

SAD is the most common pediatric anxiety disorder, causing difficulty with separation and interfering with daily activities and developmental tasks. It manifests from 5 to 16 years old and the mean age for clinical presentation is 9 years old. SAD is a risk factor for the future development of panic disorder and depression in adolescence or adulthood and evolves from a poor attachment relationship or the interaction among physiologic, cognitive, and overt behavioral factors in response to life events that threaten safety or primary relationships, or both. Among infants and young children, only about 10% of those affected by separation anxiety are referred for care despite the concerns of the majority of parents. Often, older children are brought to the PCP when the disorder results in school refusal or somatic symptoms. A significant number of children with school refusal have SAD, and many of these have comorbid depression. Sleep problems and impaired social interactions are also common.

Clinical Findings. The following are found in SAD:
- Developmentally inappropriate or excessive anxiety about separations
- Unrealistic worry about harm to self or loved ones, or fears about abandonment during periods of separation
- Reluctance to sleep alone or sleep away from home
- Persistent avoidance of being alone
- Nightmares about separation
- Physical complaints and signs of distress in anticipation of separation
- Social withdrawal during separations
- Environmental stress, parental dysfunction, and maternal depression are risk factors especially with panic disorder or agoraphobia, the fear of being outside the home, in crowds, or places they won't be able to easily leave

The Spielberger State-Trait Anxiety Inventory for Children (STAIC) is a 20-item, self-report scale useful with children 9 to 12 years old; it can also be used with high reading–skill younger children and low reading–skill adolescents. The Screen for Child Anxiety Related Disorders (SCARED) is a 41-item self-report scale in the public domain for use in 8- to 18-year-olds.

Differential Diagnosis. Anxiety disorder not associated with separation is a differential diagnosis. Anxiety may occur as a response to trauma or as a manifestation of PTSD. It is essential to identify cues that a traumatic experience or situation (e.g., sexual or physical abuse) is the source of the anxiety symptoms. Depression, social phobia/anxiety, and ADHD are also common comorbidities. Problems at home can cause or exacerbate school refusal. For instance, a child may want to stay at home if the child worries about the caregiver's safety when she is alone.

Management. Anxiety disorder is best treated as a family system or relationship-based problem. Symptom relief is the first priority in school-age children. Identifying and treating the source of the problem is the first line of treatment for infants and young children and a secondary focus of treatment for school-age children and adolescents. Note the role of attachment figures, and refer the child to a therapist for psycho-educational, behavioral, and cognitive-behavioral interventions. Eighty to ninety percent of children respond to a combination of psychoeducation and parental education/training. PCPs can help children identify their anxious feelings and physical responses to their anxiety. Caregivers benefit from learning how to help their children identify feelings of anxiety and by supporting them during exacerbations. Pharmacotherapy is not particularly helpful in reducing symptoms and should only be used if the child fails to respond to nonpharmacologic intervention and has considerable impairment in function, thus meriting referral to a pediatric behavioral health provider.

Generalized Anxiety Disorder

GAD is cognitive and obsessive in nature and causes excessive anxiety, worry, and apprehension generalized to a number of events or activities. These anxieties do not focus on a specific person, object, or situation, nor are they the result of a recent stressor. Children with GAD are characterized as "worriers" or as being "overwhelmed." The diagnosis is most often made in late middle childhood and adolescents aged 9 to 18 years old. GAD is one of the most prevalent psychiatric disorders, affecting as many as 15% of older children and adolescents and is the second most common pediatric anxiety disorder. However, only 22% of adolescents who meet diagnostic criteria for GAD are diagnosed by PCPs (McBride, 2015). There are clear genetic influences of GAD, especially in females.

Clinical Findings. Major symptoms of GAD are:
- Worry about future events and/or preoccupation with past behavior
- Poor-quality sleep and unexplained fatigue
- Irritability and tantrums in young children
- Overconcern about competence and marked preoccupation with performance

- Significant self-consciousness and unusual need for reassurance
- Restlessness, difficulty concentrating
- Somatic complaints without a physical basis
- Comorbidity with other anxiety disorders, ADHD, or mood disorder

Differential Diagnosis. Differential diagnoses are separation anxiety, adjustment disorder associated with a specific stressor, substance abuse, and ADHD. It is important to pay attention to cues that point to traumatic experiences or conditions as the source of anxiety symptoms and to symptoms suggestive of the presence of pediatric acute onset neuropsychiatric syndrome (PANS) (see OCD).

Management. The treatment of preschool children and toddlers generally focuses on behavioral and family interventions with the best response coming with interventions that incorporate cognitive behavior therapy with a caregiver component (Fig 30.1). Preschoolers may benefit from play therapy. Refer the older child or adolescent to a pediatric mental health therapist for treatment of symptoms using mindfulness, psychodynamic therapy, or cognitive-behavioral therapy (CBT). Individual and/or family counseling can be used to identify the source of anxiety and to help with family discord. Treatment outcomes are more positive when parents are involved in interventions that target familial contextual processes. Younger school-age children seem to benefit from a combination of cognitive-behavioral strategies and family intervention. Individual and group treatments or child- and

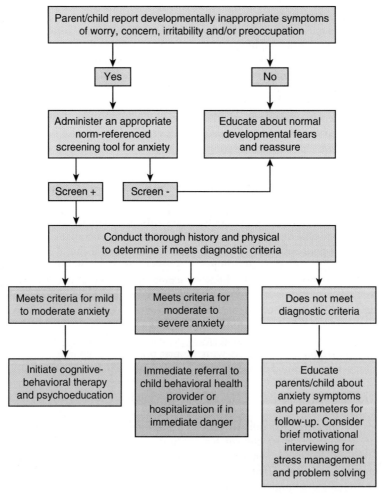

• **Fig 30.1** Primary care management of pediatric anxiety disorders.

family-focused treatments are equally effective, and follow-up data demonstrate that treatment gains are maintained up to several years after treatment.

Pharmacologic intervention in combination with psychotherapy is advisable for older children and adolescents (see Fig 30.1). Evidence points to the safety and efficacy of the selective serotonin reuptake inhibitors (SSRIs), especially sertraline, and fluoxetine; serotonin and norepinephrine reuptake inhibitors (SNRIs), especially venlafaxine and duloxetine; and other medications like buspirone (Table 30.1). Benzodiazepines are not recommended because of cognitive impairment and concerns about tolerance and dependency.

Obsessive-Compulsive Disorder

Obsessions are recurrent thoughts, images, or impulses that are disturbing to the child and difficult to dislodge. They often involve a sense of risk or fear of harm to the child or family members; concerns about contamination are common. Compulsions are repetitive behaviors or mental acts that the child feels driven to perform with the aim of reducing the anxiety associated with obsessions and include behaviors such as washing (e.g., hands, objects, or body), counting, or arranging objects. Recurrent worries, rituals, and superstitious games are common in children at various stages of development; these behaviors result in mild anxiety but

---

TABLE 30.1   Evidence-Supported Drug Therapy for Common Mental Health Conditions in Childhood

Drug Class and Examples	Conditions Treated	Primary Care Drug Interactions	Common Side Effects
Selective Serotonin Reuptake Inhibitor			
Fluoxetine (FDA approved 8+)	Anxiety; MDD, OCD, selective mutism	Multiple drug interactions Contraindicated drugs: MAOIs, tryptophan, St. John's wort, thioridazine, and TCAs	Headache, nervousness, insomnia or sedation, fatigue, nausea, diarrhea, dyspepsia, appetite loss Diet: Avoid grapefruit juice and alcohol
Escitalopram (FDA approved 7+)	Depression, anxiety	Same as above but better drug interaction profile	Same as above
Fluvoxamine (FDA approved 8+)	MDD, OCD	Increased risk of bleeding: NSAIDs, aspirin, warfarin	Same as above
Sertraline (FDA approved 6+)	MDD, OCD	Same as above Diet: May interact with grapefruit juice	Same as above
Serotonin Norepinephrine Reuptake Inhibitor			
Duloxetine (FDA approved 7+)	MDD, GAD	Multiple drug interactions. Risk for toxic levels: SSRIs, amphetamines, guanfacine- potentiates BP effects	Nausea, headache, dizziness, diaphoresis, behavior activation Diet: Avoid grapefruit juice and alcohol
Venlafaxine (FDA approved 8+)	MDD, GAD	Same as above	Same as above
Mood Stabilizer			
Lithium	Bipolar disorder, CD	Multiple drug interactions Risk for toxic drug levels: NSAIDs, metronidazole, and a wide range of antihypertensives	Weight gain, acne, sedation, tremors, GI upset, hair loss Diet: Limit caffeine, alcohol; ensure good fluid intake; maintain salt intake
Second-Generation Antipsychotics			
Risperidone (FDA approved 5+ ASD with aggression, 11+ BPD, 14+ schizophrenia)	Aggression CD ODD Schizophrenia Tourette syndrome	Multiple drug interactions Avoid: St. John's wort Potentiates: Antihypertensives	Orthostatic hypotension, sedation, syncope, tachycardia, insomnia, agitation, headache, dizziness, seizures, rash, weight gain, nausea, vomiting, diarrhea, polyuria, weight gain, elevated lipids, hyperglycemia, rhinitis, suicidal ideation
Aripiprazole (FDA approved 6+ ASD, 11+ BPD, 14+ schizophrenia)	BPD Schizophrenia Aggression with ASD	Same as above	Same as above
Olanzapine (FDA approved 14+)	BPD Schizophrenia	Same as above	Same as above
Quetiapine (FDA approved 11+ BPD, 14+ schizophrenia)	BPD Schizophrenia	Same as above	Same as above Hypertension

ASD, Autism spectrum disorder; *BPD*, bipolar disorder; *CD*, conduct disorder; *FDA*, U.S. Food and Drug Administration; *GAD*, generalized anxiety disorder; *GI*, gastrointestinal; *MAOI*, monoamine oxidase inhibitor; *MDD*, major depressive disorder; *NSAID*, nonsteroidal anti-inflammatory drug; *OCD*, obsessive-compulsive disorder; *ODD*, oppositional defiant disorder; *SSRI*, selective serotonin reuptake inhibitor; *TCA*, tricyclic antidepressant.

do not cause distress. OCD differs from normal child behavior in that it results in marked distress; is time consuming (individuals often spend a minimum of 1 hour a day engaged in the behavior); and interferes with the child's social, familial, or academic function. Abnormal compulsive behavior is distinguished by a sense of urgency or a profound discomfort until the ritual is completed. Children often deny the fear and lack recognition of the "senselessness" of the ritual and try to hide their illness often out of embarrassment. Obsessive thoughts are intrusive, recurrent, and disturbing, and unlike anxious worries, are generally unrelated to events or situations.

OCD has environmental and genetic influences, and international prevalence estimates are 1% to 2% (French, Boydston & Varley, 2016). OCD is more common in males (3:2) prior to adolescence, but gender-based differences disappear after puberty. Most adults with OCD report experiencing initial symptoms in late childhood or adolescence. Like most psychiatric conditions, OCD is a chronic disease, and if untreated can result in lifelong disease and significant loss of quality of life.

There are strong familial patterns of transmission, and the link between genetics and OCD is strong (French et al., 2016). A subgroup of pediatric patients with OCD and Tourette syndrome is diagnosed with PANS, also known as pediatric autoimmune neuropsychiatric disorders associated with streptococcal infection (PANDAS), a condition believed to be the result of autoimmune responses following group A β-hemolytic streptococci (GABHS) infection. PANDAS diagnostic criteria include dramatic onset of OCD or tic disorder in children between 3 years old and puberty shortly following GABHS infection and symptom exacerbation. However, it is important to note that this diagnosis has been controversial since it was first established in the mid-1990s, although recent evidence indicates this is a validated illness. OCD is a chronic condition, and about half of all affected individuals have comorbid psychiatric conditions, typically other anxiety disorders, major depression, ADHD, or substance abuse disorder (French et al., 2016). Disruptive behavior disorders and learning disorders are also common comorbidities.

Clinical Findings

OCD is characterized by obsessions and compulsions, as previously defined. Children may not recognize that their obsessions or compulsions are excessive or unreasonable, so insight into the behaviors is important. These are time consuming and significantly interfere with the child's daily functioning. The most common obsession is fear of contamination that results in compulsive washing and avoidance of "contaminated" objects. Other common obsessive worries include fears about safety (their own or their parents), exactness or symmetry, and religious sinfulness (scrupulosity). Common compulsions include repetitive counting, arranging or touching patterns, and compulsive rechecking (doors, homework, and exam items). High anxiety levels are common if they are unable to perform their obsession "until I get it right." Children with PANS/PANDAS often have additional symptoms like enuresis, emotional irritability, aggression, separation anxiety, and nightmares.

Differential Diagnosis

In order to assess context and severity of symptoms, PCPs should obtain information from the child, parents, family members, and teachers. A diagnosis of OCD is warranted if the content of the obsessions and compulsions is unrelated to another mental health disorder (e.g., social phobia, trichotillomania (pulling out hair),

pervasive developmental disorder, and body dysmorphic disorder). Medical conditions that mimic OCD include autism, carbon monoxide poisoning, tumors, encephalitis, traumatic brain injury, Prader-Willi (compulsive eating), drug side effects (stimulants), and rheumatic fever. Providers should assess developmental history to determine delays and/or difficulties. School performance may be impaired, and OCD may mimic learning disorders when children have compulsions to reread or rewrite or have pathologic perfectionism. Caregivers of children with secretive rituals may bring their child to primary care with complaints of skin rashes (dermatitis, chapped hands), temper tantrums, declining school performance, or sudden food or activity aversions. Individuals with self-injurious behavior (see Chapter 13) physically harm themselves in order to decrease mental anguish; however, this disorder is distinct from the rituals of OCD.

Assessment should include symptom description and context, frequency, and effect on daily functioning. It is important to note how these behaviors contribute to difficulties in home, school, and other domains. Six screening questions can be used to determine OCD pathology (Box 30.1). Children with suspected PANS/PANDAS and unclear history of recent upper respiratory tract infection should have confirmation of streptococcal infection either by throat culture or ASO titer.

Management

Decisions regarding treatment of OCD should center on the degree of child impairment. If the child's symptoms do not interfere with the child's life and do not cause undue distress, medications and intensive therapy can be deferred (see Chapter 15 for alternative strategies to promote mental health). Optimal treatment involves an individualized and developmentally appropriate approach that centers on child and family therapy to help the child learn to manage his or her anxiety and distress. CBT provides the best long-term effectiveness for OCD and is considered first-line therapy for all children and adolescents with mild to moderate OCD (French et al., 2016). Individuals with moderate to severe disease (e.g., causes excessive distress, leads to significant social isolation or inability to perform developmentally normal tasks, or that occurs with significant comorbid psychopathology) should receive pharmacologic management. SSRIs are first-line pharmacologic agents and have the most effectiveness of all drug classes. Individuals who fail to respond to CBT, who experience increasing symptom severity during treatment, who show signs of psychosis and/or suicidality, and who fail to respond to SSRI should be emergently referred to a child behavioral health provider.

Research in a subgroup of children with PANS/PANDAS indicates that antibiotic treatment can help rapidly diminish tics; however, routine penicillin prophylaxis is not recommended.

• BOX 30.1 Quick Screening Questions for Obsessive-Compulsive Disorder

Do you wash yourself or clean more than most people?
Do you feel the need to check or double-check things often?
Do you have thoughts that bother you that you would like to get rid of but can't?
Do you find yourself spending a lot of time doing things (brushing teeth, getting dressed)?
Does it bother you when things are not lined up or are not in order?
Do these problems bother you?

Individuals with mild to moderate symptoms may benefit from oral corticosteroids, whereas moderate to severe cases have more controversial treatment options including intravenous immuno-globulin or plasma exchange (Frankovich et al., 2017). Children with suspected PANS/PANDAS are best managed by referring to a PANS/PANDAS specialist.

Tic Disorders

Tic disorders are characterized by repetitive, fast, unconscious movements or vocalizations. Motor and verbal tics that persist for more than one year are called *Tourette syndrome.* All children have some repetitive habits (such as finger sucking or hair twirling), and many of these are adaptive behaviors that help decrease stress or provide a sense of calm. Habits are considered pathologic when they have no clear purpose and result in physical or social impairment. Tic disorders cause significant anxiety for affected children and often result in impaired self-esteem, bullying, and emotional or academic problems.

Chronic tic disorders affect 1% to 2% of the population, and transient tic disorders affect 5% of the population. For children with OCD, prevalence rates for tics are 20% to 59% (Hojaard et al., 2017). Half of all motor tics begin by age seven, and half of all vocal tics begin by age nine (Murphy et al., 2013). There is some evidence that children with developmental disorders have greater risk of developing tics than their nonaffected peers.

Clinical Findings and Diagnostic Studies

Motor tics can be simple (involving a single muscle group) or complex (complicated movements like jumping or a series of simple tics). Common simple tics include blinking, twitching of hands or limbs, shoulder shrugging, tongue thrusting, or squinting. Verbal tics include vocalizations or pushing air through the nose. Grunting sounds and/or clearing the throat are common. Obscene gestures and swearing are rare. Symptoms generally worsen during periods of stress, fatigue, or anxiety. Most children with tic disorders can suppress vocal tics when they intensely concentrate on other things like homework, games, and so on or when social pressure against verbalizations is high. Other common tic disorders include trichotillomania, bruxism (tooth grinding), skin pulling, and nail biting.

There are a number of potential organic causes of new onset tic disorders, especially with disorientation and/or loss of fine motor skills (e.g., loses ability to draw figures or penmanship becomes impaired). Laboratory testing for hemoglobin, ferritin, renal function, hepatic function, thyroid function, and substance use are appropriate at the time of diagnosis (Murphy et al., 2013).

Management

Mild tics do not require treatment. Children with moderate to severe tics that disrupt self-esteem or impair socialization best respond to psychotherapy, specifically comprehensive behavioral intervention for tics (CBIT). The focus of treatment is to extinguish the tic, to increase children's awareness of the behaviors, and to teach another behavior to engage in when they feel they are about to have a tic behavior. Best responses are often obtained with older children and adolescents. Common reminder strategies include using an elastic bandage over a digit to discourage thumb sucking, using an elastic hair band to make it difficult to grasp hair, or placing a rubber band that can be gently pulled when a child is aware of engaging in a tic behavior. Positive reinforcement is another effective extinguishing strategy. It is important to note that tics cannot be extinguished when the child is not interested

in stopping the habit. For moderate to severe symptoms, common psychopharmaceuticals include SSRIs, atypical antipsychotics (e.g., risperidone), and antihypertensives (e.g., clonidine).

Posttraumatic Stress Disorder

PTSD describes a characteristic set of symptoms that develops following actual or threatened exposure to a severe stressor or trauma. The trauma may result from a single event ("one sudden blow" trauma) or variable, multiple long-standing events, such as ongoing maltreatment. According to the *Diagnostic and Statistical Manual of Mental Disorders,* fifth edition (DSM-5), the criteria for PTSD include (American Psychiatric Association [APA], 2013):
- Witnessing or experiencing a traumatic event(s) that resulted in risk of death or serious injury to oneself or a loved one
- Event(s) that resulted in fear, helplessness, recurrent distress, agitation, or irritable behavior (the latter two are part of the diagnostic criteria for children younger than 6 years old)
- Symptoms that cause increased arousal, excessive startle, altered mood and emotional response, or intrusive thoughts or recurrent dreams and continued avoidance of reminders of the trauma
- Symptoms that last at least 1 month and cause significant impairment in social, cognitive, or school functioning
- Acute symptoms that last less than 3 months and chronic symptoms that last more than 3 months

Exposure to trauma is a key feature of the diagnosis of PTSD. Unfortunately, there are those who are skeptical about whether children suffer from PTSD. Parents and teachers frequently minimize traumatic effect, perhaps to relieve themselves of vicarious distress or to reassure themselves that their children have not suffered harm.

Substantial PTSD rates are documented for children who experience maltreatment. Children can experience PTSD following exposure to any traumatizing experience including natural disasters and witnessed violence. Three factors consistently influence the severity of the response: (1) severity of the trauma exposure, (2) parental distress related to the trauma, and (3) temporal proximity to the event. Approximately 60% of children experience trauma before age 18, and about 15% of them develop PTSD (Hall, 2016). The rate of PTSD is high among those who have been physically and sexually abused. The closer the perpetrator is in relation to the victim, the greater the trauma (e.g., PTSD is more likely when the perpetrator is a member of the immediate family as opposed to an extended family member, family friend, or stranger).

Clinical Findings

A diagnosis of PTSD requires that the child demonstrate specific behaviors following trauma, as follows (APA, 2013):
1. The child repeatedly re-experiences a set of symptoms from each of the three following categories:
   - Recurrent and intrusive memories of the trauma
   - Nightmares of monsters or threats to self or others or distressing dreams about a specific event
   - Distress caused by cues that symbolize or resemble an aspect of the trauma, including physiologic reactivity
2. The child demonstrates three of the following symptoms, reflecting avoidance of stimuli associated with the traumatic event(s) and numbing of general responsiveness. These symptoms must not have been present before the trauma:
   - Avoidance of reminders of the trauma
   - Efforts to avoid thoughts, feelings, or conversations linked to the trauma

- Amnesia for an important aspect of the trauma
- Detachment or estrangement from others
- Emotional constriction (restricted range of affect)
- Diminished interest in or participation in usual activities
- A sense of a foreshortened future

3. Two persistent symptoms of increased arousal must be new to the child, present for at least 1 month, and cause clinically important distress or negatively affect functioning. These symptoms include the following:
   - Sleep disturbances
   - Hypervigilance
   - Difficulty concentrating
   - Exaggerated startle response
   - Agitated or disorganized behavior
   - Irritability or angry outbursts, extreme fussiness or tantrums

Among infants, toddlers, and preschoolers, symptoms must be understood within the context of the trauma itself, the child's temperament and personality, and the caregiver's ability to support the child and provide a sense of safety and protection. Table 30.2 includes a listing of PTSD symptoms by age group.

PTSD assessment in children requires careful and direct clinical interviews with the child and caregivers. If the identified traumatic event involves a caregiver as the perpetrator of child maltreatment or domestic violence, the nonoffending caregiver or other caretaker should be interviewed. During assessment, do not use prompting or leading questions. Instead ask questions about whether someone has invaded the child's privacy, how it happened, and how the injuries came to be. Assessment should ascertain that a trauma has occurred, the nature of the trauma, and the consequent symptom pattern. Screen by identifying **TRAUMA** symptoms:

Trauma—known traumatic experience
Re-experience—includes flashbacks and nightmares
Avoidance—avoids stimuli associated with the event
Unable to function
Month or longer
Arousal—is hypervigilant, has sleep disturbances, concentration difficulties, or an exaggerated startle response.

TABLE 30.2	Posttraumatic Stress Disorder Symptoms by Age Group
Age Group	**Common Symptoms**
Infancy	Feeding problems, failure to thrive, sleep problems, irritability
Preschool age	Sleep problems, nightmares, developmental regression, aggression, extreme temper tantrums, anxiety symptoms, sudden worsening of fears, irritability, avoidance symptoms
School age	Sleep problems, nightmares, developmental regression, repetitive themes in play, social withdrawal, may have partial amnesia of events, new onset anxiety or fears, panic attacks, impaired concentration, impaired school performance, avoidance symptoms or hypervigilance, somatic complaints
Adolescence	"Acting out," nightmares, insomnia, extreme startling, social withdrawal, fears, anxiety, panic attacks, depression, anger or rage, internalizing, suicidal ideation, impaired concentration, impaired school performance, hypervigilance

Differential Diagnosis

The stressor must be of an extreme nature to warrant a diagnosis of PTSD. However, the stressor can be of any severity in an adjustment disorder (e.g., moving, starting a new school, birth of a sibling, divorce). Anxiety disorders, the most common differential diagnosis, are distinguished by not being precipitated by a traumatic event. Acute stress disorder is distinguished by the symptom pattern occurring and resolving within a 4-week period after the traumatic event. Recurrent intrusive thoughts occur in OCD but are experienced as inappropriate and are not related to an experienced trauma as they are in PTSD. Flashbacks also connect to the event and involve a feeling of reliving the event in PTSD, whereas hallucinations and other perceptual disturbances are unrelated to exposure to trauma. Comorbid conditions in preschoolers differ from those of adults and older children. Oppositional defiant disorder (ODD) is most common, followed by SAD and ADHD. Major depressive disorder (MDD) is very unlikely.

Management

Referral to a pediatric behavioral health specialist is crucial and a report to social service agencies is essential for children younger than 18 years who have witnessed or experienced violence. Many child abuse intervention centers are prepared to accept referrals, assess, and direct management of children who have witnessed violence. Psychotherapy is the core of PTSD treatment with trauma-focused CBT (TF-CBT) showing the most promise (Hall, 2016). Eye movement desensitization and reprocessing therapy (EMDR) is not as well studied in children as adults, but shows promise as an effective therapy strategy.

Medication management for PTSD is not well supported in children (Hall, 2016). β-blockers like propranolol may be effective at decreasing somatic symptoms (e.g., racing heart rate and hyperpnea) associated with posttraumatic stress responses. Anxiety and depressive symptoms respond well to SSRIs. As such, children who fail therapy should be referred to a behavioral health provider prior to starting medication.

Crisis intervention is often necessary for the child as well as the parents. The PCP should educate themselves about trauma and PTSD so they can provide good psychoeducation to parents and pediatric patients. The National Child Traumatic Stress Network has lots of evidence-based information about childhood trauma (www.nctsn.org).

Mood Disorders

Depression

There are three categories of depression that occur during childhood and adolescence: (1) MDD, (2) dysthymic disorder, and (3) adjustment disorder with depressed mood. MDD is defined as either a depressed or irritable mood or a markedly diminished interest and pleasure in almost all of the usual activities, or both, for a period of at least 2 weeks. A dysthymic disorder is characterized by depressed or irritable mood for the majority of days in the past 2 years that is less intense but more chronic than major depressive episodes. Adjustment disorder with depressed mood typically occurs within 3 months after a major life stressor, involves less-severe symptoms, and is relatively mild and brief.

There are multiple subtypes of MDD. Children and adolescents with psychotic depression (e.g., affected individuals hallucinate or have delusions) have a greater incidence of adverse long-term outcomes, resistance to psychopharmacotherapy, and a much higher risk of developing bipolar depression. Atypical depression affects approximately 15% of children with depression and is characterized by hypersomnia, increased appetite, psychomotor retardation, and weight gain. Seasonal affective disorder is most common during the fall and winter months when there is less daylight. Premenstrual dysphoric disorder occurs within a week of menstruation and lasts until a few days after menstruation.

Only half of depressed youth are identified prior to adulthood and there are estimates that as many as two-thirds of youth with depression are identified by their PCPs (Zuckerbrodt et al., 2018). Depression rates increase with age. Although depression occurs in children younger than 5 years old, the true incidence is unknown given the limits of cognitive and language skills to communicate feelings. Approximately 9% of adolescents experience depression at any given point, and about 20% of youth experience depression prior to age 18 (Cheung et al., 2018). Adolescent depression has biologic (e.g., sexual maturation and the influence of the sex hormones), social environment (e.g., greater social and academic expectations, greater exposure to negative events), and developmental (e.g., increased autonomy and abstract thinking) factors. Vulnerability to depression involves interplay of genetic, biologic, biochemical, and psychosocial forces. Genetic factors underlie the risk for major depression, especially for earlier onset. Children of depressed parents are three to four times more likely to be diagnosed with depression than their peers.

Three biologic theories of depression are used to understand the psychopharmacology of depression: (1) impaired neurotransmission, (2) endocrine dysfunction, and (3) biologic rhythm dysfunction. Given a biologic predisposition, certain life events may trigger the onset of depression. These include loss of a parent or significant other, losses that accompany a disability or injury, family dysfunction, chronic adversity, exposure to traumatic events, and physical or sexual abuse. There is a high risk of recurrent depression persisting into young adulthood.

An important feature of early-onset depressive illness is the potential for the condition to switch from unipolar depression to bipolar depression (see below). As many as one-third of preadolescent children who meet criteria for major depression develop bipolar depression. Psychiatric comorbidity with depression is common. The most common comorbidity with depression is an anxiety disorder (up to 70%). Other comorbid conditions include dysthymia, disruptive behavior disorders, eating disorders, substance abuse and/or dependence, learning disorders, stress disorders, and ADHD. Comorbid conditions may also occur with a variety of medical conditions, especially those with a neurologic component, such as brain injury, learning disorder, migraine headaches, and epilepsy.

Clinical Findings. Older children and adolescents with depression usually present with symptoms similar to those of adults. School-aged children rarely spontaneously admit to depression symptoms. Parents and teachers may report decreased mood, impaired concentration, inattention, irritability, fluctuating mood, temper tantrums, social withdrawal, somatic complaints, agitation, separation anxiety, or behavioral problems (Calles, 2016). Males are more likely to have externalizing symptoms (e.g., aggression, acting-out, anger), and females are more likely to have internalizing symptoms (e.g., somatic complaints, feelings of sadness). Females have two times higher depression rates than males after puberty, but prepubertal gender rates are roughly equal. Major depression symptoms represent a persistent change that occurs across settings, activities, and relationships and causes the child distress, impaired functioning, or developmental alteration. Infants and young children may present with failure to thrive,

speech and motor delays, repetitive self-soothing behaviors, withdrawal from social interaction, poor attachment, and loss of developmental skills. Infants may not respond to extra efforts to soothe or engage them.

Toddlers and preschoolers may lack energy, be too eager to please others, be excessively or unusually clingy or whiny, and have developmentally inappropriate problems with separation. Preschoolers with MDD may present with sad or grouchy mood, lack of pleasure in play or activity, poor appetite and weight loss, sleep problems, low energy and activity levels, low self-esteem, or increased death or suicide play or talk.

School-age children may be irritable, angry, or hostile or have externalizing behavior, such as hyperactivity, difficulty handling aggression, or reckless behavior. Frequent absences from school, perhaps because of school phobia, or poor performance and other school problems are common. On the other hand, school-age children may have internalizing symptoms, such as boredom, lack of interest in playing with friends, social withdrawal, somatic complaints (e.g., stomachaches, headaches, muscle aches, or tiredness), eating or sleeping disturbances, enuresis, or encopresis. Some children with depression describe themselves in negative terms, whereas others, in an effort to compensate for feelings of poor self-worth, become preoccupied with attempting to please others.

Depression symptoms in adolescents include impulsivity, fatigue, hopelessness, antisocial behavior, substance use, restlessness, grouchiness, aggression, hypersexuality, and problems with family members or at school. Social withdrawal, manifested as shyness, boredom, or a lack of motivation, is common. Substance abuse is a significant comorbidity, and some substances (alcohol and cannabis, and MDMA ["ecstasy"] and stimulant withdrawal) exacerbate or cause depressive symptoms (Calles, 2016).

Talking directly with the child or adolescent is essential because it is thought that half of depression cases are missed when only parents are interviewed. The following symptoms are common:
- Depressed mood: Sad, "blue," down, angry, bored
- Loss of interest and pleasure in usual activities
- Change in appetite or weight (loss or increase)
- Insomnia or hypersomnia
- Low energy and fatigue
- Difficulty concentrating; indecision
- Feelings of worthlessness or inappropriate or excessive guilt
- Recurrent thoughts of death or suicidal ideation

A diagnosis of MDD is made if there have been at least 2 weeks of depressed mood or loss of interest and at least four additional symptoms of depression. The symptoms cause considerable distress and impairment in social and academic functioning and cannot be caused by bereavement. Therefore, it is important to assess the following:
- Recent life events and losses
- Family history of depression or other psychiatric disorders
- Family dysfunction
- Changes in school performance
- Risk-taking behavior, including sexual activity and substance use
- Deteriorating relationships with family
- Changes in peer relations, especially social withdrawal

Mild depression causes impact in daily life, but affected individuals are still able to function and complete normal tasks although doing so requires a lot of energy because of lack of motivation. Mild MDD causes lower scores on standardized assessments, shorter symptoms duration, and results in 5 to 6 MDD symptoms with mild functional impairment. In moderate depression, what began as a decreased interest in engaging in activities becomes a complete lack of interest, and affected individuals often express concern about their inability to function and complete tasks. Its severity lies between mild and severe disease. Severe depression is demonstrated by increased agitation, psychosis, and suicidality and will often demonstrate all the depression symptoms. Current clinical practice guidelines state all adolescents with a minimum of five symptoms who have clear suicidality and a plan or recent attempt, who are psychotic, have a first-degree relative with bipolar disorder, or who have significant impairment including being unable to leave the home should be considered as having severe depression (Zuckerbrodt et al., 2018). Undiagnosed and untreated/undertreated depression can be fatal. Suicide is the second leading cause of death for 14- to 24-year-olds (Centers for Disease Control and Prevention [CDC], 2016). Possible warning signs for suicide are listed in Table 30.3.

Both patient self-report and clinician-completed rating scales are available. Table 30.4 contains a listing of these scales.

Differential Diagnosis. Some medications and certain chronic illnesses (hypothyroidism, adrenal insufficiency, epilepsy, metabolic disease, sleep disorders, hepatitis, multiple sclerosis, inflammatory bowel disease, and type 1 diabetes) predispose children and adolescents to depression. If a substance (e.g., medication, toxin, or drug of abuse) is related to the mood disturbance, a substance-induced mood disorder is diagnosed. Medications that commonly cause depressive symptoms include β-blockers, benzodiazepines, nonsteroidal antiinflammatory drugs (NSAIDs), stimulants, clonidine, corticosteroids, oral contraceptives, and isotretinoin. Infections, lead intoxication, anemia, eating disorders, mitral valve prolapse, premenstrual syndrome, and neurologic disorders can mimic depression in children and adolescents. In general, a physical examination and screening laboratory tests are necessary to rule out organic causes. Suggested diagnostic testing for an individual with new symptoms of depression include complete blood count (CBC), vitamin D, pregnancy testing, Epstein-Barr titers, thyroid panel, liver function testing, urinalysis, and drug screening.

Depressive symptoms in response to a psychosocial stressor are diagnosed as adjustment disorder, which has a good short-term prognosis and does not predict later dysfunction. With SAD, depressive symptoms usually arise only in the context of separation and resolve quickly with reunion; however, concomitant depressive disorder is not uncommon. A depressive episode with irritable mood can be difficult to distinguish from a manic episode with irritable mood; careful evaluation of the presence of manic symptoms (e.g., excessive activity, inflated self-esteem, little need for sleep, talkativeness) is required. Many adolescents and adults who develop mania had preponderantly depressive symptoms in childhood. Family history of bipolar depression is an important risk factor. Depression can be differentiated from the irritability and inattention of ADHD in that children with MDD are not usually impulsive. In addition, they typically have a normal attention span before the onset of symptoms.

Management. The first goals of management are to determine suicidal risk and intervene to prevent suicide. Suicidal risk is greatest during the first 4 weeks of a depressive episode. Patients with acute suicidal intent that includes a plan, psychosis, risk of abuse, and unstable behavior require immediate psychiatric evaluation. Cumulative suicidal risks—prior suicidal behavior or attempts, depression, and alcohol, tobacco, or drug abuse/dependence—require behavioral health intervention as well, and immediate referral must be made. Attention must also be paid to establish a safe environment (e.g., removal of firearms, knives, and lethal medications, including tricyclic antidepressants [TCAs]). Families of adolescents with depression may be noncompliant with recommendations to remove guns from the home in spite of compliance with other aspects of treatment. Vigilant follow-up in this regard

TABLE 30.3	**Warning Signs for Suicide**
Area of Functioning	**Signs**[a]
Changes in behavior	Accident prone or risk taking Drug and alcohol abuse Physical violence toward self, others, or animals Loss of appetite Sudden alienation from family, friends, coworkers Worsening performance at work or school Putting personal affairs in order Loss of interest in personal appearance Disposal of possessions Writing letters, notes, or poems with suicidal content; talking about suicide Buying a gun or other weapon
Changes in mood	Expressions of hopelessness or impending doom Explosive rage Dramatic swings in affect Crying spells Sleep disorders Talking about suicide
Changes in thinking	Preoccupation with death Difficulty concentrating Irrational speech Hearing voices, seeing visions Sudden interest (or loss of interest) in religion
Major life changes	Death of a family member or friend (especially by suicide) Separation or divorce Public humiliation or failure Serious illness or trauma Loss of financial security Recent relationship loss (e.g., first love)

[a]These signs must be interpreted in context. Many of them are common outside the realm of pre-suicidal behavior.

TABLE 30.4	**Diagnostic Rating Scales for Depression Diagnosis**
Scale	**Appropriate Ages**
Child Behavior Checklist (CBCL)	1.5-5 and 6-18 years old
Children's Depression Rating Scale-Revised (CDRS-R)	6-12 years old
Children's Depression Inventory (CDI)	6-18 years old
Center for Epidemiologic Studies-Depression Scale (CES-D)	Adolescents
Depression Self-Rating Scale	Adolescents
Pediatric Symptom Checklist (PSC)	4 years old to adolescent
Patient Health Questionnaire-9 (PHQ-9) and PHQ-9 Modified for Teens	6-10 years old and 11 years old to adolescent

is crucial. Other management strategies by the PCP include referral to community resources, such as hotlines, and to identify an emergency plan for the family should the patient become actively suicidal, psychotic, or a danger to others. It is important to note that suicidal ideation often increases during the treatment phase known as *emergence.* Emergence occurs in the first week to month of treatment when the patient's energy levels increase, but feelings of hopelessness and helplessness have not yet receded.

A major depressive episode requires intervention by a behavioral health specialist. Unfortunately only about half of all individuals with depression achieve full remission of their symptoms. Therapies typically include CBT in a group or individual psychotherapy format. Group CBT may help adolescents. Often, family therapy or psychoeducation is indicated. See Fig 30.2 for primary care management of pediatric depression.

Available studies do not support the efficacy of TCAs and older medications for depression in young children, and they may actually be harmful (Cheung et al., 2018). Although the 2004 "black box" warning for SSRIs occurred because of concerns of increased suicidality with use of these medications, randomized controlled trials of pediatric depression consistently demonstrate that best treatment responses come from combinations of CBT and SSRIs. CBT appears to have a protective effect against suicide. Currently,

there are only a few antidepressants the U.S. Food and Drug Administration (FDA) approves for use in children and adolescents (see Table 30.1). The FDA specifically recommends against the use of paroxetine in children and adolescents because of the 3.5-fold increased risk for suicide. A general rule of antidepressant dosing is to start low and slowly increase. It takes 4 to 6 weeks to see maximum response, but medication doses can be adjusted to improve response every 2 to 4 weeks as long as significant side effects are absent. Activation (e.g., elevated energy without mood change) and mania can occur in patients secondary to treatment with antidepressants. Therefore, it is critical that parents be taught about symptoms that merit immediate evaluation, including decreased impulse control, marked elevated mood, acting out, fearlessness, and risk taking. For children with psychosis, child behavioral health specialists often add antipsychotics like risperidone or olanzapine to the therapeutic drug plan.

Close follow-up is recommended for all children and adolescents with depression, especially when symptoms are significant enough to merit pharmacotherapy. Providers should make phone contact with the patient and/or family within 3 days and see the patient weekly until stable with the first 4 weeks of treatment being critical (Calles, 2016). Once stable, maintenance visits can occur at 3-month intervals.

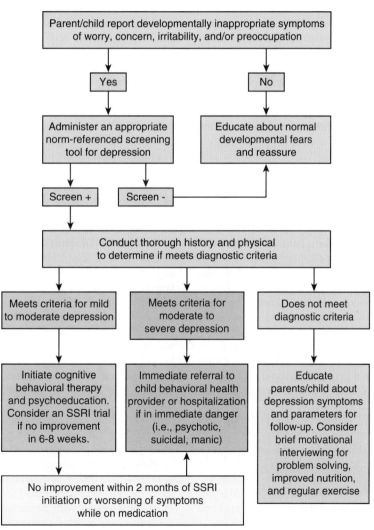

• **Fig 30.2** Primary care management of pediatric depression. *SSRI,* Selective serotonin reuptake inhibitor.

Prognosis. MDD is a chronic condition with a high rate of recurrence. Although most children and adolescents recover from an MDD episode, the probability of recurrence is 60% within 2 years and 75% by 5 years. Poor long-term outcomes are associated with severe or frequent disease, and in patients with significant family dysfunction, low socioeconomic status, and history of abuse or family strife.

Bipolar Disorder

Bipolar disorder, formerly known as *manic depression,* is characterized by unusual shifts in mood, energy, and functioning and may begin with manic, depressive, or a mixed set of manic and depressive symptoms. The majority of adults with bipolar disorder report their initial symptom was depression, and those who develop symptoms in childhood are significantly more likely to develop severe disease, to be hospitalized frequently, and to have a less favorable life course. It is a recurrent disorder, and nearly all of those (90%) who have a single manic episode will have future episodes. Approximately 1% to 2% of children younger than age 18 meet the diagnostic criteria for bipolar disorder (West & Pavuluri, 2016). The risk of suicide in bipolar depression is the highest of all the psychiatric disorders.

A characteristic pattern usually evolves for a particular person, with manic episodes preceding or following major depressive episodes. Most individuals with bipolar disorder return to a full level of functioning between episodes; 20% to 30% experience persistent mood lability and interpersonal difficulties (APA, 2013). Sometimes psychotic symptoms develop after several days or weeks of manic symptoms. Such features tend to predict that the individual with subsequent manic episodes will again experience psychotic symptoms.

Multiple theories explain the cause of bipolar disorder, but no definitive cause is known. Biologic influences include structural changes in the third ventricle, the white matter, the prefrontal cortex, the amygdala, and the basal ganglia (Frias, Palma & Farriols, 2015). There is evidence of a genetic influence for bipolar disorder from twin studies and adoption studies; bipolar disorder tends to cluster in families. Parents who are bipolar are at greater risk for having bipolar children. The most common onset of symptoms occurs between 15 and 19 years old. There is no differential incidence based on race, ethnicity, or gender. Children with ADHD seem to be vulnerable to bipolar illness, or it may be that ADHD is a misdiagnosed early sign of the mania to come. If children are also bipolar, treatment of ADHD with psychostimulants or antidepressants may precipitate a manic episode. Antidepressants in depressed children may also precipitate mania and the onset of bipolar illness.

Clinical Findings. Bipolar disorder in childhood or early adolescence appears to be a different, more severe form of the illness than occurs with late adolescent or adult onset. The early-onset form is characterized by irritability and continuous, rapid-cycling, and mixed-symptom state that may also co-occur with disruptive behavior disorders (e.g., ADHD or CD); features of ADHD or behavior disorder are often early symptoms. Prepubertal and early adolescent bipolar disorder is fairly consistent with no differences according to gender, puberty, or comorbid ADHD. In the late adolescent or adult form, the hallmark features include classic manic episodes, episodic patterns of mania and depression, and relative stability between episodes. Symptoms include the following (West & Pavuluri, 2016):

- Severe mood changes—extreme irritability or overly elated and silly
- Inflated self-esteem or grandiosity—"I am the best in the world at X"
- Increased energy and physical agitation

- Decreased need for sleep (sleeps few hours or no sleep for days without tiring)
- Talkativeness or compulsion to talk; frequent topic changes or cannot be interrupted
- Racing thoughts
- Distractibility, with attention moving constantly from one thing to another
- Increase in goal-directed activity (socially or at school)—get "stuck" on activities and can't stop doing them
- Risk-taking behaviors or activities; taking "more dares"
- Hypersexuality in talk, thoughts, feelings, or behaviors
- Psychosis—visual or auditory hallucinations
- Suicidal thoughts and behaviors in 76% of cases and suicidal attempts in 31% of cases

Most adolescents experience depression as their initial symptom. The most common symptoms of mania include irritable mood and grandiosity, elevated mood, decreased sleep, racing thoughts, poor judgment, flight of ideas, and hypersexuality. With mania, children appear to be the happiest of people, but the happiness and laughter do not match the situation or context. Grandiosity may manifest in efforts to correct teachers or critique their efforts, seeing themselves as above rules and laws, or devoting time to an activity for which they have no talent. Children's sleep difficulties (a hallmark sign) are reflected in high activity levels before bed (e.g., rearranging the furniture), whereas adolescents need little sleep at all. Risk-taking behavior ranges from children climbing excessively high trees or hopping between rooftops to adolescents driving recklessly and speeding. In adolescents, manic episodes are more likely to include psychotic features and may be associated with school truancy, school failure, substance use, or antisocial behavior. The child or adolescent who has depression but also manifests symptoms of ADHD that seem severe (e.g., extreme temper outbursts and mood changes) should be evaluated by a child behavioral health specialist with experience in bipolar disorder. Symptoms are manifested in relatively age-specific ways.

Assessment for comorbid conditions is important. Anxiety disorders, including panic disorder, affect about half (54%) of patients with bipolar disorder. Other common comorbidities include ADHD (48%), disruptive behavior disorders (31%), and substance abuse (31%) (Frias, Plama & Farriols, 2015).

Differential Diagnosis. A manic episode must be distinguished from a mood disorder caused by a medical condition (e.g., brain tumor) and a substance-induced mood disorder (e.g., laughing fits with marijuana, amphetamine highs followed by withdrawal "crashes," perceptual distortions or hallucinations of hallucinogens). Distinguishing bipolar disorder from ADHD can be a challenge. ADHD, like mania, is characterized by excessive activity, poor impulse control and judgment, and denial of problems. However, ADHD lacks a clear onset or episodes, mood disturbances, and psychotic features. Recent evidence suggests that children with ADHD are vulnerable to bipolar disorder and that pharmacological treatments may precipitate manic episodes, so providers should carefully evaluate and refer any child treated for ADHD who does not respond to therapy or who experiences a sudden worsening of agitation while using ADHD medications.

Management. Referral to a child behavioral health provider is critical. Current recommendations for pharmacologic treatment include the use of mood stabilizers, such as lithium, alone or in combination with antiseizure medications (e.g., valproate, divalproex) and atypical antipsychotics (e.g., risperidone). Neither antidepressants nor stimulants have proven effective. Antidepressant use may potentiate manic responses. The use of lithium must be carefully monitored. The best clinical responses occur when pharmacotherapy is combined with individual and family psychotherapy. Therapy should focus on minimizing comorbidities, enhancing problem-solving and communication skills, and reducing negative self-thoughts. Other nonpharmacologic interventions with proven effectiveness include stress reduction, healthy diet, routine exercise, and developing good sleep hygiene.

Attention-Deficit/Hyperactivity Disorder

Definition and Diagnostic Criteria

ADHD is one of the most commonly diagnosed disorders in childhood. It is considered a neurodevelopmental disorder because it has a clear neurologic base with symptoms that can profoundly affect the behavior of individuals across many settings in their lives. It is a chronic condition that persists for many into adolescence and adulthood. The symptoms of ADHD affect cognitive,

educational, behavioral, emotional, and social functioning and core symptoms include inattention, hyperactivity, and impulsivity occurring at a developmentally inappropriate level observed in at least two settings (home, school, or work) with clear evidence of clinical impairment in social, academic, or occupational functioning. There is a range of severity of symptoms from one individual to the next (mild, moderate, and severe), and the scope and severity of behaviors may change within an individual as maturation occurs. ADHD criteria are listed in Table 30.5 with information about how to differentiate between types in Box 30.2.

ADHD affects executive functions and self-regulation and can have a significant impact on social relationships. Children may present with struggles in the classroom, difficulties with peers, or trouble regulating their behavior or emotions. Because ADHD symptoms cross over so many settings and often persist into adulthood, this condition has a major effect on the individual, as well as

TABLE 30.5	DSM-5 Criteria for Attention-Deficit/Hyperactivity Disorder
A. A persistent pattern of inattention and/or hyperactivity-impulsivity that interferes with functioning or development, as characterized by (1) and/or (2)	
Symptom	**Criteria**

Inattention (1)	Six (or more) of the following symptoms have persisted at least 6 months to a degree that is inconsistent with developmental level and that negatively impacts directly on social and academic/occupational activities:
	Note: The symptoms are not solely a manifestation of oppositional behavior, defiance, hostility, or failure to understand tasks or instructions. For older adolescents and adults (age 17 and older), at least five symptoms are required.
	  a. Often fails to give close attention to details or makes careless mistakes in schoolwork, at work, or during other activities (e.g., overlooks or misses details, work is inaccurate)
	  b. Often has difficulty sustaining attention in tasks or play activities (e.g., has difficulty remaining focused during lectures, conversations, or lengthy reading.
	  c. Often does not seem to listen when spoken to directly (e.g., mind seems elsewhere, even in the absence of any obvious distraction.
	  d. Often does not follow through on instructions and fails to finish schoolwork, chores, or duties in the workplace (e.g., starts tasks but quickly loses focus and is easily sidetracked).
	  e. Often has difficulty organizing tasks and activities (e.g., difficulty managing sequential tasks; difficulty keeping materials and belongings in order; messy, disorganized work; has poor time management; fails to meet deadlines).
	  f. Often avoids, dislikes, or is reluctant to engage in tasks that require sustained mental effort (e.g., schoolwork or homework; for older adolescents and adults, preparing reports, completing forms, reviewing lengthy papers).
	  g. Often loses things necessary for tasks or activities (e.g., school materials, pencils, books, tools, wallets, keys, paperwork, eyeglasses, mobile telephones).
	  h. Is often easily distracted by extraneous stimuli (for older adolescents and adults, may include unrelated thoughts).
	  i. Is forgetful in daily activities (e.g., doing chores, running errands; for older adolescents and adults, may include unrelated thoughts).

Hyperactivity/ impulsivity (2)	Six or more of the following symptoms have persisted for at least 6 months to a degree that is inconsistent with developmental level that negatively impacts directly on social and academic/occupational activities:
	Note: The symptoms are not solely a manifestation of oppositional behavior, defiance, hostility, or a failure to understand tasks or instructions. For older adolescents and adults (age 17 and older), at least five symptoms are required.
	  a. Often fidgets with or taps hands or feet or squirms in seat.
	  b. Often leaves seat in situations when remaining seated is expected (e.g., leaves his or her place in the classroom, in the office or other workplace, or in other situations that require remaining in place).
	  c. Often runs about or climbs in situations where it is inappropriate. (**Note:** In adolescents or adults, may be limited to feeling restless.)
	  d. Often unable to play or engage in leisure activities quietly.
	  e. Is often "on the go" acting as If "driven by a motor" (e.g., is unable to be or uncomfortable with being still for extended time, as in restaurants, meetings; may be experienced by others as being restless or difficult to keep up with).
	  f. Often talks excessively.
	  g. Often blurts out an answer before a question has been completed (e.g., completes people's sentences; cannot wait turn in conversation).
	  h. Often has difficulty waiting his or her turn (e.g., while waiting in line).
	  i. Often interrupts or intrudes on others (e.g., butts into conversations, games, or activities; may start using other people's things without asking or receiving permission; for adolescents and adults, may intrude into or take over what others are doing).

B. Several inattentive or hyperactive-impulsive symptoms were present prior to age 12 years.	
C. Several inattentive or hyperactive-impulsive symptoms are present in two or more settings (e.g., at home, school, or work; with friends or relatives: in other activities).	
D. There is clear evidence that the symptoms interfere with, or reduce the quality of, scial, academic, or occupational functioning.	
E. The symptoms do not occur exclusively during the course of schizophrenia or another psychotic disorder and are not better explained by another mental disorder (e.g., mood disorder, anxiety disorder, personality disorder, substance intoxication or withdrawl).	

Attention-Deficit/Hyperactivity Disorder Diagnostic Presentations

ADHD, Combined Type

Significant number of symptoms from both inattention and hyperactivity/impulsivity are present

Accounts for the majority of ADHD cases

ADHD, Predominantly Inattentive

Significant number of inattentive symptoms identified, but not significant number in hyperactivity/impulsivity

Accounts for about one-third of ADHD cases

ADHD, Predominantly Hyperactive/Impulsive

Significant number of hyperactivity/impulsivity symptoms identified, but not significant number in inattention category

Accounts for the fewest ADHD cases

ADHD, Attention-deficit/hyperactivity disorder.

TABLE 30.6 **Summary of Attention-Deficit/Hyperactivity Disorder Impairments Across the Life Span**

Life Stage	Impairment
Childhood	Academic difficulties including: • Needs for special education (high comorbidity with learning disabilities) • Grade retention • Classroom behavior management issues • Difficulties with friendships and peer relationships • Behavioral difficulties at home and other settings (child care, sports, after-school programs) • High comorbidity with other childhood psychiatric problems • Associated difficulties (at higher rates than non-ADHD children) with sleep disorders, enuresis, encopresis
Adolescence	Academic difficulties including: • Needs for special education (high comorbidity with learning and emotional disabilities) • School failure and dropout • Social difficulties with peer relationships • Substance abuse (in untreated ADHD) • High comorbidity with other psychiatric disorders (depression, anxiety, conduct disorder) • High-risk behaviors leading to greater accident rates • Involvement in juvenile criminal activities
Adulthood	Difficulties include: • Fewer employment possibilities and higher rates of unemployment • Higher risk of tobacco, drug, and alcohol abuse • Higher risk of motor vehicle accidents • Marital discord and higher divorce rates • Increased incidence of criminal involvement

ADHD, Attention-deficit/hyperactivity disorder.

on the family and community (Table 30.6). Families report significantly higher levels of stress; individuals have difficulties with peer relationships, increased nonfatal injuries, and issues with driving (traffic violations and accidents). There are significant direct and indirect costs, including days of missed work due to the child's school and medical appointments, evaluation and treatment that are often not covered by health insurance (e.g., psychological or educational testing beyond that done at the school), and cost of medication and mental health care.

ADHD prevalence rates vary depending on the source, criteria used to make the diagnosis, and the ages sampled. It is more common in males than females, and females tend to have more problems with inattention. The National Survey of Children's Health reports a 6.1% overall prevalence of ADHD in children 2 to 17 years of age in the United States (Danielson et al., 2018). This study also showed that children in rural areas are more likely to be diagnosed and less likely to receive behavioral therapy for their ADHD; that 62% take medication and represent 1 of every 5 children in the United States; 47% receive behavioral treatment; and 64% have another emotional, mental, or behavioral disorder (52% behavior or conduct problem, 33% anxiety, 17% depression, 14% autism spectrum disorder (ASD), 1% Tourette syndrome).

Children who have ACEs are more likely to have ADHD and are more likely to have moderate to severe disease (Brown et al., 2017). It is important to ascertain if the symptoms are caused by ADHD with comorbidity or if the comorbid disorder is masquerading as ADHD as the approach to treatment may be very different. Additionally, some coexisting conditions manifest over time, so monitoring for these conditions after assessment is critical.

Genetics, Neurobiologic Pathophysiology, and Environmental Factors. Attention is a complex and multilayered neurologic activity requiring the function and interconnection of a number of different brain areas. Structural and functional imaging demonstrate smaller brain volume in the accumbens, amygdala, and hippocampus in addition to the caudate and putamen regions (Hoogman, et.al, 2017). Anomalous brain development (reductions in gray matter) in preschoolers 4 and 5 years of age (youngest studied) correlated with behavioral symptoms (Jacobson et al., 2018).

There is no single cause for ADHD; research indicates that it is primarily a genetic disorder with environmental factors that modulate the biochemical predisposition. Genetic variations include deletions and duplications of DNA segments (copy number variants) involved with manufacture and regulation of the catecholamine (noradrenergic) neurotransmitters, noradrenaline and dopamine. Individuals with ADHD have less neurotransmitters in certain brain regions. Dopamine and noradrenaline help alert, maintain attention and appropriate internal arousal, and inhibit external distraction.

Identified risk factors include alcohol and tobacco use during pregnancy, premature and low birth weight, exposure to environmental toxins (lead) in pregnancy or in early childhood, brain injury, and ACEs. Maternal inflammation during pregnancy is theorized to cause reduced infant brain circuitry thus affecting key pathways connecting the executive hub and deeper emotional processing regions and affecting working memory (NIMH, 2018).

The faster pace and demands of society also impact the child with ADHD. Schools have longer school days, increasingly complex tasks, a higher pupil to teacher ratio, more lecture versus active learning, increased homework, emphasis on timed tasks and tests, and reduced art, music, and physical education classes. Untreated, children with ADHD can struggle with learning, social relationships, self-management and self-esteem, employment (lower socioeconomic status, higher unemployment rates), more traffic violations and higher motor vehicle accident rates, difficult family interactions including marital discord and divorce, and increased risk of substance abuse, depression, and anxiety.

Clinical Findings and Assessment

Often, the child presents after being referred by a child care provider, the school, or the parent/guardian. Concerns may include the inability to sustain attention, curb activity level, or inhibit impulsivity (core symptoms). However, concerns may be related to memory, emotional control, organization, planning or inhibiting thoughts or actions (executive functions or cognitive control), and/or difficulty with peers, following classroom rules, or regulating behavior. ADHD symptoms affect the domains where children and adolescents work on developmental mastery—school, peers, family life, sports, and recreational activities. It is important for the provider to inquire about all of these areas.

The components of the ADHD assessment include interviewing the parent and youth, physical examination, standardized ADHD assessment scales from several different sources (parents, caregivers, teachers, child care programs, and/or sports coaches) to ensure impairment in multiple domains, and other pertinent evaluations, such as school testing and psychological or other mental health evaluations. A comprehensive history for ADHD assessment is outlined in Table 30.7.

A complete physical examination should be done with a focus on the following:

- Vital signs—weight, height, body mass index (BMI), blood pressure, pulse, and head circumference in young children
- Vision and hearing screening
- General observation of child's behavior (may or may not present with ADHD symptoms in the clinical setting); observations of parent-child interaction
- General—dysmorphic stigmata suggestive of genetic syndrome or prenatal exposure to drugs or alcohol
- Skin—café au lait spots; signs of abuse
- Ear, nose, and throat (ENT)—signs of past recurring otitis media (scarring of tympanic membranes), signs of respiratory allergies, enlarged tonsils, sleep apnea
- Cardiovascular—heart sounds and rhythm, murmur, pulses
- Neurologic—general screening examination—mental status, speech and language, motor skills, and general cognition and mental process as appropriate for age
- Screening for iron deficiency, lead, and thyroid dysfunction, if indicated

Attention Deficit/Hyperactivity Disorder, Scales and Diagnostic Tools, Differential Diagnosis, and Comorbidities

Use of ADHD-specific behavior rating scales provides the most objective data to assess the scope and severity of the symptoms and are useful to monitor change once treatment begins. A number of different behavioral scales evaluate ADHD symptoms, and some also screen for executive function and comorbidities. Common screeners include the Vanderbilt ADHD Scales, the ADHD Rating Scale IV, Conner Parent and Teacher Rating Scales, and the Child Attention Profile. All can be found online, some at no charge. Consistent use of one scale is recommended in order to become familiar with the scoring and interpretation. Scales should be completed independently by individuals who know the youth and should be obtained from at least two different domains (e.g., home, school, and day care). As children get older, obtain information from teachers who work with the student; this information provides valuable insight into symptom variation at different hours of the day and clues about learning difficulties.

Management

Diagnosis and Initial Meeting With Families. Once the PCP collects all data from the history and physical examination,

behavioral rating scales from various domains, and any other evaluations (school reports, psychoeducational testing, mental health assessment), it is important to assess the onset, duration, the settings where impairment is present, and the nature and degree of symptoms and functional impairment. Use clinical judgment to determine the effect of symptoms on academic achievement and classroom performance; family, peer, and authority relationships; sports and recreation participation; and behavioral and emotional regulation with thoughtful consideration of the possibility of coexisting conditions. These data should be compared to the diagnostic criteria to identify if ADHD is present and which subtype best describes the symptoms.

It is imperative to set aside sufficient time to discuss the findings in detail with the family. This discussion should be comprehensive to help the parents understand their child's attentional difficulties as part of an inclusive picture of his or her functioning. Families need education about developmental concerns, academic performance issues, learning disabilities, medical diagnoses, social concerns, family issues and stressors, and associated coexisting mental health diagnoses. For those children not meeting the criteria for ADHD and who do not have another condition identified, it is equally important to meet with their families to review findings and establish a plan that includes close monitoring and further evaluation of their learning or behavior problems.

It is imperative for PCPs to identify the child's and family's strengths and to build on those during the entire diagnostic and treatment process. It is also worthwhile to share the perspective that, although some of these traits are a problem in childhood, the high energy, creativity, humor, and flexibility in ideation can actually lead to a successful career—note some of the very famous and successful people with ADHD (e.g., Albert Einstein, Bill Gates, Michael Phelps, and Walt Disney).

PCPs act as care coordinators with strong family-school partnerships. The plan of care focuses on the areas of functional impairment: academic achievement; relationships—parent, peer, sibling, and adult authority; social skills—sports and recreational participation; and behavior and emotional regulation. A key element is having three specific, measurable short-term target goals at a time from the areas that are most impaired, incorporating the child's strengths and resiliency (Box 30.3).

Family Education and Support. Education focuses on parent-child management techniques. The chronic nature of ADHD affects family functioning and treatment compliance. Parents often have to educate others about their child's special needs. Likewise, education of the child or adolescent, the parents, teachers, and other caregivers is critical. Providers should have several resources available that they are familiar with and comfortable recommending to families.

It is necessary to help parents understand the diagnosis complexity, to deal with feelings of shock, confusion or guilt, if present. The diagnosis of a child is often the first clue to the eventual diagnosis of a sibling or parent who has similar difficulties. ADHD symptoms impact the already complex relationships within a family, so ongoing support is important. As a culture we value attention and control of impulsivity with educational standards centered on these values. Perceptions about parenting and childrearing, beliefs about medication and the healthcare system in general, family and social networking roles in managing child behavior problems, and parents' own experiences with school are all factors that shape the approach to seeking care, diagnosis, and treatment. Families may have differing understanding of what constitutes a

TABLE 30.7 Attention-Deficit/Hyperactivity Disorder History

Assessment Area	Suggested Topics to Explore
Chief complaint and history of present problem	Major areas of concern and beliefs about causation of problem First awareness of problem and previous evaluations and results Medication history for behavioral, emotional, or learning problems
Birth history	Prenatal history: maternal health; use of medications, recreational drugs, alcohol, and tobacco during pregnancy Birth and postpartum complications, prematurity, low birth weight or intrauterine growth retardation, anoxia, difficult delivery, birth defects Neonatal behavior: Feeding, sleep, temperament problems
Family and environmental history	ADHD, neurologic problems, learning difficulties Mental health history of close family members, health or behavior problems in other family members Genetic disorders: Cognitive disabilities, growth disorders, neurofibromatosis Drug or alcohol abuse (current and/or past), involvement with law enforcement, weapons in the home
Medical history	Chronic diseases, ongoing medications, environmental allergies Hospitalizations, prolonged illness Trauma history (head injury, frequent injuries) Poisoning or lead or environmental exposures Neurologic status, seizures, tics, habit spasms, uncontrolled twitches, outbursts of uncontrollable sounds or words Cardiovascular history
Developmental history	Milestones: Motor, personal/social, language, cognitive Strengths (e.g., personality, activities, friendliness) and weaknesses
Behavioral history	Frequency with which child complies when told to do something Methods used at home to improve behavior and effectiveness Parenting skills and style, cultural beliefs, and agreement about child management Counseling history for child or family (or both)
ADHD history	Attention: Paying attention, sustaining attention, listening, following through, organization, reluctant to engage in activities that need sustained attention, hyperfocusing on activities of interest, loses things, forgetful, ability to follow three or four step commands Activity: Fidgets, leaves seat, runs or climbs when inappropriate, has difficulty with quiet games, talks excessively, has problems waiting turn, interrupts, "on the go"
Academic history	Child's progress at each grade level (strengths seen) Adjustment problems at school, child's history with peers, friendships Difficulties with specific skills: Reading, writing, spelling, math, concepts Performance problems: Attention, grades, participation, excessive talking, disturbing others, fighting, bullying, teasing, abusive language, not completing work School assistance: Tutoring, counseling, special help
Activities of Daily Life	
Feeding	Ability to sit through a complete meal, messy and clumsy with utensils, dishes, and glasses Inadequate caloric intake can be result of symptoms
Elimination	Enuresis, encopresis
Sleeping	Difficulty falling asleep, night waking, needs less sleep than other family members Complains about fatigue interfering with completion of tasks
Activity	Amount and activity or exercise Amount and details of screen time
Family relationships	General family relationships (child and parents/siblings) Home, day care, and school environments Births, deaths, marriage, and family transitions, recent moves; parental deployment, separation, divorce, remarriage Violence: domestic, current, or past abuse of parent or child; problems with the law; weapons in the home Inadequate social and relational skills: lies, steals, plays with fire, hurts animals, is aggressive with other children, talks back to adults
Mental health, coping and stress tolerance	Difficulty maintaining routines Struggles with self-concept and low self-esteem Family stress (e.g., parent job loss or change, financial problems) and coping patterns Outbursts of temper, low tolerance for frustration Moody, worried, sad, quiet, destructive, fearful or fearless, self-deprecating Somatic complaints
School & teacher history	Level of performance (below potential for achievement) Tends to miss the point of conversations and activities Often does things the hard way in absence of established routines Information from school about child's strengths, weaknesses, difficulties, academic management of issues

ADHD, Attention-deficit/hyperactivity disorder.

• BOX 30.3 Potential Goals for Family Support

Family Support

- *Routines, rules, and family relationships* are key. Home should be a safe place where one feels valued. Life with ADHD is stressful for the child and the family, and keeping family ties strong helps ease the stress.
- *Family meetings* provide opportunity to discuss structure, rewards, and consequences, as well as to plan and problem solve.
- *Support and advocacy groups* help with managing daily problems that come from living with ADHD.
- *Family therapy or counseling* is frequently used short term with specific family situational goals. It is especially helpful if there is aggressive behavior or problems related to anxiety, self-esteem, and depression or if other family members (especially siblings) need psychological assessment or support.
- *"Coaching"* helps a child or adolescent develop difficult skills. Helps with problem solving, time management, organizational skills, and learning strategies (how to be an active learner, learning to learn, and learning how to organize learning).

Home Management

- *Environmental management:* A calm, predictable home with clear, consistent morning and evening routines is extremely helpful for the child with ADHD. An organized place for everyday things to go is another way to provide structure.
- *Homework support* is essential (see Box 30.5). Monitor for mental fatigue.
- *Exercise:* Aerobic exercise improves clinical, cognitive, and scholastic performance because it increases dopamine, serotonin, and norepinephrine levels. Scheduling daily time to be active and expend energy, especially in the morning before school, is extremely important to help children with ADHD stay regulated. Martial arts, which demand discipline and self-control, are especially useful.
- *Downtime or senseless fun:* Children with ADHD need more time for normal childhood activities, including time to do nothing and daydream. Time in less-structured activities improves self-directed executive function.
- *Computers:* Many children with ADHD love computers; they produce neat results, never criticize, offer second and third chances, can help with spelling and organization, and provide opportunities for relaxation.

Keep an open mind to their use to ensure they are not used to the point of social isolation.

- *Nutrition:* Regular mealtimes with normal portion sizes provide healthy eating that provides necessary energy. Small meals with the morning dose of stimulant medication can decrease stomachaches. Instant breakfast drinks and other high-calorie foods supplement calories when the child has low caloric intake because of difficulty sitting through meals or side effects of medications.
- *Sleep:* Many children and adults with ADHD do not require as much sleep as other people or have trouble falling or staying asleep. It is important to ask if the child is sleeping well and staying in bed the entire night. Ritualized bedtime routines are important; massage, deep breathing, and relaxation techniques are sometimes helpful. Melatonin (2-6 mg/day), low-dose clonidine, or an antihistamine may be helpful; however, long-term use of these agents is not recommended.
- *Patience, unconditional love, and support* are especially important for children with ADHD, because they face so many challenges getting through their day. Plan a daily "time in" for 15-20 min with undivided parent attention focused on a child-selected activity.
- Complementary treatments may also have some benefit (see Chapter 27).

Friends and Activities

- *Areas of strength* should be developed (music, sports, computer) rather than always focusing on areas of weakness. Camps, clubs, and appropriate work provide avenues for development of skills and new friendships.
- *Activities* of the child's choosing in areas of strength or developmentally appropriate work can help build peer relationships and self-esteem.
- *Friendships* may come more easily if structure is provided (going to a movie or a sporting event) and the time frame is consistent with what the child can handle.
- *Musical training* facilitates development and maintenance of certain executive functioning skills that may be helpful to children with ADHD.

ADHD, Attention-deficit/hyperactivity disorder.

---

behavior problem. Providers should be open and honest in the discussion of diagnoses and all treatment options and include key family members in collaborative decision-making, striving to become more aware of the community and cultural values of patients.

Children with ADHD often struggle with self-esteem as they strive to meet expectations placed on them. It is crucial to identify their areas of strength and promote mental health in order to develop those areas rather than constantly focusing on remediating areas of weakness (see Chapter 15). Help parents focus on the many positive attributes, sometimes called "superpowers," of ADHD: they are innovators, dreamers, creative thinkers and problems solvers, highly sensitive, humorous, doers, risk takers, and persistent.

Behavior Management, Parent Skills Training, and Counseling. Behavior management modifies behavior and physical and social environments. These modalities are not as powerful as medication in reducing core ADHD symptoms, but they are effective. Behavior management alone should be used if the child is younger than 6 years old, symptoms are mild, and/or DSM criteria are not met. Medication paired with behavior management

is used when there is a poor response to medication alone, there are psychosocial stressors or coexisting conditions, or when the parents desire it. Reports on children receiving both medication and behavior management show greater parent and teacher satisfaction and lower medication dosages than reports on children receiving monotherapy.

Calm parenting is very successful with an ADHD child. This takes positive parenting and adds the essential component of deepening the bond between parent and child. Strategies are: staying cool, thinking like a cop ("Do you realize...?) instead of reacting and yelling; looking for the parent role in the issue; knowing how the child is hardwired and differentiating between what is hypersensitivity and what is truly rebellion; and remembering to play and connect. Parenting programs can help caregivers set up rewards and reinforcers for positive behavior, give clear and effective commands and structure, and establish safe and consistent discipline strategies. The goal of parent skills training is for parents to learn ways to optimize child success by giving the child direction, setting goals and limits to improve compliance, increasing self-esteem, enhancing the parent-child relationship, and reducing struggles in the home. Three essential components include: (1) increasing positive parent-child interactions, (2) practicing different scenarios with the child, and (3) learning time-out/disciplinary consistency. If parents disagree about management or do not get along, this approach is not likely to work.

Therapy can help parents learn to parent effectively, to foster improved communication, and help children learn self-regulation skills. As a child with ADHD approaches middle school, high school, and college age, new approaches are needed as the child assumes more control. These may be times of strain for the family, and counseling may be needed.

Educational and Adaptive Supports. It is essential that the PCP works with the family and the school to set reasonable expectations and develop a plan for the child to be successful in school. The PCP can provide information on common features of ADHD and how they relate to the child's previous and current problems in school, as well as future expectations of the clinical course and intervention strategies. For the child, a developmentally appropriate explanation and demystification of ADHD are essential—knowing how attention works and identifying their own strengths and attributes, as well as the areas of weakness that need support. The importance of teacher selection each year should be emphasized. Communication with the school personnel is imperative to provide specific teacher-focused information about diagnosis

and difficulties in all identified areas and to address appropriate intervention strategies and modifications. Many teachers are familiar with ADHD and many schools have behavior management programs or interventions to enhance academic and social functioning. Most children benefit from either a 504 plan with accommodations or an IEP for academic learning or behavior (see Chapter 7 and Box 30.4).

Classroom behavior management helps improve attention to instruction and work productivity as well as decrease disruptive behavior. Common techniques include: increased structure with the use of behavior contracts with goals and reinforcement; token economy (earning or losing points that can be exchanged for privileges or items); creating a periodic behavior report card (e.g., daily or weekly progress notes); and/or study or organizational skills training. Other considerations are brain/energy breaks (a set time to stretch, get up and walk around), secret signals to indicate need for a break, and allowing a child not to be still (bouncy balls, standing or pacing while working). Peer intervention strategies, either in groups or as a pair, help reduce inappropriate or disruptive behavior.

Adaptive technology (AT) can assist the child with ADHD and should be in any 504 or IEP. Examples of AT that are readily available include: voice-activated and word prediction software to

---

• BOX 30.4 Suggestions for Classroom Accommodations for Children with Attention-Deficit/Hyperactivity Disorder

Memory and Attention

Seat the child close to the teacher away from heavy traffic areas (e.g., doorways).
Keep oral instructions brief with repetitions; avoid multiple commands.
Provide written directions—broken down or simplified if needed.
"Walk" the child through assignments to be sure they are understood.
Break tasks and homework into small tasks.
Use visual aids, hands-on, and experiential teaching methods rather than strict lecture style.
Teach active reading with underlining and active listening with note taking.
Provide remedial help in small sessions.
Teach sub vocalization (saying words in your head while reading) to aid memorizing.
Establish a signal that reminds the child to focus and return to task.
Allow nondistracting motor activity during tasks requiring concentration (e.g., squeezing a ball or fingering Velcro to replace pencil tapping).
Allow earplugs for auditory processing issues.

Impulse Control

Allow for freedom of movement as much as possible (e.g., classroom helper).
Never punish the child by taking away physical education, recess, or other physical activity outlets.
Teach the child to monitor quality of work before turning it in.

Classroom Atmosphere

Provide a structured classroom with clear expectations.
Use moderate, consistent discipline.
Rely on positive reinforcement for good behavior.
Provide a quiet place to work in the classroom (headsets with select music may block out distractions).

Organizational Skills

Establish a daily checklist of tasks.
Use a daily planner. List homework assignments with due date and needed resources.

Divide notebook into three sections: work to be completed, work completed, and work to be saved.
Color code class material to help organize.
Follow up on homework not turned in.
Allow extra time for gathering necessary items, packing backpack, and so on.
Provide an extra set of textbooks for use at home.
Teach strategies for time management and basic study skills.
Develop preview and planning skills.

Productivity Problems

Divide worksheets into sections.
Reduce the amount of homework and written classwork.
Modify the number of math problems to be completed.
Provide test modification—quiet location and extra time.
Use assistive technology—word processor, calculator, audio books, and note-taker pen.

Written Expression

Give extra time to complete written tests and assignments.
Provide help with handwriting.
Allow child to dictate reports and take tests orally.
Reduce the quantity of written work required.
Grade papers on content rather than untidy work, spelling errors, or poor handwriting.

Self-Esteem

Reward progress.
Encourage performance in areas of child's strength.
Avoid humiliation.
Give hand signals only the child can see as private reminders of appropriate behavior.

Social Relationships

Provide feedback about behavior involving other children.
Make sure other children do not believe that the child is doing less or is allowed unacceptable behavior; change the rules for all children if necessary.

help with writing papers, note-taking pens that download into a computer, visual thinking tools, electronic organizers, cell phones or iPads with timers and reminders, and a multitude of apps.

Homework is often a challenge for parents (who want their children to do well) and children who have trouble focusing after a long day at school. Helping parents plan a home routine is essential (Box 30.5). Children with ADHD often work best in nontraditional study areas—upside down off a couch, under a table, or memorizing while jumping on a trampoline (see Chapter 15 for sensory techniques). Parents should monitor how much homework is given and how the child deals with it, at times stepping in to work with teachers if modifications are needed. The PCP should recognize homework struggles may be a sign of learning disability and may need further evaluation. It is important to give time off while still structuring summer plans to provide stress-free activities and hands-on learning.

Pharmacologic Management. Medications effectively reduce core symptoms and are recommended for children who meet the ADHD diagnostic criteria. Medication alone is usually not as effective as medication combined with behavior therapy (Catala-Lopez, Hutton, Nunez-Beltran, et al., 2017). Stimulants are the most effective medications, but three nonstimulants (one selective norepinephrine-reuptake inhibitor and two α_2-adrenergic agonists) are also efficacious. Medication selection depends on the age of the child, the desired timing and length of coverage, coexisting conditions, and insurance coverage. Information on current available and approved medications is readily available online, however, one of the most up-to-date sources is the ADHD Medication Guide available at http://adhdmedicationguide.com. The PCP should focus on finding the medication and dosage that best fits the child's needs. Evidence indicates that methylphenidate was better for children and adolescents, while adults did better on amphetamines (Cortese et al., 2018).

Stimulants. The first-line medications for uncomplicated ADHD treatment are methylphenidate and amphetamine compounds which are equally effective and available in a variety of forms. These work by increasing the availability of neurotransmitters at the neuron synapses by blocking the transporters that remove dopamine and norepinephrine in key areas of the brain. This action is theorized to allow the child to exhibit more purposeful, goal-oriented behavior by focusing attention, lessening impulsiveness, and decreasing motor activity. Between 70% and 90% of children respond positively to stimulant medications although

there is no predictor for which one will work best. If treatment at the highest tolerated dose of one stimulant group does not help (the child is a non-responder), then the recommendation is to try a medication from the other group, or a different medication from the same group. Amphetamines are dosed at 0.3 to 1.0 mg/kg/day, with a maximum dose of 1.5 mg/kg/day (or 40 mg, except for lisdexamfetamine [Vyvanse] at 70 mg/day). Methylphenidates are dosed at 0.3 to 2.0 mg/kg/day, with a maximum dose of 2.0 mg/kg/day (or 60 mg, except for Concerta at 72 mg/day and dermal methylphenidate at 30 mg/day); dexmethylphenidates at about half that dose, with a maximum dose of 20 mg for Focalin and 30 mg for Focalin XR.

Both stimulant compounds are efficacious and the side effect profiles are similar, so consider the impairment severity, coexisting conditions, and if an extended-release or short-acting form is the best fit. Children with inattentive presentation often respond well to lower doses, whereas children with hyperactive presentation have a more positive response at moderate to high doses. In general, the long-acting forms are preferred because no midday school dosing is required, thus providing smoother coverage, greater convenience, improved compliance, and less stigma. A short-acting medication might be chosen for initial dosing or if dosage titration or side effects are of concern.

When working with the adolescent, it is important to assess for substance abuse and, if identified, refer for treatment prior to prescribing stimulants. If no risk is detected but there are concerns about stimulant diversion (e.g., selling the drug to other students), lisdexamfetamine or dermal methylphenidate should be considered as they are less likely to result in diversion; alternatively, a nonstimulant drug could be chosen. PCPs must consider the risks that an adolescent driver with ADHD faces and the long and late hours when studying, and consider which medications best provide coverage for these situations.

Preschoolers, 4 to 5 years old, need special consideration and care with diagnosis. Symptoms in preschoolers are often related to other conditions, such as language disorders, hearing loss, low intellectual functioning, or another psychopathology. Behavioral therapy, especially group parent training, is the recommended first line of treatment. However, medication can be considered for a child with moderate to severe dysfunction, who has at least 9 months of symptoms, with dysfunction in more than one domain (e.g., home, daycare, preschool), and/or who has an inadequate response to behavioral therapy. Adderall is the only FDA-approved stimulant for children as young as 3 years old. This age group has slower drug metabolism thus necessitating a lower starting dose (2.5 mg twice per day).

When dosing stimulants, it is important to remember that:
- Dose response is unique to each child/teen and should be adjusted for age, body weight, degree of impairment, and specific symptoms
- Begin dosing at the low end and titrate up every 1 to 3 weeks with monitoring for symptom improvement and side effects
- Approximately one-third of children/teens respond at the low dose, one-third at mid-dose range, and one-third require the higher doses for maximum benefit
- The dosing goal is maximum reduction of ADHD core symptoms with minimal side effects
- Change to a different medication, the other stimulant group, or a nonstimulant medication if the child is at the maximum dose without adequate response or is having significant side effects
- Instruct families to monitor for benefit and adverse effects to identify the lowest effective dose

---

• BOX 30.5 Tips for Home-Based Homework Support

1. Provide a quiet location where work will be done with minimal distractions. Set up a work station equipped with necessary materials.
2. Establish a homework time as early as possible to prevent the child from being too tired, but allow a break after school.
3. Establish a homework plan: Review assignments and make a schedule for completion, breaking into small, manageable pieces.
4. Help the child to get started. Monitor without taking over. Praise effort; do not insist on perfection.
5. Use a timer to help with time management. Structure time for breaks as often as every 15 min if needed. Encourage movement during breaks.
6. Permit time for editing so the child does not lose points due to editing errors. Help to study for tests.
7. Provide incentives to help motivation.
8. Identify another student to contact for clarification.

When a change in medication is needed, consider the following:
- An amphetamine is approximately 1.5 times as potent as methylphenidate
- Focalin products are approximately two times more potent than regular methylphenidate products, and dermal methylphenidate is approximately 1.5 times more potent than immediate release methylphenidate
- Vyvanse potency is less than other amphetamine products with estimated 30 mg = Adderall 10 mg; Vyvanse 50 mg = Adderall 20 mg; Vyvanse 70 mg = Adderall 30 mg

Common adverse effects of the stimulants include decreased appetite, weight loss, insomnia, stomachache, and headache. Adjustments to the time that medication is given and the relationship to food intake can sometimes help. With time, these symptoms often resolve but must be monitored. If they persist, decreasing the dose, switching the medication, or adding a medication may help. Emotional lability and irritability, especially if persistent and not just the result of the medication wearing off, can indicate the need to adjust the dose, change the medication, or revisit the diagnosis. Contraindications to stimulants include psychosis or any previous untoward reactions to stimulant medication. If using transdermal methylphenidate, the skin may be irritated where the patch is applied; alternating sites, good skin care, and moisturization usually take care of the irritation. The use of a topical steroid may help irritation or itching.

The FDA published a study (USFDA, 2011), currently being updated, that showed no association between the use of ADHD medications, including stimulants and atomoxetine, and adverse cardiovascular effects—stroke, myocardial infarction, or sudden cardiac death. In general, stimulants and atomoxetine should not be given to anyone with serious heart problems or in those whom increased blood pressure or heart rate is problematic. Screening for cardiovascular risk prior to initiating treatment with any of the ADHD medications includes: (1) detecting a cardiac history of shortness of breath with exercise, exercise intolerance, fainting or seizures with exercise, palpitations, elevated blood pressure, previously detected cardiac abnormalities, rheumatic fever, cardiomyopathy, and/or dysrhythmia; (2) a family cardiac history of sudden unexplained or cardiac death before age 50, or any familial rate, rhythm, or structural cardiac problems; and (3) complete physical examination with special attention to the cardiovascular system. If the cardiac history and examination are negative, no further tests are recommended prior to starting ADHD medication. If there are any positives in the history or examination, a consultation with a pediatric cardiologist is necessary before initiating medication.

Approximately 20% of all children develop tics, although often these are mild and simple in complexity and typically resolve within a year. Up to 20% of children with ADHD develop a chronic tic disorder, and over half of children with Tourette syndrome or chronic tic disorder have coexisting ADHD. Typically ADHD emerges before tic onset. The FDA issued a contraindication for methylphenidate and a warning for amphetamine in patients with preexisting tic disorders or those with a family history of Tourette syndrome; however, stimulant medication is unlikely to evoke or exacerbate tics and may improve tic symptoms and reduce oppositional behaviors. Stimulants may exacerbate anxiety disorders. Options for children with tics include low-dose, short- or long-acting stimulants, α-agonists, or atomoxetine. If tics emerge after medication, are not severe or disturbing to the child or adolescent, and the medication is beneficial, it is acceptable to continue stimulant treatment.

Non-Stimulant Medications. Atomoxetine is a noncontrolled, norepinephrine reuptake inhibitor, nonstimulant medication approved for ADHD for children older than age 6 years. Unlike the stimulants, it may take up to 6 weeks of regular use before effects are noted. It should be given with food and is usually dosed once a day, but it can be given twice daily. Although it is not as effective as the stimulants, atomoxetine may be a preferable first choice if the family prefers a nonstimulant medication, a substance abuse concern exists in the family, or the child has significant side effects with the stimulants including tics, anxiety, or sleep initiation difficulties. It provides 24-hour coverage, but it must not be discontinued abruptly. Common adverse effects of atomoxetine include decreased appetite, gastrointestinal complaints (nausea, anorexia), somnolence and dizziness, and mild hypertension or tachycardia. Most side effects resolve with time—headaches are the most likely to persist—and can be managed with dose reduction or medication change. There are a few reports of liver toxicity in patients taking atomoxetine. There is no need to do liver studies prior to treatment; however, if evidence of jaundice or elevated liver function is found, stop the medication. Caution patients to report dark urine, flulike illness, fatigue, abdominal pain, or nausea. Increased risk of suicidal ideation or attempts may occur in children and adolescents being treated with atomoxetine. Although the risk is small, parents and patients should be advised that if there is any change in mood—depression, mood lability, agitation, suicidal thoughts or gestures—they must get care immediately. Preexisting and development of suicidal thoughts, hallucinations, psychosis, or mania are absolute contraindications and these children need referral to a qualified behavioral health clinician. Finally, because of the possibility of clinically significant increased blood pressure or heart rate (for example, a 15 to 20 mm Hg blood pressure rise or 20 beats per minute pulse increase), the FDA recommends that atomoxetine should not be used in those individuals with tachyarrhythmias or hypertension.

Extended-release guanfacine (Intuniv) and extended-release clonidine (Kapvay) are α-agonists approved for ADHD treatment in children 6 years old and older, although their efficacy is not as strong as for the other medications. Guanfacine improves oppositional symptoms in addition to ADHD core symptoms, especially impulsivity. Clonidine helps children with sleep issues. These medications do not worsen tics, are typically not abused, and may help children with trouble sleeping or conduct disorder symptoms. It takes 1 to 2 weeks to appreciate any effect. Both are FDA approved as adjunctive therapy to stimulant medications and provide additional symptom reduction. A cardiovascular history and full physical examination are recommended prior to initiating these medications. The most common adverse effects include sedation, bradycardia, and abdominal pain. With guanfacine, these effects tend to resolve over time. Monitoring blood pressure and heart rate is important but medications should not be discontinued unless the child becomes symptomatic (e.g., hypotensive or bradycardic). Instruct the family not to abruptly discontinue the medication because of the possibility of rebound hypertension.

Complementary Therapies. Outdoor exercise, aerobic exercise, adequate sleep, and good nutrition are key. Ensure a healthy diet with high-quality macronutrients—protein, fats, and carbohydrates. A clean, uncluttered environment and learning to manage stress are helpful. Only prescribe zinc and iron in patients with a proven deficiency. Omega-3 fatty acids are considered most effective given with ADHD medication, with the largest effect at 560 mg EPA. Vayarin is a prescription-strength form of omega-3 fatty acids classified as a medical food for use in dietary management of ADHD. It is not FDA regulated, approved, or registered, but it may be used as a supplement or for families who resist traditional pharmacotherapy. In early 2019, the FDA approved a trigeminal nerve stimulator to treat nonmedicated children with ADHD. Evidence for this approach is limited to a small study of 62 children (FDA, 2019) https://www.fda.gov/news-events/press-announcements/fda-permits-marketing-first-medical-device-treatment-adhd. There are a multitude of other complementary therapies but none have clear scientific efficacy (Goode, et.al, 2018).

Follow-up and Referral

Regular child and family follow-up includes reassessment of core symptoms, functioning, and target goals; review of medication regimen; education; care coordination and advocacy; and assessment of family functioning and need for family support or other resources (Box 30.6). Refer to specialists if things don't go as expected, or there is poor medication response or emergent comorbidities. At times, transitions are overwhelming and referral to behavioral health for coping skills training helps.

As the child matures, so does the brain, and symptomatology and coexisting conditions may change. PCPs must be attuned to these changes and provide anticipatory guidance and modify treatment plans as needed. Empowering children/adolescents to understand and comanage their condition and impairments is essential. Include management strategies, clarifying that ADHD is not a lack of intelligence, and help them build on strengths. Equip parents with proactive strategies for the home and for dealing with transitions to middle school, high school, and college or vocational studies. Families are often under stress because of the ongoing challenges and helping them learn how to cope with the stress or access behavioral health services is important. As the child nears the end of adolescence, plan for transition to adult care. Got Transition (www.gottransition.org) is a model developed to guide this practice.

When initiating medication treatment and any time there is a dose or medication change, the PCP should meet with the family to assess the effectiveness within 2 to 3 weeks of the change and monthly until all is stable to assess for core symptoms changes. It is important to note that sometimes a change in medication from brand name to generic may result in symptom changes. Regular reassessment of the child's core symptoms and functioning should occur every 3 to 6 months if stable with feedback from the family, the school, and anyone else involved. In addition to assessment of medication effectiveness, it is important to comprehensively look at the child's functioning in school, at home, with peers, and in activities. Assess family functioning, including the reasonableness of parental expectations with a focus on areas where additional resources or support is needed. The Vanderbilt Scale has a follow-up version for parents and teachers that collects information about the core ADHD symptoms, level of impairment, potential side effects, and comorbid symptoms. Often families think things are going fairly well when they may actually benefit from modifications or other support. Monitor height, weight, blood pressure, sleep, appetite, and the development of any significant symptoms such as aggression or tics. Perform an abbreviated physical examination with a focus on the cardiac system. Medication modification may include dose adjustment, a change in the timing of the dose, or adding an adjunct medication.

Many of the medication side effects can be minimized by having children and teens eat a healthy meal before taking their medication, ensuring medications are taken by 9 am, taking the medication with food, or eating soon after the dose. Assess and advise about sleep hygiene. Some children taking stimulants experience "rebound" moodiness as the medication wears off, often in the afternoon after school. These symptoms can be treated by giving the child a low dose of the same short-acting stimulant in the afternoon. A trial without medications may be considered if the child is stable and doing well. It is best done at a time when there will be few transitions, and definitely not at the beginning of the school year, especially the junior/senior year of high school. If there is a decision to take the child off medication, there should be close follow-up during the first 4 weeks.

Specific Learning Disorders

Definition and Diagnostic Criteria

The DSM-5 defines SLD as a biologic neurodevelopmental disorder that causes learning and academic skills acquisition problems in the early school years, lasting for at least 6 months, not attributed to intellectual developmental disorders, external factors such as economic or environmental disadvantage, vision or hearing problems, neurological condition, or motor disorders (APA, 2014). SLD is classified as mild, moderate, or severe and results in reading, written expression, or math involvement (Box 30.7). Key skills impacted include reading single words, reading

---

> **• BOX 30.6** **Questions to Consider When Developing the Plan of Care for a Child/Adolescent with Attention-Deficit Hyperactivity Disorder**
>
> - Does the family understand the core ADHD symptoms and their child's/adolescent's target symptoms and coexisting conditions?
> - Does the family need support to establish, measure, and monitor target goals?
> - Have the family's goals been identified and addressed in the care plan?
> - Does the family understand effective behavior management techniques for responding to tantrums, oppositional behavior, or poor compliance to requests and commands?
> - Is help needed for normalizing peer and family relationships?
> - Does the child/adolescent need help in academic areas? If so, has a formal evaluation been performed and reviewed to distinguish work production problems secondary to ADHD from coexisting learning or language disabilities?
> - Does the child/adolescent need help in achieving independence in self-help or schoolwork production?
> - Does the child/adolescent or family require help with optimizing, organizing, planning, or managing schoolwork flow?
> - Does the family need help in recognition, understanding, or management of coexisting conditions?
> - Is there a plan in place to systematically educate the child/adolescent about ADHD and its treatment as well as the child's/adolescent's own strengths and weaknesses?
> - Is there a plan in place to empower the child/adolescent with the knowledge and understanding that will increase his or her adherence to treatments and has that begun as early as possible and been addressed at the child's/adolescent's developmental level?
> - Does the family have a copy of a care plan that summarizes findings and treatment recommendations that can be updated and used in school settings and other professional settings so that the history and treatment plan does not need to be constantly reinvented?
> - Is the follow-up plan sufficient to provide comprehensive, coordinated, family-centered, culturally competent, and ongoing care?
>
> *ADHD, Attention-deficit hyperactivity disorder.*
> *Adapted from American Academy of Pediatrics (AAP).* Implementing the Key Action Statements: An Algorithm and Explanation for Process of Care for the Evaluation, Diagnosis, Treatment, and Monitoring of ADHD in Children and Adolescents. *Available from: http://pediatrics. aappublications.org/content/suppl/2011/10/11/peds.2011-2654.DC1/zpe611117822p.pdf. Accessed October 3, 2018.*

comprehension, writing, spelling, math calculation, and math problem solving. Reading difficulties include reading rate or fluency, reading accuracy and comprehension, and foreign language. *Dyslexia* refers to difficulties with word recognition, decoding, and spelling. Difficulties in writing include spelling, punctuation, grammar, organization, and clarity of written expression. *Dysgraphia* describes difficulty with handwriting (forming letters, writing within a defined space). Math difficulties include number sense, memorizing math facts, math calculations or math reasoning, and problem solving. *Dyscalculia* describes difficulties with learning math facts and performing calculations, including making change in cash transactions.

It is not clear what causes learning disorders, but problems are often present from birth, and often inherited. Known environmental factors include alcohol and drug use, exposure to toxins, poor nutrition, abnormal family involvement, emotional disturbances, and cultural differences. Dyslexia, the most common SLD, includes structural brain differences in the language area. SLD affects 5% to 15% of school-aged children and is more common in males. Issues with learning and attention affect one in every five children in the United States; about one-third have both disorders. SLDs affect children from all socioeconomic, racial, and ethnic groups, but they are less common in upper-income children and children who are not of color. One in 16 public school students have an IEP for SLD (ADHD or Dyspraxia, a motor disorder that results in uncoordination); 1 in 50 have accommodations through a 504 plan (Horowitz, 2017).

Coexisting neurodevelopmental (e.g., ADHD) issues are not uncommon, and social, emotional, and behavioral challenges may result in lower academic achievement, school distress (avoidance, acting-out, disengagement, or alienation), school failure (retention, expulsion, and dropping out), lower self-esteem, involvement in the justice system, and anxiety and depression. Other comorbidities include chronic health problems such as fetal alcohol syndrome, lead or other toxic exposure, and fragile X syndrome.

Clinical Findings and Assessment

Children with SLD have test scores and grades significantly below what is expected given cognitive ability. In early childhood, delays in attention, language, or motor skills may emerge. Early school-aged children may not be able to recognize or write letters, or have trouble breaking words into syllables or recognizing rhyming words. Later elementary children have difficulty connecting letters with sounds, read slowly and inaccurately, and have trouble with spelling or math facts. Adolescents may still read slowly, with much effort, and have difficulty understanding what they read or solving math problems. Behaviors may include reluctance to engage in learning (e.g., it's boring) or oppositional behavior.

Screening and Specialty Referral for Diagnosis

Developmental surveillance is a routine part of health care and includes monitoring a child's school attendance and performance to identify difficulties that may not arise until the child faces challenges. The Level I school performance prescreening questionnaire (Box 30.8) is a five-item instrument that can be administered at every well-child check. If school problems are suspected, a Level II school performance screener (see Box 30.8) provides a more comprehensive assessment to be used in conjunction with samples of school work, report cards, and previously administered tests. The National Center for Learning Disabilities has a free Learning Disabilities Checklist (www.ncld.org/), organized by skill set and age group. If delays are suspected, it is extremely important to get the child evaluated and into early-intervention services quickly. The family may need support and direction through the assessment process, which is often lengthy and emotional and involves interprofessional collaboration with colleagues in healthcare and educational fields.

The history provides clues to SLD presence and consideration of other causes of the learning problems. Important items in the family history include dyslexia or other learning disability, decreased academic achievement, attention deficits, and grade retention or school dropout. Assess for prematurity or low birthweight, early developmental concerns or delays (especially speech/language issues), head injury, seizure disorder, and chronic health conditions. Assess for child connectedness to school (feels accepted, valued, respected, and included); description of school and effort; perception of the problem's cause; experiences with teachers, peers, and homework; social competence, temperament, and coping skills. Teacher reports of academic performance, absences, engagement, behavioral information, and educational testing results should be evaluated. Also investigate home versus school functioning; behavioral and stress responses to problems; ability to attend to and complete tasks; and child strengths and weaknesses.

The physical examination is typically normal and includes behavioral observations, hearing and vision evaluation, sensory processing screening, neurologic changes, dysmorphic features, and assessment for minor congenital anomalies. The psychoeducational evaluation includes identification of strengths and weaknesses, determination of cognitive ability, assessment of perceptual strengths and weaknesses, examination of communicative ability, and assessment of social and emotional adaptation and is completed by a specialist within the school system or privately. Unfortunately, this process is costly and often not covered.

Management

Most children with academic struggles have more than one dysfunction. Identified strengths balance out the difficulties. Although the educational system focuses primarily on linguistic and logical-mathematical intelligence, and many cultures esteem highly articulate or logical people, there are other types of intelligence. The theory of multiple intelligences (Table 30.8) offers

Level I School Performance Prescreening Questionnaire

1. Do you have any concerns about your child's learning or school performance?
2. Do you have any concerns about your child's attention, concentration, impulsivity, and/or overactivity?
3. Do you have any concerns about how your child is doing in certain subjects at school? If yes, is it reading? Writing? Math? Other?
4. Do you have any concern about how much your child is enjoying school compared with friends or classmates?
5. Does your child have any problems completing homework?

Level II School Performance Screener

1. In what area(s) does your child have problems in school performance? Learning/achievement? Attention/concentration/memory? Behavior?
2. Subjects/activities of difficulty: Reading? Math? Spelling? Writing? Speaking? Listening? Remembering? Science? Social studies? Language/grammar? Following directions? Inconsistency? Transferring knowledge from one situation to another? Organizing?
3. Current grade? What grade did problems become evident? Did child repeat a grade? Was the child ever in danger of repeating a grade?
4. Grades on report card? Performance on standardized testing? Is excessive amount of help needed to do homework? Is excessive amount of homework due to child not completing in school? Would grades be lower without a great amount of extra work being done at home with parents? Is homework a battle each night?
5. Stressors? None? Current? At time of onset of school problems? With family? Peers? At school?
6. Medical concerns? Frequent ear infections? Hearing problem? Vision problem? Prenatal/perinatal problems? Allergies? Loss of consciousness? Sleep problem? Describe.
7. Strengths? Reading? Math? Spelling? Writing? Speaking? Listening? Remembering? Science? Social studies? Language/grammar? Other? Learns better by seeing versus hearing or vice versa?
8. How does the child get along with peers? Involved in extracurricular activities? Type? If so, how does he or she do?
9. Emotional issues: Lack of motivation? School avoidance? Homework avoidance? Seems lazy? Irritable? Anxious? Volatile? Down on self? Aggressive? Gives up easily? Refuses to work in class? Doesn't turn work in? Oppositional? Angry?
10. Tested by school system? If yes, eligible for services? Receives services (types)? Found ineligible? Has received services, but they have been discontinued?

TABLE 30.8 Multiple Intelligences

Intelligence	Description
Linguistic	Sensitivity to language; language-based function (word smart)
Logical/mathematical	Abstract reasoning, manipulation of symbols, detection of patterns, logical reasoning (number/reasoning smart)
Musical	Detection and production of musical structures and patterns; appreciation of pitch, rhythm, musical expressiveness (music smart)
Spatial	Visual memory, visual-spatial skills, visualization (picture smart)
Body/kinesthetic	Representation of ideas, feeling in movement; use of body, coordination, goal-directed activities (body smart)
Naturalistic	Classification and recognition of animals, plants (nature smart)
Social/interpersonal	Sensitivity and responsiveness to moods, motives, intentions, and feelings of others (people smart)
Personal/intrapersonal	Sensitivity to self, feelings, strengths, desires, weaknesses, and understanding of intention and motivation of others (self-smart)

- Organize information about your child's learning disability—a folder with letters and material, copies of school files, samples of work that demonstrate difficulty as well as strengths; a contact log; a log of own observations.
- Know your child's strengths and make sure they are utilized.
- Have your child evaluated as needed and monitor your child's progress.
- Establish realistic expectations and provide opportunities to assume responsibility.
- Improve social skills and provide for successful interaction.
- Work as an advocate for your child and find reasonable accommodations that work.
- Talk to your child about learning disabilities.
- Know your legal rights.

that perspective. Unfortunately, many children with non-linguistic and non-logical-mathematical intelligence do not receive much reinforcement in school, and end up being labeled learning disabled or underachievers, when in actuality their unique ways of thinking and learning are not addressed by the typical classroom.

Family Education and Support. Once a child receives a diagnosis, they should receive children with special healthcare needs (SHCN) status. The PCP can help identify child and family strengths, affinities, and interests in order to develop passions and areas of expertise. Assisting the family with interpretation of evaluations, describing lagging skills and treatment and accommodations, and monitoring for co-occurring conditions are part of the PCP role. Encouraging the parents to do research and become experts on their child's needs proves helpful, especially in

planning for school. This may include helping parents and children understand the implications of a particular learning disability and its effects on peer interactions; exploring ideas and acting as a conduit to help parents find reliable resources and others who solved similar problems; and assisting them to devise an organized approach to respond to their child's struggles (Box 30.9). PCPs may also coach parents about demystifying the diagnosis, reminding children of their intelligence and special way of learning.

Behavior Management and Counseling. School challenges and having to work harder and longer to achieve in school may affect the child's self-esteem, ability to cope, and mental health. Participation in activities outside of school, especially those in which the child can excel, provide benefit. Remind parents that their relationship with the child, their attitude and emotional support influence the child more than anything else. Providing social-emotional skills training and being alert to issues with self-esteem, self-regulation, and emerging emotional problems allows early intervention and referral for counseling to deal with the demands and stresses before they become overwhelming.

Educational System and Adaptive Supports. Children with neurodevelopmental problems are entitled to special education opportunities to maximize their learning potential. These are detailed in an IEP or a 504 plan with appropriate plans and accommodations. Specific, individualized, intensive instruction helps the child improve or find strategies to compensate. Project-based learning can be a welcome alternative (www.bie.org). Assistive technologies should be part of the plan. Acknowledge a child's aptitude, initiative, spirit, industry, and self-efficacy to provide tangible strengths support. The PCP may be involved in discussion about school placement of the child (mainstream classroom, special classroom, or combination of settings); may be asked to provide relevant information related to the child's development; may advocate for the child's rights and needs; or may serve as mediator, consultant, or resource to the school.

Follow-up and Referral

Routine well care includes ongoing evaluation of the school setting, performance, and accommodations. Maintain a heightened awareness of the possibility of mental health issues and screen for any comorbidities. Additional visits and referrals may be recommended in order to ensure the child achieves maximal potential.

Intellectual disability and Global Developmental Delay

Intellectual functioning, the general mental capacity to learn or understand and deal with new situations, is often measured by intellectual quotient (IQ) tests that evaluate problem-solving, language, attention, memory, and information processing. Adaptive functioning defines how well a person is able to care for themselves (conceptual, social, and practical skills) and how independent they are compared with others their same age.

Definition and Diagnostic Criteria

The DSM-5 defines intellectual disability (ID) as a neurodevelopmental disorder that results in deficits in intellectual and adaptive functioning (APA, 2014). Adaptive functioning encompasses (1) conceptual: language, reading, writing, math, reasoning, knowledge, memory; (2) social: empathy, social judgment, communication skills, the ability to follow rules, and the ability to make and keep friends; and (3) practical: independence in personal care, job responsibilities, managing money, recreation, and organizing school and work. ID severity is defined as mild, moderate, severe, or profound based on adaptive functioning, not IQ score, and the diagnosis is usually not given before age 5 years (Box 30.10). The term *global developmental delays (GDD)* is used to describe children younger than age 5 who have significant delays in 2 or more areas of development. Not all children with GDD go on to be diagnosed with ID, but two-thirds will (Purugganan, 2018). ID is also often classified as syndromic ID or nonsyndromic ID of unknown etiology.

There are many ID causes, but genetic disorders such as Down syndrome, fragile X, and Rett syndrome are most common. Environmental causes such as fetal alcohol spectrum disorder,

---

> ### • BOX 30.10   Severity Score for Intellectual Disability
>
> **Mild (85%)**
> Presents early school years; difficulties in academic setting; more socially immature than peers; thinking and communication concrete; function adaptively but need support for complex daily living; reach 6th grade level
>
> **Moderate (10%)**
> Presents earlier than mild; learning and language difficulties in preschool; deficits in social and communication requiring support; may be able to function adaptively with training and support; may be able to be employed in jobs with minimal communication and cognitive skills needed; reach 2nd grade level
>
> **Severe (3%-4%)**
> Limited ability to understand written language, numbers, and time; needs significant support throughout life; understanding of verbal and gestural communication and spoken language limited; requires extensive support and supervision for all daily living activities; may reach pre-K level
>
> **Profound (1%-2%)**
> Use of objects in a goal-directed manner for self-care or recreation; communication very limited with limited understanding and nonverbal expression; requires pervasive support and dependent in all levels of care and living

intrauterine infections (including Zika), hypoxic-ischemic injury in the neonate, toxin exposure (mercury, lead, maternal drugs), inborn errors of metabolism, and head trauma are also noted.

Incidence is more common in males and cited as 1% to 3% of the population with 85% of those mildly affected (Parekh, 2018).

Co-occurring conditions are common, including sensory processing difficulties, sleep difficulties, seizure disorders, cerebral palsy, and respiratory and gastrointestinal issues. Other neurodevelopmental disorders occur in about a third of children with ID (ASD, ADHD, anxiety and depression, aggression, and self-injury) (Purugganan, 2018). Issues needing extra attention include nutrition, the potential for obesity, exercise and activity, safety, dental issues and care, sexuality and abuse, and pain management.

Clinical Findings and Assessment

Presentation varies depending on impairment severity, with the more severe recognized earlier and the milder at times not until school age. Delays in receptive and expressive language, adaptive skills, fine motor deficits, problem-solving difficulties, social immaturity, and behavioral difficulties may be presenting concerns. Gross motor delays are the least likely to occur.

Screening and Specialty Referral for Diagnosis

Diagnosis begins with a thorough developmental, educational, medical, and family history (including a three-generation family history focused on neurodevelopmental issues, genetic conditions, and consanguinity). A complete physical and neurologic exam including vision and hearing testing is needed with a focus on head circumference, skin evaluation, and any dysmorphic features. If syndromic form is suspected, laboratory, chromosomal studies, and neuroimaging may be indicated, and referral to a genetics specialist initiated. If nonsyndromic, chromosomal microarray, fragile X testing, and karyotyping may be indicated as first-line tests, but referral to genetics is recommended as further evaluation may be needed. See the AAP Committee on Genetics (Moeschler & Shevell, 2014), the American Academy of

Neurology practice parameter and evidence report for global developmental delay (AAN, 2013), and Sherr & Shevell (2018) for diagnostic algorithms.

Neurocognitive diagnostic evaluation includes intelligence testing and adaptive testing with standardized measures and interview usually done by a psychologist or other certified clinician. Intelligence testing is most reliable after 5 years of age using standardized tests such as Wechsler Intelligence Scale or Stanford-Binet Intelligence Scales. A majority of people (68%) have an IQ between 85 and 115 (Parekh, 2017). Scores of 70 (2 standard deviations [SD] below the mean [mean IQ score of 100 and SD of 15]) are considered ID, with an incidence of 2.5% (Purugganan, 2018). Individuals with scores between 70 and 84 are considered borderline or "slow learners." Assessment of adaptive functioning is done with standardized tests such as Vineland Adaptive Behavior Scales or Adaptive Behavior Assessment System. Impairment in one of the three domains (conceptual, social, or practical) requiring ongoing support is needed in order to qualify as impairment.

Management

Early identification and intervention benefits the child in cognition, language, academics, and behavior, enabling maximum potential and minimizing functional decline. Timely identification and management of other conditions are key.

Family and Social Support. Family support starts with knowing the child's strengths, learning to appreciate their uniqueness, offering hope, and encouraging patience. Parents need resources to learn about the disability and connect with other parents. Assisting the family with home environmental management helps maintain a smoother, more controlled family life where calm instead of chaos is the rule. Community services and educational resources are available for social, recreational, and sports opportunities (Special Olympics, Best Buddies). Though schools often manage transitional support plans, the PCP should be actively involved in assisting the family with advocacy and issues related to medical care.

Behavioral Management and Counseling. As any child, the child with ID benefits from secure emotional attachment, warm parental interaction, and developing social-emotional skills to allow enhanced peer interactions. Parents or other family members may need counseling as they deal with the diagnosis (guilt) and manage the extra burdens (financial, fatigue, isolation) required to care for a child with ID. Siblings may need support as they are relied upon to help or are overlooked in the complexity of the situation. Parent classes and education provide the family with behavioral management strategies (see Chapter 15). Group sessions can be helpful for those with mild severity functioning at age 6 or 7. Some comorbid behaviors that do not respond to behavioral and environmental management may require use of medication to enhance participation and function. This should be a part of the psychosocial plan for the child that the PCP may be involved in.

Educational and Adaptive Support. Early intervention and support as provided through an IFSP or IEP are essential. Mainstreaming with special education support teachers or aides is common for children with milder severity. Self-contained classrooms with small student-teacher ratios are helpful for those with moderate to profound severity. Components may include OT, PT, and speech/language therapy; accommodations may include special instruction, personnel, equipment, or strategies. By age 16, every child should have a transitional plan in place looking toward employment, adult living skills, and recreation.

Follow-up and Referral

Management of the child with ID includes routine well child care for the SHCN child, with special attention, follow-up, and referral as needed for co-occurring or comorbid issues. As children grow and mature, needs change and lags appear more significant so staying attuned to child and family needs is important.

Aggression and Disruptive Behavior Disorders

Social Aggression

Social aggression is a pattern of social behavior with the intent to harm others. Onset may occur as early as toddlerhood. It can be overt (e.g., hitting or pushing) or covert (e.g., gossiping or socially ostracizing). Disruptive behavior disorders include CD, ADHD, and ODD.

Approximately 5% to 6% of American children have behavioral problems with aggression and 2% to 8% of children meet criteria for ODD (Calles, 2016b). Males are more likely to be aggressive than females, and aggression peaks during adolescence. Females are more likely to be socially or covertly aggressive, whereas males are more likely to be physically aggressive. Acute, stressful life events or transitions can precipitate a brief period of social aggression. Aggression has neurobiologic and socioenvironmental influences. Biologic changes noted include alterations in dopamine, serotonin, and GABA, and multiple genes have been identified that contribute to aggressiveness (Austerman, 2017). Significant risk factors include a history of maltreatment or trauma with or without PTSD; inconsistent or harsh discipline, or both; lack of maternal responsiveness; separations from parents; weak social ties; bullying; peer influences (especially for older children and adolescents); and parental figure changes or parental rejection. Social aggression can be a precursor to CD or ODD.

Clinical Findings. During preschool, social aggression manifests as oppositional or defiant behavior and is considered clinically significant if it interferes with normal developmental functioning. The pervasiveness, intensity, and persistence of irritable, argumentative, defiant, and easily annoyed behaviors identify a pathologic condition and may be precursors to ODD. Preschool children have a basic understanding of the effect of their behavior on others and can control their behavior on the basis of internalized norms and developing self-regulation. When social aggression becomes a pattern, peer rejection is common. Aggressive behavior involves the following: property destruction; name-calling; physically pestering and deliberately annoying others; hitting, biting, kicking, fighting; frequent peer conflict; temper tantrums; misinterpreting social cues and responding aggressively; lack of problem-solving in social situations; swearing, obscene language and gestures; excessive arguing; and/or inappropriate or aggressive sexual behaviors

Screening should include suicidality, homicidality, child and family behavioral health disorders, abuse by a caregiver or peer, and substance abuse history. Table 30.9 includes screening tools for youth aggression.

TABLE 30.9 Screening Tools for Aggression

Scale	Appropriate Ages
Child Aggression Scale	5-18 years old
The Modified Overt Aggression Scale	Not defined
Buss-Perry Aggression Questionnaire	9 years-old to adulthood

Adapted from Austerman J. Violence and aggressive behavior. *Pediatr Review* 2017;38(2):69–78.

Differential Diagnosis. ODD is a pattern of problems with rules and authority figures. ODD symptoms emerge during the preschool years and persist for a minimum of 6 months. CD is a clear pattern of behavior established over a 6-month period, typically diagnosed at school age. CD differs from ODD in that it involves serious aggression toward people or animals, willful destruction of property, or theft. However, there is growing evidence that preschool children manifest clinically significant disruptive behavior problems, and valid diagnoses of ODD and CD can be made even in young children. Typical and atypical problems can be differentiated, and children with these problems can be identified with a developmentally based DSM-5 framework (APA, 2013).

Management. It is important to ascertain whether a difficult temperament underlies the behavioral difficulty, especially in conjunction with a parental temperament lack of fit. A difficult temperament may account for a child's being difficult to discipline, having social behavior problems in school (e.g., poor fit with the teacher), or having poor academic achievement. In these situations, the use of positive parenting strategies does not have to change, but supportive counseling for the parents should be provided regarding temperament, its manifestations, and strategies for managing transitions and other difficult times or behaviors. A teacher conference may provide similar information and explore strategies to facilitate the child's learning and positive behavior.

When social aggression is a response to acute stress, the problem usually resolves if parents use positive parenting strategies and facilitate developmentally appropriate coping efforts. If peer relationship development is hampered, close monitoring of and intervention with peer interactions by day care, preschool, and school personnel, especially with the parents present for observation, enhances appropriate social behavior and competence. Changing schools in an effort to lessen problems is not advised because children carry their social difficulties with them and assume the same roles in new groups. It is helpful to work with teachers to ensure that they are supportive and facilitative.

When social aggression becomes a pattern of social behavior, referral for intervention to a behavioral health specialist is critical. Negative behavior in preschool playgroups is predictive of externalizing behavior problems in kindergarten. Research supports the stability and persistence of disruptive behavior and aggression from toddlerhood to school age. Early intervention is essential. Parental education should focus on reestablishing positive parent-child interactions, use of consistent limit setting, and teaching parents to use effective discipline. Strategies employed to manage inappropriate aggression include individual and family therapy, and school- and community-based programs.

Conduct Disorder

CD is a repetitive and persistent pattern of behavior in which the basic rights of others or major age-appropriate societal norms and rules are violated (APA, 2013). The onset of aggressive behavior is observed in toddlerhood. Early-onset conduct problems are diagnosed from 4 to 6 years old, and a formal diagnosis is typically made when the child is 7 years old or older. The cause of the disorder rests in chronic negative circumstances, as described for social aggression. CD is frequently associated with a history of harsh discipline, abuse, or neglect. Prevalence rates are approximately 2% in the general population (Calles, 2016b). CD is more common in males than females (3:1). However, it is thought that the prevalence data do not accurately reflect the occurrence of CD for females, because the diagnostic criteria emphasize physical aggression.

Behavioral dysregulation usually becomes notable during the transition from early to middle childhood and is mediated by changes in the structure and demands of the social environment—peers and school settings. There is a high rate of comorbidity with major depression, and the joint presence of CD and depression increases the risk for substance abuse and suicide. ADHD negatively influences the development, course, and severity of CD.

Clinical Findings. Clinical features fall into four main subgroups: (1) aggressive behavior that threatens or results in physical harm to other people or animals, (2) nonaggressive behavior that causes property damage, (3) lying or stealing, and (4) serious violation of rules or laws. Several factors are relevant to practitioners for their prognostic importance:

- How atypical the behaviors are for age or gender
- How overt versus covert the behaviors are
- The nature of any aggression
- The presence of early antisocial or psychopathic-related symptoms

Most commonly, referrals for clinical treatment are for aggressive behavior patterns. Physical aggression toward others includes the following: hitting, kicking, fighting; physical cruelty to animals or people; property destruction (including fire setting); frequent temper tantrums; high rates of annoying behavior, such as yelling, whining, or threatening; disobedience to adults; lying, cheating, covert stealing; truancy and running away from home; blaming others for mistakes; using or selling illegal drugs; engaging in inappropriate or violent sexual behaviors (e.g., sexual assault); and/or academic problems.

There is growing evidence that preadolescent and adolescent girls manifest CD more indirectly through verbal and relational aggression, including alienation, ostracism, and character defamation directed at the relationships between friends. With CD, social role functioning tends to be impaired with poor academic performance, poor family and peer relationships, and poor self-management. Childhood CD may predict antisocial personality disorder in adulthood. Poorer prognoses are associated with increased symptom severity.

Differential Diagnosis. ODD is characterized by more disobedience than aggressiveness and is evidenced in preschool or early school age. ADHD is characterized by inattention, impulsiveness, and hyperactivity, but willful destruction is uncommon. CD is distinguished from isolated acts of aggressive behavior by degree of aggression exhibited, the presence of willful defiance, and by the persistence of symptoms for a minimum of 6 months (APA, 2013). A thorough physical examination is essential to rule out organic causes of behavior and to identify evidence of abuse, neglect, and substance abuse disorders.

Management. If aggressive behavior is identified before a CD develops, preventive efforts can be implemented. Successful programs are multifaceted, including a parent-directed component (e.g., parent education and support for positive parenting strategies and healthy, consistent approaches to discipline), social-cognitive skills training, proactive classroom management and teacher training, and group therapy (Calles 2016b; Austerman, 2017). Effective education includes conflict resolution strategies and development of coping and resiliency skills. Once a CD is evident, referral for child and family intervention is crucial.

Safety is a priority in caring for children with aggressive and oppositional disorders. Because of the strong association of child abuse and neglect with CD, it is critical to determine if the child is in safe living conditions. If there is evidence of abuse or neglect, prompt referral to child protective agencies is mandatory. The practitioner must also determine whether other family members are safe from the child's or adolescent's aggressive behavior. Potential interventions when family safety is at risk include referral for inpatient psychiatric evaluation, police notification of criminal activity, supporting the family to petition the juvenile court for services, and referral to community health services.

Family therapy can be helpful for adolescents with CD. Collaboration between the family and the school is of critical importance, and the PCP can assist with strategies. Isolated individual treatment is not superior to parent intervention programs. Education about problem-solving skills may also be effective.

Psychopharmacologic intervention is reserved for explosive aggression and includes mood stabilizers, typical and atypical antipsychotics, clonidine, and stimulants. However, PCPs should refer patients to a behavioral health specialist for drug therapy given the high risk for substance abuse in those with CD.

Oppositional Defiant Disorder

ODD is a pattern of negative, hostile, and defiant behavior that is excessive compared with other children of the same age (APA, 2013). Symptoms often occur in early childhood, from 3 to 7 years old with the disorder typically beginning by 8 years old.

Etiologic factors include many of the parenting and family dysfunctions identified for social aggression. Precursors to the disorder are common in early childhood, especially defiance and negativism. More common in boys before puberty, the gender distribution is approximately equal thereafter.

Clinical Findings. The essential feature of ODD is a recurrent pattern of behavior that is negative, defiant, disobedient, and hostile toward authority figures. Behavior is typically directed at family members, teachers, or peers that the child knows well. The child manifests the following behaviors to an extent that leads to impairment (APA, 2013):

- Actively defies or refuses adult requests or rules
- Is argumentative, angry, resentful, touchy, or easily annoyed
- Easily loses temper; is vindictive
- Blames others for own mistakes or difficulties
- Deliberately does things to annoy others
- Children often see their own behavior as justifiable, not oppositional or defiant

Differential Diagnosis. CD involves more serious violations of the rights of others and a more willful disregard of authority.

Management. Attend to the early signs of defiant and oppositional behavior or aggression, or both, and educate parents about positive parenting strategies and exercising consistent, healthy discipline, which is similar to the management of CDs. Because these children typically do not perceive themselves as having a problem and cause distress within the family system, referral for intervention is indicated. As described for CD, parent training programs are more successful if they include information about child behavior in multiple environments (e.g., school and home) and target dysfunctional family processes. Child training groups provide added benefit if combined with parent training groups. Again, collaboration with the school is important. These multiple approaches, conducted simultaneously, are most effective.

Autism Spectrum Disorder

Definition and Diagnostic Criteria

ASD is a complex neurodevelopmental disorder that affects communication and behavior beginning in the first two years of life. According to the DSM-5, ASD causes impairment in social interaction with additional impairment in communication and restrictive, repetitive, stereotyped patterns of behaviors, interests, and activities. This is a spectrum disorder with a wide variation in symptom severity. Affected individuals must show symptoms from early childhood even if the symptoms are not recognized until later in life. DSM-5 criteria for ASD (Box 30.11) and severity levels (Table 30.10) guide diagnosis. ASD is a lifelong disorder but symptoms can be improved with early and appropriate services.

The etiology of ASD is unclear but greatest consensus lies with genetic etiology with familial inheritance patterns (the 4:1 male dominance, increased prevalence in siblings and concordance in twins, and increased risk in relatives) and the association of certain genetic disorders (fragile X syndrome [most common single gene cause of ASD], neurofibromatosis, tuberous sclerosis, Angelman syndrome, and Rett syndrome). A number of genes are associated with ASD and affect the function of the chemical connections between neurons or synapses. Inherited genetic variations are important, as are *de novo*, or spontaneous, mutations (NINDS, 2018). Biologic causes implicated include differences in gray and white matter volumes, sulcal and gyral anatomy, brain chemical concentrations, neural networks, cortical structure and organization, brain lateralization, and cognitive processing (Augustyn, 2017). Interaction between multiple genes and environmental modifiers contribute to variable expression. Environmental factors are considered a "second hit" in that they modulate existing genetic factors increasing ASD predisposition: these include extreme prematurity, meconium aspiration, breech delivery, and low 5-minute Apgar scores; maternal medications (valproic acid and thalidomide) and advanced parental age; autoimmune and toxin exposure (Hirtz et al., 2018).

The prevalence of ASD is 2.47%, a nonsignificant increase over the previous period, and greater in boys (3.63%) than girls (1.25%) (Zablotsky, Black & Blumberg, 2018). Non-Hispanic white children (2.76%) are more likely to be diagnosed than Hispanic children (1.82%) and children aged 8 to 12 years (2.88%) are more likely to be diagnosed than children 3 to 7 years (2.23%). Parents who have a child with an ASD have a 2% to 18% chance of having an affected second child; ASD occurs more frequently in certain genetic or chromosomal conditions (e.g., Down syndrome, fragile X syndrome); 44% have average to above average intelligence; 83% have one or more co-occurring neurodevelopmental diagnosis; and 10% have co-occurring psychiatric disorders (CDC, 2018).

Clinical Findings and Assessment

Children with ASD demonstrate problems with social interactions, communication, and language skills; unusual ways of relating to people, objects, and events; abnormal responses to sensory stimuli, usually sound; and restricted, repetitive, or stereotypical behaviors and echolalia (meaningless repetition of others' speech). Children with ASD may only demonstrate unusual behavior 11% of the time making it easy to miss (Weill, Zavodny & Souders, 2018). *Infants* may be passive, non-engaging, quiet, floppy or difficult, colicky, stiff, have poor eye contact, or fail to respond to name or gestures. During *early childhood*, parents often become convinced that something is wrong with their child as language delays (especially expressive), lack of social relatedness, and severe behavior problems are common. If speaking, echolalia is present or the child primarily talks about specific interests and has trouble modulating their voice. Language delays include lack of meaningful speech, decreased gestures, and gaze disturbances. Socially, the child exhibits detachment, decreased eye contact, a lack of reciprocity or initiating conversation, lack of fear, poor creative

• BOX 30.11 DSM V Diagnostic Criteria for Autistic Disorders

A. Persistent deficits in social communication and social interaction across multiple contexts, as manifested by the following currently or by history (examples are illustrative, not exhaustive, see text):

1. Deficits in social-emotional reciprocity, ranging, for example, from abnormal social approach and failure of normal back-and-forth conversation; to reduced sharing of interests, emotions, or affect; to failure to intiate or respond to social interactions.
2. Deficits in nonverbal communicative behaviors used for social interaction, ranging, for example, from poorly integrated verbal and nonverbal communication; to abnormalities in eye contact and body language or deficits in understanding and use of gestures; to a total lack of facial expressions and nonverbal communication.
3. Deficits in developing, maintaining, and understanding relationships. Ranging, for example, from difficulties adjusting behavior to suit various social contexts; to difficulties in sharing imaginative play or making friends; to absence of interest in peers.
   Specify current severity: **Severity is based on social communication impairments and restricted, repetitive patterns of behavior** (See Table 30.10)

B. Restricted, repetitive patterns of behaviour, interests, or activities, as manifested by at least two of the following, currently or by history (examples are illustrative, not exhaustive, see text):

1. Stereotyped or repetitive movements, use of objects, or speech (e.g., simple motor stereotypies, lining up toys or flipping objects, echolalia, idiosyncratic phrases).
2. Insistence on sameness, inflexible adherence to routines, or ritualized patterns of verbal or nonverbal behaviour (e.g., extreme distress at small changes, difficulties with transitions, rigid thinking patterns, greeting rituals, need to take same route or eat same food every day).
3. Highly restricted, fixated interests that are abnormal in intensity or focus e.g., strong attachment to or preoccupation with unusual objects, excessively circumscribed or perseverative interests).

4. Hyper- or hyporeactivity to sensory input or unusual interest in sensory aspects of the environment (e.g., apparent indifference to pain/temperature, adverse response to specific sounds or textures, excessive smelling or touching of objects, visual fascination with lights or movement).
   Specify current severity: **Severity is based on social communication impairments and restricted, repetitive patterns of behavior** (See Table 30.10)

C. Symptoms must be present in the early developmental period (but may not become fully manifest until social demands exceed limited capacities, or may be masked by learned strategies in later life).

D. Symptoms cause clinically significant impairment in social, occupational, or other important areas of current functioning.

E. These disturbances are not better explained by intellectual disability (intellectual developmental disorder) or global developmental delay. Intellectual disability and autism spectrum disorder frequently co-occur; to make comorbid diagnoses of autism spectrum disorder and intellectual disability, social communication should be below that expected for a general developmental level.

Note: Individuals with a well-established DSM-IV diagnosis of autistic disorder, Asperger's disorder, or pervasive developmental disorder not otherwise specified should be given the diagnosis of autism spectrum disorder. Individuals who have marked deficits in social communication, but whose symptoms do not otherwise meet criteria for autism spectrum disorder, should be evaluated for social (pragmatic) communication disorder. Specify if:

With or without accompanying intellectual impairment
With or without accompanying language impairment
Associated with a known medical or genetic conditions or environmental factor
Associated with another neurodevelopmental, mental, or behavioural disorder
With catatonia (refer to the criteria for catatonia associated with another mental disorder)

TABLE 30.10 Severity Levels for Autism Spectrum Disorder

Severity Level	Social Communication	Restricted, Repetitive Behaviors
Level 3 "Requiring very substantial support"	Severe deficits in verbal and nonverbal social communication skills cause severe impairments in functioning; very limited initiation of social interactions; and minimal response to social overtures. For example, a person with few words of intelligible speech who rarely initiates interaction and, when he or she does, makes unusual approaches to meet needs only and responds to only very direct social approaches.	Inflexibility of behavior, extreme difficulty coping with change, or other restricted/repetitive behaviors markedly interfere with functioning in all spheres. Great distress/difficulty changing focus or action.
Level 2 "Requiring substantial support"	Marked deficits in verbal and nonverbal social communication skills; social impairments apparent even with supports in place; limited initiation of social interactions; reduced or abnormal responses to social overtures from others. For example, a person who speaks simple sentences, whose interaction is limited to narrow special interests, and who has markedly odd nonverbal communication.	Inflexibility of behavior, difficulty coping with change, or other restricted/repetitive behaviors appear frequently enough to be obvious to the casual observer and interfere with functioning in a variety of contexts. Distress and/or difficulty changing focus or action.
Level 1 "Requiring support"	Without supports in place, deficits in social communication cause noticeable impairments. Difficulty initiating social interactions, and clear examples of atypical or unsuccessful response to social overtures of others. May appear to have decreased interest in social interactions. For example, a person who is able to speak in full sentences and engages in communication but whose to-and-fro conversation with others fails, and whose attempts to make friends are odd and typically unsuccessful.	Inflexibility of behavior causes significant interference with functioning in one or more contexts. Difficulty switching between activities. Problems of organization and planning hamper independence.

• BOX 30.12 Red Flags for Autism Spectrum Disorder

Social

Lack of social smile and eye contact at 2-3 months of age
Lack of joint attention (shared spontaneous enjoyment) around 9 months
Does not respond to his or her name by 12 months old
Does not follow a point to a picture or object and look back at pointer by 12 months
Does not point at objects to show interest (pointing at an airplane flying over) by 14 months old
Does not pretend (feed a doll) by 18 months old
Avoids eye contact and wants to be alone
Trouble understanding other people's feelings or talking about their own feelings
Gives unrelated answers to questions
Loss of social abilities at any age

Language

Delayed speech and language skills (no babbling or gesturing by 12 months old; no single words by 16 months old; no two-word [not echolalic] phrases by 24 months old)
Repeats words or phrases over and over (echolalia)
Monotone intonation, rhythm, rate, pitch, volume, and quality of sound issues
Speech that sounds scripted
Difficulty with conversation where each person adds information
Parental concern about hearing due to lack of response
Loss of language at any age

Patterns of behavior or interests

Gets upset by minor changes
Has obsessive interests
Flaps hands, rocks body, or spins in circles
Unusual reactions to the way things sound, smell, taste, look, or feel
Self-injurious behaviors (head-banging, biting, pinching)

---

play, invasion of others' space, preference to be alone, and lack of social awareness. Persistent and insistent behaviors, excessive temper tantrums, repetitive movements, and a preference to line, stack, or spin toys occur. The child may have precocious or average development of rote memory skills but often without concept comprehension. By *school age,* children with autism often lack reciprocal friendships, have ritualistic behaviors, and continue with language, social, and behavioral problems. Transitions between places and activities can be difficult. *Adolescents* have similar behaviors. Rote learning is possible, but comprehension lags. High-functioning autistic children do well in regular classrooms and mildly affected persons can be academically successful but have social relationship problems.

Development is uneven (dissociated), with occasional talent in a limited area, such as music or mathematics, coupled with severe deficits in other areas. Many autistic children have other impairments, such as sleep problems, gastrointestinal problems (diarrhea, constipation, and abdominal pain), and irritability. Co-occurring diagnoses of ID (32% to 60%), ADHD (33%), anxiety or depression, disruptive disorders (aggression, tantrums, and self-injury), and seizures (20% to 25%) are common (Weill, Zavodny, & Souders, 2018).

Screening and Specialty Referral for Diagnosis

Routine developmental surveillance in early childhood helps identify red flags for ASD (Box 30.12), and PCPs should be sensitive to parental concerns. The AAP recommends screening for autism at both 18 and 24 months, as a negative screen at 18 months may be abnormal at 24 months. The Modified Checklist for Autism in Toddlers revised with follow-up *(M-CHAT-R/F)* is the most used tool. Readily available online in multiple languages (http://mchatscreen.com; https://m-chat.org), it screens children 16 to 30 months of age and identifies those who need further evaluation. Other available tools include: Screening Tool for Autism in Two-Year-olds *(STAT)* (24 to 35 months); Childhood Autism Screening Test *(CAST)* (3+ years-old); Social Communication Questionnaire *(SCQ)* (4+ years-old); and Autism Spectrum Screening Questionnaire *(ASSQ)* (7 to 16 years). The gold standard diagnostic tools are the second edition of the Autism Diagnostic Observation Schedule (ADOS-2) and the Autism Diagnostic Interview (ADI-R) which are costly and require training. The ADOS takes 45 to 60 minutes to administer, the ADI 90 to 150 minutes. Some settings use the ADOS without the ADI.

Children who fail routine developmental screening should begin an early identification process including analysis of family and provider concerns and descriptions of behavior. Family history may reveal other members with ASD, speech delay or language deficits, mood disorders, or mental retardation. Identify seizures, hearing loss, head injury, and meningitis. Perform a complete physical examination with a focus on findings suggestive of genetic syndromes (e.g., skin findings) or neurologic abnormalities (e.g., macrocephaly, hypotonia), and test for iron levels and lead exposure. Comprehensive diagnostic assessment should be done by a multidisciplinary team, ideally at a specialty center, and address core symptoms, cognition, language, and adaptive, sensory, and motor skills. Specialty assessment includes developmental, behavioral, and IQ testing; audiologic evaluation; and genetic testing with microarray. Neuroimaging, EEG, and metabolic testing may be done if indicated by examination and history. The differential diagnosis includes pragmatic social disorder, language disorder with ADHD, ID with visual impairment, and harsh psychosocial conditions (PTSD, reactive attachment disorder, and abuse in childhood).

Management

ASD diagnosis and severity determination is just the beginning. The PCP must assist the parent with ongoing routine care, developmental changes, and day-to-day behavior management as well as the typical problems with sleep, feeding, gastrointestinal issues, and irritability. The child must be identified as child with special healthcare needs (CSHCN) with a comprehensive plan and appropriate interventions developed.

Diagnostic and Initial Meeting with Families. After a diagnosis of autism is made, it is important to take time to meet with the family and ensure they understand the diagnosis and have resources and a management plan. Care of the child with ASD is tailored to disease severity and can be complex, requiring a multidisciplinary approach including a behavioral-developmental pediatrician or nurse, an applied behavior analysis (ABA) therapist, gastroenterologist or allergist, a dietician, and/or speech and occupational therapists. Levels of severity change over time and an ongoing relationship with someone who knows the child helps modify the plan to ensure the child receives the correct services.

When establishing the initial plan of care, detailing essential therapies and plans for diet, gastrointestinal issues, exercise, sleep, and safety are essential. Ensure that the following therapies are in place: ABA therapy supervised by a Board Certified Behavior Analyst (BCBA), speech therapy, occupational therapy with a sensory processing focus (modulation for self-regulating and soothing) and assistance with play and self-help skills, and physical therapy if needed. Referring the child for dental care with a provider who is familiar with ASD issues is helpful. Children with ASD are often picky eaters with limited diets due to atypical food preferences, food selectivity, and disruptive mealtime behaviors. Children are often overweight, but can be underweight, and may have issues with pica. The bottom line is to optimize well-balanced nutrition. The PCP can suggest different foods and techniques as well as behavioral tips, but referral to a nutritionist and/or an occupational therapist with an emphasis in feeding (often combined in a feeding clinic) is worthwhile. Gastrointestinal issues such as abdominal pain, constipation, and diarrhea are common (Harrington & Bora, 2017). The PCP should acknowledge these difficulties and work with families to monitor and find strategies to minimize issues. Exercise decreases self-stimulating behaviors and improves academic performance in children with neurodevelopmental disorders. Physical therapy and/or shoe inserts help with weak ankles or flat feet. Sleep problems are common, so working with parents to develop good child sleep hygiene is important. An evidenced-based Sleep Tool Kit for children and teens is available from the Autism Treatment network (www.autismspeaks.org). If difficulties persist, melatonin can be used. Safety concerns must be considered especially for nonverbal children or children with low IQ. They should have identification with them at all times and local authorities should be aware of their presence. Consideration of risks related to water and fire, and safety around the house, needs to be addresses. The Autism Speaks website also has a Safety Tool Kit.

A helpful, free resource created for families with children age 4 and under is the *100 Day Kit* available at Autism Speaks. It provides families with information about diagnosis, services, and treatment, and a week by week plan for the first 100 days. The Autism Evidenced-Based Practice Review Group (Wong et al., 2015) investigated thousands of studies to determine which were worthy of being called evidence-based. Twenty-seven interventions were identified with substantial research to confirm their findings; another 24 had some support. The full report is available online (http://cidd.unc.edu/Registry/Research/Docs/31.pdf).

Family Education and Support. Families need support and education to manage children with autism, and siblings need help dealing with the time and attention focused on the child with ASD. Groups and mentors provide support and concrete management ideas. Helping the family find ways to enjoy the child, promoting positive routine, creating a calm environment, and coordinating with specialists to improve quality of life for everyone are helpful. Although the prognosis for children with autism is highly variable, long-term care needs to be addressed to help those who can be fully independent, employed adults.

Behavior Management, Parent Skills Training, and Counseling. Behavioral management is the most important aspect of ASD management. Target behaviors vary according to age, developmental level, and disruptiveness. PCPs can utilize the ABC approach, considering gaps in the child's skills (Chapter 15) to help parents work through behaviors. Utilizing the child's "rigidity" to establish routine is another strategy to help the child regulate while learning flexibility with the normal variations in family life (Howard, 2017). Social stories, short descriptions of an activity, event, or situation (e.g., getting dressed, what to do in a thunderstorm), and simple visual representation of social interactions are learning tools that assist children to learn skills and behaviors (National Autistic Society, 2018).

ABA therapy is an optimal strategy and focuses on the development of socially appropriate behaviors while decreasing challenging behaviors. ABA requires extensive parental education, is very time intensive and expensive, and is often not covered by insurance,

thereby limiting its use by many families. Social skills training (one on one or in small groups), early and intense developmental work, and parenting strategies are also helpful. Parents are important collaborators at all stages—from assessment through goal development and treatment delivery. Following the family regularly allows identification of stressful times when referral for counseling might be helpful. Because comorbidity is common, the PCP needs to maintain ongoing surveillance for new symptoms or concerns.

Educational and Adaptive Supports. Early intense intervention is necessary to maximize educational abilities and enhance learning for children with autism. Early intervention programs for preschoolers, school-based special education, and information and assistance for school personnel are essential components of care. Educational needs may range from resource rooms or personnel to part- or full-time special education. Care planning requires cognitive testing to identify the child's strengths and weaknesses in addition to social, behavioral, and language assessment. Every child with ASD needs an IEP or 504 plan. When special abilities are discovered in children with autism, attempts should be made to encourage opportunities for success in those areas. Parents should be skilled advocates for the child and protect them from unrealistic expectations of social competence when necessary. The long-term goal is to help the child to function as effectively and comfortably as possible in the least restrictive environment.

AT is available for use at home and in the school setting. Autism groups and online sites are often the best place to find these resources. Other AT devices are under development, such as: computerized smart glasses as a social and behavioral aid (Sahin et al., 2018) and Fitbit-like devices to predict oncoming aggressive outbursts allowing better intervention and prevention (Kalter, 2018).

Pharmacologic Management. Though there is no medication to treat the core symptoms of autism, medications are moderately successful at treating ASD associated behaviors. The AACAP position statement on ASD states that there is limited benefit and significant limitations to medication use, although it may be offered for specific symptoms of co-occurring mental health conditions (Volkmar et al., 2014). The most common symptoms addressed by pharmacotherapy are attentional difficulties, hyperactivity, affective difficulties (e.g., anxiety or depression), compulsive behaviors or interfering repetitive activity, irritability, aggression, self-injurious behavior, and sleep disruption. Autistic children do not benefit from stimulant medications unless they also suffer from an attention deficit (about half do); they are more sensitive to stimulants so the "start low, go slow" approach should be adhered to. Alpha agonist (guanfacine or clonidine) or norepinephrine reuptake inhibitors (atomoxetine) may prove more effective. Atypical antipsychotics, risperidone or aripiprazole, are FDA approved for irritability and explosive behaviors but are not routinely recommended. Fluoxetine, an SSRI, may be used in lower doses for anxiety, phobias, and compulsions, and requires monitoring for agitation, increased energy, and poor sleep. Citalopram is not recommended (Volkmar et al., 2014). About one-quarter of autistic children also need anticonvulsants for seizures. Disproven treatments include antifungal medication, chelation, secretin, and immunotherapy (Harrington & Bora, 2017).

Nutrition, Complementary and Alternative Therapies. PCPs should be familiar with complementary or alternative therapies and ask families what they are using or considering. While maintaining a nonjudgmental approach, encourage the family to thoroughly research the approach they are considering, know what specific behavior they hope to affect, and attempt only one treatment at a time.

There are many studies looking at nutrition and its effects on ASD, although to date none have strong enough data to be evidence-based. Nonetheless, it is useful for the PCP to be familiar with some of the information that families may hear or ask about. *Nutritional strategies* are either additive (supplementing with vitamins [A, C, B$_6$, B$_{12}$, D$_3$], minerals [magnesium, iron, zinc, copper], folic acid, amino acids, omega-3 fatty acids) or they are subtractive (eliminating based on food intolerance, allergy, yeast-free, gluten-free, casein-free, ketogenic, or specific carbohydrate). Not only is there lack of evidence-based research to support the effectiveness of these diets, but they also are costly, take time to prepare, have an effect on other family members, and a few studies show amino acid depletion and bone loss. Special diets also complicate school participation. Mind-body therapies (biofeedback and neurofeedback, music therapy, yoga) and body-based practices (acupuncture, auditory integrative training, transcranial magnetic stimulation, hippotherapy, massage, Qigong) are other options (Harrington & Bora, 2017). There is new evidence on the gut microbiome and autism.

Follow-up and Referral

In addition to ensuring the child with ASD receives regular well-child care, additional visits may be required to monitor medication, work on behavioral concerns, or assist the family with establishing or modifying school plans. Monitoring family and child coping and need for additional referrals are components of care. Beginning transitional care planning is also recommended in the teen years.

Eating Disorders

Eating disorders cause abnormal eating behaviors that are secondary to altered body image (dysmorphism). Anorexia nervosa (commonly called *anorexia*) and bulimia nervosa (commonly called *bulimia*) are the primary eating disorders of concern; however, there are other conditions in this diagnostic cluster, including eating disorders not otherwise specified, rumination disorders, pica, and feeding disorders of infancy. Some believe obesity should be classified as an eating disorder because of the correlation between self-soothing and eating, and because many obese individuals have feelings of loss of control over their eating and symptoms of body dysmorphism. Eating disorders are complex conditions that are very difficult to treat and are associated with significant medical and mental health comorbidities. Anorexia has the highest mortality rate of all the mental health conditions. The 5-year mortality rate for anorexia is 15% to 20%, and the majority of these deaths are caused by electrolyte imbalance, malnutrition, and suicide. Due to the complexity of these disorders, specialty care is needed; however, PCPs play a critical role through detection and early intervention, case coordination, and monitoring for complications.

Lifetime prevalence rates for anorexia and bulimia are approximately 1% each (Mehler & Andersen, 2017). Both disorders affect females at much greater rates than males (9:1). Symptom onset usually occurs during mid to late adolescence, but preadolescent cases do occur and are associated with significantly higher morbidity and mortality. Athletes are more likely to develop eating disorders, especially those who compete in sports that are based on weight divisions (e.g., wrestling), long distance running, and those with emphases on aesthetic lines and flexibility (e.g., dancers, gymnasts, and ice skaters). Other individual risk factors include middle to high socioeconomic status, divorced families, chronic disease (e.g., diabetes mellitus, cystic fibrosis, depression, obesity, and substance abuse), recent weight loss in a previously obese person, personality disorders (e.g., borderline, narcissistic, and antisocial), strong will, and history of child abuse. Children

and adolescents with eating disorders are more likely to have parents who have a weight or fitness focus, are substance abusers, have high achievement expectations, who comment on their child's physical appearance, have difficulty expressing emotions, or who are overprotective or enmeshed with their children. Like most mental illness, there is an increasing body of evidence suggesting a strong genetic component to anorexia and bulimia that results in altered serotonin and dopamine receptors.

Clinical Findings

Diagnosing anorexia or bulimia can be difficult. Some clinical findings characteristic of these disorders occur in the healthy adolescent. For example, it is not uncommon for a 14-year-old girl who is neither anorexic nor bulimic to express concern about her body appearance, stating that she is too fat or ugly. Additionally, anorexic or bulimic adolescents and their families commonly hide their condition and actions, deny problems, or present a mature, self-sufficient, and successful facade. Early in the disease process, the family system may appear to be coherent, making it difficult to collect accurate data about family relations and behavior patterns that contribute to eating disorders.

Many consider anorexia and bulimia to be part of a disease continuum with categories that are more arbitrary than actual. Clinical presentations vary depending on the disease severity. Both anorexia and bulimia are associated with disordered eating and body dysmorphism with or without purging (e.g., laxative abuse, enemas, diuretics, and induced vomiting). Generally, there is no loss of appetite or sense of hunger. Affected individuals often link feelings of self-worth with weight or the ability to restrict food intake despite being hungry. Diagnostic criteria for anorexia are (APA, 2013):
- Refusal to maintain body weight at least 85% expected for age and height or failure to gain weight during growth periods so that weight drops below 85% expected
- Intense fear of weight gain and "being fat"
- Body dysmorphism
- Binge eating/purging subtype, which is associated with frequent purging although bingeing episodes are rare
 Diagnostic criteria for bulimia are (APA, 2013):
- Consuming large quantities of food in a short period of time (within 2 hours)
- Loss of control during binge episodes (e.g., cannot control the amount of food they eat or are shocked at amount consumed)
- Engaging in repeated behaviors to lose weight, including purging, excessive exercise, or fasting
- Bingeing or purging behaviors that occur at least once a week for at least 3 months

Individuals with anorexia are underweight, but children and adolescents with bulimia are often average weight or overweight. In addition to the regular primary care monitoring of weight and growth, it is important to include routine screening to detect the red flags (Table 30.11). Also helpful is the SCOFF questionnaire. This five-item screen asks the following questions:
1. Do you make yourself **S**ick because you feel uncomfortably full?
2. Do you worry that you have lost **C**ontrol over what you eat?
3. Have you lost **O**ver 10 pounds in the last 3 months?
4. Do you believe you are **F**at when others say you are thin?
5. Would you say **F**ood dominates your life?

Patients with suspected eating disorders need a thorough history and physical examination and evaluation for comorbid depression, anxiety, suicidality, and risk of physical harm. Common history findings include:
- Menstrual irregularity
- Body dysmorphism

TABLE 30.11	Red Flags and Signs That Indicate Need for Eating Disorder Treatment	
Red Flags	**Needs Treatment Signs**	
Reads diet books or clips dieting articles	Regularly fasts or skips meals	
Visits pro-anorexia or bulimia websites (pro Anna or pro Mia)	Stops eating with family or friends	
Intense focus on diet or regular dieting	Misses two or more periods during weight loss	
Sudden desire to be a vegetarian	Reports binge eating	
Sudden picky eating	Reports purging	
Visits bathroom regularly during or after meals	Parents find laxatives or diet pills	
Showers multiple times a day	Excessive exercise	
Skips meals because "I ate at school" or other place away from home	Refuses to eat non-diet foods	
Large amounts of missing food	Refuses to eat meals prepared by others	
	Extreme calorie counting or portion controls	

- Preoccupation with food; often fixes elaborate meals but does not eat; rituals associated with food
- Desire to lose weight and history of dieting
- Weight fluctuation or loss
- Guilt about eating
- Hides eating or lies about having eaten or amount eaten
- Social isolation, mood changes, suicidal ideation
- Fixed, highly structured schedule; inflexible to change
- Cold intolerance, fatigue, myalgias
- Constipation, diarrhea, abdominal bloating, gastrointestinal (GI) distress
- Sore throat
- Dizziness, syncope
- Substance abuse, self-harm
- Family history of chaos, abuse, sexual abuse

Common physical findings that may indicate an eating disorder are:

- Altered growth
- Parotid gland enlargement
- Fluid retention, facial edema
- Thin body type, low body temperature
- Hypotension, bradycardia, orthostatic hypotension, shallow respirations
- Dental enamel erosion, dental caries
- Russell sign (e.g., knuckle cuts/calluses/abrasions from inducing vomiting)
- Thinning hair, alopecia, decreased deep tendon reflexes
- Abdominal distention, altered bowel sounds
- Lanugo, dry skin
- Muscle atrophy
- Mental torpor

Differential Diagnosis

Inflammatory bowel disease and peptic ulcer disease result in chronic pain and microscopic or gross bleeding. Central nervous system lesions cause focal neurologic signs. Hormonal and metabolic diseases cause symptoms like polyphagia, polydipsia, polyuria, abnormal hair growth, and goiter. Immune disorders are associated with frequent, rare, and opportunistic infections. Other mental health differential diagnoses include OCD, SUD, and major depression.

Diagnostic Studies

Laboratory testing is done to ascertain the degree of electrolyte imbalance and malnutrition and to rule out other causes of weight loss and amenorrhea. Suggested diagnostic testing for an individual with a newly diagnosed eating disorder includes CBC (anemia), serum electrolytes (potassium, sodium, and acid-base imbalance), fasting glucose (diabetes), thyroid studies (hyperthyroidism), liver function testing, follicle-stimulating hormone (FSH), luteinizing hormone (LH), urinalysis, electrocardiogram (ECG for premature ventricular contractions and QT elongation), and bone density (if amenorrheic to look for osteopenia).

Management

Management of children and adolescents with anorexia or bulimia is difficult, in part because the child, family, and even the health care provider often deny the significance of the problem. Therefore, referral to behavioral health specialists is needed. Even though early detection and treatment are helpful in reducing physical complications, diagnosis can be delayed and treatment may be inadequate. Because the issue is not food, but rather sociopsychological dynamics of control in the child's life, effective treatment is complex and long term. Eating disorders are managed with a multifaceted approach with emphasis on nutritional rehabilitation, pharmacotherapeutics (e.g., antidepressants, atypical antipsychotics), and individual, family, and group therapy. Intensive, inpatient management is warranted for medical instability, psychosis or self-destructive behavior, and failure to improve with outpatient therapy.

Many children and adolescents with eating disorders require inpatient management, especially if there are fluid and electrolyte imbalances, cardiovascular instability, or significant mental illness. Individual and family therapy is critical. Pharmacologic approaches include antidepressants and atypical antipsychotics, but their use is controversial in many cases. The role of the PCP in the management of eating disorders is primarily that of screening and early identification. Weight gain during refeeding is expected to occur at 1.1 pounds (0.5 kg) per week (Mehler & Andersen, 2017). Close monitoring for refeeding syndrome is warranted. This is a rare, potentially life-threatening condition that occurs in the first days of enteral or parenteral feeding and results in severe fluid and electrolyte imbalance. Symptoms include confusion, severe irritability, organ dysfunction, and seizures.

Complications

Anorexia has the highest mortality rate of all mental health disorders. The complications of anorexia or bulimia include death, usually secondary to cardiac arrhythmia, hypokalemia, congestive heart failure, or suicide; altered metabolism (chronic); alcohol and drug addictions; osteoporosis; GI disturbance: ulcers; motility disorders; fertility problems; gynecologic problems related to prolonged amenorrhea; growth retardation; and dehydration.

Substance Abuse Disorder

Substance use is a precursor to abuse or dependence, and regular use clearly increases the risk for developing a SUD. However, the use of substances per se is not sufficient for a diagnosis of SUD.

Substance abuse is a maladaptive pattern of the use of alcohol or drugs manifested in significant impairment or distress. The criteria for substance dependence in the DSM-5 is divided into specific categories (alcohol, cannabis, inhalants, and so on), and in adults it includes tolerance, withdrawal, and compulsive substance use (APA, 2013). For children and adolescents, tolerance and loss of control are not good indicators for a diagnosis. Instead, substance-related blackouts, craving, and impulsive sexual or risk-taking behavior tend to be more important criteria.

The cause of SUD is multifaceted. Many contributing factors exist, including:

- Genetic vulnerability (family history)
- Parental substance use
- Dysfunctional family relationships (i.e., rigidity, distant relationships, neglect) and negative life events
- Psychiatric conditions (e.g., CD, ADHD, depression), low self-esteem, poor body image, ineffective coping (poor emotional regulation, poor problem-solving skills)
- Poor sleep hygiene
- School failure
- Low religiosity
- Competitive athleticism

Precipitating life events tend to center around loss of relationships (e.g., parental separation, divorce, or death; death of a close friend) and chronic negative circumstances (e.g., parental substance abuse, maltreatment).

Data from the Youth Risk Behavior Survey indicate that 30% of teens reported drinking alcohol and 20% reported using marijuana within the previous month (Kann et al., 2018). Approximately 13% of high school students binge drink, almost 15% of students drank alcohol for the first time before they were 13 years old, and about 4% reported having 10 or more drinks in a row during the past year. Nearly half of problem drinkers are thought to have tried alcohol by 10 years old and two-thirds by 13 years old. The majority of adolescents who use drugs do not progress to abuse or dependence. Peer influence seems to be less significant to the cause of substance abuse than previously thought. Boys tend to be more involved in use of both alcohol and drugs of all kinds than girls are at the same age. It is estimated that for both boys and girls, abuse of alcohol and other drugs is negligible from 10 to 13 years old, but doubles between adolescence (12 to 16 years old) and late adolescence (17 to 20 years old), peaks between 18 and 25 years old, and declines thereafter. The percentage of students reporting lifetime use of alcohol, marijuana, steroids, methamphetamines, and hallucinogenic drugs has decreased in the past decade, although the percentage of those reporting current use of cocaine and amphetamines has not changed significantly (Kann et al., 2018).

Clinical Findings

Identifying an adolescent's problem with substance abuse requires a careful assessment, conducted with an accepting, nonjudgmental, nonthreatening, matter-of-fact attitude. The covert nature of substance abuse and the dynamic of denial make it crucial to avoid a critical tone (see Chapter 13 for discussion of adolescent risk behaviors).

Interviewing the adolescent with the parents is a key strategy for obtaining information about etiologic factors and behavioral, cognitive, emotional, and physical changes that they have observed in the adolescent. However, it is essential that the adolescent also be interviewed alone at every visit to assess mental health and family issues. When talking about substance use with an adolescent, it is important to begin with general questions that are not overly personal. Begin by asking the adolescent about acquaintances or friends who smoke, drink, or use drugs; whether anyone in the family has had problems with these; and what the adolescent does with friends when they get together. It is helpful to ask about experimentation, under what circumstances it occurs, and the adolescent's feelings about it. To obtain a chronologic history of tobacco, alcohol, or drug use, it may be helpful to approach the subject by inquiring about prescription drugs and moving to illicit substances. The key is to remain nonjudgmental to elicit information that will indicate whether the adolescent is experimenting, a regular user, or dependent on substances. Ask about the adolescent's source of drugs or alcohol; the adolescent who uses substances provided by a friend or acquaintance is less advanced than one who purchases them directly. The practitioner should ask, "What? How much? How often? When? How? Where? With whom? Does the patient use substances at parties, home, school, alone, or with friends?"

Teens who screen positive should receive Screening, Brief Intervention, and Referral to Treatment (SBIRT). Information and training can be found online at https://www.integration.samhsa.gov/clinical-practice/sbirt.

The CRAFFT questionnaire (https://www.integration.samhsa.gov/clinical-practice/sbirt/CRAFFT_Screening_interview.pdf) is an appropriate screening instrument for substance abuse in the primary care setting. Positive responses to two or more items indicate a high likelihood for substance abuse and merits further evaluation and treatment.

Significant behavioral changes that may reflect drug use include the following:

- Infants and young children: Excessive crying; poor feeding or failure to thrive; irritability, jitteriness, or excessive lethargy; poor eye contact; sleep disorders
- Older children and adolescents: Decreased school performance; lethargy, hyperactivity or agitation, hypervigilance, decreased attention; disinhibition; deviant or risk-taking behavior; repeated absences or suspensions from school; loss of interest in previously enjoyed activities; withdrawal from family and usual friends, or change in friends to those involved in drugs and alcohol; irritability, fighting, or acting out; hypersexuality; exaggerated mood swings; sleep pattern changes or nightmares; altered menstruation; and change in appetite (from anorexia to unusual hunger)

Mood changes include swings from depression to euphoria, nervousness, unreasonable anger, and frequent expressions of hopelessness or failure. Low self-esteem typically characterizes those who abuse substances.

Physical signs that indicate a substance use problem include the following:

- Weight loss
- Red eyes with inhaled or smoked substances
- Hoarseness, chronic cough, wheezing, frequent "colds" or "allergy" symptoms, epistaxis, and perforations of nasal septum with cocaine and inhalant use
- Accidents, trauma, injuries
- Intoxication
- Complete or partial amnesia for events during intoxication with alcohol and date rape drug use
- Dilated or constricted pupils
- Gynecomastia, irregular periods, small testes with marijuana
- Needle tracks occur with intramuscular (IM) steroids or intravenous (IV) use
- Generalized pruritus with opiate use
- Reflux, diarrhea, gastritis, and constipation with opiate and alcohol use
- Perioral sores or pyodermas from huffing and bagging

Differential Diagnosis

Substance abuse is distinguished from social drinking or non-pathologic substance use by the presence of compulsive use, craving, or substance-related problems. SUDs are comorbid most often with CD, depression, and anxiety.

Diagnostic Studies

Urine toxicology can be helpful to verify adolescent truthfulness, although a positive drug screen result does not indicate substance abuse or dependence; it only indicates substance use. A negative drug screen result does not rule out an SUD. The approximate duration that drugs can be detected in the urine is as follows (Hadland & Levy, 2016):

- Alcohol—10 to 12 hours
- Amphetamines—2 to 4 days
- Cocaine and its major metabolite—1 to 3 days
- Benzodiazepines—1 day to 1 week
- Barbiturates—1 day to 1 week
- Opiates—2 to 5 days
- Marijuana—up to 30 days

Duration of detection from last substance use varies according to the laboratory and type of test used. All urine tests should be validated by ensuring that the specific gravity does not demonstrate very dilute urine (creatinine between 2 and 20 mg/dL) (Hadland & Levy, 2016).

Management

Exposure to tobacco and alcohol and illicit substances begins in early childhood. The pediatric PCP should discuss parental modeling for the use of alcohol, tobacco, and other substances in early childhood during routine well-child visits. It is important to educate school-age children and their parents about substance use and its consequences. For adolescents, a direct assessment and an interview about substance use are essential. Parents should be advised not to involve their child in their own substance use. Something as seemingly innocuous as "getting dad a beer from the refrigerator" gives the child practice in alcohol use.

Substance abuse must be treated, and referral to a substance abuse program is crucial. The initial goal is to help adolescents take positive steps toward changing their substance use and abuse behavior. If the adolescent denies any problem, efforts should focus on helping the adolescent acknowledge problems. Clarifying reported negative consequences, creating doubts about substance use, and raising awareness of the risks related to current use are motivational interviewing strategies that may be helpful. It is important to remain empathic and yet emphasize the adolescent's responsibility to make healthy choices. If the adolescent does not have chronic use, harm prevention is the goal of the intervention. Guide the adolescent to examine his or her substance use responsibly and identify ways to prevent harmful consequences.

If the adolescent progresses to chronic substance use, a number of options exist. Outpatient or day treatment programs are effective for those who can live and be managed at home. For adolescents with more serious addiction, comorbid psychiatric conditions, or suicidal ideation, residential treatment or hospitalization may be necessary. Given the prominence of family dysfunction and family life events in the cause of the problem, family-based treatment programs are essential. Family treatment, rather than family psychoeducation or family support groups, has been shown to be superior to other modalities. Follow-up assessments should include substance use issues and other predictors of use: stress or negative life events, depression or negative affect regulation, and the presence of positive support within or outside of the family. Self-help or 12-step groups are thought to be an essential element in the recovery process.

References

American Academy of Neurology (AAN). Guideline summary for clinicians evaluation of the child with global developmental delay. Available at http://tools.aan.com/professionals/practice/guidelines/guideline_summaries/Global_Devlopmental_Delay_Clinicians.pdf. Accessed October 10, 2018.

American Psychiatric Association (APA). *Diagnostic and Statistical Manual of Mental Disorders (DSM-5)*. 5th ed. Arlington, VA: American Psychiatric Association; 2013.

Augustyn M. Autism spectrum disorder: clinical features. 2017. Available at https://www.uptodate.com/contents/autism-spectrum-disorder-clinical-features#H22. Accessed January 20, 2018.

Austerman J. Violence and aggressive behaviour. *Pediatr Review*. 2017;38(2):69–78.

Brown NM, Brown SN, Briggs RD, et al. Associations between adverse childhood experiences and ADHD diagnosis and severity. *Acad Pediatr*. 2017;17(4):349–355.

Calles JL. Major depressive and dysthymic disorders: a review. *J Altern Med Res*. 2016;8(4):393–404.

Calles JL. A review of oppositional defiant and conduct disorders. *J Altern Med Res*. 2016b;8(4):371–378.

Catala-Lopez F, Hulton B, Nunez-Beltran A, et al. The pharmacological and non-pharmacological treatment of attention deficit hyperactivity disorder in children and adolescents: a systematic review with network meta-analyses of randomized trials. Available at https://journals.plos.org/plosone/article?id=10.1371/journal.pone.0180355. Accessed October 2, 2018.

Centers for Disease Control and Prevention (CDC). Web-based injury statistics query and reporting system (WISQARS), Atlanta, 2016, Department of Health and Human Services, Centers for Disease Control. Available at: www.cdc.gov/ncipc/wisqars. Accessed September 15, 2018.

Centers for Disease Control and Prevention (CDC). Autism spectrum disorder: data & statistics (website). 2018. Available at https://www.cdc.gov/ncbddd/autism/data.html. Accessed October 1, 2018.

Cheung AH, Zuckerbrot RS, Jensen PS, et al. Guidelines for adolescent depression in primary care (GLAD-PC): part II. Treatment and ongoing management. *Pediatr*. 2018;141(3):e20174082.

Chun TC, Mace ER, American Academy of Pediatric Committee on Pediatric Emergency Medicine, et al. Evaluation and management of children with acute mental health or behavioral problems. part II: recognition of clinically challenging mental health related conditions presenting with medical or uncertain symptoms. *Pediatr*. 2016;138(3):31–e23.

Cortese S, Adamo N, Del Giovane C, et al. Comparative efficacy and tolerability of medications for attention-deficit hyperactivity disorder in children, adolescents, and adults: a systematic review and network meta-analysis. *Lancet Psychiatry*. 2018;5(9):7270738.

Danielson ML, Bitsko RH, Ghandour RM, et al. Prevalence of Parent-Reported ADHD Diagnosis and Associated Treatment among U.S. Children and Adolescents. *J Clin Child Adolesc Psychol*. 2016. Published online before print. Accessed January 24, 2018.

Frias A, Palma C, Farriols N. Comorbidty in pediatric bipolar disorder: prevalence, clinical impact, etiology and treatment. *J Affective Disord*. 2015;174(15):378–389.

Frankovich J, Swedo S, Murphy T, et al. Clinical management of pediatric acute-onset neuropsychiatric syndrome: part II- use of immunomodulatory therapies. *J Child Adolesc Psychopharmacol*. 2017. https://doi.org/10.1089/cap.2016.0148. Last accessed September 17, 2018.

French WP, Boydston L, Varley CK. Obsessive compulsive disorder: a review. *J Altern Med Res*. 2016;8(4):431–439.

Hadland SE, Levy SL. Objective testing- urine and other drug tests. *Child Adolesc Psychiatr Clin N Am*. 2016;25(3):549–565.

Hagan JF, Shaw JS, Duncan PM, eds. *Bright Futures: Guidelines for Health Supervision of Infants, Children and Adolescents*. 4th ed. Elk Grove Village, IL: American Academy of Pediatrics; 2017.

Hall AY. Treatment of posttraumatic stress disorder. *Pediatr News*. 2016.

Harrington JW, Bora S. Autism spectrum disorder. In: Rakel D, ed. *Integrative Medicine*. 4th ed. New York: Elsevier; 2017:64–73.

Hirtz DG, Filipek PA, Sherr EH. Autism spectrum disorder. In: Swaiman K, Ashwal S, Hojaard DRM, Skarphedinsson G, Nissen JB, et al. Pediatric obsessive-compulsive disorder with tic symptoms: clinical presentation and tic outcomes. *Eur Child Adolesc Psychiatr*. 2017;26(6):681–689.

Hoogman M, Bralten J, Hibar DP, et al. Subcortical brain volume differences in participants with attention deficit hyperactivity disorder in children and adults: a cross-sectional mega-analysis. *Lancet Psychiatry*. 2017;4(4):310–319. https://doi.org/10.1016/S2215-0366(17)30049-4.

Horowitz SH, Rawe J, Whittaker MC. *The State of Learning Disabilities: Understanding the 1 in 5*. New York: National Center for Learning Disabilities; 2017.

Howard BJ. You can help with behavior of children with autism. *Pediatric News*. 2017.

Jacobson LA, Crocetti D, Dirlikov B, et al. Anomalous brain development is evident in preschoolers with attention-deficit/hyperactivity disorder. *J Int Neuropsychological Society*. 2018;24(6):531–539.

Kalter L. Fitbit-like device shows promise in predicting autism aggression. Available at https://www.disabilityscoop.com/2018/05/14/fitbit-like-autism-aggression/25085/. Accessed May 16, 2018.

Kann L, McManus T, Harris WA, et al. Youth risk behavior surveillance—United States, 2017. *MMWR Surveill Summ*. 2018;67(8):1–409.

Mahedy L, Heron J, Stapinksi LA, et al. Mother's own recollections of having been parented and risk offspring depression 18 years later: a prospective cohort study. *Depress Anxiety*. 2014;31(1):38–43.

Mehler PS, Andersen AE. *Eating Disorders A Guide to Medical Care and Complications*. 3rd ed. Baltimore: Johns Hopkins University; 2017.

McBride ME. Beyond butterflies: generalized anxiety disorder in adolescence. *Nurse Pract*. 2015;40(3):28–36.

Moeschler JB, Shevell M. Committee on genetics comprehensive evaluation of the child with intellectual disability or global developmental delays. *Pediatrics*. 2014;134(3):e903–e918.

Morey RA, Haswell CC, Hooper SR, et al. Amygdala, hippocampus, and ventral prefrontal cortex volumes differ in youth with and without chronic posttraumatic stress disorder. *Neuropsychopharm*. 2016;41:791–801.

Murphy TK, Lewin AB, Storch EA, et al. Practice parameter for the assessment and treatment of children and adolescents with tic disorders. *J Am Acad Child Adolesc Psychiatry*. 2013;52(12):1341–1359.

National Autistic Society. Social Stories and comic strip conversations. Available at www.autism.org.uk/about/strategies/social-stories-comic-strips.aspx. Accessed October 1, 2018.

National Institute of Neurological Disorders and Stroke (NINDS). autism spectrum disorder fact sheet. Available at https://www.ninds.nih.gov/Disorders/Patient-Caregiver-Education/Fact-Sheets/Autism-Spectrum-Disorder-Fact-Sheet. Accessed October 1, 2018.

National Institute of Mental Health (NIMH). Inflammation in pregnant moms linked to child's brain development. Available at https://www.nimh.nih.gov/news/science-news/2018/inflammation-in-pregnant-moms-linked-to-childs-brain-development.shtml. Accessed October 1, 2018.

Parekh R. Intellectual disability. American Psychiatric Association. Available at https://www.psychiatry.org/patients-families/intellectual-disability/what-is-intellectual-disability. Accessed October 2, 2018.

Puruggganan O. Intellectual disabilities. *Pediatrics Review*. 2018;339(6):299–307.

Sahin NT, Keshav NU, Salisbury JP, Vahabzadeh A. Second version of google glass as a wearable socio-affective aid: positive school desirability, high usability, and theoretical framework in a sample of children with autism. *JMIR Human Factors*. 2018;5(1):e1–e11.

Sherr EH, Shevell MI. Global developmental delay and intellectual disability. In: Swaiman K, Ashwal S, Ferriero D, et al., eds. *Swaiman's Pediatric Neurology*. 6th ed. New York: Elsevier; 2018:e1007–e1028.

Stevens AJ, Rucklidge JJ, Kennedy MA. Epigenetics, nutrition and mental health. Is there a relationship? *Nutritional Neurosci*. 2018;21:602–613.

Tost H, Champagne FA, Meyer-Lindenberg. Environmental influence in the brain, human welfare and mental health. *Nature Neurosci*. 2015;18:1421–1431.

U.S. Food and Drug Administration (FDA). FDA drug safety podcast for healthcare professionals: safety review update of medications used to treat attention-deficit/hyperactivity disorder (ADHD) in children and young adults, FDA (website). 2011. Available at https://www.fda.gov/Drugs/DrugSafety/ucm277770.htm. Accessed October 11, 2018.

Van den Bergh BRH, Van den Bergh MI, Lahti M, et al. Prenatal developmental origins of behavior and mental health: the influence of maternal stress in pregnancy. *Neurosci Biobehavioral Rev*. 2017. https://doi.org/10.1016/j.neubiorev.2017.07.003. Last accessed October 10, 2018.

Voight RG. Developmental and behavioral diagnoses: the spectrum and continuum of developmental-behavioral disorders. In: Voight RG, Macias MM, Myers SM, eds. *Developmental and Behavioral Pediatrics*. Elk Grove, IL: American Academy of Pediatrics; 2011:121–145.

Volkmar F, Siegel M, Woodbury-Smith M, et al. Practice parameter for the assessment and treatment of children and adolescents with autism spectrum disorder. *J Am Acad Child Adolesc Psychiatry*. 2014;53(2):237–257.

Wallman KK. America's children: key national indicators of well-being, 2015, ChildStats.gov (website). Available at: www.childstats.gov/americaschildren. Accessed February 27, 2015.

Wehry AM, Beesdo-Baum KB, Connolly SD, et al. Assessment and treatment of anxiety disorders in children and adolescents. *Curr Psychiatry Rep*. 2015. https://doi.org/10.1007/s11920-015-0591-z. Last accessed October 13, 2018.

Weill VA, Zavodny S, Souders MC. Autism Spectrum disorder in primary care. *Nurse Practitioner*. 2018;43(2):21–28.

West AE, Pavuluri MN. A review of pediatric bipolar disorder. *J Altern Med Res*. 2016;8(4):405–409.

Wong C, Odom SL, Hume KA, et al. Evidence-based practices for children, youth, and young adults with autism spectrum disorder: a comprehensive review. *J Autism Dev Disord*. 2015;45(7):1951–1966.

Zuckerbrodt RA, Cheung A, Jensen PS, et al. Guidelines for adolescent depression in primary care (GLAD-PC): part 1. Practice preparation, identification, assessment and initial management. *Pediatr*. 2018. https://doi.org/10.1542/peds.2017-4081. Last accessed October 12, 2018.

31

Infectious Diseases

SUSAN K. SANDERSON AND NAN M. GAYLORD

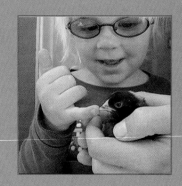

Infectious diseases are the leading causes of illness in infants and children despite advances in public and personal health, antimicrobials, and active and passive vaccination. The ability to distinguish serious infections from those that resolve with minimal or no intervention is an important skill for primary care providers (PCPs). Nearly as important as the medical care provided to the sick child is the ability to effectively communicate with, educate, and support the often frustrated and anxious parents. In addition, the provider must include preventive education, including vaccinations, in the routine delivery of primary health care.

Pathogenesis of Infectious Diseases

Researchers from the National Institutes of Health (NIH) Common Fund Human Microbiome Project (2018) are mapping the normal microbial makeup of healthy individuals. This project has found that approximately 100 trillion microorganisms (mostly bacteria, but also viruses and fungi) abound in the body (the brain, spinal fluid, blood, urine, lungs, and tissues are inherently sterile) and for the most part live in harmony with their human hosts, contributing to human survival. Bacteria outnumber human cells by 10 to 1 and can weigh 2 to 7 pounds, depending upon an individual's size (NIH, 2012), although that number is presently debated (Sender, Fuchs, and Milo, 2016). In turn, viruses outnumber bacteria 10 to 1 and are common both in and on humans and in most ecosystems (Saey, 2014).

The normal human flora, or "normal microbiota" (Table 31.1), remain throughout life unless environmental changes affect them. Studies show that humans are losing some of their microbial diversity. It is believed that this loss is in part due to the overuse of antibiotics, cesarean sections, and modern sanitation. This loss may account for the increase in asthma, allergies, diabetes, obesity, and possibly some forms of cancer (Blaser, 2014).

It is estimated that only 10% of pathogens attributed to causing human diseases are identified. Although viruses are the most frequent cause of childhood infectious illnesses, bacterial infections (particularly of the skin and mucosal surfaces) are also common. Bacteria are ubiquitous in the environment. They are intercellular microorganisms that carry all their requirements and mechanisms for growth and multiplication with them. Most can grow on nonliving surfaces and some live at temperature extremes. They have many shapes, including curved rods, spheres, rods, and spirals. Each bacterium has its own unique mode(s) of transmission and mechanisms of colonization and pathogenesis. Humans are inoculated with important bacteria on the skin (especially in moist areas) and mucosal surfaces (including the upper respiratory,

urinary, and gastrointestinal [GI] tracts) during vaginal birth or shortly afterward.

Most bacteria are harmless and are the first line of defense against the colonization by potentially pathogenic organisms. Microbiotas are required for digestion, to degrade toxins, and help mature the immune system. Infectious disease results when the balance between harmless colonization and protective immunity is disrupted in favor of harmful proliferation of a microorganism. Bacteria are adept at adapting, as evidenced by increasing resistance to antibiotics.

In comparison, viruses (Latin noun meaning *toxin* or *poison*) are submicroscopic particles that invade a host cell, redirect the normal cell's functions, and effectively transfer genetic information (deoxyribonucleic acid [DNA] and ribonucleic acid [RNA]) to replicate viral particles. Viruses need to have a living host in order to multiply. Viruses are rarely dangerous because of their inability to simultaneously meet three criteria necessary for virulence: (1) to inflict serious harm, (2) to remain unrecognized by the immune system, and (3) to spread efficiently. Viruses can also control bacteria; these are referred to as *bacteriophages,* or "eaters of bacteria." These phages are numerous in the environment and practically harmless to humans. Vaccines prevent the spread of some viruses, and antiviral medications help slow down their reproduction in some cases. Newer research focuses on human resident viruses (human virome), and there is indication that viruses play a part in the human defense system (Saey, 2014).

The human immune system is complex and provides many layers of protection from disease. Skin and mucosal surfaces provide a barrier to invasion by microorganisms, and antibodies and immune cells allow the body to defend itself in general and specific ways against pathogen invasion. Microorganisms may breach the immune barrier of the skin and mucosa by binding to cell surface structures. For example, influenza virus uses its hemagglutinin protein to attach to cell membranes and invade respiratory mucosa. Disease caused by microbial pathogens can result from infected cell and tissue destruction and from normal cell function disruption. Some disease symptoms are caused by the immune system's response to infection, resulting in local or systemic inflammatory responses. Biotechnology is developing bacterial-based treatments that harness the ability of some bacteria to enter into cells and trigger intense immune responses, much like vaccines. A variety of genetically engineered and modified bacterial strains are being studied as possible treatments for certain bacterial infections (e.g., malaria, human immunodeficiency virus [HIV]) and cancers (Trafton, 2018).

TABLE 31.1 Common Distribution Sites of Normal Microflora[a] Found in Humans

Bacterium	Very Commonly or Commonly Found in These Locations	Notes
Aerobic Bacteria		
Gram Positive		
Staphylococcus aureus	Skin, hair, naso-oropharynx, lower GI, cerumen, vagina	Rarely found in the anterior vagina and conjunctiva; trachea, bronchi, lungs, and sinuses are normally sterile; has potential for being a pathogen. High levels of MRSA bacteria in the nose may indicate MRSA colonization in other parts of the body, specifically the axilla, groin, and perineum.
Staphylococcus epidermidis	Skin, hair, naso-oropharynx, adult vagina, urethra, conjunctiva, ear (including cerumen), lower GI	Occasionally found in the vagina of prepubertal females; found in low numbers in "normal" urine, probably as a result of contamination from urethra and skin areas.
Staphylococcus saprophyticus	Skin, mucous membranes, vagina, perineum	Most common cause of UTI in sexually active women.
Streptococci • *S. mitis* • *S. mutans* • *S. pneumoniae* (Pneumococcus, Diplococcus) • *S. pyogenes* (group A)	Skin, pharynx, mouth; less commonly in adult vagina and urethra; rare lower GI Mouth, pharynx Nasopharynx, mouth; rarely found in conjunctiva, nose, vagina Mouth, pharynx; rarely skin, conjunctiva, adult vagina, lower GI	Has the potential of being a pathogen. Common cause respiratory tract and ear infections; pathogen of sepsis, pneumonia, meningitis. Common cause of skin and pharyngeal infections.
Bifidobacterium bifidum	Lower GI	
Enterococcus faecalis	Lower GI, postpubertal vagina; mouth, anterior urethra; rarely pharynx	Has potential of being a pathogen.
Propionibacterium acnes	Skin (rarely seen in children prior to age of 10 years); external ear	Commonly involved in acne vulgaris during puberty.
Gram Negative		
Acinetobacter spp.	Skin; less commonly respiratory tract, mouth, GI	Has the potential of causing pathogenic outbreaks and developing antibiotic resistance.
Corynebacterium	Skin, conjunctiva, naso-oropharynx, mouth, lower GI, anterior urethra, adult vagina	
Citrobacter diversus	Lower GI	Common cause of UTI.
Escherichia coli	Lower GI, vagina, mouth, anterior urethra; rarely found in conjunctiva, nose, pharynx	Has the potential of being a pathogen.
Haemophilus influenzae	Nasopharynx, mouth; rarely conjunctiva, ear	Cause of upper respiratory tract, ear, and eye infections.
Kingella kingae (formerly referred to as *Moraxella kingae*)	Pharynx	Has the potential of being a pathogen (cause of invasive infections in young children).
Klebsiella pneumoniae	Nose, colon, axillary area	Associated with neonatal sepsis; urinary tract infections.
Lactobacillus spp.	Pharynx, mouth, lower GI, adult vagina	
Moraxella catarrhalis	Nasopharynx	Implicated in otitis media.
Morganella morganii	Lower GI	
Mycobacterium spp.	Skin, lower GI, anterior urethra; rarely nasopharynx	
Mycoplasma	Mouth, pharynx, lower GI, vagina; rarely anterior urethra	Implicated in upper and lower respiratory tract infections.
Neisseria spp. (e.g., *N. mucosa*)	Nose, pharynx (100% of population), conjunctiva, mouth, anterior urethra, vagina	Nonpathogenic species.

Continued

TABLE 31.1	Common Distribution Sites of Normal Microflora[a] Found in Humans—cont'd	
Bacterium	**Very Commonly or Commonly Found in These Locations**	**Notes**
N. meningitidis	Nose, pharynx (100% of population), mouth, vagina	Significant cause of meningitis and sepsis in children.
Proteus spp.	Skin, nasopharynx, mouth, lower GI, vagina, anterior urethra; rarely in conjunctiva	
Pseudomonas aeruginosa	Lower GI; rarely in pharynx, mouth, anterior urethra; colonization in lungs of patients with cystic fibrosis (Murray et al., 2007); small numbers can be found on the skin	Has the potential of being a pathogen.
Anaerobic Bacteria		
Bacteroides spp.	Lower GI, anterior urethra; rarely adult vagina	Has the potential of being a pathogen.
Clostridium spp.	Lower GI; rarely mouth	Has the potential of being a pathogen.
Streptococcus spp.	Mouth, colon, adult vagina	
Spirochetes (a distinct form of bacteria)	Pharynx, mouth, lower GI	
Fungi		
Actinomycetes spp.	Pharynx, mouth	
Candida albicans	Skin, conjunctiva, mouth, lower GI, adult vagina	Can be found in voided urine, but is a contaminant.
Cryptococcus spp.	Skin	
Protozoa	Mouth, lower GI, adult vagina	

[a]Normal microflora in humans consists of indigenous microorganisms that colonize human tissues and live in a mutualistic state without producing disease. An individual's microflora depends on genetics, age, sex, stress, nutrition, and diet. A pathogen is a microorganism (or virus) that produces disease. Normal flora can become pathogens when a host is compromised or weakened (endogenous pathogen); other microorganisms invade a host during times of disease only (obligate pathogens) or lowered resistance (opportunistic pathogens). Skin microflora also includes yeast *(Malassezia furfur)*, molds *(Trichophyton mentagrophytes* var. *interdigitale)*, and mites *(Demodex folliculorum)*. The normal flora found in the vagina depends on one's age, pH, and hormonal levels. Cerumen contains some antimicrobial elements to discourage growth of pathogenic *Pseudomonas aeruginosa* and *Staphylococcus aureus*. The cervix is normally sterile but can demonstrate flora similar to those in the upper area of the vagina. Greater than 500 species of bacteria are identified in the colon. The flow of tears and inherent antibacterial lysozymes prevent the growth of flora in the conjunctiva.

GI, Gastrointestinal; *MRSA,* methicillin-resistant *Staphylococcus aureus*; *spp.,* species; *URI,* urinary tract infection.

Data from Carroll KC, Hobden JA, Miller S, et al., eds. *Jawetz, Melnick, & Adelberg's Medical Microbiology.* 27th ed. Normal human microbiota. New York: McGraw-Hill; 2016; Cystic Fibrosis Foundation. *Pseudomonas aeruginosa;* 2015. Retrieved from https://www.cff.org/Life-With-CF/Daily-Life/Germs-and-Staying-Healthy/What-Are-Germs/Pseudomonas/; and Todar K. The normal bacterial flora of humans. *Todar's Online Textbook of Bacteriology* (website), 2008–2012. Retrieved from www.textbookofbacteriology.net/normalflora.html. Accessed June 17, 2018.

Clinical Findings

History

Most pediatric infectious illnesses are diagnosed solely based on history and physical examination. A comprehensive history generates and helps prioritize the individual's differential diagnoses based on symptomatology and history. Many symptoms are shared by different illnesses, and establishing a differential diagnoses can be challenging (e.g., fever is most commonly associated with infectious illnesses but also occurs with rheumatologic or oncologic diseases). Crucial aspects of the history that help distinguish infectious illnesses from other types of diseases or assist in determining the responsible pathogen include careful questioning of:

- The history of present illness with a careful analysis of the presenting symptoms: When did the symptoms start? What other symptoms were associated with the illness? Were there periods when the patient seemed improved or even back to normal?
- A comprehensive past medical history: Determine place of birth and past acute or chronic illnesses that increase specific illness risk. A history of asthma in a teenager with fever and cough, for example, is suspicious of atypical pneumonia.
- Current and recent medications: Recent antibiotic use may negate culture results or contribute to resistant infections (e.g., methicillin-resistant *Staphylococcus aureus* [MRSA] infection). Include any nonprescription, herbal, or natural health products that were recently used.
- Immunizations: Adherence to recommended vaccine schedules (American Academy of Pediatric [AAP], 2018b), including age and spacing of vaccines, is an important consideration if the child's symptoms suggest a vaccine-preventable disease.
- Family history, particularly noting infectious illness: A history of any relative (first- or second-degree) with a known immune deficiency, with numerous infections or difficulty recovering from infections, or with a history of recurrent miscarriages. Any of these may raise suspicion for an immune deficiency. A strong history of autoimmune disease in the family may suggest possible rheumatologic diagnoses as opposed to an infectious process.
- Social history: Day care or school attendance or living in a crowded setting increases exposure to viral infections. A sexual history (Chapters 13 and 21) is important for accurate assessment of the sexually active adolescent to identify males who have sex with males and those who have high-risk sexual practices.

- Exposure history, including any known contacts with individuals with similar symptoms: A comprehensive, in-depth exposure history helps diagnose infections caused by epidemic illness (e.g., influenza) and those that might otherwise not be considered. Ask about contact with individuals with known illnesses or at high risk for certain illnesses, or contact with animals (e.g., at farms or animal markets) or animal by-products (e.g., hides, waste, blood), insects, or snakes (e.g., bites). A history of travel to tropical countries or areas with endemic illnesses is important (e.g., Lyme disease, malaria, dengue, or parasitic illnesses), as well as the lodging accommodations during travel (e.g., possible exposure to parasites). Other important exposures include environmental tobacco smoke or mold, swimming in rivers, flood waters, or other waterways.
- Complete review of symptoms: Some illness presenting features may be discounted or forgotten by children or parents and recalled only when direct questions are asked.
- Diet history: Any ingestion of raw milk or raw/undercooked meats and/or fish; history of pica.

Physical Examination

A complete physical examination is necessary; however, the differential diagnoses generated during the process of history taking can stimulate the examiner to focus on certain exam aspects. Physical findings that may be noted with infectious diseases include:
- Abnormal vital signs (e.g., fever, tachypnea, low blood pressure [concerning for dehydration and/or septic shock]).
- Irritability is nonspecific in ill children, but may raise concern for meningitis or Kawasaki disease. Lethargy raises concern for meningitis and sepsis (particularly in infants and younger children).
- A stiff or painful neck (suggestive of meningitis).
- A new murmur (may herald the possibility of endocarditis or rheumatic fever).
- Refusal to walk (can be a manifestation of deep tissue infections [e.g., pyomyositis], osteomyelitis, septic arthritis, or meningitis).
- Skin or mucous membrane changes (exanthema or enanthema, respectively) are common with viral illness, and characteristic rashes of specific illnesses (e.g., chickenpox).

Diagnostic Aids

Laboratory and Imaging Studies

Laboratory studies measure the "host-pathogen damage-response framework." Inflammation or tissue damage stimulates proinflammatory cytokines, which activate proteins referred to as *acute-phase reactants*. There is no single marker with the necessary sensitivity, specificity, or predictive values to serve as a stand-alone test upon which to initiate therapy for suspected serious infection. Likewise, testing cannot positively confirm when to stop therapy in proven infection (Long and Vozdak, 2018). New bloodstream infections/sepsis biomarkers types are under investigation.

In selected circumstances, laboratory evaluation can clarify a diagnosis or rule out a serious illness that may be under consideration. When in doubt, it may be helpful to consult with knowledgeable laboratory personnel or an infectious disease expert. The following should be taken into consideration when ordering diagnostic studies:
- The quality of the specimen sent to the lab strongly affects the reliability of the results. For example, pus aspirated from a skin

infection is generally more likely to grow the pathogen of concern than a surface swab. The collection site of the microbiologic specimen needs to be appropriately cleansed with sterile saline, 70% alcohol, and/or iodine to minimize possible skin contamination.
- Sample collection timing affects the accuracy of results. Bacterial cultures collected after the antibiotic administration may be negative even with active infection. Acute and convalescent titers or certain blood chemistries help to make a diagnosis or monitor treatment response.
- Laboratory tests require a certain volume or quantity to ensure valid and reliable results. Be prepared to prioritize test requests when a limited quantity is collected (e.g., if a catheterized urine specimen only yields 7 mL, it may be more important to get a urine culture than a urinalysis).
- Microbiologic samples may require special handling and should be transported to the laboratory promptly. Contact the laboratory if there is any question regarding the sample collection and transport.

The Centers for Disease Control (CDC) lists the notifiable infectious diseases and conditions that must be reported to local public health authorities or their agents (CDC, 2018r). In many cases, this reporting is done by the laboratory, but there are some conditions the provider may treat without obtaining a laboratory specimen (e.g., Lyme disease). Providers should be familiar with the list (https://wwwn.cdc.gov/nndss/).

Complete Blood Count

From an infectious disease standpoint, the white blood cell (WBC) count is generally the most useful piece of information obtained from the complete blood count (CBC). It is often elevated (leukocytosis) in bacterial infections and may be decreased (leukopenia) in some viral infections. A differential WBC may further focus the diagnosis. Bacterial infections often (but not always) cause increases in the neutrophil (or polymorphonuclear cell) count and may elevate bands (immature neutrophils), whereas viral infections often cause elevated lymphocyte counts and/or atypical lymphocyte production (see Chapter 39). WBCs can be affected by long-term use of certain medications (some can decrease), age, steroid use (can increase), and clinical state (e.g., overwhelming sepsis can lead to decreased WBCs). Chronic inflammatory processes can cause a decrease in red blood cells (RBCs) (e.g., anemia).

Platelet Count

The platelet count is elevated (thrombocytosis) during the active phase of acute infection and correlates with concurrent elevations in C-reactive protein (CRP) and erythrocyte sedimentation rate (ESR).

C-Reactive Protein

The CRP is among the serum acute phase reactants that increase in the presence of acute inflammation and specific pathogens. CRP is sometimes used as part of the workup for infants at risk of septicemia; however, its diagnostic value for influencing clinical judgment remains weak. The value above which CRP is most highly predictive of bacterial infection is not firmly established; normal is 0.0 to 0.05 mg/dL (Hughes and Kahl, 2018) but sepsis is much less likely to occur with a CRP of less than 10 mg/L. Serial CRPs 24 to 48 hours after the onset of symptoms are recommended and can help monitor the body's response to treatment in certain infections (e.g., in neonatal sepsis and osteomyelitis). Inflammatory processes other than infection may lead to an elevated CRP, including maternal and perinatal factors, trauma, rheumatologic diseases, and oncologic diseases. Persistent elevations of CRP may be related to treatment failure and conditions such as adiposity, use of birth control pills, and pregnancy.

Procalcitonin

Serum procalcitonin (Pro-CT) is a biomarker that differentiates certain viral infections from serious bacterial infections. Pro-CT is a protein that has activity similar to hormones and cytokines. It is produced by several cell types and many organs in response to systemic proinflammatory stimuli. Pro-CT levels tend to rise and fall quicker than CRP during onset and control of bacterial infections. It may prove to be a valuable tool when the ability to draw and process blood cultures is limited. Levels are increased in children with bacteremia and reflect the severity of the illness (Vijayan et al., 2017). Its usefulness has been studied and there is a higher sensitivity and specificity than CRP (Long and Vozdak, 2018) for predicting pyelonephritis, pneumonia, early-onset sepsis in premature infants, bacterial infection in febrile neutropenic children with cancer, diarrhea-associated hemolytic-uremic syndrome, bacterial causes of acute hepatic disease, bacterial versus aseptic meningitis, and various diseases or conditions that involve inflammatory processes (e.g., posttraumatic sepsis, Crohn disease). At this point, it should only be used with other clinical and diagnostic data when making diagnostic and management decisions. Rapid test kits are available.

Erythrocyte Sedimentation Rate

The ESR is another measure of inflammation and reflects RBCs settling faster when acute-phase proteins (such as fibrinogen) are present in serum than when they are not. Although the ESR is not a specific test for infection, it is useful in evaluating fever of unknown origin (FUO) and, like CRP, can be used to monitor therapy response. A low sedimentation rate (<10 mm/h) is unlikely in bacterial infection as a cause of prolonged unexplained fever. Viral infections result in mean ESR values around 20 mm/h (90% <30 mm/h), with the exception of adenovirus, which may be associated with values higher than 30 mm/h. An ESR more than 50 mm/h in children warrants further evaluation (Long and Vozdak, 2018).

During the waxing and waning period of infection, the ESR tends to increase and resolve more slowly than CRP values. ESR is considered a useful marker to evaluate the effectiveness of therapy when long-term antibiotics are needed. It is used when managing diseases in which treatment effectiveness is judged, in part, by the normalization of the ESR (e.g., osteomyelitis). Like CRP, the ESR is often elevated in noninfectious conditions that cause inflammation (e.g., miliary tuberculosis [TB], bacterial arthritis, head/neck abscesses for which ESRs >100 mm/h can occur). Anemia also causes a nonspecific increase in the ESR.

Cultures, Stains, and Antimicrobial Susceptibility Testing

The usefulness of microbiologic testing is dependent on the quality of the sample and on the correct choice of test for the given clinical situation. Details of appropriate tests for given infections are discussed in the sections about specific infectious agents.

The presence of pus assists in the diagnosis of some infections. Staining methods can be useful in certain clinical situations, such as when fungal or other infections are suspected. Antigen detection immunofluorescence or antibody assays (e.g., complement fixation tests [CFTs], immunofluorescence techniques, and enzyme-linked immunosorbent assays [ELISAs]) are often used in the diagnosis of viral infections. There are many diagnostic staining methods available.

Fluid and tissue specimens can be sent for bacterial, viral, or fungal cultures; however, the laboratory may need to be notified for instruction on certain pathogens for the most accurate evaluation of the sample (e.g., pertussis). Antibody bacterial susceptibility can be done on cultured samples, especially if organism resistance is suspected because of community resistance patterns.

Other Technologies

DNA and RNA testing are common in the in-patient setting and are being used more frequently in clinical practice. These tests rely on using polymerase chain reaction (PCR). Multiple organisms can be screened using one sample. Pathogens that are commonly detected by PCR include *Neisseria gonorrhoeae*, *Chlamydia trachomatis*, HIV, *Bordetella pertussis,* herpesviruses, and enteroviruses. Newer technologies also include molecular finger printing for nosocomial infection and microarrays to differentiate between viral and bacterial pathogens.

Immunoserology

In specific situations, tests that rely on the generation of an antibody response may be useful. Various methods (e.g., hemagglutination, enzyme immunoassays, latex agglutination, complement fixation, immunofluorescence, and neutralization assays) can be used to detect the presence of antibodies to specific infectious organisms (e.g., HIV, West Nile virus [WNV], *Bartonella henselae,* and *Mycoplasma pneumoniae*).

Imaging Techniques

Radiographs, computed tomography (CT) scans, magnetic resonance imaging (MRI), echocardiography, and ultrasounds can assist in the diagnosis of infections of the bone, sinus, lung, skin, viscera, brain, and heart. Several nuclear imaging techniques evaluate possible bone infections, tumors, fractures, urinary backflow blockage, heart conditions, GI bleeding, and thyroid disorders.

General Management Strategies

Preventing the Spread of Infection

Thorough and frequent hand washing is the most effective means of preventing the spread of infection. In addition to educating parents and children on the importance of proper hand washing, it is crucial that PCPs practice proper hand washing. Alcohol-based hand rubs may be substituted for soap and water in most cases, as long as the ethanol content is at least 60% (Centers for Disease Control and Prevention [CDC], 2018d). However, they are ineffective against controlling the spread of *Clostridium difficile*. It is recommended that gloves and washing hands with soap and water be used when in contact with children with *C. difficile*–associated disease and/or in outbreak settings (CDC, 2016b).

Specific guidance that should be given to children and parents includes:

- Wash hands after using the bathroom, before meals, and before preparing foods. The proper technique includes scrubbing with soap and water for at least 20 seconds (the time it takes to sing "Happy Birthday" twice), rinsing with warm water, and drying completely.
- Avoid finger-nose and finger-eye contact, particularly if exposed to someone with a cold.
- Use a tissue to cover the mouth and nose when coughing or sneezing to help prevent the spread of pathogens. If a tissue is unavailable, the upper sleeve should be used (not the hands).

Use of Antibiotics

In the United States, at least 2 million people each year become infected with antibiotic-resistant bacteria, at least 23,000 people die as a direct result of this, and others die from complications stemming from an antibiotic-resistant infection (CDC, 2018b). Antibiotics are often prescribed for conditions that do not require their use, and inappropriate prescribing patterns contribute to the emergence of resistant bacteria. This is particularly troublesome for children in group child care settings. PCPs should educate children and parents about the role and efficacy of antibiotics and to assume a more "targeted therapy" approach when prescribing. The CDC (2018c) provides brochures, posters, and information sheets that may be helpful in explaining the importance of judicious use of antibiotics. Knowledge about emerging resistance patterns, local epidemiology, and susceptibility patterns of bacterial agents within their practice communities will better arm the provider to appropriately prescribe antibiotics (see Chapter 26 for a further discussion about the overuse of antibiotics).

Prevention of Infection Through the Use of Vaccines

Immunizations are the mainstay of disease prevention in children. Vaccines reduce the burden of mortality and morbidity due to infectious diseases around the world and are cost effective. See Chapter 22 for a full discussion on immunizations.

Infections in Children in Child Care Settings

Children in child care settings are 2 to 18 times more likely to suffer from a myriad of infectious diseases, principally respiratory and GI in nature. Additionally, these children receive two to four times more antibiotic treatment and acquire antibiotic-resistant organisms more frequently than children not in child care (Sosinsky and Gilliam, 2016). Infections typically spread in these settings are listed in Table 31.2.

Specific Viral Diseases

Enteroviruses

Nonpolio Enteroviruses

Ten to 15 serotypes account for most diseases from more than 100 serotypes of nonpolio RNA enteroviruses. There are four genomic classifications: human enteroviruses (HEVs) A, B, C, and D. Coxsackieviruses and echoviruses are subgroups of HEVs. Hand-foot-mouth, herpangina, pleurodynia, acute hemorrhagic conjunctivitis, myocarditis, pericarditis, pancreatitis, orchitis, and dermatomyositis-like syndrome are manifestations of infection. These enteroviruses are the most common cause of aseptic meningitis and are

---

TABLE 31.2 Pathogens and Modes of Transmission in Child Care Settings

Modes of Transmission	Bacteria	Viruses	Parasites, Fungi, Mites, and Lice
Respiratory	Haemophilus influenzae type B Neisseria meningitides Group A Streptococcus (GAS) Streptococcus pneumonia Bordetella pertussis Mycobacterium tuberculosis Kingella kingae (also known as Moraxella kingae)	Adenovirus Coronavirus Influenza A and B Measles Mumps Varicella-zoster Metapneumovirus Parainfluenza Parvovirus B19 Respiratory syncytial virus Rhinovirus	
Fecal-oral	Campylobacter jejuni Salmonella spp. Shigella spp. Clostridium difficile Aeromonas Plesiomonas Escherichia coli O157:H7	Enteroviruses (including genus Klebsiella) Hepatitis A virus Rotavirus Calicivirus Astrovirus Norovirus (Norwalk) Enteric adenovirus	Cryptosporidium parvum Giardia lamblia Enterobius vermicularis
Person-to-person via skin contact	Group A Streptococcus (GAS) Staphylococcus aureus	Herpes simplex Varicella-zoster Molluscum contagiosum	Pediculus capitis Sarcoptes scabiei Trichophyton spp. Microsporum spp.
Contact with blood, urine, or saliva		Cytomegalovirus (CMV) Hepatitis B and C Herpes simplex Human immunodeficiency virus (HIV)	

Data from Collins JP, Pickering LK. Infections associated with group childcare. In: Long SS, Prober CG, Fisher M, eds. *Principles and Practice of Pediatric Infectious Diseases*. 5th ed. New York: Elsevier; 2018:25–32.e3; American Academy of Pediatrics (AAP) Committee on Infectious Diseases, Kimberlin DW, Brady MT, et al., eds. *Children in Out-of-Home Child Care: Red Book: 2018 Report of the Committee on Infectious Diseases*. 31st ed. Elk Grove Village, IL: American Academy of Pediatrics; 2018.

associated with paralysis, neonatal sepsis, encephalitis, and other respiratory and GI symptoms. The specific serotype may not be unique to any given disease (Abzug, 2016).

As evidenced by the name, enteroviruses concentrate on the GI tract as their primary invasion, replication, and transmission site; they spread by fecal-oral contamination, especially in diapered infants. They are also transmitted via the respiratory route and vertically either prenatally, during parturition, or during breastfeeding by an infected mother who lacks antibodies to that particular serotype. Transplacental infection can lead to serious disseminated disease in the neonate that involves multiorgan systems (liver, heart, meninges, and adrenal cortex).

Enteroviruses have worldwide distribution, occurring in temperate climates during the summer and fall and in tropical climates year round. In known cases, infants younger than 12 months old have the highest prevalence rate (>25%), and HEVs account for 55% to 65% of hospitalizations for suspected infant sepsis. Illness occurs more frequently in males; in those living in crowded, unsanitary conditions; and in those of lower socioeconomic status (Abzug, 2016). Infection ranges from asymptomatic to undifferentiated febrile illness to severe illness. Young children are more likely to be symptomatic. The incubation period is 3 to 6 days (less for hemorrhagic conjunctivitis). After infection, the virus sheds from the respiratory tract for up to 3 weeks and from the GI tract for up to 7 to 11 weeks; it is viable on environmental surfaces for long periods.

Nonpolio enteroviral infection is not a reportable disease, nor is it routinely tested for in the clinical setting, so the overall incidence rate is not known. The CDC administers the National Respiratory and Enteric Virus Surveillance System (NREVSS) and the National Enterovirus Surveillance System (NESS) to monitor detection patterns of respiratory and enteric adenoviruses. There have been 386 confirmed cases, mostly in children, between August 2014 and October 2018 of an illness referred to as *acute flaccid myelitis* which bears some similarity to infections caused by viruses, including enterovirus; epidemiologic studies are ongoing (CDC, 2018a).

Clinical Findings

History. General symptoms include:

- A mild upper respiratory infection (URI) is common and may include complaints of sore throat, fever, vomiting, diarrhea, anorexia, coryza, abdominal pain, rash, and headache.
- Nonspecific febrile illness of at least 3 days: In young children, there is an undifferentiated abrupt-onset febrile illness (101°F to 104°F [38.5°C to 40°C]) associated with myalgias, malaise, irritability; fever may wax and wane over several days.
- Onset of viral symptoms within 1 to 2 weeks after delivery for neonates infected transplacentally.

Physical Examination. General findings include mild conjunctivitis, pharyngitis, and/or cervical adenopathy. Other findings include:

- Skin: Rash may be macular, macular-papular, urticarial, vesicular, or petechial. May imitate the rash of meningitis, measles, or rubella.
- Herpangina: There is a sudden onset of high fever (up to 106°F [41°C]) lasting 1 to 4 days. Loss of appetite, sore throat, and dysphagia are common, with vomiting and abdominal pain in 25% of cases. Small vesicles (from one to more than 15 lesions of 1 to 2 mm each) appear and enlarge to ulcers (3 to 4 mm) on the anterior pillars of the fauces, tonsils, uvula, and pharynx and the edge of the soft palate. The vesicles commonly have red areolas up to 10 mm in diameter. This self-limiting infection usually lasts 3 to 7 days.

- Acute lymphonodular pharyngitis: This manifests as an acute sore throat lasting approximately 1 week.
- Hand-foot-mouth disease: This is a clinical entity with fever, vesicular eruptions in the oropharynx that may ulcerate, and a maculopapular rash involving the hands and feet. The rash evolves to vesicles, especially on the dorsa of the hands and the soles of the feet, and lasts 1 to 2 weeks (Fig 31.1).
- Aseptic meningitis: There are the usual signs of fever, stiff neck, and headache. Altered sensorium and seizures are common. Most cases appear in epidemics or as unique cases; most patients recover completely.
- Paralytic disease: A Guillain-Barré–type syndrome has been described.
- Congenital or neonatal infection: The neonatal infection often manifests as a sudden onset of vomiting, coughing, anorexia, fever or hypothermia, rash, jaundice, irritability, cyanosis, tachycardia, and dyspnea. It is often mistaken for pneumonia. The latter three symptoms can progress to myocarditis and congestive heart failure (CHF). Infants can have cardiac collapse, hepatic and adrenal necrosis, intracranial hemorrhage, and death. For those who survive severe disease, the recovery can be rapid.
- Acute hemorrhagic conjunctivitis: Characterized by sudden eye pain, photophobia, blurred vision, tearing, and conjunctival erythema and infection. Most patients recover in a few weeks.
- Pleurodynia (Bornholm disease or devil's grip): This condition usually occurs in epidemics, but some isolated cases occur. It is most often caused by type B disease, but echoviruses are implicated. There may be a prodrome before the onset of chest pain ushered in by headache, malaise, anorexia, and myalgia. The onset of chest or upper abdominal pain can be sudden, is pleuritic in nature, and is aggravated by deep breathing, coughing,

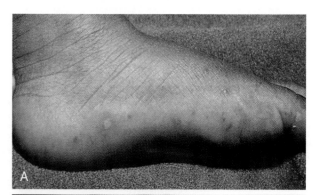
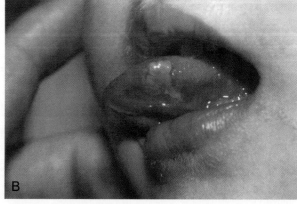

• **Fig 31.1** (A and B) Hand-foot-mouth rash.

or sudden movements. The pain occurs in waves of spasms that last several minutes to several hours and is described by individuals as feeling like being stabbed with a knife or being squeezed in a vise. It can be mistaken for coronary artery disease, pneumonia, or pleural inflammation. Low to high fever occurs, and a pleural friction rub often is heard. The disease generally lasts from 3 to 6 days (up to a few weeks).

- Orchitis: This type B infection is clinically similar to mumps.
- Myocarditis or pericarditis: HEVs are associated with 25% to 35% of cases of identified cause myocarditis and pericarditis. Symptoms range from mild to severe (sudden death), and male adolescents and young adults are particularly vulnerable (Abzug, 2018).
- Respiratory symptoms are frequently reported before the onset of fatigue, dyspnea, chest pain, CHF, and dysrhythmias. Wheezing, asthma exacerbation, apnea, respiratory distress, pneumonia, otitis media, bronchiolitis, croup, parotitis, and paroxysmal thoracic pain may be seen.

Diagnostic Studies. PCR assay is highly sensitive for all enteroviruses, results can be available in hours, and the test is more sensitive than cell culture. Cultures can be obtained from throat, stool, rectum, cerebrospinal fluid (CSF), urine, and blood; sensitivities range from 0% to 80% (Kimberlin et al., 2018). CBC is usually normal. Serology for serotype-specific IgM antibody or other testing is less useful than culture or PCR.

Differential Diagnosis and Management. The differential diagnosis includes other causes of the aforementioned conditions (e.g., viral or bacterial infections [pneumonia, meningitis, sepsis], or connective tissue diseases).

There is no specific therapy available. IGIV has been used and proven helpful in some chronic and life-threatening infections. The use of antiviral therapy is under study or development, although none are commercially available at this time (e.g., pleconaril and pocapavir) (Kimberlin et al., 2018). Enteric precautions and good hand washing are the only efficient control measures.

Poliomyelitis Virus

The poliovirus is an enterovirus with three serotypes (types 1, 2, and 3). The disease ranges from an asymptomatic illness to severe central nervous system (CNS) involvement. Humans are the only documented source of infection. Transmission is through fecal-oral and respiratory routes. Almost all cases in North America occur in individuals most likely exposed to children who had received oral poliovirus vaccine in another country (AAP, 2018a). There have been wild-type poliovirus importations into countries previously deemed polio-free (Europe, Africa, and Asia), and polio continues to be endemic in Pakistan, Nigeria, and Afghanistan. Through the efforts of the Global Polio Eradication Initiative the incidence of polio worldwide remains low; however, reemergence is a concern. Eighty percent of the world's people now live in polio-free areas, including India and WHO members in the Southeast Asia region (CDC, 2017b).

Poliomyelitis should be considered in any unimmunized or underimmunized child who has a nonspecific febrile illness, aseptic meningitis, or paralytic symptoms (paralysis occurs in <1% of infections). Asymptomatic disease occurs in about 72% of those infected (Kimberlin et al., 2018), symptomatic but nonparalytic illness occurs in approximately 5% of cases (Simões, 2016).

The diagnostic test of choice is a viral culture from stool and throat (two samples taken 24 to 48 hours apart) as soon as polio is suspected and at least within 14 days of onset of symptoms. The wild-type virus needs to be differentiated from the vaccine-acquired type. The CSF may be normal or show changes based on the degree of CNS involvement. Antibody titers vary from the acute phase and those taken 3 to 6 weeks later.

Differential Diagnosis and Management. Polio is rare. Differential diagnoses include other conditions causing flaccid muscular weakness and/or paralysis: acute flaccid myelitis, Guillain-Barré syndrome, peripheral neuritis, transverse myelitis, encephalitis, vaccine-associated paralytic poliomyelitis (VAPP) [only occurs following live virus (oral) vaccination], rabies, tetanus, botulism, demyelinating encephalomyelitis, tick-bite paralysis, WNV, spinal cord tumors, familial periodic paralysis, myasthenia gravis, and hysterical paralysis. Conditions that cause decreased limb movement or pseudo-weakness are also differential diagnoses and include unrecognized sciatic nerve trauma, toxic synovitis, acute osteomyelitis, acute rheumatic fever, scurvy, and congenital syphilitic osteomyelitis.

Management is supportive and directed at minimizing skeletal deformity in the paralytic form of the disease. Both nonparalytic and mild paralytic cases can be managed on an outpatient basis, but otherwise individuals should be hospitalized. During the early stages of the disease, individuals should be advised against increasing their physical activity, exercising, or becoming fatigued because these factors may increase the risk of paralytic disease (Simões, 2016).

Preventive measures include active and passive vaccination. The CDC Travelers' Health site provides guidelines for vaccination in individuals traveling to endemic countries.

Hepatoviruses

Hepatitis A Virus

Hepatitis A virus (HAV) is an RNA-containing virus belonging to the Picornaviridae family, comprised of five genera (enteroviruses, rhinoviruses, hepatoviruses, cardioviruses, and aphthoviruses). HAV causes primary infection in the liver. It is highly contagious and commonly spreads through person-to-person contact and fecal-oral contamination of food and water and rarely via contaminated blood transfusion. It accounts for most of the acute and benign viral hepatitis in the United States and worldwide. There is no seasonal or geographic variance.

Transmission occurs readily in households and child care centers; risk factors include personal contact with an infected individual, international travel, recognized food-borne outbreak, men who have sex with men, and illicit drug use. In children younger than 6 years old, about 30% are symptomatic; few of these have jaundice (CDC, 2018e). This high anicteric incidence allows considerable spread of disease to adult caretakers in child care settings. Infants are protected by maternal antibodies during the first few months of life. Older children and adults tend to be more symptomatic. Incidence rates are similar across all age groups and geographic regions.

The incubation period is 15 to 50 days (average 28 to 30 days). The period of contagion occurs during viral shedding, usually 1 to 3 weeks. The highest period of infectivity is up to 2 weeks before the onset of illness until 1 week after the onset of jaundice, although neonates and young children may shed the virus in their stool for longer periods.

Clinical Findings

1. Preicteric phase: This phase manifests as an acute febrile illness. Malaise, nausea, anorexia, vomiting, digestive complaints, fever (rarely higher than 102°F [38.9°C]), headache, and occasional abdominal complaints occur. This phase goes unnoticed

in many children. There may be dull right upper quadrant pain; some children may have only mild URI and GI symptoms along with a transient fever.

2. Icteric phase: Jaundice appears shortly after symptom onset (70% of older children and adults) (AAP, 2018c) and lasts from a few days to almost a month; it may be subtle in children. Urine darkens, and stools become clay colored. Often these are the only apparent signs of illness. Diarrhea is common in infants, whereas constipation is more common in older children and adults. Patients feel sick. Infants have poor weight gain during the icteric phase. Mild hepatomegaly and tenderness, posterior cervical adenopathy, and a tender spleen (10% to 20% incidence) may occur.

Fulminant disease is rare. There is no chronic disease. Complete recovery is expected within 1 to 2 months with occasional relapses lasting up to 6 months.

Diagnostic Studies. Serologic testing is widely available. IgM-specific antibodies indicate recent infection. These are replaced by IgG-specific antibodies 2 to 4 months later and serve as indicators of past infection. Elevations of AST and alanine aminotransferase (ALT) usually occur, may precede symptoms by a week or more, and indicate the degree of inflammatory injury. Elevations are also seen in γ-glutamyl transpeptidase (GGTP) and serum bilirubin (rarely above 10 mg/dL); mild lymphocytosis may be seen.

Differential Diagnosis. Any cause of jaundice is in the differential diagnosis.

- Infancy: Physiologic jaundice, hemolytic disease, galactosemia, hypothyroidism, biliary metabolic disorders, biliary atresia, α 1-antitrypsin deficiency, and choledochal cysts. Hypervitaminosis A causes a yellow pigmentation (carotenemia) of the skin often mistaken for jaundice in children. Infections, such as those referred to as TORCH (toxoplasmosis, other [syphilis, varicella-zoster, parvovirus B19], rubella, cytomegalovirus [CMV], and herpes infections), also cause hepatitis.
- Older infants, children, and adolescents: Hemolytic-uremic syndrome, Reye syndrome, malaria, leptospirosis, brucellosis, chronic hemolytic diseases with gallstone development, Wilson disease, cystic fibrosis, Banti syndrome, collagen-vascular disease (e.g., systemic lupus erythematosus [SLE]), infectious mononucleosis syndrome (IMS), CMV, coxsackievirus, toxoplasmosis, Weil disease, yellow fever, acute cholangitis, amebiasis, and hepatitis B, C, and D are in the differential diagnosis. Drugs and poisons such as pyrazinamide, isoniazid, valproic acid, acetaminophen overdose, zoxazolamine, gold, cinchophen, phenothiazines, and methyltestosterone also cause hepatitis.

Management, Complications, and Prevention. Therapy is supportive. Good hand hygiene after diaper changes is a crucial preventive measure, especially for child care personnel. The use of immunoglobulin or HAV vaccine within 2 weeks of exposure is discussed earlier in this chapter (Table 31.3). Those with acute infections who work as food handlers or in schools/child care settings should be excluded for 1 week after onset of symptoms (Kimberlin et al., 2018). Although patients can become very ill, most cases of HAV resolve completely. Fulminant hepatitis with liver failure is rare. Prevention includes good personal hygiene and safe drinking water, in addition to routine HAV vaccine for those 12 months old and older.

Hepatitis B Virus

HBV is a DNA-containing hepadnavirus. It is highly contagious and causes severe liver disease. The most common method of transmission is percutaneous or permucosal exposure to contaminated blood/serum, semen, vaginal secretions, and other bodily fluids, including but not limited to amniotic, cerebrospinal, and pleural. It is not spread by the fecal-oral route. HBV can survive in a dried state for more than 1 week, but it is highly susceptible to common household disinfectants, such as 1:10 diluted bleach. Prolonged percutaneous contact with contaminated fomites, such as toothbrushes and razors, can be a source of infection.

The major reservoirs for HBV are healthy chronic carriers and patients with acute disease. Approximately 700,000 to 1.4 million people have chronic HBV in the United States, and approximately 240 million worldwide (CDC, 2018f; WHO, 2018c). Unimmunized children who immigrated to the United States from sub-Saharan Africa and East Asia and other high endemic areas pose the highest infection risk. Transmission is rare within the United States because of the high HBV immunization coverage in children. Highest infection rates in the United States are reported in men from 25 to 44 years old (CDC, 2018f). Perinatal transmission is highly efficient during birth from female carriers (HBsAg-positive or hepatitis B e antigen [HBeAg]-positive, or both) to the newborn. In utero transmission is rare because HBV is a large molecule and rarely crosses the placenta. The infection rate is 70% to 90% if both maternal antigen markers are positive, and 5% to 20% if the mother is HBsAg-positive but HBeAg-negative (Kimberlin et al., 2018).

Whether one eventually develops chronic infection depends on the age one is infected and the rate of loss of HBeAg. More than 90% of infected infants develop chronic infection after exposure. Twenty-five percent to 50% of children who acquire the infection between 1 and 5 years old (as compared to about 5% exposed as adults) develop chronic HBV infection. Twenty-five percent of those chronically infected children die prematurely of cirrhosis or liver cancer (CDC, 2018f). Individuals who abuse IV drugs, engage in sexual activity with multiple partners, or men who have sex with men have the greatest HBV risk. Healthcare workers exposed to blood, blood products, or blood-contaminated body fluids and those working with the developmentally disabled are also high-risk, as are chronic renal dialysis patients. Tattooing or body piercing with contaminated instruments is another route of infection. Breastfeeding is not contraindicated. Screen all pediatric patients who missed the HBV birth dose, especially if their parents were born in regions of high-HBV endemicity.

Clinical Findings. The incubation period is 45 to 160 days (average of 120 days). HBV illness ranges from asymptomatic seroconversion to fulminating disease and death. HBV usually has a gradual onset. Most children who acquired HBV at an early age are asymptomatic. Some have minimal nonspecific constitutional complaints, such as fever, nausea, and minimal hepatomegaly. Arthralgia and skin problems, such as urticaria or other rashes, are often the first apparent signs. Papular acrodermatitis is described in infants. Acute HBV infection is somewhat similar to the icteric phase of HAV, but it is usually more severe. Skin, mucous membranes, and sclerae are icteric. The liver is enlarged and tender.

Diagnostic Studies. Serologic tests include HBsAg, hepatitis B core antigen (HBcAg), HBeAg, and antibodies to these antigens; the results can help determine the stage of infection (Table 31.4). Changes in liver enzymes indicate the degree of injury. There is elevation of serum transaminases (SGOT, AST, SGPT, and ALT). Prothrombin time can be elevated, especially in fulminating disease. Hybridization assays, nucleic acid amplification testing (NAAT), and gene amplification techniques (e.g., PCR) are also available.

TABLE 31.3 Immunoglobulins Used in Children in the United States

Immunoglobulin	Reference Name	Indications for Use	Comments
Botulism immune globulin intravenous	BIG-IV	Botulism toxin A or B in infants <1 year old	Available as BabyBig from California Department of Health Services (510-231-7600). A HBAT may be indicated for life-threatening food-borne botulism (other than infant botulism) but risk must be weighed against side effects (fever, serum sickness, anaphylaxis); only available from CDC (770-488-7100).
Cytomegalovirus immune globulin intravenous	CMV-IGIV	For stem cell or organ transplants; studies ongoing to evaluate use for CMV transmission to newborns	Used in combination with IV ganciclovir to treat CMV pneumonia. In hematopoietic stem cell transplant recipients, CMV-IGIV and ganciclovir administered intravenously have been reported to be synergistic in treatment of CMV pneumonia.
Diphtheria antitoxin (from equine sera)		Life-threatening *Corynebacterium diphtheriae* disease	Only available from CDC to treat life-threatening diphtheria; preferred route of administration is IV. Anaphylaxis and delayed serum sickness are possible adverse reactions and need to be weighed against risks of disease. Tests for reaction to animal sera should be performed.
Hepatitis B immune globulin	HBIG	Prophylaxis for those unvaccinated or undervaccinated; who have discrete identifiable exposure to blood; exposed to body fluids that contain blood: • Newborns whose mothers are HBsAg positive • Household contacts <12 months old who have received only one prior HBV vaccine and the second dose is not due • Sexual contact or needle-sharing with known HBsAg-positive cases, including sexual assault or abuse victims • Individuals with percutaneous or permucosal exposure to body secretions of known cases	If mother's HBsAg status is unknown before delivery, infants should receive both HBV vaccine and HBIG within 12 h of birth or 24 h of blood exposure; vaccines administered after birth should be given at different injection sites. HBIG can be given within 7 days of delivery if mother tests positive for HBsAg postpartum but it is less effective. Sexual partners of known cases: give HBIG and HBV vaccine up to 14 days after last exposure; repeat vaccine at 1 and 6 months. Household contacts <12 months old: HBIG and three doses of HBV vaccine. If >12 months old, follow index case's antibody profile (if a carrier, vaccinate all household members). If children and adolescents have documented Hep B series and unknown seroconversion status, a booster dose is indicated. Hepatitis B vaccine can be used for postexposure prophylaxis if given within 12-24 h after exposure.
Immune globulin	IG	Hepatitis A prophylaxis: • Household contacts and sexual partners of known cases • Persons accidentally inoculated with a contaminated needle • Newborn infants of infected, jaundiced mothers • People with open lesions directly exposed to body secretions of known cases • Children in schools where more than one case is reported • All children and employees of child care centers where a case is reported • Custodial care residents and staff in close contact with an active case • Persons traveling to developing countries for <3 months • Can give HAV vaccine concurrently with IG, if warranted, for those traveling internationally	Give within 2 weeks of exposure; can be used in children <2 years old; is thimerosal-free; >85% effective; dosage for those with continuous exposure to HAV differs from that given for short-term exposure. HAV vaccine is used for postexposure prophylaxis if given within 14 days of exposure.

Continued

TABLE 31.3	Immunoglobulins Used in Children in the United States—cont'd			

Immunoglobulin	Reference Name	Indications for Use		Comments
		Measles prophylaxis: • To prevent or modify infection in unvaccinated children <1 year old and others at higher risk of complications who have been exposed to measles • IGIV is recommended for pregnant women and the immunocompromised who are without immunity		Not indicated in those who have had one dose of vaccine at ≥12 months old, unless immunocompromised. Given within 6 days after exposure; the dose for those immunocompromised differs according to the type and degree of immunodeficiency, whether IGIV has been given, and prior dosage amounts of immune globulin.
		Rubella prophylaxis: • Modifies or suppresses the clinical manifestations of the disease, urine shedding, and decreases the rate of viremia • For use in: • Early pregnancy after confirmed exposure and only if termination of pregnancy is not an option • Infants after maternal exposure • Older children not vaccinated with known exposure or at serious risk (immunocompromised)		If pregnant woman is exposed to wild rubella or as a result of being accidentally vaccinated within 28 days of conception, fetus has theoretic risk of 1.3% of congenital rubella; refer to OB-GYN. Administration of immune globulin and the absence of clinical manifestation of maternal rubella infection do not guarantee the infant will be born without congenital rubella syndrome. IgM antibody (not IgG) after immune globulin can be used to determine maternal infection after exposure.
Immune globulin intravenous	IGIV	FDA-approved for treating primary immunodeficiencies, chronic lymphocytic leukemia, bone marrow transplantation, HIV in children, ITP, Kawasaki disease; IGIV contains measles antibodies sufficient for measles prophylaxis (see Immune globulin)		Off-label use, including treatment for toxic shock syndrome, has created shortages.
Rabies immune globulin (human)	HRIG, RIG	For postexposure prophylaxis for rabies; used in conjunction with rabies vaccine		Prior to use, consult with local health authorities.
Respiratory syncytial virus immune globulin	RSV-IGIV (RespiGam)	Reduces risk of RSV bronchiolitis or pneumonia in high-risk children Provides additional protection against other respiratory viral illnesses; may be preferred over palivizumab in children with immune deficiencies or for premature infants prior to discharge in the RSV season for the first month of prophylaxis		Palivizumab, a monoclonal antibody, is generally preferred over RSV-IGIV (see Chapter 29, Bronchiolitis).
Tetanus immune globulin	TIG	For individuals with tetanus-prone wounds who are undervaccinated (fewer than three tetanus toxoid vaccine doses) or whose vaccination status is unknown For individuals with tetanus infection in combination with antibiotics (metronidazole or penicillin G) For immunodeficient patients, including those with HIV; they should be considered undervaccinated regardless of actual tetanus toxoid status		Tetanus-prone wounds include those contaminated with dirt (especially if around horses), feces, or saliva; puncture wounds; avulsions; wounds acquired as a consequence of missiles, burns, crushing, or frostbite. In infants <6 months old without the initial three-dose series, decision to use TIG depends on mother's tetanus toxoid immunization history at the time of delivery and if the wound is tetanus prone (e.g., out-of-hospital delivery and umbilical cord cut with non-sterile implement). TIG is given IM plus a dose of tetanus toxoid vaccine. If TIG not available, IGIV may be considered (not licensed for this use in the United States); equine TAT is another alternative to TIG (not available in the United States)—hypersensitivity testing required before use of TAT. Smaller dose is administered for tetanus neonatorum.
Vaccinia immune globulin intravenous	VIG-IGIV	Being held in reserve to prevent or manage complications of smallpox; can be used in individuals receiving an experimental vaccine that involves a vaccinia carrier virus		Only available from CDC.

TABLE 31.3 Immunoglobulins Used in Children in the United States—cont'd

Immunoglobulin	Reference Name	Indications for Use	Comments
Varicella immune globulin	VariZIG (varicella-zoster immune globulin)	Given to those exposed to varicella infection who are most susceptible to varicella and most likely to develop the disease and in whom complications of the infection would result: • Household contacts • Playmates with face-to-face contact (5 min to 1 h) • Infant whose mother had varicella onset 5 days or less before delivery or within 48 h after delivery • Immunocompromised children and adolescents without history of varicella, varicella immunization, or known to be susceptible • Hospitalized preterm infants 28 weeks or more gestation whose mother lacks history of varicella or serologic evidence of protection • Hospitalized preterm infants <28 weeks' gestation or <1000 g birth weight exposed in neonatal period regardless of mother's history or VZV serologic evidence[a] • Other conditions: See CDC guidelines	Available from FFF Enterprises 24 h/day (1-800-843-7477); strict adherence to forms and protocols required. Administered within 96 h of exposure; may be of benefit if given within 10 days (AAP, 2015b). Not indicated in infants whose mothers had zoster infection. In the absence of VariZIG, IGIV or acyclovir may be considered.[a]

[a]Consult with an expert in infectious disease or the CDC.

CDC, Centers for Disease Control and Prevention; *CMV*, cytomegalovirus; *FDA*, U.S. Food and Drug Administration; *HAV*, hepatitis A virus; *HBAT*, heptavalent equine antitoxin; *HBsAg*, hepatitis B surface antigen; *HBV*, hepatitis B virus; *HIV*, human immunodeficiency virus; *IG*, immune globulin; *IgG*, immunoglobulin G; *IgM*, immunoglobulin M; *IM*, intramuscular; *ITP*, idiopathic thrombocytopenia purpura; *IV*, intravenous; *IVIG*, intravenous immunoglobulin; *OB-GYN*, obstetrics and gynecology; *RSV*, respiratory syncytial virus; *TAT*, tetanus antitoxin.

Data from Goddard AF, Meissner HC. Passive immunization. In: Long SS, Prober CG, Fischer M, eds. *Principles and Practice of Pediatric Infectious Diseases*. Elk Grove Village, IL: Elsevier; 2017, 37–43; and Kimberlin DW, Brady MT, Jackson MA, Long SS, eds. *Red Book: 2018 Report of the Committee on Infectious Diseases*. 31st ed. American Academy of Pediatrics. Elk Grove Village, IL: 2018.

TABLE 31.4 Interpretation of Serologic Markers for Hepatitis B Virus Infection

SEROLOGIC MARKER				
HBsAg	Anti-HBs	IgM Anti-HBc	Total Anti-HBc	Interpretation
−	−	−	−	Susceptible; never infected
+	−	−	−	Acute infection, early incubation; transient, up to 3 weeks after vaccination
+	−	+	+	Acute infection
−	−	+	+	Acute infection, resolving
−	+	−	+	Past infection, recovered, and immune
+	−	−	+	Chronic infection
−	−	−	+	False positive (i.e., susceptible) past infection, or "low level" chronic infection
−	+	−	−	Immune from vaccination

Anti-HBs, Antibody to hepatitis B surface antigen; *HBsAg*, hepatitis B surface antigen; *IgM anti-HBc*, immunoglobulin M antibody to hepatitis B core antigen; *total anti-HBc*, total antibody to hepatitis B core antigen.

From Byrd KK, Murphy TV, Hu DJ. Hepatitis B and hepatitis D viruses. In: Long SS, Pickering LK, Prober CG, eds. *Principles and Practice of Pediatric Infectious Diseases*. 4th ed. New York: Elsevier; 2012, Table 213.2.

Differential Diagnosis and Management. Any cause of jaundice is included (see HAV).

Therapy for acute infection is supportive and prevented by active and passive vaccination (Chapter 22). A pediatric hepatitis B specialist should be consulted for management of suspected HBV reactivation or for chronic hepatitis B due to the risk of developing hepatocellular carcinoma. The FDA approved five medications for treatment of children with chronic hepatitis B: Interferon-alfa (>12 months old); lamivudine (>3 years old); adefovir and tenofovir (>12 years old); and entecavir (>16 years old). The choice of who should receive medication and the duration of therapy remain controversial, however the European Society of Pediatric Gastroenterology, Hepatology and Nutrition (ESPGHAN) published a guideline with algorithms describing initial evaluation, monitoring, and treatment criteria. Those with chronic infection should receive yearly liver ultrasound, testing of liver function and α-fetoprotein concentration, and vaccination for HAV. Liver biopsies may be done to accurately monitor the effects of liver involvement. HBIG and corticosteroids are not useful (Kimberlin et al., 2018).

Complications and Prevention. Liver failure, cirrhosis, and hepatocellular carcinoma are complications of chronic infection. The initial infection can be prevented with hepatitis B vaccination. Transmission in utero or during labor to newborns and postexposure prophylaxis (PEP) is covered in Chapter 22.

Hepatitis C Virus

Hepatitis C virus (HCV), a single-stranded RNA virus with seven genotypes and multiple subtypes in the Flaviviridae family, causes the chronic form of what used to be called *non-A, non-B hepatitis*. The virus is transmitted by contact with infected blood, blood supply products, or unsafe drug injection practices. The estimated prevalence in the United States is 1.3% (about 4 million people) and 170 million people worldwide (Jhaveri and El Kamarey, 2019). The prevalence in children of all ages is difficult to establish with estimates ranging from approximately 0.1% to 0.4%. Those who do not go on to develop chronic hepatitis C (15% to 25%) spontaneously clear the virus without treatment (CDC, 2018w). However, HCV infection causes the highest rate of chronic infection and liver disease (70% to 80% of adults) than all of the hepatitis viruses; the incidence of chronic liver failure in children is low (approximately 5%) but increases with the duration of infection (Kimberlin et al., 2018).

Perinatal transmission is the major pediatric infection route: approximately 6 out of every 100 infants born to HCV-infected mothers become infected (CDC, 2018w). Mothers who are HIV-positive have a two to threefold increased risk of transmitting the virus to their infants (Mack et al., 2012). Vaginal birth and breastfeeding do not contribute to higher rates of transmission, and women with HCV alone should not be discouraged from experiencing either (American College of Obstetricians and Gynecologists, 2013). Infants who acquire HCV per vertical transmission have a high rate of spontaneous resolution, approaching 50%, usually by 24 months old but some as late as 7 years old. Older children experience spontaneous resolution at a rate of 6% to 12% (Mack et al., 2012).

The most common means of HCV transmission in the United States is from injection drug use, infecting an estimated one-third of injection drug users between the ages of 18 and 30 years old (CDC, 2018w). Men who have sex with men are also at increased risk of infection. Strict blood product screening and manufacturing practices in the United States significantly reduced the risk of transmission.

Clinical Findings. HCV has an incubation period ranging from 2 weeks to 6 months (average 45 days). Onset of symptoms is often insidious; most children are asymptomatic. Flu-like prodromal symptoms (jaundice, nausea, anorexia, upper right quadrant abdominal pain) may occur in 20% to 30% of older children and adults (Collier, Holtzman, and Homberg, 2018). Chronic hepatitis with cirrhosis is a late occurrence, often 20 to 30 years later. Fulminant infection is uncommon. Teenagers may be discovered to be HCV-positive when being screened for other reasons (e.g., a school blood donation drive).

Diagnostic Studies. There is no serologic marker for acute infection. Screening and diagnosis of HCV includes IgG antibody enzyme immunoassay for anti-HCV, enhanced chemiluminescence immunoassay (CIA), and HCV RNA PCR. Early in the infection, false negative results can occur. The majority of individuals seroconvert within 15 weeks postexposure or within 5 to 6 weeks after the onset of illness. A newborn can be anti-HCV-positive from maternal transfer for up to 18 months, so testing should ideally be done after that time. Liver function tests are indicated and liver enzymes may go up and down with some near normal levels for many years; liver biopsy is confirmatory but not recommended with newer ultrasound available (CDC, 2018w; Jhaveri and El Karava, 2019). A table with the interpretation of results of tests for HCV infection is available from the CDC at www.cdc.gov/hepatitis/HCV/HCVfaq.htm#section1 (2018w).

Differential Diagnosis and Management. Differential diagnoses include HAV and HBV and other causes of chronic hepatitis (see HAV).

Treatment of acute HCV in children is supportive. Chronic HCV infections in children 3 to 17 years old respond to therapy with nonpegylated interferon alfa-2b and ribavirin. The newer anti-HCV agents are not used to treat children at the present time (Jhaveri, 2018). HAV and HBV vaccines should be given to prevent further liver complications. Liver damage can be exacerbated by comorbid conditions such as cancer, iron overload, thalassemia, or HIV. Drugs such as acetaminophen or antiretroviral medications need to be closely monitored; patients should have serum hepatic transaminases monitored closely. Children with HCV infection need not be excluded from child care facilities (Kimberlin et al., 2018). Individuals with HCV should be discouraged from using alcohol to prevent further liver injury and from sharing razors and toothbrushes; condom use should be encouraged.

Complications and Prevention. The course of HCV is generally mild even with cirrhosis. Liver transplantation is an option in severe cases although reinfection after transplant is common and progressive. The outcome of chronic HCV disease in children is less known. Immunoglobulin is not recommended for prophylaxis after exposure. Research into developing a vaccine is ongoing.

Hepatitis D Virus

Hepatitis D virus (HDV) is caused by an RNA virus that is structurally different from HAV, HBV, and HCV. HDV infection is uncommon in children but must be considered in cases of fulminant hepatitis or hepatic failure. It cannot cause infection unless the child also is infected with HBV, which it needs to replicate. Transmission is through parenteral, percutaneous, or mucosal contact (including sexual) with infected blood and can be acquired either as a coinfection with or superinfection with chronic HBV. Incubation is 2 to 8 weeks. In the United States, it is diagnosed most commonly in drug users, individuals with hemophilia, and immigrants from southern Italy and parts of Eastern Europe, South America, Africa, and the Middle East. Mother-to-newborn transmission is rare (Kimberlin et al., 2018). Infection is detected by IgM antibody to HDV. There is no vaccine against HDV. However, HBV vaccine is preventive of HDV because of its comorbidity with HBV. Those with chronic HBV should take precautions against being infected.

Hepatitis E Virus

Hepatitis E virus (HEV) is an RNA virus in the family Hepeviridae; certain strains can also have zoonotic hosts (e.g., swine, nonhuman primates). It is passed via the fecal-oral route. Contaminated water is the most common reservoir. It is an acute infection with symptoms that resemble those of other viral hepatitis infections. Symptomatic individuals are usually older adolescents and young adults; pregnant women (notably in the third trimester) are particularly vulnerable to serious illness. Children are either asymptomatic or experience mild symptoms. If symptoms appear, they do so within 15 to 60 days (mean 40 days) after exposure. Endemic areas include India, the Middle East, parts of Africa, Southeast Asia, and Mexico. Most cases in the United States are found in immigrants or visitors from these locations. Clinical symptoms include jaundice, malaise, anorexia, fever, abdominal pain, and arthralgia; these are similar to symptoms of HAV but are often more severe. Laboratory studies include IgM and IgG anti-HEV, but these can be unreliable. Definitive diagnosis is determined by the detection of viral RNA in serum or stool using reverse transcriptase–polymerase chain reaction (RT-PCR) assay. Treatment is supportive; there is no approved vaccine in the United States. Good hand hygiene is crucial. Chronic infection is rare, and recovery is usually complete. The overall mortality rate is 4% or less; however, in pregnant women, the mortality rate can reach 25% (Teshale and Kamili, 2018).

Herpes Family of Viruses

The herpes family of viruses is large with several features in common: all infect humans, the viruses establish latency for the life of the host, and reactivation is controlled by immune function. Most active infections are self-limited. Infection becomes serious and life threatening when the cellular immune system is compromised or is naïve, such as in the newborn. This family of viruses includes herpes simplex virus (HSV) types 1 and 2; varicella zoster virus (VZV); Epstein-Barr virus (EBV); CMV; and human herpesvirus 6, 7, and 8 (HHV-6, HHV-7, and HHV-8). HSV-1, HSV-2, and VZV are members of the α-herpesvirus subfamily with neurotropic characteristics and latency in the sensory ganglia.

HSV-1, HSV-2, VZV, EBV, HHV-6, and HHV-7 are discussed in the following sections. See Chapter 29 for a discussion of perinatally acquired CMV infection and other resources for a discussion about HHV-8.

Herpes Simplex Virus

HSV is among the most widely disseminated infectious agents in humans; it is a double-stranded DNA virus and there are two types. HSV-1 is traditionally associated with orolabial lesions or oral secretion and infects the mouth, lips, and eyes and can progress to the CNS. HSV-2 is traditionally shed from genital lesions and genital secretions and is most commonly associated with genital and neonatal infection. Both HSV types can be found in oral or genital sites depending upon the extent of oral-genital contact. Although HSV-2 accounts for 70% to 85% of neonatal cases, both types are equally devastating to a newborn (Harrison et al., 2019). Type 1 virus typically is the causative agent in primary infections in children 6 months to 5 years old and most often presents as gingivostomatitis. Distribution is worldwide, but the infection is more frequent in crowded environments. It is spread by intimate, direct contact usually by an adult with or without symptoms. There is no seasonal variation.

HSV-2 infections usually occur as a result of sexual activity. Sexual molestation must always be ruled out when the infection is found in non-neonates; for this reason, determining the type of virus is always important. Neither type is transmitted by inanimate objects, such as toilet seats.

Neonatal HSV-2 infection is primarily transmitted from the mother as the infant passes through an infected birth canal with

viral migration to the neonate's conjunctiva, nose and/or mouth mucosa, or broken skin due to forceps or a scalp electrode. Infection can also occur with cesarean births. Risk of infection for an infant born to a mother with a primary genital infection is 33% to 50%. The risk is reduced to 3% to 5% to an infant born vaginally to a woman with recurrent genital HSV infections and less than 3% if born to a woman with recurrent asymptomatic shedding at the time of delivery. However, about 60% to 80% of infants with congenital HSV infection are born to women without a history or clinical findings of active infection during pregnancy. The incidence is 1 in 3000 to 20,000 live births in the United States depending upon demographics and geographic area (Harrison et al., 2019). Although rare (5%), in utero transmission can occur. Postnatal transmission is described but is less common (10%) than during the peripartum period (Harrison et al., 2019). Mothers can inoculate their babies from oral, breast, or skin lesions. Fathers also can inoculate infants with nongenital lesions from their mouths or on their hands. There can be lateral transmission from an infected baby in the nursery due to inadequate hand hygiene by hospital personnel.

The period of communicability for HSV-1 and HSV-2 (for non neonates) is 2 days to 2 weeks. Some cases of perinatal infection occur more than 6 weeks after birth depending on when the fetus was exposed. Infection can be transmitted during either primary or recurrent infections, whether symptomatic or asymptomatic.

Clinical Findings. History and physical findings are determined by the viral port of entry, age, state of health, and immune competence. Eczema alone or in combination with other manifestations is a complicating factor. Clinical findings, diagnosis, management, and treatment of some of the most commonly seen infections in children and adolescents due to HSV-1 and HSV-2 are discussed in other chapters (i.e., gingivostomatitis, neonatal herpetic infection, eczema herpeticum, herpes vulvovaginitis, herpes labialis, and herpes keratoconjunctivitis). A few general observations follow:

- Neonatal infection: The neonate is always symptomatic; infection is described by the extent and location of disease: disseminated (approximately 25% of cases); CNS (approximately 30% of cases); and skin, eye, and/or mouth (SEM) (approximately 45% of cases). Disseminated disease presents around day 10 to 12 of life with multiple organ failure; two-thirds develop concurrent encephalitis. Almost half of the infants with disseminated disease never develop the characteristic vesicular rash. CNS disease presents around 16 to 19 days of life with neurologic manifestations of focal/generalized seizures, lethargy and/or irritability, and poor feeding. The majority of these infants develop herpetic lesions during the course of the illness. SEM manifests itself around day 10 to 12 of life (Harrison, 2019) (see Chapter 29).
- Traumatic herpetic infection: This is a localized infection that occurs in a susceptible child because of an abrasion, teething, finger sucking, laceration, or burn that is inoculated with herpesvirus by an orally infected parent who kisses the "boo-boo" or from auto-inoculation. Vesicles appear at the site of the lesion. There may be fever, constitutional symptoms, and regional lymph node involvement. Athletic activities such as wrestling and rugby have been implicated in mucocutaneous herpetic lesions.
- Acute herpetic meningoencephalitis: After the neonatal period, infection with HSV-1 is a leading cause of intermittent,

nonepidemic encephalitis in children and adults in the United States. Encephalitis can be focal, mimicking a mass lesion. Diagnosis is made by brain biopsy. In contrast, HSV meningitis is usually a relatively benign disease most often caused by HSV-2.

- Recurrent infections: The body does not truly eradicate the virus; the virus lies dormant, and recurrent infections are common. Recurrent infections occur either as herpes labialis or genital herpes. Some incidence of recurrent aseptic meningitis can be attributed to HSV infection.

Diagnostic Studies. Intrapartum cultures from mother and child should be obtained no later than 12 and 24 hours after birth if neonatal infection is suspected. Tests may include viral culture, cytology-Pap smears, Tzanck stains, ELISA, fluorescent techniques, glycoprotein G assay, blood or CSF PCR in neonates, or histologic evaluation and viral culture from a brain biopsy in encephalitis. Cultures in neonates need to be taken from skin vesicles, mouth, nasopharynx, eyes, blood, rectum, and CSF. Serologic tests are not helpful in neonates. If encephalitis is suspected, an electroencephalogram (EEG) and MRI of the brain are performed. In disseminated disease, elevated transaminase and/or radiographic evidence of HSV pneumonitis may be seen.

Differential Diagnosis and Management. The diagnosis is usually not a problem if vesicles are present. Coxsackievirus can cause a vesicular stomatitis. Neonatal HSV disease should always be suspected in cases of neonatal respiratory distress or sepsis.

The management of HSV infections is discussed in other chapters (i.e., gingivostomatitis, neonatal herpetic infection, eczema herpeticum, herpes vulvovaginitis, herpes labialis, and herpes keratoconjunctivitis). Parenteral acyclovir is the treatment of choice in life-threatening illness, neonatal infection, or disease in immunocompromised patients.

Oral acyclovir suppressive therapy for 6 months after parenteral treatment of any classification of acute neonatal disease reduces the recurrence of mucocutaneous lesions and improves neurodevelopmental outcomes. The absolute neutrophil count (ANC) should be continuously monitored in infants during the 6 months of suppressive treatment. If neutropenia occurs, stop acyclovir therapy until the neutrophil count recovers, then restart therapy. Any suspected new lesion(s) should be cultured.

Infants born to women with active *recurrent* genital infection are generally not given empiric antiviral medication, but instead are closely monitored by parents/caregivers and providers over the following 6 weeks. Basic preventative measures include careful hand hygiene before and after handling newborns and refraining from kissing or nuzzling (masks can be worn until lesions crust over) by those with active herpes labialis infection.

Complications. Most HSV infections are usually mild. However, bacterial superinfection is always a potential problem. Any child with evidence of HSV ocular involvement must be referred to an ophthalmologist immediately.

The morbidity and mortality associated with neonatal herpetic infection significantly improve with aggressive antiviral therapy (acyclovir). When treated appropriately, 1-year mortality is 29% for disseminated disease and 4% for CNS disease. Poor neurologic outcomes occur in 17% of neonates with disseminated disease and 69% with CNS disease. Aggressive acyclovir therapy has resulted in SEM infections remaining limited to the mucocutaneous lesions and not causing disseminated or CNS disease (Harrison et al., 2019).

Patient and Family Education

- Toddlers and infants with primary gingivostomatitis who drool should be excluded from child care centers if they cannot control their saliva. Children with recurrent "fever blisters" may attend school. Cover recurrent HSV lesions with a bandage in children with active nonmucosal involvement.
- Wrestlers should be excluded from competition until lesions heal. (See also Chapter 19.)
- All pregnant women must be asked about HSV infection in themselves and their sexual partners. Signs and symptoms of HSV should be carefully monitored throughout pregnancy.
- During labor, all women must be questioned about HSV and carefully examined for signs and symptoms of infection. Cesarean delivery is indicated in women with apparent infection unless membranes are ruptured for more than 4 to 6 hours. Scalp monitoring should be avoided.

Infectious Mononucleosis Syndrome

More than 90% of cases are caused by EBV, a member of the γ-herpesviruses. The remaining cases are attributed to acute CMV, *Toxoplasma gondii,* adenovirus, viral hepatitis, HIV, and possibly rubella. Distribution of IMS is worldwide, infecting more than 95% of the population (Jenson, 2016). Almost all older children and adolescents in developing countries and poor urban settings of developed countries are seropositive for EBV. In these children, primary exposure occurs in infancy or early childhood, tends to produce only mild symptoms, and is subclinical. Infection in children younger than 4 years old occurs less frequently in affluent populations in developed countries; one-third of cases occur during adolescence or young adulthood (Jenson, 2016). The mode of transmission is personal contact, usually from deep kissing, by penetrative sexual contact, or from the exchange of saliva among children. The virus can live outside the body in saliva for several hours. About 20% to 30% of healthy immune individuals shed EBV at any given time. From 60% to 90% of EBV-infected individuals on immunosuppressive therapy, including those on steroids, shed virus (Jenson, 2016).

Because IMS virus is found in the saliva and blood of both clinically ill and asymptomatic infected persons for many months, the period of communicability is difficult to assess. The period of incubation is thought to be from 30 to 50 days. It is only mildly contagious.

Clinical Findings. IMS affects the primary lymphoid tissue and peripheral blood. Lymphoid tissue—regional lymph nodes, tonsils, spleen, and liver—is enlarged. Atypical lymphocytes are seen in the peripheral blood. Almost all body organs are involved, including but not limited to the lungs, heart, kidneys, adrenals, CNS, and skin. Symptoms are variable and can last up to 2 to 3 weeks. Clinical presentation typically occurs in three phases: *prodrome, acute,* and *resolution.* During the *prodrome* phase, symptoms are mild and may include malaise, fatigue, and possibly fever, and it is difficult to distinguish IMS from other viral infections. The acute phase follows with the classic symptoms of fever (100.4°F [38°C] to 104.9°F [40.5°C]), pharyngitis, malaise, and fatigue. Physical findings include discrete, nontender, non-erythematous lymphadenopathy, as well as tonsillopharyngitis (exudative in approximately half of the patients). Hepatomegaly and splenomegaly occur in about 50% to 60% of children and are more common in the younger child (Castagnini and Leach, 2019). Skin rash occurs in 3% to 15% of cases, usually on the trunk, arms, and palms. It can be maculopapular, urticarial, scarlatiniform, hemorrhagic (rarely), or nodular and usually occurs during the first few days of symptom onset and lasts 1 to 6 days. The rash occurs more frequently in those taking ampicillin or amoxicillin (up to 80%) and probably represents a form of arteritis or vasculitis rather than hypersensitivity. The rash typically starts 5 to 10 days after the drug is started. Additionally, a symmetric rash of erythematous papules with or without coalescence on the cheeks, extremities, and buttocks (looks similar to atopic dermatitis) is associated with EBV infection and is referred to as the Gianotti-Crosti syndrome (Jensen, 2011). After several days (or up to 3 to 4 weeks), the *resolution* phase begins with gradual decrease of fatigue and fever; organomegaly may take 1 to 2 months to resolve (Castagnini and Leach, 2019).

Diagnostic Studies. The CBC provides a classic picture of lymphocytosis with more than 10% atypical lymphocytes. Elevated liver enzymes are typical. Monospot and the serum heterophile test are positive in 85% of infected patients older than 4 years old (often negative in those younger than 4 years old). Children older than 4 years usually must be ill for approximately 2 weeks before seroconverting. Viral culture and Epstein-Barr–specific core and capsule antibody testing are usually used for diagnosis if the primary screening test results are negative and there is continued suspicion of IMS (e.g., in younger children). Depending on the specific EBV antigen system tested, levels can be detectable for years after infection.

Differential Diagnosis and Management. IMS is in the differential diagnosis of almost every infectious disease. Conditions and infections typically associated with a mononucleosis-like syndrome are gram-positive α-β hemolytic streptococcal pharyngitis, leukemia, lymphoreticular malignancies, adenoviruses, toxoplasmosis, CMV, rubella, HIV, hepatitis, SLE, drug reactions, and diphtheria.

Treatment is supportive with adequate bed rest for debilitated cases, over-the-counter pain relievers, fluids, and increased calories. Corticosteroids and acyclovir are not recommended for routine, uncomplicated disease; penicillin products should not be given. Contact sports and strenuous exercise should be avoided for 4 weeks and especially in those with hepatosplenomegaly (see Chapter 19 for return-to-play sports participation recommendations). Symptoms generally resolve within 2 to 4 weeks; fatigue and weakness may persist for up to 6 to 12 months after severe infection. Complete recovery can be expected in more than 95% of cases without treatment (Castagnini and Leach, 2019).

Complications and Patient and Family Education. Otherwise healthy children and youth experience few sequelae. Rare complications include splenic rupture, neurologic complications (from aseptic meningitis, encephalitis, myelitis, optic neuritis, cranial nerve palsies, Guillain-Barré syndrome), thrombocytopenia, agranulocytosis, hemolytic anemia, orchitis, myocarditis, or chronic IMS. The virus increases the risk for Hodgkin disease. Death is rare. There is no clear evidence that supports an association between EBV infection and chronic fatigue syndrome (Castagnini and Leach, 2019).

Persons with a recent history of IMS or an infectious mononucleosis-like disease should not donate blood or organs. Sharing food and drinks with infected individuals needs to be avoided in order to reduce the risk of acquiring EBV-associated IMS (Castagnini and Leach, 2019).

Roseola Infantum (Exanthem Subitum)

HHV-6 and HHV-7 are members of the *Roseolovirus* genus in the Betaherpesvirinae subfamily of HHVs. HHV-6 is responsible for the majority of cases of roseola infantum (exanthema subitum or sixth disease) and is associated with other diseases, including encephalitis, especially in immunocompromised hosts. A small percentage of children with roseola have primary infection with HHV-7 (Caserta, 2016). Humans are the only natural reservoir. The method of transmission is not completely understood, but the virus is probably spread via the oral, nasal, and conjunctival routes from close contacts. Transmission is suspected to also occur prenatally or during or after birth. The disease is most commonly seen in children between 7 and 24 months old, after protective maternal antibodies wane. It is rare in children younger than 3 months old or older than 4 years old (Cherry, 2019). Most children are HHV-6 seropositive by 4 years old, and about 85% are seropositive for HHV-7 by adulthood (Kimberlin et al., 2018). Reactivation of infection can occur in those who are immunocompromised. Visits to emergency departments by infants are common because of associated fevers, toxicity, and/or seizures. The disease occurs worldwide, year round, and shows no gender preference (Cherry, 2019). The incubation period has a mean of 9 to 10 days. The period of communicability is probably greatest during the fever phase before the rash erupts.

Clinical Findings. There is a sudden onset of fever from 101°F to more than 103°F (38.3°C to more than 39.5°C) for 3 to 7 days, but the child does not seem ill. However, during high fevers irritability and malaise may be noted. There may be URI signs; cervical and posterior occipital lymphadenopathy; lethargy; infected palpebral conjunctiva; eyelid edema; GI complaints; reddened TMs; and occasionally, a febrile convulsion (10% to 15%) (Kimberlin et al., 2018). As the fever breaks, a diffuse, nonpruritic, discrete, rose-colored maculopapular rash, 2 to 3 mm in diameter, appears (Fig 31.2). It fades on pressure and rarely coalesces. The roseola exanthema is similar to the rash of rubella. The rash lasts from hours to 2 to 3 days, begins on the trunk, and spreads centrifugally. In the rare case of CNS involvement, the anterior fontanelle may bulge (Cherry, 2019).

Diagnostic Studies. The diagnosis of roseola exanthema can usually be made clinically and diagnostic studies are not indicated. If serology is done (diagnosis is unclear or symptoms are severe or unusual), the WBC count is distinctive, showing a decrease for age initially, dropping further by the third or fourth day, and then returning to normal. It tends to follow the fever pattern.

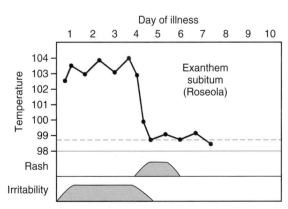

• **Fig 31.2** Schematic Diagram Illustrating the Symptoms of Roseola.

Other serologic testing may involve isolating HHV-6 for peripheral blood mononuclear cells and documenting a significant rise in antibody titer; however, test results vary widely, so diagnosing unequivocal acute infection is problematic. Serial titers 2 to 3 weeks apart are more reliable. Fourfold increases in HHV-6 or HHV-7 IgG antibodies suggest active infection. Virus cultures are helpful. A rapid HHV-6 culture is available. A RT-PCR assay distinguishes between the acute and latent infection.

Differential Diagnosis, Management, and Complications. The clinical course usually makes this illness easy to diagnose. The differential diagnoses include most viral rashes, scarlatina, and drug hypersensitivity. A roseola-like illness is also associated with parvovirus B19, echovirus 16, other enteroviruses, measles, and adenoviruses. Until the rash develops, fever without focus and bacterial sepsis are in the differential diagnosis. If a febrile seizure occurs, meningitis is added to the differential diagnosis.

Management is supportive. Acetaminophen can be used if the child is uncomfortable with the fever. There is no practical means of prevention. Complications include febrile convulsions, meningoencephalitis, encephalitis, and hemiplegia.

Varicella

VZV is a common highly contagious herpesvirus. Chickenpox is the primary illness. It derives its name not from chickens but from the propensity of the lesions to resemble chickpeas. Shingles (herpes zoster) is the reactivation infection of latent VZV acquired during varicella infection (Chapter 34).

Humans are the only infection reservoir; illness is spread by direct contact, droplets, and airborne transmission. Victims of shingles are infectious and can cause primary varicella illness. Immunity is usually lifelong; reinfection is rare and when it does occur symptoms are usually mild. Immunocompromised patients risk developing generalized zoster. The disease peaks in those aged 10 to 14 years, although the overall incidence decreased in all age groups from prevaccine levels (after licensure in 1995, incidence declined 90% by 2005 with further reduction after the second dose was made routine in 2006) (AAP, 2018a). Distribution is worldwide and endemic in most large cities. Epidemics occur at irregular intervals; the highest incidence is in late winter and spring in temperate climates. Mild varicella breakthrough infection occurs in approximately 10% to 20% of those previously vaccinated; however, the vaccine is 97% protective against severe disease (Gershon, 2019; CDC, 2016c).

The incubation period is 10 to 21 days (mean of 14 to 16 days). The period of communicability is 1 to 2 days before the rash erupts until all lesions crust over (about 3 to 7 days). Communicability is prolonged in individuals who received varicella immune globulin (VZIG) or IGIV (Kimberlin et al., 2018).

Clinical Findings

The following two phases are seen in varicella:

1. Prodrome: Not always present. It is composed of low-grade fever, listlessness, headache, backache, anorexia, mild abdominal pain, and occasionally URI symptoms. These symptoms may occur 1 to 2 days before onset of the second phase.
2. Rash: Classic appearance. It is centripetal, beginning on the scalp, face, or trunk. Crops of generally highly pruritic lesions progress from spots to "teardrop vesicles" that cloud over and umbilicate in 24 to 48 hours. After a few days, all

morphologic forms can be seen simultaneously. An average number of lesions is about 300 (LaRussa and Marin, 2016). Scabs last from 5 to 20 days, depending on the depth of the lesions. There can be fever to 105°F (40.6°C). The more severe the rash, the higher the fever. Lesions can develop on all mucosal tissues, mouth, pharynx, larynx, trachea, vagina, and anus. Breakthrough varicella disease can occur more than 42 days after vaccination and should be regarded as contagious (LaRussa and Marin, 2016).

Diagnostic Studies. As the incidence of varicella disease has decreased, many providers may be unfamiliar with the clinical presentation of the disease, especially in mild cases with few lesions. Diagnostic studies play an important role in these instances. For both unvaccinated and vaccinated persons, the most reliable method for diagnosing VZV is the PCR (preferred) or direct fluorescent antibody (DFA) done from scrapings of a vesicle base during the first 3 to 4 days post-eruption. Tzanck smears of lesions demonstrate multinucleated giant cells containing intranuclear inclusion bodies but are not specific for VZV. A positive serologic test for varicella-zoster IgM antibody is confirmatory. Serial IgG antibody titers from acute and convalescent samples can be compared to confirm diagnosis. The virus can be cultured from vesicular fluid, CSF, and biopsy of tissue, but the sensitivity of this method is less than that of the PCR. The WBC count is usually within normal limits.

Differential Diagnosis and Management. The rash is a classical symptom; therefore, the diagnosis is usually clinical. Fig 31.3 shows differences in distribution of the maculopapular eruptions and prodromal symptoms of scarlet fever, chickenpox, and smallpox. Occasionally, impetigo, cigarette burns, and insect bites cause diagnostic confusion in children with a mild rash. Other infections that can be confused with varicella include eczema herpeticum, HSV, and Stevens-Johnson syndrome.

Chickenpox is usually a benign infection in healthy children. Treatment is supportive and includes management of itching with antihistamines or oatmeal baths, acetaminophen for fever, and antistaphylococcal penicillin or cephalosporins for bacterial superinfections. Children with fever for more than several days, or increasing temperatures 4 or more days after the appearance of the rash, should be evaluated closely for invasive disease. Aspirin is contraindicated because of the possibility of Reye syndrome. The use of ibuprofen for fever is questionable because of a possible causal relationship with bacterial superinfections (Gershon, 2019).

Intravenous acyclovir is efficacious for immunocompromised individuals and for those with severe disease. See Table 31.2 regarding use of VZIG; it is not effective after the disease progresses. Oral acyclovir is expensive and is not routinely recommended for most children. When given to otherwise healthy children within 24 hours after eruption of the rash, there is a modest decrease in the symptoms and illness duration. Indication for oral acyclovir use is available from the CDC (2018t) and AAP *Red Book* (Kimberlin et al., 2018). It can be considered for use in pregnant women with varicella, especially in their second or third trimester. The safety of acyclovir to the fetus in the first trimester is uncertain; however, one large study showed that exposure to acyclovir or valacyclovir in the first trimester of pregnancy was not associated with an increased risk of major birth defects (Harrison et al., 2016).

Complications. The following complications can occur: pyodermas (about a 5% incidence, causing serious invasive disease

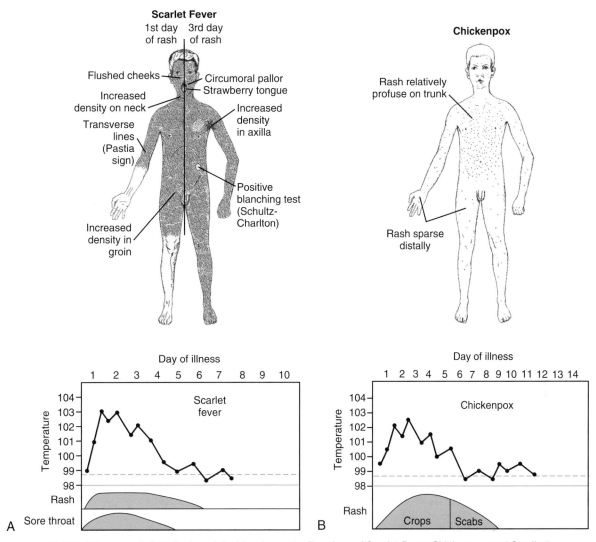

• **Fig 31.3** Differences in Distribution of the Maculopapular Eruptions of Scarlet Fever, Chickenpox, and Smallpox.

with *Streptococcus* and *Staphylococcus*); idiopathic thrombocytopenic purpura (ITP) (1% to 2%); pneumonia (smoking is a risk factor); CNS complications (e.g., encephalitis and Reye syndrome); and, rarely, glomerulonephritis, orchitis, hepatitis, toxic shock, osteomyelitis, necrotizing fasciitis, myositis, myocarditis, arthritis, and appendicitis. Primary varicella is rarely associated with mortality; since the licensure of the varicella vaccine, the highest mortality is found in newborns and immunocompromised children (Gershon, 2019). Neonatal involvement is directly tied to the timing of the maternal infection with varicella. See Chapter 29 for a discussion about congenital varicella syndrome.

Patient and Family Education

- Children exposed to chickenpox may attend school for about 1 week. If they show signs of illness, they must be kept home for 1 week. If they do not break out in a rash, they may return to school. Children with active disease are to be kept home until all lesions are dry.
- Exposed patients: Use of VZIG was discussed earlier and can cause asymptomatic infection. Individuals who receive VZIG should obtain age-appropriate varicella immunization (unless contraindicated) in 5 months. The AAP *Red Book* and the CDC website include further recommendations regarding VZIG for the immunocompromised.

Influenza Viral Infections

Influenza virus is an orthomyxovirus with three antigenic types: A, B, and C. Types A and B cause epidemic disease; type C causes sporadic mild influenza-like illness in children. Type A is further classified into two surface proteins—hemagglutinin (H) and neuraminidase (N). Three hemagglutinin subtypes and two neuraminidase types are known to cause disease in humans (e.g., H1N1, HIN2, and H3N2). Variant influenza viruses also infect humans and originate from swine and domestic or wild avian sources. Influenza is a highly contagious disease and is spread person to person by direct contact, droplet contamination, and fomites recently contaminated with infected nasopharyngeal secretions.

Typical Influenza

In temperate climates, typical influenza epidemics occur in the winter months, last approximately 4 to 8 weeks, and peak 2 weeks after the index case. Influenza illness circulates year round in countries closest to the equator. In recent years, some epidemics lasted 3 months as a result of more than one strain of virus circulating within a community. Children, particularly those of school age, can shed the virus longer than adults (10 days versus 5 days) and are particularly prolific community transmitters.

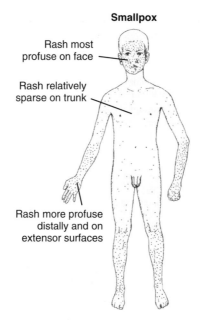

Smallpox

Rash most profuse on face

Rash relatively sparse on trunk

Rash more profuse distally and on extensor surfaces

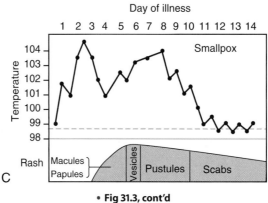

• **Fig 31.3, cont'd**

After a newly shifted subtype emerges, the highest incidence of the illness occurs in healthy children 5 to 18 years old. Children younger than 2 years old (especially infants younger than 6 months old), individuals 65 years old and older, and those with chronic diseases have high hospitalization rates. Mortality rates in the United States from 1976 to 2006 ranged from 3000 to 49,000 deaths per year (CDC, 2018l). Those 65 years and older account for the majority of deaths; children under 5 years old with high-risk conditions account for most deaths in children (Kimberlin et al., 2018). According to the CDC, approximately 80,000 persons died from influenza during the 2017 to 2018 season.

The incubation period is 1 to 4 days. Patients become infectious 24 hours before the onset of symptoms. Viral shedding usually peaks by day 3 and ceases 7 days after the onset of illness (WHO, 2018b).

Clinical Findings. Classic clinical symptoms include a sudden onset of high fever (102°F to 106°F [38.8°C to 41°C]), headache, chills, coryza, vertigo, pharyngitis, pain in the back and extremities, and a dry hacking cough that resembles pertussis. Vomiting, diarrhea, and croup occur in young children, as well as conjunctival infection and epistaxis. Infants can become septic. In severe infection, there may be involvement of the lower respiratory tract with atelectasis or infiltrates. Severe influenza-associated myocarditis (evidenced by weak heart sounds and rapid, weak pulse)

results in distention of the right side of the heart and CHF. Acute symptoms generally last 2 to 3 days, rarely over 5 days.

Diagnostic Studies. Rapid influenza diagnostic tests have limited sensitivities and predictive values. They are useful when determining the etiology of a respiratory disease outbreak in certain settings (e.g., schools, camps, hospitals) or if the child was recently exposed to pigs, poultry, or other animals, or had exposure to novel influenza A infection. A negative result should not determine the treatment course (e.g., antiviral treatment), to stop an outbreak, or to protect others at risk for complications (CDC, 2017a). Special viral cultures taken from the nasopharyngeal or nasal cavity by swab, nasal wash, or aspirate (varies by test) within 72 hours of the onset of illness can isolate the virus in 2 to 6 days and confirm the diagnosis. Other tests for influenza virus include serology (acute and convalescent sera), PCR, immunofluorescent assay (IFA), and rapid molecular assays. A CBC may show leukopenia.

Differential Diagnosis, Management, and Complications. The differential diagnosis includes other viral respiratory infections (e.g., common cold, parainfluenza, respiratory syncytial virus [RSV], rhinovirus, avian flu based on risk factors), allergic croup, epiglottitis, and bacterial pulmonary infections (e.g., *M. pneumoniae*).

Treatment is supportive (bed rest, fluids, over-the-counter antipyretics, cough medications). Children and parents need to be advised of symptoms that warrant further medical consultation (e.g., dehydration, difficulty breathing, muscle weakness). Hand hygiene, barrier protection (e.g., masks, gowns), and social distancing should be promoted. Five antiviral medications are approved for treatment or chemoprophylaxis of influenza A and B strains in the United States. However, due to viral resistance to amantadine and rimantadine, the ACIP recommends that neither be used until susceptibility is reliable (CDC, 2017c). Treatment or prophylaxis with antiviral therapy (i.e., zanamivir, oseltamivir, or peramivir [restricted to those 18 years old or older] in the United States) should be reserved for the following (CDC, 2017c):

- Children with immunosuppression
- Children younger than 2 years old
- Children with chronic illnesses (pulmonary [including asthma], cardiovascular [excludes hypertension alone], renal, hepatic, hematological [including sickle cell disease], metabolic disorders [including diabetes mellitus], neurologic and neurodevelopment conditions [including seizure disorders], intellectual disability, moderate to severe developmental delay, muscular dystrophy, or spinal cord injury)
- Women who are pregnant or postpartum (within 2 weeks after delivery)
- Individuals younger than 19 years old on long-term aspirin therapy
- American Indians/Alaska Natives
- Children who are morbidly obese (i.e., BMI is 40 or greater)
- Children in residential care facilities

When antivirals are indicated, treatment should be started within 48 hours of symptom onset and continued until the patient is asymptomatic for 24 to 48 hours. The FDA recommends oseltamivir to treat influenza in those 2 weeks old or older and for chemoprophylaxis in those 1 year old or older. The AAP and CDC endorse its use to treat influenza in those under 2 weeks old and as chemoprophylaxis in those 3 months to 1 year old (CDC, 2017c). Antiviral effectiveness varies from year to year based on the virus and strains present. PCPs can consult the CDC website "FluView Interactive" https://www.cdc.gov/flu/weekly/usmap.htm for information regarding circulating strains and antiviral resistance patterns within their geographic regions during influenza season.

Complications include Reye syndrome, respiratory infections (acute otitis media [AOM], pneumonia), acute myositis, toxic shock, myocarditis, and cystic fibrosis and asthma exacerbations followed by bacterial superinfection, usually with *H. influenzae*. Do not give aspirin to persons with influenza!

Patient and Family Education. Influenza vaccine should be widely promoted (Chapter 22). The CDC recommends the influenza vaccine for everyone 6 months of age and older. Although not mandated by any professional organization, the Infectious Diseases Society of America (IDSA), the Society for Healthcare Epidemiology of America (SHEA), and the Pediatric Infectious Diseases Society (PIDS) recommend that all healthcare providers receive yearly influenza vaccine to protect themselves and prevent the spread of this disease to their patients and families. This action is viewed as an ethical obligation of all healthcare providers and personnel (IDSA, 2013).

Highly Pathogenic Avian Influenza

The highly pathogenic avian influenza A (HPAI H5N1 or, simply H5N1) virus has the potential to acquire genes from the influenza virus that affect other species. It spreads quickly and has morphed into a more pathogenic virus than when it first emerged in 1996. There is little natural immunity in humans; fortunately the disease

in humans is uncommon, and the virus has not yet mutated to be efficiently transmitted from person to person. To date, only humans who had direct contact with sick or dead poultry, wild birds, or who visited live poultry markets are at high risk for virus acquisition. The outbreak worldwide has not diminished significantly, and healthcare providers in the United States should remain on alert. Human cases have been reported in Asia, Africa, the Pacific, Canada, Europe, and Near East. The highest number of cases occur in Indonesia, Egypt, and Vietnam (CDC, 2018g).

Humans who acquire the disease may experience a range of mild to more severe symptoms. Symptoms include fever (often >100.4°F [38°C]), cough, pharyngitis, malaise, myalgias, abdominal pain, diarrhea, and respiratory symptoms progressing to pneumonia with shortness of breath, difficulty breathing, and hypoxia. Complications of severe infection include acute respiratory and multiorgan system failure leading to death. To date, the mortality rate in humans is approximately 60% (WHO, 2018a). A vaccine for HPAI H5N1 was recently developed. If avian influenza is suspected, the CDC provides guidance in obtaining specimens, monitoring suspected cases, and advising precautions for those traveling to endemic locales. The United States banned import of birds (dead or alive) and bird products (including hatching eggs) from H5N1-affected countries (a list of countries is available from the CDC).

Other Viral Diseases

Human Immunodeficiency Virus

Human immunodeficiency viruses (serotypes HIV-1 and HIV-2) are retroviruses that cause human disease. Retroviruses are RNA viruses that must make a DNA copy of their RNA in order to replicate. HIV cells enter into a target CD4+ T cell and, using the reverse transcriptase enzyme, convert their RNA into DNA that integrates with the T-cell DNA within the cell nucleus, permanently infecting the host cell. Through the processes of transcription, translation, and maturation, the HIV genes convert into messenger RNA and leave the nucleus. Eventually new virions bud from the CD4+ T cells, infect other cells, and the cycle repeats. HIV persists in infected individuals for life; latent virus protein remains in cells of the blood, brain, bone marrow, and genital tract even when the plasma viral load cannot be detected.

Both serotypes cause clinically indistinguishable disease; most of the infections worldwide are attributed to HIV-1 (HIV-2 is generally limited to West Africa and India). In the United States, HIV-1 group M subtype B is the most prevalent, but non-subtype B and group O strains have been detected in infants whose mothers come from regions in Africa, India, Southeast Asia, or countries in proximity to these countries (U.S. Department of Health and Human Services [USDHHS], 2018b).

The worldwide burden of HIV/acquired immune deficiency syndrome (AIDS) remains high, with approximately 35 million individuals infected with HIV at the end of 2013. Sub-Saharan Africa is the most affected region and accounts for approximately 90% of all children with newly diagnosed infection (Shetty and Maldonado, 2016). Antiviral treatment is increasingly available in low- and middle-income countries; however, pediatric coverage with these drugs is lagging as compared to coverage for adults (WHO, 2018d). Limited resources in some countries also make unscreened blood products a means of transmission.

In the United States (including the six dependent territories and the District of Columbia) from 2008 through 2012, the annual estimated number of diagnoses of HIV infection remained stable while the overall estimated rate decreased. In 2015, there were an estimated 38,500 new HIV infections—down from 41,800 in 2010 (CDC, 2018h). Rates were stable for children younger than 13 years old and 15 through 19 years old but increased for children 13 and 14 years old and individuals 20 through 29 years old. The rate of female infection decreased. Eighty percent of infections occurred in adolescent and adult males with over 50% of youth unaware they were infected. Because of the long incubation period (8 to 12 years), these adolescents may not experience symptoms until they are in their 20s or 30s. Transmission was greatest for males through male-to-male sexual contact and/or injection drug use (67%), and for females through heterosexual contact (26%). Increased infection rates were seen for American Indians/Alaska Natives and Asians, whereas they decreased or were stable for all other ethnicity and race categories (CDC, 2018h, 2018j, 2015k). Vertical transmission from an infected mother to her infant occurs more often in non-Hispanic African Americans and Hispanics, although race and ethnicity alone are not risk factors (socioeconomic and injection drug use are suspected contributors).

Humans are the only known reservoir for HIV-1 and HIV-2. Although there are AIDS-like syndromes in other primates and felines, infection does not spread from pets, animals, or insects. HIV is isolated from blood (lymphocytes, macrophages, and plasma), CSF, pleural fluid, cervical secretions, human milk, feces, saliva, and urine. However, only blood, semen, cervical secretions, and human milk are implicated in transmission. Transmission is through intimate sexual contact, sharing of contaminated needles (inconclusive mode for HIV-2), transfusion of contaminated blood or blood products, perinatal exposure, and breastfeeding. HIV-2 has lower transmissibility rates than HIV-1 (Read, 2018). Accidental needlesticks in occupational settings rarely account for seroconversion with no confirmed cases of occupational transmission since 1999 in the United States. Transmission from accidental needlesticks from nonoccupational sources is not documented. Transmission of HIV from a human bite (even when saliva is contaminated with blood) or from antibody-screened blood transfusions in the United States is extremely rare (CDC, 2018i). A small number of children are reported to have acquired HIV from sexual abuse (Yogev and Chadwick, 2016).

The transmission of HIV to infants can occur in several ways. In utero transmission accounts for about 30% of infections (usually occurs by 10 weeks of gestation and is associated with early, severe newborn disease); via intrapartum transmission (at least 60%; from infected blood and cervicovaginal secretions in the birth canal or microtransfusions between mother and fetus during labor); or postpartum transmission via breast milk (15%; transmission rates range from 33% to 50% globally in resource-poor countries) (Shetty and Maldonado, 2016; UNICEF, 2015). Risk of an untreated HIV-infected woman giving birth to an infected infant with HIV-1 is 25% to 35% (4% or less for HIV-2) (Read, 2018). In vaginal twin deliveries, the firstborn twin has a greater risk of developing HIV than the second. Other risk factors for increased transmission include maternal drug use, premature rupture of membranes more than 4 hours before the onset of labor, low birthweight, and premature birth before 34 weeks (Shetty and Maldonaldo, 2016; Yogev and Chadwick, 2016). Transmission has been reported in infants who were fed premasticated food by HIV-1-infected caregivers (CDC, 2018i).

Mother-to-child transmission has been virtually eliminated in the United States and other high-income countries due to rigorous, universal antenatal HIV testing, use of combination antiretroviral treatment (cART), cesarean births (cesarean delivery reduces the risk of fetal infection by 87% if zidovudine is given to both mother and infant), and abstaining from breastfeeding (Shetty and Maldonado, 2016).

Studies confirm that transmission rates increase with breastfeeding longevity; infants exclusively breastfed until 6 months have one-third the risk of infection than those breastfed until 2 years. Exclusive breastfeeding may offer some protective immune factors, and the concentration of HIV in breast milk increases after weaning and when mixed feeding occurs (UNICEF, 2015). In developing countries where pediatric AIDS is pandemic, treatment regimens—out of nutritional necessity—traditionally included breastfeeding plus short-term antiretroviral drug treatment for women and infants.

The incubation period is variable. The onset of HIV infection symptoms in infants untreated perinatally occurs as early as 5.2 months (Shetty and Maldonaldo, 2016). The infection can also have a latency period longer than 5 years. Disease progression and earlier mortality are faster in children born to mothers with advanced infection, low CD4+ T-lymphocyte count, and who have high viral loads. In sub-Saharan Africa, approximately 30% of children untreated with antiviral medication succumb to the disease by 1 year old, and more than 50% die before they turn 2. Children untreated that live in the United States and Europe have a mortality rate between 10% and 20% (Shetty and Maldonado, 2016).

Clinical Findings. HIV infection is often experienced as an influenza-like illness (fever, rash, sore throat, lymphadenopathy, and myalgias) for 2 to 4 weeks. These symptoms can suggest a nonspecific viral process, and a provider may not consider HIV in the differential diagnosis. At this point, the asymptomatic infection may continue for a few months to up to 15 years, depending on the viral load. The CD4+ T cells start declining at an average rate of about 50 cells/μL/year.

There are four HIV clinical categories for children with HIV infection, ranging from "not symptomatic" to "severely symptomatic." These categories, paired with the degree of age-specific CD4+ T-lymphocyte count and total lymphocyte percentage, are used to determine the disease stage and management strategies. Newborn examinations are usually normal. Lymphadenopathy is often the first symptom, then hepatosplenomegaly. Some children have failure to thrive, chronic or recurrent diarrhea, pneumonia (*Pneumocystis jiroveci* peaks at 3 to 6 months of age), oral candidiasis, recurrent bacterial infections, chronic parotid swelling, and progressive neurologic deterioration. Those with high HIV loads develop symptoms earlier, including failure to thrive and encephalopathy. Other opportunistic diseases are *Mycobacterium avium* infection, severe CMV after 6 months old, EBV, VZV, disseminated histoplasmosis, RSV, *M. tuberculosis*, and measles (despite vaccination).

Children—other than infants—generally have more recurrent bacterial infections (20%), parotid gland swelling, lymphoid interstitial pneumonitis, or neurologic deficiencies that can progress to encephalopathy. *S. pneumoniae,* Hib, *S. aureus,* and *Salmonella* organisms are common infections in pediatric AIDS patients. Sinusitis, cellulitis, gingivostomatitis, herpetic zoster, glomerulopathy (especially in those of African descent), cardiac hypertrophy, anemia, CHF, and purulent middle ear infections are common. Malignancies are uncommon in pediatric AIDS (Yogev and Chadwick, 2016).

Diagnostic Studies. With newborn HIV screening, approximately 30% to 40% of those infected in utero are identified within 48 hours of birth and nearly 93% by age 2 weeks. Those infected intrapartally might become positive 2 to 6 weeks after birth (Shetty and Maldonaldo, 2016). Most infants without other exposure risks (e.g., those breastfed) lose maternal antibody between 6 and 12 months, but some take as long as 18 or more months to serorevert (Yogev and Chadwick, 2016). Table 31.5 lists recommended tests and testing times.

Lymphopenia occurs as the disease progresses. There are decreased circulating CD4+ cells (T-suppressor, T-helper cells), and the helper-suppressor ratio is less than one. The CDC defines an individual as suffering from autoimmune deficiency disease (e.g., AIDS) when their CD4+ T cell count is less than 200/mm^3. Some AIDS patients become seronegative late in the disease because the weakened immune system cannot manufacture antibodies.

Partners and other children of the HIV-infected mother need to receive appropriate HIV screening. In cases where an infant is adopted or in foster care, and when the HIV status of the mother is unknown, an appropriate HIV testing should be performed. HIV-infected pregnant women are advised to start antiretroviral treatment during pregnancy, irrespective of their CD4+ cell counts and HIV RNA levels, to help prevent vertical transmission (USDHHS, 2018a). Prior to starting a newborn on antiretroviral prophylaxis, a CBC and differential need to be obtained because anemia is a side effect of some of the drugs.

If HIV infection is suspected because of history in a child over 18 months old, screening HIV antibody assays plus a confirmatory antibody test or virologic detection test are warranted. In cases of acute HIV infection or AIDS, antibody tests may be negative and virologic testing is necessary. A pediatric HIV specialist should be consulted.

Differential Diagnosis. The differential diagnosis includes other causes of immunologic deficiency, such as recent immunosuppressive agent use, lymphoproliferative disease, congenital immunologic states, inflammatory bowel disease, DiGeorge syndrome, ITP, chronic allergies, cystic fibrosis, graft-versus-host reaction, congenital CMV, toxoplasmosis, ataxia, or telangiectasia.

Management and Complications. Treatment goals include suppressing viral replication to undetectable levels; restoring/preserving immune function; reducing HIV-associated sequelae; minimizing drug toxicity; promoting normal growth and development; promoting treatment regimen adherence; and improving quality of life. Any information about HIV and AIDS treatment in children is subject to change, and the PCP should check with the CDC or AIDSinfo regarding updated guidelines for diagnosis, treatment, monitoring drug toxicity and adherence, and specific immunization precautions and regimens. Treatment decisions and laboratory studies should be made in consultation with a pediatric HIV specialist.

Current recommended drug regimens for cART include at least three oral antiretroviral drugs from at least two drug classes. Generally two nucleoside reverse transcriptase inhibitors (NRTIs) plus either a non-nucleoside reverse transcriptase inhibitor (NNRTI) or protease inhibitor (PI), often with low-dose ritonavir, are used. Treatment regimens are individualized based on a number of factors (e.g., age, immune status, viral load, clinical categories, viral resistance, potential adherence issues, drug toxicity, and comorbid conditions). Frequent laboratory studies and possible antiretroviral changes throughout the life of the individual are required. cART regimens resulted in an 81% to 93% reduction in mortality from 1994 to 2006 in the United States and United Kingdom. Some children infected as infants are living into their third and fourth decades of life with the potential to live longer (USDHHS, 2017).

Established protocols for the HIV-infected mother and her newborn are available on the AIDSinfo website at https://aidsinfo.nih.gov/guidelines/html/3/perinatal/0. The zidovudine prophylaxis protocol (or alternatives) for the HIV-exposed newborn from birth to 6 weeks old can be accessed at the site above and seen in Table 31.5. Ensure bloodwork is done before initiating prophylaxis. The infant should be discharged from the hospital with the full 6-week course of zidovudine in hand for the parent, not just a prescription, with complete instructions for administration. This helps ensure greater compliance and prophylaxis continuity. Additionally, infants with known HIV exposure whose status remains unknown or who are HIV

TABLE 31.5 Testing Schedule for Human Immunodeficiency Virus in the Exposed, Non-Breastfeeding Infant[a] in the United States

Test[b]	Time After Birth
First HIV DNA PCR[c] or HIV qualitative RNA assay[d] from peripheral blood (not cord blood); confirm if positive using the same test on another blood sample	Within 48 hours
Optional, HIV DNA PCR[c] or HIV qualitative RNA assay[d]; confirm if positive	14-21 days (some clinicians prefer this optional testing date)
Second HIV DNA PCR[c] or HIV qualitative RNA assay[d]; confirm if positive	1-3 months
Third HIV DNA PCR[c] or HIV qualitative RNA assay[d]; confirm if positive	4-6 months
Fourth[e] HIV DNA PCR[c] or HIV qualitative RNA assay[d]; confirm if positive	12 and 24 months

[a]Infant is considered infected if two separate samples test positive by HIV DNA PCR or qualitative HIV RNA PCR. Infant greater than 18 months old and non-breastfeeding is considered *definitely negative* if two negative tests are obtained at ≥1 month and ≥4 months OR two separate negative tests are obtained at ≥6 months AND no other laboratory or clinical evidence that suggests HIV/acquired immune deficiency syndrome (AIDS).

[b]The following HIV tests are not recommended for use in those younger than 1 month old: HIV culture; HIV p24 antigen assay; immune complex dissociated (ICD) p24 antigen assay. Those older than 18 months old can be tested using an HIV antibody assay. Most tests will detect both HIV-1 and HIV-2 infection but will not discern between the two. HIV-2 infection can be confirmed using other tests.

[c]HIV DNA PCR testing may be preferable for infants who are receiving combination antiretroviral treatment (cART) prophylaxis or preemptive treatment because HIV RNA assays may be less sensitive in the presence of such treatment.

[d]The newer qualitative HIV RNA PCR assay detects HIV-1 non-type B or group O strain in infants and is recommended for infants born to mothers from Africa, India, or Southeast Asia or if infection is suspected and the initial HIV DNA PCR assay(s) are negative (HIV DNA PCR has limited sensitivity to this subtype/strain).

[e]This fourth test is an option to document loss of maternal antibodies in infants 12 to 18 months old with prior negative tests; or to definitely exclude or confirm HIV infection in infants 18 to 24 months with prior HIV-antibody positive tests.

DNA, Deoxyribonucleic acid; *HIV*, human immunodeficiency virus; *PCR*, polymerase chain reaction; *RNA*, ribonucleic acid.

Data from U.S. Department of Health and Human Services (USDHHS). Guidelines for the use of antiretroviral agents in pediatric HIV infection: diagnosis of HIV infection in infants and children; 2018b. Retrieved from http://aidsinfo.nih.gov/guidelines/html/2/pediatric-arv-guidelines/55/diagnosis-of-hiv-infection-in-infants-and-children.

infected should be prescribed trimethoprim-sulfamethoxazole (TMP-SMX) to prophylax against *Pneumocystis jirovecii* starting at 4 to 6 weeks old and until the child is 1 year old (administered either on 3 consecutive days a week or daily). If the newborn is uninfected with HIV, the prophylaxis can be stopped. Alternative prophylaxis antibiotics are available on the AIDSinfo website. Treatment of associated conditions with appropriate medical therapy is indicated using immunoglobulin (IGIV), antifungals, antivirals, antimycobacterials, and nutritional counseling. After delivery, mothers need to be encouraged to continue their cART, use a reliable method of birth control, and take precautions to prevent sexual transmission of the virus. At present, it is not clear from clinical and laboratory studies if in utero exposure to cART taken by the mother has any long-term sequelae in the child/adolescent (USDHHS, 2018a).

Treatment of a child (versus newborn) infected with HIV also requires collaboration with pediatric HIV specialists because drug regimens are complex and are constantly being revised. Adolescents present a particular noncompliance risk because of denial and fear of their infection, substance abuse and addiction, misinformation, distrust of and inexperience with the medical system, self-esteem issues, unstable living situations, and/or lack of familial and social support systems. It is important for the PCP to be nonconfrontational yet discuss risk factors and advocate for family planning services and needle exchange programs, PEP regimens, and prompt involvement in new treatments as they become available.

An important role of the PCP in HIV treatment is helping to boost adherence rates. In addition, side effects must be monitored closely because many of the antiretroviral drugs interact with other commonly prescribed medications (including oral contraceptives). The treatment regimens are highly challenging for parents because of complex dosing schedules and possible unwillingness of children to take the medications. Many preparations are not offered in liquid form or the taste is not attractive to children. See Chapter 22 for information about addressing and enhancing medication adherence rates in children and adolescents.

HIV becomes a multisystemic illness with multiorgan complications.

Prevention and Reduction of Perinatal Transmission of Human Immunodeficiency Virus. The CDC, WHO, and United Nations AIDS agencies are useful resources for current treatment regimens; recommendations may vary by country. WHO strategies for preventing the transmission of HIV to women and from mother to child include:

- Improve access to antiretroviral therapy for HIV-infected women and children. cART use to reduce perinatal transmission of HIV is the accepted treatment standard in developed and underdeveloped countries. WHO recommends using a once-daily simplified triple antiretroviral drug regimen for all pregnant and breastfeeding women with HIV, with consideration of lifelong treatment (WHO, 2018d).
- Improve access to testing (<40% of people in United Nation Member States know their HIV status); encourage use of self-testing kits for early diagnosis and treatment (one is approved by the FDA; others are under development).
- Increase blood/tissue/surgical/injection safety education.
- Expand maternal/newborn/child health care (to initiate earlier treatment and prevention education).
- Expand sexual and reproductive health education.
- Strengthen infant nutrition support.
- Use cesarean delivery if indicated.

- Promote exclusive breastfeeding by HIV-positive mothers.
- Increase availability of chemophylaxis for the neonate and infant until HIV status is known (WHO, 2018d).

In the United States, guidelines for preventing transmission by HIV-infected women include discouraging breastfeeding, even if on cART. Delivery by cesarean is recommended, depending upon the mother's viral load (CDC, 2018i). However, research in developing countries, notably South Africa, demonstrates that a combination of exclusive breastfeeding and cART by the mother or infant significantly reduces the risk of breast milk HIV transmission. Protection against HIV infection increases if the infant is breastfed exclusively prior to 6 months with continued breastfeeding to 12 months. HIV-positive women who are treated with cART in developing countries are encouraged to breastfeed their infants (WHO, 2018).

Because cART is now standard treatment for HIV-infected pregnant women and their infants, adherence to the recommended postnatal HIV prophylaxis for both the mother and her infant can be problematic. One meta-analysis demonstrated that only 73.5% of pregnant women achieved an 80% or greater adherence rate; this rate decreased in the postpartum period. Reasons for lack of adequate adherence were attributed to the following factors (Nachega et al., 2012):

- Concern about the safety of antiretroviral therapy drugs on the fetus or woman
- Advanced AIDS stage and health-related symptoms of pregnancy (nausea, vomiting, fatigue)
- HIV disease
- Other physical or economic factors
- Depression (especially postpartum)
- Presence of alcohol or drug abuse
- The complexity and length of antiretroviral therapy drug regimens for woman or infant
- Lack of social support

Recent studies reinforced those of Nachega and colleagues and also found that other mental health issues, age, homelessness, poverty, inconsistent access to antiretroviral therapy, and HIV stigma are associated with lower adherence, whereas trust and/or satisfaction with the HIV care provider are correlated with higher adherence (Langebeek et al., 2014; USD-HHSHHS, 2014b) in the United States.

The following is standard knowledge and practice for providers:

- Healthcare providers need to be alert to the potential risk of transmission of HIV infection to infants in utero, in the postpartum period, and through human milk. Counsel caregivers against giving premasticated food to infants.
- Document routine HIV education and routine testing with consent of all adolescents seeking prenatal care; ensure that each adolescent knows her HIV status and the methods available to prevent the acquisition and transmission of HIV to her newborn.
- At the time of delivery, provide education about HIV and complete a rapid HIV testing with consent if HIV status is unknown.
- Women in the United States diagnosed with HIV infection just prior to labor or soon after delivery or those who have known infection risks (e.g., injection drug users) but whose status is unknown at delivery should be advised against breastfeeding. If a woman desires to breastfeed, she can pump (and discard milk) until HIV testing is done and seronegativity is confirmed.
- There are no special precautions for handling expressed breast milk of HIV-infected women. No transmission to another

infant has been reported after a single exposure to milk expressed by an HIV-infected mother (CDC, 2017g). Pasteurization and donor screening ensures the safety of human milk banks. The nonprofit Human Milk Banking Association of North America (HMBANA) sets standards of testing for all their members' milk banks.

- Adolescents must be counseled about the risk of HIV transmission (e.g., sexual transmission, sharing of needles or syringes) and the use of condoms. Condom use during last intercourse was reported by 53.8% of adolescents, whereas only 9.3% report ever having had an HIV test (female rates are higher than for males) (Redfield et al., 2018).
- School attendance for HIV-infected children: The benefit from attendance far outweighs the risks. Factors that must be taken into account include the risk to the immunosuppressed child from "normal germs" from healthy kids and school personnel. Because casual transmission is unknown, there is no risk to other children as long as the infected child controls body secretions. Children who display biting behavior or have oozing wounds should be cared for in a setting that minimizes risk to others. The child's PCP is the only person with an absolute need to know the child's primary diagnosis. If the family decides to inform the school, those informed should maintain confidentiality. If the family chooses not to inform the school, parents should get assurance that the school will notify them of any communicable disease outbreaks (e.g., varicella, measles) or physical altercations with others.
- Routine screening of school-age children for HIV antibodies is not indicated.

Preexposure Prophylaxis for Certain High-Risk Individuals. Preexposure prophylaxis (PrEP) is now recommended in the United States and by the WHO for those at ongoing, substantial risk of being infected with HIV. Individuals who qualify for PrEP include those having male-to-male anal sex without a condom or with a diagnosed sexually transmitted disease in the past 6 months; those having sex with an HIV-positive partner; injection drug users who share equipment or who have been in a drug treatment program in the past 6 months; individuals not in a monogamous sexual relationship with partners who have not been recently tested and found to be HIV-negative; or heterosexual men or women who do not use condoms and have sex with high-risk partners (e.g., bisexual males, injection drug users). These risk factors result in HIV transmission rates from 62% to 92% (CDC, 2018t). The prophylaxis regimen involves a fixed-dose daily two-drug combination. The clinical practice guideline for PrEP is available on the CDC website (www.cdc.gov/hiv/risk/prep/index.html). The efficacy and safety for use in adolescents is not established and still being studied. A monthly inserted vaginal ring with an antiviral and two long-acting injectable antiviral agents are under development as alternatives to daily PrEP.

Postexposure Prophylaxis After Nonoccupational Exposure. The PCP may need to assess and counsel parents after their child has an accidental puncture wound from a discarded needle found in a public setting; from a bite wound, a fight, or during a sports activity; or from sexual abuse. Though transmission is extremely rare, the PCP needs to address the situation with a level of understanding of the risks and CDC recommendations.

The body fluids of an HIV-infected person do not all carry the same viral load or risk. For example, exposure to blood of a known HIV-infected person carries the highest risk, whereas blood-free saliva, semen or vaginal secretions, and human milk carry a low risk; urine, feces, and vomitus are unlikely to transmit the virus. Syringes that might have been used and discarded by an HIV-infected, injection-drug user generate the most concern of parents. The following information is useful when counseling parents (WHO, 2018t):

- HIV viability is vulnerable to drying.
- The smaller the needle bore, the more limited the amount of blood present due to a lesser intra lumen volume available, and, therefore lower the risk.
- There are no documented HIV transmission cases from an accidentally found, discarded needle.
- There is greater risk from biting an individual who is HIV-positive (saliva contaminated with HIV-infected blood) than from having been bitten by an HIV-positive person (saliva not contaminated by infected blood).

The PCP and parent must weigh the unproven safety and benefits of participating in the PEP regimen against the significant toxicity of the drugs themselves. If instituted, PEP therapy ideally needs to start within 72 hours after exposure and continue for 28 days. Close follow-up for support, medication monitoring (adherence and toxicity), and serial HIV antibody screening are needed (Box 31.1). The CDC provides an algorithm for evaluating and treating possible nonoccupational exposure and makes recommendations as to whether or not PEP is warranted (www.cdc.gov/hiv).

Measles (Rubeola)

Measles (rubeola) is a Morbillivirus in the Paramyxoviridae family, is similar to mumps and influenza, and causes serious illness in children. There is only one antigenic type. Measles has a characteristic rash, indicating viremia. Worldwide, approximately 20 million people annually are infected with measles with 146,000 deaths. In the United States, annual rates since 2000 ranged from 37 (in 2004) to 668 (in 2014); in 2018 there were 220 reported cases (2018q). Most of the U.S. cases originated in unvaccinated individuals who imported the measles after being in countries with large outbreaks (including, but not limited to, England, France, Germany, India, the Philippines, Asia, and Africa). The disease spreads within communities where there are larger numbers of unvaccinated or undervaccinated individuals and where herd immunity falls below a critical point.

Humans and primates are the only known infection reservoir. The sources of the infection include respiratory secretions, blood, and urine of infected persons. Droplet contact, fomites, and, less likely, aerosol transmission transmit virus. Peak incidence of infection in susceptible persons occurs during late winter and spring months. Once exposed, approximately 9 out of 10 susceptible individuals develop the disease (CDC, 2018o).

The incubation period for measles is 8 to 12 days; for modified measles, as long as 21 days. A person is contagious 1 to 2 days before the onset of symptoms (3 to 5 days before the rash), and 4 days after the rash appearance, or roughly 14 days (range 7 to 18 days). There is no carrier state; disease or two vaccinations usually confer lifelong immunity.

Clinical Findings. The clinical manifestations include:
1. Incubation period: There are no specific symptoms.
2. Prodromal period: This first sign of the illness lasts 4 to 5 days and consists of URI symptoms, low to moderate fever (>101°F [38.3°C]), and cough, coryza, and conjunctivitis (the "three Cs" of measles). An enanthem (Koplik spots) can

Management After Possible Exposure to Human Immunodeficiency Virus

1. Treat the exposure site.
   • Wash wounds with soap and water; flush mucous membranes with water. Give Td or Tdap booster if appropriate (see Chapter 22).
2. Evaluate the exposure source if possible to guide need for postexposure prophylaxis.
   • Determine the human immunodeficiency virus (HIV) infection status of the exposure source. If unknown, testing with appropriate consent should be offered if possible.
3. Evaluate the exposed person.
   • Perform HIV serologic testing to identify current HIV infection and hepatitis B and hepatitis C serologic testing as appropriate.
   • Provide or refer for counseling to address stress and anxiety.
   • Discuss prevention of potential secondary HIV transmission.
   • Discuss prevention of repeat exposure, if appropriate.
   • Report the incident to legal or administrative authorities as appropriate to the setting of the exposure and the severity of the incident.
4. Consider postexposure prophylaxis (not to be used for frequent exposures).
   • Explain potential benefits and risks.
   • Discuss issues of drug toxicity and medication compliance.
   • Measure complete blood cell count, creatinine, and alanine transaminase concentration as baseline for possible drug toxicity.
   • Begin postexposure prophylaxis as soon as possible after exposure, preferably within 1 to 4 h; prophylaxis begun more than 72 h after exposure is unlikely to be effective.
   • Arrange for follow-up with HIV specialist and psychologist if appropriate.
   • Educate about prevention of secondary transmission (sexually active adolescent should avoid sex, or use condoms, until all follow-up test results are negative).
5. Choose therapy (should contain three [or more] antiretroviral drugs).
   • Consider drug potency and toxicity, regimen complexity and effects on compliance, and possibility of drug resistance in the exposure source.
   • Supply 3 to 5 days of medication immediately, instructing patients to obtain remainder of medication at follow-up visit (for total of 28 days).
6. Follow-up.
   • Perform initial follow-up within 2 to 3 days to review drug regimen and adherence, evaluate for symptoms of drug toxicity, assess psychosocial status, and arrange appropriate referrals, if needed.
   • Ensure patient has enough medication to complete 28-day regimen.
   • Monitor for drug adverse effects at 4 weeks with complete blood cell count and alanine transaminase concentration.
   • Evaluate for psychological stress and medication compliance with weekly office visits or telephone calls.
   • Consider referral for counseling if needed.
   • Repeat HIV serologic testing at 6 weeks, 12 weeks, and 6 months after exposure.

From Havens PL, American Academy of Pediatrics Committee on Pediatric AIDS. Postexposure prophylaxis in children and adolescents for nonoccupational exposure to human immunodeficiency virus. Pediatrics. 2003;111(6):1475–1489, reaffirmed 2009; Kuhar DT, Henderson DK, Struble KA, et al. Updated U.S. Public Health Service guidelines for the management of occupational exposures to human immunodeficiency virus and recommendations for postexposure prophylaxis. Infect Control Hosp Epidemiol. 2013;34(9):875–892; Center for Disease Control and Prevention (CDC). Post-exposure Prophylaxis (PEP); 2018. Retrieved from https://www.cdc.gov/hiv/basics/pep.html.

be found on the oral mucosa opposite the lower molars. They are small, irregular, bluish white granules on an erythematous background, last 12 to 15 hours, and are pathognomonic of measles infection.

3. Rash stage: The rash of unmodified measles usually appears on the third or fourth day of the illness. As the rash appears, temperature rises, often to 105°F (40.5°C). The rash is maculopapular and first appears behind the ears and on the forehead. Papules enlarge, coalesce, and move progressively downward, engulfing the face, neck, and arms over the next 24 hours. By the end of the second 24 hours, the rash has spread to the back, abdomen, and thighs. As the legs become more involved, the face begins to clear. The entire process takes approximately 3 days. Respiratory symptoms are most severe on day 3 of the rash. The more severe the rash, the more severe the illness. It can become hemorrhagic, and this can be fatal because of disseminated intravascular coagulation (DIC). The rash begins to fade after the fourth day. The disease peaks; defervescence occurs. After the rash clears, a residual desquamating light-colored pigmentation occurs, lasting approximately 1 week.

Modified measles illness can present in children who are passively immunized with immunoglobulin after disease exposure, have residual maternal antibodies, or received an improperly administered measles vaccine. In these cases, the illness is an abbreviated version of the typical disease. The prodrome period can last 1 to 2 days with normal to low-grade fever. URI symptoms are minimal to absent. Koplik spots usually do not appear. The rash is so mild that it is often missed.

Diagnostic Studies. A single measles IgM antibody level is useful if drawn when symptoms appear; the reactivity is low after more than 30 days. Disease confirmation can be made by viral isolation from urine, blood, throat or nasopharyngeal secretions, or from serial IgG antibody titers that compare acute and convalescent serum specimens. Measles is a reportable disease in the United States within 24 hours of diagnosis.

Differential Diagnosis and Management. Any viral rash, toxoplasmosis, scarlet fever, Kawasaki syndrome, meningococcemia, Rocky Mountain spotted fever (RMSF), drug rashes, and serum sickness are included in the differential diagnosis.

Treatment is supportive (antipyretics, bed rest, adequate fluids, air humidification, warm room, darkened room if photophobia is present). No antiviral therapy is available, although ribavirin has been used off label to treat severe measles infections and in children who are immunocompromised (Kimberlin et al., 2018). Bacterial superinfections (e.g., ear infections, bronchopneumonia, and encephalitis) are treated with appropriate antibiotics. All children with encephalitis, severe pneumonia, or compromised immune systems should be managed in consultation with an infectious disease expert.

Children in the United States and in countries where malnutrition is an issue are at greater risk for measles morbidity or mortality. These children, and those with severe measles, have lower vitamin A levels. The WHO recommends vitamin A for all children despite their country of residence. Dose once daily for 2 days: under 6 months old, 50,000 international units; 6 through 11 months old, 100,000 international units; 12 months old or older, 200,000 international units.

Care of Exposed Individuals. The measles vaccine should be given within 72 hours of exposure to those who are vaccine-eligible and who were exposed. This is the first choice to prevent or modify the infection and may be given to infants 6 to 11 months old (AAP, 2018a). Immune globulin (IGIM or IGIV) given within 6 days of exposure can be administered to prevent or modify the disease in those susceptible (those without prior measles vaccine, infants younger than 12 months old, pregnant women, and immunocompromised individuals), regardless of their measles vaccination status.

Complications

Bacterial superinfection and viral complications can manifest as a URI, obstructive laryngitis, otitis, diarrhea, mastoiditis, cervical adenitis, bronchitis, transient hepatitis, and pneumonia (the largest cause of fatalities in infants). The causative organism is the measles virus itself or group A β-hemolytic streptococci (GABHS), pneumococci, *H. influenzae,* or *S. aureus.* Infection can exacerbate underlying TB. Other complications include myocarditis, purpura fulminans ("black measles," characterized by multiorgan bleeding), encephalitis and other neurologic sequelae, and subacute sclerosing panencephalitis (fatal complication of wild-type measles). There are usually no complications with modified measles.

Mumps

Mumps is an acute generalized viral disease with painful enlargement of one or more salivary glands (usually parotid glands). Mumps is in the Paramyxoviridae family. There is only one serotype, and humans are the only natural reservoir. The source of infection is contact with the saliva and/or respiratory tract secretions of infected persons. This illness' incidence decreased by more than 99% in the United States since the advent of the mumps vaccine (CDC, 2018p). After two doses, the effectiveness of mumps vaccine ranges from 66% to 95%; higher rates of infection occur more often in individuals who are unvaccinated or undervaccinated. Infection occurs during all seasons but is most common during late winter and spring, and in children younger than 10 years old; it affects both sexes equally. Mumps virus crosses the placenta; studies are inconsistent in determining whether or not infection during the first trimester increases the risk of spontaneous abortion or intrauterine fetal demise. Fetal malformations after prenatal mumps infection is demonstrated (Kimberlin et al., 2018).

The incubation period ranges from 12 to 25 days (usually 16 to 18 days). Disease communicability is about 1 to 2 days before glandular swelling and up to 5 days after the swelling onset. About one-third of patients are asymptomatic or only have URI symptoms. Lifelong immunity is usually conferred after one infection; rarely is a second infection seen.

Clinical Findings. There are two clinical stages:
1. Prodromal stage: Rare in children but can cause fever, headache, anorexia, neck or other muscular pain, and malaise.
2. Swelling stage: Approximately 24 hours after the prodromal stage, 31% to 65% of those affected have painful swelling of one or both parotid glands. If both glands are affected, one generally swells before the other. The gland fills the space between the posterior border of the mandible and mastoid, pushing downward and forward to the zygoma. The ear is pushed forward and upward. Swelling lasts a few hours to a few days. The enlarged glands usually return to normal size in 3 to 7 days. Rarely a maculopapular, truncal, pink discrete rash is seen. Pain on the affected side can be elicited by having the patient eat something sour. This is known as the "pickle sign." The Stensen duct is red and swollen. The Wharton duct is frequently swollen. Fever is usually moderate; 20% are afebrile. Ten percent to 15% of cases involve only the submandibular glands. Little pain is associated with submandibular infection; however, the redness subsides slower. If sublingual salivary glands are involved, there is bilateral swelling in the submental region in the floor of the mouth. Edema caused by lymphatic obstruction of the manubrium and upper chest is reported.

Orchitis may occur in individuals who contract mumps after puberty.

Diagnostic Studies. This virus can be detected from a buccal swab (Stenson duct exudate), throat washings, saliva, or spinal fluid using RT-PCR and serologic tests (mumps-specific IgM antibodies or serial acute/convalescent titers for IgG antibodies). Leukopenia with relative lymphocytosis and an elevated amylase are typical. Test results are more reliable for diagnosis when specimens are obtained within 1 to 3 days after onset of symptoms ((Kimberlin et al., 2018).

Differential Diagnosis, Management, and Complications. Cervical or preauricular lymphadenitis, CMV, HIV, enteroviruses, tumor, suppurative parotitis bacterial (e.g., nontuberculous mycobacterium) or viral (influenza A, coxsackievirus, parainfluenza 1 and 3, EBV) infection, idiopathic recurrent parotitis, parotid ductal obstruction, Mikulicz syndrome, uveoparotid fever, and cancer (especially lymphosarcoma) are included in the differential diagnosis.

Treatment is supportive (antipyretics, bed rest as needed, diet appropriate for chewing discomfort). Corticosteroids or nonsteroidal anti-inflammatory drugs (NSAIDs) are given to manage arthritic complications. Manage orchitis with bed rest and scrotal elevation. School and day care students should be kept home until 9 days after the onset of parotid swelling. Use active and passive immunization.

Complications include meningoencephalitis (mostly males older than 20 years old), orchitis and/or epididymitis (10% incidence in postpubertal males; sterility is rare), oophoritis (in postpubertal women; fertility is not affected), pancreatitis (rare), thyroiditis (uncommon), myocarditis, deafness (transient or permanent), arthritis (rare), thrombocytopenia, hemolytic anemia (usually self-limited), mastitis, and glomerulonephritis.

Erythema Infectiosum

Erythema infectiosum, or fifth disease, is caused by parvovirus B19. This virus is a member of the Parvoviridae family and is a single-stranded DNA virus that replicates in erythrocyte precursors. It is called *fifth disease* because it was the fifth childhood eruptive rash described historically. These rashes include measles, scarlet fever, rubella, Filatov-Dukes disease, erythema infectiosum, and erythema subitum (roseola infantum, sixth disease). Humans are the only reservoir. Erythema infectiosum is spread via vertical transmission from mother to fetus, by respiratory tract secretions, and percutaneous exposure to blood or blood products. Distribution is worldwide. It is a disease of childhood, highest in 5- to 15-year-olds, but infants and adults are not immune. Secondary spread to household contacts is up to 50% (Kimberlin et al., 2018). The disease occurs most commonly in late winter and early spring.

The incubation period is approximately 4 to 21 days; the rash and symptoms occur between 2 and 3 weeks after exposure. The highest period of communicability is before the rash, joint pain, or edema (the latter two seen are rare). Chronic infection can occur in those immunocompromised or with most types of hemolytic anemias.

Clinical Findings. The following two phases are seen in erythema infectiosum:
1. Prodrome: Consists of mild fever (15% to 30% of cases), myalgia, headache, malaise, and/or URI symptoms.
2. Rash: Appears 7 to 10 days after the prodromal stage and occurs in three stages: It first appears on the face as an intense

red eruption on the cheeks (slapped cheek) with circumoral pallor that lasts 1 to 4 days. Next, a lacy maculopapular eruption appears on the trunk and moves peripherally to the arms, thighs, and buttocks. Palms and soles are generally spared. This phase can last a month. Finally, the rash subsides. Older children may have mild pruritus. There may be periodic recurrences precipitated by trauma, heat, exercise, stress, sunlight, or cold (Fig 31.4). Children less commonly experience arthralgia (more often in the knees) than adults, who may complain of symmetric polyarthropathy. Arthralgia most commonly resolves in 2 to 4 weeks. Those with hemolytic anemias or who are immunocompromised may have fever, pallor, tachycardia, and symptoms of heart failure.

Diagnostic Studies. Laboratory testing is not generally indicated because it is a clinical diagnosis. Serum B19-specific IgM antibody confirms the presence of infection and persists for 6 to 8 weeks. Anti-B19 IgG confirms past infection. For immunocompromised individuals, PCR assay is the method of choice. Standard cultures are not useful.

Differential Diagnosis, Management, and Complications. This is not a difficult disease to diagnose. The differential diagnoses include rubella, enterovirus disease, lupus, atypical measles, and drug rashes.

There is no specific antiviral treatment. Consider transfusion for those with hemolytic anemia or who are immunocompromised. IGIV helps those with immunocompromised conditions. Because there is widespread undetected infection in children and adults, avoidance of known exposure can reduce, but not eliminate, the risk of infection. Children in the rash stage may attend school.

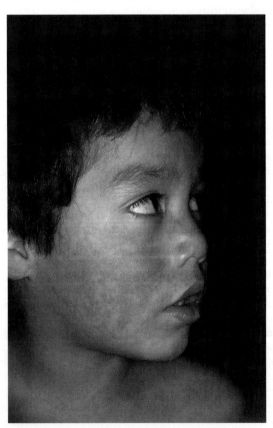

• **Fig 31.4** Erythema Infectiosum, Fifth Disease.

Complications are few and typically not significant in healthy patients; recovery is usually without sequelae. The most frequently reported complications include arthritis (hands, wrists, knees, and/or ankles occurring 2 to 3 weeks after onset of initial symptoms); chronic infection in those immunodeficient; aplastic crisis (more common in those with chronic hemolytic anemias, including sickle cell anemia, thalassemia, hereditary spherocytosis, or other types of chronic hemolysis); thrombocytopenic purpura or neutropenia; myocarditis (rare); papular-purpuric "gloves and socks" syndrome (fever, pruritus, purpura, painful edema, and erythema with a glove-and-sock distribution) followed by petechiae and oral lesions; or fetal hydrops, death, or intrauterine growth retardation if exposed in utero (no reports of congenital anomalies) (Kimberlin et al., 2018). An exposed pregnant woman should consult with her healthcare provider.

Parainfluenza Virus

Human parainfluenza virus (hPIV), a paramyxovirus, is similar to the influenza and mumps viruses and is an important cause of laryngotracheobronchitis (croup), bronchitis, bronchiolitis, and pneumonia. This virus accounts for 7% of hospital admissions of children younger than 5 years old. In the United States, epidemiologic studies attribute hPIV to two-thirds of croup cases, one-quarter of tracheobronchitis, and 50% of URIs (colds, laryngitis, pharyngitis, otitis media) in children (Yogev and Chadwick, 2016).

There are four antigenic hPIV types. Types 1 and 2 usually strike children 1 to 5 years old and are usually associated with croup; outbreaks are seen more in summer and fall and in odd-numbered years; reinfections occur at any age. Type 3 is endemic, associated more with bronchitis, bronchiolitis, and pneumonia in those younger than 12 months old, results in shorter immunity (a particular problem for immunocompromised patients), and outbreaks peak in the spring and summer (sometimes into fall months). Type 4 infections are less well pathologically and clinically understood, may be more pervasive than once thought, and can cause mild to severe respiratory illness. By the time most children are 5 years old, they have been exposed to all of the types. An individual typically has repeated infections due to hPIV as immunity is transient and limited.

This virus spreads by direct person-to-person contact through infected nasopharyngeal secretions or from fomite contamination. It replicates in the superficial ciliated epithelial lining the airways of the upper and lower respiratory tract and spreads readily. The incubation period is 2 to 6 days. Healthy children shed virus for 4 to 7 days before symptom onset and up to 7 to 21 days after resolution of symptoms. The virus lives on nonporous surfaces for up to 10 hours (Yogev and Chadwick, 2016).

Clinical Findings. Symptoms may include an acute onset of mild fever, sore throat, rhinitis, hoarseness, and cough (including a typical "croup" cough). Lower respiratory involvement symptoms include dyspnea, crackles, wheezing, and hyperaeration. In older children and adolescents, recurrent infection may manifest as a mild URI.

Diagnostic Studies. Routine testing is not needed. Specific RT-PCR assays are the standard diagnostic test when needed. The virus can be isolated from nasopharyngeal secretions; culture results are usually available within 4 to 7 days (or earlier). Sensitivities vary when rapid antigen identification is performed by IFAs and enzyme immunoassays. WBC count may be normal or slightly elevated with a mild lymphocyte elevation.

Differential Diagnosis, Management, and Complications. The differential diagnosis includes other viral URIs, allergic croup, laryngotracheitis, bacterial tracheitis, retropharyngeal abscess, epiglottitis, laryngeal diphtheria, foreign body aspiration, or GI reflux.

The treatment is supportive; recovery is uncomplicated in most cases. Reliable studies using ribavirin are lacking; therefore, aerosolized ribavirin should only be considered for high-risk patients with severe lower respiratory involvement (Yogev and Chadwick, 2016). With the newer outpatient guidelines for managing croup, few children need hospitalization (see Chapter 37). Antibiotics are reasonable in cases of severe infection when secondary bacterial invasion is suspected (e.g., otitis media, bronchitis, tracheitis, pneumonia). No vaccine is available; intravenous immune globulin is not helpful. Good hand hygiene is important.

Complications are infrequent. Immunocompromised individuals are more prone to developing secondary bacterial infections.

Rubella (German or 3-Day Measles)

Rubella is an acute disease of childhood that occurs either postnatally or congenitally. Rubella is an RNA virus of the genus *Rubivirus*, in the Togaviridae family. Humans are the only reservoir; disease is seen more in adolescents and young adults (Cherry and Baker, 2019). Infection spreads through nasopharyngeal secretions or transplacentally during either apparent or silent infection. It is worldwide in distribution. The virus has been isolated in blood, breast milk, conjunctival sac, and urine of infected individuals.

One must have prolonged and repeated contact to become infected. The incubation period is 14 to 21 days (mean 18 days). The maximum period of viral shedding (and presumed transmissibility) is believed to be 5 days before to 6 days after the rash appearance. Males and females are equally affected. Genetic factors may play a role in transmissibility. Infants infected in utero can shed virus past their first birthday (Cherry and Baker, 2019). In the United States, disease occurs during the winter and spring months, notably March, April, and May. There is lifelong immunity after naturally occurring disease; however, asymptomatic reinfection can occur. Because illness without rash exists, the actual number of reinfections is unknown. Reinfection occurs from wild-type virus and in those previously immunized.

Use of the rubella vaccine eliminated endemic rubella infections in the United States and other countries with national immunization programs. Most cases in the United States occur in those unvaccinated (including infants born to unvaccinated mothers), foreign-born, or immigrants from areas with poor vaccination coverage. Endemic rubella rates increased and congenital rubella remains high in the Western Pacific, Southeast Asia, and some African regions where vaccination programs are not universal (Cherry and Baker, 2019).

If primary maternal rubella infection occurs during the first 12 weeks of pregnancy, there is an estimated 61% risk of congenital defects (ophthalmologic, cardiac, auditory, or neurologic); the risk is 26% if maternal infection occurs in the second trimester. In pregnant women, reinfection rarely results in congenital rubella syndrome. Accidental revaccination of a pregnant woman alone is not a reason for pregnancy termination; surveillance demonstrates signs of infection in the infant but not congenital rubella syndrome (Cherry and Baker, 2019).

Clinical Findings. Approximately 25% of infections are subclinical (Cherry and Baker, 2019). Postnatal disease is marked by three stages:
1. Prodrome: The mild symptoms of fever (101.5°F [38.6°C]), lower GI upset, sore throat, eye pain, arthralgia, malaise, and headache occur about 1 to 5 days prior to onset of stage 3 and are occasionally missed.
2. Lymphadenopathy: Usually begins within 24 hours, but can begin as early as 7 days before the rash appears, and lasts for more than 1 week. The postauricular, posterior cervical, and posterior occipital are the primary lymph nodes involved. There is generalized lymph node involvement, and at times splenomegaly is noted.
3. Rash: An enanthem (known as Forchheimer spots) can appear before the general rash, consisting of small rose-colored to reddish spots on the soft palate, but is not pathognomonic. The rubella rash (discrete maculopapules that occasionally coalesce) is often the first obvious sign of illness, typically begins on the face, can fade before it spreads to the chest and caudally during the next 24 hours, and is usually gone by the third day. There can be itching without a rash or a fine, bran-like desquamation. A low-grade fever can occur during the eruptive phase and continue for up to 3 days. There is no photophobia; anorexia, headache, and malaise are rare. Exanthems occur less often in adolescents and young adults; they may have more pruritus. A facial acneiform rash is more common in adolescents (Cherry and Baker, 2019).

Diagnostic Studies. Diagnosis is usually made by clinical symptoms. Real-time RT-PCR and RT-PCR of nasal or throat (preferred) specimens can detect this virus. Serologic testing for confirmation of disease or immunity includes enzyme immunoassays and latex agglutination tests for rubella IgG and IgM antibodies. However, timing is everything; IgM may not be detectable before the fifth day after the rash appears. If the test is conducted earlier and yields negative results, it should be repeated after day 5. To detect IgG antibody, the specimen should be obtained as soon after symptom onset as possible, and then repeated in 7 to 21 days. IgG antibody levels determine immune status due to natural infection or vaccination. False-positive rubella IgM tests can occur due to the presence of rheumatoid factors or other viral infections. Leukopenia is common.

Differential Diagnosis, Management, and Complications. The disease is difficult to diagnose unless there is an epidemic. The rash is similar to scarlet fever, mononucleosis, enterovirus, roseola, rubeola, erythema infectiosum, EBV, and drug eruptions.

Treatment is supportive (e.g., antipyretics for fever control) unless complications occur. Children with rubella should be kept at home for approximately 1 week after the rash erupts. Use active and passive immunization.

Complications of postnatal rubella are uncommon. These include arthralgia, arthritis, thrombocytopenia, and encephalitis. The arthralgia/arthritis (fingers, knees, wrists) occurs in postpubertal ages with females afflicted more often than males. Onset is about a week after appearance of rash and symptoms last 3 to 28 days. Thrombocytopenia or encephalitis can occur within 4 days of onset of rash. Severe thrombocytopenic purpura can be managed with corticosteroid therapy and platelet transfusions. Myocarditis, pericarditis, follicular conjunctivitis, hemolytic anemia, and hepatitis are rare.

Mosquito-Borne Viruses

Zika Virus

Zika is a member of the Flaviviridae family of viruses and is spread by the bite of the infected Aedes mosquito. It can be transmitted through sexual encounters, passed from a pregnant woman to her fetus, and through blood transfusions although this has not been reported in the United States. The virus may impact the growing fetus's brain resulting in microcephaly or other defects. In 2018, there were no reported local mosquito-borne Zika virus transmissions; however, the virus is an international threat. A map describing the risk of Zika is available for review prior to travel (CDC, 2018y).

Clinical Findings. Persons infected with the Zika virus have either no symptoms or mild symptoms such as low-grade fever, rash, headache, joint pain, conjunctivitis, and muscle pain that last several days to a week. Current CDC research suggests that Guillain-Barré syndrome is linked with Zika virus; however only a small proportion of persons with the disease are impacted. Infection is likely protective for future infections.

Diagnostic Studies. The virus' RNA is detectable in blood and urine early in the course of the disease or when symptomatic. Zika testing is recommended only if there are symptoms of Zika and travel to or living in a Zika risk area, or for unprotected sex with a partner who lives in or traveled to a Zika risk area. Test pregnant women who are asymptomatic but have ongoing exposure by living or traveling to high-risk areas or who have an abnormal ultrasound (CDC, 2018y).

Differential Diagnosis, Management, and Complications. Mild viral or influenza infection, GI viral infection, and other mosquito-borne diseases are included in the differential diagnosis for mild disease. For these mild cases, supportive treatment is indicated: rest, fever control with acetaminophen, hydration, and nausea/vomiting control. Hospitalization is indicated for those with symptoms of meningitis, encephalitis, severe muscle weakness, paralysis, or dysphagia.

Patient and Family Education. To prevent disease, avoid mosquito bites. Institute mosquito community abatement programs to reduce mosquito breeding grounds. Counseling includes:

- Stay indoors during the mosquitoes' most active times—dawn and dusk; if you must be outdoors during these times, wear light-colored, long-sleeved shirts and long pants.
- Apply insect repellent with either N,N-diethyl-3-methylbenzamide (DEET), picaridin 5% to 10%, oil of lemon eucalyptus, or soybean oil to exposed skin (permethrin and DEET can be applied to clothing). DEET concentration depends on time length of expected mosquito or tick exposure: 10% DEET confers approximately 2 hours of protection; 30% about 5 hours. Children over 6 months old may use a concentration of no more than 30% DEET. Apply according to length of protection needed. Use sparingly and wash DEET off with soap and water when the child is inside (AAP, 2018b).
- Do not use DEET on skin or clothing of children younger than 2 months old. Do not apply to face, hands, or open wounds/cuts (AAP, 2018b).
- Do not use combination sunscreen and DEET products because sunscreen needs to be reapplied more frequently; the DEET component applied too frequently can be toxic.
- Inventory outdoor areas for standing water mosquito breeding areas (e.g., old tires, pots or containers, birdbath [change once a week], neglected swimming pools, pool or spa covers). Keep pools and spas clean and chlorinated.
- Use tight-fitting screens on all doors and windows.
- Report any dead birds, especially crows, jays, hawks, magpies, and owls, to local health department or a pest control agency.

West Nile Virus

WNV is an arbovirus (family Flaviviridae) related to St. Louis and Japanese encephalitis viruses. Previously endemic to Africa, West Asia, and the Middle East, the virus has spread globally since 1999, including to the United States (with the exception of Alaska and Hawaii). It recurs yearly during warmer weather when mosquitoes begin breeding. WNV is mainly spread to people by bites from a variety of infected mosquitoes (most often the *Culex* genus in the United States).

Mosquitoes are infected by feeding on the blood of infected birds. They transfer the virus via saliva to other birds, horses, humans, and other animals. The level of viremia amplifies in the birds and a hallmark of the presence of WNV in communities is the die-off of specific bird species, notably ravens, crows, magpies, and jays. Bird-to-human transmission is not believed to occur unless dead infected birds are handled without precautions.

Clinical Findings. Symptoms develop 2 to 14 days after infected mosquito bites. The disease more frequently affects children aged 10 and older. Neuroinvasive disease affects less than 1% of cases, and mostly older adults, but can be severe and has a mortality rate of approximately 10% (CDC, 2018x).

The PCP needs to take seasonality, presentation, and virulence into consideration because symptoms mimic those of other mosquito-borne diseases, influenza, or GI infection, leading to misdiagnosis. About 20% of individuals exhibit illness signs and symptoms (CDC, 2018x), which are nonspecific and typically include fever, headache, muscle aches, rash, lymphadenopathy, weakness, anorexia, nausea, diarrhea, abdominal pain, and vomiting. Those with mild disease are typically asymptomatic within a week, but fatigue may linger for a few weeks.

Children with severe infection may experience high fever, headache, neck stiffness, stupor, disorientation, coma, tremors, convulsions, muscle weakness, vision loss, numbness, and paralysis. Most pregnant women who contract WNV deliver infants who show no signs of congenital WNV involvement. Examine the newborn closely for congenital anomalies, neurologic and hearing deficits, and signs of viral infection.

Diagnostic Studies. Consider testing children with a febrile or acute neurologic illness whose history includes exposure to mosquitoes, or prenatal exposure with or without breastfeeding. IgM antibody capture–enzyme-linked immunosorbent assay (MAC-ELISA) from serum or CFS collected is preferred by day 7 or 8 (more likely detectable) of clinical symptom onset. Collect serial titers 2 to 3 weeks apart to compare acute and convalescent samples. Confirm positive tests by other specific WNV tests; if tested early in the disease the virus's RNA may be detectable in the serum. MRI or CT scan (or both) are indicated if the individual has neurologic findings.

Differential Diagnosis, Management, and Complications. Mild viral or influenza infection, GI viral infection, aseptic meningitis, poliomyelitis, Guillain-Barré syndrome, dengue fever, chikungunya, St. Louis encephalitis, and acute flaccid paralysis are included in the differential diagnosis.

Supportive treatment is indicated for mild disease (rest, fever control, hydration, and control of nausea/vomiting). Hospitalization is indicated for those with neurological symptoms such as those from meningitis, encephalitis, severe muscle weakness, paralysis, dysphagia, or dysarthria.

Patient and Family Education. Avoid mosquito bites to prevent disease. A vaccine for humans is under development. See discussion in Zika virus section above.

Dengue Virus

Dengue virus (DENV) is an RNA virus belonging to the Flaviviridae family with four serotypes (DENV1, -2, -3, and -4). There is no cross immunity between serotypes; in fact, cross-reactivity occurs between serotypes that often intensify the disease in subsequent infections. Lifelong immunity-specific serotypes occur following infection. Serotypes DENV1 and DENV4 cause most primary infection; DENV2 and DENV3 are more likely to cause severe dengue hemorrhagic fever. Virus transmission is by a bite from an infected *Aedes aegypti* (less commonly *Aedes albopictus* or *Aedes polynesiensis*) mosquito. Humans pass the virus through blood transfusions, organ transplants, percutaneous exposure to blood, or transplacentally. An infected person can transmit the virus 2 days before symptom onset and during the 7-day period of viremia (this can threaten the blood supply, which is not currently screened for WNV in the United States) (Rios, 2018). The incubation period is 3 to 14 days.

Due to climate change, increased travel, returning military personnel, and emigration from tropical and subtropical regions, DENV and viral hemorrhagic fever increasingly occur in the United States, Europe, and other world regions. Multiple DENV serotypes make epidemics ubiquitous, occurring in more than 100 countries in the WHO regions of Africa, the Eastern Mediterranean, Southeast Asia, the Western Pacific, and the Americas. The latter three are the most seriously impacted regions. Endemic areas in the United States include Puerto Rico, the Virgin Islands, and American Samoa. Outbreaks have occurred in Texas, Hawaii, and Florida. Worldwide, approximately 284 million to 528 million people are infected each year (WHO, 2018e).

Clinical Findings. For suspected DENV infection, it is imperative to question children and families about travel or residence outside of the United States (including any military deployment), onset of fever, vaccination records, and any prior infections with DENV, WNV, St. Louis encephalitis virus, Japanese encephalitis virus, or yellow fever virus (these have cross-reacting antibodies). Inquire about past 24-hour fluid intake, changes in mental status, dizziness, urinary output, and diarrhea. Approximately 50% of infections are asymptomatic or have undifferentiated fever (often these are seen in young children or in those experiencing their first infection) (CDC, 2014). Three phases of infection occur:

- Febrile phase: Fever rises rapidly, lasts 2 to 7 days, and is greater than 102.2°F (39°C). This phase is classified as "dengue fever" and includes acute fever plus two or more of the following: headaches, retro-orbital pain, photophobia, general body ache, myalgia, arthralgia, facial flushing progressing to maculopapular or morbilliform rash, injected oral pharynx, leukopenia, anorexia, nausea/vomiting, diarrhea, mild epistaxis, bleeding gums, ecchymosis, bleeding at venipuncture sites, hepatomegaly, menorrhagia, or conjunctival injection. After this febrile phase, a person starts the recovery phase or continues to the critical phase (WHO, 2018e).
- Critical phase (mild to severe plasma leak): Begins 4 to 7 days after viral transmission and fever abatement and lasts 3 to 10 days. The hallmark is increased capillary permeability and plasma leakage. At this point, the infection may be classified as "dengue hemorrhagic fever," which has four requirements: prior fever of 2 to 7 days; spontaneous bleeding (a tourniquet test is sufficient); platelet count 100,000/mm³ or less; and evidence of anemia or a progression to "dengue shock syndrome"

(internal bleeding, shock, platelet count <50,000/mm³, hematocrit values ≥20% of normal for age/gender) (Garcia et al., 2015). The increased hematocrit is an important early sign to indicate severe disease as plasma leaks into body tissues. Other warning signs of progressing disease include lethargy, restlessness, confusion, vomiting, severe abdominal pain (GI bleeding), respiratory distress (pleural effusion), ascites, hepatitis, encephalitis, myocarditis, and blood pressure and volume changes. The critical phase may last 24 to 48 hours. The mortality rate reaches over 20% without aggressive treatment at this stage (WHO, 2018e).

- Recovery phase: Reabsorption of extravascular compartment fluid occurs over 48 to 72 hours. As other symptoms resolve, pruritus may occur; ascites, pulmonary and cardiac issues may arise if from overhydration with IV fluids; body systems and laboratory studies normalize.

Diagnostic Studies. A CBC, platelet count, and hematocrit are crucial. Progressive leukopenia is an early sign. A rapid, progressive decrease in platelet count and hematocrit rising elevation are early signs of plasma leakage. Hematuria may occur. A serum urea more than 4.0 mmol/L (indicates dehydration) and total protein 67.0 g/L or less (indicates plasma leakage into tissues) signify a child is at greater risk for hemorrhagic fever and shock syndrome (Garcia et al., 2015).

Viral isolation, serology, and molecular tests are available. However, it is a challenge to decide which test is most efficacious based upon the timing of symptoms, course of the disease, and if a specific serotype is needed. The CDC's Dengue Branch can be consulted to help with the decision.

Differential Diagnosis, Management, and Complications. Influenza, other hemorrhagic diseases, sepsis, meningococcemia, adenoviruses, HIV, chikungunya, infectious mononucleosis, measles, rubella, severe acute respiratory syndrome (SARS), malaria, Henoch-Schönlein purpura, or other thrombocytopenic purpura syndromes may present with some similar symptoms. It is noteworthy that DENV does not involve upper respiratory symptoms. The PCP must elicit details about onset of fever and rash, and use diagnostic studies to distinguish between the differential diagnoses.

Correct diagnosis and rapid treatment are crucial. In the United States, DENV is a nationally reportable disease to the CDC (2018r). Management is supportive, consisting of fluids to prevent dehydration (evaluate child's ability to take in adequate fluids and family's ability to care for child), antipyretics, and stringent monitoring for urinary output and bleeding. Infants or children with coexisting conditions should be hospitalized. Children should be seen daily during the febrile phase of this illness. Hospitalization is warranted for those showing signs of progressive disease (see Diagnostic Studies). WHO provides a downloadable guideline and useful algorithm for diagnosis and management (https://www.cdc.gov/dengue/index.html).

Dehydration and fever in children can result in neurological disturbances and febrile seizures. Severe dengue shock syndrome is a leading cause of serious illness and death among children younger than 5 years-old in some Asian and Latin American countries. Myocarditis, pancreatitis, hepatitis, and neuroinvasive disease can occur. Aggressive treatment brought the mortality rate down to less than 1% (WHO, 2018e).

Patient and Family Education. To prevent disease, avoid mosquito bites (see Zika discussion). Community-wide efforts largely focus on controlling vectors with insecticides. There is ongoing effort to develop a dengue vaccine.

Hantavirus Pulmonary Syndrome

Hantavirus pulmonary syndrome (HPS), formerly referred to as *Hantaviru* and commonly called Sin Nombre virus (SNV) in the United States, is 1 of 23 Hantaviruses found worldwide that cause considerable morbidity and mortality (Chapman et al., 2019). The virus reservoirs include Old and New World rats, mice, voles, and lemmings, mostly in rural areas; the deer mouse is the most common reservoir in North America. Disease is spread by aerosolization of the rodent's saliva, urine, and feces excretions. Because of the widespread distribution and the role of these rodents in biodiversity, eradication is neither feasible nor desirable. Most cases in the United States occur in the spring and summer months but this can vary depending on location and rodent population.

Incidence of HPS is rare in the United States; less than 7% of cases occur in children younger than 17 years old. Thirty-four states in the United States reported cases in 2013, with 95% of those states located west of the Mississippi River (CDC, 2017f). In 2011, HPS resulted in similar mortality rates of about 35% in both the United States and the Americas (Chapman et al., 2019).

Providers should suspect HPS infection in a child with an ill-defined febrile disease (or FUO) with abdominal or back pain or myalgia; who lives in or has been in an appropriate rural, endemic geographic HPS setting; has thrombocytopenia or proteinuria; or has been exposed to rodents or engaged in an activity where rodent nests or excreta may have been disturbed (e.g., cleaning out barns or sheds). The incubation period is typically 4 to 42 days after exposure to infected rodent excreta. The illness typically involves a prodromal phase of abrupt fever, chills, headache, nausea, vomiting, diarrhea, and myalgia (notably of shoulders, lower back, and upper legs) for 3 to 7 days followed by abrupt onset of pulmonary edema, cardiac decompensation, and hypotension. On physical examination, restlessness; flushed face, neck, and upper thorax; injected conjunctiva and pharynx; bradycardia; and petechiae may be seen. There is early thrombocytopenia and leukocytosis with a shift to the left; proteinuria and hematuria may also occur.

The diagnosis is confirmed by detecting hanta-specific IgG and IgM antibodies to SNV using ELISA; RT-PCR also detects SNV RNA. A rapid diagnostic test is available. Those with suspected HPS need to be hospitalized for supportive management of pulmonary edema, hypoxemia, and hypotension. Generally, the acute illness is followed by a prolonged convalescence period of 3 to 6 weeks, then by complete recovery.

The differential diagnosis includes rickettsial diseases, leptospirosis, influenza, streptococcal pneumonia, legionellosis, *Yersinia pestis* infection (plague), meningococcemia, brucellosis, mycoplasmal and fungal pneumonias (including *Coccidioides immitis* and *Histoplasma* pneumonia), tularemia, psittacosis, and autoimmune disorders (including thrombotic thrombocytopenic purpura).

Human avoidance of rodent waste and nests is the goal with this disease. Before people work around mouse-infested basements or outbuildings, they should know the guideline about cleaning up after rodents, which is available on the CDC (2017f) website. Chemoprophylaxis or vaccines are not available.

Additional Noteworthy Viruses in Circulation

Human Pneumovirus (Metapneumovirus)

Metapneumovirus (human pneumovirus; hMPV) is a respiratory pathogen of the Paramyxoviridae family, discovered in 2001. Its antigenicity, symptomatology, and epidemiology are closely related to RSV, including a simultaneous (and expanded) seasonal pattern. This agent should be considered as a causative agent of acute respiratory infection among hospitalized children before their second birthday, especially in the late winter/early spring months in temperate climates. Incidence rates range from 5% to 25% in those with acute lower respiratory tract infections. Approximately 95% to 100% of all 5-year-old children are seropositive for this agent with the majority being seropositive by 2 years old (Schuster and Williams, 2019). Symptoms of hMPV include fever, transient maculopapular rash, vomiting/diarrhea, rhinitis, wheezing/stridor, tachypnea, abnormal tympanic membranes, pharyngitis, hoarseness, rhonchi, rales, and hypoxia. Asthma may cause exacerbation. Chest x-rays demonstrate diffuse perihilar infiltrates, peribronchial cuffing, lobar infiltrates, or hyperaeration. Viral shedding is approximately 7 to 14 days. The differential is RSV, parainfluenza, and influenza. Immunoassays, RT-PCR, and serology tests are diagnostic. Treatment is supportive; acute respiratory distress requires hospitalization. Ribavirin has had limited application in cases involving immunocompromised children (Schuster and Williams, 2019). A vaccine is under development. Complications include AOM or bacterial pneumonia.

Human Calicivirus Infections (Norovirus and Sapovirus)

Norovirus (also called *Hunter virus* and *Norwalk-like virus*) and Sapovirus belong to the Caliciviridae family. These viruses are highly contagious and occur in closed populations, such as in child care centers, schools, camps, cruise ships, hotels, or other closed facilities. Norovirus accounts for about 80% to 90% of the sporadic gastroenteritis epidemics in children younger than 5 years old and it causes 20% of diarrheal illness hospitalizations. Most children have antibodies by the time they are 5 years old (Lucero and O'Ryan, 2019). Transmission is through the fecal-oral route, through contaminated water, or by food contaminated by infected food handlers (notably salads, shellfish, ice, and a variety of ready-to-eat foods [e.g., prepared fruit, bakery products]). Children can acquire norovirus from contaminated water in public swimming pools, wading pools, water parks, and from flooding where fresh water and sewage mingle. The incubation period is 12 to 60 hours (average 24 hours); the illness duration is typically 24 to 48 hours (5 to 6 days in endemic settings); and the virus is excreted for 15 days to 2 months after symptom onset. Symptoms include nausea, vomiting, nonbloody diarrhea, abdominal cramps, chills, headache, muscle aches, and fatigue; some individuals experience low-grade fever. Vomiting is more pronounced in children over 1 year old whereas diarrhea is more prominent in infants and adults (Lucero and O'Ryan, 2019).

Stool specimens are negative for bacterial, parasitic, or fungal pathogens. Diagnosis is made with real-time quantitative RT-PCR assay. Enzyme immunoassays are readily available but useful only during gastroenteritis outbreaks. In these circumstances, negative results do not exclude *Norovirus,* and the newer RT-PCR test should be performed.

Treatment is supportive, including rehydration, as dehydration is a serious complication of norovirus infection. There is no antiviral treatment or vaccine. Preventive measures include training child care and school personnel, food handlers, and children/caregivers in good hand washing and other hygienic measures (cleaning surfaces with sodium hypochlorite solution or 70% ethanol). Precautions when in public recreational water facilities include not swimming with diarrhea; not swallowing the water; washing children's perianal area with soap and water before going into the water; and taking children for frequent bathroom breaks and diaper checks. This illness can recur.

Coronaviruses

Multiple strains of human coronaviruses (HCoVs) cause a variety of respiratory tract infections in humans. Not all of the strains are epidemiologically or clinically understood. It is postulated that a strain(s) of coronaviruses may be an enteric pathogen and play a causative role in infants with gastroenteritis and necrotizing enterocolitis (Poutanen, 2018). HCoVs are likely transmitted by a combination of droplet and direct and indirect contact. After rhinoviruses, they are the most common cause of the common cold. Depending upon the strain, some are associated with AOM, asthma exacerbations, croup, bronchiolitis, pneumonia, gastroenteritis, nausea/vomiting, and febrile seizures. The severe acute respiratory syndrome coronavirus (SARS-CoV) strain leads to more severe disease.

SARS-CoV is one of the coronaviruses that is better understood, largely due to being the causative strain of a worldwide outbreak in late 2003 (no cases since 2004). After mucosal inoculation, this virus replicates in the lung and GI tract and ultimately leads to clinical deterioration. Fortunately, children are infected less by this strain; when they are infected, their illness is milder than those of adolescents and adults. The U.S. National Select Agent Registry Program declared SARS coronavirus as having the potential to pose a severe threat to public health and safety (CDC, 2017h).

The incubation period for HCoV strains is a few days (SARS-CoV ranges from 2 to 10 days); HCoV strains typically transmit in the first 2 to 5 days of illness (it is more intense during the second week of illness). Outbreaks occur during the winter and spring in temperate climates (winter for SARS).

HCoVs are not typically diagnosed from respiratory tract specimens; however, some specialized laboratories offer comprehensive diagnostic testing based on RT-PCR and can identify HCoV. Antibody tests are available for SARS-CoV.

Management is supportive, although SARS-CoV infection involves strict isolation of the index case, respiratory precautions (hand hygiene, gloves, masks), and home isolation of index cases and their caregivers. Drug treatments are under development. Prevention of transmission is the same for other respiratory infections.

Potential Emerging and Reemerging Viruses on the Horizon

Based upon data and statistical modeling, there is speculation about what "candidate diseases" appear or reappear, taking into consideration such factors as: global climate changes, increasing international travel, known vectors, increasing drug resistance (notably to HIV, TB, malaria, and pathogens causing pneumonia, sepsis, skin and urinary tract infections), decreased vaccination levels, importation of wild animals (that serve as vectors), and bioterrorism. Among others factors to be considered are the migration of the mosquito as a vector of flaviviruses (dengue fever, Japanese encephalitis, and yellow fever), chikungunya (an alphavirus), St. Louis encephalitis, and La Crosse encephalitis. Other emerging and re-emerging viruses worldwide include Das-Congo hemorrhagic fever virus, HIV 1 and 2, monkeypox, and other hemorrhagic fever diseases.

Middle Eastern Respiratory Syndrome

Identified in 2012, all cases of Middle Eastern respiratory syndrome coronavirus (MERS-CoV) are linked to countries in and near the Arabian Peninsula. Few cases have been diagnosed in the United States; those identified were in healthcare workers exposed to the virus in Saudi Arabia. The CDC continues to monitor and study this virus in efforts to better understand it because of its potential to spread to the United States. In the Middle Eastern countries, the illness occurs in all ages. Symptoms are predominately fever, cough, and shortness of breath progressing to acute respiratory illness. The mortality rate ranges from 30% to 40% (CDC, 2016e).

Monitoring the Global Spread of Viruses

Global Viral (GV) (formerly the Global Viral Forecasting Initiative) is an international organization that monitors the emergence of deadly viruses spread from animals to humans to address the most important global infectious disease threats and detect emerging pandemics. Among its current activities, this organization supports international research, public health development and education, and scientific leadership. One GV goal is to increase the "bank of genetic information" from known viruses in order to develop vaccines to stop the disease spread. Newer technologies are being developed to more quickly sequence and identify the genetic identity of viruses. GV and global partners have numerous "viral listening posts" in sub-Saharan Africa and Southeast Asia, where pandemics often start. Air travel and road development increase the transmission of these potentially dangerous viruses.

Parasitic-Caused Disease: Malaria

Malaria is spread worldwide by the bite of the nocturnal-feeding female *Anopheles* genus of mosquito. This mosquito is the vector for the five different species of the intraerythrocytic parasite, *Plasmodium,* that infects humans. Poorer tropical and sub-tropical areas of the world experience malaria in epidemic proportions. In the United States, infection is typically acquired from travel or residence abroad, although anopheline mosquitoes are present in temperate regions of the country. Globally, an estimated 198 million cases of malaria were identified in 2013; 500,000 people died of malaria, mostly children in the African region (CDC, 2018m). Infection relapses occur because of dormant liver stage parasites (hypnozoite) or chronic asymptomatic parasitemia.

Malaria presents as a febrile nonspecific illness without localizing signs from 7 to 30 days after exposure. Malaria should be suspected in a person with a fever who recently traveled to an endemic area. Symptoms typically include high fever with chills, rigor, sweats, and headache, and may appear suddenly and in a 2- to 3-day cyclic pattern. Nausea, vomiting, diarrhea, cough, pallor, jaundice, tachypnea, arthralgia, myalgia, abdominal and back pain, and hepatosplenomegaly may occur. The disease progresses in severity and ends in death as a result of neurologic compromise, renal and respiratory failure, metabolic acidosis, severe anemia, or vascular collapse and shock.

Diagnostic studies may show anemia, thrombocytopenia, elevated bilirubin, and aminotransferases. Diagnosis is confirmed by identifying the parasite microscopically. Negative smears should be retested every 12 to 24 hours during a 72-hour period. PCR, DNA probes, and RNA testing are also used. A rapid test for antigen detection is available.

Choice of treatment is dependent upon the identified species, possible drug resistance, and severity of disease. Assistance with diagnosis and management is available from the 24-hour CDC Malaria Hotline (770-488-7788). Research focuses on using imidazopyrazine chemicals to disable an enzyme necessary for replication. Vaccines and new drugs to combat malaria are under development and in clinical trials.

In malaria-epidemic regions, treatment and preventive efforts involve four measures: (1) case management (diagnosis and treatment), (2) insecticide-treated nets (ITNs), (3) intermittent preventive treatment of malaria in pregnant women (IPTp) and infants (IPTi), and (4) indoor residual spraying (IRS). Larval and other vector control, mass drug administration, and mass fever treatment may also be used (see WHO in Additional Resources). The CDC offers useful information regarding traveler risk assessment, antimalarial drug prophylaxis selection for children and adults, a malaria country map, and preventive measures.

Tick-Borne Diseases

Lyme disease, ehrlichiosis, anaplasmosis, RMSF, tick-borne relapsing fever, babesiosis, tularemia, and African tick bite fever are common tick-borne diseases in the United States. It is important for providers to know the specific tick vectors and vector epidemic geographic areas. Only the first three diseases are discussed here (tularemia is a potential bioterrorism agent). PCPs should be suspicious of and include tick-borne diseases in the differential diagnosis for individuals with influenza-like symptoms (fever, headache, myalgia) during summer (an unusual time for such symptoms), especially if they live and recreate outdoors in endemic areas.

Lyme Disease

Borrelia burgdorferi (Bb), a spirochete, is the causative agent that is transmitted to humans by infected species of *Ixodes* ticks. Lyme disease is the most commonly reported vector-borne infection in the United States and Europe.

The ticks infected with *Bb* in the United States are predominantly found in the northeast, the mid-Atlantic states, Wisconsin, Minnesota, and Northern California (Moore, 2015). Scandinavian countries and central Europe (Germany, Austria, and Switzerland) also report Lyme disease (LD). It is estimated that as many as 300,000 people are diagnosed in the United States each year (CDC, 2017g). When eastern black-legged deer tick *(Ixodes scapularis)* or western black-legged deer tick *(Ixodes pacificus)* larvae hatch in early summer, they are usually not infected. During their life cycle (nymphal and adult molt stages), the tick feeds on an infected host and becomes infected with *Bb*. In the east, the natural host for *Bb* is the white-footed mouse or deer; in the west, it is the western gray squirrel or western fence lizard, less so chipmunks and some bird species (they are poor reservoirs). Tick vectors in Europe include ground-feeding birds and small to medium-sized mammals. The infected tick transmits the organism to humans, more commonly by immature ticks in the nymphal stage. The size of the tick in the nymphal stage is about 1 mm (poppy seed size); in the adult stages from 2.5 mm to 4 mm (sesame seed size).

There is varied risk of transmission, depending on the percentage of ticks infected with *Bb*. Annual confirmed incidence rates vary (in 2014, a high of 87 per 100,000 cases was reported in Maine) (CDC, 2015a). Boys 5 to 9 years old have higher incidence rates than all other ages (CDC, 2015b). Coinfection with other tick-borne pathogens must be considered in endemic regions. The risk of human infection after an *Ixodes* tick bite is low, even in endemic areas (1.2% to 4.4%) (Sood and Krause, 2019) and is related to how long the tick feeds. It takes hours for the tick to fully implant its mouth into the host's skin and days to become fully engorged. Nymphal ticks must feed for 36 to 48 hours or more and adult ticks for 48 to 72 hours before the risk of transmission of *Bb* is significant; many human victims remove the tick before this time. Because of the small size of the tick and body location where it lodges (e.g., scalp), an engorged tick may not be noticed before it drops off. The disease is not teratogenic as long as the mother receives the appropriate antibiotic treatment (CDC, 2015b). The majority of infections occur from June to August, less so from December through March.

Clinical Findings. Lyme disease presents with a variety of symptoms. Only 25% to 30% of people diagnosed recall having a tick bite (CDC, 2018m). Classic Lyme disease has three stages:

1. Stage 1 (early localized disease): Generally within 1 to 2 weeks after the bite, a typical rash appears at the inoculation site (range from 1 to 31 days; mean 10 days). Erythema migrans (EM) rash begins as a red, annular macule or papule at the tick bite site that progresses over 24 to 48 hours to being surrounded by a clear ring and then a larger annular erythematous outer ring. It may appear as a "bull's-eye" and needs to be at least 5 cm in size to meet diagnostic criteria for EM (Fig 31.5). Multiple lesions may occur in different sites; however, 10% of children do not demonstrate EM (Sood and Krause, 2019). EM typically is warm and pruritic, but not painful. The rash remains for a few weeks and fades even if untreated. In many cases, the rash does not follow this classic pattern but instead may resemble nummular eczema, tinea, granuloma annulare, an insect bite, or cellulitis; the rapid enlargement of EM helps distinguish it. Those without EM and 50% with EM present with flu-like symptoms including fever, malaise, headache, arthralgia, myalgia, and stiff neck (CDC, 2018m). Without treatment, these symptoms, including the rash, become intermittent, lasting for weeks to months.

2. Stage 2 (early disseminated disease): Through spirochetemia, the organism disseminates through hematologic or lymphatic channels. Secondary annular lesions (1 to 3 cm) appear that are morphologically similar to, but smaller than, the EM lesion. Symptoms in children with disseminated disease present as neurologic (frequent headaches; lethargy; neck pain; mood swings; irritability; neuralgia; paresthesia; and motor or sensory impairment, mostly affecting cervical and thoracic dermatomes; cranial neuropathies [especially seventh nerve palsy in children]), cardiac (Lyme carditis, presenting as syncope and malaise), and generalized illness (stomachaches, urinary symptoms, migratory musculoskeletal pains). Stage 2 lasts from weeks to 2 years without treatment. Most of the symptoms (including the rash) wax and wane during this time.

3. Stage 3 (late disease): Stage 3 usually begins with pauciarticular or monoarticular arthritis that occurs weeks to months after the initial tick bite; chronic neurologic symptoms occur in 5% of those untreated (cognitive and memory loss, paresthesias in hands and feet). The knees are most commonly affected. The joints are erythematous, hot, and edematous, but not as painful as other types of bacterial arthritis. Untreated, the arthritis initially resolves in a few weeks but becomes recurrent, migratory (but rarely to small joints), and chronic. Adolescents experience more severe arthritis for longer periods of time (Sood and Krause, 2019). Untreated, late manifestation of the disease appear months to years after the initial infection.

Diagnostic Studies. The IDSA and CDC (2018m) provide guidelines for the diagnosis and treatment of LD. It is best

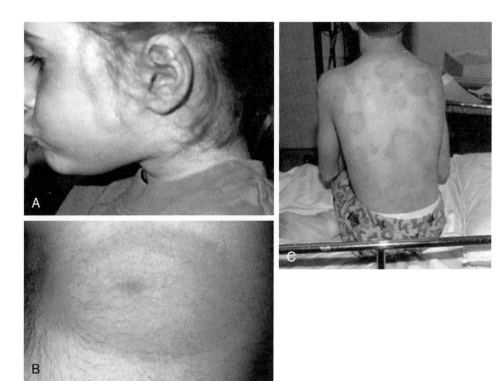

• **Fig 31.5** Erythema Migrans (EM) of Lyme Disease. (A) Erythema migrans (EM) scalp lesion only partially visible on the face. (B) EM oval lesion. (See companion Expert Consult website for color version.) (C) EM dark annular lesion. (From Cherry, JD, Demmler-Harrison G, Kaplan S, et al. *Feigin and Cherry's Textbook of Pediatric Infectious Diseases.* 8th ed. Philadelphia: Saunders/Elsevier; 2019. [A -C] Courtesy Vijay Sikand, MD. All images reproduced from Sood SK, editor. *Lyme Borreliosis in Europe and North America: Epidemiology and Clinical Practice.* Hoboken, NJ: John Wiley and Sons; 2011.)

diagnosed by clinical and epidemiologic history and physical findings. The presence of EM is diagnostic; no serologic test is necessary. If the provider suspects LD without EM, they should keep in mind several factors: First, serologic tests for IgM antibodies become positive 2 to 4 weeks (4 to 6 weeks for IgG) after a bite. Because of false-positive results, serological tests should not be routinely used for screening. Finally, serologically positive results may indicate prior infection rather than present acute infection because IgM antibodies do not decline until 4 to 6 months after disease onset, and IgG antibodies remains elevated for years (CDC, 2018m).

The CDC (2018m) recommends a two-step approach to serologic testing. The first step is enzyme immunoassay (ELISA) or (rarely) indirect IFA. If results are negative, the second step is not needed. If the first test results are positive or equivocal, a second test using an IgM and IgG Western blot for *Bb* antibodies is done for an individual with symptoms for less than 30 days. If symptoms are present more than 30 days, an IgG Western blot test alone is performed. A positive Western blot test is interpreted as reacting with 5 to 10 scored bands on the IgG assay and 2 to 3 on the IgM assay. The number of bands necessary for confirmation of LD is controversial. The ELISA produces many false-positives because of cross-reactions with other spirochetes, lupus, and varicella organisms. After 4 weeks of symptoms, the IgG result should only be used to support the diagnosis (CDC, 2018m).

Differential Diagnosis, Management, and Complications. The rash, if present, may suggest eczema, tinea, granuloma annulare, cellulitis, or an insect bite. Other differential diagnoses include osteomyelitis, WNV, parvovirus B19, relapsing fever, syphilis, leptospirosis, *Mycoplasma*, septic arthritis, infectious

hepatitis, nonresponsive lymphadenopathy, meningitis, multiple sclerosis, amyotrophic lateral sclerosis, juvenile arthritis, Bell palsy, other spirochete-caused diseases, thyroid disease, heavy metal toxicity, and vasculitis. Primary psychiatric disorders should be considered in recalcitrant cases after appropriate Lyme treatment.

Clinical judgment determines whether to treat a patient. The earlier in the EM stage that treatment starts, the better the long-term outcome. In suspicious LD cases, delaying treatment until laboratory results are known decreases the chances of successful disease treatment. The provider should study the literature from the CDC and IDSA, or consult with an infectious disease specialist if uncertain how to proceed.

Give prophylactic doxycycline, amoxicillin, or cefuroxime in children when the history includes the following (Moore, 2015):
- Tick bite only: The tick is reliably identified as a nymph or adult *I. scapularis* species (providers in endemic areas should have expertise identifying, and most commercial and public health laboratories in endemic areas can make this determination), the tick was attached for at least 36 to 72 hours (as indicated by engorgement size or known exposure time), *and* the tick was acquired in an endemic area. For treatment, see drugs and dosages under early, localized disease or EM.
  - If a tick was removed but cannot be identified as an *Ixodes* nor the attachment timeline verified, prophylaxis should not be given. Give the child and caregivers guidance about the signs and symptoms of EM and localized disease. Should these develop within 30 days, the child should be considered for diagnostic tests and treatment of the disease (Moore, 2015).
- Early localized disease (stage 1) or EM usually resolves within several days of starting treatment. Drugs and dosages

(Kimberlin et al., 2018) can be found at https://www.cdc.gov/lyme/treatment/index.html and presently are:

- Younger than 8 years old: Amoxicillin 50 mg/kg/day, orally, divided into 3 doses for 14 days (maximum 1.5 g/day)
- 8 years or older: Doxycycline: single 200 mg dose daily or 4 mg/kg/day divided into two doses PO for 14 days (maximum 200 mg/day). Give a small snack with doxycycline to reduce nausea.
- For children unable to take amoxicillin or doxycycline: cefuroxime 30 mg/kg/day, orally, divided into two doses for 14 days (maximum 1000 mg/day) is preferable.
- Early or late disseminated disease: Consult with a Lyme disease specialist.

Post-Lyme disease syndrome causes persistent subjective symptoms that some experience after treatment. Some providers speculate that this is a chronic form of the infection with its own diagnostic criteria and treatment approaches (CDC, 2018m). In children, lingering fatigue, musculoskeletal pain, or cognitive or short-term memory difficulties occur and may be due to persistent immune-mediated inflammation rather than continued *Bb* infection b. A child with chronic symptoms whose family attributes them to LD should be questioned about prior treatment adherence, reevaluated for reinfection, and referred to appropriate specialists as indicated by symptomatology. A positive serologic finding without other symptoms of clinical disease does not warrant the use of antibiotics (Sood and Krause, 2019).

Complications include Lyme meningitis, myocarditis, myopericarditis, left ventricular dysfunction, or cardiomegaly. Other tick-borne diseases can be co-transmitted with Lyme disease (human babesiosis and human granulocytic anaplasmosis).

Patient and Family Education. Avoid tick-infested areas whenever possible. If in such areas, follow previously described tick repellent strategies using DEET. Shower after being outdoors, and inspect the entire body carefully every day during the tick season (special attention to armpit, groin, back, and scalp areas). Spray permethrin on clothing and wear light-colored long pants (tucked into socks or shoes), long sleeves, and a hat. Chronic absorption of insecticides can produce toxicity, especially in children; however, when used according to directions, children older than 2 months can safely use DEET. Picaridin (KBR 3023) and plant-based oil of eucalyptus are alternative repellents. Families should know how to remove ticks safely; removed ticks should be saved in a dry container and brought with the child for identification. Pets should be checked each day and ticks removed if found.

Ehrlichiosis and Anaplasmosis

Both ehrlichiosis and anaplasmosis are caused by distinct species of obligate intracellular bacteria carried by the lone star tick (*Amblyomma americanum,* of which there are two species, for ehrlichial infections) and the black-legged or deer tick (*I. scapularis,* for anaplasmosis). The southeast, south-central, and west Texas are common ehrlichiosis endemic areas in the United States. Anaplasma infections are reported more commonly in the northeast, Midwest states, and the same regions in which Lyme disease occurs; the provider must always consider a coinfection with Lyme disease or babesiosis and anaplasmosis. Any individual with a history of tick exposure in an endemic area, a nonspecific rapid onset febrile illness from May through October, and some of the following symptoms should be evaluated for ehrlichiosis or anaplasmosis. Children increasingly acquire these diseases, which are most likely underreported (Lantos and McKinney, 2019). The

incubation period for both diseases ranges from 7 to 14 days after a tick bite.

Both infections produce similar acute, systemic symptoms in about half of cases: fever, headache, myalgia, malaise, chills, nausea, and anorexia. Less common symptoms include diarrhea and vomiting, weight loss, arthralgia, cough, and mental status changes. A rash occurs in about 60% of infected ehrlichiosis children and rarely occurs with *Anaplasma* (CDC, 2018v). The rash (petechial, macular, or maculopapular and distinguishable from that of RMSF) varies in appearance, generally involves the trunk with sparing of the hands and feet, and appears about a week after the onset of other symptoms.

Diagnosis is made using an IFA assay to determine IgG antibody specific titers on a blood sample tested during the acute and convalescent periods (2 to 4 weeks apart). Titers are then compared. The gold standard is a fourfold increase in the antibody titer between assays; titers may be negative in the first 7 to 10 days of the illness. DNA by PCR assay titer can also be used. Other laboratory tests show similar results: leukopenia (relative and absolute lymphopenia and a left shift), neutropenia, anemia, or thrombocytopenia with elevated hepatic transaminases in the first week of clinical illness. Pleocytosis with predominance of lymphocytes and increased total protein is commonly seen in CSF samples.

The differential diagnosis for ehrlichiosis and anaplasmosis includes RMSF, Lyme disease, other tick-borne illnesses (e.g., babesiosis, Colorado tick fever, relapsing fever, and tularemia), dengue, malaria, enteroviruses, adenoviruses, sepsis, and toxic shock syndrome.

The treatment of choice for both infections, to be started before laboratory confirmation, is doxycycline *for all* ages given the life-threatening nature of these illnesses: 100 lb (45.4 kg) or more: 100 mg twice daily PO or IV for 10 to 14 days to cover Lyme disease; less than 100 lb, 2.2 mg/kg per dose twice daily PO/IV (maximum dose is 100 mg). Data suggest that discoloration of permanent teeth is not significant if doxycycline is taken for 14 days or less (CDC, 2018v). Treatment response should occur within 1 week.

Systemic complications include pulmonary infiltrates, bone marrow hypoplasia, respiratory failure, encephalopathy, meningitis, DIC, spontaneous hemorrhage, and renal failure. The mortality rate for ehrlichiosis is about 3%, and anaplasmosis is about 0.5% (Lantos and McKinney, 2019). Recovery is usually complete after 1 to 2 weeks; some children with systemic disease have residual neurologic difficulties. Prevention is the same as that for Lyme disease. Prophylaxis is not recommended due to the low risk of infection.

Rocky Mountain Spotted Fever

Rickettsia rickettsii, a nonmotile, pleomorphic, weakly gram-negative coccobacillus, is the etiologic agent of RMSF. In the United States, it is the most severe rickettsial disease and most common vector-borne disease after Lyme disease (Reller and Dumler, 2016). Vectors for *R. rickettsii* include the American dog tick (*Dermacentor variabilis*) found in the eastern and central United States, the Rocky Mountain wood tick (*Dermacentor andersoni;* also the vector for Colorado tick fever and tularemia) found in the Rocky Mountain states and west, and the brown dog tick (*Rhipicephalus sanguineus*) recently reported in eastern Arizona. Southwestern Canada, Mexico, and Central and South America also have reported cases.

In the United States, RMSF was historically centered in northern Rocky Mountain states but it is now found in all contiguous states except Maine and Vermont. Sixty percent of cases are located in North Carolina, Tennessee, Arkansas, Missouri, and Oklahoma (CDC, 2018u). The incidence continues to increase (6 cases per million in 2010 [CDC, 2018u]). RMSF is most common in spring and summer months when ticks are most active (peak is June and July). The incubation period is 2 to 14 days. The longer the tick is attached, the more likely *R. rickettsii* is to be transmitted. Prompt removal of a tick is important to lower the chance of infection.

Clinical Findings. Symptoms include the following: fever (104°F [40°C]; occurs in up to 98% of children), chills, severe headache, myalgias, malaise, GI upset/tenderness, diarrhea, cough, conjunctival injection, photophobia, and altered mental status. Focal neurologic deficits (e.g., paralysis, transient deafness) appear with disease progression. Most individuals (90%) develop a maculopapular rash, typically 2 to 5 days after fever onset (CDC, 2018u). The rash begins as small, flat, nonpruritic, faintly pink spots on the wrists, forearms, and ankles, then spreads to the trunk (sometimes to palms and soles). It may be easily missed in dark-skinned individuals. On day 6 or later, a petechial rash, a sign of progressive disease, may appear. Only 60% of individuals recall having removed a tick (Reller and Dumler, 2016).

Diagnostic Studies. The most rapidly available diagnostic aid is immunohistochemical staining or PCR testing performed on a skin biopsy of petechial or macular lesions to look for *R. rickettsii*. The diagnostic gold standard is IFA on paired serologic samples taken in the first week and 2 to 4 weeks later. A fourfold change in IgG-specific antibody titer is typical. However, antibody titers may be negative in the first 7 to 10 days of the illness.

Diagnostic studies also show diffuse vascular injury characterized by thrombocytopenia (<150,000 platelets/μL), mild to moderate hyponatremia (<130 mEq/mL), leukocytosis as the disease progresses (a left-shift), and anemia. Mildly elevated hepatic transaminase levels may be found.

Differential Diagnoses. The differential diagnoses include enteroviral infections, adenoviral infections, meningococcemia, influenza, gram-negative bacterial sepsis, toxic shock syndrome, measles, rubella, secondary syphilis, leptospirosis, typhoid fever, disseminated gonococcal infection, immune thrombocytopenic purpura, thrombotic thrombocytopenic purpura, immune complex vasculitis (e.g., SLE), infectious mononucleosis, hypersensitivity reaction to drugs, murine typhus, rickettsialpox, recrudescent typhus, and sylvatic *R. prowazekii* infection (Lantos and McKinney, 2019).

Management. It is important to start antibiotic treatment prior to the onset of the rash and within the first 5 days if other clinical symptoms suggest RMSF, especially because of possible early false-negative serology. Without early treatment, the disease rapidly progresses to death. Lantos and McKinney (2019) provide the following guidance:

- If the child appears in the summer in an endemic area (with or without history of exposure to a tick or dog) with an acute fever of less than 2 days but without profound malaise/myalgia/headache, obtain a CBC and chemistry panel and monitor the child.
- If the fever progresses to the third day and laboratory studies suggest RMSF, or if the child appears toxic, empiric antibiotics should be started. Although conjunctival injection and

peripheral edema may appear at the same time as the rash, their presence points toward a diagnosis of RMSF.

Treatment consists of doxycycline *for all* ages for 7 to 10 days. Children under 100 lb (45.4 kg): 2.2 mg/kg per dose given twice daily PO or IV; children over 100 lb: 100 mg twice daily PO or IV (maximum dose for all is 100 mg per dose). Doxycycline does not pose a significant risk considering the mortality associated with this disease (CDC, 2018u).

Complications and Patient and Family Education. Complications include short- or long-term neurologic deficits (e.g., speech and swallowing dysfunction, global encephalopathy, gait disturbances, and cortical blindness). Digit loss due to autoamputation can occur. Untreated, the fatality rate is about 20%; for those treated, the rate is about 5% (Lantos and McKinney, 2019). For prevention, see prior discussion under Lyme disease.

Bacterial Infections

Although less common than viral diseases, bacterial infections allow for interventions (including antibiotics) that decrease the course of an illness and prevent subsequent complications. Many bacterial infections are diagnosed clinically and treated empirically. A good understanding of the pathophysiology of common bacterial infections, and knowledge of the most likely organisms, allows for efficient and effective treatment. Bacterial infections of the skin and soft tissues, lymphadenitis, osteomyelitis, fasciitis, pneumonia, meningitis, infectious diarrhea, and UTI are discussed in other chapters; fungal infections and parasitic infections are also discussed in other chapters.

Community-Acquired Methicillin-Resistant Staphylococcus aureus

PCPs should know the prevalence of community-acquired methicillin-resistant *S. aureus* (CA-MRSA) to effectively treat severe pneumonia, cellulitis, osteomyelitis, myositis, bacteremia, endocarditis, empyema, meningitis, scalded skin syndrome, toxic shock syndrome, deep tissue abscesses (especially those that come on quickly), spider bites, skin and soft tissue infections, and necrotizing fasciitis. CA-MRSA is often the cause of purulent skin and soft tissue infections in the United States (CDC, 2016d). It is increasingly implicated as the causative agent in pneumonia in younger age groups and in those without other underlying risk factors for pneumonia. CA-MRSA has novel elements. It has an altered penicillin-binding protein with decreased sensitivity to all β-lactam antibiotics except for ceftaroline. With a combination of this protein and specific genetic encoding for cytotoxicity (affects the degree of virulence), the *S. aureus* strains are invading the tissues with toxin release that triggers the inflammatory cascade and causes tissue necrosis (Daum, 2018; Liu et al., 2011).

The following history and physical findings place healthy individuals at risk of acquired CA-MRSA infection:

- Boil, furuncle, or abscess without draining pus that is erythematous, warm, painful; onset may be rapid (key finding).
- Treatment failure with a β-lactam agent. If individual has been in contact with a cat, consider cat-scratch disease as a differential diagnosis.
- Other family members have similar skin infections.
- Recent history of skin infection, even if it was responsive to a β-lactam agent.
- Neonate with skin or soft tissue infection.

- Skin lesion looks like a spider bite; larger lesions are suspicious for MRSA.
- Pus is present.
- History of recurrent small, nontender, nonpruritic maculopapular lesions that become pruritic or painful; multiple lesions present.
- Participation in contact sports (e.g., wrestling, football) where turf burns and abrasions are common, and athletes share lockers, bars of soap, towels, other equipment.
- Ethnic minority, lower socioeconomic status, in the military, homeless, recently incarcerated, living in a crowded environment, using illicit drugs, or participates in high-risk sexual behaviors.
- Nonpregnant or pregnant woman has a breast abscess.
- A history in the past year of hospitalization, surgery, or a percutaneous permanent indwelling medical device placement.
- Attends child care; is younger than 2 years old.
- Cystic fibrosis or progressive respiratory tract infection.
- Head or neck infection (retropharyngeal abscess, mastoiditis, AOM, sinusitis, periorbital and orbital infections),

osteomyelitis, myositis, pneumonias with empyema, sepsis, pustulosis in neonates.

PCPs can safely treat many superficial skin lesions without obtaining a culture, outside of neonatal period (e.g., impetigo) using topical bacitracin or mupirocin ointment three times daily for 7 to 10 days. Consider oral or IV antimicrobial therapy for widespread impetigo (Daum, 2018). In all cases, PCPs need to assess each case carefully and provide instructions to parents to return if the child is unresponsive to treatment. Anticipate complications and consider the clinical clues previously mentioned for skin and soft-tissue infection. The selection of a drug that covers MRSA should be made on the basis of the community prevalence of MRSA, if infection was nosocomial, and the severity of the infection.

Recommended management strategies (Fig 31.6) include:
- Incision and drainage (I&D) with culture is the treatment of choice for any non-draining but fluctuant abscess; antibiotics alone are ineffective (performing I&D prior to localization of pus is not effective and may promote more serious infection). Antibiotics are not needed after draining the abscess in mild

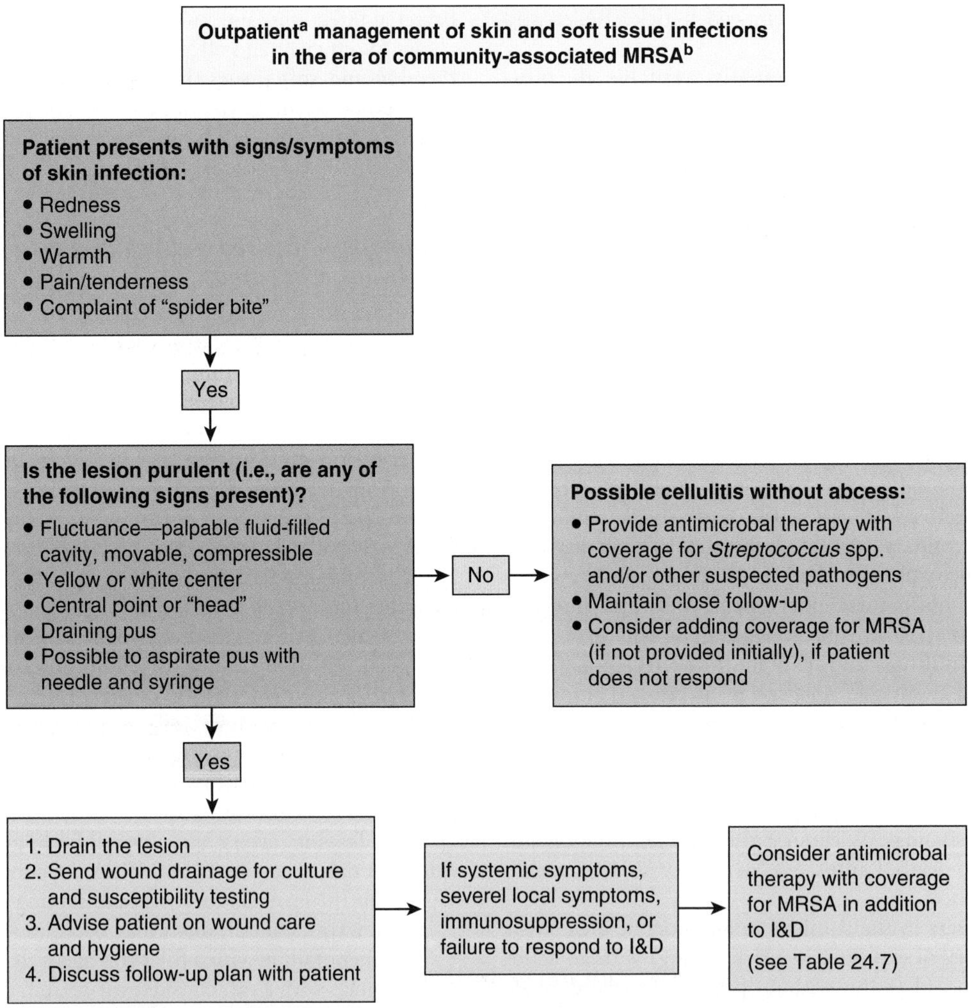

• **Fig 31.6** Algorithm for Outpatient Management of Skin and Soft Tissue Infections. [a]Severe infections (appears toxic, has unstable comorbidity or limb-threatening infection; sepsis or life-threatening infection [e.g., necrotizing fasciitis]) require inpatient management; consult an infectious disease specialist. [b]Visit www.cdc.gov/mrsa for more information. *I&D,* Incision and drainage; *MRSA,* methicillin-resistant *Staphylococcus aureus; SSTI,* skin and soft tissue infection.

cases. Consider empiric treatment (PO or IV) for MRSA for those with severe local infection, those with signs of systemic toxicity, or those who failed to respond to prior oral treatment (Stevens et al., 2014). Those with a temperature higher than 100.4°F (38°C), heart rate higher than 90, tachypnea more than 24 breaths/min, or WBC count more than 12,000 or less than 400, who are immunocompromised or at risk of endocarditis may require IV antibiotics. Refer to an infectious disease consult.

- Send specimens to the laboratory for a Gram stain, culture and sensitivity, and "d-test" (indicates possible inducible clindamycin resistance). Cultures should not be taken from superficial open surface wounds due to contaminating skin bacteria.
- For deep-seated infections without fluid fluctuation and signs of bacteremia (e.g., fever, chills, malaise), use warm compresses, and oral antibiotics can be considered. The individual should return for further evaluation in 24 to 36 hours for I&D as indicated (providers need to have a way to contact patient regarding status).
- For uncomplicated soft tissue infection (e.g., bullous and non-bullous impetigo; secondarily infected eczema, ulcers, or lacerations) without fluid fluctuation, empiric topical mupirocin 2% is usually sufficient. Using moist heat on small furuncles to promote draining may be sufficient. Treat ecthyma and impetigo with an oral antimicrobial for 7 days (Stevens et al., 2014).
- The use of oral antibiotic treatment for suspected methicillin-sensitive *S. aureus* infection is appropriate under the following circumstances, and providers should contact the child/family within 2 to 3 days to determine treatment response (Table 31.6):
  - Presence of abscesses (one or multiple sites) or rapidly progressing local infection with signs of cellulitis; systemic symptoms; comorbidities or immunosuppression; abscess is

in an area difficult to incise/drain (e.g., face, hand, genitalia); or lack of response to incision/drainage (Stevens et al., 2014).
- Prevention measures for athletes and return to play guidelines are included in Box 13.6 and Table 13.9.
- For recurrent MRSA soft tissue infections:
  - Review hygiene and wound care.
  - Institute environmental hygiene measures (clean surfaces in contact with skin [e.g., doorknobs, bathtubs, counters, and toilet seats]).
  - Decolonization techniques (consider where ongoing transmission is occurring within a household despite adherence to hygiene and wound care strategies). May include nasal decolonization with mupirocin 2% twice daily for 5 days (apply to groin and around rectal area of diapered infants/children); daily antiseptic body wash with a skin antiseptic solution (e.g., chlorhexidine) for 5 to 14 days or diluted bleach baths (¼ cup bleach for ¼ tub of water) for 15 minutes twice weekly for about 3 months. Oral antibiotics are not routinely recommended for decolonization. Consider an infectious disease consult for individuals with recurrent MRSA infections (Liu et al., 2011).

Other Emerging Drug-Resistant Bacterial Infections

- At least 2 million people in the United States acquire a serious bacterial infection that is resistant to one or more antibiotics, and approximately 23,000 deaths are attributed to those infections (CDC, 2016a). Multiple drug resistant gram-negative bacteria are a major concern. Enterobacteriaceae, *Pseudomonas aeruginosa,* and *Acinetobacter* are resistant to virtually all antibiotics in hospital settings. Multi-drug resistance is emerging to gram-positive

TABLE 31.6	Initial Outpatient Treatment Options for Mild to Moderate Suspected Community-Acquired Methicillin-Resistant *Staphylococcus aureus* Infections	
Antibiotic[a]	**Comments**	**Precautions**
Clindamycin	Treats serious infections (nonpurulent [mild] or purulent) due to *Staphylococcus aureus*. Additional d-test should be done on specimen by lab to ensure clindamycin susceptibility. Resistance seen in deep-seated infections (osteomyelitis, endocarditis, pneumonia). Do not use if local resistance rates exceed 10%-15%.	Although uncommon, may cause *Clostridium difficile*-associated disease.
Doxycycline	For children 8 years old and older; treats *S. aureus*, but activity against GAS less well known.	Can cause photosensitivity; do not use in pregnancy.
Minocycline	For children 8 years old and older.	Limited recent clinical experience.
Linezolid	For complicated skin/soft tissue infections, pneumonia.	Is associated with myelosuppression, neuropathy, and lactic acidosis during prolonged therapy. Before using, consult with infectious disease specialist.
Trimethoprim-sulfamethoxazole (TMP-SMX)	Limited efficacy data for treating GAS so avoid using for initial treatment of cellulitis (Kimberlin, 2018).	Do not use in infants under 2 months old; do not use in third trimester of pregnancy.

[a]Treatment recommendations do not apply to neonates. Antibiotic treatment is for 7 days, depending upon response. If response is low, treat for up to 10 to 14 days.

Serious systemic symptoms (sepsis), severe local symptoms, immunosuppression, or failure to respond to incision and drainage (I&D) require hospitalization. In typical cases, Gram stain and culture of pus or exudates from skin lesions of impetigo and ecthyma are recommended to identify *Staphylococcus aureus* and/or a β-hemolytic streptococcus; treatment without these studies is reasonable (AAP, 2015b).

GAS, Group A streptococcus; *PO, per os* (by mouth, orally).

Data from Stevens DL, Bisno AL, Chambers HF, et al. Practice guidelines for the diagnosis and management of skin and soft tissue infections: 2014 update by the Infectious Disease Society of America. *Clin Infect Dis.* 2014;59(2):e10–e52; Stewart EE, Fernald D, Staton EW. A toolkit to improve the treatment of CA-MRSA. *Fam Pract Manag.* 2012;19(5):21–24; and Kimberlin DW, Brady MT, Jackson MA, et al., eds. *Red Book: 2018-2021 Report of the Committee on Infectious Diseases.* 31st ed. Elk Grove Village, IL: American Academy of Pediatrics; 2018.

organisms as well (e.g., *Staphylococcus* and *Enterococcus*) but to a lesser degree. Resistance to anti-malarials, multiple drug-resistant tuberculosis (MDR-TB), and extensively drug-resistant tuberculosis (XDR-TB) are increasing (CDC, 2016a).

- Antibiotics are among the most commonly prescribed drugs for people, with up to 50% of all prescribed antibiotics either dosed ineffectively or unnecessarily (CDC, 2016a). More than 70% of antibiotics are prescribed in ambulatory pediatrics for respiratory conditions; 23% of the prescribed antibiotics are for conditions without an indication for antibiotic treatment (e.g., asthma, viral conditions) (Hersh et al., 2011). Improving antibiotic prescribing/stewardship is an essential part of decreasing antibiotic resistance influenced by inappropriate and/or overuse of antibiotics (see Chapter 26).

Cat-Scratch Disease

B. henselae, a slow-growing, gram-negative bacillus, causes cat-scratch disease. It is a common infection and cause of chronic persistent (>3 weeks) lymphadenopathy in children. In 90% of cases, a cat (usually a kitten) is involved (occasionally a dog). The organism is transmitted to humans through a cat bite or scratch or from hands contaminated with flea feces that touch an open skin lesion or eye. The incidence is greater than 22,000 cases annually in the United States, the highest incidence occurs in the Southern states and in children younger than 5 years old (Howard and Edwards, 2019). The disease is most prevalent in fall and winter except in tropical areas, where it shows no seasonal predilection. The incubation period between injury and primary skin lesion is 7 to 12 days. The lymphadenopathy may take 5 to 50 days to develop but averages 12 days.

Clinical Findings. Systemic illness is present in approximately one-third of cases although the majority of patients are afebrile without constitutional symptoms (Han and Jacobs, 2018). The illness typically presents with cutaneous findings and other characteristics that include:

- Erythematous papules (2 to 5 mm) arise in two-thirds of individuals approximately 7 to 12 days after inoculation and persist for up to 4 weeks. They follow a linear pattern that parallels the cat scratch. The rash may be misdiagnosed as impetigo. The cutaneous lesions heal spontaneously. One to 4 weeks after the inoculation, the axillary, cervical, submandibular, preauricular, epitrochlear, inguinal, and femoral nodes closest to the lesion begin to swell (in that general order). Single or multiple nodes may be involved and swell to 1 to 5 cm. The area around the infected node is usually warm, tender, indurated, and erythematous during the first 2 to 4 weeks. Cellulitis is uncommon, but large nodes may suppurate up to 30% of the time (Han and Jacobs, 2018). The lymphadenopathy usually lasts 4 to 6 weeks without treatment (AAP et al., 2015b). Mucous membrane ulcers may occur. A fever of 100.4°F to 102.2°F (38°C to 39°C), malaise, anorexia, fatigue, and headache also accompany the lymphadenopathy in one-third of patients.
- A small percentage of children present with Parinaud oculoglandular syndrome (a painful nonsuppurative conjunctivitis) with preauricular lymphadenopathy. Inoculation is surmised to be from rubbing the eye(s) following handling a cat. Recovery is spontaneous and without sequelae in 2 to 4 months (Kimberlin et al., 2018; Howard and Edwards, 2019).
- Immunocompromised hosts can have persistent or relapsing fevers, bacteremia, weight loss, and other systemic symptoms.

Diagnostic Studies. An IFA for serum antibodies is available from commercial labs, state health departments, or the CDC and shows good correlation with this disease (Kimberlin et al., 2018). *B. henselae* is rarely recovered from cultures. A *Bartonella* DNA PCR can be performed on tissue and body fluids (pleural and CSF). CT or ultrasonography identify hepatic or splenic abscesses and granulomas. The CBC may be normal or show mild leukocytosis. The ESR and CRP is elevated early in the disease process; hepatic transaminases may increase with systemic disease. Lymph node biopsy may show nonspecific bacilli.

Differential Diagnosis, Management, and Complications. The differential diagnosis includes any cause of lymphadenopathy, but most commonly includes bacterial and viral infections (e.g., streptococci [especially group A β-hemolytic], staphylococci, anaerobic bacteria, atypical mycobacteria, tularemia, brucellosis, CMV, HIV, EBV, systemic fungal infections, toxoplasmosis). Malignancy and neck masses from other sources (e.g., cystic hygromas, bronchogenic cysts, tumors) are in the differential.

Most cases of cat-scratch disease resolve spontaneously within 2 to 4 months, so symptomatic treatment is usually sufficient. Use antipyretics for moderate fever. Treat painful nodes with moist wraps or needle aspiration. Needle aspiration yields material for diagnostic testing. Avoid I&D of nonsuppurative lesions because of the high risk of chronic draining sinuses. Antibiotics are not generally used unless there is concern for systemic cat-scratch disease or bacterial involvement of lesions. Azithromycin, clarithromycin, TMP-SMX, rifampin, ciprofloxacin, and doxycycline are commonly used (Kimberlin et al., 2018). A 5-day course of oral azithromycin is of moderate benefit and can be given for localized disease to speed recovery (Howard et al., 2014). Treatment is recommended for the immunocompromised and may be beneficial for those with acute or severe systemic sequelae (e.g., hepatic or splenic involvement or painful adenitis). Treatment with one of the oral agents and parenteral gentamicin are effective. Optimal length of therapy is not known, but several weeks may be needed (Kimberlin et al., 2018).

Discourage children from playing roughly with cats. Wash cat scratches thoroughly with soap and water. Immunocompromised individuals should stay away from cats that scratch or bite and avoid stray cats and cats younger than 1 year old. A small percentage of individuals manifest systemic illness. This is associated with fever up to 106°F (41.2°C), malaise, fatigue, anorexia, weight loss, emesis, headache, hepatosplenomegaly, sore throat, exanthema, blindness secondary to stellate macular retinopathy, neurologic changes (bizarre behavior), seizures, and arthralgia. Enlarged mediastinal or pancreatic nodes can cause pleurisy, obstructive phenomena, and splenic and hepatic abscesses (may be associated with prolonged fevers). Other complications include encephalopathy (5% incidence after 1 to 3 weeks of lymphadenopathy), aseptic meningitis, severe chronic systemic disease, erythema nodosa, neuroretinitis, thrombocytopenic purpura, primary atypical pneumonia, relapsing bacteremia, breast mass, endocarditis, angiomatoid papules, and osteomyelitis. Almost all of these problems generally resolve completely over several months, rarely as long as a year (Han and Jacobs, 2018).

Kingella kingae Infection

Kingella kingae is an important cause of invasive infections in children younger than 4 years old, but is not reported in infants younger than 6 months old. The organism is part of the normal flora of the pharynx in children (over 6 months old) more than in adults; it is easily transmitted in childcare settings. The onset is usually insidious, which can result in delay of diagnosis (Murphy, 2015). The history often includes recent or concomitant gingivostomatitis or URI. Suspect *K. kingae* in culture-negative skeletal infections of young children; it is the most common cause of septic arthritis in children younger than 3 years old (Yagupsky, 2018). Septic arthritis usually involves the knee, hip, or ankle. Other invasive disease includes osteomyelitis (distal femur is the most common site), endocarditis in those with underlying cardiac disease (HACEK group of organisms [*Haemophilus* spp., *Actinobacillus actinomycetemcomitans, Cardiobacterium hominis, Eikenella corrodens, Kingella kingae*]), meningitis, occult bacteremia, and pneumonia. *Kingella kingae* is the most common cause of spondylodiskitis in the 6 to 48 months age group (Yagupsky, 2018). The organism is difficult to isolate in solid culture media. Recent studies show PCR dramatically enhances detection in bone and joint fluid samples (Porsch and Geme, 2019). The organism is susceptible to many antibiotics (penicillins, aminoglycosides, ciprofloxacin, and erythromycin) but is resistant to vancomycin with 40% of clindamycin isolates showing resistance (Yagupsky, 2016). Most strains are susceptible to TMP-SMX despite resistance to trimethoprim alone. Standard hygienic preventive measures should be in place in child care settings to decrease risk of transmission (Porsch and Geme, 2019).

Meningococcal Disease

Many organisms cause meningitis (group B streptococcus, *E. coli, Listeria monocytogenes,* enterococci, *S. pneumoniae, N. meningitidis,* and *H. influenzae*). The causative organism varies with age. Only *N. meningitidis* is discussed here (see Chapter 46).

N. meningitidis is a gram-negative diplococcus. It is a common commensal organism in the human nasopharynx. Serotypes A, B, C, W (previously designated W-135), X, and Y (polysaccharide encapsulated organisms) are largely the causes of invasive disease worldwide. In the United States, serogroups B, C, and Y account for the majority of cases of disease after one year of age and share equal incidence (Pollard and Sadarangani, 2016). Infants and adolescents 11 to 23 years old have the highest incidence, although it occurs in all ages (CDC, 2018s). Serogroup B causes 60% of disease in infants and children under 5 years old. Serogroups C, Y, and W-135 affect the majority of cases in adolescents and young adults (Kimberlin et al., 2018). The organism spreads from person to person via respiratory tract secretions (large droplets) or contact with saliva (kissing). Asymptomatic carriers are the most common source of transmission, as 10% of the population at any given time is a carrier (Pollard and Sadarangani, 2016). Disease occurs most often during the winter season, but can occur sporadically; rates increase in sub-Sahara Africa during the dry season. Epidemics occur in semi-closed communities (e.g., child care centers, schools, college dormitories [especially among college freshmen], and military barracks) and account for about 2 to 3 percent disease cases (CDC, 2017c). Children or youth with functional or anatomic asplenia, complement deficiencies (e.g., nephritic syndrome, SLE, hepatic failure), or properdin deficiency are at increased risk for invasive or recurring meningococcal disease (Pollard and Finn, 2018). The incubation period is 1 to 14 days. Individuals are contagious until 24 hours after initiating treatment. Carriage persists for weeks to months, although disease onset is usually days to a week after colonization (Pollard and Sadarangani, 2016).

Clinical Findings. Meningococcal disease presentation varies widely from mild viral symptoms with fever to severe disease. Recognized patterns of disease include bacteremia without sepsis, meningococcemic sepsis without meningitis, meningitis with or without meningococcemia, meningoencephalitis, and specific organ infection. Presenting symptoms can include:

- Occult bacteremia: This appears in a febrile child with a URI or GI-like symptoms. There may be a maculopapular rash. Often these children are treated for a viral illness. Bacteremia may resolve without antimicrobial intervention, but approximately 66% of cases with sustained bacteremia progress to meningococcal meningitis (Pollard and Finn, 2018).
- Meningococcemia: Fulminant meningococcemia progresses rapidly over several hours, starting with fever onset, and may be accompanied by signs of septic shock. Initial symptoms include fever, headache, myalgia, chills, cold hands and feet, influenza symptoms, vomiting, and abdominal pain. Skin changes are characterized by prominent petechiae (Fig 31.7) that quickly progress to purpura fulminans. Other signs include hypotension, DIC, acidosis, adrenal hemorrhage, renal failure, myocardial failure, and coma. In fulminant cases, death can occur within hours of onset despite appropriate therapy (Kimberlin et al., 2018). Meningitis is present in 5% to 20% of meningococcemia cases (Hamborsky et al., 2015).
- Meningococcal meningitis: The most common clinical findings are fever, headache, and stiff neck. Fever and irritability may be the only initial symptoms in young children, whereas fever and headache are more typical in older children and adolescents. Other symptoms include nausea, vomiting, photophobia, and altered mental status. Bacteremia is present in 75% of meningococcal meningitis (Hamborsky et al., 2015).

Diagnostic Studies. The diagnosis is confirmed with a positive culture or Gram stain from normally sterile sites (blood, CSF, synovial fluid), sputum, or petechial or purpural lesion scraping. Blood and CSF cultures may be negative if the child was pretreated with antibiotics. PCR assays can be used with CSF, serum, and plasma to detect meningococcal DNA; results are available in 4 to 8 hours. PCR is more sensitive than blood culture and increases detection by 30% to 40% when antibiotics are given before testing and organism growth is suppressed (Pollard and Finn, 2018). In a probable case, a positive latex agglutination test

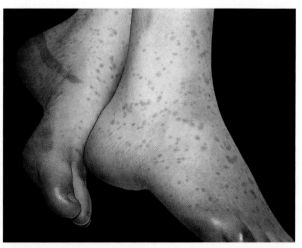

• **Fig 31.7** Meningococcemia. (From Zitelli BJ, McIntire SC, Nowalk AJ. *Atlas of Physical Diagnosis.* 7th ed. Philadelphia: Elsevier; 2018. Slides B and C from 13.39)

of CSF supports the clinical diagnosis of meningitis. However, this test has poor sensitivity and specificity, especially for serogroup B, and is not recommended if the PCR (in addition to culture) is available. Other laboratory findings include leukopenia or leukocytosis with increased bands and neutrophils, hypoalbuminemia, hypocalcemia, metabolic acidosis with increased lactate levels, decreased platelets, and elevated ESR and CRP. Decreased prothrombin and fibrinogen and prolonged coagulation times are seen with DIC.

Differential Diagnosis. The list of differential diagnoses is long and includes septicemia caused by other invasive bacteria (e.g., *Pneumococcus* or *H. influenza*), viral meningitis, TB brain abscess, chronic otitis media, and sinusitis. Collagen-vascular diseases, primary hematologic and oncologic disease, erythema nodosa, erythema multiforme, RMSF, *Mycoplasma*, lead encephalopathy, coxsackievirus, echovirus, rubella and rubeola infections, Henoch-Schönlein purpura, ITP, viral exanthems, typhus, typhoid, toxic shock syndrome, rat bite fever, gonococcemia, *S. aureus* endocarditis, and Kawasaki syndrome are also in the differential diagnosis.

Management, Control Measures, and Complications. If the child is suspected of having meningococcemia, hospitalization is mandatory and IV antibiotics started pending culture results. A 5- to 7-day treatment course is usually adequate in children.

Exposed contacts must be carefully monitored. Household, school, or child contacts who develop a febrile illness must be promptly evaluated for invasive disease. Household contacts have 500 to 800 times the risk factor of individuals in the general community (Kimberlin et al., 2018). Control measures include:

- Chemoprophylaxis is ideally given within 24 hours of index case identification regardless of immunization status (vaccines are not 100% effective). Individuals (including children in child care and preschool) who had close contact with the index case 7 days before the onset of symptoms are at increased risk of invasive disease and should receive prophylaxis. Airline travel of more than 8 hours while sitting next to an infected individual qualifies one for prophylaxis (Kimberlin et al., 2018). Casual contact with the index case or with a high-risk contact is usually not considered high risk. Medical staff (unless they performed mouth-to-mouth resuscitation, intubation, or suctioning before antibiotics) are also not at high risk. Oral rifampin or ciprofloxacin are the antimicrobials of choice for infants and children. If the community has ciprofloxacin-resistance to *N. meningitidis*, azithromycin as a single oral dose is effective (Kimberlin et al., 2018).
- Prophylaxis during outbreak: Vaccination, in conjunction with chemoprophylaxis, is advisable to prevent extended outbreaks only if the identified strain is contained in the vaccine (see Meningococcal vaccine). Vaccines are available for serogroups A, B, C, Y, and W-135.

Complications are caused by inflammation, intravascular hemorrhage, necrosis in multiple organ systems, and shock. Skeletal deformities and limb amputations are not infrequent. Meningitis can lead to ataxia, seizures, pneumonia, deafness (5% to 10%), arthritis and pericarditis, visual field defects, palsies and paralysis, developmental delays, and hydrocephalus. The fatality rate is about 10%. Even with aggressive treatment, meningococcemia has a fatality rate of approximately 5%. Survivors may experience such permanent sequelae as hearing loss (2% to 15%), neurologic damage (7%), or loss of a limb (3%) (Pollard and Finn, 2018).

Streptococcal Disease

Streptococci are gram-positive spherical cocci that are broadly classified based on their ability to hemolyze RBCs. Complete hemolysis is known as *β-hemolytic*. Partial hemolysis is *α-hemolytic*; non-hemolysis is *γ-hemolytic*. Cell wall carbohydrate differences further subdivide the streptococci into Lancefield antigen subgroups A-H and K-V. Subgroups A-H and K-O are associated with human disease. Group A β-hemolytic streptococcus is the most virulent, although group B β-hemolytic streptococcus causes bacteremia and meningitis in infants younger than 3 months old (rarely older). Group A streptococcus (GAS) are subdivided into more than 100 subtypes based upon their cell surface M protein antigen and fimbriae on the cell's outer edge. The virulence of GAS depends upon their M protein. If the M protein is present, GAS strains can resist phagocytosis; if the M protein is weak or absent, the strains are basically avirulent (e.g., chronic GAS pharyngeal carriers). GAS also produces many varieties of enzymes and toxins that stimulate specific antitoxin antibodies for immunity or serve as evidence of past infection but do not confer immunity. There is not cross-immunity between antibodies for different GAS strains (e.g., scarlet fever is caused by three different pyrogenic exotoxins, so the illness can recur). Some general remarks about specific illnesses due to GAS and non-group A and B streptococcus infection are discussed in this chapter; cross-references to specific chapters are noted for other GAS caused infections.

Group A Streptococcus

Streptococci usually invade the respiratory tract, skin, soft tissues, and blood. Transmission is primarily through infected upper respiratory tract secretions or, secondarily, through skin invasion. Fomites and household pets are not vectors. Food-borne outbreaks from contamination by food handlers are reported. Both streptococcus pharyngitis and impetigo are associated with crowding, whether at home, school, or other institution. Streptococcal pharyngitis is rare in infants and children younger than 3 years old, but the incidence rises with age and is most common in the winter and early spring in temperate climates. Carrier rates in asymptomatic children are up to 20% (Arnold and Nizet, 2018). By contrast, streptococcus skin infection (impetigo, pyoderma) is more common in toddlers and preschool-age children. Those at increased risk for invasive GAS are individuals with varicella infection, IV drug use, HIV, diabetes, chronic heart or lung disease, infants, and older adults.

The incubation period is 2 to 5 days for pharyngitis and 7 to 10 days for skin infection. In untreated individuals, communicability is from the onset of symptoms up to a few months. Children are considered non-infectious 24 hours after the start of appropriate antibiotic therapy.

Clinical Findings and Diagnostic Studies. The following may be seen:

- Respiratory tract infection: Streptococcal tonsillopharyngitis (GABHS) and pneumonia are described in Chapter 37. Peritonsillar abscess, cervical lymphadenitis, retropharyngeal abscess, otitis media, mastoiditis, and sinusitis may be clinical features.
- Scarlet fever: This is caused by erythrogenic toxin. It is uncommon in children younger than 3 years old. The incubation period is approximately 3 days (the range is 1 to 7 days). There is abrupt illness with sore throat, vomiting, headache, chills, and malaise. Fever reaches 104°F (40°C). Tonsils are erythematous, edematous, and usually exudative. The pharynx

is inflamed and can be covered with a gray-white exudate. The palate and uvula are erythematous and reddened, and petechiae are present. The tongue is usually coated and red, desquamation of the coating leaves prominent papillae (strawberry tongue). The typical scarlatina rash appears 1 to 5 days following symptom onset but may be the presenting symptom. The exanthema is red, blanches to pressure, and is finely papular, making the skin feel coarse, with a sandpaper feel. The rash generally begins on the neck and spreads to the trunk and extremities becoming generalized within 24 hours. The face may be spared (cheeks may be reddened with circumoral pallor), but the rash is denser on the neck, axilla, and groin. Pastia lines, transverse linear hyperpigmented areas with tiny petechiae, are seen in the joint folds (see Fig 31.3). In severe disease, small vesicles (miliary sudamina) are found on the hands, feet, and abdomen. There is circumoral pallor and the cheeks are erythematous. The rash fades and desquamates after 3 to 4 days, starting on the face and slowly moving to the trunk and extremities, and may include fingernail margins, palms, and soles; this process can take up to 6 weeks. Sore throat and constitutional symptoms resolve in approximately 5 to 7 days (average 3 to 4 days).

- Bacteremia: This occurs after respiratory (pharyngitis, tonsillitis, AOM) and localized skin infections. Some children have no obvious source of infection. Meningitis, osteomyelitis, septic arthritis, pyelonephritis, pneumonia, peritonitis, and bacterial endocarditis are rare but associated with GAS bacteremia. (Neonatal sepsis due to group B streptococcus is discussed in Chapter 29.)
- Vaginitis and streptococcal toxic shock syndrome (Chapter 42).
- Perianal streptococcal cellulitis: Symptoms include local itching, pain, blood-streaked stools, erythema, and proctitis. Fever and systemic infections are uncommon. Although infection is usually the result of autoinoculation, sexual molestation is in the differential.
- Skin infections (Chapter 34); rheumatic heart disease (Chapter 38); and necrotizing fasciitis (Chapter 34).

Differential Diagnosis, Management, and Complications. Many viral pathogens are in the differential for acute pharyngitis, including influenza, parainfluenza, rhinovirus, coronavirus, adenovirus, and RSV. EBV is common and is usually accompanied by other clinical findings (e.g., splenomegaly, generalized lymphadenopathy). Other causes of bacterial upper respiratory disease include (though rare) tularemia, *Yersinia*, gonorrhea, *Chlamydia*, and *Mycoplasma*. Diphtheria is rare with universal vaccination but is a serious cause of acute pharyngitis (Gerber, 2016). Staphylococcal impetigo must be differentiated from GABHS pyoderma. Septicemia, meningitis, osteomyelitis, septic arthritis, pyelonephritis, and bacterial endocarditis cause similar symptoms but result from other bacteria.

Antimicrobial therapy is recommended for GABHS pharyngitis to decrease the risk of acute rheumatic fever, decrease the length of the illness, prevent complications, and reduce transmission. See appropriate aforementioned site-specific chapters for recommendations for managing specific infections.

Complications are usually caused by disease spread from the localized infection. Upper respiratory complications include cervical lymphadenitis, retropharyngeal abscess, otitis media, mastoiditis, and sinusitis if the primary infection is unrecognized or treatment is inadequate. Acute poststreptococcal glomerulonephritis occurs following skin or upper respiratory GAS infection, whereas acute rheumatic fever only occurs following GAS URIs.

Poststreptococcal reactive arthritis occurs following GAS pharyngitis. Skin infection with GAS may progress to cellulitis, myositis, or necrotizing fasciitis. Other complications associated with invasive infections include pneumonia, pleural empyema, meningitis, osteomyelitis, and bacterial endocarditis.

Pediatric autoimmune neuropsychiatric disorders associated with streptococcal infections (PANDAS) is a group of neuropsychiatric disorders thought to result from the production of autoimmune antibodies; these include obsessive-compulsive disorders, tic disorders, and Tourette syndrome (Chapter 30).

Non–Group A or B Streptococci

Lancefield group streptococci (principally groups C and G) cause invasive disease in all age groups. They may cause septicemia, UTIs, endocarditis, respiratory disease (upper and lower), skin soft tissue infection, pharyngitis, brain abscesses, and meningitis in newborns, children, adolescents, and adults. The incubation period and communicability times are unknown. Positive culture from normally sterile body fluids is adequate for diagnosis. Penicillin G is the drug of choice with modification based on culture sensitivities. Pneumonia with empyema or abscess may respond slowly despite effective antimicrobial therapy with fevers lasting more than 7 days (Haslam and St. Geme, 2018).

Tuberculosis

TB is caused by *M. tuberculosis* and is a very slow-growing organism, taking up to 10 weeks to grow on solid media and 1 to 6 weeks in liquid media. The degree of infectivity depends on the exposure intensity and length and the burden of bacilli carried by the index case. For this reason, TB is moderately infectious under most situations (Fitzgerald et al., 2015). The bacilli are spread primarily by droplet contamination from coughing, sneezing, or talking. Droplets stay suspended in the air for hours. Fomite transmission is uncommon; the portal of entry is most often the respiratory tract from mucus droplets from a person infected with pulmonary TB (Chiang and Starke, 2018).

TB may be either latent (latent tuberculosis infection [LTBI]; the individual is infected but not contagious) or active (active disease is present and individual is contagious). Generally about 3% to 4% of those infected with the bacilli progress to active disease during the first year after infection; thereafter, an additional 5% progress to disease (Fitzgerald et al., 2015). These estimates are based on heavy exposures during disease-prone periods of life.

Globally, one-third of the world's population is infected with the mycobacteria (Chiang and Starke, 2018). Ninety-five percent of active TB cases occur in countries where HIV/AIDS infection is epidemic and health care is poor or inaccessible. Individuals in the United States with the highest incidence of active TB live in urban, low-income areas. Approximately 60% of reported TB cases in the United States are foreign-born, 80% are Hispanic and non-Caucasian. High-risk groups include immigrants, international adoptees, those from or travelers to high-prevalence regions (Asia, Africa, Latin America, and former Soviet Union countries), the homeless, alcoholics, IV drug users, and individuals in correctional facilities or other close communal settings (Kimberlin et al., 2018).

Infection is typically detected by a positive Mantoux TST or a positive interferon γ release assay (IGRA) in a high-risk child. In certain circumstances a child may have findings suggestive of TB infection and not have a positive TST or IGRA. These tests are reactive within 2 to 10 weeks after initial exposure to an active TB case. Risk of progression to disease is highest in the first 6 months after infection. The risk remains high for the subsequent 2 years after infection, but the infection may remain latent for years before progressing to disease. After treatment starts, infectivity in active cases may cease within days or take several weeks depending on the drugs prescribed, response of the organisms, and other disease characteristics (e.g., for cavitary disease, response takes longer). In children younger than 10 years old, there is usually minimal cough and bacilli expulsion and, therefore, less contagion. Most infections in children are from adults.

The age at the time of infection is predictive of the likelihood an infection evolves into disease. Progression to disease is highest in infants, individuals 15 to 25 years old, and older adults; those older than 14 years have the highest risk of developing clinical disease. Children younger than 5 years account for about 60% of American childhood cases; children 5 to 14 years old have the lowest rate of disease. Other factors that make an individual prone to active disease include having another TB infection within the prior 2 years; immune status (immunocompromised individuals [from a disease (e.g., HIV) or immunosuppressive drugs] are at higher risk); IV drug use; those with chronic diseases (e.g., Hodgkin disease, lymphoma, diabetes mellitus, chronic renal failure, malnutrition); and those receiving tumor necrosis factor-α antagonists to treat arthritis, inflammatory bowel disease, or other diseases.

Congenital TB is extremely rare. Infants most likely become infected after delivery from contact with an infected person. Exposure in utero occurs from exposure to maternal bacteremia, seeding of the placenta by disseminated (miliary) TB in the fetal circulation, fetal aspiration of amniotic fluid at delivery, or in utero infected amniotic fluid ingestion (Chiang and Starke, 2018).

Clinical Findings Primary Pulmonary Tuberculosis

Table 31.7 describes the clinical findings and interventions for TB stages. Most children ages 3 to 15 years with primary pulmonary TB are asymptomatic except for a positive TB skin test

or IGRA. An effective immune response eliminates most of the bacilli, although small numbers of bacilli spread throughout the body during the bacteremic phase.

Any symptoms in children are generally minor and slightly more evident in infants; up to 50% exhibit radiographic changes but have no physical findings. Most children with disease first develop hilar lymphadenopathy then focal hyperinflation and atelectasis (Hatzenbuehler and Starke, 2016). Signs and symptoms typically occur 1 to 6 months after infection and include low-grade fever, nonproductive cough and dyspnea (more common in infants), malaise, decreased appetite, weight loss (failure to thrive in infants), night sweats, chills, erythema nodosum, and phlyctenular keratoconjunctivitis (a hypersensitivity reaction marked by elevated clear nodules with surrounding hyperemia near the limbus). Approximately 25% to 30% of children present with extrapulmonary TB symptoms (e.g., meningitis and/or granulomatous inflammation of the lymph nodes, bones, joints, skin, and middle ear and mastoid) (Hatzenbuehler and Starke, 2016). Rarely, enlarging lymph nodes compress and obstruct regional bronchus, causing respiratory distress; this is more commonly seen with infants. Esophageal compression (causing dysphagia or aspiration) and vasoconstriction of major arteries and veins (causing edema) can occur. Recurrent cough, stridor, and wheezing are signs of increasing pulmonary infection.

Screening Tests for Infection. Low-risk groups do not need to be routinely screened for TB. Children are considered at high risk for TB if they meet any of the following criteria:
- Have close contact with others with suspected or confirmed TB
- Were born in, or traveled for more than 1 week to, TB-prevalent parts of the world (Asia, Middle East, Africa, Latin America, countries formerly part of the Soviet Union) (it is reasonable to wait 10 weeks after return from areas to screen if the child is well and has no history of exposure)
- Live in an area where there is a rise in TB infection
- Have clinical signs suggestive of TB on chest radiograph or other clinical evidence suggestive of TB infection

TABLE 31.7 Characteristics of Tuberculosis in Children

| | STAGE | | |
	Exposure	Infection (LTBI)	Disease
Mantoux skin test or IGRA (for children 3 years and older and in those who have received BCG); use Mantoux if HIV infected	Negative (results not reliable in infants younger than 3 months)	Positive (TST: in 60%-90% of cases)	Positive (TST: in 60%-90% of cases)
Physical examination	Normal	Normal	Usually abnormal[a]
Chest radiograph	Normal	Usually normal[b]	Usually abnormal[c]
Treatment	If <4 years old or with impaired immunity (e.g., HIV)	Always	Always
Number of drugs	One	One (additional regimens available)	Four

[a]More than 50% of infants and children with pulmonary tuberculosis have a normal physical examination.

[b]May reveal healed lesions (calcification in the lungs, hilar lymph nodes, or both).

[c]Some children with extrapulmonary tuberculosis have a normal chest radiograph.

BCG, Bacille Calmette-Guérin vaccine; *HIV,* human immunodeficiency virus; *IGRA,* interferon-gamma release assay; *LTBI,* latent tuberculosis infection.

Data from American Academy of Pediatrics, Kimberlin DW, Brady MT, et al., eds. Tuberculosis, *Red Book: 2018 Report of the Committee on Infectious Diseases.* 31st ed. Elk Grove Village, IL: American Academy of Pediatrics; 2018:829–852; and Hatzenbuehler LA, Starke JR. Tuberculosis (*Mycobacterium tuberculosis*). In: Kliegman RM, Stanton BF, St. Geme III JW, et al., eds. *Nelson Textbook of Pediatrics.* 20th ed. Philadelphia: Saunders; 2016:1445–1461.

- Are HIV positive (beginning at 3 to 12 months of age; TST only), have an immunosuppressive disorder, or are being treated with immunosuppressive drugs
- Are homeless, reside in correctional or other residential institution, are a member of a migrant farm family
- Consider in children with Hodgkin disease, diabetes mellitus, chronic renal failure, malnutrition, and those receiving tumor necrosis factor antagonists.

Mantoux Tuberculin Skin Test. Tuberculin skin testing is based on the delayed hypersensitivity to *M. tuberculosis* antigens. The Mantoux skin test is used, which is a purified protein derivative (PPD). If the child becomes infected with TB, the test usually becomes positive 4 to 8 weeks (between 3 weeks and 3 month) after bacilli inhalation (Hatzenbuehler and Starke, 2016). All children with positive TST need quick clinical and radiographic evaluation.

The Mantoux test uses 0.1 mL of 5 tuberculin units (TU) of PPD, is injected intradermally into the volar surface of the forearm, and produces a palpable wheal with 6 to 10 mm of induration (crucial for accurate testing). A multipuncture skin test should not be used. Read the Mantoux test 48 to 72 hours later by an experienced healthcare professional. Measure the induration, not the erythema. Sensitivity to the TST persists for years, even after effective antitubular drug treatment.

Children with prior BCG vaccination can receive the TST, and interpretation of the test is the same as for non-recipients. Prior BCG vaccination produces a mild to severe hypersensitivity reaction, depending on several factors: the age of the BCG vaccine, its quality, the strain of *M. bovis* used, the number of BCG doses received, nutritional status, immunologic factors, infection with environmental mycobacteria, and the frequency of skin testing (boosts the response). The degree of positivity decreases over time, depending on the age at vaccination.

All children with positive TST need quick clinical and radiographic evaluation. A Mantoux skin test is defined as positive for LTBI or TB disease if the following reactions occur (Kimberlin et al., 2018):

- Induration (5 mm or greater) in children who are in close contact with an individual with active or previously active TB cases, have a chest radiograph consistent with active or previously active TB, clinical TB findings, have an immunosuppressive disorder or HIV infection, or are receiving immunosuppressive drugs
- Induration (10 mm or greater) in children younger than 4 years old with any high-risk factors
- Induration (15 mm or greater) in children 4 years old or older without any risk factors
- If the skin test shows induration onset after 72 hours, it should be interpreted as positive

Skin testing is not always valid and can be negative in 10% to 40% of children with positive cultures. This decreased reactivity occurs in immunocompromised children (e.g., with HIV), infants younger than 3 months of age, those with poor nutrition, or those with other viral infections (notably measles, varicella, and influenza). Ten percent of those with progressive TB (up to 50% with disseminated disease or meningitis) do not react until several months after receiving drug treatment (Kimberlin et al., 2018; Hatzenbuehler and Starke, 2016). Additionally, a poor response to the skin test can occur due to inadequate handling of the Mantoux solution, improper injection technique, or interpretation error. Individuals sensitized to nontuberculous mycobacteria can cross-react and have a less than 10- to 12-mm reaction to TB skin testing.

Interferon γ Release Assays. IGRAs include QuantiFERON-TB Gold In-Tube and T-SPOT.TB. IGRAs are FDA-approved screening tests for detecting T-cell response to specific *M. tuberculosis* antigens. They have the advantage over the Mantoux test of not being affected by prior BCG vaccination. TST is the preferred test for children less than 5 years of age. Children with indeterminate IRGA may need to have the test repeated. IGRAs are recommended for the following circumstances (Kimberlin et al., 2018; CDC, 2017f):

- Immunocompetent children 5 years old or older to confirm suspected LTBI or active disease. A positive result indicates TB infection; a negative IGRA does not rule-out infection or disease if clinical signs and symptoms suggest otherwise
- Children 5 years old or older who received BCG vaccine
- Children 5 years old or older who are unlikely to return for TST reading
- If the initial TST is positive in children 5 years old or older who received BCG vaccine, in whom additional evidence is needed to improve compliance, or if nontuberculous mycobacterial disease is suspected
- Might be used with other diagnostic tests in an infant suspected of having congenital TB

Diagnostic Studies. Chest radiography early in the disease may show only localized, nonspecific infiltrates. Inflammation of lung tissue and hilar lymph nodes continues as the disease progresses; this quickly resolves in most children, but increased hilar adenopathy is usually seen in infants. The hallmark is disproportionately enlarged regional lymph nodes compared with a relatively small pleural focus (Chiang and Starke, 2018).

Radiography in older children shows inconspicuous pneumonitis in the lower and middle lung fields. In adolescents, apical or subapical infiltrates are seen, often with cavitations, and no hilar adenopathy (Fitzgerald et al., 2015). Extensive pulmonary infiltrates and cavitation occur if there is erosion and necrosis from disseminated bacilli. Lesions may be the size of millet seeds; hence the name "miliary" TB.

Hilar adenopathy suggests TB, but culture of the organism is essential to establish the diagnosis. Culture specimens may be obtained from gastric aspirates, sputum, bronchial washings, pleural fluid, CSF, urine or other body fluids, or biopsies. However, mycobacteria are isolated in less than 50% of children and 75% of infants with pulmonary TB (Kimberlin et al., 2018). Those older than 5 years old can be induced to cough to produce sputum with aerosolized hypertonic saline. When age or ability to produce sputum is a factor, early morning gastric aspirates, collected on three separate mornings and analyzed by fluorescent staining, is an effective and sensitive testing method. Histologic examination for acid-fast bacilli (AFB) from biopsies is helpful. Solid media cultures can take up to 10 weeks to grow with an additional 2 to 4 weeks for susceptibility testing, whereas liquid cultures take 1 to 6 weeks. Rapid DNA probes or high-pressure liquid chromatography of cultured organisms differentiate between *M. tuberculosis* and *M. bovis* based on pyrazinamide resistance that is characteristic of *M. bovis*.

If an isolate from an index case is positive for TB, culture material is not needed from an exposed child. However, a culture is necessary in the following circumstances: the index case is unavailable, the child has HIV infection or is immunocompromised, drug-resistant TB is suspected, or the child has extrapulmonary symptoms (Kimberlin et al., 2018). A NAAT on respiratory secretions is the standard practice for suspected TB; it does not exclude TB. It aids in the diagnosis of TB when symptoms suggest active TB infection, but it does not supplant an AFB smear and culture. Results are known 1 or more weeks earlier than a culture. Its use expedites the appropriate initiation of treatment. Additional research needs to be done before NAATs can be approved for use in extrapulmonary or primary TB in children who cannot produce sputum (Kimberlin et al., 2018).

Differential Diagnosis. PCPs should consider TB in children with symptoms of basilar meningitis, hydrocephalus, cranial nerve palsy, or stroke. Permanent neurologic dysfunction can result and has a worse prognosis in infants than in older children. The differential diagnosis also includes mycotic infections, staphylococcal pneumonia, sarcoidosis, chronic pneumonia, and Hodgkin lymphoma. Differential diagnosis in lymph node diseases includes cat-scratch disease, tularemia, toxoplasmosis, tumor, brachial cysts, cystic hygroma, and pyogenic infection.

Management. A TB specialist should be consulted when a child has a positive TST, when TB is suspected, or a child is a contact. TB is a reportable infectious disease. After index and contact cases are identified and diagnostic studies are done, the state and/or local health department often initiate treatment and follow-up. The treatment regimens are often in flux. It is advised that providers consult a pediatric TB specialist before initiating treatment for any type of TB infection to ensure that the most current treatment is prescribed; different regimens will be used if the child also has concurrent HIV infection.

Antitubercular drug treatment focuses on eradicating the bacilli and inhibiting their multiplication in LTBI and early pulmonary disease. Rapid resolution of caseous or granulomatous lesions will not occur. It is imperative to have strict adherence to drug combination to minimize drug resistance. This may need to be done under directly observed therapy (DOT). If the treatment regimen is prescribed by a TB specialist or health department, the PCP should know the child's specific antitubercular drug regimen. The first-line drugs are administered orally and include isoniazid (INH), rifampin (RIF), pyrazinamide (PZA), and ethambutol (EMB). The typical treatment regimens for children/families include (Chiang and Starke, 2018; Hatzenbuehler and Starke, 2016; Kimberlin et al., 2018):

- For prophylaxis after contact with person with active TB or for LTBI: INH, taken once daily or twice weekly for 9 months; RIF, taken once daily for 4 to 6 months; INH and RIF daily for 2 to 3 months; or INH and rifapentine for 12 doses once weekly.
- For pulmonary disease and extrapulmonary disease (except CNS, bone, and joint): All four drugs are taken once daily for 2 months. INH and RIF then continue for 4 months, administered 2 to 3 times a week (duration of treatment with HIV co-infection is 6 to 9 months or 6 months from sterile sputum culture—whichever is longest).
- For bone, joint infection, and disseminated disease: same as pulmonary except is given for 9 to 12 months since 6 months is inadequate.
- For hilar adenopathy only, or no other abnormalities and minimal risk for resistant disease: some experts recommend INH and RIF for 6 months but may need to extend to 9 months if slow improvement or culture is positive 2 months after starting treatment.
- For meningitis: INH, RIF, and PZA are given with either ethionamide, an aminoglycoside, or levofloxacin as the fourth drug. The fourth drug may be stopped if cultures are susceptible to INH and RIF. PZA can be stopped after 2 months

if good clinical response. Total treatment time is 9 to 12 months.
- Newborns suspected of having congenital TB: INH, RIF, PZA, and an aminoglycoside are used.

The treatment regimens are often in flux, and there are alternative regimens in use. Under some alternative regimens the drugs may be administered twice a week under DOT, provide for shortened durations of treatment, or use different combinations of drugs depending upon age, drug-resistance, extent of TB infection, and concurrent infections. The CDC, AAP *Red Book*, and WHO are excellent resources for drug regimens and recommended dosages.

Pregnant women diagnosed with TB disease, who have signs and symptoms or abnormal findings on chest x-ray consistent with TB, should be promptly treated and tested for HIV. If the pregnant woman has LTBI and a normal chest x-ray, she should start on LTBI treatment for 9 months after the postpartum period, and the newborn needs no further evaluation or therapy (Kimberlin et al., 2018). If she has active disease, isolation may be recommended and the newborn evaluated for congenital TB disease. If congenital TB is excluded, the infant should be started on treatment for LTBI after birth for 3 or 4 months (at which time a Mantoux skin test should be given) even if breastfeeding and the mother is on concurrent therapy.

The exclusively breastfed infant receiving isoniazid should be given pyridoxine, although it is not routinely recommended for children and adolescents. It is also recommended for use in children whose diets are either deficient in meat or milk, if they have HIV, and for pregnant adolescents; the tablets can be pulverized for easier administration. For children with meningeal, endobronchial, pleural and pericardial effusion, abdominal TB, and miliary TB, corticosteroids decrease the inflammation that is detrimental to organ function; it also decreases mortality rates and neurologic disability.

Monitoring Response to Treatment. Tracking of index and contact cases is under the jurisdiction of state and local health departments. Initial evaluation, drug management, and follow-up may also take place in these centers. However, the PCP plays a crucial role in monitoring response to treatment. The following are general monitoring guidelines (Kimberlin et al., 2018):

- See all individuals monthly who are being treated for any stage of TB. Evaluate for antitubercular drug adherence and side effects, notably for symptoms of hepatitis if on isoniazid (a rare finding in healthy infants, children, and adolescents). Educate patients to call immediately if experiencing signs of hepatoxicity (e.g., vomiting, abdominal pain, and jaundice), peripheral neuritis, diarrhea, or GI irritation. Those on pyrazinamide may experience hepatoxicity, arthralgia, or GI disturbances. Rifampin may cause orange secretions in urine, vomiting, hepatitis, flulike symptoms, thrombocytopenia, and pruritus; those on oral contraceptives need to use a back-up birth control method.
- Routine lab monitoring is not recommended in children unless they have severe TB disease, meningitis, or disseminated disease. In these cases, check transaminases monthly for the first several months. Other indications for laboratory studies include current or recent liver or biliary disease, use of hepatotoxic drugs (e.g., HIV, seizure medications), clinical evidence of hepatotoxicity, and/or pregnant or within 12 weeks postpartum.
- Collect sputum for AFB smear and culture after 2 months of drug therapy to evaluate response; if sputum culture is positive

after 3 months of therapy, the bacilli need to be rechecked for drug susceptibility.

- If cavitation is present on initial chest x-ray and a 2-month sputum culture is positive, treatment with INH and RIF should be extended an additional 3 months for a total treatment duration of 9 months.
- Repeat chest radiograph after 2 months; it is good practice to take one after therapy is completed as a baseline for comparison against any subsequent films. Hilar adenopathy can persist for 2 to 3 years despite adequate therapy. Residual calcification of the primary focus or regional lymph nodes may be evident on x-ray.
- Extrapulmonary disease: Follow clinical symptoms.
- For those taking ethambutol, ask about presence of any visual disturbances (screen visual acuity and red-green color vision if dosages exceed 20 mg/kg/day or if on more than 2 months of treatment); if unable to test visual acuity, consider an alternate drug.
- Children can be given measles and other attenuated live-virus vaccines at age-appropriate times, unless they are on high-dose corticosteroids, are severely ill, or have another contraindication.
- If therapy is interrupted, treatment length should be extended. Consult with a TB specialist.

Complications. The following complications with their clinical findings can occur with TB:

- Progressive primary pulmonary disease: Rarely, primary TB progresses and disseminates. This occurs more frequently in infants and children younger than 5 years old, a result of their immune systems being immature or inadequate to the task of eliminating bacilli. The primary pleural focus enlarges and develops a large caseous center, and liquefaction forms a cavity that contains large numbers of bacilli. Symptoms in children with progressive disease are more acute and include high intermittent fevers, night sweats, severe cough, and weight loss. Pleural effusion, peritonitis, or meningitis occurs in as many as two-thirds of individuals (Fitzgerald et al., 2015). In young adults, the infection is usually more chronic and onset is subtle. Nonspecific symptoms include fever, anorexia, weakness, and weight loss. The physical examination should include a careful skin examination, looking for cutaneous eruptions, sinus tracts, scrotal masses, and lymphadenopathy; hepatomegaly, splenomegaly, tachypnea, dyspnea, rales, wheezes, and stridor are often found. Inflamed nodes may erode through the endobronchial wall; fistulas can occur between the lymph node and the bronchial lumen and cause fibrosis, bronchiectasis, and pneumonia.
- Reactivation of pulmonary TB: There is potential for reactivation of pulmonary TB in those who acquire their initial infection when they are older than 7 years old. Reactivation is more likely after the child reaches adolescence and can present with either few symptoms, or fever, anorexia, malaise, weight loss, night sweats, productive cough, hemoptysis, and chest pain. These individuals are highly contagious until effective treatment is started, but full recovery is likely with appropriate treatment (Chiang and Starke, 2018).
- Miliary disease: During the early stages of the primary disease, bacilli disseminate and reach the bloodstream directly from the initial focus or by way of the regional lymph nodes. Prior to effective drug therapy, this primary pulmonary disease complication occurred more commonly in infants, children, and adolescents. It now appears more in racial minorities, in those

with underlying conditions that may compromise the immune system, and in older adults (Fitzgerald et al., 2015). Systemic signs such as anorexia, weight loss, and low-grade fever progress over weeks to lymphadenopathy, hepatosplenomegaly, higher fever, dyspnea, cough, rales, wheezing, frank respiratory distress, and pneumothorax or pneumomediastinum. Headache suggests meningitis; abdominal pain suggests tuberculous peritonitis (Hatzenbuehler & Starke, 2016).

- Lymph node disease: This is an extrapulmonary form of TB affecting the superficial lymph nodes; it is known as *scrofula*. It can be caused by drinking raw milk contaminated with *M. bovis* or after initial infection with *M. tuberculosis*. The head, trunk, neck, and inguinal and lower extremity nodes are firm (but not hard), fixed to underlying tissue, and nontender. The lymphadenopathy is usually initially unilateral and progresses to multinode involvement. Tuberculin skin testing is usually positive; a chest x-ray is normal 70% of the time; cultures from lymph node biopsies reveal mycobacteria in about 50% of cases (Hatzenbuehler and Starke, 2016).
- Pleural effusions: Pleural effusion frequently occurs in primary disease, caused by an extension of the bacillus into the pleural space by subpleural foci or hematogenous spread, or both. It can occur months to years after the primary infection. Symptoms include abrupt onset of low to high fever, shortness of breath, chest pain on deep inspiration, and decreased breath sounds. Response to treatment takes several weeks; radiographic changes can be evident for months following treatment (Chiang and Starke, 2018).
- Tuberculous meningitis: Meningitis is the most serious complication of TB. It generally follows primary pulmonary disease in 0.5% to 3% of untreated infants and young children 6 months to 4 years old (rare in infants younger than 4 months old). Meningeal infection is common in miliary TB. Bacilli migrate to the subarachnoid space. Caseous lesions enlarge, encapsulate, and form a tuberculoma that acts just like any other CNS mass. Tuberculomas are rare and usually occur in children younger than 10 years old. Symptoms evolve slowly or rapidly; infants and children generally experience rapid onset. Tuberculin skin testing is negative in 45% of cases with up to 30% also having negative chest x-rays (Chiang and Starke, 2018). Diagnosis is via CSF AFB stain and culture. Symptoms include headache, fever, malaise, irritability, drowsiness, decreased developmental milestones, nuchal rigidity, positive Kernig or Brudzinski signs, hypertonia, vomiting, seizures, and other neurologic symptoms. The provider should consider TB in the differential diagnosis for any child who presents with basilar meningitis and hydrocephalus, cranial nerve palsy, or stroke without other apparent cause.
- Cutaneous TB: This variant occurs in 1% to 2% of all TB cases worldwide, but is rare in the United States (Hatzenbuehler and Starke, 2016). Individuals at high risk include those with HIV, living in poor sanitary conditions, of low socioeconomic status, and the malnourished.
- Hematogenous spread of TB to other organs or body systems: Every body system can be affected by TB. Spread occurs to endocrine and exocrine glands, urogenital tract, heart and pericardium, skeleton, eyes, abdomen, tonsils, adenoids, larynx, middle ear, and mastoids.
- MDR-TB is defined as resistance to isoniazid and rifampin. XDR-TB is defined as resistance to isoniazid and rifampin,

one fluoroquinolone, and at least one aminoglycoside (capreomycin, amikacin, or kanamycin). Over the last few years drug resistance rates in the United States have been around 1% to 9% (Chiang and Starke, 2018).

Helminthic Zoonoses

Greater than 50% of infectious diseases originate with animals, and approximately 60% of all human pathogens are zoonotic (transmitted from an animal to a human host) in origin (CDC, 2017e). Transmission of zoonotic infections occurs by several routes:

- Direct infection by ingestion of eggs or the larvae penetration into the body (infections such as tapeworms and roundworms are acquired from their eggs; hookworms penetrate the skin)
- Indirect infection by ingestion of larvae in food (e.g., fish, meat, snails, freshwater shrimp, land crabs)
- Exposure to an intermediary vector (e.g., mosquitoes, flies, fleas, ticks)

A large percentage of households in the United States have domestic pets; an estimated range of 50.4% to 70.8% of U.S. homes have a dog or cat, therefore, close contact is inevitable (American Veterinary Medical Association, 2018). Domesticated dogs, cats, and wild animals (e.g., raccoons) kept as pets can be infected with intestinal helminth parasites. Mild to severe illness results when a helminth transmits to children, most often by fecal contamination. Only toxocariasis larva migrans is discussed here. (See Chapter 40 for discussion on intestinal parasites.)

Toxocariasis

Toxocariasis, or larva migrans, is caused by a parasitic helminth larvae (of the roundworm) found in dogs (*T. canis*) and cats (*T. catis*). The larvae live for extended periods in human and animal organs and tissues and cause an inflammatory condition. The most common clinical syndromes are visceral larva migrans (VLM), ocular toxocariasis (formerly called ocular larva migrans), and covert disease. *Toxocara* larvae rarely migrate to the CNS causing eosinophilic meningoencephalitis or granuloma formation (CDC, 2013). They are further classified as *asymptomatic* or *clinically unapparent*. *T. catis* causes less VLM than *T. canis*; *T. canis* causes VLM, OLM, and, in severe cases, neural larva migrans.

Dogs or cats of any age can carry the *Toxocara* roundworm; worldwide, dogs (especially puppies) are a more common vector than kittens. Puppies are infected prior to birth (not true for kittens) or from their mother's milk. Ingestion of these hardy eggs (they remain viable for months and in inclement weather conditions) occurs from contact with excreta in contaminated soil (e.g., in sandboxes, parks, playgrounds, schoolyards, public places where dogs and cats visit), hands, toys, or in food. Once the eggs are ingested and hatch, the larvae penetrate the intestines and migrate to the liver, lungs, heart, brain, and muscles. With initial or mild infestations, the larvae reach other locations, such as the brain and eye, more easily. In humans, the larvae cannot mature into adult worms (as they do in animals), so infected individuals do not pass eggs or larvae in their excreta.

The most recent study in the United States showed a prevalence rate of 14% for toxocariasis with 4.6% to 7.3% of children infected (Dent and Kazura, 2016). Young children and those younger than 20 years old are most commonly infected

(CDC, 2013). VLM occurs in older children and adolescents but is most commonly seen in children 2 to 7 years old and in those with a history of pica. Ocular toxocariasis occurs more often in older children and adolescents (Kimberlin et al., 2018).

Clinical Findings. Symptoms result from the migrating larvae and from the induced eosinophilic granulomatous inflammation of organs and tissues. Symptom severity depends on the number of larvae ingested and degree of allergic response. Assess exposure history for pica or geophagia; exposure to dogs, cats, or environments where animals are known to frequent (parks, sandboxes); and recent travel. In the case of ocular toxocariasis, there may be history of pica or previous VLM.

Toxocariasis should be considered in any child with a nonspecific history of recurrent abdominal pain, reactive airway disease, and allergies of unknown cause. The clinical history of VLM includes rash, abdominal and/or limb pain, anorexia, nausea/vomiting, lethargy, or respiratory symptoms (cough, wheezing). Ocular toxocariasis is usually associated with a history of a "wandering eye" or squinting, light sensitivity, a white pupil, swelling around an eye, or eye pain. Neural larva migrans often presents 2 to 4 weeks after larvae ingestion. The child's history can include weakness, incoordination, ataxia, irritability, seizures, altered mental status, stupor, and/or coma.

Physical Examination.
- Ocular toxocariasis: Posterior or peripheral subretinal mass, decreased vision, pain, strabismus, or leukocoria
- VLM: Abdominal pain, hepatomegaly, irritability, respiratory symptoms (coughing, wheezing, pneumonia), cervical adenitis, urticaria, pruritic skin lesions or nodules, macular rash
- Neural larva migrans: Neurologic impairment
- Covert larva migrans: Chronic weakness, abdominal pain, allergic signs (asymptomatic eosinophilia or wheezing may be the only indicators of disease)

Diagnostic Studies. Eosinophilia (>20%) is present in 50% to 75% of cases; a normal count does not rule out this infection (Dent and Kazura, 2016).
- VLM: CBC reveals leukocytosis, marked eosinophilia (>500/μL), hypergammaglobulinemia (IgG, IgM, IgE), and elevated A and B blood group isohemagglutinin titers. *Toxocara* ELISA antibody is confirmatory; it does not, however, distinguish from past and active disease. Most symptomatic children have titers of 1:32 or greater (Dent and Kazura, 2016).
- Ocular toxocariasis: Serologic VLM testing is not reliable because it is less sensitive. Diagnosis is usually based on the typical clinical findings of retinal scarring or granuloma formation and elevated antibody titers. Vitreous-aqueous fluid *Toxocara* titers are usually higher than serum titers. CT and MRI detect granulomatous lesions.
- Overt larva migrans: May demonstrate eosinophilia and increased IgE.

Differential Diagnosis. Other helminths, hypereosinophilic syndromes, retinoblastoma, autoimmune disease, and allergic conditions are included in the differential diagnoses.

Management and Complications. Most individuals do not require treatment because symptoms are usually mild with spontaneous recovery occurring over a period of weeks to months (Dent and Kazura, 2016). Pediatric infectious disease referral for evaluation and treatment is indicated for patients with symptomatic VLM, ocular toxocariasis, or CNS disease. Management is based on controlling inflammatory reactions (corticosteroids) and using appropriate anthelmintic therapy.

Albendazole is the drug of choice, mebendazole is an alternative. Longer courses of 3 to 4 weeks are needed to treat disease with CNS and ocular involvement; systemic and intraocular corticosteroid therapy should be considered for ocular toxocariasis (managed by qualified ophthalmologist and infectious disease specialist). Family pets need evaluation by a veterinarian. Permanent ocular structural damage may result from ocular toxocariasis. Neural larva migrans may cause acute eosinophilic meningoencephalitis.

Patient and Family Education. Prevention of zoonotic infestations includes identifying possible sources of exposure, encouraging routine helminth testing for pets, decontamination of soiled environments, and further exposure prevention. The last intervention includes education about safe pet fecal cleanup, the regular deworming of pets, good hand washing, behavioral modification in cases of pica and geophagia, and covering sandboxes when not in use. Communities should be encouraged to promote leash laws and responsible pet ownership (e.g., cleaning up pet fecal waste), to disallow dogs from playgrounds and parks, and to restrict open access to sandboxes.

The Child Presenting With Fever

Fever is defined as an abnormally elevated rectal temperature of 100.4°F (38°C) or greater.

The normal physiologic hypothalamic set-point for body temperature is altered by many different agents (see Chapter 28). Neonatal febrile illnesses are usually the result of congenital infections or infections acquired at delivery (e.g., late-onset group B, streptococcal infection), in the nursery (especially in premature infants), at home (e.g., pneumococcal or meningococcal infection), and as a result of anatomic or physiologic dysfunction (e.g., renal). Fever causes in children are related to bacterial and viral infections, vaccines, biologic agents, tissue damage, malignancy, drugs, collagen-vascular disorders, endocrine disorders, inflammatory disorders, and other disease states. Temperatures higher than 105.8°F (41°C) are rarely of infectious origin but are due to CNS dysfunction (e.g., malignant hyperthermia, drug fever, heat stroke).

There are two situations of invasive bacterial or viral infections that are a particular challenge for any provider dealing with neonates, infants, and children 36 months old or younger—*fever without focus*—and in all ages—*FUO*. Each of these situations is discussed separately, and guidelines for their management are given. A fairly objective diagnosis can be reached by completing a careful history and physical examination and following diagnostic, assessment, and management guidelines based on age, symptoms, estimated risks, associated diseases, and immune status. A few general epidemiologic points are helpful for this discussion (Nield and Kamat, 2016):

- The majority of infants less than 3 months old with fever have a viral infection. A workup for bacterial disease is still necessary. The younger the infant, the greater the uncertainty about the possibility of a serious bacterial infection, and the greater the need to rule out this possibility.
- Viruses have a seasonal pattern: RSV and influenza A in winter; enterovirus in summer and fall.
- Bacteremia occurs in approximately 5% of previously well infants younger than 3 months old.
- Bacteremia can be an occult infection in young infants and children (i.e., nontoxic-appearing child whose blood culture is positive for a pathogenic organism).

- Occult bacteremia occurs in less than 0.5% of children between 3 and 36 months old who are vaccinated with both conjugated Hib and *S. pneumoniae* vaccines. Otitis media, pneumonia, URIs, enteritis, UTIs, osteomyelitis, and meningitis more commonly account for infections in this age range.

Fever Without Focus in Infants and Young Children

Fever without focus is an acute febrile illness with nonapparent fever etiology after careful history and physical examination. Approximately 30% of febrile children 1 month to 36 months old do not have localizing signs of infection. In the vast majority of these children, the etiology is viral (Nield and Kamat, 2016). However, children between birth and 24 months old are at greatest risk for unsuspected occult bacteremia; it is less common in those older than 36 months. Table 31.8 lists the most common pathogens causing bacteremia in infants

TABLE 31.8	Age-Related Causes of Serious Bacterial and Viral Infections in Very Young Infants
Age	**Bacterial and Viral Infections**
Meningitis	
<1 month	Group B streptococcus
	Escherichia coli (and other enteric gram-negative bacilli)
	Listeria monocytogenes
	Streptococcus pneumoniae
	Haemophilus influenzae
	Staphylococcus aureus
	Neisseria meningitidis
	Salmonella spp.
	Herpes simplex
	Enteroviruses
1-3 month	*S. pneumoniae*
	Group B streptococcus
	N. meningitidis
	Salmonella spp.
	H. influenzae
	L. monocytogenes
	S. aureus
Osteoarticular Infections	
<1 month	Group B streptococcus
	S. aureus
1-3 month	*S. aureus*
	Group B streptococcus
	S. pneumoniae
Urinary Tract Infection	
0-3 month	*E. coli*
	Other enteric gram-negative bacilli
	Group D streptococcus (including *Enterococcus* spp.)

In decreasing order of frequency.

Data from Nield LS, Kamat D. Fever without a focus. In: Kliegman RM, Stanton BF, St. Geme III JW, et al, eds. *Nelson Textbook of Pediatrics*. 20th ed. Philadelphia: Saunders; 2016:1281–1287; and Jhaveri R, Shapiro ED. Fever without localizing signs. In: Long SS, Pickering LK, Prober CG, eds. *Principles and Practice of Pediatric Infectious Diseases*. 5th ed. New York: Elsevier; 2018:115–117.

younger than 3 months old. Since the advent of the Hib conjugate vaccine, this pathogen is a rare cause of bacteremia in children 3 to 36 months old; the incidence of *S. pneumoniae* bacteremia decreased substantially since conjugate vaccine has been routinely in use (Nield and Kamat, 2016; Jhaveri and Shapiro, 2018).

Clinical Findings

History and Physical Examination. The following should be included in the history of the illness:

- Duration and degree of fever (rectal temperature was 100.4°F [38°C] or greater)
- Associated symptoms: Vomiting, diarrhea, respiratory symptoms, rash (especially petechiae or purpura), feeding pattern, irritability, inconsolability, change in play activities, lethargy (level of consciousness characterized by poor or absent eye contact, failure to recognize parents or interact with persons or objects in the environment)
- Review of known exposures (family illness, contacts with other ill children, day care contacts); recent travel history
- Recent vaccination
- Past medical history of malignancy, splenectomy, shunt, indwelling catheter, immunologic disorders, recurrent bacterial infections, serious bacterial infection
- Neonatal history of complications, prior antibiotics, prior surgeries, hyperbilirubinemia
- Chronic illness
- Current medications, including antipyretics, antibiotics, herbs, and dietary supplements
- Immunization history, particularly with Hib conjugate and pneumococcal conjugate vaccines

A complete physical examination should be done. Of special note are symptoms suggestive of serious bacterial illness (e.g., fever, bulging anterior fontanelle, respiratory system changes, lethargy and other CNS symptoms, evidence of skin infection or rashes, skin perfusion and turgor).

Diagnostic Studies. An algorithm for determining the diagnostic studies based upon specific age groups is in Fig 31.8. Febrile infants younger than 1 month old or any febrile toxic-appearing child 0 to 36 months old should be admitted to the hospital for a complete sepsis workup and given appropriate antibiotic treatment. The need for CSF analysis from infants 1 month to 3 months old varies between different management guidelines if empiric antibiotics are being considered (Palazzi, 2019).

A negative, low-risk ambulatory workup is characterized by:

- CBC: WBC count less than 15,000/mm³, absolute band count of fewer than 1500/mm³; non-elevated ESR and/or CRP (included in some standard guidelines)
- Catheterized urinalysis: Fewer than 10 WBCs/hpf spun sediment, negative leukocytes and nitrites
- When diarrhea is present: Fewer than 5 WBCs/hpf in stool
- If cough is present: Negative chest x-ray

Appropriate cultures should be obtained and monitored every 24 hours until results are finalized. Viral testing should be done based on seasonality. Obtain HSV PCR from blood and CSF and PCR/culture from skin sites (mouth/throat, eyes, umbilicus, perirectal) if infant is 42 days old or less, has vesicular skin lesions, abnormal CSF, or seizures.

Differential Diagnosis. The differential diagnoses include upper respiratory tract disease (e.g., viral URI, otitis media, and sinusitis); lower respiratory tract disease (e.g., bronchiolitis, pneumonia); GI disease; musculoskeletal infections (e.g.,

cellulitis, septic arthritis, osteomyelitis); urinary tract infection (especially due to *E. coli*); and occult bacteremia due to other pathogens in children 3 to 36 months old. In those immunized with both Hib and pneumococcal conjugate vaccine, the rate of occult bacteremia is much lower (Nield and Kamat, 2016). Serious bacterial agents are identified in approximately 7% of previously well neonates with fever and sepsis, meningitis, UTI, enteritis, osteomyelitis, or suppurative arthritis diagnosis. Other possible illnesses to consider in this age group include pyelonephritis (more often occurring in uncircumcised boys, neonates, those with urinary tract anomalies, and females), otitis media, omphalitis, mastitis, and other skin or soft tissue infections (Nield and Kamat, 2016).

Management

Applying Risk Criteria. There are several criteria or protocols for identifying infants younger than 3 months old who have serious bacterial illness (e.g., bacteremia, UTI, meningitis, bacterial gastroenteritis, or pneumonia) that require empiric antibiotics and possibly hospitalization. The most widely cited guidelines include the Boston, Philadelphia, Milwaukee, and Rochester; all are based upon clinical assessment and laboratory studies (Moher et al., 2012; Smitherman and Macias, 2018). (See Fig 31.8.)

High risk is regarded as any of the following:

- Any febrile infant younger than 1 month old; any toxic-appearing neonate, infant, or child regardless of age, risk factors, or degree of fever
- An infant 1 to 3 months old with a rectal temperature of 101.5°F (38.6°C) or greater
- An infant 1 to 3 months old with a chronic illness or underlying condition (including prematurity) with unreliable caretakers
- An infant younger than 3 months old even if diagnosed with otitis media
- Gestational age less than 37 weeks—history of prematurity
- Given antibiotic in the past week
- Infants and children 3 to 36 months old with a rectal temperature of 102.2°F (39°C) and laboratory results that place the child in a high-risk category
- Any aged child with fever and petechiae who appears ill

Immediate hospitalization and workup are indicated for high-risk cases. Any child younger than 36 months old who appears well with rectal temperature more than 102.2°F (39°C), WBC more than 15,000/mm³, and who is not vaccinated with Hib and *S. pneumoniae* conjugate vaccines should be started on empiric antibiotic therapy (Nield and Kamat, 2016).

Low risk is regarded as any of the following:

- An infant 1 to 3 months old who is nontoxic-appearing with no clinical evidence of ear, skin, joint, or bones infections and who has low-risk diagnostic study results.
- An infant 3 to 6 months old with a rectal temperature more than 100.4°F (38°C) but less than 102.2°F (39°C) who does not appear ill.
- An infant or child 3 to 36 months old with a fever more than 102.2°F (39°C), who is nontoxic-appearing, previously healthy with a non-focal bacterial infection and a positive rapid influenza A test.
- An infant or child 3 to 36 months old who is mildly ill appearing with rectal temperature greater than 102.2°F (39°C) but less than 104°F (40°C) and low-risk diagnostic study results. There should be documented immunizations to at least two doses of both *H. influenzae* conjugate vaccine and pneumococcal conjugate vaccine (PCV7 or PCV13).

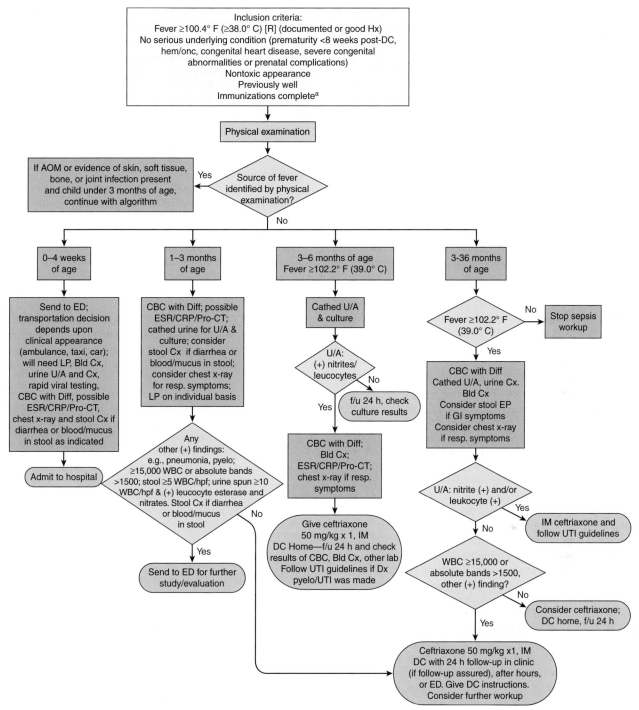

• Fig 31.8 Fever Without Focus Algorithm. [a]Occult bacteremia can be as high as 5% if immunizations are incomplete (<1% if complete). *AOM,* Acute otitis media; *Bld Cx,* blood culture; *Cathed,* catheterized; *CBC,* complete blood count; *CRP,* C-reactive protein; *Cx,* culture, *DC,* discharge; *Diff,* differential; *Dx,* diagnosis; *ED,* emergency department; *EP,* enteric pathogens (culture); *ESR,* erythrocyte sedimentation rate; *f/u,* follow-up; *GI,* gastrointestinal; *h,* hours; *hem/onc,* hematologic/oncology issue; *hpf,* high power field; *Hx,* history; *IM,* intramuscular; *LP,* lumbar puncture; *Pro-CT,* procalcitonin; *pyelo,* pyelonephritis; *resp.,* respiratory; *U/A,* urinalysis; *UTI,* urinary tract infection; *WBC,* white blood cell count; *wk,* week. From Hui C, Neto G, Tsertsvadze A, et al. *Diagnosis and management of febrile infants (0–3 months): Evidence Report/Technology Assessments, No. 205.* Rockville, MD: Agency for Healthcare Research and Quality; 2012; and Nield LS, Kamat D. Fever without a focus. In Kliegman RM, Stanton BF, St. Geme III JW, et al., eds. *Nelson Textbook of Pediatrics.* 20th ed. Philadelphia: Elsevier; 2016:1280–1287.

In light of the decrease in bacteremia caused by *H. influenzae* and *S. pneumonia,* a well-appearing nontoxic infant from 1 to 3 months old with no foci of infection, who meets low-risk criteria, has reliable caregivers, and close follow-up does not need empirical antibiotics (nor a lumbar puncture) (Nield and Kamat, 2016).

Follow-up management criteria for any child not being hospitalized includes:

- Reevaluation in the clinic in 24 hours and access to emergency care if condition worsens.
- Daily follow-up on culture results (blood, urine, CSF) until results are final.
- If cultures become positive, infant/child needs to be seen for evaluation and appropriate antibiotic treatment based on organism and additional workup as needed.
- Parents of infants managed as outpatients need detailed instructions on signs and symptoms that indicate a worsening of their infant's illness. Symptoms that prompt emergency care include: a change in or new rash; duskiness, cyanosis, or mottling; coolness of extremities; poor feeding or vomiting; irritability; cries with positional changes; difficulty in comforting or arousing; seizure activity (eye rolling or jerking of extremities); or bulging anterior fontanelle.

Fever of Unknown Origin

The definition of *FUO* in children is: (1) a documented fever (rectal temperature more than 101°F [38.3°C] or oral temperature more than 100°F [37.8°C]) present most days for 3 weeks or more without an etiology, despite 3 weeks of outpatient visits and extensive studies, and (2) no etiology after 1 week of evaluation in the hospital or as an outpatient (Manthiram et al., 2018; Nield and Kamat, 2016). The PCP must frequently rethink and reevaluate historical, clinical, and laboratory data from a child with a FUO. An infectious disease consultation is recommended.

Many FUOs are atypical presentations of common disorders, notably infections (accounting for more than one-third of cases) or rheumatologic and connective tissue diseases (e.g., juvenile rheumatoid arthritis, SLE). In the United States, infectious diseases associated with most diagnoses of FUO include EBV, cat-scratch disease *(B. henselae),* complicated UTIs, and vertebral and pelvic osteomyelitis (Manthiram et al., 2018). Other causative agents include salmonellosis, TB, rickettsial diseases, syphilis, Lyme disease, prolonged viral infections, CMV, viral hepatitis, coccidioidomycosis, histoplasmosis, malaria, toxoplasmosis, tularemia, brucellosis, rat-bite fever, leptospirosis, drug fever, Kawasaki disease, inflammatory bowel disease, and rheumatic fever. Neoplastic conditions and AIDS generally have symptoms other than just fever. Fevers lasting more than 6 months occur in those with granulomatosis or autoimmune disease (Nield and Kamat, 2016). In children younger than 6 years old an infectious cause of fever is more likely than older children. Older children are more likely to have auto inflammatory or autoimmune disorders. The most common causes of FUO are UTI/pyelonephritis, respiratory illnesses, localized infections (abscess, osteomyelitis), juvenile arthritis, and, rarely, leukemia and lymphoma (Manthiram et al., 2018).

Clinical Findings

History. A careful history helps distinguish between recurrent fever episodes and those that need further evaluation. Recurrent fevers resolve with well periods between them, suggesting an etiology of multiple self-limiting infections. History includes:

- A careful analysis of symptoms or signs, a meticulous review of systems, history of the fever pattern, and patient's age. An adolescent with complaints of low-grade fevers, or whose fever resolved but who feels ill and is unable to attend school or social activities may have "fatigue of deconditioning" (Box 31.2). These children require the same careful medical evaluation, but rarely have a serious infection or medical condition (Manthiram et al., 2018).
- Note of past medical history of recurrent infections, surgery, transfusions, and contact with ill individuals
- Medication use, including over-the-counter and herbal/natural/dietary supplements
- Family medical history, including autoimmune disease or inflammatory bowel disorder; genetic background (inherited periodic fever syndromes [e.g., familial Mediterranean fever, hyperimmunoglobulinemia D with periodic fever syndrome], tumor receptor–associated periodic syndrome)
- Family pets including reptiles, pet immunization history, or exposure to wild or other domestic animals
- Unusual dietary habits (eating squirrel, rabbit, or other unusual animal meat)
- History of pica; history of travel (location; travel immunizations; water/food ingested; if returned home with travel souvenirs containing dirt, rocks, or earth-contaminated artifacts)

Physical Examination. Special attention needs to be paid to these areas:

- Skin: Presence of rashes, lesions, nailfold capillary abnormalities; presence or absence of sweating
- Mouth: Note a smooth tongue with absence of fungiform papillae; presence of candidiasis
- Throat: Exudate, erythema
- Local or generalized lymphadenopathy or hepatosplenomegaly
- Joint examination, and palpation of bones for tenderness, edema
- Palpation/percussion of sinus and mastoid areas for tenderness; tap upper teeth

---

> ● **BOX 31.2** **Typical Findings in Patients With Fatigue of Deconditioning**

- Older than 12 years old
- Pre-illness achievement high (academic and social)
- Family expectations high (performance)
- Acute febrile illness with onset easily dated
- Family and outside attention high
- Multiple but vague complaints
- Odd complaints (e.g., 10-s "shooting" pains at multiple sites; 30-s "blindness"; stereotypic, sporadic, brief unilateral tremors, jerks, or "paralysis" lasting <1 min)
- Tiredness, but no daytime sleep (or reversal of daytime and nighttime sleep)
- There is a model of chronic illness in family, recent loss of important person, and/or change in family dynamics
- Unusual cooperation and interest during interview and examination (or unusual fearfulness and dependency on parent)
- Preserved or increased weight
- Normal physical and neurologic examination
- Normal results of screening laboratory tests syndromes

In Long SS, Pickering LK, Prober CG, eds: Principles and Practice of Pediatric Infectious Diseases. 5th ed. New York: Elsevier; 117–128.

Manthiram, K., Edwards, K., & Long, S. Prolonged, recurrent & periodic fever syndromes. 2018.

- Eye examination noting exudate, palpebral or bulbar conjunctivitis, conjunctival hemorrhages, papillary reaction; a complete ophthalmologic examination is indicated to fully evaluate for uveitis, chorioretinitis, proptosis
- Pelvic examination in adolescent females
- Rectal examination and guaiac test
- Deep tendon reflexes

Diagnostic Studies. Laboratory studies depend on a history and physical examination that point to a specific infection or area of suspicion. Studies might include:

- CBC with differential, ESR (>30 mm/h needs further evaluation), CRP, or procalcitonin
- Serologic tests for specific diseases suggested by history and examination
- Blood cultures obtained aerobically (may require serial specimens to rule out endocarditis, osteomyelitis, or deep abscesses)
- Urinalysis plus urine cultures
- Mantoux skin test or IGRA
- Chest, sinus, mastoid, and GI tract radiographs may be indicated
- Liver chemistries
- If bone marrow biopsy is obtained, send cultures for bacteria, AFB, and fungus
- Echocardiogram if subacute endocarditis is suspected
- Other tests may involve radionuclide scans, total body CT, MRI, ultrasounds, or biopsies

Differential Diagnosis and Management. Infectious diseases, collagen-vascular disease (e.g., juvenile arthritis, SLE), malignancies, drug fever (can be any drug), nosocomial, HIV-associated illnesses, diabetes insipidus, hyperthyroidism, inflammatory bowel disease, hematoma in a confined space, anhidrotic ectodermal dysplasia, and Munchausen syndrome by proxy are included in the differential diagnosis of an FUO.

An infectious disease consultation is advised with consideration of hospitalizing the child if there is evidence of systemic illness or failure to thrive, the child is very young, the parent(s) anxiety is extreme, or an extensive workup is planned. Otherwise, the child should be followed with frequent visits, documented fever pattern, and other specialized tests if screening tests, as indicated, or if other physical findings develop. Treatment is based on the underlying diagnosis. Empiric use of antibiotics should be avoided unless the child is critically ill and suspected to have disseminated TB (Nield and Kamat, 2016).

Infectious Agents Used in Bioterrorism

Agents of biologic warfare are categorized by the CDC according to their potential for aerosol transmission, susceptibility of the population, degree of person-to-person transmission, expected high morbidity and mortality rates, the likelihood for delayed diagnosis, and the lack of effective and efficacious treatments. Agents at highest risk to the populace are known as *category A weapons of bioterrorism*. These include specific bacteria (e.g., *Bacillus anthracis* [anthrax]; *Clostridium botulinum* [botulism]; *Francisella tularensis* [tularemia]; *Yersinia pestis* [plague]) and viruses (e.g., variola virus [smallpox]; viruses of hemorrhagic fever [Ebola, Marburg, Lassa fever]). Most of these diseases are rarely, if ever, seen in clinical practice settings. Refer to the CDC website for specific details about agents. The CDC established a Laboratory Response Network to provide standardized diagnostic testing for selected agents and link state and local public health laboratories with other advanced-capacity laboratories (see Additional Resources).

Children are at particular risk for exposure to and absorption of biologic warfare agents (e.g., anthrax and botulinum toxin). Factors that predispose them to such risk include being within closer proximity to the ground, having faster ventilation rates and thinner skins, having an increased risk of dehydration, and having greater undeveloped cognition.

Providers can join other community healthcare providers to develop pediatric readiness plans to any large disaster (e.g., storms, earthquakes, acts of bioterrorism). These readiness plans should include triage, isolation and treatment/care facilities, transportation, communication, housing, and the establishment of vaccination clinics on a massive scale for children, especially in communities where health departments and/or emergency departments may not have the procedural skills to address a severely ill pediatric population. Health alerts can be requested by email from the CDC.

Additional Resources

Infectious Diseases Society of America (IDSA). www.idsociety.org
American Academy of Pediatrics. www.aap.org
AIDSinfo (U.S. Department of Health and Human Services). www.aidsinfo.nih.gov/guidelines
Centers for Disease Control and Prevention. www.cdc.gov
FluView Interactive. www.cdc.gov/flu/weekly/fluviewinteractive.htm
Hepatitis C Laboratory Studies Table. www.cdc.gov/mmwr/preview/mmwrhtml/mm6218a5.htm
Travelers' Health: Malaria Prophylaxis. wwwnc.cdc.gov/travel/yellowbook/2014/chapter-3-infectious-diseases-related-to-travel/malaria#1939
World Health Organization. www.who.int/en/
Intermittent Preventive Treatment of Malaria in Pregnancy (IPTp). www.who.int/malaria/areas/preventive_therapies/pregnancy/en/
Malaria: Intermittent Preventive Treatment in Infants (IPTi). www.who.int/malaria/areas/preventive_therapies/infants/en/

References

Abzug MJ. Nonpolio enteroviruses. In: Kliegman, RM, Stanton BF, St Geme JW, Schor NF (eds): Philadelphia: Elsevier; 2016;1561–1568.e1.

American College of Obstetricians and Gynecologists (ACOG). *Hepatitis B and Hepatitis C in Pregnancy*; 2013. Retrieved from www.acog.org/Patients/FAQs/Hepatitis-B-and-Hepatitis-C-in-Pregnancy.

American Academy of Pediatrics (AAP). *Child Immunization Schedule: Why is it Like That?*; 2018. Retrieved from www.healthychildren.org/English/safety-prevention/immunizations/Pages/Child-Immunization-Schedule-Why-Is-It-Like-That.aspx.

American Academy of Pediatrics (AAP). *Choosing an Insect Repellent for Your Child*; 2018. Retrieved from www.healthychildren.org/English/safety-prevention/at-play/Pages/Insect-Repellents.aspx.

American Veterinary Medical Association (AVMA). *National Pet Week: Survey Says! Discover Top Ten Dog and Cat Owning States*; 2018. Retrieved from https://petweek.org/top-10-dog-cat-owning-states.html.

Arnold JC, Nizet V. Pharyngitis. In: Long SS, Pickering LK, Prober CG, eds. *Principles and Practice of Pediatric Infectious Diseases*. 5th ed. New York: Elsevier; 2018:202–207.

Blaser MJ. *Missing Microbes: How the Overuse of Antibiotics is Fueling Our Modern Plagues*. New York: Henry Holt and Company; 2014.

Caserta MT. Roseola (human herpes viruses 6 and 7). In: Kliegman RM, Stanton BF, St. Geme JW, Schor NF, eds. *Nelson Textbook of Pediatrics*. 20th ed. Philadelphia: Elsevier; 2016:1594–1597.

Castagnini LA, Leach CT. Epstein-Barr virus. In: Cherry JD, Harrison GJ, Kaplan SL, Steinbach WJ, Hotez PJ, eds. *Feigin and Cherry's Textbook of Pediatric Infectious Diseases*. 8th ed. Philadelphia: Elsevier; 2019:1450–1471.

Centers for Disease Control and Prevention (CDC). *Tuberculosis: Report of an Expert Consultation on the Uses of Nucleic Acid Amplification Tests for the Diagnosis of Tuberculosis*; 2012. Retrieved from www.cdc.gov/tb/publications/guidelines/amplification_tests/recco mendations.htm.

Centers for Disease Control and Prevention (CDC). Parasites—toxocariasis (also known as roundworm infection); 2013. Retrieved from www.cdc.gov/parasites/toxocariasis/.

Centers for Disease Control and Prevention (CDC). *Clinical Guidance: Dengue Virus*; 2014. Retrieved from www.cdc.gov/dengue/clinicalLa b/clinical.html.

Centers for Disease Control and Prevention (CDC). *How Many People Get Lyme Disease?*; 2015a. Retrieved from www.cdc.gov/lyme/stats/h umanCases.html.

Centers for Disease Control and Prevention (CDC). *Lyme Disease: Transmission*; 2015b. Retrieved from www.cdc.gov/lyme/transmission/ind ex.html.

Centers for Disease Control and Prevention (CDC). *Antibiotic Resistance Threats in the United States*; 2016a. Retrieved from www.cdc.gov/drug resistance/biggest_threats.html 2013.

Centers for Disease Control and Prevention (CDC). *Clostridium Difficile Infection*; 2016b. Retrieved from https://www.cdc.gov/hai/organisms /cdiff/cdiff_infect.html.

Centers for Disease Control and Prevention (CDC). *Managing People at Risk for Severe Varicella*; 2016c. Retrieved from www.cdc.gov/chicken pox/hcp/persons-risk.html.

Centers for Disease Control and Prevention (CDC). Methicillin-resistant *staphylococcus aureus* (MRSA). Information for clinicians. Retrieved from www.cdc.gov/mrsa/community/clinicians/index.html; 2016d.

Centers for Disease Control and Prevention (CDC). *Middle-Eastern Respiratory Syndrome (MERS)*; 2016e. Retrieved from www.cdc.gov/ coronavirus/MERS/about/index.html.

Centers for Disease Control and Prevention (CDC). *Tuberculosis: Interferon-Gamma Release Assays (IGRAs)—Blood Tests for TB Infection*; 2016f. Retrieved from www.cdc.gov/tb/publications/factsheets/testi ng/igra.htm.

Centers for Disease Control and Prevention (CDC). *What to do if an Infant or Child is Mistakenly Fed Another Woman's Expressed Breast Milk*; 2016g. Retrieved from www.cdc.gov/breastfeeding/recommen dations/other_mothers_milk.htm.

Centers for Disease Control and prevention (CDC). *Guidance for Clinicians on the Use of Rapid Influenza Diagnostic Tests*; 2017a. Retrieved from www.cdc.gov/flu/professionals/diagnosis/clinician_guidance_ri dt.htm#figure1.

Centers for Disease Control and Prevention (CDC). *Global Health—Polio: Our Progress Against Polio*; 2017b. Retrieved from www.cdc.gov /polio/progress/index.htm.

Centers for Disease Control and Prevention (CDC). *Influenza Antiviral Medications: Summary for Clinicians*; 2017c. Retrieved from https://www.cdc.gov/flu/professionals/antivirals/summary-clinicians. htm.

Centers for Disease Control and Prevention (CDC). *Meningococcal Disease*; 2017d. Retrieved from www.cdc.gov/meningococcal/about/ind ex.html.

Centers for Disease Control and Prevention (CDC). *National Center for Emerging and Zoonotic Infectious Diseases (NCEZID): What we do*; 2017e. Retrieved from www.cdc.gov/ncezid/what-we-do/index.html.

Centers for Disease Control and Prevention (CDC). *Reported Cases of HPS: HPS in the United States*; 2017f. Retrieved from www.cdc.gov/h antavirus/surveillance/index.html.

Centers for Disease Control and Prevention (CDC). *Lyme Disease Incidence Rates by State*; 2017g. Retrieved from www.cdc.gov/lyme/stats/c hartstables/incidencebystate.html.

Centers for Disease Control and Prevention (CDC). *Severe Acute Respiratory Syndrome (SARS)*; 2017h. Retrieved from www.cdc.gov/sars/.

Centers for Disease Control and Prevention (CDC). *AMF Investigation*; 2018a. Retrieved from https://www.cdc.gov/acute-flaccid-myelitis/afm-surveillance.html.

Centers for Disease Control and Prevention (CDC). *Antibiotic/Antimicrobial Resistance (AR/AMR)*; 2018b. Retrieved from https://www.cdc .gov/drugresistance/.

Centers for Disease Control and Prevention (CDC). *Antibiotic Prescribing and Use*; 2018c. Retrieved from https://www.cdc.gov/antibiotic-use/index.html.

Centers for Disease Control and Prevention (CDC). *Handwashing: Clean Hands Save Lives: Show me the Science—When to Use Hand Sanitizers*; 2018d. Retrieved from www.cdc.gov/handwashing/show-me-the-science-hand-sanitizer.html.

Centers for Disease Control and Prevention (CDC). *Hepatitis A Questions and Answers for Health Professionals*; 2018e. Retrieved from https://ww w.cdc.gov/hepatitis/HAV/HAVfaq.htm#B.

Centers for Disease Control and Prevention (CDC). *Hepatitis B FAQs for Health Professionals*; 2018f. Retrieved from www.cdc.gov/hepatitis/H BV/HBVfaq.htm#overview.

Centers for Disease Control and Prevention (CDC). *Highly Pathogenic Asian Avian Influenza A (H5N1) Virus*; 2018g. Retrieved from https:/ /www.cdc.gov/flu/avianflu/h5n1-virus.htm.

Centers for Disease Control and Prevention (CDC). *HIV in the United States: at a Glance*; 2018h. Retrieved from www.cdc.gov/hiv/statistics /basics/ataglance.html.

Centers for Disease Control and Prevention (CDC). *HIV Among Pregnant Women, Infants, and Children*; 2018i. Retrieved from https://ww w.cdc.gov/hiv/group/gender/pregnantwomen/.

Centers for Disease and Prevention (CDC). *HIV Among Youth*; 2018j. Retrieved from www.cdc.gov/hiv/risk/age/youth/index.html.

Centers for Disease Control and Prevention (CDC). *HIV Transmission*; 2018k. Retrieved from www.cdc.gov/hiv/basics/transmission.html.

Centers for Disease Control and Prevention (CDC). *Influenza: Estimating Seasonal Influenza-Associated Deaths in the United States*; 2018l. Retrieved from https://www.cdc.gov/flu/about/disease/us_flu-related_ deaths.htm.

Centers for Disease Control and Prevention (CDC). *Lyme Disease*; 2018m. Retrieved from https://www.cdc.gov/lyme/index.html.

Centers for Disease Control and Prevention (CDC). *Malaria*; 2018n. Retrieved from https://www.cdc.gov/parasites/malaria/index.html.

Centers for Disease Control and Prevention (CDC). *Measles (Rubeola): for Health Professionals*; 2018o. Retrieved from www.cdc.gov/measle s/hcp/index.html.

Centers for Disease Control and Prevention (CDC). *Mumps Vaccination*; 2018p. Retrieved from www.cdc.gov/mumps/vaccination.html.

Centers for Disease Control and Prevention (CDC). *Measles Cases and Outbreaks: Measles Cases in 2018*; 2018q. Retrieved from www.cdc.gov/measles/cases-outbreaks.html.

Center for Disease Control. *National Notifiable Disease Surveillance System*; 2018r. Retrieved from https://wwwn.cdc.gov/nndss/.

Centers for Disease Control and Prevention (CDC). *Meningococcal Disease: Surveillance*; 2018s. Retrieved from www.cdc.gov/meningococca l/surveillance/index.html.

Centers for Disease Control and Prevention (CDC). *Pre-Exposure Prophylaxis (PrEP)*; 2018t. Retrieved from www.cdc.gov/hiv/prevention /research/prep/.

Centers for Disease Control and Prevention (CDC). *Rocky Mountain Spotted Fever (RMSF): Epidemiology and Statistics*; 2018u. Retrieved from www.cdc.gov/rmsf/stats/.

Centers for Disease Control and Prevention (CDC). *Tickborne Diseases of the United States: A Reference Manual for Health Care Providers*; 2018v. Retrieved from https://www.cdc.gov/ticks/tickbornediseases/index.h tml.

Centers for Disease Control and Prevention (CDC). *Viral Hepatitis—Hepatitis C Information: Hepatitis C FAQs for Health Professionals*; 2018w. Retrieved from www.cdc.gov/hepatitis/HCV/HCVfaq.htm# section1.

Centers for Disease Control and Prevention (CDC). *West Nile Virus*; 2018x. Retrieved from https://www.cdc.gov/westnile/index.html.

Centers for Disease Control and Prevention (CDC). *Zika Virus*; 2018y. Retrieved from https://www.cdc.gov/zika/index.html.

Chapman LE, Peters CJ, Mills JN, McKee KT. Hantaviruses. In: Harrison GJ, Kaplan SL, Steinbach WJ, Hotez PJ, eds. *Feigin and Cherry's Textbook of Pediatric Infectious Diseases*. 8th ed. Philadelphia: Elsevier; 2019:1854–1866.

Cherry J. Roseola infantum (exanthem subitum). In: Cherry JD, Harrison GJ, Kaplan SL, Steinbach WJ, Hotez PJ, eds. *Feigin and Cherry's Textbook of Pediatric Infectious Diseases*. 8th ed. Philadelphia: Elsevier; 2019:559–561.

Cherry J, Baker A. Rubella virus. In: Cherry JD, Harrison GJ, Kaplan SL, Steinbach WJ, Hotez PJ, eds. *Feigin and Cherry's Textbook of Pediatric Infectious Disease*. 8th ed. Philadelphia: Elsevier; 2019:1601–1622.

Chiang SS, Starke JF. Mycobacterium tuberculosis. In: Long SS, Pickering LK, Prober CG, eds. *Principles and Practice of Pediatric Infectious Diseases*. 5th ed. New York: Elsevier; 2018:790–806.

Collier MG, Holtzman D, Homberg SD. Hepatitis C virus. In: Long SS, Pickering LK, Prober CG, eds. *Principles and Practice of Pediatric Infectious Diseases*. 5th ed. New York: Elsevier; 2018:1135–1142.

Daum RS. Staphylococcus aureus. In: Long SS, Pickering LK, Prober CG, eds. *Principles and Practice of Pediatric Infectious Diseases*. 5th ed. New York: Elsevier; 2018:692–706.

Dent AE, Kazura JW. Toxocariasis (visceral and ocular larva migrans). In: Kliegman RM, Stanton BF, St. Geme III JW, et al., eds. *Nelson Textbook of Pediatrics*. 20th ed. Philadelphia: Elsevier; 2016:1743–1744.

Fitzgerald DW, Sterling TR, Hass DW. Mycobacterium tuberculosis. In: Bennett JE, Dolin R, Blaser MJ, eds. *Mandell, Douglas, and Bennett's Principles and Practice of Infectious Diseases*. 8th ed. Philadelphia: Elsevier/Saunders; 2015.

Garcia RA, Chismark E, Eggert J. Dengue virus: another type of immigrant. *JNP*. 2015;11(1):34–40.

Gerber MA. Group A streptococcus. In: Kliegman RM, Stanton BF, St. Geme III JW, et al., eds. *Nelson Textbook of Pediatrics*. 20th ed. Philadelphia: Saunders/Elsevier; 2016:1327–1337.

Gershon AA. Varicella-zoster virus. In: Cherry JD, Harrison GJ, Kaplan SL, et al., eds. *Feigin and Cherry's Textbook of Pediatric Infectious Diseases*. 8th ed. Philadelphia; 2019:1476–14841.

Hamborsky J, Kroger A, Wolfe S. Epidemiology and prevention of vaccine-preventable diseases. In: Centers for Disease Control and Prevention, ed. *Pink book*. 13th ed. Washington, DC: Public Health Foundation; 2015:231–245.

Han JY, Jacobs RF. Bartonella species. In: Long SS, Pickering LK, Prober CG, eds. *Principles and Practice of Pediatric Infectious Diseases*. 5th ed. New York: Elsevier; 2018:881–886.

Harrison G, Pinsky B, Arvin AM. Herpes simplex viruses 1 and 2. In: Cherry JD, Harrison GJ, Kaplan SL, et al., eds. *Feigin and Cherry's Textbook of Pediatric Infectious Diseases*. 8th ed. Philadelphia: Elsevier; 2019:1403–1429.

Haslam DB, St. Geme III JW. Groups C and G streptococci. In: Long SS, Pickering LK, Prober CG, eds. *Principles and Practice of Pediatric Infectious Diseases*. 5th ed. New York: Elsevier; 2018:736–737.

Hersh AL, Shapiro DJ, Pavia AT, et al. Antibiotic prescribing in ambulatory pediatrics in the United States. *Pediatrics*. 2011;128(6):1053–1061.

Howard LM, Edwards KM. Bartonella infections. In: Cherry JD, Harrison GJ, Kaplan SL, Steinbach WJ, Hotez PJ, eds. *Feigin and Cherry's Textbook of Pediatric Infectious Diseases*. 8th ed. Philadelphia: Elsevier; 2019:1240–1246.

Hatzenbuehler LA, Starke JR. Tuberculosis (Mycobacterium tuberculosis). In: Kliegman RM, Stanton BF, St. Geme III JW, et al., eds. *Nelson Textbook of Pediatrics*. 20th ed. Philadelphia: Elsevier; 2016:1445–1461.

Hughes HK, Kahl LK. Blood chemistries and body fluids. *Harriet Lane Handbook*. 21st ed. Philadelphia PA: Elsevier; 2018.

Infectious Diseases Society of America (IDSA). *IDSA, SHEA, and PIDS Joint Policy Statement on Mandatory Immunization of Health Care Personnel According to the ACIP-Recommended Vaccine Schedule*; 2013. Retrieved from https://www.idsociety.org/public-health/immunization/immunization/nations-leading-infectious-diseases-experts-call-for-mandatory-flu-vaccine-for-all-healthcare-personnel/

or http://www.shea-online.org/index.php/policy/positions-statements/290-policy-statement-on-mandatory-immunization-of-health-care-personnel.

Jhaveri R, El-Kamary SS. Hepatitis C virus. In: Cherry JD, Harrison GJ, Kaplan SL, Steinbach WJ, Hotez PJ, eds. *Feigin and Cherry's Textbook of Pediatric Infectious Diseases*. 8th ed. Philadelphia: Elsevier; 2019:1723–1728.

Jhaveri R, Shapiro ED. Fever without localizing signs. In: Long SS, Pickering LK, Prober CG, eds. *Principles and Practice of Pediatric Infectious Diseases*. 5th ed. New York: Elsevier; 2018:115–117.

Kimberlin DW, Brady MT, Jackson, Long SS, eds. *Red Book: 2018-2021 Report of the Committee on Infectious Diseases*. 31st ed. Elk Grove Village, IL: American Academy of Pediatrics; 2018.

Langebeek N, Gisolf EH, Reiss P, et al. Predictors and correlates of adherence to combination antiretroviral therapy (ART) for chronic HIV infection: a meta-analysis. *BMC Med*. 2014;12:142.

Lantos PM, McKinney R. Rickettsial and ehrlichial diseases. In: Cherry JD, Harrison GJ, Kaplan SL, et al., eds. *Feigin and Cherry's Textbook of Pediatric Infectious Diseases*. 8th ed. Philadelphia: Elsevier; 2019:1963–1975.

LaRussa PS, Marin M. Varicella-zoster virus infections. In: Kliegman RM, Stanton BF, St. Geme III JW, et al., eds. *Nelson Textbook of Pediatrics*. 20th ed. Philadelphia: Elsevier; 2016:1579–1586.

Liu C, Bayer A, Cosgrove SE, et al. Clinical practice guidelines by the Infectious Diseases Society of America for the treatment of methicillin-resistant Staphylococcus aureus infections in adults and children. *Clin Infect Dis*. 2011;52(3):285–292.

Lucero YC, O'Ryan ML. Caliciviruses. In: Cherry JD, Harrison GJ, Kaplan SL, et al., eds. *Feigin and Cherry's Textbook of Pediatric Infectious Diseases*. 8th ed. Philadelphia: Elsevier; 2019:1571–1577.

Mack CL, Gonzalez-Peralta RP, Gupta N, et al. NASPGHAN practice guidelines: diagnosis and management of hepatitis C infection in infants, children, and adolescents. *J Pediatr Gastroenterol Nutr*. 2012;54(6):838–855.

Manthiram K, Long SS, Edwards KM. Prolonged, recurrent, and periodic fever syndromes. In: Long SS, Pickering LK, Prober CG, eds. *Principles and Practice of Pediatric Infectious Diseases*. 5th ed 5. New York: Elsevier; 2018:117–128.

Moher D, Hui C, Neto O, et al. *Evidence Report/Technology Assessment number 205: Diagnosis and Management of Febrile Infants (0-3 months)*; 2012. Retrieved from effectivehealthcare.ahrq.gov/ehc/products/279/1015/EvidenceReport205_Febrile-Infants_20120322.pdf.

Moore KS. Lyme disease: diagnosis, treatment guidelines, and controversy. *JNP*. 2015;11(1):64–69.

Murphy TF. Moraxella catarrhalis, Kingella, and other gram-negative cocci. In: Bennett JE, Dolin R, Blaser MJ, eds. *Mandell, Douglas, and Bennett's Principles and Practice of Infectious Diseases*. 8th ed. Philadelphia: Elsevier; 2015:2463–2471.

Nachega JB, Uthman OA, Anderson J, et al. Adherence to antiretroviral therapy during and after pregnancy in low-income, middle-income, and high-income countries: a systematic review and meta-analysis. *AIDS*. 2012;26(16):2039–2052.

Nield LS, Kamat D. Fever without a focus. In: Kliegman RM, Stanton BF, St. Geme III JW, et al., eds. *Nelson Textbook of Pediatrics*. 20th ed. Philadelphia: Saunders/Elsevier; 2016:1281–1287.

National Institute of Health [NIH]. *Human Microbiome Project*; 2018. Retrieved from https://commonfund.nih.gov/hmp.

National Institute of Health. *NIH Human Microbiome Project Defines Normal Bacterial Makeup of the Body*; 2012. Retrieved from https://www.nih.gov/news-events/news-releases/nih-human-microbiome-project-defines-normal-bacterial-makeup-body.

Palazzi DL. Fever without source and fever of unknown origin. In: Cherry J, Harrison GJ, Kaplan SL, et al., eds. *Feigin and Cherry's Textbook of Pediatric Infectious Diseases*. 8th ed. Philadelphia: Elsevier/Saunders; 2019:608–616.

Pollard AJ, Finn A. Neisseria meningitidis. In: Long SS, Pickering LK, Prober CG, eds. *Principles and Practice of Pediatric Infectious Diseases*. 5th ed. New York: Elsevier; 2018:747–759.

Pollard AJ, Sadarangani M. Neisseria meningitidis (meningococcus). In: Kliegman RM, Stanton BF, St. Geme III JW, et al., eds. *Nelson Textbook of Pediatrics*. 20th ed. Philadelphia: Elsevier; 2016:1356–1364.

Porsch EA, St. Geme JF. Kingella kingae. In: Cherry J, Demmler-Harrison GJ, Kaplan SL, et al., eds. *Feigin and Cherry's Textbook of Pediatric Infectious Diseases*. 7th ed. Philadelphia: Elsevier/Saunders; 2014:1222–1228.

Poutanen SM. Human coronaviruses. In: Long SS, Pickering LK, Prober CG, eds. *Principles and Practice of Pediatric Infectious Diseases*. 5th ed. New York: Elsevier; 2018:1148–1152.

Read JS. Epidemiology and prevention of HIV infection in children and adolescents. In: Long SS, Prober CG, Fischer M, eds. *In Principles and Practice of Pediatric Infectious Diseases*. Elsevier; 2018:659–665.

Redfield RR, Schuchat A, Dauphin L, et al. Centers for Disease Control and Prevention: youth risk behavior surveillance—United States, 2017. *MMWR Surveill Summ*. 2018;67(No. 8):68–103.

Reller ME, Dumler JS. Rocky Mountain spotted fever (Rickettsia rickettsii). In: Kliegman RM, Stanton BF, St. Geme III JW, et al., eds. *Nelson Textbook of Pediatrics*. 20th ed. Philadelphia: Elsevier; 2016:1497–1504.

Rios M, U.S. Food and Drug Administration. *Reducing threats to the blood supply from West Nile virus, dengue virus, and chikungunya virus through development of detection tools and studies of genetic evolution and pathogenesis*; 2018. Retrieved from www.fda.gov/BiologicsBlood Vaccines/ScienceResearch/BiologicsResearchAreas/ucm127094.htm.

Schuster JE, Williams JV. Human metapneumovirus. In: Cherry JD, Harrison GJ, Kaplan SL, et al., eds. *Feigin and Cherry's Textbook of Pediatric Infectious Diseases*. 8th ed. Philadelphia: Elsevier/Saunders; 2019:1797–1804.

Sender R, Fuchs S, Milo R. Revised estimates of the number of human and bacteria cells in the body. *PLoS Biology*. 2016;14(8):e1002533. Retrieved from https://doi.org/10.1371/journal.pbio.1002533.

Shetty AK, Maldonado YA. Human immunodeficiency virus/acquired immunodeficiency syndrome in the infant. In: Wilson CB, Nizet V, Maldonado YA, et al., eds. *Remington and Klein's Infectious Diseases of the Fetus and Newborn Infant*. 8th ed. Philadelphia: Elsevier/Saunders; 2016:619–674.

Sood SK, Krause PJ. Lyme disease. In: Cherry J, Harrison GJ, Kaplan SL, et al., eds. *Feigin and Cherry's Textbook of Pediatric Infectious Diseases*. 8th ed. Philadelphia: Elsevier; 2019:1246–1252.

Sosinsky LS, Gilliam WS. Childcare: how pediatricians can support children and families. In: Kliegman RM, Stanton BF, St Geme JW, Schor NF, eds. *Nelson Textbook of Pediatrics*. 20th ed. Philadelphia: Elsevier; 2016:101–106.

Stevens DL, Bisno AL, Chambers HF, et al. Practice guidelines for the diagnosis and management of skin and soft tissue infections: 2014 update by the Infectious Disease Society of America. *Clin Infect Dis*. 2014;59(2):e10–e52.

Teshale EH, Hepatitis E. virus. In: Long SS, Pickering LK, Prober CG, eds. *Principles and Practice of Pediatric Infectious Diseases*. 5th ed. New York: Elsevier; 2018:1126–1128.

U.S. Department of Health and Human Services (USDHHS). AIDS-info: Recommendations for use of antiretroviral drugs in pregnant HIV-1-infected women for maternal health and interventions to reduce perinatal HIV transmission in the United States. *AIDS-info (website)*; 2018a. Retrieved from http://aidsinfo.nih.gov/contentfiles/l vguidelines/perinatalgl.pdf.

U.S. Department of Health and Human Services (USDHHS). AIDS info: Guidelines for the use of antiretroviral agents in HIV-1-infected adults and adolescents: limitations to treatment safety and efficacy: adherence to antiretroviral therapy *AIDS-info (website)*; 2017. Retrieved from http://aidsinfo.nih.gov/guidelines/html/1/adult-and-adolescent-arv-guidelines/30/adherence-to-art.

U.S. Department of Health and Human Services (USDHHS). Guidelines for the use of antiretroviral agents in pediatric HIV infection: diagnosis of HIV infection in infants and children; 2018b. Retrieved from http://aidsinfo.nih.gov/guidelines/html/2/pediatric-arv-guidelines/ 55/diagnosis-of-hiv-infection-in-infants-and-children.

Vijayan AL, Vanimaya SR, Saikant R, Lakshmi S, Kartik R, Manoj G. Procalcitonin: a promising diagnostic marker for sepsis and antibiotic therapy. *J Intensive Care*. 2017;5:51. https://doi.org/10.1186/s40560-017-0246-8.

World Health Organization (WHO). *Handbook for Clinical Management of Dengue*; 2012. Retrieved from www.wpro.who.int/mvp/documents/ handbook_for_clinical_management_of_dengue.pdf.

World Health Organization (WHO). *March 2014 Supplement to the 2013 Consolidated Guidelines on the use of Antiretrovirals for Treating and Preventing HIV Infection: Recommendations for a Public Health Approach*; 2014. Retrieved from http://apps.who.int/iris/bitstream/1 0665/104264/1/9789241506830_eng.pdf?ua=1.

World Health Organization (WHO). *Guidance for National Tuberculosis Programmes on the Management of Tuberculosis in Children*. 2nd ed; 2014. Retrieved from. http://apps.who.int/medicinedocs/documents/ s21535en/s21535en.pdf.

World Health Organization (WHO). *Influenza: Avian and Other Zoonotic*; 2018a. Retrieved from http://www.who.int/en/news-room/fact-sheets/detail/influenza-(avian-and-other-zoonotic.

World Health Organization (WHO). *FAQs: H5N1 Influenza*; 2018b. Retrieved from www.who.int/influenza/human_animal_interface/avi an_influenza/h5n1_research/faqs/en/.

World Health Organization (WHO). *Hepatitis B*; 2018c. Retrieved from www.who.int/mediacentre/factsheets/fs204/en/.

World Health Organization (WHO). *HIV/AIDS*; 2018d. Retrieved from http://www.who.int/news-room/fact-sheets/detail/hiv-aids.

World Health Organization (WHO). *Dengue and Severe Dengue*; 2018e. Retrieved from www.who.int/mediacentre/factsheets/fs117/en/.

Yagupsky P. Kingella species. In: Long SS, Pickering LK, Prober CG, eds. *Principles and Practice of Pediatric Infectious Diseases*. 5th ed. New York: Elsevier; 2018:945–948.

Yagupsky P. Kingella kingae. In: Kliegman RM, Stanton BF, St. Geme III JW, et al., eds. *Nelson Textbook of Pediatrics*. 20th ed. Philadelphia: Elsevier; 2016:1369–1371.

Yogev R, Chadwick EG. Acquired immunodeficiency syndrome (human immunodeficiency virus). In: Kliegman RM, Stanton BF, St. Geme III JW, et al., eds. *Nelson Textbook of Pediatrics*. 20th ed. Philadelphia: Elsevier; 2016:1645–1666.e1.

32

Congenital and Inherited Disorders

MARTHA DRIESSNACK AND SANDRA DAACK-HIRSCH

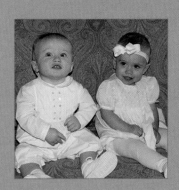

As the field of genetics and genomics continues to evolve, the pediatric primary care provider's (PCPs) scope of practice continues to expand. PCPs are now required to meet basic genetic clinical competencies, which include recognizing historical and physical features of common genetic disorders, identifying children with congenital and inherited disorders, and providing basic genetics information to children and families. The PCP is ideally situated to evaluate and co-manage children with a wide array of congenital and inherited disorders. With the support of health supervision guidelines developed for these children, PCPs provide primary care, anticipate areas of medical vulnerability, and advocate for the prevention of any secondary disability. In addition to providing ongoing primary care for children with congenital and/or inherited disorders, the American Academy of Pediatrics (AAP) also states that pediatric PCPs should consider the genetic implications of common pediatric conditions (AAP website) as disease causation of many common pediatric conditions, including asthma, allergy, autism, cancer, cardiac conditions, developmental delay, mental health disorders, and obesity, is being reconceptualized, recognizing that every disease is located on the spectrum of genetic influence (Figure 3.1).

Obtaining a complete family health history and constructing a three-generation pedigree is now part of every child's well-child record. The family health history and identification of genetic red flags, along with the identification of a child's individual risk for congenital and/or inherited disorders, are included in a child's comprehensive health and environmental assessment. The well-child physical exam should also focus on the identification of any phenotypic or physical characteristics, developmental delays, and/or cognitive neurologic deficits that could be caused by/associated with a congenital and/or inherited condition. An overview of common physical signs was introduced in the earlier chapter on genetics (Figure 3.6); additional resources for honing pediatric physical assessment skills are located in Table 32.1. If the child's history or physical exam indicates any such findings, a genetics consultation and/or referral for testing and evaluation is recommended.

Genetics Referral

A genetic consultation and/or referral should be considered when there is/are: (1) a positive history for an inherited disorder for which the child is at risk, (2) physical findings/dysmorphic features on physical exam consistent with a known syndrome, (3) known inborn errors of metabolism, and/or (4) noted developmental,

growth, and/or structural anomalies. A selection of common clinical findings and cues is summarized in Table 32.2.

Genetic specialists not only provide guidance in terms of ordering appropriate tests, but also are a trusted source of information for navigating this evolving field with expertise in diagnosis, understanding inheritance patterns and recurrence risk, genetic testing, nuanced mechanisms of congenital and inherited disorders, and evolution of clinical manifestations across the lifespan. Co-management with a genetic specialist offers many benefits, especially in terms of access to emerging evidence and high-value child and/or family support resources.

Genetic counseling is one specific aspect of the genetic specialist referral. Families often need to consider genetic information when making health-related decisions that can affect their personal physical and reproductive health, as well as the lives of their child, other children, and extended family. Additionally, genetic counseling facilitates families' understanding of the diagnosis of concern, its course, and its management. It also facilitates families' understanding of how genetics/genomics

TABLE 32.1	Resources to Hone Physical Assessment Skills

- *Diagnostic Dysmorphology* (1990), by Jon M. Aase, is one of the classic, most comprehensive, and detailed textbooks on dysmorphology.
- *Genetics and Genomics in Nursing and Health Care*, **2e** (2018), by Theresa A. Beery, M. Linda Workman, and Julia A. Eggert, includes a detailed chapter on congenital anomalies, basic dysmorphology, and genetic assessment, including measurements, drawings, and photographs.
- *Medical Genetics in Pediatric Practice* (2013), by Robert A. Saul (Editor) and the American Academy of Pediatrics (AAP) Committee on Genetics, provides focused information for clinicians on the clinical features (including pictures), laboratory diagnosis, and management needs for specific genetic conditions, from achondroplasia to Williams syndrome.
- *Positive Exposure* http://positiveexposure.org/. Positive Exposure was founded in 1998 by Rick Guidotti, an award-winning fashion photographer. He extended his talent to help transform public perceptions of children and adults living with genetic, physical, and behavioral differences. His refreshing, yet realistic images provide a different lens for health care providers.

TABLE 32.2 Selected Syndromes and Common Findings/Cues

Syndrome	Common Clinical Findings	Neurodevelopmental Cues
Down (trisomy 21)	• Short stature • Brachycephaly • Midface hypoplasia with flat nasal bridge • Brushfield spots • Epicanthal folds with upslanting palpebral fissures • Small mouth with protruding tongue • Myopia/cataracts • Small ears/narrow canals • Extra skin at nape of neck • Lax joints (atlantoaxial instability) • Short broad hands/feet/digits • Single palmar crease • Clinodactyly • Exaggerated space/plantar groove between great and second toes • Congenital heart disease • At risk for leukemia, hypothyroidism, Alzheimer disease	• Intellectual/cognitive disability/developmental delays • Hearing loss • Hypotonia (infant)
Turner (XO) Fig 32.1	• Short stature (for family) • Short neck with webbing and low posterior hair line • Posteriorly rotated ears, narrow canals • Ptosis • Short 4th/5th metacarpals • Short legs • Hyperconvex nails • Cardiac disorders (e.g., bicuspid aortic valve, coarctation of the aorta) • Hip dysplasia, scoliosis, and/or kyphosis • Horseshoe kidney • Chronic OM, with conductive hearing loss • Delayed puberty/infertility	• Nonverbal learning disabilities • Hearing loss • Strabismus
Klinefelter (XXY) Fig 32.2	• Tall, with long arm span • Dental decay • Delayed puberty • Small penis, cryptorchidism (or small testes) • Gynecomastia • Autoimmune disorders • Skin striae • Scoliosis • Increased risk of malignancies, including male breast cancer	• Delayed expressive language • Shy, withdrawn • Immature for age • ADHD
Fragile X Fig 32.3	• Prominent forehead, long narrow face, prominent jaw, high-arched palate/dental crowding, protuberant ears develop late childhood/early adolescence • Feeding problems/GER • Strabismus, refractive errors (e.g., hyperopia, astigmatism), nystagmus, ptosis. • Recurrent/chronic OM • Seizures • Short stature • Macroorchidism (puberty) • Connective tissue dysplasia (e.g., velvet-like skin, joint hypermobility especially fingers), pes planus, congenital hip dislocation, clubfoot, scoliosis • Obstructive sleep apnea • Possible in girls	• Intellectual disability • Language delays • Behavioral problems (e.g., anxiety, attention, aggression) • Stereopathies, such as hand-flapping • Autism spectrum disorder
Prader-Willi	• Decreased fetal movement/position • Failure to thrive • Short stature • Central obesity • Hypothalamic insufficiency • Strabismus • Myopia/hyperopia • Sleep apnea • Enamel hypoplasia • Scoliosis	• Motor delays • Poor coordination • Language delays • Mild intellectual disability • Compulsive hyperphagia • Behavioral phenotype: Tantrums, stubborn, rigidity, skin picking, high pain tolerance, ADHD, compulsiveness

TABLE 32.2 **Selected Syndromes and Common Findings/Cues—cont'd**

Syndrome	Common Clinical Findings	Neurodevelopmental Cues
Angelman	• Seizures • Global developmental delays • Abnormal gait, arms held high/flexed elbows • Hypotonic trunk with hypertonic limbs (commando crawl) • Feeding/growth problems • Acquired microcephaly	• Speech delay, but adequate receptive language • Intellectual disability • Spontaneous (persistent) social smile/fits of laughter • Hand flapping • Loves water • Abnormal sleep
Beckwith-Wiedemann	• Omphalocele or umbilical hernia • Macroglossia; with later onset of malocclusion/maxillary underdevelopment • Facial features: Prominent eyes, nevus flammeus, helical pits, anterior ear lobe creases • Large placenta/long umbilical cord • Hypoglycemia (newborn) • Large at birth (LGA) with increased growth after birth (macrosomia) • Abnormal enlargement of one side of the body/structure (hemi-hyperplasia/-hypertrophy)	• Normal development • Articulation issues
22q11 deletion (previously DiGeorge or velocardiofacial)	• Congenital heart defect • Palate abnormalities • Facial features: Long tubular nose, crumpled ears, hypertelorism, malar hypoplasia • Hypotonia • Early feeding problems • Constipation • Chronic otitis media/sinusitis • Polydactyly • Vertebral anomalies • Strabismus	• Developmental disability • Communication disorders, including delayed speech and hypernasality • Psychiatric disorders
Marfan Fig 32.4	• Phenotypic variability, including variable facial features (e.g., long, narrow face, downward slanting eyes, malar hypoplasia, and micrognathia) • Often tall for age, extremities disproportionately long in comparison with trunk; altered arm-span: height ratio • Paucity of muscle mass/fat stores • Aortic root dilatation, aortic tear/rupture, aortic valve prolapse/regurgitation, tricuspid vale prolapsed, mitral valve prolapse/regurgitation • Myopia, ectopia lentis (hallmark), retinal detachment, glaucoma, and early cataract formation • Spontaneous pneumothorax, reduced pulmonary reserve, and obstructive sleep apnea • Skeletal issues, including pectus deformities, scoliosis, thoracic kyphosis, and protrusion acetabuli, pes planus, reduced mobility of elbow, increased laxity of other joints • Stretch marks (lower back, inguinal, axillary regions) • At risk for dural ectasia	• Usually within normal range
Neurofibromatosis 1 (NF1)	• Two or more of the following features are required: • ≥6 café-au-lait spots 5 mm (prepubertal)/15 mm (postpubertal) • ≥2 neurofibromas or 1 plexiform neurofibroma • Axillary/inguinal freckling • Optic glioma • ≥2 Lisch nodules (iris hamartomas) • Associated osseous lesion (e.g., sphenoid wing dysplasia, cortical thickening of cortex in long bones) • First-degree relative with NF1	• Learning, speech/language, and motor abilities vary
Fetal alcohol spectrum disorder (FASD; Fig 32.5)	• Poor prenatal and postnatal growth • Hypotonia, poor coordination • Cardiac defects (e.g., VSD, ASD) • Narrow eyes, microphthalmia, large epicanthal folds, microcephaly, small upper jaw, smooth groove in upper lip, thin upper lip • Simian creases common	• Delayed development in three or more areas: cognitive, speech, motor, psychosocial

ADHD, Attention-deficit/hyperactivity disorder; *ASD*, atrial septal defect; *GER*, gastroesophageal reflux; *OM*, otitis media; *VSD*, ventricular septal defect.

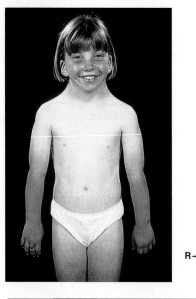

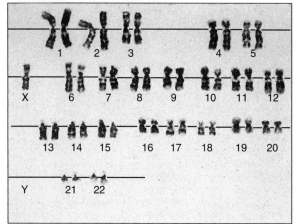

• **Fig 32.1** Turner Syndrome (A) Physical appearance. (B) Karyotype. (From Patton KT, Thibodeau GA. *The Human Body in Health & Disease.* 6th ed. St. Louis: Mosby/Elsevier; 2014.)

influence the disorder (e.g., risk of recurrence, carrier status, etc.). Identifying strategies to address recurrence risk and assisting individuals and families to choose a plan of action are part of genetic counseling. Finally, genetic counseling assists individuals and families to cope with a diagnosis, its prognosis, and the risk of recurrence. All of these are complex issues. Most families have low genetic/genomic literacy, see the genetic counselor infrequently, and/or may not be ready to take in information at the time of the initial counseling; therefore the child's PCP needs to have ongoing collaboration with child's geneticist/genetics counselor. Genetic specialists can also offer guidance to the family and the PCP when faced with difficult end-of-life conversations (e.g., post-mortem investigations). Equally important, for those children who live beyond the pediatric lifespan, genetic specialists can provide continuity in care as children with congenital and inherited disorders transition from pediatric to adult PCPs and specialists.

The AAP recommends a registry and referral tracking system for children/families who present with a potentially "positive" family history and/or clinical concerns suggestive of a congenital and/or inherited disorder (AAP website). A referral tracking system allows for documentation of tests/results, past and active referrals/consultations, and any related follow-up plan/activities.

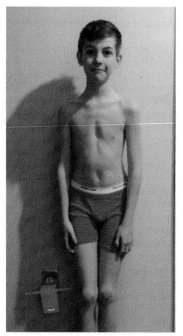

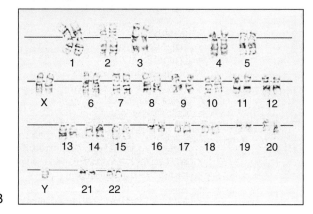

• **Fig 32.2** Klinefelter Syndrome (A) Physical appearance. (B) Karyotype. (From Patton KT, Thibodeau GA. *The Human Body in Health & Disease.* 6th ed. St. Louis: Mosby/Elsevier; 2014.)

It also serves as a point of documenting specialists' evaluations and their implications with the child/family.

Creating an Emergency Plan

Genetic specialists, in collaboration with PCPs, are also key resources for families creating an emergency plan or set of instructions that outlines when, where, who, and how to contact emergency personnel should their child need emergent care. This can be in letter form for the family to use when needed (see sample emergency letter for patients with Maple Syrup Urine Disease: Emergency letter for families [MSUD, Div Metabolic Genetics, UUHSC]). While emergency plans should identify the child's diagnosis (or diagnoses), clinical findings/status, current medications, allergies, and immunizations, they also need to highlight common presenting problems/findings with specific management strategies and professional pediatric and subspecialty contact information, especially for emergency care providers who may have limited knowledge regarding congenital and/or inherited disorders. It is important to remember that with many genetic conditions (e.g., inborn errors of metabolism), an illness or surgical procedure may become life-threatening if certain precautions are not attended to.

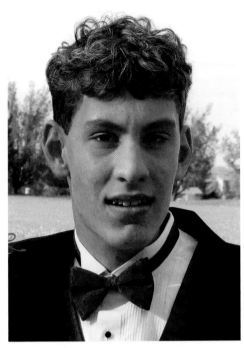

• **Fig 32.3** Fragile X Syndrome.

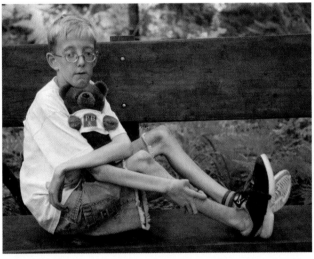

• **Fig 32.4** Marfan Syndrome (Courtesy The Marfan Foundation).

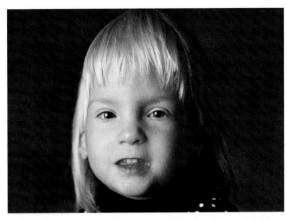

• **Fig 32.5** Fetal Alcohol Spectrum Disorder (From McKinney E. *Maternal-child Nursing.* 4th ed. Philadelphia: Saunders/Elsevier; 2013; Fortinash KM, Holoday Worret PA. *Psychiatric Mental Health Nursing.* 5th ed. St. Louis: Mosby/Elsevier; 2012.)

reinforce genetic counseling information, assess the family's need for return genetic counseling visits, refer to local specialists and support services when appropriate, and advocate for the child/family within the community as well as within the healthcare system.

Primary Care for Children with Congenital and Inherited Disorders

Most children with congenital malformations and inherited conditions fit into the category of a children and youth with special health care needs (CYSHCN), as they are at an increased risk for chronic physical, developmental, behavioral, or emotional conditions, and may require added health-related services. The needs of children with congenital and inherited conditions may require an array of subspecialty services in the hospital as well as in the community and school. The PCP assists families with upfront identification of specialists, refers when services are needed, and maintains ongoing communication, so that subspecialists' recommendations can be followed and reviewed with the child/family.

All members of the child's health care team should follow age-appropriate health supervision guidelines as per the AAP Bright Futures (2017) to provide health promotion, health education, early identification, and prevention of disease for all children, typical and atypical. In addition to the Bright Futures guidelines, the AAP Committee on Genetics developed specific health supervision guidelines that highlight the most current management guidelines for children with a specific genetic and genetic-related condition. For example, syndrome-specific health management guidelines are already available for PCPs caring for children with achondroplasia, Down syndrome, Fragile X and permutation-associated disorders, Marfan syndrome, neurofibromatosis-type I, Noonan syndrome, Prader-Willi syndrome, sickle cell disease, Turner syndrome, and Williams syndrome (See AAP website for guidelines). Each guideline is updated regularly and provides important resources that highlight assessment needs by age, cautions, syndrome-specific growth charts, vaccine considerations, and current/emerging research findings. For example, children with Down syndrome have a variety of congenital malformations and medical disorders (see Table 32.2). Not only are these variations highlighted, but there is also a tracking record for children with Down syndrome available. There are also other syndrome-specific growth charts for

The PCP's role is to help the family find a genetic specialist or counselor; to initiate referrals with screening pedigrees, medical records, and other information; and to evaluate the family's understanding of the need for a referral to genetic professionals. It is important to prepare the child and family for the consultation and/or referral so that they understand the role of the specialist in the child's overall care. The PCP can anticipate the need for the family to obtain additional family health history and records, as well as specialized neuro-developmental testing, imaging studies, and child/family photographs. The PCP is the first line, point of entry—the one who decides which children warrant attention and further testing/retesting, monitoring, and referral. Shared decision-making with the family and, when applicable, the child, is essential. Once the family has had genetic counseling, the child's PCPs should

Disorder	Primary Care Issues
Achondroplasia *Most common disorder associated with disproportion short stature*	• Monitor growth using syndrome-specific growth chart. Note that hydrocephalus is a lifelong risk, but is most likely to develop during first 2 years of life. Occipital frontal circumference (OFC) should be monitored and charted at each visit. • Achondroplasia-specific early development charts are available. Most children will have delayed motor milestones, but not social or cognitive. • Persistent or recurrent middle-ear dysfunction is common. Annual hearing evaluations are recommended. • Cranio-cervical junction compression risk—rear-facing car seat provides the best protection/positioning angle for a child with macrocephaly/skeletal dysplasia. • Bowing of the lower legs thoracolumbar kyphosis are common. Avoid devices that cause curved ("C") sitting, such as umbrella-style strollers, infant carriers, and/or soft canvas seats during first year of life. Avoid walkers, jumpers, and/or backpack carriers until child able to bear weight (which should occur no later than 2–2½ years). • Snoring is common; monitor for obstructive sleep apnea. • GER is more common. • Restrictive pulmonary disease; avoid living at high elevation. • Greater-than-average sweating is normal. • Anesthesia risk—care must be taken in manipulation of the neck. Avoid spinal anesthesia. • Ensure medication doses are appropriate for age AND size. • Spinal cord compression/stenosis (manifest in older children with numbness, weakness, and altered deep tendon reflexes).
Angelman syndrome *Rare disease*	• Monitor severe developmental delays/learning disabilities and speech, as there is often absence/near absence of speech. • Monitor characteristic behavioral cluster (happy disposition, unprovoked episodes of laughter/smiling, and fascination with water). • Increased risk of seizures, sleep disorders and feeding difficulties/GER. • May not develop expressive language, but usually can understand simple commands. Older children/teens may learn to communicate through gesturing and or using communication boards. • Easily excited, hypermotoric and hyperactive; active explorers; often may appear to be constantly in motion; increased safety concerns. • Some children may never walk; however, there is a normal progression through puberty; increased risk for scoliosis.
Beckwith-Wiedemann syndrome *Overgrowth syndrome*	• Anticipate neonatal hypoglycemia. • Assess for umbilical hernia/omphalocele requiring surgical referral. • Monitor for feeding problems, secondary to macroglossia, which can also cause difficulties in speaking and breathing. • Monitor for unequal (asymmetric) growth; limb length discrepancies; hemi-hypertrophy/-plasia. • Increased risk of developing certain childhood cancers, particularly Wilms tumor (nephroblastoma) and tumors involving the liver (hepatoblastoma); risk of malignancy is greatest before the age of 8. The trend in alpha-fetoprotein (AFP) levels over time should be followed regularly until age 4 years and abdominal ultrasounds every 3 months until age 8 years. • Increased incidence of renal anomalies (e.g., nephromegaly, renal medullary dysplasia, nephrocalcinosis, duplicated collecting system, medullary sponge kidney, and diverticula.
Down syndrome *Chromosomal disorder*	• Careful review of newborn screen for hypothyroidism. Annual and/or systematic screening for hypothyroidism. • Careful review of newborn critical congenital heart disease (CCHD) with ongoing cardiac evaluations. • Monitor growth using syndrome-specific growth chart. • Ongoing ophthalmologic exam for cataracts. • Careful review of newborn hearing screening, followed by ongoing otologic/hearing evaluation. • Monitor for obstructive sleep apnea. • Increased risk for duodenal atresia. • High risk for atlantoaxial instability; if any signs of cervical myelopathy, obtain radiograph, refer to neurosurgery. • Monitor for neurologic conditions (e.g., infantile spasms, seizures, Moyamoya malformation). • Systematic screening for celiac disease (CD). • Increased risk for leukemia.
Fragile X syndrome *Most commonly inherited form of mental retardation*	• Any male child with developmental delay, borderline intellectual ability, or mental retardation should be tested as early physical recognition is difficult as clinical phenotype (males) can be subtle prior to puberty. • Cognitive deficits can be moderate to severe. • Often experience delayed toilet training, enuresis. • Hypersensitivity to sensory stimuli is common. Avoid excessive stimulation (e.g., large crowds, loud noises); provide earphones. • Monitor for behavior problems, including ADHD, emotional lability, irritability, and temper tantrums. • Increased risk for seizure activity, decreasing at adolescence. • Language delay is common, especially conversational speech. • Infants may have congenital hip dysplasia and/or clubfoot, feeding difficulties/GER, hypotonia, and irritability. • Increased incidence of recurrent/chronic OM, sinusitis. Audiologic evaluation annually for conductive hearing loss. • Orthopedic referral for connective tissue dysplasia issues (e.g. pes planus, hypermobile joints, scoliosis). • Ophthalmologic evaluation annually for strabismus, refractive errors. • Increased risk of inguinal hernia(s). • Macro-orchidism begins ~9 years of age. Adolescent growth spurt is less. • Increased risk for autism, hypertension, mitral valve prolapse. • Females have wider phenotypic variability; however, premature ovarian failure (menopause) is common.

TABLE 32.3	Cross-Section of Congenital and/or Inherited Disorders—Primary Care Issues—cont'd	
Disorder	**Primary Care Issues**	
Klinefelter syndrome *Sex chromosome disorder*	• Monitor growth and development, especially speech. • Monitor for scoliosis. • Annual thyroid screen. • Caution—delayed puberty/gynecomastia/low testosterone, increased risk for autoimmune disorders, breast cancer.	
Marfan syndrome *Heritable, multisystem disorder of connective tissue*	• Monitor growth using syndrome-specific growth chart; Peak growth velocity occurs up to 2 years earlier. • Excessive linear growth of long (tubular) bones; typically taller than predicted for their family; altered arm-span to height ratio; bones of hands/fingers are elongated, but palm is normal, giving rise to positive thumb/wrist signs. • Monitor for orthopedic conditions/problems, including joint laxity, protrusion acetabuli, scoliosis, thoracic kyphosis, pes planus; pectus abnormalities are common. • Many clinical features are age-dependent (e.g., ectopia lentis, aortic dilation, dural ectasia, protrusion acetabuli). • Cardiac screening with echocardiogram continues throughout life; age on onset/rate of progression of aortic dilation is highly variable; β-blockers are often prescribed; decongestants and psychostimulants should be used with caution. • Ongoing BP monitoring (hypertension). • Participation in contact/competitive sports, as well as isometric exercise is restricted; aerobic activities in moderation. • Annual ophthalmology screen; myopia is common and progresses rapidly; ectopia lentis is a hallmark feature; increased risk of retinal detachment, glaucoma, and early cataract formation. • Dural ectasia often presents with postural hypotension/low-pressure headaches. • Increased risk of spontaneous pneumothorax, reduced pulmonary reserve, and sleep apnea. • Stretch marks are common across lower back, inguinal and axillary regions (perpendicular to axes of growth). • Hernias/recurrent hernias and incisional hernias are common.	
Neurofibromatosis type 1 (NF1) *Multisystem disorder primarily involving skin and nervous system*	• Monitor growth using syndrome-specific growth chart; macrocephaly and short stature are common; puberty growth spurt is reduced. • Clinical features are age-dependent; café-au-lait spots are usually the initial manifestation (birth-infancy); plexiform neurofibromas are usually congenital (on face, trunk extremities); axillary/inguinal skinfold freckling typically develops between 3 and 5 years; dermal neurofibromas typically develop prepubertally (increasing in size/number in puberty). • Monitor for learning disabilities, with deficits in visual-spatial-perceptual skills and poor fine motor coordination leading to reading, spelling, and handwriting issues. • Annual ophthalmology screen; optic glioma present with visual loss, severe proptosis, and/or hydrocephalus in young children; Lisch nodules typically develop in early adolescence (slit-lamp exam). • Precocious puberty may occur, but need to rule out optic glioma as cause. • Monitor BP (hypertension) as a screen for renal artery stenosis, aortic stenosis, and pheochromocytoma (adult). • Hypotonia and subtle neurologic changes can affect gait/balance; caution for sports/activity. • Monitor skeletal changes, including tibia dysplasia, scoliosis; increased risk for osteoporosis (adult). • Advise use of sunscreen after 6 months of age (as sun will increase pigmentation of café-au-lait spots).	
Noonan syndrome	• Monitor growth using syndrome-specific growth chart. • Annual vision/hearing screen. • Monitor for developmental delays. • Caution—increased risk for cardiac anomalies (hypertrophic cardiomyopathy), coagulopathies, and renal anomalies.	
Prader-Willi syndrome (PWS) *Disorder related to genomic imprinting*	• Monitor growth using standard growth chart, paying close attention to weight-to-height; monitor for failure to thrive (FTT) and later short stature/central adiposity. • Infants (first phase) have significant hypotonia and early feeding problems; need for assisted feeding is nearly universal from birth to 6 months (e.g., tube feedings; feeding adaptations, such as Haberman nipple). • Children (second phase) involves hyperphagia, with associated behavioral problems and obesity/obesity-related health concerns. • Anticipate/help family plan for progression of behavioral issues: temper tantrums, obsessive behaviors, perseverant speech, skin picking (peri-anal, intertriginous folds), elopement. • Hypogonadism (undescended testes; scrotal hypoplasia, small phallus/clitoris); trial of hCG is recommended for males, as anesthesia during infancy is high risk secondary to hypotonia. • Premature (isolated) adrenarche is common. • Global developmental delay; mild-moderate mental retardation; increased risk of seizures (associated with fever). • Challenges for PCP: High pain threshold complicate timely assessment of illness/injury; children with PWS rarely vomit. • Generalized hypothalamic insufficiency is characteristic, including growth hormone (GH); GH is approved for young children with PWS older than 2 years of age, but newer, promising trials are exploring starting at 2 months of age (side effects include macrocephaly, adenotonsillar hypertrophy/obstructive sleep apnea). • Reduced salivation leads to increased caries risk as early as 1 year of age; involve pediatric dentistry early; increase dental cleanings needed. • Annual vision/hearing screen.	

Continued

TABLE 32.3	Cross-Section of Congenital and/or Inherited Disorders—Primary Care Issues—cont'd
Disorder	**Primary Care Issues**
Turner syndrome *Sex chromosome disorder*	• Monitor growth using syndrome-specific growth chart; short stature is expected; GH treatment typically begun early (~4-5 years of age). • Nonverbal (e.g., math) learning disabilities are common. • Annual hearing exam; recurrent otitis media; progressive midfrequency sensorineural hearing loss. • Ongoing vision assessment; strabismus. • Early onset osteo-penia/-porosis; vitamin D supplementation; appropriate estrogen therapy; exercise. • Monitor BP (hypertension). • Annual thyroid screen (hypo-/hyperthyroidism); monitor for celiac disease. • Ongoing assessment for celiac disease (tissue transglutaminase immunoglobulin A). • Careful early monitoring for kyphosis, scoliosis, lordosis. • Increased risk of hyperlipidemia; cardiac defects (e.g., aortic root dilatation; bicuspid aortic value; coarctation of aorta) and renal anomalies (e.g., horseshoe kidney, double collecting system, increased urinary tract infection [UTI]). • Supplemental estrogen therapy for sexual development and preservation of bone mineral density (late childhood/early adolescence). • Tendency to form keloids.
Williams syndrome *Chromosomal microdeletion*	• Monitor growth using syndrome-specific growth chart. • Infantile hypercalcemia is an early hallmark contributes to irritability, vomiting, constipation, and muscle cramping; resolves in late childhood, but lifelong abnormalities (e.g., hypercalciuria, nephrocalcinosis) in calcium/vitamin D metabolism are lifelong. • Consider urinary UTI in children with fever. • Annual/close monitoring of urine (urinalysis), urinary calcium-creatinine ratio, total calcium, and serum creatinine. • Often present to PCP with difficulty feeding, GER, colic, FTT. • Can be missed in infancy, as dysmorphic facies are subtle, tending to become more distinctive with advancing age. • Do not suggest multivitamin preparations containing vitamin D. • Recommend diligent sunscreen to minimize production of vitamin D. • Ongoing cardiac evaluations; supravalvular aortic stenosis, coarctation of the aorta, renal artery stenosis, hypertension. • Cognitive, motor, and language delays. • Children can be over-friendly; personal safety issues. • Close monitoring of hearing; recurrent otitis media is common.

ADHD, Attention-deficit/hyperactivity disorder; *BP,* blood pressure; *GER,* gastroesophageal reflux; *PCP,* primary care provider.

Bull and Committee on Genetics. (2011); Committee on Genetics (2001); Fri, Davenport, and Committee on Genetics (2003); Hersh, Saul, and Committee on Genetics (2011); Hersh and Committee on Genetics (2008); McCandless and Committee on Genetics (2011); Romano et al. (2010); Tinkle, Saal, and Committee on Genetics (2013); Trotter, Hall, and Committee on Genetics (2005).

children with conditions that affect growth, including Cornelia deLange syndrome, Down syndrome, cerebral palsy, and Marfan, Prader-Willi, Turner, and Williams syndromes.

Primary care management and health supervision highlights for common syndromes are located in Table 32.3. It is recommended that PCPs refer to the AAP website for more in-depth and evolving primary care management guidelines and cautions. For each congenital and/or inherited disorder, the treatment plan is individualized to the child/family; however, it is common that treatment will require the coordinated efforts of a team of specialists. Geneticists, pediatricians, plastic surgeons, kidney specialists, dental specialists, speech pathologists, pediatric oncologists, and other health care professionals may need to systematically and comprehensively review and revise the treatment plan. At the center of this coordinated effort is the child's medical home and PCP.

General Guidelines for Primary Care Providers Caring for Children With Congenital and/or Inherited Disorders

When parents are given the diagnosis of a congenital and/or inherited disorder—whether as part of a prenatal diagnosis or after a child is born—they often react with fear, sadness, and confusion, and have many questions about their child's future (Saul

and Meridith, 2016). The first primary care visit is important for families of children with a congenital and/or inherited disorder or syndrome, as they are hoping to find support and guidance in coping with the new diagnosis and interpreting the myriad of information they have been receiving. PCPs should be aware of the regional resources on the different congenital and/or inherited disorders, so they can refer families to the available resources. Key family resources are listed in Table 32.4.

The Genetic Alliance is an especially useful PCP/family resource containing a tool called disease InfoSearch. The Info-Search database contains information on thousands of congenital or inherited disorders manifested in children (or affecting children in the future) along with links to educational materials as well as advocacy and support organizations. It is vital that the PCP remain in communication with specialists caring for the child in order to coordinate local care and to provide access to health, social, and spiritual support for the family. The PCP should also advocate for parents who can face significant challenges managing health care, daily care, and educational needs for their child. Finally, the PCP should be familiar with recurrence and occurrence risks for the child's disorder, as it may have health implications for siblings who are under the PCP's care. While parents are often the focus of genetic counseling (i.e., their recurrence risks are discussed and the affected child's recurrence risk may be discussed), the child's siblings' risks are often not

TABLE 32.4 Family Resources	
Resource for Families	**URL (Accessed August, 2018)**
Autism Speaks	https://www.autismspeaks.org/science/initiatives/autism-genome-project
Baby's First Test	http://www.babysfirsttest.org/
Centers for Disease Control and Prevention (CDC)b—Folic Acid	https://www.cdc.gov/ncbddd/folicacid/index.html
Genes In Life	http://www.genesinlife.org/
Genetic Alliance Disease InfoSearch	http://www.geneticalliance.org/
MotherToBaby	https://mothertobaby.org/
National Organization for Rare Disorders (NORD)	https://rarediseases.org/

included and siblings are not typically referred for genetic counseling. Parents may need future guidance about the appropriate time for all their children to learn about recurrence and future health risks, and may have other ongoing questions—some of which may necessitate referrals for consultation with a genetics specialist or a genetic counseling team.

References

Bull MJ, Committee on Genetics. Health supervision for children with Down syndrome. *Pediatrics*. 2011;107(2):393–404.

Committee on Genetics. Health care supervision for children with Williams syndrome. *Pediatrics*. 2001;107:1922–1204.

Fri JL, Davenport ML, Committee on Genetics. Clinical Report – Health supervision for children with Turner Syndrome. *Pediatrics*. 2003;111(3). 692–670.

Hersh JH, Saul RA, Committee on Genetics. Clinical Report – Health supervision for children with fragile X syndrome. *Pediatrics*. 2011;127(5):994–1006.

Hersh JH. Committee on Genetics. Clinical Report – Health supervision for children with neurofibromatosis. *Pediatrics*. 2008;121(3):633–642.

McCandless SE. Committee on Genetics. Clinical Report – Health supervision for children with Prader-Willis syndrome. *Pediatrics*. 2011;127(1):195–204.

Romano AA, Allanson JE, Dahlgren J, Gelb BD, Hall B, Noonan JA. Noonan syndrome: clinical features, diagnosis, and management guidelines. *Pediatrics*. 2010;126(4).

Saul RA, Meredith SH. Beyond the genetic diagnosis: providing parents what they want to know. *Pediatr Rev*. 2016;37(7):269–278. https://doi.org/10.1542/pir.2015-0092.

Tinkle BT, Saal HM, Committee on Genetics. Clinical Report – Health supervision for children with Marfan syndrome. *Pediatrics*. 2013;132(4):1059–1072.

Trotter TA, Hall JG. Committee on Genetics. Health supervision for children with achondroplasia. *Pediatrics*. 2005;116(3).

33

Atopic, Rheumatic, and Immunodeficiency Disorders

RITA MARIE JOHN AND MARGARET A. BRADY

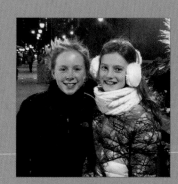

Atopic disorders, rheumatic disorders of childhood, and immunodeficiency disorders share certain characteristics. Inflammation, chronicity, and genetic predisposition are common to these groups of disorders. The most common pediatric atopic disorders that a primary care provider (PCP) is likely to encounter are atopic dermatitis (AD), allergic rhinitis (AR) (or "hay fever"), and asthma. The most common rheumatic diseases are juvenile idiopathic arthritis (JIA) and systemic lupus erythematosus (SLE). Although the incidence of rheumatic fever has diminished significantly in the United States, it is still found across the globe. Henoch-Schönlein purpura (HSP) is the most common systemic vasculitis syndrome of childhood (Ting, 2014), and Kawasaki disease (KD) is the most common cause of acquired heart disease (Cohen and Sundel, 2016). The chapter ends with a synopsis of the more common primary immune deficiency disorders, such as selective immunoglobulin A (IgA), immunoglobulin G (IgG) subclass deficiencies, and 22q11.2 deletion syndrome (DiGeorge syndrome), seen in childhood because early diagnosis and intervention are critical.

Pathophysiology and Defense Mechanisms

Allergic and Atopic Disorders

Allergies are acquired alterations in the body with an immunologic basis. An allergen acts as an antigen that triggers an immunoglobulin E (IgE) response in genetically predisposed individuals. The union of antigen and antibody creates a cascade of biochemical reactions. There are four types of allergic reactions (Coico and Sunshine, 2015):

- Type I: An IgE-mediated reaction, in which the binding region on the IgE attaches to high-affinity receptors $F_c\epsilon RI$ on basophils, mast cells, and eosinophils, resulting in inflammatory mediators and cytokine release.
- Type II: A cytotoxic reaction, occurring when IgM or IgG antibodies bind to surface antigens on normal tissue cells activating the complement cascade with resultant inflammation or causing cellular dysfunction or toxicity, leading to cell destruction.

- Type III: Immune-complex reactions result from IgG or IgM antibodies-antigen complexes that accumulate in the tissue and circulation, activating the complement cascade. This reaction also attracts granulocytes, which results in tissue damage.
- Type IV: Delayed T cell type reaction (hypersensitivity) involves the activation and proliferations of T cells and their migration to the site of specific antigen. The hypersensitivity reaction is mediated by the T cells and monocytes/macrophages rather than by antibodies. First, there is a local inflammatory and immune reaction at the antigen site that is followed by a secondary cellular response 48 to 72 hours after the initial antigen exposure. Damage to cells and tissues can result from interleukins and other lymphokines secreted by macrophages.

These four types can be easily remembered as type I (A) = Allergic, Anaphylaxis, Atopy; type II (B) = antibody; type III (C) = immune Complex; and type IV (D) = Delayed. All four types of allergic reactions are mediated by circulating cellular antibodies and generally can occur in any individual (Coico and Sunshine, 2015). Type I (IgE-mediated) is immediate and involves local and systemic manifestations, resulting in a wide range of clinical manifestations ranging from urticaria and angioedema to anaphylaxis and death. Type II (cytotoxic hypersensitivity or IgG-/IgM-mediated) reactions cause cellular death or dysfunction to target cells by means of IgG and IgM antibody-mediated autoimmunity with or without activation of the entire complement system; IgG and IgM bind to antigens present on cell surfaces with or without subsequent complement fixation. Examples of these reactions include drug-induced hemolytic anemia, immune thrombocytopenia purpura where autoantibodies are directed against platelets, ABO incompatibility transfusion reactions, and hemolytic erythroblastosis fetalis.

In type III (complex-mediated) reactions, immune complexes, normally removed by phagocytic cells, overwhelm the body, resulting in systemic or localized disease. Immune complexes can be deposited in the eye, kidney, skin, joints, and choroid plexus. An example of a local, subacute, type III reaction is an Arthus reaction, which occurs when the body is exposed to a large amount of foreign protein, such as a vaccine. Examples of a systematic reaction include lupus erythematosus (SLE), serum sickness, rheumatic fever, and rheumatoid arthritis. Type IV allergic reaction is a delayed-type hypersensitivity interaction, involving sensitized T-lymphocytic cells. Cytokines are released, which stimulate bone marrow precursors to produce more leukocytes that become macrophages. Examples of type IV reactions are tuberculin skin test reactions and contact dermatitis (Coico and Sunshine, 2015).

Atopy involves a genetic predisposition to allergic diseases of the epithelial barrier surfaces, commonly affecting the eyes, digestive tract, skin, and respiratory tract (Oetijen and Kim, 2018). Atopic disorders are immune deviations that likely result from genetic alteration in the immune response possibly from changes in the epigenome due to environmental exposures (Mastroilli, Caffarelli, and Hoffman-Somergruber, 2017). Atopy is a form of allergic reactivity that occurs only in certain susceptible individuals. Certain antigens (e.g., cat dander, ragweed) are problematic for atopic individuals, but not for others. Atopic individuals become sensitized to the offending allergen, resulting in an allergic manifestation. Development of one allergic disorder predisposes the child to another disorder, a phenomenon called the atopic march.

Development of an allergic response likely results from a combination of genetics, microbial exposure, antibiotic use, environmental and gut microbiome, diet, and lack of breastfeeding (Mastroilli et al., 2016). It involves a susceptible individual who is both exposed to an offending antigen and has a predisposition to selective synthesis of IgE when in contact with common environmental antigens. Allergic disease involves the production of IgE, activation of mast cells, eosinophil recruitment, and dysregulated sensory responses leading to pathologic reflexes such as itch, airway hyperreactivity, sneezing, and gastrointestinal (GI) discomfort (Oetigen and Kim, 2018).

In addition, epithelium-derived cytokines, including interleukin (IL)-2, IL-33, and thymic stromal lymphopoietin (TSLP), activate the immune system from cellular barriers along the GI tract, lung, and skin, calling into play adaptive T helper type-2 (Th2) cells, basophils, eosinophils, mast cells, and innate lymphoid cells (ILC2). These immune cells help product type-2 effector cytokines IL-4, IL-5, and IL-13, causing an increase in mucous production, epithelial hyperplasia, and additional inflammatory cells at the epithelial surface. Type 2 cytokines promote the production of IgE from mast cells and basophils. These granulocytes cause the release of proteins and small molecules, including histamine, cytokines, and proteases such as tryptases, which produce not only inflammatory reactions but also activation of the sensory nervous system. Tryptase activates sensory neurons via protease-activated receptors, which causes pruritus. Tissue from atopic patients demonstrates marked increases in sensory innervation at the site of inflammation. Sensory neurons also regulate motility of the immune cells (Oetijen and Kim, 2018).

Immediate allergic reactions can involve sneezing, hives, wheezing, vomiting, or anaphylaxis. Acute reactions (<30 minutes) can be followed by a late-phase response several hours (2 to 12) after the initial response. This late-phase response is due to the influx of other inflammatory cells (such as basophils, eosinophils, monocytes, lymphocytes, and neutrophils) and their inflammatory mediators that are recruited to the site of the acute allergic reaction.

The pathogenesis of atopic diseases involves a complex interrelationship of genetic, environmental, and immunologic factors. There are risk factors for development of food allergies and AD at different points in the child's life span. Prenatal factors include genetics, microbial exposure, changes in fetal growth, and antibiotic use. Avoidance of allergic foods during pregnancy does not influence the risk of atopy. In infancy, the microbial environment including alterations in the GI microbiota influences the onset of allergic disease (Mastrorilli, Posa, Cipriana, et al., 2016). Breastfeeding may expose an infant to a wide variety of food allergens and therefore may be protective against allergic disease. There are unanswered questions regarding infant dietary intake combined with a family history of atopy and whether this combination leads to the development of asthma. Exposure to antibiotics in the first 12 months of life alters the intestinal microbiota and may indirectly affect the development of asthma (Metsala, 2015).

Pharmacologic therapy reduces symptoms and checks the allergic process, but does not cure atopic disorders. For example, drugs may be used to control inflammation (corticosteroids), compete with histamine for receptor sites on target tissues (antihistamines), act as a selective leukotriene receptor antagonist (LTRA) (e.g., montelukast), and prevent mast cell degranulation and mediator release (cromolyn sodium). Recent research focuses on the use of pharmacogenomics, epigenomics, and transcriptomics to improve the management of atopic diseases such as asthma (Farzan, Vijverber, Kabesch, Sterk, and Maitland-van der Zee, 2018).

Rheumatic Disorders

Several rheumatological disorders occur in childhood. In general, they are chronic, autoimmune disorders with multisystem inflammation and circulating autoantibodies directed against the body. Inflammation is a significant factor in these diseases. There are no natural defense mechanisms, and the exact reason why these autoimmune diseases develop is not clear. In diseases like SLE, there are circulating autoantibodies, which form immune complexes that lead to complement activation and a cascade of proinflammatory markers that cause tissue damage (Sadun, Ardoin, and Schanberg, 2016).

The first-line tests commonly ordered in a child with or suspected of having an autoimmune disease include acute phase reactants, such as C-reactive protein (CRP), erythrocyte sedimentation rate (ESR), serum ferritin, platelets, and procalcitonin; a complete blood count (CBC) with differential; comprehensive, metabolic profile; and urinalysis. Urinalysis is frequently done in rheumatologic disorders known to have renal involvement. Second-line tests include antinuclear antibodies (ANAs), anti–double-stranded deoxyribonucleic acid (DNA), anti-Smith (Sm) antibody, and serum complement levels. The presence of anti-cyclic citrullinated peptide (anti-CCP) antibody is a surrogate marker, as it is only positive in patients with a positive rheumatoid factor (Sahai, Adams, Kamat, 2016). Table 33.1 describes tests commonly used in the laboratory workup of rheumatic diseases and autoimmune diseases.

Imaging studies are done to assess and manage joint abnormalities. Because of the increased risks associated with excessive radiation exposure, a reminder to "image gently" should be heeded.

Immune Deficiency

The immune system is divided into primitive (innate) immunity and adaptive (acquired) immunity. Both systems rely on effective functioning of leukocytes from the bone marrow (Toskala,

TABLE 33.1	Diagnostic Testing in Autoimmune Diseases	
Diagnostic Test	What Does It Measure/Significance	Autoimmune Disease
CBC with differential	Looks for anemia of chronic disease, leukopenia/leukocytosis and thrombocytosis/thrombocytopenia	Anemia may be seen in SLE, JIA, other autoimmune diseases Thrombocytosis
Sedimentation rate	Acute-phase reactant Can be falsely low if not measured in a timely fashion	Can be elevated in all autoimmune diseases
C-reactive protein	Acute-phase reactants Produced by the liver More reliable than sedimentation rate Goes up within 6 h and comes down quickly	Can be elevated in all autoimmune diseases
Serum ferritin	Acute-phase reactants	Very elevated (over 5000) in macrophage activation syndrome
Rheumatoid factor	Misnomer; are a measure of autoantibodies that are against the Fc portion of IgG	Elevated most commonly in children with polyarticular JIA
Anti-cyclic citrullinated peptide (anti-CCP) antibodies	Very specific for JIA but not commonly elevated; not a routine test	More likely to be elevated with severe JIA with irreversible joint damage; found more commonly in polyarticular arthritis
Antinuclear antibody (ANA)	ANAs are measured to determine activity against a variety of nuclear antigens Nonspecific; significant increase is over 1:160 Tend to become positive with age with as many as 5% of healthy adults having a positive ANA	ANA is a nonspecific test; should be done when the history points to SLE
Anti-double-stranded DNA (anti dsDNA)	Specific antibodies for SLE and are positive in 95% of patients with SLE	Very specific test for SLE; not routinely done as a first-line test
Complement levels	Can be used to monitor disease activity	Second-line test; will be low in SLE and other pediatric vasculitis

CBC, Complete blood count; IgG, immunoglobulin G; JIA, juvenile idiopathic arthritis; SLE, systemic lupus erythematosus.
Adapted from Mehta J. Laboratory testing in pediatric rheumatology. Pediatr Clin N Am. 2012;59:263–284.

2018). The *innate* immune system involves the natural barriers or surfaces of the body including the skin, mucous membrane, and the cough reflex that protects from invasion of environmental pathogens (Coico and Sunshine, 2015). Components of the innate immune system include natural barriers; phagocytes (neutrophils, monocytes, macrophages) and natural killer cells; soluble mediators (complement) and pattern recognition molecules. The complement system attracts cells to the area of inflammation via chemoattractants and enhances phagocytosis. Opsonins are molecules that coat and bind to bacterial surfaces and attract phagocytic cells to engulf or ingest the bacteria. They make the process of phagocytosis more efficient.

The *innate* immune system is responsible for alerting the adaptive immune system to the presence of infection (Coico and Sunshine, 2015). The adaptive immune system provides a more specific response to the presence of antigens or foreign substances. Lymphocytes, a key player in adaptive immunity, are divided into T cells, B cells, and natural killer cells. T-specific lymphocytes bind with antigens and also trigger a response causing the release of humoral mediators, including cytokines and B-cell–produced immunoglobulins. Antibodies block the binding of antigens to cellular receptors neutralizing microbes and microbial toxins. T cells function as the cellular immune system, whereas the less numerous B cells serve as the humoral immune system. The role of

killer cells in host defense involves killer inhibitory receptors that recognize major histocompatibility complex (MHC) antigens; however, their relationship to myeloid cells is not well defined (Buckley, 2016b).

General Management Strategies

Atopic and rheumatic disorders and immune deficiencies tend to be chronic conditions with exacerbation and remission of symptoms. Individual management strategies are based on the specific disease process. The following general measures are part of the management of atopic, rheumatoid, and immune deficiency disorders:

- Encourage self-care and learning about one's disease. The use of phone applications to remind patients about taking their medication can be effective (Ahmed et al., 2018). Examples of such applications include https://www.carespeak.com/corp/, https://medactionplan.com/, and MyMedSchedule Plus.
- Address issues associated with living with a chronic disease, such as:
  - Financial burdens associated with the disease
  - School, peer, and family dynamics along with body image
  - Pain management as needed
  - Child and adolescent engagement in his/her care leading to improved adherence

- Child-parent role in management of a long-term illness or chronic condition
- Nutrition and avoidance of obesity, if activity is limited, or foods if they are known triggers
- Social and environmental factors including healthcare disparities, cultural factors, ethnic factors, and healthcare access that may affect the disease process (Lewis et al., 2017)
- Refer to parent and/or child support groups and professional organizations and resource groups (see Chapter 7).

Atopic Disorders

Allergic diseases are growing in developing countries with AR and asthma the most common chronic diseases in children. The burden of these diseases on the child's activities of daily living as well as the social and economic cost point to a need for prevention. Recent developments in allergy prevention include feeding peanut food to infants at 4 to 6 months, making sure that vitamin D is appropriately supplemented, and avoiding environmental exposure to allergens to decrease allergies in children (Du Toit et al., 2018). Environmental exposure to peanuts or application of peanut oil on eczematous skin during infancy increases the risk of peanut allergy in children, whereas two significant studies (LEAP and EAT studies) reported that feeding infants peanut-containing food decreased peanut allergies (Perkin et al., 2016; Du Toit et al., 2015). The dual-allergen exposure hypothesis proposes that different exposures during the first year of life can prime the immune system (Du Toit et al., 2018). Viral respiratory infections in infancy also increase the risk of asthma likely through the production of cytokines IL-25 and IL-33 that also interact with inflammatory allergic pathways, inducing Th2-related inflammation (Edwards et al., 2017).

Among allergic disorders, the respiratory disorders are common and can affect about a third of the population. In patients with atopy, the allergic march progresses from AD to AR and finally asthma. This march can start in young infants, continue through childhood, worsen through adulthood, or ultimately resolve with increasing age. Because patients who are already sensitized have a greater risk of developing more allergies than those without sensitization, prevention of allergy in a patient predisposed to allergy and avoidance of new sensitization in an individual who already has allergies are key strategies (Porcaro, Corsello, Pajno, 2018).

Asthma

Asthma is a complex, chronic, multifaceted respiratory disease resulting from inflammation, airway hyperresponsiveness, and airway remodeling. It is characterized by varying degree of airflow obstruction that presents as coughing, wheezing, chest tightness, breathlessness, and respiratory distress. It can also manifest as a persistent cough without significant wheezing. It is the most common chronic pulmonary disease in children with one out of 12 children ages 0 to 17 years old diagnosed with asthma in 2016. It is more prevalent in boys (9.2%) than girls (7.4%). Children from low-income families have a higher prevalence of the disease (10.5%), which is more common among African Americans (15.7%) and children of Puerto Rican descent (12.9%). Children with asthma missed less school and had fewer hospitalizations in 2013 than in 2003 (Zahran, Bailey, Damon, et al., 2018). Advances in therapy have reduced asthma-related deaths and improved the quality of life for patients with asthma.

The first contact for many pathogens as well as environmental irritants is typically the normal airway. Alveolar epithelial cells function to protect the lung against environmental insults and also signal professional immune cells to activate. Alveolar macrophages and neutrophils neutralize foreign particles including pathogens. In airways of patients with asthma, there are eosinophils, degranulated mast cells, lymphocytes, altered goblet cells, as well as epithelial cell tight junctions. The dendritic T cells (DC) present the antigen to native T cells that triggers a Th2 response. The pathophysiology involves the activation of cytokines, which influence T cell differentiation and the intracellular signaling cascade. Toll-like receptor (TLR) and transcription factors, such as nuclear factor kappa-light-chain enhancers of activated B cells, play a key role in the pathophysiology of asthma (Mishra, Banga, Silveyra, 2018).

Persistent inflammation associated with asthma can result in irreversible changes, such as airway wall remodeling. Inflammation causes acute bronchoconstriction, airway edema, and mucous plug formation. In addition, airway inflammation can trigger a hyperresponsiveness to a variety of stimuli, including allergens, exercise, cold air, as well as physical, chemical, or pharmacologic agents. This results in bronchospasm, which presents as wheezing, breathlessness, chest tightness, and cough that can be worse at night or with exercise. Airflow obstruction is often reversible, either spontaneously or with treatment; however, remodeling of the airway can occur secondary to persistent fibrotic changes in the airway lining. Fibrosis alters the airway caliber, leading to decreased airflow with permanent changes starting in childhood that become recognizable in adults.

Asthma is a disease with multiple phenotypes that can be characterized by age of onset, severity, triggers, comorbidities, as well as differences in the inflammatory cells responsible for clinical manifestations. In the future, phenotypic classification will enable management based on the patient's phenotype (Huffaker and Phipatanakul, 2015). For example, severe asthma is likely linked to neutrophil-derived inflammation, which is more common in females, obese patients, and those with airway microbiota changes. Neutrophilic airway inflammation is uncommon in children and can be resistant to inhaled steroids. Genetics also plays a role as patients with 17q21 variants are more likely to have early onset of asthma. This locus is associated with four genes; however, the function of these genes is still unknown. Heritability of asthma ranges from 35% to 95% (Mastrorilli et al., 2016). Asthma risk is also related to the type of allergen sensitization with pollen, mold, and staphylococcal enterotoxin associated with severe asthma. Sex hormones have an impact on the immune response as progesterone promotes the T2 response. There is also an association between blood eosinophil counts and eosinophilic phenotype of asthma with an eosinophilic steroid refractory phenotype associated with uncontrolled asthma, despite the use of high-dose steroids. This type of asthma might be seen in older adolescents. In addition, there is a paucicellular asthma phenotype that has a better prognosis and is associated with low-grade inflammatory disease (Just, Bourgoin-Heck, Amat, 2017). These phenotypes of asthma are new discoveries and will potentially assist in the development of a personalized medicine approach to the treatment of asthma (Mastrorilli et al., 2016); however, more research is needed (Global Initiative for Asthma, 2018).

The 2007 National Asthma Education and Prevention Program Expert Panel Report (EPR3) classified asthma in children as intermittent, mild persistent, moderate persistent, or severe persistent depending on symptoms, recurrences, need for specific medications, and pulmonary function (Table 33.2). This stepwise

TABLE 33.2	Classification of Asthma Severity in Children: Clinical Features before Treatment		
Classification and Step	**Symptoms[a]**	**Nighttime Symptoms**	**Lung Function**
Step 1: Intermittent	Symptoms two times or less per week Asymptomatic and normal PEF between exacerbations Requires SABA 2 days/week Exacerbations brief (few hours or days); varying intensity No interference with normal activity	Two times or less per month	FEV_1 >80% predicted Normal FEV_1 between exacerbations
Step 2: Mild persistent	Symptoms more than two times per week but less than one time per day Requires SABA more than 2 days/week but not more than one per day Exacerbations may affect activity (minor)	Three to four times per month	FEV_1 >80% predicted
Step 3: Moderate persistent	Daily symptoms Daily use of inhaled SABA Some limitations Exacerbations affect activity, two times or more per week; may last days	More than one time per week but not nightly	FEV_1 >60% but <80% predicted
Step 4: Severe persistent	Continual symptoms Requires SABA several times/day Extremely limited physical activity Frequent exacerbations	Often seven times per week	FEV_1 <60% predicted

[a]Having at least one symptom in a particular step places the child in that particular classification.

FEV₁, Forced expiratory volume in 1 second; *PEF*, peak expiratory flow; *SABA*, short-acting β₂-agonist.

Adapted from National Heart, Lung, and Blood Institute (NHLBI). *Full Report of the Expert Panel: Guidelines for the Diagnosis and Management of Asthma, (EPR-3)*. Bethesda, MD: National Institutes of Health; 2007.

approach remains the key to asthma management. Children classified at any level of asthma can have episodes involving mild, moderate, or severe exacerbations. Exacerbations involve progressive worsening of shortness of breath, cough, wheezing, chest tightness, or any combination of these symptoms. The degree of airway hyperresponsiveness is usually related to the severity of asthma that can change over time.

Allergic asthma exacerbations are biphasic. The immediate or early asthmatic response (EAR) phase is characterized by bronchospasm and bronchoconstriction. The pathophysiologic mechanisms involve IgE-mediated degranulation of mast cells with the release of prostaglandin D2, histamine, and cysteinyl leukotrienes leading to smooth muscle contraction and bronchoconstriction. EAR starts within 15 to 30 minutes of mast cell activation and resolves within approximately 1 hour if the individual is removed from the offending allergen. The EAR phase typically responds well to inhaled bronchodilator agents. The late-phase asthmatic response is due to inflammatory mediators as well as DCs, eosinophils, neutrophils, helper T cells, and mast cells that cause airway constriction. The late-phase response usually follows the EAR within 6 to 26 hours after exposure to the allergen, is often associated with airway hyperresponsiveness more severe than the EAR presentation, and can last from hours to several weeks. This requires the use of corticosteroid as the response to inhaled β agonist is muted.

Exercise-induced bronchospasm (EIB) describes the phenomenon of airway narrowing during, or minutes after, the onset of vigorous activity. Most asthmatics exhibit airway hyperirritability after vigorous activity and display EIB. For some children, exercise is the trigger for their asthma. Although asthma is not always associated with an allergic disorder in children, many children with chronic asthma have an allergic component (Huffaker and Phipatanakul, 2015).

The diagnosis of asthma is often delayed in children from 0 to 4 years of age; instead they are diagnosed with reactive airway disease, wheezy bronchitis, or recurrent bronchitis. Asthma is rarely diagnosed before 12 months old due to the high rate of viral illnesses causing bronchiolitis. A diagnosis of asthma should be made with caution in a toddler who only has wheezing associated with viral infections. Using the well-known expression "all that wheezes is not asthma and all asthma does not wheeze," the EPR3 cautions providers about the diagnosis of asthma under age 4 years.

Whether hyperresponsiveness of the airways is present at birth or acquired later in genetically predisposed children is not known. However, the genetic predisposition for the development of an IgE-mediated response to common aeroallergens, known as *atopy*, remains the strongest identifiable predisposing risk factor for asthma (Dinakar, 2017). A combination of genetic predisposition and exposure to certain environmental factors are the necessary components responsible for the pathophysiologic response associated with asthma. Common triggers for an asthma exacerbation include viral respiratory infections, environmental allergens, change in the weather, stress, emotional expression, and exercise as well as comorbid conditions such as sinusitis and gastroesophageal reflux. Global warming, climate change, and air pollution also contribute to allergic asthma (Paramesh, 2018).

Allergen-induced asthma results in hyperresponsive airways. The majority of children with asthma show evidence of sensitization to any of the following inhalant allergens:

- House dust mites, cockroaches, indoor molds
- Saliva and dander of cats and dogs
- Outdoor seasonal molds
- Airborne pollens—trees, grasses, and weeds
- Food allergy, including egg and tree nut

Overview of Asthma Guidelines and Tools

The new Global Initiative Guidelines (GINA) for 2018 recommend that PCPs query about a history of wheezing, chest tightness, cough, and shortness of breath in children 6 years and older. Ask whether the symptoms vary in intensity and over time and if they are usually worse when awakening or at night. Symptoms may be triggered by a viral infection, exercise, allergens, environment, or weather. These guidelines also suggest documenting airflow limitations and include asking the patient to do a forced expiratory volume in 1 second (FEV_1).

The latest American Academy of Pediatrics (AAP) recommendations clearly advocate for the use of age-specific asthma control tools as part of assessment. In a primary care setting, asthma should be monitored using a standardized instrument, which may include the Asthma Control Test (ACT), Asthma Control Questionnaire, Asthma Therapy Assessment Questionnaire, Asthma Control Score, or the TRACK (for children 0 to 5 years) (Dinakar et al., 2017). The advantages of a standardized questionnaire are that it allows the PCP to assess changes in the patient's asthma and alter the management plan as needed. Because of the self-reporting measures, the use of these tools may underreport the patient's degree of airway inflammation as patients may accept their symptoms as the norm. ACT is reliable for uncontrolled patients with asthma; it is not as reliable in controlled patients. Additionally, the presence of AR does affect ACT accuracy (Caminati et al., 2016). Assessment of quality of life can also be done, although it is not routinely done in many clinical practices.

Objective measures of asthma control include assessment of lung function, airway hyperresponsiveness assessment, and biomarkers. Peak flow is the easiest measure to use but has variable results even when done well. Spirometry is suggested every 1 to 2 years by the EPR recommendations; unfortunately, it is not performed in over 59% of pediatric practices. The use of prebronchodilator and postbronchodilator spirometry, otherwise known as the bronchodilator reversibility flow test, can be done to see if there is significant improvement of at least 12% in the FEV_1 following a treatment. Home-based airflow measurement can be done; the use of this technology is not widespread (Dinakar et al., 2017).

Airway hyperresponsiveness is assessed by bronchial provocation test done with methacholine or exercise. A 20% reduction in FEV_1 with methacholine or a 10% reduction following exercise shows hyperresponsive airways. In terms of biomarkers, exhaled fractional concentration of nitric oxide is a measure of airway nitric oxide and the joint ATS/ERS guidelines for its use are the current standard of care (AAAAI/ACAAI Joint Statement of Support of the ATS Clinical Practice Guideline, 2012; Dweik, Boggs, Erzurum, 2011). It is a measure of eosinophilic airway inflammation and can be elevated in patients with atopy, but without asthma. While the upper limit of normal is 25 ppb, a change of 20% for values greater than 50 ppd of 10 ppb in values ≤50ppb is significant (Dinakar et al., 2017). This biomarker is not recommended in the Global Strategy 2018 guidelines.

In primary care settings and emergency departments (EDs), patients with acute asthma are assessed based on their respiratory rate, work of breathing, ability to talk in sentences, breathlessness, and alertness. The management of an acute exacerbation includes reversal of bronchoconstriction, restoration of oxygen level, and prevention of relapse (Stenson, Tchou, Wheeler, 2017).

TABLE 33.3	Physical Assessment of Asthma and Asthma Severity	
Severity of Asthma	**Physical Assessment Findings**	
Mild	Wheezing at the end of expiration or no wheezing No or minimal intercostal retractions along posterior axillary line Slight prolongation of expiratory phase Normal aeration in all lung fields Can talk in sentences	
Moderate	Wheezing throughout expiration Intercostal retractions Prolonged expiratory phase Decreased breath sounds at the base	
Severe	Use of accessory muscles plus lower rib and suprasternal retractions; nasal flaring Inspiratory and expiratory wheezing or no wheezing heard with poor air exchange Suprasternal retractions with abdominal breathing Decreased breath sounds throughout base	
Impending respiratory arrest	Diminished breath sounds over entire lung field Tiring, inability to maintain respirations Severely prolonged expiration if breath sounds are heard Drowsy, confused	

Clinical Findings

History. Critical points to cover in the history include:
- Family history of asthma or other related allergic disorders (e.g., eczema or AR)
- Conditions associated with asthma (e.g., chronic sinusitis, nasal polyposis, gastroesophageal reflux, and chronic otitis media)
- Complaints of chest tightness or dyspnea
- Cough and wheezing particularly at night and in the early morning or shortness of breath with exercise or exertion (characteristic of asthma)
- Seasonal, continuous, or episodic pattern of symptoms that may be associated with certain allergens or triggering agents
- Episodes of recurrent "bronchitis" or pneumonia
- Precipitation of symptoms by known aggravating factors (upper respiratory infections, acetaminophen, aspirin)

Physical Examination. Table 33.3 outlines the physical assessment findings correlated with asthma severity. Broadly speaking, the following may be seen on physical examination:
- Heterophonous wheezing (different pitches but may be absent if severe obstruction)
- Continuous and persistent coughing
- Prolonged expiratory phase, high-pitched rhonchi especially at the bases
- Diminished breath sounds
- Altered level of alertness; signs of respiratory distress, including tachypnea, retractions, nasal flaring, use of accessory muscles, increasing restlessness, apprehension, agitation, drowsiness to coma

- Tachycardia, hypertension, or hypotension
- Cyanosis of lips and nail beds if hypoxic
- Possible associated findings include sinusitis, AD, and AR

Diagnostic Studies. Laboratory and radiographic tests should be individualized and based on symptoms, severity or chronology of the disease, response to therapy, and age. Tests to consider include:

- Oxygen saturation (SaO_2) of hemoglobin by pulse oximetry to assess the percentage of total hemoglobin that is oxygenated to determine severity of an acute exacerbation. This should be a routine part of every assessment of a child with asthma.
- A CBC if secondary infection or anemia is suspected (also check for elevated numbers of eosinophils).
- Routine chest radiographs are not indicated in most children with asthma. Results are typically normal or only show hyperinflation. Imaging should be ordered judiciously with consideration of the long-term risk. However, chest radiographs and imaging are useful in the following situations: selected cases of asthma or suspected asthma or if the child has persistent wheezing without a clinical explanation, and children with hypoxia, fever, suspected pneumonia, and/or localized rales requiring admission. Infants with wheezing during the winter who have clinical bronchiolitis do not need imaging.
- If sinusitis is suspected as the trigger, no diagnostic radiographic testing is needed.
- Allergy evaluation should be considered; however, history and physical examination are key in this consideration. (Refer child to pediatric allergist as needed.)
- Sweat test should be considered based on history in every patient with asthma.
- Pulmonary function tests:
  - Pulmonary function testing is the best way to evaluate obstructive respiratory pathology and remains the gold standard for diagnosing asthma (Ayuk et al., 2017). It should be used on a regular basis to monitor, evaluate, and manage asthma. Exercise challenges using spirometry can also be done to evaluate the child with exercised-induced asthma. Spirometry is an underutilized tool worldwide. As previously reviewed, the GINA guidelines recommend spirometry every 1 to 2 years. Children older than 5 years can typically perform spirometry (Kaslovsky and Sadof, 2014).
  - To evaluate the accuracy of the spirometry, the volume flow loop should have an initial sharp peak with an extension down to the baseline at the end of expiration that is reproducible three times (Kaslovsky and Sadof, 2014). The normal flow-volume is when the horizontal axis shows the vital capacity and the vertical axis shows the peak flow. Compare the child's values with the predicted value for the child's age, height, sex, and race. The U.S. Department of Health and Human Services Publication number 2011-135 reviews how to correct test errors and can be retrieved online.
  - Look at forced expiratory volume in 1 second (FEV_1), which represents the amount of air exhaled in 1 second. Reversibility with a bronchodilator is an increase in FEV_1 of 12% or more or 100 mL from baseline. Interpretation of percentage predicted is:
    - >75%: Normal
    - 60% to 75%: Mild obstruction
    - 50% to 59%: Moderate obstruction
    - <49%: Severe obstruction

TABLE 33.4 Abnormal Spirometry Findings in Obstructive and Restrictive Airway Disease

	Obstructive	Restrictive
FVC	Normal or ↓	↓
FEV_1	↓	↓
FEV_1/FVC	↓	Normal or ↑

FEV_1, Forced expiratory volume in 1 second; *FVC,* forced vital capacity.

- Forced vital capacity (FVC) represents the amount of air expelled:
  - 80% to 120%: Normal
  - 70% to 79%: Mild reduction
  - 50% to 69%: Moderate reduction
  - <50%: Severe reduction
- FEV_1/FVC represents the amount of air expelled in the first second over the total amount of air expelled and should be greater than 90% of the predicted value. Spirometry testing is done prior to a breathing treatment and 10 minutes after the treatment. If the child's FEV_1 improves by 12%, asthma is likely because this illustrates hyperresponsiveness.
- Forced expiratory flow (FEF) (FEF_{25} to FEF_{75}) reflects the middle portion of the downward limb of the curve and is a good measure of smaller airway function. Interpretation of percentage predicted is:
  - >60%: Normal
  - 40% to 60%: Mild obstruction
  - 20% to 40%: Moderate obstruction
  - <10%: Severe obstruction
- Doing spirometry during well-child checks and sick visits gives the PCP an excellent indication of the amount of inflammation and bronchospasm present in the airway. Table 33.4 represents abnormal spirometry patterns.
- Consider the use of more sophisticated pulmonary laboratory studies for the child with severe asthma.
- Peak flow measurements:
  - If spirometry is not an option, peak expiratory flow (PEF) can be used in children as young as 4 to 5 years old.
  - PEF values are instrument specific; the child's personal best value is the best guide to help detect possible changes in airway obstruction. The predicted range for height and age can be substituted if personal best rate is not available (Table 33.5). Interpretation of PEF reading is as follows if PEF is in the:
    - Green zone: More than 80% to 100% of personal best signals good control.
    - Yellow zone: Between 50% and 79% of personal best signals a caution.
    - Red zone: Between 0% and 50% of personal best signals major airflow obstruction.
    - Box 33.1 describes use of peak flowmeter and interpretation of results.
- Exhaled nitric oxide
  - Fraction of exhaled nitric oxide (FE_{no}) has moderate accuracy when diagnosing children 5 and over. It is more accurate in children and in patients who have not been on steroids (Wang, 2018). Recent studies have shown that repeat measurements during the same visit are not needed (Yang et al., 2018).

TABLE 33.5 Predicted Average Peak Expiratory Flow for Normal Children and Adolescents

Height (Inches)	Males and Females (L/min)	Height (Inches)	Males and Females (L/min)	Height (Inches)	Males and Females (L/min)
43	147	51	254	59	360
44	160	52	267	60	373
45	173	53	280	61	387
46	187	54	293	62	400
47	200	55	307	63	413
48	214	56	320	64	427
49	227	57	334	65	440
50	240	58	347	66	454
				67	467

From National Heart, Lung, and Blood Institute (NHLBI). *Executive Summary: Guidelines for the Diagnosis and Management of Asthma, NIH Pub No 94-3042A*. Bethesda, MD: National Institutes of Health; 1994; and Adapted from Polger G, Promedhar V. *Pulmonary Function Testing in Children: Techniques and Standards*. Philadelphia: Saunders; 1971.

• BOX 33.1 Use of the Peak Flow Meter and Its Interpretation

Steps to follow in using a peak flow meter:
1. Have child stand up.
2. Make sure that indicator is at the base of the numbered scale.
3. Ask child to take a deep breath.
4. Have the child place the peak flow meter in the mouth with the lips sealing the mouthpiece. Tell the child not to put his or her tongue in the hole of the mouthpiece.
5. Tell the child to blow out as hard and fast as possible.
6. Record the rate, but if the child coughs, do not write down that number.
7. Repeat steps 2 through 6 two more times.
8. Record the highest of the three values.

Peak Expiratory Flow Rate
Maximum flow rate that is produced during forced expiration with fully inflated lungs.

Personal Best Value
Highest value achieved in measuring peak expiratory flow (PEF) rate over a 2-week period when child's asthma is under good control is known as one's *personal best value* or *rate*. Good control is defined as when one feels well without asthma symptoms. To determine personal best, take readings twice daily, in the morning and late afternoon or evening, and 15-20 min after taking an inhaled short-acting β_2-agonist (SABA). Using the personal best value is the most accurate gauge to use to interpret changes in peak flow measurements because the child's own scores are used as the standard for comparison.

- The test measures eosinophilic airway inflammation. The patient must have a constant expiratory flow rate while the FE_{no} is measured. It may support the diagnosis of asthma and can help determine compliance with corticosteroid therapy.
- A FE_{no} value of more than 35 ppb in children indicates eosinophilic inflammation and likely responsiveness to corticosteroids, whereas values of 25 to 35 ppb should be interpreted with caution.

Differential Diagnosis

Numerous conditions can cause airway obstruction and be incorrectly confused with asthma, especially in young children and infants. Differential diagnoses include acute bronchiolitis, laryngotracheobronchitis, bronchopneumonia, pneumothorax; inhaled foreign body; congenital malformations of the heart and pulmonary abnormalities or bronchopulmonary dysplasia or bronchiectasis; genetic disorders (e.g., cystic fibrosis and α-1-antitrypin deficiency); primary ciliary dyskinesia; tracheal or foreign body compression (e.g., vascular aortic ring, enlarged lymph nodes, or tumors); chronic lower respiratory tract infections caused by immunodeficiency disorders; congenital malformation of the GI system with resultant recurrent aspirations and gastroesophageal reflux disease; vocal cord dysfunction; exposure to toxic substance; and anaphylaxis.

Management

Management strategies are based on whether the child has intermittent, mild persistent, moderate persistent, or severe persistent asthma (see Table 33.2). A stepwise approach is recommended. If control of symptoms is not maintained at a particular step of classification and management, the PCP first should reevaluate for adherence and administration factors. If these factors are not responsible for the lack of symptom control, go to the next treatment step. Likewise, gradual step-downs in pharmacologic therapy may be considered when the child is well controlled for 3 months (GINA, 2018). Inhaled corticosteroids (ICS) may be reduced about 25% to 50% every 3 months to the lowest possible dose needed to control the child's asthma (NHLBI, 2007).

Chronic Asthma

Treatment of chronic asthma in children is based on general control measures and pharmacotherapy. Control measures can include the following:
- Avoid exposure to known allergens or irritants, especially when mold and pollen counts are at their highest.

- Use air conditioning, close windows and doors, and remain indoors as much as possible during high pollen and mold season.
- Reassure the parent that fever can be controlled with either nonsteroidal anti-inflammatory drug (NSAID) or acetaminophen, which will not make the asthma worse unless the child has a known allergic/sensitivity reaction (Sheehan, Mauger, Paul, et al., 2016).
- Control environment to eliminate or reduce offending allergen.
- Consider allergen immunotherapy (AIT). Reduction in healthcare cost and improved outcomes associated with allergy immunotherapy are reported (Porcaro, Corsello, Pajno, 2018).
- Treat rhinitis, sinusitis, or gastroesophageal reflux.
- Other pharmacologic agents that may need to be considered include:
  - Anticholinergics—to reduce vagal tone in the airways (may also decrease mucus gland secretion).
  - Cromolyn sodium—to inhibit mast cell release of histamine.
  - LTRA—to disrupt the synthesis or function of leukotrienes
  - If needed, refer to pulmonology for omalizumab, a recombinant DNA-derived, humanized IgG monoclonal antibody that binds to human IgE on the surface of mast cells and basophils. This anti-IgE monoclonal antibody is used as a second-line treatment for children older than 12 who have moderate to severe allergy-related asthma and react to perennial allergens. It is used when symptoms are not controlled by ICS (Licari et al., 2017).
- Administer yearly influenza vaccine.
- Provide a clear written asthma action plan using a traffic light approach of green, yellow, or red to manage exacerbations (see Fig 33.6). Parents should know what to do when their child has slipped into the yellow (79% to 50% of best personal peak flow) or red (<50% of personal best peak flow) zone.
- Instruct parent to advance the asthma action plan to the yellow zone if the child has an upper respiratory infection (Dinakar et al., 2014).
- Educate regarding asthma basics, including triggers and prevention with environmental modification, as well as the different treatment modalities including the techniques of administration; dispel any myths regarding asthma medication.
- Address coping and self-management issues. The child and family need to be able to understand their emotions, worries, and uncertainty, as well as when to contact their PCP. Developing and understanding the asthma action plan is an important guide that promotes self-management and provides objective criteria for decision-making.
- Follow up with PCP after an exacerbation requiring ED care.

Pharmacologic management of childhood asthma is based on the severity of asthma and the child's age. The stepwise approach to treatment (Figs 33.1 and 33.2) is based on severity of symptoms and the use of pharmacotherapy to control chronic symptoms, maintain normal activity, prevent recurrent exacerbations, minimize adverse side effects and achieve nearly "normal" pulmonary function. Within any classification, a child may experience mild, moderate, or severe exacerbations. NHLBI guidelines for assessing asthma control and initiating and adjusting asthma therapy for various pediatric age groups are found in Figs 33.3 and 33.4.

Important considerations to note in the pharmacologic treatment of asthma include:

- Control of asthma should be gained as quickly as possible by starting at the classification step most appropriate to the initial severity of the child's symptoms or at a higher level (e.g.,

a course of systemic corticosteroids or higher dose of inhaled corticosteroid). After control of symptoms, decrease treatment to the least amount of medication needed to maintain control.
- Systemic corticosteroids may be needed at any time and stepped up if there is a major flare-up of symptoms. Control of inflammation is a key management principle.
- The combination of ICS with a long-acting β_2-agonist (LABA) can further control asthma (Kaur and Singh, 2018).
- Children with intermittent asthma may have long, symptom-free periods; they can also have life-threatening exacerbations, often provoked by respiratory infection. In these situations, a short course of systemic corticosteroids should be used.
- Variations in asthma necessitate individualized treatment plans.
- β_2 agonists can be administered with metered dose inhaler (MDI) therapy via spacer for children with mild and moderate exacerbations of asthma. A nebulizer may be better for children with severe airway obstruction who may have decreased deposition of drug in the base of the lung (Kaur and Singh, 2018). A spacer or holding chamber with an attached mask enhances the delivery of MDI medications to a child's lower airways. Spacers eliminate the need to synchronize inhalation with activation of MDI. Older children can use a spacer without the mask. It is important to check technique at every asthma-related visit.
- Dry powder inhalers (DPIs) do not need spacers or shaking before use. Instruct children to rinse their mouth with water and spit afterward. DPIs should not be used in children younger than 4 years old.
- Different ICS are not equal in potency to each other on a per puff or microgram basis. Tables 33.6 and 33.7 compare daily low, medium, and high doses of various ICS used for children. Combination inhaled corticosteroid (see Table 33.7) and LABA can be used in children 4 years and older (Taketomo et al., 2018).
- For treatment of exercise-induced asthma (EIA) or EIB:
  - Warm up before exercise for 5 to 10 minutes.
  - As preventive, use an inhaled short-acting β_2-agonist (SABA) 5 to 20 minutes prior to exercise. A mast cell stabilizer such as Cromolyn can be added. Combination of both types of drugs is the more effective therapy. Adding an anticholinergic may help if the SABA is not working (Caggiano, Cutrera, DiMarco, et al., 2017).
  - If a SABA is used daily, a controller therapy should be instituted with either ICS ± LABA and/or LTRA. Antihistamine should be used for allergic symptoms.
  - Using a scarf or mask around the mouth in cold weather may decrease EIA (Caggiano et al., 2017).
  - High-risk sports for EIB include high-endurance sports, long-distance running, and track and field events.
  - Low-risk sports for EIA are those physical activities of short duration—golf, volleyball, gymnastics, baseball, wrestling, football, and short-term track and field events. While some swimming can be a high-endurance event, the warmth and humidity around the pool make breathing easier (Caggiano, 2017).

Table 33.8 identifies the usual dosages for long-term control medications (exclusive of ICS) used to treat asthma in children. Quick-relief medications are listed in Table 33.9. Practice parameters are guides and should not replace individualized treatment based on clinical judgment and unique differences among children.

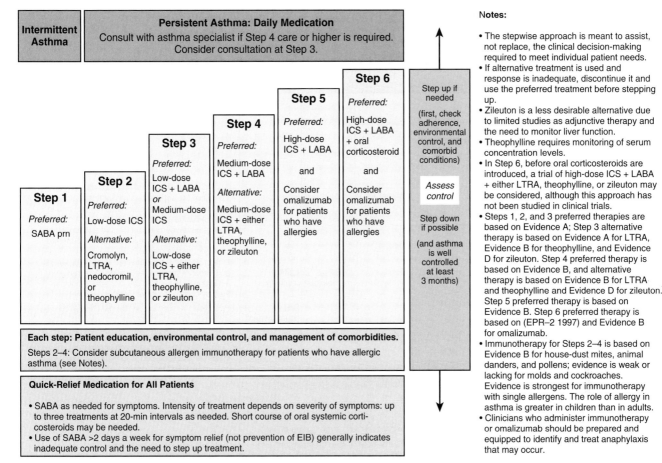

- The stepwise approach is meant to assist, not replace, the clinical decision-making required to meet individual patient needs.
- If alternative treatment is used and response is inadequate, discontinue it and use the preferred treatment before stepping up.
- Zileuton is a less desirable alternative due to limited studies as adjunctive therapy and the need to monitor liver function.
- Theophylline requires monitoring of serum concentration levels.
- In Step 6, before oral corticosteroids are introduced, a trial of high-dose ICS + LABA + either LTRA, theophylline, or zileuton may be considered, although this approach has not been studied in clinical trials.
- Steps 1, 2, and 3 preferred therapies are based on Evidence A; Step 3 alternative therapy is based on Evidence A for LTRA, Evidence B for theophylline, and Evidence D for zileuton. Step 4 preferred therapy is based on Evidence B, and alternative therapy is based on Evidence B for LTRA and theophylline and Evidence D for zileuton. Step 5 preferred therapy is based on Evidence B. Step 6 preferred therapy is based on (EPR–2 1997) and Evidence B for omalizumab.
- Immunotherapy for Steps 2–4 is based on Evidence B for house-dust mites, animal danders, and pollens; evidence is weak or lacking for molds and cockroaches. Evidence is strongest for immunotherapy with single allergens. The role of allergy in asthma is greater in children than in adults.
- Clinicians who administer immunotherapy or omalizumab should be prepared and equipped to identify and treat anaphylaxis that may occur.

• **Fig 33.1** Stepwise approach for managing asthma in patients 12 years old and older and adults. Alphabetical listing is used when more than one treatment option is listed within either preferred or alternative therapy. *EIB,* Exercise-induced bronchospasm; *ICS,* inhaled corticosteroid; *LABA,* long-acting β_2-agonist; *LTRA,* leukotriene receptor antagonist; *prn,* pro re nata (when necessary); *SABA,* short-acting β_2-agonist. (From National Heart, Lung, and Blood Institute. National Asthma and Prevention Program: expert panel report 3: guidelines for the diagnosis and management of asthma; 2007. www.nhlbi.nih.gov/guidelines/asthma/asthsumm.pdf. Accessed April 12, 2019. p. 45.)

Acute Exacerbations of Asthma

Treatment of acute episodes of asthma is also based on classification of the severity of the episode. Acute episodes are classified as mild, moderate, and severe. Signs and symptoms are summarized in Table 33.10. Early recognition of warning signs and treatment should be stressed in educating patients, parents, or both.

The initial pharmacologic treatment for acute asthma exacerbations is shown in Fig 33.5. It consists of inhaled SABAs (albuterol), two to six puffs every 20 minutes for three treatments by way of MDI with a spacer, or a single nebulizer treatment (0.15 mg/kg; minimum 1.25 to 2.5 mg of 0.5% solution of albuterol in 2 to 3 mL of normal saline).

If the initial treatment results in a good response (PEF/FEV$_1$ >70% of the patient's best), the inhaled SABAs can be continued every 3 to 4 hours for 24 to 48 hours with a 3-day course of oral steroids at 1 to 2 mg/kg/day in two divided doses to a maximum of 60 mg/day. Reassessment is important to ensure an adequate response and to further assess asthma severity.

An incomplete response (PEF or FEV$_1$ between 40% and 69% of personal best or symptoms recur within 4 hours of therapy) is treated by continuing β_2 agonists and adding an oral corticosteroid. The β_2 agonist can be given by nebulizer or

MDI with spacer. Parents should be taught to call their PCP for additional instructions. If there is marked distress (severe acute symptoms) or a poor response (PEF or FEV$_1$ <40%) to treatment, the child should have the β_2 agonist repeated immediately and should be taken to the ED. Emergency medical rescue (911) transportation should be used if the distress is severe and the child is agitated and unable to talk. If children experience recurrent acute asthma exacerbations (more than once every 4 to 6 weeks), compliance to therapy as part of a treatment plan reevaluation should be done.

This chapter focuses on the outpatient management of children with asthma. However, familiarity with other drug options used in more severe asthma is important. They include:

- Magnesium sulfate intravenous (IV) is used in EDs to decrease the intracellular calcium concentration. It causes bronchodilation due to respiratory smooth muscle relaxation. The most significant side effect is hypotension.
- The use of continuous infusion of terbutaline IV is limited to pediatric intensive care settings due to the risk of sinus tachycardia, decreases in systolic and diastolic blood pressure, and myocardial ischemia (Stenson et al., 2017).
- Theophylline, even at suboptimal doses, improves the lungs' responsiveness to steroids.

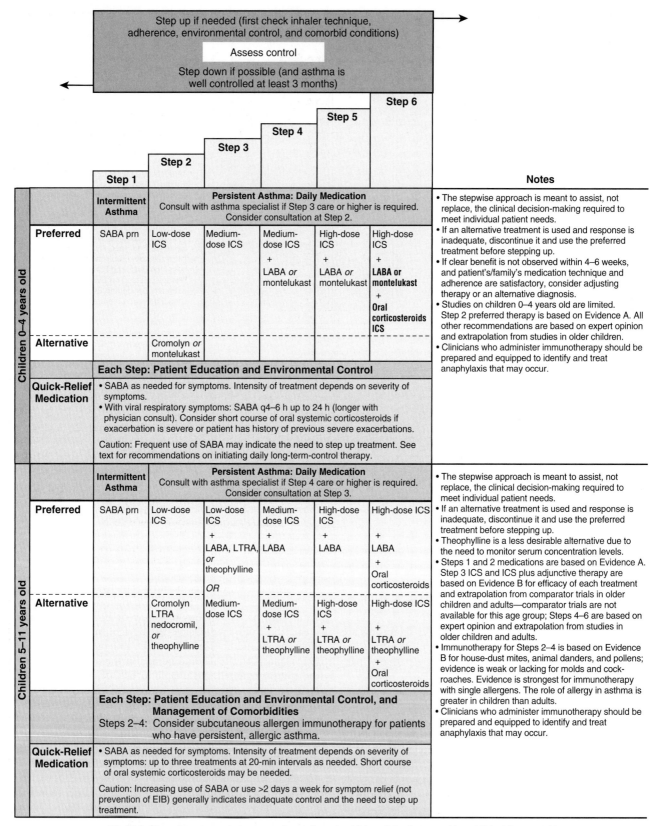

		Step 1	**Step 2**	**Step 3**	**Step 4**	**Step 5**	**Step 6**	**Notes**
Children 0–4 years old		**Intermittent Asthma**	— Persistent Asthma: Daily Medication — Consult with asthma specialist if Step 3 care or higher is required. Consider consultation at Step 2.					

Step up if needed (first check inhaler technique, adherence, environmental control, and comorbid conditions)

Assess control

Step down if possible (and asthma is well controlled at least 3 months)

Children 0–4 years old

	Step 1	**Step 2**	**Step 3**	**Step 4**	**Step 5**	**Step 6**
	Intermittent Asthma	**Persistent Asthma: Daily Medication** Consult with asthma specialist if Step 3 care or higher is required. Consider consultation at Step 2.				
Preferred	SABA prn	Low-dose ICS	Medium-dose ICS	Medium-dose ICS + LABA *or* montelukast	High-dose ICS + LABA *or* montelukast	High-dose ICS + **LABA or montelukast** + **Oral corticosteroids ICS**
Alternative		Cromolyn *or* montelukast				

Each Step: Patient Education and Environmental Control

Quick-Relief Medication	• SABA as needed for symptoms. Intensity of treatment depends on severity of symptoms. • With viral respiratory symptoms: SABA q4–6 h up to 24 h (longer with physician consult). Consider short course of oral systemic corticosteroids if exacerbation is severe or patient has history of previous severe exacerbations. Caution: Frequent use of SABA may indicate the need to step up treatment. See text for recommendations on initiating daily long-term-control therapy.

Notes (Children 0–4 years old):
- The stepwise approach is meant to assist, not replace, the clinical decision-making required to meet individual patient needs.
- If an alternative treatment is used and response is inadequate, discontinue it and use the preferred treatment before stepping up.
- If clear benefit is not observed within 4–6 weeks, and patient's/family's medication technique and adherence are satisfactory, consider adjusting therapy or an alternative diagnosis.
- Studies on children 0–4 years old are limited. Step 2 preferred therapy is based on Evidence A. All other recommendations are based on expert opinion and extrapolation from studies in older children.
- Clinicians who administer immunotherapy should be prepared and equipped to identify and treat anaphylaxis that may occur.

Children 5–11 years old

	Step 1	**Step 2**	**Step 3**	**Step 4**	**Step 5**	**Step 6**
	Intermittent Asthma	**Persistent Asthma: Daily Medication** Consult with asthma specialist if Step 4 care or higher is required. Consider consultation at Step 3.				
Preferred	SABA prn	Low-dose ICS	Low-dose ICS + LABA, LTRA, *or* theophylline *OR*	Medium-dose ICS + LABA	High-dose ICS + LABA	High-dose ICS + LABA + Oral corticosteroids
Alternative		Cromolyn LTRA nedocromil, *or* theophylline	Medium-dose ICS	Medium-dose ICS + LTRA *or* theophylline	High-dose ICS + LTRA *or* theophylline	High-dose ICS + LTRA *or* theophylline + Oral corticosteroids

Each Step: Patient Education and Environmental Control, and Management of Comorbidities

Steps 2–4: Consider subcutaneous allergen immunotherapy for patients who have persistent, allergic asthma.

Quick-Relief Medication	• SABA as needed for symptoms. Intensity of treatment depends on severity of symptoms: up to three treatments at 20-min intervals as needed. Short course of oral systemic corticosteroids may be needed. Caution: Increasing use of SABA or use >2 days a week for symptom relief (not prevention of EIB) generally indicates inadequate control and the need to step up treatment.

Notes (Children 5–11 years old):
- The stepwise approach is meant to assist, not replace, the clinical decision-making required to meet individual patient needs.
- If an alternative treatment is used and response is inadequate, discontinue it and use the preferred treatment before stepping up.
- Theophylline is a less desirable alternative due to the need to monitor serum concentration levels.
- Steps 1 and 2 medications are based on Evidence A. Step 3 ICS and ICS plus adjunctive therapy are based on Evidence B for efficacy of each treatment and extrapolation from comparator trials in older children and adults—comparator trials are not available for this age group; Steps 4–6 are based on expert opinion and extrapolation from studies in older children and adults.
- Immunotherapy for Steps 2–4 is based on Evidence B for house-dust mites, animal danders, and pollens; evidence is weak or lacking for molds and cockroaches. Evidence is strongest for immunotherapy with single allergens. The role of allergy in asthma is greater in children than adults.
- Clinicians who administer immunotherapy should be prepared and equipped to identify and treat anaphylaxis that may occur.

• **Fig 33.2** Stepwise approach for managing asthma in children 0 to 4 years old and 5 to 11 years old. Alphabetical order is used when more than one treatment option is listed within either preferred or alternative therapy. *EIB*, Exercise-induced bronchospasm; *ICS*, inhaled corticosteroid; *LABA*, long-acting β₂-agonist; *LTRA*, leukotriene receptor antagonist; *prn*, pro re nata (when necessary); *SABA*, short-acting β₂-agonist. (From National Heart, Lung, and Blood Institute. National Asthma and Prevention Program: expert panel report 3: guidelines for the diagnosis and management of asthma; 2007. www.nhlbi.nih.gov/guidelines/asthma/asthsumm.pdf. Accessed April 12, 2019. p. 42.)

Children 0–4 years old

Components of Severity		Classification of Asthma Severity			
		Intermittent	Persistent		
			Mild	Moderate	Severe
Impairment	Symptoms	≤2 days/week	>2 days/week but not daily	Daily	Throughout the day
	Nighttime awakenings	0	1–2x/month	3–4x/month	>1x/week
	SABA use for symptom control (not prevention of EIB)	≤2 days/week	>2 days/week but not daily	Daily	Several times per day
	Interference with normal activity	None	Minor limitation	Some limitation	Extremely limited
Risk	Exacerbations requiring oral systemic corticosteroids	0–1/year	≥2 exacerbations in 6 months requiring oral systemic corticosteroids, or ≥4 wheezing episodes/1 year lasting >1 day *and* risk factors for persistent asthma		
		← Consider severity and interval since last exacerbation. Frequency and severity may fluctuate over time. →			
		Exacerbations of any severity may occur in patients in any severity category			
Recommended Step for Initiating Therapy (See Fig 25-2 for treatment steps.)		Step 1	Step 2	Step 3 and consider short course of oral systemic corticosteroids	
		In 2–6 weeks, depending on severity, evaluate level of asthma control that is achieved. If no clear benefit is observed in 4–6 weeks, consider adjusting therapy or alternative diagnoses.			

Notes

- The stepwise approach is meant to assist, not replace, the clinical decision-making required to meet individual patient needs.

- Level of severity is determined by both impairment and risk. Assess impairment domain by patient's/caregiver's recall of previous 2–4 weeks. Symptom assessment for longer periods should reflect a global assessment, such as inquiring whether the patient's asthma is better or worse since the last visit. Assign severity to the most severe category in which any feature occurs.

- At present, there are inadequate data to correspond frequencies of exacerbations with different levels of asthma severity. For treatment purposes, patients who had ≥2 exacerbations requiring oral systemic corticosteroids in the past 6 months, or ≥4 wheezing episodes in the past year, and who have risk factors for persistent asthma may be considered the same as patients who have persistent asthma, even in the absence of impairment levels consistent with persistent asthma.

Children 5–11 years old

Components of Severity		Classification of Asthma Severity			
		Intermittent	Persistent		
			Mild	Moderate	Severe
Impairment	Symptoms	≤2 days/week	>2 days/week but not daily	Daily	Throughout the day
	Nighttime awakenings	≤2x/month	3–4x/month	>1x/week but not nightly	Often 7x/week
	SABA use for symptom control (not prevention of EIB)	≤2 days/week	>2 days/week but not daily	Daily	Several times per day
	Interference with normal activity	None	Minor limitation	Some limitation	Extremely limited
	Lung function	• Normal FEV$_1$ between exacerbations • FEV$_1$ >80% predicted • FEV$_1$/FVC >85%	• FEV$_1$ >80% predicted • FEV$_1$/FVC >80%	• FEV$_1$ = 60–80% predicted • FEV$_1$/FVC = 75-80%	• FEV$_1$ < 60% predicted • FEV$_1$/FVC < 75%
Risk	Exacerbations requiring oral systemic corticosteroids	0–1/year (see Notes)	≥2/year (see Notes)		
		← Consider severity and interval since last exacerbation. Frequency and severity may fluctuate over time for patients in any severity category. →			
		Relative annual risk of exacerbations may be related to FEV$_1$.			
Recommended Step for Initiating Therapy (See Fig 33-2 for treatment steps.)		Step 1	Step 2	Step 3, medium-dose ICS option	Step 3, medium-dose ICS option, or step 4
				and consider short course of oral systemic corticosteroids	
		In 2–6 weeks, evaluate level of asthma control that is achieved, and adjust therapy accordingly.			

Notes

- The stepwise approach is meant to assist, not replace, the clinical decision-making required to meet individual patient needs.

- Level of severity is determined by both impairment and risk. Assess impairment domain by patient's/caregiver's recall of previous 2–4 weeks and spirometry. Assign severity to the most severe category in which any feature occurs.

- At present, there are inadequate data to correspond frequencies of exacerbations with different levels of asthma severity. In general, more frequent and intense exacerbations (e.g., requiring urgent, unscheduled care, hospitalization, or ICU admission) indicate greater underlying disease severity. For treatment purposes, patients who had ≥2 exacerbations requiring oral systemic corticosteroids in the past year may be considered the same as patients who have persistent asthma, even in the absence of impairment levels consistent with persistent asthma.

• **Fig 33.3** Assessing asthma severity and initiating therapy in children 0 to 4 years old and 5 to 11 years old who are not currently taking long-term control medication. *EIB,* Exercise-induced bronchospasm; *FEV$_1$,* forced expiratory volume in 1 second; *FVC,* forced vital capacity; *ICS,* inhaled corticosteroid; *ICU,* intensive care unit; *SABA,* short-acting β$_2$-agonist. (From National Heart, Lung, Blood Institute. National Asthma Prevention Program: expert panel report 3: guidelines for the diagnosis and management of asthma; 2007. www.nhlbi.nih.gov/guidelines/asthma/asthsumm.pdf. Accessed April 12, 2019. pp. 40–41.)

Components of Severity		Classification of Asthma Severity				Notes
		Intermittent	Persistent			
			Mild	Moderate	Severe	
Impairment Normal FEV₁/FVC: 08–19 years old 85% 20–39 years old 80% 40–59 years old 75% 60–80 years old 70%	Symptoms	≤2 days/week	>2 days/week but not daily	Daily	Throughout the day	• The stepwise approach is meant to assist, not replace, the clinical decision-making required to meet individual patient needs. • Level of severity is determined by both impairment and risk. Assess impairment domain by patient's/caregiver's recall of previous 2–4 weeks and spirometry. Assign severity to the most severe category in which any feature occurs. • At present, there are inadequate data to correspond frequencies of exacerbations with different levels of asthma severity. In general, more frequent and intense exacerbations (e.g., requiring urgent, unscheduled care, hospitalization, or ICU admission) indicate greater underlying disease severity. For treatment purposes, patients who had ≥2 exacerbations requiring oral systemic corticosteroids in the past year may be considered the same as patients who have persistent asthma, even in the absence of impairment levels consistent with persistent asthma.
	Nighttime awakenings	≤2x/month	3–4x/month	>1x/week but not nightly	Often 7x/week	
	SABA use for symptom control (not prevention of EIB)	≤2 days/week	>2 days/week but not daily, and not more than 1x on any day	Daily	Several times per day	
	Interference with normal activity	None	Minor limitation	Some limitation	Extremely limited	
	Lung function	• Normal FEV₁ between exacerbations • FEV₁ >80% predicted • FEV₁/FVC normal	• FEV₁ >80% predicted • FEV₁/FVC normal	• FEV₁ >60 but <80% predicted • FEV₁/FVC reduced 5%	• FEV₁ <60% predicted • FEV₁/FVC reduced >5%	
Risk	Exacerbations requiring oral systemic corticosteroids	0–1/year (see Notes)	≥2/year (see Notes) ——————————————————→			
		←———— Consider severity and interval since last exacerbation. ————→ Frequency and severity may fluctuate over time for patients in any severity category.				
		Relative annual risk of exacerbations may be related to FEV₁.				
Recommended Step for Initiating Therapy (See Fig 33-1 for treatment steps.)		Step 1	Step 2	Step 3	Step 4 or 5	
				and consider short course of oral systemic corticosteroids		
		In 2–6 weeks, evaluate level of asthma control that is achieved and adjust therapy accordingly.				

(Left vertical label: **Children ≥12 years old**)

• **Fig 33.4** Assessing asthma severity and initiating therapy in children 12 years old and older and adults who are not currently taking long-term control medication. *EIB*, Exercise-induced bronchospasm; *FEV₁*, forced expiratory volume in 1 second; *FVC*, forced vital capacity; *ICU*, intensive care unit; *SABA*, short-acting β₂-agonist. (From National Heart, Lung, Blood Institute. National Asthma Prevention Program: expert panel report 3: guidelines for the diagnosis and management of asthma; 2007. www.nhlbi.nih.gov/guidelines/asthma/asthsumm.pdf. Accessed April 12, 2019. p. 43.)

- Ketamine, a potent bronchodilator, may be used as an induction agent in critically ill children with asthma and respiratory failure (Stenson et al., 2017).
- Ipratropium, an anticholinergic bronchodilator, via oral inhalation is used to treat bronchospasms.
- Epinephrine given subcutaneously or intramuscularly is an option in severe asthma where the delivery of medication to smaller airways is limited due to bronchoconstriction.
- Heliox, a mixture of oxygen and helium, can improve drug delivery in obstructed airways because it has a lower density and less airway resistance (Stenson et al., 2017).

Complications

Complications from asthma can range from mild secondary respiratory infections to respiratory arrest. Unresponsiveness to pharmacologic agents can lead to status asthmaticus and ultimately to death. Chronic high-dose steroid use leads to growth retardation and other related side effects.

Patient and Parent Education and Prevention

The PCP needs to support self-care management through indepth education as appropriate. Easy-to-understand education must be tailored to meet cultural beliefs and the individual child and family needs using a "teach back" technique. Correct administration of inhaled medication should be demonstrated during initial training sessions and reevaluated in subsequent visits. Provide instruction on the following:

- Basic understanding of what asthma is, what is effective asthma control, and what is the child's current level of symptomatology
- Environmental control of allergens or triggers (e.g., smoking and dust)
- Basic understanding of what different medications do and how to use them: Give clear, written instructions about: how to administer, how much and when to give, the need for monitoring side effects, and how long medication should be taken. A written plan is recommended based on either symptoms or peak expiratory flow rate (PEFR).
- How to use inhalers, spacer devices, or aerosol equipment (Box 33.2) along with proper cleaning of aerosol equipment
- Identifying asthma symptoms that indicate a need to change therapy or necessitate immediate reevaluation; when and where to seek emergency care
- Home PEF or symptom monitoring: What to do if symptoms worsen (what medications to add or increase; how frequently to use inhaled medication; specific indications about when to seek additional medical treatment if symptoms worsen)
- Regular physical activity such as walking as tolerated
- Avoid medications that can make asthma worse; NSAIDs and aspirin (ASA) can exacerbate asthma in some patients

TABLE 33.6 Estimated Comparative Daily Dosages for Inhaled Corticosteroids

Drug	LOW DAILY DOSE		MEDIUM DAILY DOSE		HIGH DAILY DOSE	
	Child[a]	Adult[b]	Child[a]	Adult[b]	Child[a]	Adult[b]
Beclomethasone HFA (40 or 80 mcg/puff) Redi-inhaler is breath activated	80-160 mcg Approved 4 and over	80-240 mcg	>160-320 mcg	>240-480 mcg	>320 mcg	>480 mcg
Budesonide (90 or 180, mcg/actuation) aerosol powder breath-activated inhalation	180-400 mcg	180-600 mcg	>400-800 mcg	>600-1200 mcg	>800 mcg	>1200 mcg
Budesonide inhaled suspension for nebulization (child dose) (0.25 mg/2 mL, 0.5 mg/2 mL)	≤4 years 0.25-0.5 mg 5-11 years 0.5 mg		≤4 years >.5 mg-1 mg 5-11 years 1 mg		≤4 years >1 mg 5-11 years 2 mg	N/A
Flunisolide aerosol solution inhalation (80 mcg/spray)	6-11 years 160 mcg	320 mcg	320 mcg	>320-640 mcg	>640 mcg	>640 mcg
Fluticasone HFA: 44, 110, or 220 mcg/actuation	88-176 mcg	88-264 mcg	>176-352 mcg	>264-440 mcg	>352 mcg	>440 mcg
Fluticasone aerosol powder breath-activated inhalation: 50, 100, or 250 mcg/inhalation	4-11 years 100-200 mcg	100-300 mcg	4-11 years >200-400 mcg	>300-500 mcg	>400 mcg	>500 mcg
Mometasone aerosol powder breath-activated inhalation (220 mcg/INH)[c]	N/A	200 mcg	N/A	400 mcg	N/A	>400 mcg

[a]Child 5-11 years old.

[b]Adult 12 years old and older.

[c]Note 220 mcg/inhalation provides 200 mcg of mometasone per actuation.

HFA, Hydrofluoroalkane; *INH*, inhalation; *N/A*, not approved and no data available for this age group.

Adapted from the National Heart, Lung, and Blood Institute (NHLBI). *Full Report of the Expert Panel: Guidelines for the Diagnosis and Management of Asthma (EPR-3)*. Bethesda, MD: National Institutes of Health; 2007; and Taketomo CK, Hodding JH, Kraus DM. *Pediatric Dosage Handbook*. 24th ed. Hudson, OH: Lexi-Comp; 2019.

TABLE 33.7 **Inhaled Corticosteroids in Children 0 to 4 Years Old**

	Low Daily Dose	Medium Daily Dose	High Daily Dose
Budesonide inhaled suspension for nebulization (0.25 mg/2 mL, 0.5 mg/2 mL)	0.25-0.5 mg	>0.5-1 mg	>1 mg
Fluticasone HFA: 44, 110, or 220 mcg/actuation	176 mcg	>176-352 mcg	>352 mcg

HFA, Hydrofluoroalkane.

Adapted from the National Heart, Lung, and Blood Institute (NHLBI). *Full Report of the Expert Panel: Guidelines for the Diagnosis and Management of Asthma (EPR-3)*. Bethesda, MD: National Institutes of Health; 2007; and Taketomo CK, Hodding JH, Kraus DM. *Pediatric Dosage Handbook*. 24th ed. Hudson, OH: Lexi-Comp; 2019.

TABLE 33.8 **Long-Term Control Medications for the Treatment of Asthma**

Medication	Dosage Form	Child Dosage[a]	Adult Dosage[b]	Comments
Inhaled Corticosteroids (see Tables 33.6 and 33.7)				
Systemic Corticosteroids—Applies to All Three Corticosteroids				
Methylprednisolone	2-, 4-, 8-, 16-, 32-mg tablets	0.25-2 mg/kg daily in a single dose in a.m. or every other day as needed for control; 60 mg maximum dose	7.5-60 mg daily in a single dose in a.m. or every other day as needed for control	For long-term treatment of severe persistent asthma, administer single dose in a.m. either daily or on alternate days (alternate-day therapy may produce less adrenal suppression). If daily doses are required, one study suggests improved efficacy and no increase in adrenal suppression when administered at 3 p.m.
Prednisolone	5-mg tablets, 5 mg/5 mL, 1 mg/mL	Same as above	Same as above	
Prednisone	1-, 2-, 5-, 10-, 20-, 50-mg tablets; 5 mg/mL, 1 mg/mL	Short-course "burst": 1-2 mg/kg/day in single or two divided doses a day, maximum 60 mg/day for 3-10 days	Short-course "burst" to achieve control: 40-60 mg/day as single or two divided doses for 3-10 days	Short courses or "bursts" are effective for establishing control when initiating therapy or during a period of gradual deterioration. The bursts should be continued until patient achieves 80% PEF rate personal best or symptoms resolve. This usually requires 3-10 days but may require longer treatment. There is no evidence that tapering the dose following improvement prevents relapse.
Cromolyn				
Cromolyn	20 mg/ampule for nebulization solution, inhalation	Children ≥ 2 years old: 1 ampule four times a day initially; usual dose three times a day	1 ampule three or four times a day; usual dose three times a day	≥2 years old: Single dose of 20 mg 10-15 min before exercise or allergen exposure provides effective prophylaxis for 1-2 h.
Inhaled Long-Acting β₂-Agonists—Should Not Be Used for Symptom Relief or for Exacerbations: Use With Inhaled Corticosteroids				
Salmeterol	DPI: 50 mcg/inhalation	≥4 years old: 1 activation/puff every 12 h	1 activation/puff every 12 h	Use with inhaled corticosteroid only. Do not use as a rescue inhaler for symptom relief or for exacerbations.
Formoterol	DPI: 12 mcg/single-use capsule	≥5 years old: 1 capsule every 12 h apart	1 capsule every 12 h	Do not take orally; must be used with aerolizer. Should be used with inhaled steroid.

Continued

TABLE 33.8	Long-Term Control Medications for the Treatment of Asthma—cont'd			
Medication	**Dosage Form**	**Child Dosage[a]**	**Adult Dosage[b]**	**Comments**
Leukotriene Modifiers				
Montelukast	4- or 5-mg chewable tablet, 10-mg tablet; granules 4 mg/packet	12 months to 5 years old: 4 mg a day; 6-14 years old: 5 mg a day	≥15 years old: 10 mg a day Prevention of EIB: 6-14 years old: 5 mg; ≥15 years old: 10 mg at least 2 h before exercise (no other doses should be given in 24 h)	
Zafirlukast	10- or 20-mg tablet	5-11 years old: 10-mg tablet twice a day	>12 years old: 20-mg tablet twice a day	Take zafirlukast at least 1 h before or 2 h after meals.
Zileuton	600-mg tablet and 600 mg extended release		2400 mg daily (give tablets four times a day) or 1200 mg twice a day of the extended release	Less desirable because of the need to monitor hepatic enzymes (ALT); used in children older than 12 years old.
Combined Medication				
Fluticasone/salmeterol	HFA: 45, 115, fluticasone 230 mcg/21 mcg salmeterol		HFA: ≥12 years old: Two inhalations twice a day of 45 mcg fluticasone/21 mcg salmeterol *or* 115 mcg fluticasone/21 mcg salmeterol	HFA adult dose not to exceed 2 inhalations of 230 mcg fluticasone/21 mcg salmeterol twice daily. Starting dose dependent on current steroid therapy.
	Diskus: 100, 250, or 500 mcg fluticasone/50 mcg salmeterol	Diskus: >4-11 years old: 1 inhalation twice a day of 100 mcg fluticasone/50 mcg salmeterol; dose depends on severity of asthma	Diskus: 1 inhalation twice a day of 100 mcg fluticasone/50 mcg salmeterol; dose depends on severity of asthma	Starting dose based on current steroid therapy.
Budesonide/formoterol aerosol for oral inhalation	Aerosol: 80 mcg *or* 160 mcg budesonide/4.5 mcg formoterol	5-11 years old: 2 inhalations twice a day of aerosol 80 mcg/4.5 mcg, not to exceed 4 inhalations/day	≥12 years old: 2 inhalations twice a day of aerosol 80 mcg/4.5 mcg, not to exceed 4 inhalations/day; if not controlled may increase to 160 mcg budesonide/4.5 mcg formoterol inhalation twice daily not exceeding 4 inhalations day	

[a]Infants and children <12 years old.

[b]Adult, 12 years old and older.

ALT, Alanine amino transferase; *DPI,* dry powder inhaler; *EIB,* exercise-induced bronchospasm; *HFA,* hydrofluoroalkane; *PEF,* peak expiratory flow.

Adapted from the National Heart, Lung, and Blood Institute (NHLBI). *Full Report of the Expert Panel: Guidelines for the Diagnosis and Management of Asthma (EPR-3).* Bethesda, MD: National Institutes of Health; 2007; and Takemoto CK, Hodding JH, Kraus DM. *Pediatric Dosage Handbook.* 24th ed. Hudson, OH: Lexi-Comp; 2019.

- Development of a written action/treatment plan with the child or parent to cover these issues (Fig 33.6 shows a sample form for home treatment plan)
- Need to have an adequate supply of all medications (including oral corticosteroids) at home and medications readily accessible to the child at school or other settings where the child frequents
- Eat a generally healthy diet with increase in fruits and vegetables; if obese or overweight, discuss diet using motivational interviewing techniques
- Discuss involving allergist in care to consider AIT

- Management of the child at school, camp, or other places away from home
- Need for regular follow-up every 1 to 6 months and as needed with exacerbations

Stress that asthma is a chronic disease, which can be controlled—the goal of therapy is to maintain normal activity. The absence of symptoms does not mean the disease has disappeared, rather it is well controlled. The child should wear a medical alert bracelet. Acquaint children and parents with local asthma education programs and activities, such as asthma camp. Written instructions and handouts should be provided for other

TABLE 33.9 Quick-Relief Medications for the Treatment of Asthma

Medication	Dosage Form	Child Dosage[a]	Adult Dosage	Comments
Short-Acting Inhaled β₂-Agonists				
Metered Dose Inhalers				
Albuterol HFA	90 mcg/puff, 200 puffs	Acute exacerbation: 4-8 puffs every 20 min for three doses, then every 1-4 h as needed. Maintenance: 0-4 years old, 1-2 inhalations every 4-6 h; >5 years old, 2 puffs every 4-6 h prn	Acute exacerbation: 4-8 puffs every 20 min for 4 h, then every 1-4 h as needed. Maintenance: 2 puffs every 4-6 h prn	Not generally recommended for long-term treatment. Regular use on a daily basis indicates the need for additional long-term control therapy.
Pirbuterol	200 mcg/INH, 400 INH	Acute exacerbation: 4-8 inhalations every 20 min for three doses, then every 1-4 h as needed. Maintenance: 2 inhalations three or four times/day	Acute exacerbation: 4-8 inhalations every 20 min for up to 4 h, then every 1-4 h as needed. Maintenance: 2 inhalations three or four times/day	
Levalbuterol HFA	45 mcg/puff	Acute exacerbation: 4-8 puffs every 20 min for three doses, then every 1-4 h. Maintenance: ≥5 years old: 2 inhalations every 4-6 h	Acute exacerbation: 4-8 puffs every 20 min for up to 4 h, then every 1-4 h as needed. Maintenance: 2 inhalations every 4-6 h	Not FDA approved for long-term, daily maintenance use. Use more than 2 days/week indicates need for long-term control therapy. Non-selective agents (e.g., epinephrine, isoproterenol, metaproterenol) are not recommended because of their potential for excessive cardiac stimulation, especially at high doses.
Nebulizer Solution				
Albuterol	5 mg/mL (0.5%) 0.63 mg/3 mL 1.25 mg/3 mL, 2.5 mg/3 mL	<5 years old: 0.63-2.5 mg in 3 mL NS every 4-6 h prn. >5 years: 1.25-2.5 mg in 3 mL of NS every 4-8 h prn	Adults: 1.25-5 mg in 3 mL of NS every 4-8 h prn	May mix with cromolyn or ipratropium nebulizer solutions; may double dose for mild exacerbations.
Levalbuterol	0.31 mg/3 mL 0.63 mg/3 mL 1.25 mg/3 mL	Acute exacerbation: 0.075 mg/kg (minimum dose 1.25 mg) every 20 min for three doses, then 0.075-0.15 mg/kg (not to exceed 5 mg) every 1-4 h as needed. Maintenance: 0-4 years old: 0.31-1.25 mg every 4-6 h prn; ≥5 years old and adults: 0.31-0.63 mg every 8 h prn	Acute exacerbation: 1.25-2.5 mg every 20 min for three doses, then 1.25-5 mg every 1-4 h as needed. Maintenance: 0.31-0.63 mg every 8 h as needed	Use more than 2 days/week indicates need for long-term control therapy.
Anticholinergics				
Ipratropium HFA (MDI) Ipratropium (nebulizer solution)	17 mcg/puff, 200-puff canister 0.02% (2.5 mL)	Refer to a pharmacology textbook	Refer to a pharmacology textbook	Evidence is lacking that ipratropium HFA produces added benefit to β₂-agonists in long-term asthma therapy.
Systemic Corticosteroids—Dosage Applies to All Three Corticosteroids				
Methylprednisolone	2-, 4-, 8-, 16-, 32-mg tablets	Short-course "burst": 1-2 mg/kg/day in divided doses once or twice daily, maximum 60 mg/day, for 3-10 days	Short-course "burst" to achieve control: 40-60 mg/day as single or two divided doses for 3-10 days	Short courses or "bursts" are effective for establishing control when initiating therapy or during a period of gradual deterioration.

Continued

TABLE 33.9 Quick-Relief Medications for the Treatment of Asthma—cont'd

Medication	Dosage Form	Child Dosage[a]	Adult Dosage	Comments
Prednisolone	5-mg tablets, 5 mg/5 mL, 15 mg/5 mL			
Prednisone	1-, 2.5-, 5-, 10-, 20-, 50-mg tablets: 5 mg/mL, 5 mg/5 mL			The burst should be continued until patient achieves 80% PEF rate personal best or symptoms resolve; this usually requires 3-10 days but may require longer; there is no evidence that tapering the dose following improvement prevents relapse.

[a]<12 years old.

FDA, U.S. Food and Drug Administration; *HFA,* hydrofluoroalkane; *INH,* inhalations; *MDI,* metered dose inhaler; *NS,* normal saline; *PEF,* peak expiratory flow; *prn, pro re nata* (when necessary).

Adapted from the National Heart, Lung, and Blood Institute (NHLBI). *Full Report of the Expert Panel: Guidelines for the Diagnosis and Management of Asthma (EPR-3).* Bethesda, MD: National Institutes of Health; 2007; and Taketomo CK, Hodding JH, Kraus DM. *Pediatric Dosage Handbook.* 24th ed. Hudson, OH: Lexi-Comp; 2019.

TABLE 33.10 Classifying Severity of Asthma Exacerbations

	Mild	Moderate	Severe	Respiratory Arrest Imminent
Symptoms				
Breathless	While walking	While at rest (infant—softer, shorter cry; difficulty feeding)	While at rest (infant—stops feeding)	
	Can lie down	Prefers sitting	Sits upright	
Talks in	Sentences	Phrases	Words	
Alertness	May be agitated	Usually agitated	Usually agitated	Drowsy or confused
Signs				
Respiratory rate	Increased	Increased	Often >30/min	
Use of accessory muscles; suprasternal retractions	Usually not	Commonly	Usually	Paradoxical thoracoabdominal movement
Wheeze	Moderate, often only end expiratory	Loud; throughout exhalation	Usually loud; throughout inhalation and exhalation	Absence of wheeze
Pulse/min	<100	100-120	>120	Bradycardia
Functional Assessment				
PEF percentage predicted or percentage personal best	≥70%	Approximately 40%-69%	<40% predicted or personal best, or response lasts < 2 h	<25%
PaO_2 (on room air) *and/or*	Normal (test not usually necessary)	>60 mm Hg (test not usually necessary)	<60 mm Hg: possible cyanosis	
PCO_2	<42 mm Hg (test not usually necessary)	<42 mm Hg (test not usually necessary)	≥42 mm Hg: possible respiratory failure	
SaO_2% (on room air) at sea level	>95% (test not usually necessary)	90%-95%	<90%	

TABLE 33.10 **Classifying Severity of Asthma Exacerbations—cont'd**

	Mild	Moderate	Severe	Respiratory Arrest Imminent
		GUIDE TO NORMAL RESPIRATORY AND CARDIAC RATES		

NORMAL RATES OF BREATHING IN AWAKE CHILDREN

Age	Rate
<2 months old	<60/min
2-12 months old	<50/min
1-5 years old	<40/min
6-8 years old	<30/min

NORMAL PULSE RATES IN CHILDREN

Age	Rate
2-12 months old	<160/min
1-2 years old	<120/min
2-8 years old	<110/min

The presence of several parameters, but not necessarily all, indicates the general classification of the exacerbation. Many of these parameters have not been systematically studied, so they serve only as general guides.

PaCO2, Partial pressure of carbon dioxide; *PaO2*, partial pressure of oxygen in arterial blood; *PEF*, peak expiratory flow; *SaO2*, oxygen saturation in arterial blood.

From National Heart, Lung, and Blood Institute (NHLBI). *Full Report of the Expert Panel: Guidelines for the Diagnosis and Management of Asthma (EPR-3)*. Bethesda, MD: National Institutes of Health; 2007.

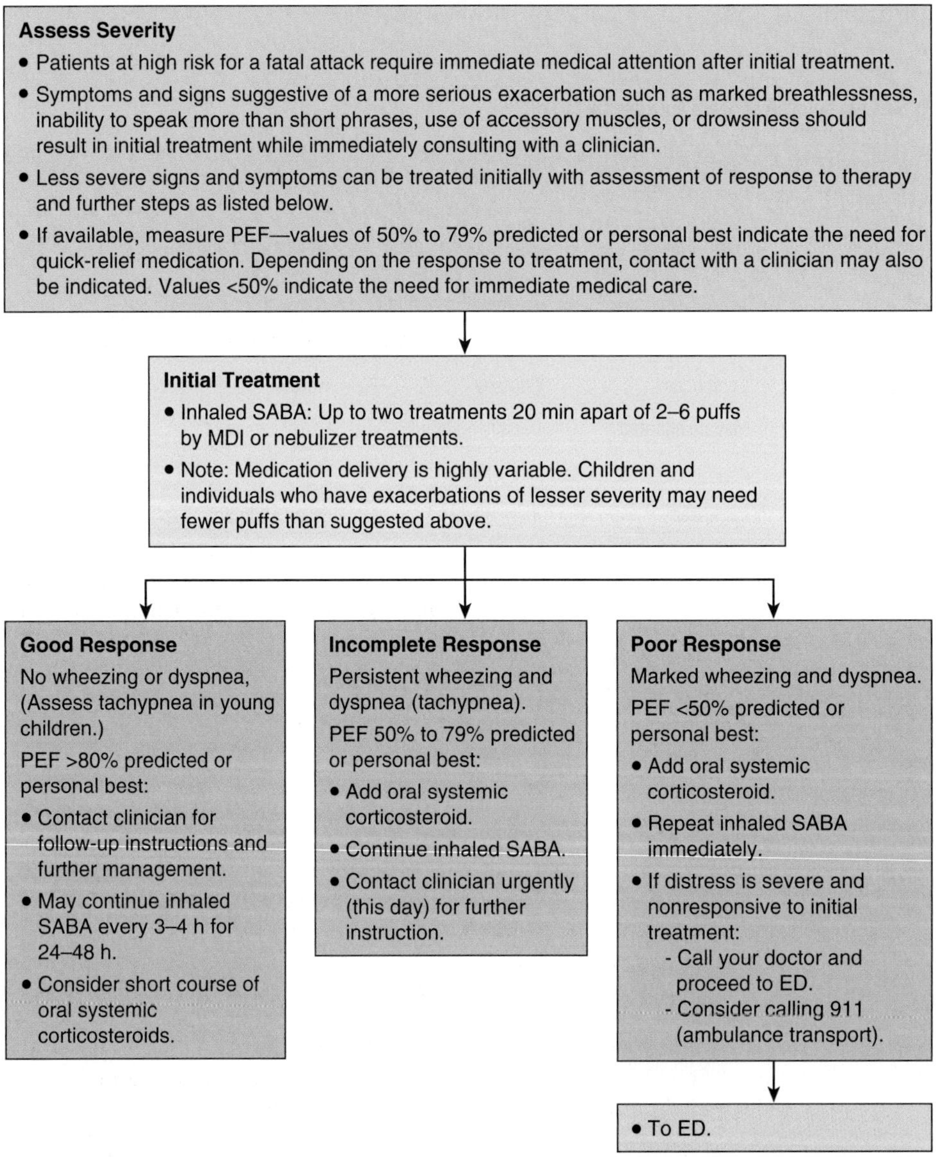

Assess Severity
- Patients at high risk for a fatal attack require immediate medical attention after initial treatment.
- Symptoms and signs suggestive of a more serious exacerbation such as marked breathlessness, inability to speak more than short phrases, use of accessory muscles, or drowsiness should result in initial treatment while immediately consulting with a clinician.
- Less severe signs and symptoms can be treated initially with assessment of response to therapy and further steps as listed below.
- If available, measure PEF—values of 50% to 79% predicted or personal best indicate the need for quick-relief medication. Depending on the response to treatment, contact with a clinician may also be indicated. Values <50% indicate the need for immediate medical care.

Initial Treatment
- Inhaled SABA: Up to two treatments 20 min apart of 2–6 puffs by MDI or nebulizer treatments.
- Note: Medication delivery is highly variable. Children and individuals who have exacerbations of lesser severity may need fewer puffs than suggested above.

Good Response
No wheezing or dyspnea, (Assess tachypnea in young children.)
PEF >80% predicted or personal best:
- Contact clinician for follow-up instructions and further management.
- May continue inhaled SABA every 3–4 h for 24–48 h.
- Consider short course of oral systemic corticosteroids.

Incomplete Response
Persistent wheezing and dyspnea (tachypnea).
PEF 50% to 79% predicted or personal best:
- Add oral systemic corticosteroid.
- Continue inhaled SABA.
- Contact clinician urgently (this day) for further instruction.

Poor Response
Marked wheezing and dyspnea.
PEF <50% predicted or personal best:
- Add oral systemic corticosteroid.
- Repeat inhaled SABA immediately.
- If distress is severe and nonresponsive to initial treatment:
  - Call your doctor and proceed to ED.
  - Consider calling 911 (ambulance transport).

- To ED.

• **Fig 33.5** Management of Asthma Exacerbations: Home Treatment. *ED*, Emergency department; *MDI*, metered dose inhaler; *PEF*, peak expiratory flow; *SABA*, short-acting β2-agonist.

Using an inhaler seems simple, but most patients do not use it correctly.

Steps for Using an Inhaler for Children Younger Than 5 Years Old

1. Use of a mask chamber with MDI allows the delivery of inhaled medications even in an uncooperative child.
2. The child should be placed in the parent's lap, and the mask placed around the child's mouth.
3. Press down on the MDI while firmly holding the mask around the child's mouth. The child will eventually take a deep breath and inhale the medication.

Steps for Using an Inhaler for Children 5 Years Old or Older
Getting Ready
1. Take off the cap and shake the inhaler.
2. Breathe out all the way.
3. Hold the inhaler as shown in steps A, B, or C.

Breathe in Slowly
1. Start breathing in slowly through the mouth, and then press down on the inhaler one time. (If a holding chamber is used, first press down on the inhaler.) Within 5 s, begin to breathe in slowly.
2. Keep breathing in slowly, as deeply as possible.

Hold Your Breaths
1. Hold breath for a slow count to 10 if possible.
2. For inhaled quick-relief medicine (β_2-agonists), wait about 1 min between puffs. There is no need to wait between puffs for other medicines.
   A. Hold inhaler 1-2 inches in front of mouth (about the width of two fingers).

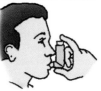

B. Use a spacer/holding chamber. These come in many shapes and can be useful to any patient.

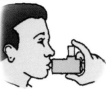

C. Put inhaler in mouth. Do not use for steroids.

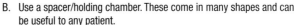

Step A or B is best, but step C can be used if patient has trouble with step A or B.

Clean Inhaler as Needed
Look at the hole where the medicine sprays out from inhaler. If "powder" can be seen in or around the hole, clean the inhaler. Remove the metal canister from the L-shaped plastic mouthpiece. Rinse only the mouthpiece and cap in warm water and let dry overnight. In the morning, put the canister back inside. Put the cap on.

Know When to Replace Inhaler
For medicines taken each day: As an example, a new canister has 200 puffs (number of puffs is listed on canister), and child is told to take 8 puffs/day; 8 puffs/day for 25 days equal 200 puffs in canister. This canister will last 25 days. If child started using this inhaler on May 1, replace it on or before May 25. Write the date on the canister. For quick-relief medicine, take as needed and count each puff. Do not put canisters in water to see if empty.

MDI, *Metered dose inhaler.*

---

significant individuals in the child's life, including caregivers and school personnel.

Prognosis
Asthma is a chronic disease that for most children can be successfully managed with proper pharmacologic therapy, allergen and environmental control, and patient education. Mild asthma is more likely to disappear with increasing age than is moderate or severe asthma.

Allergic Rhinitis

AR and asthma are increasing in prevalence and are comorbid conditions with up to 40% of individuals with AR also having asthma (Mastrorilli et al., 2016). The link between upper and lower respiratory disease causes poorly controlled AR to lead to poorly controlled asthma. AR is a disorder that results in nasal mucosal inflammation due to Th2 cell. More specifically the antigen uptake by the antigen-presenting cell leads to antigen-specific T cell activation. At the same time proteases lead to epithelia cytokine release, favoring the Th2 cell and basophil activation, releasing Th-2 cytokines that drive B cells to form plasma cells that release IgE. On re-exposure to the antigen, the IgE clings to IgE

receptors activating mast cells and basophils, leading to the release of cysteinyl leukotrienes and histamine. These substances along with the local Th2 activation cause the motor reflex of sneezing and parasympathetic reflex that stimulate vasodilation and nasal secretion. Vascular engorgement leads to obstruction of the nasal passages. Sensory nerves are also hyperresponsive in AR (Wheatley and Togias, 2015).

There are two phases of the nasal response. The immediate phase occurs 15 to 30 minutes after an exposure to an allergen and is due to mast cell mediator release. In about 60% to 70% of individuals, there is a late-phase response that occurs 6 to 12 hours after exposure and is due to inflammatory cells (i.e., T lymphocytes, basophils, eosinophils) infiltrating the nasal mucosa.

Most children with AR have significant symptoms affecting their quality of life and leading to school and work absences. It is a clinical diagnosis based on the presence of rhinorrhea, nasal pruritus and congestion, and sneezing. Manifestations can be seasonal or perennial depending on exposure to the offending agent and subsequent sensitization to the offending allergen (Siedman et al., 2015). There may be a related family or medical history of AD, AR, or asthma.

AR is second only to asthma as the most common atopic disorder. There is an increased incidence in families with an atopic

Asthma Treatment Plan

(This asthma action plan meets NJ Law N.J.S.A. 18A:40-12.8) (Physician's Orders)

The Pediatric/Adult Asthma Coalition of New Jersey
"Your Pathway to Asthma Control"
PACNJ approved Plan available at www.pacnj.org

Sponsored by
 AMERICAN LUNG ASSOCIATION® IN NEW JERSEY

 NEW JERSEY DEPARTMENT OF HEALTH AND SENIOR SERVICES

(Please Print)

Name	Date of Birth	Effective Date

Doctor	Parent/Guardian (if applicable)	Emergency Contact

Phone	Phone	Phone

HEALTHY ▬▬▶

You have _all_ of these:
- Breathing is good
- No cough or wheeze
- Sleep through the night
- Can work, exercise, and play

And/or Peak flow above _____

Take daily medicine(s). Some metered dose inhalers may be more effective with a "spacer" – use if directed.

MEDICINE	HOW MUCH to take and HOW OFTEN to take it
☐ Advair® ☐ 100, ☐ 250, ☐ 500 _____	1 inhalation twice a day
☐ Advair® HFA ☐ 45, ☐ 115, ☐ 230 _____	2 puffs MDI twice a day
☐ Alvesco® ☐ 80, ☐ 160 _____	☐ 1, ☐ 2 puffs MDI twice a day
☐ Asmanex® Twisthaler® ☐ 110, ☐ 220 _____	☐ 1, ☐ 2 inhalations ☐ once or ☐ twice a day
☐ Flovent® ☐ 44, ☐ 110, ☐ 220 _____	2 puffs MDI twice a day
☐ Flovent® Diskus® ☐ 50 ☐ 100 ☐ 250 _____	1 inhalation twice a day
☐ Pulmicort Flexhaler® ☐ 90, ☐ 180 _____	☐ 1, ☐ 2 inhalations ☐ once or ☐ twice a day
☐ Pulmicort Respules® ☐ 0.25, ☐ 0.5, ☐ 1.0 _____	1 unit nebulized ☐ once or ☐ twice a day
☐ Qvar® ☐ 40, ☐ 80 _____	☐ 1, ☐ 2 puffs MDI twice a day
☐ Singulair ☐ 4, ☐ 5, ☐ 10 mg _____	1 tablet daily
☐ Symbicort® ☐ 80, ☐ 160 _____	☐ 1, ☐ 2 puffs MDI twice a day
☐ Other	
☐ None	

Remember to rinse your mouth after taking inhaled medicine.

If exercise triggers your asthma, take this medicine_____ _____ minutes before exercise.

CAUTION ▬▬▶

You have _any_ of these:
- Exposure to known trigger
- Cough
- Mild wheeze
- Tight chest
- Coughing at night
- Other:_____

And/or Peak flow from_____ to_____

Continue daily medicine(s) and add fast-acting medicine(s).

MEDICINE	HOW MUCH to take and HOW OFTEN to take it
☐ Accuneb® ☐ 0.63, ☐ 1.25 mg _____	1 unit nebulized every 4 hours as needed
☐ Albuterol ☐ 1.25, ☐ 2.5 mg _____	1 unit nebulized every 4 hours as needed
☐ Albuterol ☐ Pro-Air ☐ Proventil® _____	2 puffs MDI every 4 hours as needed
☐ Ventolin® ☐ Maxair ☐ Xopenex® _____	2 puffs MDI every 4 hours as needed
☐ Xopenex® ☐ 0.31, ☐ 0.63, ☐ 1.25 mg _____	1 unit nebulized every 4 hours as needed
☐ Increase the dose of, or add:	
☐ Other	

➡ **If fast-acting medicine is needed more than 2 times a week, except before exercise, then call your doctor.**

EMERGENCY ▬▬▶

Your asthma is getting worse fast:
- Fast-acting medicine did not help within 15-20 minutes
- Breathing is hard and fast
- Nose opens wide
- Ribs show
- Trouble walking and talking
- Lips blue • Fingernails blue

And/or Peak flow below _____

Take these medicines NOW and call 911.
Asthma can be a life-threatening illness. Do not wait!

☐ Accuneb® ☐ 0.63, ☐ 1.25 mg _____	1 unit nebulized every 20 minutes
☐ Albuterol ☐ 1.25, ☐ 2.5 mg _____	1 unit nebulized every 20 minutes
☐ Albuterol ☐ Pro-Air ☐ Proventil® _____	2 puffs MDI every 20 minutes
☐ Ventolin® ☐ Maxair ☐ Xopenex® _____	2 puffs MDI every 20 minutes
☐ Xopenex® ☐ 0.31, ☐ 0.63, ☐ 1.25 mg _____	1 unit nebulized every 20 minutes
☐ Other	

Triggers
Check all items that trigger patient's asthma:

- ☐ Chalk dust
- ☐ Cigarette Smoke & second hand smoke
- ☐ Colds/Flu
- ☐ Dust mites, dust, stuffed animals, carpet
- ☐ Exercise
- ☐ Mold
- ☐ Ozone alert days
- ☐ Pests - rodents & cockroaches
- ☐ Pets - animal dander
- ☐ Plants, flowers, cut grass, pollen
- ☐ Strong odors, perfumes, cleaning products, scented products
- ☐ Sudden temperature change
- ☐ Wood Smoke
- ☐ Foods: _____
  _____
  _____
- ☐ Other: _____
  _____
  _____
  _____
  _____
  _____

This asthma treatment plan is meant to assist, not replace, the clinical decision-making required to meet individual patient needs.

The Pediatric/Adult Asthma Coalition of New Jersey, sponsored by the American Lung Association of New Jersey, and this publication are supported by a grant from the New Jersey Department of Health and Senior Services (NJDHSS), with funds provided by the U.S. Centers for Disease Control and Prevention (USCDCP) under Cooperative Agreement 5U59EH000206-3. Its contents are solely the responsibility of the authors and do not necessarily represent the official views of the NJDHSS or the USCDCP.

Although this document has been funded wholly or in part by the United States Environmental Protection Agency under Agreement XA97296707-2 to the American Lung Association of New Jersey, it has not gone through the Agency's publications review process and therefore, may not necessarily reflect the views of the Agency and no official endorsement should be inferred.

REVISED MAY 2009
Permission to reproduce blank form www.pacnj.org

FOR MINORS ONLY:
☐ This student is capable and has been instructed in the proper method of self-administering of the non-nebulized inhaled medications named above in accordance with NJ Law.

☐ This student is _not_ approved to self-medicate.

Make a copy for patient and for physician file. For children under 18, send original to school nurse or child care provider.

PHYSICIAN/APN/PA SIGNATURE_____ DATE_____

PARENT/GUARDIAN SIGNATURE_____

PHYSICIAN STAMP

• **Fig 33.6** Sample Asthma Treatment Plan Form. (From the Pediatric/Adult Asthma Coalition of New Jersey. Asthma treatment plan; 2009. www.pacnj.org/pdfs/asthmatreatmentenglish2010.pdf. Accessed April 18, 2019.)

history. Genetic (the presence of an abnormal sensitivity that is associated with IgE production) and environmental factors are linked to its cause. Repeated exposure to the offending allergen for a period of time is an important contributing factor necessary for sensitizing the immune system to produce an allergic IgE response. Frequently, there is pruritus of the nose, palate, and eyes. The history may also include poor sleep, generalized malaise, and behavioral issues along with impaired school performance.

The classification can be intermittent if it persists for only 4 weeks or less, or persistent if it is present for longer than 4 weeks. If it is mild, it does not impair any of the following four: daily activities, sleep, school or work activities, and the child is not troubled by the symptoms. If it is moderate to severe, there are changes in one or more of these four items (Tharpe and Kemp, 2015).

AR is rare in children under 2 years as it requires a few years to develop the allergic response. In a young child with nasal symptoms, consider other differentials such as infections, irritants, tumors, or choanal atresia (Tharpe and Kemp, 2015). Food allergens occasionally cause rhinitis. AR tends to be seasonal, perennial, or episodic.

Seasonal AR (hay fever or seasonal pollenosis) results from sensitization to airborne allergens, such as tree, grass, and weed pollen (e.g., ragweed) and outdoor molds. There can be geographic variations in seasonal AR depending on climate and when allergens are released into the environment. Perennial AR has year-round signs and symptoms that may be more severe in the winter. Onset can occur before the second year of life, and offending substances tend to be indoor allergens, including house-dust mites, cockroaches, feathers, allergens or dander of household pets, and indoor mold spores and seasonal pollens. Episodic AR occurs with intermittent exposure to an allergen with a resultant rhinitis and is related to a distinct event, such as visiting a house where a cat lives.

Clinical Findings

Common nasal symptoms and findings on physical examination include:
- Reduced patency from chronic or recurrent bilateral nasal obstruction as a result of congestion and inflammation
- Mouth breathing, snoring, nasal speech
- Pale to purplish and edema (bogginess) of nasal mucous membranes
- Clear, thin, watery to seromucoid rhinorrhea
- Nasal crease—horizontal crease across the lower third of the nose
- Itching, rubbing of nose, or "allergic salute"
- Nasal stuffiness, postnasal drip, paroxysms of sneezing, congested cough, or night cough
- Allergic shiners, Dennie lines, Morgan fold, or atopic pleats— extra groove in lower eyelid (Fig 33.7)
  Associated manifestations include the following:
- High arched palate; itching of palate, pharynx, nose, or eyes; child may make a palatal click to scratch the palate; enlarged tonsillar and adenoidal tissue
- Repeated sniffling, snorting, coughing, frequent attempts to clear the throat, or hoarseness
- Redness of the conjunctiva, tearing, lid and periorbital edema, infraorbital cyanosis, or allergic shiners (dark periorbital swelling)
- "Cobblestone" appearance of the pharynx or palpebral conjunctivae (or both) as a result of increased lymphoid tissue

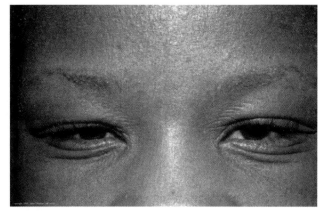

• **Fig 33.7** Dennie Line, or Morgan Line. (From Cohen B. *Pediatric Dermatology*. 3rd ed. Philadelphia: Mosby; 2005.)

- Chronic mouth breathing can lead to facial changes, dental malocclusions, and snoring
- Sleep disturbances are common in allergic disease with performance problems at school from inadequate sleep

Diagnostic Studies and Allergy Testing. History, including an evaluation of risk factors, and characteristic clinical findings are the key to diagnosis. Risk factors of pediatric AR include a positive family history, male gender, first-born child, early use of systemic antibiotics, maternal smoking, and exposure to allergens. Diagnostic testing is not needed. Allergen-specific IgE testing done by skin prick testing (SPT) is preferred and usually done by an allergist. The presence of eosinophils on nasal smear can help substantiate the diagnosis but is a nonspecific, non-universal finding. The presence of nasal eosinophilia often predicts a positive response to nasal corticosteroid sprays. Referrals for skin or serologic testing for IgE antibody to specific allergens should be reserved for children with significant symptoms that do not respond to traditional management.

The American Academy of Allergy recently recommended against ordering large panels of allergen testing and stressed the importance of only doing testing for specific allergens by history. Allergy panel can lead to the diagnosis of an allergy that the child does not have and can result in unnecessary avoidance. It can also result in false reassurance in the face of a negative test, when in fact the child's history is positive for an offending trigger. Neither positive skin testing nor positive allergen-specific IgE blood tests should be the sole basis for telling a family their child is allergic to a particular airborne antigen or food. History is critical to determine the test's accuracy (Choosingwisely.org).

Differential Diagnosis

Differential diagnoses are the common cold, purulent rhinitis, sinusitis, adenoidal hypertrophy, foreign body obstruction, nasal polyposis of cystic fibrosis, nasopharyngeal tumors, choanal atresia or stenosis, and vasomotor rhinitis. Overuse of prescription or over-the-counter topical nasal decongestants can cause drug-induced rhinitis (rhinitis medicamentosa), as can the use of cocaine. Some individuals experience idiopathic rhinitis marked by nasal hyperresponsiveness to nonspecific triggers, such as strong smells (e.g., perfumes, bleach), tobacco smoke, or changes in environmental temperature and humidity. Hormonal rhinitis occurs during pregnancy, puberty, and in hypothyroidism, and food-induced rhinitis is associated with consumption of hot and spicy foods. Patients who have unilateral discharge or blockage, severe headache, or anosmia may have an alternative diagnosis including cerebrospinal fluid rhinorrhea, sinonasal tumors, or chronic rhinosinusitis (Seidman et al., 2015).

Management

Treatment of patients with AR is tailored to the severity of the disease. For episodic symptoms, oral or nasal H_1 antihistamines with oral or nasal decongestants if needed can be used. For seasonal or perennial rhinitis with mild symptoms, there is no significant difference between inhaled nasal corticosteroids (INCS), oral or nasal H_1 antihistamine, or LTRA and any of the three can be used. For moderate to severe symptoms, INCS are the first-line agents with an alternative of oral H_1 antihistamine plus LTRA for patients who do not tolerate the side effects of INCS or who do not want to use the drug. There is no difference in use of INCS alone or with the use of oral antihistamine plus INCS in children over 12 (Dykewicz et al., 2017). AIT can be administered subcutaneously or sublingually (limited to dust mite, northern grasses, and ragweed) in patients who do not respond well to pharmacotherapy or want AIT (Wheatley, Togias, 2015). Combination therapy can be offered if patients do not respond well to monotherapy (Seidman et al., 2015).

Pharmacologic Therapy. Pharmacologic therapy depends on the severity of the symptoms and the ability of the parent or child to comply with recommendations. INCS reduce inflammation, edema, and mucus production and are typically a key component in long-term therapy to manage symptoms associated with AR. Non-sedating antihistamines are frequently used to treat the symptoms of rhinorrhea, sneezing, and nasal and eye pruritus. Pharmacologic agents should be started 1 to 2 weeks before pollen season for children with seasonal AR. For perennial AR, start with the maximum recommended dose and then taper to the minimum dose needed to control symptoms. Often children with AR benefit from a combination approach; some require only single-line therapy. Antibiotics should only be prescribed for secondary infections (sinusitis).

Oral Antihistamines

- Oral antihistamines are divided into classes based on the four different types of histamine receptors, each with a varying ability to mediate an allergic response. H_1 and H_2 receptors are found in a variety of cells and cause the early and late phase of allergic response. H_3 and H_4 receptors cause pruritus as well as a proinflammatory immune response. Different classes of drugs may be more effective for different children (Table 33.11).
- Oral antihistamines are especially helpful in seasonal AR but do little to relieve nasal obstruction. Second-generation antihistamines are particularly effective in relieving symptoms of AR (nasal itching, sneezing, and rhinorrhea) by controlling the release of chemical mediators and are often used to manage this problem.
- Drug dosage may need to be increased until there is relief of symptoms or side effects are experienced.
- Tolerance to a particular antihistamine can develop necessitating the need to rotate drugs.
- If side effects with one antihistamine are experienced, prescribe another antihistamine in a different class or one in the same class but with different actions.
- Sedating antihistamines may interfere with daytime activities and negatively affect school performance; second-generation antihistamines (e.g., cetirizine, loratadine, and fexofenadine) are associated with less sedation effect.

TABLE 33.11 Antihistamine Classes

Class	Name	Comments
First-Generation Antihistamines		
Ethanolamine	Diphenhydramine	Sedation, dizziness, thickening of bronchial secretions
	Clemastine	Dry mouth, fatigue, headache, somnolence, bradycardia
	Carbinoxamine	Drowsiness, CNS excitation, and difficulty sleeping
Ethylenediamine	Pyrilamine	Not used in children
Alkylamines	Chlorpheniramine	Drowsiness, sedation, dry mouth, GI symptoms
	Brompheniramine	Palpitations, weight gain, drowsiness, dizziness, headache
Piperazine	Hydroxyzine	Sedation, dizziness, dry mouth
Piperidine	Cyproheptadine	CNS depression or stimulation, weight gain, dry mouth
Second-Generation Nonsedating H_1 Antihistamines		
Nonsedating antihistamines	Loratadine	Dry mouth, fatigue, headache, somnolence Approved for children ≥2 years old
	Cetirizine	Dry mouth, fatigue, headache, somnolence Approved for children ≥6 months
	Fexofenadine	Dry mouth, fatigue, headache, somnolence, dysmenorrhea, flulike signs Approved for children ≥6 months for chronic urticaria and ≥2 years for allergic rhinitis

CNS, Central nervous system; *GI,* gastrointestinal.

Topical Nasal Antihistamines

- Azelastine is a nasal antihistamine spray approved for use in seasonal AR in children ≥6 months of age. Azelastine acts by competing with histamine for H_1-receptor sites; it has a bitter taste and is associated with sedation. It is available as a combination with fluticasone propionate and approved for children over 12 years.
- Olopatadine is a nasal spray approved for use in children ≥6 years of age. Like nasal azelastine, it is effective in reducing itching, sneezing, rhinorrhea, and congestion (Fitzsimons et al., 2015).

Decongestants

- Decongestants may help relieve nasal congestion; there is no evidence supporting the use of oral phenylephrine as a decongestant (Weinberger and Hendeles, 2018).

TABLE 33.12 Intranasal Corticosteroid Preparations Used for Allergic Rhinitis: Usual Dosages

Drug	Dosage	Age, Number of Inhalations or Sprays per Nostril and Daily Frequency
Beclomethasone, aerosol solution	80 mcg/actuation	≥12 years old: 320 mcg once daily (160 mcg/nostril or 2 sprays each nostril of 80 mcg)
Beclomethasone AQ, aqueous suspension	42 mcg/spray	≥6-12 years old: Initial, 1-spray/nostril (42 mcg/inhalation) twice a day (total single dose of 84 mcg); increase to 2 sprays/nostril (two 42 mcg inhalations) twice a day (total single dose of 168 mcg) if needed; decreases to 42 mcg (1 spray) each nostril twice a day with control ≥12 years old: 84 mcg (1 spray/nostril) or 168 mcg (2 sprays/nostril) twice a day
Budesonide[a]	32 mcg/actuation	≥6 years old: Initial, 1 spray/nostril once daily (64 mcg total dose) Maximum dose: <12 years old, 2 sprays/nostril once a day (daily maximum dose of 128 mcg) ≥12 years old: 4 sprays/nostril once a day (daily maximum dose of 256 mcg)
Flunisolide	25 mcg/actuation	6-14 years old: Initial, 2 spray/nostril twice daily (100 mcg twice a day), or 1 spray/nostril three times a day (50 mcg three times a day) to a maximum of 4 sprays/nostril daily (200 mcg/day); maintenance dose is 1 spray/nostril daily 15 years old: 2 sprays/nostril twice a day (total single dose of 100 mcg) to 2 sprays/nostril three times/day (total single dose of 100 mcg); max daily dose of 400 mcg); maintenance 1 spray/nostril daily
Fluticasone propionate (Flonase)	50 mcg/actuation	≥4 years old and adolescents: Initial 1 spray/nostril daily; 2 sprays daily if severe or poor response; reduce to 1 spray/nostril/day once symptoms controlled Adult: 2 sprays/nostril daily or 1 spray/nostril twice daily; may reduce to 1 spray/nostril daily once symptoms controlled
Fluticasone furoate (Veramyst)	27.5 mcg/spray	2-11 years old: Initial, 1 spray/nostril once a day (total dose of 55 mcg/day), increase to 2 sprays/nostril once a day (total 110 mcg/day); reduce to 1 spray/nostril a day with control ≥12 years old and adolescents: 2 sprays/nostril daily (110 mcg/day); reduce to 1 spray/nostril once daily (total 55 mcg/day)
Mometasone	50 mcg/actuation	2-11 years old: 1 spray (50 mcg)/nostril daily >12 years old: 2 sprays (100 mcg)/nostril daily
Triamcinolone (Nasacort AQ)	55 mcg/spray	2-5 years old: 1 spray (55 mcg)/nostril once daily 6-11 years old: Initial, 1 spray (55 mcg)/nostril once daily, can increase to 2 sprays (110 mcg)/nostril once daily; maintenance 1 spray (55 mcg)/nostril with control >12 years old: 2 sprays (110 mcg)/nostril daily; maintenance dose 1 (55 mcg) spray/nostril daily

[a]Reduce slowly every 2-4 weeks to smallest effective dose.

Data from Taketomo CK, Hodding JH, Kraus DM. *Pediatric Dosage Handbook*. 24th ed. Hudson, OH: Lexi-Comp; 2019.

- Topical decongestants can cause rebound rhinorrhea (rhinitis medicamentosa) if used for more than 3 to 5 days; errors in administration can cause systemic absorption and side effects of irritability, nervousness, and insomnia among others.
- Children younger than 4 years old should not be given decongestants.

Nasal Cromolyn

- Cromolyn is an intranasal mast cell stabilizer used for seasonal or perennial AR. It is less effective than INCS, and frequent dosing is needed. It is safe for children 2 years and older.

Intranasal Corticosteroids

- These agents are effective in reducing local cytokines and mediator release factors produced by mast cells, basophils, eosinophils, monocytes, and macrophages that lead to inflammation and subsequent nasal obstruction (Dykewicz et al., 2017). INCS are considered one of the most effective treatments to manage AR and have been safely used in long-term management of AR to relieve symptoms of nasal congestion, rhinorrhea, itching, and sneezing.
- Clear the child's nasal passages of mucus before use. Table 33.12 lists usual dosages per nostril for INCS.

- INCS can take up to 4 weeks before clinical benefit is observed (Kaur and Singh). Side effects include local burning, irritation, sneezing, or soreness (<10% experience these symptoms). Epistaxis is related to improper technique—spraying the nasal septum.

Leukotriene Modifiers

- Montelukast is the only approved LTRA for use in seasonal and perennial AR. It is approved from 6 months to 5 years at a 4 mg packet (granules) once daily. It has a moderate effect when used alone. If patient has AR, administer dose in morning or evening; if patient also has asthma, give dose in evening. Guidelines suggest the use of INCS for AR as LTRA are not as effective as nasal steroids (Dykewicz et al., 2017).

Allergy Immunotherapy and Other Treatments

AIT includes subcutaneous immunotherapy (SCIT), oral immunotherapy (OIT), epicutaneous immunotherapy (EPIT), and sublingual immunotherapy (SLIT). There are limitations to SLIT as only three sublingual tablets are presently U.S. Food and Drug Administration (FDA) approved for use—ragweed, northern pasture grasses like timothy, and dust mites' tablets with clinical trials for peanut allergy ongoing. OIT has the highest rate of allergic side effects. EPIT for peanut and milk allergy is still in the research phase.

AIT is a treatment option for allergic disease including food allergy. In patients with life-threatening reactions to foods or severe allergic asthma, treatment with AIT may negate the need for epinephrine and improve the quality of life for these patients (Burks, Sampson, Plaut, et al., 2018). There is low evidence that SCIT improves medication use, FEV_1, or quality of life (Rice et al., 2018); however, there is moderate-strength evidence that SCIT reduces allergic asthma. The goal of AIT is to induce immune tolerance and cause a change in the immune response to specific antigens and also produce longer-lasting benefits without the need for daily medication. The mechanism of action for immunotherapy is centered on modulating the immune response, changing IgE that is allergen specific to IgG4, and to decrease basophil action to allergen cross-linking, causing an increase in regulatory T cells (Burks et al., 2018).

Desensitization occurs after months of AIT. EPIT involves putting a small allergen patch to the back or upper arm with daily changes. It is well tolerated but is in early study at this time. OIT has demonstrated the best results in terms of sustained lack of reaction to food allergens. Present thinking is that some level of allergen exposure is necessary to continue the lowered levels of IgE-specific antibody. Its side effect profile is greater. AIT can induce adverse reactions that can be local, such as tingling following sublingual therapy, to systemic reactions that are life-threatening (Burks et al., 2018). The majority of the reactions occur within 30 minutes; therefore, the child should be monitored for 30 minutes afterward. AIT should be conducted in a facility that has both the necessary equipment and healthcare professionals prepared to treat anaphylaxis.

Studies investigating the use of omalizumab in patients older than 12 years old with inadequately controlled and significant AR noted significant symptom relief and improved quality of life (Dykewicz et al., 2017). Occurrences of adverse reactions were not statistically significant.

Avoidance Strategies. Determine triggering factors if possible and educate the family on the need to avoid exposure to the offending allergen or irritant as much as possible. Allergens causing seasonal rhinitis are more difficult to avoid than are the indoor allergens, such as molds, because pollens are smaller and lighter and thus remain in the air longer. Key avoidance measures for indoor allergens and irritants include the following:

- Control house dust, paying special attention to the child's bedroom.
  - Use dust mite–proof mattress and pillow covers (allergen-impermeable encasement).
  - Wash bed linens in hot water (>130°F [54.4°C]) weekly.
  - Minimize (if possible, eliminate) stuffed toys in child's bedroom.
  - Use vertical blinds instead of horizontal blinds or curtains.
  - Remove carpeting from bedroom.
  - Use plastic or wood furniture instead of cloth or upholstered furniture.
- Eliminate smoking from the child's environment; if household members still smoke despite education, emphasize smoking outside the house and never in the car.
- Consider hairless pets; pet hair collects urine, dander, and saliva; the protein in pet saliva causes the reactivity.
- Reduce mold; avoid damp basements and other sources of moisture in the home environment.
- Indoor humidity should be less than 50%; avoid vaporizers.

- Use dehumidifiers, air conditioners with efficient filters, and air-cleaning devices with an electronic precipitator or with a high-efficiency particulate air (HEPA) filter.
- Eliminate any offending substances; vector control for cockroach elimination.

Complications and Prognosis

Sinusitis may complicate AR due to secondary bacterial infection of the swollen sinus mucosal linings. The AAP guidelines on sinusitis and the AAAI do not advise imaging for confirmation of sinusitis (choosingwisely.org). Likewise, eustachian tube dysfunction and its sequel, serous otitis media, are common complications. Malocclusion, the development of a high-arched palate, and the typical allergic facies can result from long-standing AR. Chronic AR may lead to chronic cough and postnasal drip. If a child has both AR and asthma, treatment of the child's AR is essential if the asthma is to be effectively managed.

Perennial AR can be a chronic problem unless offending allergens are identified and eliminated from the environment. If this is not possible, pharmacologic therapy is usually helpful in reducing symptoms. As the child grows and nasal passages increase in size, symptoms may also lessen. Symptoms from seasonal AR often worsen from the adolescent years to mid-adulthood. Moving to a new environment often results in a short respite (1 to 3 years) from symptoms; however, the child frequently becomes sensitized to new airborne pollens and symptoms of seasonal AR return.

Patient and Parent Education and Prevention

Because AR is often a chronic problem, parents and children need to have specific information about controlling this disorder:

- Instruct on environmental control. Handouts and individualization of information are essential.
- Review pharmacologic therapy, including indications for and changes in medications, frequency of use, and common side effects and contraindications.
- Demonstrate, with return demonstration, how to use intranasal sprays or inhalers if prescribed.

Atopic Dermatitis

AD is a common chronic, pruritic, inflammatory skin disorder of childhood characterized by acute and chronic skin eruptions. The term *atopic eczema* is used interchangeably with *atopic dermatitis*. It is a complex disorder caused by the interaction of genetic susceptibility and micro- and macroenvironment, leading to tissue inflammation in the host (Ong, 2018). AD manifests a typical morphology and distribution of flexural lichenification or linearity along with acral or hand and feet distribution in adolescents and adults. In school-age children, antecubital and popliteal fossa are common places for AD; in infants, there is facial and extensor involvement. Food allergies are common with children with AD, but this does not mean there is a relationship between them. Certain foods may be a trigger or just a "fellow traveler" (Tom, 2017). Comorbid depression is common and was reported in 31.2% of adults with AD versus controls (17.3%). In general, there is a higher rate of neuropsychiatric disorders including depression, suicidal ideation, anxiety, and ADHD (Eckert et al., 2017). There is higher healthcare utilization because the itch associated with AD is severe and in some cases unbearable (Eichenfield and Gold, 2017a).

AD is frequently referred to as the "itch that rashes." With AD, the skin's ability to act as a protective barrier is impaired, resulting

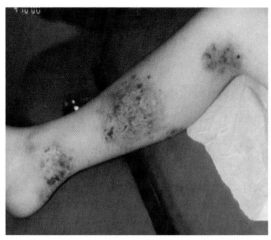

• **Fig 33.8** Acute Atopic Dermatitis. (Photograph courtesy Peggy Vernon RN, MA, CPNP, DCNP, FAANP, Creekside Skin Care, Centennial, CO.)

in xerosis (dry skin), cracking, increased skin markings, lichenification, and susceptibility to bacterial, viral, and fungal infections (Fig 33.8). Recent studies indicate the need for prevention and the use of daily moisturizer barrier therapy starting in the neonatal period to prevent the onset of AD. The prevention of AD may alter the association between early AD and other allergic manifestations such as allergic asthma and food allergy (Lowe, 2018).

The American Academy of Dermatology (Eichenfield et al., 2014) and the AAP (Tollefson et al., 2014) have published AD guidelines. There are definite similarities between their guidelines, with variations in recommendations about the frequency and length of certain treatment, such as bleach baths and skin therapy maintenance. Moisturization and topical agents are the mainstay addressed in both guidelines.

AD affects approximately 13% of the U.S. childhood population (National Eczema Association), with an increase of 5% from 1997 to 2011 (Eichenfield, 2015). AD develops before the age of 5 years in 95% of cases. There is no test to determine the diagnosis, but a history of a highly pruritic, relapsing dermatitis with erythematous papules and patches and periods of exacerbations provides the necessary information for a diagnosis of AD (Eichenfield, 2015). There is disruption in sleep and quality of life suffers (Pustisek, Vurnek, Zivkovic, and Situm, 2016). Children with mild to moderate disease can be managed by PCPs, with severe cases needing referral.

The exact etiology is unknown and may vary from individual to individual. Although many children have high IgE levels, an exact immune mechanism for this disorder is not evident. Studies investigating the pathophysiology of AD point to multifactorial interactions between environmental risk factors, immune deviation, and impaired barrier function. It is a heterogeneous disease with multiple inflammatory pathways. The identification of the filaggrin (FLG) mutation that results in loss of skin function is the strongest risk factor for AD; however, it is only present in a small number of patients (Brunner, Leung, Guttman-Yassky, 2018). The FLG is produced in the stratum granulosum and contributes to the natural moisture in the stratum corneum as well as corneum hydration and dysregulation of type 1 interferon (INF)-mediated stress response (Brunner et al., 2018). There is an impairment in the innate immune response in the skin causing increased colonization of microbes; therefore, the child is prone to recurrent skin infection. AD is a T-cell-driven disease with elevated levels of IL-4 and IL-13, causing IgE elevations. Abnormalities in histamine

production (increased in the skin), chemotaxis, monocytes, and cytokines are associated with AD. There is also a decrease in ceramides, reducing the water capacity of the skin leading to more water loss (Lyons et al., 2015). Factors that aggravate this condition include harsh soaps, heat, sweating, infections, stress, food allergies, and dry skin (Sayseng and Vernon, 2018).

A positive family history of AD is common, as is a family history of atopic disease. Sweating increases itching in atopic skin, and transepidermal water loss is increased. A predisposition to the development of pruritus is believed to be a key factor with variability in the extent of the skin involvement and severity of presentation. Pruritus and relapsing eczematous lesions in the typical morphology are essential features in making the diagnosis (Sayaseng and Vernon, 2018).

Clinical Findings

The following are seen in AD (Lyons, Milner, and Stone, 2015) (Table 33.13):

- Pruritus and eczematous changes reflecting typical age-specific morphologic patterns
- History of a chronic or relapsing skin condition
- More than one-third of cases begin before 3 months old; dry skin is the only initial sign. These infants are generally not brought in for healthcare until pruritus and the itch-scratch-itch cycle develops, generally around 2 to 3 months old.
- Pityriasis alba, cheilitis, perifollicular accentuation
- Acute manifestations (more common in infants) include:
  - Intense itching and redness
  - Papules, vesicles, edema, serous discharge, and crusts
  - Generalized dry skin (xerosis) with dry hair and scalp; diaper area usually spared
  - Lichenification is typically not seen
- Chronic manifestations (more common in children and adolescents) include:
  - Lichenification—thickened, leathery, hyperpigmented skin; scratch marks
  - Generalized xerosis with flaky and rough skin: Table 33.13 lists characteristics of AD at different ages.
- Other key features of AD:
  - Tendency to dry skin and a lowered threshold for itching (itch-scratch-itch cycle)
  - Tendency to worsen during dry winter months or with heat in the summer
  - Sweating increases pruritus
  - Chronic AD often secondarily infected with *Staphylococcus aureus* (most commonly) or *Streptococcus pyogenes* (occasionally)
  - Secondarily infection of AD with herpes simplex is called eczema herpeticum and is a dermatological emergency requiring antiviral treatment with Acyclovir or Valacyclovir (depending on age).
  - Hyperpigmentation may be noted especially in areas of lichenification
- Possible associated features:
  - Atopic pleats—extra groove in lower eyelid called *Dennie lines* or *Morgan fold* (see Fig 33.7), crease across upper bulb of nose
  - Accentuated palmar and flexural creases; keratoconus
  - Allergic shiners, mild facial pallor, or dry hair
  - Keratosis pilaris—follicular papules occurring on the extensor aspect of the arms, anterior thighs, and lateral aspects of the cheeks

TABLE 33.13   Assessment of Atopic Dermatitis

Onset/Initial Presentation	Signs and Symptoms	Comment/Prognosis
<3 months old	Dry skin first sign	Often not noticed
2-3 months old	Itch-scratch-itch cycle starts	
Infantile phase	Acute presentation—common in infants: intense itching; redness, papules, vesicles, edema; serous discharge and crusts Cheeks, forehead, scalp, extending to trunk as symmetric patches or to the extremities; lateral extensor surface of arms and legs; diaper area and groin are spared of lesion	Two-thirds of cases resolve by 2-3 years Generalized xerosis
Childhood phase (starts 2 years old to puberty)	Pruritus is severe Lesions are dry and papular with circumscribed scaly patches Involves wrists, hands, popliteal and antecubital fossa; eyebrows thin and broken off with lack of the lateral third of the eyebrow (called *Hertoghe sign*); some only have feet involved; may have allergic-atopic facies and white dermatographism Flexural involvement	One-third continue into teenage years—tendency to be chronic
Adolescent/adult phase	Begins at puberty and can commonly continue into adulthood Often involves the flexural folds (popliteal and antecubital fossae), face, neck, upper arms and back, dorsa of hands, fingers, feet, and toes Dry skin and lichenification are prominent findings Erythematous, dry-scaling papules and plaques with fewer exudates Postinflammatory hypopigmentation or hyperpigmentation that disappears	New or recurrence of a chronic condition

- Nummular eczema, dyshidrotic eczema, juvenile plantar dermatitis, nipple eczema, or ichthyosis vulgaris
- White dermatographism; some have an associated circumoral pallor (thought to be related to local edema and vasoconstriction)

Diagnostic Studies. The diagnosis of AD is based on characteristic clinical findings. A chronic or recurring rash that is pruritic and has a characteristic distribution and appearance, together with a family or personal history of atopy, are key to the diagnosis. Histologic examination of the skin is rarely needed and reserved only for difficult-to-diagnose cases and to exclude other diseases. Skin testing and desensitization are not routinely recommended for children with AD only. If secondary fungal infection is suspected, collect scrapings and use potassium hydroxide (KOH) to look for fungal hyphae.

Differential Diagnosis

Other types of dermatitis, including seborrheic dermatitis, drug reaction, nutritional deficiencies of zinc/biotin, acrodermatitis enteropathica, ichthyosis vulgaris, contact dermatitis, allergic contact dermatitis, nummular dermatitis, psoriasis, and scabies are included in the differential diagnosis. A few genetic conditions are associated with similar skin eruptions (e.g., phenylketonuria, Wiskott-Aldrich syndrome, histiocytosis X, and acrodermatitis enteropathica) as well as primary immunodeficiency diseases, cutaneous T-cell lymphoma, lymphocytic-variant hypereosinophilia syndrome (HES) (Lyons et al., 2015).

Management

Treatment strategy is based on the following key concepts:
- The itch-scratch-itch cycle must be interrupted.
- Dryness of the skin must be corrected by rehydrating the stratum corneum with lubrication as the first-line therapy to enhance skin moisturization. The choice of the moisturizer is dependent on the individual, but should be safe, free of additives, and inexpensive. Application of moisturizer should take place soon after bath to decrease transepidermal water loss.

Start skin barrier protection at birth as it may be protective against the development of AD.
- If moisturization does not control the disease, then topical corticosteroids (TCPs) are used with low-potency corticosteroids for maintenance and higher potency for exacerbations (Lyons et al., 2015).
- Use of non-soap surfactants and synthetic detergents, which are more acid, are often recommended but without good supporting evidence.
- Eliminate any known offending agents (irritants and allergic triggers).
- Secondary bacterial or viral infections must be treated.

Acute versus chronic care management is also a consideration. The following therapies are key factors in the control of AD.

Pharmacotherapy

- Antihistamine agents have little direct effect on pruritus, but sedating doses at night help relieve pruritus, which is worse at night. They have limited effectiveness as monotherapy in AD. The following agents are often used:
  - Hydroxyzine has excellent antihistaminic qualities but can cause drowsiness and behavioral changes. If an antihistamine is needed throughout the day, the usual oral dose of hydroxyzine in children (≤40 kg) is a maximum 2 mg/kg/day divided every 6 to 8 hours with some experts recommending lower daily doses (Taketomo et al., 2018).
  - Diphenhydramine hydrochloride is also a useful antihistamine, especially if sedation is also needed. The usual oral dose of diphenhydramine hydrochloride in children is 5mg/kg/day divided into 3-4 doses with a maximum of 300 mg daily or a fixed dose of 12.5-25 mg/dose 3 to 4 times daily (Taketomo et al., 2019).
  - Doxepin is a tricyclic antidepressant with strong antihistamine activity used by dermatologists to treat itching. It is not approved for use in children under 12, and the risk of suicidal ideation should be assessed if a child receives this drug.

- Nonsedating or low-sedating antihistamines may be considered (see Table 33.11).
- Topical antihistamines are not recommended.
- TCPs are a mainstay of therapy:
  - TCPs reduce inflammation and pruritus. The classification of the TCP should be known because potent and very potent TCPs are associated with more side effects (e.g., thinning of skin, striae, telangiectasia, generalized hypertrichosis, or adrenal axis suppression) than milder preparations. Most children with AD are controlled with twice-daily application for two weeks then doing twice-weekly application of a low-dose TCP for up to 4 months once the lesions are quiet. The rationale for this approach is that the child's skin is not normal and has a defect in hydration, which can be treated using an intermittent approach (Eichenfield, Ahluwalia, et al., 2017b).
  - Ointment preparations are generally stronger than all other types of preparations.
  - Gels penetrate well and are somewhat more drying so are effective in the management of acute weeping or vesicular lesions.
  - Ointments penetrate more effectively than creams or lotions and provide occlusion. They are beneficial in the management of dry, lichenified, or plaque-like areas but may occlude eccrine ducts and lead to sweating.
  - Application
    - Fingertip method: The amount of steroid to be applied should be a strip of cream from the distal interphalangeal joint to the top of the adult finger for an area equaling two adult palms. Apply a thin layer of TCP to affected areas marked with acute exacerbations twice a day or once a day if using a newer formulation (Eichenfield et al., 2014).
    - When applied over large areas of dermatitis or if occlusion (covering with plastic wrap) is used, the possibility of significant systemic absorption is greatly increased, especially in infants and young children.
  - There are seven classes of steroid with class 1 being very high potency to class 7 being the lowest potency. Greater caution is needed when applying steroids to the face, neck, and skin folds because the skin is thinner and there is higher risk of systemic absorption. Tapering of the strength of the steroids should occur only once the outbreak is fully controlled. The child is then switched to twice-weekly application of a low-dose TCS at areas of outbreak to reduce the relapse. Baseline moisturizing skin care should continue with a low-strength TCS once to twice a week to reduce inflammation (Eichenfield et al., 2014). (See Table 34.1 for a listing of TCPs by potency rating.)
- Phosphodiesterase (PDE)-4 inhibitors (Gold and Eichenfield, 2017)
  - Acts as a mediator in the conversion of cyclic adenosine monophosphate (cAMP) into AMP. In patients with AD, low cAMP levels and high PDE activity causes inflammatory hyperreactivity.
  - Crisaborole (Eucrisa), a topical PDE-4 inhibitor, is an alternative choice in mild to moderate disease.
  - Common adverse events include burning and stinging or worsening of AD.
- Topical calcineurin inhibitors (TCIs; Eichenfield, Ahluwalia, et al., 2017b; Taketomo et al., 2018)
  - TCIs are second-line therapy that is useful in both acute and chronic AD. Two agents are available—tacrolimus topical (Protopic) ointment 0.03% and 0.1% strengths and pimecrolimus topical (Elidel) 1% cream—and have been shown to be as effective as mid-strength TCS. They can be combined with TCS in the treatment of children whose AD has not responded to TCS. They are considered steroid-sparing agents. Tacrolimus 0.03% and pimecrolimus 1% are approved for use in children ≥2 yrs, whereas tacrolimus 0.1% is approved in children ≥16.
  - TCIs have black box warnings due to the higher rate of lymphoma in rats given high dosages of these drugs. These NSAIDs block calcineurin, a protein phosphatase that causes T-cell activation. Most common side effects are itching, stinging, or burning, which starts 5 minutes after the application and can last for an hour but usually decreases after 1 week. It usually occurs during the first several days of administration and in severe cases of AD. TCIs are safe steroid-sparing agents and work well on thinner skin of the face, neck, groin, and axillae. Sun protection is needed with their use.
  - Parents need to be informed of the black box warning and the pros and cons of their use should be discussed. There is an increased theoretical risk of cutaneous viral infections with the use of TCIs.
- Prescription emollient devices
  - Skin barrier repair and treatment: Drugs (i.e., EpiCeram and Eletone) that improve the skin's hydration barrier are available by prescription and are used twice a day. The preparations have unique ratios of lipids that resemble endogenous compositions. They are expensive and not covered by all insurance plans.
- Cool coal tar
  - Although these agents have been used in psoriasis, there are few studies in children with newer agents that are more cosmetically acceptable. The AD guidelines do not recommend their use.
- Wet wrap therapy (WWT)
  - WWT can be used in significant flares with recalcitrant disease. The usual topical agents are applied followed by a wet layer of tubular gauze or cotton pajama that is applied with a dry outside layer. The child sleeps overnight with the WWT (Eichenfield et al., 2014; Schneider et al., 2013).
- Topical antimicrobials and antiseptics
  - The immune dysregulation in AD results in a tendency for *S. aureus* to colonize the skin in AD, as well as viral infection, including herpes simplex. Reduction of colonization with staphylococcus, as well as treatment of infection, may be equally as important. The use of bleach baths in conjunction with intranasal topical mupirocin for 3 months may be helpful. Schneider and colleagues (2013) recommend dilute bleach baths (⅛ to ¼ cup of chlorine bleach in a full tub of bath water) twice a week in children with recurrent infection.
  - Topical antibiotic preparations are contraindicated, although the use of mupirocin does reduce colony counts of *S. aureus.*
  - Topical antibacterial scrubs are contraindicated because they dry out the skin and cause irritation.
- Oral antibiotics
  - Short courses of systemic antibiotic agents are essential if secondary skin infection with *S. aureus* or *S. pyogenes* is suspected. First-generation cephalosporins are most commonly used.

- Be cognizant that the incidence of community-based methicillin-resistant *Staphylococcus aureus* (MRSA) has rapidly increased.
- Systemic immunomodulating agents
  - Immunomodulating agents (such as cyclosporine, azathioprine, mycophenolate mofetil [MMF], and systemic corticosteroids) can provide help to patients with severe, refractory AD; due to side effect profiles, they should only be used by a specialist after all other options failed.
  - Use of biologics is still in research phase in children but is being explored for use in the patient with inadequately controlled AD (Eichenfield and Gold, 2017c).
  - Dupilumab, which targets IL-4 and IL-13, is a targeted biologic approved for adults.

Non-Pharmacological Therapy
- Skin lubrication
  - Emolliate with a moisturizer. Lubricants maintain the skin's hydration, and emollients are the treatment of choice for dry skin.
  - An ointment-based emollient (e.g., Vaseline, petrolatum jelly, vegetable oil, whipped petrolatum, Aquaphor) can be applied just before or just after getting out of bath water while still damp. If the child does not like the greasy feel of an ointment, other topical creams (e.g., Vanicream, CeraVe, Cetaphil) can be used. This is also a good time to apply TCPs, because absorption of the agent is more effective if the skin is hydrated.
  - Emollients can be applied three or four times a day as needed, such as fragrance-free Eucerin cream, Aveeno, Moisturel, Neutrogena, Dermasil, Curel, or petroleum jelly (an occlusive agent). If a child is sensitive to fragrances, scented creams, such as Nivea and Vaseline Intensive Care, should be avoided. TriCeram is a moisturizer that repairs the stratum corneum barrier function. Like CeraVe, it is a ceramide-dominant, lipid-based emollient. Avoiding products with lanolin and clothing made of wool can be helpful. Urea-containing products, such as Aquacare cream or lotion and Ureacin Crème, soften and moisturize dry skin. Stinging is a side effect when using urea-containing products on fissured or flaring skin.
  - Bathing in lukewarm but not hot water for hydration followed by applying the moisturizer is recommended by the National Institute of Allergy and Infectious Disease. An eczema management plan is available from the American Academy of Dermatology and American Academy of Allergy, Asthma, and Immunology. If a child experiences stinging when bathing during acute exacerbations, adding 1 cup of table salt into the bath may reduce the stinging sensation.
- Avoidance of triggering factors
  - Avoid common irritating substances, including toiletries, wool, and harsh chemicals.
  - Keep fingernails short to decrease additional skin trauma from scratching.
  - Consider stopping the use of fabric softeners and using a sensitive-skin detergent (e.g., All Free and Clear).
  - Evaluate for possible food triggers; if history is positive, testing is not needed (Burke et al., 2018). PCPs should *not* do an extensive battery of allergy tests or make recommendations for food elimination based on those tests without a history of food sensitivity.

Other Therapies
- Phototherapy: Ultraviolet narrow-band UVB light treatment may benefit and should only be done by dermatologists; it is rarely used because of the risk of skin cancer.

Environmental Management
- Decreased environmental humidity and an increase in antigen presentation are key causative factors. Therefore, increase environmental humidity and decrease exposure to antigens. Cool temperatures (e.g., through the use of air conditioning) help.
- Eliminate or avoid known or suspected offending agents. These include:
  - Non-breathable fabrics—nylon or wool; wool is irritating, whereas soft cotton clothing is not. Clothes should be loose fitting.
  - Overheating and overdressing (heat and perspiration are irritant triggers that increase pruritus).
  - Chlorine, turpentine, harsh soaps, fabric softeners, products with fragrances, and bleach.
  - Allergenic agents, such as feather pillows, fuzzy toys, stuffed animals, and pets.
  - House-dust mites—careful attention to the child's bedroom is important (e.g., encasing mattresses and pillows, washing bedding in hot water weekly, frequent vacuuming, removing carpets or at least frequent cleaning are recommended).

Dietary Management
- In infants, whey-protein partially hydrolyzed infant formula is not hypoallergenic and should not be given to infants who have milk allergy. Dietary restriction should only be done on the basis of a history of food allergy. Food allergens in older children and adults are not common triggers.
- The use of probiotics is recommended (Eichenfield et al., 2014).

Most children with AD can be successfully treated by PCPs. Children who are unresponsive to traditional therapy or have an unusual manifestation should be referred to a pediatric dermatologist.

Complications and Prognosis

Secondary skin infections are a frequent complication of AD due to *S. aureus*, viruses (eczema herpeticum or disseminated herpes simplex), and fungi (culture or KOH to diagnose). Lichenification, a secondary skin change marked by thickening of the skin, is associated with chronic itching. Keratoconus is occasionally seen and is associated with chronic rubbing of the eyelids. In patients with AD, nocturnal melatonin levels are lower and may be responsible for sleep disturbances (Chang et al., 2014). With appropriate treatment, AD can generally be controlled. In two-thirds of children, symptoms of AD become less severe, with complete remission in 20%; however, there is an adolescent and adult stage of AD. Self-image problems may result if AD is severe.

Patient and Parent Education and Prevention
- Emphasize that AD is often a recurrent disease that can be controlled. The goal of therapy is to prevent the itch-scratch-itch cycle and hydrate the skin. Specific written instructions and handouts should include the following as home management is complex. An action plan for eczema is available (see resources) and can aid the provider in teaching family and child about managing the child's AD. They need to understand:
  - The use of medications (when, how much, and how often to use; side effects; and proper application of topical preparations)
  - Care of the skin

- Role of environmental controls of allergens or triggers
- What to do if symptoms worsen or signs of secondary skin infection appear and when to seek additional medical treatment
- The need to avoid precipitating factors such as extreme temperatures or humidity, excess sweat, and/or emotional stress; new clothes—wash with mild detergent (with no dyes or perfumes) before wearing them to remove formaldehyde and other chemicals, harsh washing detergents—add second rinse cycle when washing clothes, wearing coarse clothes; excess soap and water, and cutaneous or systemic infection

Rheumatologic Disorders

Juvenile Idiopathic Arthritis

JIA, formerly known as juvenile rheumatoid arthritis, is the term now used to reflect the unknown cause of this condition. The estimated prevalence is 14/100,000 children (Shenoi, 2017). The diagnosis of JIA requires persistent arthritis for more than 6 weeks in a child younger than 16 years old; Table 33.14 describes the current JIA classification system by subtypes. Experts are discussing whether to group arthritis across the life span into four categories—seronegative, seropositive, systemic, and spondyloarthritis because of the similarities of human leukocytic antigen (HLA) typing and non-HLA typing associated with the risk of a variety of arthritis presentations as well as the risk of other autoimmune diseases (Nigrovic, Raychauduri, and Thompson, 2018). There may be changes based on genetics in the future.

The underlying cause of most forms of JIA is unclear; however, it is likely environmentally induced in genetically predisposed individuals (Wu, Bryan, and Rabinovich, 2016). HLA class I and II alleles have been associated with JIA (Nigrovic et al., 2018). T lymphocytes play an important role by releasing proinflammatory cytokines that cause a shift in type 1 helper T lymphocyte

response. This T lymphocyte response promotes complement activation, immune complex formation, and B cell along with synovial non-self-antigen activation. Inflammatory synovitis results with subsequent destruction of cartilage and bone (Wu et al., 2016). JIA is a complex genetic trait in which multiple genes affect disease susceptibility.

Variation of the MHC class I and class II as well as non-HLA candidates are associated with different subtypes. Environmental triggers including viruses, bacterial infection, abnormal reproductive hormones, and trauma to joint can result in an uncontrolled adaptive and innate response toward the self-antigen that activates the autoimmune reaction (Wu et. al, 2016). In contrast, systemic juvenile idiopathic arthritis (SJIA), which has no HLA gene association, is the result of an autoinflammatory response from the innate immune system, especially cytokines IL-1, IL-6, and IL-18 (Cimaz, 2016). The term autoinflammatory disease explains the difference in its pathophysiology versus other forms of JIA. The activation of aberrant phagocytes leads to the production of inflammatory cytokines as well as other inflammatory proteins (S100 A12, S100 A9, and S100 A8). The use of classifying biomarker MRP8/14, S100a12 and IL-18 enables confirmation of disease activity when the child is symptomatic; subclinical disease activity can be evaluated with the same markers (Swart, De Roock, and Prakken, 2016). This disease responds to IL-receptor antagonist Anakinra. The difference in the pathogenic processes may explain the variances in the clinical presentation of the disease.

JIA is considered an autoimmune disease with alterations in both humeral and cell-mediated immunity. In the other types of JIA, aside from SJIA, the biomarkers used to classify the disease include ANA, acute-phase reactants, RF, anti-CCP, HLA-B27, and MRP8/14 (Swart et al., 2016). The humoral response is responsible for the release of autoantibodies (especially ANAs), an increase in serum immunoglobulins, and the formation of circulating immune complexes and complement activation. The cell-mediated reaction is associated with a T-lymphocyte response that

TABLE 33.14 Juvenile Idiopathic Arthritis Subtypes and Clinical Joint Characteristics

Oligoarticular

(Most common type)

Four or less joints with persistent disease never having more than four joints involved
May present with morning limp
Up to 70% of children have an ANA, a risk factor for uveitis
Two subtypes:
Persistent oligoarticular lasting > 6 months; affecting no more than 4 joints
Extended oligoarticular with ≥ four joints after first 6 months

Polyarticular

(Up to 30-35% with JIA have this type)

Arthritis in ≥ five or more joints during first 6 months of disease with acute or insidious onset
May develop rheumatoid vasculitis; resemble adults
Acute form of uveitis occurs
Features include slowing of growth, fatigue, a low-grade fever
Large or small joints involved; typically small joints of hands, feet, ankles, wrists, knees, and cervical spine
RF negative ANA positive, polyarticular JIA may be mistaken for extended oligoarticular disease
RF negative or positive, more common in females with approximately 70% of RF positive cases being females (10-12 years at onset)
Polyarticular (RF positive)
- RF positive tests 2-3 months apart
- Children likely between ages of 8 and 10 years
- Rapidly progressive arthritis with subcutaneous rheumatoid nodules
- Adolescent late-onset differs from those with early onset as positive RF and course is similar to adults

| TABLE 33.14 | Juvenile Idiopathic Arthritis Subtypes and Clinical Joint Characteristics—cont'd |

Systemic (sJIA)

Arthritis in >1 joint for 6 weeks and younger than 16
Fever of at least 2 weeks' duration and at least 3 days of daily fever with afternoon spikes up to 104°F-106°F (40°C-41.1°C)—a quotidian fever pattern
May have any of the following
- Fleeting salmon-color rash with fever; macules or papules increased in heat areas (axilla and groin)
- Hepatosplenomegaly, generalized lymphadenopathy, polyserositis manifesting as pericarditis or pleuritis
- High inflammatory markers, marked increase in serum ferritin
- RF and ANA rarely positive
- Usually significant anemia, thrombocytosis, increased acute-phase reactants, elevated transaminase levels
- Potentially fatal complication—MAS with high levels of ferritin above 5000
- Either polyarticular or oligoarticular disease

A child with chest pain, shortness of breath, change in vocal quality suggesting Cricoarytenoid arthritis, signs of MAS, or being treated with an immunosuppressive agent with signs of infection or on NSAIDs with melena and acute anemia will need admission.

Spondyloarthropathy

Enthesitis-related arthritis

Arthritis and enthesitis or Arthritis and enthesitis plus two of the following
- Sacroiliac joint involvement with either tenderness or inflammatory lumbosacral pain
- + HLA-B27
- Male >6 years old with arthritis
- Acute anterior uveitis

First-degree relative with IBS with sacroiliitis, ankylosing spondylitis, reactive arthritis, or acute anterior uveitis
Typically, arthritis of lower limbs, especially hips and intertarsal joints with later sacroiliac joints involvement
Swelling, tenderness, warmth at insertion of tendons, ligaments, or joint capsules
Risk of ankylosing spondylitis (10-15 years later)
Occurs in late childhood and adolescence
Acute symptomatic uveitis in about 7% of cases

Psoriatic Arthritis

Asymmetric or symmetric small or large joint arthritis with psoriasis or arthritis with two or more of the following: nail pitting or onycholysis, psoriasis in a first-degree relative, or dactylitis

Undifferentiated

Arthritis that fails to fulfill one category or fulfills two or more categories

ANA, Antinuclear antibody; *HLA,* human leukocytic antigen; *IBS,* inflammatory bowel syndrome; *JIA,* juvenile idiopathic arthritis; *MAS,* macrophage activation syndrome; *NSAIDs,* nonsteroidal anti-inflammatory drugs; *RF,* rheumatoid factor.

From Cimaz R. Systemic-onset idiopathic arthritis. Autoimmun Rev. 2016;14:931–934.; Shenoi S. Juvenile idiopathic arthritis—changing times, changing terms, changing treatments. *Pediatr Rev.* 2017;38(5):221–231; Siegel DM, Gewanter HL, Sahai S. Rheumatologic Diseases (Chapter 324). In: McInerny TM, Adam HM, Campbell DE, DeWitt TG, Foy JM, Kamat DM, ed. *American Academy of Pediatrics Textbook of Pediatric Care.* 2nd ed. American Academcy of Pediatrics; 2017.

plays a key role in cytokine production, resulting in the release of tumor necrosis factor-α (TNF-α), IL-1, and IL-6. Activation of B lymphocytes by T-helper cells produces autoantibodies that link to self-antigens. B lymphocytes infiltrate the synovium producing nonsuppurative chronic inflammation of the synovium that can lead to articular cartilage and joint structure erosion.

JIA presents unique challenges to the child, family, and the provider. Approximately 1 in 1000 children are affected with oligoarticular JIA, the most common arthritic subtype. Cytokine production, proliferation of macrophage-like synoviocytes, infiltration with neutrophils and T lymphocytes, and autoimmunity are thought to be the major pathologic processes causing chronic joint inflammation. Although JIA does affect joints, there are other systems that can be affected. Enthesitis is an inflammatory reaction at sites where tendons or ligaments insert into the bone and occurs with several types of JIA. Uveitis is also associated with JIA, is more common with a positive ANA, and can be asymptomatic. Jaw involvement can also be asymptomatic; therefore, measuring the mouth opening is key to identifying temporomandibular joint (TMJ) arthritis (Shenoi, 2017).

The rate of JIA is significantly higher in girls than in boys, typically in oligoarticular and pauciarticular JIA. The female to male ratio in systemic onset is equal. Oligoarticular JIA has a late or early onset, is the most common type, and typically has knee involvement. It presents with a morning limp and a positive ANA in 70% of cases. Polyarticular JIA can be RF positive or negative and peaks at ages 1 to 3 years and during adolescence. The systemic form of JIA occurs at any age and is more complex due to high fevers. It can present with macrophage activation syndrome (MAS) with persistent fevers, seizures and drowsiness, decreased white blood cells (WBCs) and platelet counts with ferritin levels of greater than 5000, and fixed rashes (Shenoi, 2017).

Clinical Findings

History. The major complaints in all forms of JIA are from the arthritis characterized by:
- Pain—generally a mild to moderate aching
- Joint stiffness—worse in the morning and after rest; arthralgia may occur during the day

- Joint effusion and warmth
- Younger children may be irritable or have behavioral regression
- Nonspecific symptoms include decreased appetite, myalgia, nighttime joint pain, inactivity, and failure to thrive

Systemic symptoms are found more commonly in systemic and polyarticular subtypes and include anemia, anorexia, fever, fatigue, lymphadenopathy, salmon-colored rash (sJIA), and weight loss. Growth abnormalities can result in localized growth disturbances, including premature fusion of the epiphyses, bony overgrowth (rheumatoid nodules), and limb-length discrepancies.

Physical Examination. The musculoskeletal exam is key. Examine all joints including the TMJ and areas where tendons or ligament insert into bones (e.g., Achilles tendon and knees, greater trochanter, metatarsal head and plantar fascia insertion on the feet). Observe for gait abnormalities using the pediatric Gait, Arms, Legs and Spine Screen (pGALS). Abnormal positioning on the exam table or difficulty getting on and off the table may be noted. Also do vision screening (see Chapter 43).

Key musculoskeletal findings include:
- Swelling of the joint with effusion or thickening of synovial membrane, or both, noted on palpation of the joint line
- Heat over inflamed joint and tenderness along joint line
- Loss of joint range of motion and function; holds affected joints in slight flexion; may walk with limp
  Other findings that may be noted:
- Nail pits or onycholysis
- Ciliary injection (note: presence of ciliary injection or an inability to see the optic disc on fundus exam may point to uveitis, which is usually asymptomatic)
- A fleeting salmon-color rash that is more prominent on the trunk

The classification of the types of arthritis and their characteristic findings are presented in Table 33.14.

Diagnostic Studies. JIA is a diagnosis of exclusion, based on physical findings, and watchful waiting is important as joint pain must be present for greater than 6 weeks. There is no one diagnostic laboratory test for JIA. Most children with oligoarticular arthritis have negative laboratory markers. Lyme disease must be ruled out as it can present in a similar fashion. Those with polyarticular and systemic-onset typically have elevated acute-phase reactants and anemia of chronic disease. A positive result for RF by latex fixation may be present, which occurs in less than 10% of children with JIA and rarely with sJIA. ANA may be present in up to 50% of children with oligoarticular disease; its presence helps identify children at higher risk for uveitis.

Initial laboratory testing includes a CBC (to exclude leukemia), ESR and CRP (acute-phase reactants), Lyme testing (enzyme-linked immunosorbent assay [ELISA] followed by Western blot), comprehensive metabolic profile, and liver function tests (creatine phosphokinase, aldolase, and LDH). Urine analysis and antistreptolysin O (ASO) and anti-DNase B, and complements may be added depending on presenting complaints (see Table 33.1 for a description of these tests). Results may reveal lymphopenia, anemia, elevated transaminases, and hypoalbuminemia; however, laboratory studies may be normal in some children with suspicious findings requiring second-line testing.

Although anti-CCP antibody testing has a high specificity and is more likely to identify children who have more severe JIA with irreversible joint damage, its sensitivity is low (i.e., a negative result does not exclude disease). Therefore, it is not a routine first-line test as only children with RA factor positive JIA will have anti-CCP antibodies (Sahai et al., 2016). Imaging studies including

x-ray and MRI can help in managing joint pathology. Analysis of synovial fluid is not helpful in diagnosing JIA.

Differential Diagnosis

Various causes of monoarticular arthritis are included in the differential diagnosis. Lyme disease must be excluded as it can present in a similar fashion. Lyme disease and post-infectious conditions, such as post-streptococcal arthritis, rheumatic fever, and reactive arthritis from a variety of bacteria, must be considered. Other autoimmune diseases such as SLE, juvenile dermatomyositis, scleroderma, KD, inflammatory bowel disease, and HSP should be considered. Other hematological diseases such as hemophilia, sickle cell diseases, and thalassemia can present with joint pain. Thyroid disease can also present with joint pain as can serum sickness and hypertrophic osteoarthropathy. Oncological differentials include tumors (e.g., neuroblastoma) and leukemia. Pigmented villonodular synovitis (PVNS) is a rare uncontrolled cell growth around a joint with destruction of the joint; it does not spread and tends to affect the hip or knee.

Management

Children with suspected JIA should be referred to and followed by a pediatric rheumatologist. Ophthalmology referral and evaluation is needed for patients with JIA. Those with a positive ANA and oligoarticular JIA, especially females, are at high risk for uveitis, require slit-lamp examination every 3 to 4 months for 4 years, and need regular follow-up even after the arthritis has resolved. They have a greater risk of uveitis that may not be clinically apparent but can lead to blindness if not detected and treated. Uveitis often does not correspond to the severity of the arthritis (i.e., uveitis may be present despite quiescent arthritis). Uveitis needs immediate ophthalmologic management.

Specialists in pediatric orthopedics, pain management, and cardiology are consulted as needed. Therapy depends on the degree of local or systemic involvement.

Early and more aggressive pharmacotherapy is suggested for patients with JIA rather than the previously gradual step-up treatment. Treatment goals are to suppress inflammation, preserve and maximize function, prevent joint deformities, achieve remission, and prevent blindness in those patients with uveitis. Aggressive early treatment to induce a remission is a key consideration in JIA management in order to prevent deformity and improve outcomes and is the goal of the practice guidelines for both polyarticular JIA and sJIA (Shenoi, 2017). Aspirin therapy has largely been replaced with the use of NSAIDs. Pharmacologic agents commonly used in the management of JIA include the following (Taketomo et al., 2018):

- NSAIDs: Children with oligoarthritis generally respond well to NSAIDs (Taketomo et al., 2018).
  - Ibuprofen: 30 to 40 mg/kg/day three to four divided doses (maximum single dose is 800 mg; maximum daily dose 2400 mg/day)
  - Tolmetin: 15 to 30 mg/kg/day divided in three to four doses (maximum dose is 1800 mg/day)
  - Naproxen: 10 to 15 mg/kg/day in two divided doses (maximum dose is 1000 mg/day)
  - Indomethacin: Older than 2 years old, 1 to 2 mg/kg/day divided in two to four doses (maximum dose is 4 mg/kg/day); adults, 25 to 50 mg/dose two or three times/day (maximum dose is 200 mg/day)
  - Celecoxib: Older than 2 years old and adolescents (≥10 kg to ≤25 kg), 50 mg twice daily; >25 kg, 100 mg twice daily

- Disease-modifying antirheumatic drugs (DMARDs) are managed by pediatric rheumatologist.
  - Nonbiologic DMARD treatment: methotrexate, sulfasalazine, leflunomide
  - Biologic DMARD treatment. Initiation of biological agents in JIA is usually done after one nonbiologic drug indicated for JIA failed to control the disease after 3 to 6 months or if the form of JIA has a risk for poorer outcomes. Usually, biologic agents are continued for at least 6 months before weaning is attempted (Mehta and Beukelman, 2017). The risk of overwhelming infection is the most common serious adverse event. These agents are administered either subcutaneously or by IV infusion. Agents with FDA approval for use in pediatric patients include tumor necrosis factor inhibitors (TNFi), etanercept (Enbrel) and adalimumab (Humira), to treat pJIA; IL-1 inhibitors, anti-IL-1 anakinra (Kineret) and canakinumab (Ilaris), to treat sJIA; co-stimulation inhibitor, abatacept (Orencia), for pJIA; and IL-6 inhibitor, tocilizumab (Actemra), approved for sJIA and pJIA (Mehta and Beukeman, 2017).
- Oral glucocorticoids
  - Glucocorticoids are added if there is not a prompt response (typically one week) to a biologic agent and continued polyarthritis, fever, and rash
  - Steroids are added if MAS or severe serositis
  - Gradual withdrawal of glucocorticoid once symptoms controlled
- Parenteral agents and intraarticular corticosteroids:
  - Systemic arthritis: Anti-IL-1 (anakinra) and anti-IL-6 (tocilizumab or atlizumab) (Giancane, Alongi, and Ravelli, 2017)
  - All other types of arthritis: Intraarticular corticosteroid injections are used if there is severe joint involvement. Intraarticular corticosteroid injection with triamcinolone hexacetonide, which is longer acting, can be done either under anesthesia for younger children or local anesthesia for cooperative older children. The use of ultrasound to guide needle placement into the joint is common practice. The need for more than 3 intraarticular injections per year or extension of the disease requires systemic therapies with disease-modifying anti-rheumatic drugs (Shenoi, 2017).

Other treatment modalities include physical therapy—range of motion muscle-strengthening exercises and heat treatments—used for joint involvement and occupational therapy. Rest and splinting are used if indicated.

Complications and Prognosis

Systemic involvement can include iridocyclitis, iritis, uveitis, pleuritis, pericarditis, anemia, fatigue, and hepatitis. Growth failure, leg-length discrepancy, if the arthritis is unilateral, and residual joint damage caused by granulation of tissue in the joint space can occur. Children most likely to *develop* permanent crippling disability include those with hip involvement, unremitting synovitis, or positive RF test.

The course of JIA is variable with no curative treatment. Early aggressive treatment is critical, and referral to a specialist is important. After an initial episode, the child may never have another episode, or the disease may go into remission and recur months or years later. The disease process of JIA wanes with age and completely subsides in 85% of children; however, systemic onset, a positive RF, poor response to therapy, and the radiologic evidence of erosion are associated with a poor prognosis. Onset of disease in the teenage years is related to progression to adult rheumatoid disease.

Patient and Parent Education and Prevention

The following education and preventive measures are taken:

- For children on aspirin therapy (not typically given), educate parents about the risk of Reye syndrome and its signs and symptoms.
- Recommend yearly influenza vaccine.
- Offer chronic disease counseling and encourage normal play and recreation.
- Educate about side effects of medications, in addition to splinting, orthotics, and bracing requirements if needed.
- Instruct about need to follow up with an ophthalmologist. Frequency of screening for uveitis is based on subtype of JIA, protocol guidelines, and ophthalmology.
- Confirm family has a plan for giving medications. Instruct about phone reminders using phone applications.
- Ensure parent and child understand that physical therapy is a mainstay of treatment for chronic childhood arthritis and should be part of the child's daily routine, including passive, active, and resistive exercises.
- Water therapy and using heat or cold reduce pain and stiffness. Swimming is an excellent activity, except for children with severe anemia and severe cardiac disease; tricycle or bike riding and low-impact dance are other beneficial activities.
- Refer to the American Arthritis Foundation and the Juvenile Arthritis Association.
- Instruct on the need to involve school personnel in the identification of required school-related services through an individualized education plan (IEP) or a 504.
- Discuss challenges of pain management and its assessment in children with chronic arthritis and encourage parents to advocate for effective pain control for their child.

Systemic Lupus Erythematosus

SLE is a chronic, multisystem autoimmune disease characterized by autoantibodies that cause aberrant immune function with presentation of self-antigens as well as defects in clearance of apoptotic debris (Lo and Tsokos, 2017). It is associated with inflammatory damage to target organs brought on by autoantibodies attacking self-antigens and immune dysregulation. There is a strong genetic component with more than 80 loci associated with susceptibility of SLE (Chen, Morris, and Vyse, 2017). It is more prevalent in females between puberty and menopause with a 6:1 female to male predilection. The concordance rate is 10-fold higher in monozygotic twins. There is a reported 43.9% heritability with shared environmental factors versus 25.8% to 30.3% with non-shared factors playing a significant role (Kuo et al., 2015). Environmental factors thought to play a role in its pathogenesis are oral contraceptive use, pregnancy, microbials (viral agents mostly), temperate climates, exposure to ultraviolet light, hormonal changes in puberty, and certain drugs (e.g., hydralazine and procainamide). The strongest environmental evidence is for cigarettes and oral contraceptive pills along with exposure to crystalline silica. Emerging research shows that solvent exposure, household and agricultural pesticides, air pollution, and heavy metal may also play a role (Parks, de souza Espindola Santos, Barbhaiya et al., 2017).

Excess INF production and plasmacytoid dendritic cell (pDC) activation increase the inflammatory response in multiple organ systems, including the blood cells, kidneys, nervous system, and skin. Abnormalities of immune function include metabolic derangements, immune cells biochemical defects, and an impaired sensing and repair of DNA damage (Lo and Tsokos, 2017). B cells are responsible for increased activation of plasma cells with subsequent increases in autoantibody production and T cell co-stimulation. This causes immune complexes to form together with recruitment of other immune cells with subsequent tissue injury. The T cells are responsible for dysregulated T-cell receptor (TCR) signaling with a decrease in IL-2 and T cell regulatory cell (Treg) function and an increase in the mammalian target of rapamycin (MTOR) activity and Ras activity, IL-17 and IFN-α. Aside from stimulating more T cell activity, IFN-α also stimulates neutrophils leading to more production of pDC.

Childhood onset is rare with an incidence of 6 to 30 children per 100,000 children per year. In general, it is more acute and severe in children than in adults. There is a higher incidence in Asians, African Americans, Hispanics, and Native Americans. Males with Klinefelter syndrome and family members with first-degree relatives with SLE have a higher incidence of SLE (Siegel, Grewanter, and Sahai, 2017).

Clinical Findings

The butterfly or malar erythematous facial rash that increases in intensity in sunlight makes the diagnosis more obvious; however, findings vary, making the diagnosis difficult in some patients. Clinical findings depend on organ involvement. Presentation may be abrupt or have a gradual, nonspecific onset. Fever, rash, fatigue, and joint pain are the most typical presentation in children. Box 33.3 outlines the clinical criteria from the Systemic Lupus International Collaborating Clinics.

History. The history may include the following:
- Joint involvement (most common initial finding)
  - Nonerosive arthritis with tenderness, effusion, and swelling
- Arthralgia
- Constitutional and systemic manifestations:
  - Low-grade fever (intermittent or sustained), weight loss, and lymphadenopathy
  - Painless, oral ulcers typically in the mouth or nose
  - Malar or discoid rash; Raynaud phenomenon; alopecia
  - Symptoms of organ involvement, typically disorders of the renal, cardiopulmonary, immunologic, neurologic, and hematologic system

Physical Examination. The following may be seen on physical examination (Siegel et al., 2017):
- Skin manifestations
  - Pallor, livedo reticularis, petechiae, palpable purpura, and digital ulcers
  - Malar or "butterfly" rash—scaly erythematous maculopapular rash covering malar areas extending over the bridge of the nose and cheeks; may spread down the face to the chest and extremities; "butterfly" rash and other lesions can be photosensitive; seen in approximately 95% of those with SLE
  - Mucous membrane manifestations (ulceration) of the mouth and nasal septum
  - Gingivitis, mucosal hemorrhage, erosions, ulcerations
  - Silvery whitening of the vermilion border or thickening, redness, ulceration, or crusting of lips

> **• BOX 33.3** **Systemic Lupus International Collaborating Clinics Diagnostic Criteria for Systemic Lupus Erythematosus**
>
> Must have four criteria with at least one clinical criteria and one laboratory criteria
> 1. Acute cutaneous lupus
> 2. Chronic cutaneous lupus
> 3. Oral ulcers OR nasal ulcers (not attributed to another disease)
> 4. Nonscarring alopecia
> 5. Synovitis with swelling or effusion or tenderness involving 2 or more joints
> 6. Serositis including pleurisy, pericardial effusion, or pain (not attributed to another disease)
> 7. Renal: Red blood cell cast or urine protein to creatinine ratio of 500 mg protein/24 h
> 8. Neurologic—including seizures, psychosis, myelitis, acute confusional state
> 9. Hemolytic anemia
> 10. Leukopenia (<4000/mm^3) OR lymphopenia (<1000/mm^3)
> 11. Thrombocytopenia (<100,000/mm^3)
>
> **Immunologic Criteria**
> 1. ANA level above laboratory reference range
> 2. Anti-dsDNA antibody level above laboratory reference range
> 3. Positive anti-Sm: presence of antibody to Sm nuclear antigen
> 4. Antiphospholipid antibody positivity, as determined by
>   - Positive test for lupus anticoagulant
>   - False-positive test result for rapid plasma reagin
>   - Medium- or high-titer anticardiolipin antibody level (IgA, IgG, or IgM)
>   - Positive test result for anti–2-glycoprotein I (IgA, IgG, or IgM)
> 5. Low complement (C3, C4, or CH50)
> 6. Direct Coombs test (in the absence of hemolytic anemia)
>
> ANA, *Antinuclear antibody, Ig, immunoglobulin.*
>
> *Adapted from Petri M, Orbai AM, Alarcon GS, et al. Derivation and validation of the Systemic Lupus International Collaborating Clinics classification criteria for systemic lupus erythematosus. Arthritis Rheum. 2012;64(8):2677–2686.*

- Joint tenderness
- Cardiac friction rub due to pericarditis; pleural friction rubs due to pleuritis
- Hepatosplenomegaly and lymphadenopathy

Diagnostic Studies. Initial laboratory testing includes CBC, ANA, ESR, CRP, serum chemical analysis (metabolic and protein screen), and urinalysis. The ANA test is positive in more than 97% to 99% of children who have active, untreated SLE and titers above 1:1080 point to the diagnosis; however, ANA specificity is as low as 36%. A negative ANA makes SLE diagnosis less likely; however, there is always a risk of a rare false-negative test. A positive ANA with clinical findings consistent with SLE should be followed up with testing for disease-specific types of ANA (e.g., antibodies to Sm, Ro, or La). The ANA autoantibody profile screens for anti-Sm, anti-Ro, anti-La, anti-double-strand DNA, and anti-ribonucleoprotein (anti-RNP) antibodies (Siegel et al., 2017). Antibody testing for double-stranded DNA and extractable nuclear antigen panel (anti-Smith antibody) and anti-RNP antibody (RNP) should be done as it is specific for SLE and is present in up to 50% of patients with SLE (Siegel et al., 2017). Anti-Ro (anti–SSA) and anti-La (anti-SSb) antibodies are also associated with SLE.

Leukopenia or lymphopenia, hemolytic anemia, and thrombocytopenia are frequent laboratory findings. Other laboratory and radiographic studies depend on organ involvement and can include a chest x-ray, electrocardiogram (ECG), urine and serologic testing, renal ultrasound, and histopathologic studies. Proteinuria and hematuria are hallmarks of lupus nephritis. Newer biomarkers are in development as a result of advances in genomics, epigenetics, and transcriptomics that will eventually provide greater ability to diagnose SLE and determine a prognosis.

Differential Diagnosis

Differential diagnoses include infection, malignancy, or autoimmune/inflammatory disease. Infectious diseases that resemble SLE include bacterial infections such as brucellosis, leptospirosis, and sepsis; viral infections such as cytomegalovirus (CMV), Epstein-Barr virus (EBV), parvovirus, and human immunodeficiency virus (HIV); and other infectious disease such as Q fever *(Coxiella)*, tuberculosis, Lyme disease, or toxoplasmosis. Leukemia, lymphoma, neuroblastoma, and Langerhans cell histiocytosis are malignant differentials. Other autoimmune diseases that mimic SLE include acute rheumatic fever (ARF), JIA, Sjögren syndrome, systemic vasculitis, sarcoidosis, hemolytic-uremic syndrome (HUS), and autoimmune lymphoproliferative syndrome, and common variable immunodeficiency can also resemble SLE (Siegel et al., 2017). A temporary, drug-induced SLE can be caused by several pharmacologic agents, including hydantoin compounds, hydralazine, isoniazid (INH), procainamide, and sulfonamides.

Management

Children with SLE need an interprofessional approach that includes specialists in rheumatology, nephrology, adolescent medicine, pharmacology, psychiatry, nursing, physical therapy, occupational therapy, and pain management. Therapy depends on the degree of local or systemic involvement. Because sunlight is a known trigger of SLE, ultraviolet A and B sunscreen is essential both indoors due to daylight fluorescent lighting and outdoors due to sun exposure. Prompt recognition and treatment of disease flares are essential to prevent systemic complications; therefore, frequent clinical and laboratory monitoring is important. The following measures also may be helpful.

- NSAIDs are used for relief of musculoskeletal pain, arthritis, arthralgias, serositis, or pain. (If nephritis is present, use with caution.)
- Antimalarials are used for mild symptoms and maintenance.
- Oral steroids are prescribed for rapid control; however, the goal is to find a less toxic maintenance therapy. Dosage is adjusted depending on clinical and laboratory findings. Cautious tapering of steroids is often needed.
- Immunosuppressant agents, such as methotrexate and azathioprine (Imuran), may be used as steroid-sparing agents. Methotrexate is used for arthritis, whereas azathioprine is used in treating cytopenias, vasculitic rash, or serositis (Siegel et al., 2017). MMF or CellCept is used to induce remission in lupus nephritis or for maintenance therapy in other organ diseases. When other agents fail to induce a remission, calcineurin inhibitors such as tacrolimus or cyclophosphamide may suppress the calcium/calcimodulin-dependent phosphatase calcineurin, which activates T cells, with the former having a lesser side effect profile (Mok, 2017). Immunosuppressive agents have a higher risk of severe infection and malignancies.
- Use of other pharmacologic agents or therapies depends on the type and degree of organ system involvement. Rituximab (Rituxan) is a monoclonal antibody that binds and kills active B cells and is used for cytopenias. Belimumab (Benlysta) was specifically developed to treat lupus; it is only approved in adults and with mixed results in African Americans.
- Adjunctive treatment includes antihypertensive agents with angiotensin converting enzyme inhibitors used to reduce proteinuria and anticonvulsive agents prescribed for seizures. Estrogen-containing agents for contraception can be used if the patient does not have antiphospholipid antibodies. Progestin-only agents should be used if the patient has antiphospholipid antibodies.
- Parents need education about sun exposure and the use of sunscreen protection as well as the child's need for rest between activities because fatigue is a frequent problem.

There are limited studies demonstrating effectiveness of vitamin D and calcium supplements to prevent or reduce the risk of osteoporosis related to chronic corticosteroid use in children. A recent Cochrane review could not find strong evidence to recommend them in children with Duchenne muscular dystrophy who were on steroids (Bell, Shields, Watters, et al., 2017).

Complications and Prognosis

SLE is a chronic disease with periods of waxing and waning of symptoms; however, complete remission can occur. Children with mild disease do well; those with severe major organ involvement have a poorer prognosis. During disease flares, the child may experience poor sleep and daytime fatigue with decreased cardiovascular conditioning, resulting in increased pain. A diagnosis of SLE in childhood is not always lethal, especially if renal involvement or cerebritis is not present. Renal failure, central nervous system (CNS) lupus, myocardial infarction, cardiac failure, and infection are the leading causes of death in children with SLE. There is a higher risk of leukemia in younger children with SLE and a higher risk of lymphoma in older children (Choi, Flood, Bernatsky, et al., 2017). Exposure to ultraviolet light may bring out or worsen skin lesions and result in exacerbation of systemic problems. Side effects resulting from chronic use of high-dose corticosteroids (e.g., osteoporosis, avascular necrosis) are a complication of treatment.

Juvenile Fibromyalgia Syndrome

Juvenile fibromyalgia (JFM) is the term used to describe a chronic, idiopathic amplified pain syndrome characterized by widespread, diffuse, nonarticular musculoskeletal pain associated with nonrestorative sleep, unrelenting fatigue, and dysfunction in sensory, autonomic, and cognitive nervous system. New information points to an organic problem with the pain processing system, whereas previously it was thought to fall under psychosomatic domains. It is estimated that 1% to 2% of pediatric patients have significant JFM. While adolescent onset is typical, and females are more likely to have JFM, it occurs as young as 4 years of age. It is also associated with irritable bowel syndrome, daily tension headaches, and chronic fatigue (Zemel and Blier, 2016). There is a genetic component with multiple generations affected by the fibromyalgia. JFM can cause significant functional impairment in activities of daily living and interfere with normal adolescent development. Rather than pain at specific trigger points, there is a widespread abnormal sensation.

The pathophysiology of JFM involves abnormal responses to stimuli and changes in the pain mechanism where nociceptive input connects at the level of the dorsal horn. This causes hyperalgesia or increases sensitivity to painful stimuli, allodynia or pain

- Pain in at least three areas for more than 3 months without underlying cause and normal laboratory tests
- More than 5 of 18 tender points, which include occiput, low cervical spine, trapezius at the midpoint, supraspinous above the scapula near the medial border, second rib at the costochondral junctions, lateral epicondyle, upper outer quadrants of the gluteal muscle, posterior to greater trochanter prominence, and at the medial fat pad of the knee at the joint line
- Three of 10 minor criteria listed below:
  - Fatigue
  - Poor sleep
  - Irritable bowel syndrome
  - Chronic tension or anxiety
  - Soft tissue swelling
  - Pain affected by weather
  - Paresthesia
  - Pain affected by activity
  - Headache
  - Pain affected by anxiety and/or stress

being triggered by touch, or more widespread pain due to receptive field expansion or secondary hyperalgesia. The exact mechanism of pain in this disease is still being elucidated.

Pediatric diagnostic criteria were first defined by Yunus and Masi (1985). The Yunus and Masi criteria (Box 33.4) are not validated and the lack of clearly defined pediatric criteria leads to a delay in diagnosis. The adult 2010 criteria for fibromyalgia evaluate widespread pain criteria and symptom severity (SS) using the Widespread Pain Index (WPI) and a SS score (Ting, 2015). The use of these scales may be helpful in evaluating patients with JFM. Because there are no major organ system abnormalities found, the presentation of JFM can occur as a primary condition or in conjunction with other rheumatologic disorders (secondary fibromyalgia) (Kashikar-Zuck and Ting, 2014a).

Clinical Findings

The finding of 3 months of widespread pain with 3 of associated symptoms seen in Box 33.4 points to the diagnosis of JFM. The patient may complain of changes in pain with different weather conditions and levels of physical activities. Children with widespread musculoskeletal pain and painful point tenderness may have fibromyalgia and should be referred to a rheumatologist.

History. Pain history is the key finding because early on the associated symptoms of chronic fatigue, depression, or mood disorder may be lacking (Jay and Barkin, 2015). Stress may exacerbate the pain; therefore, a careful psychosocial history is a critical component to identify triggers. The history may include the following long-standing common symptoms:
- Pain at multiple sites, including muscles and soft tissues around joints
- Pain may awaken from sleep and interfere with routine activities
- Fatigue and malaise, daily tension headache
- Paresthesias, allodynia, hypersensitivity
- Insomnia or prolonged night awakenings
- Depression (a significant number exhibit depressive symptoms) and anxiety
- School absence due to pain is not uncommon but the child typically keeps up with school work

Physical Examination. Typically, there is no evidence of arthritis or muscular weakness. Trigger points around the neck, back, lateral epicondyles, greater trochanter, and knees may provide a gross measure of the patient's discomfort (Jay and Barkin, 2015). There may be hypermobility; the use of the 9-point Brighton Hypermobility Score is positive in 80% of patients with fibromyalgia (Zemel and Blier, 2016).

Diagnostic Studies. Laboratory studies are of little benefit in diagnosing JFM but may be helpful in ruling out other diagnoses. Blood count, liver functions, and muscle enzymes are normal. If secondary fibromyalgia is present, order appropriate tests to rule out a different rheumatoid disorder. Children with fibromyalgia can have a false-positive ANA, as do 20% of children without rheumatoid disorders.

Differential Diagnosis

This disease can mimic many other diseases. The classification criteria for SLE were defined by the Systemic Lupus International Collaborating Clinics (see Box 33.3). The differential diagnosis includes autoimmune, autoinflammatory, or post-infectious fatigue following a viral illness or mood disorders. In CFS, tiredness lasting longer than 6 months rather than pain is the major complaint. Primary and secondary fibromyalgia can occur, so the PCP needs to consider that fibromyalgia initially may be mistaken for other rheumatoid diseases; however, it does not have the associated rashes, weight loss, fever, or joint swelling. Lyme disease is also in the differential, but its course of illness is not characterized by pain.

Management

Children and parents need reassurance that fibromyalgia is not life-threatening, rather it is a chronic condition that can be a lifelong issue. Treatment focuses on relieving symptoms and can include the following:
- Physical therapy for range-of-motion exercises (Sherry et al., 2015), mild low-impact aerobic exercises (e.g., swimming, bicycling, and walking), and muscle strengthening
- Psychotherapy and relaxation techniques to help cope with this condition
- NSAIDs for pain control; gabapentin can be used to reduce pain sensitivity

Prognosis

The outcome of fibromyalgia in children varies, but studies demonstrate the persistence of fibromyalgia into adulthood. Fibromyalgia in children generally has a better prognosis than it does in adults (Kashikar-Zuck et al., 2014b).

Patient and Parent Education

Patients and parents should be educated about fibromyalgia and that it is not a psychosomatic disorder. Guidance should be given about sleep hygiene and the possibility that it could be a chronic problem with periods of remissions followed by exacerbations.

Myalgic Encephalomyelitis/Chronic Fatigue Syndrome or Systemic Exertion Intolerance Disease

Myalgic encephalomyelitis/chronic fatigue syndrome (ME/CFS) is a disease with specific characteristics now defined by the Institute of Medicine (2015). Systemic exertion intolerance disease is another term used for this problem. The clinical criteria include a substantial reduction or impairment in the ability to carry out normal activities of daily living persisting for more than 3 months that is accompanied by the new onset of severe, medically unexplained fatigue. This fatigue is not the result of ongoing excessive exertion and does not improve with rest. It is critical to ascertain the frequency and severity not only of the fatigue but also the post-exertional malaise and an unrefreshing sleep. In addition to fatigue, unrefreshing sleep, and post-exertional malaise, the child must complain of either cognitive impairments or orthostatic intolerance or both. Widespread or migratory myofascial joint, abdominal, or head pain and neuroendocrine (feeling feverish or cold) or immune (flu-like complaints) manifestation may be reported. These symptoms must be different from the way the child was before the onset of the illness. A primary sleep disorder does not make the diagnosis of ME/CFS impossible. The term chronic fatigue does not reflect the seriousness of the condition.

There is convincing evidence for a subset of patients that this is an autoimmune disease with immune dysregulation as well as changes in the cytokine profile and immunoglobulin levels. Decrease in natural killer cell cytotoxicity (Tomas and Newton, 2018) and changes in the T- and B-cell phenotype (Sotzny et al., 2018) were reported. Infections with pathogens such as EBV, human herpesvirus 6 (HHV-6), and parvovirus as well as intracellular bacteria are known triggers. EBV infection is a noninfectious risk factor for various autoimmune diseases. Autoantibodies can cause immune activation and dysregulation and cellular metabolic alterations. Enhanced levels of immunoglobulins and alterations in B cells are found in autoimmune diseases such as SLE, JIA, and Sjögren syndrome. As previously described in the SLE pathophysiology, the alteration in autoimmune diseases is multifaceted. Autoantibodies in ME/CFS are directed against neurotransmitters as well as nuclear and membrane structures. There is clinical heterogeneity in the disease onset likely as a result of whether the disease had a noninfectious or infectious trigger (Sotzny et al., 2018). Aggravation of the symptoms with exertion is likely a dysregulation of the autonomic parasympathetic and sympathetic nervous system and includes GI dysfunction, vasomotor instability, and increased pain sensitivity (Loebel et al., 2016).

Clinical Finding

It is important to evaluate the patient's history carefully as the physical exam findings are limited.

History

- Query about unrefreshing sleep as to how they feel in the morning, the quality of the sleep, need for naps, or problems going to or staying asleep.
- Obtain a history about possible cognitive impairments, ability to multitask, difficulty with complex tasks, or memory issues.
- Question about orthostatic intolerance (e.g., problems with standing, or symptoms when changing positions, need to study on a recliner, or preference for sitting position)
- Questions about pain and systemic manifestations (e.g., feeling feverish or cold, flu-like symptoms)
- Use questionnaires or tools to help clarify symptoms of fatigue pain, orthostatic intolerance, post-exertional malaise, or decreases in function (see ME/CFS resources).

Physical Examination.
Exam findings may be normal or painful lymph nodes may be present.

Diagnostic Studies

There is ongoing research into potential biomarkers for this disease investigating ATP levels, 5′-adenosine monophosphate-activated

protein kinase, skeletal muscle cell acidosis, and a chemical signal for ME/CFS using plasma metabolomics (Tomas and Newton, 2018).

Differential Diagnosis

Because CFS is a diagnosis of exclusion, other conditions must be investigated. Care must be taken in diagnosing this disorder in children, because other conditions (e.g., hypothyroidism, sleep apnea, hepatitis B or C, SLE, cancer, alcohol or drug abuse, Lyme disease, and major depressive and other psychiatric disorders) must first be ruled out. The child is best referred to a specialist in CFS for management.

Management

Recent studies with Rituximab in adults showed clinical improvement and further studies are still pending. Initial randomized control trials with intravenous immunoglobulin (IVIG) did not show consistent improvement (Sotzny et al., 2018). It is important to avoid referrals to multiple providers where duplication of lab work is done. Although some may not believe this is a real illness, the latest studies point to autoimmune dysfunction. The patient's complaints should be taken seriously; referrals to support groups and the CDC website may be helpful. Psychological support (stressing that this disease is not made up) with cognitive behavioral therapy may help. Cochrane review reported a graded exercise program was more effective than no treatment or passive treatment for ME/CFS (Larun, Brurberg, Odgaard-Jensen et al., 2016).

Reactive Arthritis Related to Streptococcal Infection: Acute Rheumatic Fever and Post-Streptococcal Reactive Arthritis

ARF is an exaggerated autoimmune response in a susceptible host to an anaerobic gram-positive coccus, group A streptococcus (GAS). Epitopes, the surface portion of certain subspecies of GAS, are similar to human myosin and to the tissue of the mitral annulus and chordae. These sites act as antigens, which activate the immune response that results in antibody formation and initiation of the antibody/antigen response (Maness, Martin, Mitchell, 2018). Antistreptococcal immunoglobulins, stimulated by repeated streptococcal infections, attack the heart and joints, CNS, and cutaneous tissue. Greater organism virulence is associated with specific M protein types and a more "mucoid" capsule. There appears to be a strong genetic influence for susceptibility to GAS infection, with a family history of rheumatic fever and a lower socioeconomic status as known risk factors. GABHS causes several post-infectious, nonsuppurative immune-mediated diseases including ARF, post-streptococcal reactive arthritis (PSRA), pediatric acute-onset neuropsychiatric syndrome (PANS), and post-streptococcal glomerulonephritis (Maness et al., 2018).

The incidence of ARF has declined in developing countries but is still a significant cause of heart disease worldwide. Echocardiographic techniques allow for a more accurate diagnosis of ARF. Recurrence of ARF following subsequent episodes of GAS pharyngitis (symptomatic or asymptomatic infection) is high. The most commonly affected age group in children is 5 to 15 years (Gewitz et al., 2015).

Evidence of a prior GAS infection is needed for the diagnosis of a nonsuppurative immune-mediated disease. Confirmation of a GAS infection by throat culture or rapid strep test does not differentiate carrier state from a true infection. Serologic testing for the presence of elevated or increasing antistreptococcal antibody titers (ASO test) or anti-DNase B testing confirms a recent strep infection (Gewitz et al., 2015). The ASO titer and the anti-DNase B levels rise 1 to 2 weeks following an acute GAS infection. The ASO titer peaks in 3 to 6 weeks; DNase B level peaks in 6 to 8 weeks. Both remain elevated for months after GAS infection; increasing titers are the key to the diagnosis.

Post-Streptococcal Reactive Arthritis

PSRA can develop within 7 to 10 days after GABHS pharyngitis and may present with knee, ankle, hip, or wrist arthritis in a patient who does not meet the Jones criteria for ARF (Maness et al., 2018). The acute phase reactants are generally not as elevated in PSRA. The most common age in children is 8 to 14. There are no specific criteria for PSRA, but a history of recent streptococcal infection documented using the titers discussed earlier is important. In PSRA, the arthritis may occur sooner, be more persistent, and involve small joints as well as the more common ones previously mentioned. Although there is no associated cardiac involvement in PSRA, it is suggested that prophylaxis with penicillin to prevent carditis be continued for one year after the arthritis occurs (Maness et al., 2018). This form of arthritis is more persistent and less receptive to NSAID treatment but resolves without joint damage.

Acute Rheumatic Fever

ARF is a nonsuppurative complication following a Lancefield GAS pharyngeal infection that results in an autoimmune inflammatory process involving the joints (polyarthritis), heart (rheumatic heart disease), CNS (Sydenham chorea), and subcutaneous tissue (subcutaneous nodules and erythema marginatum). Recurrent ARF with its multisystem responses can follow subsequent GAS pharyngeal infections. Guidelines recommend an echocardiogram in all confirmed or suspected cases of ARF, and the diagnostic criteria must be met in order to confirm carditis. Morphological findings of rheumatic carditis include acute or chronic mitral valve changes. Development of ARF occurs 2 weeks after an infection with S. Pyogenes (Gewitz et al., 2015). The most common ages are between 5 and 15 years (Sika-Paotonu, Beaton, Raghu et al., 2016). Long-term effects on tissues are generally minimal except for the damage done to cardiac valves that leaves fibrosis and scarring and results in rheumatic heart disease.

Clinical Findings and History

The diagnosis of an initial attack of ARF is based on the revised Jones criteria found in Box 33.5. Abdominal pain, malaise, leukocytosis, precordial pain, rapid sleeping pulse rate, and a tachycardia out of proportion to the degree of fever is not uncommon. A family history of ARF should also raise the index of suspicion because of an increased frequency in families. The most serious clinical manifestation is carditis that can lead to involvement of the endocardium, which is reflected in valvular dysfunction, or pericarditis due to involvement of the pericardium (Sika-Paotonu et al., 2016).

• BOX 33.5 Revised Jones Criteria for Rheumatic Fever (American Heart Association, 2015)

Evidence of preceding streptococcal infection by one of the following:
- Increased or rising anti-streptolysin O titer or other streptococcal antibodies (anti-DNASE B) (class I, Level of Evidence B).
  - Rise in titer is better evidence than a single titer result.
- Positive throat culture for group A β-hemolytic streptococci (class I, Level of Evidence B).
- Positive rapid group A streptococcal carbohydrate antigen test in a child whose clinical presentation suggests that the infection is caused by a streptococcal infection

Revised Criteria for Low-Risk Populations (ARF incidence <2/100,000 children ages 5-14 years old per year or ≤1/1000 population/year)
- Major criteria:
  - Carditis (clinical and/or subclinical)
  - Arthritis (polyarthritis)
  - Chorea
  - *Erythema marginatum*
  - Subcutaneous nodules
- Minor criteria:
  - Oligoarthralgia,
  - Fever (≥38.5°F)
  - Sedimentation rate ≥60 mm and/or C-reactive protein (CRP) ≥3.0 mg/dL
  - Prolonged PR interval (unless carditis is a major criterion)

Revised Jones Criteria for Moderate- and High-Risk Populations
- Major criteria:
  - Carditis (clinical and/or subclinical)
  - Arthritis (monopolyarthritis or polyarthritis, or polyarthralgia)
  - Chorea
  - *Erythema marginatum*
  - Subcutaneous nodules

- Minor criteria:
  - fever (≥38.5°F)
  - Sedimentation rate ≥30 mm and/or CRP ≥3.0 mg/dL
  - Prolonged PR interval (unless carditis is a major criterion)
    Doppler findings in rheumatic valvulitis (may be subclinical findings)
- Pathological mitral regurgitation (all 4 criteria met)
  - Seen in at least 2 views
  - Jet length of ≥2 cm in at least 1 view
  - Peak velocity >3 m/s
  - Pansystolic jet in at least 1 envelope
- Pathological aortic regurgitation (all 4 criteria met)
  - Seen in at least 2 views
  - Jet length of ≥1 cm in at least 1 view
  - Peak velocity >3 m/s
  - Pansystolic jet in at least 1 envelope
    Must have two major criteria, or one major plus two minor criteria for an initial episode of ARF
    High-risk patients who have a history of ARF or rheumatic heart disease (RHD) who get infected with Group A strep
- Two major, one major and two minor, or three minor manifestations may be sufficient for a presumptive diagnosis (class IIb, Level of Evidence C).
- When minor manifestations alone are present, exclusion of other more likely causes of the clinical presentation is recommended before a diagnosis of an ARF recurrence is made (class I, Level of Evidence C).
  If re-infected with group A streptococci:
- And a reliable past history of ARF or established RHD, and in the face of documented group A streptococcal infection, two major, one major and two minor, or three minor manifestations may be sufficient for a presumptive diagnosis (class IIb, Level of Evidence C).
- When minor manifestations alone are present, the exclusion of other more likely causes of the clinical presentation is recommended before a diagnosis of an ARF recurrence is made (class I, Level of Evidence C).

ARF, Acute rheumatic fever.

Major Manifestations

- Polyarthritis: Migratory arthritis, involving large joints including the knees, ankle, elbows, and wrist, is the most common manifestation. It responds readily to salicylates and NSAIDs and does not usually last more than 4 weeks, even without treatment. A septic monoarthritis can occur in high-risk populations and can be seen in indigenous Australian populations with ARF in 16 % to 18% of patients, but is rarely found in the United States.
- Carditis is common (pancarditis, valves, pericardium, myocardium) and can cause chronic, life-threatening disease (i.e., congestive heart failure [CHF]). ARF is more common in younger children than adolescents. The need to recognize subclinical disease stresses the importance of serial echocardiogram. Symptoms of carditis may be vague and insidious with decreased appetite, fatigue, and pains. When clinically apparent, carditis presents with tachycardia and a holosystolic murmur heard at the aortic or mitral area with radiation to the infrascapular area. Mitral and aortic valve changes occur in 95% of cases, usually within 2 weeks of RF illness, and can be subclinical. Recurrent episodes of RF lead to worsening valve disease.
- Sydenham chorea is uncommon.
- Erythema marginatum or erythema annulare manifested as nonpruritic, bright pink blanching papules or macules that spread in a serpiginous pattern on the trunk and extremities; it is nonpruritic and an uncommon finding.
- Subcutaneous nodules are painless nodules (0.5 to 2 cm) that develop on bony prominences or extensor tendons. They usually remain for 1 to 2 weeks and tend to be in groups of three to four nodules. This sign occurs in less than 10% of patients (Gewitz et al., 2015).

Minor Manifestations

- Fever (≥ 37.5°C or 99.5°F is now the cutoff), arthralgia, history of ARF

Diagnostic Studies. Diagnostic study findings include an elevated acute-phase reactant (ESR) greater than 30 and a CRP higher than the upper limit of normal, leukocytosis, and a prolonged PR interval on ECG. Additional studies should include an echocardiogram and chest x-ray. Test for confirmation of streptococcal infection by culture, serology (ASO titer and anti-deoxyribonuclease B titer). There are two situations when a diagnosis of ARF without evidence of a preceding streptococcal infection may be made: a child with Sydenham chorea or a child with a chronic, indolent rheumatic carditis (Gewitz, 2016). Approximately 80% of children with ARF have an elevated ASO titer. A combination of both DNase-B testing and ASO rising may confirm the recent infection.

Differential Diagnosis. Guidelines for echocardiogram findings in patients who present with symptoms and signs of ARF should be closely followed. The differential includes isolated congenital mitral and aortic valve anomalies as well as congenital heart disease (e.g., bicuspid aortic valve). Infective endocarditis can be mistaken for rheumatic carditis if there are no signs of vegetation and valve damage. Annular dilation from conditions associated with left-sided heart dilation as a result of a myocarditis and cardiomyopathy should be considered in the differential diagnosis.

Management

The treatment of ARF includes the following:
- Antibiotic therapy to eradicate GAS infection: Primary prevention requires that a GAS infection be treated within 10 days of onset. Benzathine penicillin G (BPG) is the drug of choice unless there is an allergic history; erythromycin then becomes the drug of choice. Azithromycin and cephalosporins are also sometimes used (AAP, 2018). A patient with a history of ARF who has an upper respiratory infection should be treated for GAS whether or not GAS is recovered because an asymptomatic GABHS infection can trigger a recurrence.
- Anti-inflammatory therapy: Aspirin usage is falling out of favor due to the risk of toxicity and Reye syndrome. There is increasing use of NSAIDs (naproxen for older patients and ibuprofen for younger patients) to reduce the need for frequent dosing (Sika-Paotonu et al., 2016). Aspirin and NSAIDs provide symptomatic relief for joint symptoms. Some experts recommend the use of corticosteroids in patients with severe carditis, reducing its morbidity and mortality. Yearly influenza immunization is critical, especially for children on aspirin therapy because of the increased risk of Reye syndrome association with aspirin usage in patients with influenza.
- Chest radiographs, ECG, and echocardiography are indicated; carditis usually develops within the first 3 weeks of symptoms.
- Referral for CHF treatment if needed: medical management and or valve replacement.
- Bed rest is generally indicated only for children with CHF. Children with Sydenham chorea may need to be protected from injury until their choreiform movements are controlled. Steroids in the absence of other symptoms are not useful in the treatment of chorea.
- Children with severe chorea may benefit from the use of antiepileptic agents, such as valproic acid or carbamazepine with the latter being the first-line agent due to liver toxicity with valproic acid.
- Education about the need for prophylaxis is key to prevent further episodes of ARF.

Primary and Secondary Prevention of Acute Rheumatic Fever

- Primary prevention of ARF includes the treatment of GAS pharyngeal infections with appropriate antibiotics, eliminating bacteria before the triggering of an autoimmune response within 9 days of the onset of a sore throat. A 10-day course of oral penicillin or amoxicillin or intramuscular Bicillin can be given (AAP Red Book, 2018). A community-based approach involves identifying a community outbreak and preventing its spread or identifying at-risk children in a community and having resources readily available to screen them for strep throat.
- Secondary prevention involves antibacterial prophylaxis for those with a prior history of ARF because of the greatly increased risk of recurrent ARF with subsequent inadequately treated GAS infections. Intramuscular Bicillin L-A, which slowly releases penicillin to prevent colonization and reoccurrences, can be given every 4 weeks for at least 10 years following ARF and in some cases, lifetime prophylaxis is suggested (Wyber et al., 2014). This method is more effective than daily penicillin V twice a day; however, adherence to either method is problematic. Pain of injections every four weeks is a real problem for children, and globally the quality of Bicillin can vary. In the majority of patients, valvular disease will resolve if they are compliant in taking antibiotic prophylaxis after the first episode of rheumatic heart disease.
- Tertiary prevention is medical and surgical intervention to prevent cardiac damage that occurs from ARF.

Complications

Chronic CHF can occur after an initial episode of ARF or follow recurrent episodes of ARF. Residual valvular damage is responsible for CHF. The risk of significant cardiac disease increases dramatically with each subsequent episode of ARF; therefore, prevention of subsequent GAS infections is critical. Family engagement in follow-up is essential to prevent the need for cardiac valvular repair.

Pediatric Vasculitis

Pediatric vasculitis represents a complex group of conditions that cause inflammatory changes in the blood vessels. Vasculitis can occur as a primary condition, primarily involving large vessels (Takayasu arteritis), medium-size vessels (childhood polyarteritis nodosa, cutaneous polyarteritis, KD), and small-vessel disease in a granulomatous form (granulomatosis with polyangiitis [formerly Wegener granulomatosis]), eosinophilic granulomatosis with polyangiitis (formerly Churg-Strauss), or small-vessel disease in a nongranulomatous form (microscopic polyangiitis, HSP, isolated cutaneous leukocytoclastic vasculitis, hypocomplementemic urticarial vasculitis). Secondary vasculitis can result from infection, malignancy, drugs, or connective tissue disease. The occurrence of primary vasculitis in childhood is approximately 23/100,000. Symptoms are variable ranging from skin eruptions to multi-organ failure. Aneurysmal dilations can occur due to neutrophil, lymphocyte, and eosinophilic infiltration (Barut, Sahin, Kasapcopur, 2016). Fever and diffuse pain associated with malaise may be early symptoms, along with elevated acute-phase reactants (ESR, CRP, platelets, ferritin, procalcitonin). As the vasculitis progresses, there may be specific clinical findings, such as organ involvement, purpuric rash, or detection of antibodies known as antineutrophil cytoplasmic antibodies (ANCAs). The most common types of vasculitis are HSP, KD, and Takayasu arteritis involving the aorta and its branches. All of these conditions require pediatric specialist care to prevent significant health problems.

Henoch-Schönlein Purpura

HSP is the most common vasculitis of children and is characterized as an IgA vasculitis. The pathophysiology involves IgA-immune deposits, neutrophil activation and infiltration, and complement factors that produce vascular inflammation (Heineke et al., 2017). The incidence of the disease is higher in fall and winter, pointing to an environmental trigger including viral infection. While an upper respiratory infection often precedes HSP, a clear association between an infectious agent and HSP has not been found (Barut, Sahin, and Kasapcopur, 2016). For the majority of children, the prognosis is excellent. It can occur anytime from infancy (as early as 6 months old) to adulthood.

The classic presentation includes abdominal pain, palpable petechial or purpuric rash on the lower extremity, non-deforming arthritis, and colicky abdominal pain. In 30% to 50% of patients, nephritis occurs 4 to 6 weeks after the initial presentation (Chen and Mao, 2015). The abdominal pain is a result of subserosal or submucosal hemorrhage and edema. Intestinal perforation is a rare but life-threatening complication (Lerkvaleekul et al., 2016). Neurological involvement (convulsions and confusion) due to vasculitis is not commonly seen.

HSP is a leukocytic vasculitis with granulocytic infiltration of tissue along with IgA deposition within the vessel walls (Heineke et al., 2017). Hemorrhage and ischemia are associated findings. With inflammation of the small blood vessels, extravasation of blood occurs into local tissue, resulting in a variety of skin manifestations, including a maculopapular rash or urticarial rash the first 24 hours, followed by purpura, bullae, or necrotic lesions. The rash along with an oligoarticular, self-limiting, and nondestructive arthritis occurs in 80% of children. The lower extremities, typically the ankles and knees, are the most common arthritic sites. The latest Chapel Hill nomenclature describes HSP as a vasculitis affecting the small blood vessels with IgA1-dominant deposits involving the skin and GI tract, with an accompanying nonerosive arthritis and an associated glomerulonephritis. GI manifestations occur in more than 50% of children and include hematochezia, colicky abdominal pain, and intussusception; glomerulonephritis occurs in 40% to 50% of patients (Heineke et al., 2017). The most common manifestation of renal disease is microscopic hematuria with or without proteinuria.

Clinical Findings

Clinical findings begin with skin manifestations; a third of children will have the aforementioned symptoms for 2 weeks, with another one-third having symptoms up to 1 month and can have reoccurring symptoms for 4 months (Eleftheriou and Brogan, 2016). Hematuria is the most common renal symptom and usually develops within 4 weeks. Hypertension can be seen at any time from the start of the disease to the recovery phase (Barut et al., 2016).

History. The history of a preceding viral illness and the clinical presentation of symptoms listed earlier support the diagnosis of HSP. It can also present with seizures, stroke, mental status change, hemoptysis due to pulmonary hemorrhage, or edema of the eyes, hands, or scrotum if the child has associated nephrotic syndrome.

Physical Examination

- Skin rash: starts as a pinkish maculopapular rash and progresses from red to purple to brown palpable purpura; lower part of the body and lower arm
- Arthritis: warmth, swelling, and erythema over the joints; periarthritis is common and involves the knees and ankles
- Other findings: diffuse abdominal pain on palpation, edema of the scrotum, eyes, or hands; hypertension

Diagnostic Studies. The diagnosis of HSP is based on clinical findings. A urinalysis must be done to check for hematuria and proteinuria (a common sign of nephritis) and needs to be repeated on follow-up due to the risk of renal disease. Other studies include a CBC with differential and platelets, metabolic profile including creatinine and blood urea nitrogen (BUN) to evaluate renal function, and stool guaiac for occult blood as the incidence of GI bleeding is high even in the absence of frank rectal bleeding. HSP is associated with a nonthrombocytopenic purpura and a normal or high platelet count, as platelet elevation is an acute-phase reactant. Other acute-phase reactants including CRP may be helpful markers of disease activity (Barut et al., 2016). If GI obstruction is a consideration, abdominal radiographs should be ordered. Diagnostic studies are useful to identify specific organ system involvement and the severity of complications. Other tests (e.g., chest radiographs, computed tomography [CT] scans, or electroencephalographs) are ordered based on signs and symptoms of complications, such as shortness of breath, seizures, mental status changes, or hypertension. Renal biopsy may be warranted if severe renal involvement.

Differential Diagnosis

Familial Mediterranean fever should be considered in patients with recurrent attacks, especially in patients of Middle Eastern or Mediterranean descent. HSP must be differentiated from other diseases that cause purpura: immune thrombocytopenic purpura, post-streptococcal glomerular nephritis, hemolytic uremic syndrome, infections, SLE, serum sickness, or hypersensitivity vasculitis. Other types of vasculitis, including microscopic polyangiitis, granulomatosis with polyangiitis (formerly Wegener granulomatosis), eosinophilic granulomatous polyangiitis (previously Churg-Strauss syndrome), and polyarteritis nodosa, although more common in adults, need to be considered (Barut et al., 2016).

Management

Children with HSP need co-management with pediatric specialists, depending on organ system involvement. Hospitalization is necessary with moderate to severe GI and renal system involvement or if pulmonary, cardiac, or CNS manifestations are present. The arthritis is generally treated with NSAIDs (Eleftheriou and Brogan, 2016). Treatment with corticosteroid can improve outcomes, especially in GI complications; however, IVIG is used for steroid-resistant complications (Lerkvaleekul et al., 2016). Prophylaxis with corticosteroids does not reduce the incidence of renal disease. In severe, life-threatening cases, treatment with immunophoresis (Chen and Mao, 2015) or other immunosuppressive agents including cyclophosphamide, azathioprine, or MMF (Eleftheriou and Brogan, 2016) may be instituted.
- Monitor for GI bleeding via stool guaiac, hematuria and proteinuria, and hypertension.
- Prescribe analgesics and NSAIDs for arthritis.
- Follow up and refer patients with HSP to nephrologist, cardiologist, and gastroenterologist as complications arise.

Complications and Prognosis

Infrequent complications of HSP seen in children include myositis, orchitis, hemorrhagic cystitis, pancreatitis, cholecystitis, bowel infarction, perforation or stricture, intussusception, acute renal failure, seizures, ataxia, pulmonary hemorrhage, carditis, anterior uveitis, and episcleritis. Ileoileal intussusception is a complication marked by severe colicky abdominal pain.

The presence of significant nephritis in the initial course of the disease (elevated BUN and persistent high-grade proteinuria) is a potentially serious complication with risk for long-term sequelae, such as hypertension or renal insufficiency. The nephritis can progress to end-stage renal disease in 1% to 7% of children with the disease (Chen and Mao, 2015).

Patient and Parent Education. The provider should educate patients and parents about the illness, its complications, and the risk of recurrence; the need to closely monitor for signs of complications and recurrent disease; and the importance of monitoring blood pressure and follow-up visits to evaluate for renal disease and hypertension (Chen and Mao, 2015).

Kawasaki Disease

KD (also known as *mucocutaneous lymph node syndrome* or *infantile polyarteritis*) presents as an acute febrile illness and is the leading cause of acquired heart disease. It is the second most common childhood vasculitis with a varying incidence from country to country, with Japan having the highest incidence of 264.8/100,000 in 2012 in children from 0 to 4 years (Son and Newburger, 2018). In contrast, the rate of KD in the United States has remained stable

at 19/100,000. Children of Asian/Pacific Islander descent have the highest rate of hospitalization in the United States, pointing to the role genetics play in the disease (Cohen and Sundel, 2016). In terms of risk factors for coronary artery disease (CAD), the rate is higher at age <6 months or >9 years and in males. Children of Asian, Pacific Islander, and Hispanic descent have poor outcomes. Laboratory parameters, such as a thrombocytopenia, hyponatremia, elevated CRP, neutrophilia, and elevated transaminases, increase the risk of CAD with poor response to IVIG (Son and Newburger, 2018).

The disease is characterized by an acute generalized systemic small and medium vessel vasculitis occurring throughout the body. The infiltration of macrophages in the vasculature is unique to KD. The disease mimics an infectious agent because of seasonal peaks and suggestion of toxin release as the rash resembles an erythroderma. However, the search for an infectious agent has remained elusive. It is proposed that a toxin acts as a superantigen that activates T cells, causing a massive release of cytokines and subsequent inflammation. The present hypothesis is that in genetically susceptible individuals, the infectious agent triggers the inflammatory cascade. Unfortunately, no single genetic marker has been found (Cohen and Sundel, 2016).

There are three vasculopathic processes in the arterial wall. The first phase is an acute arteritis with marked neutrophil infiltration within the lumen of the vessel causing necrosis of all vessel layers. A subacute or chronic vasculitis begins weeks after the fevers and can be seen months or years later. It is closely associated with a third phase marked by luminal myofibroblastic proliferation, which originates in the adventitia and involves cytotoxic T lymphocytes, and can result in coronary artery stenosis (Newburger et al., 2016).

KD exhibits geographic and seasonal outbreaks, in the late winter and early spring. Person-to-person spread is low. The original criteria for KD described in 1967 are still the same and include a persistent fever for at least 5 days plus four of the following: bilateral conjunctival injection, changes of the lips and oral cavity, cervical lymphadenopathy, polymorphous exanthema, and changes in the peripheral extremities (swelling of the hands or feet) or perineal area (Newburger, 2017a).

KD supplemental laboratory criteria were identified to help in diagnosing cases of incomplete KD. The six components that need to be present in a patient with suspected KD but an incomplete diagnosis include: (1) albumin ≤3.0 g/dL; (2) urine ≥10 WBC/HPF; (3) platelet count ≥450,000 after 7 days of fever; (4) anemia consistent with age values; (5) total white blood cell count ≥15,000/mm³; and (6) elevation of alanine aminotransferase.

Atypical KD should be reserved for children who lack some of the classic findings, have findings that are not usually present in KD, including Kawasaki shock syndrome, and have findings previously listed under clinical findings (Zhu and Ang, 2016; Pilania, Bhattarai, Singh, 2018). Children with atypical or incomplete KD have the same, if not higher, risk of cardiac involvement.

Clinical Findings

The course of the disease is triphasic with an acute phase characterized by conjunctival hyperemia sparing the limbus, erythematous rash, edema of the hands and feet, a polymorphous erythematous rash, and unilateral lymph nodes. The subacute phase begins when the fever, rash, and cervical lymphadenopathy abate. Arthralgias with desquamation of the skin over the tips of the finger, thrombocytosis, and cardiac disease then tend to occur. In the final or convalescent phase, starting at around day 25 of illness, signs of disease are absent but there is still a marked elevation of the ESR. The cardiac findings include abnormalities of the coronary vessels, and myocarditis is almost universal (Pilania et al., 2018).

In addition to criteria previously mentioned, children, particularly with atypical KD, may have other findings involving the respiratory, musculoskeletal, GI, CNS, and genitourinary systems. They may have peribronchial and interstitial infiltrates or pulmonary nodules on chest x-ray. There may be arthralgia or arthritis as well as diarrhea, vomiting, abdominal pain, hepatitis jaundice, hydrops of the gallbladder, and pancreatitis. CNS findings may include irritability, aseptic meningitis, peripheral facial nerve palsy, and sensorineural hearing loss. There may be a urethritis or meatal redness (Son and Newburger, 2018). Other findings include anterior uveitis, retropharyngeal phlegmon, desquamating rash in the groin or erythema, and induration at the site of bacilli Calmette-Guerin (BCG) vaccination (Kuo, 2017).

Diagnostic Studies. KD is a diagnosis of exclusion. Results of lab investigations are not diagnostic, but rather help rule in another diagnosis. A CBC with differential and platelet count, a comprehensive metabolic profile, ESR, and CRP should be done. It is important to use the laboratory criteria previously mentioned to elucidate the diagnosis of incomplete KD. Laboratory findings include neutrophilia with bands; an elevation of acute-phase reactions such as ESR, CRP, and platelets; elevated serum transaminase levels; hypoalbuminemia; abnormal plasma lipid levels; and anemia and leukocytosis in synovial fluid. Leukopenia and thrombocytopenia in KD may occur in association with the life-threatening MAS.

Differential Diagnosis

Differential diagnoses include viral infections (e.g., measles, adenovirus, EBV, enterovirus, influenza, or roseola); bacterial infections (e.g., cervical adenitis, scarlet fever); toxin-mediated diseases (staphylococcal scalded skin syndrome, toxic shock syndrome), hypersensitivity reactions (drug hypersensitivity reactions, Stevens Johnson Syndrome) or acrodynia (mercury toxicity); and sJIA (Son and Newburger, 2018).

Management

- Early diagnosis is essential to prevent aneurysms in the coronary and extraparenchymal muscular arteries. Treatment goals include: (1) evoking a rapid anti-inflammatory response; (2) preventing coronary thrombosis by inhibiting platelet aggregation; and (3) minimizing long-term coronary risk factors by exercise, a heart-healthy diet, and smoking prevention. The child should be referred for initial treatment that includes the following medications and agents (Cohen and Sundel; 2016):
  - IVIG therapy (a single dose of 2 g/kg over 8 to 12 hours, ideally in the first 10 days of the illness) to control vascular inflammation. IVIG has immunomodulatory effects that cause down-regulation of antibodies and proinflammatory cytokines, augmentation of suppressor T-cell activity, as well as saturation of Fc receptors. Retreatment with immunoglobulin is done when the initial IVIG does not reduce the inflammation.
  - While ASA has no effect on coronary artery aneurysm (CAA) formation, it does have an antiplatelet effect. The American Heart Association recommends high-dose aspirin be given for its anti-inflammatory properties (80 to 100 mg/kg/day in four divided doses, every 6 hours initially) until afebrile for at least 48 to 72 hours, then lowering the aspirin dose to 3 to 5 mg/kg/day for 6 to 8 weeks with discontinuation if the echocardiogram is normal. If significant coronary artery abnormalities develop and do not resolve, aspirin or other antiplatelet therapy is used indefinitely.

- If a second treatment of IVIG at 2 mg/kg over 12 hours is not successful, then prednisolone (corticosteroids) has been used (with greater success in Japan than in the United States). Other agents such as cyclophosphamide, anakinra, rituximab, and plasmapheresis may be administered.
  - If coronary aneurysm is present, then antiplatelet agents and anticoagulants, such as warfarin or clopidogrel, may be used as an adjuvant to aspirin (Cohen and Sundel, 2016).
- A baseline echocardiogram should be obtained as soon as the diagnosis is established, with subsequent studies at 2 weeks and 6 to 8 weeks after onset of illness. Cardiac MRI may give a better view of anatomy and cardiac function; CT angiography, while an alternative, involves too much radiation (Dietz et al., 2017).
- All children on chronic aspirin therapy should receive inactivated influenza vaccination. If varicella or influenza develops, aspirin treatment should be stopped for 6 weeks and another antiplatelet drug substituted to minimize the risk of Reye syndrome.
- Live virus vaccines should be delayed until 11 months after administration of IVIG (AAP Red Book, 2018).
- Children without coronary or cardiac changes should be followed by a cardiologist during the first year after the onset of KD. If there are no cardiac changes during that first year, then the PCP may follow the patient with no activity restrictions imposed at that point.
- Patients with any range of transient coronary artery dilation (including giant aneurysms) should be followed by a cardiologist for years; physical activity limitations may be imposed.
- Follow and counsel all KD patients about a heart-healthy diet.

Complications and Prognosis

The acute disease is self-limited; however, during the initial stage (acute phase), inflammation of the arterioles, venules, and capillaries of the heart occurs and can progress to CAA in 15% to 25% of untreated children (<5% when treated appropriately). The process of aneurysm formation and subsequent thrombosis or scarring of the coronary artery may occur as late as 6 months after the initial illness. Other possible complications include recurrence of KD (<2%); CHF or massive myocardial infarction; myocarditis or pericarditis, or both (30%); pericardial effusion; and mitral valve insufficiency. Children with a giant CAA can have thrombosis within the CAA as well as stenosis distal or proximal to the CAA calcifications (Dietz et al., 2017).

Although around 50% of the aneurysms of the coronary artery tend to regress after two years, there is myointimal thickening and stenosis seen in the segment adjacent to the giant aneurysm and in areas of resolved aneurysms. While the stenosis regresses over years, collateral arteries develop that prevent symptoms. The use of percutaneous coronary intervention and coronary artery bypass grafting can be used if there is ischemic heart disease (Newburger, 2017b). Prompt treatment of chest pain, dyspnea, extreme lethargy, or syncope is always warranted.

Pediatric Primary Immunodeficiency Disorders

Immunodeficiency is a failure of one part of the body's defense mechanism resulting in recurrent infection of variable degrees and associated with morbidity and mortality. Primary immunodeficiency disorder (PIDD) is caused by hereditary or genetic defects.

They may be present at birth or in early childhood and affect a single part of the immune system or one or more of its components. These disorders or diseases differ in presentation depending on the type of defect that alters the functions of the body's normal immune system.

The World Health Organization currently recognizes over 350 inborn errors of immunity, with others emerging (Picard et al., 2018). The rapid expansion in this field is due to next-generation sequencing, which has increased the identification of inborn errors of immunity, which underlie the development of PIDDs. A free application can be found as "PID phenotypical diagnosis" or "PID classification" from iTunes and Android app stores. New PIDD classifications (Picard et al., 2018) include immunodeficiencies affecting cellular and humoral immunity, combined immunodeficiencies associated with syndromic features, predominantly antibody deficiencies, diseases of immune dysregulation, congenital defects of phagocyte number or function, defects in intrinsic and innate immunity, autoinflammatory diseases, complement deficiencies, and phenocopies of inborn error of immunity.

Physiology of the Immune System

In order to understand immunodeficiency, one needs to understand the immune system. There are three lines of defense against antigens: *external barriers*, *innate immunity*, and *adaptive immunity*. *External barriers* that assist the immune defense system are physical and mechanical and include skin and the epithelial lining of the GI tract, genitourinary tract, and respiratory tract. The biochemical barriers include perspiration, tears, saliva, surfactant, hydrochloric acid in the stomach, and normal bacterial flora in our body.

Innate immunity destroys pathogens. The inflammatory reaction occurs after the pathogen-associated molecular patterns (PAMPS) on immune cells recognize invading antigens. The pattern recognition receptors or PRRs are found on epithelial cells and innate immune cells (Hirayama, Iida, and Nakase, 2018). PRRs respond without prior exposure and are activated when there is direct contact with specific microbial products, such as lipopolysaccharides, cell wall components, and microbial nucleotides. Innate immunity is utilized by receptors such as the TLR, which cannot discern the cell from the nonself which trigger defenses that are imprecise and can cause damage to healthy tissue (Yatim and Lakkis, 2015). TLR are germline-encoded PRR and play an import role in host cell recognition and response to microbial pathogens. TLR specifically recognize different kinds of components of antigens and cause a cascade through adapter molecules, which ultimately leads to a greater inflammatory response (Hirayama et al., 2018). Phagocytes including neutrophils, macrophages, and dendritic cells (DCs) have several PRR that specifically bind to certain PAMPs. Macrophages and DCs act as antigen-presenting cells in *adaptive immunity*.

The complement and cytokines signal specific cellular and humoral immunity to aid in host defenses. Complement amplifies the innate immune response by providing critical factors to enhance phagocytosis via opsonin and attracts white cells to the site of inflammation, thereby acting as chemoattractives. Neutrophils form a first line of defense and ingest the infecting organisms, internalizing the organism into an intracellular compartment and releasing bactericidal products. The role of neutrophils in the early inflammation process is primarily phagocytic, resulting in the creation of pus at the site of infection. Monocytes appear at the site of inflammation 1 to 7 days after the initial neutrophil infiltration

and turn to macrophages ingesting and disposing of foreign material, including bacteria. Eosinophils have mild phagocytic activity and help in the regulation of vascular mediators released by mast cells. They play an important role in the hypersensitive allergic response seen in anaphylaxis (Mishra et al., 2018).

Adaptive immunity is a specific process of recognition in which the host responds specifically to a foreign substance, such as a bacterium antigen. DCs are found all over the body and activate adaptive immunity by packaging antigenic peptides into human leukocyte antigens (MHC proteins). This is presented to the T lymphocyte to optimize TCR affinity and specificity. DCs also send out signals to allow for full differentiation of the T lymphocyte. The B and T cells play a major role in this system with T lymphocytes forming the cellular arm and B lymphocytes producing specific antibodies or immunoglobulins. In the initial primary exposure, the antigen exposure to B cells results in antibody formation. This reaction stimulates memory T cells to recognize the antigen for future exposures. Antibodies provide protection against bacterial infections and promote the ingestion of bacteria, as well as the neutralization of bacterial toxins and inactivation of virus. There are different classes of antibodies, with IgM and IgG providing protection against systemic infections and IgA providing protection at mucosa surfaces in the GI, genitourinary, and respiratory tract (Yatim and Lakkis, 2015).

Although cytokines primarily act locally, they mediate innate and adaptive immunity and stimulate T-lymphocyte formation. The T-helper cells recognize antigen by binding to the antigenic fragment displayed by the HLA molecules. T-helper type 1 (Th1) cells are the arm of cellular immunity and activate macrophages, enhance cytotoxic T-cell function, produce cytokines, and recognize the infecting agent. T-helper type 2 cells (Th2) enhance antibody formation by B cells, releasing cytokines, increasing IgE production, and mediating eosinophil recruitment and activation (Yatim and Lakkis, 2015).

The soluble protein components of the immune system, aside from antibodies IgA, IgG, and IgM, include cytokines, chemokines, and complement activation products (blood and cell surface proteins that help antibodies clear pathogens). *Cytokines*, such as interleukin and INF, are critical in the differentiation and maturation of immune cells. Interleukins are biochemical messengers produced by macrophages and lymphocytes and promote the production of leukocytes, induce leukocyte chemotaxis, and cause alteration of adhesion molecule expression on many cells. Interferons protect against viral infection but do not directly kill the antigen; rather they attempt to prevent further infection. They have no effect on cells already infected. Other cytokines, such as TNF-α, are secreted by mast cells and macrophages and initiate fever by the production of prostaglandins and other inflammatory serum proteins. *Chemokines* also promote leukocyte chemotaxis.

Primary and Secondary Immunodeficiency Disorders

Immunodeficiency can be a primary or secondary disorder. PIDDs are rare genetic disorders that typically run in families and can result in chronic debilitating disease. Of the primary immunodeficiency diseases, the B cell line that produces antibodies is the one most commonly associated with these disorders, with IgA deficiency as the most common antibody defect with 1 in 333 to 1 in 18,000 people affected. These patients present with recurrent infections of the respiratory, GI, and urogenital tract (Buckley, 2016a). Table 33.15 shows the immune deficiency and the common clinical presentation.

TABLE 33.15 Selected Pediatric Primary Immunodeficiencies and Their Clinical Presentation

Immunodeficiency	Clinical Presentation
Severe combined immunodeficiency (SCID)	In infancy, persistent thrush, failure to thrive, pneumonia, diarrhea, recurrent difficult-to-treat unusual infections
Wiskott Aldrich syndrome	Thrombocytopenia, bloody stools, draining ears, atopic eczema, recurrent infections with encapsulated organisms, EBV-associated malignancy (Burkitt lymphoma)
Hyper-IgE syndrome	Staphylococcal abscess, pneumatoceles, osteopenia, unusual infection, recurrent otitis and sinusitis, recurrent pneumonias
DiGeorge syndrome	With partial thymic hypoplasia, may have normal course; if no thymus, resemble patients with SCID
Common variable immunodeficiency	Normal or enlarged tonsils, splenomegaly, alopecia areata, thrombocytopenia, sprue-like disease, 438-fold increase in lymphoma
Selective IgA	Infections of respiratory, GI, and genitourinary tracts

EBV, Epstein-Barr virus; *GI,* gastrointestinal; *IgA,* immunoglobulin A; *IgE,* immunoglobulin E.
Adapted from text in Buckley RH. Evaluation of suspected immunodeficiency. In: Kliegman RM, Stanton BF, St. Geme JW, et al, eds. *Nelson Textbook of Pediatrics.* 19th ed. Philadelphia: Saunders/Elsevier; 2016:715–722; Buckley RH. Primary defects of antibody production. In: Kliegman RM, Stanton BF, St. Geme JW, et al, eds. *Nelson Textbook of Pediatrics.* 19th ed. Philadelphia: Saunders/Elsevier; 2016:722–728; and Buckley RH. T lymphocytes, B lymphocytes, and natural killer cells. In: Kliegman RM, Stanton BF, St. Geme JW, et al, eds. *Nelson Textbook of Pediatrics.* 19th ed. Philadelphia: Saunders/Elsevier; 2016:722.

• BOX 33.6 Warning Signs of Primary Immunodeficiency Disorders

Jeffrey Modell Foundation
- Four or more new ear infections within 1 year
- Two or more serious sinus infections within 1 year
- Two or more months on antibiotics with little effect
- Two or more pneumonias within 1 year
- Failure of an infant to gain weight or grow normally
- Recurrent, deep skin or organ abscesses
- Persistent thrush in mouth or fungal infection on skin
- Need for intravenous antibiotics to clear infections
- Two or more deep-seated infections including septicemia
- Family history of primary immunodeficiency

Common PIDDs include selective IgA, IgG subclass deficiencies, transient hypogammaglobulinemia of infancy, and 22q11.2 deletion syndrome (DiGeorge syndrome). Uncommon PIDDs include X-linked agammaglobulinemia (XLA), severe combined immunodeficiencies, complement deficiencies, as well as phagocytic disorders like combined granulomatous disease. Secondary immunodeficiencies can occur due to infections, drugs (e.g., corticosteroids), renal failure, HIV, and leukemia and lymphoma.

The first immunodeficiency described was an XLA. The condition causes deficiency of B cell production that leads to a lack of all types of immunoglobulins. The infant is generally well for the first 1 to 2 months of life: as maternal antibodies start to wane, the child becomes infected with extracellular pyogenic bacteria. Therefore, there is an increased incidence of otitis media, pneumonia, sinusitis, and infections with encapsulated bacteria such as *Haemophilus influenzae* and *Streptococcus pneumoniae* (Buckley, 2016a). While children and adults with XLA can develop severe, life-threatening bacterial infections, they are not particularly vulnerable to infections caused by viruses.

Clinical Presentation

History. A history of unusual, frequent, or recurrent infections is crucial to identify children with PIDDs. It is important to remember that these children do not typically have dysmorphology. While children with B cell disorders have *recurrent* infections, those with defects in T-cell function have a history of *severe* infections. Onset of infection is important and suggests type of cell-line defect: before 6 months of age (T cell); 12 months or later (B cell or a secondary immunodeficiency); and between 6 and 12 months (combined B and T cells or B cell). There may be a sibling who died from sepsis or meningitis, but no workup for immune deficiency was done. A complete family history should be obtained. The child may present with congenital infections but also may present later in infancy, childhood, or adulthood. Box 33.6 contains a list of the 10 warning signs of immunodeficiency (Modell et al., 2018).

Physical Assessment. The child with an immunodeficiency may not have any distinguishing characteristics. Small or absent cervical lymph nodes, adenoids, and/or tonsils may be a sign of XLA. A child with defects of the great vessels, cleft palate, hypognathia, and low, cupped ears may have 22q11.2 deletion syndrome (DiGeorge syndrome). Patients with cutaneous telangiectasia may develop ataxia in early childhood and have recurrent infections.

Diagnostic Studies. The child with an immunodeficiency disorder may present with a low lymphocyte count, low neutrophil count, or a low leukocytes count. It is important to calculate the total neutrophil count. A low IgA is likely to be the most common deficiency. The initial workup includes a complete history and physical examination, a CBC with differential and platelet count, and quantitative immunoglobulins, including IgG, IgA, and IgM. Referral to a specialist in immunology may be needed for further testing, including IgG subclass; candida, pneumococcal, and tetanus skin tests; lymphocyte surface markers—CD3, CD4, CD8, CD19, CD15, and CD16—along with a neutrophil oxidation burst and mononuclear lymphocyte proliferation studies. Table 33.15 addresses the more common immunodeficiency disorders and their clinical presentation. Using the 10 warning signs, the PCP can refer to immunology with stage 1 workup already done (Modell et al., 2018).

Management

Children with immunodeficiency disorders have a higher risk of oncologic disorders as a result of their treatment, which in some cases requires granulocyte stimulation factor. The role of the PCP is to consider immunodeficiency disorders in children with recurrent, persistent, unusual infections and refer to specialists. These children and their families need coordinated health services in a pediatric healthcare home with providers who will support them and act as their advocate and educator for health supervision and health promotion services. It is also important to recognize that infections in children with immunodeficiency may require consultation due to the unusual nature or more persistent course of the infection.

Additional Resources

Advancing Global Immunology Education - Immunopaedic.org. https://www.immunopaedia.org.za/

Allergy and Network—Mothers of Asthmatics, Allergy and Asthma Network—Mothers of Asthmatics, Inc. www.aanma.org

American Academy of Allergy, Asthma, and Immunology. www.aaaai.org

American Academy of Dermatology (Atopic Dermatitis Action Plan). https://www.aad.org/public/diseases/eczema/eczema-resource-center/controlling-eczema/eczema-action-plan

American Autoimmune Related Diseases Association, Inc. 1-800-598-4668 (literature requests). www.aarda.org

American College of Allergy, Asthma, and Immunology. www.acaai.org

American Lung Association. www.lung.org

Arthritis Foundation. www.arthritis.org

Asthma and Allergy Foundation of America. www.aafa.org

Centers for Disease Control and Prevention- ME/CFS. https://www.cdc.gov/me-cfs/healthcare-providers/index.html

Genetic Home Reference. https://ghr.nlm.nih.gov/primer/mutation-sanddisorders/predisposition

Jeffrey Modell Foundation: Primary Immunodeficiency Resource Center. http://jmfworld.com

Lupus Foundation of America, Inc. www.lupus.org

National Asthma Education and Prevention Program. www.nhlbi.nih.gov/about/org/naepp/

National Eczema Association. www.nationaleczema.org

National Heart, Lung, and Blood Institute. www.nhlbi.nih.gov

National Institute of Allergy and Infectious Diseases. www.niaid.nih.gov

National Jewish Health Science Transforming Life. www.nationaljewish.org/healthinfo

Primary Immune Deficiency Foundation. https://primaryimmune.org/about-primary-immunodeficiencies

U.S. Environmental Protection Agency (EPA). www2.epa.gov/asthma

References

AAP and the Committee on Infectious Diseases. Summaries of infectious diseases. In: Kimberlin DW, ed. *Red Book 2018 Report of the Committee on Infectious Diseases*. 30th ed. Elk Gove Villages, IL; 2018.

AAAAI/ACAAI Joint Statement of Support of the ATS Clinical Practice Guideline. *Interpretation of Exhaled Nitric Oxide for Clinical Applications*. 2012. Available at: www.aaaai.org/Aaaai/media/MediaLibrary/PDF%20Documents/My%20Membership/FeNOJointStatement3-6-12.pdf .

Ahmed I, Ahmad NS, Ali S, et al. Medication adherence apps: review and content analysis. *JMIR mHealth uHealth*. 2018;6(3):e62. https://doi.org/10.2196/mhealth.6432.

Ayuk AC, Uwaezuoke SN, Ndukwu CI. Spirometry in asthma care: a review of the trends and challenges in pediatric practice. *Clin Med Insights*. 2017;11:1–6.

Barut K, Sahin S, Kasapcopur O. Pediatric vasculitis. *Curr Opin Pediatr*. 2016;28:29–38.

Bell JM, Shields MD, Watters J, et al. Treatments to prevent and treat thinning of bones and prevent fractures caused by corticosteroids in Duchenne muscular dystrophy. *Cochrane Rev*. 2017. Retrieved from: http://www.cochrane.org/CD010899/NEUROMUSC_treatments-prevent-and-treat-thinning-bones-and-prevent-fractures-caused-corticosteroids-duchenne.

Brunner PM, Leung D, Guttman-Yassky E. Immunologic, microbial, and epithelial interactions in atopic dermatitis. *Ann Allergy Asthma Immunol*. 2018;120:34–41.

Buckley RH. Primary defects of antibody production. In: Kliegman RM, Stanton BF, St. Geme JW, et al., eds. *Nelson Textbook of Pediatrics*. 19th ed. Philadelphia: Saunders/Elsevier; 2016a:715–721.

Buckley RH. Primary defects of cellular immunity. In: Kliegman RM, Stanton BF, St. Geme JW, et al., eds. *Nelson Textbook of Pediatrics*. 19th ed. Philadelphia: Saunders/Elsevier; 2016b:722–738.

Burks AW, Sampson HA, Plaut M, et al. Treatment for food allergy. *J Allergy Clin Immunol*. 2018;141(1):1–9.

Caggiano S, Cutrera R, Di Marco A, et al. Exercise-induced bronchospasm and allergy. *Front Pediatr*. 2017;5:1–9.

Caminati M, Daimmi C, Dama A, et al. What lies beyond asthma control test: suggestions for clinical practice. *J Asthma*. 2016;53(6):559–562.

Chang YS, Chou YT, Lee JH, et al. Atopic dermatitis, melatonin, and sleep disturbance. *Pediatrics*. 2014;134(2):e397–e405.

Chen JY, Mao JH. Henoch-Schonlein purpura nephritis in children: pathogenesis and management. *World J Pediatr*. 2015;11(1):29–34. https://doi.org/10.1007/s12519-014-0535-5.

Chen L, Morris DL, Vyse T. Genetic advances in systemic lupus erythematosus: an update. *Curr Opin Pediatr*. 2017;29:423–433.

Choi M, Flood K, Bernatsky S, et al. A review on SLE and malignancy. *Best Pract Res Clin Rheumatol*. 2017;31:373–396.

Cimaz R. Systemic-onset juvenile idiopathic arthritis. *Autoimmunity Rev*. 2016;15:931–934.

Cohen E, Sundel R. Kawasaki disease at 50 years. *JAMA Pediatr*. 2016;170(11):1093–1099.

Coico R, Sunshine G. *Immunology: A Short Course*. 7th ed. John Wiley: Sons Ltd; 2015.

Dietz SM, van Stijn D, Burgner D, et al. Dissecting Kawasaki disease: a state-of-the-art review. *Eur J Pediatr*. 2017;176:995–1009.

Dinakar C, Chipps BE. Section on allergy and immunology, section on pediatric pulmonology and sleep medicine: clinical tools to assess asthma control in children. *Pediatrics*. 2017;139(1):1–9.

Dinakar C, Oppenheimer J, Portnoy J, et al. Management of acute loss asthma control in the yellow zone: a practice parameter. *Ann Allergy Asthma Immunol*. 2014;113:143–159.

Du Toit G, Roberts G, Sayre P, et al. Randomized trial of peanut consumption in infants at risk for peanut allergies. 372(9):803–813.

Du Toit G, Sampson H, Plaut M, et al. Food allergy: update on prevention and tolerance. *J Allergy Clin Immunol*. 2018;141(1):30–40.

Dweik RA, Boggs PB, Erzurum SC, et al. An official ATS clinical practice guideline: interpretation of exhaled nitric oxide levels (FENO) for clinical applications. *Am J Respir Crit Care Med*. 2011;184(5):602–615.

Dykewicz MS, Wallace DV, Baroody F, et al. Treatment of seasonal allergic rhinitis: an evidence based focused 2017 guidelines update. *Ann Allergy Asthma Immunol*. 2017;17(4):286–294.

Eckert L, Gupta S, Amand C, et al. Impact of atopic dermatitis on health-related quality of life and productivity in adults in the United States: an analysis using the national health and wellness Survey. *J Am Acad Dermatol*. 2017;77(2):274e–279e.

Edwards M, Strong K, Cameron A, et al. Viral infections in allergy and immunology: how allergic inflammation influences viral infections and illness. *J Allergy Clin Immunol*. 2017;140(4):909–920.

Eichenfield LF, Gold LF. The disease burden of atopic dermatitis. *Semin Cutan Med Surg*. 2017a;36(S4):S92–S94.

Eichenfield LF, Ahluwalia J, Waldman A, et al. Current guidelines for the evaluation and management of atopic dermatitis: a comparison of the Joint Task force Practice Parameter and American Academy of Dermatology guidelines. *J Aller Clin Immunol*. 2017b;139(4S):S49–S57.

Eichenfield LF, Gold LF. Systemic therapy of atopic dermatitis: welcome to the revolution. *Semin Cutan Med Surg*. 2017c;36(S4):S103–S107.

Eichenfield LP, Boguniewicz M, Simpson EL, et al. Translating atopic dermatitis management guidelines into practice for primary care providers. *Pediatrics*. 2015;136:554–565.

Eichenfield LF, Tom WL, Berger TG, et al. Guidelines of care for the management of atopic dermatitis with topical therapies. *J Am Acad Dermatol*. 2014;71(1):116–132.

Eleftheriou D, Brogan PA. Therapeutic advances in the treatment of vasculitis. *Pediatr Rheum*. 2016;14:26–36.

Farzan N, Vijverber S, Kabesch M, et al. The use of pharmacogenomics, epigenomics, and transcriptomic to improve childhood asthma: where do we stand?. *Pediatr Pulmonol*. 2018:1–10. Epub ahead of print.

Fitzsimons R, van der Poel L, Thornhill W, et al. Antihistamine use in children. *Arch Dis Child Educ Pract Ed*. 2015;100:122–131.

Gewitz MH, Baltimore RS, Tani LY, et al. on behalf of the American Heart Association Committee on Rheumatic Fever, Endocarditis, and Kawasaki Disease of the Council on Cardiovascular Disease in the Young. Revision of the Jones Criteria for the diagnosis of acute rheumatic fever in the era of Doppler echocardiography: a scientific statement from the American Heart Association. *Circulation*. 2015;131(20):1806–1818.

Giancane G, Alongi A, Ravelli A. Update on the pathogenesis and treatment of juvenile idiopathic arthritis. *Curr Opin of Pediatr*. 2017;29:523–529.

Global Initiative for Asthma. *Global Strategy for Asthma Management and Prevention*. 2018. Available from: www.ginasthma.org.

Gold LF, Eichenfield LF. Topical therapy for atopic dermatitis: new and investigational agents. *Semin Cutan Med Surg*. 2017;36(S4):S99–S100.

Heineke MH, Ballering AV, Jamin A. New insights in the pathogenesis of immunoglobulin A vasculitis (Henoch-Schonlein purpura). *Autoimmunity Rev*. 2017;16:1246–1253.

Hirayama D, Iida T, Nakase H. The phagocytic function of macrophage-enforcing innate immunity and tissue homeostasis. *Int J Molecular Sci*. 2018;19:1–14.

Huffaker M, Phipantanakul W. Pediatric asthma: guidelines-based care, omalizumab and other potential biologic agents. *Immunol Allergy Clin N Am*. 2015;35:129–144.

IOM (Institute of Medicine). *Beyond myalgic Encephalomyelitis/Chronic Fatigue Syndrome: Redefining an Illness*. Washington, DC: The National Academies Press; 2015.

Jay GW, Barkin RL. Fibromyalgia. *Dis Month*. 2015;61:66–111.

Just J, Bourgoin-Heck M, Amat F. Clinical phenotypes in asthma during childhood. *Clin Exp Allergy*. 2017;47:848–855.

Kashikar-Zuck S, Ting TV. Juvenile fibromyalgia: current status of research and future developments. *Nat Rev Rheumatol*. 2014a;10(2):89–96.

Kashikar-Zuck S, Cunningham N, Sil S, et al. Long-term outcomes of adolescents with juvenile-onset fibromyalgia in early adulthood. *Pediatrics*. 2014b;133(3):e592–e600.

Kaslovsky R, Sadof M. Spirometry for the primary care Pediatrician. *Pediatr Rev*. 2014;35(11):465–475.

Kaur S, Singh V. Asthma and Medicines – Long-term side-effects, monitoring and dose titration. *Ind J Pediatr*. 2018. Epub ahead of print.

Kuo CF, Grainge MJ, Valdes AM, et al. Familial aggregation of systemic lupus erythematosus and coaggregation of autoimmune diseases in affected families. *JAMA Int Med*. 2015;175(9):1518–1526.

Kuo H. Preventing coronary artery lesions in Kawasaki disease. *Biomed J*. 2017;40:141–146.

Larun L, Brurberg KG, Odgaard-Jensen J, et al. Exercise therapy for chronic fatigue syndrome. *Cochrane Database Syst Rev*. 2016;2:CD003200.

Lerkvaleekul B, Treepongkaruna S, Saisawat P, et al. Henoch-Schonlein purpura from vasculitis to intestinal perforation: a case report and literature review. *World J Gastroenterol*. 2016;22(2):6089–6094.

Lewis KA, Brown SA, Tiziana S. Sociocultural considerations in juvenile arthritis: a review. *J Pediatr Nurs*. 2017;37:13–21.

Licari A, Castagnoli R, Panfili E, et al. An update on Anti-IgE therapy in pediatric respiratory diseases. *Curr Respir Med Rev*. 2017;13:22–29.

Lo MS, Tsokos GC. Recent developments in systemic lupus erythematosus and applications for therapy. *Curr Opin Pediatr*. 2017;29:1–7.

Loebel M, Grabowski P, Heidecke H, et al. Antibodies to β adrenergic and muscarinic cholinergic receptors in patients with chronic fatigue syndrome. *Brain Behav Immun*. 2016;52:32–39.

Lowe AJ, Leung D, Tang M. The skin as a target for prevention of the atopic march. *Ann Allergy Asthma Immunol*. 2018;120:145–151.

Lyons JJ, Milner JD, Stone K. Atopic dermatitis in children: clinical features, pathophysiology, and treatment. *Immunol Allergy Clin N Am*. 2015;35:161–183.

Maness D, Martin M, Mitchell G. Poststreptococcal illness: recognition and management. *J Amer Fam Physician*. 2018;97(8):517–522.

Mastrorilli C, Posa D, Cipriani F, et al. Asthma and allergic rhinitis in childhood: what's new. *Pediatr Allergy Immun*. 2016;27:795–803.

Mehta J, Beukelman T. Biologic agents in the treatment of childhood-onset rheumatic disease. *J Pediatr*. 2017;189:31–39.

Metsala J, Lundqvist A, Virta LJ, et al. Prenatal and post-natal exposure to antibiotics and risk of asthma in childhood. *Clin Exp Allergy*. 2015;45:137–145.

Mishra V, Banga J, Silveyra P. Oxidative stress and cellular pathways of asthma and inflammation: therapeutic strategies and pharmacological targets. *Pharm Ther*. 2018;181:169–182.

Modell V, Orange JS, Quinn J, Modell F. Global report on primary immunodeficiencies: 2018 update from the Jeffrey Modell Centers Network on disease classification, regional trends, treatment modalities, and physician reported outcomes. *Immunol Res*. 2018;66(3):367–380. https://doi.org/10.1007/s12026-018-8996-5.

Mok CC. Calcineurin inhibitors in systemic lupus erythematosus. *Best Practice Res Clin Rheumatol*. 2017;31:429–438.

National Heart, Lung, and Blood Institute (NHLBI). *Full Report of the Expert Panel: Guidelines for the Diagnosis and Management of Asthma*. 2007. Available at: www.nhlbi.nih.gov/files/docs/guidelines/asthgdln.pdf.

Newburger JW. Kawasaki disease: state of the art. *Cong Heart Dis*. 2017a;12:633–635.

Newburger JW. Kawasaki disease: medical therapies. *Cong Heart Dis*. 2017b;12:641–643.

Newberger JW, Takahashi M, Burns J. Kawasaki disease. *J Amer College of Cardiol*. 2016;67:1737–1749.

Nigrovic P, Raychaudhuri S, Thompson SD. Genetics and the classification of arthritis in adults and children. 2018;70(1):7–17.

Ong PY. Moving toward a more precise treatment of atopic dermatitis. *Ann Allergy Asthma Immuno*. 2018;120:3–4.

Oetijen LK, Kim BS. Interactions of the immune and sensory nervous systems in atopy. *FEBS J*. 2018. https://doi.org/10.1111/febs.14465.

Paramesh H. Air pollution and allergic airway disease: social determinant and sustainability in the control and prevention. *Indian J Pediatr*. 2018;85(4):284–294.

Parks CG, de souza Espindola Santos A, Barbhaiya M, et al. Understanding the role of environmental factors in the development of systemic lupus erythematosus. *Best Pract Res Clin Rheumatol*. 2017;31:306–320.

Perkin MR, Logan K, Tseng A. EAT Study Team: randomized trial of introduction of allergenic foods in breast-fed infants. *N Engl J Med*. 2016;374:1733–1743.

Picard C, Gaspar HB, Al-Herz W, et al. International Union of Immunological Societies, 2017 Primary Immunodeficiency Disease Committee Report on Inborn error of Immunity. *J Clin Immunol*. 2018;38:96–128.

Pilania RK, Bhattarai D, Singh S. Controversies in the diagnosis and management of Kawasaki disease. *World J Clin Pediatr*. 2018;7(1):27–35.

Porcaro F, Corsello G, Pajno G. SLIT's prevention of the allergic march. *Curr Allergy Asthma Rep*. 2018;18:31. https://doi.org/10.1007/s1182-018-0785-7.

Pustisek N, Yurnek Zivkovic M, Situm M. Quality of life in families with children with atopic dermatitis. *Pediatr Derm*. 2016;33(1):28–32.

Rice JL, Diette GB, Suarez-Cuervo C, et al. Allergen-specific immunotherapy in the treatment of pediatric asthma: a systematic review. *Pediatr*. 2018;141(5):e20173833.

Sadun RE, Ardoin SP, Schanberg LE. Systemic lupus erythematosus (pp1176-1180). In: Kliegman RM, Stanton B, St. Geme J, Schor NF, ed. *Nelson Textbook of Pediatrics*. 20th ed. Philadephia: Elsevier; 2016.

Sahai S, Adams M, Kamat D. A diagnostic approach to autoimmune disorders: clinical manifestations: part 1. *Pediatr Ann*. 2016;45(6):e223–e271.

Sayaseng K, Vernon P. Pathophysiology and management of mild to moderate pediatric atopic dermatitis. *J Pediatr Healthcare*. 2018;32(8):S1–S13.

Schneider L, Tiles S, Lio P, et al. Atopic dermatitis: a practice parameter update 2012. *J Allergy Clin Immunol*. 2013;131(2):295–299.

Seidman MD, Gurgel RK, Lin SY, et al. Clinical practice guideline: allergic rhinitis. *Otolaryng—Head Neck Surg.* 2015;152(IS):S1–S43.

Sheehan WJ, Mauger DT, Paul IM, et al. Acetaminophen versus ibuprofen in young children with mild persistent asthma. *N Engl J Med.* 2016;375:619–630.

Shenoi S. Juvenile idiopathic arthritis—changing times, changing terms, changing treatments. *Pediatr Rev.* 2017;38(5):221–231.

Siegel DM, Gewanter HL, Sahai S. Rheumatologic Diseases (Chapter 324). In: McInerny TM, Adam HM, Campbell DE, DeWitt TG, Foy JM, Kamat DM, ed. *American Academy of Pediatrics Textbook of Pediatric Care.* 2nd ed. American Academcy of Pediatrics; 2017.

Sika-Paotonu D, Beaton A, Raghu A, et al. Acute rheumatic fever and rheumatic heart disease, (2-016). In: Ferretti JJ, Stevens DL, Fishetti VA, eds. *Streptococcus Pyogenes: Basic Biology to Clinical Manifestations [Internet].* Oklahoma City University of Health Science Center; 2016.

Sherry DD, Brake L, Tress J, et al. The treatment of juvenile fibromyalgia with an intensive physical and psychosocial program. *J Pediatr.* 2015;167(3):731–737.

Sotzny F, Blanco J, Capelli E, et al. myalgic encephalomyelitis/chronic fatigue syndrome – evidence for an autoimmune disease. *Autoimmunity Rev.* 2018. pii: S1568-9972(18)30088-0. Epub ahead of print.

Son MF, Newburger JW. Kawasaki disease. *Pediatr Rev.* 2018;39:7990.

Stenson EK, Tchou MJ, Wheeler DS. Management of acute asthma exacerbations. *Curr Opin Pediatr.* 2017;29:205–310.

Swart JF, deRoock S, Prakken B. Understanding inflammation in juvenile idiopathic arthritis: how immune biomarkers guide clinical strategies in the systemic onset subtype. *Euro J Immunol.* 2017;46:2068–2077.

Taketomo CK, Hodding JH, Kraus DM. *Pediatric & Neonatal Dosage Handbook.* 24th ed. Hudson, OH: Lexi-Comp; 2018.

Tharp CA, Kemp SF. Pediatric allergic rhinitis. *Immuno Allergy Clin N Am.* 2015;35:185–198.

Tollefson MM, Bruckner AL. Section on dermatology: atopic dermatitis: skin-directed management. *Pediatrics.* 2014;134(6):e1735–e1744.

Tom WL. Food allergy and atopic dermatitis: fellow travelers or triggers? *Semin Cutan Med Surg.* 2017;36(S4):S95–S97.

Tomas C, Newton J. Metabolic abnormalities in chronic fatigue syndrome: a mini review. *Biochem Soc Transactions.* 2018. pii: BST20170503. Epub ahead of print.

Toskala E. Immunology. *Inter Forum Allerg Rhino.* 2018;4(52):S21–S26.

U. S. Department of Health and Human Services. Publication No 2011-135 Get Valid Spirometry Results Every Time. Assessed May 4, 2018: https://www.cdc.gov/niosh/docs/2011-135/pdfs/2011-135.pdf

Wang Z, Pianosi PT, Keogh KA, et al. The diagnostic accuracy of fractional exhaled nitric oxide testing in asthma: a systematic review and meta-analyses. *Mayo Clin Proc.* 2018;93(2):191–198.

Weinberger M, Hendeles L. Nonprescription medications for respiratory symptoms: facts and marketing fictions. *Allergy Asthma Proc.* 2018;39(3):169–173.

Wheatley LM, Togias A. Allergic rhinitis. *NEJM.* 2015;372(5):450–463.

Wyber R, Zuhlke L, Carapetis J. The case for global investment in rheumatic heart-disease control. *Bull World Health Organ.* 2014;92(10):768–770.

Yang SY, Kim YH, Byun MK, et al. Repeated measurement of fractional exhaled nitric oxide is not essential for asthma screening. *J investing allergol Clin Immunol.* 2018;28(2):98–105.

Yatim KM, Lakkis FG. A brief journey through the immune system. *Clin J Am Soc Nephrol.* 2015;10:1274–1281.

Yunus MB, Masi AT. Juvenile primary fibromyalgia syndrome: a clinical study of thirty-three patients and matched normal controls. *Arthritis Rheum.* 1985;28(2):138–145.

Zahran HS, Bailey CM, Damon S, et al. Vital signs: asthma in children—United States, 2001–2016. *MMWR.* 2018;67:1–4.

Zemel L, Blier PR. Juvenile fibromyalgia: a primary pain, or pain processing, disorder. *Sem Pediat Neurol.* 2016;23:231–241.

Zhu RH, Ang JY. The clinical diagnosis and management of Kawasaki disease: a review and update. *Curr Infec Dis Rep.* 2016;18:32–40.

34
Dermatologic Disorders

TAMI B. BLAND

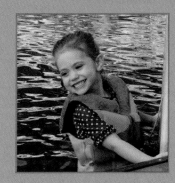

The skin is the body's largest organ and one of its most important as alterations in skin appearance can not only reflect overall health but also give clues to underlying conditions.

Anatomy and Physiology

The skin is composed of two layers with an underlying subcutaneous layer (Fig 34.1). The *epidermis*, a thinner outer layer, functions as a protective barrier between the body and the environment and is composed of five layers of stratified squamous epithelium. Most epidermal cells are keratinocytes, and the replication and maturation of the keratinocytes is called *keratinization*. New keratinocytes of the basal layer mature and are shed approximately every 28 days. The outer horny layer is called the *stratum corneum* and is responsible for much of the barrier protection against microorganisms and irritating chemicals. It impedes the exchange of fluids and electrolytes with the environment and provides strength for the skin. Ambient moisture influences the epidermal barrier, with either excess or inadequate amounts contributing to microscopic and macroscopic breaks. Melanin protects deoxyribonucleic acid (DNA) from damage by ultraviolet (UV) light irradiation. It is produced in the basal layer of the epidermis and contributes to the color of the skin, eyes, and hair.

The *dermis* is the thicker middle layer that contributes strength, support, and elasticity to the skin. It is a tough, leathery mechanical barrier that also regulates heat loss, provides host defenses of the skin, and aids in nutrition and other regulatory functions. The dermis is primarily composed of fibrous connective tissue (made up of fibroblasts and collagen), with some elastic fibers and a mucopolysaccharide gel. It includes mast cells, inflammatory cells, blood and lymph vessels, and cutaneous nerves that elicit sensations. These specialized receptors are a defense mechanism to protect the skin surface from environmental trauma.

Underlying the dermis is subcutaneous tissue primarily composed of adipose tissue. It contains arteries and arterioles that assist in skin thermoregulation. The subcutaneous tissue insulates and cushions the body from trauma, provides energy, and metabolizes hormones.

Skin appendages include the hair, nails, sweat glands, and sebaceous glands. Hairs are threads of keratin. Hair follicles are found over the entire body except for the palms, soles, knuckles, distal and interdigital spaces, lips, glans and prepuce of the penis, and areolae and nipples of the breast. Two types of hair can be found on the body. Terminal hair is thick, visible, and found on the scalp, axillae, and pubis. Very fine vellus hair is found over the remainder of the body. The visible portion of the hair is the shaft.

The hair root is embedded in the dermis as a pilosebaceous unit, consisting of a hair follicle and a sebaceous gland. The hair shaft may be straight, wavy, helical, or spiral. *Sebaceous glands* are usually attached to hair follicles. They are distributed over the entire body except the soles, palms, and dorsa of the feet and are most abundant on the scalp and face. These glands secrete *sebum* (an oily, lipid substance) when stimulated by androgen and function to prevent excessive water evaporation, minimize heat loss, and lubricate the skin and hair.

Nails are epidermal cells converted to keratin that grow continually. The nailbed, underneath the nail plate, is composed of layers of epidermis and dermis, which serve as structural support. The nail root lies just under the epidermis.

There are three types of sweat glands. *Eccrine glands* are distributed over the entire body. They help maintain fluid and electrolyte balance and body temperature and provide some excretory function. *Ceruminous glands* are located in the external ear canal and secrete a waxy pigmented substance called cerumen. *Apocrine glands* are located primarily in the axillary, genital, and periumbilical areas. They open into hair follicles, require androgens to stimulate their secretions, and are thought to be responsible for body odor.

Pathophysiology and Defense Mechanisms

Disruption of the skin and subcutaneous tissue can result from:
- Bacterial, fungal, and viral infections
- Allergic and inflammatory reactions
- Infestations
- Vascular reactions
- Papulosquamous/bullous eruptions
- Congenital lesions
- Hair and nail disorders

There are three cutaneous reactions to trauma, infection, or inflammation. *Pigment lability* occurs as postinflammatory hypopigmentation or hyperpigmentation. If superficial, with changes in the epidermis only, normal pigmentation returns in about 6 months (e.g., in diaper rash, seborrhea, tinea, or pityriasis alba). If dermal changes happen, dermal tattooing may occur, causing long-term or permanent changes (e.g., excoriated acne, impetigo, varicella, and contact dermatitis). A *follicular response* results in prominent papule and follicle formation, especially with atopic dermatitis, pityriasis rosea, syphilis, or tinea versicolor. A *mesenchymal* response, which often follows varicella, ear piercing, burns, or any surgical procedure may cause scars and/or keloids. Keloids are scars that thicken and extend beyond the margins of the initial injury.

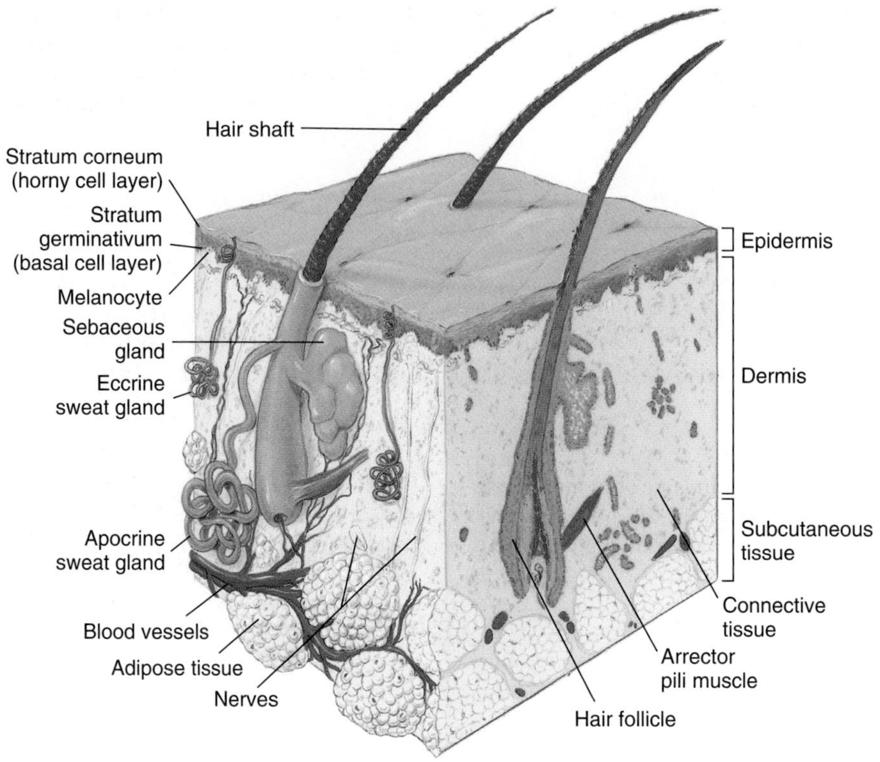

• **Fig 34.1** Structure of the Skin. (From Jarvis C. *Physical Examination and Assessment.* 7th ed. St. Louis: Elsevier; 2016.)

Normal Variations and/or Common Skin Problems

Normal variations in children with variations in skin color include:
- Variation in color and texture of skin from one part of the body to another
- Pigmentation of gingiva, mucous membrane, sclera, and nails correlates with degree of cutaneous pigmentation (pigment lability)
- Increased areas of melanin in thicker-skinned areas (elbow, knee)
- The terms *Futcher line* or *Ito line* describes the vertical line that separates the hyperpigmented dorsal and extensor surfaces from less pigmented ventral surfaces; this line of differentiation follows Voigt lines and is most noticeable on the extremities
- Congenital dermal melanocytosis
- Increased numbers of café au lait spots
- Exfoliation can produce a fine layer of gray scales
- Color alterations (jaundice, anemia, cyanosis) are important to assess
- Erythema may appear as a purplish, rather than reddish tinge
- Significant postinflammatory hypopigmentation and hyperpigmentation

Assessment of the Skin and Subcutaneous Tissue

History

The history should assess the following:
  History of present illness
- Onset and duration of present or recent illness
- Related concerns (e.g., pruritus, scaling, cosmetic appearance)

- Symptom analysis:
  - Appearance/progression
    - What did the rash or lesion(s) originally look like? How has it changed in appearance?
    - Is the way it looks today typical of its appearance?
    - Where did the eruption first begin?
    - Has the rash or lesion spread to other locations (pattern of spread)?
    - Has the lesion blistered, bled, or had discharge?
    - Parts of the body not affected by the rash or lesions (e.g., face, soles, palms)
  - Timing
    - How long has the rash been present?
  - Does it come and go? Systemic symptoms (e.g., fever, malaise, pain) associated with lesion or eruption
    - Pruritus
    - Factors that alleviate, trigger, or worsen skin symptoms
  - Exposures
    - Foods, animals, plants, new substances, people with similar symptoms or illness, soaps, hair products, lotions, detergents
    - Allergies to things that could cause skin reactions
    - Medication (prescription and over the counter) taken over the past few days, including creams, ointments, powders, or lotions (It is often helpful to have patients bring medications that they have used to the appointment.)
  - Historical context
    - Prior incidents of a similar rash
    - Recent travel
  How much is the problem affecting your life or feelings about yourself? Review of systems/past medical history
- Usual state of health and recent illnesses
- Skin, hair, and nails: Skin type (dry or oily), recent and long-term changes, previous incidence of skin disease

- Eyes, ears, nose, and throat: Swelling, itching, crusting, discharge or circles around eyes, nasal mucus discharge, patency or irritation, dry mouth, lesions, or pain
- Chest: Wheezing, coughing, or respiratory difficulty
  Chronic illnesses with related dermatologic findings
- Family review of systems
  - Any family member with similar symptoms
  - Skin/atopy disorders/(e.g., asthma, seasonal/drug allergies, atopic dermatitis)
  - Chronic illnesses with dermatologic findings

Physical Examination

The dermatologic examination includes a thorough look at the skin, scalp, hair, palms and soles, nails, and anogenital region. It is important to remember that the entire body, not just exposed skin, needs to be examined.

Good light is essential. Natural daylight is best; however a direct light, such as a gooseneck lamp, is the best alternative. Other helpful tools include a magnifying glass, a ruler, a glass slide, and a Wood's lamp (UV light). A glass slide gently pressed on the skin (diascopy) allows viewing of the skin with and without capillary filling. A Wood's lamp is used to examine fluorescent-positive fungal infections and depigmenting skin disorders, such as vitiligo.

Essential documentation includes:
- Location and type of lesion
- Color/color changes, size, and shape
- Arrangement (e.g., isolated, grouped, linear, annular, zosteriform)
- Pattern (e.g., sun-exposed area, symmetry)
- Distribution (e.g., regional, generalized, crops)
- Border (e.g., indistinct, well-circumscribed)
- Consistency (e.g., firm, soft, mobile)

Primary skin lesions (Box 34.1) arise from previously normal skin. *Secondary* skin lesions (Box 34.2) result from changes in primary skin lesions. *Vascular* skin lesions (Box 34.3) involve the blood supply. Other useful descriptive terms are listed in Box 34.4.

Diagnostic Studies

Proper sample procurement is important. Lesions can be scraped with a No. 15 blade or toothbrush. Scrapings can be obtained from the edges of skin lesions, from plucked hair (getting the root is essential), from the nail plate, or from subungual debris. Scales or debris are then placed on a glass slide or in culture material. The No. 15 blade is also useful for draining blisters. It is important to scrape under scabs to access organisms present. (NOTE: Moistening the lesion may facilitate this.)

• BOX 34.1 Primary Skin Changes to Lesions

Bulla: Vesicle larger than 1 cm
Comedo: Plugged, dilated pore; open (blackhead), closed (whitehead)
Cyst: Palpable lesion with definite borders filled with liquid or semisolid material
Macule: Flat, nonpalpable, discolored lesion, 1 cm or smaller
Nodule: Raised, firm, movable lesion with indistinct borders and deep palpable portion, 2 cm or smaller
Papule: Solid, raised lesion of varied color with distinct borders, 1 cm or smaller
Patch: Macule, larger than 1 cm
Plaque: Solid, raised, flat-topped lesion with distinct borders, larger than 1 cm
Pustule: Raised lesion filled with pus, often in hair follicle or sweat pore
Tumor: Large nodule, may be firm or soft
Vesicle: Blister filled with clear fluid
Wheal: Fleeting, irregularly shaped, elevated, itchy lesion of varied size, pale at center, slightly red at borders

• BOX 34.2 Secondary Skin Changes to Lesions

Atrophy: Thinning skin, may appear translucent
Crusts: Dried exudate or scab of varied color
Desquamation: Peeling sheets of scale
Erosion: Oozing or moist, depressed area with loss of superficial epidermis
Excoriation: Abrasion or removal of epidermis; scratch
Fissure: Linear, wedge-shaped cracks extending into dermis
Keloid: Healed lesion of hypertrophied connective tissue
Lichenification: Thickening of skin with deep visible furrows
Scales: Thin, flaking layers of epidermis
Scar: Healed lesion of connective tissue
Striae: Fine pink or silver lines in areas where skin has been stretched
Ulcer: Deeper than erosion; open lesion extending into dermis

• BOX 34.3 Descriptive Terms for Vascular Skin Lesions

Angioma or hemangioma: Papule made of blood vessels
Ecchymosis: Bruise, purple to brown, macular or papular, varied in size
Hematoma: Collection of blood from ruptured blood vessel, larger than 1 cm
Petechiae: Pinpoint, pink to purple macular lesions that do not blanch, 1-3 mm
Purpura: Purple macular lesion, larger than 1 cm
Telangiectasia: Collection of macular or raised dilated capillaries

• BOX 34.4 Descriptive Terms for Dermatologic Lesions

Acral: Involving extremities (hands, feet, ears, and so on)
Annular: Ring-shaped
Arcuate: Arc-shaped
Circinate: Circular
Confluent: Running together
Contiguous: Touching or adjacent
Diffuse or generalized: Scattered, widely distributed
Discrete: Distinct and separate
Eczematous: Referring to vesicles with oozing crust
Grouped: Arranged in sets
Guttate: Small, droplike
Herpetiform: Referring to grouped vesicles resembling those of herpes
Iris: Arranged in concentric circles, one inside the other
Linear: Arranged in a line
Localized: In a limited area
Nummular: Coin-shaped
Pedunculated: Having a stalk
Polycyclic: Oval with more than one ring
Reticular: Netlike
Serpiginous: Snakelike, creeping
Symmetric: Balanced on both sides
Target lesion (iris or targetoid): Erythematous papule or plaque characterized by a red to violet dusky center surrounded by a raised, edematous pale ring and red periphery
Telangiectatic: Referring to dilated terminal vessels
Umbilicated: Depressed or shaped like a navel
Verrucous: Wartlike
Zosteriform: Resembling shingles, following a nerve root or dermatome

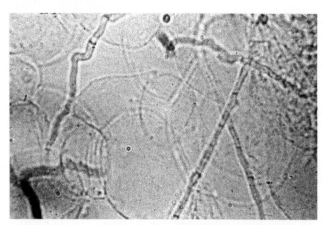

• **Fig 34.2** Fungal elements (hyphae: long septae, branching rods) as seen on microscopic examination of a potassium hydroxide (KOH) preparation. (From Paller A, Mancini, A. *Hurwitz Clinical Pediatric Dermatology: A Textbook of Skin Disorders of Children and Adolescence.* 5th ed. Philadelphia: Elsevier; 2016.)

Laboratory tests can include:
- Complete blood count (CBC) and differential; C-reactive protein (CRP) or erythrocyte sedimentation rate (ESR)
- Microscopic examination of skin scrapings:
  - Potassium hydroxide (KOH) for fungal disorders (hyphae or spores; Fig 34.2).
- Wright, Giemsa, or Wright-Giemsa stains for bacteria, white cells, and multinucleated giant cells (or Tzanck cells found in viral lesions, such as herpes, varicella, or zoster). Microbial culture of lesions for bacteria, viruses, or fungi. Referral for patch/ skin testing for allergic/contact reactions.
- Referral for skin biopsy (punch or shave method).

Management Strategies

Hydration and Lubrication

Adequate skin hydration is essential to prevent and treat skin conditions. If the skin is overhydrated, the bonds between cells at the stratum corneum loosen. If the skin is too dry, it cracks. Both involve breaking the skin barrier. Excessive (greater than 90%) or deficient (less than 10%) humidity can cause disruption of the skin. Macerated skin benefits from less humidity, while itchy dry skin is often relieved by increasing ambient humidity (e.g., using a vaporizer or humidifier). In hot temperatures, itching can be alleviated by air conditioning.

Bathing and Moisturizers

Moisturizers and lubricants treat chronic dryness and inflammation of the skin by retaining water in the skin. There is little evidence to suggest that bathing alone will hydrate skin. Applying emollients/moisturizers immediately after a bath may help to retain the skin moisture, but moisturizers alone may be of the same benefit in most children (Oranje, 2016). Regular bathing reduces scale and debris, cleanses, and eradicates causative organisms of many skin infections, including staphylococcus which is commonly found in individuals with atopic dermatitis. Baths containing baking soda or colloidal oatmeal may relieve pruritus. Bathing and other heat exposures can make a rash seem worse temporarily. Non-allergic, mild soaps or soap substitutes are best. Known irritants, such as bubble bath solutions, should be avoided.

Other Considerations
- Common irritants and sensitizing agents (i.e., wool, sweat, saliva) should be avoided.
- Children with food allergies (such as milk, egg, and peanuts) are more likely to experience eczematous skin manifestations than the general population (Tom, 2017).

Dressings

Wet Dressings

For acute oozing, crusting, or itching skin, wet dressings help dry the skin, decrease itching, and remove crusts. Thin cloths, such as diapers, handkerchiefs, or strips of sheets, make the best wet dressings. Dressings should be moderately wet but not dripping, with lukewarm water and applied for 10 to 20 minutes 2 to 4 times daily over a period of 48 to 72 hours. Alternative solutions include saline (1 teaspoon salt with 1 pint of water) or Burow solution (1 Domeboro tablet [aluminum acetate; calcium acetate] with 1 pint of cool or tepid water). Topical medications applied following wet dressings are absorbed more effectively. Short-term (up to 10 days) topical corticosteroids under the dressing may alleviate pruritus or burning sensations. Care must be taken to prevent excessive steroidal absorption by focused application of steroid only to the affected areas (Paller and Mancini, 2016).

Occlusive Dressings

Occlusive dressings decrease water evaporation from the skin and enhance hydration and absorption of topical medications. Plastic wrap is placed over the affected area after hydrating the skin and/ or applying cream/ointment; these dressings should not be left on longer than 8 hours. Ointments, oils, urea compounds, and propylene glycol used alone may be considered occlusive. Lichen simplex chronicus, dyshidrotic eczema, and psoriasis are skin conditions that benefit from occlusion.

Sunscreens and Sunblocks

Sunscreens and sunblocks protect the skin from UV light. UV radiation is part of the electromagnetic (light) spectrum that reaches the earth from the sun with longer wavelengths that penetrate the skin deeper (UVA) and shorter wavelengths (UVB) with less penetration that cause sunburn. Both wavelengths contribute to premature skin aging, eye damage (including cataracts), and skin cancers as well as immune system suppression. Sunscreens are graded by their ability to provide sun protection. Because skin damage from the sun begins in childhood and is cumulative, daily application of a fragrance-free sunscreen with a sun protection factor (SPF) of 30 is recommended for older infants and up (American Academy of Dermatology [AAD], 2018). Newborns are to be kept out of direct sun exposure. Children who are extremely photosensitive should use sunscreen with levels of SPF 30 or higher. Sunscreens that act by absorbing UVB (burning) light include para-aminobenzoic acid (PABA) or PABA esters, cinnamates, salicylates, benzophenones, and anthranilates. Emerging evidence shows the negative consequences of some chemicals found in sunscreens on our coastal areas, particularly the coral reef biota (Mccoshum, Schlarb, and Baum, 2016).

Sunscreen is never a substitute for sensible sun protection, which includes limiting exposure to intense sun rays. Other protective strategies include wearing protective clothing, hats with visors, and sunglasses with UV protection. Chemical-containing sunscreens should be applied 30 minutes before exposure to the sun to allow binding of the agents to the stratum corneum. Reapply sunscreens after swimming, excessive periods of perspiration, or after washing or showering. To protect the environment, do not wash off sunscreen in lakes or oceans.

Medications

General Considerations

Thought must be given not only to the medication but also to its preparation (Box 34.5) and vehicle (Fig 34.3), including stabilizers, preservatives, and perfumes. Occasionally an individual is sensitive to a medication vehicle or preparation, and symptoms are aggravated rather than relieved. Common agents that cause sensitization include ethylenediamine, lanolin, parabens, thimerosal, diphenhydramine, propylene glycol, "caines," and neomycin. The following guidelines for use of preparations may be helpful:

- Acute inflammation—wet dressings, powders, suspension lotions, alcohol- or water-based lotions, aerosols, or foams
- Chronic inflammation—creams, oil-based lotions or gels, ointments, or foams

---

• BOX 34.5   Preparations of Topical Medications

Creams: Contain more water than oil and therefore are less occlusive; better used with less dry skin, in high-humidity areas, in summertime, and on parts of body that naturally cause occlusion (body folds); often accepted better by patient but must be applied every 2-3 h

Gels: Alcohol based, provide good penetration of skin but can burn on application; primarily used for acne and in hairy areas

Lotions: Mixtures of powder and water, useful for drying, cooling, and soothing actions; *emulsion lotions* contain some oil, so are not as drying as lotions; lotions come in suspension or solution

Oils: Fluid fats that hold medication to the skin as barriers or occlusive agents

Ointments: Best used with dry skin; composed primarily of oil with little or no water; provide most potent concentration of medication because of their occlusive action on skin; generally need to be used only every 12 h; tend to leave a greasy feeling and can cause heat retention from decreased evaporation

Pastes: Made of a combination of powder and oil, which makes them somewhat difficult to apply and remove, but effective in providing dryness and protection for skin

Powders: Absorb moisture and reduce friction, provide cooling, decrease itching, increase evaporation

Shampoos: Liquid soaps or detergents for cleaning the hair and skin (e.g., tar for psoriasis or seborrhea, antifungal shampoos for tinea versicolor or tinea corporis)

Foam: Gas dispersed in a lotion containing one or more active substances; shown to have effective drug delivery; well accepted by most patients and increasing in use

---

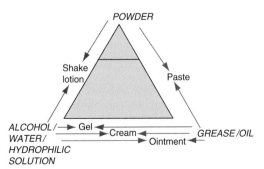

• **Fig 34.3** Vehicles for Dermatologic Therapy. See Box 34.5 for description.

- Patient's tolerance for and willingness to use certain vehicles
- Patient's environment (dry or humid)

All topical medications except powders have enhanced absorption if applied to skin immediately after it has been saturated with water. Occlusion enhances absorption (see previous discussion). Application of the topical medication is best done in one direction, preferably along the hair follicles, without rubbing, applied with a single motion. Use an adequate but not excessive amount.

Antibacterial Agents

Soap, antibacterial soap, and topical antiseptics thoroughly cleanse the skin and reduce the number of bacteria on the skin. Topical antibiotics are applied to treat minor skin infections. Products containing neomycin should be avoided because of the high incidence of contact sensitization. Oral antibiotics may be necessary to treat more significant bacterial skin infections. If methicillin-resistant *Staphylococcus aureus* (MRSA) is suspected, obtain a culture and sensitivity of the drainage (see Chapter 31).

Antifungal Agents

Many topical antifungals are over-the-counter medications. Oral antifungals are used for hair and nail infections or refractory skin infections. Because of concerning side effects and minimal clinical experience in children, oral antifungals should be used with caution in children; many of these drugs are not US Food and Drug Administration (FDA) approved for pediatric use (antifungal agents are listed in Table 34.4).

Antiviral Agents

Topical antivirals are used to control cutaneous herpes infections. Oral antivirals, such as acyclovir, can shorten the course of the infection and can be used in children with acute or recurrent herpetic skin infections.

Wart therapy agents destroy keratinocytes. These include salicylic acid and lactic acid collodion, salicylic plaster, salicylic solution, liquid nitrogen, cantharidin, podophyllum, and trichloroacetic acid.

Anti-Inflammatory Agents

Topical glucocorticoids are frequently used to reduce inflammation, decrease itching, and promote vasoconstriction without causing the widespread systemic effects of oral steroids. They are subdivided into three categories: high potency, moderate potency, and low potency (Table 34.1); and they are classified as fluorinated or nonfluorinated. Nonfluorinated steroids are less potent and have fewer side effects.

The key to using topical steroids is to be familiar with a few low-, medium-, and high-potency steroids and use them consistently. Brand-name preparations often have a more consistent base and potency. Ointments are more potent than creams, creams are more potent than lotions, and foams are more effective in hairy areas. Absorption is enhanced in areas that are traumatized or denuded.

Primary care providers should rarely use high-potency topical steroid preparations. Always use the lowest potency available, use them sparingly, and for the shortest length of time possible. Only low-potency steroids should be used on the face, buttocks, groin, and axillae. Potential side effects of prolonged topical steroid use include skin atrophy, striae, increased fragility of the skin, hypopigmentation, secondary infection, acneiform eruption, folliculitis, miliaria, hypertrichosis, telangiectasia, and purpura. Oral glucocorticoids (prednisone) are used only in acute situations and

TABLE 34.1 Topical Corticosteroids

Class/Potency	Generic Name/Trade Name	Class/Potency	Generic Name/Trade Name
1. High potency ↑↑↑↑	Betamethasone dipropionate augmented 0.05% *Diprolene O/L/G* Clobetasol propionate 0.05% *Clobex L/S/Sp; Cormax O/S; Olux F; Olux-E F; Temovate C/O/G/S; Temovate-E C;* Halobetasol propionate 0.05% *Ultravate C/O* Fluocinonide 0.1% *Vanos C* Flurandrenolide 4 µg/cm² *Cordran tape* Diflorasone diacetate 0.05% O	4. ↑	Flurandrenolide 0.025% *Cordran C* Triamcinolone acetonide 0.1% *Kenalog C* Triamcinolone acetonide 0.2% *Kenalog Sp* Desoximetasone 0.05% C Fluocinolone acetonide 0.025% *Synalar O* Hydrocortisone valerate 0.2% O Mometasone furoate 0.1% *Elocon C/L*
2. ↑↑↑	Amcinonide 0.1% O Betamethasone dipropionate 0.05% *Diprolene AF C, Diprolene C* Diflorasone diacetate 0.05% *ApexiCon E C* Halcinonide 0.1% *Halog C/O* Fluocinonide 0.05% C/O/G/S Desoximetasone 0.25% *Topicort EC/O* Desoximetasone 0.05% *Topicort G* Mometasone furoate 0.1% *Elocon C/O/L* Triamcinolone acetonide 0.5% O	5. ↓↑	Fluocinolone acetonide 0.025% *Synalar C* Clocortolone pivalate 0.01% *Cloderm C* Hydrocortisone valerate 0.2% C Hydrocortisone butyrate 0.1% *Locoid C/O/L/S* Hydrocortisone probutate 0.1% *Pandel C* Prednicarbate 0.1% *Dermatop O/C* Triamcinolone acetonide 0.1% L
3. ↑↑	Fluticasone propionate 0.05% *Cutivate C/L* Fluticasone propionate 0.005% *Cutivate O* Betamethasone valerate 0.1% C/O/L Betamethasone valerate 0.12% *Luxiq F* Amcinonide 0.1% C/O/L Triamcinolone acetonide 0.1% C/O/L Triamcinolone acetonide 0.5% C Desoximetasone 0.05% C Flurandrenolide 0.05% *Cordran C/L*	6. ↓↓	Desonide 0.05% *Verdeso F; DesOwen O/L; Desonide G; Tridesilon C* Hydrocortisone 2.5% C/O/L Fluocinolone acetonide 0.01% *Dermotic Oil; Synalar S; Derma-Smooth/FS oil;* Alclometasone dipropionate 0.05% C/O
		7. ↓↓↓	Triamcinolone acetonide 0.025% C Hydrocortisone 1.0% C/O
		8. Low potency	Hydrocortisone 0.5% C

C, Cream; *EC*, emollient cream; *F*, foam; *G*, gel; *L*, lotion; *O*, ointment; *S*, solution; *Sp*, spray.

From Cohen BA. *Pediatric Dermatology.* 4th ed. Philadelphia: Saunders/Elsevier; 2013, p 11; Bolognia JL, Schaffer, JV, Duncan KO, et al. *Dermatology Essentials.* Saunders/Elsevier; 2014, p 985; Paller, AS, Mancini, AJ. *Hurwitz Clinical Pediatric Dermatology.* 5th ed. Elsevier; 2016, p 51; Karch, AM. *Lippincott Nursing Drug Guide.* Philadelphia: Wolters Kluwer Health; 2015.

are limited to short courses. Intralesional steroid injections may be used by a dermatologist to control localized eczema, lichen planus, or psoriasis. 🖐

Antipruritic Agents

Antihistamines are used both for sedation and to relieve itching. The most commonly used antihistamines are hydroxyzine, cetirizine, fexofenadine, and diphenhydramine. Topical antihistamines, especially diphenhydramine HCl and "caine" medications, should be avoided because of the possibility of contact sensitization.

Calcineurin Inhibitors

This class of immunosuppressive, nonsteroidal anti-inflammatory topical medication is used for short-term or intermittent long-term

treatment of atopic dermatitis when conventional therapy is inadvisable, ineffective, or not tolerated. Immunomodulators are expensive and cannot be used in children younger than 2 years old.

Scabicides and Pediculicides

These agents are toxic to mites and lice. Spinosad, permethrin, and pyrethrin plus piperonyl butoxide are used in children but should be used sparingly. Lindane is no longer recommended for use in children.

Hair and Scalp Preparations

Antimicrobial, tar, keratolytic, and detergent shampoos are used on the hair and scalp when needed for infection, psoriasis, dandruff, dermatitis, or general cleansing.

Bacterial Infections of the Skin and Subcutaneous Tissue

Diagnosis and treatment of common bacterial infections are listed in Table 34.2.

Impetigo

Impetigo is a common contagious bacterial infection of the superficial layers of the skin. It has two forms: nonbullous, with honey-colored crusts on the lesions, and bullous (Fig 34.4). Impetigo is usually caused by group A *streptococcus (Streptococcus pyogenes), S. aureus,* or MRSA. Often streptococcus and staphylococcus can be cultured from an impetigo lesion. Nonbullous impetigo accounts for more than 70% of cases, with *S. aureus* as the most common pathogen. Nonbullous impetigo usually follows some type of skin trauma (e.g., bites, abrasions, or varicella) or another skin disease, such as atopic dermatitis. Bullous impetigo occurs sporadically, develops on intact skin, and is more common in infants and young children. Certain epidermal types of *S. aureus* produce a toxin that causes bullous skin lesions.

Bacterial colonization of the skin occurs several days to months before lesions appear; the organism usually spreads from autoinoculation via hands, towels, clothing, nasal discharge, or droplets. Impetigo occurs more frequently with poor hygiene; during the summer months; in warm, humid climates; and in lower socioeconomic groups. Streptococci that cause pharyngitis rarely cause impetigo and vice versa. Secondary bacterial infections of underlying skin problems (dermatitis, varicella, psoriasis) are most commonly caused by staphylococci (Cohen, 2013).

Clinical Findings

History
- Pruritus, spread of the lesion to surrounding skin, and earlier skin disruption at the site
- Weakness, fever, and diarrhea may accompany bullous impetigo

Physical Examination. The following can be found:
- Nonbullous, classic, or common impetigo—begins as 1- to 2-mm erythematous papules or pustules that progress to vesicles or bullae, which rupture, leaving moist, honey-colored, crusty lesions on mildly erythematous, eroded skin; less than 2 cm in size; little pain but rapid spread
- Bullous impetigo—large, flaccid, thin-wall, superficial, annular, or oval pustular blisters or bullae that rupture, leaving thin varnish-like coating or scale
- Lesions are most common on face, hands, neck, extremities, or perineum; satellite lesions may be found near the primary site, although they can be anywhere on the body
- Regional lymphadenopathy

TABLE 34.2 Diagnosis and Treatment of Common Bacterial Infections

	Causative Organism	Presentation	Area of Involvement	Treatment	Prevention
Impetigo	*Staphylococcus aureus* or *Streptococcus pyogenes*	Honey-colored crust on erythematous base, or blisters that rupture, leaving varnish-like coat	Superficial layers of skin (epidermis)	Topical antibiotic if minor; oral antibiotics (amoxicillin/clavulanate, cephalexin, dicloxacillin, cloxacillin, or clindamycin) if more significant infection	Moisturize skin; thoroughly cleanse any break in skin
Cellulitis	Most commonly group A streptococcus (GAS) or *S. aureus*	Erythema, swelling, tenderness; irregular borders with significant induration resembling an orange peel is associated with GAS	Dermis and subcutaneous tissue	Oral antibiotic depending on likely organism; amoxicillin clavulanate (first-line) or cephalexin or dicloxacillin	Same as above
Folliculitis	*S. aureus*	Pruritus, erythematous papule or pustule at hair follicle	Hair follicle	Warm compresses, topical keratolytics, topical antibiotics, or antistaphylococcal antibiotic if severe	Same as above; good hygiene and antibacterial soap

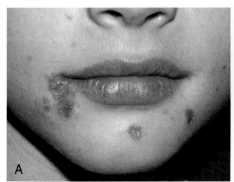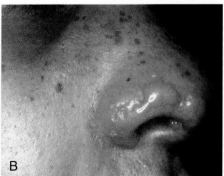

• **Fig 34.4** (A) Nonbullous impetigo. (B) Bullous impetigo. (From Bologia J, Schaffer JV, Duncan KO, et al. *Dermatology Essentials.* Philadelphia: Saunders/Elsevier; 2014.)

Diagnostic Studies. Gram stain and culture are ordered if identification of the organism is needed in recalcitrant or severe cases.

Differential Diagnosis

Herpes simplex, varicella, nummular eczema, contact dermatitis, tinea, kerion, and scabies are included in the differential diagnosis.

Management

Management involves the following:

- Topical antibiotics are preferred if the impetigo is superficial, nonbullous, or localized to a limited area. In localized regions, topical antibiotics such as bacitracin, polymyxin B, and neomycin may be used, but, given the increasing resistance to traditional topical antibiotics, mupirocin and retapamulin are considered better choices for topical treatment (Paller and Mancini, 2016; Weston and Morelli, 2017). Oral antibiotics are recommended for multiple lesions or nonbullous impetigo with infection in multiple family members, child care groups, or athletes. Treat for *S. aureus* and *S. pyogenes* because coexistence is common (Cohen, 2013).
- For widespread infection with constitutional symptoms and deeper skin involvement, use an oral antibiotic active against β-lactamase–producing strains of *S. aureus,* such as amoxicillin/clavulanate, dicloxacillin, cloxacillin, or cephalexin.
  - Cephalexin: 40 mg/kg/d for 7 to 10 days
  - Amoxicillin/clavulanate: 50 to 90 mg/kg/d for 7 to 10 days
  - Dicloxacillin: 15 to 50 mg/kg/d for 7 to 10 days
  - Cloxacillin: 50 to 100 mg/kg/d for 7 to 10 days
  - Clindamycin: 10 to 25 mg/kg/d for 7 to 10 days
- If an infant has bullous impetigo, use parenteral beta-lactamase–resistant antistaphylococcal penicillin, such as methicillin, oxacillin, or nafcillin.
- If there is no response in 7 days, swab beneath the crust, and do Gram stain, culture, and sensitivities. Community-acquired MRSA should be considered. This organism is more susceptible to clindamycin and trimethoprim-sulfamethoxazole (TMP-SMX) (see Chapter 31 for treatment of MRSA).
- Educate regarding cleanliness, hand washing, and spread of disease.
- Exclude from day care or school until treated for 24 hours.
- Schedule a follow-up appointment in 48 to 72 hours if not improved.

Complications

- Cellulitis may occur with nonbullous impetigo and present in the form of ecthyma (infection involving entire epidermis) or erysipelas (spreading cellulitis with induration). Lymphangitis, suppurative lymphadenitis, guttate psoriasis, erythema multiforme, scarlet fever, or glomerulonephritis may occur following infection with some strains of *Streptococcus*. Acute rheumatic fever is a rare complication of streptococcal skin infections.
- Staphylococcal scalded skin syndrome (SSSS) is a blistering disease that results from circulating epidermolytic toxin–producing *S. aureus*. SSSS is most common in neonates (Ritter disease), infants, and children younger than 5 years. It manifests abruptly with fever, malaise, lethargy, poor feeding, and tender erythroderma, especially in the neck folds and axillae, rapidly becoming crusty around the eyes, nose, and mouth. Nikolsky sign (peeling of skin with a light rub to reveal a moist red surface) is a key finding. Treatment may include hospitalization and parenteral antibiotics, especially for young children

(Strom, Hsu and Silverberg, 2017). Antibiotics of choice are intravenous (IV) or oral dicloxacillin, a penicillinase-resistant penicillin, first- or second-generation cephalosporins, or clindamycin. Quicker healing without scarring results if steroids are avoided, there is minimal handling of the skin, and ointments and topical mupirocin are used at the infection site (Bolognia, 2014; Paller and Mancini, 2016). Severe cases may need treatment similar to extensive burn care.

Patient and Family Education

- Thorough cleansing of any breaks in the skin helps prevent impetigo.
- Postinflammatory pigment changes can last weeks to months.
- The patient should not return to school or day care until 24 hours of antibiotic treatment is completed.

Cellulitis

Cellulitis is a localized bacterial infection often involving the dermis and subcutaneous layers of the skin. It is commonly seen following a disruption of the skin surface from an insect or animal bite, trauma, or a penetrating wound. Cellulitis is more common in children with diabetes and immunosuppression. Periorbital cellulitis is discussed in Chapter 35.

In children, cellulitis is often periorbital, perivaginal, perianal, or buccal, or it involves a joint or an extremity. *Streptococcus pneumoniae* and *S. aureus* are the most common causes. Buccal cellulitis and infections over joints are most commonly caused by *Haemophilus influenzae* and occur in children 3 months to 3 years old, but the incidence has decreased since the introduction of the *H. influenza* vaccine (Bolognia et al, 2014). Periorbital and orbital cellulitis are most commonly caused by streptococcal species (*S. pneumoniae* and group A β-hemolytic streptococci [GABHS]). Most cases of cellulitis of the extremities and perianal area are caused by streptococci or *S. aureus*. MRSA can also cause cellulitis with pus accumulation. Rarely, other aerobic, anaerobic, and fungal organisms can cause cellulitis in immunocompromised individuals.

Clinical Findings

History

- A previous skin disruption at the site or recent upper respiratory infection *(H. influenzae)*. Note that edema that occurs within 24 hours of an insect bite is most likely to be inflammatory, whereas edema that occurs between 48 to 72 hours is more likely to be infectious.
- Fever, pain, malaise, irritability, anorexia, vomiting, and chills can be reported.
- Recent sore throat or upper respiratory infection.
- Anal pruritus, stool retention, constipation, and blood-streaked stools.

Physical Examination

- Erythematous, indurated, tender, swollen, warm areas of skin with poorly demarcated borders
- Buccal cellulitis often appears with a blue to purple tinge and is associated with *H. influenza.*
- Regional lymphadenopathy
- Well-demarcated perianal erythema up to 2 cm around the anus; vulvovaginitis is common in females and balanoposthitis in males.
- Erysipelas—a superficial (dermis and epidermis) variant of cellulitis—presents with rapidly advancing lesions that are tender, bright red, have sharp margins and an "orange peel" look and feel.

Diagnostic Studies. Most cellulitis cases are treated empirically. CBC and blood culture are done if the child is febrile, appears ill or toxic, or is younger than 1 year old. Leukocytosis is common. Positive blood cultures are low, ranging from 1% to 18% of cases. Perform Gram stain and culture of the erythematous area if unusual organisms are suspected, pus is present (which is more typical of MRSA), or the child looks toxic. An aspirate at the point of maximum inflammation is more likely to yield a causative organism than one taken from the leading edge, although the bacterial counts tend to be low with either method. Cultures are generally not helpful and little evidence exists to support this practice (Bystritsky, 2018).

Differential Diagnosis

Pressure erythema, giant urticaria, contact dermatitis, popsicle panniculitis (reaction to cold exposure), early erythema nodosum, subcutaneous fat necrosis, herpetic whitlow, and diaper dermatitis are included in the differential diagnosis.

Management

Immediate antibiotic therapy is required.
- Hospitalization is recommended if the child is a neonate or febrile infant, is acutely ill or toxic, or has periorbital cellulitis.
  - Neonates with cellulitis require a full septic workup and initiation of empiric therapy with methicillin or vancomycin and gentamicin or cefotaxime (Paller and Mancini, 2016).
- Antibiotic therapy
  - As noted earlier, prompt administration of antibiotics is essential.
  - If a streptococcal infection is suspected:
    - A hospitalized febrile acutely ill infant or child should have penicillin, up to 2 million units per day.
    - Penicillin VK: 20 to 50 mg/kg/d orally every 6 to 8 hours for 10 days or dicloxacillin 12.5 to 50 mg/kg/day for mild infections (50 to 100 mg/kg/d for severe infections) orally every 6 hours if <40kg and 125 to 500 mg every 6 hours if >40 kg (Stevens, et al., 2014).
    - If allergic or concern for multiple organisms a third-generation cephalosporin is usually effective. Can consider topical mupirocin.
  - If suspected organism is staphylococcus:
    - Trimethoprim-sulfamethoxazole 8 to 12 mg/kg/d (TMP) given BID if child >2 months.
    - Doxycycline 4.4 mg/kg/d given BID in children 8 years of age or older and weighing ≤45 kg.
    - If MRSA suspected, clindamycin 10 to 30 mg/kg/day orally divided 3 times a day for 10 days. Max dose =1.8 gm in 24 hours.
  - If suspected organism is *H. influenzae:*
    - Amoxicillin clavulanate 50 to 90 mg/kg/d orally for 10 days.
    - Methicillin or a third-generation cephalosporin is also an option.
- Follow up in 24 hours to assess response and observe toxicity. Continue daily visits until child is recovering. Counsel parents to call the provider immediately or return for an urgent visit if the infection is not improving or is getting worse.

Complications

Recurrent perianal streptococcal infection, septicemia, necrotizing fasciitis (NF), and toxic shock syndrome (TSS) are possible complications and all require immediate referral for care and hospitalization.
- NF is a rare infection in children and has two subtypes. Type I is generally a polymicrobial infection that usually affects children who have an underlying disease. Type II, commonly referred to as *flesh-eating strep,* is an acute, rapidly progressing necrotic invasion of GABHS through the skin and subcutaneous tissue to the fascial compartments. It is more common in otherwise healthy children or children with varicella. NF is more common in boys younger than 5 years old and children with diabetes, skin injury, surgery, immunodeficiency, IV drug use, malnutrition, and obesity. NF begins as cellulitis (usually on the leg or abdomen in infants) with severe pain, edema, fever, and bullae on an erythematous surface. It quickly progresses to ulcer, eschar, and gangrene within 2 days. Prompt treatment (hospitalization, surgical debridement, and fluid management), prolonged antibiotic treatment (penicillin), and intravenous immunoglobulin (IVIG) may be lifesaving, because the overall mortality rate is high (Fig 34.5).
- TSS is an acute febrile illness with rapid onset that causes significant fever, vomiting and diarrhea, engorged mucous membranes, hypotension, a diffuse macular or sunburn-like rash, conjunctival injection, and multiple organ system involvement. *S. aureus* or *S. pyogenes* (group A streptococci) are the causative agents associated with TSS, and incubation can be as little as 14 hours. Both organisms can be associated with invasive infection (e.g., pneumonia, osteomyelitis, bacteremia, or endocarditis) or focal tissue invasion that is rapidly progressive. Initially recognized in menstruating adolescents, TSS is also found in males and younger children. *S. aureus* is usually the causative agent in menstruating females. Nasal packing, surgical procedures, and postpartum condition are some factors linked to nonmenstrual TSS. Treatment is intensive, requires hospitalization, and consists of fluid management, antibiotics, and other supportive measures. The mortality rate of all TSS in children 0 to 18 years is 1.9% with a significantly higher mortality in staphylococcal TSS (Strom, Hsu, and Silverberg, 2017). It is a reportable disease in most states (Fig 34.6).

Patient and Family Education

- Thorough cleansing of any break in the skin helps prevent cellulitis.
- Keep bites, scrapes, and rashes clean and bandaged until healed to prevent them from being infected by staphylococcal bacteria.

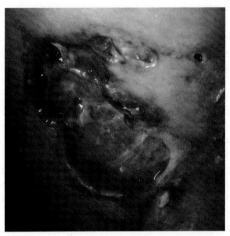

• **Fig 34.5** Necrotizing Fasciitis. (From Bologia J, Schaffer JV, Duncan KO, et al. *Dermatology Essentials*. Philadelphia: Saunders/Elsevier; 2014.)

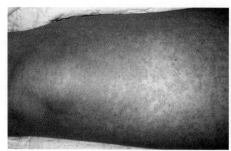
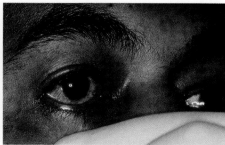

• **Fig 34.6** Toxic Shock Syndrome. (From Bologia J, Schaffer JV, Duncan KO, et al. *Dermatology Essentials*. Philadelphia: Saunders/Elsevier; 2014.)

- Frequent hand washing is essential.
- Immunize against *H. influenzae.*
- Perianal spread can occur through shared bath water.
- See Chapter 31 regarding treatment of children and families with MRSA infection.

Folliculitis and Furuncle

A superficial bacterial inflammation of the hair follicle is called *folliculitis* (Fig 34.7); a deeper infection with involvement of the base of the follicle and deep dermis is called a *furuncle* (boil).

Obstruction of the follicular orifice is the most important factor contributing to the development of folliculitis, but a moist environment, maceration, poor hygiene, occlusive emollients, and prolonged submersion in contaminated water are also factors. *S. aureus* is the common causative organism. *Pseudomonas aeruginosa* may be found with hot-tub folliculitis. *Escherichia coli* is also implicated. These infections are more common in males than in females.

Clinical Findings

History
- Pruritus with folliculitis; tenderness with furuncle
- Hot-tub exposure
- Irritating surface agent
- Occasional fever, malaise, or lymphadenopathy

Physical Examination. The child often is asymptomatic, but the following can be seen:
- Discrete, erythematous 1- to 2-mm papules or pustules on an inflamed base centered around a hair follicle
- Involvement of face, scalp, extremities (typically thighs and upper arms), buttocks, and back
- Nodules with larger areas of erythema and tenderness (furuncle)
- Pruritic papules, pustules, or deep red to purple nodules, most dense in areas covered by swimsuit 8 to 48 hours after exposure (hot-tub folliculitis)

Diagnostic Studies. Gram stain and culture are occasionally ordered. In the case of persistent or difficult-to-treat folliculitis, consider the possibility of MRSA.

Differential Diagnosis

Cellulitis, *Candida* infection, tinea, acne pustules, and chemical folliculitis constitute the differential diagnosis.

Management

The following steps are taken:
- Warm compresses after washing with soap and water several times a day

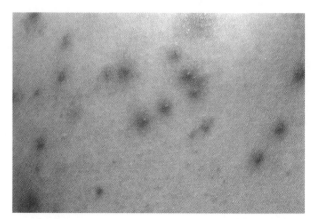

• **Fig 34.7** Staphylococcal Superficial Folliculitis. (From Zitelli BJ, McIntire S, Nowalk AJ. *Zitelli and Davis' Atlas of Pediatric Physical Diagnosis.* 7th ed. Philadelphia: Elsevier; 2018.)

- Topical keratolytics, such as benzoyl peroxide 5% to 10% twice a day for 5 days, especially if chronic or recurrent
- Fluctuant lesions should be incised and drained, which may be sufficient for many lesions
- If lesion is superficial, topical antibiotic, such as erythromycin or clindamycin, in cream, gel, solution, or ointment twice a day for 10 to 14 days
- Antistaphylococcal β-lactamase–resistant antibiotics, such as dicloxacillin 15 to 50 mg/kg/d divided 4 times a day for 7 to 10 days, or cephalexin 40 to 50 mg/kg/d divided 3 times a day for 7 to 10 days in severe or widespread cases
- Review of good personal hygiene habits; avoid shaving until resolved
- Follow-up treatment in 1 week for folliculitis, in 1 day for furuncle or abscess, which may need incision and drainage
- Identify and eliminate predisposing factors
- If recurrent, look for nasal or skin carrier state

Complications

Deep abscess formation or carbuncles can occur. *Sycosis barbae* occurs on the chin, upper lip, and jaw, especially in adolescent African American males.

Patient and Family Education

Good personal hygiene and an antibacterial soap minimize spread to other household members. Hot-tub folliculitis resolves in 5 to 14 days but can recur up to 3 months after exposure.

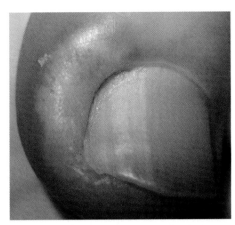

• **Fig 34.8** Paronychia. (From Bologia J, Schaffer JV, Duncan KO, et al. *Dermatology Essentials.* 1st ed. Philadelphia: Saunders/Elsevier; 2014.)

Paronychia

Paronychia is a chronic or acute inflammation and infection around a fingernail or toenail. It is a common disorder in childhood and adolescence caused by bacteria (often *S. aureus,* occasionally *Streptococcus* or *Pseudomonas), Candida* (in infants with thrush or thumb sucking or when hands are frequently immersed in water), or herpes (see Fig 34.8). It is more common with tight shoes, or when nails are malaligned, or cut too short or with rounded edges.

Clinical Findings

History. Tenderness, drainage, and discomfort (especially with walking) are reported.

Physical Examination
- Proximal nailfold is erythematous, swollen, and tender; if chronic, may not be tender
- Purulent exudate expressed
- Cuticle broken or absent
- Nontender erythema and edema with thickened, disrupted nail (*Candida* infection, often with secondary bacterial infection)

Diagnostic Studies. A culture of the exudate is occasionally done.

Differential Diagnosis

Herpetic whitlow (grouped vesicles on an erythematous base) and eczematous inflammation should be ruled out.

Management

Management includes the following:
- Systemic oral antibiotic if acute infection; coverage for staphylococcal infection may be required.
- If *Candida* is suspected, nystatin cream under occlusion (a plastic glove covered by a cotton stocking) every night for 3 to 4 weeks.
- If purulent area is full, loosen cuticle from nail with a No. 11 blade to allow exudate to escape.
- Frequent warm soaks, after which cotton pledgets are inserted beneath the nail to lift it.
- Instruction on proper trimming of nails and care of toenails:
  - Wear wide-toed shoes.
  - Trim nails straight across and not too short.
  - If condition is recurrent, refer for surgical removal of lateral portion of nail.
  - Do a follow-up visit in 1 month, as recurrent infection is possible.

Fungal Infections of the Skin

Diagnosis and treatment of common fungal infections are listed in Table 34.3.

Candidiasis (Moniliasis)

Candidiasis is a fungal infection of the skin or mucous membranes commonly called a *yeast infection* or *thrush.* See Chapter 42 for discussion of vaginal candidiasis.

Candida albicans, a yeast-like fungus, is commonly found on skin and oral, vaginal, and intestinal mucosal tissue. Although *Candida* is part of the normal flora, overgrowth and penetration of inflamed skin or mucous membranes can occur when there is a localized or systemic alteration in host defenses. Candidiasis is more common in infants, obese children, adolescents, and chronically ill or immunocompromised children. It also is often seen as a secondary infection in persistent diaper rashes or with antibiotic, oral steroid, or oral contraceptive use. Systemic infection with candidiasis is not discussed in this text (Figs 34.9 to 34.11).

Clinical Findings

History. The history often includes antibiotic or steroid use over the previous weeks and occurrence of a rash in a moist, warm area.

Physical Examination
- Mouth—friable, adherent white plaques on an erythematous base on the mucous membranes (thrush); cracked lips (cheilitis); fissured and inflamed corners of the mouth (angular cheilitis)
- Intertriginous areas (neck, axillae, or groin)—bright erythema in flexural folds
- Diaper area—moist, beefy-red macules and papules with sharply marked borders and satellite lesions; erosions may also be present
- Vulvovaginal area—thick, cheesy, yellow discharge; erythema; edema; and itching
- Nail plates—transverse ridging of the nail plate, loss of cuticle, and mild proximal lateral periungual erythema (chronic paronychia)

Diagnostic Studies. If treatment failure or questionable diagnosis occurs, KOH-treated scrapings of satellite lesions or mucosa reveal yeast cells and pseudohyphae (see Fig 34.2).

Differential Diagnosis

The differential diagnoses include erythema toxicum, miliaria, staphylococcal pustulosis, transient neonatal pustulosis, neonatal herpes simplex, and congenital syphilis.

Management

The following steps are taken (Table 34.4):
- Thrush: Oral nystatin suspension 4 times a day, or gentian violet 1% to 2% aqueous solution applied twice a day until 1 to 2 days after white adherent patches are gone. If breastfeeding, the mother should put the solution on her nipples to eliminate reinfection. A second course is sometimes needed to clear the infection.
- If resistant to treatment, oral fluconazole 6 mg/kg the first day in a single dose; then 3 mg/kg/dose daily for 14 days (Paller and Mancini, 2016).
- Thrush (in older children), cheilitis, and angular cheilitis: Clotrimazole troche 10 mg dissolved slowly 5 times a day for 14 days (Balognia, 2014).

TABLE 34.3	Diagnosis and Treatment of Common Fungal Infections			
Infection	Causative Organism	Clinical Findings	Management	Complications
Candidiasis	*Candida albicans*	Moist, bright-red diaper rash with sharp borders, satellite lesions; may have associated white spots in mouth, mucous membranes, or corner of mouth	Topical or oral antifungal, generally nystatin; diaper area hygiene	Paronychia or onycho-mycosis
Tinea corporis	*Trichophyton tonsurans, Trichophyton rubrum, Microsporum canis*	Pruritic, slightly erythematous circular lesion with a slightly raised border and central clearing; well demarcated	Topical antifungals; identify and treat source; exclude from day care until treated; use oral medications for resistant cases	Tinea incognita from steroid treatment
Tinea cruris	*Epidermophyton floccosum, T. rubrum, Trichophyton mentagrophytes*	Raised-border, scaly lesion on upper thighs and groin; penis and scrotum spared; symmetric	Same as for tinea corporis; loose clothes, absorbent medicated powder	Possible secondary infection
Tinea pedis	*T. rubrum, T. mentagrophytes*	Vesicles and erosions on instep; fissure between toes with scaling and erythema; diffuse scaling on weight-bearing surfaces with exaggerated scaling increases; pruritus	Same as for tinea corporis; absorbent medicated powder; cotton socks; open-toed shoes; moisturize	Reinfection common
Tinea versicolor	*Malassezia furfur (Pityrosporum orbiculare, Pityrosporum ovale)*	Multiple scaly, discrete oval macules on neck, shoulders, upper back, and chest; hypopigmented to hyperpigmented areas; fail to tan in summer	Selenium shampoo; ketoconazole shampoo; topical imidazoles; oral itraconazole or fluconazole for severe or recurrent disease	50% recurrence rate

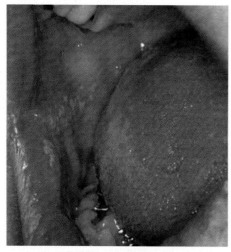

• **Fig 34.9** Thrush. (From Bologia J, Schaffer JV, Duncan KO, et al. *Dermatology Essentials.* Philadelphia: Saunders/Elsevier; 2014.)

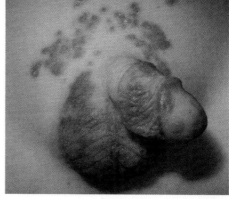

• **Fig 34.10** Candidiasis of the Suprapubic Area. (From Bologia J, Schaffer JV, Duncan KO, et al. *Dermatology Essentials.* Philadelphia: Saunders/Elsevier; 2014.)

- Skin infection: Topical antifungals (such as nystatin, miconazole, clotrimazole, ketoconazole, ciclopirox, or econazole) applied to skin at every diaper change until the rash is gone plus an additional 1 to 2 days (Weston and Morelli, 2017). Avoid antifungal/corticosteroid combination medications.
- If inflammation is severe, 1% hydrocortisone can be applied simultaneously to the diaper area for 1 or 2 days (Bolognia et al., 2014).
- Keep area dry and cool. Minimize skin irritation:
  - Frequent diaper changes.
  - Leave diaper area open to air as much as possible.

- Blow-dry with warm air (low setting) for 3 to 5 minutes at diaper change (especially helpful in intertriginous areas in infants and obese children).
- Avoid rubber pants.
- Use mild soap and water; rinse well; avoid diaper wipes.
- Avoid powders and other medications not prescribed, such as baby powder.
- Discontinue oral antibiotics and steroids when possible.
- Discard or sterilize pacifiers.
- Educate about avoiding underlying predisposing factors (e.g., lip licking).
- Add topical or oral antibiotic if secondary infection is suspected.

TABLE 34.4 **Antifungal Medications**

Drug Generic Name	Strength and Formulation	Application	Mode of Action, Indications, Side Effects, and Comments
Topical Medications			
Imidazoles			
Clotrimazole	1% cream, lotion, solution and powder	Twice daily	Fungistatic; erythema, stinging, blistering, peeling, edema, pruritus, hives, burning
Econazole nitrate	1% cream	Daily or twice daily	Fungistatic; burning, pruritus, stinging, erythema; may have antibacterial effects
Ketoconazole	2% cream and shampoo	Daily or twice daily	Fungistatic; irritation, dry skin, pruritus, stinging
Miconazole nitrate	2% cream, powder, and lotion	Daily or twice daily	Fungistatic; irritation, maceration, urticaria, allergic contact dermatitis, pruritus; economical
Allylamines			
Naftifine HCl	1% cream and gel	Daily or twice daily	Fungicidal; burning, stinging, erythema, pruritus, irritation
Terbinafine HCl	1% cream and solution	Daily or twice daily	Fungicidal; pruritus, irritation, burning
Ethanolamine			
Ciclopirox olamine	1% cream, lotion, gel, and nail lacquer (8% solution)	Twice daily; nail lacquer applied daily at bedtime	Fungicidal; irritation, erythema, burning
Others			
Gentian violet	1%-2% solution	Twice daily	Topical antiseptic/germicide; staining, burning, vesicle formation
Nystatin	100,000 units/gram cream, powder, and ointment	Twice or 4 times a day	Fungistatic; rare adverse reactions; effective against yeast only
Selenium sulfide shampoo	1% and 2.25% shampoo, 2.5% lotion	Daily for lotion Twice weekly for shampoo for 2 weeks then once every 1-4 weeks as needed	Used for tinea capitis (reduces transmission), tinea versicolor, and seborrheic dermatitis (shampoo may be used as lotion); thought to block the enzymes involved in growth of epithelial tissues; discoloration of hair, alopecia
Tolnaftate	1% cream, powder, and solution; aerosol powder and solution also available	2-3 times daily	Fungistatic; rare adverse reactions; pruritus, stinging
Oral Medications			
Clotrimazole	10 mg troche	1 troche 5 times a day dissolved slowly in mouth	Treatment of oral candidiasis; gastrointestinal symptoms; hepatotoxicity
Fluconazole	10 mg/mL and 40 mg/mL; 50, 100, 150, and 200 mg tablets	3-6 mg/kg/d in single dose for 2 weeks for oropharyngeal candidiasis; day 1 dosage is 6 mg/kg (children) and 200 mg/dose (adults) followed by daily therapy of 3 mg/kg/dose (pediatric) and 100 mg/dose (adults); dosage for tinea capitis is 3-6 mg/kg/d	Possible drug interactions; caution with liver or kidney dysfunction and arrhythmias
Griseofulvin	Ultramicrosized: 250 mg ultramicrosized = 500 mg microsized Microsized: 125 mg/mL 500 mg tablets	>2 years old: 10-15 mg/kg in single or in two divided doses; maximum dose 750 mg/d 10 to 20 mg/kg/d given daily or two divided doses (consider 20 to 25 mg/kg/d for tinea capitis); maximum dose 1 g/d	Fungistatic; mainstay of therapy; excellent safety profile and extensive use Duration of treatment: Tinea corporis: 2-4 weeks; tinea capitis: 4-6 weeks or longer; tinea pedis: 4-8 weeks; tinea unguium: 4-6 months or longer Evaluate clinical status frequently, and consider CBC, LFTs, renal function after 8 weeks of therapy or with status change while on treatment; possible drug interactions

Continued

TABLE 34.4 Antifungal Medications—cont'd

Drug Generic Name	Strength and Formulation	Application	Mode of Action, Indications, Side Effects, and Comments
Nystatin	100,000 units/mL	Infants: 2 mL 4 times a day after meals. Children/adolescents: 400,000 to 600,000 units 4 times a day—swished about in mouth	Treatment of oral candidiasis
Terbinafine	125 mg/packet of granules 250 mg tablets	Granules: Tinea capitis in children >4 years old: <25 kg: 125 mg once daily for 6 weeks; 25-35 kg: 187.5 mg once daily for 4-6 weeks; >35 kg: 250 mg once daily for 6 weeks. Onychomycosis dosage once daily for 6 weeks (fingernails) or 12 weeks (toenails) as follows: 10-20 kg: 62.5 mg; 20-40 kg: 125 mg; >40 kg: 250 mg	Treatment of tinea capitis in children >4 years old; costly; possible drug interactions; CBC and liver LFT recommended at baseline and if therapy continues past 6 weeks; more effective for tinea capitis due to *Trichophyton tonsurans*

CBC, Complete blood count; *LFT,* liver function test.

Data from Paller AS, Mancini AJ. *Hurwitz Clinical Dermatology: A Textbook of Skin Disorders of Childhood and Adolescence.* 5th ed. Philadelphia: Elsevier; 2016; Chen X, Jiang X, Yang M, et al. Systemic antifungal therapy for tinea capitis in children. *Cochrane Database Syst Rev.* 2016; (5): CD004685; Weston WL, Lane AT, Morelli JG. *Color Textbook of Pediatric Dermatology.* 4th ed. St. Louis: Mosby; 2007.

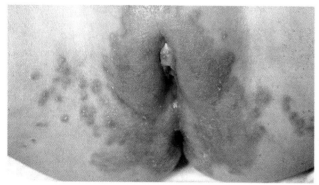

• **Fig 34.11** Diaper Candidiasis. (From Zitelli BJ, McIntire S, Nowalk AJ. *Zitelli and Davis' Atlas of Pediatric Physical Diagnosis.* 7th ed. Philadelphia: Elsevier; 2018.)

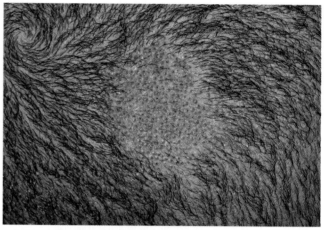

• **Fig 34.12** Tinea Capitis. (From Paller AS, Mancini AJ. *Hurwitz Clinical Pediatric Dermatology: A Textbook of Skin Disorders of Children and Adolescence.* 5th ed. Philadelphia: Elsevier; 2016.)

• Nail involvement (chronic paronychia) can be treated with topical application of antifungal cream twice daily, but it will take several months for the nail plate to grow out normally; oral fluconazole may be needed for severe or resistant involvement.

Complications

Chronic mucocutaneous candidiasis resulting from immunologic deficit can occur and is heralded by widespread involvement (oral, skin, nails). Paronychia may occur with thumb sucking.

Patient and Family Education

Emphasize good hand washing. Treatment failure is usually due to lack of compliance.

Tinea

Tinea Capitis

Ringworm of the scalp and hair may be seen in four different manifestations: (1) diffuse fine scaling without obvious hair breaks and with subtle to significant hair loss; (2) discrete areas of hair loss with stubs of broken hairs (black-dot ringworm) (see Fig 34.12); (3) "classic" patchy hair loss and scaly lesions with raised borders; and (4) scaly, pustular lesions, or kerions. Tinea capitis occurs in a noninflammatory stage for 2 to 8 weeks and then becomes inflammatory.

The fungus invades the scalp and hair shaft, causing an inflammatory response and hair shaft fragility. *Trichophyton tonsurans* and *Microsporum canis* are the most common organisms associated with tinea capitis (Weston and Morelli, 2017). Tinea capitis is transmitted by fomites when humans share hats, combs, and brushes, or by cats, dogs, or rodents. Tinea capitis is the most common dermatophyte infection of childhood, typically found in children 2 to 10 years old (Cohen, 2013; Paller and Mancini, 2016). It is more common in boys and African American children.

Clinical Findings

History. Hair loss, itching, and contact with another person or pet with ringworm are sometimes reported.

Physical Examination

- Scaling, erythema, or crusting usually occurs.
- Bald patches or areas of broken hairs are noted.
- *T. tonsurans* manifests as black-dot tinea, with tiny black dots that are the remainder of hair that has broken off at the shaft; no scalp scale is present (most common).
- *M. canis* leaves the hair broken and lusterless with a fine gray scale on the scalp.
- Occipital or posterior cervical adenopathy may be significant.
- A kerion is a boggy, inflamed mass filled with pustules. It results from a delayed inflammatory reaction. There may be regional lymphadenopathy, fever, and leukocytosis. The contents of the kerion are sterile.

Diagnostic Studies. Examine hair scrapings as follows:

- Wood's light fluoresces yellow-green (positive with *M. canis*, negative with *T. tonsurans*).
- KOH examination of scraped hair: Wait 20 to 40 minutes after application of KOH to examine. If Wood's light was positive, under microscopy the KOH-prepared outer surface of hair is coated with tiny mats of spores; if Wood's light was negative, hyphae and spores are present in hair shaft.
- Fungal culture of a completely plucked hair with its root (use a Kelly clamp) is most reliable.

Differential Diagnosis

Traumatic alopecia, alopecia areata, hypothyroid and hyperthyroid hair loss, seborrhea, atopic dermatitis, psoriasis, impetigo, and folliculitis are included in the differential diagnosis.

Management

Topical antifungals are ineffective. Antibiotic treatment is not indicated. The following steps are taken:

- Griseofulvin ultramicrosize at 10 to 15 mg/kg/d once daily or in two divided doses or griseofulvin microsize at 20 to 25 mg/kg/d once daily or in two divided doses for 6 to 8 weeks; taken with fatty food, such as ice cream, to enhance absorption. Treatment should be continued until clinical and mycologic cure (Chen et al., 2016).
- In addition to griseofulvin therapy, shampoo with selenium sulfide 2.5% or econazole or ketoconazole 2% (2 or 3 times per week for 4 weeks) to decrease spore viability and keep other household members from being infected.
- If a long-standing kerion with severe inflammation is present, give prednisone 1 to 2 mg/kg/d for 5 to 14 days and consider systemic antibiotics for secondary bacterial infection (Paller and Mancini, 2016).
- Family members and pets should be checked for infection by fungal culture and treated if positive. Do not rely on lack of symptoms, as asymptomatic carriers are common.
- A follow-up visit should be scheduled after 2 weeks to evaluate response to treatment. Medication should be continued until 2 weeks after culture is negative. Follow-up should be continued every 2 to 4 weeks until new hair growth is evident.
- Monitoring of CBC, liver function tests (LFTs), and renal function is no longer required in children treated with oral griseofulvin due to its favorable safety profile; however, clinical monitoring is required with laboratory evaluation considered with a change in clinical status (Paller and Mancini, 2016). In extended therapy with the medication, over 8 weeks, laboratory evaluation may be considered.
- Oral itraconazole and fluconazole are also approved antifungals for use in children. New evidence suggests that terbinafine may

be more effective if causative organism is *T. Tonsurans*. (Chen et al., 2016) Dosing guidelines found in Table 34.4.

Complications

An idiosyncratic (id) reaction to the fungus, not to the medication, can occur. It manifests either as a red, superficial edema or as scaly, red plaques and papules on the scalp and is treated with 1 to 2 weeks of topical or systemic steroids. Permanent hair loss and scarring can occur with an untreated kerion.

Patient and Family Education

- Sites and modes of transmission are identified (*M. canis*, animal source; *T. tonsurans*, human source) and treated.
- Side effects of medication should be explained and monitored; griseofulvin typically may result in gastrointestinal disturbances, photosensitivity, skin eruptions, and headache.
- Hair regrowth is slow (3 to 12 months) and, if a kerion was present, hair loss can be permanent.
- Laundering sheets and clothes in a hot water wash and hot dryer cycle and vacuuming may decrease spread in the family.
- Grooming practices (e.g., hair traction, greasy pomades, infrequent shampooing) may be predisposing factors.
- There is a high rate of asymptomatic carriers; culture is the only definitive means of identification.

Tinea Corporis

Tinea corporis, commonly called *ringworm*, is a superficial fungal skin infection found on the non-hairy skin of the body. It is also identified by the part of the body affected (e.g., tinea manuum [hand], tinea barbae [beard], tinea faciei [face]) (Fig 34.13). Tinea corporis is most commonly caused by the dermatophytes *Microsporum canis, Trichophyton, Microsporum,* and *Epidermophyton* species (Bolognia et al, 2014; Cohen, 2013). Transmission comes as the stratum corneum is invaded following direct contact with infected humans, animals, or fomites. The exact mechanism is unknown but is probably due to a toxin causing an inflammatory response. Infection is common in children. Contact sports (especially wrestling), hot and humid climates, crowded living conditions, day care, school settings, and immunosuppression increase the risk of tinea corporis. Autoinoculation accounts for spreading lesions (Cohen, 2013).

Clinical Findings

History. Contact with a person or animal with tinea is sometimes reported.

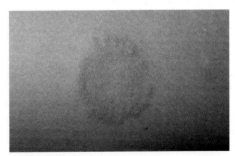

• **Fig 34.13** Tinea Corporis, Ringworm. (From Zitelli BJ, McIntire S, Nowalk AJ, *Zitelli and Davis' Atlas of Pediatric Physical Diagnosis.* 7th ed. Philadelphia: Elsevier; 2018.)

Physical Examination

- Classical appearance of lesions: Annular, oval, or circinate with one or more flat, scaling, mildly erythematous circular patches or plaques with red, scaly borders
- Lesions spread peripherally and clear centrally or may be inflammatory throughout with superficial pustules
- Often prominent over hair follicles
- Multiple secondary lesions may merge into a large area several centimeters in diameter

Diagnostic Studies. If treatment failure or questionable diagnosis occurs:

- KOH-treated scrapings of border of lesion reveal hyphae and spores (see Fig 34.2)
- Wood's lamp will fluoresce most tinea corporis
- Fungal culture of the lesion

Differential Diagnosis

Pityriasis rosea herald patch, nummular eczema, psoriasis, seborrhea, contact dermatitis, tinea versicolor, granuloma annulare, and Lyme disease are in the differential diagnosis.

Management

- For superficial or localized tinea corporis, topical antifungals (see Table 34.4) (such as miconazole or clotrimazole) are generally effective. Antifungal and steroid combinations should be avoided. Apply cream to the lesion, including a zone of normal skin, twice a day until clinical resolution, which can take 1 to 4 weeks. Prescription antifungals (e.g., econazole, ciclopirox) penetrate the skin more effectively but are more expensive.
- Tinea faciei (face), extensive infection, immunosuppression, coexisting tinea infections on scalp or nails, or infection that is unresponsive to topical treatment may require systemic treatment. Griseofulvin (see Table 34.4) is the systemic drug of choice for children older than 2 years old. Treatment typically lasts for 2 to 4 weeks for areas other than the scalp. Griseofulvin should be taken with fatty foods for better absorption. Because of the risk of hepatotoxicity, nephrotoxicity, and neutropenia, patients requiring extended therapy should have a CBC and liver and renal function 8 weeks after initiating therapy and every 8 weeks until treatment is stopped. Tinea corporis gladiatorum may require systemic therapy, because it is endemic among wrestling team members.

Complications

Tinea incognito is a dermatophyte infection that has been altered by the use of topical calcineurin inhibitors (e.g., tacrolimus and pimecrolimus) or steroid creams, either alone or in combination with a topical antifungal. The lesions improve but there is a rapid relapse when the creams are stopped and chronic infection persists. Occasionally a pruritic papulovesicular rash on the trunk, hands, or face that is caused by a hypersensitivity response to the fungus may occur and is known as an *id response* (Bolognia et al, 2014).

Patient and Family Education

- Find the source of infection and treat or eliminate it to prevent recurrence. Keep skin dry following application of antifungal.
- Identify and treat contacts.
- Educate about communicability of lesions and length of treatment.
- Exclude from day care or school until 24 hours after treatment has begun.

- Follow up in 2 weeks or sooner if lesions are not responding. If unresponsive, diagnosis is incorrect or resistance is possible. Culture to confirm diagnosis and change class of antifungal used.

Tinea Cruris

Tinea cruris, commonly called *jock itch,* is a superficial fungal skin infection found on the groin, upper thighs, and intertriginous folds. Caused by the dermatophyte *Epidermophyton floccosum, Trichophyton rubrum,* or *Trichophyton mentagrophytes,* tinea cruris rarely occurs before adolescence and is more common in males, obese individuals, or those with hyperhidrosis or experiencing chafing from tight clothes or moisture. It is extremely common.

Clinical Findings

History

- Hot, humid weather, tight clothing, vigorous physical activity and chafing, or contact sport, such as wrestling
- Often associated with tinea pedis

Physical Examination

- Erythematous to slightly brown, sharply marginated plaques with a raised border of scaling, pustules, or vesicles; central clearing may be present
- Usually bilateral and symmetric, but not always
- Occurs on inner thighs and inguinal creases; penis, scrotum, and labia majora generally spared
- Occasionally occurs in perianal region or on the buttocks and/or abdomen

Diagnostic Studies. If treatment failure or questionable diagnosis occurs:

- KOH-treated scraping reveals hyphae and spores
- Fungal culture

Differential Diagnosis

Psoriasis, candidiasis, contact dermatitis, seborrhea, intertrigo, and erythrasma are in the differential diagnosis.

Management

Management is the same as for tinea corporis. Duration of topical treatment is usually 4 to 6 weeks. Antifungal and steroid combinations are to be avoided. Do not use steroids because of risk of atrophy and striae. Advise the patient to wear cotton underwear and loose clothing and to use absorbent antifungal powder. If tinea pedis is suspected, advise the patient to put socks on before underwear to prevent the spread of the infection. Maintain good hygiene following a wrestling event (e.g., bathing as soon as possible, sole use of towel; dry thoroughly).

Tinea Pedis

Tinea pedis is a superficial fungal skin infection found on the feet, commonly called *athlete's foot.* There are three clinical forms: (1) vesicles and erosions on the instep of one or both feet; (2) an occasional fissure between the toes with surrounding scale and erythema; and (3) rare diffuse scaling on the weight-bearing surface of the foot with exaggerated scaling increases (moccasin foot) often extending to lateral foot margins (Fig 34.14A).

Caused by the dermatophytes *T. rubrum* or *T. mentagrophytes,* tinea pedis is uncommon in preadolescent children and is more common in males. It is acquired through direct contact with

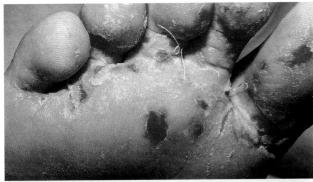
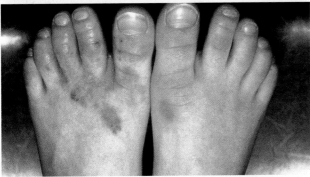
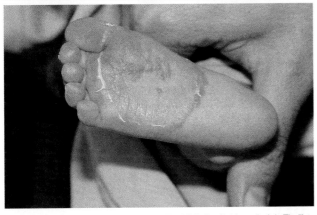

• **Fig 34.14A** Tinea Pedis. (From Zitelli BJ, McIntire S, Nowalk AJ. *Zitelli and Davis' Atlas of Pediatric Physical Diagnosis.* 7th ed. Philadelphia: Elsevier.)

contaminated surfaces (e.g., warm moist environment of showers and locker room floors) and often occurs with tinea cruris (see Fig 34.11).

Clinical Findings

History
- Sweaty feet
- Use of nylon socks or nonbreathable shoes
- Exposure in family or at school
- Itching, intense burning, stinging, foul odor
- Microtrauma to feet—cracks, abrasions, nicks, cuts
- Contact with damp areas (e.g., swimming pools, locker room, showers)

Physical Examination
- Red, scaly, cracked rash on soles or interdigital spaces and instep, especially between the third, fourth, and fifth toes
- Infection initially presents as white peeling lesions becoming erythematous, vesicular, macerated, fissured, and scaly
- Dorsum of foot remains clear

- Chronic infection manifested by diffuse scaling (plantar hyperkeratosis) and mild erythema

Diagnostic Studies. Laboratory studies are the same as those for tinea corporis.

Differential Diagnosis

Contact dermatitis, atopic dermatitis, dyshidrotic eczema, psoriasis, pitted keratolysis, and juvenile plantar dermatosis (red, dry fissures of weight-bearing surface) are in the differential diagnosis.

Management

Management is the same as that for tinea corporis. Antifungal medication should be applied 1 cm beyond the borders of the rash twice daily until 7 days after clearing. Usual treatment is 3 to 6 weeks. In rare cases, griseofulvin may be required, and treatment for 6 to 8 weeks is usually recommended.

Patient and Family Education

- Advise patient to keep feet dry, use absorbent antifungal powder or sprays, wear cotton socks, avoid scratching, and wear shoes that allow the feet to breathe or go barefoot when home. Thoroughly dry feet and between toes after using a commercial showering facility.
- Rinse feet with plain water or water and vinegar; dry carefully, especially between the toes. Moisturize and protect feet to prevent splitting and cracking.
- Aluminum chloride (Drysol, Certain Dri, Xerac AC, or Arrid Extra Dry antiperspirant sprays) may be used for hyperhidrosis.
- Acute vesicular lesions can be treated with wet compresses 2 to 4 times daily for 10 to 15 minutes in addition to application of topical antifungals.
- Tinea pedis may need the addition of a keratolytic agent (lactic acid or urea) with the application of antifungals.
- Tennis shoes may be washed in the machine with soap and bleach.
- Physical education or sports may be continued.
- Follow up in 2 to 3 weeks or sooner if lesions are not responding.

Complications

A secondary bacterial infection, indicated by foul odor, can occur. An allergic reaction to fungus, called an *id response,* is manifested by a vesicular eruption on the palms and sides of fingers and occasionally on the trunk and extremities.

Onychomycosis

Onychomycosis is a fungal infection of the nail(s) typically with *T. rubrum* or *Candida* (see Fig 34.14B). When the nail infection is due to a dermatophyte, it is often called *tinea unguium.* One or two nails are often involved. The infection may be superficial, hypertrophic (onychauxis), or cause separation of the nail plate from the tissue (onycholytic).

The infecting organism invades the nail, proliferates, and destroys the nail integrity, causing separation of the nail plate from the nailbed. The infection originates at the distal edge of the nail. It is uncommon during the first two decades of life, limited most commonly to adolescents and adults. When it occurs in children, there is often a concurrent tinea pedis or tinea manuum. There may be a relationship to the use of occlusive shoes. The causative organisms include *T. rubrum, T. mentagrophytes, E. floccosum,* and *C. albicans.* However, 50% of the time another condition is responsible for dystrophic nail.

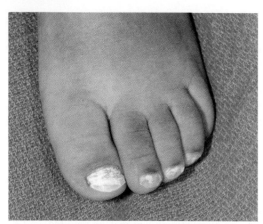

• **Fig 34.14B** Onychomycosis. (From Paller AS, Mancini AJ. *Hurwitz Clinical Pediatric Dermatology: A Textbook of Skin Disorders of Children and Adolescence.* 5th ed. Philadelphia: Elsevier; 2016.)

Clinical Findings

History. The patient may report a thickened, discolored nail.

Physical Examination

• Opaque white or silvery nail that becomes thick, yellow, with subungual debris.
• Toenails are involved more often than fingernails with tinea.
• Fingernails are involved more often than toenails with *Candida.*
• Seldom symmetric; it may be one to three nails on one extremity.

Diagnostic Studies. KOH preparations and fungal cultures of the material under the nail are helpful in confirming the diagnosis.

Differential Diagnosis

Psoriasis (involves all nails and includes pitting), hereditary nail defects, dystrophy secondary to eczema or chronic paronychia, lichen planus, and trauma are the differential diagnoses.

Management

1. Successful treatment is difficult and requires oral medication. Griseofulvin can be used, but side effects, length of treatment, low cure rates, and high recurrence rates following treatment make successful management uncommon (Paller and Mancini, 2016).
2. Oral terbinafine, fluconazole, and itraconazole have a better short-term success rate than griseofulvin and a lower relapse rate. Treatment recommendations for onychomycosis are based on the site of infection (Feldstein, Totri, and Friedlander, 2015):
   • Toenails
      • Itraconazole: 5 mg/kg/d for 12 weeks; or as pulse therapy, 5 mg/kg/d for 1 week each month for 3 months. Generally 2 to 3 pulses are commonly needed for fingernails and 3 to 4 pulses for toenails.
      • Terbinafine: 62.5 mg for children <20 kg, 125 mg for children 20 to 40 kg, and 250 mg for children >40 kg. Treatment is generally for 6 weeks for fingernails and up to 12 weeks for toenails.
      • Fluconazole: 6 mg/kg/wk with slower resolution time (6 to 9 months for fingernails and 8 to 18 months for toenails).
3. Ciclopirox in nail lacquer has been used as monotherapy and adjunctive therapy (Paller and Mancini, 2016). Topical monotherapy generally requires extended treatment, usually 6 to 12 months. Those best suited for topical monotherapy have few effected nails, no matrix involvement, and limited nail plate involvement or a contraindication to oral therapy.

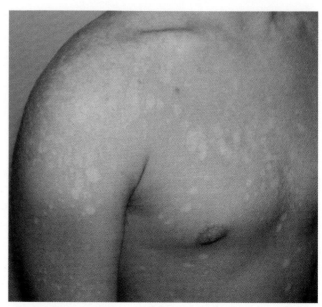

• **Fig 34.14C** Tinea Versicolor. (From Zitelli BJ, McIntire S, Nowalk AJ. *Zitelli and Davis' Atlas of Pediatric Physical Diagnosis.* 7th ed. Philadelphia: Elsevier; 2018.)

4. If triazoles (i.e., efinaconazole) are used, a careful history of current medications must be taken, because there are many interactions. Monitoring of CBC and hepatic function is recommended at onset of therapy and every 4 to 6 weeks.
5. Follow-up visits at 1-month intervals to monitor laboratory values are recommended; long-term follow-up every 6 months is suggested.

Patient and Family Education

The unfortunate truth to communicate is that cure is difficult to obtain and relapse is common.

Tinea Versicolor

Tinea versicolor is a superficial fungal infection, also called *pityriasis versicolor,* that tends to be persistent and occurs predominantly on the trunk. The lesions do not tan in the summer and become relatively darker in winter months (Fig 34.14C).

This infection is caused by a yeastlike organism, *Malassezia furfur* (referred to as *Pityrosporum orbiculare* and *Pityrosporum ovale*) and occurs more commonly in adolescents than in younger children, in chronically ill and immunocompromised children, and in warmer seasons and humid climates. Breastfeeding infants can acquire the organism from their mother and exhibit facial lesions.

Clinical Findings

History. The infection is associated with warm, humid weather. Occasional mild itching may occur.

Physical Examination. Multiple, annular, scaling, discrete macules or patches, ranging from hypopigmented in dark-skinned individuals to hyperpigmented (salmon-colored to brown) in light-skinned individuals, are seen on the neck, shoulders, upper back and arms, chest midline, and face (especially in children). They tend to have a guttate or raindrop pattern.

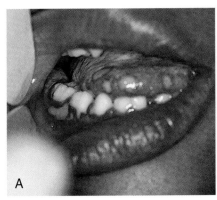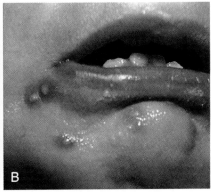

• **Fig 34.15** (A) Herpetic stomatitis. (B) Labialis. (From Zitelli BJ, McIntire S, Nowalk AJ. *Zitelli and Davis' Atlas of Pediatric Physical Diagnosis.* 7th ed. Philadelphia: Elsevier; 2018.)

Diagnostic Studies. KOH scrapings, though not necessary, reveal short curved hyphae and circular spores ("spaghetti and meatballs"). Scrapings fluoresce yellow-orange under Wood's lamp if not cleansed recently.

Differential Diagnosis

Pityriasis alba, pityriasis rosea, vitiligo, postinflammatory hypopigmentation or hyperpigmentation, seborrhea, and secondary syphilis are included in the differential diagnosis.

Management

The following steps are taken (Bolognia et al, 2014):
• Selenium sulfide 2.5% lotion or 1% shampoo (over the counter) applied in a thin layer several hand-widths beyond lesions for 30 minutes twice a week for 2 to 4 weeks followed by monthly applications for 3 months to help prevent recurrences. Older adolescents can use ketoconazole 2% shampoo as directed earlier or for smaller areas of infection, topical imidazoles (e.g., clotrimazole, miconazole, ciclopirox, or terbinafine solution) or topical azoles (e.g., ketoconazole or oxiconazole) applied twice daily for 2 to 4 weeks.
• Resistant or severe cases in older adolescents sometimes require oral antifungal treatment with fluconazole 400 mg by mouth once or itraconazole 400 mg once. Follow up in 1 month.

Patient and Family Education

• Sun exposure makes lesions appear hypopigmented as the surrounding skin tans.
• Repigmentation takes several months.
• If the patient is taking oral antifungal medication, encourage exercise to induce sweating, because this may enhance concentration of medication in the skin.
• Skin irritation occurs with overnight application.
• Absence of flaking when skin is scraped is a sign of effective treatment.

Viral Infections of the Skin

Herpes Simplex

In the active state, herpes simplex virus (HSV) causes contagious infections of the skin and mucous membranes ranging from mild to life threatening. HSV infection can be either primary or recurrent. Primary infection occurs in individuals without circulating antibodies after direct contact with secretions or mucocutaneous lesions of an infected individual. Incubation takes days to weeks and then manifests itself anywhere from subclinical to severe infection. The virus then becomes dormant in certain nerve cells until reactivated by triggering factors, such as stress, menses, illness, sunburn, windburn, and fatigue. Recurrent infection occurs in individuals previously infected who had either clinical or subclinical manifestations of infection.

HSV type 1 (HSV-1) usually affects the oral mucosa, pharynx, lips, and occasionally the eyes, causing a herpes labialis infection, commonly called *cold sores* or *fever blisters* (see Fig 34.15A). HSV-2 infection commonly occurs as a neonatal infection (see Chapter 29) or herpetic vulvovaginitis (see Chapter 42) or progenitalis. Type 1 can also be found in the genital area, and type 2 can be found on the lips and mouth. Herpetic keratoconjunctivitis is discussed in Chapter 35; other information may be found in Chapter 31.

Herpetic whitlow, occurring on a finger or thumb, is a swollen, painful lesion with an erythematous base and ulceration resembling a paronychia. It occurs on fingers of thumb-sucking children with gingivostomatitis or adolescents with genital HSV infection.

HSV is transmitted by close contact with skin, mucous membranes, and body fluids, often through a break in the skin or by autoinoculation. Lesions occur in children of all ages, are contagious as long as they are present, and have an incubation period of 2 to 12 days. Primary lesions usually occur before 5 years old, are more painful and extensive, and last longer.

Clinical Findings

History. In primary herpes, fever, malaise, sore throat, and decreased fluid intake can occur. Primary genital HSV presents with painful vesicles in genital areas. In recurrent HSV infection, there is often a painful prodrome of burning, tingling, paresthesia, and itching at the involved site. Recent acute febrile illness or sun exposure may also be reported.

Physical Examination. The following are seen on physical examination:
• HSV-1
  • Gingivostomatitis: Pharyngitis with grouped vesicles on an erythematous base that ulcerate and form white plaques on mucosa, gingiva, tongue, palate, lips, chin, and nasolabial folds; lymphadenopathy and halitosis are present (Fig 34.15A)
  • Herpes labialis: Cluster of small, clear, tense vesicles with an erythematous base that become weepy and ulcerated, progressing to crustiness, usually only on one side of the mouth and on the vermillion border—classic cold sore (see Fig 34.15B)

- Herpetic whitlow on hand or fingers: Deep-appearing vesicles (Fig 34.16)
- Common sites of involvement: Lips, hand, fingers, nose, cheek, forehead, and eyes; can also occur in the genital area
- HSV-2
  - Grouped vesicopustules and ulceration with edema
  - Primary lesions on vaginal mucosa, labia, or perineum in females and on the penile shaft or perineum in males; females may have cervical involvement; oral lesions are possible
  - Recurrent lesions on labia, vulva, clitoris, or cervix in females and on the prepuce, glans, or sulcus in males; generally less severe cutaneous lesions
  - Regional lymphadenopathy

Diagnostic Studies. A Tzanck smear can be done on fluid from the lesions to identify epidermal giant cells; however, it does not distinguish HSV-1 from HSV-2. Viral cultures are the gold standard for definitive diagnosis. Direct fluorescent antibody (DFA) tests, enzyme-linked immunosorbent assay (ELISA) serology, and polymerase chain reaction (PCR) tests are usually only used with severe forms of HSV infection.

Differential Diagnosis

The differential diagnosis includes aphthous stomatitis, coxsackie virus or hand-foot-and-mouth disease, varicella, impetigo, folliculitis, and erythema multiforme.

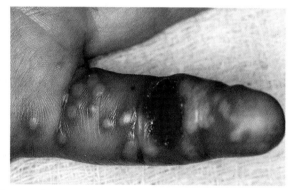

- **Fig 34.16** Herpetic Whitlow. (From Zitelli BJ, McIntire S, Nowalk AJ. *Zitelli and Davis' Atlas of Pediatric Physical Diagnosis.* 7th ed. Philadelphia: Elsevier; 2018.)

Management

Management can be guided by considering the host (e.g., age, area and extent of involvement, and immune status) and the drug needed (Table 34.5). Treatment includes:

1. Burow solution compresses tid to alleviate discomfort
2. Acyclovir 20 to 40 mg/kg/dose orally 5 times a day for 5 days, or 200 mg 5 times a day for 7 to 10 days (maximum pediatric dose 1000 mg/d) may be indicated to help shorten the course and alleviate symptoms for children older than 2 years old with the following conditions:
   - Any underlying skin disorder (e.g., eczema)
   - An immunocompromised disease
   - Systemic symptoms with primary genital infection
   - Occasionally for initial severe gingivostomatitis Acyclovir is most effective if started within 3 days of disease onset. Famciclovir or valacyclovir are additional antiviral agents approved for use in adults.
3. Topical antivirals may help for initial genital herpes infections and recurrent herpes labialis. Most are not approved for children under 12.
4. Oral acyclovir 200 mg 5 times a day for 5 to 10 days may speed healing of herpetic whitlow (see Fig 34.15).
5. Antibiotics for secondary bacterial (usually staphylococcal) infection:
   - Mupirocin: Topically 3 times a day for 5 days
   - Erythromycin: 40 mg/kg/d for 10 days
   - Dicloxacillin: 12.5 to 50 mg/kg/d for 10 days
6. Oral anesthetics for comfort; use with caution in children (the child needs to be able to rinse and spit):
   - Viscous lidocaine 2% topical
   - Liquid diphenhydramine alone or combined with aluminum hydroxide or magnesium hydroxide as a 1:1 rinse (maximum of 5 mg/kg/d diphenhydramine in case it is swallowed); it can also be applied to the lesions with cotton-tipped swabs
7. Newborn infant, immunosuppressed child, child with infected atopic dermatitis, or child with a lesion in the eye or on the eyelid margin; consult with or refer to an appropriate provider.
8. Offer supportive care, such as antipyretics, analgesics, hydration, and good oral hygiene
9. Exclude from day care only during the initial course (gingivostomatitis) and if the child cannot control secretions
10. Recurrent, frequent, and severe HSV infection may be treated with acyclovir prophylaxis for 6 months

TABLE 34.5	Diagnosis and Treatment of Herpes Simplex and Herpes Zoster			
	Presentation	**Clinical Findings**	**Treatment**	**Education**
Herpes simplex	Gingivostomatitis as primary infection; herpes labialis or herpes facialis as recurrent infection	Pharyngitis with erythematous vesicles, near, on, and/or in mouth; small, clear vesicles on erythematous base progressing to crusting	Burow solution; acyclovir in primary case or underlying disorder; antibiotics if secondary infection; oral anesthetics; supportive care	Degree and duration of contagion; triggers to infection
Herpes zoster	Reactivation of latent varicella virus, especially after mild cases or in infants younger than 1 year old or immunocompromised host	Two or three clustered groups of vesicles on erythematous base, especially over 2nd cervical to 2nd lumbar and 5th to 7th cranial nerve dermatomes; does not cross the midline; pain (can be severe), itch, tingle is minimal in children	Burow solution; antihistamine; drying lotions; possible acyclovir; silver sulfadiazine; antibiotics if secondary infection	New vesicles occur for up to 1 week; takes 2-3 weeks to resolve; contagious until lesions stop erupting and are crusted over; varicella vaccine to prevent

Complications

Eczema herpeticum or Kaposi varicelliform eruption is discussed in Chapter 31. HSV has also been implicated as a possible cause of erythema multiforme and Stevens-Johnson syndrome (SJS).

Patient and Family Education

Recurrence of infection, possible triggering factors, and avoidance measures should be discussed. Triggers can include physical and psychological stress, trauma, fever, exposure to UV light, illness, menses, and extreme weather. Contagiousness of lesions and oral secretions must be understood. Explanation of the course of primary disease, with fever lasting up to 4 days and lesions taking at least 2 weeks to heal, is important.

Herpes Zoster

Herpes zoster (HZ) is a recurrent varicella infection commonly called *shingles* (Fig 34.17). Caused by reactivation of the latent varicella zoster infection from the sensory root ganglia, HZ occurs in 10% to 20% of all individuals, is rare in childhood, and occurs more frequently with increasing age (three times more common in adolescents than preschoolers). HZ is more common following mild cases of varicella infections before 1 year old (threefold to twentyfold increased risk) and in immunocompromised children.

Clinical Findings

History. Burning, stinging pain, tenderness to light touch, hyperesthesia, or tingling precedes eruption by about 1 week, although this is less common in children. The lesions can be extremely itchy and painful.

Physical Examination

- Two or three clustered groups of macules and papules progress to vesicles on an erythematous base. These vesicles become pustular, rupture, ulcerate, and crust.
- Lesions develop over 3 to 5 days and last 7 to 10 days. Lesions may develop for up to 1 week followed by crusting and healing during the next 2 weeks. In children, delayed chronic pain, known as *postherpetic neuralgia,* is rare.
- Lesions commonly follow the dermatomes of the second cervical to lumbar nerves and the fifth to seventh cranial nerves with scattered lesions outside these areas.

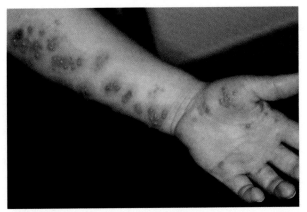

• **Fig 34.17** Herpes Zoster. (From Weston WL, Lane AT, Morelli JG. *Color Textbook of Pediatric Dermatology.* 4th ed. St. Louis: Mosby/Elsevier; 2007, p 134.)

- Lesions do not cross midline (key to diagnosis); sharp demarcation at the midline with occasional contralateral involvement.
- Lymphadenopathy may occur.

Diagnostic Studies. The diagnosis is clinical. If needed, Tzanck smear or viral culture can distinguish HZ from HSV infection. Bacterial culture or Gram stain can be used to distinguish from impetigo. A DFA stain of vesicle base scrapings is beneficial in the difficult-to-diagnose case and results are timely.

Differential Diagnosis

Local cutaneous HSV infection and impetigo are differential diagnoses.

Management

Management steps include the following:

1. Burow solution compresses three times a day to alleviate discomfort
2. Warm, soothing baths
3. Antihistamines for itching
4. Analgesics for discomfort; do not use salicylates
5. Ointment (such as Aquaphor or Vaseline) to moisturize the lesions and decrease itching
6. Antiviral medications are not recommended for use in all children with HZ:
   - Acyclovir 30 mg/kg/d divided 4 times a day for 5 days may be useful for children who are immunosuppressed, have ocular herpes, or have Ramsay-Hunt syndrome (Weston and Morelli, 2017)
7. Antibiotics for secondary bacterial (usually staphylococcal) infection:
   - Mupirocin topically twice daily
   - Dicloxacillin 12.5 to 25 mg/kg/d for 7 to 10 days
8. Refer for immediate ophthalmologic examination if eyes, forehead, or nose is involved.

Complications

Complications are rare except in immunocompromised children. Occasionally HZ is the initial finding in acquired immunodeficiency syndrome (AIDS), especially if more than one dermatome is involved. Eczema herpeticum may occur.

Patient and Family Education

- New vesicles appear for up to 1 week and take 2 to 3 weeks to resolve. Illness is usually mild.
- The child is contagious for varicella until lesions are crusted. If the lesions can be covered, the child does not need to be excluded from school or child care. If the lesions cannot be covered, the child should avoid contact with others until the lesions are crusted (Cohen, 2013).

Molluscum Contagiosum

A benign common childhood viral skin infection with little health risk, molluscum contagiosum often disappears on its own in a few weeks to months and is not easily treated (Fig 34.18). This poxvirus replicates in host epithelial cells. It attacks skin and mucous membranes and is spread by direct contact, by fomites, or by autoinoculation (typically scratching). It is commonly found in children and adolescents. The incubation period is about 2 to 7 weeks but may be as long as 6 months. Infectivity is low but the child is contagious as long as lesions are present.

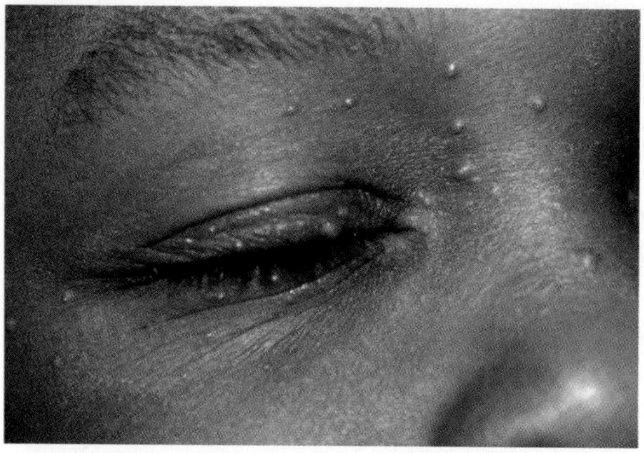

• **Fig 34.18** Molluscum Contagiosum. (From Weston WL, Lane AT, Morelli JG. *Color Textbook of Pediatric Dermatology.* 4th ed. St. Louis: Mosby/Elsevier; 2007, p 144.)

Clinical Findings

History
- Itching at the site
- Possible exposure to molluscum contagiosum

Physical Examination
- Very small, firm, pink to flesh-colored discrete papules 1 to 6 mm in size (occasionally up to 15 mm)
- Papules progressing to become umbilicated (may not be evident) with a cheesy core; keratinous contents may extrude from the umbilication
- Face, axillae, antecubital area, trunk, popliteal fossae, crural area, and extremities are the most commonly involved areas; palms, soles, and scalp are spared
- Single papule to numerous papules; most often numerous clustered papules and linear configurations
- Sexually active or abused children can have genitally grouped lesions
- Children with eczema or immunosuppression can have severe cases; those with human immunodeficiency virus (HIV) infection or AIDS can have hundreds of lesions

Differential Diagnosis

Warts, closed comedones, small epidermal cysts, blisters, folliculitis, and condyloma acuminatum are included in the differential diagnosis.

Management

- Untreated lesions usually disappear within 6 months to 2 years but may take up to 4 years to completely disappear. There is no consensus on the management of molluscum contagiosum (Forbat, Al-Niaimi, and Ali, 2017). The decision to treat may be based on discomfort, reduction of itching, minimization of autoinoculation, limitation of transmission, and for cosmetic reasons. Genital lesions may need to be treated to prevent spread to sexual partners. Dermatology specialists can assist the family in determining the best treatment option based on pain and side effects of treatment and known efficacy in the molluscum presentation. Current treatment options with larger supporting controlled studies include:
- Curettage
- Salicylic acid
- KOH

- Imiquimod
- Cantharidin
- Lemon myrtle oil (Forbat, Al-Niaimi, and Ali, 2017)

Patient and Family Education

- Sexual abuse of children with genitally grouped lesions should be suspected and evaluated.
- Evaluate for HIV infection if hundreds of lesions are found.
- Wait and see approach—spontaneous clearing generally occurs.

Complications

Molluscum dermatitis, a scaly, erythematous, hypersensitive reaction, can occur and will respond to moisturizer; avoid hydrocortisone because it causes molluscum to flare. Impetiginized lesions, inflammation of the eyes or conjunctiva, and scarring can occur.

Patient and Family Education

Patients are contagious, but there is no need to exclude them from day care or school. Children with impaired immunity, atopic dermatitis, or traumatized skin are at greater risk for broader spread. Severe inflammation is possible several hours after application of cantharidin. Scarring is unusual.

Warts

Warts are common childhood skin tumors characterized by a proliferation of the epidermis and mucosa infected by the human papillomavirus (HPV). There are over 100 HPV types, and each one produces characteristic lesions in specific locations (e.g., verruca vulgaris, verruca plana, verruca plantaris, and condyloma acuminatum). Trauma promotes inoculation of the HPV (Koebner phenomenon); as a result, most warts are on the hands, fingers, elbows, and plantar surfaces of the feet.

The transmission of warts from person to person depends on viral and host factors, such as quantity of virus, location of warts, preexisting skin injury, and cell-mediated immunity. Transmission is from fomites or skin-to-skin contact, and autoinoculation is frequent. Incubation is from 1 to 6 months, possibly years.

Although a large percentage of all warts resolve spontaneously within 3 to 5 years, there is a high recurrence rate. Cutaneous warts are rarely a serious health concern but present cosmetic problems for children and their families (Cohen, 2013).

Clinical Findings

History. The history can include exposure to someone with warts. Though most common on the extremities, warts can occur anywhere on the body, including the face, scalp, and genitalia.

Physical Examination
- Common warts (verruca vulgaris) are usually elevated flesh-colored single papules with scaly, irregular surfaces and occasionally black pinpoints, which are thrombosed blood vessels. They are usually asymptomatic and multiple and are found anywhere on the body, although most commonly on the hands, nails, and feet. They may be dome shaped, filiform, or exophytic (Fig 34.19). Filiform warts project from the skin on a narrow stalk and are usually seen on the face, lips, nose, eyelids, or neck. Periungual warts are common, occurring around the cuticles of the fingers or toes.

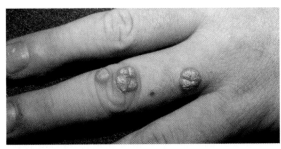

• **Fig 34.19** Multiple Common Warts (Verruca Vulgaris). (From Weston WL, Morelli JG. *Pediatric Dermatology DDx Deck*. Philadelphia: Elsevier/Saunders; 2013.)

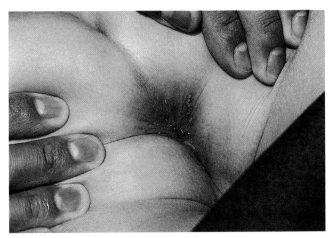

• **Fig 34.20** Condylomata Acuminata. (From Paller AS, Mancini AJ. *Hurwitz Clinical Pediatric Dermatology: A Textbook of Skin Disorders of Children and Adolescence*. 5th ed. Philadelphia: Elsevier; 2016.)

- Plantar warts (verrucae plantaris or mosaic) are commonly found on weight-bearing surfaces of the feet. They grow inward and disrupt skin markings.
- Flat warts (verruca plana or juvenile warts) are seen commonly on the face, neck, and extremities. They are small, slightly elevated papules and number from few to several hundred.
- Condylomata acuminata on genital mucosa and adjacent skin are multiple, confluent warts with irregular surfaces, light color, and cauliflower-like appearance (Fig 34.20).

Differential Diagnosis

The differential diagnosis includes calluses, corns, foreign bodies, moles, comedones, and squamous cell carcinoma.

Management

There is no single effective treatment for warts; watchful waiting is an option. The recurrence rate is high; they typically do not resolve with just a single treatment. No treatment is necessary if the warts are asymptomatic. The decision to treat should be based on location, number and size of lesions, discomfort, and whether they are cosmetically objectionable. Treatment should not be harmful, and scarring should be avoided. Genital warts found in young children or in adolescents who are not sexually active should create suspicion of sexual abuse. Specific treatment options are outlined in Box 34.6. Follow up in 2 to 3 weeks to evaluate response.

• BOX 34.6 Treatment Options for Warts

- Keratolytics eliminate the wart by causing an inflammatory response and topical peeling. They are often available over the counter, cause little pain, and are low in cost and risk, but they are slow to work.
  - Salicylic acid paints with a concentration of greater than 20% are applied with a toothpick once or twice a day for 4-6 weeks. On thick skin, a combination of 16.7% salicylic acid and 16.7% collodion is more effective. This method is useful for common or periungual warts, but it is not effective with warts larger than 5 mm in diameter. Both products may be more effective if combined with duct tape occlusion.
  - Salicylic acid plasters with 40% concentration are cut to size and taped in place for 3-5 days. After the plaster is taken off, the area should be soaked for 45 min and the dead epidermis removed. A new plaster is then applied. Treatment can last 3-6 weeks. This method is useful for plantar warts.
  - Retinoic acid gel 0.025%-0.05% applied once or twice daily brings resolution in 4-6 weeks. This method is useful for flat warts, but it does not work for common, plantar, or periungual warts.
- Occlusion with duct tape: Place on for 12 h a day for 6 days in a row, followed by soaking and scraping of epidermis; is easy, painless, and inexpensive.
- Destructive agents eliminate the wart by causing necrosis and blister formation. Most techniques are painful and require patient cooperation.
  - Cryotherapy: Liquid nitrogen, available over the counter as well as for in-office use, is applied for 2-10 s until an area 1-3 mm beyond the wart turns white or patient complains of pain; goal is to induce blister formation above the dermal-epidermal junction. Take care not to freeze the wart too vigorously. Caution should be used when freezing warts over joints and the lateral aspects of digits. This method is uncomfortable and often not tolerated by children. Retreatment is often necessary. Cantharidin 0.7% is applied directly to the wart with a toothpick and covered with tape for 24 h. This is a potent blistering agent that creates a blister in 2-3 days that is sloughed after 7-14 days. This method is useful for periungual and some plantar warts. Do not use on other body surfaces.
  - Podophyllum 25% solution in compound benzoin tincture is applied to the wart with a toothpick; it should be washed off in 4 h; may be repeated in 1 week. Podofilox, available over the counter for home use, is applied twice a day for 3 days. After a 4-day rest period, the 3-day cycle may be repeated as necessary. This technique is useful for common or genital warts.
  - Surgical excision of warts can lead to scarring that can be more painful than the wart itself, but can be highly effective for large individual warts. Surgery by snipping with scissors, not scalpel, is useful for filiform warts.
  - Laser treatments are often as effective as cryosurgery, but can be painful and require several treatments for complete resolution.
- Immunotherapy modalities stimulate an immune response to HPV. These newer treatment modalities do not have controlled studies evaluating their effectiveness.
  - Oral cimetidine, a histamine 2–receptor-blocking agent, may improve immunity to HPV. It is used in conjunction with other modalities at a dose of 20-30 mg/kg divided twice a day for 3-4 months.
  - Imiquimod cream creates cell-mediated immunity in surrounding areas and is often effective as a home treatment. It is approved for children over 12 years of age and is applied daily for 1-2 months.
  - Contact sensitization and interferon injection are methods used by dermatologists, usually in adult patients.

HPV, Human papillomavirus.

Complications

Scarring from removal can occur. A ring of satellite warts may develop at the edge of the blister following treatment with cantharidin. Immunocompromised hosts can have extensive involvement.

Patient and Family Education

A blister, sometimes hemorrhagic, may form 1 to 2 days after liquid nitrogen treatment. Redness and itching may herald regression of a wart. Parents and patients must be warned that multiple or prolonged treatment is often necessary.

Infestations of the Skin

Pediculosis

Pediculosis (lice infestation) can affect the scalp (most common), body, or pubic area (considered a sexually transmitted disease). Infestation is defined by some as the presence of either nits (eggs) or lice and by others as presence of lice alone.

Lice infestation is caused by three subspecies, *Pediculus humanus capitis* and *corporis* (head and body) or by *Phthirus pubis* (pubic). The adult female louse, which survives by sucking human blood, deposits 6 to 10 eggs per day on a gluelike substance within 4 mm from the scalp on the hair shaft in a waterproof shell. Nits incubate for about 1 week, hatch and grow into adult lice over another 1 to 2 weeks, then begin laying eggs. Head lice live approximately 30 days on a host and lay up to 10 eggs per day. Transmission is by direct or indirect contact, often by sharing hairbrushes, caps, clothing, or linen or through close living quarters, or sexual activity (pubic lice).

Pediculosis capitis is common in children. Head lice are not considered a health hazard, because they do not spread disease. All socioeconomic groups are affected, but lice are most common in school-age children, with the peak season occurring from August to November. Lice are uncommon in African American children (Guenther, 2018).

Pediculosis corporis is uncommon in childhood. The louse is rarely seen on the body; rather it attaches to clothing and intermittently pierces the skin. It is the only louse that can carry human disease (e.g., epidemic typhus and trench fever).

Pubic lice may involve the scalp, eyebrows, or eyelashes but primarily are found in the pubic area. Clothing and bed linens are a source of residence. If pediculosis pubis is found in a child, sexual abuse must be considered.

Clinical Findings

History
- A history of infestation in a family, friend, or day care contact
- Dandruff-like substance in the hair
- Itching of the scalp, scratching, and irritability if infestation has been present for a few weeks
- Reports of a crawling sensation in the scalp

Physical Examination
- Head lice
  - Lice can be visualized; nits can be seen as small white oval cases attached tightly to a hair shaft. Nits are usually laid within 4 mm of the scalp; as the hair grows, the nits and empty shells are found farther from the scalp, indicating more long-term infestation.
  - Care must be taken to differentiate hair casts, epithelial cells, and other debris from nits.
  - Common sites are the back of the head, nape of the neck, and behind the ears; eyelashes can be involved. Scalp excoriations and occipital or cervical adenopathy can be present.
  - Rinse topical pediculosides in sink rather than shower in order to reduce skin exposure and in warm water rather than hot water to reduce absorption through vasodilation (Devore, Schutze, Council on School Health and Committee on Infectious Disease, 2015).
- Body lice
  - Excoriated macules or papules may be present (secondary bacterial infection of the skin may develop).
  - Belt line, collar, and underwear areas are common sites.
  - A hemorrhagic pinpoint macule is seen where the louse extracted blood.
  - Axillary, inguinal, or regional lymphadenopathy can be present.
- Pubic lice
  - Excoriation and small bluish macules and papules may be present.
  - Eyelashes can be involved; spread to other short-haired areas (thighs, trunk, axillae, beard) may occur.

Diagnostic Studies
- Microscopic examination of a hair shaft can more clearly identify nits.
- Test for other sexually transmitted infections if pubic lice found; specifically gonorrhea and syphilis.

Differential Diagnosis

Scabies, dermatitis herpetiformis, and necrotic excoriations are in the differential diagnosis. Rule out sexual abuse if pubic lice are found.

Management

Correct diagnosis is imperative to effective management. Treatment is recommended when live lice and viable nits are observed, because nonviable nits (which do not necessarily indicate the presence of lice) can persist on the hair shaft for several months.

Treatment options are varied and controversial. Treatment failure is common, whether as a result of poor technique or because of increasing drug resistance to available pharmacologic treatment options in children who have been treated multiple times. Over the counter Permethrin 1% and pyrethrins are inexpensive but resistance is widespread (Drugs for Head Lice, November 21, 2016). The increasing treatment failure has led to the trial of many alternative treatments such as over-the-counter medications, and dangerous substitutes (e.g., kerosene) may be used by parents. It is recommended that providers follow local resistance patterns when determining treatment. Table 34.6 outlines recommended treatment.

Pediculicides are a first-line treatment option. They are toxic substances, however, and should be used only as directed and with care. Proper pediculicide application is key to success. Prior to use, do not use a shampoo that contains conditioner or cream rinse, or petrolatum products on the hair or scalp. Keep the pediculicide out of the eyes. If applying to damp hair, make sure the hair is damp, not wet (dilutes the pediculicide). Do not rewash the hair for 1 to 2 days following treatment. Most treatments call for reapplication in 7 to 10 days with 9 days being the optimal interval based on the life cycle of lice (Devore et al., 2015).
- Permethrin 1% cream rinse is the treatment of choice for head lice because of its safety (can be used in children older than 1 month old), efficacy, and 10-day residual. Hair should be shampooed and towel dried (damp), permethrin applied,

TABLE 34.6 Diagnosis and Treatment of Pediculosis and Scabies

	Clinical Findings	Treatment
Pediculosis (head lice)	History of infestation; itchy scalp, scratches; postoccipital nodes; occasional visualization of lice or nits (small white oval cases), commonly on back of head, nape of neck, behind ears, possibly eyelashes	Key to treatment is proper technique! *First step:* Apply pediculicide: permethrin *or* pyrethrin plus piperonyl butoxide *Second step:* Remove nits: comb hair with fine-toothed comb in 1-inch sections with special attention to nape of neck and behind ears *Third step:* Cleanse the environment: check family, friends, day care/school contacts; clean sheets, towels, clothing, and headgear; store other items in plastic for 2 days; vacuum; soak brushes and combs; follow up in 2 weeks with daily recheck at home by parent May return to school after pediculicide treatment; "no nit" policies are not recommended
Scabies	Key finding: Itching, worse at night, and complaints are more significant than physical findings; fitful sleep, crankiness; curving burrows, especially in webs of fingers, sides of hands, folds of wrist, armpits, forearms, elbows, belt line, buttocks, proximal half of foot and heel; secondary excoriation; infants may have lesions on palms, soles, scalp, face, posterior auricle and axilla, folds, red-brown; may be <10 lesions total or may be dozens (typical of infants); lesions may occur in the form of firm nodules in infants	Treat with permethrin 5%, repeated in 1 week; use antihistamine, hydrocortisone, or nonsteroidal anti-inflammatory drugs (NSAIDs) for itching; simultaneously treat family members (even if asymptomatic), friends, and school/day care contacts Cleanse environment: Linens and clothing, vacuum, store anything else in plastic bags for 2 days; rash and itch persist for up to 3 weeks after treatment; return to school 24 hours after treatment

left on for 10 minutes, and then rinsed. Hair should not be rewashed for at least 24 to 48 hours. Resistance to permethrin 1% has been reported but prevalence is unknown. Reapplication is recommended (Devore et al., 2015).

- Spinosad is approved for use in patients 6 months of age and older. Superiority of spinosad over permethrin has been well documented. It is applied to dry hair and left on for 10 minutes before rinsing. Reapplication is recommended only if live lice are seen.
- Pyrethrin, a natural extract from the chrysanthemum plant, is effective as a pediculicide but not as an ovicide. Pyrethrin is formulated with piperonyl butoxide to form a 10-minute shampoo or mousse that is applied to dry hair, with a repeat reapplication in 7 to 10 days. Pyrethrin is contraindicated in children with allergy to ragweed. Because pyrethrin does not kill both lice and eggs, treatment failures are more common than with permethrin. Highly variable resistance is found with pyrethrin.
- Topical ivermectin lotion is a single-dose, 10-minute application to dry hair. It is approved for children 6 months old and older. Caution is advised for use during pregnancy. Repeat application is not necessary as the lice of treated eggs are not viable.
- Lindane is no longer recommended by the American Academy of Pediatrics (AAP) or the Medical Letter due to potential neurotoxic effects (Devore et al., 2015).
- Malathion lotion 0.5% is an organophosphate with a pine-needle–oil base that is available only by prescription. It is a potent lice killer that binds to the hair shaft for 4 weeks and it is considered the most effective therapy for killing lice and nits. It is not recommended in children younger than 2 years old. The drug is flammable, and if ingested causes severe respiratory distress. Malathion 0.5% lotion should be applied to dry hair, be allowed to dry, and then carefully rinsed off 8 to 12 hours later (Guenther, 2018). Avoidance of hair dryers, curling irons, and flat irons will reduce the risk of burns. A single application is adequate for most patients but a repeat

application in 7 to 10 days is appropriate if live lice are seen (Devore et al., 2015).

Many providers and families choose to forgo the use of pediculicides in favor of a manual removal of lice and nits. Although combing may not always be necessary, this step is usually taken in order to remove nits after a pediculicide is used. Proper technique is the key to success. A good light, a magnifying glass, and tweezers are useful. A wide-toothed comb may be used initially to straighten the hair, but a fine-toothed nit-removal comb is necessary to remove nits.

- Some products claim to dissolve the substance (cement) that attaches the nit to the hair to facilitate removal. A 1:1 vinegar-to-water solution applied along the proximal hair shaft and allowed to rest for 3 minutes prior to combing has not been shown to be effective. In fact, there are no effective products available to loosen the "glue" of lice nits.
- Use a proper nit-removal comb with fine teeth (included in most pediculicide kits).
- Comb damp hair for a minimum of 20 to 30 minutes, working from the top of the scalp down in 1-inch sections. Pay special attention to the nape of the neck and behind the ears.
- If eyelashes are involved, coat with petroleum jelly two or three times a day for 8 to 14 days and manually remove nits.
- Comb-outs and inspection should be repeated every night for 2 to 3 weeks to ensure cure.

The third step in lice treatment is thorough cleansing of the environment.

- Examine family members, friends, school, and day care contacts. Do not treat family members if nothing is found because of the emergence of treatment-resistant lice and pediculicide toxicity.
- Launder sheets, towels, clothing, and headgear in hot water and machine dry on hot cycle for 20 minutes, iron, or dry clean.
- Although rarely needed, any other item in close contact with others that cannot be washed or dry-cleaned should be stored in a plastic bag for 2 weeks.

- Family may choose to vacuum play areas, floors, rugs, and furniture. This type of exhaustive cleaning is rarely needed (Devore et al., 2015).
- Soak brushes, combs, and hair accessories in pediculicide, alcohol, or Lysol for 1 hour, followed by a hot-water rinse.
- Spraying or fumigating the house is not recommended.

Alternative treatments include herbal or essential oils, and occlusive methods such as olive oil, pine oil, tea-tree oil, margarine, mayonnaise, dog shampoo, styling gels, and petroleum jelly, all of which suffocate and kill the lice. Further evidence-based studies are needed regarding these practices. Definitely avoid wrapping the hair in plastic and putting the child under a hair dryer or washing the hair with gasoline or kerosene.

Treatment failure is not unusual. Common mistakes that lead to recurrence of lice include dilution of pediculicide by applying to wet, not damp hair; use of a shampoo with conditioner or cream rinse before treatment; inadequate combing techniques; not cleansing personal care items; and not screening and treating family members and close contacts. However, with proper use of a pediculicide, if lice reappear, reinfection from contact with an untreated individual is a more likely cause.

Prevalence to particular products is not known and appears to be regional. There are neither formal recommendations nor FDA approval for dealing with resistance. Some methods for treating resistant lice include the following:

- Benzoyl alcohol 5% if the child is older than 6 months
- Malathion 0.5% if the child is older than 2 years
- Manual removal by wet combing
- Occlusive method with careful technique for 2 to 4 lice life cycles

Body lice are treated by improving hygiene and cleaning clothes. Wash infested clothing and dry at hot temperatures on a weekly basis for several weeks. Pediculicides are not necessary (Guenther, 2018). Pubic lice are treated as pediculosis capitis.

Complications

Secondary bacterial infection can occur.

Patient and Family Education

Items for discussion include the following:

- Daily to weekly checks or combing for lice or nits should be carried out at home.
- Educate family members about the expected course, that lice infestation is not a social disease, and about the need to avoid excessive or unnecessary retreatment. Do not use extra amounts; do not treat more than three times with the same medication without being seen by a care provider; do not mix pediculicides.
- Children should not be excluded or sent home from school because of lice. Parents should be notified and informed that the child should be treated. The AAP discourages "no-nit" policies in schools, because such policies have been ineffective in controlling head lice transmission and result in excessive lost school and workdays (Devore et al., 2015).

Scabies

Scabies is caused by the mite *Sarcoptes scabiei,* which is an obligate human parasite that burrows into the epidermis and causes intense itching (Figs 34.21A and B). Scabies is a highly contagious infestation spread through close contact and shared clothing or linen. The female mite burrows into the skin, laying up to three eggs a day as she travels. The eggs hatch in about 3 to 4 days and mature into adult mites in 10 to 14 days. The female mite has a life span of 15 to 30 days. Sensitization, which causes intense itching, occurs approximately 3 weeks after infestation. Scabies occurs in all socioeconomic groups and in all age groups.

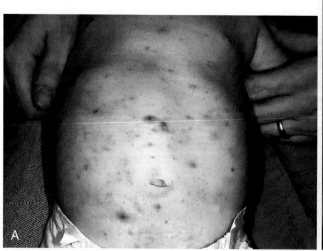
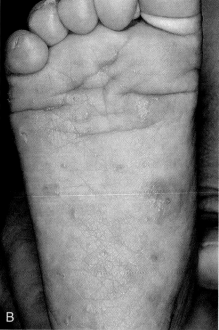

• **Fig 34.21** Scabies. (A) Erythematous papules and crusting. (B) Erythematous papules and linear burrows. (From Paller AS, Mancini AJ. *Hurwitz Clinical Pediatric Dermatology: A Textbook of Skin Disorders of Children and Adolescence.* 5th ed. Philadelphia: Elsevier; 2016.)

Clinical Findings

History
- Key finding: Itching, worse at night, initially mild but progressively more intense
- Fitful sleep, crankiness, or rubbing of hands and feet (infants)

Physical Examination
- Complaints are significantly greater than examination findings.
- Characteristic lesions include curving S-shaped burrows, especially on webs of fingers and sides of hands, folds of wrists and armpits, forearms, elbows, belt line, buttocks, genitalia, or proximal half of foot and heel.
- Vesiculopustular lesions tend to be found in infants and young children. They classically have vesicular lesions on palms, soles, scalp, face, posterior auriculae, and axillae, concentrated in the folds; head and neck lesions typically are red-brown vesicopustules or nodules. However, any child younger than 2 years old can have an unusual manifestation.
- Secondary lesions include itchy papules, red-brown nodules from inflammatory response, crusting, excoriation, and other signs of secondary infection.
- Infants classically have dozens of lesions; older children may have fewer than 10.
- Crusted, or Norwegian scabies, presents as scaly papules or plaques and is more often found in immunocompromised patients. This form of scabies is much more contagious due to large number of mites present.

Diagnostic Studies
- Microscopic examination of scrapings from an unscratched burrow in saline or mineral oil can reveal an eight-legged mite, eggs, or feces. Do not use KOH because it dissolves the mites, eggs, and feces. Burrows and fresh papules are best for specimen collection.

Differential Diagnosis

Papular urticaria; atopic, seborrheic, or contact dermatitis; insect bites; folliculitis; lichen planus; and dermatitis herpetiformis are included in the differential diagnosis.

Management

Management involves the following:
1. Pharmacologic treatment begins with applying a thin layer of scabicide to the entire body, excluding the eyes. Areas of special importance are under the fingernails, the scalp, behind the ears, all folds and creases, and the feet and hands. In general, the scabicide should be reapplied in 7 days on all symptomatic patients.
2. Permethrin 5% cream remains the drug of choice for the treatment of scabies. Despite frequent use over the past two decades, there is no clear evidence of resistance to permethrin 5% cream for the treatment of classic scabies (Paller and Mancini, 2016). It is indicated for use in children as young as 2 months old (Cohen, 2013). Parents and patients should be educated on proper application of a thin layer of cream to the entire body from the neck down, and rinsing after 8 to 14 hours. Application may be repeated in 1 week (Paller and Mancini, 2016). Unlike adults and older children, infants generally present with lesions on the face, neck, scalp, and hands and feet; be sure to include these areas on application, avoiding the areas around the eyes and mouth (Bethel, 2014). The treatment of crusted or Norwegian scabies has proven to be more difficult due to common misdiagnosis. Ivermectin 200 µg/kg is recommended orally on days 1, 2, 8, 9, and 15 of treatment, in conjunction with full body application of permethrin 5% cream for 7 days, then twice weekly until resolved (Workowski, 2015). Due to a lack of safety data, ivermectin is not recommended for children younger than 5 years old, or less than 15 kg (Cohen, 2013). Antihistamines (hydroxyzine or diphenhydramine) or topical 1% hydrocortisone can be helpful for itching, which can last for several weeks after successful treatment.
3. Simultaneous treatment of family members, friends, and school and day care contacts, even if asymptomatic, is essential.
4. At time of treatment, linens and any clothing worn during the past 48 hours should be washed with hot water, put into a hot dryer for 20 minutes, or dry-cleaned. The house should be vacuumed.
5. Store nonwashable items in sealed plastic bags for a 1 week. Mite survival when separated from the human host is only a few days.

Resistance to medication is not common and continued infestation is usually due to treatment failure rather than resistance. Reasons for treatment failure include an incorrect diagnosis, not applying medication to the whole body, or not treating all members of the household. The child may develop postscabetic eczema that can be misdiagnosed as treatment failure. Evaluate and treat with topical corticosteroids.

Complications

A secondary bacterial infection is possible and should be treated. Postscabetic syndrome is common, with visible lesions and pruritus persisting for days to weeks following treatment; nodular lesions can persist for weeks to months.

Patient and Family Education

Educate the family about the course of disease. Rash and itching persist for up to 3 weeks following treatment. Avoid overbathing and further irritation of the skin. The child should not be infectious 24 hours after treatment and may return to school or day care.

Allergic and Inflammatory Skin Conditions

Acne Vulgaris

Acne is an inflammatory disorder of the pilosebaceous unit in which excess sebum, keratinous debris, and bacteria accumulate, producing microcomedones. The microcomedones may be noninflamed (comedones) or inflamed lesions (papules, pustules, or nodules). Although rarely a serious disorder, acne may cause permanent scarring and decreased self-esteem, and occasionally heralds underlying disease. It is often of significant concern to the adolescent, having a serious effect on social development (Fig 34.22). Acne is the most common skin disorder and affects approximately 85% of adolescents in the United States (Paller and Mancini, 2016). Four mechanisms contribute to this sebaceous follicle disorder:
- Sebaceous follicles become plugged with keratinous material.
- Colonies of anaerobic bacteria grow deep in the follicle, primarily *Propionibacterium acnes,* but coagulase-negative staphylococci and *M. furfur* can be involved.
- Sebum is overproduced and androgen production increases, resulting in expansion of the follicle.

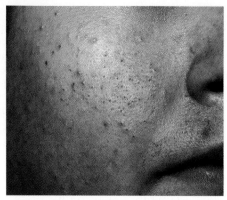

- **Fig 34.22** Acne Vulgaris. Open comedones present as blackheads. (From Paller AS, Mancini AJ. *Hurwitz Clinical Pediatric Dermatology: A Textbook of Skin Disorders of Children and Adolescence.* 5th ed. Philadelphia: Elsevier; 2016.)

- Inflammation occurs and pustules form secondary to trapped *P. acnes* and sebum. The bacteria release chemotactic factors that attract neutrophils to ingest the bacteria and release hydrolytic enzymes.

Acne usually begins at the onset of puberty, occurring earlier in girls (12 to 13 years old) than boys (14 to 15 years old). It tends to improve in the summer and worsens with menses and stress. The pathogenesis of acne is multifactorial; gender, age, neuroendocrine regulation, genetic factors, and environment are significant factors. Although not a serious physical disorder, acne has been associated with psychosocial morbidity and decreased emotional well-being. "Patients with even mild to moderate acne have demonstrated high scores on the Carrol Rating Scale for Depression and an increased prevalence of suicidal ideation" (Paller and Mancini, 2016, p. 175).

Clinical Findings

History
- Family history of acne
- Stage of pubertal development and menstrual history
- Facial and hair products used, especially occlusive products or pomades
- Oral and topical prescription medication, especially oral contraceptives, antibiotics, or steroids
- Current or previous acne treatment and results
- Sports participation, especially if wearing football pads, helmets, headbands, or other protective devices
- Jobs, such as cooking at a fast-food grill or working at a gas station
- Other medical conditions

Physical Examination. Lesions most commonly are found on the face, back, and chest.
- Noninflammatory lesions:
  - Microcomedone—a follicular plug as a result of obstruction of the pilosebaceous unit (hair follicle and sebaceous gland) typically localized on the face and trunk.
  - Open comedone (blackhead)—a noninflammatory lesion or papule, firm in consistency, caused by blockage at the mouth of the follicle and occurring on the face, upper back, shoulders, and chest. The black color is thought to come from oxidized keratinous material at the follicular opening. This is the main lesion in early adolescence.
  - Closed comedone (whitehead)—a noninflammatory lesion, semisoft in consistency, caused by blockage at the neck of the follicle. This is a precursor to inflammatory acne.

- Inflammatory lesions occur secondary to rupture of noninflamed lesions into the dermis and can include papules, pustules, excoriation, lesion crusting, nodules, cysts, scars, and sinus tracts (confluent nodules likely to scar).

The severity of acne is determined by the quantity, type, and spread of lesions. It is helpful to use a diagram of the face or a grading graph to identify the number and type of lesions to allow more precise patient follow-up. If only open and closed comedones are found, the disorder is called *comedonal acne.* Most adolescents have a combination of comedones, red papules, and pustules called *papulopustular acne,* which can be mild or severe. *Nodulocystic acne* is the most severe form and requires more intensive intervention. Specific types of acne include *frictional,* occurring from rubbing of bras, tight clothes, or headbands; *pomadal,* along the temple and forehead, as a result of pomades or oil-based cosmetics; *athletic,* on forehead, chin, or shoulders, caused by helmets and pads; and *hormonal,* with a beard distribution.

Differential Diagnosis
Cosmetic, mechanical, environmental, or drug-induced acne; rosacea; flat wart; milia; perioral dermatitis; and folliculitis are included in the differential diagnosis.

Management
The goals of acne management are to (1) reduce the excess production of sebum, (2) counteract the abnormal desquamation of epithelial cells, (3) decrease the proliferation of *P. acnes,* and (4) prevent or decrease scarring. Choice of treatment depends on the extent, severity, and duration of disease; type of lesions; and psychological effects the adolescent is experiencing. Table 34.7 shows the treatment algorithm established by the AAD. Box 34.7 lists some of the common medications used.
- Medications used in treatment of acne vary by action, route of administration, and strength. They include topical and systemic preparations; keratolytic or comedolytic agents; those with antibacterial or antibiotic effects; hormonal agents; and preparations that have a combination of actions.
- Topical keratolytic or comedolytic agents, used to minimize follicular obstruction and break up microcomedones, are the first line of acne treatment. They may be dispensed in a combination form with a topical antibacterial agent. Many strengths and forms are available, the strongest being the gels, if tolerated; creams are the least drying. A general rule is to start low (in strength) and slowly (in frequency) and advance as tolerated or needed. A useful technique to decrease the incidence of irritation is to start therapy only for 3 nights a week and slowly increase to a nightly application over a few weeks. A minimum of 4 to 6 weeks of treatment is required before improvement is seen. There are three topical retinoids (tretinoin, adapalene, and tazarotene) and two agents that possess both antibacterial and keratolytic properties (benzoyl peroxide and azelaic acid). Each works by a different mechanism. They can be used together and interchangeably. Dryness, erythema, irritation, and scaling can occur with these products, and the strength and frequency of use must be adjusted for this.
- Tretinoin is a keratolytic that causes sun sensitivity. A pea-sized application should be made 20 minutes after washing the face. Initially it is used every other night, advancing to every night. Sensitivity to tretinoin is worst in the first 2 weeks of use and decreases thereafter.
- Adapalene seems to cause less irritation and less photosensitivity, and it has better efficacy.

TABLE 34.7	Treatment Algorithm for the Management of Acne		
	Mild	**Moderate**	**Severe**
First-line treatment	Benzoyl peroxide (BP) or topical retinoid -or- topical combination therapy[a] BP + antibiotic or retinoid + BP or retinoid + BP + antibiotic	Topical combination therapy[a] BP + antibiotic or retinoid + BP or retinoid + BP + antibiotic -or- oral antibiotic + topical retinoid + BP -or- oral antibiotic + topical retinoid + BP + topical antibiotic	Oral antibiotic + topical combination therapy[a] BP + antibiotic or retinoid + BP or retinoid + BP + antibiotic -or- oral isotretinoin
Alternative treatment	Add topical retinoid or bp (if not on already) -or- consider alternate retinoid -or- consider topical dapsone	Consider alternate combination therapy -or- consider change in oral antibiotic -or- add combined oral contraceptive or oral spironolactone (females) -or- consider oral isotretinoin	Consider change in oral antibiotic -or- add combined oral contraceptive or oral spironolactone (females) -or- consider oral isotretinoin

[a]Indicates that the drug may be prescribed as a fixed combination product or as a separate component.

From Zaenglein AL, Pathy AL, Schlosser BJ, et al. Guidelines of care for the management of acne vulgaris. *J Am Acad Dermatol.* 2016;74(5):945–973.

BOX 34.7 Medications Commonly Used in Treating Acne

Topical Keratolytic or Comedolytic Agents
Retinoids
  Tretinoin: 0.01%-0.025% gel; 0.025%-0.1% cream; 0.1% microgel
  Tretinoin/clindamycin (combination topical)
  Tazarotene: 0.05%-0.1% cream; 0.05%-0.1% gel
  Adapalene: 0.1% gel or cream; 0.3% gel; 0.1% with 2.5% BP gel
Benzoyl peroxide: 2.5%-20% gel; 5% and 10% cream; 5%-20% lotion or wash
Azelaic acid: 20% cream; 15% gel

Topical Antibiotics
Clindamycin: 1% solution, lotion, gel, pledget, foam
Clindamycin: 1% with 5% benzoyl peroxide
Erythromycin: 1.5% to 2% solution, 3% gel or swabs
Erythromycin: 3% with benzoyl peroxide 5% gel

Oral Antibiotics
Tetracycline: 250-500 mg per dose twice a day
Minocycline: 50-100 mg per dose twice a day (associated with more side effects)
Doxycycline: 50-100 mg per dose twice a day
Erythromycin: 250-500 mg per dose twice a day

Combination Oral Contraceptions
Ethinyl estradiol/norgestimate
Ethinyl estradiol/norethindrone acetate/ferrous fumarate
Ethinyl estradiol/drospirenone
Ethinyl estradiol/drospirenone/levomefolate

- Tazarotene is a keratolytic to be used once daily.
- Azelaic acid is antibacterial and keratolytic. It is useful in individuals with sensitive or dark skin and is also effective in treating acne rosacea.
- Benzoyl peroxide, the most frequently used topical preparation for acne, is used once or twice a day, depending on the severity of acne and dryness of skin. It is a powerful antimicrobial with comedolytic and anti-inflammatory effects. Use in combination with topical antibiotics causes less antibiotic resistance.
- Topical antibiotics are used to control the inflammatory process, usually most helpful in moderate inflammatory acne. They are also used to maintain control after treatment with oral antibiotics, and are applied to the entire skin surface, not just to problem areas. They should not be applied within 30 minutes of shaving. Due to developing bacterial resistance, topical antibiotics are not recommended as monotherapy. Topical clindamycin may be preferred over erythromycin due to resistance in *Staphylococcus* and *P. acnes* (Paller and Mancini, 2016).
  - Topical clindamycin or erythromycin is used once or twice a day in combination with other topical medications.
  - Topical clindamycin with benzoyl peroxide and erythromycin with benzoyl peroxide are combination products that are more effective than either drug alone and have less resistance from *P. acnes.* This combination is especially effective in mild to moderate inflammatory acne or as an adjunct to oral therapy (Paller and Mancini, 2016).
- Oral antibiotics are used in addition to topical agents to decrease the concentration of *P. acnes* and to decrease the degree of inflammation if there is no response to topical agents. Systemic antibiotics should be used for the shortest time possible, rarely longer than 6 months, and often require 3 to 4 weeks to see improvement. Once improvement is noted, the dose should be tapered to a daily dose, and then discontinued. Combination use with benzoyl peroxide or retinoid is recommended with continuation of topical medication after stopping the oral antibiotic. The tetracycline class of antibiotics (tetracycline, minocycline, doxycycline) are considered first-line oral antibiotic therapy (Zaenglein et al., 2016).
  - Tetracycline should be taken with 8 ounces of water 1 hour before or 2 hours after eating. Tetracycline should not be

used by pregnant or breastfeeding females or in children younger than 9 years old. Photosensitivity reactions can occur. The usual dose is 250 to 500 mg twice daily.

- Erythromycin use should be limited to those who cannot take tetracycline because of increasing resistance to erythromycin. Erythromycin can be taken with food, but gastrointestinal upset is common, and vulvovaginal candidiasis can be problematic. The usual dose is 250 to 500 mg twice daily.
- Minocycline can be taken with food, although dairy products decrease absorption. Side effects include blue-black discoloration in scars, photosensitivity, and hypersensitivity reactions. The usual dose is 50 to 100 mg twice daily.
- Doxycycline can be taken with food (dairy products decrease absorption), but has the highest rate of photosensitivity reactions. The usual dose is 50 to 100 mg twice daily.
- Oral retinoids are used for severe, recalcitrant nodulocystic acne. Isotretinoin is contraindicated in pregnancy (pregnancy Category X drug known for its teratogenic effect) and requires evaluation by a dermatologist before use. Its association with depression and suicide is controversial. The usual course is 20 weeks; there are many side effects, and LFTs, serum cholesterol, triglycerides, human chorionic gonadotropin (hCG), and urinalysis for pregnancy must be monitored every month while the patient is taking the medication. The iPledge program creates a registry for all patients being treated with isotretinoin. The FDA requires healthcare providers, female patients, and pharmacists to access the iPledge website monthly after office visits and before filling their prescription for documentation regarding pregnancy, blood donation, and contraceptive counseling. Providers should also monitor for any signs of inflammatory bowel disease.
- Hormonal and other therapies: Hormonal therapies can be used in females to oppose effects of androgen on sebaceous glands, such as antiandrogens (e.g., spironolactone) and androgen receptor blockers; oral contraceptive pills (OCPs) provide estrogen and a progestin, and some are FDA approved to treat acne vulgaris. Intralesional steroid therapy for large cysts or nodules is sometimes used; resurfacing lasers and dermabrasion are used for acne scarring.
- Noncomedogenic moisturizers can be used for dryness, which is common with treatment. Noncomedogenic makeup is also available and helpful in treating these patients.

Patient and Family Education

- Education is the first priority. The adolescent must have realistic expectations and understand the pathophysiology and the process of treatment, including the fact that the acne often worsens before improving. Reading materials about acne and its treatment provide support for self-management efforts.
  - Wash face twice a day with a mild soap, such as Dove, Neutrogena, or Aveeno Cleansing Bar. Avoid scrubbing, rubbing, picking, and squeezing. Medication should be applied lightly.
  - Use of a comedone extractor can cause scarring and should be discouraged. Hot soaks applied to pustules may help their resolution.
- All products used on the face should be labeled as *noncomedogenic.*
- Identify and discontinue use of aggravating substances, such as oil-based cosmetics, pomades, hair spray, mousse, and face creams.
- Identify possible aggravating factors, such as stress; hot, humid weather; and jobs involving frying oil or grease.
- Limited evidence supports a strong connection between foods and acne; however emerging evidence supports an association with high glycemic index foods. A well-balanced diet is important to maintaining healthy skin.
- Discuss psychosocial concerns and provide support.
- Remind the adolescent that results take months and that adherence to treatment is essential to improvement.
- Sun exposure helps clear acne for some adolescents but may worsen it for others. Sunscreen use is recommended, and caution about sun exposure should be given if a medication that increases photosensitivity is being used.

Follow-up visits should occur at least every 4 to 6 weeks until control is established, defined as when lesions clear or only a few new lesions appear every 2 weeks. Refer to a dermatologist for nonresponsive or severe cases.

Mild cases of neonatal cephalic pustulosis and infantile acne are best treated with a plan of watchful waiting and gentle daily cleansing with soap and water. In mild comedonal acne, sparing use of topical tretinoin is recommended. Use 2.5% benzoyl peroxide or topical antibiotics for mild inflammatory acne. Have the parents apply these agents every other night. Careful examination for growth and signs of androgen excess is warranted.

Complications

Failure can be due to lack of patient motivation, lack of education, inappropriate treatments, initial treatment that was too strong, or expectations of a quick fix. Psychological effects include decreased self-esteem and poor body image, problems with interpersonal relationships, self-consciousness, embarrassment, depression, and decreased athletic participation, especially in gymnastics, swimming, and wrestling. Resistance of *P. acnes* to tetracycline, erythromycin, and minocycline is increasing.

Atopic Dermatitis

See Chapter 33.

Contact Dermatitis

Contact dermatitis is an acute or chronic inflammation resulting from a hypersensitive reaction to a substance (either irritants or allergens). Common types of contact dermatitis include the following:

- Dry skin dermatitis caused by extremely low humidity (less than 30%), excess soap or cleansing cream use, or inadequate rinsing of soap products
- Nickel dermatitis from contact with jewelry, belts, snaps, or eyeglasses
- Lip-licker dermatitis caused by frequent lip licking, most often in dry, cold weather
- Phytophotodermatitis from sun exposure following contact with plants or juices, such as limes, lemons, carrots, celery, figs, parsnips, or dill; manifests as a blistered lesion on an erythematous base and may be confused with a burn

- Plant oleoresins, such as poison ivy, oak, or sumac; contact can be direct or indirect (exposure to burning plant material); oils may be inhaled, causing damage to lung tissue. (Urushiol, the allergen in poison ivy, oak, and sumac can remain on contaminated items, such as clothing, animal hair, toys, and sports equipment resulting in sequential outbreaks due to reexposures.)
- Juvenile plantar dermatosis, manifested as dryness, cracking, and erythema of weight-bearing surfaces of the feet, initially the big toes; it mimics tinea pedis, often found in children with atopic dermatitis
- Latex dermatitis, associated with the use of products containing latex, such as protective gloves

Substances such as saliva, urine, and feces; baby wipes; bubble bath; agents that dry the skin; and adhesives often cause contact dermatitis. Diaper dermatitis is the most common form (see following section). Contact dermatitis can also be caused by allergens. Allergic reactions occur as an immunologic response to an antigen penetrating the skin. There are two phases: sensitization and elicitation. Allergic dermatitis is seen only after sensitization to an allergen has occurred and a subsequent type IV delayed hypersensitivity response has activated an immune cascade. Common causes are contact with shoes (components, such as rubber and potassium dichromate); nickel; clothes with woolen or rough textures; topical medications (e.g., neomycin and lanolin); perfumed soaps or cosmetics (including lanolin); preservatives; or poison ivy, oak, or sumac. Sometimes the cause is obvious; often no specific cause can be identified. Although it occurs at any age, contact dermatitis is extremely common in children (Tan et al, 2014).

Clinical Findings

History
- Contact with any new or unusual substances
- Repeated exposure to any substance or item
- Diarrhea or infrequently changed diapers
- Rash localized to specific area(s)

Physical Examination. The area of involvement offers clues to the causative agent. Often the rash is localized to one area and has sharp borders. Common examples include a linear-type rash secondary to wearing a necklace or bracelet, circular areas from snaps on clothing, or inflammation of the earlobes from jewelry or a reaction pattern on the toes and dorsum of the foot from shoes. The severity of the rash depends on the length of exposure and the concentration of the irritant. Minimal contact may produce only mild erythema, whereas prolonged or concentrated contact may produce significant erythema, edema, and blistering with possible crusting and secondary infection. Irritant reactions tend to be immediate, whereas allergic ones are delayed.
- A chafed appearance with shiny, mild to severely erythematous, peeling, or dry, fissured skin or red patches and plaques with secondary scales may be seen if the reaction is due to an irritant. For example, the dorsum of the hand may exhibit the above characteristic appearance with frequent hand washing with irritating soaps.
- Erythema, vesicles, and weeping may be present in the acute stage of allergic contact dermatitis. The lesions are pruritic.
- Hyperpigmentation and lichenification are seen in chronic conditions.
- A generalized idiosyncratic (id) reaction can develop to an allergen. An id reaction occurs as a secondary or "sympathy" rash distant from the primary site of exposure.

Differential Diagnosis
The differential diagnosis includes atopic dermatitis, impetigo, herpes simplex, psoriasis, and seborrhea.

Management
Appropriate skin care, recognizing and eliminating offending agents, and treating inflammation are key to managing contact dermatitis successfully. Identify and avoid the substance (irritant or allergen) causing the dermatitis. General treatment measures include:
- Burow solution soaks or oatmeal baths and cool compresses (1 teaspoon salt/pint water) applied for 20 minutes every 4 to 6 hours to soothe vesicular rashes.
- Water and either petrolatum-based or lanolin-and-petrolatum–based emollients applied to the skin to restore moisture to areas of dryness and chafing.
  - Petrolatum-based emollients include dimethicone, white petrolatum, and Vaseline Dermatology Formula.
  - Lanolin-and-petrolatum–based emollients should not be used if there is inflammation.
- Topical corticosteroids used 2 or 3 times daily give relief in 2 or 3 days, although it may take 2 or 3 weeks for complete healing. Occasionally oral corticosteroids are used for short periods if the area of allergic involvement exceeds 10% of the skin surface (10 to 14 days, tapered the last 7 days).
- Do not use flavored lip creams in cases of lip-licker dermatitis. Emollient lotions and petroleum-based emollients can moisturize the skin and discourage lip licking because of their bad taste.
- Oral antihistamines are helpful if itching and scratching are problems.

Resolution may take 2 to 3 weeks. Refer to a dermatologist or an allergist for patch testing if the dermatitis worsens, fails to respond, or recurs. Allergic contact dermatitis can develop into chronic dermatitis if left untreated. Psoralen and UVA treatment, narrow-band UVB treatment, systemic treatment with immunomodulators, and targeted biologic therapy may be considered if unresponsive to other measures.

Diaper Dermatitis

Diaper dermatitis is the most frequent contact dermatitis seen in children and one of the most common skin disorders of infants (Table 34.8; Fig 34.23). The initial rash is termed *irritant contact diaper dermatitis*. A variation of this is called *tidewater* or *tidemark dermatitis* and is found at the diaper edges. *Jacquet dermatitis,* a severe form manifested by punched-out lesions or erosions primarily on the labia and buttocks, is especially prone to secondary infection.

Factors contributing to diaper dermatitis include the following:
- Improper hygiene and cleansing methods
- Chemical irritation caused by prolonged contact with skin products, urine, feces, or breakdown products. Feces and its breakdown products are the major factors
- Mechanical irritation from diapers or skinfolds
- Occlusion of skin with use of diapers and plastic or rubber pants
- Other skin dermatoses aggravated by wearing diapers (e.g., seborrhea, atopic dermatitis, or psoriasis)
- In the diaper area around the anus, the rash is often due to diarrhea; if the skin is affected but the folds are spared, urine is often responsible

TABLE 34.8   Diagnosis and Treatment of Diaper Dermatitis

Type	Cause	Presentation and Location	Other Characteristics	Treatment
Irritant contact dermatitis	Related to wearing diapers; contact with urine and feces	Chapped, shiny, erythematous, parchment-like skin with possible erosions on convex surfaces; creases spared	Peaks at 9-12 months old; may progress to involve creases; skin may be dry	Frequent diaper changes, gentle cleansing; greasy lubricant; sitz bath, air-dry; 0.5%-1% hydrocortisone for inflammation
Candidiasis	Related to wearing diapers; a superinfection with *Candida*	Shallow pustules, fiery-red scaly plaques on convex surfaces, inguinal folds, labia, and scrotum	Satellite lesions, oral thrush; recent antibiotic or diarrhea; occurs at any age	Antifungal cream plus same measures as for contact dermatitis
Miliaria or intertrigo	Related to wearing diapers; a result of heat and occlusion	Discrete vesicles or papules (miliaria); erythematous, scaly, maceration in skinfolds	Sweat retention or friction associated	Self-limited (miliaria); avoid precipitating factors; care as for contact dermatitis
Seborrhea	Exaggerated by wearing diapers; overgrowth of *Malassezia* yeast in areas of sebaceous gland activity	Greasy, erythematous scales, well circumscribed in creases of skin, groin; spared convex surfaces	Onset at 3-4 weeks old; also occurs on face or body; often superinfected with *Candida*	Ketoconazole and/or hydrocortisone is treatment of choice
Atopic dermatitis (AD)	Exaggerated by wearing diapers; exact cause unknown	Increased number of lines in skin; areas of excoriation in folds and convex surfaces and buttocks; less widespread	AD in other areas; usually begins in first year of life; scratches skin with diaper change; hyperlinear skinfolds with diffuse borders	Skin care as for contact dermatitis and as indicated for AD (see Chapter 33); antibiotics for bacterial infection
Psoriasis	Exaggerated by wearing diapers; psoriasis evolves in response to chronic trauma	Erythematous, well-defined sharp, scaly plaques on convex surfaces and inguinal folds; less widespread	Psoriasis affects other places; rare occurrence if found, usually at 6-18 months old	Treatment often required for weeks or until toilet trained; steroids; ketoconazole if *Candida* present
Bacterial dermatitis	Usually caused by staphylococcal or streptococcal infection	Red, denuded areas or fragile blisters; crusting and pustules in suprapubic area and periumbilicus	Usually in newborn, can occur anywhere	Nystatin if yeast is present as well; mupirocin if minimal; amoxicillin clavulanate or cephalexin

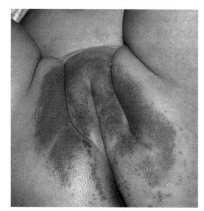

• **Fig 34.23** Diaper Dermatitis. (Adapted from White G, Cox N. *Diseases of the Skin.* 2nd ed. St. Louis: Mosby/Elsevier; 2006.)

Clinical Findings

History
- Type of diapers and diaper covering used; recent change in brand or laundering products
- Frequency of wet diapers and stools
- Frequency of diaper changes and methods of cleansing used
- Any new baby care products used

- Medication taken (particularly antibiotics) or used on rash
- Present or recent use of antibiotics

Physical Examination. Erythema, edema, and vesiculation are typically the first characteristic changes observed. Chronic changes include scale, lichenification, and increased or decreased pigmentation. Other findings associated with specific causative factors can include the following:
- Chemical causes
  - Shiny, peeling, erythematous macular or papular rash confluent in the diaper area, sparing folds
  - Head of penis erythematous and dry
  - Erythema primarily on buttocks and around anus (fecal irritation)
- Mechanical causes
  - Erythematous, macerated (acute) or dry (chronic), hyperpigmented area prominent along edges of diaper or plastic or rubber pants
  - Erythematous, macerated folds caused by overlapping skin
- Hygiene problems
  - Any finding listed previously
  - Poor hygiene in general

Differential Diagnosis
Differential diagnoses include contact dermatitis; bacterial, viral, or monilial infection; atopic dermatitis; psoriasis; seborrhea; scabies; and congenital syphilis.

Management

The best treatment is prevention!

1. Keep diaper area dry, clean, and aerated.
- Frequent diaper changes are essential; every 1 to 2 hours is recommended with one change at night and a minimum of eight changes in a 24-hour period for infants. Cleanse the area well with water at every diaper change and use mild soap, rinsing well following a stool. Avoid vigorous cleansing because this can worsen matters. Avoid using wipes.
- Use a protective barrier ointment or cream, such as Desitin (cod liver oil with zinc oxide), A&D Ointment, Aquaphor, petrolatum, or zinc oxide at the first sign of irritation.
2. Proper use of diapers
- In addition to frequent changes, use thick or absorbent diapers.
- Cloth diapers should be soaked, prerinsed, washed in a mild soap, double rinsed with ¼ cup of vinegar, and dried in the sun if possible.
- Disposable diapers must be large enough not to bind and should never be worn with rubber pants.
3. Treatment of diaper rash
- Sitz baths in warm water for 10 to 15 minutes 4 times a day.
- Expose diaper area to air by leaving diaper off or by blow-drying with low heat three or 4 times a day.
- Burow solution soaks or compresses 4 times a day if skin is weepy.
- Diaper cream containing undecylenic acid or zinc oxide to decrease the friction and exposure to moisture.
- Hydrocortisone 0.5% or 1% applied as a thin layer 3 times a day for no more than 5 days, especially if skin is dry, for moderate to severe diaper dermatitis. Do not use fluorinated steroids.
- Increase intake of fluids to dilute urine. In older infants, 2 to 3 ounces of cranberry juice acidifies the urine.
- Any recalcitrant rash should be referred to a dermatologist.
- Follow up by phone in 1 to 2 days. If not improved, reassess within 1 week.

Complications

Secondary infection with bacteria, viruses, or fungi can occur (see previous sections). Red flags that could indicate systemic disease or require consultation with a dermatologist include severe erosions or ulcers; bullae or pustules; large papules or nodules, purpura, or petechiae; and redness or scaliness over entire body.

Seborrheic Dermatitis

Seborrhea is a chronic inflammatory dermatitis commonly called *cradle cap* in infants or *dandruff* in adolescents. The condition is thought to be related to overproduction of sebum because it commonly occurs in areas with large numbers of sebaceous glands. It may be an overgrowth of *Malassezia ovalis* (formerly *P. ovale*), a saprophytic yeast, which is universally present on the human body. Seborrhea occurs most often in early infancy and adolescence, is associated with blepharitis, and is more common in spring and summer.

Clinical Findings

History. Note age of onset (infancy or adolescence).

Physical Examination. In infants, erythematous, flaky to thick crusts of yellow, greasy (waxy appearance) scales occur predominantly on the scalp, but also on the face, behind the ears, on the neck and trunk, and in the diaper area (Fig 34.24). In adolescents there are mild flakes with some erythema and yellow, greasy scales on the scalp, forehead, nasal bridge, and eyebrows; behind the ears; on the face and flexural surfaces; and in intertriginous areas. The dermatitis is not pruritic and has no pustules.

Differential Diagnosis

Atopic dermatitis, psoriasis, *Candida* infection, contact dermatitis, tinea, scabies, and pityriasis rosea are included in the differential diagnoses.

Management

Three categories of agents may be helpful in the treatment of seborrheic dermatitis in both infants and adolescents. These include antifungal agents, anti-inflammatory agents, and keratolytic agents:
- Antifungal: Azoles, selenium sulfide
- Anti-inflammatory: Topical steroids, topical calcineurin inhibitors
- Keratolytic (remove excess scale): Topical salicylic acid, urea
Seborrhea in infants may be self-limited, typically resolving spontaneously in the first year of life (Cohen, 2013).
- Mineral oil may be applied to the scalp for 5 to 10 minutes before shampooing with a mild shampoo. Scales can be removed with a soft brush or toothbrush (Weston and Morelli, 2017). Frequent shampooing is generally effective. There are no medicated or prescriptive shampoos approved for children under 2 years old (Clark, Pope, and Jaboori, 2015).
- Treatment for adolescents with seborrheic dermatitis includes (Clark, Pope, and Jaboori, 2015):
  - Facial dermatitis
    - Daily ketoconazole 2% topical preparations (cream, shampoo, gel, or foam)
    - Intermittent use of low-potency topical corticosteroids (0.05% desonide cream or lotion)
    - Calcineurin inhibitors are good for face and ears
  - Scalp dermatitis
    - Medicated shampoos (tar, salicylic acid, ketoconazole, or selenium sulfide) 2 or 3 times a week (1 to 4 times per month for African Americans) alternated with prescription-strength shampoos (ketoconazole 2.5%, selenium sulfide 2.5%) (Clark, Pope, and Jaboori, 2015). Shampoo should be left on the scalp for 5 to 10 minutes before scrubbing crusts and then rinsing.
    - Topical corticosteroids added weekly for recalcitrant dermatitis (leave-in foams or solutions work best)
- Body and skinfold seborrheic dermatitis: The same regimens mentioned previously can be used on the body.
- Educate parents about the etiology, control measures, and the need to continue treatment for a few days after resolution, and arrange for follow-up in 1 to 2 weeks.

Complications

Secondary infection with bacteria or *Candida* can occur. Severe, generalized seborrhea is commonly found in persons infected with HIV.

Drug Eruptions

Drugs taken systemically can result in a variety of skin reactions. The two most common types of drug-related eruptions found in children are a morbilliform (measles-like) rash (also called an

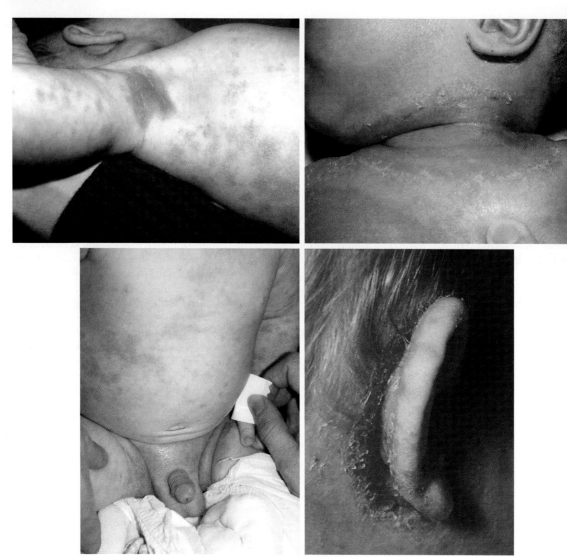

• **Fig 34.24** Seborrheic Dermatitis. (From Zitelli BJ, McIntire S, Nowalk AJ. *Zitelli and Davis' Atlas of Pediatric Physical Diagnosis*. 7th ed. Philadelphia: Elsevier; 2018.)

exanthematous reaction manifested by erythematous macules and/or papules) and urticaria typified by erythematous wheals (Table 34.9). Morbilliform rash is discussed here and urticaria is discussed later in the section on vascular reactions. Although not described in this chapter, other drug-related dermatologic reactions include acute generalized exanthematous pustulosis, drug hypersensitivity syndrome, serum sickness-like reaction, vasculitis, fixed drug eruption, acneiform eruptions, and SJS.

The morbilliform, or exanthematous, rash is the most common allergic skin reaction to a drug (Fig 34.25). The rash may be an immunologic or nonimmunologic reaction to the drug. The most common drugs causing reactions are penicillins, cephalosporins, sulfonamide antibiotics (including TMP-SMX combinations), nonsteroidal anti-inflammatory drugs (NSAIDs), anticonvulsants, and oral fluconazole or ketoconazole antifungal drugs (Weston and Morelli, 2017). The risk of this type of eruption is increased if the child also has a viral infection (e.g., the rash that appears after giving penicillin to a child with Epstein-Barr virus). Exanthematous rashes typically have their onset within 1 to 2 weeks of starting a new medication and can occur after the medication has been stopped. Repeated exposure can lead to faster reactions and progress to anaphylaxis.

Clinical Findings

History
- Medication taken within the past 3 weeks
- Varying degrees of itching—can be intense
- Rash worsens even after medicine is discontinued for up to 5 days
- Possible systemic symptoms—low-grade fever, arthralgia, arthritis, lymphadenopathy, edema

Physical Examination
Findings include the following:
- Condition often begins as a fairly symmetric, macular erythematous rash that becomes papular and confluent.
- Patches of normal skin are scattered throughout areas of involvement.
- Rash begins on the trunk, where it is a brighter red, more confluent, and extends distally to the extremities, including the palms and soles.
- Rash may turn brownish red and desquamate in 7 to 14 days.
- The face often has confluent areas of erythema.
- Mucous membranes are typically spared.

TABLE 34.9	Differentiating Drug Eruptions, Urticaria, and Erythema Multiforme		
	Drug Eruption	**Urticaria**	**Erythema Multiforme**
Etiology	Reaction to medication, especially penicillin, cephalexin, erythromycin, sulfa drugs, NSAIDs, barbiturates, isoniazid, carbamazepine, phenytoin	Hypersensitive reaction; immunologic antigen-antibody response to release of histamines; often unknown cause; possible reaction to food, drug, insect bite or sting, pollen; possible reaction to infection, especially streptococcal, sinus, mononucleosis, hepatitis	Immune-mediated hypersensitivity reaction often to infection, especially HSV; also to many other agents
Clinical findings	Symmetric, macular, erythematous to papular, confluent morbilliform rash; intense itching; patches of normal skin throughout; begins on trunk, extends distally, including palms and soles; face with confluent erythema	Key finding: Appears suddenly, fades in 20 minutes to 24 hours. Family history of hives; possible atopy; intense itching; mild erythema, annular, raised wheals with pale centers; lesions scattered or coalesced; blanch with pressure; associated edema of eyelids, lips, tongue, hands, feet	Key finding: Target or iris lesions: Lesions fixed, symmetric, typical distribution on hands, feet, elbows, knees, also face, neck, trunk. History of infection, especially herpes labialis; variety of lesions on skin and mucous membranes—macules, papules, vesicles, early lesions, such as, urticaria; possible oral mucous membrane involvement
Treatment	Stop drug and label as allergen to the child; give antihistamine, antipruritic, prednisone if severe; lubricate skin; rash can last 7-14 days; use medical alert bracelet	Quick resolution; identify and remove offending agent if possible and treat; stop antibiotic; give oral antihistamines; topical antipruritics; epinephrine or prednisone if anaphylactic, angioedema, or refractory; refer if >6 weeks' duration	Identify, treat, discontinue trigger if possible; treat infection; supportive measures for hydration, prevention of secondary infection, relief of pain; oral antihistamines, cool compresses; oral lesions—mouthwash, topical anesthetics; lesions last 5-7 days, recur in batches over 2-4 weeks, resolve without scarring or sequelae

NSAID, Nonsteroidal anti-inflammatory drugs; *HSV,* herpes simplex virus.

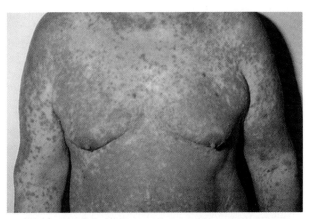

• **Fig 34.25** Allergic Drug Reaction. (From Lookingbill DP, Marks JG. *Principles of Dermatology.* 2nd ed. Philadelphia: Saunders; 1993, p 218.)

Diagnostic Studies

The following are ordered if necessary for differential diagnosis: CBC, monospot test, CRP, antinuclear antibodies, anti-streptolysin O (ASO), cold agglutinins.

Differential Diagnosis

Viral exanthem; measles; toxic erythema, such as in scarlet fever, staphylococcal scarlatina, or Kawasaki disease; TSS; roseola; and erythema infectiosum are included in the differential diagnosis.

Management

Decisions about whether a drug is to be implicated depend on the patient's previous history of taking the drug, the experience of the general population with the drug, the morphology and timing of the rash, and other possible explanations for the rash (e.g., viral illness). The following steps are taken:

1. Discontinue the suspected drug.
2. Label the patient's medical record with the potential allergen.
3. Prescribe antihistamines if itching is present; recommend a lubricant and antipruritics as adjuncts.
4. Systemic steroids are not usually indicated in a morbilliform drug eruption. If severe reaction, give prednisone 1 to 2 mg/kg/d for 5 to 7 days (Paller and Mancini, 2016).
5. Schedule follow-up visit as determined by severity of reaction and other illness.

Refer to an allergist for skin testing to confirm allergy if there are limited or no alternative medications, for desensitization, to clarify drug allergy, for severe parental anxiety, or if symptoms are severe and life threatening.

Complications

Body heat and water loss can occur if the rash is severe. Progression of the rash if medicine is continued can lead to toxic epidermal necrolysis (TEN) or SJS (see Erythema Multiforme, Stevens-Johnson Syndrome, TEN section) or allergic interstitial nephritis.

Patient and Family Education

• The rash can last 7 to 14 days with itching, and it may worsen before getting better.
• There is potential risk from further exposure to that drug or related ones; alternative therapies should be explained.
• Identification and communication of the child's allergy are imperative. If the child has a life-threatening allergy, wearing a medical alert bracelet or necklace is essential.

Vascular Skin Conditions

Urticaria and Angioedema

Urticaria and angioedema are hypersensitivity reactions (usually a type I reaction—immunoglobulin E [IgE] mediated) commonly called *hives* (Fig 34.26). Urticaria involves the superficial dermis; in contrast, angioedema involves the deeper dermis and subcutaneous tissue.

Urticaria and angioedema are the result of a complex interplay of immunologically mediated antigen-antibody responses to the release of histamine from mast cells and other vasoactive mediators, such as leukotrienes and prostaglandins. Vasodilation and increased vascular permeability cause erythema and the characteristic wheal of urticaria. Onset is usually rapid, and resolution occurs within a few days of onset. Possible causative factors include the following:

- Reactions to foods (e.g., nuts, eggs, shellfish, strawberries, tomatoes), stings (e.g., bees, wasps, scorpions, spiders, jellyfish), bites (e.g., mosquitoes, fleas, mites), parasites (scabies), or pollen
- Reaction to skin contact with antigens, such as chemicals, latex, fish, or caterpillars
- The most common cause is a response to bacterial, viral, or fungal infections, especially streptococcal or sinus infection, mononucleosis, hepatitis, adenoviruses, and enteroviruses
- Cholinergic response to physical stimuli (e.g., heat or cold, sun or water [aquagenic urticaria], tight clothing, vibrations) or stress
- Reaction to drugs (about 10% of urticaria, usually acute in nature; salicylates, penicillins, and sulfonamides are the most common) (Bolognia, 2014)
- Genetic origin
- Concurrent with inflammatory systemic diseases (e.g., collagen-vascular or inflammatory bowel disease)
- Immunologic (rare)
- Approximately 50% of urticarial is idiopathic or unknown

Portals of entry for the causative agent include infection (most common), ingestion, injection, or inhalation. Urticaria and angioedema are more common in children than adults, and about 50% of patients with urticaria also have angioedema. Children who get both angioedema and urticaria tend to have more severe reactions. Urticaria occurs sometime in the lives of about 15% of the population. Transient or acute urticaria lasts less than 6 weeks; chronic, recurrent, or persistent urticaria lasts more than 6 weeks.

Angioedema is an extension of the reaction into the subcutaneous tissue with indistinct borders, and tends to involve the face (especially the eyes), hands, and feet (Weston and Morelli, 2017). It is gradual in onset and often involves reactions to medication. Hereditary angioedema is a rare autosomal dominant disorder that results from either a deficiency or dysfunction of the first component of complement (C-esterase inhibitor). It is life threatening and usually manifests before 10 years old, typically with exacerbations in adolescence, often following trauma (e.g., dental work, surgery, or accident). It is manifested by repeated episodes of swelling of the extremities, face, and throat, accompanied by abdominal pain that becomes progressively more severe (Bolognia, 2014). Severe airway edema, if untreated, is often the cause of death.

Clinical Findings

History
- Family or previous history of hives, angioedema, connective tissue disease, juvenile arthritis
- Possibility of atopy
- Intense itching and scratching
- Ingestion (within 4 hours) of nuts, shellfish, chocolate, berries, spices, egg white, milk, fish, sesame
- Ingestion or injection of medicines (e.g., penicillin, sulfa drugs, sedatives, diuretics, analgesics, acetylsalicylic acid), additives, or preservatives
- Injection of diagnostic agents, vaccine, insect venom, blood
- Infection with upper respiratory infectious agent, virus, streptococcus, mononucleosis; hepatitis; parasites
- Inhalation of animal dander, pollen, dust, smoke, or aerosols
- Flea or mite bites
- Cold, heat, exercise, sun, water, pressure, or vibration

Physical Examination. Location of lesions may help determine the cause (e.g., a lesion around the mouth or tongue is likely due to an ingested agent). Findings can include the following:
- Urticaria is seen as mildly erythematous, annular, raised wheals or welts with pale centers from 2 mm to several centimeters in diameter; however, they can be of various shapes. Such lesions typically:
  - Are scattered or coalesced but generalized
  - Appear suddenly as individual lesions and fade in anywhere from 20 minutes to less than 24 hours, reappearing in other areas later; if fixed more than 48 hours, it is not urticaria
  - Blanch with pressure
  - Seem to be intensified with heat
  - Appear as wheals after rubbing or stroking the skin (dermatographism)
  - Occur most commonly as papulovesicular lesions with central punctate lesion and wheals in toddlers (papular urticaria)
  - Can appear as large, blotchy, erythematous lesions with 1- to 3-mm central wheals (cholinergic urticaria)
- Angioedema is seen as asymmetric, localized, nondependent, and transient edema.
  - Typically less pruritic than urticaria
  - May involve the upper airway and progress to life-threatening obstruction
  - Can cause associated edema of eyelids, lips, tongue, hands, feet, and genitalia

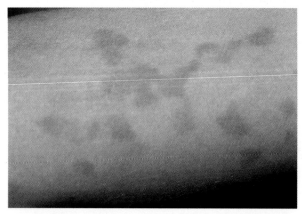

• **Fig 34.26** Urticaria. (From Weston WL, Lane AT, Morelli JG. *Color Textbook of Pediatric Dermatology.* 4th ed. St. Louis: Mosby/Elsevier; 2007, p 259.)

Diagnostic Studies. If urticaria with possible anaphylaxis from an insect bite is suspected, refer to an allergist for testing and hyposensitization. If fever is present, evaluate for underlying disease.

Differential Diagnosis
Contact dermatitis, atopic dermatitis, scabies, erythema multiforme (lesions are fixed with dusky centered target-like lesions that appear within 72 hours; Fig 34.27), mastocytosis, reactive erythemas, vasculitis, psoriasis, and juvenile arthritis are also included in the differential diagnosis (see Table 34.9).

Management
Control of symptoms is the main goal of treatment. The following steps are taken:
1. Identify and remove the offending substance if possible. Stop all antibiotics. Avoid any possible food or environmental trigger.
2. Test for dermatographism by stroking the skin, for cholinergic urticaria by applying heat or observing immediately after exercising, for cold urticaria by applying cold packs, for pressure urticaria by applying weighted bands for several minutes, and for water urticaria by applying wet compresses.
3. Administer medications as indicated.
- Oral antihistamines, such as diphenhydramine 0.5 to 1 mg/kg/dose every 4 to 6 hours as needed (maximum 50 mg/dose and 300 mg/d) or hydroxyzine 0.6 mg/kg/dose every 6 hours as needed (400 mg/d maximum) until itching and urticaria are resolved. Nonsedating antihistamines are less effective, but if needed, astemizole, cetirizine, or loratadine are best. Urticaria is less likely to recur if the antihistamine is continued for 1 to 2 weeks after resolution.
- Topical antipruritics may be helpful.
- Aqueous epinephrine 1:1000 (subcutaneously 0.01 mL/kg up to 0.3 mL) may be needed if anaphylaxis or significant angioedema with swelling of the face, mucous membranes, and airway is present.
- Prednisone: 1 to 2 mg/kg/d for 1 week with rapid taper only if refractory to other measures or if angioedema is present with swelling of lips and face.
4. Follow-up visit if not improved within 24 to 48 hours.

Chronic urticaria persisting longer than 6 weeks needs evaluation for infection or systemic causes or referral for further evaluation.

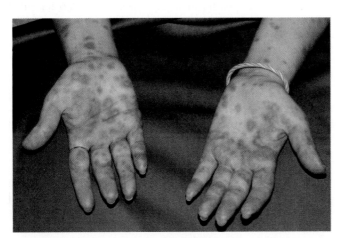

• **Fig 34.27** Erythema Multiforme. (From Paller AS, Mancini AJ. *Hurwitz Clinical Pediatric Dermatology: A Textbook of Skin Disorders of Children and Adolescence.* 5th ed. Philadelphia: Elsevier; 2016.)

An emergency epinephrine kit (EpiPen Jr, 0.15 mg; or adult, 0.3 mg) should be prescribed for children after the first episode or with recurrent episodes of life-threatening urticaria or angioedema.

Complications
Angioedema or anaphylaxis occurs by the same mechanism as urticaria.
- Anaphylactic symptoms require emergency intervention.
- Serum sickness begins with hives, but has other systemic symptoms (e.g., fever, arthralgias, malaise, lymphadenopathy, or proteinuria).
- If urticaria is from a drug reaction, rechallenge with the drug is more likely to cause anaphylaxis.

Patient and Family Education
The following are needed:
- Explanation of causes (often unknown), course, and treatment. The entire episode usually resolves in 24 to 48 hours, rarely extending beyond 3 to 4 weeks. Further evaluation is needed only if urticaria lasts longer than 8 weeks.
- Papular urticaria hypersensitivity often declines within 6 to 12 months.
- Physical urticarias last 2 to 4 years in most cases, but occasionally persist into adulthood.
- Occasionally macular blue-brown lesions are found on resolution of urticaria.
- Avoid allergen if known; wear a medical alert bracelet in case severe reaction occurs. Refer for hyposensitization if life-threatening symptoms occur.
- Carry an epinephrine kit if indicated.

Erythema Multiforme, Stevens-Johnson Syndrome, Toxic Epidermal Necrolysis
In the past, erythema multiforme minor, SJS (also known as *erythema multiforme major*), and TEN were thought to be related disorders. However, erythema multiforme minor is a distinct disorder that does not progress to SJS or TEN. Erythema multiforme is an acute, usually benign, self-limited eruption characterized by target lesions and minor mucosal involvement (papules and varying bullae); it is rarely associated with complications. SJS and TEN are considered to represent a distinct syndrome that occurs with variable expression along a continuum. SJS and TEN are associated with significant risk of morbidity and mortality.

Erythema multiforme usually follows an infection, with approximately 80% of cases of classic erythema multiforme attributed to HSV, in particular, herpes labialis or progenitalis lesion(s) (see Fig 34.31). The herpetic lesion may have healed or had a subclinical presentation but led to an immune response in the body. Erythema multiforme tends to be recurrent as do herpes lesions. Erythema multiforme may also be associated with other viruses, such as EBV, cytomegalovirus (CMV), and other herpesviruses (Weston and Morelli, 2017).

Clinical Findings
History
- With erythema multiforme
  - Recent or current infection with herpes virus (herpes labialis or progenitalis)
  - Exposure to UV light or trauma to area
  - Low-grade fever, malaise, and myalgia

- With SJS or TEN
  - SJS is usually caused by medication or viral illness
  - SJS can have a prodrome of high fever, cough, sore throat, vomiting, diarrhea, chest pain, and arthralgia that usually lasts 1 to 3 days (but can last from 1 to 14 days) followed by the onset of lesions
  - TEN is nearly exclusively caused by medication (Paller and Mancini, 2017)
  - TEN begins with a fever, sore throat, malaise, and generalized sunburn-like erythema

Physical Examination. It is important to differentiate the clinical findings of erythema multiforme from SJS and TEN.
- In erythema multiforme
  - Lesions vary from patient to patient, within a single episode, and with recurrence.
  - Lesions initially appear dusky, as red macules or edematous papules that evolve into target lesions with multiple, concentric rings of color change.
  - Lesions are fixed (another diagnostic clue), tend to be symmetric, and have a typical distribution predominantly on the face, extensor surface of the arms and legs, dorsum of the hands and feet, and the palms and soles.
  - The oral mucosa is commonly involved, and 50% of children will present with shallow oral lesions (Weston and Morelli, 2017).
- In SJS or TEN
  - SJS skin lesions typically are erythematous macules on the head and neck and can spread to the trunk and extremities with blister formation (within hours) that is often hemorrhagic, extensive, and confluent; mucosal involvement of eyes, nose, and mouth is widespread.
  - The TEN rash has rapidly coalescing target lesions and widespread bullae that become full-thickness epidermal peeling or sloughing within 24 hours; Nikolsky sign (peeling of skin with a light rub that reveals a moist red surface) is present. Conjunctivae, urethra, rectum, oral and nasal mucosa, larynx, and tracheobronchial mucosa may or may not be involved with TEN.

Diagnostic Studies. Studies are ordered as indicated by the clinical condition of the child.

Differential Diagnosis

Urticaria can be differentiated by lack of itching, lability of lesions, and shorter-lasting hives that are pale centrally, not target or iris lesions (see Table 34.9). Viral exanthems are more centrally located, confluent, and less erythematous. Purpura is present in vasculitis. In SSSS, the skin peels superficially (not full thickness) and is significantly red. Kawasaki disease and lupus erythematosus are also included in the differential diagnosis.

Management

Care for erythema multiforme is generally supportive because the condition is self-limited.
- Symptomatic and supportive care: Maintain hydration, prevent secondary infection, and relieve pain.
  - Mild analgesics, cool compresses, and oral antihistamines, such as diphenhydramine
  - Soothing mouthwashes or topical anesthetics, such as Kaopectate or Maalox, mixed in equal parts with diphenhydramine
  - Topical intraoral anesthetics, such as dyclonine liquid or viscous lidocaine, are sometimes used with caution in older children and adolescents
  - Débridement of oral lesions with half-strength hydrogen peroxide
  - Wound care
  - IV fluids if oral hydration is not adequate
  - Systemic antihistamines, analgesics, and antimicrobials as needed
- Prevention of herpes simplex: Avoid sun exposure and use sunscreen and protective clothing.
- Prophylaxis for recurrent erythema multiforme treatment:
  - Oral acyclovir, for child weighing less than 40 kg, 20 mg/kg/d divided twice daily, or weighing more than 40 kg, 400 mg/d divided twice daily, for a 6- to 12-month trial with periodic stopping to reassess.
  - Acyclovir during an acute episode of erythema multiforme does not alter its course.

SJS and TEN are potentially life-threatening diseases. Children are typically admitted to the pediatric intensive care unit (PICU) or burn unit for wound care, management of hydration and electrolyte issues, nutritional support, and pain control. IVIG should be started as quickly as possible in order to reverse the blistering and sloughing (Paller and Mancini, 2016).

Complications

SJS and TEN are associated with significant morbidity including pneumonitis, sepsis, gastrointestinal bleeding, renal disease, keratitis, and other ophthalmologic disorders.

Patient and Family Education

Erythema multiforme lesions can erupt in crops that last 1 to 3 weeks, but resolve without scarring or sequelae, except for transient desquamation, scaling, or hyperpigmentation. Recurrence of erythema multiforme is common.

Papulosquamous Eruptions of the Skin

Pityriasis Rosea

Pityriasis rosea, meaning rose-colored flaking, is a common, mild, self-limited papulosquamous disease (Fig 34.28).

The etiology of pityriasis rosea has not been established. There is debate as to whether it is caused by human herpesvirus 6 or 7 (HHV-6 or HHV-7). It is minimally contagious and occurs most commonly in the fall, early winter, and spring in temperate climates. Fifty percent of all cases occur before 20 years old, most commonly in adolescence, with males and females equally affected. Approximately 98% of cases result in lifelong immunity (Van Ravenstein and Edlund, 2017).

Clinical Findings

History. Although most are otherwise well, a small percentage (5%) of patients experience a prodrome of mild symptoms including malaise, pharyngitis, lymphadenopathy, and headache before onset of rash. Those that have prodromal symptoms tend to have a more florid rash.

Physical Examination
- Herald spot or patch (70% of presentations): a 2- to 5-cm solitary, ovoid, slightly erythematous lesion with a finely scaled slightly elevated border that enlarges quickly with central clearing); typical locations for the herald patch include the trunk, upper arm, neck, or thigh.
- Secondary generalized lesions appear that are symmetric, small macular to papular, thin and round to oval. The lesions have

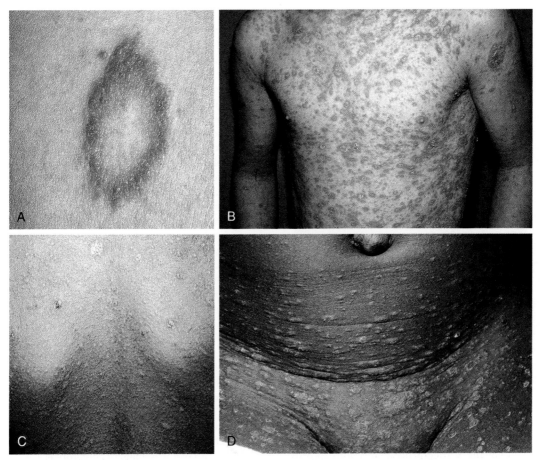

• **Fig 34.28** Pityriasis Rosea. (A) Herald patch. (B) Numerous oval lesions on chest of white teenager. (C) Christmas tree pattern on the back of a black adolescent. (D) Small, papular lesions as well as larger scaly patches most prominent on abdomen and thighs of 5-year-old female. (From Cohen B. *Pediatric Dermatology.* 4th ed. Philadelphia: Saunders/Elsevier; 2013.)

thin scales centrally with thicker scales peripherally ("collarette" scales surround the lesions). They are also pale pink; more common on trunk and proximal extremities from neck to knees; typically spare the face, scalp, and distal extremities; and usually occur 2 to 21 days after the appearance of the herald patch (key finding).
- Christmas tree pattern—rash, especially on back, follows dermatome skin lines with oval lesions running parallel and wrapping around the trunk horizontally.
- Itching occurs in about 75% of cases particularly with secondary lesions.
- Oral lesions have punctate hemorrhages, erosions or ulcerations, erythematous macules, or annular plaques; such lesions occur in about 16% of patients.
- An atypical presentation, limb-girdle pityriasis rosea, can occur with lesions involving areas that are usually spared (e.g., the face, axilla, and/or groin). The face and neck are frequent areas of involvement in young children, especially African American children (Paller and Mancini, 2016).

Diagnostic Studies. If needed, a KOH preparation of a skin scraping is done to rule out tinea.

Differential Diagnosis

Include psoriasis, guttate psoriasis, nummular eczema, scabies, tinea (especially the herald patch), secondary syphilis, drug eruptions, or viral exanthems in the differential diagnosis.

Management

The following steps are taken:
- Application of calamine lotion (or other lotions containing menthol and/or camphor or pramoxine), tepid baths with Aveeno, antihistamines, and emollients may provide relief from itching.
- Topical steroids do not change the lesions or hasten recovery. Oral steroids can exacerbate symptoms (VanRavenstein and Edlund, 2017).
- Minimal sun exposure can help lesions resolve more quickly. Prevent sunburn.
- Oral erythromycin 250 mg 4 times a day for 2 weeks may hasten the resolution of the eruption (VanRavenstein and Edlund, 2017).

Patient and Family Education

Pityriasis rosea is a benign, self-limited, and noncontagious disease that has three cycles (emerging, persisting, and fading) with spontaneous resolution in 6 to 12 weeks. Transient pigmentary changes can occur, especially in African Americans. Recurrence is common.

Psoriasis

Psoriasis, a chronic papulosquamous skin disorder with spontaneous remissions and exacerbations, is characterized by thick silvery

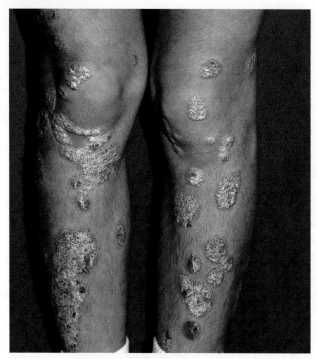

• **Fig 34.29** Psoriasis. (From Paller AS, Mancini AJ. *Hurwitz Clinical Pediatric Dermatology: A Textbook of Skin Disorders of Children and Adolescence.* 5th ed. Philadelphia: Elsevier; 2016.)

scales, varied distribution patterns, and an isomorphic (Koebner phenomenon) response (Fig 34.29). Types of psoriasis include guttate psoriasis (following a streptococcal infection), psoriasis vulgaris, napkin psoriasis (occurring in the diaper area), inverse psoriasis (limited to areas that are normally spared), localized pustular psoriasis, generalized pustular or psoriatic erythroderma, and psoriatic arthritis.

Psoriasis is an immune-mediated disorder associated with genetic predisposition and environmental risk factors. Though the exact cause is unknown, chromosome 6p21.3 is linked to the development of psoriasis, and the contributing gene is termed PSORSI. The disease results from keratinocyte proliferation and dermal vascular abnormalities. Trigger factors include infection, local trauma, stress (physical and psychological), and certain drugs (corticosteroids, lithium, beta-blockers, NSAIDs).

Psoriasis occurs at all ages; 30% of cases have onset in childhood. There is a common co-morbidity of obesity in both children and adults. Guttate psoriasis, often triggered by a group a beta hemolytic strep (GABS) infection, may be the first sign of psoriasis in children (Paller and Mancini, 2016).

Clinical Findings

History
- The etiology of psoriasis includes both genetic and environmental factors; more than one-third of patients have a family history of psoriasis (Paller and Mancini, 2016)
- Streptococcal infection of the oropharynx or perianal area before onset (guttate)
- Trauma before onset
- Itching (variable)

Physical Examination
- The scalp (encircling the hairline and external ears), elbows, knees, and buttocks (especially the diaper area in infants) are the most common sites of involvement. In children, the face may also be involved. Lesions are often found around areas of trauma (e.g., genitalia, palms, soles).
  - Plaque psoriasis: Discrete, initially erythematous, symmetric, well-marginated rash becoming papular with silver scales that may be trivial to widespread.
  - Guttate (teardrop) psoriasis: Widespread, symmetric, round, or oval 0.5- to 2-cm lesions occurring primarily on the trunk and proximal extremities, occasionally on the face, scalp, and ears and rarely on the palms or soles. There is less scaling than in psoriasis vulgaris.
  - Psoriasis vulgaris: Well-circumscribed, erythematous plaques with thick, silvery white scales concentrated on elbows, knees, scalp, and hairline, but also seen on eyebrows, around ears, and in intergluteal fold and genital area.
  - Koebner phenomenon (isomorphic response): Psoriatic lesions occur in areas of local injury, such as scratches, surgical scars, or sunburns.
  - Auspitz sign: Bleeding occurs when a scale is removed.
  - Nail signs: Nails have "ice pick" pits and ridges, are thick and discolored (yellowing), can have splinter hemorrhages or subungual hyperkeratosis, and can be separated from the nailbed (Paller and Mancini, 2016).
  - Napkin or diaper area psoriasis: Appears eczematous with sharply defined plaques, bright red coloration, shiny with large drier scales, affecting inguinal and gluteal folds.

Diagnostic Studies
- ASO if guttate pattern
- KOH-treated scrapings and culture to rule out fungal infection
- Venereal Disease Research Laboratory (VDRL) to rule out secondary syphilis

Differential Diagnosis

Pityriasis rosea, seborrhea, *Candida* infection, contact or irritant dermatitis, atopic dermatitis, tinea, dyshidrosis, secondary syphilis, and other nail-pitting conditions such as tinea and mold infections of the nail.

Management

In children, treatment should be as conservative as possible. Medications and treatments should be rotated for best effectiveness. The following are treatment options:
- Sun exposure in moderate amounts alleviates lesions. Prevent sunburn.
- Emollient creams (such as petrolatum, Eucerin, Aquaphor, or Cetaphil) for dry skin can minimize trauma and subsequent psoriasis and may improve psoriasis.
- Apply topical steroids 2 or 3 times a day for 2 to 3 weeks. They should be used intermittently but not discontinued spontaneously, because worsening can occur. Monitoring of the child during use is important. Small, localized lesions can be treated with topical fluorinated steroids. A moderate-potency steroid can be used on thick plaques and larger areas. Severe plaques on the elbows and knees may need a higher-potency steroid (see Table 34.1). Systemic steroids are not indicated and may worsen the condition, causing pustular flare.
- Tar or keratolytic shampoos (ketoconazole, anthralin, salicylic acid) can be used on the scalp.
- Follow up every 2 weeks until psoriasis is controlled and during exacerbations and then as needed.

A child with psoriasis necessitates a referral to the dermatologist and additional treatments that may be prescribed include (Paller and Mancini, 2016):

- Keratolytic agents, such as sulfur 3% or salicylic acid 3% to 6%, to reduce thick, unresponsive plaques. Salicylic acid blocks UVB and should not be used in combination with phototherapy.
- Anthralin ointment for plaques that are resistant to steroids and tar. Apply ointment in high strengths (1% and higher) for 10 to 30 minutes once a day, then wash off. In lower strengths, leave on for 8 hours. Strength used is determined by tolerance. Anthralin stains skin and clothing and can irritate skin.
- Calcipotriol, a vitamin D analogue, is effective for mild to moderate plaque psoriasis in adults and children. Available in cream, ointment, and lotion, it is safe, effective, and well tolerated for short- and long-term treatment. Hypercalcemia is reported with application of excessive quantities over large areas.
- Tazarotene is a retinoid that may be effective in management of plaque psoriasis, but is often too irritating for use in childhood psoriasis.
- Tacrolimus ointment, a calcineurin inhibitor, has demonstrated benefit when used for facial and intertriginous psoriasis in children.
- UV light therapy may be used for disseminated, chronic, or recalcitrant disease. Narrowband UVB light therapy is preferred in children due to safety and efficacy.
- Cyclosporine and methotrexate are systemic therapies used for recalcitrant and severe disease.
- Other treatment options include psoralens, intralesional steroids, retinoids, cyclosporine, biologic therapy, and immunotherapy.

Complications

The following complications are possible and require referral to a dermatologist:

- *Candida* infection: May be a secondary infection in the diaper area.
- Erythrodermic and pustular psoriasis: Unusual in childhood; characterized by generalized or local multiple 1- to 2-mm pustules with erythema and scaling also involving palms and soles; accompanied by malaise, fever, electrolyte and fluid imbalances, temperature instability, and leukocytosis; can be fatal.
- Exfoliative erythroderma: Rare manifestation, including desquamation and loss of hair and nails with previous history of psoriasis.
- Psoriatic arthritis: An inflammatory arthritis that is rare but increasing in frequency, most common in females 9 to 12 years old. Prognosis is good but should be referred to a rheumatologist.

Patient and Family Education

Emotional support and education are the most important aspects in dealing with psoriasis. Areas for discussion include the following:

- Psoriasis is chronic and involves spontaneous remissions and exacerbations. Control and relief are sought, but cure is not available. Treatment may require up to 1 month to determine effectiveness.
- Guttate psoriasis often resolves with antibiotic treatment for streptococcal infection. Psoriasis vulgaris may persist for months to years.
- Lifestyle changes help prevent recurrence. These include avoiding cutaneous injury, streptococcal infection, sunburn, stress, itching, bites, tight clothes and shoes, some medications (e.g., oral steroids, NSAIDs), and occlusive dressings. Good skin care, including regular use of emollients and avoiding irritating underarm deodorants and harsh soaps, may improve psoriasis and minimize recurrences. With nail involvement, avoid long fingernails or toenails and use of nail polish. Do not vigorously brush or comb hair if scalp area is affected.
- Psoriasis tends to improve during summer and with pregnancy.
- Psoriasis is considered stable if there are either no new plaques or if existing plaques are not enlarging.
- Refer patients to the National Psoriasis Foundation (see "Additional Resources").

Lichen Striatus

Lichen striatus (LS) is peculiar to childhood, characterized by unilateral shiny papules along embryonic lines, or lines of Blaschko. Although the etiology is unknown, it is thought to be related to a cutaneous defect from an embryologic mutation of somatic cells. It is most common in school-age children and affects girls more than boys. LS is typically located on the extremities, upper back, or neck, but can be found on the palms, soles, nails, genitals, or face. Lesions spontaneously disappear after 3 to 12 months, but they may last up to 3 years. Short relapses occur on occasion.

Clinical Findings

History. Lesions appear spontaneously without prodrome.
Physical Examination

- Linear, shiny hypopigmented or flesh-colored, flat-topped papules with adherent scale
- Limited to one extremity, initially lesions coalesce in a linear distribution down an extremity
- Lesions involving a nailbed result in nail deformity
- Rarely are lesions noted on the face
- May be asymptomatic or may be intensely pruritic
- May resolve with hypopigmentation that lasts several months

Differential Diagnosis

The unilateral linear lesions are characteristic. However, differential diagnosis includes lichen planus, lichen nitidus, psoriasis, epidermal birthmarks, and linear Darier disease.

Management

Lesions generally resolve without treatment in 1 to 2 years. Lubricants and topical steroids do not hasten resolution (Paller and Mancini, 2016).

Patient and Family Education

LS is a benign, self-limited, noncontagious disorder that results in complete resolution.

Keratosis Pilaris

Keratosis pilaris is a common finding on the extensor aspects of the extremities, buttocks, and occasionally the cheeks. The skin has a typical appearance of "chicken skin" with small bumps at the hair follicle. The etiology is unknown. It is common from early childhood onward. Some believe it to be a disorder of abnormal keratinization; others believe it is a response to drying of the skin surface. Keratosis pilaris is more common in children with atopic disorders; in those living in cold, dry climates; and in winter months.

Clinical Findings

History. Keratosis pilaris appears spontaneously, without prodrome. It is usually asymptomatic, although most patients are bothered by the appearance and seek treatment.

Physical Examination
- Rough dry skin on the posterior upper arms, anterior thighs, buttocks, and cheeks
- Small papules with follicular plugs of stratum corneum
- Occasional diffuse eruption with small sterile pustules

Diagnostic Studies. Skin biopsy reveals inflammation outside the hair follicle; however, this is typically not needed because the diagnosis is easy to determine.

Differential Diagnosis

Microcomedones of acne, molluscum contagiosum, warts, milia, and folliculitis are often confused with keratosis pilaris.

Management

It is important to recognize keratosis pilaris as a benign disorder to avoid detrimental treatment. Management includes the following:
- In mild cases, lubricants and emollients to moisturize skin are sufficient for improvement.
- Topical keratolytics combined with lactic acid 12%, salicylic acid, urea creams, retinoids, and lubricants are applied several times daily.
- Antibiotics active against *S. aureus* are useful for folliculitis.

Patient and Family Education

The chronic but benign nature of keratosis pilaris should be stressed. Treatment takes weeks to months, and recurrence is common.

Congenital Skin Conditions

Vascular and Pigmented Nevi

Nevi are a common finding in children. The two most common types are vascular nevi (vascular malformations and hemangiomas) and pigmented nevi (e.g., dermal melanocytosis, café au lait spots, acquired melanocytic nevi, atypical nevi, and lentigines).

Vascular nevi are caused by a structural abnormality (malformations) or by an overgrowth of blood vessels (hemangiomas) and are flat, raised, or cavernous. Flat lesions or vascular malformations include salmon patches (also called *macular stains*), an innocent malformation that is a light red macule appearing on the nape of the neck, upper eyelids, and glabella. Approximately 60% to 70% of newborns have a salmon patch on the back of the neck. Port-wine stains occur in 0.2% to 0.3% of newborns (Cohen, 2013). At 1 year old, 10% to 12% of Caucasian infants have a hemangioma—females three times more likely than males. There is also an increased incidence of hemangioma in premature neonates. Vascular malformations are always present at birth and do not resolve spontaneously. Precursor lesions of hemangiomas are present at birth 50% of the time. They undergo rapid growth

(proliferative stage), stability (plateau phase), and regression (involution phase); 90% are completely resolved in children 9 to 10 years old (Paller and Mancini, 2016).

Pigmented nevi are caused by an overgrowth of pigment cells. Pigmented nevi most commonly seen are dermal melanocytosis (found in up to 90% of African Americans, 62% to 86% of Asians, 70% of Hispanics, and less than 10% of Caucasians), café au lait spots (found in up to 33% of normal children and in 50% of patients with McCune-Albright syndrome), and acquired melanocytic nevi, the most common tumor of childhood. Atypical nevi, also called *dysplastic nevi,* are potential precursors for malignant melanoma. Dysplastic nevi are uncommon under 18 years old but have a higher incidence in melanoma-prone families (Paller and Mancini, 2016).

Clinical Findings

History
- Presence from birth, or age first noted
- Progression of lesion
- Familial tendencies for similar nevi, especially for history of melanoma

Physical Examination. Findings include the following (Box 34.8):
- Vascular malformations or flat vascular nevi are present at birth and grow commensurate with the child's growth.
- Hemangiomas are classified as superficial, deep (cavernous), or mixed. They may or may not be present at birth, but they usually emerge by 2 to 3 weeks of life. They may manifest initially as a pale macule, a telangiectatic lesion, or a bright red nodular papule. After appearing, hemangiomas go through a proliferative phase during which they grow rapidly and form nodular compressible masses, ranging in size from a few millimeters to several centimeters. Occasionally they may cover an entire limb, resulting in asymmetric limb growth. Rapidly growing lesions may ulcerate. The final phase of involution occurs slowly (10% per year) but spontaneously (30% by 3 years old, 50% by 5 years old, 70% by 7 years old, and 90% by 9 to 10 years old). Average involution begins between 12 and 24 months old, heralded by gray areas in the lesion followed by flattening from the center outward. Most hemangiomas appear as normal skin after involution, but others may have residual changes, such as telangiectasias, atrophy, fibrofatty residue, and scarring (Paller and Mancini, 2016).
- Pigmented nevi may be present at birth or acquired during childhood.
- Atypical nevi are larger than acquired nevi; have irregular, poorly defined borders; and have variable pigmentation.

Differential Diagnosis

Hematomas or ecchymoses of child abuse are occasionally confused with some nevi.

Management

1. Flat vascular nevi
- Salmon patches: Fade with time, usually by 5 or 6 years old; no treatment is needed.
- Port-wine stains: A permanent defect that grows with the child, so cosmetic covering is often used. If forehead and eyelids are involved, there is potential for multiple syndromes, including Sturge-Weber, Klippel-Trenaunay-Weber, and Parkes Weber. Neurodevelopmental and ophthalmologic follow-up is needed. Referral to a dermatologist for possible laser treatment or cosmesis is required.

• BOX 34.8 Common Vascular and Pigmented Lesions

I. Vascular malformations or flat vascular nevi
  A. Salmon patch or nevus flammeus: Light pink macule of varying size and configuration. Commonly seen on the glabella, back of neck, forehead, or upper eyelids.
  B. Port-wine stain: Purple-red macules that occur unilaterally and tend to be large. Usually occur on face, occiput, or neck, although they may be on extremities.
II. Hemangiomas
  A. Superficial (strawberry) hemangiomas are found in the upper dermis of the skin and account for the majority of hemangiomas.
  B. Deep cavernous hemangiomas are found in the subcutaneous and hypodermal layers of the skin; although similar to superficial hemangiomas, there is a blue tinge to their appearance. With pressure, there is blanching and a feeling of a soft, compressible tumor. Variable in size, they can occur in places other than skin.
  C. Mixed hemangiomas have attributes of both superficial and deep hemangiomas.
III. Pigmented nevi
  A. Dermal melanocytosis: Blue or slate-gray, irregular, variably sized macules. Common in the presacral or lumbosacral area of dark-skinned infants; also on the upper back, shoulders, and extremities. The majority of the pigment fades as the child gets older and the skin darkens. Solitary or multiple, often covering a large area.
  B. Café au lait spots: Tan to light brown macules found anywhere on the skin; oval or irregular shape; increase in number with age.
  C. Acquired melanocytic nevi are benign, light brown to dark brown to black, flat, or slightly raised, occurring anywhere on the body, especially on sun-exposed areas above the waist.
    1. Junctional nevi represent the initial stage, with tiny, hairless, light brown to black macules.
    2. Compound nevi—a few junctional nevi progress to more elevated, warty, or smooth lesions with hair.
    3. Dermal nevi are the adult form, dome shaped with coarse hair.
    4. Atypical nevi usually appear at puberty, have irregular borders, variegated pigmentation, are larger than normal nevi (6-15 mm); usually found on trunk, feet, scalp, and buttocks.
    5. Halo nevi appear in late childhood with an area of depigmentation around a pigmented nevus, usually on trunk (see Fig 34.30).
  D. Acanthosis nigricans is velvety brown rows of hyperpigmentation in irregular folds of skin, usually the neck and axilla; tags may also be present (see Fig 34.31).
  E. Lentigines are small brown to black macules 1-2 mm in size appearing anywhere on the body in school-age children.
  F. Freckles: 1-5 mm light brown, pigmented macules in sun-exposed areas.

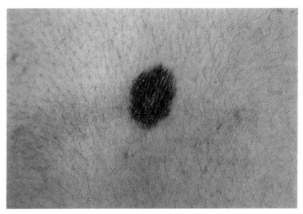

• **Fig 34.30** Atypical nevus with irregular borders and pink background. (From Weston WL, Morelli JG. *Pediatric Dermatology.* St. Louis: Elsevier; 2013, p 129.)

2. Hemangiomas
  • Reassure and educate the family about the nature and course of these nevi and that they are not related to anything the mother did during pregnancy.
  • Follow up frequently, especially during the proliferation phase. Sequential photographs are helpful.
  • If the lesions are strategically placed (eye, lip, oral cavity, ear, airway, diaper area), ulcerating, multiple, very large, or grow very quickly, prompt referral to a dermatologist is indicated because early treatment is most effective.
  • Current standard of care for infantile hemangiomas is the β-blocker propranolol. Treatment is the most effective in the proliferation phase but may help in later stages. Potential side effects include hypotension, bradycardia, bronchospasm, hypoglycemia, and hypothermia. The topical β-blocker timolol has been used with some success in small, primarily superficial, uncomplicated, and functionally insignificant hemangiomas (Paller and Mancini, 2016).
  • Steroids (intralesional and oral) may be prescribed during the proliferation phase until growth is stabilized, then gradually tapered. Their use has decreased in favor of propranolol but may be effective in smaller more localized lesions. Subcutaneous interferon-α may also be used in cases of severe treatment-resistant or life-threatening lesions. Treatment by surgery, cryotherapy, radiation, or injecting sclerosing agents often leads to scarring. Large, deep lesions can cause cardiovascular complications, disseminated intravascular coagulation, or compression of internal organs.
  • Involution (without treatment) occurs at a rate of 10% per year. Scarring may be present if ulceration occurs; fibrofatty masses, atrophy, and telangiectasis can occur following involution. Laser therapy is effective management for residual telangiectasias (Paller and Mancini, 2016).
3. Pigmented nevi: Educate family about the nature of these lesions.
  • Dermal melanocytosis: Document to distinguish from bruise; fade with time, usually no traces by adulthood.
  • Blue nevus: Heavily pigmented melanocytes in papule or nodule that can develop melanoma.
  • Café au lait spots: If six or more lesions larger than 5 mm in diameter are present in children younger than 15 years old and more than 1.5 cm in diameter for older individuals, or if axillary freckling (Crowe's sign), neurofibromas, or iris hamartomas is also present, refer child to rule out neurofibromatosis, McCune-Albright syndrome, tuberous sclerosis, LEOPARD (acronym for: **L**entigines [multiple], **E**lectrocardiographic conduction abnormalities, **O**cular hypertelorism, **P**ulmonary stenosis, **A**bnormalities of genitalia, **R**etardation of growth, **D**eafness) syndrome, epidermal nevus syndrome, Bloom syndrome, ataxia-telangiectasia, and Silver-Russell syndrome (Cohen, 2013).
4. Other disorders of hyperpigmentation that can appear in early childhood:
  • Acquired melanocytic nevi: Giant nevi (e.g., bathing trunk nevus). These children are at increased risk of developing melanoma and need referral to a dermatologist.
  • Atypical nevi appear most commonly in adolescents and require regular follow-up because of increased risk for melanoma. However, melanoma often manifests with new lesions rather than from transformation of current ones (see section on burns in Chapter 44) (Fig 34.30).

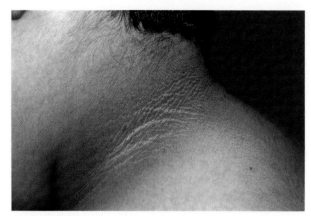

• **Fig 34.31** Acanthosis Nigricans. (From Weston WL, Lane AT, Morelli JG. *Color Textbook of Pediatric Dermatology.* 4th ed. St. Louis: Mosby/ Elsevier; 2007, p 331.)

- Halo nevus: A depigmented ring around a pigmented nevus.
- Spitz nevus: A smooth, pink to brown, dome-shaped papule often occurring on head and neck.
- Nevus spilus: A light-brown speckled lentiginous nevus with darker papules within it can be congenital or acquired and has potential to develop into melanoma.
5. Guidelines for when a child with a nevus should be referred to a dermatologist are listed in Box 34.9.

Complications

Ulceration, infection, platelet trapping, airway or visual obstruction, or cardiac decompensation can occur with large vascular nevi. Kasabach-Merritt syndrome occurs when thrombocytopenic hemorrhage occurs in a large, deep hemangioma. Melanoma in congenital nevi is possible. An autosomal dominant, familial, atypical mole and melanoma syndrome has been identified genetically. Children with multiple atypical nevi and family members with melanoma are at risk for childhood melanoma.

Patient and Family Education

Monitoring nevi that are at risk for developing melanoma is important as is teaching the family to watch nevi for any changes. Changes of particular concern are development of an off-center nodule or papule, color change, bleeding, persistent irritation, erosion, ulceration, and rapid growth.

Cutaneous Manifestations of Underlying Disease

Acanthosis Nigricans

Acanthosis nigricans is not a skin disease per se; rather it is typically a sign of an underlying problem. It may be related to:
- Heredity (autosomal dominant trait with no associated obesity): It may appear at birth or during childhood with proliferation during adolescence. Children of Native American, African American, Hispanic, Asian American, and Pacific Islander descent are at increased risk (Paller and Mancini, 2016).
- Endocrine disorders (e.g., insulin resistance, hypothyroidism, hyperandrogenic states, Cushing syndrome)
- Obesity (more commonly seen in darker-pigmented individuals)
- Drug administration (e.g., oral contraceptives, stilbestrol use in young males, high levels of nicotinic acid)
- Malignancy (e.g., adenocarcinoma, Wilms tumor, and less commonly lymphoma)

All but the malignant form of acanthosis nigricans result in papillary hypertrophy, hyperkeratosis, and an increase in the number of melanocytes from keratocyte and dermal fibroblast changes. There is no gender predominance.

Clinical Findings

Acanthosis nigricans is characterized by symmetric, brown thickening of the skin. As time progresses the skin develops a velvety, leathery, warty, or papillomatous surface. The axillary areas (most commonly), neck, groin, belt line, dorsal surfaces of the fingers, in the mouth, around the areola of the breast, and umbilicus can be affected. In areas of maceration, odor or discomfort may be reported (see Fig 34.31).

Differential Diagnosis

Terra firma-forme dermatosis, a condition with lamellar hyperkeratosis, can occur anywhere on the body. Although it can look like dirt, terra firma-forme dermatosis is not related to hygiene and cannot be washed off with soap and water. Unlike acanthosis nigricans, however, the darkened skin of terra firma-forme dermatosis can be removed with vigorous rubbing with isopropyl alcohol. It is important to diagnose terra firma-forme dermatosis in order to avoid an extensive and expensive workup for an endocrine or metabolic disorder.

Management

Treatment consists of addressing the underlying causes. This most commonly includes management of overweight (diet changes and weight loss) and correction of metabolic abnormality (hyperinsulinemia). In nonoverweight individuals, an underlying malignancy must be considered. The skin lesions themselves are benign, usually asymptomatic, and do not require intervention. Thicker lesions may cause discomfort and respond to topical retinoic acid cream or gel once daily. Dermabrasion and long-pulsed alexandrite laser therapy have also been used. Lac-Hydrin (12% lactic acid cream) can help soften lesions.

Patient and Family Education

It is important for patients to understand that acanthosis nigricans may be a cutaneous marker for an underlying condition such as insulin resistance and type 2 diabetes in obese individuals or for a malignancy. Associated tumors include gastric carcinoma, lymphoma, Hodgkin disease, and osteogenic sarcoma (Cohen, 2013). The condition may completely resolve with adequate treatment of the underlying disorder.

Lentigines

Lentigines are small, tan, dark brown or black, flat, oval or circular, sharply circumscribed lesions that appear in childhood and may increase in number until adulthood. They may also be seen on mucous membranes and may fade or disappear with time. Lentigines can be associated with various syndromes including LEOPARD syndrome and Peutz-Jeghers syndrome (Weston and Morelli, 2017).

Vitiligo and Hypopigmentation Disorders

Lack of skin pigment, leaving white or light-colored areas, can be either hypopigmentation or vitiligo. It is congenital or acquired and appears in a diffuse or localized pattern. Vitiligo is presumed to be an immune disorder that has a genetic component. A patterned pigmentation loss with great variation in location, size, and shape of individual lesions, vitiligo occurs in 1% to 2% of the population worldwide, with 50% of cases appearing before 18 years of age. Generalized vitiligo occurs most commonly in children, and it is generally associated with other autoimmune disorders, most commonly hypothyroidism (Weston and Morelli, 2017).

Hypopigmentation follows inflammation or injury to the melanocytes in the skin resulting from diseases (such as atopic dermatitis, psoriasis, or pityriasis rosea), or from abrasions, burns, injury from liquid nitrogen, or severe sunburn.

Clinical Findings
History
- Family history of vitiligo, halo nevi, traumatic depigmentation of skin, or markedly premature graying of the hair (Paller and Mancini, 2016)
- Onset of depigmentation (birth or more recent)
- Presence of any systemic or skin diseases
- Any recent trauma to the skin; Koebner phenomenon is noted in about 15% of children with vitiligo
Physical Examination
- Vitiligo
  - Flat milk-white macules or papules with scalloped, distinct borders of varied size
  - Symmetric or asymmetric, possibly following a nerve segment
  - Few to multiple, seen most commonly on face and trunk
- Hypopigmentation
  - Macules and patches with irregular mottling and borders
  - Linear or patterned
  - May be associated hyperpigmented areas

Diagnostic Studies. For vitiligo, a skin biopsy and CBC, fasting glucose, thyroid function and antithyroid antibodies, early-morning serum cortisol, and VDRL are sometimes indicated. A Wood's light may be helpful in fair-skinned individuals to delineate a contrast between the normal and depigmented skin.

Differential Diagnosis
Pityriasis rosea, pityriasis alba, tinea versicolor, and albinism (which is seen at birth and affects eye color) are included in the differential diagnosis.

Management
The following steps are taken:
- Vitiligo
  - Broad-spectrum sunscreens are used to decrease the tanning of normal skin.
  - Cover-up agents, such as skin dyes and walnut oil, may be used.
  - Mild to moderate steroids may show success in some patients. Topical calcineurin inhibitors (e.g., tacrolimus ointment, pimecrolimus cream) eliminate atrophy, with 40% to 90% of pediatric patients showing a response to these treatments (Paller and Mancini, 2016).
  - Refer for treatment with psoralens, which may be used in combination with UVA radiation (best used in children younger than 9 years old). UVB may also be used.
  - Support groups help families because this can be a highly disfiguring condition, especially for those with dark complexions.
- Hypopigmentation
  - Reassure family that repigmentation will occur. Postinflammatory hypopigmentation is self-limited and lasts only a few months.

Complications
Vitiligo may be associated with other immune disorders or their symptoms, such as thyroid disease, diabetes mellitus, pernicious anemia, Addison disease, uveitis, and alopecia areata. Patients are at risk for severe sunburn.

Hair Loss

Alopecia, hair loss from areas of skin that normally produce hair, can be limited to one area or scattered over the scalp and can be complete or leave residual hairs of differing lengths. The three main causes of hair loss are tinea capitis, traumatic alopecia, and alopecia areata (Table 34.10).

Traumatic Alopecia

Traumatic hair loss, characterized by incomplete hair loss with hair of varying lengths, can be due to chemical exposure, thermal damage, traction, or friction. The most common forms are traction alopecia and trichotillomania. Traction alopecia, commonly seen in African American females, is due to hair styling. Common causes are cornrows, ponytails, or braids; tight curlers; or excessive brushing Fig 34.32.

Trichotillomania is a common disorder seen in children of all ages after infancy. Hair loss is varied and is caused by repeated pulling and/or excessive twisting of hair with fracturing of the longer hair shafts. Research indicates etiology is multifactorial, including genetic predisposition and environmental and behavioral variables. In preschoolers it is associated with habitual behaviors and situational stress. It can also be associated with obsessive-compulsive psychiatric disease in older children (Cohen, 2013). Trichotillomania after the preschool years is classified as an impulse control disorder.

Clinical Findings
History
- Various methods of hair styling with tight pull on hair
- Habits, such as nail biting, finger sucking, or hair twirling
- Any recent life changes or stressors
- Medications (e.g., anticonvulsants, antithyroid medications, β-blockers, isotretinoin, lithium, oral contraceptives, vitamin A supplements, warfarin)
- Excess time spent lying supine
Physical Examination. The following findings are present:
- Possible erythema and pustules
- Thinning and breaking of hair in certain areas, tending to occur in a linear pattern related to hairstyle

TABLE 34.10	Diagnosis and Treatment of Alopecia		
	Etiology	**Clinical Findings**	**Treatment**
Tinea capitis	*Trichophyton tonsurans* 90%-95%; *Microsporum canis;* others	Fine diffuse scaling without obvious hair breaks and subtle to significant hair loss; hair loss discrete with stubs of broken hair; patchy hair loss with scaling and raised borders to lesions; scaly, pustular lesions or kerions	Griseofulvin taken with fatty food until 2 weeks after negative culture; prednisone if kerion present; culture family members; sporicidal shampoo; follow up in 2 weeks; launder sheets, clothes, vacuum house
Traumatic alopecia	Chemical, thermal, traction (hairstyling), friction (trichotillomania)	Traumatic: Incomplete hair loss with varying lengths Traction: Erythema and pustules, hair thins and breaks in certain areas, especially linear Trichotillomania: Circumscribed hair loss with irregular borders and broken hair of varied lengths, no erythema or scarring, especially frontal, parietal, or temporal	Traction: Avoid hairstyles that precipitate; use mild shampoo, gentle brushing; short course of antibiotics if pustules are present Trichotillomania: Discussion with parents, oil at night, counseling, behavioral modifications
Alopecia areata	Autoimmune mechanism	Family history; single or multiple round or oval patches of complete or near-complete hair loss; no erythema or scaling, scalp smooth with fine new hair growth, usually frontal or parietal; "exclamation hairs" present; nail ridging or pitting; occasional loss of body or pubic hair	Discussion and support; often self-limited course; if extensive, refer to dermatologist for alternative treatments; supportive care; prescription for wig; refer to National Alopecia Foundation

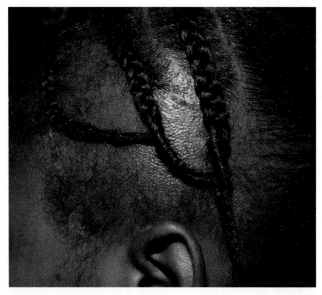

• **Fig 34.32** Traction Alopecia. (From James WD, Berger TG, Elston DM. *Andrews' Diseases of the Skin: Clinical Dermatology.* 11th ed. Philadelphia: Saunders/Elsevier; 2011.)

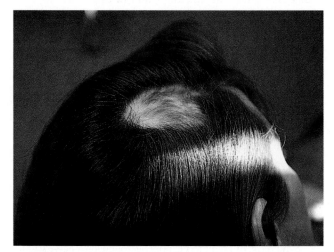

• **Fig 34.33** Alopecia Areata. (From Thibodeau GA, Patton KT. *The Human Body in Health & Disease.* 5th ed. St. Louis: Mosby/Elsevier; 2010.)

- Circumscribed hair loss with irregular borders and broken hairs of varied length
- No erythema or scaling of the scalp
- Hair loss is commonly found on frontal eyelashes, parietal, and temporal areas with peripheral sparing, but also eyebrows

Differential Diagnosis

The differential diagnosis includes tinea capitis, alopecia areata, neonatal occipital alopecia, and child abuse (make sure no one but the child is pulling out the hair).

Management

The following steps are taken:
1. Traction alopecia
- Avoid any hairstyle or device that causes traction on the hair, including cornrows, ponytails, braids, and curlers.
- Use only mild shampoo, shampoo infrequently, use wide-toothed combs with rounded ends, and brush gently.
- A short course of antibiotics is prescribed if pustules are present.
2. Trichotillomania
- A straightforward discussion and ongoing support of the child and parents are essential. In very young children, trichotillomania is usually benign and resolves spontaneously. Older children and adolescents may require individual and family therapy. Attempt to relieve stress and cope with any traumatic events.
- Applying oil to the hair at night makes it slippery and harder to pull.
- Behavior modification programs may be needed for children with more severe trichotillomania. Cognitive-behavioral therapy and/or pharmacologic therapy may be indicated if behavior modification strategies prove unsuccessful (Krooks, 2017).

Complications

Trichobezoars (hairballs) in the child with trichotillomania can cause gastrointestinal symptoms. Some children with trichotillomania have extensive psychopathologic conditions.

Patient and Family Education

The cause of the hair loss must be discussed and support offered to resolve issues. New hair growth can take 3 to 6 months.

Alopecia Areata

Alopecia areata is an asymptomatic, complete hair loss occurring primarily in frontal or parietal areas (Fig 34.33). *Ophiasis* is a form of alopecia areata that begins in the frontal or occipital hairline and spreads along the hair margins.

The cause of alopecia areata is unknown, but it is thought to be an autoimmune mechanism. Twenty-seven percent to 60% of patients experience their first episode before 20 years of age (Castelo-Soccio, 2014). Twenty-five percent of patients have a family history of alopecia areata (Weston and Morelli, 2017).

Clinical Findings

History. The history can include other family members with alopecia areata.

Physical Examination
- Single or multiple (up to three) round or oval patches of complete or nearly complete hair loss without erythema or scaling. Scalp is smooth with fine new hair growth.
- The frontal and parietal areas are involved 90% of the time.
- "Exclamation hairs" are narrower at the base, short, and broken off.
- Nail ridging or pitting (a helpful distinguishing factor).
- Occasional loss of body or pubic hair, or eyelashes or eyebrows.
- Possible atopic dermatitis or vitiligo.

Diagnostic Studies. The following are sometimes performed:
- KOH examination or fungal culture to rule out tinea
- Skin biopsy
- Thyroid screening, because it can be associated with autoimmune thyroiditis

Differential Diagnosis

Tinea capitis (see fungal infections) versus traumatic alopecia is the differential diagnosis.

Management

The following steps should be taken:
1. Open discussion and support of the child and parents. If only one or two patches are present, reassure that regrowth will occur.
2. If extensive involvement, refer to a dermatologist for treatment options. Treatment options include topical corticosteroids, local irritants, topical minoxidil, topical sensitizers, and UV light therapy (Cohen, 2013).
3. Recommend wearing a wig, depending on the severity of involvement; prescribing the wig as a medical treatment helps defray the cost. Locks of Love is an organization that provides hairpieces to financially disadvantaged children younger than 21 years old and the National Alopecia Areata Foundation (see "Additional Resources") is a national support group for affected children and families.

Complications

Self-esteem issues are common. *Alopecia totalis* is a loss of all the hair on the scalp. *Alopecia universalis* is a loss of all the hair on the body.

Patient and Family Education

All families should be put in touch with the National Alopecia Areata Foundation. The condition is self-limited in most school-age children and adolescents. Full recovery, often within 1 year, is more likely if three or fewer areas are involved and if onset is in late childhood. However, the greater the hair loss, the longer it takes for regrowth. Prognosis is guarded in infants and toddlers. Approximately one-third of patients have a recurrence within months to years, with a worsening prognosis with each episode.

Body Modifications

Tattoos, Body Piercing, and Scarification

A tattoo is an indelible mark fixed on the body by inserting pigment under the skin. Body piercing is the creation of a hole anywhere in the body (typically the ear, eyebrow, lip, naris, tongue, navel, nipple, or genitalia) to insert jewelry. Scarification is the practice of intentionally irritating the skin in order to cause a permanent pattern of scar tissue. All are considered forms of *body modification* that have been practiced throughout the ages in many cultures as rites of passage. These practices are used today to describe loyalty, interests, and lifestyle choices (Breuner, Levine, and AAP Committee on Adolescence, 2018). While often associated with high-risk behaviors in the past, the scientific link between tattooing and high-risk behaviors is less consistent today.

Many states have legislation that prevents practitioners from tattooing or piercing minors or that requires parental consent before a procedure is done on a minor. Consequently, many teens seek out unlicensed tattoo artists or social contacts for tattoos and piercing. Studies have shown that young people are often unaware of the risks associated with these behaviors (e.g. HIV, Hepatitis B, Hepatitis C, tetanus) (Breuner, Levine, and AAP Committee on Adolescence, 2018).

While much scarification is self-performed, there are increasing numbers of providers. Common techniques include hot and cold branding, cutting with a scalpel, and laser branding. Few states have any regulations for this activity.

The incidence of tattooing and piercing has been increasing, especially in the adolescent population. In one study of youth 12 to 22 years of age, 10% to 23% had a tattoo and 27% to 42% had a body piercing other than the earlobe. Girls had a higher rate than boys. There are no studies in the United States to indicate the prevalence of scarification.

Clinical Findings

History. Questions to discuss include the following:
- When and where was the body art obtained?
- Where is it located, and what care is being given?
- Were there any complications?

Physical Examination. Look for any symptoms of infection, erythema, crusting, or scabs.

Differential Diagnosis

Non-suicidal self-injury (NSSI) is often an impulsive or compulsive behavior with the intent of self-harm and without suicidal intent. NSSI is often associated with mental health disorders with most individuals seeking relief from emotional pain. As with all adolescents, teens who practice body modifications should receive a careful psychosocial assessment.

Management

1. Aftercare for tattoos:
- Antiseptic and a bandage is applied immediately after the tattoo and is not be removed for 24 hours. After 24 hours, leave tattoo open to air.

- A moderate amount of oozing and local swelling is normal for 48 hours. Keep skin moist with antibiotic ointment, thick skin cream, or vitamin E.
- Scab should be left alone except for the application of antibiotic ointment.
- Protect from rough surfaces that can traumatize; protect from sunburn.
- Tattoos generally take 2 weeks to heal.
- Review signs and symptoms of infection.

2. Aftercare for body piercings
- Wash hands before touching; cleanse area twice a day with antibacterial soap.
- A moderate amount of oozing and swelling is normal; if crusts appear, remove with wet swab.
  - Tongue
    a. Use ice to minimize swelling.
    b. Rinse mouth 10 to 12 times a day with half-strength Listerine, twice a day with carbamide peroxide.
    c. No deep kissing for 48 hours; once healed, use dental dams for dental work, and avoid smoking.
  - Navel
    a. Slowest to heal, most likely area to reject jewelry.
    b. Cleanse twice a day with antibacterial soap.
    c. Avoid handling; avoid clothing that rubs for up to 1 year.
  - Nipples and genitalia
    a. Cleanse twice a day with antibacterial soap.
    b. Avoid manipulation and tight garments; cotton clothes are ideal.
    c. Use latex barriers with sexual activity. Jewelry may compromise barrier contraceptive methods.

3. Healing times are variable and should be considered. A tattoo may take 2 to 3 weeks to heal. Body piercing, depending on the site, can take from 4 to 8 weeks for ears to 6 to 12 months for navel and genital piercings (Table 34.11).
4. Infection can be treated with dicloxacillin 500 mg 4 times a day for 10 days. The decision to remove jewelry during an infection should be based on whether leaving it in place will provide a route for drainage, become an obstacle to healing, or be an ongoing source of infection.
5. Screen for high-risk behaviors.
6. Discuss the need to remove dangling ornaments during contact sports.

Complications

Common complications of tattooing or body piercing include infections, allergic reactions to the dyes or jewelry, and the transmission of blood-borne diseases, primarily hepatitis B and C, but potentially HIV. Other reported complications of tattoos include skin neoplasms, syphilis, leprosy, cutaneous tuberculosis, tetanus, hyperplasia, and granuloma annulare. Complications of piercings also include excessive bleeding, nerve damage, keloids, dental fracture, soft-tissue damage, and speech impediments.

Patient and Family Education

Provide information and encourage teenagers to thoroughly research and consider the idea of getting a tattoo or body piercing. Removing tattoos is expensive, not necessarily completely successful, and fraught with complication (e.g., scarring, rashes) (Box 34.10). Maintaining an open, nonjudgmental attitude when discussing the options and caring for adolescents who have body art is essential. Alternatives to discuss include temporary stick-on tattoos and use of henna or other body paints.

TABLE 34.11 Healing Time for Body Piercings

Type of Piercing	Time to Heal
Navel	4 weeks-12 months
Ear cartilage	6 weeks-9 months
Nostril	6 weeks-4 months
Earlobe and eyebrow	4-8 weeks
Nipple	6 weeks-9 months
Lip	6-8 weeks
Tongue	3-8 weeks
Outer labia	4 weeks-4 months
Inner labia	2-8 weeks
Clitoris	2-10 weeks
Male genitalia	2 weeks-4 months

Data from Hoover CV, Rademayer CA, Farley CL. Body piercings: motivations and implications for health. *J Midwifery Womens Health.* 2017;62:521–530.

• BOX 34.10 Know the Facts about Getting a Tattoo or Body Piercing

Make an Informed Decision

- Be sure equipment/needles have been sterilized and dye was not previously used on another individual to decrease risk of infections, hepatitis, or possibly even HIV.
- The law in many states prohibits the tattooing of minors.
- Asking a friend to apply a tattoo may ruin a friendship if the tattoo does not look like you thought it would.
- Tattoos and permanent makeup are not easily removed and in some cases may cause permanent discoloration.
- Tattoo removal is very expensive. Blood donations cannot be made for 1 year after getting a tattoo, body piercing, or permanent makeup.

Before You Get a Tattoo or Body Piercing: Think Carefully

- First: Talk to your friends or others who have been tattooed or pierced. Ask them about their experience, the cost, pain, healing time, and so on. Ask them what they would do if they had a chance to do it over again.

- Second: Understand that you do not have to tattoo or pierce your body to belong. Remember that you are directly involved in decisions that affect your health and body. You can always change your mind or wait if you are not sure.
- Third: Because of potential complications, if you decide to get a tattoo or body piercing, never tattoo or pierce your own body or let a friend do it.

Health Risks to Consider Before You Act

- Both tattooing and piercing involve puncturing the skin to introduce a foreign material, jewelry, or ink, and the procedures carry similar risks. The primary health concern is introducing blood-borne germs or viruses into your body.
- Blood-borne illnesses, such as hepatitis B and C, tetanus, tuberculosis, and HIV infection, can lead to serious health problems or death.
- Make sure you have had the three series hepatitis B vaccination and a tetanus booster within the past 10 years.
- Localized infections, such as *Staphylococcus* or *Pseudomonas*, can lead to illness, deformity, and scarring.

- Tattoo troubles: *Tattoos are open wounds that may become infected.* Keep the new tattoo clean and moist with an ointment to prevent a scab from forming. If you are allergic to the inks in the tattoo, the site will not heal properly and scarring may occur.
- Piercing problems: Complications depend on the location of the piercing. Navel infections are the most common; it takes approximately 1 year for navel piercings to heal. Ear cartilage heals slowly. Tongue piercings may lead to tooth and enamel damage from biting on the jewelry and jewelry knocking against a tooth, partial paralysis if the jewelry pierces a nerve, and extreme inflammation during the first few days.

Selecting a Tattoo Artist or Piercer

- Visit several piercers or tattooists. The work area should be kept clean and have good lighting. If they refuse to discuss cleanliness and infection control with you, go somewhere else.
- Consent forms (which the customer must fill out) should be handled before tattooing. Reputable piercing and tattoo studios will not serve a

minor without signed consent from parents. Check the laws in your state about tattooing of minors if you are younger than 18 years old.
- The tattooist or piercer should have an *autoclave*—a heat sterilization machine used to sterilize equipment between customers.
- Packaged, sterilized needles should be used only once and then disposed of in a biohazard container.
- Immediately before tattooing or piercing, the tattooist or piercer should wash and dry his or her hands and wear latex gloves. These gloves should be worn at all times while the tattoo or piercing is being done. If the tattoo artist or piercer leaves or touches other objects, such as the telephone, new gloves should be put on before the procedure continues.
- Only jewelry made of a noncorrosive metal, such as surgical stainless steel, niobium, or solid 14-karat gold, is safe for a new piercing.
- Leftover tattoo ink should be disposed of after each procedure. Ink should never be poured back into the bottle and reused.

HIV, Human immunodeficiency virus.

Additional Resources

American Academy of Dermatology. www.aad.org
Association of Professional Piercers. www.safepiercing.org
Dermatology Online Journal. https://escholarship.org/uc/doj
Electronic Textbook of Dermatology. www.telemedicine.org/stamfor1.htm
FIRST: Foundation for Ichthyosis and Related Skin Types. www.firstskinfoundation.org
International OCD (Obsessive-Compulsive Disorder) Foundation. https://iocdf.org/
iPledge Program. www.ipledgeprogram.com
Locks of Love. www.locksoflove.org
Loyola University Dermatology. www.meddean.luc.edu/lumen/meded/medicine/dermatology/melton/atlas.htm
National Alopecia Areata Foundation. www.naaf.org
National Organization for Albinism and Hypopigmentation. www.albinism.org
National Pediculosis Association, Inc. www.headlice.org
National Psoriasis Foundation. www.psoriasis.org
National Vitiligo Foundation, Inc. www.mynvfi.org
Nevus Network. www.nevusnetwork.org
Prevent Cancer Foundation. www.preventcancer.org
Skin Cancer Foundation. www.skincancer.org
Tattooing And Body Piercing | State Laws, Statutes And Regulations. http://www.ncsl.org/research/health/tattooing-and-body-piercing.aspx
Trichotillomania Learning Center (TLC). https://rarediseases.org/organizations/trichotillomania-learning-center/

References

American Academy of Dermatology (AAD). *How to prevent skin cancer,* (website); 2018. Available at https://www.aad.org/dermatology-a-to-z/for-kids/about-skin/skin-cancer/how-to-prevent-skin-cancer. Accessed April 3, 2018.
Bolognia JL, Schaffer JV, Duncan KO, et al. *Dermatology Essentials.* Philadelphia: Elsevier/Saunders; 2014.
Breuner CC, Levine DA. AAP Committee on Adolescence. Adolescent and young adult tattooing, piercing, and scarification. *Pediatrics.* 2017;140(4):96–111.
Bystritsky R, Chambers H. Cellulitis and soft tissue infections. *Ann Intern Med.* 2018;168(3):ITC17–ITC32.
Chen X, Jiang X, Yang M, Bennett C, González U, Lin X, et al. Systemic antifungal therapy for tinea capitis in children. *Cochrane Database Syst Rev.* 2016. Issue 5. Art. No.: CD004685.
Clark GW, Pope S, Jaboori KA. Diagnosis and treatment of seborrheic dermatitis. *Am Fam Physician.* 2015;91(3):185–190.
Cohen BA. *Pediatric Dermatology.* 4th ed. Philadelphia: Saunders/Elsevier; 2013.
Devore CD, Schutze GE. Council on School Health and Committee on Infectious Diseases, American Academy of Pediatrics: head lice. *Pediatrics.* 2015;135(5):e1355–e1365.
Drugs for Head Lice. *The Medical Letter on Drugs and Therapeutics.* 2016;58:150–152.
Feldstein S, Totri C, Friedlander SH. Antifungal therapy for onychomycosis in children. *Clin Dermatol.* 2015;33(3):333–339.
Forbat E, Al-Niaimi F, Ali F. Molluscum contagiosum: review and update on management. *Pediatric Dermatology.* 2017;34(5):504–515.
Guenther L. *Pediculosis and phthiriasis (lice infestation);* 2018. Available at https://emedicine.medscape.com/article/225013-overview. Accessed April 3, 2018.
Krooks JA, Weatherall AG, Holland PJ. Review of epidemiology, clinical presentation, diagnosis, and treatment of common primary psychiatric causes of cutaneous disease. *J Dermatolog Treat.* 2017. https://doi.org/10.1080/09546634.2017.1395389.
Mccoshum S, Schlarb A, Baum K. Direct and indirect effects of sunscreen exposure for reef biota. *Hydrobiologia.* 2016;776(1):139–146.
Oranje AP. Proactive therapy in atopic dermatitis. In: Oranje A, Al-Mutairi N, Shwayder T, eds. *Practical Pediatric Dermatology.* Cham: Springer; 2016.
Paller AS, Mancini AJ. *Hurwitz Clinical Pediatric Dermatology: A Textbook of Skin Disorders of Children and Adolescence.* 5th ed. Philadelphia: Elsevier; 2016.
Stevens D, Bisno A, Chambers H, et al. Practice guidelines for the diagnosis and management of skin and soft tissue infections: 2014 update by the Infectious Diseases Society of America. *Clin Infect Dis.* An Official Publication of the Infectious Diseases Society of America. 2014;59(2):E10–E52.
Strom MA, Hsu DY, Silverberg JI. Prevalence, comorbidities and mortality of toxic shock syndrome in children and adults in the USA. *Microbiol Immunol.* 2017;61:463–473.
Tom WL. Food allergy and atopic dermatitis: fellow travelers or triggers? *Pediatric News.* 2017;51(12):S7–S9.
VanRavenstein K, Edlund BJ. Diagnosis and management of pityriasis rosea. *The Nurse Practitioner.* 2017;42(1):8–11.
Weston WL, Morelli JG. *Pediatric Dermatology DDx Deck 2e.* Philadelphia: Elsevier/Saunders; 2017.
Workowski KA, Bolan G. Sexually transmitted diseases treatment guidelines, 2015. *MMWR Recomm Rep.* 2015;64(RR-03):1–137.
Zaenglein AL, Pathy AL, Schlosser BJ, et al. Guidelines of care for the management of acne vulgaris. *J Am Acad Dermatol.* 2016;74(5):945–973.
Zitelli BJ, McIntire S, Nowalk AJ. *Zitelli and Davis' Atlas of Pediatric Physical Diagnosis.* 7th ed. Philadelphia: Elsevier; 2018.

35

Eye Disorders

TERI MOSER WOO

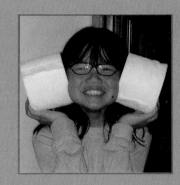

Ophthalmic diseases occur most often in the very young or very old, although exceptions include eye trauma, refractive errors, and other chronic conditions and disorders (e.g., retinoblastoma). Infants and children are particularly susceptible to permanent central visual loss (amblyopia), opacities (congenital cataracts), refractive errors not associated with amblyopia, strabismus (ocular misalignment), and other conditions that interfere with visual acuity (ptosis, anisometropia). With early detection and correction, these conditions do not lead to permanent loss in the mature central visual system of the older child or adult (American Academy of Pediatrics [AAP], America Association of Pediatric Orthoptists [AAPO], American Association for Pediatric Ophthalmology and Strabismus [AAPOS] and American Academy of Ophthalmology [AAO], 2016). When children with eye problems are being cared for, priorities include promoting optimizing growth and development of the ocular structures and maximizing visual acuity. To this end, primary care providers (PCPs) seek to promote good vision and health, detect abnormalities, and treat those conditions that fall within their scope of practice. They will refer patients with conditions requiring an ophthalmologist's expertise and provide education and reassurance to parents and children.

Standards for Visual Screening and Care

Standards and guidelines for visual screening and eye care in children are set by a number of agencies and professional groups. Pediatric-focused objectives related to vision in the U.S. Department of Health and Human Services (HHS) Healthy People 2020 (2014) propose to

- Increase the proportion of preschool children (≤5 years of age) who receive vision screening
- Reduce blindness and visual impairment in children and adolescents (≤17 years of age)
- Reduce uncorrected visual impairment due to refractive errors
- Increase the use of personal protective eyewear in recreational activities and hazardous situations around the home

The US Preventive Services Task Force (USPSTF) recommendations for vision screening for children 6 months to 5 years of age (2017) note that screening tests have reasonable accuracy in identifying strabismus, amblyopia, and refractive errors in children 3 to 5 years of age. Providers should be alert for signs of ocular misalignment when they are examining infants and children. Treating strabismus and amblyopia early greatly reduces long-term amblyopia and improves visual acuity.

The AAP, American Association of Certified Orthoptists (AACO), AAPOS, and the AAO jointly recommend that well-child

examinations should include ocular history, vision assessment, and external inspection of the eyes (including pupils and red light reflex), lids, and ocular mobility (2017c). This also includes an evaluation of fixation and following starting at birth, with visual acuity screening starting at 3 years of age (Table 35.1). Instrument-based vision screening (i.e., photoscreening) for amblyopia, high refractive error, and strabismus can start in the pediatric office as early as 6 months and continue regularly between 18 months and age 5 years, when Snellen vision screening can be performed. If the child is uncooperative, retesting should occur 6 months later. Inability to fix and follow after 3 months of age warrants a referral to a pediatric ophthalmologist or an eye specialist trained to treat pediatric patients. Subsequent testing should occur at ages 4 and 5 years and yearly or biannually until age 18 years (AAO, 2017). A subjective historical assessment should occur during visits at all other ages. Children who are difficult to screen after two attempts or who demonstrate any other eye abnormality should undergo photoscreening to detect amblyopia, medial opacities, and treatable ocular disease processes and referral to an ophthalmologist considered (AAO, 2017a; AAPOS, 2017a).

For high-risk children, the AAO (2017a) recommends that asymptomatic children have a comprehensive examination by an ophthalmologist if they have any of the following:

- Failed vision screening or inability to be screened in primary care
- A vision complaint or observed abnormal visual behavior
- Health or developmental problems that places the child at risk for developing eye problems (e.g., prematurity, Down syndrome, juvenile idiopathic arthritis (JIA), neurofibromatosis, or diagnostic evaluation of a complex disease with ophthalmologic manifestations)
- A family history of conditions that cause or are associated with eye or vision problems (e.g., retinoblastoma, significant hyperopia, strabismus [particularly accommodative esotropia], amblyopia, congenital cataract, or glaucoma)

Development, Physiology, and Pathophysiology of the Eye

Development of the Ocular Structures

At 21 days of gestation, ocular tissue is visible on each side of the head. By the end of the eighth week of pregnancy, the eyelids are completely formed and the upper and lower lids fuse to seal the eye while it develops. At 16 weeks of gestation, the eyes are fully anterior. By the seventh month of pregnancy, the fetus can open

TABLE 35.1	Visual Acuity Norms (Snellen Equivalents)	
Age	Forced-Choice Preferential Looking (FPL)	Visual Evoked Potential (VEP)
Birth	20/400	20/800
2 months old	20/400	
4 months old	20/200	20/600
6 months old	20/150	20/400
12 months old	20/50	20/20
18–24 months old	20/25 or 20/20	
5 years old	20/25 or 20/20	

Adapted from Eustis HS, Guthrie ME. Postnatal development. In: Wright KW, Spiegel PH, eds. *Pediatric Ophthalmology and Strabismus*. New York: Springer; 2003. Stout A. Pediatric eye examination. In: Wright KW, Spiegel PH, eds. *Pediatric Ophthalmology and Strabismus*. New York: Springer; 2003.

TABLE 35.2	Recommended Ages and Methods for Pediatric Eye Evaluation Screening	
Recommended Age	Method	Indications for Referral to an Ophthalmologist
Newborn to 3 months old	Ocular history Red reflex Inspection	Abnormal or asymmetric Structural abnormality
3-6 months old (approximately)	Ocular history Fix and follow	Failure to fix and follow in a cooperative infant
	Red reflex Inspection	Abnormal or asymmetric Structural abnormality
6-12 months old and until child is able to cooperate for verbal visual acuity	Ocular history Fix and follow with each eye	Failure to fix and follow
	Alternate occlusion	Failure to object equally to covering each eye
	Corneal light reflex Red reflex Inspection Photoscreening	Asymmetric Abnormal or asymmetric Structural abnormality Abnormal finding
3 years of age and older and every 1-2 years after 5 years of age	Ocular history Visual acuity[a] (monocular)	36-47 months of age: 20/50 or worse 48-59 months of age: 20/40 or worse >5 years of age: 20/30 or worse, or two lines of difference between the eyes 36-47 months of age: Must correctly identify the majority of the optotypes on the 20/50 line to pass 48-59 months of age: Must correctly identify the majority of the optotypes on the 20/40 line to pass
	Corneal light reflex/cover-uncover reflex	Asymmetric/ocular refixation movements
	Red reflex Inspection Photoscreening or autorefraction Attempt ophthalmoscopy	Abnormal or asymmetric Structural abnormality Abnormal findings

[a]Pictures (Lea Hyvärinen [LH/LEA] symbols or Allen cards for 2- to 4-year-olds), "tumbling E" or HOTV for ≥4-year-olds, or vision-testing machines.

Derived from American Academy of Pediatrics (AAP), American Association of Certified Orthoptists (AACO), American Association for Pediatric Ophthalmology and Strabismus (AAPOS), American Academy of Ophthalmology (AAO). Visual system assessment in infants, children and young adults by pediatricians. *2016 Pediatrics*. 2003;137(1):28–30. https://doi.org/10.1542/peds.2015-3596. Retrieved from http://pediatrics.aappublications.org/content/137/1/e20153596.

its eyes. Development of the eye as a visual organ is not complete at birth, yet newborns have the ability to fix their gaze, follow an object to midline, and react to a change in the intensity of light. Over the first 2 to 3 months of extrauterine life, the ability to focus at any range develops as the eyes become coordinated horizontally and vertically. By 3 months of age, infants can follow moving objects; and by 4 months of age, they can indicate visual recognition of familiar objects. The shape and contour of the eyeball changes, and visual acuity and binocularity gradually increase with age (Table 35.2). The volume of the orbits doubles by the time the child is 1 year of age and almost doubles again by 6 to 8 years of age. Eye growth is completed at 10 to 13 years of age. The corneal dimension, however, changes minimally from full-term newborn to adulthood.

During early childhood the visual pathways that ensure central vision are developing. The brain must receive equally clear, bilaterally focused images at the same time for this development to occur. The adult visual field is obtained by 10 years of age. The visual pathways are amenable to the greatest corrective influences (e.g., adequate treatment of amblyopia) until 7 to 8 years of age.

Anatomy and Physiology of the Eye

The eyeball consists of three layers of tissue: the fibrous tunic, the vascular tunic, and the inner tunic or retina. The fibrous tunic consists of the sclera and the cornea. The vascular tunic, the middle layer, is composed of the choroid, the ciliary body, and the iris (Fig 35.1). All the structures of the eye are dedicated to accurate and efficient functioning of the innermost layer of the eyeball, the retina. The optic disc consists only of nerve fibers (no rods or cones), so no visual images are formed here. Thus it is referred to as the *blind spot*.

The inside of the eyeball consists of the anterior and posterior cavities (see Fig 35.1). The anterior cavity is divided into anterior and posterior chambers. The anterior chamber lies between the cornea and the iris. The posterior chamber lies between the iris and the suspensory ligament. Aqueous humor circulates throughout these chambers to maintain intraocular pressure (IOP) and link the circulatory system with the avascular lens and cornea. The other cavity within the eyeball, the posterior cavity, lies between the lens and the retina. The gelatinous vitreous humor found in

this cavity contributes to the maintenance of IOP and holds the retina in place. The lens, which separates the cavities, hangs by the suspensory ligament. Six muscles guide movement of the globe. Four rectus muscles (superior, inferior, lateral, and medial) move the eyeball up, down, in, and out, respectively. Two oblique

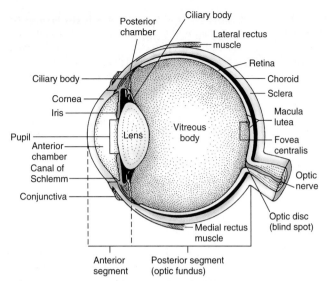

• **Fig 35.1** Anatomy of the eye. (From Ignatavicius D, Workman L. *Medical-Surgical Nursing: Patient-Centered Collaborative Care.* 8th ed. Philadelphia: Saunders/Elsevier; 2016.)

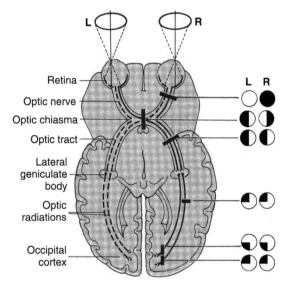

• **Fig 35.2** Visual pathway. On the right are diagrams of the visual fields with areas of blindness darkened to show the effects of injuries in various locations. (From Patton K, Thibodeau G. *Anatomy and Physiology.* 9th ed. St Louis: Mosby/Elsevier; 2016.)

muscles (superior and inferior) rotate the eyeball on its axis. Cranial nerve (CN) III (oculomotor), CN IV (trochlear), and CN VI (abducens) innervate these muscles.

The focusing of light rays involves four basic processes: (1) refraction of light rays, (2) accommodation of the lens, (3) constriction of the pupil, and (4) convergence of the eyes. *Refraction* is the bending of light rays as they pass from one transparent medium (air) to another (cornea or lens). The lens modifies the degree of refraction to create the sharpest image on the retina. *Accommodation* is the ability of the lens to focus on close objects by increasing its curvature. The normal eye refracts light rays from an object 20 feet away to focus a clear image onto the retina; hence the fraction 20/20 is used to denote the accepted standard of normal vision. The circular muscle fibers of the iris, which contract in response to light, cause constriction of the pupil. Regulating the light entering the eye can also facilitate production of a precise image. To maintain single binocular vision, close objects require the eyes to rotate medially so that the light rays from the object hit the same points on both retinas. This rotation is called *convergence*. A normal neonate demonstrates disconjugate fixation, but convergence and accommodation normally develop by 3 to 4 months of age, with parallel alignment without nystagmus or strabismus by 5 to 6 months of age. Jerky eye movements can be seen until 2 months of age, after which time smooth tracking movements are expected.

After an image is formed on the retina, light impulses are converted into nerve impulses and transmitted to the visual centers located in the occipital lobes of the cerebral cortex. Lesions in various places along the neural tracts from the eye to the cortex cause different types of loss of visual fields (Fig 35.2).

Pathophysiology of the Eyes

Potential problems with the eyes or visual system can take the form of specific disorders, infections, or injuries to the eye. The most common disorders of the eye interfering with vision are refractive errors (myopia, hyperopia, astigmatism, and anisometropia). Less common disorders include strabismus, amblyopia, ptosis, nystagmus, cataracts, glaucoma, retinopathy of prematurity (ROP), and retinoblastoma. Infections and injuries may be

relatively minor and superficial or critical, involving deep tissues of the eye. Certain systemic diseases (e.g., juvenile rheumatoid arthritis) and medications (e.g., steroids) can also affect the eyes and warrant extra assessment measures.

Assessment

Assessment of the eye, as with all body systems, requires a thoughtful history, careful physical examination, and certain specialized screening tests.

History

- General medical history including birth weight; pertinent prenatal, perinatal, and postnatal factors (e.g., prematurity, infections); past hospitalizations and surgery; general health and development
- Family medical history of ocular problems (including eye surgeries) such as glaucoma, blindness, poor vision, difficulty walking in dim light, photophobia, use of thick glasses, lazy eye, strabismus, nystagmus, leukokoria, retinoblastoma, congenital cataracts
- History of chronic systemic disease in patient or family (e.g., inflammatory bowel disease; connective tissue disorders; cardiac defects of Marfan syndrome; midfacial hypoplasia; abnormalities of teeth, umbilical cord, or urinary tract; neurologic or skin anomalies; developmental delay; mental retardation; diabetes; sickle cell hemoglobinopathies; Tay-Sachs disease; tuberculosis)
- Presence of allergies and specific allergens
- Current medications (e.g., steroids); past or present substance abuse
- Child's ocular history, including
  - Date (and results) of the last vision screening and prior eye problems or diseases, including diagnoses and treatments
  - If history of eye injury: Unilateral or bilateral injury? Associated visual changes or photophobia? What treatment was received?

- Prescription and use of eyeglasses or contact lenses: Does the child have glasses that were prescribed? Are they used? If not, why?
- Use of sunglasses with ultraviolet (UV) protection or protective eyewear for sports activities
- Symptoms or indications of eye dysfunction or disease including the following:
  - Older children may report visual loss or change in vision, such as blurring, diplopia, spots, and halos. Younger children may be observed to have problems with fixing or focusing (holding objects up close to see), or tracking, eye-hand coordination, grasp, gait, balance, behavior, or changes in the ability to maintain eye contact as well as eyelid droop, squinting, and head tilt
  - Photophobia may present as irritability, shielding, or rubbing of the eyes
  - Swollen eyelids, pruritus, excessive tearing or discharge, erythema, burning, eye fatigue, strabismus
  - Constant blinking, chronic bulbar conjunctival injection

Physical Examination

The physical examination can be challenging, depending on the child's age. The components must be done quickly to accommodate the child's short attention span and tolerance. Knowledge of visual developmental milestones is essential in assessing a child's visual capabilities (Table 35.3).

- With a penlight, gross inspection should be made of the external structures (lids, bulbar and palpebral conjunctiva, cornea, lacrimal structures, and the size, symmetry, and reactivity of the pupils), orbits, eye muscle balance, and mobility.
- The red reflex is tested at all ages. It must be assessed for color, intensity, and clarity (opacities or white spots). A rule of thumb is that if the examiner cannot see into the eye (e.g., absent red light reflex), the patient cannot see out.

TABLE 35.3	Normal Visual Developmental Milestones
Age	
Birth to 2 weeks of age	Infant sees and responds to change in illumination; refuses to reopen eyes after exposure to bright light; increasing alertness to objects; fixes on contrasts (e.g., black and white); jerky movements; pupillary reaction present.
By 2-4 weeks of age	Infant fixes and follows on an object, though sporadically.
By 3-4 months of age	Infant recognizes parent's smile; looks from near to far and focuses close again; beginning development of depth perception; follows 180-degree arc; reaches toward toy; few exodeviations; esotropia abnormal.
By 4 months of age	Color vision near that of an adult; tears are present.
By 6-10 months of age	Infant fixes on and follows toy in all directions; movements smooth.
By 12 months of age	Vision is close to fully developed.

- In children beginning at 5 years of age, funduscopic examination may allow for visualization of the retina, choroid, fovea, macula, optic disc and cup, and entry and exit of the vessels and nerves.
- Examination of the conjunctiva and sclera is sometimes facilitated by using a cotton-tipped applicator to evert the eyelid. Eyelid eversion is accomplished by having the patient look down while the examiner grasps the lashes with the thumb and index finger, places the applicator in the middle of the lid, pulls the eyelid down and out, and everts it over the applicator.
- Growth parameters (especially head growth and shape) and the head and neck or other structures should be examined if a systemic condition is suspected.

Screening Tests

Conducting Screening Tests

Fatigue, hunger, anxiety, and environmental distractions can interfere with vision testing in children and adolescents. Testing should always precede the administration of immunizations or any procedure that might cause discomfort. While testing vision, observe children for behavior indicating that they are having difficulty, such as straining, squinting, excessive blinking, head tilting or shaking, or thrusting the trunk or head forward. The tendency to peek out from behind the eye shield may or may not reflect difficulty; the child may do so out of a desire to be successful and to please the tester. The examiner should resist the tendency to correct a mistake or give the child nonverbal clues that can influence the results. Three-year-old children who have difficulty performing any of the vision tests in the PCP's office should be tested again within 6 months; those unable to perform when 4 years of age or older should be retested in 1 month. A child who is uncooperative on the second attempt should be referred for a formal visual examination (AAO, 2017a).

Red Reflex

The red reflex should be tested at every well examination, including the initial newborn examination. An adequate red reflex test (Bruckner test) allows the clinician to detect the presence of asymmetric refractive errors, strabismic deviations, and abnormalities in the ocular media (e.g., cataracts, corneal abnormalities, retinoblastoma). Disease processes involving the cornea, lens, vitreous, or retina block the light from entering or exiting the pupil and result in an abnormal red reflex. The recommended technique follows:

- Darken the examination room, as it is easier to detect more subtle asymmetries between the red reflexes. Stand an arm's length away from the infant or child with the ophthalmoscope's light set at 0 or +1 to illuminate the face. Look at both pupils simultaneously and separately. NOTE: In children with fair skin pigmentation, the red reflex is bright red-orange; in those with darker pigmentation, the red reflex is dark red-brown or pale yellow.
- The red reflexes should be symmetric; any asymmetry, dark or white spots, opacities, or leukokoria (white pupillary reflex) requires prompt referral to an ophthalmologist.

Visual Acuity Testing

Visual acuity screening for both near and distance vision should be performed on all children during routine physical examinations, when problems with visual acuity are suspected, and/or when eye trauma occurs. Children who are not reading at grade level after 5 years of age should also have formal visual acuity screening (AAPOS, 2014a). If the child or adolescent wears eyeglasses or contact lenses, visual acuity measurement must be obtained using corrective devices.

Color Vision Testing

The human retina contains 6 million red and green cones and approximately 1 million blue cones. Alterations in color vision occur when the normal photopigments in the photoreceptor cones are replaced by different ones. Color ranges are then interpreted or perceived differently.

Red-green color deficiency is an X-linked inherited disorder or may indicate optic nerve disease. Inherited (X-linked) color deficiencies are more common in males, affecting less than 5% of females. Color vision deficiency may also be acquired. A patient with acquired deficiency may have had normal color vision and then experienced color changes and losses. Diabetes, infections, optic neuritis, and toxins are systemic conditions that can lead to such losses. *Blue-yellow deficiency* is the most common type of acquired color deficiency.

A significant color vision deficiency can affect school performance, have safety implications if the child is unable able to distinguish traffic or vehicle brake lights, and affect career choices. Color vision is tested by using the Richmond pseudoisochromatic plates or Ishihara plates (AAO, 2017a). Children 3 to 4 years of age are usually able to comply with testing directions, but the test is not routinely administered. Parents may request testing when their child is young and makes errors when asked to identify colors.

Peripheral Vision Testing

Examination of peripheral visual fields provides information about retinal function, the neuronal visual pathway to the brain, and the function of CN II (the optic nerve). In an infant, assessment is limited to a rough estimate of peripheral visual fields by watching the child's response to a familiar object (e.g., bottle, toy) as it is brought into each of the four quadrants (AAO, 2017a). In children mature enough to cooperate, peripheral visual fields can be measured by confrontation or by finger counting. Peripheral visual fields should be approximately 50 degrees upward, 70 degrees downward, 60 degrees medially (toward the nose), and 90 degrees laterally.

Testing for Ocular Mobility and Alignment

The Hirschberg test (also called the *corneal light reflex*) evaluates extraocular muscle function by projecting a small light source onto the cornea of the eye with the child looking straight ahead. A normal test reveals the reflected light as a small white dot symmetrically located in the same position of each eye (often slightly nasal of center) (AAO, 2017a). The cover-uncover test and the alternating cover test should be performed with the child fixating straight ahead, first on a near-point object and then on a far-point object about 20 feet away (Fig 35.3). The process is sometimes aided by asking the child questions about the object (e.g., "How many cows do you see?" in a picture that has been placed for this purpose on the wall). During the alternating cover test, the examiner rapidly covers and uncovers the eye while shifting between the two eyes. Any orbital movement is an indication of misalignment.

Assessment of Visual Loss

If significant visual disturbance is suspected, the following functional vision assessments should be performed and the child referred immediately to an ophthalmologist:

- Shine a penlight into the eye from a lateral position and turn the light off and on several times to assess light perception. If the child can identify when the light is on or off, vision is described as "LP" (light perception).
- Move a hand back and forth with periodic cessation 12 inches from the child's face. Indication of search and recognition is documented as "H/M at 1 ft" (hand motion).
- Ask the child to count the number of fingers (C/F) seen when one, two, or three fingers are held up 12 inches from the child's face. If the child is correct, document the vision as "C/F at 1 ft."

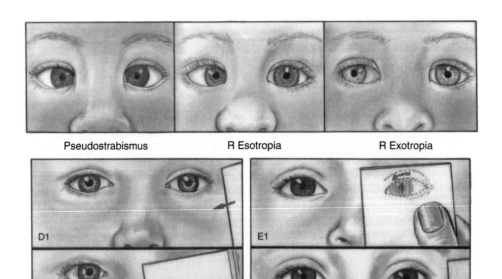

Pseudostrabismus R Esotropia R Exotropia

Right, uncovered eye is weaker   Left, covered eye is weaker

• **Fig 35.3** Extraocular muscle function testing (corneal light reflex and cover test). (From Jarvis C. *Physical Examination and Health Assessment*. 2nd ed. Philadelphia: Saunders; 1996.)

Diagnostic Studies

Photoscreening and Autorefractors

Photoscreeners and autorefractors are used to screen for optical and physical abnormalities of the eyes and at preventive visits in the pediatric office (AAP, AAPO, AAPOS, and AAO, 2016). Photoscreeners assess the red light reflex and high refractive error and screen for amblyopia and strabismus. Autorefractors may be used to determine the refractive error of each eye. Medial opacities and refractive errors can be discerned using instrument-based screening in preverbal or developmentally delayed children. Instrument-based vision screening is a valid and reliable alternative method for visual screening in children under 5 years of age or who are not able to use vision charts.

Laboratory and Imaging Studies

Cultures and Gram staining of eye discharge are done if identification of infection or particular organisms would be helpful in guiding management. Ultrasound (not to be used in cases of a suspected ruptured globe), computed tomography (CT), or magnetic resonance imaging (MRI) is sometimes useful in determining a diagnosis of orbital cellulitis, trauma, or tumor or in substantiating a concern about the central nervous system (CNS). An MRI should not be used in the case of a suspected intraocular metal foreign body.

Fluorescein Staining

Fluorescein staining may be used to determine the extent of damage to the corneal or conjunctival epithelium as a result of trauma, infection, or exposure to a foreign body. After applying fluorescein, examine the cornea with a cobalt blue filter light in a darkened room; any injury will take up the fluorescein stain and appear as a greenish area. Too much of the stain will cloud the entire cornea.

Management Strategies

Referral for Ophthalmologic and Specialty Management

Although any child with an eye pathology should be referred to an ophthalmologist, optometrists are also a valuable resource in caring for children with refractive errors or certain common eye conditions (e.g., corneal abrasions, foreign bodies). Pediatric providers should acquaint themselves with the statutory guidelines for scope of practice and prescription privileges as designated by the state board of optometry within their state to optimize referral possibilities. See Table 35.4 for guidance on when to refer for a more comprehensive examination.

Occlusion

Patching, occlusive contact lens (a last resort), optical penalization (overplussing the lens on the sound eye), or pharmacologic penalization with 0.5% or 1% atropine (not used in infants) may be used to treat strabismus and improve or prevent amblyopia by blocking vision in the sound eye.

Corrective Lenses

In children, eyeglasses or contact lenses are used to correct refractive errors. Gas-permeable or soft contact lenses can be successfully worn by children as young as 8 years of age with no higher incidence of corneal problems than noted in adults (Bullimore, 2017). Silsoft silicon polymer lenses may be used in aphakic infants and can be

TABLE 35.4	Indications for a Comprehensive Pediatric Eye Evaluation	
Indication	**Specific Examples**
Risk factors (general health problems, systemic disease, or use of medications that are known to be associated with eye disease and visual abnormalities)	Prematurity (birth weight <1500 g or gestational age 30 weeks or less) Retinopathy of prematurity Intrauterine growth retardation Perinatal complications (evaluation at birth and at 6 months of age) Neurologic disorders or neurodevelopmental delay (at diagnosis) Juvenile idiopathic arthritis (at diagnosis) Thyroid disease Cleft palate or other craniofacial abnormalities Diabetes mellitus (5 years after onset) Systemic syndromes with known ocular manifestations (at 6 months of age or at diagnosis) Chronic systemic corticosteroid therapy or other medications known to cause eye disease Suspected child abuse
A family history of conditions that cause or are associated with eye or vision problems	Retinoblastoma Childhood cataract Childhood glaucoma Retinal dystrophy/degeneration Strabismus Amblyopia Eyeglasses in early childhood Sickle cell anemia Systemic syndromes with known ocular manifestations Any history of childhood blindness not due to trauma in a parent or sibling
Signs or symptoms of eye problems by history/report	Defective ocular fixation or visual interactions Abnormal light reflex (including both the corneal light reflections and the red fundus reflection) Abnormal or irregular pupils Drooping eyelid Lumps or swelling around the eyes Ocular alignment or movement abnormality Nystagmus Persistent tearing, ocular discharge Persistent or recurrent redness Persistent light sensitivity Squinting/eye closure Persistent head tilt Learning disabilities or dyslexia

aHeadache is not included because it is rarely caused by eye problems in children. This complaint should first be evaluated by the primary care physician.

From American Academy of Pediatrics (AAP), American Association of Certified Orthoptists (AACO), American Association for Pediatric Ophthalmology and Strabismus (AAPOS), American Academy of Ophthalmology (AAO). Visual system assessment in infants, children and young adults by pediatricians. *2016 Pediatrics.* 2003;137(1):28–30. https://doi.org/10.1542/peds.2015-3596. Retrieved from http://pediatrics.aappublications.org/content/137/1/e20153596.

worn 24 hours a day for as long as a week (Stewart, 2017). Keratorefractive (laser-assisted in situ keratomileusis [LASIK]) surgery is undergoing worldwide research for its applicability in children with low to moderate myopia, severe anisometropia, bilateral high ametropia, and refractive amblyopia; however, its use remains controversial. The AAO discourages LASIK surgery in children younger than 18 years of age and provides guidelines regarding suitable candidates for the procedure (AAO, 2017b). LASIK and photorefractive keratectomy (PRK) lasers are not approved by the US Food and Drug Administration (FDA) for use in individuals under 21 years of age (AAO, 2017b). General guidelines for glasses and contact lenses can be found in Box 35.1. Glasses must be changed frequently in children because of head growth and visual acuity changes. Parents should assess the fit of the eyeglasses on a monthly basis and watch for behavior indicating discomfort in a preverbal child (e.g., constantly removing glasses, rubbing at the frames or face).

Contact lenses (includes daily wear [hard lenses] and soft, extended- and/or disposable-wear lenses), in addition to the cosmetic benefit, can provide better refractive error correction than eyeglasses, thereby enhancing visual acuity and the total corrected field of vision. Studies have also shown that their use improves how children feel about their appearance, athletic abilities, and what friends think of them (Bullimore, 2017). Daily disposable soft lenses are convenient and eliminate the need for cleaning and storage, making their use appealing for children and adolescents. Eye health can be promoted by reinforcing instructions regarding proper contact lens care and reminding the child and parent that contact lenses should not be worn when the eye is inflamed or topical ophthalmic medications are being used. The Centers for Disease Control and Prevention (CDC) has recommendations for parents considering contact lenses for their children (www.cdc.gov/contactlenses) (CDC, 2015).

Plano lenses are noncorrective contact lenses or glasses used for fashion or cosmetic purposes, sports protection, or theatre. They are available for purchase from nonvision care resources. Severe eye injuries (including blindness) result when people bypass the usual regulatory safeguards (proper fit, adequate instruction on use, and hygiene). Such cases prompted the AAO to sponsor legislation that required the FDA to regulate the lenses as medical devices. The law requires that these types of lenses be properly fitted and dispensed by prescription only from a qualified eye care professional. Another type of plano lens includes those with light-filtering tints. These block or enhance certain colors and are designed for sports use by tennis players, golfers, baseball players, spectators, trapshooters, and skiers. The AAO provides information regarding the risks posed by nonprescription contacts, including corneal abrasions and ulcers, infection, and scarring leading to blindness.

• BOX 35.1 Recommendations for Use of Corrective Lenses

Eyeglasses

Polycarbonate lenses are lightweight, strong, and shatterproof; scratch-resistant coating is recommended.

Silicone nose pads with nonskid surfaces prevent glasses from slipping.

Comfort cables secure frames by wrapping around the child's ears and are available for children 1 to 4 years of age. Straps are recommended for infants below 1 year of age, allowing them to roll and lie down.

Flexible hinges allow outward bending for easy removal by the child.

Match the frame to the child's facial shape and features to encourage compliance; if old enough, allow the child to choose the frame.

To encourage compliance with infants and children, do not fight them when they remove glasses; be persistent, replace the glasses, and provide distraction. Parents may have to set the glasses aside for a few hours before trying again. Seek counsel from the prescribing provider for further help.

Tinted lenses can be used for photosensitivity; ultraviolet (UV) light filters are helpful with aphakia (absence of lens), congenital absence of iris, and albinism.

Do not place the glasses down with lenses in contact with hard surfaces.

Clean glasses daily with liquid soap and a soft cloth. (Do not use paper products.)

Contact Lenses

Contact lenses are appropriate for children 8 years of age and older; children must be able to demonstrate ability to manage lens hygiene, including insertion and removal.

Contact lenses are helpful for an aphakic child who would otherwise need very thick glasses that distort images.

Provide protective outer eyewear for sports.

Do let the child wear contact lenses if one or both eyes are inflamed or when topical ophthalmic medications are being used. Children with recurrent conjunctival or corneal infections, inadequate tears, severe allergies, or excessive exposure to dust or smoke should not wear contact lenses.

Extended-wear contact lenses (usually worn overnight) should not be worn for 1 night a week in order to perform lens hygiene procedures.

Ophthalmic Medications

Caution and precision must be exercised when ocular medications are being administered to children because their smaller body mass and faster metabolism may potentiate the action of the drugs and result in adverse ocular and systemic side effects. Topical ophthalmic medications—such as antibiotics, mydriatics, and corticosteroids—are frequently found in ointment or solution vehicles. These topical agents are primarily used to treat disorders affecting the anterior segment of the eye. Solubility is one of several factors that influence the absorption of topical ophthalmic medications. Those that are water-soluble (e.g., anesthetics, steroids, and alkaloids) penetrate the corneal epithelium easily. Fat-soluble preparations (e.g., most antibiotics) do not penetrate the epithelium of the cornea unless it is inflamed.

Topical Antibiotics

Prescription of topical antibiotics is ideally based on empiric evidence of infection. The best choice of a topical antibiotic is one that is not often prescribed for problems in other body systems. Topical ophthalmologic preparations—such as fluoroquinolones, sulfacetamide, bacitracin, and bacitracin/polymyxin B—are effective and rarely produce a hypersensitivity reaction. Topical penicillins, on the other hand, are to be avoided. The pros and cons of these antibiotics are addressed in later sections of this chapter. Ophthalmic ointments may be preferred over solutions for use in children, especially infants, because they last longer, do not sting, do not have to be given as often, and are less likely to be absorbed into the lacrimal passage.

Ophthalmic Corticosteroids

Although ophthalmic corticosteroids are effective in the treatment of ocular inflammation and traumatic iritis (excluding ocular allergy), a patient with a condition severe enough to warrant consideration of corticosteroid use should be referred to an ophthalmologist. Steroids are associated with numerous complications, such as an increased incidence of herpes simplex keratitis and corneal ulcers, fungal keratitis, corneal perforation and intraocular sepsis, glaucoma, slowed healing of corneal abrasions and wounds, increased IOP, cataract formation, and permanent loss of sight. A child receiving long-term ophthalmologic steroids should be assessed frequently for signs of adrenal suppression or other side effects. Encourage parents to keep scheduled ocular tonometry appointments at 2- to 3-month intervals to assess intraocular pressures.

Other Topical Preparations

Topical decongestants or antihistamines or a combination of the two, mast cell stabilizers, and nonsteroidal antiinflammatory drugs (NSAIDs) are used in treating various ophthalmologic conditions. Over-the-counter vasoconstrictors or vasoconstrictor-antihistamine preparations can be tried first for mild allergic conjunctivitis. Cycloplegic agents are used for iritis.

Systemic Medications

In ocular infections involving the posterior segment and the orbit, systemic antibiotic preparations are necessary. A combination of topical and systemic antibiotics can also be used. These conditions warrant referral to an ophthalmologist. Systemic drugs may also cause damage to the eyes (Table 35.5).

Prevention of Eye Injury

Ocular trauma accounts for one-third of all cases of acquired blindness in children. The male-to-female ratio of trauma incidence is 4:1, with males 11 to 15 years of age outnumbering all other age groups. Many of these injuries could be prevented by using protective eyewear, as half are the result of sports-related accidents. Other causes include battered child syndrome (40% have ocular findings), birth trauma, fingers/fists/other body parts in the eye, fireworks (firecrackers, sparklers, rockets), and auto airbags. Eye injuries often occur in the home. The areas most affected by superficial trauma include the cornea, conjunctiva, and sclera; the most serious eye injuries involve the cornea, iris, lens, and optic nerve and may result from anterior chamber hyphema, vitreous hemorrhage, or retinal tear or detachment.

Prevent Blindness (2018) recommends parental supervision and child education regarding the prevention of eye injury as essential to minimize eye injuries. Prevention includes fundamental concepts such as understanding the dangers to sight, finding and removing hazards, and watching children closely. Specific prevention steps include the following:

- Using safety gates and cushions/pads at sharp corners, storing sharp utensils/tools out of reach of children, and storing chemicals securely
- Restraining children properly in the car, not allowing children under 12 years of age to sit in the front seat
- Limiting/supervising the use of laser pointers, BB guns, air rifles, paintball devices, darts, and fireworks

Sunglasses

Ultraviolet A (UVA) and B (UVB) radiation from the sun can damage the lens and retina of the eye, causing cataracts and other conditions harmful to vision later in life (e.g., macular degeneration). Sunlight has more UVA than UVB, but UVB is more damaging. Sunglasses should be used to minimize such damage by absorbing these light wavelengths, even if UV-treated contact lenses are being worn. It is never too early to start wearing sunglasses. Wearing a hat with a wide (3-inch) brim with sunglasses reduces the UV rays that reach the eyes by half (Prevent Blindness, 2018b).

Sunglasses should fit well and have large-framed wraparound lenses with side shields to provide the best protection. They should provide 99% to 100% protection from UVA and UVB short waves (Prevent Blindness, 2018b). The lens and frame should be made of nonbreakable plastic or polycarbonate. The protection comes from the chemical coating on or incorporated in the lenses. Gray, brown, and green colors are sufficient for general purposes and lead to minimal color distortion. Darker colors or polarized lenses alone do not offer the protection that is needed unless they specifically state otherwise. Sunglasses that are for fashion purposes or that do not list the UV protective wave spectrum should be avoided, including inexpensive novelty store glasses. Lenses should be purchased only if they carry the American National Standards Institute (ANSI) label or American Optometric Association (AOA) notation. ANSI communicates their standards by labeling their lenses Z80.3 and "general purpose," "special purpose" (for snow and water sports), and "cosmetic use" (lowest protection) (Kelechava, 2016). In addition to the requisite UVA and UVB protection, the AOA recommends purchasing only lenses that state that they screen out 75% to 90% of visible light, are gray (for best color perception), and cause no distortion in vision (AOA, 2018a).

Sports Protection

Protective glasses or goggles are mandatory for all functionally one-eyed individuals or for any athlete who has had eye surgery or trauma or whose ophthalmologist recommends eye protection (Prevent Blindness, 2018b). Additionally, these children or adolescents should not participate in boxing or full-contact martial arts. Caution is also recommended for these individuals if they choose to wrestle, even though there is a low rate of reported injury.

Eye protection is recommended for any child or adolescent participating in sports that have a high eye injury rate, specifically hockey, fencing, boxing, full-contact martial arts, racquetball, lacrosse, squash, basketball, baseball, tennis, badminton, soccer, volleyball, water polo, fishing, golf, field hockey, paintball games, pool activities, and football. Specific protective eyewear is available; however, there are no standards for eyewear in these sports.

Protective eyewear should be properly fitted and selected specifically for the sport. A complete list of recommended eyewear for each sport is available online from the AAO website (www.aao.org). The list serves as a useful handout for parents. A headband or wraparound earpieces should be used to secure the glasses (AAO, 2013b). Sports eye guards should have protective lenses designed to stay in place or pop outward in case of a blow to the eye (Prevent Blindness, 2018b). Athletes who need prescription eyewear can either choose polycarbonate lenses in a sports frame that is rated for the specific sport, wear polycarbonate contact lenses plus the appropriate protective eyewear, or wear an attached over-the-glasses eye guard that also meets sport specifications. Younger children who do not fit into manufactured protective eyewear may be fitted with 3-mm polycarbonate lenses, although adequate protection cannot be guaranteed and perhaps another choice of sport should be discussed.

Laser Pointers

Lasers are rated on a scale of I to IV, with class I lasers used in laser printers and class IV used in research lasers. The FDA strengthened its message to manufacturers regarding the labeling and safety of laser pointers, stating that class IIIa lasers may be used as pointers but class IIIb (laser light shows, industrial lasers) and class

TABLE 35.5 **Systemic Drugs, Herbs, and Nutritional Supplements That Can Cause Ocular Side Effects**

Drug	Ocular Side Effects	Intervention
Corticosteroids (prednisone at dosage of 15 mg/day for ≥1 year, inhaled corticosteroids)	Cataracts, increased IOP	Monitor with ophthalmologic examinations.
Chemotherapy drugs 5-fluorouracil (5-FU)	Visual changes, lacrimation, photophobia	No long-term damage.
Digoxin at moderately toxic ranges	Snowy, flickering, yellow vision	Resolves when drug is administered in correct range.
Hydroxychloroquine	Potential retinal toxicity	
Isoniazid in greater than recommended dosages	Loss in color vision, decreased visual acuity, and visual field changes	Effects are reversible only if discovered early. Ophthalmologic examination is indicated before treatment and every 6 months; any changes warrant stopping isoniazid and referring to an ophthalmologist.
Isotretinoin	Pseudotumor cerebri (after initiating treatment) with resultant blurred vision, visual field loss, and varying visual acuity changes, including optic neuritis, dry eye, decreased night vision, and transitory myopia	Monitor for symptoms. Annual eye examination recommended while on isotretinoin.
Minocycline hydrochloride	Pseudotumor cerebri and orthostatic blackouts, evidenced by blurred vision, visual field loss, varying visual acuity changes, diplopia; scleral pigmentation	Monitor for symptoms; scleral pigmentation may not resolve.
Phenytoin and carbamazepine	Blood levels in moderately toxic ranges can produce diplopia, blurred vision, nystagmus; sensitivity to glare	Resolve when therapeutic doses are within normal ranges.
Sildenafil	Nonarteritic anterior ischemic optic neuropathy (NAION) reported in adults	
Topiramate	Acute angle closure glaucoma; mydriasis; ocular pain; decreased visual acuity (myopia)	Onset of symptoms within 3-14 days after medication started. Stop medication. Treatment may include cycloplegics, hyperosmotic therapy, and topical antiglaucoma medications.
Quetiapine	Cataracts	Monitor with ophthalmologic examinations.
Oral contraceptives (estrogen and/or progesterone)	Optic neuritis, pseudotumor cerebri, dry eyes	Monitor.
Fluoxetine/SSRIs	Dry eye, blurred vision, mydriasis, photophobia, diplopia, conjunctivitis, and ptosis	Monitor.
Herbs		
Canthaxanthin (taken to produce artificial suntan; food coloring)	Decreased visual acuity; retinopathy	
Cassava (with prolonged usage)	Decreased visual acuity; retinopathy	Contains natural cyanide, so it is important that this plant has been processed correctly.
Datura (may be used by those with asthma, influenza, coughs)	Mydriasis	
Ginkgo biloba	Retrobulbar and retinal hemorrhage; hyphema	
Licorice	Decreased visual acuity	
Vitamin A	Intracranial hypertension	

IOP, Intraocular pressure; *SSRI,* selective serotonin reuptake inhibitor.

Dellabella A, Andres J. Ophthalmic toxicities of systemic drug therapy. *U.S. Pharmacist.* 2015;40(6):HS19–HS24. Retrieved from https://www.uspharmacist.com/article/ophthalmic-toxicities-of-systemic-drug-therapy. Accessed March 9, 2018; and Wellik S. Ocular toxicity associated with systemic drug therapy. 2017. American Academy of Ophthalmology. Retrieved from https://www.aao.org/annual-meeting-video/ocular-toxicity-associated-with-systemic-drug-ther. Accessed March 9, 2018.

IV lasers should not be used (FDA, 2017). Lasers traditionally available to the public currently have a maximum output of from 1 to 5 mW. Although harmless when used as intended by lecturers, potential injury from direct, intentional, prolonged exposure to the retina is of concern if the pointers are used as toys.

Computer Use

The aging eye can develop "computer vision syndrome," leading to eyestrain, headaches, blurred vision, dry eyes, and neck and shoulder pain (AOA, 2018b). Children's eyes have more flexibility of the lens, allowing them to adapt to different visual environments without eyestrain (AAPOS, 2017). A policy statement from the AAPOS states that there is no evidence that the use of computer, phone, or video screens increases the incidence of visual problems (AAPOS, 2017a). However, the AOA still recommends following the 20-20-20 rule as a guideline to ensure regular screen breaks and avoid eye fatigue, meaning after every 20 minutes of screen time, individuals should look away from the screen, focusing on something at least 20 feet away for at least 20 seconds.

Vision Therapy, Lenses, and Prisms

Vision therapy, lenses, and prisms are controversial methods of treatment claimed by some to be effective therapy for those with learning disabilities and dyslexia. These interventions consist of (1) visual training, including muscle exercises, ocular pursuit, tracking exercises, or "training" glasses (with or without bifocals or prisms); (2) neurologic organizational training (laterality training, crawling, balance board, perceptual training); and (3) the wearing of colored lenses.

In a joint statement, the AAP and other organizations indicate that there is insufficient evidence to support the contention that vision abnormalities cause disabilities, including dyslexia (AAP et al., 2016). The joint statement further notes that the literature supporting vision therapy is "poorly validated," anecdotal, and consists of poorly controlled studies. Recommendations regarding vision care for children with learning disabilities include (AAP et al., 2014) the following:

- PCPs should perform periodic eye and vision screening for all children according to national standards and refer those who do not pass screening to ophthalmologists.
- Children with a suspected or diagnosed learning disability in which vision may play a role should be referred to an ophthalmologist.
- Ophthalmologists should identify and treat any significant ocular or visual disorder present.
- PCPs should recommend only evidence-based treatments and educational accommodations to school district staff.
- Diagnostic and treatment approaches for dyslexia that lack scientific evidence of efficacy (such as behavioral vision therapy, eye muscle exercises, or colored filters and lenses) are not endorsed or recommended.

When parents who inquire about vision therapy are being counseled, the clinician should be aware of the pressure parents may be under from optometrists who may be advocating vision therapy for learning disabilities and the divergent opinions held by educators and the ophthalmologic community about this modality of treatment. Managing a child with academic difficulties requires a multidisciplinary approach involving education and psychologic and other medical specialists.

Visual Disorders

Refractive Errors and Amblyopia

Alterations in the refractive power of the eye include myopia, hyperopia, astigmatism, accommodation, and anisometropia. In a normal eye, light from a distant object focuses directly on the retina. When there are variations in axial length of the eyeball or curvature of the cornea or lens exists, light focuses in front of or behind the retina. This abnormal focusing produces an alteration in the refractive power of the eye that results in a visual acuity deficit. Box 35.2 provides more complete definitions.

Refractive errors are the most common visual disorders seen in children. Approximately 9% of children between the ages of 5 to 17 years have significant refractive errors (0.75 diopters or more) (AAO, 2017b). Myopia may be present at birth; however, it is more likely to develop between 6 and 9 years of age, with increased prevalence after the adolescent growth spurt (AAO, 2017b). Mild hyperopia is normal in a young child and should decrease rapidly between 7 and 14 years of age. Genetic and environmental factors appear to be associated with the development of myopia, with the prevalence of myopia up to 80% in East Asian countries (AAO, 2017). Based on studies indicating increased myopia with more time spent indoors, the AAO practice guidelines recommend that children spend increased time outdoors to protect against myopia.

Amblyopia affects approximately 1% to 5.5% of children in the general population (AAO, 2017c). It is usually a unilateral deficit in which there is defective development of the visual pathways needed to attain central vision. Clear focused images fail to reach the brain, resulting in reduced or permanent loss of vision. The condition is labeled (or typed) according to the structural or refractive problem that is causing the poor visual image to reach the brain: *deprivational*, or obstruction of vision (e.g., caused by ptosis, cataract, nystagmus), *strabismic* (caused by strabismus or lazy eye), or *refractive* (myopia, hyperopia, astigmatism, anisometropia). Diagnosis of amblyopia prevents permanent loss of vision in the affected eye.

Clinical Findings

- Squinting, tendency to cover or close one eye when concentrating
- Abnormal vision, cover/uncover, and/or fundoscopic exam
- Pain in or around eyes and/or headaches (rare)
- Fatigue, dizziness
- Developmental delay
- Family history of refractive errors, strabismus, or amblyopia

---

• BOX 35.2   Descriptive Terms for Refractive Errors

Myopia, or nearsightedness, exists when the axial length of the eye is increased in relation to the eye's optical power. As a result, light from a distant object is focused in front of the retina rather than directly on it. A myopic child sees close objects clearly but distant objects are blurry.

Hyperopia, or farsightedness, exists when the visual image is focused behind the retina. As a result, distant objects are seen clearly but close objects are blurry.

Astigmatism exists when the curvature of the cornea or the lens is uneven; thus the retina cannot appropriately focus light from an object regardless of the distance, which makes vision blurry close up and far away. Rarely, astigmatism can be caused by an alteration in the corneal sphere caused by a soft tissue mass on the inner aspect of the eyelid, such as a chalazion or hemangioma.

Anisometropia is a different refractive error in each eye. It may consist of any combination of refractive errors discussed earlier, or it may occur with aphakia.

Management

- Refer to an ophthalmologist or optometrist for prescription corrective lenses. School-age children and teenagers should participate in the selection of frames; contact lenses may be considered.
- Once a refractive error has been determined or if a child is wearing glasses, annual evaluations are recommended.
- Moderate amblyopia usually responds to 2 hours of daily patching or weekend atropine (produces cycloplegia of non-amblyopic eye).
- Support and reassurance according to the child's developmental level are needed during the period of adjustment to contact lenses or eyeglasses. Infants and toddlers need distraction with consistent replacement of glasses once removed. Verbal children may be aided by the use of positive reinforcement, such as sticker charts.
- Untreated or inadequately treated amblyopia in young childhood results in irreversible and lifelong visual loss (AAO, 2017).

Strabismus

Strabismus is a defect in ocular alignment, or the position of the eyes in relation to each other; it is commonly called *lazy eye*. In strabismus, the visual axes are not parallel because the muscles of the eyes are not coordinated; when one eye is directed straight ahead, the other deviates. As a result, one or both eyes appear crossed. In children, strabismus may appear as a phoria or tropia (Box 35.3). Pseudostrabismus is present when the sclera between the cornea and the inner canthus is obscured by closely placed eyes, a flat nasal bridge, or prominent epicanthal folds (see Fig 35.3). In children older than 7 to 9 years of age who have acquired tropia, double vision occurs. In those younger than 6 to 7 years of age, cortical suppression of vision in the deviated eye results, which stops the diplopia but leads to amblyopia. Exo-deviations may be constant or intermittent—the intermittent type occurs more often. Both types of strabismus may be hereditary or the result of various eye diseases (e.g., neuroblastoma), trauma, systemic or neurologic dysfunction that paralyzes the extraocular muscles, uncorrected hyperopia, craniofacial abnormalities, accommodation, and accommodative convergence (Coats and Paysse, 2018). Esotropia can also be seen in those with a history of prematurity, low birth weight, cerebral palsy, hydrocephalus, and maternal substance or tobacco use (Schliesser, Sprunger, and Helveston, 2016).

• BOX 35.3 **Descriptive Terms for Strabismus**

A **phoria** is an intermittent deviation in ocular alignment that is held latent by sensory fusion. The child can maintain alignment on an object. Deviation occurs when binocular fusion is disrupted, most often during the cover/uncover test.

A **tropia** is a consistent or intermittent deviation in ocular alignment. A child with a tropia is unable to maintain alignment on an object of fixation. Intermittent tropia may occur when a child is tired.

Phorias and tropias are classified according to the pattern of deviation seen, as follows:

- *Hyper-* (up) and *hypo-* (down) are used to classify vertical strabismus.
- *Exo-* (away from the nose) and *eso-* (toward the nose) describe horizontal deviations.
- *Cyclo-* describes a rotational or torsional deviation.

The incidence of ocular misalignments is approximately 1% to 6%, and each type varies by population (e.g., there are more exo-deviations in Japan and more eso-deviations in Ireland). Accommodative esotropia is most visible when the child is looking at a near object, occurs between 1 and 8 years of age (average between 2 and 3 years of age), may occur intermittently, and children generally have hyperopia.

Variable alignment is common in the newborn, and up to 70% can exhibit transient exotropia, which should resolve by 6 months of age, with 0.5% to 2% having esotropia. Up to 25% of esotropia occurring between 3 and 6 months of age resolves over time (AAO, 2012). Congenital esotropia is ascribed to an infant with an onset before 6 months of age who did not have a deviation as a newborn. Accommodative esotropia is an inward deviation caused by hyperopia (Schliesser et al., 2016).

Clinical Findings

- Intermittent exotropia in children (6 months to 4 years of age) who are ill, tired, exposed to bright light, or with sudden changes from close to distant vision. It is more often seen when the child is looking with distant fixation.
- When only one eye is affected (i.e., child always fixates with the unaffected eye).
- When both eyes are affected, the eye that looks straight at any given time is the fixating eye.
- The angle of deviation may be inconsistent in all fields of gaze.
- Persistent squinting, head tilting, face turning, overpointing, awkwardness, marked decreased visual acuity in one eye, or nystagmus may be seen.
- Cataracts, retinoblastoma, anisometropia, and severe refractive errors are rare.

Diagnostic Techniques. The corneal light reflection technique and the cover-uncover and alternating cover tests are used to screen for strabismus. Asymmetry of light reflection on the cornea is indicative of a deviation in ocular alignment. The cover-uncover test is used to detect tropias, whereas the alternating cover test detects phorias (see Fig 35.3). The photoscreener can also be used to detect strabismus.

Management

- Any ocular misalignment seen after the age of 4 months is considered suspicious, and the child should be referred. Hyper-, hypo-, and exotropia, acquired esotropia or exotropia, cyclo-vertical deviation, or any fixed deviations is an indication for referral as soon as first observed.
- The unaffected ("good") eye is occluded (using an adhesive bandage eyepatch, an occlusive contact lens, or an overplussed lens), which forces the child to use the deviating eye. Patching for 2 hours a day is as successful as patching for 6 hours a day (DeSantis, 2014). Surgical alignment of the eyes may be necessary, but this does not preclude additional amblyopia therapy.
- Corrective lenses alone improve amblyopia in 27% of patients (DeSantis, 2014). Assessment for amblyopia should be done at every visit, even after straightening the eyes, because changes in alignment can occur through the fifth year.
- The ocular status of an affected child's siblings is monitored.

Botulinum toxin (Botox) may be used as an alternative to surgery in patients with mild esotropia (Schliesser et al., 2016). Although response to treatment is more rapid in younger children, age should not be used as the deciding factor for referring a child with amblyopia.

Complications

Amblyopia occurs in 30% to 50% of children with strabismus (Coats and Paysse, 2018).

Blepharoptosis

Blepharoptosis or ptosis is drooping of the upper eyelids affecting one or both eyes. It can be congenital or acquired, secondary to trauma or inflammation. Congenital ptosis is caused by striated muscle fibers of the levator muscle being replaced by fibrous tissue. It can be transmitted as an autosomal dominant trait. Other possible etiologies include trauma to CN III during the birthing process, trauma to the eyelid or neck, chronic inflammation (particularly of the anterior segment of the eye), or a neurologic disorder (myasthenia gravis, botulism, muscular dystrophy) (Alsuhaibani, Burkat, Stelzner, and Marcet, 2018). Parents may remark that one eye appears smaller. In severe cases, children may have a chin-up head position or adapt by raising their brow.

Management

- Correct any underlying systemic disease.
- Evaluate for anisometropia (unequal refractive errors in each eye), anisocoria, and decrease in pupillary light reflex.
- If vision is compromised, surgery is performed. Surgical correction depends on the degree of levator muscle compromise (Alsuhaibani, Burkat, Stelzner, and Marcet, 2018).

Nystagmus

Nystagmus is the presence of involuntary, rhythmic movements that may be pendular oscillations or jerky drifts of one or both eyes. Movement is horizontal, vertical, rotary, or mixed, and is classified as congenital or acquired. Congenital nystagmus is present between 6 weeks and 3 months of age; acquired nystagmus occurs at a later age (AAPOS, 2016). Nystagmus can occur in association with albinism, high refractive errors, CNS abnormalities, vitamin B_{12} deficiency, tumors, after infection (e.g., coxsackievirus B, cytomegalovirus [CMV], *Haemophilus influenzae* meningitis), various diseases of the inner ear and retina, middle ear trauma, visual loss before 2 years of age, and pharmacologic toxicity. The child may have a birth history of prematurity, intraventricular hemorrhage, intrauterine psychogenic drug exposure, developmental delays, hydrocephaly, or the mother may have had gestational diabetes. Nystagmus can be inherited, sometimes with a strong family history.

Clinical Findings

The clinician should observe the nystagmus closely and note the type of movement (up, down, sideways), frequency (number of oscillations per a time unit), distance of movement, fields of gaze within which the nystagmus is evident (e.g., field of gaze straight ahead, left, or up), and any compensatory head or neck postures of the child. The movements may be constant or varied, depending on the direction of gaze and head position. Latent nystagmus manifests only when one eye is covered (Kim and Koda, 2018). Oscillation of the newborn's eyes (infantile idiopathic nystagmus) is common and exists for a short time during the neonatal period. Involuntary oscillation (opsoclonus) that persists or occurs beyond the initial weeks of life indicates a pathologic condition.

Management and Prognosis

Management consists of treating any underlying systemic disorder and referring the patient to an ophthalmologist. An acquired nystagmus is most worrisome and requires prompt evaluation. Prognosis is varied, with sometimes only a slightly decreased acuity (20/50 or better) and at other times severe disability (20/200) (AAPOS, 2016).

Cataracts

Cataract, a partial or complete opacity of the lens affecting one or both eyes, is the most common cause of an abnormal pupillary reflex. Some cataracts are considered clinically significant, others insignificant. They are categorized as congenital or acquired and are most commonly isolated findings not associated with other abnormalities (AAPOS, 2017b).

Cataracts may occur spontaneously or be genetic (e.g., Down syndrome, albinism). If there is a family history of cataracts, present in multiple family members, referral to a geneticist is indicated. Cataracts can be the result of infection (e.g., congenital rubella, CMV, toxoplasmosis), trauma to the eye (including physical abuse, airbag deployment), metabolic disease (e.g., galactosemia, hypocalcemia), long-term use of systemic corticosteroids or ocular corticosteroid drops, prematurity, CNS anomalies (e.g., craniosynostosis, cranial defects), and demyelinating sclerosis and ataxia-telangiectasia (Heidar, 2017). They may also be seen in children who have other ocular abnormalities, such as strabismus or pendular nystagmus, and in those with diabetes mellitus, atopic dermatitis, or Marfan syndrome.

The incidence of cataracts is approximately 3 to 4 out of 10,000 children, with a variable incidence worldwide (AAPOS, 2017; Heidar, 2017). Incidence rates vary between industrialized nations (lower) and undeveloped countries (believed to be higher) (Bashour et al., 2014).

Clinical Findings

- Positive history of prenatal maternal infection, drug exposure, or hypocalcemia.
- Cataract appears as an opacity on the lens—unilateral or bilateral. A pale red reflex in people of color should not be confused with a cataract.
- Visual acuity deficits vary.

Management

Management depends on the size, density, and location of the cataract. The recommended lab workup of a child with bilateral congenital cataracts includes titers for TORCH (toxoplasmosis, other, rubella, cytomegalovirus, herpes), syphilis (the Venereal Disease Research Laboratory [VDRL] test), serum calcium and phosphorus levels, and urine testing for reducing substances (Heidar, 2017). Genetic testing is recommended if there are dysmorphic features. A small or partial congenital or infantile cataract can be monitored over several years for a progression that could produce amblyopia; some types of cataracts do not progress. Patients should be monitored by an ophthalmologist as amblyopia may develop. Surgical removal of the lens optically clears the visual axis. The resultant aphakic refractive error can be corrected with a permanent intraocular implant, the use of a contact lens, or glasses, although the lenses are often very thick, causing magnification and limitation of the visual fields. Ophthalmic surgeons may insert an intraocular lens into the posterior chamber to partially correct aphakia, with residual refractive error corrected with spectacles.

Complications

Complications include amblyopia, residual anisometropia, and aniseikonia (unequal ocular image between eyes). Complications of surgery include infection, retinal detachment, glaucoma, displacement of the intraocular lens, or the development of vitreous cloudiness (AAPOS, 2017).

Prognosis and Prevention

The ultimate degree of visual function depends on the cataract type, age at time of surgery, underlying diseases, age of onset and duration, and presence of amblyopia or other ocular abnormalities. If the cataract is dense and present at birth, outcomes are better if it is removed within the first few weeks of life or before 2 months of age because amblyopia may occur due to visual deprivation (Heidar, 2017). Visual outcomes are variable, with poorer results seen with congenital unilateral cataracts than with congenital incomplete bilateral cataracts. Children with histories of cataract surgery may exhibit later inflammatory sequelae, glaucoma, retinal detachment, secondary membranes, and orbital architectural distortions. The use of UV protectant sunglasses is essential in the prevention of cataract formation.

Glaucoma

Glaucoma is a disturbance in the circulation of aqueous fluid that results in an increase in IOP and subsequent damage to the optic nerve. It can be classified according to age at the time of its appearance and type of structural abnormality or other associated conditions. Primary congenital glaucoma is present at birth; infantile glaucoma develops in the first 1 to 2 years of life; juvenile glaucoma occurs after age 3. Most glaucoma has no identifiable cause and is considered primary. Primary glaucoma occurs because of a congenital abnormality of the structures that drain the aqueous humor. Fortunately it is rare and generally caught early. The incidence is approximately 1 in 10,000 live births in the United States, and it is more common in males (Clark, 2017).

Ten percent of cases are present at birth, with 80% diagnosed by 1 year of age. About 10% of primary cases are hereditary, and a high carrier rate of the CYP1B1 gene (2p21) is associated with a higher prevalence of glaucoma (AAPOS, 2014; Clark, 2017). Glaucoma is also seen in association with dominantly inherited conditions, such as neurofibromatosis or aniridia; diffuse facial nevus flammeus (port wine stain); Sturge-Weber, Marfan, Hurler, or Pierre Robin syndromes; intraocular hemorrhage; or intraocular tumor. There is a higher incidence in children with a history of cataract removal (AAPOS, 2014).

Secondary or juvenile glaucoma occurs when the drainage network for aqueous humor becomes obstructed after ocular infection, trauma, systemic disease, or long-term corticosteroid use.

Clinical Findings

Parents may report that something is unusual about their child's eyes, especially with unilateral glaucoma, as the orbital size discrepancy is more noticeable. Clinicians should look for
- The classic triad—tearing, photophobia, and excessive blinking/blepharospasm
- Whether their infant tends to turn away from light
- Hazy corneas, corneal edema

Corneal and ocular enlargements are common in infants and young children. Bulbar conjunctival erythema and visual impairment may occur. If the condition is bilateral, parents may not notice any difference in the size of the corneas.

Symptoms of secondary glaucoma include the following:
- Extreme pain, vomiting
- Blurred, lost, or tunnel vision

- Pupillary dilation and/or erythema (often in only one eye)
- Change in configuration of optic nerve cupping with asymmetry between the eyes and loss of vision over time

Management

Early diagnosis is important. The goal is the normalization of IOP and prevention of optic nerve damage along with correction of associated refractive errors and prevention of amblyopia. The following are recommended:
- Prompt recognition and referral to an ophthalmologist. Examination under anesthesia may be required to obtain an accurate IOP reading. Primary treatment is surgery as early as possible (often multiple surgeries are required). Medications may be used as part of the medical management. Systemic (azetazolamide or methazolamide) or topical (dorzolamide or brinzolamide drops) carbonic anhydrase inhibitors will reduce IOP. Beta blocker (timolol) or combined beta blocker/carbonic anhydrase inhibitor drops may be used (Clark, 2017). Drug therapy may be difficult owing to its prolonged nature, side effects, and adverse systemic effects.
- Parent and patient education must emphasize the importance of medication compliance and discourage excessive physical or emotional stress as well as straining during defecation.
- A medical identification tag worn at all times.
- Follow-up is for life, often every 3 to 6 months.
- Ophthalmoscopic examination (including ocular tonometry) for every member of the family.

Complications and Prognosis

Myopia, amblyopia, and strabismus are common in children with glaucoma. Additionally, permanent vision loss secondary to stretching of the cornea and sclera—with resultant scarring and glaucomatous optic nerve damage—can also occur. Some 80% to 90% of infants who receive prompt surgery and long-term monitoring will do well, but blindness occurs in 2% to 15% of childhood patients (Clark, 2017).

Retinopathy of Prematurity

ROP is a multifactorial retinal vascular pathologic disease primarily caused by early gestational age with low birth weight. It involves abnormal growth of the retinal vessels in incompletely vascularized retinas of premature infants. An international classification system provides guidance for understanding this disease and predicting outcome. ROP is classified according to the distance to which the vascularization has progressed away from the optic nerve (zone I, II, or III), severity of inflammatory changes (stages 1 through 5), duration (clock hours), presence of Plus disease (marked vascular dilation and tortuosity), scarring patterns, prethreshold and threshold ROP (clinical subclassification), and the presence of Rush disease (aggressive posterior ROP, or AP-ROP) (Heidar et al., 2018).

Developing retinal vessels grow outward from the optic nerve. The immature and incompletely vascularized retina is in a state of hypoxia, which stimulates the production of vascular endothelial growth factor (VEGF). Requisite levels of VEGF are needed to maintain the integrity of retinal vessels and stimulate their growth. Exposure to supplemental oxygen presents an additional risk factor. Higher oxygen concentrations produce lower VEGF levels, which slow vessel growth. Over several weeks, an avascular retina becomes ischemic and, in turn, stimulates renewed VEGF production. The increase in VEGF stimulates vessel growth but not necessarily in an ordered manner. Multiple studies have established a target oxygen saturation of 90% to 95% to lower the risk of ROP they are associated with the lowest patient morbidity and mortality (Jordan, 2014). ROP occurs primarily in premature infants born at or less than 28 weeks of gestation or weighing less than 1500 g. The overall incidence of ROP in all newborns is 0.14% (Jordan, 2014), with incidence inversely proportional to weight. The risk in infants under 1250 g is approximately 50% (Heidar et al., 2018). Other risk factors for ROP in premature infants include poor weight gain, dopamine-resistant hypotension, white race, hyperglycemia, insulin treatment, corticosteroid treatment, and insufficient intake of docosahexaenoic acid (Jordan, 2014). Hypoxia, hemolytic disease, necrotizing enterocolitis, maternal preeclampsia, breast milk, and adequate intake of lipids and calories may protect against developing ROP (Jordan, 2014).

Clinical Findings
ROP is initially diagnosed by a pediatric ophthalmologist while the infant is in the neonatal intensive care unit (NICU) or nursery, with the first exam based on gestation at birth (at 31 to 36 weeks postconception) and chronologic age (Heidar et al., 2018). All infants born at gestational age 32 weeks or earlier require an ophthalmologic examination.

An infant (especially if born at full or near term) not previously diagnosed with ROP with detached retinas or leukocoria needs an ophthalmologic evaluation to rule out genetic disorders (e.g., Norrie syndrome, familial exudative vitreoretinopathy).

Management
ROP progresses at variable rates. Initial ophthalmologic examinations should be done on all infants born at less than 32 weeks' gestation or weighing 1500 g or less or those born at more than 1500 g or at 29 to 34 weeks with an unstable course during hospitalization (Heidar et al., 2018). The PCP's role in managing ROP is to ensure that all infants fitting these criteria (even those whose ROP resolved or who did not have ROP) receive the initial and follow-up ophthalmologic examinations (within 2 weeks after discharge) by a specialist experienced in examining preterm infants. The PCP must further do the following:
- Discuss with parents the implications of their child's disease.
- Monitor for late sequelae or ROP progression (e.g., strabismus, pseudostrabismus, amblyopia, myopia, anisometropia, leukokoria, and cataracts).
- Assist children who have sequelae so as to maximize their potential by referring to early intervention services for low-vision children, to low-vision community support services, and to family support groups.
- Refer all children for yearly ophthalmologic follow-up if ROP required any treatment (even if ROP has resolved); less frequent follow-up is needed if no treatment was required.

Cryosurgery or laser photocoagulation is used to arrest the progression of abnormally growing blood vessels; argon and diode laser is the treatment of choice (Heidar et al., 2018). Intravitreal anti-VEGF monoclonal antibodies including bevacizumab (Avastin), ranibizumab (Lucentis), and aflibercept (Eylea) have been used successfully off label in the treatment of ROP and may be used in conjunction with laser treatment (Coats, 2018).

Complications
Complications can arise secondary to ROP or the treatment. Retinal detachment, strabismus, amblyopia, cataracts, serious myopia, nystagmus, astigmatism, anisometropia, uveitis, hyphema, macular burns, occlusion of the central retinal artery, glaucoma, and cicatrix (residual retinal scars) leading to later vision loss are possible (Heidal et al., 2018).

Prevention
Minimizing or preventing ROP can be accomplished by decreasing the occurrence of premature births and closely monitoring oxygen needed to keep oxygen saturation at 90% to 95%.

Retinoblastoma
Retinoblastoma is an intraocular tumor that develops in the retina. Although it is rare, this malignant retinal tumor is the most common tumor in childhood (some 4% of cancers in children younger than 15 years of age) (US National Library of Medicine [NLM], 2018). Approximately 300 children per year are diagnosed in the United States and Canada and 6000 children worldwide (AAPOS, 2016). Age-adjusted incidence is 1 in 15,000 to 18,000 live births with two-thirds diagnosed before 2 years of age and 95% diagnosed before 5 years of age (Skalet et al., 2018). Single or multiple tumors may be found in one or both eyes. Most children have unilateral tumors (60%), but 40% have bilateral tumors (Choe et al., 2017).

Hereditary and nonhereditary forms occur, and carrier and prenatal diagnosis is possible. Mutation of the retinoblastoma susceptibility gene *RB1* occurs in hereditary retinoblastoma (40%) and is known as *germinal retinoblastoma*. All bilateral disease is considered hereditary, and 15% of unilateral disease involves germline mutation (Choe et al., 2017). It is critical to determine whether the initial mutation is germline, as the ongoing management of the patient and family members is determined by whether there is such a mutation. Patients with *RB1* germline mutation are at risk for additional retinoblastoma tumors and second primary malignancies throughout life (Skalet et al., 2018). There is some evidence that human papillomavirus (HPV) contributes to retinoblastoma development in children in developing countries, with HPV 16 and 18 both contributing to the development of retinoblastoma in children in India who have no family history (Shetty et al., 2012; Naru et al., 2016).

The diagnosis of retinoblastoma in developing countries can be delayed and the care may be suboptimal due to poor education, poor socioeconomic conditions, and inadequate access to health care. The extraocular spread of retinoblastoma due to delayed diagnosis increases the risk of death.

Screening Guidelines
The AAP, AACO, AAPOS, and AAO recommend that all infants and children should have a red reflex exam before discharge from the newborn nursery and thereafter at every health maintenance visit (2016). The American Association of Ophthalmic Oncologists and Pathologists (AAOOP) with support from the AAPOS and AAP have developed screening guidelines for children at risk of retinoblastoma (Skalet et al., 2018). They are as follows:
- All children at high risk require serial dilated fundus examinations by an ophthalmologist familiar with retinoblastoma monthly for the first 12 months of life, every 2 months from age 12 to 24 months, every 3 months from ages 24 to 36 months, every 4 months from age 36 to 48 months, and then every 6 months from ages 48 months to 7 years.
- Children at intermediate risk of retinoblastoma should be screened monthly for the first 3 months of life, every 2 months from ages 3 to 12 months, every 3 months from ages 12 to 36 months, every 4 to 6 months from ages 36 to 60 months, and every 6 months from ages 5 to 7 years.

- At-risk children should be screened from birth to age 7 years. Children who are known carriers of the *RB1* mutation should be screened every 1 to 2 years after age 7 years.
- Genetic testing should be conducted on the child with retinoblastoma and his or her first-degree relatives.

Clinical Findings

- Strabismus is the most common finding.
- There is decreased visual acuity.
- Uni- or bilateral white pupil (leukocoria), described often as an intermittent "glow, glint, gleam, or glare" by parents, is usually seen in low-light settings or noted in photographs taken with a flash (e.g., *cat's eye reflex*).
- Other symptoms include an abnormal red reflex, nystagmus, glaucoma, orbital cellulitis and photophobia (causes pain), hyphema, hypopyon (pus in anterior chamber of eye); signs of global rupture are also possible.

Diagnosis is made via ophthalmic exam (under anesthesia), ultrasound, or MRI. CT is no longer recommended due to the increased risk of radiation-induced second cancers.

Management

Refer a child with any abnormal findings suspicious of retinoblastoma for diagnosis and management by a multidisciplinary team. An international classification system for intraocular retinoblastoma lists the criteria of tumors based on their size, location, number, and degree of invasiveness or seeding. Depending on the diagnosis, treatment may involve cryotherapy, laser photocoagulation, episcleral plaque brachytherapy, systemic chemotherapy, or enucleation (Kaufman, Kim, and Berry, 2017). Early detection and advances in treatment have led to less enucleation and the preservation of sight. In those with advanced tumors requiring enucleation, a hydroxyapatite implant is placed at the time of enucleation.

Frequent follow-up (adhering to the AAOP, AAPOS, and AAP screening guidelines) to assess treatment and monitor for recurrence is critical to optimizing vision. Close to half of children with retinoblastoma will develop new or recurrent ocular tumors that require further treatment.

Complications and Prognosis

Retinoblastoma has a high (95%) cure rate in US children, with unilateral retinoblastoma having the best prognosis (Choe et al., 2017; Kaufman, Kim, and Berry, 2017). In countries with poor resources, the survival rate may be less than 30%. Children with germinal retinoblastoma have an increased risk of other cancers outside the eye and require lifelong follow-up. These subsequent neoplasms are the most common cause of death, accounting for more than 50% of deaths in children with bilateral disease. Pinealoma, osteosarcoma, cancers of the soft tissues, and melanoma are the most common second cancers. Those who survive are at high risk for cataracts, vitreous hemorrhage, neovascular glaucoma, lacrimal duct or gland injury, impaired orbital bone growth, radiation retinopathy, optic neuropathy, or bone marrow suppression. Late effects of retinoblastoma therapy include diminished orbital growth, visual-field deficits, and hearing loss.

Infections

Conjunctivitis

Conjunctivitis is an inflammation of the palpebral and occasionally the bulbar conjunctiva (Fig 35.4). It is the most frequently

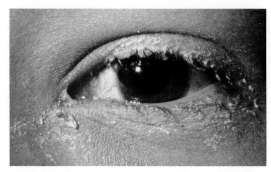

- **Fig 35.4** Bacterial conjunctivitis. (From Palay DA, Krachmer JH. *Primary Care Ophthalmology*. 2nd ed. Philadelphia: Mosby; 2005.)

seen ocular disorder in pediatric practice, and bacteria are the most common cause of infection (50% to 75%) in children, typically occurring from December to April. Pathogens include *H. influenzae, Streptococcus pneumoniae,* and *Moraxella* species, with both gram-negative and gram-positive organisms implicated (Jacobs, 2017a; Lopez Montero, 2017). Conjunctivitis also occurs as a viral or fungal infection or as a response to allergens or chemical irritants.

Bacterial conjunctivitis is often unilateral, whereas viral conjunctivitis is most often bilateral. Unilateral disease can also suggest a toxic, chemical, mechanical, or lacrimal cause. The management of conjunctivitis is based on etiology, clinical findings and diagnostic studies Table 35.6. Patient age may also indicate the likely etiology.

Conjunctivitis in the Newborn (Ophthalmia Neonatorum)

Conjunctivitis in the newborn, also known as *ophthalmia neonatorum* or *neonatal blennorrhea,* is a form of conjunctivitis that occurs in the first month of life. In most states, conjunctivitis of the newborn is a reportable infectious disease. It occurs in 0.3% to 11% of newborns. A prior common cause of chemical conjunctivitis was prophylactic instillation of silver nitrate at birth, which is one reason the product is no longer recommended. *Chlamydia trachomatis* is the most common cause of ophthalmia neonatorum, and 25% to 50% of newborns with a mother positive for *C. trachomatis* at the time of delivery will contract the disease (AAP, 2015a). Various bacteria account for 30% to 50% of cases (*Staphylococcus, Streptococcus, Pseudomonas, H. influenzae, Escherichia coli, Corynebacterium* species, *Moraxella catarrhalis, Klebsiella pneumoniae, Pseudomonas aeruginosa*). *Neisseria gonorrhoeae* and HSV are also seen (AAP, 2015a). Gonococcal conjunctivitis is the most serious cause of ophthalmia neonatorum owing to concerns of the bacteria causing blindness (AAP, 2015b).

Clinical Findings

History and Physical Examination

- Chemical conjunctivitis usually occurs in the first 24 to 72 hours of life.
- Septic conjunctivitis caused by
  - Bacteria usually occurs between 5 and 14 days of life.
  - *C. trachomatis* usually begins between 5 and 14 days of life; it can also occur in newborns born via cesarean section with intact membranes.
  - *N. gonorrhoeae* usually appears in the first 3 to 5 days of life (up to 29 days).
  - HSV presents at birth or in the first 4 weeks of life.

TABLE 35.6 Types of Conjunctivitis

Type	Incidence/Etiology	Clinical Findings	Diagnosis	Management
Ophthalmia neonatorum	Neonates: *Chlamydia trachomatis, Staphylococcus aureus, Neisseria gonorrhoeae*, HSV (silver nitrate reaction occurs in 10% of neonates)	Erythema, chemosis, purulent exudate with *N. gonorrhoeae*; clear to mucoid exudate with *Chlamydia*	Culture (ELISA, PCR), Gram stain, R/O *N. gonorrhoeae, Chlamydia*	Saline irrigation to eyes until exudate gone; follow with erythromycin ointment For *N. gonorrhoeae*: ceftriaxone or IM or IV For chlamydia: erythromycin or possibly azithromycin PO For HSV: antivirals IV or PO
Bacterial conjunctivitis	In neonates 5-14 days of age, preschoolers, and sexually active teens: *Haemophilus influenzae* (nontypeable), *Streptococcus pneumoniae, S. aureus, N. gonorrhoeae*	Erythema, chemosis, itching, burning, mucopurulent exudate, matter in eyelashes; worse in winter	Cultures (required in neonate); Gram stain (optional); chocolate agar (for *N. gonorrhoeae*) R/O pharyngitis, *N. gonorrhoeae*, AOM, URI, seborrhea	Neonates: Erythromycin 0.5% ophthalmic ointment ≥1 year of age: Fourth-generation fluoroquinolone For concurrent AOM: Treat accordingly for AOM Warm soaks to eyes three times a day until clear No sharing of towels or pillows No school until treatment begins
Chronic bacterial conjunctivitis (unresponsive conjunctivitis previously treated as bacterial in etiology)	School-age children and teens: Bacteria, viruses, *C. trachomatis*	Same as above; foreign body sensation	Cultures, Gram stain; R/O dacryostenosis, blepharitis, corneal ulcers, trachoma	Depends on prior treatment, laboratory results, and differential diagnoses Review compliance and prior drug choices of conjunctivitis treatment Consult with ophthalmologist
Inclusion conjunctivitis	Neonates 5-14 days of age and sexually active teens: *C. trachomatis*	Erythema, chemosis, clear or mucoid exudate, palpebral follicles	Cultures (ELISA, PCR), R/O sexual activity	Neonates: Erythromycin or azithromycin PO Adolescents: doxycycline, azithromycin, EES, erythromycin base, levofloxacin PO
Viral conjunctivitis	Adenovirus 3, 4, 7; HSV, herpes zoster, varicella	Erythema, chemosis, tearing (bilateral); HSV and herpes zoster: unilateral with photophobia, fever; zoster: nose lesion; spring and fall	Cultures, R/O corneal infiltration	Refer to ophthalmologist if HSV or photophobia is present Cool compresses three or four times a day
Allergic and vernal conjunctivitis	Atopy sufferers, seasonal	Stringy, mucoid exudate, swollen eyelids and conjunctivae, itching (key finding), tearing, palpebral follicles, headache, rhinitis	Eosinophils in conjunctival scrapings	Naphazoline/pheniramine, naphazoline/antazoline ophthalmic solution (see text) Mast cell stabilizer (see text) Refer to allergist if needed

AOM, Acute otitis media; *EES*, erythromycin ethylsuccinate; *ELISA*, enzyme-linked immunosorbent assay; *HSV*, herpes simplex virus; *IM*, intramuscular; *IV*, intravenous; *PCR*, polymerase chain reaction; *PO*, (by mouth, orally); *R/O*, rule out; *URI*, upper respiratory infection.

Symptoms most commonly seen include the following:
- Chemically induced conjunctivitis frequently manifests as nonpurulent discharge and edematous bulbar and palpebral conjunctiva (AAP, 2015c).
- *C. trachomatis* specifically causes moderate eyelid swelling and palpebral or bulbar conjunctival injection and moderate thick, purulent discharge.
- *N. gonorrhoeae* specifically causes acute conjunctival inflammation, lid edema, erythema, and excessive, purulent discharge.
- Bacteria present with conjunctival erythema, purulent discharge.

- HSV specifically causes mild conjunctivitis, erythema, corneal opacity, serosanguineous discharge, and vesicular rash on eyelids and is often unilateral.

There may be a maternal history of vaginal infection during pregnancy or current sexually transmitted infection (STI).

Diagnostic Studies. Swabs and scrapings must be done. Gram and Giemsa staining, direct immunofluorescent monoclonal antibody staining, cultures, enzyme-linked immunosorbent assay (ELISA), or polymerase chain reaction (PCR) testing can be used. Any infant younger than 2 weeks with ophthalmia neonatorum should be tested for gonorrhea. A culture for gonorrhea (on chocolate agar or Thayer-Martin medium) or aggressive scraping for a

Gram stain is used for diagnosis. Culturing purulent discharge is not sufficient. If gonorrhea is suspected, also check for *C. trachomatis*.

Management
- Irrigate the eyes, after obtaining cultures, with sterile normal saline until clear of exudate.
- Gonococcal conjunctivitis: In the newborn, gonococcal conjunctivitis requires intramuscular (IM) ceftriaxone (25 to 50 mg/kg, not to exceed 125 mg) given once (AAP, 2015b). If there are extraocular manifestations, a 7-day course of intramuscular or intravenous ceftriaxone is warranted. Ceftriaxone is not given to neonates with hyperbilirubinemia; cefotaxime is an alternative (AAP, 2015a). Ocular morbidity (corneal infection with possible scarring or perforation) can result if infection is missed.
- Nongonococcal conjunctivitis: A topical ophthalmic antibiotic preparation, such as erythromycin 0.5% ointment, trimethoprim-polymyxin B, or fluoroquinolone drops, is indicated (Jacobs, 2017a). The eyes should be cleansed with water or saline applied with cotton balls before instilling the ointment into the lower conjunctival sac.
- Herpes simplex conjunctivitis: Immediate referral for hospitalization and topical and systemic antivirals are needed. Spread of virus to the CNS, mouth, and skin is of concern.
- *Chlamydia*: Assess for systemic infection (pharyngitis, ear infection, pneumonia). Chlamydial conjunctivitis is treated with systemic erythromycin (50 mg/kg/day in four divided doses for 14 days) or azithromycin (20 mg/kg for 3 days) (AAP, 2015a). Topical treatment is not indicated because it does not lower the risk for a subsequent pneumonia caused by *Chlamydia* (see "Inclusion Conjunctivitis" in the next section).
- Chemically induced conjunctivitis resolves spontaneously within 3 to 4 days without specific treatment.
- Mothers and their sexual partners should receive treatment if gonococcal and/or chlamydial infections occur in their newborns.

Prevention. To prevent ophthalmia neonatorum, prophylactic administration of antibiotic eye medication within 1 hour of vaginal delivery or delivery via cesarean is recommended (AAP, 2016a). The antibiotic of choice is erythromycin ointment 0.5% (a 0.25- to 0.5-inch strip to each eye). Prophylaxis may be delayed for up to an hour to facilitate parent-infant bonding (AAP, 2015b). Prophylaxis is required by law in most states and territories to prevent gonococcal conjunctivitis in the newborn. However, prophylaxis does not prevent neonatal chlamydial conjunctivitis or extraocular infection. It should be determined at the time of the first well child visit whether infants born at home have received this prophylaxis.

Inclusion Conjunctivitis (Chlamydia)

Inclusion conjunctivitis is usually caused by one of eight known strains of *C. trachomatis* and is most often seen in a neonate or sexually active adolescent. Neonates usually demonstrate symptoms within the first 5 to 14 days of life (to 6 weeks), whereas *N. gonorrhoeae* symptoms are usually detected earlier. Nasopharyngeal infection with *C. trachomatis* is found in 50% of infants with inclusion conjunctivitis, whereas inclusion cysts in sexually active teens and adults (54% of males; 74% of females) are associated with a genital chlamydial infection (Azari and Barney, 2013).

Clinical Findings
History and Physical Examination
- Maternal history of an STI or a history of a sexual partner with an STI
- Conjunctival erythema and mild to severe mucopurulent to bloody discharge, usually bilateral

- Follicular reaction (large, round elevations) in the conjunctiva of the lower eyelids; conjunctiva may bleed if stroked
- Associated cervicitis, urethritis, or rectal infection
- Infants may have symptoms suggestive of chlamydial pneumonia at 1 to 3 months of age.

Diagnostic Studies. Definitive diagnosis of *Chlamydia* can be made by isolating the organism by tissue culture (AAP, 2015a). Direct fluorescence antibody (DFA) tests are the only FDA-approved test for conjunctival swabs; nucleic acid amplification tests (NAATs) are not approved for conjunctival testing (CDC, 2015). Conjunctival scrapings for Giemsa staining are indicated. Scrapings must contain epithelial cells because *Chlamydia* is an obligate intracellular organism (CDC, 2015). A specimen should also be gathered to test for gonorrhea because of the comorbidity of these two organisms and ocular morbidity if gonorrhea is missed.

Management. Owing to the high incidence of concurrent nasopharyngeal, lung, and genital tract infections in infants and genital infections in adolescents, systemic therapy is required for the treatment of conjunctivitis caused by *C. trachomatis* (AAP, 2015a). Treatment options have expanded from the traditional use of oral erythromycin ethylsuccinate (EES) to azithromycin. There is an increased incidence of idiopathic hypertrophic pyloric stenosis (IHPS) in infants younger than 6 weeks of age following administration of systemic EES. However, this has not altered the recommendation of EES as the preferred treatment. The risk of using azithromycin has not been fully established, although there have been reports of IHPS after the use of azithromycin (CDC, 2015). Medical providers who treat newborns with EES should discuss with parents the signs and potential risks of developing IHPS.

Treatment recommendations include the following:
- A 14-day course of oral EES. Sometimes a second 14-day course is required because the failure rate with EES is 10% to 20%. EES may be repeated, although oral azithromycin is also effective (AAP, 2015a). Providers are encouraged to use systemic EES with caution; if no other alternatives are viable, they must have a high index of suspicion for the development of IHPS.
- Doxycycline, azithromycin, ofloxacin, or levofloxacin can be used in young adults.
- Topical ointment (erythromycin, moxifloxacin) is sometimes recommended despite systemic drug treatment; the AAP notes that such concurrent treatment is unnecessary and ineffective (AAP, 2015a).
- Mothers of infants with *C. trachomatis* conjunctivitis, partners of such mothers, and partners of sexually active adolescents also need examination and treatment for 2 weeks with tetracycline or erythromycin.

Complications. Complications include chlamydial pneumonia (5% to 20% of infants will develop pneumonia if their mother has a chlamydial infection at delivery), nasopharyngeal colonization (in up to 50% of infants treated for inclusion conjunctivitis), or gastroenteritis in infants (AAP, 2015a). Complications may occur 6 to 8 weeks following the conjunctivitis.

Bacterial Conjunctivitis

Acute bacterial conjunctivitis (commonly called *pinkeye*) is a contagious and easily spread disease. *H. influenzae* is the most common organism isolated in children who are below 7 years of age (Jacobs, 2017a; Lopez Montero, 2018). *S. pneumoniae, M. catarrhalis,* and adenovirus are also common pathogens. Bacterial conjunctivitis is most common in the winter and in toddlers and preschoolers (see Fig 35.4).

Clinical Findings
- Erythema of one or both eyes, usually starting unilaterally and becoming bilateral (key finding)
- Yellow-green purulent discharge (key finding)
- Encrusted and matted eyelids on awakening (key finding)
- Burning, stinging, or itching of the eyes and a feeling of a foreign body
- Photophobia
- Petechiae on bulbar conjunctiva
- Symptoms of upper respiratory infection, otitis media, or acute pharyngitis
- Vision screen should be normal and documented in the patient's record

Diagnostic Studies. Routine culture testing is *not necessary*. Gram stain and culture can be done if the conjunctivitis is chronic, recurrent, or difficult to treat. An in-office rapid antigen test with high sensitivity and specificity for adenovirus is available and may be warranted to decrease inappropriate prescribing of antibiotics for viral conjunctivitis.

Differential Diagnosis. Bacterial conjunctivitis requires consideration of nasolacrimal duct obstruction in infants, ear infection, Kawasaki disease, foreign body, corneal abrasion, uveitis, herpetic conjunctivitis, poor compliance, or wrong choice of drug. Cultures or scrapings are appropriate for unresolved infection.

Management. Bacterial conjunctivitis is considered a self-limited disease (unless caused by *Neisseria gonorrhoeae* or *Chlamydia*) that usually resolves within 8 to 10 days. However, because both gram-negative and gram-positive organisms have been implicated, children who receive topical antibiotics demonstrate faster clinical improvement, can return to day care or school faster, and cause less parental work loss (Jacobs, 2017a). The common practice of prescribing antibiotics for conjunctivitis, however, has led to an increasing rate of drug resistance. It is imperative that providers make their diagnosis judiciously and then treat with an effective drug that is more likely to be tolerated and taken as directed. For this reason, older children and teens may be treated conservatively without using antibiotics. This prevents the overuse of antibiotics and takes into consideration the self-limited nature of this disease.

Choose broad-spectrum coverage that has the lowest resistance rate, greatest compliance, and best penetration of tissues. The cost of ophthalmic antibiotics varies significantly. If patients have a large copayment for brand-name drugs or if they lack paid drug coverage, cost should be factored in when treatment for this self-limited disease is being prescribed.

Parents can be instructed to put pressure over the lacrimal duct when they are instilling the medication to prevent drainage into the nasolacrimal system. If improvement is not seen within 3 days after treatment is initiated, refer to or consult as appropriate with an ophthalmologist. Contact lenses should not be worn during conjunctivitis treatment. Disposable lenses should be discarded and permanent contacts sterilized before being reinserted.

For uncomplicated bacterial conjunctivitis, treatment includes (Jacobs, 2017a; Lopez Montero, 2018) the following:
- Sodium sulfacetamide 10% ophthalmic solution or ointment; not effective against *H. influenzae;* stings; can cause allergic reactions (including Stevens-Johnson syndrome)
- Trimethoprim sulfate plus polymyxin B sulfate ophthalmic solution

- Erythromycin 0.5% ophthalmic ointment for patients with sulfa allergy and infants Azithromycin drops for children older than 12 months
- Fluoroquinolone ophthalmic drops including besifloxacin, ciprofloxacin, gatifloxacin, levofloxacin, moxifloxacin, or ofloxacin for children older than 12 months

The aminoglycosides (neomycin, tobramycin, and gentamicin) are to be avoided because of possible hypersensitization, severe allergic reactions, and increasing resistance.

Conjunctivitis-Otitis Syndrome. This syndrome is usually caused by *H. influenzae*. The PCP should treat for the otitis media. Concurrent use of a topical antibiotic is not necessary.

Patient Education. If only one eye is involved, it is likely that the infection will spread within a day or two to involve both eyes. The patient (or parent) is instructed to do the following:
- Cleanse the eyelashes several times a day with a weak solution of no-tears shampoo and warm water. The importance of wiping from the inner canthus outward and using a different cloth or cotton ball for each eye should be emphasized.
- Use warm soaks three or four times a day to relieve itching and burning.
- Instill the prescribed ophthalmic solution or ointment into the lower conjunctival sac. A moistened cotton swab may be used to facilitate instillation of ointments. Dosing while the child is sleeping greatly increases compliance and therefore effectiveness.
- Wash hands frequently and avoid shared linens to limit spread of the infection.

Also treat seborrheic dermatitis on the scalp and face if present. Day care center exclusion policies vary. Some allow return once the treatment is started, whereas others allow return only after the completion of 1 to 2 days of treatment. Improvement in the child's condition should be seen within 48 hours. If improvement is not seen within 72 hours, the patient can be referred to an optometrist or ophthalmologist (Jacobs, 2017a).

Complications. If the infection proves recalcitrant to treatment, eye pain is present, vision is blurred, or ophthalmoscopic examination reveals a bulging iris and a contracted, fixed pupil, suspect more serious inflammation of the uveal tract (iritis, cyclitis, or choroiditis). Refer immediately to an ophthalmologist to avoid ocular morbidity.

Viral Conjunctivitis

Viral conjunctivitis is usually caused by an adenovirus but can also be caused by herpes simplex, herpes zoster, enterovirus, molluscum contagiosum, or varicella virus. It is more common in children older than 6 years of age and in the spring and fall (see Table 29.6). In-office testing is available for adenovirus, which can cause up to 80% of acute conjunctivitis cases (Azari and Barney, 2013).

Clinical Findings
- Tearing and profuse clear, watery discharge (key findings)
- Fever, headache, anorexia, malaise, upper respiratory symptoms (pharyngitis-conjunctivitis-fever triad with adenovirus [key findings])
- Pharyngitis with enlarged preauricular nodes (key findings)
- Itchy, red, and swollen conjunctiva
- Hyperemia and swollen eyelids
- Photophobia with measles or varicella rashes
- Herpetic vesicles on the eyelid margins and eyelashes (marginal blepharitis) or on the conjunctiva and cornea (keratoconjunctivitis)

Management

- Good hygiene is essential. Viral conjunctivitis is self-limited and should resolve in 7 to 14 days. Conjunctivitis is often difficult to distinguish from keratitis. If there is any question about diagnosis, refer for ophthalmologic assessment.
- Warm or cold compresses and artificial tears can be used.
- Prophylaxis with antibiotics is not recommended.
- Antihistamine or vasoconstrictive ophthalmic solutions may be used for symptomatic relief.
- If HSV infection is suspected, immediate referral to an ophthalmologist is indicated. Topical corticosteroids should be avoided because they may worsen the course.

Conjunctivitis-Pharyngitis Syndrome. This syndrome is more likely to be caused by adenovirus than by a bacterium and should be treated accordingly.

Complications. Involvement of deeper layers of the cornea (keratitis) can occur and must be differentiated from conjunctivitis. Scarring of the cornea resulting in blindness is a significant complication of HSV infection. If in any doubt, refer to an ophthalmologist for a slit-lamp examination.

Allergic Conjunctivitis

Allergic conjunctivitis usually occurs in childhood and into adulthood (Fig 35.5). Four types of allergic conjunctivitis have been identified:

- *Acute allergic conjunctivitis* has a sudden onset of symptoms (within 30 minutes) after exposure to an environmental allergen, such as animal dander. There is usually itching, tearing, chemosis, and eyelid edema; the condition resolves within 24 hours once exposure to allergen ends (Hamra and Dana, 2017).
- *Seasonal allergic conjunctivitis* (hay fever) is characterized by mild injection and swelling and is associated with exposing the eyes to outdoor pollens and may be associated with generalized allergic reaction including nasal congestion (allergic rhinoconjunctivitis). Seasonal allergens (e.g., grass pollens, ragweed) cause 90% of allergic conjunctivitis in the United States.
- *Perennial conjunctivitis* is chronic conjunctivitis related to year-round exposure to allergens such as dust mites, animal dander, and molds. Perennial conjunctivitis is usually mild and waxes and wanes throughout the year.
- *Vernal conjunctivitis* is more severe, with peak incidence in 10- to 12-year-olds; it occurs in boys twice as commonly as in girls and has an increased prevalence in warm weather.
- Atopic keratoconjunctivitis occurs in those with atopic dermatitis and/or asthma, affecting the lower tarsal conjunctiva; it usually occurs in late adolescence and is notable for significant (beyond that seen in allergic conjunctivitis) itching, burning, and tearing that is often chronic.

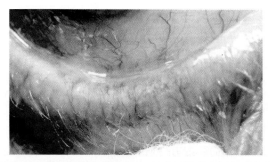

- **Fig 35.5** Allergic conjunctivitis. (From Palay DA, Krachmer JH. *Primary Care Ophthalmology*. 2nd ed. Philadelphia: Mosby; 2005.)

- Giant papillary conjunctivitis occurs most often in contact lens wearers, occurring 10 times more frequently in those wearing soft contacts than hard contacts.

Clinical Findings

- Severe itching, tearing (key findings)
- Rhinitis
- Family or current history of atopy (eczema, asthma) and/or seasonal allergies
- Acute attacks precipitated by allergens (e.g., pollen, animals, molds, dust, dust mites, occasionally food)
- Redness and swelling of the conjunctiva or eyelid (or both)
- Follicular reaction of the conjunctiva
- Stringy, mucoid discharge
- Bilateral involvement most common
- Cobblestone papillary hypertrophy in the tarsal conjunctiva
- Vision screening generally normal and should be documented in patient's record

Diagnostic Studies. Conjunctival or nasal smears (using Wright stain) reveal numerous eosinophils.

Management

- Prevention is best; avoid allergens.
- For mild cases, saline solution or artificial tears are administered along with cool compresses. Refrigerated eye drops are more soothing. Pharmacologic treatment includes topical decongestants, oral or topical antihistamines, topical mast cell stabilizers, or topical NSAIDs (Hamra and Dana, 2017). The decongestants do not decrease the allergic response but do relieve erythema, injection, and lid edema.
- A combination antihistamine-decongestant is more effective than either agent alone; naphazoline hydrochloride plus antazoline ophthalmic solution can be used sparingly to reduce ocular congestion, irritation, and itching.
- Topical mast cell stabilizers may be helpful for maintenance therapy, chronic allergies, or vernal conjunctivitis and are available over the counter.
  - Cromolyn sodium 4% on a regular basis.
  - Nedocromil sodium 2% or lodoxamide tromethamine 0.1%.
- Topical olopatadine hydrochloride 0.1% is a mast cell stabilizer combined with an antihistamine for children above 3 years of age.
- Topical NSAIDs, like ketorolac tromethamine 0.5%, provide relief of itching and burning.
- Ophthalmic histamine 1 (H_1) blockers such as ketotifen or levocabastine can be prescribed for allergic conjunctivitis and ocular pruritus.
- Topical steroids should not be used because of possible side effects (increased IOP, potential for viral infection, contraindication with herpes, potential to cause cataracts, and poor corneal healing). An ophthalmologist should be consulted if a patient's condition warrants considering topical corticosteroids.

  Patients may be treated with systemic antihistamines (fexofenadine, loratadine, or cetirizine) if systemic symptoms are present.
- Refer to an allergist for allergen immunotherapy when rhinitis is present because therapy can lead to better control without the need for medication.
- Refer to an ophthalmologist if there is no response to treatment or if any of the following is present: corneal abrasions, impaired vision, need for corticosteroids, severe keratoconjunctivitis, or atypical manifestations.
- Maintain a high threshold of suspicion for herpes-induced blepharitis or atopic keratoconjunctivitis if pain is present.

Complications. Some forms of allergic conjunctivitis (e.g., vernal conjunctivitis) can lead to corneal ulceration, scarring and vision loss, corneal degeneration, and changes in the corneal curvature.

Blepharitis

Blepharitis is an acute or chronic inflammation of the eyelash follicles or meibomian sebaceous glands of the eyelids (or both). It is usually bilateral. The two types of blepharitis are anterior and posterior. *Anterior* blepharitis may be caused by seborrhea or staphylococcal bacteria that colonize the eyelid (Shtein, 2017). *Demodex folliculorum* is a parasite that may cause chronic anterior blepharitis, presenting with cylindrical sleeves of dandruff around the eyelashes. *Posterior* blepharitis occurs when there is inflammation at the inner portion of the eyelid at the meibomian glands. Diseases with chronic inflammation, such as rosacea or seborrheic dermatitis, may be source of posterior blepharitis. Blepharitis may also be caused by allergic contact dermatitis, eczema, or psoriasis.

Clinical Findings
- Swelling and erythema of the eyelid margins and palpebral conjunctiva
- Flaky, scaly debris over eyelid margins on awakening
- Gritty, burning feeling in eyes
- Mild bulbar conjunctival injection
- Ulcerative form: Hard scales at the base of the lashes (if the crust is removed, ulceration is seen at the hair follicles, the lashes fall out, and an associated conjunctivitis is present)

Differential Diagnosis
Pediculosis of the eyelashes.

Management
Instructions include the following:
- Scrub the eyelashes and eyelids with a cotton-tipped applicator or clean washcloth containing a weak (50%) solution of no-tears shampoo to maintain proper hygiene and debride the scales. Rinse well after washing.
- Use warm compresses for 5 to 10 minutes at a time two to four times a day and wipe away lid debris.
- Massage the lids two to four times a day to express meibomian secretions.
- Sometimes an antistaphylococcal antibiotic (e.g., bacitracin or erythromycin 0.5% ophthalmic ointment) is used once daily at bedtime until symptoms subside and for at least 1 week thereafter. Ointment is preferable to eye drops because of increased duration of contact with the ocular tissue. Azithromycin 1% ophthalmic solution for 4 weeks may also be used for posterior blepharitis (Shtein, 2017).
- Treat associated seborrhea, psoriasis, eczema, or allergies as indicated.
- Remove contact lenses and wear eyeglasses for the duration of the treatment period. Sterilize or clean lenses before reinserting.
- Purchase new eye makeup; minimize use of mascara and eyeliner.
- Use artificial tears for patients with inadequate tear pools.

Chronic staphylococcal blepharitis and meibomian keratoconjunctivitis respond to oral antibiotics. Doxycycline or tetracycline can be used chronically in children older than 8 years of age. Azithromycin for 5 days may be used in younger children.

Hordeolum (Stye)

A hordeolum, or *stye*, is an infection of either the sebaceous glands, the eyelids (external hordeolum) or the meibomian glands (internal hordeolum). The causative organism is *S. aureus* or, rarely, *P. aeruginosa*.

Clinical Findings
A tender, swollen red furuncle is seen. In an external hordeolum, the swelling is generally smaller, superficial, and located along the lid margin (Fig 35.6). An internal hordeolum is larger and may point through the skin or conjunctival surface. The patient complains of a foreign body sensation. An internal hordeolum on the palpebral conjunctiva can be inspected by rolling back the eyelid.

Differential Diagnosis
Cellulitis of the lid or orbit, sebaceous cell cancer, or pyogenic granuloma should be considered.

Management
- Rupture often occurs spontaneously when the furuncle becomes large and a point develops. Removal of an eyelash near the furuncle frequently promotes rupture.
- Warm, moist compresses three or four times daily, 10 to 15 minutes each time, facilitate the process of rupturing.
- Hygiene for the eye can be maintained by scrubbing the eyelashes and eyelids with a cotton-tipped applicator or clean washcloth containing a weak (50%) solution of no-tears shampoo once or twice a day.
- Antistaphylococcal ointment (e.g., 0.5% erythromycin) can also be an effective treatment.
- Steroids are not indicated.
- If the hordeolum does not rupture on its own after coming to a point or for multiple or recurrent hordeolum, refer to an ophthalmologist for incision and drainage.

Chalazion

Chalazion is a chronic sterile inflammation of the eyelid resulting from a lipogranuloma of the meibomian glands, which line the posterior margins of the eyelids (see Fig 35.6). It is deeper in the

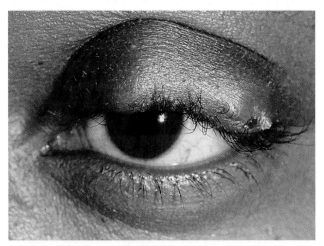

• **Fig 35.6** Chalazion and external hordeolum. (From Neff AG, Carter KD. Benign eyelid lesions. In: Yanoff M, Duker JS, eds. *Ophthalmology.* 4th ed. Philadelphia: Elsevier/Saunders; 2014. Fig. 12.9.22, A.)

eyelid tissue than a hordeolum and may result from an internal hordeolum or retained lipid granular secretions.

Clinical Findings

Initially mild erythema and slight swelling of the involved eyelid are seen. After a few days the inflammation resolves and a slow-growing, round, nonpigmented, painless (key finding) mass remains. It may persist for a long time and is a commonly acquired lid lesion seen in children.

Management

- Acute lesions are treated with hot compresses.
- Refer to an ophthalmologist for surgical incision or topical intralesional corticosteroid injections if the condition is unresolved or the lesion causes cosmetic concerns. A chalazion can distort vision by causing astigmatism as a result of pressure on the orbit.

Complications

Recurrence is common. Fragile vascular granulation tissue called *pyogenic granuloma*, which enlarges and bleeds rapidly, can occur if a chalazion breaks through the conjunctival surface.

Nasolacrimal Duct Conditions: Dacryostenosis and Dacryocystitis

Nasolacrimal duct obstruction, or dacryostenosis, is an abnormal obstruction (imperforate valve of Hasner) of the nasolacrimal duct that prevents tears from flowing into an opening in the nasal mucosa. Dacryocystitis is an inflammation of the involved nasolacrimal duct; infection can result (Fig 35.7). Nasolacrimal duct obstruction is fairly common (up to 6%) in neonates (Paysse and Coats, 2017). It is thought to be due to a membrane that covers the nasolacrimal duct, which then fails to break down quickly. It may also occur at any age secondary to trauma to the duct or to a chronic duct obstruction complicated by an upper respiratory infection. The condition is also found more frequently in those with craniofacial disorders and Down syndrome. Congenital failure of the duct to canalize may be unilateral or bilateral, and clinical signs appear 2 to 6 weeks after birth when tear production develops. Duct blockage usually resolves spontaneously in 90% of infants by 6 months of age and 96% of infants by 12 months (Paysse and Coats, 2017). Bacterial overgrowth may occur, resulting in excessive mucous production.

Clinical Findings

- Continuous or intermittent tearing, stickiness, and mucoid discharge at the inner canthus that can become purulent, with possible expression of purulent material
- Blepharitis in lids and lashes
- Occasional nasal obstruction and drainage
- Expression of a thin mucopurulent exudate from the punctum lacrimale
- Tenderness and swelling over the lacrimal duct (can be exquisitely painful)
- Eyelids closed with dried mucous on awakening
- Edema and erythema of the tear sac (most prominent in the triangular area just below the medial canthus)
- Excoriation and thickening of the periorbital skin
- Conjunctival injection is not common
- Mucocele of inner canthal tendon (unusual; presents as a bluish mass)
  Diagnostic Studies
- Fluorescein dye, instilled bilaterally in the inferior conjunctival sac and checked in 2 and 5 minutes with a cobalt blue light source, will disappear if duct is patent.
- A white blood cell (WBC) count (elevated) and cultures are obtained from the expressed exudate if the inflammation is severe.

Differential Diagnosis

Punctual or canalicular atresia, ophthalmia neonatorum, conjunctivitis, foreign body, corneal abrasion, congenital glaucoma, dacryocele, intraocular inflammation, and nasal mucosal edema are differential diagnoses (Paysse and Coats, 2017).

Management

The treatment goals are to minimize stagnation in the tear duct and prevent infection.

- Daily massage of the lacrimal sac may be performed to facilitate canalization of the duct. The technique involves placing a clean finger over the medial canthus and pressing in a posterior direction until the fingertip enters the space behind the inferior bony orbital ridge. Gentle pressure applied in a downward and medial direction transmits hydrostatic force through the nasolacrimal duct to the obstruction (Fig 35.8). This technique should be performed two or three times a day. The eyelid should be cleaned with plain water after massage (Paysse and Coats, 2017).

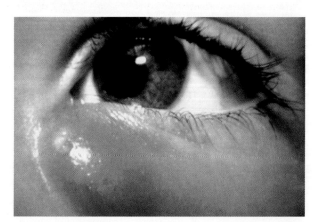

• **Fig 35.7** Dacryocystitis. (From Sharma R, Brunette DD. Ophthalmology. In: Marx JA, Hockberger RS, Walls RM, eds. *Rosen's Emergency Medicine*. 8th ed. Philadelphia: Elsevier; 2014. Fig. 71.20.)

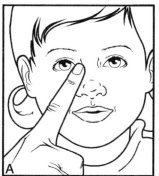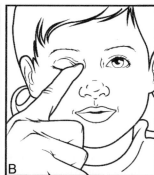

• **Fig 35.8** Technique to clear nasolacrimal duct obstruction. (A) Incorrect technique. (B) Correct technique. The finger is pushing behind the bone, "in and up." Note that the fingertip is not visible in the proper technique.

- Bacterial conjunctivitis or excessive mucopurulent exudate is most commonly *S. pneumoniae* (35%) or *H. influenzae* (20%) and may be treated with erythromycin ophthalmic ointment, or a fluoroquinolone (moxifloxacin, ciprofloxacin, ofloxacin, norfloxacin) for 1 to 3 weeks with massage and frequent cleansing of secretions (Paysse and Coats, 2017). The duct may open spontaneously with resolution of the bacterial infection.
- Saline drops into the nose, followed by aspiration before feeding and at bedtime, help to relieve any concurrent nasal congestion.

If the mucopurulent exudate persists for 1 to 2 weeks despite the previously mentioned interventions, refer the child to an ophthalmologist regardless of age. Some ophthalmologists may probe the duct in an infant as early as 6 months of age, whereas others wait until the child is 9 to 12 months old. Early in-office probing is less expensive and does not require anesthesia, but it does require a skilled ophthalmologist (Paysse and Coats, 2017). If probing fails to alleviate the problem (which is unusual), surgery may be required for placement of a tube stent or for a dacryocystorhinostomy (DCR). Dacryocystitis may be acute or chronic and is evidenced by erythematous swelling below the medial canthal area. Treatment of dacryocystitis is warm compresses and oral or parenteral antibiotics (Örge and Boente, 2014). When fever, marked erythema, swelling, tenderness, and toxic appearance occur, hospitalization for parenteral antibiotics is indicated. Periorbital or orbital cellulitis is a complication of chronic dacryocystitis.

Preseptal (Periorbital) Cellulitis

Preseptal cellulitis is often associated with trauma or focal infection near the eye, an eyelid abscess, or sinusitis (Gappy et al., 2017). *Preseptal* (rather than *periorbital*) cellulitis is the preferred term to reflect the fact that the infection is anterior to the orbital septum and does not involve the orbit or other eye structures (Fig 35.9). Orbital cellulitis is a more serious infection involving tissues posterior to the orbital septum (Gappy et al., 2017).

Preseptal cellulitis is most commonly seen in children up to 6 years of age. It can also occur with infected lacerations, abrasions, insect stings or bites, impetigo, or a foreign body where the infection is spread via venous or lymphatic channels. It may also be secondary to paranasal sinusitis (Gappy et al., 2017). The etiology is often unknown. The bacteria most commonly responsible for periorbital

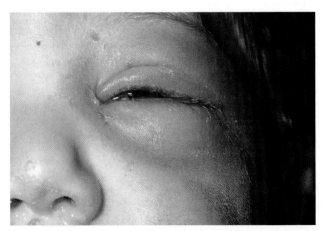

- **Fig 35.9** Preseptal cellulitis due to *Haemophilus influenzae* in a 6-month-old infant. (From Hoyt C, Taylor D. *Pediatric Ophthalmology and Strabismus*. 4th ed. Philadelphia: Elsevier/Saunders; 2013.)

cellulitis are streptococcal organisms, and *S. aureus. H. influenza* is uncommon now with the introduction of the Haemophilus influenza type B (Hib) vaccine. *S. aureus,* Community-acquired methicillin-resistant *Staphylococcus aureus* (MRSA) has been reported as a cause of periorbital cellulitis, and such infections appear to be on the rise.

Clinical Findings

- The patient is usually afebrile. If fever is present, consider orbital cellulitis.
- Swelling and erythema of tissues surrounding the eye; the upper lid is affected more often than the lower lid. Deep red eyelid (the color is purple-blue with *H. influenzae* infection).
- Orbital discomfort or pain, proptosis, or paralysis of the extraocular muscles can occur with orbital cellulitis.
- History of sinusitis, insect bite or eye trauma.
- Bacteremia may indicate orbital cellulitis.
  Diagnostic Studies. Diagnostic studies are not usually required for preseptal cellulitis. Depending on the severity and speed of progression of the cellulitis, the following are useful in evaluating for orbital cellulitis (Paysse and Coats, 2017):
- Visual acuity, extraocular movement, and pupillary reaction testing
- Complete blood count (CBC) with differential
- Blood cultures
- CT scan to rule out sinusitis, orbital cellulitis or subperiosteal abscess

Differential Diagnosis

Conjunctivitis, cavernous sinus thrombosis, and orbital cellulitis (proptosis, limited extraocular movement, and reduced visual acuity) are in the differential diagnoses in children; consider conjunctivitis, dacryocystitis, and ruptured dacryocystocele in neonates.

Management

Management must be planned on a case-by-case basis. Referral to an ophthalmologist is needed when proptosis, ophthalmoplegia, or changes in visual acuity occur; these conditions are suggestive of orbital cellulitis. Moderate to severe cellulitis, cellulitis in a child less than 1 year of age, a poor response to outpatient management, or a purulent wound near the eyelid require hospitalization and intravenous administration of antibiotics followed by a 10-day course of oral antibiotics (Gappy et al., 2017).

The child may be managed as an outpatient if older than 1 year, the cellulitis is mild, the orbit is not involved (full eye movements are present, no pain with eye movement, visual changes, or ptosis), and the child exhibits no symptoms of systemic bacterial sepsis.

Outpatient management consists of:

- Oral antibiotics to complete a 7- to 14-day course. Amoxicillin with clavulanic acid, cefdinir, and cefpodoxime are first-line choices for treatment.
- If MRSA is suspected, treat with clindamycin or a combination regimen of trimethoprim/sulfamethoxazole (TMP-SMX) *plus* amoxicillin *or* cefpodoxime *or* cefdinir (Gappy et al., 2017).
- Warm soaks to the periorbital area every 2 to 4 hours for 15 minutes may provide comfort and also speed healing.
- If a rapid clinical response is not seen, further evaluation and treatment are required. The parent is advised to call immediately if there is any change in condition.
- Reexamine the patient in 24 hours. Failure to improve in 24 hours indicates a need for hospitalization and parenteral antibiotics, usually ceftriaxone. The child is monitored daily until blood cultures are negative for 48 hours or clinical improvement is seen.

Complications

Complications include orbital cellulitis or extension of the infection into the orbit, subperiosteal or orbital abscess, optic neuritis, retinal vein thrombosis, panophthalmitis, meningitis, epidural and subdural abscesses, and cavernous sinus thrombosis.

Keratitis and Corneal Ulcers

Inflammation of the cornea (keratitis) can cause a dramatic alteration in visual acuity and may progress to corneal ulceration and blindness. It is a medical emergency and requires prompt referral to an ophthalmologist. A corneal ulcer begins as a well-defined infiltration at the center or edge of the cornea and subsequently suppurates and forms an ulcer that may penetrate deep into the corneal tissue or spread to involve the width of the cornea. Involvement is usually unilateral. The causative agents include viruses (HSV-1, varicella zoster, hepatitis C), bacteria (*H. influenzae, Moraxella, S. aureus, S. pneumoniae, Pseudomonas, N. gonorrhoeae,* Enterobacteriaceae [including *Klebsiella, Enterobacter, Serratia,* and *Proteus*]), fungi (rare), and protozoa. Less common causes include an allergic reaction, conjunctivitis, systemic infections, toxic chemicals, and the use of corticosteroids. The use of improperly fitted decorative contact lenses, popular with teenagers, has also been implicated; these lenses are often purchased over the counter from outlet stores.

The most common risk factor for keratitis is trauma, which can also result from wearing extended-wear contact lenses or having poor contact lens hygiene. Age (younger than 30 and older than 50 years), sex (males more than females [secondary to increased ocular trauma]), smoking, low socioeconomic status, and vitamin A deficiency are other risk factors.

Clinical Findings

Symptoms vary in intensity according to the depth and extent of ulceration. The following are often reported or seen:
- Exposure to an infected individual
- History of illness, eye trauma, extended contact lens wear, foreign body, or history of recent antibiotic treatment for conjunctivitis that was unresponsive
- White lesions on cornea; occasional corneal opacification
- Vesicles on the skin or eyelids; herpes lesions elsewhere on the body
- Severe pain, sensation of a foreign body ("gritty"), inflamed eye
- Photophobia, tearing, blurred vision, erythema, and spasms of the eyelid
- Area staining green with a fluorescein strip (if herpes, a dendritic ulcer is seen)

Management

When a corneal ulcer is suspected, the child should be referred immediately for a slit-lamp examination 🔍. Delay can result in loss of vision in the eye. Do not attempt to treat. Visual acuity outcome is good when these ulcers are treated aggressively with the appropriate agent.
- Steroids should never be used.
- Treatment with antivirals, such as trifluridine or vidarabine, may speed healing in herpes simplex infections.
- If treatment is delayed, complications include corneal opacification, scarring, and loss of vision.

Inflammation of the Uveal Tract

Inflammation of the uveal tract (iris, ciliary body, choroids) and other ocular structures is often called *uveitis* (Fig 35.10).

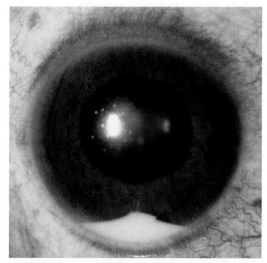

• **Fig 35.10** Uveitis. (From Palay DA, Krachmer JH. *Primary Care Ophthalmology.* 2nd ed. Philadelphia: Mosby; 2005.)

The inflammation may be anterior (affecting the iris, ciliary body, or both) or posterior (affecting the choroid). Adjacent ocular structures can also be involved, including the retina, vitreous, sclera, lens, and optic nerve. The inflammation may be acute or chronic. In the United States, 2% to 13% of patients with uveitis are children; prevalence in children with JIA is 4% to 38% (Wentworth et al., 2014). Many processes have been implicated; they are broadly divided into infectious and noninfectious types. Known etiologies include viral or bacterial infections, ocular trauma, and infection elsewhere in the eye. Other causes include allergy, malignancy, and systemic diseases such as JIA, inflammatory bowel disease, Kawasaki disease, herpes simplex, tuberculosis, Lyme disease, CMV, toxoplasmosis, syphilis, acquired immunodeficiency syndrome (AIDS), ulcerative colitis, rubella retinitis, and Stevens-Johnson syndrome.

Clinical Findings

- Acute onset of pain (key finding)
- Red eye, photophobia, and blurred or decreased vision (key findings)
- Excessive tearing and eyelid edema
- Conjunctival erythema, circumcorneal injection
- Hypopyon (pus layer in the bottom of the anterior chamber)
- Cloudy appearance of the eye with a bulging iris and a contracted, irregular, or fixed pupil
- If chronic, there may be no ocular pain, photophobia, redness, or tearing
- There may be a history of prior viral infection, joint pain, trauma, or gastrointestinal problems

Management

Evaluate and treat any underlying systemic disease. Refer the patient to an ophthalmologist; definitive diagnosis is made by slit-lamp examination. The prognosis is improved with early treatment. Cycloplegics and topical or systemic corticosteroids (depending on the cause of the inflammation) are often used in treatment. Cycloplegic mydriatics are used regularly to prevent posterior synechiae (adhesions of iris to lens and cornea); NSAIDs may be used as adjunctive treatment.

Complications

Anterior and posterior synechiae, changes in IOP, corneal edema, various degrees of visual impairment, papillary scarring, retinal detachment, glaucoma, enucleation, and cataracts are possible complications.

Trachoma

Trachoma is a chronic infectious disease of the eye characterized by follicular keratoconjunctivitis with neovascularization of the cornea. It is contagious—often spread by direct contact with eye, nose, or throat secretions of infected persons; by contact with towels or washcloths contaminated by secretions; or by flies that are attracted to the eyes. Although rare in the United States, trachoma is the second leading cause of blindness in the world, with 7.2 million people having advanced trachoma (Wright et al., 2017). It is caused by one of the two existing *C. trachomatis* biovars and is endemic in Africa, the Middle East, Asia, the Pacific Islands, and among the Aboriginals in Australia. The peak incidence of active infection is in children 4 to 6 years of age, with scarring and blindness occurring in adults.

Clinical Findings

Clinical findings include inflammation, pain, photophobia, excessive tearing, granulation follicles (large white or pale yellow follicles 0.5 to 2 mm in size on the upper tarsal conjunctiva), and, in adults, eventual entropion—inversion of the eyelid leading to corneal trauma, scarring, and blindness. The Simplified World Health Organization (WHO) Trachoma Grading System is used to grade the severity of the infection https://www.who.int/trachoma/diagnosis/en/.

Management

Consult with an ophthalmologist, because trachoma treatment is difficult and recommendations vary. The WHO recommends mass antibiotic treatment within a region when the prevalence of trachoma in children is greater than 10%. Trachoma may be treated with a single dose of azithromycin (20 mg/kg) (AAP, 2015b). Steroids are contraindicated.

Trachoma is spread by close personal contact, so education reinforcing the need for frequent hand washing and careful cleansing of the eyes as well as discouraging sharing of towels and handkerchiefs is important. The WHO and the CDC have set a goal of eliminating trachoma by the year 2020 through a public health campaign known as *S.A.F.E.: Surgery to correct advanced disease, Antibiotics to treat active disease, Facial cleanliness, and Environmental improvements in water and sanitation.*

The Injured Eye

Subconjunctival Hemorrhage

Subconjunctival hemorrhage is seen as a splotchy bulbar conjunctival redness that occurs spontaneously or is secondary to increased intrathoracic pressure (from coughing, sneezing, straining, or trauma) that results in the bursting of conjunctival vessels. It is commonly found in neonates as a benign occurrence after a vaginal delivery. The hemorrhages are painless and usually resolve spontaneously within 2 to 3 weeks. No treatment is indicated unless there is pain, vision loss, or photophobia, which indicate a referral to an ophthalmologist. Spontaneous hemorrhages can (rarely) occur with hypertension, diabetes mellitus, and blood dyscrasias or, if there is a history of trauma, they can be a sign of a ruptured globe (Gardiner and Kloek, 2017).

Eyelid Contusion ("Black Eye")

An eyelid contusion is usually a result of blunt injury to the eye and surrounding tissues. The result is bruising, swelling, and often an impressive appearance ("black eye"). If the child complains of increased pain or swelling, decrease in visual acuity, double vision, flashing lights or "floaters," or develops a bilateral "raccoon eyes" appearance, an ophthalmologic evaluation is needed to rule out a more serious eye injury (e.g., ruptured globe, basilar skull fracture, detached retina, hyphema). All eye structures should be examined before excessive swelling sets in. Treatment consists of elevating the head and intermittent ice compresses for 48 hours (Gardiner, 2017).

Corneal Abrasion

Damage to or loss of the epithelial cells of the cornea in the form of a corneal abrasion or tear is relatively common. Scratches from forceps delivery, paper, brushes, fingernails, contact lens overuse, improperly fitted cosmetic contact lenses, airbag deployment, plants, or foreign body in the conjunctival sac are often responsible.

Clinical Findings

- Evidence and sensation of a foreign body; conjunctival erythema
- Severe pain, photophobia, and decreased vision
- Tearing, blepharospasm
- Disrupted tear film over the corneal epithelium (seen with a penlight)
- Fluorescein staining with superficial uptake indicative of a minor corneal abrasion

If the fluorescein staining goes deeply into the cornea, subepithelial corneal damage (e.g., corneal ulceration or corneal tear) is possible. Vertical striations on the cornea suggest a foreign body embedded under the eyelid.

Management

- Refer severe corneal injuries or possible subepithelial damage to an ophthalmologist.
- Refer those who wear contact lenses and have an abrasion to an ophthalmologist to rule out bacterial corneal infection (a prophylactic topical antibiotic [e.g., gentamicin or ciprofloxacin] may be prescribed in these circumstances to cover *Pseudomonas*).
- If there are no symptoms of corneal infection, topical antibiotics (0.5% erythromycin ointment [preferred as more lubricating] or polymyxin/trimethoprim, ciprofloxacin or ofloxacin drops) four times daily for 3 to 5 days may be prescribed (Jacobs, 2017b). The use of a patch does not improve healing or decrease pain and a poorly applied patch can cause a corneal abrasion. If a patch is used, it should be worn for no longer than 24 hours. An abrasion generally heals in 24 to 48 hours. Advise the patient to return daily for follow-up evaluation or refer him or her for slit-lamp examination within 24 to 36 hours. If the patient is responding, continue the ointment for 2 to 3 days. If no improvement is seen after 24 to 48 hours or if symptoms worsen, the patient should be seen by an ophthalmologist.
- Elbow restraints may be used for an infant to ensure that the eye is not rubbed or further irritated.
- Oral analgesics or ophthalmologic NSAIDs (e.g., ketorolac 0.5%) may be used to ease discomfort. Topical anesthetics should not be used because they are toxic to the epithelium; topical steroids should also be avoided (Jacobs, 2017b).

Foreign Body

A superficial foreign body in the eye is usually lodged on the surface of the eye or superficially in the cornea. It rarely results in serious trauma but may penetrate the globe (may be intraocular), with more serious consequences. Foreign bodies are commonly introduced in younger children during play and in older children during sports; they can include dirt, dust, metallic particles, or alkaline products from the deployment of an airbag.

Clinical Findings

Be sure to inquire into the history to determine whether the individual was working on a metal-on-metal activity. The following may be noted:

- Pain and foreign body sensation, foreign body visible in the conjunctival sac, perforating wound to the cornea or iris
- Tearing, photophobia, inflammation
- Irregular or peaked pupil, opaque lens
  Diagnostic Studies. Fluorescein staining may be useful if no foreign body is visualized. Ultrasonography or CT scan may be needed, depending on the foreign body and its location. An MRI is contraindicated.

Management

- Never remove an intraocular foreign body. In all such instances, refer the patient immediately to an ophthalmologist, particularly if the history indicates the injury was caused by a projectile object or if the patient has had a LASIK procedure.
- View the upper bulbar conjunctiva by having the patient look down while the upper lid is pulled away from the globe and the upper recess is illuminated. Evert the eyelid to visualize the superior tarsal conjunctiva.
- Use of a topical anesthetic facilitates cooperation.
- If an extraocular foreign body is not visualized but suspected, remove it via irrigation with sterile saline or sterile eye solution.
- If the object is visualized, either irrigate or gently lift the object away with a moistened cotton-tipped swab (after instillation of topical anesthetic). The latter technique should be used only with cooperative individuals and for small foreign bodies in order to avoid further trauma to the epithelial surface.
- If any difficulty is encountered, stop all efforts and refer the patient immediately to an ophthalmologist 🌐. Treat with antibiotic ointment (erythromycin four times a day) until seen by an ophthalmologist (Jacobs, 2017b).
- After removing any extraocular object, instill fluorescein stain and inspect the cornea with cobalt-blue light for corneal abrasion; check visual acuity.
- Reschedule the patient in 24 hours or refer to an ophthalmologist for follow-up.
- In the case of an airbag deployment (i.e., talc, cornstarch, and/or baking soda released), irrigate the eyes with sterile saline or sterile eye solution and carefully examine the eyes for further evidence of trauma.

Complications

Sympathetic ophthalmia, chronic siderosis, or a uveitis of the injured eye can occur at any time from 10 days to many years after a penetrating injury of the globe.

Burns

Burns to the eyes and surrounding tissues can be thermal (caused by exposure to steam, flame, intense heat [e.g., touching cornea with a curling iron], cinders, or cigarettes), chemical (e.g., cleaning agents, fertilizers, pesticides, battery fluid, or laboratory products), or induced by UV light (e.g., from bright snow, laser pointers, or a sunlamp). The amount of damage to the eye is directly related to the length of exposure and the nature of the source of the burn (Solano, 2013). Chemical burns are true emergencies because of the progressive damage that can occur. Alkaline solutions are especially damaging. Burns on the eyelids are classified and treated the same as burns elsewhere on the body.

Clinical Findings

- Pale or necrosed appearance of the surrounding skin and eyelids
- Opacity of corneal tissue, swollen corneas
- Visual impairment (decreased acuity)
- Initial exquisite pain or delayed complaints of pain (e.g., in UV burns, pain emerges about 6 hours after exposure)
- Photophobia; tearing within 12 hours of exposure
- Fluorescein stain revealing pinpoint uptake

Management

- Instill a topical anesthetic if available.
- Chemical burns require immediate, ongoing, copious irrigation (Solano, 2013). With the eyelids held apart, instill a steady, gentle solution of tepid water, saline, or Ringer irrigation for 20 to 30 minutes or until the pH of the tear film is 7.3 to 7.7. The pH should be rechecked after 30 minutes to make sure that it maintains this level. Refer to an ophthalmologist after irrigation to determine the extent of the damage. Do not patch the eye; allow tearing to continue to cleanse the eye. Cool compresses applied to the surrounding skin may be comforting. Hospitalization may be needed for sedation and analgesia.
- Thermal burns are often treated as corneal abrasions.
- UV burns are treated by using topical antibiotic prophylaxis, patches, and analgesics. Healing should occur in 1 to 2 days.

Lacerations of the Orbit

Lacerations from injuries cause perforation of the cornea and lead to uveal prolapse. Lacerations may occur on the anterior segment (cornea, anterior chamber, iris, and lens) or posterior segment (sclera, retina, vitreous) of the eye.

Clinical Findings

The clinical findings vary, depending on which segment is involved.

- Anterior segment: irregular pupil (retracted or peaked), iris prolapsed
- Posterior segment: poor red light reflex, decreased vision, black tissue or fluid seen under the conjunctiva

Management

Apply an eye shield (can be made from a cup) to protect the eye. Refer the patient immediately to an ophthalmologist to rule out damage to the globe and surrounding structures.

Traumatic Hyphema

A hyphema is an accumulation of visible blood or blood products in the anterior chamber of the eye and is the result of blunt trauma to the globe without penetration or perforation. This condition is most often caused by balls, fists or fingers, elbows, rocks, exploding airbags, and sticks. High-risk sports associated with hyphema include baseball, hockey, racquetball, and squash, with the stick or racket often responsible for the injury (Andreoli and Gardiner, 2016). It may also occur in infants with birth trauma or in patients with retinoblastoma, abnormal iris vessels (rubeosis), leukemia, juvenile xanthogranuloma of the iris, or abnormal hematologic profiles, such as sickle cell trait or disease, or secondary to child abuse.

Clinical Findings

Vision, pupillary motility, the lids and adnexa, the cornea and anterior segment, and the red light reflex should be assessed. An open globe must be excluded before any examination that would increase IOP (Andreoli and Gardiner, 2016). The following may be noted:

- History of traumatic eye injury; somnolence (associated with intracranial trauma)
- Blood (appearing as a dark red fluid level between the cornea and iris) on gross examination or as a hazy-appearing iris
- Inability to detect a bilateral red light reflex
- Pain, photophobia, and tearing; abnormal pupillary reflex
- Visual acuity changes and impaired vision (light perception and hand motion perception)

Management

The goals of treatment include resolving the hyphema, making the patient comfortable, and preventing complications. There is a risk of recurrent bleeding. The following steps should be taken:

- Refer the patient immediately to an ophthalmologist. A slit-lamp examination is indicated.
- Restrict oral intake until the child has been seen by an ophthalmologist.
- Place a perforated eye shield (not a patch) over the eye; avoid pressure to prevent reinjury.
- If a hematologic disorder is detected, ensure quick intervention and close follow-up.

The following steps are commonly recognized for treatment of a traumatic hyphema:

- Outpatient management is acceptable for those with a small (grade I) hyphemas. Parents should be told to elevate the head of the bed 30 degrees. The child should wear a Fox eye shield. Bed rest with bathroom privileges must be maintained for 5 days; no strenuous activities for 10 days; daily eye examinations required to check for blood staining and IOP.
- Cycloplegic agents may be used (Andreoli and Gardiner, 2018).
- Children who should be hospitalized include those with a grade II or III hyphema, with sickle cell disease, with an increase in IOP, or if there is a question about adherence to outpatient treatment.
- Acetaminophen is the analgesic of choice; avoid aspirin and NSAIDs because they may add to the risk of a rebleed. Sedatives may be necessary in pediatric patients.
- Treat nausea and prevent vomiting.
- Surgery may be necessary to remove trapped blood from the chamber for the following reasons: (1) if it is causing an increase in IOP; (2) in sickle cell patients, to prevent corneal blood staining; (3) if the hyphema remains without some clearing in the first 4 days; or (4) if a clot is pressing against the corneal epithelium.
- After hospital discharge, the child should be followed closely by an ophthalmologist because long-term monitoring is necessary to detect possible traumatic cataract, retinal detachment, or glaucoma.

Complications

A second hemorrhage can occur within 3 to 5 days of the first, increasing the risk of glaucoma, amblyopia, or corneal blood staining, which can result in permanent visual loss. The larger the hyphema, the more likely the child is to rebleed. Patients with abnormal hematologic profiles (e.g., sickle cell) are more likely to have visual loss because of optic atrophy (Andreoli and Gardiner, 2016).

Success in treatment is determined by the recovery of visual acuity. A small grade I hyphema will lead to permanent visual loss (worse than 20/50) in less than 10% of cases. When less than one-third of the anterior chamber is filled with blood, approximately 80% of these patients regain acuity of 20/40 or better. When more than half (but less than total) of the chamber is filled, this same visual acuity is regained in about 60%. However, only 35% of those with total hyphema will have this return in acuity. Patients should be followed by an ophthalmologist due to an elevated risk of developing glaucoma (Andreoli and Gardiner, 2016).

Retinal Detachment

Retinal detachment occurs when the neurosensory retina separates from its retinal pigment epithelium base within the globe. It is rare in children, so suspicion should be high for traumatic causes (e.g., child abuse), a congenital abnormality or syndrome (aphakia, cataracts, Ehlers-Danlos, Stickler, Marfan, Norrie syndromes), or specific disease (ROP, viral retinitis, retinoblastoma, or various retinopathies) (Iqbal and Klein, 2018). Traumatic retinal detachments occur relatively late due to the support of a well-formed vitreous (Wenick and Barañano, 2012). Children who had prior cataract surgery are at increased risk of retinal detachment, with an overall 20-year risk of 7% and a median time of 9.1 years after surgery (Haargaard et al., 2014). There may be concurrent ocular disease or a family history of retinal detachment.

Clinical Findings

- Blurry vision that becomes progressively worse
- Dark cloud in one visual field, flashing lights, or a "shower of floaters"
- Darkening of retinal vessels on funduscopic examination
- Gray elevation at the site of detachment

Management

Instruct the patient not to eat and refer him or her to an ophthalmologist for emergent evaluation.

Orbital Hematoma and Contusion of the Globe

This condition is usually the result of a blow to the globe. The degree of damage depends on the energy of the object hitting the globe. Such injuries commonly occur as a result of sports activities, motor vehicle accidents, assault, BB gun accidents, or airbag deployment.

Clinical Findings

- Milky white appearance of the retina
- Visual acuity changes
- Severe bruising of the eyelids and periorbital tissues
- Lens dislocation, retinal detachment or edema, rupture of the eyeball
- Vitreous, retinal, or choroid hemorrhage

Management

Refer the patient immediately to an ophthalmologist. A closed head injury, damage to the skull, and facial bone fractures must be ruled out via CT scan, MRI, or ultrasound radiography. Occasionally cryopexy or laser photocoagulation surgery is needed for contusions of the globe.

Complications

Possible complications include permanent visual loss, retinal necrosis, subretinal hemorrhage, and retinal or macular holes.

Orbital Fractures

An orbital fracture is a fracture of the walls of the orbit secondary to blunt trauma to the orbital rim or eyes. Orbital fractures are most common among adolescent and young adult males (Neuman and Bachur, 2017). The orbital floor is thin and subject to fracture. The inferior rectus muscle may become caught in the fracture site. The usual cause of an orbital fracture is a blow or blunt trauma to the orbit (e.g., ball, fist, motor vehicle accident [hitting the dashboard], or fall).

Clinical Findings

- Pain, numbness below the orbit; trouble chewing; nosebleed
- Diplopia, irregular pupil, limited ocular movement (especially upward)
- Corneal laceration, hyphema, and/or absent red light reflex
- Globe displacement (sunken or protruding) or enophthalmos (recession of the eyeball within the orbit)
- Bony discontinuity or "step-off"
- Ecchymosis of the lids; subcutaneous emphysema in surrounding tissues, and edema

Diagnostic Studies. Plain film radiography and CT scan are the best imaging modalities. A CT is preformed if the patient has evidence of fracture upon examination, limited extraocular motility, decreased visual acuity, pain, or if the examiner is unable to perform an accurate examination (Neuman and Bachur, 2017).

Management

- An orbital fracture is an ophthalmologic emergency requiring immediate intervention and referral. Diagnostic studies are performed to rule out injury to the skull and cranial contents. Open reduction may be necessary if any of the orbital bones are displaced or to rule out displacement of the globe or enophthalmos.
- Ice the injury for 48 hours and have the patient sleep with the head of bed elevated (Neuman and Bachur, 2017). Antibiotic prophylaxis to cover nasal pathogens is recommended if the patient has an orbital fracture into the sinus.
- Nasal decongestants may also be used to reduce nose blowing and sniffling.

Deformities of the Eyelids

Entropion

Entropion is a condition in which the eyelids invert so that the cilia or epithelium rubs against the corneal surface, causing abrasion or irritation. The upper and lower eyelids may be involved. There is a rare congenital form. Pain or irritation and photophobia are typical symptoms. Examination reveals evidence of lid laxity. Management involves surgical intervention and referral to an ophthalmologist (Weber, Chundury, and Perry, 2017). Complications include corneal scarring and corneal infections.

Ectropion

Ectropion is a rare condition in which the eyelid margins evert. The condition may be congenital; seen after infection; or secondary to scarring after trauma, radiation, or prior surgery. It can be confused with euryblepharon. Management involves lubrication for mild cases; surgery is indicated for chronic or symptomatic cases. The patient should be referred to an ophthalmologist for management (Billiveau, 2017).

Euryblepharon

Euryblepharon appears as a wide palpebral fissure with the appearance of a sagging half of the lower eyelid (temporal side) or a pulling away of the lid from the orbit. It can have a genetic etiology (e.g., Down syndrome), be associated with other ocular anomalies (e.g., congenital cleft lip, strabismus, congenital ptosis), or be seen in association with nonocular anomalies (e.g., hypospadias, inguinal hernias, dental anomalies). It is often confused with ectropion. It is usually a mild cosmetic condition that the child may outgrow. No treatment is indicated unless chronic tearing or exposure keratitis occurs; in such cases, reconstruction can be done.

Pterygium

A pterygium is a fibrovascular mass of thickened bulbar conjunctiva that extends beyond the limbus onto the cornea. Elastic and hyaline degenerative changes occur. The lesion is usually triangular and more commonly found on the nasal side of the orbit. It is caused by irritation of the bulbar conjunctiva from sunlight, wind, dust, fumes, or airborne allergens; it can also be hereditary. Growth rates of the lesions vary. A pinguecula may precede the pterygium, which occurs as a yellow-white, slightly raised mass on the bulbar conjunctiva. The lesion is usually painless, may itch, and may be accompanied by occasional complaints of blurred vision if the lesion enlarges (Jacob, 2018).

Because a pterygium is uncommon in children, the clinician must consider other causes: papillomas, dermoids, keratoacanthomas, an epithelial inclusion or a dermoid cyst, or a rare malignancy (Caldwell et al., 2017). Treatment involves protecting against irritants (use of goggles, sunglasses, or topical lubricants such as artificial tears) and using mild vasoconstrictors or short-term steroids for inflammation. Surgical removal may be needed if the pterygium impedes vision. Recurrence after surgical removal, restricted ocular mobility (especially with abduction), and diplopia may be complications. Because exposure to UV light is a risk factor for the development of pterygium, children should wear sunglasses and a hat to protect their eyes from exposure to UV light (Jacobs, 2018).

Visual Impairment

Visual impairment affects an individual's ability to engage in the activities of everyday life. It may be congenital or acquired; however, visual memory is retained in the latter case. The impact of the visual impairment is tied to the onset, severity, and type of visual loss as well as to any coexisting conditions. A number of other vision problems may also affect visual functioning, including sensitivity to light or glare, blind spots in visual fields, or problems with contrast or certain colors. Factors such as lighting, the environment, fatigue, and emotional status also affect visual functioning.

Vision impairment is defined as having vision that is 20/40 or worse in the better eye even with eyeglasses. *Partial or low vision* is defined as best corrected visual acuity between 20/70 and 20/200, whereas *legal blindness* is distant visual acuity of 20/200 in the better eye or a visual field that includes an angle not greater than 20 degrees. *Amaurosis* is the medical term for partial or total loss of vision.

More than half of the children with significant loss of vision have comorbid chronic or neurologic conditions. Congenital cataracts, congenital glaucoma, high refractive errors, ROP, detached retina, neurologic conditions involving CN II, cortical blindness, and optic atrophy are causative factors, as are retinoblastoma, trauma, infection, hydrocephaly, and genetic conditions. There is an increased risk for low-birth-weight, small-for-gestational age, and large-for-gestational age babies.

According to the WHO, the number of blind children in the world is approximately 1.4 million; however, prevalence varies according to socioeconomic development and mortality rates in children under 5 years of age. In low-income countries with high under-5 mortality rates, the prevalence is about 1.5 per 1000 children, whereas in high-income countries with low under-5 mortality rates, it is about 0.3 per 1000. Approximately three-quarters of the world's blind children live in the poorest regions of Africa and Asia.

The major causes of blindness in children around the world are determined by socioeconomic development and the availability of primary healthcare and eye care services. Approximately half of these children have underlying causes that could have been prevented or eye conditions that could have been treated to preserve vision. All countries deal with cataracts, glaucoma, congenital abnormalities, and hereditary retinal dystrophies. In high-income countries, lesions of the optic nerve and higher visual pathways are most common; in middle-income countries, ROP is the most common; and in low-income countries, corneal scarring from measles, vitamin A deficiency, the use of harmful traditional eye remedies, and ophthalmia neonatorum are most common.

Clinical Findings and Developmental and Behavioral Effects

The age at which vision is lost is important because children with even a brief experience of vision perceive the environment as a place of varying dimensions. Loss of vision interferes with social interactions and may delay bonding. Gross and fine motor functions, balance and spatial concepts, language and learning, and sleep are all impaired. Children with visual impairment plus other handicapping conditions have even greater developmental delays.

Assessment

Important assessment components include the prenatal and birth history, especially prematurity with diagnosis of ROP; family history of genetic visual impairments; developmental history (attachment, midline play, reaching, gross motor skills, language skills); and sleep patterns. It is wise to pay close attention to parental concerns about a child's vision because the parents may note concerns that could otherwise be missed. Hearing screening and routine developmental assessment are important in order to maximize other aspects of the visually impaired child's life.

Providing special cues for these children helps them to understand their environment and what is going on around them. Talking softly, warning before gently touching, and paying attention to body cues rather than visual or facial signals are helpful. For older children, the following tactics are helpful:

- Address the child by name
- Describe what you plan to do and how, warning the child prior to any hands on exam or intervention
- Let the child touch or examine instruments

Management

The child with visual impairment should be in a healthcare home and the PCP is ideal to serve as case manager, ensuring that all team members and needed pieces are in place for the best care. The interprofessional team should include the PCP, ophthalmologist, special certification teacher, and orientation and mobility specialist. Once a vision problem is diagnosed, the next step should be a low vision examination focused on function in order to determine appropriate interventions. The PCP can play a vital role in providing emotional support and help to parents, encouraging discussion of development, assessing the effect on siblings, and helping the family with developmental transitions, such as beginning school, adolescence, and independent living. Additionally, providing information about relevant parent support groups and national/local organizations, sharing knowledge related to school-based and community resources and eligibility requirements for special services, and communicating regularly with the specialists can be key roles.

From an information-processing perspective, much of the management of the visually impaired child is directed at providing stimuli that the child can use to understand and interact with the environment. Communication is less affected than adaptive motor skills, and language serves as a main bridge toward helping children to understand the world they live in. Sensory compensation is not automatic but must be developed and taught. For example, parents may find that smiles in infants are muted or fleeting, so they must identify other cues that their baby wants and needs them, such as reaching out to touch.

Habilitation and Assistive Devices. Sleep patterns are likely to be disturbed because visually impaired children take longer to get to sleep and have longer and more frequent night awakenings than their normally sighted peers. Many visually impaired children benefit from taking melatonin at bedtime. Difficulty with daily living skills may include dressing, eating, hygiene, use of the telephone, and the handling of money. An orientation and mobility specialist can teach the visually handicapped child to travel with a sighted guide, use a cane, and use public transportation. Physical education and fitness are as important to visually impaired children as they are to other children. Generally individual sports, such as gymnastics and swimming, are more successful endeavors for a blind child than team sports, even if the child is partially sighted. The Special Olympics and Junior Blind Olympic organizations hold competitions for the visually impaired in an array of sports activities.

A variety of technologic devices are available for children with visual impairment with the goal of improving function through the use of devices and/or adaptive skills. Glasses, high-powered spectacles or handheld magnifiers, a telescope, or a spectacle-mounted telescope may be used to assist with low vision. Special optical devices, Braille devices, low vision devices, phone accessibility, screen readers and magnifiers, voice synthesizers, reading systems, digital books, and mobility devices are some options. The internet provides easy access to many different options. For children who have visual and hearing loss, the National Deaf-Blind Equipment Distribution Program provides great alternatives.

Educational System. Early intervention for children with visual impairment should be implemented with an appropriate Individual Family Service Plan (IFSP) or Individual Educational Plan (IEP) 504 educational plan in place as appropriate to ensure proper educational services as soon as possible after a child is identified. Infant early education and developmental preschool programs are essential, and an IFSP with parent involvement provides the structure for this. When children are ready to enter elementary school, specific psychologic assessments for visually impaired children should be completed to ensure correct educational placement and appropriate educational support systems. From this, the IEP or 504 plan is developed and reviewed annually, with input from parents and school officials.

Educational programs for visually handicapped children may include some of the following components: Children with peripheral losses may have to be taught to scan with the head and eyes to gain more awareness of the environment. Accommodations may include a preferred seat in class or supplying larger print materials. Both parents and teachers may have to be educated to expect and encourage the child to hold reading materials close enough to see them. Learning to read Braille begins when sighted children learn to read, and learning to write Braille involves learning to use a special keyboard in the early elementary grades. By fourth grade, visually impaired children should also learn to use a regular keyboard. Developing additional listening skills and gaining proficiency in the use of computers with aids are also essential skills. Full-time classes for visually impaired children may be available and taught by teachers with special certification—these are teachers of visually impaired (TVIs). Some schools have resource room programs in which the child spends part of the day with a specially trained teacher and the remainder of the day in a regular classroom. Some school districts provide itinerant programs in which a specially trained teacher works with several teachers in regular classrooms, consulting with them about the learning needs of the visually impaired children. An orientation and mobility specialist can be used to help the child learn to navigate independently. Schools for the blind are generally reserved for children with multiple handicaps.

Family Support. As with other disabling conditions, parents want to be told as soon as possible about their child's visual impairment, and they want not only the diagnosis but also resources and direction about where to get more information. Because visual cues are so important in language and social interactions, there may be difficulties with attachment resulting from failure of eye contact and facial expressiveness. Families of children with visual impairment benefit from education and specialized anticipatory guidance designed to facilitate development throughout childhood. Families learn to adapt in a variety of ways. Parent support groups are valuable, and national organizations provide helpful resources. Some families also benefit from counseling.

Additional Resources

American Academy of Ophthalmology.
www.aao.org

American Association for Pediatric Ophthalmology and Strabismus.
www.aapos.org

Grajewski Lyra (GL) Foundation for Children with Glaucoma.
www.gl-foundation.org

InfantSEE.
www.infantsee.org

National Center for Children's Vision and Eye Health.
http://nationalcenter.preventblindness.org/

National Eye Institute.
www.nei.nih.gov

Prevent Blindness.
www.preventblindness.org

References

AAP, AAPOS, AACO and AAO Hoskins Center for Quality Eye Care. *Joint Statement: learning disabilities, dyslexia, and vision—reaffirmed*; 2014. https://www.aao.org/clinical-statement/joint-statement-learning-disabilities-dyslexia-vis. Accessed February 23, 2018.

Alsuhaibani, A, Burkat, CN, Stelzner, SK, Marcet, MM. Blepharoptosis. *EyeWiki. (website)*; *American Academy of Ophthalmology.* http://eyewiki.org/Blepharoptosis. Accessed March 3, 2018

American Academy of Ophthalmology (AAO). *Protective eyewear for young athletes—2013, ONE Network. (website)*; 2013b. Available https://www.aao.org/clinical-statement/protective-eyewear-young-athletes. Accessed February 23, 2018.

American Academy of Ophthalmology (AAO). *Pediatric Eye Evaluations Preferred Practice Pattern*; 2017a. Retrieved from https://www.aao.org/preferred-practice-pattern/pediatric-eye-evaluations-ppp-2017.

American Academy of Ophthalmology (AAO). Refractive errors and refractive surgery PPP—2017. *Ophthalmol.* 2017b;125(1):P1-P104. Retrieved from http://www.aaojournal.org/article/S0161-6420(17)33028-2/fulltext.

American Academy of Ophthalmology (AAO). *Amblyopia Preferred Practice Pattern*; 2017c. Retrieved from https://www.aao.org/preferred-practice-pattern/amblyopia-ppp-2017. Accessed February 23, 2018.

American Academy of Pediatrics. Chlamydia trachomatis. In: Kimberlin DW, Brady MT, Jackson MA, Long SS, eds. Red Book: 2015 Report of the Committee on Infectious Diseases. *American Academy of Pediatrics.* 2015a:288–294.

American Academy of Pediatrics. Gonococcal Infections. In: Kimberlin DW, Brady MT, Jackson MA, Long SS, eds. Red Book: 2015 Report of the Committee on Infectious Diseases. *American Academy of Pediatrics.* 2015b:356–367.

American Academy of Pediatrics. Nongonococcal, Nonchlamydia Ophthalmia. In: Kimberlin DW, Brady MT, Jackson MA, Long SS, eds. Red Book: 2015 Report of the Committee on Infectious Diseases. *American Academy of Pediatrics.* 2015c:974.

American Academy of Pediatrics (AAP), American Association of Certified Orthoptists (AACO), American Association for Pediatric Ophthalmology and Strabismus (AAPOS), American Academy of Ophthalmology (AAO). Visual system assessment in infants, children and young adults by pediatricians. *Pediatrics.* 2016;137(1):28–30. https://doi.org/10.1542/peds.2015-3596. Retrieved from http://pediatrics.aappublications.org/content/137/1/e20153596.

American Association for Pediatric Ophthalmology and Strabismus (AAPOS). *Computer Vision Syndrome in Children, AAPOS. (website)*; 2017a. Available at https://aapos.org//client_data/files/2017/608_computervisionsyndromeandchildren.pdf. Accessed February 23, 2018.

American Association for Pediatric Ophthalmology and Strabismus (AAPOS). *Cataract, AAPOS. (website)*; 2017b. Available at www.aapos.org/terms/conditions/31. Accessed March 3, 2018.

American Association of Pediatric Ophthalmology and Strabismus (AAPOS). *Vision Screening Recommendations, AAPOS. (website)*; 2014a. Available at www.aapos.org/terms/show/131. Accessed February 22, 2018.

American Association for Pediatric Ophthalmology and Strabismus (AAPOS). *Glaucoma for Children, AAPOS. (website)*; 2014b. Available at www.aapos.org/terms/conditions/55. March 3, 2018.

American Association for Pediatric Ophthalmology and Strabismus (AAPOS). *Nystagmus, AAPOS. (website)*; 2016. Available at www.aapos.org/terms/conditions/80. Accessed March 3, 2018.

American Association for Pediatric Ophthalmology and Strabismus (AAPOS). *Retinoblastoma, AAPOS. (website)*; 2016. Available at www.aapos.org/terms/conditions/93. Accessed March 4, 2018.

American Association of Pediatric Ophthalmology and Strabismus (AAPOS). AAPOS policy statement: Medically necessary eye examinations for children who have failed vision screening. *AAPOS. (website)*; 2017a. https://aapos.org//client_data/files/2017/328_510_medically_necessary_eye_examinations.pdf.

American Optometric Association (AOA). *Sunglasses Shopping Guide, AOA. (website)*; 2018a. Available at https://www.aoa.org/patients-and-public/caring-for-your-vision/uv-protection/sunglasses-shopping-guide. Accessed February 28, 2018.

American Optometric Association (AOA). *Computer vision syndrome, AOA. (website)*; 2018b. Available at www.aoa.org/patients-and-public/caring-for-your-vision/protecting-your-vision/computer-vision-syndrome?sso=y. Accessed February 23, 2018.

Andreoli CM, Gardiner MF. Traumatic hyphema: clinical features and management. *UpToDate. (website)*; 2016. Available at www.uptodate.com/contents/traumatic-hyphema-clinical-features-and-management. Accessed March 4, 2018.

Bullimore M. The safety of soft contact lenses in children. *Optom Vis Sci.* 2017;94(6):636–646. Retrieved from https://journals.lww.com/optvissci/Fulltext/2017/06000/The_Safety_of_Soft_Contact_Lenses_in_Children.2.aspx.

Caldwell, M. Hirst, L Woodward, MA. Pterygium. EyeWiki. *(website) American Academy of Ophthalmology.* http://eyewiki.org/Pterygium. Accessed March 4, 2018.

Centers for Disease Control and Prevention (CDC). *Healthy contact lens wear and care: children and contact lenses. (website)*; 2015. https://www.cdc.gov/contactlenses/children-and-contact-lenses.html. Accessed February 23, 2018.

Choe C, O'Brien JM, Miller AM, et al. Retinoblastoma. *EyeWiki. (website). Am Acad Ophthalmol*; 2017. http://eyewiki.org/Retinoblastoma. Accessed March 3, 2018.

Clark RA. Glaucoma, Congenital or Infantile. *EyeWiki. (website). Am Acade Ophthalmol*; 2017. http://eyewiki.org/Glaucoma,_Congenital_Or_Infantile. Accessed March 3, 2018.

Coats DK. Retinopathy of prematurity: treatment and prognosis. *UpToDate. (website)*; 2018. Available at www.uptodate.com/contents/retinopathy-of-prematurity-treatment-and-prognosis. Accessed March 3, 2018.

Coats DK, Paysse EA. Evaluation and management of strabismus in children. *UpToDate. (website)*; 2018. Available at www.uptodate.com/contents/evaluation-and-management-of-strabismus-in-children. Accessed March 3, 2018.

DeSantis D. Amblyopia. *Pediatr Clin North Am.* 2014;61(3):505–518.

Gappy C, Archer S, Barza M. Preseptal cellulitis. *UpToDate. (website)*; 2017. Available at www.uptodate.com/contents/preseptal-cellulitis. Accessed March 4, 2018.

Gardiner, MF, Kloek, CE. Conjunctival injury. *UpToDate. (website)*; www.uptodate.com/contents/conjunctival-injury. Accessed March 4, 2018.

Haargaard B, Andersen EW, Oudin A, et al. Risk of retinal detachment after pediatric cataract surgery. *Invest Ophthalmol Vis Sci.* 2014;55(5):2947–2951.

Hamra P, Dana R. Allergic conjunctivitis: clinical manifestations and diagnosis. *UpToDate. (website)*; 2017. www.uptodate.com/contents/allergic-conjunctivitis-clinical-manifestations-and-diagnosis. Accessed March 3, 2018.

Heidar K. Cataracts in children, congenital and acquired. *EyeWiki. (website). Ame Acade Ophthalmol*; 2017. http://eyewiki.org/Cataracts_in_Children,_Congenital_and_Acquired. Accessed March 3, 2018.

Heidar K, Miller AM, Stevenson E, Epley KD, Pihlblad MS. Retinopathy of prematurity. *EyeWiki. (website). Am Acad Ophthalmol*; 2018. http://eyewiki.org/Retinopathy_of_Prematurity. Accessed March 3, 2018.

Iqbal S, Klein BL. *Approach to acute vision loss in children. UpToDate*; 2018. Available at www.uptodate.com/contents/approach-to-acute-vision-loss-in-children. Accessed March 4, 2018.

Jacobs DS. Conjunctivitis. *UpToDate. (website)*; 2017a. Available at www.uptodate.com/contents/conjunctivitis. Accessed March 3, 2018.

Jacobs DS. *Corneal abrasions and corneal foreign bodies: management. UpToDate. (website)*; 2017b. Available at www.uptodate.com/contents/corneal-abrasions-and-corneal-foreign-bodies-management. Accessed March 4, 2018.

Jacobs DS. *Pterygium. UpToDate. (website)*. 2018. Available at www.uptodate.com/contents/pterygium. Accessed March 4, 2018.

Jordan CO. Retinopathy of prematurity. *Pediatric Clinics of North Am.* 2014;61(3):567–577.

Kaufman PL, Kim J, Berry JL. Retinoblastoma: Treatment and outcome. *UpToDate. (website)*; 2017. www.uptodate.com/contents/retinoblastoma-treatment-and-outcome. Accessed March 3, 2018.

Kelechava B. ANSI Z80.3—Sunglasses Requirements. *American National Standards Institute*; 2016. https://blog.ansi.org/2016/05/ansi-z803-sunglasses-requirements/#gref. Accessed February 23, 2018.

Kim J, Konda S. Nystagmus. EyeWiki. *Am Acad Ophthalmol*; 2018. http://eyewiki.org/Nystagmus. Accessed March 3, 2018.

Lopez Montero, MC. EyeWiki. American Academy of Ophthalmology. Available at: http://eyewiki.org/Conjunctivitis. Accessed March 3, 2018

Neuman MI, Bachur RG. Orbital fractures. *UpToDate. (website)*; 2017. Available at www.uptodate.com/contents/orbital-fractures. Accessed March 4, 2018.

Naru J, Aggarwal R, Singh U, Kakkar N, Bansal D. HPV-16 detected in one-fourth eyes with retinoblastoma: a prospective case-control study from North India. *J Pediatr Hematol Oncol. [serial online]*. 2016;38(5):367–371. Available from: MEDLINE, Ipswich, MA. Accessed March 3, 2018.

Örge FH, Boente CS. The lacrimal system. *Pediatr Clin North Am.* 2014;61(3):529–539.

Paysse EA, Coats DK. Congenital nasolacrimal duct obstruction (dacryostenosis) and dacryocystocele. *UpToDate. (website)*; 2017. Available at www.uptodate.com/contents/congenital-nasolacrimal-duct-obstruction-dacryostenosis-and-dacryocystocele. Accessed March 4, 2018.

Prevent Blindness. *Choosing UV Protection, Prevent Blindness. (website)*; 2018b. Available at www.preventblindness.org/choosing-uv-protection. Accessed February 23, 2018.

Prevent Blindness. *Protect Your Child from Eye Injuries, Prevent Blindness. (website)*; 2018a. Available at www.preventblindness.org/protect-your-child-eye-injuries. Accessed February 23, 2018.

Schliesser J, Sprunger D, Helveston E. Strabismus: Infantile Esotropia. *American Academy of Ophthalmology. (website)*; 2016. https://www.aao.org/disease-review/strabismus-infantile-esotropia. Accessed March 3, 2018.

Shetty OA, Naresh KN, Banavali SD, et al. Evidence for the presence of high risk human papillomavirus in retinoblastoma tissue from nonfamilial retinoblastoma in developing countries. *Pediatr Blood Cancer.* 2012;58(2):185–190.

Shtein RM. Blepharitis. *UpToDate. (website)*; 2017. Available at www.uptodate.com/contents/blepharitis. Accessed March 3, 2018.

Skalet AH, Gombos DS, Gallie BL, et al. Screening children at risk for retinoblastoma. *Ophthalmol.* 2018;125(3):453–458. Retrieved from http://www.aaojournal.org/article/S0161-6420(17)31784-0/fulltext#sec1.1. Accessed March 3, 2018.

Solano J. Ocular burns. *Medscape. (website)*; 2013. Available at http://emedicine.medscape.com/article/798696-overview. Accessed March 4, 2018.

Stewart A. Infant aphakia: putting study results into practice. *AAO. EyeNet Magazine*; 2017. Retrieved from https://www.aao.org/eyenet/article/infant-aphakia-putting-study-results-into-practice.

U.S. Department of Health and Human Services (HHS). Office of Disease Prevention and Health Promotion: 2020 topics & objectives: vision. *HealthPeople.gov. (website)*; 2014. Available at www.healthypeople.gov/2020/topics-objectives/topic/vision/objectives. Accessed March 7, 2018.

U.S. Food and Drug Administration (FDA). Important information for laser pointer manufactures. *FDA. (website)*; Retrieved from https://www.fda.gov/Radiation-EmittingProducts/RadiationEmittingProductsandProcedures/HomeBusinessandEntertainment/LaserProductsandInstruments/ucm116373.htm. Accessed March 7, 2018

U.S. National Library of Medicine (NLM). Retinoblastoma, Genetics Home Reference. *(website)*; 2018. Available at http://ghr.nlm.nih.gov/condition/retinoblastoma. Accessed March 3, 2018.

U.S. National Library of Medicine (NLM). Color Vision Deficiency, Genetics Home Reference. *(website)*; 2018. Available at http://ghr.nlm.nih.gov/condition/color-vision-deficiency. Accessed March 3, 2018.

U.S. Preventive Services Task Force. Vision screening in children aged 6 months to 5 years: US Preventive Services Task Force Recommendation Statement. *JAMA.* 2017;318(9):836–844. https://doi.org/10.1001/jama.2017.11260. Retrieved from https://jamanetwork.com/journals/jama/fullarticle/2652657. Accessed March 7, 2018.

Weber AC, Chundury RV, Perry JD. Entropion. *EyeWiki. (website). American Academy of Ophthalmology.* http://eyewiki.org/Entropion. Accessed March 4, 2018

Wenick AS, Barañano DE. Evaluation and management of pediatric rhegmatogenous retinal detachment. *Saudi J Ophthalmol.* 2012;26(3):255–263.

Wentworth BA, Freitas-Neto CA, Foster CS. Management of pediatric uveitis. *F1000Prime Rep.* 2014;6(41). http://f1000.com/prime/reports/m/6/41. Accessed March 4, 2018.

Wright HR, Taylor HR. O'Kearney, E. Overview of trachoma. *UpToDate. (website)*; 2017. Available at www.uptodate.com/contents/overview-of-trachoma. Accessed March 4, 2018.

36

Ear and Hearing Disorders

ADEBOLA M. OLAREWAJU

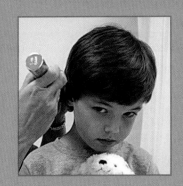

The ear serves two functions—hearing and equilibrium. Malfunction of any of the ear structures can impact the external or internal ear, as well as the surrounding tissues. Additionally, ear dysfunction can cause global developmental delays with lifelong effects. Adequate hearing is important for speech and language acquisition, academic performance, and socialization. Pediatric primary care providers (PCPs) must have an understanding of normal ear anatomy and physiology and be able to identify, assess, and diagnose ear disorders in children. The acute and chronic management of ear disorders is also discussed in this chapter.

Embryonic Development

Ear development begins during the third week of gestation and is complete by the third month of embryonic life. Insult to the fetus during this time can cause irreparable damage to the ear and negatively affect hearing. Because ear development occurs at the same time as kidney development, malformation or dysfunction in one system should alert the health care provider to look for problems in the other.

Anatomy and Physiology

The ear has three main structures: the external ear, middle ear, and inner ear.

The external ear consists of the pinna (or auricle), the auditory canal, and the tympanic membrane (TM). The external ear transmits sound waves from outside the ear to the middle ear and requires patency of the external auditory canal (EAC). The canal contains glands that secrete sweat, sebum, and cerumen that help lubricate the hair follicles and aid in debris removal. The ear canal starts at the outer ear, stops at the TM, and moves sound waves from the pinna to the TM at the proximal end of the EAC. The TM separates the external ear from the middle ear.

The middle ear consists of the structures between the TM and the oval window and includes the ossicles, oval window, round window, and eustachian tube. The ossicles—the malleus, incus, and stapes—transmit sound waves from the EAC to the inner ear. The malleus lies against the TM and the stapes rests against the oval window. Vibrations across the TM, ossicles, and oval window cause the fluids of the inner ear to stimulate the cochlea resulting in sound perception.

The eustachian tube links the middle ear with the posterior aspect of the palate and the function of the eustachian tube is to: (1) ventilate the middle ear to equalize middle ear pressure with atmospheric pressure and (2) drain secretions from the middle ear into the nasopharynx.

The inner ear functions to transmit sound and aid balance. The sound waves that reach the cochlea are transmitted by the organ of Corti to the auditory nerve (cranial nerve VIII) and then the auditory cortex of the brain's temporal lobe. There are equilibrium receptors in the semicircular canals and vestibule of the inner ear that respond to changes in movement direction and help maintain equilibrium.

Pathophysiology

Defense Mechanisms

The processes that negatively affect the ear are usually localized; however, pathologic ear conditions can be related to systemic dysfunction or disorders. Common localized pathologic conditions include viral, bacterial, or fungal infections; foreign bodies; and trauma. Neurologic dysfunction, poor immunologic competence, and congenital anomalies can affect the ear and its function. Debris produced by keratinizing cells in the ear form *cerumen,* or "ear wax," which is lubricated and extruded by the cilia in the EAC. Normally, an acidic pH in the ear canal prevents the growth of pathogenic bacteria. Additionally, the surface lining of the external ear is water resistant and has ample blood and lymph supplies. These characteristics and the antibacterial properties of cerumen help protect against invading microorganisms.

The proximal end of the EAC has more nerve fibers, which cause discomfort when touched; this serves a protective function by deterring the insertion of foreign bodies into the ear, thus preventing damage to the middle ear. The structures for both hearing and equilibrium are deep within the skull and provide additional protection to the inner ear. External influences, such as excessive environmental noise, can cause irreparable damage to the hearing structures.

Assessment of the Ear

Clinical Findings

History
The health history of a child presenting with ear symptoms or an ear disorder should include:
- Pain (onset, location, quality, duration, alleviating or aggravating factors)
- Associated symptoms (e.g., fever, upper respiratory infection, cough symptoms)
- Itching or discharge

• BOX 36.1   Red Flags for Hearing Loss

Infancy
- Does not startle at loud noises
- Does not turn to the source of a sound after 6 months of age
- Does not say single words, such as "dada" or "mama" by 1 year of age
- Turns head when he or she sees you but not just to voice
- Seems to hear some sounds but not others

Childhood
- Delayed or unclear speech
- Difficulty following instructions
- Teacher concerns about paying attention
- Often saying "Huh?" or "What?"
- Turning the volume on television or radio up very high

- Exposure to risk factors for ear infection: Environmental tobacco smoke (ETS), bottle propping, pacifier use, child care attendance, swimming
- Ear conditions (e.g., effusion in middle ear, otitis media, trauma)
- History of meningitis due to prevalence of associated hearing loss
- Tinnitus or hearing loss (see Box 36.1 for Red Flags of Hearing Loss)
- Craniofacial abnormalities (e.g., cleft palate) or syndromes associated with craniofacial anomalies (e.g., Down syndrome or 22q11 deletion syndromes)
- Family history of ear dysfunction or history of kidney malformation
- Prematurity
- Developmental milestones for speech and hearing-impaired children (Table 36.1).

Physical Examination

The physical examination includes the following:
- Start with visual inspection of the ear without an otoscope. Inspect the external ear structures for symmetry, ear shape (presence of helix, antihelix, fully formed pinna), skin abnormalities (ear pits or tags), or discharge. The inner and outer canthi of the eye should form a straight line with the superior portion of the pinna. If the pinna inserts below this line, the ear is considered low-set, which can be associated with genetic syndromes. Assess for preauricular ear pits and auricular skin tags, which can be an isolated finding or associated with hearing loss, renal disorders, and genetic syndromes (e.g., Branchio-oto-renal syndrome).
- Palpate the external ear and the mastoid process for tenderness and inflammation.
- Otoscopic examination is best accomplished in a young child at the end of the physical examination with the child seated on the parent's lap or examination table for older children. Pull the helix of the ear downward, outward, and backward to enhance visualization of the EAC and TM in infants and small children. In older children and adolescents, lift the ear upward and backward, slightly away from the head. Examine the EAC for redness, edema, or discharge. Assess the entire TM surface, the bony processes, and the cone of light (Fig 36.1). Look for air-fluid level or bubbles behind the TM. Note any retraction, bulging, perforation, fibrosis, redness, or other color alteration.
- Assess TM mobility using pneumatic otoscopy.

TABLE 36.1   Developmental Milestones for Hearing-Impaired Children

	Developmental Milestones
Infants (0-1 year)	Sensorimotor stage is normal Language development: Deaf children exposed early to sign language develop language similarly to hearing children exposed to spoken language. Deaf children exposed to both spoken and sign language learn both and progress as hearing children. Deaf children exposed only to spoken language have language delays. Language output is decreased around 6-9 months old.
Toddlers (12 months-2 years)	Sensorimotor stage is normal Language output decreased
Preschoolers (3-5 years)	May have early processing delays Symbolic play may be delayed if language skills are decreased
School-age (6-12 years)	May have concrete processing delays Decreased self-concept
Adolescents (13-19 years)	Increased adjustment problems and decreased social maturity Decreased self-concept May have formal processing delays

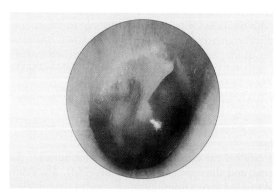

• **Fig 36.1** Normal Tympanic Membrane. (Photograph courtesy Sylvan Stool, MD, The Children's Hospital, Denver, CO.)

Cerumen Removal

The removal of impacted cerumen is essential when it impedes ear examination or alters hearing. This can be accomplished by mechanical removal or by cerumenolytics with or without irrigation. Infants or young children may need to be swaddled during manual cerumen removal. Movement during manual extraction can cause injury to the external canal, so proper restraint is essential during the procedure. The best results occur with water ear irrigation following the instillation of a cerumenolytic agent. Common cerumenolytics include docusate sodium or mineral oil. Irrigation is accomplished by using a bulb syringe, ear irrigation bottle, or "water jet" (on low setting). Water-based cerumenolytics disintegrate the wax, whereas oil-based products soften the wax. Irrigation should not be attempted if there is suspected TM perforation or patent pressure-equalizing tubes. Providers and parents typically prefer the irrigation technique over manual removal of cerumen (Loveman et al., 2011).

Mechanical cerumen removal requires skill and special instrumentation. Blunt plastic ear curettes may be less traumatic than the metal variety. Always carefully explain the procedure to parents and inform them that the ear canal is extremely sensitive and fragile and bleeds easily when touched. This may prevent an adverse parent reaction when there is blood on the curette or in the ear canal. For children with chronic cerumen impactions that affects hearing, routine otic drops containing carbamide peroxide may be needed to keep the EACs clear of cerumen.

Standards for Hearing Screening

All infants should receive hearing screening before 1 month of age. Any infant with abnormal findings should be referred for additional evaluation and early intervention. Children identified with hearing loss through newborn screening have earlier referral, diagnosis, and management than those identified later in infancy or early childhood (Pimperton et al., 2016). The National Center for Hearing Assessment and Management (NCHAM) reports that the detection and treatment of hearing loss at birth saves $400,000 in special education costs by the time the child finishes high school (NCHAM, 2011). Infants who pass newborn screening but have other risk factors for hearing loss should have at least one diagnostic audiology assessment by 24 to 30 months of age (AAP, The Joint Committee on Infant Hearing, 2007).

In addition to newborn hearing screening, the American Academy of Pediatrics (AAP) Bright Futures guidelines recommend pure-tone audiometry at 3, 4, 5, 6, 8, 10, 13, 16, and 20 years of age, with subjective assessment at other ages (AAP, 2017). More frequent hearing, speech-language, and communication screenings are indicated for children at high risk for hearing loss, including those with craniofacial anomalies, persistent or recurrent acute otitis media (AOM), middle ear effusion (MEE), and those with chronic exposure to loud noises.

Diagnostic Studies

- **Evoked otoacoustic emission** (EOAE) testing is the method of hearing screening used for universal newborn screening. The normal-hearing ear emits detectable sounds called *spontaneous otoacoustic emissions* when stimulated. EOAE shows the cochlea's outer hair cells are functioning appropriately and hearing is likely intact. EOAE is efficient, highly sensitive, and easy to perform in a quiet room with a cooperative child, which makes it conducive for newborns. EOAE does not quantify hearing deficit and may not identify auditory nerve dysfunction. The EOAE and auditory brainstem response (ABR) tests have highly sensitivity and specificity at relatively low cost.
- **Auditory brainstem response** (ABR) measures sound-induced electrical signals in the cochlea and the functioning of the peripheral auditory system and neurologic pathways related to hearing. Although it is not a direct measure of hearing, ABR indicates hearing thresholds. The ABR is useful in identifying hearing loss in a young infant or in children unable to cooperate with EOAE or audiometry. Occasionally, sedation is required for infants and children who are unable to successfully complete the test. Neurologic abnormalities may make interpretation of an ABR impossible.
- **Audiometry** assesses hearing loss in older children and measures hearing in decibels (dBs) at varying frequencies (Tables 36.2 and 36.3). Twenty dB is about as loud as a whisper, 40 dB is normal speaking loudness, and 90 dB produces pain. The frequencies of normal speaking range from 250 to 4000 Hz. Hearing loss, especially in the higher frequencies (2000 to 6000 Hz), can cause significant problems in understanding speech. Screening audiograms test hearing at 20 dB and frequencies of 500, 1000, 2000, and 4000 Hz and are useful in office settings. If a more detailed audiogram is needed, refer to a qualified audiologist.
- **Conditioned Play Audiometry** (CPA) can be used for children with a developmental age of at least 2.5 years. The child is taught to perform a simple task such as placing a block in a bucket when they are presented with a sound.
- **Pneumatic otoscopy** helps assess TM mobility. A good seal with the ophthalmoscope speculum is required. Brisk movement of the membrane should be seen; altered mobility suggests MEE or possible perforation.
- **Tympanometry** evaluates the function of the middle ear by assessing the movement of the TM. TM movement is translated into a graph called a *tympanogram* (Fig 36.2). The type A tympanogram has a compliance peak between ±100 mm H_2O and reflects a normal TM. The type B tympanogram has no peak or a flattened wave and suggests effusion, perforation, or the presence of a pressure-equalizing tube (Fig 36.3). The type C tympanogram has a sharp peak between −100 and −200 mm H_2O and reflects negative ear pressure.

Laboratory tests of blood and urine are rarely indicated unless questions remain regarding perinatal infection, systemic illness, or concomitant kidney dysfunction. Exudate from AOM with perforation may be cultured.

Hearing Impairment: Sensorineural, Conductive, and Mixed Hearing Loss

Normal hearing threshold is between 0 to 20 dB. Hearing loss is defined as pure-tone hearing loss greater than 20 dB at any frequency. Hearing loss can range from mild to profound (deaf), affect one or both ears, and from low to high frequencies. The overall prevalence of congenital deafness is estimated to be one to three in 1000 births, 1.1 per 1000 children 3 to 10 years old, and 14.9% of children 6 to 19 years old (CDC, 2015). Seventy percent of genetic hearing loss is nonsyndromic (Casazza, 2017). More than 300 genetic conditions cause deafness (Alford et al., 2014). Fifty percent to 60% of congenital deafness is genetic and referral for genetic testing is key if genetic hearing loss is suspected (CDC, 2015). Twenty-five percent of hearing loss in newborns is due to environmental causes, such as maternal infection during pregnancy or complications at the time of delivery. A combination of genetics and environmental factors may cause hearing loss. Mutations of the GJB2 gene cause about 40% of genetic hearing loss in children without a syndrome (CDC, 2015).

There are three types of hearing loss or impairment: sensorineural, conductive, and mixed.

Sensorineural hearing loss (SNHL) is most commonly associated with dysfunction or damage to the inner ear (e.g., the cochlea) or the auditory nerve (cranial nerve VIII). It can be congenital or acquired, mild or severe, and is almost always permanent. Environmental causes include exposure to excessive noise over time. Prenatal and perinatal causes include intrauterine infections (e.g., cytomegalovirus), toxic chemicals, and erythroblastosis fetalis.

TABLE 36.2	Audiologic Tests for Infants and Young Children			
Test	Characteristics	Age Range	Advantages	Disadvantages
Behavioral observation audiometry (BOA)	Behavioral test: Responses to noisemakers or calibrated sounds are observed	0-5 months	Low cost	Insensitive to unilateral or less than severe hearing loss; highly subject to observer bias; child tires rapidly when subjected to repeated stimuli
Visual reinforced audiometry (VRA)	Behavioral test: Child is given an animated toy for turning to sounds	5-24 months	Low cost; child responds at softer levels and for longer periods compared with BOA	Insensitive to unilateral loss (unless earphones used); need two examiners to reduce bias
Play audiometry	Behavioral test: Child is trained to respond to tones by playing a game	2-5 years	Low cost; can detect unilateral and mild hearing loss	Requires cooperation of child
Screening audiometry	Behavioral test: Child raises hand or responds verbally to tones at fixed levels (20-25 dB)	4 years and older	Can be performed by trained paraprofessional in most children 4 years and older; can detect unilateral and mild hearing loss	Further tests required if failed
Evoked otoacoustic emission (EOAE)	Physiologic test: Response of inner ear to brief clicks or tones is measured with specialized instrument	Any	Child's response not needed; takes less than 2 min if child is quiet; can be performed by a trained paraprofessional; low cost; can detect unilateral and mild hearing loss	Cannot tell type or degree of loss; further tests required if failed
Auditory brainstem response (ABR) audiometry	Physiologic test: Averaged number of responses of brainstem to brief tones or clicks	Any	Child's response not needed; can detect unilateral and mild loss; can determine degree and slope of loss (with tone bursts and bone conduction testing)	Requires audiologist and equipment to administer and interpret; expensive; requires sedation beyond about 6 months old

TABLE 36.3	Evaluation of Audiometric Results	
Average Threshold at 500-2000 Hz (Decibels)	Description	Significance
−10 to +15	Normal	
16-25	Slight loss (minimal)	Difficulty hearing faint speech, slight verbal deficit
26-40	Mild loss	Auditory learning dysfunction, language, or speech problems
41-55	Moderate loss	Trouble hearing conversational speech; may miss 50% of class discussion
56-70	Moderately severe loss	
71-90	Severe loss	Educational retardation, learning disability, limited vocabulary
90+	Profound loss	

Conductive hearing loss (CHL), either congenital or acquired, is caused by a problem in the outer ear or middle ear. It results from blocked sound wave transmission from the EAC to the inner ear and the causes include AOM, OME, foreign body, aural canal stenosis or atresia, ossicular malformations, cerumen impaction, TM perforation, cholesteatoma, and otosclerosis. The cochlea and auditory nerve function normally in CHL, usually in the range of 20 to 60 dB.

Mixed hearing loss involves a combination of SNHL and CHL. Abnormalities occur in the outer, middle, and/or inner ears. Central hearing loss occurs when the nerves or nuclei of the central nervous system (CNS) are impaired either in the pathways to the brain or in the brain.

Clinical Findings

History

Hearing loss is often a "silent disease." Pay careful consideration and attention to identified risk factors.

The risk factors for SNHL in newborns include the following:
- Birth weight less than 1500 g
- Severe respiratory depression at birth (e.g., Apgar score of 0 to 3 at 5 minutes, failure to initiate a response by 10 minutes, or hypotonia at up to 2 hours old)
- Neonatal intensive care unit admission for 2 days or longer
- Prolonged mechanical ventilation for greater than 10 days
- Persistent pulmonary hypertension

A normal tympanogram is depicted below. Four features of the tympanogram can be used to evaluate the ear under test:

❶ **Static admittance (Peak Y_a)** is a measure of the height of the tympanometric peak. Given appropriate norms, static admittance is a useful indicator of middle ear disease.

❷ **Equivalent ear canal volume (+200 Vea)** is the admittance value determined with an ear canal air pressure of +200 d_aP_a (dekapascals). An abnormally high equivalent ear canal volume suggests the presence of a tympanic membrane perforation, or a patent tympanostomy tube.

❸ **Tympanometric peak pressure (TPP)** is the position of the tympanometric peak on the pressure axis. TPP is an imprecise measure of the middle ear pressure. By itself, TPP is not an accurate indicator of middle ear disease.

❹ **Tympanometric gradient (GR) or tympanometric width** is a measure of the width of the tympanometric peak. Defined as the pressure interval required for a 50% reduction of peak eardrum admittance, tympanometric width is a good indicator of the presence of **middle ear effusion**.

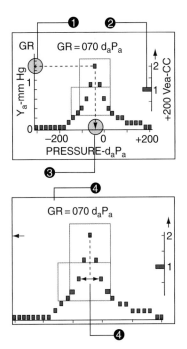

• **Fig 36.2** A Normal Tympanogram.

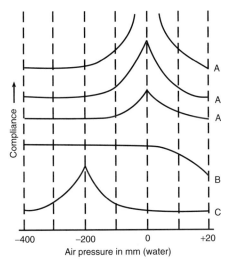

• **Fig 36.3** Five Types of Tympanogram Curves. Generally, an *A curve* indicates a normal tympanic membrane, a *B curve* is abnormal, a *C curve* may be abnormal, and a *D curve (not shown)* indicates hypermobility. An A_s curve (not shown) may be normal in infants.

- Long QT syndrome (usually profound hearing loss)
- Congenital infections, such as toxoplasmosis, bacterial meningitis, syphilis, rubella, cytomegalovirus, and herpes
- Metabolic disorders, such as phenylketonuria (PKU) and galactosemia
- Endocrine disorders, such as adrenal hyperplasia and hypothyroidism
- Craniofacial anomalies, including morphologic abnormalities of the pinna and ear canal
- Genetic syndromes, such as sickle cell disease, Usher syndrome, neurofibromatosis, Waardenburg syndrome, osteopetrosis, or findings associated with other genetic syndromes known to include hearing loss
- Hyperbilirubinemia requiring exchange transfusion or causing kernicterus

- Family history of hereditary childhood SNHL
- Ototoxic drug exposure
  In addition, risk factors for hearing loss in children 1 month to 3 years old include:
- Parental or caregiver concern regarding hearing, speech, language, or developmental delay (Harrison et al., 2016; Woolfenden et al., 2016)
- Kidney malformation
- Neurodegenerative disorders (such as, Hunter syndrome) or sensorimotor neuropathies (such as Friedreich ataxia and Charcot-Marie-Tooth disease)
- Head trauma with loss of consciousness or skull fracture
- Bacterial meningitis
  Other risk factors or indicators of hearing loss in children include the following (Box 36.1):
- Failure to respond to auditory stimuli, delayed speech development, speech that is monotone and difficult to understand, speaking avoidance
- Failed school screening audiogram; decreased note taking; seeming to misunderstand, ignore, confuse, or miss what is being said
- Aggression, increased physical complaints, difficulty in school and social situations
- Environmental exposure to loud noises like firecrackers, pistols, firearms, loud music, and machines (e.g., snowmobiles, farm equipment, lawn mowers)
- History of head or neck irradiation

Physical Examination

- Ears: Preauricular pits, auricular malformation, abnormal TM, or impaired mobility with pneumatic otoscopy.
- Eyes: Cataracts, corneal opacities, coloboma, blindness, nystagmus, exophthalmos, night blindness, heterochromia iridis, or blue sclerae (associated with genetic disorders that can cause SNHL).
- Note craniofacial abnormalities, low-set ears or abnormalities of the pinna and ear canal associated with SNHL or note a white forelock on hairline as seen in Waardenburg syndrome.

Diagnostic Studies

Evoked otoacoustic emission or EOAE testing and ABR testing are diagnostic for newborn hearing loss and ABR testing is used routinely prior to newborn discharge. Behavioral testing using a conditioned response or ABR testing is recommended for children older than 6 months. After early childhood, pure tone audiometry screening is the preferred hearing testing.

Differential Diagnosis

Differential diagnoses for conductive loss include cerumen impaction, OME, AOM or AOM with TM perforation. Differential diagnoses for congenital SNHL are infection, malformation, perilymph fistula, genetic (hereditary, prematurity, hyperbilirubinemia, infection, ototoxic drug exposure, noise exposure, trauma, tumor (rare in children without neurofibromatosis type 2), or heavy metals. For the child with significant hearing loss, comorbidities may exist, including developmental and speech and language delays, family disruptions, depression, and associated genetic disorders.

Management

For suspected hearing loss, the PCP should:
- Evaluate and treat AOM and OME if present.
- Screen for hearing loss if bilateral MEE is present for 3 months or longer and refer to otolaryngology as indicated.
- If suspected hearing loss, refer to an audiologist for full evaluation as soon as possible. If hearing impairment or hearing loss is identified, then referral to otolaryngology is indicated.
- Refer families for genetic counseling if heritable causes suspected.
- Encourage the use of amplification devices early as appropriate to improve school readiness.

Cochlear implants with an external speech processor are used for profound SNHL. Cochlear implants provide direct electrical stimulation to the auditory nerve. They are usually used in children with bilateral, severe SNHL, and require a dedicated family and educational support system. Children with cochlear implants may not be able to undergo standard magnetic resonance imaging (MRI) so consult with an otolaryngologist before ordering one. Bone-anchored hearing implants may be used when auricular or postauricular aids cannot be used. They increase audibility in noisy situations, improve speech understanding, and help with sound localization through temporal bone sound conduction.

- Ensure a family-centered approach in making decisions regarding interventions for the child.
- Refer to the public school district for evaluation for special education and classroom support for hearing impairment and preferential classroom seating.

Optimizing the care of a child with hearing loss or hearing impairment requires a multidisciplinary team including the PCP, otolaryngologist, audiologist, speech and language pathologist, sign language specialist if indicated, a developmental linguist to provide training in listening and proper use of assistive devices, and a supportive learning environment with a teacher who is trained to work with the deaf and hearing impaired. From an information-processing perspective, management of the deaf child is directed at providing stimuli that the infant and child can use to understand and interact with the environment.

Complications

Significant hearing loss impedes speech, language, cognitive development, and social interaction skills.

Developmental and Behavioral Effects

Developmental milestones for hearing-impaired children can be found in Table 36.1. Most hearing-impaired children have some functional hearing. Factors affecting the behavioral and developmental outcomes include the type and degree of hearing loss, the etiology of the loss (with comorbidities), the age of hearing loss onset and identification, the timing and appropriateness of educational interventions, and the family environment. The four main areas affected by hearing loss are: (1) delay in the development of receptive and expressive communication skills, (2) reduced academic achievement due to language deficit causing learning problems, (3) communication difficulties causing social isolation and poor self-concept, and (4) impact on vocational choices. Children who experience difficulty with language development due to hearing deficits may also exhibit a decreased ability to communicate their needs and thoughts. They generally do well on nonverbal and performance measures of intelligence but score below average in abstract concepts and language abilities. In early childhood, schooling focuses on communication development, which may cause less focus on instruction in other areas, and lower scores in reading comprehension and math (Box 36.2).

Hearing-impaired children may manifest more behavioral and emotional problems than normal-hearing children, with impulsivity and aggression most commonly seen. Unless their families focus on methods for joint communication, children with hearing loss may not receive the same nurturing and social support as their hearing cohorts receive from their parents. For example, if a child learns American Sign Language (ASL) but his or her parents do not, that communication opportunity is lost. Teens with hearing loss often face identity confusion because they compare themselves to their hearing peers, have academic challenges because they miss information and have a difficult time in class discussion, and experience depression or low self-esteem from feelings of being different.

Habilitation and Assistive Devices and Amplification Devices. Many technologic advances help those who have hearing impairments. Alert and warning devices such as strobe lights and vibrating wake-up alarms; text messaging and email; closed-captioned television, videos, and phones; service animals; and social network sites are helpful. If children use sign language, they should have an interpreter during healthcare visits. Children with hearing loss may have inadequate health literacy because of poor communication between provider and child.

Amplification from a very early age is crucial in improving speech, language, and cognitive abilities of hearing-impaired children. Different types of hearing amplification have different purposes, and wireless and Bluetooth technologies have vastly improved the flexibility and use of these devices.

Hearing assistive technology systems (HATS), including teacher microphone systems, frequency modulation (FM) systems, infrared systems, induction loop systems, and one-to-one communicators, may be used with or without amplifiers. Sound field systems amplify sound throughout a room, not just to an individual. The body-worn hearing aids with a lead to ear phones may be used for children younger than 3 years old, and those in need of more powerful or durable amplification. Postauricular, or behind-the-ear, devices may be used as early as 4 weeks of age, and postauricular external canal devices are frequently used in early childhood and as children grow. For external ear devices, ear molds are used and must fit well. Ear molds must be revised initially every 3 to 6 months, then annually after 4 to 6 years of age. Ear molds for external ear devices should be washed with

Effects of Hearing Loss on Development

Vocabulary

- Vocabulary develops more slowly
- Learns concrete words more easily (e.g., "cat," "jump," "five," and "red") than abstract words (e.g., "before," "after," "equal to," and "jealous").
- Difficulty with function words (e.g., "the," "an," "are," and "a").
- The gap in vocabulary between children with normal hearing and those with hearing loss widens with age; there is no catch up without intervention.
- Has difficulty understanding words with multiple meanings (e.g., "bank" can mean the edge of a stream or a place where we put money).

Sentence Structure

- Comprehends and produces shorter and simpler sentences.
- Has difficulty understanding and writing complex sentences—for example, relative clauses ("The teacher whom I have for math was sick today.") or passive voice ("The ball was thrown by Mary.").
- Often cannot hear word endings, such as "-s" or "-ed," leading to misunderstandings and misuse of verb tense, pluralization, nonagreement of subject and verb, and possessives.

Speaking

- Often cannot hear quiet speech sounds, such as "s," "sh," "f," "t," and "k," and may not include them in their speech, making the child difficult to understand.
- May not hear their own voices when they speak, thus speaking too loudly or not loud enough, speak in too high a pitch, or sound like they are mumbling because of poor stress, poor inflection, or poor rate of speaking.

Academic Achievement

- Difficulty with all areas, especially reading and mathematical concepts.
- Children with mild to moderate hearing losses, on average, achieve one to four grade levels lower than their peers with normal hearing, unless appropriate management occurs.
- Those with severe to profound hearing loss usually achieve skills no higher than the third- or fourth-grade level, unless appropriate educational intervention occurs early.
- The gap in academic achievement between children with normal hearing and those with hearing loss widens as they progress in school.
- Level of achievement is related to parental involvement and the quantity, quality, and timing of the support services children receive.

Social Functioning

- Severe to profound hearing loss children often report feeling isolated, without friends, and unhappy in school, particularly when their socialization is limited with other children whose hearing loss is limited.
- Social problems appear more frequently in children with a mild or moderate hearing loss than severe to profound loss.

Data from the American Speech-Language-Hearing Association: effects of hearing loss on development, American Speech-Language-Hearing Association (website), available at http://www.asha.org/public/hearing/disorders/effects.htm. Accessed October 17, 2017.

soap and water each night and cleaned carefully to avoid clogging. Continuous high-pitched sounds from the hearing aid may be a sign that the ear molds do not fit properly. Avoidance of infection in the external ear canal includes ear-adjusting molds to reduce irritation and using petroleum jelly to decrease friction. If an *otitis externa* infection occurs, ear molds should be left out for 1 to 2 days in bacterial infection and 3 to 5 days for fungal infections.

Prevention of Noise-Induced Hearing Loss

Noise is defined as any sound, but is usually considered loud, harsh, unpleasant, or unwanted. Noise pollution is the presence of irritating, distracting, or physically dangerous noise. Sound has qualities of frequency or pitch (measured in cycles per minute and stated in hertz [Hz]), intensity or loudness (measured in dB sound pressure levels [SPLs]), periodicity, and duration (either continuous, short-term, or episodic). The human voice is approximately 50 to 60 dB SPL, blow dryers or food processors are 80 to 90 dB SPL, and jackhammers are 130 dB SPL. The National Institute for Occupational Safety and Health (NIOSH) defines hazardous noise as 85 dB for an average of 8 hours of sound exposure (CDC, 2017). Hazardous noise is a common cause of SNHL in children, and the pattern of damage depends on the frequency, intensity, and duration of the noise. Any structure in the ear can be permanently damaged by noise at a 140-dB SPL or greater.

Humans are subject to noise-induced hearing loss (NIHL) and tinnitus from exposure to continuous noise or to sudden acoustic trauma that causes damage to the hair cells of the cochlea due to excessive vibration; extreme noise can rupture the TM. Noise of more than 85 dB but less than 140 dB leads to temporary hearing loss—most often in the 4000 Hz range. Permanent hearing loss can result from one exposure to a sudden, extreme noise (greater than 120 dB in children) of short duration, or from ongoing lower levels of noise. Permanent loss is often in the 3000 to 6000 Hz range. Music listened to with headphones, ear buds, and at concerts; firecrackers; electrical tools; and airport noise can cause hearing loss. Chronic, everyday noise causes sleep disturbance, distraction, impairment of cognitive function (e.g., poor reading comprehension, decreased memory), and an increased stress response (e.g., increased heart rate, blood pressure, adrenaline, and cortisol production); these in turn result in irritability, poor coping, and lower achievement in children. Newborn infants are a particularly vulnerable. It is important to recognize that excessive noise in nurseries and intensive care units may impact growth and development in infancy.

Clinical Findings

History

A careful history looks at the following:
- Type of noise in the child's environment
- Exposure to chronic noise
- Episodic acoustic trauma
- History of ear disease
- History of prematurity or exposure to ototoxic drugs

Physical Examination

Visual examination of the TM with insufflation should be done at every well-child visit. Tympanography can help rule out chronic MEE.

Management

NIHL is virtually 100% preventable. The goals of management are to:
- Increase awareness of hazardous noise in the child's environment. Well-child visits should include targeted history related to the child's noise environment, and both children and parents should be given information on excessive noise, its relationship to the auditory system, and how to avoid exposure to hazardous noise.

Parents and children should be encouraged to minimize noise in the child's environment, including efforts to:
- Reduce excessive noise from television and car radios.
- Use ear buds and headphones cautiously; volume should allow the child or teen to hear normal conversation.
- Avoid hazardous loud music, firecrackers, and other sources of episodic, extreme noise.
- Create a "quiet" place in the home setting.
- Mitigate exposure to noise. Wear earplugs to protect against "unavoidable" occupational noise. Commercial-quality earplugs are available for use in the home (e.g., when electrical saws or other loud tools are used).
- Prevention is possible by reducing hazards in the environment and increasing awareness of hazardous noise among children, teens, and families.

Foreign Body in the Ear Canal

External ear foreign bodies are frequently seen by PCPs in clinic, in emergency departments, and by otolaryngologists. Foreign bodies are usually placed into the ear canal by the child or thrown by another child and can include insects. Leaves and other plant materials can be intentionally inserted into the EAC as a form of native remedy.

Clinical Findings

History

The PCP elicits history including:
- Child reports putting something into the ear or having something thrown at him or her
- Complaints of itching, buzzing, fullness, or an object in the ear
- Persistent cough or hiccups
- Unilateral otalgia and otorrhea (bloody or purulent)
  Some children may be asymptomatic despite the presence of a foreign body in the EAC.

Physical Examination

A foreign body is visible with the naked eye or by otoscopic examination.

Management

Adequate visualization in a cooperative child is key to successful removal of the foreign body in the EAC. Foreign bodies in the lateral one-third of the ear canal are the easiest to remove, and those in the medial two-thirds of the ear canal are more difficult to remove because the canal is narrower, lined with bone, quite vascular, and is exquisitely sensitive.
- Soft, irregularly shaped objects are generally graspable with a bayonet forceps, alligator forceps, or curved hook.
- Round or breakable objects can be removed using a wire loop, a curette, or right-angle hook slowly advanced beyond the object and withdrawn carefully.
- Irrigation can only be done if the TM is intact. Use body temperature fluid and a commercial irrigator or 60-mL syringe with an angiocatheter on the end. Irrigation can push the object farther into the ear canal.
- Do not irrigate if the object is a disk battery, the TM is not intact, or if it is made of organic material (corn, peas, and so on), because moisture may cause the object to expand and become more difficult to remove.

- Disk, coin-shaped, or button batteries must be removed emergently as disc batteries exposed to moisture leak corrosive material causing severe tissue damage and possible hearing loss.
- Spherical objects are the most difficult to remove and require referral to an otolaryngologist.
- If the object is made of iron, nickel, or cobalt, a magnet may be used for retrieval.
- Insects in the ear canal should be suffocated with mineral oil, then the ear can be irrigated or the child can be referred for otolaryngology for removal.
- If the foreign body cannot be extracted on the first few attempts or cannot be removed without risking damage to the external canal or TM, or there is worsening pain, then refer the child to an otolaryngologist. Also, refer if the child is uncooperative or the object is lying on the TM or has been in the EAC more than 24 hours.
  Post removal, topical antibiotic drops with steroid are recommended for drainage/infection, to prevent infection if the canal is damaged during the removal, and to decrease inflammation.

Complications

Infection, perforation of the TM, and damage to the ossicles are possible if the object is not removed.

Ear Conditions in Children

Otitis Externa

Otitis externa (OE), commonly called *swimmer's ear,* is a diffuse inflammation of the EAC and can involve the pinna or TM. Inflammation is evidenced as (1) simple infection with edema, discharge, and erythema; (2) furuncles or small abscesses that form in hair follicles; or (3) infection of the superficial layers of the epidermis. OE can also be classified as mycotic OE, caused by fungus, or as chronic external otitis, a diffuse low-grade infection of the EAC. Severe infection or systemic infection can occur in children who have diabetes mellitus, are immunocompromised, or who received head and neck irradiation.

OE results when the protective barriers in the EAC are damaged by mechanical or chemical mechanisms. OE is usually caused by retained moisture in the EAC that changes the usually acidic environment to a neutral or basic environment, thereby promoting bacterial or fungal growth. Chlorine in swimming pools adds to the problem because it kills the normal ear flora, allowing the growth of pathogens. Regular cleaning of the EAC removes cerumen, an important water and infection barrier. Soapy deposits, alkaline topical medications, debris from skin conditions, local trauma, sweating, allergy, stress, and hearing aids can also cause OE (Rosenfeld et al., 2014).

OE is most often caused by *Pseudomonas aeruginosa* and *Staphylococcus aureus,* but it is not uncommon for the infection to be polymicrobial. Furunculosis of the external canal is generally caused by *S. aureus* and *Streptococcus pyogenes.* Otomycosis is caused by *Aspergillus* or *Candida* and can result from systemic or topical antibiotics or steroids. Otomycosis is more common in children with diabetes mellitus or immune dysfunction, and in these cases is most commonly caused by *Aspergillus niger, Escherichia coli,* or *Klebsiella pneumonia. Group B streptococci* are a more common cause in neonates.

Long-standing ear drainage may suggest a foreign body, chronic middle ear pathology (such as cholesteatoma), or granulomatous tissue. Bloody drainage may indicate trauma, severe otitis media, or granulation tissue. Chronic or recurrent OE may result from eczema, seborrhea, or psoriasis. Eczematous dermatitis, moist vesicles, and pustules are seen in acute infection, whereas crusting is more consistent with chronic infection.

Clinical Findings

History
- Itching and irritation
- Pain that is disproportionate to what is seen on examination
- Pressure and fullness in ear
- Conductive or SNHL, or otorrhea
- EAC or periauricular edema, and preauricular and postauricular lymphadenopathy with more severe disease
- Extension to the surrounding soft tissue results in the obstruction of the canal with or without cellulitis.

Physical Examination
Findings on physical examination include the following:
- Pain, often quite severe, with movement of the tragus (when pushed) or pinna (when pulled) or during otoscopic examination
- Swollen EAC with debris, making visualization of the TM difficult or impossible
- Occasional regional lymphadenopathy
- Tragal tenderness with a red, raised area of induration that can be deep and diffuse or superficial and pointing, which is characteristic of furunculosis
- Red, crusty, or pustular spreading lesions
- Pruritus associated with thick otorrhea that can be black, gray, blue-green, yellow, or white, and black spots over the TM are indicative of mycotic infection
- Dry-appearing canal with atrophy or thinning of the canal and virtually no cerumen visible with chronic OE
- Presence of tympanostomy or pressure-equalizing (PE) tubes or TM perforation

Diagnostic Studies
Culturing the discharge from the ear is not customary but may be indicated if clinical improvement is not seen during or after treatment, severe pain persists, in neonates and immunocompromised children, or chronic or recurrent OE is suspected. Culturing requires a swab premoistened with sterile nonbacteriostatic saline or sterile water.

Differential Diagnosis
AOM with perforation, tympanostomy tube otorrhea (TTO), chronic suppurative otitis media (CSOM), necrotizing OE, cholesteatoma, mastoiditis, posterior auricular lymphadenopathy, dental infection, and eczema are all possible differential diagnoses.

Management
The following steps outline the management of OE:
- Eardrops are the mainstay of OE therapy (Table 36.4). Eardrops containing acetic acid or antibiotic with and without corticosteroid drops are the treatment of choice. Symptoms should markedly improve within 7 days, but resolution of the infection may take up to 2 weeks. Use drops until all symptoms resolve.
  - Choose antibiotic agents based on efficacy, resistance patterns, low incidence of adverse effects, cost, and likelihood of compliance. Neomycin-containing drops should not be used if the TM is not intact, because these drugs are known to cause damage to the cochlea and may cause hypersensitivity (Rosenfeld et al., 2014).
  - The quinolone products are effective against *Pseudomonas, S. aureus,* and *Streptococcus pneumoniae,* which may be a factor if the OE is a complication of AOM.
- Systemic antibiotics should not be used unless there is extension of infection beyond the ear or host factors that require more systemic treatment (severe OE, systemic illness, fever, lymphadenitis, or failed topical treatment).

TABLE 36.4 Commonly Used Topical Preparations for Otitis Externa and Analgesia

Product Name (Manufacturer)	Antibiotic	Steroid	Acid	Comments
Antibiotics (Not Ototoxic)				
Ciprodex (Alcon)	Ciprofloxacin	Dexamethasone		Use ≥6 months old Contains steroid
Floxin Otic (Daiichi Pharmaceutical)	Ofloxacin	None	Acetic and boric	Does not contain steroid
Vasocidin ophthalmic (Ciba Vision Ophthalmics)	Sulfacetamide sodium	Prednisolone sodium phosphate		No documented ototoxicity with either agent Excellent broad-spectrum coverage Contains steroid
Antibiotics (Ototoxic)				
Cortisporin Otic Susp Pediotic (King Pharmaceutical)	Polymyxin B and neomycin	Hydrocortisone	Hydrochloric acid	May be painful on instillation Neomycin may cause cutaneous irritation Not to be used if TM integrity unknown
Cipro HC Otic (Alcon Labs)	Ciprofloxacin	Hydrocortisone	Glacial acetic acid	Use ≥1 year old Contraindicated with TM perforation
Cleansing and Antipruritic Agent (Ototoxic)				
Domeboro Otic (Bayer Pharmaceutical Division)	None	None	Acetic acid	Excellent choice for cleansing of the EAC Aluminum acetate helps to prevent itching Not to be used if TM integrity is unknown

EAC, External auditory canal; *TM,* tympanic membrane.

- OE treatment must include parent education regarding the instillation of otic drops. The drops should be administered with the child lying down with the affected ear upward and instilled until the EAC is filled. Pump the tragus to remove any trapped air and ensure filling (Rosenfeld et al., 2014). The child should remain lying down for 3 to 5 minutes, leaving the ear open to the air.
- If the infection is severe and not improving in the first 5 to 7 days, aural irrigation with water, saline, or hydrogen peroxide may be tried, or refer to the otolaryngologist for debridement and suction (Rosenfeld et al., 2014).
- Avoid cleaning, manipulating, and getting water into the ear. Swimming is prohibited during acute infection.
- Administer analgesics for pain.
- Debridement with calcium alginate swabs is indicated once the inflammatory process subsides and enhances the effectiveness of the ototopical antibiotic drops. Lance a furuncle that is superficial and pointed with a 14-gauge needle. If it is deep and diffuse, a heating pad or warm oil-based drops can speed resolution.
  - If infection is present, clear the canal by using water or an antiseptic solution followed by a warm-water rinse. Apply an antibiotic ointment (mupirocin) twice a day for 5 to 7 days, or retapamulin in children over 9 months of age if resistant to mupirocin. The child should avoid touching the ear. Fingernails should be short, and hands should be cleansed with soap and water.
  - Fungal OE is uncommon and more likely related to chronic OE or follows treatment with topical and/or systemic antibiotics. *Aspergillus* and *Candida* species are most commonly seen in mycotic OE (Rosenfeld et al., 2014). Treatment consists of antifungal solutions, such as clotrimazole-miconazole or nystatin.

If the child is not improved within 72 hours (relief of otalgia, itching, and fullness), recheck to confirm diagnosis. Lack of improvement may be due to obstructed ear canal, foreign body, poor adherence, or contact sensitivity among other things. Routine follow-up is not needed. If symptoms worsen after treatment or there is no improvement in a week, a referral to an otolaryngologist is indicated.

Complications

Infection of surrounding tissues, irritated furunculosis, and malignant OE with progression and necrosis caused by *Pseudomonas* are possible complications. Involvement of the parotid gland, mastoid bone, and infratemporal fossa is rare (Rosenfeld et al., 2014).

Prevention

The patient should be instructed to do the following:
- Avoid water in the ear canals.
- Use alcohol vinegar otic mix (two parts rubbing alcohol, one part white vinegar, and one part distilled water) 3 to 5 drops daily, especially after swimming or bathing, to prevent recurrence of OE (Waitzman, 2015).
- Use a blow dryer on warm setting to dry the EAC.
- Avoid persistent scratching or cleaning of the external canal.
- Avoid prolonged use of cerumenolytic agents.

Acute Otitis Media

AOM is an acute infection of the middle ear (Fig 36.4). It is important that clinicians accurately diagnose otitis media to

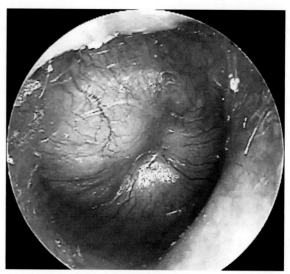

• **Fig 36.4** Acute Otitis Media of the Right Ear.

reduce overtreatment and antibiotic resistance (Schilder, Marom, and Bhutta, 2017). The AAP Clinical Practice Guideline requires the presence of the following three components to diagnose AOM (Kaur et al., 2017; Lieberthal et al., 2013):
- Recent, abrupt onset of middle ear inflammation and effusion (ear pain, irritability, otorrhea, and/or fever)
- MEE confirmed by bulging TM, limited or absent mobility by pneumatic otoscopy, air-fluid level behind TM, and/or otorrhea
- Signs and symptoms of middle ear inflammation confirmed by distinct TM erythema or ear pain (holding, tugging, rubbing the ear)

Characteristics of different types of AOM are defined in Table 36.5. AOM often follows eustachian tube dysfunction (ETD). Infants and children are prone to ETD because of the proximity to the adenoids, the horizontal orientation of the eustachian tube (takes an adult orientation in late childhood), and narrow diameter of the tube. Common causes of ETD include upper respiratory infections, craniofacial anomalies (cleft palate), allergies, adenoid hypertrophy, and tobacco smoke exposure. ETD leads to functional eustachian tube obstruction and inflammation that decreases the protective ciliary action in the eustachian tube. Eustachian tube obstruction causes negative pressure as air absorbs in the middle ear (see Fig 36.4). The negative pressure pulls fluid from the mucosal lining and causes a sterile fluid accumulation that may be colonized by bacteria and result in purulent fluid. Young children have shorter, more horizontal, and more flaccid eustachian tubes that are easily disrupted by viruses, which predisposes them to AOM. Respiratory syncytial virus and influenza are two of the viruses most responsible for the increase in the incidence of AOM seen from January to April. Other risk factors associated with AOM are listed in Box 36.3.

S. pneumoniae, nontypeable *Haemophilus influenzae*, *Moraxella catarrhalis*, and *S. pyogenes* (group A streptococci) are the most common infecting organisms in AOM (Conover, 2013). *S. pneumoniae* continues to be the most common bacteria responsible for AOM, and the strains of *S. pneumoniae* in the heptavalent pneumococcal conjugate vaccine (PCV7) have virtually disappeared from the middle ear fluid of children with AOM (Palmu et al., 2018). With the introduction of the 13-valent *S. pneumoniae* vaccine, the bacteriology of the middle ear is likely to continue to

TABLE 36.5 Types of Acute Otitis Media

Type	Characteristics
AOM	Suppurative effusion of the middle ear
Bullous myringitis	AOM in which bullae form between the inner and middle layers of the TM and bulge outward
Persistent AOM	AOM that has not resolved when antibiotic therapy has been completed or AOM recurs within days of treatment
Recurrent AOM	Three separate bouts of AOM within a 6-month period or four within a 12-month period; often a positive family history of otitis media and other ENT disease

AOM, Acute otitis media; *ENT,* ear, nose, and throat; *TM,* tympanic membrane.

BOX 36.3 Risk Factors for Otitis Media, Chronic Otitis Media, or Otitis Media With Effusion

Genetic susceptibility/sibling with history of otitis media
Native Americans and Native Alaskans
Non-Hispanic Caucasian
Prematurity
Younger than 2 years of age
Unimmunized
Day care attendance
Sharing a bedroom
Breastfeeding for less than 6 months
Parental smoking and other ETS exposure
Environmental pollution exposure
Overweight or obese
Feeding in supine position
Autumn season
Male gender
Early onset otitis media
Bilateral OME
Lower socioeconomic status

ETS, Environmental tobacco smoke; OME, *otitis media with effusion.*

evolve. Bullous myringitis is almost always caused by *S. pneumonia.* Nontypeable *H. influenza* remains a common cause of AOM. It is the most common cause of bilateral otitis media, severe TM inflammation, and otitis-conjunctivitis syndrome. *M. catarrhalis* obtained from the nasopharynx is increasingly more beta-lactamase positive, but the high rate of clinical resolution in children with AOM from *M. catarrhalis* makes amoxicillin a good choice for initial therapy (Venekamp et al., 2015). *M. catarrhalis* rarely causes invasive disease. *S. pyogenes* is responsible for AOM in older children, is responsible for more TM ruptures, and is more likely to cause mastoiditis.

Although a virus is usually the initial causative factor in AOM, strict diagnostic criteria, careful specimen handling, and sensitive microbiologic techniques have shown that the majority of AOM is caused by bacteria or bacteria and virus together (Van Dyke et al., 2017).

Clinical Findings

History

Rapid onset of:
- Ear pain that may interfere with activity and/or sleep, especially when lying flat
- Irritability and ear pulling in an infant or toddler
- Otorrhea
- Fever

Other key risk factors or symptoms include prematurity, craniofacial anomalies or congenital syndromes associated with craniofacial anomalies, daycare attendance, disrupted sleep or inability to sleep, lethargy, dizziness, tinnitus, unsteady gait, diarrhea and vomiting, sudden hearing loss, stuffy nose, rhinorrhea, and sneezing.

Physical Examination

- Presence of MEE, confirmed by pneumatic otoscopy, tympanometry, or acoustic reflectometry, as evidenced by:
  - Bulging TM (see Fig 36.4)
  - Decreased TM translucency
  - Absent or decreased TM mobility
  - Air-fluid level behind the TM
  - Otorrhea

Signs and symptoms of middle ear inflammation indicated by TM (amber color is usually seen in otitis media with effusion [OME]; white or yellow may be seen in either AOM or OME) (Schilder et al., 2017).

In addition, the following TM findings may be present:
- Increased vascularity with obscured or absent landmarks (see Fig 36.4).
- Red, yellow, or purple TM. (Redness alone should not be used to diagnose AOM, especially in a crying child.)
- Thin-walled, sagging bullae filled with straw-colored fluid seen with bullous myringitis

Diagnostic Studies

Pneumatic otoscopy is the simplest and most efficient way to diagnose AOM. Tympanometry reflects effusion (type B pattern). Tympanocentesis identifies the infecting organism and is helpful in the treatment of infants younger than 2 months old. In older infants and children, tympanocentesis is rarely done and is useful only if the patient is toxic or immunocompromised, or in the presence of resistant infection or acute pain from bullous myringitis. If a tympanocentesis is warranted, refer the patient to an otolaryngologist for this procedure.

Differential Diagnosis

OME, mastoiditis, dental abscess, sinusitis, lymphadenitis, parotitis, peritonsillar abscess, trauma, ETD, impacted teeth, temporomandibular joint dysfunction, and immune deficiency are differential diagnoses. Any infant 2 months old or younger with AOM should be evaluated for fever of unknown etiology and not just treated for an ear infection.

Management

Many changes have been made in the treatment of AOM because of the increasing rate of antibiotic-resistant bacteria related to the injudicious use of antibiotics. Ample evidence demonstrates that symptom management may be all that is required in children with MEE without other symptoms of AOM (Schilder et al., 2017). Treatment is based on the child's age, illness severity, and the

TABLE 36.6	Treatment Guidelines for Acute Otitis Media	
Diagnosis	**Treat**
Any child with moderate/severe bulging TM with otorrhea not associated with AOM	Yes
Any child with mild bulging of the TM with recent (<48 h) onset pain (holding, tugging, and so on) or intensely erythematous TM	Yes
Babies ≥6 months of age with severe signs of AOM (fever >102.2°F [39°C], otalgia for ≥48 h)	Yes
Any child 6-23 months old with acute bilateral otitis media without severe symptoms, without fever, and sick less than 48 h	Yes
Young children with unilateral AOM without severe symptoms and fever <102.2°F [39°C]	Provide prescription and/or wait Close follow-up
Children ≥24 months old without severe symptoms	Provide prescription and/or wait Close follow-up
Children not treated and no improvement in 48-72 h	See the patient again Clinician discretion whether or not to treat

AOM, Acute otitis media; *TM,* tympanic membrane.

From Lieberthal AS, Carroll AE, Chonmaitree T, et al. The diagnosis and management of acute otitis media. *Pediatrics.* 2013;131(3):e964–e999. Adapted from Clinical Practice Guidelines.

certainty of diagnosis. Table 36.6 shows the recommendation for the diagnosis and subsequent treatment of AOM.

1. Pain management is the first principle of treatment with weight-appropriate doses of children's ibuprofen or acetaminophen to decrease discomfort and fever. Distraction, oil application, or external use of heat or cold may be of some use.

2. Antibiotics are also effective (Table 36.7).

- Amoxicillin remains the first-line antibiotic for AOM if there has not been a previous treated AOM in the previous 30 days, there is no conjunctivitis, and no penicillin allergy (Schilder et al., 2017). *β-lactam* coverage (amoxicillin/clavulanate, third-generation cephalosporin) is recommended when the child has been treated with amoxicillin in the previous 30 days, there is an allergy to penicillin, or the child has concurrent conjunctivitis or has recurrent otitis that has not responded to amoxicillin.

- If the child is younger than 2 years of age, treatment with amoxicillin or amoxicillin/clavulanate for 10 days, or for children older than 2 years of age, treatment for 5 to 7 days.

- Ceftriaxone may be effective for the vomiting child, the child unable to tolerate oral medications, or the child who has failed amoxicillin/clavulanate.
  - Clindamycin may be considered for ceftriaxone failure but *should only* be used if susceptibilities are known.
  - Prophylactic antibiotics for chronic or recurrent AOM are *not* recommended.

3. Observation or "watchful waiting" for 48 to 72 hours (see Table 36.6) allows the patient to improve without antibiotic treatment. Pain relief should be provided, and a means of

follow-up must be in place. Recommendations for follow-up include: parent-initiated visit or phone call for worsening or no improvement; scheduled follow-up appointment; routine follow-up phone call; or give a prescription to be started if the child's symptoms do not improve or if they worsen in 48 to 72 hours (see Table 36.6).

4. Routine follow-up is not needed if the child improves within 48 hours. If the child has not shown improvement in ear symptomatology after 48 to 72 hours, the child should be seen to confirm or exclude the presence of AOM. If the initial management option was an antibacterial agent, the agent should be changed.

Management of Persistent and Recurrent Acute Otitis Media

- Persistent AOM occurs when antibiotic therapy is completed and AOM is still present or AOM recurs within days of treatment. Retreatment with a broader-spectrum antibiotic is suggested.

- Persistent MEE is common after resolution of acute symptoms and should not be seen as a need for continuing antibiotics (see Otitis Media with Effusion section).

- Recurrent AOM is defined as more than three distinct and well-documented bouts of AOM in 6 months or four or more episodes in 12 months.

An otolaryngology referral is indicated when appropriate therapy for otitis media fails. Placement of tympanostomy or PE tubes can help relieve discomfort, reduce time with OME, improve hearing, and decrease the likelihood of further infection (Wallace et al., 2014). Indications for tympanostomy and the insertion of pressure-equalizing tubes is discussed below.

Other Treatment Issues

- The PCP is encouraged to maintain understanding of current recommendations for AOM management because of rapid changes in resistance patterns and newly developed treatments.

- Decongestants and antihistamines are not indicated.

- Antimicrobial ototopical drops (ofloxacin or ciprofloxacin) or ophthalmic drops (tobramycin or gentamicin) are indicated if the TM is perforated (Fig 36.5), the child has otorrhea, or the child has patent, draining PE tubes.

- Xylitol, a sugar found in fruits and birch bark, has bacteriostatic effects against *S. pneumoniae* and interferes with bacterial adhesion to mucous membranes. It appears to have some suppressive effects in preventing ear infections. Xylitol is available in an oral solution, lozenges, and chewing gum. The lozenges and chewing gum are more effective than the oral solution. Children younger than 2 years old cannot have chewing gum or lozenges. Xylitol must be given three to five times a day on a regular basis to be effective.

- There is no safe or effective herbal treatment for AOM or OME.

Complications

Persistent AOM, persistent OME, TM perforation, OE, mastoiditis, cholesteatoma, tympanosclerosis (Fig 36.6), hearing loss of 25 to 30 dB for several months, ossicle necrosis, pseudotumor cerebri, cerebral thrombophlebitis, and facial paralysis are possible complications.

TABLE 36.7	Medications Used to Treat Acute Otitis Media	
Drug	**Dosage**	**Comments**
Amoxicillin	80-90 mg/kg/day divided twice a day (maximum dose 2 to 3 gm daily)	First choice unless allergy
Amoxicillin-clavulanate	80-90 mg/kg/day divided twice a day (maximum dose depends on formulation of drug)	Clavulanate <10 mg/kg/day Good beta-lactamase coverage Costly and more likely to cause diarrhea
Azithromycin	10 mg/kg/day on day 1 (maximum dose 500 mg/day) then 5 mg/kg/day on days 2-5 given daily (maximum dose 250 mg/day)	Children older than 6 months need 5-day treatment course Macrolide primarily used because of penicillin allergy Should not be used as first-line treatment due to high resistance
Cefdinir	14 mg/kg/day daily or divided twice a day (maximum dose 600 mg/day)	Broad-spectrum Third-generation cephalosporin Causes red stool
Cefixime	8 mg/kg daily or divided twice a day (maximum dose 400 mg/day)	Broad-spectrum Third-generation cephalosporin Reduced efficacy against *Streptococcus pneumoniae*
Cefpodoxime	10 mg/kg/day daily divided twice a day (maximum dose 400 mg/day)	Broad spectrum of coverage Third-generation cephalosporin
Ceftriaxone	50 mg/kg/day IM (maximum dose 1 gm/day) 1-3 doses over 5 days	Costly Third-generation cephalosporin
Cefuroxime	15-30 mg/kg/day divided twice a day (maximum dose 500 mg/day) 250 mg every 12 h for 2-12 years old 250-500 mg every 12 h for 12 years or older	Broad spectrum of coverage Costly Most potent second-generation cephalosporin Poor taste
Clindamycin	30-40 mg/kg/day given divided three times a day (maximum dose 1.8 gm/day)	Should not be used unless culture and sensitivities are done

IM, Intramuscular.

Data from Taketomo CK, Hodding JH, Kraus DM. *Pediatric Dosage Handbook.* 21st ed. Hudson, OH: Lexi-Comp; 2014.

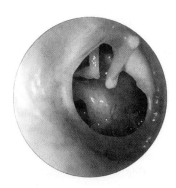

• **Fig 36.5** Perforated Tympanic Membrane. (Photograph courtesy Sylvan Stool, MD, The Children's Hospital, Denver, CO.)

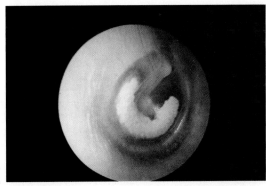

• **Fig 36.6** Tympanosclerosis of the Right Ear. (Photo courtesy Sylvan Stool, MD, The Children's Hospital, Denver, CO.)

Prevention and Education

The following interventions, shown to be helpful in preventing AOM, should be encouraged:
• Exclusive breastfeeding until at least 6 months of age protects against AOM (Bowatte et al., 2015)
• Avoid bottle propping, feeding infants lying down, and passive smoke exposure
• Pneumococcal vaccine; specifically, PCV13, which contains subtype 19A
• Annual influenza vaccine helps prevent otitis media
• Xylitol liquid or chewing gum as tolerated

• Choose licensed day care facilities with fewer children
• Educate regarding the problem of drug-resistant bacteria and the need to avoid antibiotic use unless absolutely necessary. If antibiotics are used, the child needs to complete the entire course of the prescription and follow up if symptoms do not resolve.

Otitis Media With Effusion

The diagnosis of OME is made in the presence of MEE without signs or symptoms of acute ear infection (see Fig 36.7). MEE decreases the mobility of the TM and interferes with sound conduction.

OME can occur spontaneously with ETD caused by an inflammatory process after AOM, viral illness, anatomic abnormalities, barotrauma, allergies, or a combination of these conditions (Figs. 36.7 and 36.8). ETD changes the middle ear mucosa in the following sequence: (1) the mucosa becomes secretory with increased mucus production, (2) the mucus absorbs water as the mucosa becomes viscous, and (3) fluid becomes stuck behind the TM. Bacterial biofilms may explain the persistence of OME. Biofilms are mixed microorganisms enclosed in a polymeric matrix that adhere to surfaces, such as the middle ear mucosa.

Risk factors for chronic OME are listed in Box 36.4.

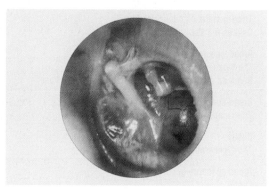

• **Fig 36.7** Left Ear With Posterior Retraction. (Photo courtesy Sylvan Stool, MD, The Children's Hospital, Denver, CO.)

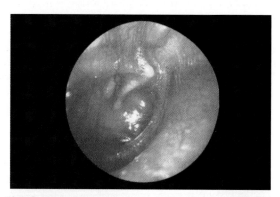

• **Fig 36.8** Severely Retracted, Opaque Right Tympanic Membrane in Otitis Media With Effusion. (From Bluestone CD, Klein JO. *Otitis Media in Infants and Children*. 2nd ed. Philadelphia: Saunders; 1995.)

• BOX 36.4 **Risk Factors for Hearing Loss Caused by Otitis Media with Effusion**

Bilateral OME for 4 months or longer
If two or more present:
    OME present for longer than 8 weeks
    Speech development slower than peers
    Speech less clear than previously
    Child decreases amount of talking
    Child less responsive to name and other familiar sounds
    Child says "Huh?" or "What?" frequently
    Child sits close to TV or wants volume louder
    Child has difficulty learning (reading, spelling)
    Child is hyperactive or overly inattentive

OME, Otitis media with effusion.

Clinical Findings

History

Children with OME are often afebrile and asymptomatic. However, some children may present with intermittent complaints of mild ear pain, fullness in the ear ("popping" or feeling of "talking in a barrel"), dizziness or impaired balance. The older child may complain of hearing loss. The young child may request that you speak louder or require a higher volume than usual for the radio or television.

Physical Examination

Pneumatic otoscopy reveals decreased TM mobility. An abnormal-appearing TM, often described as dull, varying from bulging and opaque with no visible landmarks to retracted and translucent with visible landmarks and an air-fluid level or bubble may be seen (Figs. 36.7 to 36.9). Examine head and neck structures for abnormalities.

Diagnostic Studies

The tympanogram is flat-type B. The audiogram can show hearing loss ranging from mild to moderate (25 to 60 dB).

Differential Diagnosis

Differential diagnoses include AOM, all causes of hearing loss and anatomic abnormalities, and persistent unilateral OME can indicate a nasopharyngeal lesion or mass.

Management

Recommendations for management of OME in children 2 months to 12 years of age include (Rosenfeld et al., 2016):

1. Pneumatic otoscopy should be performed to document OME, particularly in children with ear pain and/or hearing loss. Tympanometry may be indicated in children to confirm OME diagnosis.
2. Manage the child with OME with watchful waiting for 3 months from date of diagnosis.
3. Intranasal steroids or systemic steroids, system antibiotics, antihistamines, and decongestants are not recommended for treatment of OME.
4. Children with OME who are at risk for speech, language, and learning problems should be identified. An age-appropriate hearing test should be performed if OME persists for 3 months or longer.
   - At-risk children are defined as having developmental delays because of sensory, physical, cognitive, or behavioral factors (e.g., hearing loss independent of OME, speech or

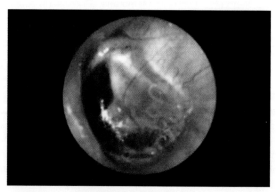

• **Fig 36.9** Serous Effusion.

language delays, pervasive or other developmental disorders, syndromes or craniofacial disorders, blindness, and/or cleft palate). These children should be promptly referred for hearing, speech, and language evaluation.

5. Reevaluate a child with OME every 3 months until the effusion resolves, or every 3 to 6 months for children with chronic OME. When managing a child with OME, clinicians should document resolution of OME in the medical record.

6. Communication is key to families understanding the duration and course of OME, the need for follow-up, and the associated sequelae including potential hearing impairment and impact on speech and language development.

7. Referral to an otolaryngologist is recommended when otoscopy suggests possible or impending structural damage of the TM, significant hearing loss is identified, and/or for chronic or persistent OME for more than 6 months. The need for referral should be clearly communicated to the family.

8. In a child younger than 4 years old, insertion of tympanostomy tubes is performed for persistent or chronic OME with associated sequelae; adenoidectomy is not recommended unless an indication exists other than OME. In a child 4 years old or older, insertion of tympanostomy tubes and/or adenoidectomy is recommended for OME.

Complications

Recurrent AOM and hearing loss that may be transient CHL, or with persistent OME, permanent high-frequency SNHL.

Perforated Tympanic Membrane

Perforated TMs are most commonly associated with AOM. Perforation occurs in approximately 30% of children with a middle ear infection (Conover, 2013). Children with a perforation are more likely to have had otitis media in the past.

The pain associated with the AOM generally improves significantly once the rupture occurs and there is usually profuse otorrhea. The fluid that drains from the ruptured TM usually contains the same virus and bacteria that is associated with TTO. In older children with ruptured TM, the most common bacteria are *P. aeruginosa* and *S. aureus* (Conover, 2013). Most ruptures heal without intervention in 1 to 3 months.

Traumatic TM perforations are caused by blows to the ear, blasts (fireworks), improper attempts at ear cleaning, and children putting things in their ears. Perforating the TM is not necessarily painful, and most children will present with acute onset of bleeding from the ear. Traumatic perforations are less likely to heal spontaneously and can be prone to infection and hearing loss.

Clinical Findings

History, Physical Examination, and Diagnostic Studies

- The child may be asymptomatic. After perforation, the child may feel immediately better. Children may present with whistling sounds during sneezing or nose blowing, or hearing loss.
- TM perforation is evident on otoscopic examination. Profuse otorrhea from the perforation may decrease TM visibility.
- Tympanogram will be flat. Perform a hearing test once the acute infection clears or the traumatic perforation heals.

Differential Diagnosis

Included are AOM, TTO, or nonaccidental trauma (boxed ears).

Management

The goal of therapy is to control the otorrhea and watchful waiting to ensure healing of the perforation.

Medications

If the perforation was caused by an AOM, treat the ear with otic drops (see Table 36.4), analgesics if needed, and oral antibiotics (Table 36.7). There is no evidence that medicated eardrops improve traumatic perforation healing (Conover, 2013).

Other Treatment Considerations

- Perforation makes the ear more susceptible to infection if water enters the EAC. Thus, having a TM perforation is an absolute contraindication to swimming, getting water into the ears when shampooing, and irrigation for cerumen removal (Hardman, 2015).
- Small perforations are not usually repaired unless there is a quality-of-life issue. Perforations caused by acute infection tend to heal spontaneously. Primary care follow-up is important to assure there are no sequelae from the perforation. Hearing loss is the most common sequelae of a TM perforation. The degree of hearing loss can range from mild to severe depending on the size and location of the perforation.
- Referral to the otolaryngologist is indicated if there is significant hearing loss or structure damage noted on otoscopy.

Auricular Hematoma

Auricular hematoma is also commonly referred to as "wrestler's ear" or cauliflower ear. Blunt trauma to the ear from activities such as wrestling, martial arts, or boxing results in a tear in the perichondrial blood vessels causing hematoma formation. The hematoma in the subperichondrial space stimulates asymmetrical cartilage formation resulting in ear deformity. Prompt drainage of the blood and ear bolstering to prevent reaccumulation of blood is needed.

Clinical Findings

History and Physical Examination

The history should elicit the details of the mechanism of the blunt trauma and document safety of home and school environment for the child or adolescent. It is important to note that children on anticoagulants may develop a hematoma after minor trauma. Other symptoms include:
- Auricular tenderness
- Auricular swelling
- Blood on the outside of the ear
- Erythema or ecchymosis to the overlying skin

Differential Diagnosis

Infections of the middle ear cartilage or inflammation from the autoimmune condition relapsing polychondritis may look similar on physical exam.

Management and Complications

Patients with an auricular hematoma should be referred to otolaryngology as soon as possible and within 7 days of the trauma to prevent the formulation of granulation tissue and asymmetrical cartilage growth in the ear. Reaccumulation of the hematoma or an untreated hematoma can result in permanent deformity, scar formation, perichondritis, infection, and/or necrosis.

Cholesteatoma

Cholesteatoma is usually the result of a chronic ear infection and involves the formation of an epidermal inclusion cyst of the middle ear or mastoid consisting of desquamated debris from the keratinizing, squamous epithelial lining of the middle ear (Fig 36.10). As the cholesteatoma grows in size, it can destroy the surrounding structures. Chronic otorrhea, ossicular erosion, and hearing loss are common sequelae. Any child with chronic ear drainage that does not resolve with appropriate antibiotic treatment should be referred to an otolaryngologist to rule out cholesteatoma. Permanent hearing loss, facial nerve paralysis, meningitis, and brain abscess are rare but potential complications of untreated cholesteatoma.

Cholesteatomas can be congenital, primary acquired, or secondary acquired. Congenital cholesteatomas are small and self-contained at birth and initially appear as a pearly white mass behind the TM. Primary acquired cholesteatomas arise from negative middle ear pressure that causes TM retraction and subsequent accumulation of an erosive keratin-filled cyst. Secondary acquired cholesteatomas are the result of skin ingrowth from a perforated TM or trapped epithelium due to ear trauma or a procedure.

Clinical Findings

History and Physical Examination

The history may be negative with congenital cholesteatomas. The history with an acquired cholesteatoma might include:

- Chronic otitis media with malodorous purulent otorrhea
- Vertigo and hearing loss
- History or presence of tympanostomy or PE tubes
- A pearly white lesion is present on or behind the TM. Aural polyps are considered cholesteatomas unless proven otherwise. Congenital cholesteatomas are often in the most anteroinferior position behind the TM (see Fig 36.10).

Differential Diagnosis

Tympanosclerosis (Fig 36.6), debris from chronic OME, malignant rhabdomyosarcoma, and aural polyps are some of the differential diagnoses.

Management and Complications

Cholesteatoma is managed surgically. Accurate diagnosis and immediate referral to an otolaryngologist for surgical excision are needed. Complications include irreversible structural damage, permanent bone damage, facial nerve palsy, hearing loss, and intracranial infection, especially in untreated cases.

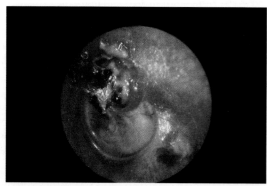

• **Fig 36.10** Cholesteatoma of the Left Ear. (Photograph courtesy Sylvan Stool, MD, The Children's Hospital, Denver, CO.)

Mastoiditis

Mastoiditis is a suppurative infection of the mastoid cells that may occur with AOM or follow an AOM. The mucoperiosteal lining of the mastoid air cells becomes inflamed, with subsequent progressive swelling and obstruction caused by drainage from the mastoid. It is now rare in children since the introduction of the *H. influenzae* (HIB) and the *S. pneumoniae* or pneumococcal (Prevnar or PCV13) vaccine. Other causative invasive organisms identified include *M. catarrhalis, S. aureus, S. pyogenes,* and *Mycobacterium tuberculosis* (rare). Gram-negative *E. coli, Proteus,* and *Pseudomonas* are more common in chronic mastoiditis, more virulent infections, and young infants. Intracranial complications of mastoiditis are common and may develop despite treatment.

Clinical Findings

History, Physical Examination, and Diagnostic Studies

- Concurrent or recurrent AOM
- Fever and otalgia
- Persistent otitis media unresponsive to antibiotic therapy
- Postauricular swelling: Infants may have edema above the ear, displacing the pinna inferiorly or laterally. Older children have edema that pushes the earlobe superiorly and laterally.
- Computed tomography (CT) or MRI provide definitive anatomical information and should be ordered by otolaryngology either before or after hospitalization.
- Tympanocentesis with culture and gram stain help identify the offending organism.

Differential Diagnosis

Postauricular inflammation or swelling such as lymphadenopathy, periauricular cellulitis, perichondritis of auricle, mumps, or mastoid tumors.

Management

Urgent ENT referral is imperative. Hospitalization, intravenous antibiotics, and often surgical intervention with myringotomy, pressure-equalizing tube placement, and mastoidectomy are required.

Tympanostomy or Pressure-Equalizing Tubes

Insertion of tympanostomy tubes is the most common ambulatory surgery performed on children in the United States (Rosenfeld et al., 2013). Tympanostomy tubes are most often inserted because of persistent middle ear fluid, frequent ear infections, or ear infections that persist after antibiotic therapy (see the previous discussion on referral for OME). Criteria for referral to otolaryngology when managing children 6 months to 12 years of age include:

- Bilateral OME for 3 months or more, unilateral OME for 6 months or more, or recurrent episodes of OME with cumulative duration of OME for more than 6 of the previous 12 months
- CHL associated with MEE
- Recurrent or recurrent AOM
- Prevention of acquired cholesteatoma due to a retraction pocket of the TM

It is important to clearly communicate to families the importance of referral and possible long-term sequelae of hearing loss from persistent MEE.

Management

Viral myringitis or early AOM without otorrhea in a child with tympanostomy or PE tubes usually resolves spontaneously. TTO can occur within the first few weeks of ear tube placement and should self-resolve (Rosenfeld et al., 2013). Approximately 7% of children experience recurrent otorrhea (Rosenfeld et al., 2013). It usually occurs when a child with tubes has an upper respiratory infection. TTO usually involves the same bacterial pathogens seen in AOM. Combination antibiotic and corticosteroid otic drops are the preferred treatment for TTO (van Dongen et al., 2014). Otic medications are listed in Table 36.4.

A child with tympanostomy or PE tubes does not need to take precautions during bathing, showering, or surface swimming, unless instructed otherwise by their otolaryngologist (Wilcox and Darrow, 2014). Swimming in lake water should be avoided due to the inherent bacteria level of stagnant water.

Most tympanostomy or PE tubes come out spontaneously. If the tube is extruded and there are persistent ear complaints, or if it remains in the TM for more than 2 or 3 years, the child should see an otolaryngologist (Rosenfeld et al., 2013). Complications of tympanostomy or PE tubes include otorrhea, OE, granuloma, cholesteatoma, tube obstruction, persistent TM perforation, and tympanosclerosis. Bacterial biofilms can form on implanted prostheses and tend to be antibiotic resistant. If the biofilm is antibiotic resistant, the PE tubes will likely have to be replaced by the otolaryngologist if the child has persistent symptoms.

Additional Resources

American Cleft Palate-Craniofacial Association (ACPA). www.cleftline.org
American Society for Deaf Children (ASDC). www.deafchildren.org
Beginnings for Parents of Children With Hearing Loss and Their Families. http://ncbegin.org/
Cochlear Implant Awareness Foundation. www.ciafonline.org/
Dolly Parton's Imagination Library. www.imaginationlibrary.com/
Family Voices. www.familyvoices.org
Imagery Language and Visual Communication. www.handspeak.com
My Baby's Hearing. www.babyhearing.org
National Association of the Deaf (NAD). https://www.nad.org/
National Family Association for Deaf-Blind (NFADB). www.nfadb.org
National Institute on Deafness and Other Communication Disorders (NIDCD). www.nidcd.nih.gov

References

Alford RL, Arnos KS, Fox M. American College of Medical Genetics and Genomics guideline for the clinical evaluation and etiological diagnosis of hearing loss. *Genet Med.* 2014;16(4):347–355.
American Academy of Pediatrics Committee on Practice and Ambulatory Medicine. Bright Futures Guidelines Periodicity Schedule Update 2017. Available at: https://www.aap.org/en-us/Documents/periodicity_schedule.pdf. Accessed October 30, 2018.
American Academy of Pediatrics. Joint Committee on Infant Hearing: year 2007 position statement: principles and guidelines for early hearing detection and intervention programs. *Pediatrics.* 2007;120(4):898–921.
Bowatte G, Tham R, Allan KJ, et al. Breastfeeding and childhood acute otitis media: a systematic review and meta-analysis. *Acta Paed.* 2015;104(S467):85–95.
Casazza G, Meier JD. Evaluation and management of syndromic congenital hearing loss. *Curr Op in Otolaryngol Head Neck Surg.* 2017;25(5):378–384.

Centers for Disease Control and Prevention (CDC). *Hearing loss in children, (website)*; 2015. Available at www.cdc.gov/ncbddd/hearingloss/genetics.html. Accessed August 10, 2015.
Center for Disease Control and Prevention (CDC). *What noises cause hearing loss? (website)*; 2017. Available at https://www.cdc.gov/nceh/hearing_loss/what_noises_cause_hearing_loss.html. Accessed November 5, 2018.
Conover K. Earache. *Emerg Med Clin North Am.* 2013;31(2):413–442.
Harlor AD, Bower C, Committee on Practice and Ambulatory Medicine, et al. Hearing assessment in infants and children: recommendations beyond neonatal screening. *Pediatrics.* 2009;124(4):1252–1263.
Hardman J, Muzaffar J, Nankivell P, et al. Tympanoplasty for chronic tympanic membrane perforation in children: systematic review and meta-analysis. *Otol Neurotol.* 2015;35(5):796–804.
Harrison LJ, McLeod S, McAllister L, et al. Speech sound disorders in preschool children: correspondence between clinical diagnosis and teacher and parent report. *Australian J Learning Difficulties.* 2016;22(1):35–48.
Ho D, Rotenberg BW, Berkowitz RG. The relationship between acute mastoiditis and antibiotic use for acute otitis media in children. *Arch Otolaryngol Head Neck Surg.* 2008;134(1):45–48.
Interdisciplinary Council on Developmental and Learning Disorders. *Diagnostic Manual for Infants and Early Childhood: Mental Health, Developmental, Regulatory-Sensory Processing, Language and Learning Disorders (ICDL-DMIC).* Bethesda, MD: ICDL; 2005.
Kaur R, Morris M, Pichichero ME. Epidemiology of acute otitis media in the postpneumococcal conjugate vaccine era. *Pediatrics.* 2017;140(3):e20170181.
Lieberthal AS, Carroll AE, Chonmaitree T, et al. The diagnosis and management of acute otitis media. *Pediatrics.* 2013;131(3):e964–e999.
Loveman E, Gospodarevskaya E, Clegg A, et al. Earwax removal interventions: a systematic review and economic evaluation. *Br J Gen Pract.* 2011;61(591):e680–e683.
Available at emedicine.medscape.com/article/856116-overview#showall.html. Accessed October 13, 2017.
National Center for Hearing Assessment and Management (NCHAM). *EHDI legislation becomes law, (website)*; 2011. Available at http://www.infanthearing.org/legislation/federal.html. Accessed September 20, 2017.
Palmu AA, Lahdenkari M. Early vaccine-type pneumococcal acute otitis media does not predispose to subsequent otitis when compared with early acute otitis media due to other bacterial etiology. *Pediatr Infec Dis J.* 2018;37(6):592.
Pimperton H, Blythe H, Kreppner J, et al. The impact of universal newborn hearing screening on long-term literacy outcomes: a prospective cohort study. *Arch Dis Child.* 2016;101:9–15.
Prentice P. American Academy of Otolaryngology: Head and Neck Surgery Foundation clinical practice guideline no acute otitis externa 2014. *Arch of Dis Child: Educ Prac Ed.* 2015;100:197.
Pimperton H, Blythe H, Kreppner J, et al. The impact of universal newborn hearing screening on long-term literacy outcomes: a prospective cohort study. *Arch Dis Child.* 2016;101:9–15.
Roth DA, Hildesheimer M, Bardenstein S, et al. Preauricular skin tags and ear pits are associated with permanent hearing impairment in newborns. *Pediatrics.* 2008;122(4):e884–e890.
Rosenfeld RM, Schwartz SR, Cannon CR, et al. Clinical practice guideline: acute otitis externa. *Otolaryngol Head Neck Surg.* 2014;150(suppl 1):S1–S24.
Rosenfeld RM, Schwartz SR, Pynnonen MA, et al. Clinical practice guideline: tympanostomy tubes in children. *Otolaryngol Head Neck Surg.* 2013;149(suppl 1):S1–S35.
Rosenfeld RM, Shin JJ, Schwartz SR, et al. Clinical practice guideline: otitis media with effusion (update). *Oto Otolaryngol Head Neck Surg.* 2016;154(IS):S1–S41.
Schilder AGM, Marom T, Bhutta MF. Panel 7: otitis media: treatment and complications. *Otolaryngol Head Neck Surg.* 2017;156(suppl 4):S88–S105.

Simon F, Haggard M, Rosenfeld RM, et al. International consensus (ICON) on management of otitis media with effusion in children. *Eur Ann of Otorhinolaryn, Head, and Neck Dis.* 2018;135(1):S55–S57.

U.S. Department of Education (USDE). National Center for Education Statistics: fast facts. *Institute of Education Sciences (website)*; 2013. Available at http://nces.ed.gov/fastfacts/display.asp?id=64. Accessed October 10, 2017.

U.S. Department of Health and Human Services (HHS): Healthy People 2020, (website), Available at www.healthypeople.gov. Accessed October 17, 2017.

U.S. Preventive Services Task Force (USPSTF). *Recommendations for primary care practice, (website)*; 2017. Available at www.uspreventiveservicestaskforce.org/Page/Name/tools-and-resources-for-better-preventive-care. Accessed October 17, 2017.

van Dongen TM, van der Heijden GJ, Venekamp RP, et al. A trial of treatment for acute otorrhea in children with tympanostomy tubes. *N Engl J Med.* 2014;370(8):723–733.

Van Dyke MK, Pircon JY, Cohen R, et al. Etiology of acute otitis media in children less than 5 years of age: a pooled analysis of 10 similarly designed observational studies. *Ped Infec Dis J.* 2017;36(3):274–281.

Venekamp RP, Sanders SL, Glasziou PP, et al. Antibiotics for acute otitis media in children. *Cochrane Database of Sys Rev.* 2015;6:1–85.

Waitzman AA. Otitis externa medication, Medscape (website), updated 2015. Available at http://emedicine.medscape.com/article/994550-medication. Accessed October 13, 2017.

Wallace IF, Beckman ND, Lone KN, et al. Surgical treatments for otitis media with effusion, a systematic review. *Pediatrics.* 2014;133(2):296–311.

Wilcox LJ, Darrow DH. Should water precautions be recommended for children with tympanostomy tubes? *Laryngoscope.* 2014;124(1):10–11.

Woolfenden S, Eapen V, Jalaludin B, et al. Prevalence and factors associated with parental concerns about development detected by the Parents Evaluation of Development Status (PEDS) at 6-month, 12-month and 18-month well child checks in a birth cohort. *BMJ Open.* 2016;6(9):e012144.

37

Respiratory Disorders

RITA MARIE JOHN

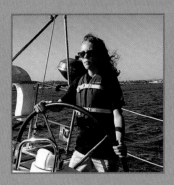

Respiratory problems including viral upper respiratory infections (URIs), pharyngitis, and otitis media are leading causes of illness in children. Caregivers seek health care to confirm the appropriate management of upper respiratory disorders and also use a variety of over-the-counter (OTC) cold medications, leading to overdosage of antipyretics and decongestants. The efforts by the Centers for Disease Control (CDC) and the American Academy of Pediatrics (AAP) for antibiotic stewardship encourages providers to avoid the use of antibiotics for viral infections (CDC, 2017; Hersh, Jackson, Hicks, and the Committee on Infectious Diseases, 2013). While there has been progress in antibiotic stewardship, recent data suggest that 30% of antibiotics used in an outpatient setting are unnecessary (CDC, 2017). There are United States geographic differences with lower rates of antibiotic prescriptions in the Pacific regions and the highest rate in the East South Central regions (Hersch et al., 2018).

It is critical that children with lower respiratory tract disorders (e.g., asthma or bacterial pneumonia) receive careful evaluation to identify a potentially life-threatening illness that demands prompt attention. Providers need to ask key questions about the history of respiratory symptoms; do a systematic and complete examination of upper and lower airways; and, if indicated, order specific laboratory tests and radiographic examinations. This systematic approach helps determine an accurate diagnosis and aids in developing a successful treatment plan.

Anatomy and Physiology

Upper Respiratory Tract

The upper respiratory tract includes the nostrils, nasopharynx, larynx, upper track of the trachea, eustachian tubes, and sinuses. Air is warmed and humidified as it travels through the nasal passages, and coarse nasal hairs filter out particles. The airway is coated with mucus with a complex mixture of water, mucins, proteins, lipids, and ions secreted by the respiratory epithelium. This mucus contains gel-forming mucins. MUCS B and particularly the MUC5AC mucins determine the viscoelastic properties of the mucus. Other host defense mechanisms in the mucus include cytoprotective molecules, including IgA, defensins, low-molecular-weight antioxidants, superoxide dismutase, catalase, and lactoperoxidase. These secretions shield the epithelial layer. The coordinated cilia move noxious stimuli such as viruses, bacteria, and allergens out of the lung and sinuses. The mucociliary clearance system is critical to prevention of airway mucus obstruction and represents the innate defense system within the lung.

When malfunction or destruction of the mucociliary clearance system occurs, a physical barrier forms, making it difficult for ions and macromolecules to function. Decreased mucociliary clearance and mucus obstruction cause small airway dysfunction leading to the accumulation of nutrient-rich mucus that allows bacteria to flourish (Zhou-Suckow et al., 2017).

The bronchoepithelium is pseudostratified, with multiciliated columnar epithelial cells, mucous-producing goblet cells, and undifferentiated cells positioned on top of smaller basal cells that can self-renew. Also, there are occasional pulmonary neuroendocrine and brush or tuft cells that play a role in neurosensory and chemosensory function. In addition to protection from mucus, the bronchial epithelium forms a sheet-like structure that acts as a physical barrier to protect the internal tissue within the airways. Epithelial cells also modulate innate lymphoid cells that function as natural killer cells (Loxham and Davies, 2017). The respiratory epithelium has approximately 200 cilia per cell; almost 250 proteins are involved in their protective function (Damseh et al., 2017).

The mucociliary action of the paranasal epithelium moves secretions from the sinuses to the nasal cavity. The frontal, maxillary, and anterior parts of the ethmoid sinuses drain into the middle meatus of the nose, whereas the sphenoid and posterior parts of the ethmoid sinuses drain into the superior meatus of the nose. Secretions then move through the patent ostia into the nose. Inflammation of nasal mucosa causes edema and disruption of mucociliary clearance. Any significant swelling of the ostia, due to a URI, allergic inflammation, or mechanical or local obstruction results in ostial obstruction and blockage of sinus secretions.

Maxillary sinuses are present by the second trimester of gestation but are not fully air-filled cavities or pneumatized until age 4 years. They reach 50% of their size around 8 years of age (Lorkiewicz-Muszynska et al., 2015). Ethmoid sinuses develop by the fourth month of gestation and form the thin lateral walls of the orbit of the eye. They are pneumatized at birth and can be visualized on plain radiographs when the child is 1 to 2 years old. Sphenoid sinuses are present by 5 years of age and frontal sinuses begin development at ages 7 to 8, completing their development by adolescence (Pappas and Hendley, 2018). A mnemonic to remember the order of sinus development is Maxillaries Early, Sphenoids Follow, which translates to the following order: (1) Maxillary (2) Ethmoids, (3) Sphenoids, and (4) Frontal. The sinuses become clinically significant sites of infection around the following ages: maxillary and ethmoid sinuses, 1 to 2 years old; sphenoid sinuses, 3 to 4 years old; and frontal sinuses, 7 to 10 years old.

There are several anatomical differences in the child's airway that make it prone to obstruction. The tongue is larger and the epiglottis is vertically positioned, omega shaped, and soft. The epiglottis deflects swallowed material toward the esophagus to protect the larynx. The larynx is anterior and superior in location at the level of the third and fourth cervical vertebrae (Darras et al., 2015). The vocal cords form a V-shaped opening known as the *glottis*. The subglottic space is beneath the vocal cords, and its walls converge toward the cricoid ring to form a complete ring of cartilage around the larynx. The cricoid ring is the narrowest part of the airway in infants and young children, whereas in adolescents and adults, the glottis is narrowest (Darras et al., 2015). The rings of tracheal cartilage support the trachea and the main stem bronchi. Marginal decreases in the caliber of the pediatric airway can cause obstruction to airflow. Thus, if upper airway radius decreases, resistance to airflow greatly increases. When a child inspires, the intraluminal pressure in the upper respiratory airway is negative. The airway is then more susceptible to collapsing resulting in turbulent airflow and stridor, a harsh high-pitched inspiratory sound. Upper airway obstruction is characterized by stridor (Mandal et al., 2015), which can lead to a medical emergency.

The trachea and airways of the infant and young child are more compliant than those of an adult. Hyperextension of the neck can constrict the infant's airway. Consequently, changes in intrapleural pressure lead to greater changes in an infant's or young child's airway compared to the effect that it exerts on adult airways, thereby causing an increased risk of airway collapse. Similarly, increased chest wall compliance in young infants makes them more vulnerable to adverse events, and their respiratory muscles cannot effectively handle sustained, intense respiratory workload that occurs during severe pulmonary illnesses. Due to weak intercostal and diaphragmatic muscles along with lower cardiac and pulmonary reserves, the ability to compensate is difficult when there is airflow obstruction (Darras et al., 2015). Upper airway obstruction needs rapid evaluation and management. The child who presents with respiratory distress and noisy breathing may indicate almost complete obstruction.

Lower Respiratory Tract

Primitive airways appear at approximately week 4 of gestation. Around week 16 of gestation, the number of bronchial branches equals that in adults. Subsequent growth continues by increasing the length of the respiratory tract. During weeks 16 to 26 of gestation, vascularization of the future respiratory portion of the lung occurs. Cartilage, glands, and muscles of the airways and type II alveolar cells are formed by week 28. Type II cells allow the fetus to produce a phospholipid called *surfactant*. Airways continue to grow, and terminal sac formation occurs. At approximately week 36, the terminal sacs divide, and alveoli are formed. Approximately 50 million primitive alveoli are present at birth. After birth, the alveolar ducts branch out from the respiratory bronchioles. Alveoli continue to form and number 100 to 200 million in older children and 200 to 600 million in adolescents. Alveolar sacs continue to increase in size. The adult lung contains approximately 300 million alveoli.

The neonatal airway has alveolar macrophages that are the predominant cell type at birth and an important first line of defense (Lambert and Culley, 2017). Most viruses replicate within the respiratory epithelium, which is in close communication with alveolar macrophages that signal the production of inflammatory mediators including interferons, mucus, and antimicrobial proteins. Antimicrobial proteins are also produced by innate leukocytes found in the lung, particularly neutrophils. Neutrophils are found in abundance in infants with severe respiratory syncytial

virus (RSV). An adult-like lung microbiota is established by around 3 years of age but is acquired from the mother at the time of birth (Lambert and Culley, 2017). Airway resistance is higher in newborns and young children than in adults. The airways of young infants and children are easily obstructed by inflammation, foreign bodies (FBs), or mucus. The maximal inspiratory pressure generated by an infant is equal to that of an adult. The infant's chest wall and supporting structures are softer and more flexible with chest wall retraction greatest in young infants. The chest wall of a newborn is highly compliant.

The lower respiratory tract passages begin at the trachea and include the right and left lungs that branch out—first to the bronchi, then the bronchioles, and end at the alveoli. The right lung has three lobes—upper, middle, and lower—with the upper and middle being separated by a minor fissure. The left lung has two lobes—upper and lower—separated by a major fissure. The upper left lobe has an area called the *lingula* that corresponds to the right middle lobe. The right main stem bronchus is shorter and wider than the left bronchus. It forms a smaller angle away from the trachea than the left bronchus does. This anatomic variation explains why FBs usually lodge in the right main stem bronchus.

Although the body surface and the number of respiratory airways and alveoli increase tenfold from birth to adult life, the tissue available for gas exchange increases approximately twentyfold. The newborn's chest is cylindrically shaped and has relatively horizontal ribs, which limits the infant's ability to expand his or her chest. Because there is greater transverse growth in the lower part of the chest wall, the shape of the chest changes during the first few years of life. This differential growth results in the ribs being positioned lower anteriorly than posteriorly. The change in rib positioning adds rigidity to the thorax of older children.

The diaphragm is the main muscle of respiration, and during normal tidal breathing, it moves about 1 cm but can move 10 cm during forced breathing (Bhalla, 2017). The external intercostal muscles are responsible for upward rib movement, increasing the anteroposterior and lateral movement of the rib cage. The sternocleidomastoid elevates the sternum and the scalene (anterior, medius, and posterior) muscles elevate the first two ribs. They are utilized during exercise or to maintain ventilation during respiratory disease and are two common accessory muscles of inspiration. While normal exhalation occurs from elastic recoil of the lung, the internal intercostal and abdominal muscles play a role in forcing air out of the lung during expiration and decrease the thoracic volume (Bhalla et al., 2017).

Pathophysiology

All lung disorders cause some form of airway obstruction. Narrowing of the airway lumen results from one or more of the following: presence of intraluminal material (e.g., secretions, tumors, or foreign matter); mural thickening (e.g., edema or hypertrophy of the glands or mucosa); contraction of smooth muscle (e.g., spasm); and extrinsic compression. These factors rarely occur in isolation. They cause pulmonary malfunction by impairing tracheobronchial hygiene and impeding normal airflow.

Obstructive Processes

Airway obstruction is the underlying etiology for the most common forms of pediatric lung diseases. The two major types of airway obstruction are complete and partial. In complete obstruction, neither airflow nor drainage of secretions occurs. Such occlusion leads to lobar atelectasis after the residual gas diffuses into the pulmonary circulation. In partial airway obstruction, airflow and secretion drainage occur but are impaired. Partial obstruction can be further divided into two separate classifications. The first causes bypass obstruction by narrowing the lumen and producing wheezing. Although resistance to flow is increased, air can still flow in during inspiration and out during expiration. The second is a check-valve or ball-valve obstruction; air entry is possible, however, during expiration the lumen is completely occluded so that escape of air is impossible. Bronchial FBs and emphysema are associated with bypass, check-valve, or ball-valve obstructions that result in over inflation of lung airways.

Upper Airway Obstruction

Airway obstruction that occurs above the level of the secondary bronchi generally interferes more with inspiration than expiration. If the obstruction is complete and above the bifurcation of the trachea, asphyxia and death can result. Partial obstruction results in severe dyspnea, stridor, and subcostal retractions. Coughing removes nonfixed, high airway obstruction. Poor inspiratory airflow limits coughing effectiveness. The sound produced by coughing may indicate the level of airway obstruction and assists in making a diagnosis. Laryngeal obstructions produce a cough that sounds croupy or barking. Obstruction in the trachea or major bronchi produces a brassy sound.

Lower Airway Obstructions

Lower airway obstruction result from peripheral lesions that are usually diffuse in location and involve bronchioles smaller than 3 mm. The usual mechanism of narrowing is spasm, accumulation of secretions, edema of the mucous membrane, extrinsic compression, or any combination of these factors. Complete airway obstruction causes atelectasis. A large percentage of the lung volume needs to be involved before symptoms become apparent; a small area of atelectasis does not produce obvious clinical manifestations.

The primary clinical manifestation of lower airway obstruction occurs during expiration. Wheezing is the principal sound made if the obstruction allows enough air to pass through the narrowed lumen. Chest excursion diminishes, and the expiratory phase prolongs. Increased airway resistance during exhalation results in over inflation of the lungs, which in turn eventually increases the anteroposterior diameter of the chest. Chronic over inflation results in a "barrel chest" typically noted in a child with chronic lung disease, such as cystic fibrosis (CF) or emphysema. The accumulation of fluids and inflammation in the lower airways usually result in a repetitive hacking, ineffectual cough. Percussing an overinflated chest elicits hyperresonance.

Symptoms worsen as the obstruction increases. The body attempts to compensate by using accessory muscles to assist in breathing. Dyspnea can result and may include orthopnea, relief from dyspnea when upright, and exercise intolerance. Cyanosis, an ominous sign, appears as the oxygen saturation drops below 85%. Mild obstruction is marked by reduced respiratory rate and increased tidal volume; severe obstruction is characterized by increased respiratory rate, increased retractions with the use of accessory muscles, anxiety, and cyanosis.

Fine crackles (formerly called *rales*) are intermittent, nonmusical, short, explosive, clicking, or rattling sounds, best heard on mid- to late inspiration and occasionally on expiration. These sounds are gravity dependent, not transmitted to the mouth, and are unaffected by cough. They are heard in pneumonia and interstitial lung disease and are caused by airways suddenly opening after having been previously closed. The gas pressure between the compartments equalizes and creates the crackling sound. Coarse crackles are nonmusical, short, and explosive sounds that are heard on early inspiration and throughout expiration. They are intermittent bubbling or brief popping sounds that are longer in duration than fine crackles. Course crackles may be affected by cough and are more common during inspiration. They may indicate intermittent airway opening and may be related to excessive airway secretions.

Restrictive Processes

Restrictive disease is less common in pediatric patients and is characterized by airflow limitation and decreased total lung capacity (TLC). The etiology is diverse and includes interstitial inflammation and fibrosis; respiratory muscle weakness as seen in spinal muscular atrophy; decrease in outward recoil of the chest wall as seen in scoliosis; alveolar destruction such as pneumonia or acute lung injury; and space occupying problems such as lung tumors, air, effusions, or cysts. Key findings of restrictive lung disease are rapid respiratory rate and decreased tidal volume/capacity (Bhalla et al., 2017).

Defense Systems

The respiratory defense system includes mechanical and biologic processes. Mechanical defenses include mucociliary clearance, sheetlike structure that forms a physical barrier to protect internal tissues within the airways, warming and humidifying inspired air, airway clearing through coughing, and spasm and breathing changes.

Approximately 75% of inspired air is warmed as it passes through the nose, paranasal sinuses, pharynx, larynx, and upper portion of the trachea. Final warming and humidifying of the airstream take place in the trachea and large bronchi. Heat and moisture are removed during the expiratory phase of respiration. The nose has a large surface area on which particles larger than 5 mm are trapped and filtered to prevent them from entering the lower airways. The trachea and bronchioles are lined with various defensive cells and mucus glands. Goblet cells secrete the mucous layer that lies on the tip of cilia. Particles entering the conducting airway are quickly cleared by the mucociliary defenses. Coughing is a reflex mechanism that has three phases: (1) inspiratory, (2) compressive, and (3) expiratory. Through forceful expiration, foreign bodies (FBs) and other materials can be removed from the airways; coughing propels particles. Young infants and children cannot effectively expectorate mucus, so they swallow it. Loss of the cough reflex leads to aspiration and pneumonia. Temporary breathing cessation, reflex shallow breathing, laryngospasm, and even bronchospasm are compensatory efforts aimed at stopping foreign matter from further entry into the lower respiratory tract. However, these respiratory efforts offer limited protection and have significant drawbacks.

Biologic processes that protect the respiratory system include phagocytosis, absorption of noxious gases in the vasculature of the upper airway, and absorption of particles by the lymph system. The work of phagocytosis is aided by neutrophils, innate lymphoid cells, gel-forming mucins, and cytoprotective molecules including defensins secretory IgA, lactoperoxidase, catalases, and low molecular weight antioxidants (Zhou-Suckow et al., 2017). Particles reaching the alveoli can be phagocytized by a variety of white blood cells, cleared from the lung by the mucociliary system, or carried by lymphocytes into regional nodes or the blood. These particles can take days to months to clear.

The respiratory defense system is at risk for compromise from numerous environmental factors. Damage to epithelial cells is caused by a variety of substances and gases, such as sulfur, nitrogen dioxide, ozone, chlorine, ammonia, and cigarette smoke. Hypothermia, hyperthermia, morphine, codeine, and hypothyroidism can adversely alter mucociliary defenses. Dry air from mouth breathing during periods of nasal obstruction, tracheostomy placement, or inadequately humidified oxygen therapy results in dryness of the mucous membrane and slowing of the cilia beat. Cold air is irritating to the lower airways.

Phagocytic ability is reduced by many substances, including ethanol ingestion and cigarette smoke. Hypoxemia, starvation, chilling, corticosteroids, increased oxygen, narcotics, and some anesthetic gases also impair phagocytosis. Recent acute viral infections can reduce antibacterial killing capacity. Damage from infection and chemical irritants may or may not be reversible.

Recurrent respiratory infections in children merit investigation for immunodeficiency or other underlying diseases, such as primary ciliary dyskinesia or CF. The mnemonic SPUR (Bush, 2009) helps remind which children need further workup: **S**evere infection, **P**ersistent infection and poor recovery, **U**nusual organisms, and **R**ecurrent infection.

There are 10 warning signs for an immunodeficiency and the diagnosis should be considered if the child has (1) four or more new ear infections in a year, (2) two or more serious sinus infections, (3) 2 or more months on antibiotics without improvement, (4) two or more pneumonias in a year, (5) failure to gain weight or grow normally, (6) recurrent deep-seated skin or organ abscesses, (7) persistent oral candidiasis or fungal infection on the skin, (8) the need for intravenous (IV) antibiotics to clear infections, (9) two or more deep-seated infections including septicemia, and (10) a family history of immunodeficiency (Jeffrey Modell Foundation, 2017).

Assessment of the Respiratory System

History

The history provides valuable information about the causes, progression, and potential complications of a child's respiratory condition. The physical examination and diagnostic testing allow the provider to determine the extent of respiratory distress.
- Onset: When did the disease start, what was the onset of symptoms? Was there any recent travel within the past 6 months?
- Promoting, preventing, precipitating, palliating factors:
  - *Contacts:* Are any family members or close contacts (e.g., day care, school) ill with similar signs and symptoms?
  - *Prevention:* Do you give your child any medications or supplements (e.g., herbs, botanicals, or vitamins) to try to prevent a cold? What are your hand-washing practices? Do you encourage fluids when your child has a URI? Are immunizations up to date?
  - *Progression:* Are the respiratory signs or symptoms increasing in severity, lessening, or about the same? Is the child easily fatigued, less active, having trouble sleeping, or working harder to breathe?
  - *Treatment:* Have any OTC, prescription drugs, herbs, supplements, or botanicals been used? Have any other treatment modalities been used, including folk cures or home remedies?
- Quality or quantity: How severe are the symptoms? Is the illness interfering with school attendance or play? Are breathing problems affecting the child's ability to sleep?
- Region or radiation: Does the child complain of chest pain?
- Severity, setting, simultaneous symptoms, or similar illnesses in the past:
  - *Key signs and symptoms:* Has the child had symptoms or signs of a daytime or nighttime cough, fever, vomiting, malaise, rhinorrhea, sore throat, lesions in the mouth, retractions, cyanosis, dyspnea, or increased respiratory effort? Table 37.1 lists key characteristics and causes of cough.

- *Associated symptoms:* Has there been a decrease in appetite or eating? Any rashes, headaches, or abdominal pain? Does the child drink well but not want to eat?
  - *Similar illnesses in the past:* Does the child have a history of respiratory tract infections, allergies, or asthma? How many similar infections has the child had (e.g., croup, pneumonia, rhinosinusitis, streptococcal tonsillopharyngitis, or frequent colds)?
- Temporal factors: When did the illness begin? Was the onset acute or insidious or proceeded by the common cold? How long has it lasted? How has it changed over time?
- Family history:
  - Do others in the family have a history of allergies or asthma?
  - Is there any family history of immunodeficiency, ear-nose-throat, or respiratory problems?
  - Does anyone in the family have genetic diseases, such as CF or α 1-antitrypsin deficiency?
  - Are other family members ill?
- Review of systems: Note any infections, constitutional diseases, or congenital problems that might have a respiratory component.
- Environment:
  - Does anyone in the family or in the day care setting smoke? Does the child live or attend school in an urban or industrial area subject to air pollution (e.g., near a major highway, industrial plant, or bus terminal)? Has the child or a family contact traveled recently and where?

Physical Examination

When determining respiratory distress, think about the total presentation and not just individual isolated findings. Consider the anxiety level, respiratory rate and rhythm, use of accessory muscles, color, breath sounds, grunting, and pulse oximetry results. Information pertinent to the physical examination of a child with suspected respiratory disease includes the following:
- Measurement of vital signs and observation of general appearance:
  - Normal respiratory rate is age dependent and, if elevated, is a key indicator of lower respiratory tract involvement (see Box 37.1).
  - Anxiety level, nasal flaring, and "prefers to stay upright" are useful indicators of respiratory distress. Changes in skin color may be subtle or obvious, depending on the level of deoxygenation. Grunting is a sign of small airway disease.
- Inspection:
  - Nose: Look for rhinorrhea—clear, mucoid, mucopurulent; FBs, erosion, polyps, lesions, bleeding, septal position, and mucous membrane color.
  - Throat, pharynx, and tonsils: Look for lesions, vesicles, exudate, enlargement of any structure, or other abnormalities. It is important to see the entire tonsil to make sure there are no abscesses in a child with a severe sore throat; however, if epiglottitis is a consideration, do not inspect the mouth or attempt to elicit a gag reflex.
  - Chest: Look at respiration depth, symmetry, and rythm of respiration. These are key indicators of lower respiratory tract involvement. Note the use of accessory muscles and the presence of retractions. In infants, early retractions are best seen on the chest along the posterior axillary line. A prolonged expiratory phase is associated with lower airway respiratory obstruction.
- Palpation or percussion of the chest:
  - Percuss for signs of dullness or hyperresonance caused by consolidation, fluid, or air trapping.

TABLE 37.1	Key Characteristics of Cough, Common Causes, and Questions to Ask in a Pediatric History
Key Characteristics to Consider	**Description and Questions to Ask**
Age	Infants less than 1 mo with pneumonia may not have a cough
Quality	Staccato-like (*Chlamydia trachomatis* in infants); barking or brassy (croup, tracheomalacia, habit cough); paroxysmal or inspiratory whoop (pertussis or parapertussis); honking (psychogenic). Is the cough wet or dry?
Duration	*Acute* (most causes are infectious and last less than 2 wk), *subacute* (cough lasts from 2 to 4 wk); *recurrent* (associated with allergies and asthma), or *chronic* (lasting greater than 3 mo [e.g., CF, asthma]). Is the cough continuous or intermittent?
Productivity	Mucous-producing or nonproductive? Younger children do not expectorate
Timing	During the day, night (associated with asthma), or both? Associated with exercise?
Family history	Is there a history of CF in the family? What genetic diseases run in the family?
Effect on caregiver and child	What are caregiver's responses to cough? Is it causing loss of sleep and work time? Are there concerns that the child may have something seriously wrong?
Associated symptoms	High fever in an acutely ill child: Can be bacterial or viral infection (pneumonia). Rhinorrhea, sneezing, wheezing, atopic dermatitis, pale boggy mucosa: Associated with asthma and allergic rhinitis. Malaise, sneezing, watery nasal discharge, mild sore throat, no or low fever, not ill appearing: Typical of URI. Tachypnea: Pneumonia or bronchiolitis in infants (infants may not have a cough).
Exposure to infection or travel	Travel history (areas of tuberculosis or novel coronaviral infection)? Is there a member of the household being treated for a cough illness?
Causes	
Congenital anomalies	Tracheoesophageal fistula, vascular ring, laryngeal cleft, vocal cord paralysis, pulmonary malformations, tracheobronchomalacia, congenital heart disease
Infectious agent	Viral (RSV, adenovirus, parainfluenza, HIV, metapneumovirus, human bocavirus), bacterial (tuberculosis, *B. pertussis*, *Streptococcus pneumoniae*, *Haemophilus influenza*, *Moraxella catarrhalis*), fungal, and atypical bacteria (*C.* and *M. pneumoniae*)
Allergic condition	Allergic rhinitis, asthma
Other	FB aspiration, gastroesophageal reflux, psychogenic cough, environmental triggers (air pollution, tobacco smoke, wood smoke, glue sniffing, volatile chemicals), CF, drug induced, tumor, congestive heart failure

CF, Cystic fibrosis; *FB*, foreign body; *HIV*, human immunodeficiency virus; *RSV*, respiratory syncytial virus; *URI*, upper respiratory infection.

BOX 37.1 Normal Respiratory Rates in Children

Age (years)	Respiratory Rate (breaths/minutes)
0-1	24-38
1-3	22-30
4-6	20-24
7-9	18-24
10-14	16-22
15-18	14-20

- Auscultation of the chest:
  - Upper tract: Pathology frequently causes noisy breathing, snoring, stridor, and musical or wheezing tracheal breath sounds and can be a source of referred breath sounds. Make sure to go from cheek to chest to distinguish these sounds.

Have the child take a deep breath by having him blow out the light on the otoscope or blow paper off your hand.
- Lower tract: Pathology is suggested by fine crackles, coarse crackles, rhonchi, pleural friction rub, wheezing, and bronchial breath sounds.

Diagnostic Studies

Diagnostic procedures used to evaluate respiratory illness in children managed as outpatients include the following:
- Monitoring oxygenation. Pulse oximetry can be used to spot check or continuously measure pulse rate and is a noninvasive method of monitoring arterial oxygen saturation. The oxyhemoglobin saturation percentage (SpO_2) is digitally displayed (Bhalla et al., 2017). Results generally correlate well with simultaneous arterial oxygen saturation (SaO_2). Continuous outpatient measurement of oxygen saturation in diseases like bronchiolitis is no longer recommended and may be responsible for the increasing

admission rate for bronchiolitis (Quinonez et al., 2017). With anoxia, there is a rise in organic phosphate content within the red blood cells (RBCs) resulting in more oxygen (O_2) available to tissues. People living at higher elevations suffer from chronic hypoxia. When first arriving at a high elevation, many individuals experience a transient mountain sickness with symptoms that include headache, insomnia, irritability, breathlessness, nausea, and vomiting. This phenomenon lasts approximately 1 week before acclimatization begins. The affected person begins to increase production of RBCs. Finally, functional nonpathologic right ventricular hypertrophy occurs. These effects last as long as the person remains at high elevation. Severe altitude sickness can lead to cerebral and pulmonary edema and can be life-threatening.

- Monitoring carbon dioxide (CO_2). Monitoring CO_2 can be done by a transcutaneous measurement (TCOM) or nasal cannula/endotracheal end tidal CO_2 monitoring. TCOM involves a small patch placed on the abdomen or chest measuring CO_2 diffusing to the surfaces. It can be affected by extreme obesity or if there is poor peripheral perfusion. Nasal cannula provides a noninvasive way of monitoring for hypoventilation or apnea but may underestimate the actual CO_2 so elevated readings need further investigation (Bhalla et al., 2017).
- Blood gas studies. These studies are used in acute care settings to assess possible respiratory collapse. A rising partial arterial pressure of carbon dioxide ($Paco_2$) is an ominous sign.
- Rapid diagnostic testing. Testing for bacteria, viruses, and fungal infections performed by CLIA-waved tests now include more accurate second-generation antigen assays, newer molecular testing with real-time polymerase chain reaction (PCR), and increased antigen detection sensitivity at the point of care (Gonzalez and McElvania, 2018). The Food and Drug Administration (FDA) approved molecular tests for the pediatric population include testing for *Group A Beta hemolytic Streptococcus* (GABHS), respiratory viruses panels including *RSV, influenza, Bordetella pertussis, Chlamydophila pneumoniae, Mycoplasma pneumonia, Bordetella parapertussis,* and *Bordetella holmesii.* The rapid digital immunoassays and molecular testing for influenza A and B have a higher sensitivity and can improve management for selected populations (Merchx, Wali, Schiller, 2017). The newer GABHS molecular point of care tests have specificity and sensitivity over 95%; therefore, back-up cultures are not needed if these tests are negative. Of note, this testing should be done only if doing so contributes to the child's treatment decision (Gill, Richardson, Ostrow et al., 2017).
- Radiographic imaging to assess respiratory disease should be done in accordance with clinical guidance and the principles of imaging with consideration of risks of radiation exposure (Levine, 2018). Imaging can include radiographs, ultrasonography, magnetic resonance imaging (MRI), and computed tomography (CT) of the sinuses, soft tissues of the neck, and chest. Abnormalities of the nasal mucosa, such as thickening, may reflect inflammation. Imaging in acute rhinosinusitis (ARS) is not indicated as CT demonstrates abnormality in 80% of patients with uncomplicated URI (Magit, 2014). Chest radiographs should be done in both posteroanterior and lateral positions, because lesions may only be seen in one of the two views. Pulmonary function tests are discussed in Chapter 33 in the section on asthma.
- Other specialized tests, including sweat testing, cultures, and blood work, are addressed under the specific illness. Children with unusual signs and symptoms should be referred to

a pulmonary specialist for further evaluation and diagnostic work-up. Fluoroscopy is useful in the evaluation of stridor and abnormal movement of the diaphragm. Endoscopy (bronchoscopy and laryngoscopy), bronchoalveolar lavage, percutaneous tap, lung biopsy, and microbiology studies can be helpful if used appropriately. Contrast studies (e.g., barium esophagogram) are useful for patients with recurrent pneumonia, persistent cough, tracheal ring, or suspected fistulas. Other imaging studies that might be needed to assess these children include bronchograms (useful in delineating the smaller airways), pulmonary arteriograms (evaluation of the pulmonary vasculature), and radionuclide studies (evaluation of the pulmonary capillary bed).

Basic Respiratory Management Strategies

General Measures

There are several essential and basic measures related to the prevention of respiratory illnesses that should be emphasized. They include avoidance of smoke and exposure to secondhand smoke, good hand-washing practices, and immunization coverage for age. Children who are significantly ill or have unusual manifestations need referral to or consultation with a pediatrician or pediatric subspecialist. For those with mild or moderate respiratory illnesses, the following general management measures are applicable:

- *Fluid:* Hydration is important to keep mucous membranes and secretions moist. Intake of fluids should be encouraged, and caregivers should be given guidelines regarding the type, amount, and frequency of fluids and feedings.
- *Oxygen administration:* The use of supplemental oxygen is important to help relieve hypoxemia in most children who have acute respiratory distress. Depression of the respiratory drive is possible with supplemental oxygen administration if central nervous system (CNS) chemoreceptors are blunted by hypercapnia. Children at risk for blunting are those with issues related to chronic hypercapnia and are generally easily recognized, because they tend to have chronic severe respiratory diseases, such as CF and bronchopulmonary dysplasia (also called neonatal chronic lung disease). In acute situations, administer oxygen using an appropriately sized mask or a high-flow oxygen source held near the child's face if a mask frightens the child. While ideally a child's oxygen should range between 95% to 100%, new guidelines for bronchiolitis allow an infant to go home when the oxygen ranges between 90% to 95%. (Ambalavanan, 2014; Quinonez, Coon et al., 2017). Children with oxygen saturations less than 85% and those with significant distress who need to be seen in an ED should be transported via emergency medical services for management 🔊.
- *Humidification:* A cold-mist humidifier helps provide moisture to the nares and oropharynx in a dry environment during a common cold. The tank and parts exposed to water should be cleaned every 2 to 3 days of operation in a 10% bleach solution. Vaporizers are no longer recommended.
- *Bulb syringe:* Infants are preferential nose breathers; therefore, caregivers should be instructed in gentle and intermittent use of the nasal bulb syringe to relieve obstruction of the infant's nares. Improper use can cause irritation, inflammation, and respiratory obstruction from tissue damage. To improve understanding, providers need to give written instructions about suctioning the infant's nose with a bulb syringe (see resources for guidelines).

- *Normal saline (NS) nose drops, nasal rinses, or spray:* Use before feedings and when mucus is thick or crusted. Follow by suctioning the nares with a bulb syringe. Saline nasal rinses are widely available commercially and are helpful for older children and adolescents (Box 37.2).

Medications

The following pharmacologic agents may be needed to treat symptoms of respiratory illnesses:
- *Analgesics and antipyretics:* Acetaminophen and ibuprofen may be prescribed for relief of pain or fever.
- *Decongestant, antihistamines, and cough medicine:* The use of decongestants, antihistamines, and cough medicine does not shorten the course of a disease. Due to the risk of overdose, unsupervised ingestions, potential for harm, and little evidence of efficacy, the use of decongestants and/or cough medication is no longer recommended for children younger than 6 years. Extreme caution is recommended in prescribing them to children less than 6 years (Ballengee and Turner, 2014; Weintraub, 2015). The FDA issued warnings not to prescribe any cold medications containing codeine or hydrocodone to pediatric patients under 18 years of age due to serious side effects, deaths, and addiction potential (FDA, 2018).
- *Expectorants:* Water is one of the most effective expectorants. OTC agents provide some symptomatic relief, but do not shorten the course of respiratory illnesses. Although expectorants like guaifenesin are approved for use in children over 2 years of age, they are not recommended for use in children less than 6 years old (Ballengee and Turner, 2014). While guaifenesin has a safety profile with over 50 years of use in the United States, common side effects include gastrointestinal upset, dizziness, and headache (Albrecht, Dicpinigaitis, and Guenin, 2017).
- *Cough medication:* There is lack of evidence to recommend any OTC cough medication for children (Bergamini, Kantar, Cutrera et al., 2017). The use of honey over the age of 2 years has been suggested by some authors. Recent guidelines on chronic cough of greater than 4 weeks requires further evaluation. Antihistamines and cough and cold medications are not recommended for persistent cough (Chang, Oppenheimer, and Weinger, 2017).
- *Zinc and vitamin C:* The use of zinc is not recommended in children due to potential side effects and questionable efficacy. Similarly, studies investigating the effect of large dosages of vitamin C in either the prevention or treatment of the common cold have demonstrated little to no benefit (Ballengee and Turner, 2014).
- *Probiotics:* The use of probiotics is being explored as a possible option for prevention of common cold illnesses in young children, with a recent study showing moderate effectiveness in reducing URIs (Lauren et al., 2018).

Patient and Family Education

Frequent hand washing and avoiding touching the eyes and nose can help prevent the spread of infection. Always educate about the dangers related to exposure to smoke and secondhand smoke exposure and the need to avoid this respiratory trigger. Teach the child and other family members how to cough/sneeze into sleeve, dispose of tissues, and use hand sanitizers, because these measures may decrease the spread of infections. Caregivers should be educated about assessment and management of changes in the child's condition. Significant educational issues are identified in Box 37.2.

• BOX 37.2 Education for At-Home Care of the Child with a Respiratory Tract Infection

General Management Issues to Discuss
Fluid: Give guidelines on type, amount, and frequency of fluids.
Humidification: For acute laryngotracheitis, take the child out into the cold night air or open a freezer door. In dry climates, humidifiers help in common colds; instruct about cleaning of nebulizers and humidifiers (see bullet about care of nebulizers and humidifiers).
Bulb syringe: Instruct to use the bulb syringe gently and intermittently for suctioning the nares.
Normal saline nose drops or spray: Use before feedings and when mucus is thick or crusted. Follow by suctioning nares with bulb syringe.
Good hand washing and avoidance of exposure to smoke or secondhand smoke.

Other Educational Topics to Cover
- Indications for immediate reevaluation of child:
  - Signs and symptoms of respiratory distress
  - Other indicators of worsening of illness (e.g., (toxic appearance [mild or moderately ill looking], malaise, feeding difficulty)
- Give information on when to expect improvement in the child's symptoms and what to do if symptoms do not improve as expected.
- Clear instructions about medications: Give instructions regarding how much medication to give, when to give it, what side effects to watch for, how long to give the medication, and the necessity of completing the course of antibiotics.
- Infection control information if needed: Give information regarding hand washing and disposal of infected secretions; the CDC has excellent written and video education materials available on hand washing at www.cdc.gov/Features/HandWashing.
- Care of nebulizers and humidifiers: To prevent the growth of organisms, nebulizers and humidifiers should be cleaned daily with soapy water, rinsed thoroughly, soaked for one half hour in a solution of one part vinegar to two or three parts distilled water, and then air-dried. Control III disinfectant is a commercial product that can be substituted for vinegar; however, it is expensive.
- Give instructions regarding next return visit.

CDC, Centers for Disease Control and Prevention.

Disorders of Respiratory Function

Upper Respiratory Tract Infection

A URI or the common cold is a frequent problem seen in pediatric practice, and caregivers often seek information from their child's primary healthcare provider as to whether their child's symptoms represent a typical URI or indicate the beginning or advancing signs of a more serious illness. Children have on average 2 to 10 URIs, or colds, per year with daycare attendance increasing the amount up to 14 URI per year (Weintraub, 2015). The typical course of these illnesses is an initial low-grade fever with a sore throat that progresses to rhinorrhea, cough, and congestion (Weintraub, 2015). The average duration is 7 to 9 days; the peak is generally on the third day when purulent discharge may be noted. There is a slow resolution with clear nasal discharge by day 10.

Viruses cause most URIs, with 50% resulting from infection by the more than 100 serotypes of rhinoviruses. The incidence of rhinovirus peaks in the spring and fall. It is most contagious in the first 3 days of illness and can shed for up to 2 weeks (Miller and Williams, 2016). Parainfluenza viruses, RSV, adenoviruses, coronavirus, human bocavirus, and human metapneumovirus are also common agents (Weintraub, 2015). Day care and preschool attendance are associated with an increased number of URIs in young children that spread to school-age children in the family. The acquisition of viruses occurs by hand contact of the infected surface to the nose or conjunctiva, inhalation of small airborne particles that are airborne, or by deposition of large particles that land directly on the conjunctiva or nasal mucosa. Transmission by direct contact is most efficient pathway for infection with rhinovirus and RSV (Miller and Williams, 2016).

The viral infection of the nasopharyngeal mucosa initiates a host response that produces the symptoms of a URI. Once the virus is deposited on the nasal mucosa, it attaches to cell receptors and enters the cells. Potent cytokines including interleukin (IL)-8 attract large number of neutrophil cells by 6 hours after infection. As a result, vascular permeability increases, causing the leak of plasma proteins into nasal secretions. Bradykinins cause the pharyngitis and rhinitis. The presence of polymorphonuclear leukocytes (PMN), rather than bacterial colonization, changes the color of nasal mucus, with yellow to green mucus due to PMN enzymatic activity and yellow mucus caused simply by PMN presence. The presence of neutrophils attracts interleukins 1 and 6, tumor necrosis factor, and chemoattractant ultimately leading to cell death. Adenovirus and influenza have a significant destructive effect on the respiratory epithelium (Camp and Jonsson, 2017).

Clinical Findings

Symptoms of a viral URI include nasal congestion, cough, sneezing, rhinorrhea, fever, hoarseness, and pharyngitis (Miller and Williams, 2016). Sleep disturbances do occur with URIs, but vomiting and diarrhea are uncommon. The symptoms should decrease at the end of 10 days.

History. The following may be reported:
- Gradual onset, low-grade fever especially in younger children
- Prominent nasal symptoms of rhinorrhea (key finding)
- Sore throat and dysphagia; mild cough and poor sleep
- After a variable period of 1 to 3 days, nasal secretions are thicker and more purulent, leading to nasal excoriation

Physical Examination. Virus-specific findings include:
- Mild conjunctival injection; red nasal mucosa with secretions of varying colors depending on the degree of nasal mucosa destruction and PMN activity; mild erythema of the pharynx
- Anterior cervical lymphadenopathy with freely movable nodes less than 2 cm
- Chest clear to auscultation and without adventitious sounds

Diagnostic Studies. A throat culture is not recommended if there are nasal symptoms with complaints of throat pain. If the presenting symptom is a sore throat rather than rhinitis, a rapid antigen detection test (RADT), or a rapid strep test, should be done.

Differential Diagnosis

The most common differentials are allergic rhinitis, rhinosinusitis, and adenoiditis (Table 37.2).

Management

Only supportive care is needed for a viral URI. See the Respiratory Management Strategies section and Box 37.2. Antibiotics are not appropriate treatment. The child should receive symptomatic relief for fever, pain, and nasal congestion using NS and an antipyretic. Although topically applied menthol may improve nighttime cough, there is a risk of chemical irritation and accidental ingestion, causing CNS and gastrointestinal (GI) side effects. Fluid intake should be encouraged.

Complications

Common colds are self-limiting, but secondary bacterial infections including otitis media, pneumonia, and sinusitis can occur along with secondary wheezing.

Pharyngitis, Tonsillitis, and Tonsillopharyngitis

Pharyngitis is an inflammation of the mucosa lining the structures of the throat, including the tonsils, pharynx, uvula, soft palate, and nasopharynx. It can be due to infectious agents or noninfectious causes, such as environmental exposures, allergic responses, referred pain, or oncological causes. Most children with pharyngitis have an acute illness involving an inflammatory response, including erythema, exudate, or ulceration.

If there are nasal symptoms with pharyngitis, it is called *nasopharyngitis,* but if there are no nasal symptoms, the illness is called *pharyngitis* or *tonsillopharyngitis.* Most cases of pharyngitis are caused by viruses (Bochner et al., 2017) and typically include adenovirus, Epstein-Barr virus (EBV), parainfluenza, influenza, herpes simplex virus (HSV), cytomegalovirus (CMV), enterovirus, and human immunodeficiency virus (HIV). While adenoviruses are more likely to cause pharyngitis as a prominent symptom, other viruses (e.g., rhinovirus) cause rhinorrhea or cough as predominant features. Adenoviruses are generally self-limiting illnesses in children under 5 years old (Ghebremedhim, 2014). Enterovirus (coxsackievirus, echovirus), herpesvirus, and EBV are also common. Viral infections occur year-round, but adenovirus presenting as pharyngoconjunctival fever occurs in outbreaks during the summer due to contaminated swimming pools and school exposure, particularly kindergartens (Ghebremedhim, 2014). Hoarseness, cough, coryza, conjunctivitis, and diarrhea are classic features of a viral infection (Bochner et al., 2017). It is helpful to know what agents are currently infecting children in the community.

When a patient has only a sore throat, it is difficult to differentiate viral from bacterial causes and RADT is positive in acute illness and carriage states (Shapiro et al., 2017).

The most common bacterial cause of pharyngitis and tonsillitis in all pediatric patients, typically between 5 and 11 years of age, is GABHS. It accounts for about 15% to 30% of infections in children with acute sore throat and fever (Sande and Flores, 2014).

There are other less common causes of bacterial pharyngitis in children. *Group C* and *group G streptococci* can cause pharyngitis as well as more severe infections but are less common. *M. pneumoniae* and *C. pneumoniae* are associated with cough along with pharyngitis. *M. pneumonia* can cause a significant sore throat and most commonly is accompanied with lower tract symptoms. *A. haemolyticum* is more common in adolescents, resembles EBV infection, and causes pharyngitis (100% of the time), a fine, scarlatiniform rash (40% to 70%), pruritus (50%), fever (75%), and cough (40%); however, it can have a variable presentation characterized by mild or marked pharyngeal erythema, with or without tonsillar exudate, or cervical adenopathy (Ching, 2014). *N. gonorrhoeae* is a cause of pharyngitis if the patient engages in oral to genital sex with individuals who have *N. gonorrhoeae* of the genital region. *C. diphtheria* is an extremely rare cause of pharyngitis and is not endemic in the United States with only five cases reported between 2006 and 2016 (CDC, 2018a). *Corynebacterium diphtheria* and *H. influenza B* are uncommon in developing countries. *Francisella tularensis* is found in patients who ingest undercooked game meat (Bochner et al., 2017).

TABLE 37.2 Differentiations of Common Upper Respiratory Infections in Children

Site of Infection	Symptoms	Duration of Symptoms	Etiologic Agent	Management	Duration of Treatment	Comments
The common cold (viral URI)	Malaise, sneezing, watery nasal discharge, mild sore throat, may have a fever, not ill appearing	0-10 days	Adenovirus, rhinovirus, RSV, parainfluenza, adenovirus	No antibiotics; symptomatic treatment (e.g., saline nose drops, increased fluids); for infants, bulb-syringe the nose before meals and bedtime; for older children, use a humidifier	As long as symptoms last	If lasts longer than 10-14 days, consider other diagnosis (e.g., rhinosinusitis).
Acute rhinosinusitis (ARS)	Persistent nasal symptoms for more than 10 days with URI, nasal drainage (purulent or discolored), cough Acute presentation with high fever, purulent rhinitis	10-30 days	*Streptococcus pneumoniae, Moraxella catarrhalis,* nontypeable *Haemophilus influenza*	Amoxicillin, or amoxicillin-clavulanic acid	10 days	By 7 days, should be asymptomatic; change antibiotics 48-72 h after start of treatment if no response.
Subacute rhinosinusitis	Same as above but persistent for at least 30 days	30-84 days	Same as above; may be β-lactamase producing	Amoxicillin-clavulanic acid		If initial acute infection did not clear, need to switch antibiotics.
Chronic/recurrent rhinosinusitis	Malaise, easy fatigability, unilateral or bilateral nasal discharge, postnasal discharge, nasal obstruction if middle turbinate significantly obstructed	Recurrent >10 to <28 days but symptom free for at least 10 days in between bouts Chronic >84 days	Same as above plus α-hemolytic streptococci and *Staphylococcus aureus*	Amoxicillin-clavulanic, azithromycin, staph coverage	3-6 wk	May need endoscopic sinus surgery if CRS does not respond to prolonged medical management; investigate differential diagnoses or underlying issues (e.g., allergic rhinitis).

CRS, Chronic rhinosinusitis; *RSV,* respiratory syncytial virus; *URI,* upper respiratory infection.

Clinical Findings

History. A history of pain, myalgia and arthralgia, fever, sore throat, and dysphagia may be reported in viral or bacterial presentations.

In viral illnesses the following is commonly reported:
- Rhinitis, cough, hoarseness, stomatitis, stridor and conjunctivitis, nonspecific rash, or diarrhea (Bochner et al., 2017)

The following characterize GABHS infection (Bochner et al., 2017; Sande and Flores, 2014):
- Most commonly found in 5- to 13-year-old children; infrequent in children younger than 3 years old
- Abrupt and acute onset without nasal symptoms
- Tender lymph nodes, although not necessarily enlarged
- Constitutional symptoms, such as arthralgia, myalgia, headache
- Moderate to high fever, malaise, prominent sore throat, dysphagia
- Nausea, abdominal discomfort, vomiting, headache
- Presentation in late winter or early spring

Physical Examination

Common findings include:
- Erythema of the tonsils and the pharynx
- Reactive tender cervical lymphadenopathy

Virus-specific physical findings include the following:
- EBV can produce exudate on the tonsils, soft palate petechiae, and cervical lymphadenopathy.
- Adenovirus can cause pharyngoconjunctival fever associated with fever, pharyngitis, rhinitis, cervical lymphadenopathy, and bulbar and palpebral follicular conjunctivitis (Ghebremedhim, 2014).
- Enterovirus can produce vesicles or ulcers on the tonsillar pillars and posterior fauces; coryza, vomiting, or diarrhea may be present.
- Herpesvirus produces gum erythema, small erupted vesicles in the mouth anteriorly, and marked adenopathy (Goldman, 2016).
- Parainfluenza and RSVs cause more lower respiratory tract disease (e.g., croup, pneumonia, and bronchiolitis) with their typical respiratory signs of stridor, rales, or wheezing.

- Influenza usually is associated with a cough, fever, and multiple systemic complaints.

The following may be seen in GABHS:

- Petechiae on soft palate and pharynx, swollen beefy-red uvula, red enlarged tonsillopharyngeal tissue
- Tonsillopharyngeal exudate that is yellow, blood-tinged (frequently)
- Tender and enlarged anterior cervical lymph nodes; bad breath
- Stigmata of scarlet fever may be seen—scarlatiniform rash, strawberry tongue, circumoral pallor

Lack of a cough or nasal symptoms, along with an exudative, erythematous pharyngitis with a follicular pattern and typical historical findings point to GABHS.

Diagnostic Studies

It is important to use RADT for patients with clinical features consistent with GABHS to diagnose acute illnees and avoid false-positive tests on patients who are carriers of streptococcus and do not need treatment. Testing for GABHS should be performed in children 3 years and older with pharyngitis, because it is difficult to distinguish viral and streptococcal infections by history and physical examination. Testing for GABHS in children younger than 3 years and in asymptomatic household contact is not recommended (Bochner et al., 2017). Whether back-up cultures are done following a negative RADT depends on the type of rapid strep testing as the newest molecular tests do not need a back-up culture. At present, the first- and second-generation testing does need back-up throat culture if the RADT is negative. Judicious use of RADT is needed to avoid overuse of antibiotics and maintain antimicrobial stewardship (Shapiro et al., 2017).

Serological tests, such as anti-streptolysin O (ASO) and anti-deoxyribonuclease B tests (anti-DNase B), are not useful in the diagnosis of acute pharyngitis, because antibody response takes 1 to 3 weeks after infection and the titers remain elevated for months after an acute infection. While anti-streptolysin O (ASO) is the most common test used to document past GABHS infection, it is also positive in Group C and G infections (Sande and Flores, 2014). ASO and anti-DNase B testing involves identifying antibody titers in response to streptolysin O or deoxyribonuclease B, respectively; these tests are often done together. The ASO titer rises 1 week post infection and peaks 3 to 5 weeks after infection. Measurement of anti-streptococcal antibody titers is useful in the diagnosis of the nonsuppurative complications of GABHS, such as rheumatic fever or acute glomerulonephritis. The anti-DNase B test rises 2 weeks after infection, peaks 6 to 8 weeks following infection (later than ASO), and remains elevated for months and longer than ASO.

Rare bacterial causes of pharyngitis that need treatment with antibiotics include *C. diphtheria* and *N. gonorrhoeae*. Adolescents who have oral to genital sex and pharyngitis need to be cultured as should adolescents and young adults with a sore throat, and a scarlatiniform rash similar to scarlet fever may be infected with *A. haemolyticum*. Their specimens need to be sent out for a culture with specific instructions to evaluate for these organisms.

If infectious mononucleosis is suspected in a child, a complete blood count (CBC) identifies lymphocytosis with atypical lymphocytes. This is a nonspecific test, because reactive (atypical) lymphocytes can occur in EBV, acquired CMV (Pinninti, Hough-Telford, Pati et al., 2016), as well as viral hepatitis, rubella, roseola, and mumps. Heterophile antibody testing (Mono Spot) for infectious mononucleosis can be helpful in school-age children and adolescents after the first week of infection but commonly yields false negatives.

Management

For viral infection, only supportive care is needed including dietary modifications. With fever and sore throat pain acetaminophen or ibuprofen are recommended. Adequate fluid intake should be encouraged.

Antibiotics should only be used in a symptomatic child with GABHS when the RADT or throat culture is positive. Antibiotic stewardship is needed to decrease the rise of antibiotic resistance associated with overuse (Bochner et al., 2017). The goal of antibiotic therapy is to shorten the course and severity of bacterial illness, prevent its spread to others, and prevent the development of suppurative and nonsuppurative complications. Treatment must be initiated within 9 days to prevent the nonsuppurative complications of rheumatic fever. The use of β-lactam antibiotics during an acute CMV or EBV infection is not needed and can cause a diffuse, morbilliform skin eruption (Pinninti et al., 2016). The management plan includes the following:

- Antimicrobial therapy shortens the length of the fever, decreases infectivity, lowers toxicity, and is based on positive bacterial testing results in a symptomatic patient (Sande and Flores, 2014)
  - Penicillin (drugs of choice due to cost, efficacy, and infrequent adverse reactions):
    - Penicillin V potassium: Children (<27 kg): 250 mg twice daily or three times daily for 10 days; children (greater than 27 kg) and adolescents: 500 mg twice daily or three times daily for 10 days; can do 250 mg four times a day with teens (Taketomo et al., 2018)
    - Amoxicillin suspension is more palatable (efficacy seems equal to penicillin): 50 mg/kg once daily (maximum dose = 1000 mg); alternate: 25 mg/kg (maximum dose = 500 mg) twice daily for 10 days
    - Benzathine penicillin G intramuscular (IM): 600,000 units as a single dose if less than 27 kg; 1.2 million units as a single dose for larger children and adults
  - If allergic to penicillin:
    - Cephalexin: 20 mg/kg/dose twice daily (maximum dose = 500 mg/dose) for 10 days but should be avoided in patients with moderate hypersensitivity reaction to penicillin
    - Cefadroxil: 30 mg/kg/day divided twice daily (maximum daily dose = 1 gm/day) for 10 days but should be avoided with moderate hypersensitivity reaction to penicillin
    - Clindamycin: 7 mg/kg/dose three times daily (maximum dose = 300 mg/dose) for 10 days
    - Azithromycin: 12 mg/kg once a day to a maximum of 500 mg for 5 days. It should be noted that macrolide resistance is variable in the United States (American Academy of Pediatrics and the Committee on Infectious Diseases Red Book, 2018 [AAP, 2018]).
    - Clarithromycin: 7.5 mg/kg/dose to a maximum of 250 mg twice per day for 10 days
- Supportive care: Antipyretics, fluids, and rest.
- Use of corticosteroids is not indicated (Bochner et al., 2017).
- Repeat culture is not needed except in situations where it is necessary to ensure eradication of the organism.
- Fomites, such as bathroom cups, toothbrushes, or orthodontic devices, may harbor GABHS and should be cleaned or discarded.
- Children can return to school when they are afebrile and have been taking antibiotics for at least 12 hours to 24 hours.

Continued symptoms of streptococcal pharyngitis and a positive culture for streptococcus may represent an actual treatment failure or a new infection with a different serologic type of streptococcus (DeMuri and Wald, 2014). Noncompliance with pharmacologic therapy can explain treatment failure, and in these instances, an injection of benzathine penicillin is recommended.

The mean carriage rate of GABHS is around 16%. To avoid overusing antibiotics, it is not recommended to do a follow-up culture in asymptomatic children nor to do a RADT on a patient with primarily nasal symptoms. The degree of communicability is less in carriage state due to difference in the M protein surrounding GABHS. The published guidelines do not recommend routine treatment of the carriage state except in special circumstances: (1) An outbreak in a closed community, (2) family or personal history of rheumatic fever, (3) ping pong spread in family members for several weeks, (4) if a tonsillectomy is being considered due to continued carriage, or (5) a local outbreak of rheumatic fever or invasive group A strep disease (DeMuri and Wald, 2014).

Treatment of chronic symptomatic carriage of GABHS:
- Clindamycin: 20 to 30 mg/kg/day in three doses (maximum dose = 300 mg/dose) for 10 days
- Amoxicillin-clavulanic acid: 40 mg/kg/day in three doses (maximum daily dose = 2000 mg/day) for 10 days
- Penicillin V: 50 mg/kg/day in four doses for 10 days (maximum dose = 2000 mg/day) with the use of rifampin: 20 mg/kg/day in one dose (maximum dose = 600 mg/day) during the last 4 days of treatment
- Benzathine penicillin G: 600,000 units for less than 27 kg and 1,200,000 units for 27 kg or greater; rifampin: 20 mg/kg/day in two doses (maximum dose = 600 mg/day)

If clinical relapse occurs, a second course of antibiotic is indicated, as discussed earlier. If recurrent infection is a problem, culturing of the family for the chronic carrier state is advised. Erythromycin is the drug of choice for *A. haemolyticum*.

Complications

Nonsuppurative complications of streptococcal infections include rheumatic fever, poststreptococcal reactive arthritis, Sydenham chorea (St. Vitus Dance), and acute glomerulonephritis. Suppurative complications include cervical adenitis, rhinosinusitis, otitis media, pneumonia, mastoiditis, and retropharyngeal or peritonsillar abscess. Retropharyngeal abscess is more common in children younger than 6 years old, whereas peritonsillar abscess peaks in adolescence with an average age of 13.6 (Bochner et al., 2017). Most peritonsillar abscesses are caused by streptococcus and Fusobacterium and are polymicrobial.

Other poststreptococcal sequela include poststreptococcal arthritis and pediatric autoimmune neuropsychiatric disorder syndrome (PANDAS). Pediatric Acute-onset Neuropsychiatric Syndrome (or PANS) is a condition in which there is a sudden onset of obsessive-compulsive symptoms and/or severe restriction of eating with at least two of seven different categories including cognitive, neurological, or behavioral symptoms (Swedo et al., 2017). PANS can result from different disease mechanisms ranging from psychological trauma to underlying neurological autoimmune, neuroinflammatory, endocrine, and post-infectious etiology. When a recent streptococcal infection is the cause, it is called PANDAS. The treatment of PANS and PANDAS is similar. New guidelines have a threefold approach: (1) Cognitive behavioral or family therapy and/or psychotropic medications to treat the psychiatric symptoms, (2) antimicrobial therapy to treat the underlying cause of inflammation if the source can be identified, and (3) use of immunomodulatory or anti-inflammatory medications to treat the immune system disturbance (Thienenman et al., 2017).

Indications for Tonsillectomy and Adenoidectomy

Current guidelines for tonsillectomy and adenoidectomy (T&A) clearly define the indications for tonsillectomy (Baugh, Archer, Mitchell, 2011). They include having more than seven episodes of throat infections in the past year, or more than five episodes of throat infection in the past 2 years or at least three episodes per year for the past 3 years. The definition of throat infections includes a temperature of higher than 100.9°F (38.3°C), cervical lymphadenopathy with tonsillar exudate, or a positive GABHS culture or if antibiotics had been administered in suspected or proved cases of GABHS. A recent systematic review of tonsillectomy versus watchful waiting found that the benefits of tonsillectomy do not persist over time and the quality of life was not different in either group. (Morad, Sathe, Francis et al., 2017). Sleep apnea is the most common reason for T&A. Other indications include recurrent tonsillitis, peritonsillar abscesses, periodic fever with aphthous ulcers, and adenopathy (Bochner et al., 2017).

The chief indication for an adenoidectomy is severe nasal obstruction for more than one year and unresponsiveness to medical therapy including antibiotics and nasal steroids. Severe nasal obstruction presents with hyponasal speech, olfaction difficulties, and chronic mouth breathing. Refractory otitis media, chronic otitis media with effusion, and recurrent otitis media in children who had tympanostomy tubes placed are relative contraindications (Bochner et al., 2017).

Rhinosinusitis

Sinusitis is an inflammatory condition that may or may not be infectious. Bacteria form biofilms, which are a matrix of polysaccharides, proteins, and nucleic acids. These films allow bacteria to aggregate in a protective environment, such as the sinuses, and are responsible for antimicrobial resistance (Magit, 2014). The maxillary and anterior ethmoid sinuses are most frequently involved in children because they are present at birth, but only the ethmoidal sinuses are pneumatized.

Rhinosinusitis can be divided into acute or chronic designations. *Acute rhinosinusitis (ARS)* involves inflamed mucosal lining of the nasal passages and paranasal sinuses. Sinusitis presents in three ways: (1) onset of severe upper respiratory symptoms, (2) onset of upper respiratory symptoms with persistent symptoms, and (3) a "double sickening" with initial improvement followed by onset of severe disease (Magit, 2014). *Chronic rhinosinusitis (CRS)* symptoms must persist for 12 weeks or longer (Brietzke et al., 2014). Acute bacterial sinusitis is a complication of a viral URI; approximately 8% of URIs are complicated by sinusitis (Marom et al., 2014). Sinusitis results because of several anatomical factors including inflammation of the sinus mucosa obstructing the sinus ostia, nasal polyps, allergic rhinitis, and underlying conditions such as ciliary dyskinesia, CF, and immunodeficiency.

The microorganisms responsible for ARS include *Streptococcus pneumoniae,* nontypeable (30%), *Haemophilus influenza* (20% to 30%), *Moraxella catarrhalis* (10% to 20%), and rarely by *Staphylococcus aureus* (Butler and Myer, 2018; Fang, England, Gausche-Hill, 2015). Although there is no consensus about the bacteriology of CRS, it is believed that CRS is a multifactorial inflammatory disease instead of a persistent bacterial infection. Predisposing factors for CRS include a preceding viral, bacterial, and/or fungal infection; environmental irritants; allergies; anatomic problems, including septal deviation, nasal polyps, trauma, FB, or abnormality of the ostiomeatal complex; gastroesophageal reflux; cigarette smoking; CF; primary ciliary dyskinesia; and immunodeficiencies (Brook, 2017). Persistent swelling of the sinonasal mucosa impairs sinus drainage, which is associated with sinusitis.

The adenoids are believed to be a reservoir for bacterial infections that lead to nose and nasal sinus infections. That is why adenoidectomy may be recommended as "a cleansing procedure" in rhinosinusitis as it has been shown to be of benefit in children (Stenner and Rudack, 2014).

The presence of antibiotic-resistant organisms is associated with the production of cephalosporinase and β-lactamase and is more common in patients in day care or with recent exposure to antibiotics (Brook, 2017). The role of viruses in rhinosinusitis is not clear. Children with immunodeficiency disorders need to be treated with antibiotics that cover Pseudomonas spp; children with CF are predisposed to sinus infections with *Aspergillus* and *Zygomycetes*.

Clinical Findings

The duration of symptoms determines the classification of rhinosinusitis. The history of acute sinusitis differs from an uncomplicated URI. A child with an uncomplicated URI presents with a thick, yellow discharge on the third or fourth day without fever or with low-grade fever followed by improvement. Headache, bad breath, fatigue, and decreased appetite are nonspecific symptoms and, therefore, not helpful in the diagnosis. Table 37.3 shows major and minor criteria for sinusitis. ARS is a clinical diagnosis and should not be confirmed by any diagnostic testing including imaging. Transillumination and percussion of the sinuses are not recommended (Fang et al., 2015).

Diagnostic Studies. Imaging studies should only be done if a complication is suspected. If the child is suspected of having an orbital or CNS extension of sinusitis, then contrast-enhanced CT of the brain sinuses and orbits is generally done due to speed and ease. An MRI with contrast is an excellent option if readily available (Fang et al., 2015).

TABLE 37.3	Criteria for Bacterial Sinusitis
Major criteria	• Facial pain or pressure (second major criteria is needed) • Facial congestion or fullness • Nasal congestion/obstruction • Nasal discharge, purulence, or discolored postnasal discharge • Hyposmia or anosmia • Fever (acute sinusitis requires a second major criteria) • Purulence on intranasal exam
Minor criteria	• Headache • Fever • Halitosis • Fatigue • Dental pain • Cough • Ear pain, pressure, or fullness

Differential Diagnosis

The differential diagnosis of sinusitis includes a viral URI, allergic rhinitis, nasal polyps, nasal tumors, and tension, migraine, or cluster headache. Remember that sinusitis may exacerbate asthma. Ethmoiditis can occur after a child is 6 months old, in contrast to frontal rhinosinusitis, which is first seen around 10 years old.

Management

The healthcare provider must be cautious to not over diagnose rhinosinusitis and subsequently indiscriminately use antibiotics. Chronic or recurrent rhinosinusitis may result in referral to an otolaryngologist and/or allergist.

To aid in decision-making about when to treat, the AAP developed clinical guidelines for the treatment of ARS based upon three different clinical presentations in children (Wald et al., 2013):
- A URI with persistent nasal discharge or daytime cough lasting for more than 10 days without clinical improvement
- A URI that worsens or there is a new onset of fever, nasal discharge, or daytime cough after initial improvement
- A fever higher than 102.2°F (39°C) with purulent nasal discharge for at least 3 days in a child who also has sinusitis

Severe onset or a worsening course requires oral antibiotics. If the child has a persistent illness suggestive of rhinosinusitis, antibiotics can be given or a watchful waiting for 3 days can be offered. Symptomatic pain relief with acetaminophen or ibuprofen has been shown to be helpful. The sinusitis guidelines suggest treatment with amoxicillin with or without clavulanate as a first-line treatment (Wald et al., 2013). Treatment length varies from 10 to 28 days. An alternative to this is to continue treatment for 7 days after the child is completely free of any signs or symptoms. After starting treatment with antibiotics or watchful waiting, reassessment is needed after 72 hours.

Treatment considerations include the following:
- Amoxicillin at a standard dose of 45 mg/kg/day divided in two doses is the first-line treatment in communities with low incidence of nonsusceptible *S. pneumoniae*. In communities with more than 10% of resistant *S. pneumonia,* amoxicillin should be used at 80 to 90 mg/kg/day divided every 12 hours (maximum dose: 1000 mg/dose).
- In patients younger than 2 years old, day care attendees, recent antimicrobial use, or in patients with moderate to severe illness, amoxicillin-clavulanate at 80 to 90 mg/day of amoxicillin component divided every 12 hours and only use the 600 mg/5 mL formulation.
- In children with vomiting, a single dose of 50 mg/kg of ceftriaxone can be given either IV or IM.
- In patients with allergy to amoxicillin, the type of allergic reaction determines the antibiotic:
- If the child has a serious type 1 immediate or accelerated reaction, the cephalosporins cannot be used. However, if they have a non-type 1 hypersensitivity reaction, they can safely be treated with one of the third-generation, cephalosporin antibiotics—cefdinir, cefpodoxime, or cefuroxime.

The management of CRS is more complicated because bacteria are generally only one of other contributing factors. Referral to an otolaryngologist is often needed as an adenoidectomy is an effective first-line procedure for children under 12. Surgical drainage by an otolaryngologist, treatment of allergies and control of allergic rhinitis by an allergist, or both may be necessary.

Additional management considerations include the following:
- *Decongestants and antihistamines:* There is no randomized controlled trial (RCT) to support the use of topical decongestants

(Wald et al., 2013). Similarly, there are no data to support the use of either topical or oral antihistamines as an adjuvant therapy (Snidvongs and Thanaviratananich, 2017).

- *Intranasal corticosteroids:* Due to the increased evidence of inflammation as a cause of chronic rhinosinusitis, there is increased evidence that supports the use of intranasal steroids adjunctive medication in both ARS and CRS (Snidvongs and Thanaviratananich, 2017).
- *Saline irrigation:* NS is used to mechanically clean the nasal passages of mucus, biofilms, antigens, cytokines, inflammatory mediators, and thin secretions, and moisturize the nasal passages. While the 2013 clinical guidelines do not support or negate the use of saline (Wald et al., 2013), there is initial evidence to support the use of NS (Snidvongs and Thanaviratananich, 2017).
- *Analgesics:* Comfort measures include the use of acetaminophen and ibuprofen for severe pain. Adequate hydration is important.
- Diving is contraindicated with rhinosinusitis.

Complications

Orbital complications are common and usually occur following ethmoid sinusitis (Fang, et al., 2015). Complications of eye involvement include preseptal cellulitis, orbital cellulitis, and subperiosteal and orbital abscess. While orbital cellulitis is manifested by swelling and erythema of the eyelids, proptosis, decreased extraocular movements, and altered vision, an orbital abscess can lead to proptosis, ophthalmoplegia, and ultimately vision loss. Further extension can lead to a cavernous sinus thrombosis (CST). A CST starts with periorbital edema with chemosis and headaches and can advance to cranial nerve palsies as the infection invades the cavernous sinus (Fang et al., 2015).

Intracranial complications are more likely from frontal sinusitis and include Pott's puffy tumor, epidural abscess, subperiosteal abscess, brain abscess, venous thrombosis, and meningitis. The child with Pott's puffy tumor or osteomyelitis of the frontal bone presents with frontal bone tenderness and swelling on the forehead ●. A neurosurgical consult should be obtained. An infectious disease and otolaryngology consult is important with these complications.

Prevention

Prevention of sinusitis includes allergy and gastroesophageal reflux management, influenza vaccine, and relief of nasal airway obstruction.

Diphtheria

Diphtheria is a rare infection of the respiratory tract caused by toxigenic strains of gram-positive *C. diphtheria* or, less commonly, *Corynebacterium ulcerans*. The toxigenic strains produce two exotoxins—enzymatically active A domain and binding B domain. The binding B domain promotes entry of A into the cell. The bacterium has four biotypes (mitis, intermedius, belfanti, and gravis) that can be toxigenic or nontoxigenic. The ability of a strain of *C. diphtheria* to produce toxin is related to bacteriophage infection of the bacterium, not to colony type.

Humans are the only reservoir, and the organism is spread by respiratory droplets as well as contact with skin lesions. There have been no cases in the United States since 2003 (AAP, 2018). The bacteria can be shed for 2 to 6 weeks in an untreated patient. Disease may be mild or asymptomatic in partially or fully immunized individuals and severe if unimmunized. With toxin production, the primary infection can become lethal.

The disease is transmitted through respiratory droplets, touching the open sores of someone with diphtheria (rare) or via fomites (CDC, 2018a). Asymptomatic carriers can transmit the organism. The incubation period averages from 2 to 5 days with a range of 1 to 10 days (AAP, 2018). The incidence of respiratory diphtheria is greater in the fall and the winter; skin infections are more common in the summer. Endemic areas include Africa, Latin America, Asia, and the Middle East. In developing countries, a diphtheria-like illness caused by *C. ulcerans* is emerging (AAP, 2018).

Clinical Findings

History. Infection is associated with a history of low-grade fever and gradual onset of symptoms over 1 to 2 days with bacterial shedding for 2 to 6 weeks if untreated. Fully immunized individuals can carry the bacteria asymptomatically and may present with a mild sore throat.

Physical Examination. Signs of primary infection include:
- A thick, grayish, adherent pseudomembrane found in either the nasopharynx, pharynx, or trachea that bleeds on removal is the hallmark of diphtheria (Mandal et al., 2015)
- Bloody nasal discharge (with membranous pharyngitis) is highly suggestive of diphtheria (AAP, 2018)
- Sore throat, serosanguineous or seropurulent nasal discharge, hoarseness, cough
- Extensive neck swelling with cervical adenitis (bull neck) characterizes severe disease (AAP, 2018) and causes airway obstruction (due to membranous obstruction of the upper airway)
- Cutaneous lesions (nonhealing ulcers with dirty gray membrane or colonization of preexisting dermatoses) infected with diphtheria (seen less often)
- Possible otic and/or conjunctival infection findings

Clinical indications of toxin production include the following: myocarditis and electrocardiographic changes, respiratory compromise, cranial nerve and local neuropathies, and peripheral neuritis.

Diagnostic Studies. A confirmatory diagnosis is based on a positive culture of *C. diphtheria*. Specimens should be obtained from the nose, throat, any skin lesions, and either beneath the membrane or from a portion of the membrane. Because a special culture medium is needed, the lab needs to be notified if *C. diphtheria* is suspected. Toxigenicity tests are performed if *C. diphtheriae* is confirmed. Culture results take 8 to 48 hours; however, treatment begins when diphtheria is suspected (AAP, 2018). Do not wait for laboratory confirmation. Results of the CBC may be normal or show a slight leukocytosis and thrombocytopenia.

Differential Diagnosis. Acute streptococcal pharyngitis and infectious mononucleosis are included in the differential diagnosis of pharyngeal diphtheria. A nasal FB or purulent rhinosinusitis can resemble nasal diphtheria; epiglottitis, laryngeal diphtheria, and viral croup can also cause obstruction.

Management

Children with diphtheria require hospitalization with early tracheostomy for airway stabilization (Mandal et al., 2015) ●. Treatment consists of the following:
- *Antitoxin administration (hyperimmune equine antiserum):* A single dose needs to be administered if there is a high index of suspicion prior to a positive culture result. Allergic reaction to the serum occurs in 5% to 20%, so a scratch test should be performed prior to administration. Dosages range from 20,000

to 40,000 units for pharyngeal or laryngeal disease of 2 days duration to a high of 80,000 to 120,000 units for a bull neck. IV immunoglobulin is not FDA approved for use (AAP, 2018).

- *Antimicrobial therapy:* Erythromycin given orally or parenterally for 14 days, penicillin G for 14 days either IM or IV, or penicillin G procaine IM for 14 days. This is not a substitute for antitoxin administration.
- Supportive care for respiratory, cardiac, and neurologic complications as appropriate.
- Standard and droplet precautions until two cultures are negative (AAP, 2018).
- Immunization after recovery because disease does not necessarily confer immunity.
- Monitoring and antimicrobial prophylaxis of contacts regardless of immunization status.
- Care for respiratory, cardiac, and neurologic complications.

Complications and Prevention

Cranial and peripheral neuropathy, myocarditis with heart block, and upper airway obstruction occur with severe disease. Universal immunization against diphtheria with regular booster injections is the only effective method of control. Infection can occur in immunized or partially immunized children, but the disease severity is greatly diminished in these individuals. Disease generally occurs in nonimmunized children; the frequency of severe life-threatening complications in this group is high. Care of a child exposed to diphtheria includes a booster dose of a diphtheria toxoid containing vaccine that is age appropriate and close surveillance. If the contact cannot be followed, penicillin G benzathine is recommended (AAP, 2018).

Recurrent Epistaxis

Recurrent epistaxis is common in children, with an incidence of 30% in children from birth to 5 years old and over 50% in children older than 5 years (Shay, Shapiro, Bhattacharyya, 2017). While it is classified into anterior and posterior epistaxis, anterior bleeding is far more common in children. Only 10% of epistaxis originates in the posterior area and these are more likely to be arterial bleeds. Primary epistaxis represents about 85% of the cases (Yau, 2015). Etiologies include medication and local, systemic, environmental, and idiopathic factors. A recent study found that pediatric epistaxis incidence was highest in the spring and summer months (Shay et al., 2017). Local factors that can cause mucosal irritation resulting in bleeding include nasal trauma, allergies, septal abnormalities, neoplasia, juvenile nasopharyngeal angiofibroma in an adolescent, and inflammation. However, in children, local trauma is commonly due to digital trauma or irritation. Systemic causes include coagulopathies, allergies, polyps, hemangiomas, FB, and viral or bacterial infections of nasal tissue. Known environmental risk factors are living in dry climates or dryness from artificial heat during winter months. Use of medications such as nonsteroidal antiinflammatory drugs (NSAIDs), anticoagulants, chronic use of topical nasal sprays containing corticosteroids or antihistamine decongestants, and topical cocaine abuse can all lead to epistaxis.

The bleeding originates from the anterior portion of the nasal septum, called *Little's area* where a plexus of vessels (called *Kiesselbach plexus*) meet under the thin nasal mucosa. The blood supply of the Kiesselbach area comes from branches of the internal carotid, which break up into the facial and internal maxillary arteries, which supply most of the face. Two of the six branches of the internal maxillary artery, the palatine and sphenopalatine arteries, supply 80% of the

blood supply with an additional 20% coming from the facial artery (Yau, 2015). A coagulopathy, generally von Willebrand disease or platelet aggregation disorders, can manifest as recurrent epistaxis; a careful history will reveal hallmark clinical signs of mucocutaneous bleeding beyond epistaxis that includes easy bruisability, menorrhagia, and gastrointestinal bleeding (Schinco et al., 2018).

Clinical Findings

History. The following may be reported:
- Recent nasal trauma, including nose-picking; allergies; or a recent URI
- Unexpected bruising or bleeding from other sites; frequent nosebleeds (unilateral or bilateral)
- Tarry stools (the result of swallowed blood)

The provider should always ask about a family history of excessive bleeding episodes or bleeding disorders. Oral anticoagulants and topical nasal medication use, including topical steroid spray, nasal decongestants, or in the case of the teen, cocaine or other inhaled recreational drugs should be explored.

Physical Examination. Nares visualization using the otoscope without a tip may reveal fresh or old clots, nasal masses, FB, polyps, and/or raw, red Little's area (Patel et al., 2014; Siddiq and Grainger, 2015). The nasal mucosa on the medial surface of the anterior septum may be dry, cracked, excoriated, or scabbed. It is important to evaluate *Little's area* in children. Signs of nasal allergy including allergic shiners, Dennie-Morgan lines, adenoidal facies, and pale boggy mucosa should be assessed.

Diagnostic Studies. A baseline hematocrit may be indicated in severe or chronic epistaxis. It can reveal anemia secondary to the bleeding. Unless the history points to a coagulopathy or the nosebleeds are recurrent and refractory to treatment, coagulation studies are not indicated (Siddiq and Grainger, 2015).

If a coagulopathy is suspected, order a CBC, platelet count, prothrombin time, and activated partial thromboplastin time (aPTT). If the labs are normal but the diagnosis is strongly suspected, further workup for von Willebrand disease is needed.

Differential Diagnosis

Differential diagnoses as to causes of epistaxis include tumors, long-standing nasal FB, congenital bleeding disorders, idiopathic thrombocytopenia purpura (ITP), vasculitis, nasal hemangioma, hereditary hemorrhagic telangiectasia, and allergic rhinitis (Siddiq and Grainger, 2015). A bleeding disorder is characterized by epistaxis that is severe, prolonged, and recurrent. Nonaccidental injury or coagulopathy should be considered in children younger than 2 years of age with spontaneous epistaxis. If epistaxis is associated with a traumatic injury, evaluate for the presence of a nasal fracture and/or septal hematoma. A nasal neoplasm may present with facial swelling, pain, nasal obstruction, Eustachian tube dysfunction with effusion, and cranial neuropathies with severe epistaxis. Wegener granulomatosis, a small vessel vasculitis, can present in adolescents with nasal bleeding (Siddiq and Grainger, 2015).

Management

There is a lack of studies regarding the optimal management for epistaxis; however, nasal mucosal hydration techniques were found to be effective in the management of pediatric patients. Nasal cautery is a useful adjuvant for those who do not respond to the measures below (Patel et al., 2014). The following steps are recommended (Siddiq and Grainger, 2015):
- Have the child sit upright and lean forward to prevent swallowing the blood.

- Apply direct pressure at the nasal ala (pinch the nares together at the bony structure) for 10 to 15 minutes (watch the time, because perceptions of time are subjective).
- Packing and topical vasoconstrictor drugs are occasionally needed.
- Use a bedside humidifier to moisten the air in dry climates or in winter with forced-air heating. NS nose sprays can add moisture to dry nasal mucosa.
- Apply topical antibiotic to the site of the septal scab for 2 weeks to reduce nasal colonization with *S. aureus* crusting and inflammation.
- Topical agents such as BleedCease, WoundSeal, or NasalCease are hydrophilic polymers that form an artificial scab when in contact with blood. These can be applied via a swab to the *K. plexus* area. Local applications of a solution of oxymetazoline or Neo-Synephrine (0.25% to 1%) can also be used.
- Silver nitrate sticks can be used to cauterize exposed vessels if bleeding persists; however, the site must be easily accessible, visible, and not bleeding briskly. Silver nitrate has a high failure rate and is associated with nasal septum atrophy.
- Nasal packing with absorbable oxycellulose material can be used if bleeding continues or the site cannot be localized; the child should be referred to an ear, nose, and throat (ENT) specialist for further evaluation and management.
- Treat the underlying cause of the problem (e.g., trauma from nose-picking, dry air, and/or topical nasal sprays).
- Teach caregivers to leave blood scabs alone, because removal may precipitate further bleeding.

McGarry (2013) found that the use of antiseptic cream (containing chlorhexidine hydrochloride plus neomycin sulfate) plus silver nitrate cautery to be more effective at reducing the frequency and severity of nosebleeds than antiseptic cream alone. In addition, the effectiveness of petroleum jelly in promoting the resolution of recurrent bleeding has not been well documented.

Prevention

Preventive measures include instructions on an effective nasal regimen to keep the nasal mucosa moist, such as humidifier use and NS nose drops or sprays. If nasal corticosteroids are used, make sure that the child directs the spray laterally rather than toward the septum. This reduces epistaxis associated with nasal spray (Siddiq and Grainger, 2015).

Nasal Foreign Body

Young children tend to insert all types of FBs into body orifices. A recent review found that children with psychological problems, but not peer relationship problems, were more prone to foreign body insertion (Bakhshaee, Habrani, Shams et al., 2017). Objects can be noted immediately by the caregiver or lie undetected until classic symptoms appear. Jewelry beads are the most common reported FB in North America (Svider et al., 2014).

Clinical Findings

History. A persistent or recurrent unilateral purulent nasal discharge is reported. Foul odor, epistaxis, nasal obstruction, and mouth breathing are less commonly reported symptoms (Haddad and Keesecker, 2016). Young children often deny inserting an FB.

Physical Examination

The classic symptom of a nasal FB is unilateral, purulent, foul-smelling nasal discharge. If the FB is embedded in granulation tissue or mucosa, it may take on the appearance of a nasal mass. Other symptoms include mouth breathing, epistaxis, and nasal obstruction.

Differential Diagnosis

Nasal polyps, purulent rhinitis, adenoiditis, rhinosinusitis, and nasal tumors are conditions that cause bilateral or unilateral discharge.

Management

Management involves the following (Haddad and Keesecker, 2016):
- Properly restrain the child in order to avoid movement during the examination. Use a head light or overhead light when possible to free up your hands for examination.
- Elevate the child's head and suction out blood and secretions.
- Detection of an FB in the nasal cavity establishes the diagnosis.
- Removal of the nasal FB depends on its location, its composition, and the skill of the practitioner. A curette, alligator forceps, suction with narrow tips, and cotton-tipped applicators with collodion with or without topical vasoconstrictor drugs (to reduce swelling) can be used. If the object is small and 5-French catheter with a balloon can be advanced past the FB, the balloon can be inflated and gently withdrawn with the object. A Katz Extractor can be used to remove oto-rhino FB.
- Otolaryngology referral is merited for young children who cannot cooperate or when the FB is extremely difficult or dangerous to remove, such as paper clips or staples. On a cautionary note, an FB can be forced deeper into the nose if the practitioner is inexperienced at nasal FB removal.

Airway Disorders

Croup (Laryngotracheobronchitis) and Spasmodic Croup

Croup (laryngotracheobronchitis) is the most common cause of upper airway obstruction in children. It is an acute, inflammatory disease of the larynx, trachea, and bronchi that clinically presents with a brassy cough that sounds like a bark and is associated with varying degrees of inspiratory stridor, hoarseness, and respiratory distress. The clonus elasticus, the lower portion of the laryngeal membrane that is plastic and thicker, is prone to edema due to its lax mucosal attachment, which is the reason why the subglottic region is the most narrowed area despite edema of upper airway and trachea.

Laryngotracheobronchitis (LTB) causes disease in children younger than 6 years old. The Westley scale developed in the 1970s is still used as an objective way to assess severity. It is categorized into mild, moderate, severe, and impending respiratory failure. Spasmodic croup is short lived and thought to be related to allergic reaction or viral antigens. It is unclear as to whether it is part of the same disease spectrum (Beiner and Lecuyer, 2017) but symptoms improve on exposure to night air (Petrocheilou et al., 2014).

Human parainfluenza types 1 and 2 (less so) are the most common viral agents responsible for fall outbreaks in children 1 to 6 years old, typically in odd-numbered years. Other agents include other human parainfluenza types (notably HPIV-3), influenza A and B, human coronavirus HL-63, coxsackieviruses, echoviruses, metapneumovirus, adenoviruses, RSV, and rhinovirus (Petrocheilou et al., 2014). Coinfection is common.

Viral croup is most common in children between 6 and 36 months old (60% are younger than 24 months) and occurs most often in fall and winter. HPIV-3 is endemic in children younger than 6 months old and occurs in the spring and summer months, less commonly in the autumn if other parainfluenza viruses are absent (Fox and Christenson, 2014). Viral shedding of parainfluenza viruses occurs for up to 1 week before the onset of the disease and continues for 1 to 3 weeks. Males are affected more often than females (Petrocheilou et al., 2014). Recurrent croup and recurrent laryngitis can develop in children until they are 6 years old. A positive family history has been noted in a small percentage of children in whom croup develops. Croup lasts approximately 5 days. With growth, the child's laryngeal tracheal airway is less vulnerable to the effects of viral infections and less susceptible to obstruction.

Clinical Finding

Clinical manifestations depend on the infectious agent responsible for the croup and the extent of the upper airway involvement.

History. The history typically includes the following:
- URI prodromal symptoms (rhinorrhea, conjunctivitis, or both) are sometimes present before stridor
- Acute onset of a hoarse, barking-like cough
- Mild to severe laryngeal obstruction
- Mild to severe inspiratory stridor with dyspnea
- Gradual onset of symptoms (2 to 3 days)
- Sleep disturbance since symptoms are worse at night (Yang et al., 2017)
- May or may not have sore throat
- Duration is generally 3 to 5 days for viral croup
- Presence of fever without reoccurrence differentiates LTB from spasmodic croup (Fox and Christenson, 2014)

Physical Examination. The following can be seen:
- Slight dyspnea, tachypnea, and retractions
- Mild, brassy, or barking cough (harsh sounding)
- Stridor—a high-pitched, harsh sound from turbulent airflow that is generally inspiratory, but may be biphasic
- Fever is typically low grade, but may be elevated to 104°F (40°C)
- If visualized on examination of the mouth, the epiglottis appears normal
- Substernal and chest wall retraction in severe cases
- Prolonged inspiration
- Wheezing and rales may be heard if there is additional lower airway involvement

Diagnostic Studies. Croup is a clinical diagnosis and imaging is not recommended unless there is doubt about the diagnosis (Darras et al., 2015). Radiography of the soft tissues of the neck and chest displays a classic pattern of subglottic narrowing ("steeple sign") on posteroanterior views. Microbiology cultures of the pharynx are done only when bacterial tracheitis is suspected and the child has a high fever, toxic appearance, dysphagia, and respiratory distress (Mandal et al., 2015).

Differential Diagnosis

Differential diagnoses include acute epiglottitis; acute spasmodic croup (no signs of infection); FB aspiration; toxic shock syndrome; retropharyngeal or parapharyngeal abscess; extrinsic compression from tumors, trauma, or congenital malformations; angioedema (anaphylaxis), bacterial tracheitis, infectious mononucleosis; and psychogenic stridor (Blot et al., 2017).

Croup is different from bacterial tracheitis, a bacterial infection of the trachea that occurs rarely and results in inflammatory cell infiltration of the larynx, trachea, and bronchi causing epithelial lining sloughing and mucopurulent membranes (Mandal et al., 2015). Bacterial tracheitis is a rapidly progressive disease of children 3 weeks to 16 years old accompanied by high fever. The most common age is around 5 years and, due to exudative pseudomembranes that line the airway, there is a risk of obstruction (Mandal et al., 2015). *Staphylococcus* is the most common organism, but *Streptococcus* and *Streptococcus pyogenes*, *M. catarrhalis*, nontypeable *H. influenzae*, and, less commonly, gram negative organisms such as *Pseudomonas* and *Klebsiella* have been implicated in bacterial tracheitis (Kuo and Parikh, 2014). Unlike viral croup, bacterial croup results in thick pus within the trachea and lower airways. These patients do not respond to the standard croup treatment and get clinically worse.

Retropharyngeal abscess occurs when a suppurative lymph node ruptures into the retropharyngeal area; a penetrating FB enters the area; or diskitis, osteomyelitis, or a mediastinal infection spreads to the area (Darras et al., 2015). CT scan is the standard study for diagnosis; it is important that part of the mediastinum is imaged to pick up spread from this area.

Table 37.4 differentiates acute laryngotracheitis from other common causes of stridor.

Management

Therapy depends on the cause, severity, and location of the disease. The aim of therapy is to provide adequate respiratory exchange. Table 37.5 shows management of the child based on the degree of severity of croup.
- *Humidified air:* There is no evidence that the use of steam or cold humidification is harmful; however, there is no evidence to support its use (Johnson, 2014). For children with LTB, taking the child out into the cold night air may be beneficial. Occasionally, vomiting relieves the bronchospasm.
- *Corticosteroids:* Corticosteroids decrease inflammation and cell damage without prolonging viral shedding. A single dose of dexamethasone, orally (0.15 mg to 0.6 mg/kg), is beneficial, decreasing return visits and resulting in shorter hospital stay (Petrocheilou et al., 2014). Whether high or low dosing is better is not yet clearly defined (Johnson, 2014), although starting at a lower dosage may be appropriate in mild to moderate croup. Intramuscular dexamethasone can be used in a vomiting child. There is no difference in efficacy between oral and IM therapy (Mandal et al., 2015). Antibiotics are not indicated.
- *Cold medications:* Cough and cold medicines are not indicated in croup.
- *Bronchodilators:* If bronchospasm is also suspected, the use of bronchodilators in the usual doses prescribed for relief of asthma (as discussed in Chapter 33) may be advantageous.
- *Oxygen:* Blow-by oxygen is only used if the oxygen saturation falls below 92%.
- *Other acute care modalities:* Nebulized epinephrine can reduce airway edema by vasoconstriction of subglottic mucosa and has shown benefit in treatment of croup (Petrocheilou et al., 2014). Heliox has unknown effectiveness in croup as there are limited studies regarding its usage (Johnson, 2014).

Indications for Hospitalization

Children with severe respiratory distress, with severe retraction, exhibiting stridor at rest, signs of other conditions, or not

TABLE 37.4 Differentiating Common Respiratory Diseases That Can Cause Stridor or Similar Signs

Characteristic	Acute Laryngotracheitis	Epiglottitis	Laryngotracheobronchitis	Diphtheria	Foreign Body
Peak age	3-36 mo old	1-5 years old	3-36 mo old	Any age/unimmunized	Toddlers
Onset	Gradual, acute onset at night	Rapid	Acute	Gradual onset over 1-2 days	Acute symptoms or gradual onset
Common findings	URI, seal-bark cough, mild to moderate dyspnea, symptoms worse at night	Sore throat, dysphagia, anxiety with inspiratory distress without significant stridor, drooling, muffled speech, looks toxic, tripod position	Hoarseness with barking cough, inspiratory stridor and toxic presentation with purulent sputum	Membranous nasopharyngitis, obstructive laryngotracheitis with local infection presenting as sore throat, nasal discharge, hoarseness	Coughing and/or choking episode, dyspnea, wheezing, cyanosis, signs and symptoms of secondary infection
Respiratory efforts	Rate generally < 50	Marked distress	Marked distress	Minor to significant signs and symptoms of obstruction	Minor to significant distress
Fever	Common—low grade	High (ranges from 101.8° to 104°F [38.8° to 40°C])	High (102.2°F [39°C])	Low grade	Normal to low grade
CBC	Generally normal	High, left shift	High, left shift	Normal to slight leukocytosis, decreased thrombocyte count	Normal unless secondary infection
Organism(s)	Usually viral: parainfluenza, adenovirus, RSV	Usually HIB	Usually *Staphylococcus aureus*	*Corynebacterium diphtheria*	
Specific laboratory tests	None	None	None	Positive culture	None
Radiographic view with findings	Lateral or AP of neck/subglottic narrowing	Lateral of neck/thumb sign	Lateral of neck/subglottic narrowing	Signs of obstruction in severe cases	May see localized hyperinflation, mediastinal shift, atelectasis
Treatment	Humidification, corticosteroids in selected cases	Hospitalization, cephalosporin, corticosteroids	Hospitalization, staphylococcus coverage	Hospitalization, erythromycin/penicillin, antitoxin	FB removal, treatment of secondary infection or bronchospasm
Intubation	Rare	Usually necessary	Frequently necessary	May be necessary	Endoscopy to remove FB
Prevention	None	Immunization—HIB	None	Immunization—DTaP	Education on childproofing home and monitoring child

AP, Anteroposterior; *CBC*, complete blood count; *DTaP*, diphtheria-tetanus-acellular pertussis; *FB*, foreign body; *HIB*, *Haemophilus influenzae* type B; *RSV*, respiratory syncytial virus; *URI*, upper respiratory infection.

improving with the standard treatment should be hospitalized. Increasing obstruction of the airways causes continuous stridor, nasal flaring, and suprasternal, infrasternal, and intercostal retractions. With further obstruction, air hunger and restlessness occur and are quickly followed by hypoxia, weakness, decreased air exchange, decreased stridor, increased pulse rate, and eventual death from hypoventilation. Racemic epinephrine by aerosol can be used every 6 hours in conjunction with corticosteroids to limit rebound swelling. Hydration is important and IV fluids may be needed in patients who cannot tolerate feedings (Yang et al., 2017).

Complications

Bacterial superinfection is the main complication of viral croup. High fever in an acutely ill child with significant airway obstruction indicates acute epiglottitis or bacterial tracheitis. Immediate intervention is needed ●. Viral pneumonia complicates about 1% to 2% of croup cases.

Acute Spasmodic Croup

The onset of spasmodic croup occurs in the early morning hours as a result of laryngopharyngeal reflux accompanied by transient

TABLE 37.5	Croup Severity and Treatment Based on Severity			
Symptoms and Treatment	Mild	Moderate	Severe	Impending Respiratory Failure
Symptoms	Occasional croupy cough No retractions No chest wall retractions	Frequent croupy cough Audible stridor and suprasternal and sternal retractions at rest No agitation	Frequent croupy cough Tachypnea Prominent inspiratory and occasional expiratory stridor Agitation and distress	Audible stridor at rest Sternal retractions Lethargy Decreased level of consciousness with dusky color
Treatment				
Education of caregiver	X	X	X	X
Corticosteroid	X	X	X	X
Nebulized epinephrine			X	X
Blow-by oxygen			X	X until intubation
Intubation				X

Data from Alberta Clinical Practice Guidelines Working Group. *Guidelines for Diagnosis and Management of Croup.* Alberta, ON; 2003.

laryngospasm and laryngeal edema (Roosevelt, 2016). The etiologic agents are similar to those in laryngotracheitis (Roosevelt, 2016), and the condition occurs in families with a history of croup. Spasmodic croup presents with minimal coryza and acute onset of nighttime croup in a child that is well or a child with very mild cold symptoms. There is no fever, no pharyngitis, and a normal epiglottis. The episode is usually milder and of short duration, but symptoms may be recurrent. The treatment plan is the same as indicated for acute LTB. Spasmodic croup tends to respond well to exposure to cool air.

Epiglottitis

Epiglottitis is a life-threatening illness characterized by inflammation of the epiglottis, the aryepiglottic folds, and the ventricular bands at the base of the epiglottis. The causative organisms have changed from *H. influenza* to *Group A Streptococcus, Streptococcus pneumonia, Klebsiella* sp., and *Staphylococcus aureus* (Richards, 2016). Since the introduction of the *H. Influenzae* B (HIB) vaccine, fewer cases of epiglottitis are seen in both children and adults.

Clinical Findings

History. There is an abrupt onset of fever, irritability, muffled voice, severe sore throat, dyspnea, dysphagia leading to drooling, and increasing respiratory distress (Richards, 2016). The child looks acutely ill and toxic.

Physical Examination. If epiglottitis is suspected, do not examine the throat .

Findings include the following:
- Inspiratory and sometimes expiratory stridor
- Drooling, aphonia (muffled voice), and high fever
- Rapidly progressive respiratory obstruction and prostration
- Flaring of the ala nasi and retraction of the supraclavicular, intercostal, and subcostal spaces
- Child assumes a position of hyperextension of the neck
  In older children, one may find:
- Complaints of sore throat and dysphagia
- Stridor, irritability, restlessness, and brassy cough (uncommon)

- Airway obstruction follows within 2 to 24 hours; the child sits up with arms back, trunk forward, neck hyperextended, and chin thrust forward (tripod position)
- A rare, unusual finding is that of just a hoarse cough and a cherry-red epiglottis

Diagnostic Studies. Blood cultures should be ordered. If the possibility of epiglottitis is thought to be remote in a patient with croup, a lateral neck radiograph may be obtained before the physical examination is undertaken. Absence of the "thumb" sign on the radiograph rules out the condition. A healthcare professional capable of supporting the airway and skilled in intubation must accompany the child to the radiology department and back.

Management

Airway management is key as the time from the onset of symptoms until death can be only a matter of hours. Due to the risk of sudden airway obstruction, early consultation with a pediatric otolaryngologist and anesthesiologist is key . The goal of therapy is to establish an airway and start appropriate antimicrobials. Do not place the child in the supine position, and immediately transport the child to the hospital via emergency medical services. The child should be examined in the operating room by a skilled provider who can perform an emergency tracheostomy. An airway must be established, either a nasotracheal airway or a tracheostomy. The diagnosis is confirmed in the operating room by depressing the tongue to view the swollen cherry-red epiglottis. An expert in establishing an airway needs to be present because there is a risk of reflex laryngospasm, with acute and complete airway obstruction.

Treatment includes the following:
- Establish an airway, preferably by nasotracheal intubation
- Administer IV broad-spectrum antibiotics, which can include ampicillin/sulbactam, cefotaxime, ceftriaxone, or clindamycin if penicillin allergic with the addition of vancomycin if MRSA is suspected.
- Administer oxygen and respiratory support.

The acute infection rarely lasts more than 48 to 72 hours. However, idiopathic pulmonary edema can follow (in up to 9% of patients) after the establishment of an airway due to the changes in pulmonary microvascular pressure subsequent to relieving the obstruction. As improvement occurs, the child can be extubated with antibiotic therapy continuing for 10 days. If *H. influenzae* is identified as the causative agent, rifampin prophylaxis (20 mg/kg in a single dose [maximum, 600 mg] for 4 days for infants and children and 600 mg once a day for adults for 4 days) should be given to all household contacts of the patient whose household has:

- At least one child younger than 4 years old who is unimmunized or incompletely immunized
- Children less than 12 months old who have not received the primary series of HIB vaccine
- Immunocompromised children (AAP, 2018)

In addition, if there are two cases of invasive HIB disease in a day care center or preschool within 60 days, all members of the nursery need to receive prophylaxis.

Complications

Complications from epiglottis involve systemic spread of the organism causing epiglottis and include cervical lymphadenitis, pneumonia, otitis media, or less commonly septic arthritis or meningitis (Richards, 2016).

Prevention

Routine immunization is the primary means of prevention. Hand washing is also an effective method of preventing spread of infection. See prior discussion regarding rifampin prophylaxis.

Bronchiolitis

Bronchiolitis is the most common respiratory infection in infancy, causing cell death and necrosis of respiratory epithelial cells lining small airways. There is increased destruction in the lining of the bronchioles along with bronchospasm and copious mucous production (McNaughten, Hart, Shields, 2017). Bronchiolitis is characterized by the insidious onset of URI symptoms, decreased feeding, and mild fever, with apnea as a possible presentation in the younger infant. Usually after 1 to 2 days of URI symptoms, wheezing and course crackles are heard with tachypnea and mild to severe chest retractions that last as long as 12 days (Kyler and McCulloh, 2018; McNaughten et al., 2017). Usually, the child improves by the 6th day of illness. While older children can have viral induced wheezing, the classic picture of bronchiolitis is an infant to 2 years old with upper respiratory prodrome followed by wheezing and mild to severe respiratory distress (Kyler and McCulloh, 2018). The peak incidence of this disease is in infants less than 6 months old; it is the most common cause of hospital admission in children less than 1 year (Ralston et al., 2014). In severe cases, cyanosis, air hunger, retractions, and nasal flaring with symptoms of severe respiratory distress can appear within a few hours. Apnea can occur with a wide range of prevalence reported (Ralston et al., 2014) and may require mechanical ventilation.

The pathophysiology in bronchiolitis is due to shedding of bronchiole epithelium and alveolar epithelial cells (AEC), types I and II, airway edema, and resultant dysfunction of the cilia. The presence of necrotic epithelium and mucus can lead to various degrees of airway obstruction, ventilation/perfusion mismatch, and atelectasis. This pathophysiology along with increased mucous production leads to hypoxemia. Because bronchospasm is minimal, bronchodilators have limited effect. Corticosteroids and epinephrine are not effective as tissue inflammation is minimal. Membranous pneumatoceles, or AEC type I, are dominant and cover 96% of the respiratory tree. Their role is in gas exchange,

whereas AEC type II are important for surfactant production. It is a disease of the small bronchioles that are 2 mm in size with sparing of basal cells in the bronchiole.

In 50% to 80% of patients with bronchiolitis, the causative agent is RSV (Kyler and McCulloh, 2018; McNaughten et al., 2017). Human enterovirus/rhinovirus, human metapneumovirus, influenza, parainfluenza, bocavirus, and adenovirus are other causal agents. Coinfection with multiple viruses occurs in up to 10% to 30% of infants with severe bronchiolitis (Kyler and McCulloh, 2018). The incubation period for RSV ranges from 2 to 8 days but more commonly is 4 to 6 days. The disease occurs during the winter and early spring.

Respiratory viruses are spread by close contact with infected respiratory secretions or fomites. The most frequent mode of transmission is hand carriage of contaminated secretion. The source of infection is an older child or adult family member with a "mild" URI. Older children and adults have larger airways and tolerate swelling associated with this infection better than infants do. Most cases of bronchiolitis resolve completely, but recurrence of infection is common, and symptoms tend to be mild.

Infants who are at higher risk of severe RSV include children with major chronic pulmonary disease, such as CF, neuromuscular disorders, or bronchopulmonary dysplasia; premature birth before 35 weeks of gestational age; age less than 12 weeks; and infants with significant hemodynamic difficulties due to congenital heart disease (Ralston et al., 2014). Other risk factors for more severe disease include cigarette smoke exposure both in utero and postnatally and limited breastfeeding duration (Kyler and McCulloh, 2018).

Clinical Findings

History. The following are reported:
- Initial presentation: URI symptoms of cough, coryza, and rhinorrhea for 1 to 2 days prior to lower respiratory disease (McNaughten et al., 2017)
- Gradual development of respiratory distress with persistent coughing, tachypnea, chest retractions, and wheezing
- Low-grade to moderate fever up to 102°F (38.9°C); decrease in appetite
- No prodrome in some infants; rather they have apnea as the initial symptom
- Usually the course is the worst by 48 to 72 hours after wheezing starts. The disease peaks at around 5 to 7 days (McNaughten et al., 2017). If the child has a bacterial illness, the child will continue to worsen with a high fever.

Physical Examination. Findings include the following:
- Upper respiratory findings of coryza, mild conjunctivitis in 33%, and pharyngitis
- Lower respiratory findings of:
  - Tachypnea (approximately 40 to 80 breaths per minute)
  - Substernal and/or intercostal retractions
  - Heterophonous expiratory wheezing (i.e., different pitches of wheezing in different lung fields)
  - Fine or coarse crackles may be heard throughout the breathing cycle
  - Varying signs of respiratory distress and pulmonary involvement (e.g., nasal flaring, grunting, retractions, cyanosis, prolonged expiration)
  - Abdominal distention; palpable liver and spleen, pushed down by hyperinflated lungs and a flattened diaphragm

Diagnostic Studies. A diagnosis of bronchiolitis should be based on the history and physical examination (McNaughten, 2017). Overuse of diagnostic testing persists in clinical practice despite available guidelines on the diagnosis and management of bronchiolitis (Librizzi et al., 2014; Turner et al., 2014). Chest radiographs in previously healthy infants with mild RSV bronchiolitis are not indicated (Kyler and McCulloch, 2018). In severe illness, a chest x-ray may be ordered to rule out pneumonia or pneumothorax; however, its use must be weighed against the dangers of radiation exposure. The findings of chest radiography can vary, and even with severe illness the x-ray can be clear with a flattened diaphragm and an increase in anteroposterior diameter. Early bacterial pneumonia can be difficult to detect and cannot be ruled out by a chest x-ray.

Routine virologic testing is not recommended (Gill et al., 2017). In selected situations (hospitalization or if an infant has received monthly palivizumab [Synagis]), enzyme-linked immunosorbent assays or fluorescent antibody techniques to look for RSV are diagnostic procedures of choice in most laboratories. Viral culture of nasal washings can be done in severe cases to confirm RSV, parainfluenza viruses, influenza viruses, and adenoviruses. PCR testing is helpful in deciding about isolation of cohorts with the same infection in the hospital setting. The use of viral testing may not add to the management plan (Gill et al., 2017).

Hematologic testing is not recommended (Kyler and McCulloch, 2018). If a CBC is done for another reason, a mild leukocytosis may be seen with 12,000 to 16,000/mm^3. In infants under 90 days with bronchiolitis, a serious bacterial infection is unlikely (Kyler and McCulloh, 2018).

Differential Diagnosis

The diagnosis of bronchiolitis can be confused with asthma, although there are some differences that may be helpful. Asthma is an acute process due to airway hyperreactivity and inflammation, whereas the onset of bronchiolitis is insidious. The response to the usual asthma therapies of β agonist and steroids is poor in infants with bronchiolitis. In contrast, certain viral illnesses in young children can induce wheezing that will respond to a β-agonist with good results.

FB aspiration is usually found in a toddler with a history of choking who then develops focal areas of wheezing. Although children with congestive heart failure can wheeze, they also show symptoms of sweating and signs of failure to thrive with a murmur and an S$_4$ gallop rhythm. Other differentials include airway irritants, gastroesophageal reflux, pneumonia, allergic pneumonitis, vascular rings, lung cysts, and lobar emphysema.

Management

At present, no evidence shows pharmacologic therapy is effective in the management of bronchiolitis (Caballero et al., 2017; McNaughten et al., 2017). Supportive care remains the primary therapy and includes fever control, maintaining hydration and nutrition while keeping oxygen levels ≥90% (Smith et al., 2017). Evidence-based guidelines published by the AAP no longer support a trial of bronchodilators as an option for infants and children with bronchiolitis because of the risk associated with their use and the lack of evidence of an effect (Ralston et al., 2014; Schroeder and Mansbach, 2014). The use of epinephrine is also not recommended for infants and children. The use of hypertonic saline in the outpatient department is not recommended and in hospitalized children may show transient improvement in clinical scores without changing length of stay (McNaughten et al., 2017; Morikaw et al., 2018). Systemic corticosteroids should *not* be administered in the treatment of bronchiolitis in infants; chest physiotherapy is contraindicated in infants and children.

Antibiotics have no place in the treatment of a viral disease (such as, bronchiolitis), unless there is a concomitant bacterial infection or strong suspicion.

Most infants with mild signs of respiratory distress can be treated as outpatients if their oxygen level is within a normal range (Ralston et al., 2014; Schroeder and Mansbach, 2014):

- Supportive care consists of adequate hydration, nutrition, fever control, and maintaining oxygen.
- Need for supplemental oxygen administration is based on oxyhemoglobin saturation levels. If an infant's or child's oxyhemoglobin level is greater than 90%, the decision to administer oxygen is left up to the provider.
- Transcutaneous oxygen saturation monitoring (continuous pulse oximetry) is also an individual provider's choice. A recent study showed that continuous oxygen monitoring leads to overdiagnosis of hypoxemia and delayed discharge. While recurrent desaturations are common among infants with bronchiolitis, delayed discharge is not needed due to these episodes and these infants can safely be sent home (Quinonez et al., 2017).
- Fluid intake is strongly recommended to prevent dehydration.
- Nasal suctioning to clear the upper nasal passages is recommended.

The inpatient management of bronchiolitis may include using heated, humidified oxygen via nasal cannula. Oxygen should be used if oxygen saturation falls under 90% (Kyler and McCulloh, 2018). Oxygen's mechanism of action is to improve mucous ciliary clearance and avoid nasal dryness. The use of high-flow nasal cannula oxygen or continuous airway pressure needs further research to confirm benefit from these methods (McNaughten et al., 2017).

The use of deep airway suctioning is avoided, though continuing to keep the nasal airway clear on a regular basis may improve airflow. Ribavirin is no longer recommended routinely (Caballero, Polack, Stein, 2017). Although leukotriene levels are high in bronchiolitis, the use of antileukotriene inhibitors has not been adequately studied and is not recommended (Caballero et al., 2017).

Caregivers of infants and children at home need to understand:

- The management of rhinitis (use of saline drops and suctioning of nares)
- Indications for the use of antipyretics
- Signs of increasing respiratory distress or dehydration that call for hospitalization
- Guidelines for feeding an infant with signs of mild respiratory distress (amount of fluid needed per 24 hours; smaller, more frequent feedings; monitoring of the respiratory rate; and guarding against vomiting)
- Education that infants and children with bronchiolitis may cough for 2 to 3 weeks

Infants younger than 2 months old and older infants with signs of severe respiratory distress should be hospitalized. Indications for admission include the following (McNaughten et al., 2017):

- Apnea
- Oxygen saturation of less than 92% on room air
- Inadequate oral intake less than 75% to 50% of usual volume
- Respiratory distress signs including grunting, respiratory rate over 60, stridor, cyanosis, rising carbon dioxide, progressive stridor, or stridor at rest
- Restlessness or markedly decreased activity
- Guardian unable to care for child at home

In-hospital management focuses on supportive care, focusing on suctioning of nares, humidified supplemental oxygen, and elevation of the child to a sitting position at a 30- to 40-degree angle.

IV hydration (or nasogastric hydration in infants) is needed when respiratory distress interferes with nursing or bottle feeding.

Complications

Complications of bronchiolitis include apnea, respiratory failure, aspiration, and secondary bacterial infections. The child is ill-appearing and toxic but gradually improves. The fatality rate associated with bronchiolitis is less than 0.05% and only 2% of infants who require hospitalization need to be intubated (Kyler and McCulloch, 2018). Infants younger than 12 weeks old and those with underlying cardiorespiratory or immunodeficiency are at risk for severe disease.

Prolonged apnea, uncompensated respiratory acidosis, and profound dehydration secondary to loss of water from tachypnea and an inability to drink are the factors leading to death in young infants with bronchiolitis. In some children, bronchiolitis can cause minor pulmonary function problems and a tendency for bronchial hyperreactivity that lasts for years. Estimates of the risk of school-aged asthma and history of severe bronchiolitis in infancy range from 20% to 60% (Gaffin and Phipantanakul, 2017) with a recent study showing a rate of 27.6% (Balekian et al., 2017).

Prevention

Educate caregivers about decreasing exposure to and transmission of RSV, especially those with high-risk infants. Advice should include limiting exposure to child care centers whenever possible; use of alcohol-based hand sanitizers or hand washing, if hand sanitizer is not available; avoiding tobacco smoke exposure; and scheduling RSV prophylaxis vaccination, when indicated. Recent literature support wearing a face mask to reduce the risk of respiratory infections which, while common in Asia, is not a common practice in Western cultures (Papadopoulos et al., 2017). Palivizumab (Synagis) is an RSV-specific monoclonal antibody used to provide some protection from severe RSV infection for a very small population of high-risk infants (see Chapter 31).

Foreign Body Aspiration

The symptoms and physical findings associated with aspiration of an FB depend on the nature of the material aspirated, plus the location and degree of the obstruction. The cough reflex protects the lower airways, and most aspirated material is immediately expelled with coughing. Onset of a sudden episode of coughing without a prodrome or signs of respiratory infection should make the provider suspicious of FB aspiration.

Objects that are either too large to be eliminated by the mucociliary system or cannot be expelled by coughing eventually lead to some form of respiratory symptomatology. Obviously a large FB occluding the upper airway can cause suffocation. A small object in the lower respiratory tree may not produce symptoms for days to weeks. Obstruction results from either the FB itself or edema associated with its presence. Hot dogs are one of the most common causes of fatal aspiration. Other foods associated with choking are meats, sausages, fish with bones, popcorn, pretzel nuggets, candy (hard or sticky), whole grapes, raw vegetables (peas, carrots, celery), fruits with skins, nuts, seeds, cheese cubes, ice cubes, and peanut butter (spoonfuls or with soft bread). Examples of household items and toys that pose a choking risk to young children include latex balloons, coins, marbles, toys with small parts, small balls, pen or marker caps, button-type batteries, screws, rings, earrings, crayons, erasers, safety pins, small stones, and tiny figures.

Although toddlers commonly aspirate FBs, aspiration occurs in children of all ages.

Most FB aspirations occur under the age 4 with a peak incidence in toddlers between 1 and 2 years of age. In 50% of cases, there is no history of choking. In laryngeal FB aspiration there is a rapid onset of hoarseness and the development of a chronic croupy cough with aphonia is reported. Be suspicious of an FB aspiration in children with sudden episode of cough, unilateral wheezing, and/or recurrent pneumonia. The child with an FB lodged in the trachea presents with a history of a brassy cough, hoarseness, dyspnea, and possibly cyanosis. The most characteristic signs of tracheal FB aspiration are the homophonic wheeze and the audible slap and palpable thud sound produced by the momentary expiratory effect of the FB at the subglottic level.

Occasionally the FB will be lodged in the bronchus or lung. Most objects are aspirated into the right lung. A careful medical history may reveal a forgotten episode of choking.

Clinical Findings

History. There may or may not be a history of an initial episode of coughing, gagging, and choking. Blood-streaked sputum may be expectorated, but hemoptysis rarely occurs as an early symptom. On rare occasions hemoptysis does occur as an initial symptom months or years after the aspiration event took place.

Physical Examination. Children with an upper airway FB present with cough, stridor, or in respiratory or cardiorespiratory arrest. If the FB goes into the lower airway they develop cough, wheezing, retractions, and have decreased breath sounds (Richards, 2016). Initial clinical findings are similar in either tracheal or laryngeal FB aspiration. If the object is nonobstructive and nonirritating, few or no initial symptoms may be seen. The child may have limited chest expansion, decreased vocal fremitus, atelectasis, or emphysema-like changes with resulting hyporesonance or hyperresonance. Diminished breath sounds are often found. A small object can act as a bypass valve, and homophonic wheezes can be heard. Crackles, rhonchi, and wheezes can be present if air movement is adequate. If the acute episode is missed or not appreciated, a latent period of mild "wheezing" or cough may be evident.

Diagnostic Studies. Neck and chest radiographs in posteroanterior and lateral views should be ordered. Only radiopaque FB are seen, but secondary signs include over inflation, atelectasis, or opacification of the distal lung (see Fig 37.1). Virtual bronchoscopy (CT), as well as a flexible bronchoscopy, can provide a noninvasive way to diagnose an FB. If the FB cannot be removed, then a rigid bronchoscopy is done (Richards, 2016).

Management

As noted, the history may not be positive. Therefore, if a child has symptoms of an FB, a referral to a pulmonary specialist is needed 🔊. If the object is removed via bronchoscopy before permanent damage occurs, recovery is usually complete. Secondary lung infections and bronchospasms should be treated as suggested in the section on management of pneumonia in this chapter and asthma in Chapter 33.

Complications

If the FB is vegetable matter, vegetal or arachidic bronchitis can occur. Characteristics of this severe condition can include sepsis-like fever, dyspnea, and cough. If the material has been there for a long time, suppuration can occur. Lobar pneumonia, intractable wheezing, and status asthmaticus can develop. Atelectasis or emphysema, a rare occurrence, can also occur as the result of a large obstruction caused by a bronchial FB.

Prevention. Anticipatory education regarding prevention of FB aspiration should be part of well-child supervision guidance. Caregivers should be cautioned about high-risk foods (e.g., whole carrots, nuts, popcorn, and hot dogs). Young children need to be supervised closely as they put small objects into their mouths as well as when they cry, shout, run, and play with food or other objects in their mouths (see Chapter 44).

Bronchitis

The presence of a chronic wet cough may reflect a serious disease and requires a careful evaluation. Acute bronchitis is defined as a nonspecific inflammation of the bronchioles and can be classified as *acute* or *chronic*. Most cases of acute bronchitis are due to viral infections (with adenoviruses, influenza viruses, parainfluenza, and RSV being the most common) and the atypical bacteria, *M. pneumoniae* (Carolan and Sharma, 2017). *S. pneumoniae, B. pertussis,* and *H. influenzae* are the most commonly cultured bacterial organisms (Bergamini et al., 2017). *Pseudomonas aeruginosa* is the most common agent in children with CF. Protracted bacterial bronchitis (PBB) is the most common diagnosis for prolonged cough lasting longer than 4 weeks in children less than 6 years of age. The incidence of the disease peaks in midwinter and declines by midsummer with an increase in the fall.

PBB is associated with inflammation of the large airways, including the trachea and the large- and medium-sized bronchi (Chang et al., 2016). There is associated destruction of the ciliated epithelium by the causative agent. This illness is associated with pharyngitis as well as rhinitis. Although a virus is the most common cause of acute bronchitis, weakened tissue can succumb to a secondary bacterial infection. The longer the symptoms persist, the greater is the neutrophil inflammation. The uncontrolled neutrophilic response causes the release of tissue damaging substances leading to bronchiectasis (Chang et al., 2016).

Chronic bronchitis is characterized by a productive cough lasting for more than 3 months and is well defined clinically in adults. In children, this condition per se is ill defined, because it is usually a symptom of another chronic disorder, such as allergies, asthma, CF, and/or exposure to cigarette smoke.

Clinical Findings

History. Bronchitis usually presents with symptoms of a persistent cough and fever, and the larynx and trachea are not involved (which is the opposite of croup). The usual course of illness starts as an URI, evolves into a cough illness with or without fever, and then resolves over 1 to 2 weeks.

The following are reported:
- A dry, hacking, unproductive cough that begins a few days after the onset of rhinitis and fever.
- Complaints of low substernal discomfort or burning chest pain aggravated by coughing.
- Initially the cough is dry, harsh, and sometimes brassy in younger children. However, as it progresses, the cough becomes productive. Because younger children swallow sputum, vomiting and gagging can occur.
- A family history of asthma, CF, atopy, and infections as well as a history of environmental irritants, such as tobacco smoke and pollution, should be obtained.
- A history of prematurity, gastroesophageal reflux, or exposure to infection in day care should be elicited.

- The nature of the cough, timing, previous history of cough, and responses to therapy, wheezing, or stridor should be obtained.
- Check for tobacco or marijuana use in teenagers.

Physical Examination. Findings can vary and include the following:
- Variable degrees of URI symptoms
- Low-grade or no fever
- Coarse breath sounds changing rhonchi and rales

Diagnostic Studies. Chest x-ray is not routinely done unless the child is worsening or there is a suspicion of FB.

Differential Diagnosis

Pertussis should be considered in patients with a cough lasting 2 to 3 weeks because it is found in 10% of patients with a new onset of a chronic cough. Children with recurrent acute bronchitis must be evaluated for underlying pathologic conditions. Respiratory tract anomalies, FB aspiration, bronchiectasis, immunodeficiency, allergy, rhinosinusitis, anatomic problems (e.g., gastroesophageal reflux and tracheoesophageal fistulas), tonsillitis, exposure to air pollutants, adenoiditis, and CF must be considered in the differential diagnosis. In *C. bronchitis*, consider primary ciliary dyskinesia, CF, FB, congenital anomalies, reflux, aspiration, asthma, allergies, autoimmune diseases, immune deficiency, and bacteria pathogens (e.g., *B. pertussis, M. pneumoniae,* and *C. pneumoniae*). If the cough continues beyond 4 weeks and the child is less than 6 years of age, PBB should be a consideration.

Management

For acute bronchitis, no specific therapy is known, and most patients require none. Care is primarily supportive.
- *Analgesia:* Use for pain.
- *Hydration:* Intake of fluids to avoid dehydration (helps to thin mucus generally in 5 to 10 days, and the cough decreases).
- *Antiviral/antibiotics:* If *influenza A* is the likely etiologic agent and there are underlying pulmonary diseases, antiviral therapy should be used. Because most cases of acute bronchitis are from viral sources, antibiotics are not indicated. If *M. pneumoniae* or *C. pneumoniae* is suspected, macrolides can be used. Treatment for PBB is a 2-week course of amoxicillin-clavulanate to cover *S. pneumoniae, H. influenza,* and *M. catarrhalis* (Chang et al., 2017). A response to this antibiotic is one of the criteria for the disease. It is important to make sure that no systemic signs of cardiac abnormalities, immunodeficiency, feeding difficulties, TB contacts, medications associated with chronic cough, or neurodevelopmental anomalies are present (Chang et al., 2017).
- *Cough suppressants:* There is no evidence to support the use of cough suppressants. Antihistamines should not be used because of their excessive drying effect; these agents tend to prolong the symptoms.
- *Bronchodilators:* There is no evidence to support the use of inhaled β-agonists, unless there is obstruction and wheezing at the onset of illness. If there is a suspicion of asthma, a trial of bronchodilators can be used.

For *C. bronchitis*, treatment depends on whether an underlying cause is found. Bronchodilators, cromolyn sodium, corticosteroids, and anticholinergic agents are used for the treatment of chronic cough associated with asthma or underlying chronic lung disease. If reflux is the cause, underlying treatment of the reflux is indicated. Avoidance of tobacco smoke, dust exposure, and air pollution is important.

Complications

In normal, healthy children, the condition is not serious; however, malaise continues for another week or so after the cough lessens. In undernourished or chronically ill children, otitis, rhinosinusitis, and pneumonia are common.

Common Types of Childhood Pneumonia

Pneumonia is a lower respiratory tract infection associated with fever and respiratory symptoms most commonly caused by bacteria and viruses. It often involves both the conducting airways and alveoli. It can be lobar, interstitial, or bronchopneumonia. *Lobar pneumonia* involves infection of the alveolar space that results in consolidation; it is described as "typical" pneumonia. Atypical pneumonia describes patterns of consolidation that are not localized. In *interstitial pneumonia*, cellular infiltrates attack the interstitium, which makes up the walls of the alveoli, the alveolar sacs and ducts, and the bronchioles. This type of pneumonia is typical of acute viral infections but may also be a chronic process. *Bronchial pneumonia* is associated with bacterial infection with multiple areas of consolidation involving one or more pulmonary lobules. *Pneumonitis* is a general term used to describe lung inflammation that may or may not be associated with consolidation. Community-acquired pneumonia is acquired in the community as opposed to hospital-acquired or nosocomial pneumonia.

Viral infection affects the lung defenses by altering normal secretions, inhibiting phagocytosis, modifying the normal bacterial flora, and disrupting the epithelial layer. Many childhood viruses set the stage for secondary bacterial infection that can result in a serious bacterial illness (SBI). Children with immunologic problems or chronic illnesses are prone to primary bacterial pneumonia and experience recurrent pneumonias or fail to clear the initial infection completely.

In neonates, risk factors for early onset pneumonia include prolonged rupture of membranes, maternal amnionitis, premature delivery, fetal tachycardia, or maternal intrapartum fever. Risk factors for late onset pneumonia include having anomalies of the airway, severe underlying disease, prolonged hospitalization, neurologic impairment, or nosocomial infection from poor hand washing or overcrowding. Risk factors for moderate to severe childhood pneumonia include bacterial pneumonia, delayed care, household smoking, altered mental status, and multilobar or nonlobar interstitial infiltrates. Decreasing blood pressure, young age, and increasing heart and respiratory rate are associated with more severe pneumonia outcomes in children (Williams et al., 2016).

The introduction of the pneumococcal and HIB vaccines changed the etiology of pneumonia with the EPIC study demonstrating that viruses were identified in over 70% of children and bacteria were identified in only 15%. RSV, rhinovirus, metapneumovirus, and adenoviral infections occurred in over 10% of children (Jain et al., 2015). The most common bacterial pathogen noted was *M. pneumoniae*. In 19% of children in the EPIC study, there was no pathogen identified. Certain bacterial pneumonias have a specific pattern of disease (e.g., *S. pneumoniae* causes a lobar pneumonia). Community-associated methicillin-resistant *S. aureus* (MRSA) is associated with empyema and necrosis and is also linked to influenza A infection (Scheffer et al., 2016). Identification of the infecting organism is difficult and, particularly in young children, leads to overuse of antibiotics.

Atypical bacterial pneumonia is caused by *M. pneumoniae, C. pneumoniae,* and in neonates and young infants, *Chlamydia. trachomatis. M. pneumoniae,* an organism without a cell wall, is transmitted by droplet spread from one symptomatic patient to another. The incubation period is 2 to 3 weeks, and asymptomatic carriage after infection can last for weeks. Wheezing in a child over 5 years of age without a history of wheezing may point to an atypical pneumonia. This disease is usually mild and self-limited.

C. trachomatis pneumonia is a characteristic pneumonia resulting from the transmission of *C. trachomatis* from the mother's infected genital tract to the infant. It does not become apparent until the infant is 2 to 19 weeks old. Due to prenatal screening, the incidence of *C. trachomatis* infection of the newborn has decreased but should be considered in a mother with inadequate prenatal care. *C. trachomatis* is an organism that has many subtypes within the species. Approximately 50% of infants born to infected mothers acquire *C. trachomatis*, but only 5% to 20% of these infants develop pneumonia with a typical onset between 1 and 3 months of age.

Age influences the clinical manifestations of pneumonia and differing infectious agents cause varied presentations and symptoms. Table 37.6 differentiates the various forms of pneumonia commonly found in infants, children, and adolescents. Table 37.7 shows the most common infecting organisms associated with pneumonia by age. Treatment is often empirical and varies with age.

Clinical Findings in Infants and Young Children

The hallmark of pneumonia is fever and cough except in the neonate where there may be an absence of cough (Richards, 2016). Tachypnea and increased work of breathing may precede coughing. Cough, hypoxia, nasal flaring, rales, retractions, and rhonchus lung sounds are specific but not as sensitive for pneumonia. Viral pneumonia tends to have an insidious onset that is associated with more wheezing than what is typically noted with bacterial pneumonia. In contrast, lobar pneumonia (caused by pneumococcal pneumonia) typically presents with fever, cough, and decreased breath sounds in the area of the pneumonia. However, the child may present with a mixture of symptoms. Pneumonia can cause referred symptoms, such as abdominal pain, which may be present in a child with a diaphragmatic pneumonia or radiating shoulder pain that may be associated with upper lobe pneumonias. Irritation of the pleura causes chest pain in children with pneumonia.

History. The following may be reported (Katz and Williams, 2018; Richards, 2016):

In neonates:
- History of group B streptococcal or *C. trachomatis* infection in the mother
- Prenatal drug use or lack of prenatal care as risk factors for SBI in the neonate
- Poor feeding and irritability
- With *C. trachomatis,* the infant is typically afebrile; prior, concurrent, or no history of inclusion conjunctivitis reported
In infants:
- Slower onset of respiratory symptoms, cough, wheezing, or stridor with less prominent fever suggests viral pneumonia (bacterial pneumonia is less likely in a wheezing child)
- Determine mother's HIV status or infant's exposure to tuberculosis
In children and adolescents:
- Obtain immunization history and travel history of the family
- Tuberculosis status
- Evaluate for sick contacts at home and possible FB aspiration
- Initial history of a mild URI for a few days—similar for both bacterial and viral
- Abrupt high fever with temperatures greater than 103.3°F (39.6°C), chills, cough, lethargy, and dyspnea suggest bacterial pneumonia

TABLE 37.6	Differentiating Various Forms of Pneumonia in Infants, Young Children, and Adolescents				
Characteristic	Bacterial	Viral	Mycoplasma pneumonia and Chlamydophila pneumonia	Chlamydia trachomatis
Common age	All ages	All ages	>5 years old	2-19 wk old (typically 1-3 mo old)
Onset	Acute; gradual	Acute; gradual	Slow	Gradual
Clinical findings	Depends on age; starts with URI, cough, dyspnea, tachypnea, rales, decreased breath sounds, grunting, retractions, toxic look; potential progression to severe respiratory distress	Depends on age; cough, coryza, hoarseness, crackles, wheezing, stridor	Persistent cough, malaise, headache	Tachypnea, staccato cough, crackles, wheezing rare, 50% have signs or history of conjunctivitis
Fever	Acute onset of fever (≥102.2°F [≥39°C])	Present (less prominent)	>102.2°F (>39°C)	Afebrile
CBC	WBCs often elevated >15,000/mcL	Normal or slight elevation of WBC	Normal	Eosinophilia in 75% of cases
Organism(s)	90% caused by Streptococcus pneumoniae	RSV, parainfluenza, influenza	M. pneumonia C. pneumoniae	C. trachomatis
Radiographic findings	Lobar consolidation	Transient lobar infiltrates	Varies, interstitial infiltrates	Hyperinflation, infiltrates
Treatment	Depends on bacteria and age of child; amoxicillin, penicillin, methicillin, cefuroxime, gentamicin, vancomycin	Supportive care	Erythromycin Azithromycin Clarithromycin	Erythromycin

CBC, Complete blood count; *RSV,* respiratory syncytial virus; *URI,* upper respiratory infection; *WBC,* white blood cell.

- Shoulder pain radiating to the upper chest, upper arm, and neck can be a presentation of upper lobe bacterial pneumonia (Scheffer et al., 2016)
- Other manifestations include restlessness, shaking chills, apprehension, shortness of breath, malaise, and pleuritic chest pain; irritation of the pleura causes chest pain

Physical Examination. Pay close attention to the general appearance, looking at the work of breathing, assessing for hypoxia, and evaluating tachypnea, which is considered to be the most valuable sign for ruling out pneumonia. To encourage preschoolers and school-age children to breathe deeply, ask them to blow crumbled papers off your hands or use a phone application that allows them to "blow up a balloon."

Early onset pneumonia in the neonate presents within the first 3 days of life with:
- Respiratory distress, apnea, tachycardia, poor perfusion
- No fever, or fever only with subtle or no physical findings
Typical findings seen in all types of pneumonia include:
- Nasal flaring, grunting, retractions
- Tachypnea (may be the only clue), generally more than 60 breaths per minute in infants younger than 2 months old, more than 50 breaths per minute in children 2 to 11 months old, or more than 40 breaths per minute at rest in children 1 to 5 years old
- Tachycardia, air hunger, and cyanosis are significant findings
- Fine crackles, dullness, diminished breath sounds
Additional findings associated with bacterial pneumonia:
- Fever and hypoxia
- Splinting the affected side to minimize pleuritic pain or lying on the side in a fetal position helps compensate for decreased air exchange and improves ventilation

- Tachypnea and retractions
- Progression to delirium, circumoral cyanosis, and posturing
- Signs of a pleural effusion and signs of congestive heart failure
- Abdominal distention, downward displacement of the liver or spleen
In viral pneumonia:
- Wheezing
- Downward displacement of the liver or spleen
In primary atypical bacterial pneumonia *(C. trachomatis)* is it characterized by:
- Repetitive, staccato cough with tachypnea, cervical adenopathy, crackles, and rarely wheezing
- Conjunctivitis is associated with *C. trachomatis* in infants (AAP, 2018)

Diagnostic Studies. A chest x-ray should not be routinely performed in children with pneumonia. In a wheezing child, it is hard to differentiate atelectasis seen in asthma or bronchiolitis from an infiltrate seen in pneumonia (Bradley et al., 2011; Katz and Williams, 2018). Follow-up films are not needed in patients who have an uneventful recovery. Chest ultrasound is often used to detect effusions and empyema; however, studies show sensitivity of 92% to 98% and specificity of 92% to 100% for lobar pneumonia. Larger-scale studies are needed before any recommendation can be made (Katz and Williams, 2018).

Blood cultures should not be routinely used in outpatient settings unless the child fails to improve or deteriorates on antibiotic therapy. Blood cultures should be done on children who are admitted with moderate to severe pneumonia. Sputum cultures can be used in hospitalized children who can produce sputum. Urine antigen detection tests for *S. pneumonia* are not

TABLE 37.7	Age Variants in Pneumonia Microorganisms	
Age	**Viral Organisms**	**Bacterial Organisms**

Neonatal	Cytomegalovirus (CMV)	More common
		    Group B streptococci
		    Gram-negative enteric
		      bacteria
		    Listeria
		    Chlamydia trachomatis
		Uncommon organisms
		    Streptococcus
		      pneumoniae
		    Group D streptococcus
		    Anaerobes

Infants	Most common
	    Respiratory syncy-
	      tial virus (RSV)
	    Parainfluenza
	    Influenza
	    Adenoviruses
	    Metapneumovirus
		Less common
		    S. pneumoniae
		    Haemophilus influenzae
		    Mycoplasma pneumonia
		    Mycobacterium tuber-
		      culosis
		    Bordetella pertussis
		    Pneumocystis jiroveci

Preschool children	Most common
	    RSV
	    Parainfluenza
	    Influenza
	    Adenoviruses
	    Metapneumovirus
	    Bocavirus role is
	      not clear
		Less common
		    S. pneumoniae
		    H. influenza
		    M. pneumoniae
		    M. tuberculosis
		    Chlamydophila pneu-
		      moniae

School-age children	Respiratory viruses as above	*M. pneumoniae* *C. pneumoniae* *S. pneumoniae* *M. tuberculosis*

Adapted from Ranganathan SC, Sonnappa S. Pneumonia and other respiratory infections. *Pediatr Clin North Am.* 2009;56(1):140.

• BOX 37.3 Criteria for Hospital Admission for Pneumonia

Neonate to 3 Months Old
- Fever
- Poor oral intake with signs of dehydration
- Pulmonary complications noted on radiographs—abscess, empyema, pneumatocele

Infants and Children Older Than 3 Months
- Hypoxemia with oxygen less than 90%
- Tachypnea: >60 breaths/min in infants younger than 2 months old; >50 breaths/min in children 2-11 months old; or >40 breaths/min at rest in children 1-5 years old
- Respiratory rate >70 breaths/min in infants or older children >50 breaths/min indicates more severe community-acquired pneumonia
- Grunting, dyspnea, or apnea
- Poor feeding with tachycardia and signs of dehydration (slow capillary refill of >2 s) in infants
- Severe respiratory distress
- Oxygen saturation <90% with the need for supplemental oxygen (pulse oximetry reading or arterial blood gas)
- Toxic appearance
- Failure to respond to appropriate oral antibiotic

All Age Groups
- Social issues at home that indicate caregiver cannot appropriately monitor and/or care for the child

---

recommended, because the false-positive rate is high due to nasopharyngeal carriage of the organism (Katz and Williams, 2018).

Rapid tests for influenza and RSV viruses are helpful; a CBC showing a leukocytosis is a nonspecific sign and its specificity in diagnosing bacterial pneumonia is poor (Katz and Williams, 2018). Acute phase reactants do not differentiate between viral and bacterial pneumonia and are not recommended for fully immunized children who are being treated as an outpatient. A recent review of the use of procalcitonin to distinguish serious LRT infections did not support its effectiveness (Baumann, Baer, Bonhoeffer et al., 2017). These tests may be useful for more seriously ill patients. Based on current studies, testing for *M. pneumonia* using currently available PCR tests may pick up carriage as well as disease, and caution must be used in the interpretation of these results (Katz and Williams, 2018).

Differential Diagnosis

The child's age and characteristic signs and symptoms as discussed previously can help distinguish between a viral and a bacterial pneumonia. Differential diagnoses to consider with pneumonia include bronchiolitis, congestive heart failure, acute bronchiectasis,

FB aspiration, pulmonary abscess, parasitic pneumonia, and endotracheal tuberculosis. Right lower lobe pneumonia can present with abdominal pain and be confused with appendicitis. Right upper lobe pneumonia can often closely resemble meningitis as it may present with a stiff neck.

Management

Most otherwise healthy children can be managed as outpatients. Guidelines for admission are identified in Box 37.3. Neonates must always be admitted to the hospital if diagnosed with pneumonia regardless of infecting pathogen. Young infants may also need hospitalization unless *C. trachomatis* is suspected.

All children with pneumonia require supportive care with antipyretics, hydration, and rest. Antibiotics should be reserved for those with suspected bacterial infection only. Serious infections may require hospitalization for respiratory therapy, including humidified oxygen, pulmonary therapy, and/or intubation.

Guidelines for outpatient and inpatient treatment of bacterial pneumonia by age and certain specific pathogens follow (Barson, 2018; Bradley et al., 2011; Taketomo et al., 2018). Local resistance rates may need to be taken into consideration.
- *Outpatient antibiotic treatment*: Oral antibiotics are considered safe for most children older than 3 months with pneumonia.
  - *2 months to 3 months old*: If chlamydia is suspected, treat with oral azithromycin for 5 days or erythromycin base or ethyl succinate for 14 days (AAP, 2018). Admission may be needed depending on clinical presentation.
  - *3 months to 18 years old*: Amoxicillin 90 mg/kg/day, divided every 12 hours for 10 days (maximum daily dose: 4000 mg/day). If a history of a non-type I hypersensitivity reaction to penicillin, a second- or third-generation cephalosporin (e.g., cefdinir) can be used; or if a history of type I hypersensitivity reaction, clindamycin can be used.

- If *C. pneumonia* or *M. pneumonia* (community-acquired) is suspected, azithromycin is an appropriate choice. Azithromycin 10 mg/kg/day once on day 1 (maximum dose = 500 mg) and then 5 mg/kg daily for the next 4 days (maximum dose = 250 mg). Local macrolide resistance may need to be considered.
- For influenza, oseltamivir (Tamiflu) is recommended; zanamivir (Relenza) can be used in children older than 7 years.
- *Inpatient treatment:* Testing to identify the pathogen is important for selection of appropriate antimicrobial therapy.
  - *Neonate:* Ampicillin and cefotaxime, ceftriaxone, or gentamicin.
  - Ampicillin or penicillin G in a fully-immunized infant or school-age child with community-acquired pneumonia unless there is a high incidence of *S. pneumoniae.*
  - Empiric therapy with a third-generation cephalosporin (ceftriaxone or cefotaxime) if there are high rates of penicillin-resistant *S. pneumoniae.*
  - The addition of macrolide to a β-lactam therapy if *M. pneumonia* and *C. pneumonia* are present or considered likely to be present.
  - Vancomycin or clindamycin in addition to β-lactam therapy if *S. aureus* is strongly considered, keeping in mind that community-acquired MRSA may require more than 10 days of therapy (Barson, 2018; Bradley et al., 2011).

Education about medication administration, hydration, fever control, and worrisome signs and symptoms is important. In addition, the child should be seen for follow-up at the conclusion of antibiotic treatment or sooner if there is no improvement or worsening of symptoms. Children with recurrent pneumonias should be referred for further pulmonary evaluation.

Prognosis

By the second to third day of treatment, auscultation should reveal a change in respiratory sounds as the infection begins to consolidate. Increased fremitus, tubular breath sounds, and the disappearance of crackles may be noted. Most children have an uneventful recovery, and it is important to inform caregivers that the cough can last for several weeks. Routine rechecks with chest x-rays are not recommended. If pneumonia recurs or persists for longer than 1 month, further evaluation for underlying immunodeficiency disease is indicated.

Complications

Complications associated with community-acquired pneumonia can involve other systems and include meningitis, CNS abscess, endocarditis, pericarditis, osteomyelitis, and/or septic arthritis. Pulmonary complications include parapneumonic effusion, more common in staphylococcal and *S. pneumonia* infections (Cashen and Person, 2017). Pneumothorax, bronchopleural fistula, and/or abscess of the lung can also occur. Scarring of the airways and lung tissue can cause dilated bronchi, which results in bronchiectasis. *M. pneumoniae* can spread to the blood, CNS, heart, skin, or joints. A child with an underlying immunodeficiency or sickle cell disease experiences more severe pulmonary disease than the average child does.

Prevention

Identify and treat pregnant women with *C. trachomatis.* Universal vaccination against influenza, HIB, and pneumococcal infection is essential. Current guidelines limit the use of palivizumab (Synagis) prophylaxis (see Chapter 31).

Valley Fever (Coccidioidomycosis)

Coccidioidomycosis is an infection caused by a fungal spore, Coccidioides, found in southwest desert areas. Although it usually presents as a primary pulmonary infection, it can range from an asymptomatic exposure to a life-threatening disease (Twarog and Thompson, 2015). Infants and young children are more likely to develop disseminated infection. Coccidioidomycosis is caused by two species, *C. immitis* and *C. posadasii,* found from California to the southwestern United States, as well as Mexico, Central America, and South America. States with the highest incidence are California and Arizona. When a drought occurs, the hyphae develop into arthrospores then disarticulate into airborne spores when the soil is disrupted. The incubation period ranges from 7 to 28 days (Gabe et al., 2017). Person-to-person transmission only occurs in congenital infection or in patients with draining skin lesions. A single infection gives lifelong immunity; however, immunosuppressed individuals can reactivate months to years after travel to an endemic area (Gabe et al., 2017).

The incidence of this disease has increased in the southwestern United States. Persons at risk include those with consistent exposure to the soil, immunosuppressed, pregnant females in the third trimester, and patients of African or Filipino descent (Twarog and Thompson, 2015). The increasing incidence of coccidioidomycosis is likely due to environmental factors (such as drought, which may cause an increase in spore dispersal) and the increase in construction. There is marked under-reporting of the disease because of the voluntary nature of reporting and under testing by providers who fail to consider coccidioidomycosis in the differential of an influenza-like illness.

Clinical Findings in Infants and Children

Coccidioidomycosis presents with a flulike disease with cough and fever and some develop a skin reaction following several weeks of illness. Erythema nodosum or erythema multiforme are the result of an immunological phenomena. The disease commonly presents as a lobular or segmental pneumonia. The classic triad of fever, erythema nodosum, and arthralgia seen in adults is not a common presentation in infants and children (Gabe et al., 2017).

History. Typical history findings include fatigue, fever, weight loss, rash on upper body or legs, cough and headache, malaise, chest pain (with pulmonary infection), myalgia or joint pain, and neck stiffness (with meningitis).

Physical Examination. Characteristic findings are fever, crackles (with respiratory infection), and cutaneous abnormalities including erythema multiforme and erythema nodosum.

Diagnostic Studies. Serologic tests are commonly used. Antibody production lags behind illness for several weeks and the response is even weaker and more delayed in the immunocompromised. Serial testing is needed to avoid false-negative results (Gabe et al., 2017). Enzyme immunoassay (EIA) tests assess IgM and IgG; there is controversy about their accuracy and reference lab confirmation is needed. Immunodiffusion tube precipitin and immunodiffusion complement fixation can be used to confirm EIA tests or as a primary test. In primary infection, IgM can be found in the first and third weeks. Complement fixation tests, immunodiffusion, and EIA tests evaluating IgG response are used; complement fixation tests and immunodiffusion are more specific. Persistent titers of 1:16 or greater occur with severe disease that is likely disseminated. The *Coccidioides* species can be seen under a microscope when infected body fluids are examined. Clinical correlation with diagnostic tests is critical for the appropriate diagnosis (Gabe et al., 2017). It is important to evaluate the patient clinically despite significant elevation of these titers (Twarog and Thompson, 2015).

Differential Diagnosis

Differential diagnoses include a variety of respiratory conditions, such as pneumonias from other organisms, bronchitis, and influenza.

Management

While all cases of disseminated disease are treated, observation is appropriate in mild cases with an absence of pulmonary nodules and improving clinical symptom. Patients with severe symptoms or high-risk immune-suppressed children, young children, pregnant teens in their final trimester, children with underlying cardiac disease, CF, or diabetes are generally treated. Postpartum women may be at the greatest risk for dissemination of the disease (Gabe et al., 2017). Outpatient management is treatment with fluconazole or itraconazole for one year at a minimum. Severe life-threatening infection requires admission and IV amphotericin B (severe skeletal or pulmonary disease) or intrathecal amphotericin B (CNS disease).

Indications for Hospitalization

Hospitalizations for patients with severe pulmonary involvement and low oxygen level may be necessary for oxygen therapy and fluids. Patients with CNS disease may require lifelong therapy with azoles since the disease reoccurs once therapy is stopped. They must be monitored for obstructive hydrocephalus, abscess, vasculitis, and infarction.

Prevention

Immunocompromised patients should avoid activities that expose them to aerosolized spores in dust-laden areas in the southwestern United States, Mexico, Central America, and South America. Control of dust in construction sites, archaeological digs, or in locations of soil disturbances can prevent disease. There is no available vaccine (Twarog and Thompson, 2015).

Pertussis

Pertussis is caused by a tiny, gram-negative bacillus, *Bordetella pertussis*, and can be a primary infection or a reinfection. The three most common types of *Bordetella* species causing respiratory disease are *B. parapertussis*, *Bordetella holmesii*, and *Bordetella bronchiseptica* (Souder and Long, 2015). *B. bronchiseptica* infrequently causes respiratory infection; *B. holmesii* causes bacteremia. The infection caused by *B. pertussis* is also known as *whooping cough* because of the high-pitched inspiratory whoop following spasms of coughing. The cough is an attempt to dislodge plugs of necrotic bronchial epithelial tissue and thick mucus followed by a whoop to draw in oxygen.

B. pertussis produces a variety of components that are highly antigenic as well as biologically active. These include pertussis toxin (PT), adenylate cyclase toxin, dermonecrotic toxin, fimbriae, filamentous hemagglutinin, pertactin, and autotransporters. Pertactin, filamentous hemagglutinin, and fimbriae allow for bacterial adhesion, whereas PT causes a lymphocytosis that irritates and inflames the ciliated epithelium lining, leading to epithelial cell damage (Carbonetti, 2015; Souder and Long, 2015).

While the new acellular vaccines are safer and more efficacious than whole cell DTP vaccine, there has been a steady increase in pertussis rates with outbreaks occurring across the United States and the globe. Factors attributed to the increase include a shift in pertussis epidemiology, lower immunization rates, waning immunity of the acellular vaccine, lack of healthcare providers' knowledge of the clinical presentation of the disease, and changes in *B. pertussis* bacteria along with spread of other species of *Bordetella* (Faulkner, et al., 2016).

B. pertussis is highly contagious and transmission occurs by respiratory aerosols and airborne droplets; patients with a cough are more likely to be vectors (Trainer, Nicolson, Merkel, 2015). Contaminated droplets are inhaled and adhere to the ciliated epithelium of the nasopharynx. The incubation period is usually 7 to 10 days but can last as long as 28 days (Kilgore et al., 2016). Children are most contagious during the catarrhal stage, the first stage of illness that lasts 2 weeks (Souder and Long, 2015). The usual and most common source of transmission of *B. pertussis* infection to an infant is a mother with the disease (Healy et al., 2015). The highest incidence of mortality occurs in infants less than 6 months old (Kilgore et al., 2016).

Clinical Findings

The clinical presentation of the disease depends on the length of time from the last vaccination (if vaccinated), age and gender of the child, the infectious species of pertussis (*Bordetella pertussis* is more severe than *B. parapertussis*), and the amount of infectious load. The range of symptoms in children varies from an asymptomatic infection to upper respiratory tract disease to severe, progressive coughing that can last for months. There are three consecutive stages of pertussis—catarrhal, paroxysmal, and convalescent, each lasting 1 to 3 weeks without complete recovery for 2 to 3 months. Table 37.8 shows the stages of pertussis with accompanying symptoms.

In infants, particularly neonates, the clinical presentation is generally severe, and includes:
- Apnea (common) often with seizures caused by hypoxemia; tachypnea
- Cough without an inspiratory whoop; poor feeding
- Leukocytosis with a marked lymphocytosis (in the presence of illness marked by persistent cough points to *B. pertussis*)

Reinfections are common as disease immunity does not provide long-lasting protection. Coinfection with other respiratory pathogens including RSV, parainfluenza virus, *M. pneumoniae*, adenovirus, and influenza occurs (Kilgore et al., 2016).

Diagnostic Studies

PCR is the primary diagnostic test used in most commercial and state laboratories for confirmation. Starting in the mid-1990s, pertussis diagnostic test options included culture, serology, direct fluorescent antibody testing (DFA), and more recently PCR. While culture is the gold standard since it is 100% specific, it needs to be done by nasopharyngeal swab (NP) within 2 weeks of onset of symptoms (CDC, 2018b). NP collection is done with a Dacron or calcium alginate fiber-tipped swab inserted into the nasal passage and advanced to the nasopharynx then immediately placed into a special transport medium. Culture can be negative if the person had been ill for 2 weeks or more, was previously vaccinated, or if antibiotics were started (AAP, 2018). Bacteria are found in high number in the airways early in infection but decrease markedly in the paroxysmal stage (Trainer et al., 2015).

PCR testing provides faster results and earlier treatment, allowing public health officials to identify pertussis cluster cases and

TABLE 37.8 **Stages of Pertussis**

Stage of Pertussis	Length of Time	Manifestation
Catarrhal	2-3 wk	**Infant and child** Upper respiratory infection symptoms with mild progressive dry cough. Low-grade fever (to 101°F [38.3°C]). Cough worsens as child progresses to the paroxysmal stage.
Paroxysmal	2-4 wk	There is intense and violent coughing with 5-10 coughs with an inspiratory whoop. The cough can lead to eye proptosis and tearing, thick mucous production, and salivation. Cyanosis, sweating, prostration, and exhaustion after coughing. Sleep is disturbed but fever is absent or minimal. **Adolescents** Classic paroxysm of coughing is missing in up to a third of patients. Clinicians should consider pertussis if there is a persistent cough beyond 3 wk.
Convalescent	3 wk to 6 mo	Symptoms wane over a variable period that can last months. Waning of paroxysmal coughing episodes but a nonparoxysmal cough can last as long as 6 wk with coughing paroxysm occurring when child gets another viral infection.

Data from Kilore, P, Salim A., Zervos, M, et al. Pertussis: Microbiology, disease, treatment and prevention. *Clin Microbiology Rev.* 2016;29(3):449–481.

encourage faster response to outbreaks. Although there were problems with diagnostic specificity, the newer tests incorporate a parapertussis-specific molecular target, decreasing the false positive rate (Faulkner et al., 2016). These tests require an NP culture and must be done within 3 weeks of the cough onset. PCR testing is increasingly popular due to its improved sensitivity (70% to 99%) and specificity (86% to 100%).

The CDC and the FDA developed serological tests that can be done up to 12 weeks after the onset of symptoms; however, the optimal time for testing is from 2 weeks to 8 weeks. This testing has utility in identifying outbreaks (CDC, 2018b).

A CBC is nonspecific with leukocytosis and lymphocytosis common findings in infants and young children but rare in adolescents (Souder, Long, 2015). A chest x-ray may be normal or have nonspecific findings such as atelectasis, peribronchial cuffing, or perihilar infiltrates.

Differential Diagnosis

There are a number of infectious diseases that can present with a cough including RSV, *B. parapertussis*, adenoviruses, bocaviruses, human metapneumovirus, influenza A and B, parainfluenza, and rhinovirus. Noninfectious disease triggers of coughs include gastroesophageal reflux, CF, sinusitis, aspiration pneumonia, and asthma. FBs should be included in the differential diagnosis.

Management

Treatment:

- Antibiotic treatment should be started within 6 weeks of disease onset in infants and in children and adults within 21 days (Souder and Long, 2015). The macrolide class of drugs including azithromycin, clarithromycin, and erythromycin is recommended for all ages. However, there is an association between the development of pyloric stenosis and erythromycin in infants younger than 1 month (AAP, 2018; Souder and Long, 2015).
  - Azithromycin: the drug of choice for infants less than 1 month at 10 mg/kg in a single dose for 5 days. This same dose is used from 1 to 6 months.
  - Azithromycin: For infants over 6 months, children, and adolescents, a 5-day treatment course is also recommended but the first day only, a single dose of 10 mg/kg/day (maximum dose of 500 mg) is given, then a single dose of 5 mg/kg/day (maximum dose of 250 mg) on days 2 to 5.
  - Clarithromycin: For infants over 1 month, children, and adolescents, 15 mg/kg/day divided every 12 hours divided for 7 days with a maximum dose of 1 g/day.
  - Erythromycin: For infants over 1 month to 5 months, 10 mg/kg/dose, 4 times a day for 14 days; >6 months and children, 10 mg/kg/dose, 4 times a day for 7 to 14 days, maximum daily dose 2 gm/day; adolescents 500 mg 4 times a day for 7 to 14 days.
  - Sulfamethoxazole (SMX) and Trimethoprim (TMP): Can be used as an alternative in infants older than 2 months who cannot tolerate macrolides; dose at TMP 8 mg/kg/day and SMX 40 mg/kg/day in divided doses every 12 hours (maximum single dose 160 mg TMP).
- The use of corticosteroids or albuterol and other β 2-adrenergic medications are not supported by controlled, prospective studies (Bocka, 2017).

Care of Exposed Children

Post-exposure prophylaxis with a macrolide is recommended for household and close contacts irrespective of immunization status. Close contact includes household members, caretakers, healthcare workers, and any person who was within 3 to 4 feet of a symptomatic person, shared a closed space for 1 hour or more, or had direct contact with secretions of the nasal, oral, or respiratory tract. Early prophylaxis limits secondary transmission as untreated infants can have a positive NP culture 6 weeks after the start of illness; other persons can shed the bacteria for 3 to 4 weeks (Souder and Long, 2015). The value of chemoprophylaxis is limited after 21 days elapse but should be considered in high-risk household contacts (young infant, pregnant woman, or person who is in contact with infants) (AAP, 2018):

- Immunization coverage with diphtheria-tetanus-acellular pertussis (DTaP) or Tdap depending on age group needs to be reviewed and appropriate acellular pertussis vaccine given
- Students and staff in schools need to be monitored for any respiratory symptoms with exclusion and evaluation for anyone with a cough illness.
- Close monitoring of respiratory symptoms for 21 days after last contact with an infected individual.

Complications

One out of 100 infants die from pertussis. Other complications include apnea, secondary pneumonia, convulsions, insomnia, sinusitis, otitis media, syncope, rib fracture, and weight loss (Kilgore et al., 2016).

Prevention

The concept of "cocooning" around the infant is designed to protect infants from dangerous or unwanted environmental hazards (Kilgore et al., 2016; Souder and Long, 2015). Cocooning recommendations include targeted immunization strategies to immunize adults around the infant, including caretakers, grandparents over 65 years old, fathers, and mothers who were not immunized in the last trimester. In addition, all adolescents 11 to 18 years old should receive the Tdap vaccine.

In addition, the recommended guidelines for the initial series of DTaP vaccines and booster doses should be followed. Just one DTaP immunization can reduce the severity of symptoms in an infant infected with pertussis. The clinician needs to be mindful of valid contraindications to receiving pertussis vaccine. Immunity following either natural pertussis infection or illness or vaccination is *not* long lasting. Due to the wide range of clinical presentations in children, adolescents, and adults, persons who are either asymptomatic or think it is "just a cold" can transmit the infection to an unimmunized infant resulting in life-threatening illness. Universal immunization of children and adolescents is crucial to pertussis control.

Cystic Fibrosis

CF is a multisystem genetic disorder manifested by chronic obstructive pulmonary disease (COPD), GI disturbances, and exocrine dysfunction; it is the most common autosomal-recessive disease. Newer therapies that target the genetic defect are likely to further increase the life span of patients with CF, however, pulmonary manifestations will need active preventive treatments. CF occurs in approximately 1 in 4000 white births, 1 in 15,000 to 20,000 African American, and 1 in 4000 to 10,000 Latin Americans (Farrell et al., 2017; Sanders and Fink, 2016).

CF involves mutation of the CF transmembrane conductance regulator (CFTR) protein, which is expressed in epithelial and blood cells. The gene is on chromosome 7 with more than 2000 CFTR mutations identified (Goetz and Singh, 2016). Mutations are categorized into six distinct classes, although the functional importance of only a few mutations is known. CFTR functions in sodium transport through the epithelial sodium channel, regulates the adenosine triphosphate (ATP) channels, and is involved in bicarbonate chloride exchange. The CFTR gene defect causes defective ion transport, airway surface liquid depletion, and defective mucociliary clearance. Table 37.9 shows the different types of mutations.

The diagnosis is based on evidence of CFTR dysfunction and signs and symptoms of the disease. Infants in the United States with a positive newborn screening (NBS) with inconclusive diagnostic testing are identified as having CF related metabolic syndrome (CRMS); the term CF Screen Positive, Inconclusive Diagnosis (CFSPED) is used in other countries. This classification is given when there is a positive NBS and either a sweat chloride value <30 mmol/L and 2 CFTR mutations, at least one of which has unclear phenotypic consequences, or an intermediate sweat chloride value of 30 to 59 mmol/L and 1 or 0 CF-causing mutations. The CFTR-related disorder is a monosymptomatic clinical entity associated with CFTR dysfunction that does not meet the diagnostic criteria for CF. The use of atypical and nonclassical terms is not recommended (Farrell et al., 2017).

The most common defect, found in 70% of cases, is a deletion of phenylalanine in position 508 (D508) (Paranjape and Mogayzel, 2014). Polymorphism in non-CFTR genes may explain the

TABLE 37.9	Cystic Fibrosis Transmembrane Conductance Regulator Mutation Classes	
Class of Defect	Abnormalities of Cystic Fibrosis Transmembrane Conductance Regulator Synthesis, Structure, and Function	Risk Category
I	No functional CFTR protein made due to defective or absent biosynthesis	High risk: pancreatic insufficiency
II	CFTR defect in trafficking as a result of mutation of protein variants that are improperly processed to the apical cell membrane Delta-508 is a class II mutation	
III	Affects CFTR channel regulation that impairs the chloride conduction through the channel	
IV	Defects in channel conducting with a decreased amount of CFTR with decrease in function of the apical cell membrane	Low risk: pancreatic sufficiency
V	Reduced protein quantity	
VI	Stability of CFTR at the cell surface is decreased	Risk not classified

CFTR, Cystic fibrosis transmembrane conductance regulator.

difference in the manifestations of the genetic change within different families (Sosnay, Raraigh, Gison, 2016). Ultimately, the resulting mucus obstruction causes inflammation and infection. Failure to conduct ions across epithelial cell membranes leads to problems in the lungs, biliary tree, pancreas, intestines, vas deferens, and sweat glands. This results in mucus thickening and target organ damage in the lungs and exocrine glands. There is airway surface liquid depletion with inhibited transport of bicarbonate causing decreased mucociliary transport. The deficiency in mucociliary transport causes chronic inflammation and infection and, as a result of environmental insults and host defense defects, leads to bacterial colonization in trapped mucous secretions (Goetz and Singh, 2016). The mucus is adhesive and stringy leading to tenacious secretions that have poor cough clearance. There is osmolar fluid depletion leading to a loss of water and increased concentration of ions. In the exocrine system, subsequent pancreas, liver, and intestinal tract adhesive secretions lead to malabsorption of fat and proteins as a result of pancreatic insufficiency.

Clinical Findings

CF is a multisystem progressive illness with varying levels of severity. Table 37.10 outlines clinical manifestations seen in children at various ages. They may include the following:
• *Pulmonary:* CF is a major cause of severe chronic lung disease in children. Lungs of children with CF are normal at birth but become inflamed with chronic airway infection shortly after birth. The respiratory epithelium exhibits marked impermeability to chloride and excessive sodium reabsorption. Mucus is adherent and stringy with a need for periciliary fluid to aid in expectoration, leading to dysfunctional mucociliary transport, airway obstruction, and chronic infections. Pulmonary system

TABLE 37.10	Clinical Manifestations of Cystic Fibrosis: from Neonatal Period to Adolescence
Stage of Childhood	**Clinical Manifestations**
Fetal ultrasound	Hyperechoic bowel is suggestive of meconium ileus and is present in 10% of fetuses with CF
Neonatal period	Meconium ileus, delayed meconium passage, meconium plug Prolonged jaundice Intestinal atresia Edema, hypoproteinemia, and acrodermatitis enteropathica due to malabsorption Hemorrhagic disease of newborn due to vitamin K deficiency
Infancy	Cough Colonization with bacteria in mucus Bacterial pneumonia Failure to thrive Hypoproteinemia, hypochloremic dehydration Abdominal distention Cholestasis Rectal prolapse Steatorrhea DIOS Hemolytic anemia
Childhood	Respiratory manifestations: Chronic recurrent infection of sinuses and respiratory tract/nasal polyposis/poorly controlled asthma Bronchiectasis Allergic bronchopulmonary aspergillosis Digital clubbing GI manifestations: Poor weight gain and growth Steatorrhea Chronic constipation Rectal prolapse DIOS Idiopathic pancreatitis/liver disease
Adolescence	ABPA Chronic pansinusitis Nasal polyposis Bronchiectasis/hemoptysis Idiopathic pancreatitis Osteoporosis Diabetes Obstructive azoospermia

ABPA, Allergic bronchopulmonary aspergillosis; *CF,* cystic fibrosis; *DIOS,* distal intestinal obstruction syndrome; *GI,* gastrointestinal.

Adapted from Rosenfield M, Sontag, M, Ren, C. Cystic fibrosis diagnosis and newborn screening. *Pediatr Clin N Am,* 2016;63:602 and Paranjape SM, Mogayzel PJ. Cystic fibrosis. *Pediatr Rev.* 2014; 35(5):194–205.

manifestations run the clinical spectrum from chronic, dry, frequent cough and sputum production to respiratory failure. Bronchitis, bronchiolitis, bronchiectasis, and pneumonia occur frequently. Bronchospasm resembling acute or chronic asthma may be present. Airways become colonized with *S. aureus, H. influenzae,* and, finally, *P. aeruginosa. Burkholderia cepacia* is a slower-growing organism found in children with CF. Infection can present in infancy. Pulmonary disease usually becomes progressive and leads to cor pulmonale, respiratory failure, and death by adulthood. Other respiratory problems associated with CF include recurrent ARS, nasal polyps, and allergic bronchopulmonary aspergillosis, which starts by childhood and continues into adulthood. Digital clubbing is common.

- *GI tract and nutrition:* During infancy, meconium ileus, pancreatic insufficiency, and rectal prolapse can be manifestations of CF. Meconium ileus develops in up to 15% of newborns born with CF. Meconium ileus syndrome equivalent can also develop in older patients, with desiccated fecal material causing GI obstruction. Eighty-five percent of affected children have failure to thrive because of pancreatic enzyme insufficiency, which leads to bulky, malodorous stools resulting in failure to thrive. Edema with hypoproteinemia may also be present. Children have thick fat-laden stools (steatorrhea), poor muscle mass, and delayed maturation. Infants with CF who are fed soy-based formulas do very poorly, and severe hypoproteinemia and anasarca quickly result. During childhood, intussusception, hepatic steatosis, biliary fibrosis, and rectal prolapse can occur. Childhood problems continue into adulthood. Clinically apparent cirrhosis occurs in 15% of patients with subsequent risk of portal hypertension. Adenocarcinoma of the digestive tract can occur. Other GI problems associated with CF include volvulus, duodenal inflammation, gastroesophageal reflux, bile reflux, fibrosing colonopathy, and poor fat absorption that leads to vitamin A, K, E, and D deficiencies with resulting anemia, neuropathy, night blindness, osteoporosis, and bleeding disorders. Distal intestinal obstructive syndrome (DIOS) occurs when viscous fecal matter causes blockage in the distal intestine and presents with abdominal pain and distention with pain. This occurs as a result of poor fat absorption, pancreatic insufficiency, and dehydration.
- *Hepatobiliary tract:* Biliary cirrhosis occurs in 2% to 3% of children with CF and is characterized by jaundice, ascites, hematemesis from esophageal varices, portal hypertension, cirrhosis, hepatomegaly, and splenomegaly. Hepatic steatosis is also a known complication of CF. Adolescent patients may experience biliary colic and cholelithiasis.
- *Endocrine:* Recurrent acute pancreatitis is not uncommon. CF–related diabetes (CFRD) with relative insulin deficiency develops as the child ages due to autolysis of the pancreas as the pancreas body becomes fatty due to thick viscous secretions. CF patients need annual blood glucose screening with up to 30% of patients developing CFRD by adulthood (Paranjape and Mogayzel, 2014).
- *Musculoskeletal:* Vitamin D deficiency may result in osteoporosis when bone reabsorption exceeds bone formation.
- *Reproductive:* Affected children have delayed sexual development. The vas deferens is nonfunctional and atrophied due to CFTR dysfunction, leading to azoospermia and male sterility. The incidence of inguinal hernia, hydrocele, and undescended testes is also high. Females experience secondary amenorrhea, cervicitis, and decreased fertility. A pregnancy is usually carried to term if pulmonary function is not severely compromised.
- *Sweat glands:* Excessive salt loss can lead to hypochloremic alkalosis, especially in warm weather or after gastroenteritis. Children with CF often taste salty because of elevated amounts of sodium chloride lost in endogenous sweat. Dehydration and heat exhaustion are concerns.

Diagnostic Studies. NBS enables early identification of CF and referral to CF centers. Children with access to earlier routine care due to early diagnosis do better than those with a later diagnosis (VanDevanter et al., 2016). NBS detects over 60% of new diagnoses. Many NBS algorithms done by states identify immunoreactive trypsinogen or trypsin (IRT) as the main test with an IRT/IRT protocol. State guidelines typically require either 2 IRT measurements (IRT/IRT), a DNA CFTR mutation panel if the IRT is elevated (IRT/CFTR), or two IRT concentrations with a follow-up DNA CFTR mutation panel. If the IRT is elevated or the child has one CFTR mutation, the primary provider is notified and the child is referred for sweat testing. There are false-negative screens, so if an infant has symptoms and signs of CF, a sweat test should be performed. This protocol is less sensitive than the IRT/DNA algorithms (96.2% to 76.1%). False positives and false negatives do occur (VanDevanter et al., 2016).

A 139 mutation panel via next-generation sequencing has increased identification of African Americans with CF by 20% (Savant and McColley, 2017). A limited number of CF centers also test for nasal potential difference measurement. Although the cornerstone for diagnosis is the pilocarpine iontophoresis sweat test, criteria for the diagnosis have changed due to genetic testing (Rosenfield et al., 2016).

Sweat testing should be done even if the newborn screen was negative when a child has pulmonary symptoms such as chronic cough, recurrent pneumonia, nasal polyps, and digital clubbing or systemic signs such as failure to thrive, jaundice, rectal prolapse, intussusception, prolonged jaundice, or pancreatitis. Sweat tests should be done at a laboratory that routinely does these tests. Sodium chloride concentration increases with age. A concentration of sweat chloride greater than 60 mmol/L is suggestive of CF; a range of 30 to 59 mmol/L for infants less than 6 months or 40 to 59 mmol/L for older individuals suggests the need for further genetic testing. If the sweat test is less than 30 mmol/L, CF is unlikely. It is rare for someone with two mutations to have a negative sweat test. A result of greater than 60 mEq/L of chloride on two specimens is in the diagnostic range for CF. Children with CF who have hypoproteinemia may elicit false-negative sweat test results. Results of the genetic testing should be compared to the most current knowledge found at https://www.CFTR2.org/.

Other diagnostic testing is indicated depending on secondary complications of CF. Glycosylated hemoglobin levels may be elevated in older children because of impaired pancreatic functioning. Pulmonary function tests are used to follow the clinical course. Liver function tests abnormalities on three tests in a 12-month period, ultrasound, and liver tissue biopsy are used to diagnose liver disease.

Management

Children with CF have complicated treatment regimens and should be monitored by an interprofessional team at a CF-accredited center. Because lung disease is the most common cause of morbidity and mortality, it is important to educate families and develop a shared treatment plan that will optimize lung functioning, prevent disease progression, and avoid complications. Treatment of CF-related lung disease requires control of airway infections, clearance of airway secretions, and decreasing lung inflammation. Pulmonary, nutritional, physical, and pharmacologic (antibiotic and antiinflammatory) therapy and psychological counseling must be individualized for children at each stage of their illness.

- Pulmonary
  - To promote airway clearance, inhaled dornase alfa (recombinant human deoxyribonuclease) selectively cleaves the DNA and reduces mucus viscosity. Hypertonic saline works by drawing water into secretions and is used to thin secretions to allow their removal. The use of postural drainage, active cycle of breathing, autogenic drainage, percussion, positive expiratory pressure, exercise, and high-frequency chest wall oscillation are done twice a day to facilitate secretion removal.
  - CFTR modulators are approved for use in about 50% of the population. Ivacaftor, a CFTR potentiator, is approved for children over 2 years with the 551D mutation. CRFT correctors like lumacaftor are approved for use in pediatrics (Martiniano et al., 2016). The combination of ivacaftor/lumacaftor (Orkambi) is approved for children 6 and over with F508 Del mutations and will partially restore CFTR activity. This drug must be used with caution in children with advanced liver disease.
  - To reduce chronic airway inflammation, high-dose ibuprofen and oral azithromycin, dosed three times a week, are used. Children must be screened for atypical mycobacterial infection before starting long-term azithromycin. Although high-dose ibuprofen decreases neutrophil migration in children ages 6 to 17 years, the therapy is not widely used due to risk of GI bleeding and frequent drug blood level measurements. Hemoptysis can be scant (<5 mL), moderate (5 to 240 mL), or massive (>240 mL) and is associated with advancing lung disease as well as vitamin K deficiency. It results from the hypertrophy and proliferation of the bronchial arteries rupturing into airways as a result of disease progression. The management includes antibiotic therapy, cessation of the anti-inflammatory drugs, and limiting therapies for airway clearance (Goetz and Singh, 2016).
  - Pneumothorax presents as acute onset of chest pain and dyspnea and is confirmed by chest x-ray. Smaller pneumothoraces are managed by observation and discontinuation of positive pressure. Surgical or chemical pleurodesis is used in recurrent large pneumothoraces.
  - Lung transplantation is a viable therapy for selected patients with terminal lung disease and is used more in Canada than in the United States.
- Gastrointestinal
  - Replacement with exogenous pancreatic enzyme replacement therapy (PERT) with every meal and snack along with a fat-soluble vitamin supplement is done. PERT capsules are opened up but should not be crushed. Dosing ranges from 2000 to 2500 units/kg of lipase to a maximum of 10,000 units/kg/day. Higher dosing of lipase can lead to fibrosing colonopathy in a small number of patients.
  - Fat malabsorption causes deficiency of vitamins A, D, E, and K; therefore, replacement must be started along with serum monitoring of the levels annually. Vitamin D deficiency can occur, resulting in osteopenia, osteoporosis, or rickets.
  - CF liver disease (CFLD) is managed with optimizing nutritional intake and avoiding hepatotoxic drugs (Sathe and Freeman, 2016).
  - DIOS is managed using IV hydration, polyethylene Glycol solution, and oral laxatives to promote lower bowel clearance. Sodium meglumine diatrizoate (Gastrografin) enemas can be used by an experienced radiologist in instances of a complete obstruction (Sathe and Freeman, 2016).
- Endocrine disorder
  - At age 10, an oral glucose tolerance test is done annually to screen for CF-related diabetes. Hemoglobin A_{1C} is not

recommended because it underestimates overall glycemic control. Prevention of microvascular complication of diabetes including renal disease, retinopathy, and neuropathy associated with hyperglycemia is key. Ketoacidosis is rare.

- Insulin is used to treat CFRD.
- Transition from pediatric to adult care
  - More than 50% of patients with CF are adults. It is important to provide reproductive health care as well as to initiate care within an interprofessional team and make sure there is a transition to an adult care clinic (West and Mogayzel, 2016).

Pectus Deformity

Pectus excavatum (PE) deformity accounts for more than 95% of all thoracic abnormalities and is a depression of the lower sternum and lower ribs (Koumbourlis, 2015). PE is caused by costochondral cartilage growth abnormalities and can develop as a result of other problems. They include congenital diaphragmatic hernia or muscular diseases, such as spinal muscular atrophy and muscular dystrophy, and can also be seen in patients with subglottic stenosis. There is a male preponderance and in 40% of children with PE, family members have a pectus deformity. It is believed to be an autosomal dominant trait (Koumbourlis, 2015) and is also associated with inheritable connective tissue disease such as Marfan and Ehlers-Danlos syndromes. Consequences of this deformity vary from no effect to self-image concerns and, if severe, it can impair pulmonary and cardiac function or cause precordial pain following exercise (de Oliveira Carvalho et al., 2014).

PE deformity can interfere with respiratory function; lung volumes, although often normal, may be decreased. The chest has a smaller anteroposterior diameter, which can lead to a decrease in cardiac stroke volume and output. When it is severe, the heart can be compressed, or displaced to the left causing the great vessel to rotate. There is an additional risk of cardiac dysrhythmias due to lower oxygen supply to the heart. The length of the sternum abnormalities and the adjacent ribs determine the degree of pulmonary and cardiac dysfunction.

Pectus carinatum is much less common than PE. It also progresses during puberty. In pectus carinatum, there is a bowing out of the sternum (also called "pigeon chest"). Although this shape may be cosmetically unattractive, there are fewer complaints about shortness of breath, chest pain, or dyspnea. Both deformities have a male predominance (Koumbourlis, 2015).

Clinical Findings

History. The history may include exercise intolerance, easy fatigability, wheezing, chest tightness, chest pain, palpitations, or dizziness. Psychological effects can be marked as children are teased by their peers, which intensifies during puberty. Poor self-image can interfere with social activities and cause isolation.

Physical Examination. PE: There are three main types of PE. The "cup-shaped" or classic deformity is limited to the lower part of the sternum. The flat or saucer-shaped is a long pectus that involves most of the sternum. In the asymmetric type, there is asymmetry between the left and right hemithorax with the right side more affected. The sternum is also slightly rotated in this deformity, with more than a 30-degree rotation considered a significant torsion.

Pectus carinatum: In pectus carinatum, the sternum has a forward symmetric protrusion. There are four variants—chondrogladiolar, costomanubrial, horseshoe chest, or asymmetric.

Diagnostic Studies

Diagnostic testing can include chest x-ray, chest CT, or MRI.

Management. Patients with severe deformity and physiological effects should be referred to a cardiologist for pulmonary function tests and exercise testing with an echocardiogram for further evaluation. If the excavatum deformity is significant, surgical repair may be indicated. Indications for surgery are based on the degree of psychological and physical impairment rather than the severity of the pectus carinatum or PE. It is important to consider the quality of life as children want to look like their peers (Koumbourlis, 2015). A recent systematic review failed to show any superiority of minimally invasive approach versus conventional surgery (de Oliveira et al., 2014). The timing of the surgery is usually at the start of puberty. The healthcare provider needs to evaluate for a possible genetic etiology of PE and make appropriate referral to a geneticist.

Brief Resolved Unexplained Events

The normal definition of *apnea* is a cessation of air flow or effort for ≥20 seconds accompanied by bradycardia. Apnea in preterm infants is due to immature physiology and is likely to resolve by 40 to 44 weeks of post conceptual age whereas apnea in a term infant is more concerning (Patrinos and Martin, 2017). A BRUE is defined as a resolved, brief, sudden, and unexplained event of either (1) cyanosis or pallor; (2) absent, decreased, or irregular breathing; (3) marked change in tone; or (4) an altered level of responsiveness in an infant under 1 year (Tider et al., 2016). It was previously described as an apparent life-threatening event or ALTE. The guidelines for BRUE are designed to categorize patients into high risk and low risk, and this helps to determine what diagnostic work-up is needed. BRUE should only be diagnosed if the history and physical do not explain the event. Lower-risk patients include infants ≥60 days, infants with a gestational age of ≥32 weeks and a postconceptional age or ≥45 weeks, no history of a previous BRUE episode, short duration of event of ≤60 seconds, no need for CPR, and no concerning history or physical examination findings.

Clinical Findings

In infants with a potential BRUE, it is important to consider child abuse and any inconsistencies in history or developmental stage. A general history of the event including witnesses, state immediately before during and after the event, and a general family and medical history should be obtained. A complete physical exam with negative findings are consistent with low-risk BRUE.

Diagnostic Studies

Laboratory studies including a viral panel, electrolytes, blood glucose, CBC, and blood gas determination should be considered based on the history. Polysomnography, EEG, and echocardiogram should be considered depending on the history. Continuous home monitoring is not recommended.

Differential Diagnosis

Differential diagnoses of BRUE include gastroesophageal reflux disease; child abuse; cardiac conduction or ion channelopathies, arrhythmias, cardiac structural problems; anaphylaxis; bacterial infection; upper airway obstruction or obstructive sleep apnea; anemia; poisonings; or inborn errors of metabolism (Patrinos and Martin, 2017).

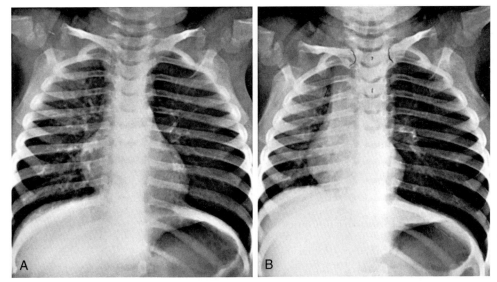

• **Fig 37.1** (A) Normal inspiratory chest radiograph in a toddler with a peanut fragment in the left main bronchus. (B) Expiratory radiograph of the same child showing the classic obstructive emphysema (air trapping) on the involved *(left)* side. Air leaves the normal right side, allowing the lung to deflate. The medium shifts toward the unobstructed side. (From Hollinger LD. Foreign bodies of the airway. In: Kliegman RM, Stanton BF, St. Geme JW, et al., eds. *Nelson Textbook of Pediatrics.* 19th ed. Philadelphia: Saunders/Elsevier; 2011.)

Management

If the infant is at lower risk, education with shared decision-making is the best course of action. Offering CPR training to caretakers of low-risk infants may be considered. Monitoring the child briefly with continuous pulse oximetry and observation can be done along with an ECG and testing for pertussis. There is no need for hospitalization, diagnostic laboratory evaluation, acid suppression therapy, or anti-epileptic medication (Tate and Sunley, 2017; Tieder et al., 2016).

Additional Resources

Cincinnati Children's Hospital Medical Center. www.cincinnatichildrens.org
Cystic Fibrosis Foundation. www.cff.org
Sounds of Pertussis. https://www.youtube.com/watch?v=wuvnvp5InE&feature=youtu.be
Suctioning the Nose with a Bulb Syringe. www.cincinnatichildrens.org/health/s/suction

References

Albrecht HH, Dicpinigaitis PV, Guenin EP. Role of guaifenesin in the management of chronic bronchitis and upper respiratory tract infections. *Multidiscip Respir Med.* 2017;12:31–37.

Ambalavanan N. Bronchopulmonary dysplasia treatment & management. Medscape (website). http://reference.medscape.com/article/973717-treatment. Last updated March 28, 2014.

American Academy of Pediatrics (AAP) and the Committee on Infectious Diseases. Summaries of infectious diseases. In: Kimberlin DW, ed. *Red Book 2018 Report of the Committee on Infectious Diseases.* 31th ed. Elk Grove Village, IL: American Academy of Pediatrics; 2018.

Bakhshaee M. Psychological status in children with ear and nose foreign body insertion. *Int J Pediatr Otorhinolaryngol.* 2017;103–107.

Balekian DS, Linnemann RW, Hasegawa K, et al. Cohort study of severe bronchiolitis during infancy and risk of asthma by age 5 years. *J Allergy Clin Immunol Pract.* 2017;5:92–96.

Ballengee CR, Turner RB. Supportive treatment for children with the common cold. *Curr Opin Pediatr.* 2014;26(1):114–118.

Barson, W. (2018). Community-acquired pneumonia in children: Outpatient treatment; *Up to Date.* Accessed 6/16/2019 https://www-uptodate-com.eu1.proxy.openathens.net/contents/community-acquired-pneumonia-in-children-outpatient-treatment?search=community%20acquired%20pneumonia%20children&source=search_result&selectedTitle=1~150&usage_type=default&display_rank=1.

Baugh R, Archer S, Mitchell R. Clinical practice guideline: tonsillectomy in children. *Otolaryngol Head Neck Surg.* 2011;144(1S):S1–S30.

Baumann P, Baer G, Bonhoeffer J, et al. Procalcitonin for diagnostics and treatment decisions in pediatric lower respiratory tract infections. *Front Pediatr.* 2017;5:1–6. Retrieved from https://www.frontiersin.org/articles/10.3389/fped.2017.00183/full.

Beiner J, Lecuyer M. *Management of Airway Obstruction and Stridor in Pediatric Patients.* EB Med. Retrieved from www.ebmedicinenet/topics

Bergamini M, Kantar A, Cutrera R, et al. Analysis of the literature on chronic cough in children. *Open Resp J.* 2017;11:1–9.

Bhalla A, Khermani RG, Newth CJL. Paediatric applied respiratory physiology—the essentials. 2017;27(7):301–310.

Blot M, Bonniaud-Blot P, Favrolt N, et al. Update on childhood and adult infectious tracheitis. *Med Mal Infect.* 2017;47:443–452.

Bochner RE, Gangar M, Belamarich P, et al. A clinical approach to tonsillitis, tonsillar hypertrophy, and peritonsillar and retropharyngeal abscesses. *Pediatr Rev.* 2017;38(2):81–91.

Bocka JJ. *Pertussis.* Medscape (website): http://emedicine.medscape.com/article/967268-overview. Updated October 20, 2017. Accessed July 27, 2018.

Bradley JS, Byington CL, Shah SS, et al. The management of community-acquired pneumonia in infants and children older than 3 months of age: clinical practice guidelines by the Pediatric Infectious Diseases Society and the Infectious Diseases Society of America. *Clin Infect Dis.* 2011;53(7):e25–e76.

Brietzke SE, Shin JJ, Choi S, et al. Clinical consensus statement: pediatric chronic rhinosinusitis. *Otolaryngol Head Neck Surg.* 2014;15(4):542–553.

Brook I. The role of antibiotics in pediatric chronic rhinosinusitis. *Laryngoscope Invest Otolayryngol.* 2017;2(3):104–108.

Bush A. Recurrent respiratory infections. *Pediatr Clin North Am.* 2009;56(1):67–100.

Butler DF, Myers AL. Changing epidemiology of *Haemophilus influenza* in children. *Infect Dis Clin N Am.* 2018;32(1):119–128.

Caballero MT, Polack FP, Stein RT. Viral bronchiolitis in young infants: new perspectives for management and treatment. *J Pediatr.* 2017;93:75–83.

Camp JV, Jonsson CB. A role for neutrophils in viral respiratory disease. *Front Immunol.* 2017;8:550–555.

Carbonetti NH. Contribution of pertussis toxin to the pathogenesis of pertussis disease. *FEMS Pathogens Dis.* 2015;73:1–8.

Carolan T, Sharma GD. *Pediatric Bronchitis.* Updated December 27, 2017. Retrieved on July 27, 2018 from https://emedicine.medscape.com/article/1001332-overview#a4

Cashen K, Petersen TL. Pleural effusions and pneumothoraces. *Pediatr in Rev.* 2017;38(4):170–180.

CDC. *Antibiotic Use in the United States, 2017: Progress and Opportunities.* Atlanta: US Department of Health and Human Services, CDC; 2017. Retrieved from https://www.cdc.gov/antibiotic-use/stewardship-report/pdf/stewardship-report.pdf.

CDC. *About Diphtheria*; 2018a. Retrieved on July 20, 2018 from https://www.cdc.gov/diphtheria/about/index.html. (page last reviewed January 15, 2016).

CDC. *Diagnosis Confirmation of Pertussis.* 2018b. Retrieved on July 20, 2018 from https://www.cdc.gov/pertussis/clinical/diagnostic-testing/diagnosis-confirmation.html. (page last reviewed August 7, 2017).

Chang AB, Upham JW, Master BI. Protracted bacterial bronchitis: the last decade and the road ahead. *Pediatric Pulm.* 2016;51:225–242.

Chang AB, Oppenheimer JJ, Weinberger MM. Management of children with chronic wet cough and protracted bacterial bronchitis CHEST Guidelines and expert panel report. *Chest.* 2017;151(4):884–890.

Ching N. *Arcanobacterium Haemolyticum in Feigin and Cherry's Textbook of Pediatric Infectious Diseases.* Chapter 93. 2014:1322–1327.e2.

Damseh N, Rumman Quercia N, et al. Primary ciliary dyskinesia: mechanisms and management. *Appl Clin Genet.* 2017;10:67–74.

Darras KE, Roston AT, Yewchuck LK. Imaging acute airway obstruction in infants and children. *Radiographic.* 2015;35:2064–20179.

DeMuri G, Wald ER. The Group A streptococcal carrier state reviewed: still an enigma. *J Pediatr Inf Dis Soc.* 2014;3(4):336–342.

de Oliveira Carvalho PE, da Silva MV, Rodriques OR, et al. Surgical Interventions for treating pectus excavatum. *Cochrane Database syst. Rev.* 2014;(10):CD008889.

Fang A, England J, Gausche-Hill M. Pediatric acute bacterial sinusitis. *Pediatr Emerg Care.* 2015;31(11):789–792.

Farrell PM, White TB, Ren CL, et al. Diagnosis of cystic fibrosis: Consensus guidelines from the Cystic Fibrosis Foundation. *J Pediatr.* 2017;181S:S4–S15.

Food and Drug Administration. FDA acts to protect kids from serious risks of opioid ingredients contained in some prescription cough and cold products by revising labeling to limit pediatric use. 2018. Retrieved from https://www.fda.gov/NewsEvents/Newsroom/PressAnnouncements/ucm592109.htm.

Fox TG, Christenson JC. Influenza and parainfluenza viral infections in children. *Pediatr Rev.* 2014;35(6):217–227.

Faulkner AE, Skoff TH, Tondella ML, et al. Trends in pertussis diagnostic testing in the United States, 1990–2012. *Pediatr Infect Dis J.* 2016;35(1):39–44.

Gabe LM, Malo J, Knox KS. Diagnosis and management of coccidioidomycosis. *Clin Chest Med.* 2017;38:417–433.

Gaffin JM, Phipantanakul W. The calculated risk of childhood asthma from severe bronchiolitis. *J Allergy Clin Immunol Pract.* 2017;5:97–99.

Gill P, Richardson SE, Ostrow O, et al. Testing for respiratory viruses in children: to swab or not to swab. *JAMA Pediatr.* 2017;171(8):798–8.

Ghebremedhin B. Human adenovirus: viral pathogen with increasing importance. *Eur J Microbiol Immunol (Bp).* 2014;4(1):26–33.

Goetz DM, Singh S. Respiratory system disease. *Pediatr Clin N Am.* 2016;63:637–659.

Goldman RD. Acyclovir for herpetic gingivostomatitis in children. *Can Fam Physician.* 2016;62(5):403–404.

Gonzalez MD, McElvania E. New developments in rapid diagnostic testing for children. *Infect Dis Clin N Am.* 2018;32(1):19–34.

Haddad J, Keesecker S. Nasal foreign body. In: Kliegman RM, Staton BF, Schor NF, et al., eds. *Nelson Textbook of Pediatric.* 20th ed. Philadelphia: Elsevier; 2016:2008–2011.

Healy MC, Rench MA, Wooton SH, et al. Evaluation of the impact of the pertussis cocooning program on infant pertussis infection. *Pediatric Inf Dis J.* 2015;34:22–26.

Hersh A, Jackson M, Hicks LA, et al. Principles of judicious antibiotic prescribing for upper respiratory tract infections in pediatrics. *Pediatrics.* 2013;132(6):1146–1154.

Hersch A, Shapiro DH, Pavia AT, et al. Geographic variability in diagnosis and antibiotic prescribing for acute respiratory tract infections. *Infect Dis Ther.* 2018;7(1):171–174.

Jain S, Williams DJ, Arnold SR, et al. Community–acquired pneumonia requiring hospitalization among U.S. children. *N Engl J Med.* 2015;372(9):835–845.

Jeffrey Modell Foundation. 10 Warning signs of primary immunodeficiency. 2017. Retrieved from http://downloads.info4pi.org/pdfs/10-Warning-Signs---Generic-Text--2-.pdf.

Johnson DW. Croup. *BMJ Clin Evid.* 2014:2014.

Katz SE, Williams DJ. Pediatric community-acquired pneumonia in the United States: changing epidemiology, diagnostic and therapeutic challenges, and areas for future research. *Infect Dis Clin N Am.* 2018;32(1).

Kilgore P, Salim A, Zervos M, et al. Pertussis: microbiology, disease, treatment, and prevention. *Clin Microbiology Rev.* 2016;29(3):449–481.

Kuo CY, Parkh SR. Bacterial tracheitis. *Pediatr Rev.* 2014;35(11):497–499.

Koumbourlis AC. Pectus deformities and their impact on pulmonary physiology. *Paediatr Resp Rev.* 2015;16:118–124.

Kyler KE, McCulloh RJ. Current concepts in the evaluation and management of bronchiolitis. *Infect Dis Clin N Am.* 2018;32(1):35–45.

Lambert L, Culley FJ. Innate immunity to respiratory infection in early life. *Front Immunol.* 2017;8:1570.

Laursen RP, et al. Probiotics for respiratory tract infections in children attending day care centers—a systematic review. *Eur J Pediatrics.* 2018;117(7):979–994. Epub.

Levine T. Pediatric imaging: Radiation exposure and how we image. *Pediatr Rev.* 2018;39(1):50–53.

Librizzi J, McCulloh R, Koehn K, et al. Appropriateness of testing for serious bacterial infection in children hospitalized with bronchiolitis. *Hosp Pediatr.* 2014;4(1):33–38.

Lorkiewicz-Muszynska D, Kociemba W, Rewekant A, et al. Development of the maxillary sinus from birth to age 18. Postnatal growth pattern. *Internat J Pedatr Otorhinolaryngol.* 2015;79:1393–1400.

Loxham M, Davies DE. Phenotypic and genetic aspect of epithelial barrier function in asthmatic patients. *J Allergy Clin Immunol.* 2017;139(6):1736–1751.

Magit A. Pediatric rhinosinusitis. *Otolaryngol Clin N Am.* 2014;47:733–746.

Mandal A, Kabra S, Lodha R. Upper airway obstruction in children. *Indian J Pedatr.* 2015;82(8):737–744.

Marom T, Alvarez-Fernandez P, Jennings K, et al. Acute bacterial sinusitis complicating viral upper respiratory tract infection in young children. *Pediatr Infectious Dis J.* 2014;33(8):803–808.

Martiniano SL, Sagel SD, Zemanick ET. Cystic fibrosis: a model system for precision medicine. 2016;28(3):312–318.

McGarry GW. Recurrent epistaxis in children. *BMJ Clin Evid.* 2013. 0311.2013.

McNaughten B, Hart C, Shields M. Management of bronchiolitis in infants: key clinical questions. *Paediatr Child Health.* 2017;27(7):324–327.

Merchx J, Wali R, Schiller I, et al. Diagnostic accuracy of novel and traditional rapid tests for influenza infection compared with reverse transcriptase polymerase chain reaction. *Annals Int Med.* 2017;167:394–409.

Miller EK, Williams JV. The Common Cold. In: Kliegman RM, Staton BF, Schor NF, et al., eds. *Nelson Textbook of Pediatric.* 20th ed. Philadelphia: Elsevier; 2016:2011–2014.

Morad A, Sathe N, Francis DO, et al. Tonsillectomy versus watchful waiting for recurrent throat infection: a systematic review. *Pediatrics.* 2017;139(2):139–150.

Morikawa Y, Miura M, Furuhata M, et al. Nebulized hypertonic saline in infants hospitalized with moderately severe bronchiolitis due to RSV infection: a multicenter randomized controlled trial. *Pediatr Pulm.* 2018;53(3):358–365.

Papadopoulos NG, Megremis S, Kitsioulis NA, et al. Promising approaches for the treatment and prevention of viral respiratory illness. *J. Allergy Clin Immunol.* 2017;140:921–1032.

Pappas DE, Hendley JO. Sinusitis. In: Kliegman RM, Staton BF, Schor NF, et al., eds. *Nelson Textbook of Pediatric.* 20th ed. Philadelphia: Elsevier; 2018:2014–2017.

Paranjape SM, Mogayzel PJ. Cystic fibrosis. *Pediatr Rev.* 2014;35(5):194–205.

Patel N, Maddalozzo J, Billings KR. An update on management of pediatric epistaxis. *Int J Pediatr Otorhinolargol.* 2014;78(8):1400–1404.

Patrinos ME, Martin RJ. Apnea in the term infant. *Sem Fetal Neon Med.* 2017;22:240–244.

Petrocheilou A, Tanou K, Kalampouka E, et al. Viral croup: diagnosis and a treatment algorithm. *Pediatr Pulm.* 2014;49:421–429.

Pinninti S, Hough-Telford C, Pati S, et al. Cytomegalovirus and Epstein-Barr virus infection. *Pediatr Rev.* 2016;37:223–233.

Quinonez R, Coon ER, Schroader AR. When technology creates uncertainty: pulse oximetry and overdiagnosis of hypoxaemia in bronchiolitis. *BMJ.* 2017;358:j3850.

Ralston SL, Lieberthal H, Meissner HC, et al. Clinical practice guideline: the diagnosis, management, and prevention of bronchiolitis. *Pediatrics.* 2014;134(5):e1474–e1502.

Richards AM. Pediatric respiratory emergencies. *Emer Med Clin.* 2016;34(1):77–96.

Roosevelt GE. Acute inflammatory upper airway obstruction (croup, epiglottitis, laryngitis, and bacterial tracheitis. In: Kliegman RM, Staton BF, Schor NF, et al., eds. *Nelson Textbook of Pediatric.* 20th ed. Philadelphia: Elsevier; 2016:2031–2036.

Rosenfield M, Sontag MK, Ren CL. Cystic fibrosis diagnosis and newborn screening. *Pediatr Clin N Am.* 2016;63:599–615.

Sande L, Flores A. Group A, Group C, Group G. Beta hemolytic. In: *Feigin and Cherry's Textbook of Pediatric Infectious Diseases.* 82:1140–1152.

Sanders DB, Fink AK. Background and epidemiology. *Pediatr Clin N Am.* 2016;63:567–584.

Sathe MN, Freeman AJ. Gastrointestinal, pancreatic, and hepatobiliary manifestations of cystic fibrosis. *Pediatr Clin North Am.* 2016;63(4):679–698.

Savant AP, McColley SA. Cystic fibrosis year in review 2016. *Pediatr Pulm.* 2017;52:1092–1102.

Scheffer AL, Patel PR, Manloor JJ. Shoulder pain in a 7 year old. *Pediatr Rev.* 2016;37(11):494–565.

Schinco P, Castaman G, Coppola A, Cultrera D, Federici AB. Current challenges in the diagnosis and management of patients with inherited von Willebrand's disease in Italy: an Expert Meeting Report on the diagnosis and surgical and secondary long-term prophylaxis. *Blood Transfus.* 2018;16(4):371–381.

Schroeder AR, Mansbach JM. Recent evidence on the management of bronchiolitis. *Curr Opin Pediatr.* 2014;26(3):328–333.

Shapiro D, Lindgreen C, Neuman M, et al. Viral features and testing for streptococcal pharyngitis. *Pediatr.* 2017;139(5):e20–e28.

Shay S, Shapiro N, Bhattacharyya N. Epidemiological characteristics of pediatric epistaxis presenting to the emergency department. *Int J Pediatr Otorhinolaryng.* 2017;103:121–124.

Siddiq S, Grainger J. Fifteen-minute consultation. investigation and management of childhood epistaxis. *Arch Dis Child Educ Pract Ed.* 2015;100(1):2–5.

Smith DK, Seales S, Budzik C. Respiratory syncytial virus bronchiolitis in children. *Amer Fam Physician.* 2017;95(2):94–99.

Snidvongs K, Thanaviratananich S. Update on intranasal medications in rhinosinusitis. *Curr Allergy Asthma Rep.* 2017;17:47–59.

Sosnay PR, Raraigh KS, Gison R. Molecular genetics of cystic fibrosis transmembrane conductance regulator: genotype and phenotype. *Pediatr Clin N Am.* 2016;63:585–598.

Souder E, Long S. Pertussis in the era of new strains of Bordetella pertussis. *Infect Dis Clin N Am.* 2015;29:699–713.

Stenner M, Rudack C. Diseases of the nose and paranasal sinuses in childhood. *Laryngorhinootologie.* 2014;93(suppl 2014;1):S24–S48.

Svider PF, Sheyn A, Folbe E, et al. How did that get there? A population-based analysis of nasal foreign bodies. *Int Forum Allergy Rhinol.* 2014;4(11):944–949.

Swedo SE, Frankovich J, Murphy TK. Overview of treatment of pediatric acute-onset neuropsychiatric syndrome. *H child and Adole psychopharm.* 2017;27(7):562–565.

Taketomo CK, Hodding JH, Kraus DM. *Pediatric Dosage Handbook.* 24th ed. Hudson, OH: Lexicomp; 2018.

Tate C, Sunley R. Brief resolved unexplained events (formerly apparent life-threatening events) and evaluation of lower-risk infants. *Arch Dis Child Educ Pract Ed.* 2017;0:1–4.

Thienemann M, Murphy T, Leckman J. Clinical management of pediatric acute-onset neuropsychiatric syndrome: part 1-psychiatric and behavioral intervention. *J Child Adole Psychopharm.* 2017;27(7):566–573.

Tieder JS, Bonkowsky JL, Etzel RA, et al. Brief resolved unexplained events (formerly apparent life-threatening events) and evaluation of lower-risk infants. *Pediatr.* 2016;137(5):e1–e30.

Trainer EA, Nicholson TL, Merkel TJ. Bordetella pertussis transmission. *FEMS Pathogens Dis.* 2015;73:1–8.

Turner TL, Kopp BT, Paul G, et al. Respiratory syncytial virus: current and emerging treatment options. *Clinicoecon Outcomes Res.* 2014;6:217–225.

Twarog M, Thompson GR. Coccidioidomycosis. Recent updates. *Semin Respir Crit Care Med.* 2015;36:746–755.

VanDevanter DR, Kahle JS, O'Sullivan A. Cystic fibrosis in young children: A review of disease manifestation, progression and response to treatment. *J Cystic Fibrosis.* 2016;15:147–157.

Wald ER, Applegate KE, Bordley C, et al. Clinical practice guideline for the diagnosis and management of acute bacterial sinusitis in children aged 1 to 18 years. *Pediatrics.* 2013;132(1):e262–e280.

Weintraub B. Upper respiratory tract infections. *Pediatr Rev.* 2015;36(12):554–556.

West NE, Mogayzel PJ. Transitions in health care: what can we learn from our experience with cystic fibrosis. *Pediatr Clin N Am.* 2016;63:887–897.

Williams DJ, Zhu Y, Grijalva CG, et al. Predicting severe pneumonia outcomes in children. *Pediatrics.* 2016 Oct;138(4). pii: e20161019.

Yang W, Lee J, Chen C, et al. Westley score and clinical factors in predicting the outcome of croup in the pediatric emergency department. *Pediatr Pulm.* 2017;52:1329–1334.

Yau S. An update of epistaxis. *Australian J Fam Prac.* 2015;44(9):653–656.

Zhou-Suckow Z, Duerr J, Hagner M. Airway mucus, inflammation and remodeling: emerging links in the pathogenesis of chronic lung disease. *Cell Tissue Res.* 2017;367:537–550.

38

Cardiovascular Disorders

JENNIFER NEWCOMBE

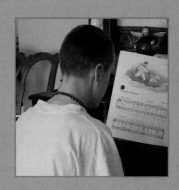

Most cardiovascular problems in the pediatric population are due to congenital heart disease (CHD), which affects nearly 1% of all live births—or approximately 40,000 babies per year. Greater numbers of these children are surviving to adulthood, increasing the total population of adults and children with CHD. CHD is the leading cause of morbidity and mortality within the first year of life in children with congenital malformations (Centers for Disease Control and Prevention [CDC], 2014).

The primary care provider (PCP) must maintain a high index of suspicion regarding any signs or symptoms of cardiovascular disease in young children. Many congenital heart defects may be recognized by a detailed fetal ultrasound and known before delivery. Critical congenital heart defects may be detected in the immediate postdelivery period by using pulse oximetry screening (Ailes, Gilboa, Honein, and Oster, 2015). Early identification significantly decreases the morbidity and mortality associated with cyanotic and ductal dependent structural heart defects (Ryan, Mikula, Germana, Silva, and Derovin, 2014).

This chapter presents information on both congenital and acquired heart disease in the pediatric population. A thorough discussion of the examination and assessment of the cardiac system is included, as well as guidance for screening, identifying, and managing specific cardiovascular disorders during the course of delivering primary health care.

Anatomy and Physiology

Fetal Circulation

Knowledge of fetal circulation is essential for understanding the circulatory changes that occur in the newborn at delivery (Fig 38.1). Fetal circulation has four unique features that differ from postnatal circulation:

- Oxygenation of the blood occurs in the placenta, not the lungs.
- Fetal pulmonary vascular resistance is high, and systemic vascular resistance is low (high pressure on the right side of the heart, low pressure on the left side).
- The foramen ovale, the opening in the septum between the two atria, permits a portion of the blood to flow from the right atrium directly to the left atrium.
- A patent ductus arteriosus (PDA) provides a connection between the pulmonary artery and the aorta that allows blood to flow from the pulmonary artery to the aorta and bypass the fetal lungs.

Oxygen from the maternal uterine arteries is diffused into the fetal circulation via the placenta. The placenta delivers oxygenated

blood through the umbilical vein to the fetus by diverting blood through the liver to the inferior vena cava (IVC) by the ductus venosus. When this well-oxygenated blood reaches the right atrium, it flows preferentially toward the atrial septum, through the foramen ovale, and into the left atrium. Oxygenated blood then flows into the left ventricle and out the aorta. Approximately two-thirds of the blood from the aorta flows toward the head and neck to ensure the fetal brain constantly receives well-oxygenated blood (Murray and McKinney, 2014).

Venous blood returns from the head and upper extremities via the superior vena cava (SVC) to the right atrium. This blood preferentially flows toward the tricuspid valve into the right ventricle. From the right ventricle, the blood enters the pulmonary artery. Because pulmonary vascular resistance is high and systemic resistance is low, most blood in the pulmonary artery flows through the ductus arteriosus into the descending aorta to supply oxygen and nutrients to the trunk and lower extremities. Only a small amount of blood flows into the pulmonary circuit to perfuse the lungs (Murray and McKinney, 2014).

The fetal circulation is best described as two parallel circuits, with the left ventricle supplying blood to the upper extremities and the right ventricle serving the lower extremities and the placenta. At the time of transition to extrauterine life, these separate blood flow circuits become a serial circuit.

Neonatal Circulation

A number of complex events occur at birth that rapidly shift the fetal circulation toward the neonatal circulation pattern. Clamping of the umbilical cord, with subsequent removal of the placenta as the oxygenating organ, causes an immediate circulatory change requiring the lungs to be the new mechanism of oxygenation. Clamping the cord also causes an increase in systemic vascular resistance (systemic blood pressure [BP]). With the first breath, mechanical inflation of the lungs and an increase in oxygen saturation bring about a dramatic fall in pulmonary vascular resistance and, consequently, increase pulmonary blood flow. The increased oxygen saturation begins the process of constricting the ductus arteriosus. As the pressures within the heart become relatively higher on the left side and lower on the right, the foramen ovale closes. Functional closure of the ductus arteriosus and foramen ovale usually occurs within the first few hours to days of life, and a serial circuit forms out of the once-parallel pulmonary and systemic circulation (Murray and McKinney, 2014).

The transition toward complete anatomic closure, or obliteration of fetal structures by tissue growth or constriction, is more

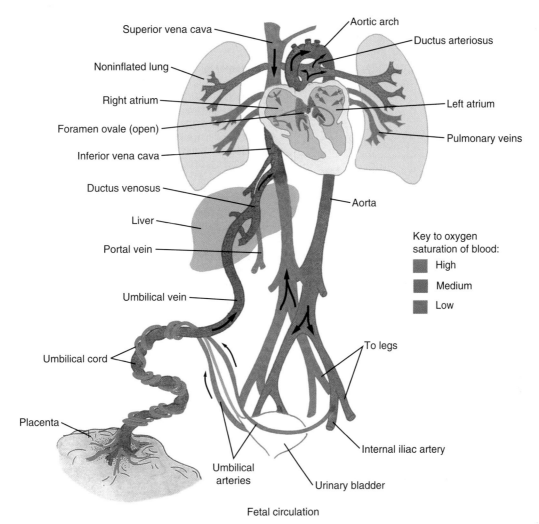

- **Fig 38.1** Fetal Circulation. (From Murray S, McKinney E. *Foundations of Maternal-Newborn and Women's Health Nursing.* 6th ed. Philadelphia: Saunders/Elsevier; 2014.)

gradual. Pulmonary vascular resistance drops gradually over the first 6 to 8 weeks of life, which can protect the pulmonary circulation against volume overload in some congenital heart anomalies. If not noted earlier, shunt murmurs or symptoms of congestive heart failure (CHF) gradually become apparent as the infant approaches 8 weeks old. At this time, pulmonary vascular resistance drops and shunting to the pulmonary bed increases.

Conditions that cause persistence of fetal shunts allow unoxygenated blood to flow from the right side of the heart to the left. Any murmur or cyanosis in a newborn should be carefully monitored and evaluated to detect cardiac abnormalities.

Normal Cardiac Structure and Function

The heart is a four-chambered muscular organ located in the mediastinum, the space in the chest between the lungs. The four chambers are divided into two larger muscular pumping chambers, the ventricles, and two smaller receiving chambers, the atria. The heart has one-way valves that open and close in response to pressure changes within the heart, thus controlling blood flow from chamber to chamber. Desaturated systemic blood returns to the right atrium by way of the inferior and superior venae cavae. The blood passes from the right atrium through the tricuspid valve to the right ventricle. The tricuspid value has three cusps held in

place by the chordate tendineae. The right ventricle pumps the blood through the pulmonic valve into the pulmonary artery, which bifurcates into right and left arteries to allow flow into both lungs. Here, the blood is oxygenated. Blood returning from the lungs enters the left atrium by way of the pulmonary veins (which contain no valves to allow easy blood flow into the atrium) and then passes through the mitral valve into the left ventricle. The high-pressured left ventricle pumps the blood through the aortic valve into the aorta to provide oxygenated blood for the systemic circulation (Park, 2016).

Conduction System

Myocardial contraction is stimulated by electrical depolarization along the conduction tract within the heart. Depolarization begins at the sinoatrial (SA) node, which is high in the wall of the right atrium. This node acts as the pacemaker of the heart by regularly beginning the depolarizing impulses of each heartbeat. The wave of depolarization travels from the SA node throughout the atria and produces contraction of the atrial muscle. The impulses reach the atrioventricular (AV) node, which is located in the lower portion of the right atrium at the junction of the atrium and ventricle. From the AV node, the depolarization wave passes through the bundle of His, the fibers extending from the AV node along the intraventricular septum. Depolarization spreads through the left and right branches of the bundle of His and through the Purkinje fibers extending into the ventricular muscle. Impulses then spread throughout the ventricles and cause contraction. The electrocardiogram (ECG) demonstrates this pattern of changing electrical impulses (Park, 2016).

Assessment of the Cardiovascular System

History

Cardiac evaluation includes review of the family, maternal, fetal, neonatal, and infant medical history, in addition to growth and development (see Box 38.1 for risk factors for CHD).

Physical Examination

Physical assessment of a child with suspected CHD should be adapted to the age of the child. Be flexible yet thorough in any evaluation, and include all aspects of the physical examination in an order that best suits the comfort and needs of the infant, child, or adolescent.

Vital Signs

Heart rate, respiratory rate, and BP vary considerably throughout childhood.

- Heart rate (Table 38.1): Heart rates should always be obtained by auscultation. Assessment should include rate and rhythm variations. An increased heart rate can be caused by excitement, anxiety, hyperthyroidism, heart disease, anemia, or fever. Irregularity may be caused by a normal sinus arrhythmia (the normal variation in heart rate that occurs with inhalation and exhalation; it is more common in children than adults).
- Pulses: Pulses should be palpated in the upper and lower extremities and evaluated for character (strength) and variation between the different sites. A bounding pulse may indicate a PDA or aortic insufficiency. Weak or "thready" pulses may indicate CHF or an obstructive lesion, such as severe aortic stenosis. Strong brachial pulses in conjunction with weak or absent femoral pulses may indicate coarctation of the aorta (COA).
- Blood pressure: In healthy children, BP should be measured annually, beginning at 3 years old rather than at every health encounter (Flynn, 2017). However, children with obesity, renal disease, diabetes, or known aortic arch disease should have BP taken at every appointment (Flynn, 2017). Auscultation remains the preferred method; BP tables are based upon this technique (National Heart, Lung, and Blood Institute [NHLBI], 2012). If the index of suspicion of heart disease is high, providers should check BPs in younger children. It is important to always use a BP cuff that is appropriate for the child's size. For arm pressure, the width of the cuff should be two-thirds the length of the upper arm measured from the axilla to the antecubital space. A cuff that is too narrow, too wide, or does not fit around an arm may cause an erroneous reading. Cuff sizes of 3, 5, 7, 12, and 18 cm should be on hand to accommodate the array of pediatric sizes. Initial evaluation should compare the pressure in all four extremities; these should be equal, with pressure in the legs being slightly higher (10 to 20 mm Hg) in a child who walks. Lower extremity pressure is measured with the stethoscope placed over the popliteal artery. The NHLBI publishes norms for BP by gender, age, and

height; they are found in Tables 38.2 and 38.3. Hypertension (HTN) is discussed later in this chapter.
- Respiratory rate: Respiratory system evaluation includes the respiratory rate, assessment of effort, and breath sounds in all

---

• BOX 38.1 Risk Factors Suggestive of Congenital Heart Disease

Perinatal Risk Factors

Maternal infections and exposures (CMV, rubella, other viral syndromes)
Maternal use of tobacco, alcohol, street drugs, retinoic acid, hydantoins, lithium, valproates, ibuprofen, naproxen, ACE inhibitors, tricyclic antidepressants, sulfonamides, sulfasalazines
Maternal chronic disease (CHD, lupus, insulin-dependent diabetes, phenylketonuria)
Maternal age at child's birth (increase in chromosomal abnormalities after 40 years old)
Maternal pregnancy history (excessive weight gain, gestational diabetes)

Neonatal Risk Factors

Fetal or newborn distress (aspiration, hypoxia, cyanosis)
Prematurity (increased incidence of CHD in premature infants)
Presence of associated anomalies (genetic or chromosomal abnormalities or syndromes)
Neonatal infections (GBS)
Birthweight (term infants <2500 g; SGA, less than two standard deviations from the mean for gestational age)

Newborn Risk Factors

Murmur at birth or early infancy
Hypertension (at birth or beyond)
Feeding difficulty (shortness of breath, easily fatigued, diaphoresis, poor intake)
Cyanosis (increase with crying, feeding, exertion)
Tachypnea (persistent, with crying, feeding)

Toddler, School-Age, and Teenage Risk Factors

Deviation from individual's normal growth and development
Deviation from an activity level appropriate for chronologic age (unable to keep up with peers; unable to run or ride bike)
Frequent respiratory tract infections (pneumonia, URIs that last longer than normal)
Prior murmurs, blue spells
Documented GABHS infection
Hypertension (documented on a minimum of three separate visits)
Chest pain with exertion
Shortness of breath with exertion (beyond normal peers)
Syncope or dizziness (especially associated with noted heart rate change)
Tachycardia or bradycardia (fluttering in chest, racing heart)

Family History Risk Factors

CHD (especially siblings, parents, first-degree relatives)
Sudden death or premature myocardial infarction (before 50 years old; includes any deaths by drowning)
Hypertension
Rheumatic fever
Genetic syndromes
Hypercholesterolemia

ACE, *Angiotensin-converting enzyme;* CHD, *congenital heart disease;* CMV, *cytomegalovirus;* GABHS, *group A β-hemolytic streptococci;* GBS, *group B streptococcus;* SGA, *small for gestational age;* URI, *upper respiratory infection.*

Data from Richards A, Garg V. Genetics of congenital heart disease. Curr Cardiology Rev. *2010;6:91–97; and Sayasathid J, Sukonpan K, Somboonna N. Epidemiology and etiology of congenital heart diseases. In: Syamasundar P, Vidyasagar D, ed.* Congenital Heart Disease: Selected Aspects, *Cardiotext Publishing, Minneapolis, MN, 2011.*

TABLE 38.1	Normal Heart Rates in Infants and Children		
Age	Resting (Awake)	Resting (Asleep)	Exercise/ Fever
Newborn	100-180 bpm	80-160 bpm	Up to 220 bpm
1 week to 3 months old	100-220 bpm	80-200 bpm	Up to 220 bpm
3 months to 2 years old	80-150 bpm	70-120 bpm	Up to 220 bpm
2 to 10 years old	70-100 bpm	60-90 bpm	195-215 bpm
10 to 20 years old	55-90 bpm	50-90 bpm	195-215 bpm

bpm, Beats per minute.

five lung lobes. It is important to evaluate the respiratory rate in a quiet infant or child. A respiratory rate greater than 40 in a young child or 60 in a newborn who is quiet, resting, and afebrile warrants further evaluation. An infant with CHD may be happily tachypneic and not show significant signs of grunting, intercostal retractions, nasal flaring, or tracheal tug (up and down movement of the trachea with each inspiration).

- Oxygen saturation: Oxygen saturation is considered to be an essential vital sign. It is important to obtain oxygen saturations in newborns or children suspected of having a cardiac condition because cyanosis is not always readily perceptible. A joint statement by the American Academy of Pediatrics (AAP) and the American Heart Association (AHA) recommends that pulse oximetry screening be automatically done for all newborns at 24 to 48 hours of life (Ailes et al., 2015).

General Appearance and Growth Parameters

The PCP should observe an infant while obtaining the history and before proceeding with the complete physical examination. Observe general nutritional state, respiratory effort, color, physical abnormalities, and distress or discomfort level.

- Look for the presence of unusual facial characteristics (e.g., malformed ears, wide-spaced eyes, noticeable anomalies) or extracardiac anomalies (e.g., cleft lip or palate, polydactyly, microcephaly) that may be associated with a syndrome or chromosomal abnormalities. Some children with conditions that are associated with CHD have obvious stigmata, such as those seen with Down syndrome, Marfan syndrome (unusually tall with an arm span wider than the head-to-toe height), Turner syndrome (webbed neck, prominent ears), or fetal alcohol spectrum disorder (microcephaly and pinched facies).
- Assess overall skin color for signs of mottling or central cyanosis while the infant is at rest. Cyanosis caused by heart disease is recognized as a pale blue or ruddy red color of the mucous membranes (lips, tongue, and nailbeds). The tongue is the best indicator because it lacks pigmentation and is abundantly served by the vascular system. Peripheral cyanosis or acrocyanosis, a blueness or pallor noted around the mouth and on the hands or feet, can be a normal variant, especially if it intensifies when the infant is cold. Clubbing of the fingers and toes may be seen in children with long-standing cyanosis.
- Note any wheezing, nasal flaring, retractions, prominent neck veins, or head bobbing with respirations.

- Note peripheral or periorbital edema. Edema around the eyes may be evident in an infant with CHF even in the absence of peripheral edema of the hands or feet. True pitting edema of the feet is an unusual finding in an infant with CHF.
- At each assessment, measure and plot height and weight on standardized charts, including Down syndrome and Turner syndrome charts as appropriate. Although many children with CHD fall within the normal height, weight, and development ranges, a large number of infants and children with heart disease experience poor weight gain, less than normal linear growth, and delays in achieving developmental milestones.

Palpation

Palpate all five areas of the chest: the aortic, pulmonic, tricuspid, and mitral areas and Erb point (Fig 38.2). Chest palpation is best accomplished by using the open palm of the hand near the base of the fingers. The hand should be gently moved across the chest to assess abnormal precordial activity, including pulsations, lifts, heaves, or thrills, and to determine the location of the apical impulse. The apical impulse is used to determine the size of the heart and is the most lateral point at which cardiac activity can be palpated. In infants and children, the impulse is normally palpated at the apex of the heart in the fourth intercostal space just to the left of the midclavicular line. At approximately 7 years old, the point shifts to the fifth intercostal space. Cardiomegaly causes the apical impulse to shift laterally or downward (Park, 2016).

- Thrills are a palpable vibration caused by turbulent blood flow through abnormal structures or defects in the heart. The turbulent flow may be due to valvular narrowing or stenosis or defects, such as a ventricular septal defect (VSD).
- Assess peripheral pulses (radial, brachial, carotid, dorsalis pedis, and posterior tibial) for amplitude and intensity. In COA, there may be decreased or absent femoral pulses and impulse lag if the radial pulse is palpated simultaneously. A fast pulse rate may indicate arrhythmia or CHF.
- The liver and spleen should be assessed for enlargement. Hepatomegaly is an important finding. Infants may have a palpable liver edge as a normal finding.
- The back should be examined for scoliosis, a finding that may be associated with CHD.

Auscultation of Heart Sounds

- Auscultate the heart in the same manner for every child by beginning at the base or apex of the heart. Ideally, assess heart sounds in a quiet environment when the child is cooperative.
- Four individual heart sounds can be heard: S_1, S_2, S_3, and S_4. S_1 and S_2 represent normal heart sounds, whereas the presence of S_3 or S_4 may indicate cardiac enlargement or volume overload.
- At each area of examination, the provider should accurately identify the first (S_1) and second (S_2) heart sounds.
- S_1 has the following characteristics:
  - It is heard in the beginning of systole and indicates closure of AV valves (mitral and tricuspid). It is the "lubb" of the lubb-dupp.
  - Often detected as a single sound. Even though the left side of the heart reacts slightly before the right side, the closure of the two values occurs so closely together that a single sound may be heard.
  - It may be differentiated from early systolic clicks by the low frequency of the sound (clicks have a higher frequency). It is best heard with the diaphragm of the stethoscope.

TABLE 38.2 Blood Pressure Levels in the 90th and 95th Percentiles for Girls 1 to 17 Years Old by Percentiles of Height

BP LEVELS FOR GIRLS BY AGE AND HEIGHT PERCENTILE

Age	BP Percentile	SBP (mm Hg) HEIGHT PERCENTILE OR MEASURED HEIGHT							DBP (mm Hg) HEIGHT PERCENTILE OR MEASURED HEIGHT						
		5%	10%	25%	50%	75%	90%	95%	5%	10%	25%	50%	75%	90%	95%
1	Height (in)	29.7	30.2	30.9	31.8	32.7	33.4	33.9	29.7	30.2	30.9	31.8	32.7	33.4	33.9
	Height (cm)	75.4	76.6	78.6	80.8	83	84.9	86.1	75.4	76.6	78.6	80.8	83	84.9	86.1
	50th	84	85	86	86	87	88	88	41	42	42	43	44	45	46
	90th	98	99	99	100	101	102	102	54	55	56	56	57	58	58
	95th	101	102	102	103	104	105	105	59	59	60	60	61	62	62
	95th + 12 mm Hg	113	114	114	115	116	117	117	71	71	72	72	73	74	74
2	Height (in)	33.4	34	34.9	35.9	36.9	37.8	38.4	33.4	34	34.9	35.9	36.9	37.8	38.4
	Height (cm)	84.9	86.3	88.6	91.1	93.7	96	97.4	84.9	86.3	88.6	91.1	93.7	96	97.4
	50th	87	87	88	89	90	91	91	45	46	47	48	49	50	51
	90th	101	101	102	103	104	105	106	58	58	59	60	61	62	62
	95th	104	105	106	106	107	108	109	62	63	63	64	65	66	66
	95th + 12 mm Hg	116	117	118	118	119	120	121	74	75	75	76	77	78	78
3	Height (in)	35.8	36.4	37.3	38.4	39.6	40.6	41.2	35.8	36.4	37.3	38.4	39.6	40.6	41.2
	Height (cm)	91	92.4	94.9	97.6	100.5	103.1	104.6	91	92.4	94.9	97.6	100.5	103.1	104.6
	50th	88	89	89	90	91	92	93	48	48	49	50	51	53	53
	90th	102	103	104	104	105	106	107	60	61	61	62	63	64	65
	95th	106	106	107	108	109	110	110	64	65	65	66	67	68	69
	95th + 12 mm Hg	118	118	119	120	121	122	122	76	77	77	78	79	80	81
4	Height (in)	38.3	38.9	39.9	41.1	42.4	43.5	44.2	38.3	38.9	39.9	41.1	42.4	43.5	44.2
	Height (cm)	97.2	98.8	101.4	104.5	107.6	110.5	112.2	97.2	98.8	101.4	104.5	107.6	110.5	112.2
	50th	89	90	91	92	93	94	94	50	51	51	53	54	55	55
	90th	103	104	105	106	107	108	108	62	63	64	65	66	67	67
	95th	107	108	109	109	110	111	112	66	67	68	69	70	70	71
	95th + 12 mm Hg	119	120	121	121	122	123	124	78	79	80	81	82	82	83

TABLE 38.2 Blood Pressure Levels in the 90th and 95th Percentiles for Girls 1 to 17 Years Old by Percentiles of Height—cont'd

BP LEVELS FOR GIRLS BY AGE AND HEIGHT PERCENTILE

Age	BP Percentile	SBP (mm Hg) HEIGHT PERCENTILE OR MEASURED HEIGHT							DBP (mm Hg) HEIGHT PERCENTILE OR MEASURED HEIGHT						
		5%	10%	25%	50%	75%	90%	95%	5%	10%	25%	50%	75%	90%	95%
5	Height (in)	40.8	41.5	42.6	43.9	45.2	46.5	47.3	40.8	41.5	42.6	43.9	45.2	46.5	47.3
	Height (cm)	103.6	105.3	108.2	111.5	114.9	118.1	120	103.6	105.3	108.2	111.5	114.9	118.1	120
	50th	90	91	92	93	94	95	96	52	52	53	55	56	57	57
	90th	104	105	106	107	108	109	110	64	65	66	67	68	69	70
	95th	108	109	109	110	111	112	113	68	69	70	71	72	73	73
	95th + 12 mm Hg	120	121	121	122	123	124	125	80	81	82	83	84	85	85
6	Height (in)	43.3	44	45.2	46.6	48.1	49.4	50.3	43.3	44	45.2	46.6	48.1	49.4	50.3
	Height (cm)	110	111.8	114.9	118.4	122.1	125.6	127.7	110	111.8	114.9	118.4	122.1	125.6	127.7
	50th	92	92	93	94	96	97	97	54	54	55	56	57	58	59
	90th	105	106	107	108	109	110	111	67	67	68	69	70	71	71
	95th	109	109	110	111	112	113	114	70	71	72	72	73	74	74
	95th + 12 mm Hg	121	121	122	123	124	125	126	82	83	84	84	85	86	86
7	Height (in)	45.6	46.4	47.7	49.2	50.7	52.1	53	45.6	46.4	47.7	49.2	50.7	52.1	53
	Height (cm)	115.9	117.8	121.1	124.9	128.8	132.5	134.7	115.9	117.8	121.1	124.9	128.8	132.5	134.7
	50th	92	93	94	95	97	98	99	55	55	56	57	58	59	60
	90th	106	106	107	109	110	111	112	68	68	69	70	71	72	72
	95th	109	110	111	112	113	114	115	72	72	73	73	74	74	75
	95th + 12 mm Hg	121	122	123	124	125	126	127	84	84	85	85	86	86	87
8	Height (in)	47.6	48.4	49.8	51.4	53	54.5	55.5	47.6	48.4	49.8	51.4	53	54.5	55.5
	Height (cm)	121	123	126.5	130.6	134.7	138.5	140.9	121	123	126.5	130.6	134.7	138.5	140.9
	50th	93	94	95	97	98	99	100	56	56	57	59	60	61	61
	90th	107	107	108	110	111	112	113	69	70	71	72	72	73	73
	95th	110	111	112	113	115	116	117	72	73	74	74	75	75	75
	95th + 12 mm Hg	122	123	124	125	127	128	129	84	85	86	86	87	87	87

Continued

Blood pressure table — first block (values by height percentile)

Age		1	2	3	4	5	6	7
9	Height (in)	49.3	50.2	51.7	53.4	55.1	56.7	57.7
	Height (cm)	125.3	127.6	131.3	135.6	140.1	144.1	146.6
	50th	95	95	97	98	99	100	101
	90th	108	108	109	111	112	113	114
	95th	112	112	113	114	116	117	118
	95th + 12 mm Hg	124	124	125	126	128	129	130
10	Height (in)	51.1	52	53.7	55.5	57.4	59.1	60.2
	Height (cm)	129.7	132.2	136.3	141	145.8	150.2	152.8
	50th	96	97	98	99	101	102	103
	90th	109	110	111	112	113	115	116
	95th	113	114	114	116	117	119	120
	95th + 12 mm Hg	125	126	126	128	129	131	132
11	Height (in)	53.4	54.5	56.2	58.2	60.2	61.9	63
	Height (cm)	135.6	138.3	142.8	147.8	152.8	157.3	160
	50th	98	99	101	102	104	105	106
	90th	111	112	113	114	116	118	120
	95th	115	116	117	118	120	123	124
	95th + 12 mm Hg	127	128	129	130	132	135	136
12	Height (in)	56.2	57.3	59	60.9	62.8	64.5	65.5
	Height (cm)	142.8	145.5	149.9	154.8	159.6	163.8	166.4
	50th	102	102	104	105	107	108	108
	90th	114	115	116	118	120	122	122
	95th	118	119	120	122	124	125	126
	95th + 12 mm Hg	130	131	132	134	136	137	138
13	Height (in)	58.3	59.3	60.9	62.7	64.5	66.1	67
	Height (cm)	148.1	150.6	154.7	159.2	163.7	167.8	170.2
	50th	104	105	106	107	108	108	109
	90th	116	117	119	121	122	123	123
	95th	121	122	123	124	126	126	127
	95th + 12 mm Hg	133	134	135	136	138	138	139

Blood pressure table — second block (values by height percentile)

Age		1	2	3	4	5	6	7
9	Height (in)	49.3	50.2	51.7	53.4	55.1	56.7	57.7
	Height (cm)	125.3	127.6	131.3	135.6	140.1	144.1	146.6
	50th	57	58	59	60	60	61	61
	90th	71	71	72	73	73	73	73
	95th	74	74	75	75	75	75	75
	95th + 12 mm Hg	86	86	87	87	87	87	87
10	Height (in)	51.1	52	53.7	55.5	57.4	59.1	60.2
	Height (cm)	129.7	132.2	136.3	141	145.8	150.2	152.8
	50th	58	59	59	60	61	61	62
	90th	72	73	73	73	73	73	73
	95th	75	75	76	76	76	76	76
	95th + 12 mm Hg	87	87	88	88	88	88	88
11	Height (in)	53.4	54.5	56.2	58.2	60.2	61.9	63
	Height (cm)	135.6	138.3	142.8	147.8	152.8	157.3	160
	50th	60	60	60	61	62	63	64
	90th	72	74	74	74	73	75	75
	95th	75	77	77	77	76	77	77
	95th + 12 mm Hg	87	89	89	89	88	89	89
12	Height (in)	56.2	57.3	59	60.9	62.8	64.5	65.5
	Height (cm)	142.8	145.5	149.9	154.8	159.6	163.8	166.4
	50th	61	61	61	62	64	65	65
	90th	74	75	75	75	76	76	76
	95th	76	78	78	78	79	79	79
	95th + 12 mm Hg	88	90	90	90	91	91	91
13	Height (in)	58.3	59.3	60.9	62.7	64.5	66.1	67
	Height (cm)	148.1	150.6	154.7	159.2	163.7	167.8	170.2
	50th	62	62	63	64	65	65	66
	90th	75	75	75	76	76	76	76
	95th	79	79	79	79	80	80	81
	95th + 12 mm Hg	91	91	91	91	92	92	93

TABLE 38.2 Blood Pressure Levels in the 90th and 95th Percentiles for Girls 1 to 17 Years Old by Percentiles of Height—cont'd

BP LEVELS FOR GIRLS BY AGE AND HEIGHT PERCENTILE

Age	BP Percentile	SBP (mm Hg) HEIGHT PERCENTILE OR MEASURED HEIGHT							DBP (mm Hg) HEIGHT PERCENTILE OR MEASURED HEIGHT						
		5%	10%	25%	50%	75%	90%	95%	5%	10%	25%	50%	75%	90%	95%
14	Height (in)	59.3	60.2	61.8	63.5	65.2	66.8	67.7	59.3	60.2	61.8	63.5	65.2	66.8	67.7
	Height (cm)	150.6	153	156.9	161.3	165.7	169.7	172.1	150.6	153	156.9	161.3	165.7	169.7	172.1
	50th	105	106	107	108	109	109	109	63	63	64	65	66	66	66
	90th	118	118	120	122	123	123	123	76	76	76	76	77	77	77
	95th	123	123	124	125	126	127	127	80	80	80	80	81	81	82
	95th + 12 mm Hg	135	135	136	137	138	139	139	92	92	92	92	93	93	94
15	Height (in)	59.7	60.6	62.2	63.9	65.6	67.2	68.1	59.7	60.6	62.2	63.9	65.6	67.2	68.1
	Height (cm)	151.7	154	157.9	162.3	166.7	170.6	173	151.7	154	157.9	162.3	166.7	170.6	173
	50th	105	106	107	108	109	109	109	64	64	64	65	66	67	67
	90th	118	119	121	122	123	123	124	76	76	76	77	77	78	78
	95th	124	124	125	126	127	127	128	80	80	80	81	82	82	82
	95th + 12 mm Hg	136	136	137	138	139	139	140	92	92	92	93	94	94	94
16	Height (in)	59.9	60.8	62.4	64.1	65.8	67.3	68.3	59.9	60.8	62.4	64.1	65.8	67.3	68.3
	Height (cm)	152.1	154.5	158.4	162.8	167.1	171.1	173.4	152.1	154.5	158.4	162.8	167.1	171.1	173.4
	50th	106	107	108	109	109	110	110	64	64	65	66	66	67	67
	90th	119	120	122	123	124	124	124	76	76	76	77	78	78	78
	95th	124	125	125	127	127	128	128	80	80	80	81	82	82	82
	95th + 12 mm Hg	136	137	137	139	139	140	140	92	92	92	93	94	94	94
17	Height (in)	60	60.9	62.5	64.2	65.9	67.4	68.4	60	60.9	62.5	64.2	65.9	67.4	68.4
	Height (cm)	152.4	154.7	158.7	163	167.4	171.3	173.7	152.4	154.7	158.7	163	167.4	171.3	173.7
	50th	107	108	109	110	110	110	111	64	64	65	66	66	67	67
	90th	120	121	123	124	124	125	125	76	76	77	77	78	78	78
	95th	125	125	126	127	128	128	128	80	80	80	81	82	82	82
	95th + 12 mm Hg	137	137	138	139	140	140	140	92	92	92	93	94	94	94

Use percentile values to stage blood pressure (BP) readings according to the scheme in Table 3 (elevated BP: ≥90th percentile; stage 1 hypertension (HTN): ≥95th percentile; and stage 2 HTN: ≥95th percentile + 12 mm Hg). The 50th, 90th, and 95th percentiles were derived by using quantile regression on the basis of normal-weight children (body mass index <85th percentile).[77]

Height percentile determined by standard growth curves.

BP percentile determined by a single measurement.

Flynn JT, Kaelber DC, Baker-Smith CM, et al. Clinical practice guideline for screening and management of high blood pressure in children and adolescents. *Pediatrics.* 2017;140(3):1–72.

DBP, Diastolic blood pressure; *SBP,* systolic blood pressure.

TABLE 38.3 Blood Pressure Levels in the 90th and 95th Percentiles for Boys 1 to 17 Years Old by Percentiles of Height

BP LEVELS FOR BOYS BY AGE AND HEIGHT PERCENTILE

Age	BP Percentile	SBP (mm Hg) HEIGHT PERCENTILE OR MEASURED HEIGHT							DBP (mm Hg) HEIGHT PERCENTILE OR MEASURED HEIGHT						
		5%	10%	25%	50%	75%	90%	95%	5%	10%	25%	50%	75%	90%	95%
1	Height (in)	30.4	30.8	31.6	32.4	33.3	34.1	34.6	30.4	30.8	31.6	32.4	33.3	34.1	34.6
	Height (cm)	77.2	78.3	80.2	82.4	84.6	86.7	87.9	77.2	78.3	80.2	82.4	84.6	86.7	87.9
	50th	85	85	86	86	87	88	88	40	40	40	41	41	42	42
	90th	98	99	99	100	100	101	101	52	52	53	53	54	54	54
	95th	102	102	103	103	104	105	105	54	54	55	55	56	57	57
	95th + 12 mm Hg	114	114	115	115	116	117	117	66	66	67	67	68	69	69
2	Height (in)	33.9	34.4	35.3	36.3	37.3	38.2	38.8	33.9	34.4	35.3	36.3	37.3	38.2	38.8
	Height (cm)	86.1	87.4	89.6	92.1	94.7	97.1	98.5	86.1	87.4	89.6	92.1	94.7	97.1	98.5
	50th	87	87	88	89	89	90	91	43	43	44	44	45	46	46
	90th	100	100	101	102	103	103	104	55	55	56	56	57	58	58
	95th	104	105	105	106	107	107	108	57	58	58	59	60	61	61
	95th + 12 mm Hg	116	117	117	118	119	119	120	69	70	70	71	72	73	73
3	Height (in)	36.4	37	37.9	39	40.1	41.1	41.7	36.4	37	37.9	39	40.1	41.1	41.7
	Height (cm)	92.5	93.9	96.3	99	101.8	104.3	105.8	92.5	93.9	96.3	99	101.8	104.3	105.8
	50th	88	89	89	90	91	92	92	45	46	46	47	48	49	49
	90th	101	102	102	103	104	105	105	58	58	59	59	60	61	61
	95th	106	106	107	107	108	109	109	60	61	61	62	63	64	64
	95th + 12 mm Hg	118	118	119	119	120	121	121	72	73	73	74	75	76	76
4	Height (in)	38.8	39.4	40.5	41.7	42.9	43.9	44.5	38.8	39.4	40.5	41.7	42.9	43.9	44.5
	Height (cm)	98.5	100.2	102.9	105.9	108.9	111.5	113.2	98.5	100.2	102.9	105.9	108.9	111.5	113.2
	50th	90	90	91	92	93	94	94	48	49	49	50	51	52	52
	90th	102	103	104	105	105	106	107	60	61	62	62	63	64	64
	95th	107	107	108	108	109	110	110	63	64	65	66	67	67	68
	95th + 12 mm Hg	119	119	120	120	121	122	122	75	76	77	78	79	79	80

TABLE 38.3 Blood Pressure Levels in the 90th and 95th Percentiles for Boys 1 to 17 Years Old by Percentiles of Height—cont'd

BP LEVELS FOR BOYS BY AGE AND HEIGHT PERCENTILE

Age	BP Percentile	SBP (mm Hg) HEIGHT PERCENTILE OR MEASURED HEIGHT							DBP (mm Hg) HEIGHT PERCENTILE OR MEASURED HEIGHT						
		5%	10%	25%	50%	75%	90%	95%	5%	10%	25%	50%	75%	90%	95%
5	Height (in)	41.1	41.8	43	44.3	45.5	46.7	47.4	41.1	41.8	43	44.3	45.5	46.7	47.4
	Height (cm)	104.4	106.2	109.1	112.4	115.7	118.6	120.3	104.4	106.2	109.1	112.4	115.7	118.6	120.3
	50th	91	92	93	94	95	96	96	51	51	52	53	54	55	55
	90th	103	104	105	106	107	108	108	63	64	65	65	66	67	67
	95th	107	108	109	109	110	111	112	66	67	68	69	70	70	71
	95th + 12 mm Hg	119	120	121	121	122	123	124	78	79	80	81	82	82	83
6	Height (in)	43.4	44.2	45.4	46.8	48.2	49.4	50.2	43.4	44.2	45.4	46.8	48.2	49.4	50.2
	Height (cm)	110.3	112.2	115.3	118.9	122.4	125.6	127.5	110.3	112.2	115.3	118.9	122.4	125.6	127.5
	50th	93	93	94	95	96	97	98	54	54	55	56	57	57	58
	90th	105	105	106	107	109	110	110	66	66	67	68	68	69	69
	95th	108	109	110	111	112	113	114	69	70	70	71	72	72	73
	95th + 12 mm Hg	120	121	122	123	124	125	126	81	82	82	83	84	84	85
7	Height (in)	45.7	46.5	47.8	49.3	50.8	52.1	52.9	45.7	46.5	47.8	49.3	50.8	52.1	52.9
	Height (cm)	116.1	118	121.4	125.1	128.9	132.4	134.5	116.1	118	121.4	125.1	128.9	132.4	134.5
	50th	94	94	95	97	98	98	99	56	56	57	58	58	59	59
	90th	106	107	108	109	110	111	111	68	68	69	70	70	71	71
	95th	110	110	111	112	114	115	116	71	71	72	73	73	74	74
	95th + 12 mm Hg	122	122	123	124	126	127	128	83	83	84	85	85	86	86
8	Height (in)	47.8	48.6	50	51.6	53.2	54.6	55.5	47.8	48.6	50	51.6	53.2	54.6	55.5
	Height (cm)	121.4	123.5	127	131	135.1	138.8	141	121.4	123.5	127	131	135.1	138.8	141
	50th	95	96	97	98	99	99	100	57	57	58	59	59	60	60
	90th	107	108	109	110	111	112	112	69	70	70	71	72	72	73
	95th	111	112	112	114	115	116	117	72	73	73	74	75	75	75
	95th + 12 mm Hg	123	124	124	126	127	128	129	84	85	85	86	87	87	87

Continued

Age		(5%)	(10%)	(25%)	(50%)	(75%)	(90%)	(95%)	(5%)	(10%)	(25%)	(50%)	(75%)	(90%)	(95%)
9	Height (in)	49.6	50.5	52	53.7	55.4	56.9	57.9	49.6	50.5	52	53.7	55.4	56.9	57.9
	Height (cm)	126	128.3	132.1	136.3	140.7	144.7	147.1	126	128.3	132.1	136.3	140.7	144.7	147.1
	50th	96	97	98	99	100	101	101	57	58	59	60	61	62	62
	90th	107	108	109	110	112	113	114	70	71	72	73	74	74	74
	95th	112	112	113	115	116	118	119	74	74	75	76	76	77	77
	95th + 12 mm Hg	124	124	125	127	128	130	131	86	86	87	88	88	89	89
10	Height (in)	51.3	52.2	53.8	55.6	57.4	59.1	60.1	51.3	52.2	53.8	55.6	57.4	59.1	60.1
	Height (cm)	130.2	132.7	136.7	141.3	145.9	150.1	152.7	130.2	132.7	136.7	141.3	145.9	150.1	152.7
	50th	97	98	99	100	101	102	103	59	60	61	62	63	63	64
	90th	108	109	111	112	113	115	116	72	73	74	74	75	75	76
	95th	112	113	114	116	118	120	121	76	76	77	77	78	78	78
	95th + 12 mm Hg	124	125	126	128	130	132	133	88	88	89	89	90	90	90
11	Height (in)	53	54	55.7	57.6	59.6	61.3	62.4	53	54	55.7	57.6	59.6	61.3	62.4
	Height (cm)	134.7	137.3	141.5	146.4	151.3	155.8	158.6	134.7	137.3	141.5	146.4	151.3	155.8	158.6
	50th	99	99	101	102	103	104	106	61	61	62	63	63	63	63
	90th	110	111	112	114	116	117	118	74	74	75	75	75	76	76
	95th	114	114	116	118	120	123	124	77	78	78	78	78	78	78
	95th + 12 mm Hg	126	126	128	130	132	135	136	89	90	90	90	90	90	90
12	Height (in)	55.2	56.3	58.1	60.1	62.2	64	65.2	55.2	56.3	58.1	60.1	62.2	64	65.2
	Height (cm)	140.3	143	147.5	152.7	157.9	162.6	165.5	140.3	143	147.5	152.7	157.9	162.6	165.5
	50th	101	101	102	104	106	108	109	61	62	62	62	62	63	63
	90th	113	114	115	117	119	121	122	74	75	75	75	75	76	76
	95th	116	117	118	121	124	126	128	77	78	78	78	78	78	79
	95th + 12 mm Hg	128	129	130	133	136	138	140	89	90	90	90	90	90	91
13	Height (in)	57.9	59.1	61	63.1	65.2	67.1	68.3	57.9	59.1	61	63.1	65.2	67.1	68.3
	Height (cm)	147	150	154.9	160.3	165.7	170.5	173.4	147	150	154.9	160.3	165.7	170.5	173.4
	50th	103	104	105	108	110	111	112	61	60	61	62	63	64	65
	90th	115	116	118	121	124	126	126	74	74	74	75	76	77	77
	95th	119	120	122	125	128	130	131	78	78	78	78	80	81	81
	95th + 12 mm Hg	131	132	134	137	140	142	143	90	90	90	90	92	93	93

TABLE 38.3 Blood Pressure Levels in the 90th and 95th Percentiles for Boys 1 to 17 Years Old by Percentiles of Height—cont'd

BP LEVELS FOR BOYS BY AGE AND HEIGHT PERCENTILE

Age	BP Percentile	SBP (mm Hg) HEIGHT PERCENTILE OR MEASURED HEIGHT							DBP (mm Hg) HEIGHT PERCENTILE OR MEASURED HEIGHT						
		5%	10%	25%	50%	75%	90%	95%	5%	10%	25%	50%	75%	90%	95%
14	Height (in)	60.6	61.8	63.8	65.9	68	69.8	70.9	60.6	61.8	63.8	65.9	68	69.8	70.9
	Height (cm)	153.8	156.9	162	167.5	172.7	177.4	180.1	153.8	156.9	162	167.5	172.7	177.4	180.1
	50th	105	106	109	111	112	113	113	60	60	62	64	65	66	67
	90th	119	120	123	126	127	128	129	74	74	75	77	78	79	80
	95th	123	125	127	130	132	133	134	77	78	79	81	82	83	84
	95th + 12 mm Hg	135	137	139	142	144	145	146	89	90	91	93	94	95	96
15	Height (in)	62.6	63.8	65.7	67.8	69.8	71.5	72.5	62.6	63.8	65.7	67.8	69.8	71.5	72.5
	Height (cm)	159	162	166.9	172.2	177.2	181.6	184.2	159	162	166.9	172.2	177.2	181.6	184.2
	50th	108	110	112	113	114	114	114	61	62	64	65	66	67	68
	90th	123	124	126	128	129	130	130	75	76	78	79	80	81	81
	95th	127	129	131	132	134	135	135	78	79	81	83	84	85	85
	95th + 12 mm Hg	139	141	143	144	146	147	147	90	91	93	95	96	97	97
16	Height (in)	63.8	64.9	66.8	68.8	70.7	72.4	73.4	63.8	64.9	66.8	68.8	70.7	72.4	73.4
	Height (cm)	162.1	165	169.6	174.6	179.5	183.8	186.4	162.1	165	169.6	174.6	179.5	183.8	186.4
	50th	111	112	114	115	115	116	116	63	64	66	67	68	69	69
	90th	126	127	128	129	131	131	132	77	78	79	80	81	82	82
	95th	130	131	133	134	135	136	137	80	81	83	84	85	86	86
	95th + 12 mm Hg	142	143	145	146	147	148	149	92	93	95	96	97	98	98
17	Height (in)	64.5	65.5	67.3	69.2	71.1	72.8	73.8	64.5	65.5	67.3	69.2	71.1	72.8	73.8
	Height (cm)	163.8	166.5	170.9	175.8	180.7	184.9	187.5	163.8	166.5	170.9	175.8	180.7	184.9	187.5
	50th	114	115	116	117	117	118	118	65	66	67	68	69	70	70
	90th	128	129	130	131	132	133	134	78	79	80	81	82	82	83
	95th	132	133	134	135	137	138	138	81	82	84	85	86	86	87
	95th + 12 mm Hg	144	145	146	147	149	150	150	93	94	96	97	98	98	99

Use percentile values to stage blood pressure (BP) readings according to the scheme in Table 3 (elevated BP: ≥90th percentile; stage 1 hypertension [HTN]: ≥95th percentile; and stage 2 HTN: ≥95th percentile + 12 mm Hg). The 50th, 90th, and 95th percentiles were derived by using quantile regression on the basis of normal-weight children (body mass index <85th percentile).[77]

Height percentile determined by standard growth curves.

BP percentile determined by a single measurement.

Flynn JT, Kaelber DC, Baker-Smith CM, et al. Clinical practice guideline for screening and management of high blood pressure in children and adolescents. *Pediatrics.* 2017;140(3):1–72.

DBP, Diastolic blood pressure; *SBP,* systolic blood pressure.

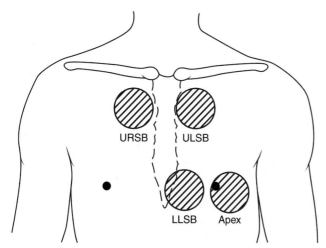

- **Fig 38.2** Direction of heart sounds for clicks and murmurs (auscultatory areas circled) with associated cardiac conditions. *Upper right sternal border (URSB)*: aortic valve clicks of aortic stenosis, venous hum. *Upper left sternal border (ULSB)*: Pulmonary valve clicks of pulmonary stenosis, pulmonary flow murmurs, atrial septal defect, patent ductus arteriosus, venous hum. *Lower left sternal border (LLSB)*: ventricular septal defects, Still murmur, tricuspid valve regurgitation, hypertrophic cardiomyopathy, subaortic stenosis. *Apex:* aortic or mitral valve clicks, mitral valve regurgitation. *Erb point: (left sternal border between 2nd and 3rd intercostal space)* aortic ejection click or aortic stenosis, or dilated aortic root.

S1 characteristic, continued
- It is usually loudest at the apex.
- It is synchronous with the apical and carotid pulses.
- S_2 has the following characteristics:
  - It is composed of the aortic (A_2) and pulmonic (P_2) components and marks the end of systole and onset of diastole. It is the "dupp" of lubb-dupp.
  - S_2 is normally split with inspiration in children because pulmonic valve closure lags behind aortic valve closure. S_2 becomes single with expiration. The intensity of splitting of S_2 is one of the most important parts of the cardiac examination.
  - S_2 is best assessed at the upper left sternal border in the pulmonic area.
  - Pulmonary HTN causes early closure of P_2 and accentuation of S_2, which may sound like a loud, single second heart sound.
  - Absence of one of the semilunar valves (as in pulmonary atresia) causes single S_2.
  - Wide splitting of S_2 without becoming a single sound on expiration may indicate increased pulmonary flow (typical of atrial septal defect [ASD]).
- S_3 and S_4 have the following characteristics:
  - S_3 is associated with rapid ventricular filling; it may be heard in a quiet infant or child with a rapid heart rate.
  - S_3 "gallop" is best heard at the apex with the bell of the stethoscope during early diastole. When combined with S_1 and S_2, it gives the impression of the word "Kentucky." S_3 is easier to appreciate when the child is in the left lateral decubitus position.
  - S_4 is always pathologic; it represents increased force of atrial contraction and ventricular distention.
  - S_4 "gallop" sounds like the word "Tennessee." It is best heard in late diastole just before S_1.
  - S_4 is low-pitched and is best heard at the apex with the bell of the stethoscope.

- Clicks: Ejection clicks are heard early in systole, immediately after S_1, and may sound like a split first heart sound. Pulmonic ejection clicks are high in frequency, vary with respiration, and disappear with inspiration. An aortic ejection click, heard best at Erb point, is constant in intensity with a sound of a "snap" or a "click." Nonejection clicks are heard best in midsystole, or midway between S_1 and S_2 in the cardiac cycle at the apex. These clicks are best heard in those who are leaning forward or standing, may disappear with inspiration, and are due to mitral valve prolapse. Fig 38.2 describes cardiac conditions associated with each of these clicks.

Murmurs

Up to 80% of children may have an innocent or "functional" murmur at some time during childhood. These are caused by normal blood flow through normal cardiac structures rather than by turbulent blood flow caused by a defect or abnormal cardiac structures. All murmurs may be intensified by factors that increase cardiac output (e.g., anemia, fever, exercise). It is important to remember significant heart defects may *not* have a murmur because there may not be turbulent blood flow (e.g., a large septal defect or nonrestrictive patent ductus) (Park, 2016). Fig 38.2 shows auscultatory areas for different murmurs.

Criteria for Describing a Heart Murmur. Every murmur is assessed according to the criteria listed in Table 38.4. These are further illustrated in Fig 38.3. Characteristics of pathologic murmurs needing referral are listed in Box 38.2. The presence of a murmur causes great anxiety for a family. If the diagnosis is uncertain or there is a suspicion of heart disease, a referral to pediatric cardiology is warranted.

Innocent or Functional Murmurs. Functional or innocent cardiac murmurs are common in children and can be evident in newborns. Table 38.5 describes common types of innocent murmurs; Box 38.2 describes the characteristics of an innocent murmur compared with a pathologic murmur. Families and older children with innocent murmurs should be reassured there is no cardiac pathology. They should be informed the murmur may come and go and may be louder at times of fever, anxiety, pain, or exercise and that activities do not need to be limited or any special precautions taken.

Common Diagnostic Studies

If the PCP intends to refer for a pediatric cardiology consult, performing any of the following routine diagnostic studies is not cost effective. The pediatric cardiology consultant is able to determine with greater discrimination which, if any, tests should be ordered (Park, 2016).
- Chest radiograph provides the following information: cardiac size and size of specific chambers and great vessels, cardiac contour, status of pulmonary blood flow, and status of the lungs and other surrounding tissue (Fig 38.4).
- Electrocardiogram: The ECG monitors the electrical activity of the heart from different locations and in different planes of the body giving information about forces of ventricular contraction, hypertrophy, chamber dilation, and rhythm.
- Complete blood count (CBC): CBC rules out severe anemia or polycythemia as a cause of a murmur.
- Hyperoxia test: Supplementation of 100% oxygen results in "pinking" and increased arterial oxygen saturation when the disease is primarily pulmonary; minimal or no color improvement indicates the disease is cardiac. More commonly, simple pulse oximetry saturations are used to evaluate for cyanosis.

TABLE 38.4	Describing a Heart Murmur
Heart Murmur	**Description**
Grade or intensity: Does not necessarily indicate severity of the problem May be altered with positional change from supine to sitting	Grade I: Barely audible; heard faintly after a period of attentive listening Grade II: Soft but easily audible Grade III: Moderately loud; no thrill Grade IV: Loud, present over widespread area; palpable thrill Grade V: Loud, audible with stethoscope barely on the chest; precordial thrill present Grade VI: Heard without stethoscope (rare)
Timing with cardiac cycle	Systolic Diastolic Continuous
Location on chest where murmur is loudest	Aortic or pulmonic listening areas, URSB, ULSB, Erb point, LLSB, apex
Radiations or transmission to other locations	To back To apex To carotids
Quality	Musical Harsh blowing
Duration	Point of onset and length of time systole and diastole murmurs last (e.g., "early systole, heard throughout cardiac cycle")
Pitch	Low Middle High

LLSB, Left lower sternal border; *ULSB,* upper left sternal border; *URSB,* upper right sternal border.

Other diagnostic studies usually done by cardiology may include the following:

- Echocardiogram: Echocardiography uses reflected sound waves to identify intracardiac structures and their motion. The types of recordings include two-dimensional, M-mode, contrast, Doppler, and tissue Doppler studies (Fig 38.5). Fetal echocardiography can diagnose CHD as early as 16 to 18 weeks' gestation (high-frequency transvaginal echocardiography as early as 10 weeks' gestation), as well as arrhythmias and hemodynamic changes (Park, 2016).
- Cardiac catheterization: This provides information regarding the heart's anatomy, pulmonary vascular resistance, and cardiac output. This procedure can also be done to obtain a sample of heart tissue, open up narrow arteries or valves, or deploy devices that can close holes in the heart or extra vessels.
- Magnetic resonance imaging (MRI): This technique yields an image of the heart structures and information about chamber volumes and function.
- Exercise testing: A graded treadmill or bicycle ergometer is used to determine cardiac output (myocardial blood flow and rhythm) response to exercise for endurance and capacity measurement.

Primary Health Care Management Strategies

The goals of primary health care for a child with cardiovascular disease include the following:

- Adequate nutritional intake and optimal growth: Depending on the child's condition, the diet may need modification to provide maximum calories or limit various types of foods. The young infant with CHF may need 24, 27, or 30 kcal per ounce formula or fortified breast milk (breast milk with added calories). The child may need a nasogastric or gastric tube to obtain adequate calories because of an inadequate suck or fatigue with feeding. Children with cyanotic conditions may initially have adequate weight gain. The PCP should refer to a nutritionist if available for assistance with complex diets. (See Chapter 17 for further information on altered patterns of nutrition.)
- Optimal psychosocial development and functioning: Discuss with the family the need to treat the child as normally as possible. Direct parents to support groups that provide informational and emotional support for all family members. Poor sibling bonding and unexpressed fears and anger in young siblings toward an infant with a severe or chronic disease can affect their relationships and family dynamics for years to come. A multicenter prospective study concluded that psychological functioning and quality of life of children and adolescents with serious congenital heart defects decreased significantly as the number of cardiac interventions increased (Knowles et al., 2014).
- Preventive vaccines: Live virus vaccines should be delayed until 6 months after cardiopulmonary bypass and exposure to red blood cells and plasma (CDC, 2011). This most often affects 1-year-old infants who are due for varicella and measles, mumps, and rubella vaccines. Other vaccines can be given on a regular schedule. The AAP also recommends provision of respiratory syncytial virus (RSV) prophylaxis for infants younger than 1 year old who have cyanotic or complicated CHD, especially those with CHF or pulmonary HTN. Per AAP guidelines, infants should receive a maximum of five doses (15 mg/kg intramuscularly every 30 days) during RSV season (AAP Committee on Infectious Diseases and AAP Bronchiolitis Guidelines Committee, 2014). Anyone older than 19 years old spending time with infants should have the Tdap vaccine, regardless of the the interval since the last Td vaccine to prevent pertussis (Curtis et al., 2017).
- Prevention of avoidable complications: Emphasize prevention of respiratory infections through good hand washing and avoiding contact (if possible) with others with upper respiratory infection (URI) symptoms. Vaccination against seasonal influenza is prudent for infants and family members/caregivers per CDC guidelines.
- Prevention of infective endocarditis (IE): Although uncommon in children, IE (also called *subacute bacterial endocarditis [SBE]*) is associated with significant morbidity and mortality rates and warrants primary prevention whenever indicated. Standards for prophylaxis against SBE for children undergoing dental procedures are available in Box 38.3 and Table 38.6. A high index of suspicion for IE should be maintained if any unusual clinical findings (e.g., petechiae, fever) are present after any procedure (Baltimore et al., 2015). Children with CHD appear to have more severe gingival inflammatory conditions, with a concomitant increase in *Haemophilus* species, *Actinobacillus actinomycetemcomitans*, *Cardiobacterium hominis*, *Eikenella corrodens*, and *Kingella* species (HACEK) and other microbes known to cause endocarditis, compared with other

SYSTOLIC MURMURS

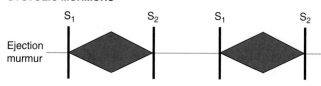

- Comprise most murmurs heard and occur between S_1 and S_2.
- Are either regurgitation murmurs (e.g., the holosystolic murmur of a VSD that begins with S_1 and continues throughout systole) or ejection murmur caused by flow of blood through narrowed or stenotic areas (e.g., AS).
- Best heard at second left or right intercostal space (ICS).
- Begin with or after S_1 and end with or before S_2.
- Include all innocent and physiologic murmurs.

DIASTOLIC MURMURS

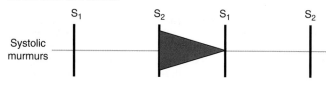

- Typically occur between S_2 and before or at S_1.
- Always indicate cardiac pathology.
- Murmur that starts with S_2 and has a decrescendo quality is most commonly due to aortic or pulmonic regurgitation.
- Mid-diastolic "rumble," a short low-pitched rumble heard best at the apex, is commonly due to atrioventricular valve stenosis or increased flow across a nonstenotic valve, such as seen with a large VSD or PDA.

CONTINUOUS MURMURS

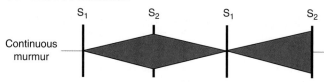

- Start at S_1 and go completely through systole and diastole.
- Most common cause is PDA.
- These murmurs need to be differentiated from the coexistence of separate systolic and diastolic murmurs and venous hums.

• **Fig 38.3** Timing of Heart Murmurs. *AS,* Aortic stenosis; *PDA,* patent ductus arteriosus; *VSD,* ventricular septal defect. (From Cassidy SC, Allen HD, Phillips JR. History and physical examination. In: Allen HD, Driscoll DJ, Shaddy RE, et al, eds. *Moss and Adams' Heart Disease in Infants, Children, and Adolescents Including the Fetus and Young Adult.* 8th ed. Philadelphia, Lippincott Williams & Wilkins; 2013, Fig 5.1, p 89.)

• BOX 38.2 Auscultatory Findings—Innocent Versus Pathologic Murmur

Innocent Murmur

Usually grade I to III/VI in intensity and localized
Changes with position (sitting to lying)
May vary in loudness or presence from visit to visit
May increase in loudness (intensity) with fever, anemia, exercise, or anxiety
Musical or vibratory in quality, sometimes blowing
Systolic in timing (except for venous hum, which is continuous), peaking in first half of systole
Duration is short
Best heard in LLSB or pulmonic area (except for venous hum)
Rarely transmitted
May disappear with Valsalva maneuver, position, or gentle jugular pressure
Vital signs: Normal
ECG: Normal
General health status: Good

Possible Pathologic Murmur

A murmur in a child with a syndrome associated with CHD (e.g., trisomy 21)
Any diastolic murmur
Any systolic murmur associated with a thrill
Pansystolic murmurs
Continuous murmurs that cannot be suppressed
Systolic clicks
Opening snaps
Fixed splitting of the second heart sound not associated with bundle branch block
An accentuated S_2
S_4 gallops
Not positional
Grade IV/VI or higher
Harsh quality

CHD, *Congenital heart disease;* ECG, *electrocardiogram;* LLSB, *left lower sternal border.*

---

children. The reason for this is not clear. Good dental hygiene is extremely important for these children, and evidence shows parents have poor knowledge about the dental risk of IE in children with CHD (Suma et al., 2011).

- Optimal fitness: Parents and children should be counseled on the importance of daily physical activity and limiting sedentary behavior. The initial goal is to develop habitual physical activity, including all types of physical movement, not just organized exercise designed to increase fitness. Certain children, such as those with ventricular arrhythmias, need complete activity restrictions (see Chapter 19, Table 20.6 for the parameters for sports participation for children with various forms of cardiac diseases or conditions). Children who have motor skill delays, often due to perioperative morbidity, tend to have more sedentary lifestyles and need encouragement to be more active.

- Prior to discussing physical activity, child assessment should include a detailed history of exertional symptoms, such as angina, excessive dyspnea, palpitations, dizziness, and syncope (see Chapter 19, Box 19.3 for the 14-element cardiovascular screening checklist for congenital and genetic heart disease).

- The assessment of capacity for physical activity should also include current behavior, current motor skills (and expected skill development that will be required), motivation, anticipated time to be spent in the physical activity, and type of activity. Reassure the parents that the child generally "self-limits" activity according to ability. If the child can comfortably talk during the activity, he/she will automatically limit their activity intensity. The cardiology provider should be consulted regarding exercise limitations before entrance into sports or any activities that require strenuous physical exertion.

TABLE 38.5	Common Innocent Murmurs			
	Stills	**Pulmonary Flow Murmur of Childhood**	**Pulmonary Flow Murmur of Infancy**	**Venous Hum**
Other names	Innocent Vibratory Functional Physiologic "Head start" murmur	Flow murmur	Peripheral pulmonary stenosis	
Description	Midsystolic, louder in supine position or with inspiration	Early systolic to midsystolic; decreases or disappears with standing; increases with cardiac output or in supine position	Short, midsystolic ejection murmur	Constant swishing sound, disappears with head turning, compression of jugular vein(s), or supine position; varies with respirations
Age	Any age but most common between 2 and 6 years old	Any age but more commonly heard in thin-chested adolescents between 8 and 14 years old	Common during newborn period, especially in preterm infants	Any age but commonly between 2 and 8 years old
Best heard	Midpoint, left lower/apex and midsternal border; does not radiate	Pulmonary outflow area; radiates to lung fields	Murmur radiates from left upper sternal border to both axilla and back, usually gone by 6 months old	In upright position, left and right upper chest below clavicles
Quality	Short, vibratory, musical, "twangy string," medium-pitched	Soft, blowing with normally split S_2; no click or thrill	Soft with middle to high pitch	Soft, high pitch; does not radiate
Intensity	Grades II (rarely III)	Grades I to II	Grades I to II	Grades II to III
Differential diagnosis	Small VSD, IHSS	ASD, pulmonic stenosis	Supravalvular pulmonic stenosis or aortic stenosis	PDA

ASD, Atrial septal defect; *IHSS,* idiopathic hypertrophic subaortic stenosis; *PDA,* patent ductus arteriosis; *VSD,* ventricular septal defect.

Adapted from Cassidy SC, Allen HD, Phillips JR. History and physical examination. In: Allen HD, Driscoll DJ, Shaddy RE, et al, eds. *Moss and Adams' Heart Disease in Infants, Children, and Adolescents Including the Fetus and Young Adult.* 8th ed. Philadelphia: Lippincott Williams & Wilkins; 2013:82–92; Bernstein D. Evaluation of the cardiovascular system. In: Kliegman RM, Stanton BF, Schor NF, et al, eds. *Nelson Textbook of Pediatrics.* 19th ed. Philadelphia: Saunders; 2011:1529–1536.

Note: Innocent murmurs typically increase with cardiac output (excitement, fever, anemia).

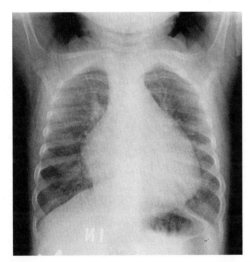

• **Fig 38.4** Chest radiogram of a 3 month old with ventricular septal defect and congestive heart failure. Cardiomegaly with increased pulmonary vascular markings from pulmonary venous congestion is visible.

• Optimal neurodevelopmental adaptation to school and life tasks: Children who require heart surgery in the first year of life can have significant neurodevelopmental impairment (Knowles et al., 2014). Those undergoing a first operation after 1 year generally have subtle or no impairment if they do not have a cyanotic heart lesion (Marino et al., 2012). Risk factors that predict worse neurodevelopmental outcomes include genetic syndromes, low birth weight, single ventricle physiology, low socioeconomic status, low maternal education, the need for cardiopulmonary resuscitation (CPR), duration of mechanical ventilation, duration of intensive care unit (ICU) stay, gestational age at time of surgery, and preoperative intubation. Only a few of these are amenable to modification in the surgical period. However, early recognition of and intervention for developmental and cognitive delays lead to improved neurodevelopmental outcomes. Most children with neurocognitive impairment have average intelligence scores, but many have difficulties with visuospatial tasks, fine motor functions, higher-order language skills, memory, and/or attention. They may have impaired ability to coordinate lower-order skills or perform higher-order tasks.

Referral

If a PCP suspects cardiac disease or is unsure about findings, it is best to refer the patient to a pediatric cardiologist. Findings suggestive of cardiac disease are the presence of oxygen saturation less

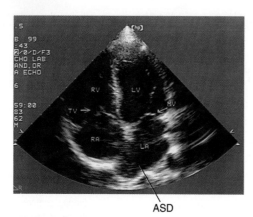

• Fig 38.5 Echocardiogram of a 2 year old with an atrial septal defect *(ASD). LA,* Left atrium; *LV,* left ventricle; *MV,* mitral valve; *RA,* right atrium; *RV,* right ventricle; *TV,* tricuspid valve.

• BOX 38.3 **Cardiac Conditions Associated With the Highest Risk of Endocarditis: Prophylaxis for Dental Procedures Recommended**

- Prosthetic cardiac valve(s) or prosthetic material used for cardiac valve repair
- Previous infective endocarditis
- Congenital heart disease (CHD)
  - Unrepaired cyanotic CHD including palliative shunts and conduits
  - Completely repaired CHD with prosthetic material or device(s) by surgery or interventional catheterization, for 6 months after repair (due to the endothelialization of prosthetic material within that period)
  - Repaired CHD with residual defects (e.g., residual VSD) at the site or adjacent to the site of a prosthetic patch or device
- Cardiac transplantation recipients who have valve disease

VSD, *Ventricular septal defect.* Data from http://www.heart.org/idc/groups/heart-public/@ wcm/@hcm/documents/downloadable/ucm_307644.pdf. Accessed May 27, 2018.

---

than 95%, symptoms of CHF, a pathologic murmur, or a murmur that is difficult to differentiate in the presence of poor growth and development. A child with a murmur who is otherwise doing well should be referred to a pediatric cardiologist for further evaluation in a timely but not urgent manner. Newborns should be evaluated within 1 or 2 days of noticeable signs or immediately (change in breathing patterns, increased irritability and poor feeding, and/ or cyanosis), depending on the severity of their symptoms. An older child with dizziness, chest pain with exertion, arrhythmia, dyspnea, syncope, signs of CHF, or abnormal vital signs should be referred as soon as possible 🌐 (Park, 2016). Some defects, such as small VSDs or bicuspid aortic valves, escape early detection and may cause no disability to a child. However, such defects pose a risk for bacterial endocarditis and thrombotic cerebrovascular accident (CVA) and should be identified.

Genetic Testing

A referral for genetic testing should be done in children who have, in addition to CHD, other congenital anomalies, dysmorphic features, neurocognitive deficits, growth retardation, mothers with a history of multiple miscarriages, or siblings with congenital defects. Approximately 35% of CHD are attributed to genetic factors. There are several testing modalities offered. However, patients' clinical findings and family history determine which genetic test is most appropriate.

Family Support

Families need the support of the PCP to help them understand the diagnosis and cope with short- and long-term consequences. Because of the stress at the time of diagnosis, many parents do not absorb the information presented and may need multiple opportunities to ask questions.

Parents and their designated support people should clearly understand the diagnosis, have diagrams of the defect, and general

---

TABLE 38.6 **Prophylactic Regimens for Dental Procedures**

ANTIBIOTIC PROPHYLACTIC REGIMENS FOR DENTAL PROCEDURES			
Situation	**Agent**	**Regimen—Single Dose 30–60 Minutes Before Procedure**	
		Adults	**Children**
Oral	Amoxicillin	2 g	50 mg/kg
Unable to take oral medication	Ampicillin **OR**	2 g IM or IV[a]	50 mg/kg IM or IV
	Cefazolin or ceftriaxone	1 g IM or IV	50 mg/kg IM or IV
Allergic to penicillins or ampicillin—oral regimen	Cephalexin[b,c]	2g	50 mg/kg
	OR		
	Clindamycin	600 mg	20 mg/kg
	OR		
	Azithromycin or clarithromycin	500 mg	15 mg/kg
Allergic to penicillins or ampicillin and unable to take oral medication	Cefazolin or ceftriaxone[c]	1 g IM or IV	50 mg/kg IM or IV
	OR Clindamycin	600 mg IM or IV	20 mg/kg IM or IV

[a]*IM,* Intramuscular; *IV,* intravenous.

[b]Or other first- or second-generation oral cephalosporin in equivalent adult or pediatric dosage.

[c]Cephalosporins should not be used in an individual with a history of anaphylaxis, angioedema or urticaria with penicillins or ampicillin.

Data from https://www.heart.org/en/health-topics/congenital-heart-defects/congenital-heart-defects-tools-and-resources. Accessed May 27, 2018.

information to take with them for future reference. Should medication be necessary, parents should understand the reason for the drug, regimen for administration, and potential side effects. They should understand the signs and symptoms of deterioration (e.g., CHF) and have clear information regarding how to proceed should symptoms develop. Infant and child CPR certification is critical for anyone caring for a child with a heart condition.

Congenital Heart Disease: General Information

When CHD is diagnosed in an infant or child, parents may incorrectly assume they are somehow responsible for the child's defect. Health care professionals must be clear about what is and what is not known about CHD to help allay needless worry and guilt.

CHD is caused by a developmental alteration in or failure of the embryonic heart to progress beyond an early developmental stage. This alteration occurs in the 2nd to 8th weeks of gestation, due to genetic, environmental, or multifactorial influences. Most cases of CHD have no identifiable cause. With the publication of the human genome and advances in molecular techniques, more genetic factors have been identified as playing a possible role in CHD. This is increasingly important as more children with CHD survive to their own childbearing years.

Two percent to 4% of CHD is caused by teratogens, maternal conditions, or environmental influences. Drugs or teratogens linked to CHD include lithium, retinoic acid, antiepileptics, ibuprofen and naproxen, angiotensin-converting enzyme (ACE) inhibitors, tricyclic antidepressants, sulfonamides, sulfasalazine, tobacco, alcohol, cocaine, and marijuana (Park, 2016). Environmental exposures to organic solvents, pesticides, and air pollution are also implicated in CHD. Exposure to these agents during the vulnerable period (2 to 8 weeks of gestation) is best avoided, although often women do not know they are pregnant this early. Maternal illnesses (e.g., diabetes mellitus, connective tissue disorders, phenylketonuria, rubella, and febrile illnesses—especially influenza) are associated with CHD (van der Bom et al., 2011) (see Box 38.1).

Many genes have etiologic roles in the development of human CHD. Most infants born with CHD do not have other birth defects, but CHD occurs in association with other anomalies or syndromes in 25% to 40% of cases. Children with an abnormal chromosomal number (aneuploidy) account for a significant percentage of these children (Simmons and Brueckner, 2017). Table 38.7 lists the most common known genetic syndromes, aneuploidies, single gene defects, and microdeletions associated with heart disease.

Specific Congenital Heart Diseases

Congestive Heart Failure

CHF is a progressive clinical and pathophysiologic syndrome found in many children with heart problems. The symptoms vary with age of the child and the root cardiac problem (Box 38.4). Besides functional changes, CHF is marked by neurohormonal and molecular changes within the heart.

Pediatric CHF can be caused by congenital malformations leading to ventricular dysfunction, pressure, or volume overload (Hussey and Weintraub, 2016). CHF also occurs in children with structurally normal hearts due to cardiomyopathy, arrhythmias, ischemia, toxins, or infections (Table 38.7). CHF is estimated to affect 12,000 to 35,000 children each year (Averbach, Everitt, Butts, and Rosenthal, 2017).

• BOX 38.4 Signs and Symptoms of Congestive Heart Failure

Infants

Tachypnea
Tachycardia
Rales or wheezing
Cardiomegaly and hepatomegaly
Periorbital edema
Poor feeding/tires easily when feeding
Poor weight gain
Diaphoresis

Children and Teens

Tachypnea
Tachycardia
Rales or wheezing
Cardiomegaly and hepatomegaly
Orthopnea
Shortness of breath or dyspnea with exertion
Peripheral edema
Poor growth and development

TABLE 38.7 Conditions Associated With Congestive Heart Failure in Children

Age	Condition
Premature infant	Patent ductus arteriosus (PDA)
Birth to 1 week old	Hypoplastic left heart syndrome (HLHS)
	Coarctation of the aorta (COA)
	Critical aortic stenosis
	Interrupted aortic arch
	Arteriovenous malformations
	Tachycardia
	Cardiomyopathy
1 week to 3 months old	Ventricular septal defect (VSD)
	Truncus arteriosus
	Atrioventricular (AV) canal (endocardial cushion defect)
	Total anomalous pulmonary venous return
	Coarctation
	Tachycardia
	PDA
	Aortic stenosis
	Tricuspid atresia
Older than 1 year	Bacterial endocarditis
	Rheumatic fever
	Myocarditis

The largest group of infants and children with CHF are those with excessive left-to-right shunting through unrepaired congenital defects. CHF is somewhat of a misnomer in these cases because the myocardium generally responds quite well to the challenge of excessive blood volume for a long time, and cardiac output remains adequate. However, the compensatory response to this excessive workload for the lungs and some heart chambers includes electrolyte and fluid imbalances, and neurohormonal changes. Children with heart failure from systolic or diastolic cardiac dysfunction caused by infections, obstruction, or arrhythmias also need treatment to ameliorate fluid and electrolyte imbalances, increase contractility, and decrease cardiac afterload.

Depending on the underlying pathophysiology, children with CHF have elevated neurohormonal and inflammatory mediators (aldosterone, norepinephrine, natriuretic peptides, tumor necrosis factor, and renin). Large-scale studies in adult populations show the value of blocking some of these changes with agents such as aldosterone inhibitors, angiotensin inhibitors, and sympathetic inhibitors (β-blockers). Various studies show the use of neurohormonal agents is more complex in children than adults. The benefits and risks of neurohormonal agents depend on the underlying cause of CHF (CHD, infection, or other) and the degree of heart failure (Simpson and Canter, 2012).

The traditional heart failure therapies (i.e., diuretics, inotropes, and afterload reducers) are still used in many cases, although further elucidation of the neurohormonal responses in children with the different conditions listed in Table 38.8 may change management strategies (Hussey and Weintraub, 2016). Pulmonary vasodilators (e.g., sildenafil) have been shown to help in single

TABLE 38.8 Congenital Malformation Syndromes Associated with Selected Congenital Heart Disease

Disorders	Resultant Heart Defect(s)/Occurrence
Syndromes with Aneuploidy (Abnormal Chromosome Number) or Microdeletion (≈10% of Congenital Heart Disease)	
Trisomy 21 (Down syndrome)	AV septal defect, VSD, ASD, PDA, TOF (50%)
Trisomy 18 (Edwards syndrome)	VSD, ASD, PDA, COA, bicuspid aortic or pulmonary valve (99%)
Trisomy 13 (Patau syndrome)	VSD, PDA, dextrocardia (90%)
Monosomy X (Turner syndrome)	Bicuspid aortic valve, COA (35%), pulmonic stenosis
Klinefelter variant (XXY)	PDA, ASD (15%)
22q11.2 deletion (DiGeorge syndrome)	Interrupted aortic arch, truncus arteriosus, TOF, perimembranous VSD, aortic arch anomalies
7q11.23 deletion (Williams syndrome)	Pulmonic stenosis, supravalvular aortic stenosis
Syndromes with Congenital Heart Disease from Single Gene Defects	
Marfan syndrome (FBN1, TGFBR1, TGFBR2)	Mitral valve prolapse, aortic root dilation
Noonan syndrome (PTPN11)	Valvular pulmonic stenosis, HCM
Costello syndrome (HRAS)	Pulmonary stenosis, HCM, conduction abnormalities
Alagille syndrome (JAG1, NOTCH2)	Pulmonic stenosis, TOF, ASD, peripheral pulmonic stenosis
Heterotaxy syndrome (ZIC3, CFC1)	DILV, DORV, d-TGA, AVSD
CHARGE (CHD7, SEMA3E)	Truncus arteriosus, interrupted aortic arch
Jacobsen (11q23 deletion)	HLHS, COA
Holt-Oram syndrome (TBX5)	ASD, VSD
Cri du chat syndrome (5p)	VSD, PDA, ASD (25%)
Neurofibromatosis	Pulmonic stenosis, COA
Leopard syndrome (PTPN11, RAF 1)	Pulmonic stenosis, conduction abnormalities
Nonhereditary Syndromes (Fetal Exposure)	
Fetal alcohol syndrome	VSD, PDA, ASD, TOF (25% to 30%)
Fetal hydantoin syndrome	Pulmonic stenosis, aortic stenosis, COA, PDA, VSD, ASD (<5%)
Fetal trimethadione syndrome	TGA, VSD, TOF (15% to 30%)
Infant of diabetic mother	TGA, VSD, COA (3% to 5%); cardiomyopathy (10%–20%)

ASD, Atrial septal defect; *AVSD,* atrioventricular septal defect; *AV,* atrioventricular; *COA,* coarctation of the aorta; *DILV,* double inlet left ventricle; *DORV,* double outlet right ventricle; *d-TGA,* dextrotransposition of the great arteries; *HCM,* hypertrophic cardiomyopathy; *HLHS,* hypoplastic left heart syndrome; *PDA,* patent ductus arteriosis; *TGA,* transposition of the great arteries; *TOF,* tetralogy of Fallot; *VSD,* ventricular septal defect.

Data from Richards A, Garg V. Genetics of congenital heart disease. *Curr Cardiol Rev.* 2010;6:91–97; van der Bom T, Zomer C, et al. The changing epidemiology of congenital heart disease. *Nat Rev Cardiol.* 2011;8(1):50–60.

ventricle heart failure. Monitoring B natriuretic peptides (amino acid polypeptides secreted by the *ventricles* in response to stretching) may be helpful in biventricular heart failure but not recommended in single ventricle disease (Simpson and Canter, 2012). Future promising approaches to heart failure include agents to decrease or block myocardial fibrosis, myocardial cell regeneration, and use of stem cell and microRNA to facilitate remodeling of the heart (Burns et al., 2014).

Left-to-Right Shunting Congenital Heart Disease (Acyanotic)

Pulmonary overflow lesions have communication between the two sides of the heart through which extra blood shunts from the high-pressure, oxygenated left side of the heart to the low-pressure, deoxygenated right side of the heart. The result is an increase in pulmonary blood flow. These lesions are acyanotic in nature. Fig 38.6 lists the various left-to-right versus right-to-left shunting disorders.

Atrial Septal Defect

An ASD is a defect or hole in the atrial septum and accounts for 5% to 10% of all CHD (Park, 2016). ASD can occur alone or as part of more complex heart disease. Of the four types of ASD, the most common involves the midseptum in the area of the foramen ovale and is called an *ostium secundum–type defect* (Fig 38.7). Defects of the sinus venosus type are high in the atrial septum, near the entry of the SVC, or low near the IVC and are frequently associated with anomalous pulmonary venous return. A primum ASD is in the lower portion of the septum and is most often seen in children with Down syndrome. The rarest form of ASD is

an unroofed coronary sinus occurring in less than 1% of ASDs (McRae, 2015a). Usually ASDs occur spontaneously; however, there are a few identified genetic mutations that cause familial ASDs (Park, 2016).

Clinical Findings

History. The child is often completely asymptomatic and may fatigue easily or have exertional dyspnea, be somewhat thin, and have a history of frequent upper respiratory tract infections or pneumonia. Symptoms may become more common in late adolescence or early adulthood.

Physical Examination

- Typically, a murmur may not be noticed until the child is 2 to 3 years old.
- Possible mild left anterior chest bulge or palpable lift at the left sternal border.
- S_1 is normal or split, with accentuation of the tricuspid valve closure sound.
- S_2 is often split widely and is relatively fixed.
- A grade I to III/VI, widely radiating, medium-pitched, not harsh, systolic crescendo-decrescendo murmur is heard best at the pulmonic area. This murmur is not due to flow across the atrial septum but is due to increased flow across the pulmonary valve.

Diagnostic Studies

- Chest radiography may reveal cardiac enlargement, especially of the right atrium and right ventricle. The main pulmonary artery may be dilated and pulmonary vascular markings increased.
- The ECG shows right axis deviation with right atrial enlargement. Lead V_1 usually shows a right bundle branch block with an rSR' pattern. P wave may be tall, showing right atrial enlargement. The PR interval may be prolonged. However, the ECG can be normal in small left-to-right defects. The ECG should be assessed for AV prolongation.
- The echocardiogram identifies the specific location of the defect in the atrial septum and will show right-sided chamber enlargement.
- Cardiac catheterization is rarely necessary unless the diagnosis is in doubt, the site of pulmonary venous return is questionable, or when transcatheter device closure is planned (Park, 2016).

Management

- Small defects found in infancy may close spontaneously.

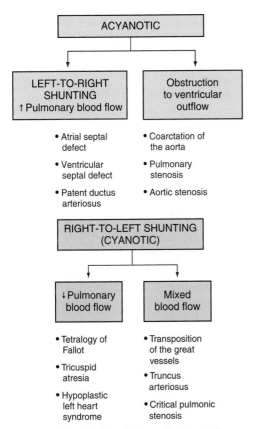

• **Fig 38.6** Classification of Congenital Heart Disease.

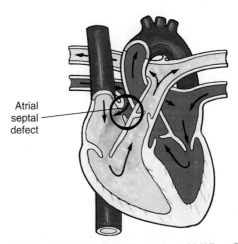

• **Fig 38.7** Atrial Septal Defect. (From Hockenberry M, Wilson D. *Nursing Care of Infants and Children.* 10th ed. St. Louis: Mosby/Elsevier; 2015.)

- Larger defects require intervention, usually after the child is 1 year old, before school entry, or when the defect is identified in an older child. Most small to moderate ostium secundum ASDs can be closed percutaneously in the cardiac catheterization laboratory if the child weighs more than 15 kgs and there are adequate margins to anchor the device. If the defect is large or unfavorable for device closure, cardiac surgery is indicated. Surgical mortality rate is less than 0.5% (Park, 2016).
- SBE prophylaxis (see Table 38.6) precautions are necessary only in the first 6 months after cardiac surgery or device closure. Low-dose aspirin is prescribed for 6 months after transcatheter device closure. In adolescents, other antiplatelet agents may be used such as clopidogrel (McRae, 2015a).
- Long-term outcome is excellent after ASD repair. However, there is a small incidence of atrial arrhythmias due to the atriotomy scar (Contractor and Mandapati, 2017).
- Left untreated, with time ASDs can result in right ventricular enlargement, fibrosis, and failure. Although rare in children, paradoxical emboli can occur (a thrombus transverses the intracardiac defect and enters the systemic circulation).
- Some with uncorrected ASDs develop severe irreversible pulmonary HTN that is disabling and life shortening.
- Exercise restriction is unnecessary (Park, 2016).

Ventricular Septal Defect

A VSD is a hole or defect in one of the areas of the ventricular septum and accounts for between 37% of all CHDs (Fig 38.8). (Dakkak and Bhimji, 2017). There are four types of VSDs: perimembranous, supracristal (occurs in the outflow part of the right ventricle above crista supraventricularis), inlet, and muscular. The most common type is the perimembranous VSD. VSDs are associated with many congenital defects, but 95% demonstrate no chromosomal anomaly (see Table 38.7). Approximately 30% to 50% of these defects are small; the vast majority of these spontaneously close by 4 years old (Park, 2016).

Clinical Findings
History

- Often, a murmur is not heard immediately after birth. When pulmonary vascular resistance falls (normally at 2 to 8 weeks old), more blood shunts across the VSD from left ventricle to right ventricle, and to the pulmonary circulation. This causes a classic loud murmur. Early signs and symptoms of CHF also begin at this time.

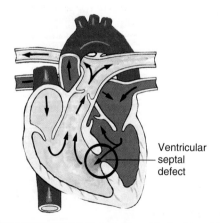

• Fig 38.8 Ventricular Septal Defect. (From Hockenberry M, Wilson D. *Nursing Care of Infants and Children.* 10th ed. St. Louis: Mosby/Elsevier; 2015.)

- Parents may note signs and symptoms of CHF (Box 38.4).
- Small defects may be completely asymptomatic at birth, appearing by 6 months old.

Physical Examination

- Small VSD
  - Harsh, high-pitched, grade II to IV/VI holosystolic murmur at left lower sternal border (LLSB)
  - All other findings within normal limits
- Large VSD
  - Low-pitched, grade II to V/VI holosystolic murmur at LLSB
  - VSD murmur that becomes higher pitched over time indicates that the defect is becoming smaller
  - Diastolic rumble at the apex
  - Thrill along the left sternal border
  - Signs of progressing CHF after the first weeks of life
  - S_3 or S_4 gallop if CHF is present

Diagnostic Studies

- Chest radiography findings vary depending on the shunt's size. Children with small shunts have a normal heart size and pulmonary vascular markings that are just beyond the upper limits of normal. Those with large shunts have cardiac enlargement involving both left and right ventricles and left atrium, as well as pulmonary vascular markings that are significantly increased (see Fig 38.4).
- The ECG is normal with small defects and may show left ventricular hypertrophy (LVH) or biventricular hypertrophy (BVH) with large shunts.
- Echocardiography provides visualization of defects and pinpoints the exact anatomic location. In "pinhole" VSDs, a murmur may be present; however, a defect may not be visualized on the echocardiogram.
- Cardiac catheterization is rarely necessary except when there is a question of elevated pulmonary vascular resistance or when transcatheter closure of a muscular VSD is expected. A transcatheter device can only be used in children weighing more than 6 kg (McRae, 2015a).

Management

- Infants with small defects and no CHF symptoms are monitored every 6 months throughout the first year of life, then biannually to assess for closure of the VSD. Some defects may never close and cause no difficulty. SBE prophylaxis is not recommended.
- Larger defects with signs of CHF are managed as follows:
  - Lanoxin, diuretics, ACE inhibitors, or β-blockers may be prescribed by cardiology.
  - Nutritional intake and weight gain must be monitored in infants and children. It is important to teach families to fortify an infant's calories to 24, 27, or 30 kcal/oz, as needed. Arrange for enteric nutritional support via nasogastric tube for young infants struggling to meet their caloric needs.
  - Families should be taught the signs and symptoms of developing or progressing CHF.
  - Surgery or percutaneous device closure can be performed if no improvement is seen over weeks or months. The long-term outcome is excellent after repair (Park, 2016). Some potential complications after VSD repair include: residual VSD, aortic insufficiency secondary to aortic cusp prolapse, or arrhythmias (McRae, 2015a).
  - SBE prophylaxis precautions are necessary for 6 months after surgery (see Box 38.3 and Table 38.6).

Atrioventricular Septal Defect (Atrioventricular Canal Defect or Endocardial Cushion Defect)

The endocardial cushion is a central cardiac structure including the septal portions of the mitral and tricuspid valves and the lower portion of the atrial septum and upper portion of the ventricular septum. Variable portions of the endocardial cushion are absent. Complete AV septal defect implies the absence of this cushion, leading to a primum ASD, a single AV valve (composed of leaflets of the intended mitral and tricuspid valves), and an inlet VSD. There may also be partial, transitional, and intermediate defects with less profound abnormalities and usually less severe CHF symptoms (Fig 38.9). Complete or partial AV canal defects account for 4% to 5% of all CHDs (Park, 2016). Complete atrioventricular canal defect (CAVC) is more commonly seen in children with Down syndrome (McRae, 2015a).

Clinical Findings

History. Children with only a primum ASD (partial AV canal) may manifest without symptoms. In infants with complete AV canal defects, parents may note signs and symptoms of CHF and failure to thrive (see Box 38.4).

Physical Examination

- Partial AV canal (primum ASD) findings are the same as those with secundum ASD. There may also be a soft blowing murmur of mitral regurgitation in the apex and/or infrascapular area.
- Complete AV canal defect findings:
  - Low-pitched, grade II to V/VI holosystolic murmur at LLSB. A murmur may not be evident at birth but increases in loudness at 2 to 8 weeks after pulmonary vascular resistance falls.
  - Diastolic rumble at the apex; thrill along the left sternal border.
  - Signs of progressing CHF after the first weeks of life; S_3 or S_4 gallop if CHF is present.
  - Some infants, particularly those with trisomy 21, maintain neonatal high pulmonary vascular resistance and show no signs of CHF. Instead, they may manifest signs of pulmonary HTN with loud single S_2, precordial heave, minimal murmur, and desaturation with agitation or effort (Park, 2016).

Diagnostic Studies

- Chest radiography findings vary depending on the size of the shunt. Children with small shunts have a normal heart size and pulmonary vascular markings just beyond the upper limits of normal. Those with large shunts (complete AV canal defect) have cardiac enlargement involving both left and right ventricles and left atrium, with increased pulmonary vascular markings (see Fig 38.4).
- The ECG usually shows superior axis between –40 and –160 degrees. Right ventricular hypertrophy is usually present, and large shunts may cause LVH or BVH in large shunts. In 50% of children, the PR interval is prolonged.
- Echocardiography (two-dimensional, Doppler, or transesophageal) provides visualization of the size of ASD and VSD defects, size and other characteristics of the AV valve(s), and relative sizes of the ventricles.
- Cardiac catheterization may be performed if there is a question of elevated pulmonary vascular resistance or discrepancy in ventricular size.

Management

- Children with a partial AV canal defect consisting of a primum ASD and possibly a cleft mitral valve are monitored every 3 to 6 months throughout the first year of life and then biannually until the defect is closed surgically during toddler or preschool years. They usually do not have signs of CHF but may gain weight slowly. They rarely manifest difficulty with pulmonary HTN after surgery.
- Infants with a complete AV canal defect usually need surgical correction before they reach 6 months of life. Infants who desaturate or develop CHF should see a cardiologist to determine surgical timing. Medical management before surgery may include:
  - Digoxin, diuretics, ACE inhibitors, and β-blockers.
  - Monitoring nutritional intake and weight and fortifying breast milk or infant formulas; enteric nutritional support via nasogastric tube may be needed.
  - Educating families on signs and symptoms of developing or progressing CHF.
- Surgical repair consists of closure of the defect and reconstruction of the common AV valve into separate tricuspid and mitral valves. Surgical mortality is between 3% and 10% for those with complete AV defects and 3% for those with partial defects (Park, 2016).
- Long-term complications include: regurgitant or stenotic AV valve, arrhythmias, and pulmonary HTN (McRae, 2015b).
- SBE prophylaxis is indicated before surgery and 6 months after surgical repair (Wilson et al., 2008).

Patent Ductus Arteriosus

Normal functional closure of the ductus arteriosus occurs in the first 12 to 72 hours after birth. Permanent closure occurs in 2 to 3 weeks in term infants. However, the ductus arteriosus may remain patent in some infants, leaving a connection between the aorta and the pulmonary artery. As pulmonary vascular resistance falls, aortic blood is shunted into the pulmonary artery and recirculates through the lungs (Fig 38.10). The incidence is 5% to 10% of all CHDs, with a female to male ratio of 3:1. The frequency of a PDA increases with decreasing gestational age of premature infants; it is as high as 45% to 80% in very young infants less than 1750 g (Park, 2016). This condition occurs with many congenital malformation syndromes (see Table 38.7).

Clinical Findings

History. The infant or child may be asymptomatic if the PDA is small. Increasing signs of CHF may appear in the first weeks of life in larger PDAs. PDA is evident usually by 3 months old.

Physical Examination

- In the immediate postnatal period, the murmur is soft, systolic, and heard along the left sternal border, under the left clavicle, and in the back.

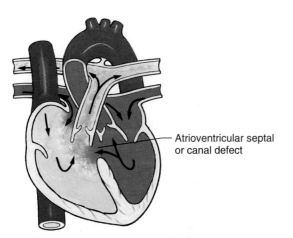

• **Fig 38.9** Complete atrioventricular (AV) septal defect (also known as AV canal defect or complete endocardial cushion defect). (From Hockenberry M, Wilson D. *Nursing Care of Infants and Children.* 10th ed. St. Louis: Mosby/Elsevier; 2015.)

Atrioventricular septal or canal defect

- After the first weeks of life, a typical grade II to V/VI, harsh, rumbling, continuous "machinery murmur" is heard in the left infraclavicular fossa and pulmonic area with a thrill at the base.
- Physical findings of CHF may be present with a large shunt.

Diagnostic Studies

Chest radiographic findings: With a small to moderate shunt, the heart is not enlarged; with larger shunts, both the left atrium and left ventricle can show enlargement. Pulmonary vascular markings may be increased.

ECG: Large shunts show LVH; QRS axis is normal or rightward.

Echocardiogram: Demonstrates the patent ductus and usually enlargement of the left atrium.

Management

- Indomethacin or ibuprofen may be given to preterm infants to effect closure when there is a significant left-to-right shunt. It is contraindicated and ineffective in term or older infants (Park, 2016).
- Asymptomatic infants with a small left-to-right shunt are followed for spontaneous closure or transcatheter device closure, preferably before 1 year old. Infants with large shunts or pulmonary HTN should have their PDA surgically closed within the first few months of life to prevent the development of progressive pulmonary vascular obstruction. Surgical ligation of the ductus is a low-risk procedure because cardiopulmonary bypass is not necessary (Park, 2016).
- Currently, interventional cardiologists close many PDAs in children older than 8 months old by inserting coils or closure plugs into the shunt in the cardiac catheterization laboratory.
- Families should be reassured their child will live an active, normal life.
- SBE prophylaxis precautions are recommended for the 6-month period after device closure (Wilson et al., 2008).

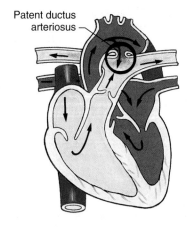

• **Fig 38.10** Patent Ductus Arteriosus. (From Hockenberry M, Wilson D. *Nursing Care of Infants and Children.* 10th ed. St. Louis: Mosby/Elsevier; 2015.)

Right-to-Left Shunting Congenital Heart Disease (Cyanotic)

Cyanotic CHD represents 10% to 18% of all congenital heart lesions. Cardiac cyanosis is due to obstruction of pulmonary blood flow or mixing of oxygenated and unoxygenated blood. Visible cyanosis occurs when oxygen saturation in blood reaches approximately 85%. Cyanosis is more readily apparent with polycythemia and less readily apparent with anemia or the presence of fetal hemoglobin. Polycythemia is a compensatory mechanism to increase the oxygen-carrying capacity in cyanotic patients; however, it increases the risk for cerebral thrombosis (Park, 2016). The most common heart conditions causing cyanosis in the immediate newborn period are listed in Fig 38.6.

Tetralogy of Fallot

Tetralogy of Fallot (TOF; also referred to as TET) is a combination of four anatomic cardiac defects resulting in right ventricular outflow tract (RVOT) obstruction: (1) pulmonary valve stenosis, (2) right ventricular hypertrophy, (3) VSD, and (4) an aorta that overrides the ventricular septum (Fig 38.11). It is the most common cyanotic cardiac lesion (approximately 10% of all CHDs), occurs slightly more in males, and has a spectrum of severity (Mancini, 2017). The most severe forms involve nonpatent pulmonary valve and artery atresia. This is referred to as *TOF pulmonary atresia,* and these infants are quite cyanotic as newborns. In the mildest form, "pink TETs," infants may not display signs of cyanosis because the valvular stenosis is mild, and their symptoms may be similar to a large VSD. However, in most cases of TOF, right-to-left shunting across the VSD and cyanosis increase over the first months of life. This is a result of increasing obstruction in the RVOT. Children with chromosome 22q11.2 deletion syndrome or Down syndrome have a higher risk of this defect (Park, 2016).

Clinical Findings

History. The severity of symptoms with TOF depends on the degree of right ventricular outflow obstruction and presence of a PDA. Symptoms include:

- Cyanosis in cases with mild RVOT obstruction may be so slight it is not initially evident or may be present at birth (with severe obstruction). Cyanosis is usually present by 6 months of age.
- Dyspnea and cyanosis (including hypercyanotic episodes, or "TET spells") increase by 2 to 4 months old, especially with crying, feeding, and/or defecation. The infant may also have a history of poor weight gain.

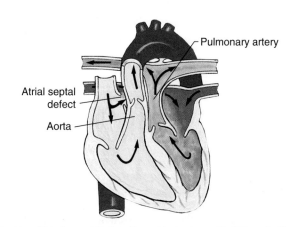

• **Fig 38.11** Tetralogy of Fallot. (From Hockenberry M, Wilson D. *Nursing Care of Infants and Children.* 10th ed. St. Louis: Mosby/Elsevier; 2015.)

Physical Examination. The following findings may be evident:

- Cyanosis of the mucous membranes and dyspnea
- A grade III to V/VI, harsh systolic ejection murmur at the left mid- to upper sternal border (VSD murmur and symptoms of a large VSD). There may be a palpable thrill and a holosystolic murmur at the LLSB.
- Sternal lift secondary to right ventricular hypertrophy.

Diagnostic Studies

- Chest radiography may show a boot-shaped heart with decreased pulmonary vascular markings.
- ECG shows right ventricular hypertrophy and right axis deviation and may show a conduction delay in V_1.
- An echocardiogram shows the extent of the pulmonary obstruction and demonstrates the anatomy of the overriding aorta and VSD.
- Pulse oximetry values decrease over time, with resultant increase in hemoglobin and hematocrit values.
- Cardiac catheterization may be performed to delineate location of coronary arteries prior to surgical correction.

Management

- In neonates with severe pulmonary obstruction, the ductus arteriosus is maintained or reopened with prostaglandin E_1 (PGE_1) until more definitive repair or palliation is possible.
- For hypercyanotic episodes, the child should be cradled in a knee-chest position, soothed, and given oxygen and perhaps morphine sulfate subcutaneously until the spell subsides. The knee-chest maneuver increases systemic resistance, decreases right-to-left shunting, and increases pulmonary blood flow, alleviating the symptoms. Immediate intervention is required for infants who are "spelling," especially if the previously mentioned maneuvers do not end the spell. Most children are surgically repaired before hypercyanotic spells begin.
- Complete repair with open-heart surgery is usually performed in infancy by closing the VSD and relieving the RVOT obstruction.
- Long-term complications after repair include pulmonary valve regurgitation and atrial and ventricular arrhythmias and require lifelong cardiology follow-up. Recent studies indicate progressive right ventricular dilation leads to increasing QRS duration on ECG. QRS duration of 180 mm significantly increases the risk of ventricular tachycardia and sudden death. A cardiology consult is indicated before clearing for sports participation (Park, 2016).
- SBE prophylaxis is indicated for 6 months after repair. Patients who have pulmonary valve replacement required prophylaxis for their entire life (Wilson et al., 2008).

Transposition of the Great Arteries

Dextro-transposition of the great arteries (d-TGA) results from incomplete septation and migration of the truncus arteriosus during fetal development. In d-TGA, the aorta arises from the right ventricle and the pulmonary artery arises from the left ventricle. The aorta receives the deoxygenated systemic venous blood and returns it to the systemic arteries. The pulmonary artery receives oxygenated pulmonary venous blood and returns it to the pulmonary circulation (Fig 38.12). There may be a number of comorbid heart malformations with d-TGA—most commonly VSD, PDA, and coronary artery defects. The incidence is 5% to 7% of all CHDs, with a male to female ratio of 3:1 (Park, 2016).

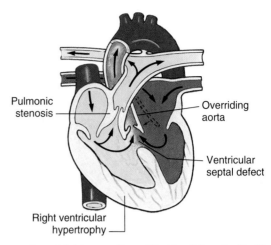

- **Fig 38.12** Complete Transposition of the Great Vessels. (Modified from Hockenberry M, Wilson D. *Nursing Care of Infants and Children.* 10th ed. St. Louis: Mosby/Elsevier; 2015.)

Clinical Findings

History

- Cyanosis is immediately evident by 1 hour of birth (approximately half) or within the first day after birth. Because d-TGA allows mixing of oxygenated and unoxygenated blood, occasionally less cyanotic infants may present as late as 3 months old.
- CHF symptoms may be present.
- Affected infants are often large for gestational age with retardation of growth and development after the neonatal period.

Physical Examination. Infants may have no murmur at birth or may have a murmur characteristic of associated lesions, such as VSD, ASD, or PDA. The S_2 is loud and single because of the anatomic placement of the great arteries.

Diagnostic Studies

- Chest radiography and ECG findings may be normal in the early newborn period, or the heart may appear egg shaped.
- ECG findings show right axis deviation and right ventricular hypertrophy.
- Echocardiography shows the pulmonary artery arising from the left ventricle and the aorta arising from the right.

Management

- Immediate referral to a pediatric cardiac center is necessary. Correction of electrolyte and acid-base imbalance may be necessary.
- Intravenous PGE_1 is given to delay closure or reopen the ductus arteriosus.
- A balloon atrial septostomy may be performed to promote mixing of oxygenated and unoxygenated blood in the atria.
- The arterial switch (Jatene procedure) is usually performed in the first few days of life. If this is not possible, a number of other operations may be performed, such as the Nakaidoh, Damus-Kaye-Stansel, or réparation à l'étage ventriculaire (REV) procedures.
- Children are monitored closely throughout life with annual echocardiogram follow-up.
- SBE prophylaxis precautions are indicated for life.

Prognosis

Without treatment, there is a 50% mortality rate in the first month of life and 90% by the first year. Operative mortality is

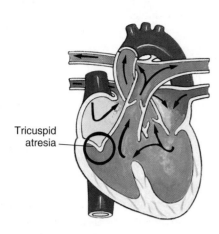

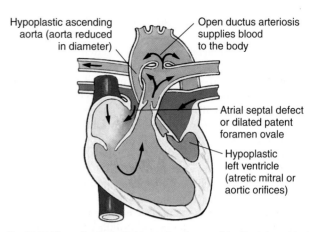

Hypoplastic ascending aorta (aorta reduced in diameter)

Open ductus arteriosis supplies blood to the body

Atrial septal defect or dilated patent foramen ovale

Hypoplastic left ventricle (atretic mitral or aortic orifices)

• **Fig 38.14** Hypoplastic Left Heart Syndrome. (Modified from Hockenberry M, Wilson D. *Nursing Care of Infants and Children.* 10th ed. St. Louis: Mosby/Elsevier; 2015.)

Tricuspid atresia

• **Fig 38.13** Tricuspid Atresia. (Modified from Hockenberry M, Wilson D. *Nursing Care of Infants and Children.* 10th ed. St. Louis: Mosby/Elsevier; 2015.)

from 5% to 17%; there are excellent long-term results after surgery (Tabbutt et al., 2012). However, close monitoring for long-term patency and growth of the coronary arteries is warranted. Neopulmonic stenosis, neoaortic regurgitation, or aortic root dilatation may occur after the arterial switch (McRae, 2015b). Refer any patient with a history of arterial or atrial switch to a pediatric cardiologist, especially with a history of palpitations, syncope, and/or shortness of breath with exertion.

Tricuspid Atresia, Hypoplastic Left Heart Syndrome, and Other Single Ventricle Defects

Tricuspid atresia, pulmonary atresia/intact ventricular septum, and hypoplastic left heart syndrome (HLHS) are the most common types of single ventricle defects. In most cases, there is functionally only one ventricle of either right or left morphology that must do the work of pumping blood to both the systemic and pulmonary circulations. Oxygenated and deoxygenated blood mix in this ventricle, and the child is cyanotic. Most of these children require palliative cardiac procedures to survive.

Tricuspid atresia results in a small right ventricle without access from the right atrium. Blood returning from the systemic circulation must pass over an ASD to the left atrium and then left ventricle before being pumped to either the lungs or the body (Fig 38.13). TGA also occurs in 50% of these patients. Less than 3% of all children with CHD have tricuspid atresia; the etiology is unknown (Park, 2016).

HLHS occurs in less than 1% of congenital heart defects (Park, 2016). Intrauterine stenosis of either the mitral or aortic valves or both, results in a small left ventricle and hypoplasia of the ascending aorta and arch (Fig 38.14). The cause is unknown although it is linked to some genetic syndromes, such as Jacobsen syndrome and Turner syndrome in 10% of cases. Central nervous system abnormalities have also been associated with HLHS (Knirsh, et al., 2016).

Clinical Findings

History. Cyanosis occurs soon after birth with increased respiratory rate, fatigue with the effort of crying, or feeding with subsequent poor weight gain. This often progresses to cardiorespiratory shock as the ductus arteriosus closes.

Physical Examination

• A grade I to III/VI early systolic murmur may be present; usually a single S_2 is heard.
• Cyanosis is generally evident as soon as the ductus arteriosus closes.
• Hepatomegaly (may or may not be present)

Diagnostic Studies

• Heart size on chest radiography is generally normal initially. Cardiomegaly and decreased pulmonary blood flow occur over time.
• ECG findings depend on the type of single ventricle disease but are always abnormal for age. Right ventricular forces are diminished in tricuspid atresia.
• Two-dimensional echocardiography is diagnostic and shows the specifics of the anatomy.

Management

• Intravenous PGE_1 may be indicated in newborns. Most children are initially palliated with aortopulmonary shunts or other procedures depending on their anatomy. At 4 to 6 months old, palliation is continued with a bidirectional anastomosis of the SVC to the pulmonary artery. The third stage of palliation (Fontan procedure) occurs at 2 to 4 years old; the IVC is connected to the pulmonary artery. Some children are considered for cardiac transplantation early in life if their anatomy is not amenable to the Fontan pathway or heart function and pulmonary vascular resistance do not allow completion of palliative staging (Park, 2016).
• Families require support throughout the child's life. Frequent surgeries and hospitalizations can interfere with normal social development. Early recognition and intervention for developmental delays are important.
• SBE prophylaxis is recommended while the child remains cyanotic (see Box 38.3 and Table 38.6).

Complications. Complications include development of collateral arterial and venous vessels, protein-losing enteropathy, arrhythmias, thromboembolic events including strokes, and many others. A decrease in exercise tolerance throughout life can be expected, in addition to left or right ventricular dysfunction. There may be fewer complications with surgical palliation at earlier ages. For those with severe long-term complications, heart transplantation can be an option (McRae, 2015b).

Obstructive Cardiac Lesions

Aortic Stenosis and Insufficiency

Aortic stenosis or narrowing may occur at the aortic valvular, subvalvular, or supravalvular level. Valvular stenosis is the most common form (Fig 38.15). The stenotic aortic valve is usually bicuspid rather than tricuspid. Stenosis causes increased pressure load on the left ventricle leading to LVH and, ultimately, ventricular failure. The imbalance between increased myocardial oxygen demand of hypertrophied myocardium and coronary blood supply may lead to ischemia and fatal ventricular arrhythmias. The bicuspid aortic valve generally becomes more stenotic and often regurgitant (insufficient) over time. Some infants are born with critical aortic stenosis and require urgent intervention, usually a balloon valvuloplasty early in life. Children with only a congenital bicuspid aortic valve and no stenosis or regurgitation are at risk of developing symptoms by adolescence. Aortic stenosis occurs in 3% to 8% of all CHDs, with a male to female ratio of approximately 4:1 (Park, 2016).

Clinical Findings

History

- Growth and development may be normal.
- Activity intolerance, fatigue, chest pain (angina pectoris), or syncope can develop or increase with age.
- CHF, low cardiac output, and shock may be evident in newborns with severe aortic stenosis.
- Sudden death, presumably due to arrhythmias, can occur with increasing severity of stenosis and exertion.

Physical Examination

- BP may reveal a narrow pulse pressure. The apical impulse may be pronounced with moderate to severe stenosis.
- A grade III to IV/VI, loud, harsh systolic crescendo-decrescendo murmur is best heard at the upper right sternal border with radiation to the neck, LLSB, and apex.
- With a valvular lesion, a faint, early systolic click at the LLSB may be heard.
- With aortic insufficiency, an early diastolic blowing murmur is heard at the LLSB to apex.
- In the most severe lesions, S_2 is single or closely split; S_3 or S_4 heart sounds may also be heard.
- A thrill may be present at the suprasternal notch.

Diagnostic Studies

- Chest radiographs are usually normal or may show LVH. Adults frequently develop radiographic evidence of calcification on the aortic valve over time.

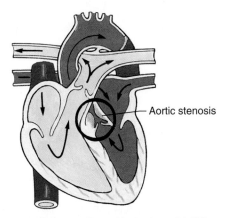

- **Fig 38.15** Aortic Stenosis. (From Hockenberry M, Wilson D. *Nursing Care of Infants and Children.* 10th ed. St. Louis: Mosby/Elsevier; 2015.)

- ECG can be normal or reveal LVH and inverted T waves.
- A 24-hour Holter monitor or 30-day event monitor demonstrates ventricular arrhythmia.
- Echocardiogram is the diagnostic examination of choice.

Management

- The type and timing of treatment depend on the severity of the obstruction.
- Balloon valvuloplasty of the stenotic valve is the initial palliative treatment in the newborn. However, the aortic valve generally needs further intervention.
- In older children, surgical division of fused valve commissures may relieve stenosis but often valve replacement is necessary for severe aortic stenosis and/or insufficiency. Unfortunately, none of the current replacement options are ideal or enduring for children. Mechanical valves are prothrombotic and require anticoagulation with warfarin. Heterograph and homograft valves have limited durability in the aortic position, and the Ross procedure requires placement of the homograft in the pulmonic position, leading to future replacements of that valve as it becomes stenosed (Parks, 2016).
- Children with subaortic stenosis require surgical resection when the gradient is greater than 35 mm Hg.; patients with supravalvar aortic stenosis require resection of the narrowed area with patch material.
- Children with mild aortic stenosis can participate in all sports but should have annual cardiac examinations. Those with moderate aortic stenosis should choose low-intensity sports (such as, golf, bowling, table tennis, or softball) as guided by their cardiologist. Children with severe aortic stenosis or moderate aortic stenosis with symptoms should avoid competitive or intensive sports because of the risk of sudden death from ventricular arrhythmias ⬤ (Park, 2016) (see Chapter 19, Table 19-7-6).
- Any aortic root dilation (commonly seen with bicuspid or stenotic aortic valves) may require intervention to prevent aortic dissection.
- Anticoagulation is necessary with mechanical valve replacement (Park, 2016).

Pulmonic Stenosis

Normally the pulmonary valve opens to allow the flow of blood from the right ventricle into the pulmonary artery. In pulmonic stenosis, there is narrowing at the subpulmonic, valvular, or supravalvular area. Right-sided pressure is increased as the ventricle pumps against the obstruction. Right ventricular hypertrophy occurs as a result of this increased load. Pulmonary stenosis can also occur in the main and/or branch pulmonary arterial system. Mild pulmonic stenosis is usually identified on routine examination. Many of these children also develop poststenotic dilation of the pulmonary artery. Isolated pulmonic stenosis occurs in 8% to 12% of all CHDs (Park, 2016). (See Table 38.7 for associated congenital malformation syndromes.)

Clinical Findings

History

- The child is usually asymptomatic, with a murmur noted on routine physical examination in the newborn to school-age child.
- Exertional dyspnea and fatigue are noticeable as stenosis progresses.
- Cyanosis from right-to-left shunting over the foramen ovale may be evident with critical pulmonic stenosis in the newborn.
- Growth and development are usually normal except in cases of Turner or Noonan syndrome in which short stature is common (Park, 2016).

Physical Examination

- A grade II to IV/VI, harsh, mid- to late systolic ejection murmur is heard at the upper left sternal border over the pulmonic region with transmission along the left sternal border, neck and back, and into both lung fields.
- An intermittent systolic ejection click may be evident in the pulmonic area decreasing with inspiration and increasing with expiration.
- Cyanosis and symptoms of right-sided CHF can occur in severe pulmonic stenosis in the newborn.

Diagnostic Studies

- Chest radiographs may be within normal limits in infants or show prominent main pulmonary artery segments. Right-sided cardiac enlargement and decreased peripheral pulmonary vascular markings may be evident if heart failure develops.
- ECG may be normal with mild stenosis; with moderate to severe pulmonic stenosis, right axis deviation and right ventricular hypertrophy occur.
- Echocardiograms confirm the diagnosis, identifying the gradient and monitoring progression of the stenosis.
- Cardiac catheterization may be used to delineate location of the main and branch pulmonary artery stenosis.

Management

- Balloon valvuloplasty in neonates and older children with stenosis greater than 50 mm Hg are performed. If unsuccessful, surgical valvuloplasty or replacement may be indicated. Stents and balloons are also used for branch stenosis.
- With mild stenosis, families must be encouraged to treat their children normally and not limit their activity. Moderate stenosis can progress to severe narrowing during periods of rapid growth, such as during infancy or adolescence (Park, 2016).
- SBE prophylaxis is not considered necessary except in the 6-month postoperative period or if prosthetic material is used (see Box 38.3).

Coarctation of the Aorta

COA is a narrowing of a small or long segment of the aorta (Fig 38.16). Coarctation may occur as a single defect caused by a disturbance in the development of the aorta or may be secondary to constriction of the ductus arteriosus. The severity of the coarctation, its location, and the degree of obstruction determine the clinical presentation. Systolic and diastolic HTN exists in vessels proximal to the narrowing, whereas hypotension is present in vessels below the narrowing. COA accounts for 8% to 10% of all congenital heart defects and occurs slightly more in males (Park, 2016). Most children with CoA have a bicuspid aortic valve. Other CHD can occur with CoA including abnormalities of the left side of the heart (O'Brien and Marshall, 2015).

Clinical Findings

History. In newborns, COA is not always apparent until the ductus closes and decreases blood flow to the lower body. Severe coarctation in infants is apparent in the first 6 weeks; symptoms include tachypnea, poor feeding, and possibly cool lower extremities. In children 3 to 5 years old, coarctation may go unnoticed until HTN or a murmur is detected. Retrospectively, children with coarctation may have had complaints of headaches or leg pain with exercise (O'Brien and Marshall, 2015).

Physical Examination

- Upper extremity HTN with lower extremity hypotension are present, although milder cases may cause only a minimal discrepancy between upper and lower extremity BPs. In severe cases, poor lower extremity perfusion may be noticed with lower body mottling or pallor.
- Delayed timing and absent or weak arterial and other distal arterial pulses may occur.
- Bounding brachial, radial, and carotid pulses may occur.
- Signs of CHF may be evident.
- A systolic ejection murmur may be detected in the left infraclavicular region with transmission to the back.
- A ventricular heave at the apex may be palpated.
- A gallop rhythm may occur in infants with CHF.

Diagnostic Studies

- Chest radiography may reveal a normal or slightly enlarged heart and normal to increased pulmonary vascular markings; rib notching may be seen.
- ECG findings depend on the severity of the lesion and the age of the child. In infants, right ventricular hypertrophy may be seen; in older children, LVH develops secondary to HTN.
- Echocardiography is helpful in confirming the diagnosis and locating the constricted aortic segment. It may also show associated cardiac abnormalities. In newborns with a PDA, diagnosis by echocardiogram can be challenging.
- MRI can define location, severity, and anatomy of the aortic arch.

Management

- In critical neonatal coarctation, PGE_1 is used to maintain or reopen the ductus.
- If possible, surgical resection of the constricted area and anastomosis of the upper and lower portions of the aorta are performed. Restenosis is more likely to occur if repair was before 1 year of age. Cardiologists may dilate or stent the coarcted area in recoarctation or mild coarctation. Other procedures, including bypass grafting, may be necessary with unusually long coarcted segments. Surgical mortality is rare. Some centers choose balloon valvuloplasty or stent procedures for initial coarctation management (Park, 2016).

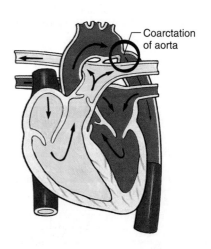

• **Fig 38.16** Coarctation of the Aorta. (From Hockenberry M, Wilson D. *Nursing Care of Infants and Children.* 10th ed. St. Louis: Mosby/Elsevier; 2015.)

- In older children with long-standing HTN, antihypertensive medication may be required for several months after repair (O'Brien and Marshall, 2015). Long-term prognosis is excellent unless there are associated intracardiac defects. BP should be monitored postoperatively for recoarctation.
- Children with previous coarctation repairs may participate in competitive sports if residual BP gradient between arm and legs is less than 20 mm Hg and peak systolic BP is normal at rest and with exercise. However, during the first year after surgery, high-intensity static exercises, such as weight lifting and wrestling, should be avoided (Park, 2016).
- Lifelong follow-up is necessary due to risk of recoarctation, residual HTN, aortic aneurysms, and problems associated with having a bicuspid aortic valve.
- SBE prophylaxis is no longer considered necessary except in the 6-month postoperative period or if prosthetic material is used (see Box 38.3).

Sudden Cardiac Death

The PCP has a responsibility to screen for causes of sudden cardiac death (SCD) whenever performing a sports physical examination or assessing a complaint of chest pain, syncope, or palpitations. This can be a daunting challenge because none of the common causes of SCD are easily diagnosed by history or examination. In the United States, the incidence of SCD (excludes sudden infant death syndrome) for ages 1 to 35 years is 0.8 to 2.8 per 1,000,000 person-years (Aro and Chugh, 2017). The most frequent cause of exercise-related SCD is cardiomyopathy, especially hypertrophic cardiomyopathy (HCM), and, to a lesser extent, arrhythmogenic right ventricular cardiomyopathy (Chandra et al., 2013). Both are inherited, structural abnormalities of the myocardium resulting in ventricular arrhythmias leading to death.

Other congenital structural abnormalities that can cause sudden death include coronary artery anomalies, aortic dissection/rupture (usually seen in children with Marfan syndrome), mitral valve prolapse, and aortic stenosis. Congenital, electrical cardiac abnormalities can also cause SCD, including Wolff-Parkinson-White syndrome, congenital long QT syndromes, and Brugada syndrome (Aro and Chugh, 2017).

Sudden death from acquired cardiac abnormalities include commotio cordis from blunt, nonpenetrating trauma to the midchest (e.g., blow by a baseball or other object), myocarditis, performance-enhancing drugs, and premature coronary artery disease due to familial hypercholesterolemia (Aro and Chugh, 2017). Commotio cordis triggers ventricular fibrillation and SCD as a result of the blow during the timing of the T wave in the cardiac cycle.

Clinical Findings

Hypertrophic and arrhythmogenic right ventricular cardiomyopathy present with a history of syncope and a family history of either of these conditions. Most individuals are asymptomatic, and arrhythmogenic right ventricular cardiomyopathy is more likely to occur in males beginning around age 15 years. There may be reports of shortness of breath with activity, palpitations, dizziness/lightheadedness, fatigue, and chest pain/pressure with or without activity. Arrhythmias and shortness of breath with exertion may be found in both conditions. Patients with HCM may have a dynamic murmur (late systolic ejection) and forceful apical beat. See Chapter 19 ⬤Box 19.8 for the 14-element cardiovascular

screening checklist to use during the pre-participation physical examination for sports.

Diagnostic Studies

- Hypertrophic cardiomyopathy: Abnormal ECG (greater than 90% have an abnormal resting ECG), sustained or nonsustained ventricular tachycardia on Holter or 30-day event monitor, severe LVH on echocardiogram, and an attenuated BP response to exercise.
- Arrhythmogenic right ventricular cardiomyopathy: Changes seen with resting/ambulatory ECG and on echocardiographic and cardiac MRI studies.

Management

Cardiology referral is indicated for all children with a family history of SCD; inheritable cardiomyopathies; Marfan syndrome; chest pain of concern; syncope; acquired cardiac disease, such as Kawasaki disease; and those with known CHD, cardiac rhythm disturbances, or palpitations.

Long-Term Complications for Children and Young Adults With Congenital Heart Disease: Transitioning to Adult Care

As children grow into adulthood, they are vulnerable to a host of long-term complications depending on their particular disease, repair, and residual lesions. Because of the success of pediatric cardiac surgery, 90% of children born with CHD live to adulthood. As a result, there are currently more adults with CHD than children. The adult congenital heart disease (ACHD) population exceeds 1.4 million individuals in the United States and is expected to grow by 5% annually (Thakkar, Chinnadurai, and Lin, 2017).

Not all surgeries performed during childhood are corrective. Many surgeries are palliative or incompletely corrective with residual problems. Thus these individuals continue to require close supervision to assess their cardiac function and need for further interventions. Despite published guidelines by the AAP and AHA concerning the need for transition of care, research indicates adults with CHD are lost to follow-up due to lack of resources and accessibility (Thakkar et al., 2017). The particular problems faced by adolescents or adults with CHD are beyond the scope of this text; however, key points in the evaluation of an older child, adolescent, or young adult with CHD are detailed in Box 38.5 (Zaidi and Daniels, 2013).

Acquired Heart Disease

Chest Pain

Chest pain in children is a common complaint but represents a serious cardiovascular problem in no more than 5% of cases (Park, 2016). Although children of all ages can have chest pain, it is the young adolescent who most frequently presents to the emergency department or PCP with this complaint. The first goal of chest pain evaluation is to rule out cardiac causes, which are also the main concern of most children and their parents. Table 38.9 lists possible cardiac causes of chest pain, history, and examination findings.

The most frequent cause of chest pain is musculoskeletal, originating in the chest wall or chest cage, is benign, and rarely requires any treatment. Chest wall pain, particularly with exercise, may indicate exercise-induced bronchospasm but rarely indicates

• BOX 38.5 **Key Points in the Evaluation of Congenital Heart Disease in the Older Child, Adolescent, and Young Adult**

- Left-sided lesions: Those with a history of bicuspid aortic valves, subaortic stenosis, aortic valve stenosis, coarctation, or aortic aneurysm may worsen over time and present with significant stenosis or regurgitation. Symptoms include exercise intolerance, dyspnea on exertion, or atypical chest pain. Problems include arrhythmias, sudden death, endocarditis, syncope, and angina.
- Left-to-right shunt lesions: Repaired or unrepaired atrial or VSDs, AV septal defect, aortopulmonary window (a hole between the aorta and the pulmonary artery), or coronary sinus fistulas may be hemodynamically significant and lead to elevated pulmonary vascular resistance (right-to-left shunting through a lesion due to elevated pulmonary vascular resistance). Symptoms include arrhythmias, dyspnea on exertion, unexplained deterioration of left ventricular function, and/or left ventricular dilation. If left untreated, left-to-right shunts lead to overloading and remodeling of the pulmonary vasculature and eventually pulmonary arterial hypertension (PAH) (Thakkar et al., 2017). The type of PAH determines the operability of shunt lesions. If PAH is fixed (Eisenmenger syndrome), patients are not surgical candidates.
- Chronic cyanosis: In addition to left-to-right shunt lesions causing Eisenmenger syndrome, chronic cyanosis can also result from defects causing right ventricular outflow obstruction, baffle leaks (can occur after certain surgical procedures to correct TGA), or palliation for a single ventricle. Chronic hypoxia to vital organs, hyperviscosity, and hematologic problems (e.g., thrombocytopenia, erythrocytosis, thromboemboli, iron deficiency, and bleeding) can result.
- Valvar problems: Besides aortic stenosis, other long-term valve abnormalities can include mitral valve prolapse (causes mitral regurgitation) and/or pulmonary valve stenosis or regurgitation (more frequent in those with repaired TOF). Pulmonic stenosis or regurgitation can cause right ventricular remodeling, decreased exercise intolerance, arrhythmias, and sudden death (Thakkar et al., 2017).
- Heart failure: Can occur via many different pathways depending on the underlying disease and previous interventions. It is the leading cause of death in patients with ACHD (Thakkar et al., 2017). Prolonged aortic or pulmonic valvar stenosis or regurgitation is a common mechanism for failure. In single ventricle patients, the development of systemic venous collateral vessels or arteriovenous pulmonary fistulas can increase ventricular volumes. Over time, these hemodynamic problems can lead to chronic cyanosis, myocardial ischemia, poor ventricular compliance, and serious ventricular arrhythmias. Management of each problem is challenging; ultimately, a heart transplant may be required.
- Arrhythmias and heart blocks: The risk of sudden cardiac death (SCD) is the most significant complication facing adults with CHD. Congenital diagnoses at greatest risk for subsequent SCD include coarctation of the aorta, TOF, aortic stenosis, and d-TGA with aortic stenosis, and TGA. Single ventricle patients with a Fontan procedure are also at increased risk for arrhythmias. Rhythm disturbances can occur as a result of long-standing cyanosis, the aforementioned chamber dilation, increased atrial pressures, dysfunction of the sinus node, and extensive fibrotic suture lines (Thakkar et al., 2017). Management is complex. Although episodes of palpitations or chest pain may bring those with CHD into care, they need to be referred to cardiology specialists.

ACHD, *Adult congenital heart disease;* AV, *atrioventricular;* d-TGA, *dextro-transposition of the great arteries;* SCD, *sudden cardiac death;* TOF, *tetralogy of Fallot;* VSD, *ventricular septal defect.*

cardiac disease. Chronic chest pain that is vague and occurs over many months in a variety of circumstances, particularly around stressful events, may be psychogenic (anxiety or hyperventilation). Chest pain associated with syncope, exertional dyspnea, or irregularities in heart rhythm needs careful evaluation for a cardiac

cause. Children or adolescents who have pain of cardiac origin usually describe a specific history with details that are consistent from event to event (Park, 2016).

Clinical Findings

History. A careful history and a thorough physical examination are especially important in assessing this complaint.
- Past medical history or family history of sudden death (including drownings), heart disease or condition, asthma, eczema, Marfan syndrome, sickle cell disease
- Sports, exercise, and activity history
- Previous trauma or muscle strains
- Characteristics of chest pain:
  - Relationship of pain to exercise; any syncope, exertional dyspnea, or wheezing
  - Any burning, substernal pain that worsens with reclining or with spicy foods (gastrointestinal etiology)
  - Pain that is sharp or stabbing, lasting several seconds to minutes, located over the midsternum or infranipple area, and occurring with nonexertion or deep inspirations (more likely musculoskeletal in origin)
  - Pain that awakens the patient (more likely organic)
- Any other associated symptoms, such as fever, nausea, vomiting, headaches, or choking episodes
- Any recent, major stressful events
- Medication, tobacco, or other drug use, including oral contraceptives (embolism)

Physical Examination. A complete chest (lungs and heart) and abdominal examination should be performed. Key findings to focus on include the presence of the following:
- Cardiac murmur, rubs, or clicks
- Point tenderness of one or more costochondral joints exaggerated with physical activity or deep inspirations (suggests costochondritis or Tietze syndrome [if associated with warmth, swelling, or tenderness over costochondral junction]): Use the middle fingertip to palpate each costochondral and chondrosternal junction for tenderness to avoid missing this finding. Tenderness and swelling may also be found in pectoral and shoulder carriage muscles due to overuse by excessive weight lifting or excessive electronic game playing.
- Irregular heart rhythm (cardiac disease)
- Rales, wheezing, tachypnea, decreased breath sounds (pulmonary disease)

Diagnostic Studies. In most cases the history and physical are necessary to make the diagnosis; other tests are not indicated unless the following problems are suspected:
- Febrile, cardiac, or pulmonary condition: Obtain a chest radiograph.
- Exercise-induced asthma: Perform a pulmonary function test with exercise.
- Rhythm disturbance: Order a 24-hour Holter or 30-day event monitor or stress test (or both).
- Signs of CHD, pericarditis, or myocarditis: Order an ECG and perhaps a chest radiograph.

Differential Diagnosis

Chest pain of musculoskeletal origin includes costochondritis, Tietze syndrome, idiopathic chest pain, precordial catch syndrome, slipping rib syndrome, hypersensitive xiphoid syndrome, trauma, and muscle strain. Esophagitis, esophageal foreign body ingestion, and exercise-induced bronchospasm are additional differential diagnoses.

TABLE 38.9	Cardiac Causes of Chest Pain and Associated Findings			
Condition	History	Physical Exam	Electrocardiogram	Chest Radiograph
Abnormal coronaries due to Kawasaki disease or other coronary artery disease	Previous history consistent with disease; typical exercise anginal pain	Usually normal; continuous murmur or possible fistulae	ST segment elevation ± myocardial infarction findings	Normal
Cocaine abuse	History of substance abuse	Hypertension; tachycardia	ST elevation ±	Normal
Pericarditis and myocarditis	History of URI ± sharp chest pain	Friction rub; muffled heart sounds	Low QRS voltages; ST segment shift	Cardiomegaly
Postpericardiotomy syndrome	Recent heart surgery; pain positional	Muffled heart sounds; rub	ST segment elevation	Cardiomegaly
Arrhythmia	May have history of Wolff-Parkinson-White or long QT syndrome	Normal to irregular heart rate	Preexcitation, long QT, or normal QT	Normal
Aortic stenosis (severe)	History of aortic stenosis	Loud SEM at USB radiating to neck	LVH with or without strain	Prominent ascending aorta and aortic knob
Pulmonary stenosis (severe)	History of pulmonary stenosis	Loud SEM at ULSB	RVH with or without strain	Prominent PA segment
Hypertrophic cardiomyopathy (HCM)	Positive family history (in ⅓ of patients)	Variable murmur	LVH; deep Q/small R or QS in LPLs	Mild cardiomegaly
Mitral valve prolapse	Positive family history	Midsystolic click; thin; thoracic skeletal abnormalities	Inverted T waves in aVF	Normal except skeletal anomalies
Eisenmenger syndrome (untreated or untreatable congenital heart disease [CHD])	History of congenital heart disease	Cyanosis, clubbing, loud S₂	Right ventricular hypertrophy	Prominent PA; normal heart size

aVF, Augmented vector right; *LPL,* lateral precordial leads; *LVH,* left ventricular hypertrophy; *PA,* pulmonary artery; *RVH,* right ventricular hypertrophy; *SEM,* systolic ejection murmur; *ULSB,* upper left sternal border; *URI,* upper respiratory infection; *USB,* upper sternal border.

Adapted from Park M. *Park's Pediatric Cardiology Handbook.* 5th ed. Philadelphia: Mosby/Elsevier; 2016.

Management

When chest pain has no clear etiology, the child appears well, and all aspects of the evaluation are normal, reassurance can be the most important treatment. Refer any child to a pediatric cardiology with chest pain that worsens with exercise or suggests angina, where there are positive findings on examination, ECG, or chest radiograph, or a concerning personal or family history. Musculoskeletal causes usually respond to nonsteroidal antiinflammatory drug (NSAID) treatment and rest.

Hypertension

Normal BP in children younger than 13 years of age is defined as systolic and diastolic BP less than the 90th percentile for age, sex, and height. HTN in children younger than 13 years of age is defined as a systolic or diastolic (or both) BP in the 95th or higher percentile for age, sex, and height on at least three separate occasions. Elevated BP is defined as average systolic or diastolic BP greater than 90th and 95th percentile. For adolescents older than 13 years of age, systolic and/or diastolic BP ≥120/80 to 129/<80 mm Hg is considered elevated, whereas ≥130/80 mm Hg is considered hypertensive. For children younger than 13 years of age, stage 1 HTN is BP between the 95th and 99th percentiles for age, sex, and height. Stage 2 HTN is BP 5 mm Hg or higher or greater

than the 99th percentile. For adolescents 13 years or older: Stage I is systolic and/or diastolic BP ≥130/80 to 139/89 mm Hg and stage II is systolic and or diastolic BP ≥140/90 mm Hg (Flynn et al., 2017).

HTN is a significant problem affecting more males (15% to 19%) than females (7% to 12%) (Flynn et al, 2017). HTN is higher in Hispanic and African-American children. Increasingly, children have high BP associated with obesity, sedentary lifestyles, and stress. Secondary HTN is more common in children younger than 6 years old (usually at significant or severe HTN levels). The primary cause of secondary, severe HTN is renovascular or parenchymal renal diseases. Other causes include coarctation of aorta, endocrine disorders, genetic disorders such as Williams syndrome, neurofibromatosis and tuberous sclerosis, drugs, and central nervous system tumors. Primary HTN onset is more likely to occur after 10 years old. Neonates with HTN are generally severely ill with neurologic, cardiac, and renal symptoms (Flynn et al., 2017).

Clinical Findings

The goal of the clinical history and physical examination is to assess whether HTN is primary or secondary to renal disease or other causes. If secondary HTN is ruled out, then the evaluation must focus on the comorbidities of primary HTN. With both types of HTN, the PCP must assess for signs of end-organ damage from prolonged HTN (Flynn et al., 2017).

History. Inquire about:
- Neonatal history of prolonged mechanical ventilation, umbilical catheterization, prematurity, or small for gestational age at birth. Poor maternal nutrition and high stress appear to have an epigenetic effect on the embryo, making HTN more likely for the child (Cowley et al., 2012).
- Cause of any prior hospitalizations
- Trauma
- Diet, physical activities, and other habits (e.g., smoking, drinking, substance abuse)
- Sleep history, particularly symptoms of sleep apnea
- Medications taken, including oral contraceptives, cold medications, steroids, and diet aids
- Chronic illness, especially renal disease, past history of urinary tract infections, diabetes, or seizures
- Headache, chest pain, dyspnea, muscle weakness, palpitations, abdominal pain, facial palsy, decreased vision, excessive sweating
- Family history of a first-degree relative with myocardial infarction (especially before 50 years old), stroke, HTN, diabetes, hyperlipidemia, SCD, polycystic kidney disease, neurofibromatosis, pheochromocytoma, or obesity (Flynn et al., 2017).

Physical Examination. Note the following:
- Body habitus, especially overweight (body mass index [BMI]), poor growth (height, weight), signs of metabolic syndrome
- Dysmorphic features
- Edema, pallor, flushing, or skin lesions suggestive of tuberous sclerosis, systemic lupus erythematosus, neurofibromatosis
- Upper and lower extremity central pulses; absent, diminished, or pounding pulses in all extremities
- Fundi abnormalities, enlarged thyroid gland, abdominal mass, flank bruit; decreased visual acuity, facial palsy
- Elevated BP on at least three separate occasions

Diagnostic Studies
- Laboratory evaluation of stage 1 or 2 HTN should focus on searching for causes of secondary HTN, comorbidities of primary HTN, and target organ damage of either primary or secondary HTN. The search for secondary causes of HTN needs to be individualized based upon age, history, physical examination, and extent of BP elevation. Because the majority of children have renal or renovascular causes for BP elevation, initial laboratory studies should include tests for renal function and plasma renin levels (Flynn et al., 2017).
- Children younger than 10 years old with stage 2 HTN require more aggressive laboratory evaluation compared with older children with stage 1 HTN and obesity. CBC, erythrocyte sedimentation rate (ESR), C-reactive protein (CRP), urinalysis and culture, electrolytes, blood urea nitrogen, creatinine, and plasma renin levels are screening studies for the most common secondary causes of HTN. If renal vascular disease is suspected, the work-up is best managed by a nephrologist with renal nuclear medicine scans and renal ultrasound or newer technologies, such as MRI and spiral computed tomography (CT), which are replacing angiography.
- Additional organ assessments include echocardiography for LVH and COA and a thorough ophthalmologic examination.

Management

Algorithms that categorize and illustrate management of children with high BP are found in Figs 38.17 and 38.18.

- BP measurements should be done annually on all children 3 years and older, with baseline and serial measurements documented in the child's record. Standardized BP norms are available (see Tables 38.2 and 38.3).
- Elevated BP: At least two follow-up BP measurements should be taken within 1 to 2 months of the initial reading to determine whether a high reading is a single, isolated event. If subsequent readings fall to less than the 95th percentile, the child should continue with routine BP checks during annual visits.
- HTN secondary to overweight can be as serious as HTN secondary to other organic disease and should be treated as such. For those with high-normal BP without any indication of organic disease, treatment should consist of nonpharmacologic intervention—diet, exercise, and weight management. Caloric restriction with exercise is more effective than caloric restriction alone (Flynn et at., 2017). Recommendations should include the following:
  - Dietary intervention to control or reduce overweight (Flynn et al., 2017). High-sodium foods and sodium supplements should be eliminated.
  - Increase physical exercise and sports participation to 30 to 60 minutes a day balanced with relaxation techniques. Aerobic, not static or isometric exercise, is recommended.
  - Avoid smoking, caffeine, alcoholic beverages, and illicit drug consumption.
- If the BP elevation persists, referral should be made to a nephrologist or cardiologist experienced in using antihypertensive agents in children. Children with confirmed BP equal to or greater than the 99th percentile should have immediate referral (Flynn et al., 2017).
- The goal is to reduce systolic or diastolic BP to less than the 95th percentile. If a concurrent condition exists, the goal becomes reducing BP to the 90th percentile.
- Medication initiation is usually done by cardiology. Management starts with a single drug (usually an ACE inhibitor, angiotensin receptor blocker [ARB], β-blocker, long-acting calcium channel blocker, or a thiazide diuretic) at the lowest recommended dose and advanced until the desired BP is reached. If maximum dose or adverse side effects are reached, a second medication should be added. Step-down therapy may be possible for overweight children who lose weight and achieve BP goals. Studies of antihypertensives in children indicate racial differences may exist in the medication effect of ACE inhibitors (Flynn et al., 2017).

Complications

Long-term BP elevation leads to an increase in left ventricular mass, increased carotid intimal medial thickness, and coronary artery calcification, especially if combined with overweight, lipid and lipoprotein abnormalities, and tobacco use. There are some indications of cognitive impairments in children with HTN as well (Flynn et al., 2017). Yearly echocardiograms are recommended to evaluate LVH.

Patient and Family Education

Because much of HTN is related to lifestyle, prevention through optimal health promotion and maintenance is essential. Regular health maintenance including evaluation of BP and health education regarding risk factors is critical. Counseling should emphasize both behavioral modification and parental involvement. Decreasing BMI and increasing aerobic fitness have been shown to reduce

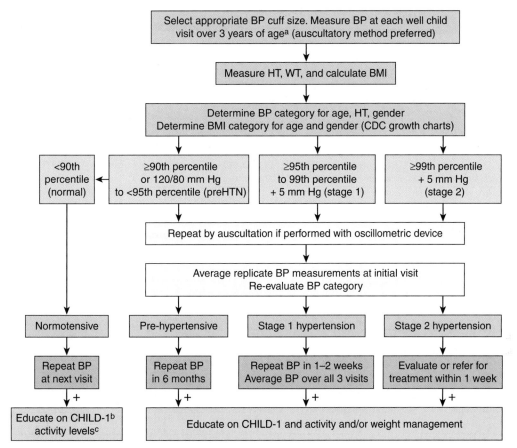

• **Fig 38.17** Blood pressure *(BP)* measurement and categorization algorithm. [a]See Tables 38.2 and 38.3. [b]Cardiovascular health integrated lifestyle diet *(CHILD-1)* recommended (see Section 5, "Nutrition and Diet" in the NHLBI reference for these nutrition and diet recommendations). [c]See Section 6, "Physical Activity" in the NHLBI reference for physical activity recommendations. [d]See Section 10, "Overweight and Obesity" in the NHLBI reference for discussion regarding overweight and obesity. *BMI,* Body mass index; *CDC,* Centers of Disease Control and Prevention; *HT,* height; *HTN,* hypertension; *WT,* weight. (From National Heart, Lung, and Blood Institute [NHLBI]. *Expert Panel on Integrated Guidelines for Cardiovascular Health and Risk Reduction in Children and Adolescents: Full Report;* 2012. www.nhlbi.nih.gov/files/docs/guidelines/peds_guidelines_full.pdf. Accessed January 20, 2018, Fig 8.1, p 84.)

elevations in age-related BP. Preventive measures include the following:

- Good nutrition with a decrease in dietary fat and sodium
- Prevention of overweight with diet and aerobic exercise for at least 30 minutes daily
- Stress management
- Avoidance of caffeine, tobacco use, and prescription or over-the-counter medications that can exacerbate high BP (e.g., cold medications with ephedrine or phenylephrine, steroids)
- Monitoring BP if oral contraceptives are used

Infective Endocarditis

IE (also known as SBE) is a condition in which a bacterial or fungal infection invades endocardial surfaces of the heart. Turbulence caused by stenotic cardiac valves, previous surgical repairs, or high-velocity jets (from blood flowing under force through a structural heart defect) traumatizes cardiac endothelium and leads to thrombogenesis. Clumps of platelets and fibrin provide a nidus for circulating bacteria or rarely fungi. The bacteria or fungi multiply, shielded from circulating white cells by the platelet-fibrin matrix.

These vegetations cause further damage by destroying nearby valve tissue and extend into surrounding endothelium (Park, 2016).

Infection can occur in any age group but is rare in those without structural heart disease. The incidence of IE has increased as more children with CHD are surviving due to improved surgical interventions. In developing countries where there is a high prevalence of rheumatic heart disease (RHD), there is a concurrent increase in IE (Bizmark, Chang, Tsugawa, Zangwill, and Kawachi, 2017). Gram-positive cocci cause 80% of cases of IE in children. *Staphylococcus aureus* is the most common causative organism, followed by *Streptococcus viridans* (Dixon and Christov, 2017). A group of gram-negative bacilli referred to as *HACEK* (**H**aemophilus species [*H. parainfluenzae, H. aprophilus,* and *H. paraphrophilus*], **A**ctinobacillus actinomycetemcomitans, **C**ardiobacterium hominis, **E**ikenella corrodens, and **K**ingella species) are less common (Park, 2016). Children with CHD have more severe gingival inflammatory conditions, increased plaque accumulation, and more HACEK microbes, which lead to endocarditis. Fungal endocarditis is the most severe form, with increased mortality rates in immunocompromised children and neonates (Gewitz and Taubert, 2013).

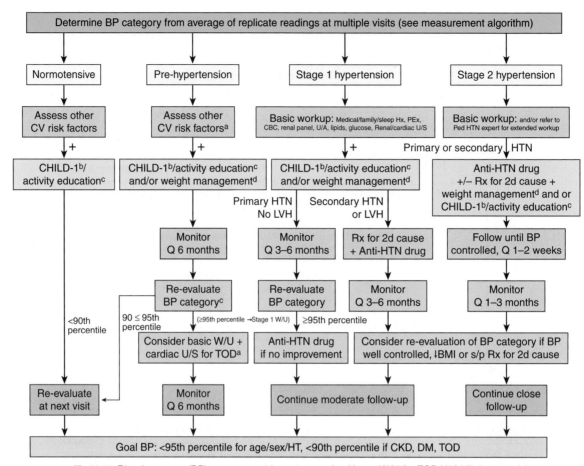

• **Fig 38.18** Blood pressure *(BP)* management by category algorithm. [a]W/U for TOD/ LVH if obese or (+) for other CV risk factors. [b]Cardiovascular health integrated lifestyle diet *(CHILD-1)* (see Section 5, "Nutrition and Diet" in the NHLBI reference). [c]Activity education (see Section 6, "Physical Activity" in the NHLBI reference). [d]Weight management for overweight and obesity (see Section 10, "Overweight and Obesity" in the NHLBI reference). *2d,* Secondary; *Anti-HTN,* antihypertensive; *BMI,* body mass index; *CBC,* complete blood count; *CKD,* chronic kidney disease; *CV,* cardiovascular; *DM,* diabetes mellitus; *HT,* height; *HTN,* hypertension; *Hx,* history; *LVH,* left ventricular hypertrophy; *Ped,* pediatric; *PEx,* physical examination; *Q,* every; *Rx,* prescription; *s/p,* status post; *TOD,* target organ damage; *U/A,* urinalysis; *U/S,* ultrasound; *W/U,* work-up. (From National Heart, Lung, and Blood Institute [NHLBI]. *Expert Panel on Integrated Guidelines for Cardiovascular Health and Risk Reduction in Children and Adolescents: Full Report;* 2012. www.nhlbi.nih.gov/files/docs/guidelines/peds_guidelines_full.pdf. Accessed November 3, 2014, Fig 8.2, p 84.)

Clinical Findings

History and Physical Examination

- History of underlying structural cardiac abnormality(ies), palliative surgery for cyanotic heart disease, prosthetic aortic valve replacements, or indwelling catheters and devices (these may have been used for oncologic or neonatologic purposes)
- Any dental procedures or oral surgery that may have caused gingival or mucosal bleeding in the past
- Intravenous drug use
- Acute manifestations: Short duration of illness, prolonged low-grade fever (101°F to 103°F [38.3°C to 39.4°C]), myalgias, night sweats, arthralgias, headache, general malaise, decreased appetite, increase in intensity of preexisting murmur, or new onset murmur (Park, 2016).
- Subacute manifestations: Low-grade or relapsing fever, progressive nonspecific symptoms (e.g., myalgias, arthralgias, headache, and general malaise)

- Neonates: Symptoms may range from relatively few to systemic hypotension, respiratory distress or other generalized signs of sepsis, and neurologic findings
- Evidence of dental caries and/or periodontal or gingival disease
- Embolization symptoms: Hematuria, acute onset of respiratory distress, splenomegaly, neurologic changes (stroke, brain abscesses, hemorrhage, meningitis), petechiae (in conjunctiva, buccal mucosa, palatal area, nailbeds, palms, and soles). The classical findings—Janeway lesions (flat, nontender lesions on palms and soles), Osler nodes (small raised lesions on pad of fingers and toes), Roth spots (retinal hemorrhages with a central white spot), and splinter hemorrhages—occur rarely in children (Park, 2016).

Diagnostic Studies

- The diagnosis is based on clinical findings and results of blood cultures. A persistent low-grade fever in a child with known cardiac abnormalities should be evaluated immediately with three sets of blood cultures over 24 hours from different sites before the administration of empirical antibiotic therapy (Dixon and Chrisov, 2017) ●. When three cultures are positive for the same organism, IE must be considered and treatment instituted. Greater than 90% of those without prior antibiotic treatment will have a positive blood culture (Park, 2016).

- Some children have blood culture–negative endocarditis due to prior antibiotic administration, poor culture techniques, or fastidious organisms (Dixon and Chrisov, 2017).
- The ESR, CRP, and white blood cell (WBC) count are elevated in the acute stage; anemia may be evident.
- Two-dimensional echocardiography is the main modality for detecting infection (Dixon and Christov, 2017).

Differential Diagnosis

The differential diagnoses include postoperative fever, collagen vascular diseases, and childhood cancers.

Management and Complications

●All children with suspected IE should be hospitalized and referred to pediatric cardiology. Treatment should begin as soon as IE is suspected, to decrease the morbidity and mortality associated with untreated bacteremia. Give high doses of appropriate antibiotics intravenously for 4 to 6 weeks (Park, 2016).

IE can lead to destruction of heart valves or disseminated sepsis. Septic and thrombotic emboli from bacterial or fungal vegetations can cause abscesses and ischemic damage to distant areas, such as the brain, abdominal viscera, and extremities (Dixon and Christov, 2017).

Patient and Family Education

For children with high-risk cardiac conditions (previous endocarditis; unrepaired or palliated cyanotic CHD; prosthetic or bioprosthetic valve, shunt, or conduit; repaired CHD with residual defects adjacent to the site of the prosthetic patch or device; and heart transplant recipients), prophylactic antibiotic therapy is given before all dental procedures involving manipulation of gingival tissue (see Box 38.3 and Table 38.6) (Dixon and Christov, 2017).

Myocarditis

Myocarditis is a rare inflammatory illness of the muscular walls of the heart. It may go unrecognized in children whose inflammatory process resolves spontaneously, or it may progress to fulminant disease resulting in chronic cardiomyopathy or death. Myocarditis is often caused by viral infections, most commonly adenoviruses, coxsackievirus A and B, parvovirus B19, echoviruses, and poliovirus. Influenza, cytomegalovirus (CMV), varicella, mumps, human immunodeficiency virus (HIV), RSV, and rubella are other viral causes. Nonviral infections (fungal, bacterial, protozoal, and rickettsial), various medications, autoimmune or inflammatory disorders (e.g., acute rheumatic fever, systemic lupus erythematosus), toxic reactions to infectious agents, or other disorders (e.g., Kawasaki disease) can also be causative factors; however, the etiology is often unknown. Myocarditis may occur in epidemics, usually in infants in association with coxsackievirus B. In Central and South America, myocarditis is commonly caused by Chagas' disease, a protozoal infection with *Trypanosoma cruzi* (Canter and Simpson, 2014).

The inflammatory process in the myocardium leads to dilation of all cardiac chambers, especially the left ventricle, which results in poor function and stretching of mitral annulus with regurgitation. The healing process may lead to replacement of myofibers with fibroblasts and scar formation. Scarring decreases elasticity and performance and creates the substrate for ventricular arrhythmias. Myocarditis causes approximately 9% of sudden death in young athletes (Canter and Simpson, 2014).

Clinical Findings

History. As the interstitial inflammation process progresses, cardiac function decreases and symptoms of CHF become evident. The following history is characteristic:

- Infants (may be manifesting intrauterine exposure): Fever, irritability or listlessness, episodes of pallor, diaphoresis; tachypnea or respiratory distress; poor appetite and vomiting
- Children and adolescents: Recent flulike or gastrointestinal viral illness (10 to 14 days previously); lethargy, low-grade fever, pallor; decreased appetite and abdominal pain; exercise intolerance, rashes, palpitations, respiratory distress (late finding)

Physical Examination

- Pallor, mild cyanosis, skin cool and mottled with poor perfusion (in infants)
- Rapid, labored respirations, grunting, decreased pulse oximetry reading
- Tachycardia, gallop rhythm, muffled heart sounds, apical systolic murmur, weak pulses
- Hepatomegaly, jugular venous distention (older children and adolescents)

Diagnostic Studies. ●Refer children with symptoms suggestive of myocarditis to a pediatric cardiologist. Diagnostic testing involves chest radiography, ECG, two-dimensional echocardiography, MRI, CBC, ESR, CRP, cardiac and liver enzymes, B-type natriuretic peptide, viral titers, blood cultures, metabolic studies (e.g., thyroid and carnitine), and viral cultures or polymerase chain reaction (PCR) from the myocardial tissue (Canter and Simpson, 2014).

Differential Diagnosis

Sepsis, asthma, recurrent vomiting, and chronic viral illness are in the differential diagnosis.

Management

Treatment is supportive with bed rest and medications, such as diuretics, ACE inhibitors, and carvedilol. Occasionally, anticoagulation and antiarrhythmia medications may be used. New modes of therapies, including the use of immunomodulators and antiviral therapy, are under investigation (Canter and Simpson, 2014). Severe cases may require mechanical ventilation, inotropic support, and mechanical circulatory assistance (Xiong, Xia, Zhu, Li, and Huang, 2017). Recovery often takes 2 to 3 months; follow-up is lifelong.

Complications and Prognosis

Pericardial effusion and pericarditis can occur concurrently. Scarring of the myocardium can be a complication and cause persistent heart failure and ventricular arrhythmias. Cardiac transplantation may be necessary in some children with myocarditis. However, approximately 50% of children progress to complete recovery (Canter and Simpson, 2014).

Pericarditis

Pericarditis refers to an inflammation or other abnormality of the pericardium, the sac surrounding the heart. Excess fluid accumulates in the pericardial space and causes the normally compliant pericardium to distend. As intrapericardial pressure increases, the heart becomes compressed and limits its ability to fill. Pericarditis may be seen in children without a history of cardiac disease. Viral infection (especially with coxsackievirus and adenovirus) is the most common cause of pericarditis in infants and children. Other etiologic agents include infections (tuberculosis, other bacteria), trauma, hypersensitivity to medication (isoniazid [INH], hydralazine), collagen-vascular and connective tissue diseases (acute rheumatic fever, juvenile rheumatoid arthritis, and systemic lupus erythematosus), Kawasaki disease, postsurgical complications, and complications of systemic infection (Park, 2016).

Pericarditis is a serious illness that may have rapidly fatal consequences if not diagnosed and treated in a timely manner. The following findings should alert the provider to refer the patient to a pediatric cardiologist:

- History of: precordial or substernal chest pain altered by respiration, coughing, or position (may not be found in small children); lethargy, loss of appetite, abdominal pain; fever, irritability; tachycardia; viral illness 10 to 14 days before onset of symptoms
- Physical examination findings: Distended neck veins; tachycardia, pericardial friction rub (an early sign heard best along the left sternal border with the child leaning forward) or muffled heart sounds (if the effusion is large); Kussmaul sign (slow, deep respirations); pulsus paradoxus, a decrease in BP of greater than 10 mm Hg during inspiration when in a supine position; hepatomegaly
- ECG shows diffuse ST segment elevation (80%), PR depression, and T wave inversion
- Chest x-ray may show enlargement of cardiac silhouette
- Echocardiogram shows relative quantities of pericardial fluid and compression of cavities if large effusion is seen

Pericarditis requires inpatient management. Cardiac tamponade can occur with large or rapid effusions. There is a relapse rate of 15% if the causative agent was viral. Most children recover fully within 3 to 4 weeks. Myocarditis is the main differential diagnosis (Park, 2016).

Heart Conduction Disturbances

Cardiac Arrhythmias

Arrhythmias can manifest as a primary disorder or as a consequence of cardiac or other systemic disorders. Some of the more common arrhythmias are described in Box 38.6. (Table 38.1 has normal heart rates.)

Clinical Findings

Slow or fast heart rate; rhythm—regular, irregular, or regularly irregular. Arrhythmias can be accompanied by symptoms of feeding difficulties in infants and exercise intolerance in older children (Baruteau, Perry, Sanatani, Horie, and Dublin, 2016).

- Long QT syndrome: The child may be asymptomatic until experiencing syncope or sudden death from a torsade de pointe ventricular tachycardia. Family history may include syncope, sudden death, or known long QT syndrome. Congenital

• BOX 38.6 Common Arrhythmias in Children

- Sinus arrhythmia—variable heart rate that increases with inspiration and decreases with expiration. This is a normal finding in children.
- Bradycardia or slow heart rate for age:
  - Sinus bradycardia is the most common cause of bradycardia in children and can be due to hypoxia, acidosis, increased intracranial pressure, abdominal distention, hypothermia, hypoglycemia, eating disorders, or athletic conditioning. Bradycardia can also be caused by drugs, such as β-blockers or digoxin (Park, 2016).
  - Complete AV block can either be congenital or acquired after cardiac surgery. Ninety percent of congenital cases are secondary to maternal connective tissue disorders or complex CHD (levo- or L-looped transposition of the great arteries [L-TGA]) heterotaxy (Smith, 2016).
- Tachycardias:
  - Sinus tachycardia is caused by predisposing factors that increase cardiac output, including fever, anxiety, infection, drug exposure, dehydration, pain, hyperthyroidism, or anemia among many others. Treatment is directed at the underlying disorder.
  - SVTs are the most common pathologic tachycardias in children.
  - AV reentrant tachycardia is the most common SVT. In AV reentrant tachycardia, there is an additional (accessory) pathway for impulse transmission from atria to ventricles besides the normal AV node. Less commonly this may be through a dual AV node (nodal reentrant AV tachycardia). AV reentrant tachycardias often first present in infants younger than 4 months old and again in young adolescents (Park, 2016).
- Long QT syndrome–induced ventricular tachycardia: Long QT syndrome is linked to 13 different genes. The clinical manifestation is delayed repolarization (the long QT interval). Genetic prolongation of the QT segment increases the susceptibility to further drug-induced long QT interval. Such drugs include antiarrhythmics (e.g., amiodarone and sotalol), psychotic drugs (e.g., haloperidol and ziprasidone), and antibiotics (such as, ciprofloxacin, clarithromycin, and erythromycin). Lists of medications that should be avoided are available on the Internet.
- Premature atrial contraction (PAC): This arrhythmia occurs in children and adults. The PAC depolarization may or may not be conducted through the AV node. PACs in a child with an otherwise normal heart is usually benign. It is not unusual to see multiple PACs on the ECG of a newborn.
- Premature ventricular contraction (PVC): PVCs are premature QRS complexes with a prolonged duration or morphologic difference from the preceding QRS. Occasional PVCs are also seen in otherwise normal infants and children. PVCs that are uniform in appearance, which means they have the same QRS complex appearance every time, are usually of no consequence.

AV, *Atrioventricular;* CHD, *congenital heart disease;* ECG, *electrocardiogram;* SVT, *Supraventricular tachycardia.*

deafness is an additional family characteristic in one type of long QT syndrome.

Diagnostic Studies

- A 12-lead ECG is essential to document the arrhythmia
- Supraventricular tachycardia (SVT): Wolff-Parkinson-White is one subtype of AV reentrant tachycardia in which there are markers on the resting (non-SVT) ECG that indicate an accessory pathway. These markers are delta waves, short PR interval, and prolonged QRS duration. Diagnosis is usually made when capturing SVT on ECG, Holter monitor, or other device. A QT interval corrected for the heart rate (QTc) of greater than 0.44 second in males and 0.46 second in females is worthy of investigation (Park, 2016).

- Long QT syndrome: 12-lead ECG (shows a long QT interval); genetic testing
- An echocardiogram may be ordered to rule out complex forms of CHD and to assess ventricular function. A Holter monitor can be ordered to determine the average heart rate over a 24-hour period and to establish rhythm related symptoms (Baruteau, et al., 2016).

Management and Complications

- Bradycardia: Treat the underlying cause. Symptomatic children and those with high-grade AV block may require temporary or permanent pacing. A permanent pacemaker may be indicated if bradycardia is persistent after the underlying cause is treated or if there is high-grade AV block (Baruteau et al., 2016).
- SVT: Vagal maneuvers, intravenous adenosine, or, if necessary, synchronized cardioversion. Long-term management involves prevention of recurrence with β-blockade or, in the absence of Wolff-Parkinson-White, digoxin. Radiofrequency ablation of accessory pathway is attempted if medical therapy fails and the child is old enough for the procedure.
- Long QT syndrome: If long QT syndrome is suspected, the child should be referred to a pediatric electrophysiologist. Treatment options include β-blockers and placement of an implantable defibrillator. These children are at high risk of SCD.

Syncope

Syncope is a transient loss of consciousness due to a decrease in cerebral blood flow; recovery is relatively prompt. Most syncope or near syncope in children is benign, unlike older adults where cardiac causes are predominant. In assessing a syncopal episode, the provider must distinguish between a simple fainting event versus one that is a red flag for a serious cardiovascular or other medical condition (Singhi and Saini, 2017).

Simple or common fainting occurs in approximately 15% of children from 8 to 18 years old. The relatively high incidence of syncope contrasts with a low incidence of aborted and cardiac-related sudden death in the pediatric and young adult population (Park, 2016).

Syncope related to cardiac causes occurs as a result of obstruction to left ventricular filling (e.g., mitral stenosis), obstruction to left ventricular ejection (e.g., aortic stenosis), or ineffective contraction along with an underlying structural, functional, or electrical heart disturbance. Syncope may be due to primary pulmonary HTN, which is an often clinically silent disease until severe symptoms are present. Syncope due to a cardiac cause often comes without prodromal symptoms or may be associated with palpitation or chest pain (angina).

In contrast, noncardiac syncope (also called *neurocardiogenic syncope [NCS]*, or simple fainting) is neurally mediated and involves systemic vasodilation, vagally induced bradycardia, and hypotension which result in decreased cerebral blood flow and fainting. NCS includes different overlapping subtypes, such as vasovagal syncope, vasodepressor syncope, cardioinhibitory syncope, pallid breath-holding spells (or reflex anoxic seizures), postural orthostatic tachycardia syndrome, or others. Ninety-five percent of syncope is vasodepressive or vasovagal. The incidence of simple fainting in female adolescents supersedes that of males (Park, 2016).

Additional causes of syncope include neurologic (headache, seizure, transient ischemic attack), psychiatric (depression, panic

TABLE 38.10	Relative Frequency of Premonitory Symptoms and Residual Findings With Common Neurally Mediated Syncope versus More Serious Cardiac Syncope	
	Neurally Mediated	**Cardiac Syncope**
Symptoms		
Premonitory symptoms	+++	±
Lightheadedness	+++	+/±
Palpitations	+	++
Occurs while upright	+++	+
Occurs while sitting	+/±	+
Emotional trigger	++	++
Exercise trigger	+	++
Residual Findings		
Pallor	+++	+/±
Incontinence	–	+
Disorientation	–	+
Fatigue	++	±
Diaphoresis	++	±
Injury	+	++

+++, Very common (>50%); ++, common (>20%); +, not rare (>≈5%); ±, uncommon (<5%); –, rare (<≈1%).

From Newburger JW, Alexander ME, Fulton DR. Innocent murmurs, syncope, and chest pain. In: Keane JF, Lock JE, Fyler DC, eds. *Nadas' Pediatric Cardiology*. 2nd ed. Philadelphia: Saunders; 2006. Reprinted with permission.

attack, conversion reaction), and metabolic (drugs, carbon monoxide, electrolyte imbalance/problems). Toddlers may faint with breath-holding spells, most commonly between 6 months and 3 years old. Many of these cases resolve by 5 years old and the majority by 8 years old (after this time, they are usually classified as convulsive syncope) (Park, 2016).

Clinical Findings

History

A thorough history that focuses on triggers and presyncopal symptoms is the most critical "test" of syncopal causation (Table 38.10). Key history elements to review include:

- Triggering factor, such as exercise, pain, or an emotional event (e.g., anxiety, panic)
- Prior incident(s) of syncope or fainting (e.g., venipuncture, seeing blood, experiencing an injury)
- Associated injury, clonic-tonic movements, or vertigo
- Associated chest pain, palpitations, tachycardia, or bradycardia
- Family history of sudden death before age 40, congenital deafness, long QT syndrome, cardiomyopathy, and/or recurrent adolescent or toddler syncope that was outgrown
- Possibility of pregnancy or the use of illicit drugs; list all medications taken (including diet supplements, herbs, other botanicals, energy drinks)
- History of exercise-induced bronchospasms, respiratory distress, or other concomitant medical disorder

- Known psychological stress or stressors at home, school or in social environments
- Standing for any length of time prior to the episode (indicates orthostasis); history of "head rushes" when standing up
- In a hot environment, sweating, dehydration; hunger
- Nausea, constriction of visual fields ("world going dark") prior to episode
- Any postepisode symptoms, such as dizziness, pallor, clammy feeling, exhaustion, headache
- History of otherwise being well, active, with minimal medical issues
- Arousal after fainting within 1 to 2 minutes; recovery to full baseline state may have taken more than 1 hour (many patients, though awake and alert, may not totally feel "like themselves" for a while)
- Stiffening, jerking motions during unconsciousness (tonic-clonic muscular contractions of face [including fixed upward deviation of eyes], trunk, and extremities mimicking epilepsy occurs in approximately half of individuals experiencing a syncopal episode)
- Other activities prior to episode: hair grooming, coughing, micturition, neck stretching

Physical Examination

A detailed neurologic examination is needed if the syncopal episode suggests a seizure disorder. A cardiovascular examination is especially important. In most cases the physical examination is completely normal.

Diagnostic Studies

The majority of individuals with cardiac syncope are identified either by a history of associated presyncopal symptoms with exercise, abnormal ECG, family history of arrhythmia, or abnormal physical examination. The diagnosis of neurally mediated syncope can confidently be made based on history, normal examination, and normal ECG (Singhi and Saini, 2017). The diagnostic workup to distinguish between the two consists of:

- Orthostatic vital signs: More than a 30 mm Hg drop in BP after standing for 5 to 10 minutes, or a baseline systolic pressure of less than 80 mm Hg in an adolescent.
- Hemoglobin, if anemia is suspected: CBC, random glucose, and glucose tolerance tests have low yields and are not recommended routine tests for syncope.
- 12-lead ECG (looking for LVH, Wolff-Parkinson-White syndrome, AV and interventricular conduction defects, electrical myopathies [e.g., long QT syndrome]): If ECG results are borderline or family history is highly suggestive of cardiac etiology, ECGs on siblings and parents may be useful. Twenty-four-hour Holter monitoring and portable 30-day event monitoring can also be beneficial.
- Echocardiography: Can be useful when history, physical, ECG, or family history suggests cardiac disease or cardiac syncope.
- Tilt table testing is not recommended for use in primary care due to poor reliability.
- Treadmill exercise testing may be used in cases of exercise-related syncope.

Management and Differential Diagnosis

If cardiac syncope is suspected, restrict the child from sports participation until referral to a pediatric cardiologist is completed. For neurally mediated syncope, education is key (cause, prevention, and how to abort a syncopal event). Prevention involves

ensuring good hydration (along with decreasing caffeine and increasing sodium intake) and initiating antigravity techniques at the onset of presyncopal sensations (isometric leg or arm contractions; squatting or lying down; possibly using compression socks). The individual should rest for 5 to 10 minutes either supine or with legs up if prodromal symptoms occur or after fainting. Concomitant cognitive-behavioral therapy is indicated if the episodes are psychogenic in etiology (Park, 2016).

In refractory cases, pharmacologic management by cardiology specialists may play a role, although this should not be the first line treatment. These therapies may involve use of volume enhancement (fludrocortisone); limiting excessive catecholamine drive (using β-blockers, such as atenolol); vagolytic agents (disopyramide); and/or selective serotonin reuptake inhibitors (SSRIs). If drug therapy is used, the typical duration is 1 year, followed by weaning. Pacemaker implantation has been used in rare cases (Singhi and Saini, 2017).

Differential diagnoses include migraine with confusion or stupor, seizures, hypoglycemia, hysteria, hyperventilation, vertigo, carbon monoxide poisoning, electrolyte imbalance, drugs, and cardiovascular disease, including underlying arrhythmia.

Additional Resources

American Heart Association.
    www.heart.org/HEARTORG/
Congenital Heart Information Network.
    www.tchin.org
Mended Hearts, Inc.
    www.mendedhearts.org
National Center for Biotechnology Information.
    www.ncbi.nlm.nih.gov
PediHeart (requires a paid membership).
    www.pediheart.org

Genetic Tests, Information About Genetic Defects or Syndromes, and Resources for Families
National Institutes of Health.
    www.genetests.org
Online Mendelian Inheritance in Man.
    www.ncbi.nlm.nih.gov/omim

References

Ailes EC, Gilboa SM, Honein MA, Oster M. Estimated number of infants detected and missed by critical congenital heart defect screening. *Pediatrics*. 2015;135(6):1000–1008.
American Academy of Pediatrics (AAP) Committee on Infectious Diseases, AAP Bronchiolitis Guidelines Committee. Updated guidance for palivizumab prophylaxis among infants and young children at increased risk of hospitalization for respiratory syncytial virus infection. *Pediatrics*. 2014;134(2):415–420.
Aro AL, Chugh SS. Prevention of sudden cardiac death in children and young adults. *Prog Pediatr Cardiol*. 2017;45:7–42.
Averbach SR, Everitt MD, Butts RJ, et al. The Pediatric Heart Failure Workforce: An International Multicenter Survey, *Pediatric Cardiology*; 2017. Available at http://doi.org/10.1007/s00246-017-1756-9.
Baltimore RS, Gewits M, Baddour LM, et al. Infective endocarditis in childhood: 2015 update. *Circulation*. 2015;132:1487–1515.
Baruteau AE, Perry JC, Sanatani S, et al. Evaluation and management of bradycardia in neonates and children. *Eur J Pediatr*. 2016;175:151–161.
Bizmark RS, Change RK, Tsugawa Y, et al. Impact of AHA's 2007 guideline change on incidence of infective endocarditis in infants and children. *Am Heart J*. 2017;189:100–119.

Burns KM, Byrne BJ, Gelb BD, et al. New mechanistic and therapeutic targets for pediatric heart failure: report from a national heart, lung, and blood institute working group. *Circulation.* 2014;130(1):79–86 .

Canter CE, Simpson KP. Diagnosis and treatment of myocarditis in children in the current era. *Circulation.* 2014;129(1):115–128.

Cassidy SC, Allen HD, Phillips JR. History and physical examination. In: Allen HD, Driscoll DJ, Shaddy RE, et al., eds. *Moss and Adams' Heart Disease in Infants, Children, and Adolescents Including the Fetus and Young Adult.* 8th ed. Philadelphia: Lippincott Williams & Wilkins; 2013:82–92.

Centers for Disease Control and Prevention (CDC). General recommendations on immunization—recommendations of the Advisory Committee on Immunization Practices (ACIP). *MMWR Recomm Rep.* 2011;60(2):1–64.

Centers for Disease Control and Prevention (CDC). *Congenital Heart Defects (CHDs): Data & Statistics, CDC (website);* 2014. Available at www.cdc.gov/ncbddd/heartdefects/data.html.

Chandra N, Bastiaenen R, Papadakis M, et al. Sudden cardiac death in young athletes: practical challenges and diagnostic dilemmas. *J Amer Coll Cardiol.* 2013;61(10):1027–1040.

Contractor T, Mandapati R. Arrhythmias in patients with atrial defects. *Card Electrophsiol Clin.* 2017;9:235–244.

Cowley AW, Nadeau JH, Baccarelli A, et al. *Report of the National Heart, Lung and Blood Institute working group on Epigenetics and Hypertension.* Available at https://www.ncbi.nlm.nih.gov/pmc/articles/PMC3885905/; 2012.

Curtis CR, Baughman Al, Debolt C. Risk factors associated with Bordetella pertussis among infants <4 months of age in the pre-Tdap era: United States, 2002-2005. *Pediatr Infect Dis J.* 2017;36(8):726–735.

Dakkak W, Bhimji S. Ventricular septal defect. NCBI stat pearls. Available at https://www.ncbi.nlm.nih.gov/books/NBK470330/.

Dixon G, Christow G. Infective endocarditis in children: an update. *Curr Opin Infec Dis.* 2017;30(3):257–267.

Flynn JT, Kaelber DC, Baker-Smith CM, et al. Clinical practice guideline for screening and management of high blood pressure in children and adolescents. *Pediatrics.* 2017;140(3):1–72.

Gewitz M, Taubert KA. Infective endocarditis and prevention. In: Allen HD, Driscoll DJ, Shaddy RE, et al., eds. *Moss and Adams' Heart Disease in Infants, Children, and Adolescents Including the Fetus and Young Adult.* 8th ed. Philadelphia: Lippincott Williams & Wilkins; 2013:1363–1376.

Hussey AD, Weintraub RG. Drug treatment of heart failure in children. *Paediatr Drugs.* 2016;18(2):89–99.

Knirsh W, Mayer KN, Scheer I. Structural cerebral abnormalities and neurodevelopmental status in single ventricle congenital heart disease before Fontan procedure. *Eur J Cardio-Thorac Surg.* 2016;51(4):740–746.

Knowles RL, Day T, Wade A, et al. Patient-reported quality of life outcomes for children with serious congenital heart defects. *Arch Dis Child.* 2014;99(5):413–419.

Marino BS, Lipkin PH, Newburger JW, et al. Neurodevelopmental outcomes in children with congenital heart disease: evaluation and management. A scientific statement from the American Heart Association. *Circulation.* 2012;126(9):1143–1172.

McRae ME. Long-term outcomes after repair of congenital heart defects: part 1. *AJN.* 2015a;115(1):24–35.

McRae ME. Long-term outcomes after repair of congenital heart defects: part 2. *AJN.* 2015b;115(2):34–45.

Mancini M. *Tetralogy of Fallot.* NORD. Available at https://rarediseases.org/rare-diseases/tetralogy-of-fallot/.

Murray S, McKinney E. *Foundations of Maternal Newborn and Women's Health Nursing.* 6th ed. Philadelphia: Saunders/Elsevier; 2014.

National Heart, Lung, and Blood Institute (NHLBI). *Expert panel on integrated guidelines for cardiovascular health and risk reduction in children and adolescents: full report;* 2012. Available at www.nhlbi.nih.gov/files/docs/guidelines/peds_guidelines_full.pdf. Accessed February 6, 2018.

O'Brien P, Marshall AC. Coarctation of the aorta. *Circulation.* 2015;131:e363–e365.

Park M. *Park's the Pediatric Cardiology Handbook.* 5th ed. Philadelphia: Mosby/Elsevier; 2016.

Ryan DJ, Mikula EB, Germana S, Silva S, Derouin A. Screening for critical congenital heart disease in newborns using pulse oximetry. *Adv Neonatal Care.* 2014;14(2):19–128.

Singhi P, Saini AE. Syncope in pediatric practice. *Indian J Pediatr.* 2017 Nov 9. https://doi.org/10.1007/s12098-017-2488-9.

Simmons A, Brueckner M. The genetics of congenital heart disease… understanding and improving long-term outcomes in congenital heart disease: a review for the general cardiologist and primary care physician. *Curr Opin Pediatr.* 2017;29(5):520–528.

Simpson KE, Canter CE. Can adult heart failure regimens be applied to children: what works and what does not? *Curr Opin Cardiol.* 2012;27(2):98–107.

Smith AH. Arrhythmias in cardiac critical care. *Pediatr Crit Care Med.* 2016;17(8 suppl 1):S146–S154.

Suma G, Usha MD, Ambika G, et al. Oral health status of normal children and those affiliated with cardiac diseases. *J Clin Pediatr Dent.* 2011;35(3):315–318.

Tabbutt S, Gaynor JW, Newburger JW. Neurodevelopmental outcomes after congenital heart surgery and strategies for improvement. *Curr Opin Cardiol.* 2012;27(?):82–91.

Thakkar AN, Chinnadurai P, Lin CH. Adult congenital heart disease: magnitude of the problem. *Current Opinion.* 2017;32(5):467–474.

van der Bom T, Zomer AC, Zwinderman AH, et al. The changing epidemiology of congenital heart disease. *Nat Rev Cardiol.* 2011;8(1):50–60.

Wilson W, Taubert KA, Gewitz M, et al. Prevention of infective endocarditis: guidelines from the American Heart Association: a guideline from the American Heart Association Rheumatic Fever, Endocarditis and Kawasaki Disease Committee, Council on Cardiovascular Disease in the Young, and the Council on Clinical Cardiology, Council on Cardiovascular Surgery and Anesthesia, and the Quality of Care and Outcomes Research Interdisciplinary Working Group. *J Amer Dental Assoc.* 2008;139(suppl):3S–24S.

Xiong H, Bingqing X, Zhu J, et al. Clinical outcomes in pediatric patients hospitalized with fulminant myocarditis requiring extracorporeal membrane oxygenation: a meta-analysis. *Pediatr Cardiol.* 2017;38(2):209–214.

Zaidi AN, Daniels CJ. The adolescent and adult with congenital heart disease. In: Allen HD, Driscoll DJ, Shaddy RE, et al., eds. *Moss and Adams' Heart Disease in Infants, Children, and Adolescents Including the Fetus and Young Adult.* 8th ed. Philadelphia: Lippincott Williams & Wilkins; 2013:1463.

Zaidi S, Brueckner M. Genetics and genomics of congenital heart disease. *Circ Res.* 2017;120:923–940.

39

Hematologic Disorders

TEREA GIANNETTA

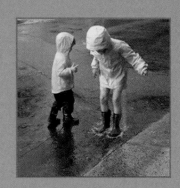

The hematologic system is a massive fluid organ that permeates the entire body, delivering nutrients and other vital elements throughout. Essential body functions carried out by blood include the transfer of respiratory gases, hemostasis, phagocytosis, and the provision of cellular and humoral agents to fight infection. Abnormalities of blood cells are seen in various disease states and with alterations in nutrition. The use of diagnostic hematologic studies is necessary to differentiate common nutritional deficiencies with straightforward treatments from rare diseases with a genetic or chronic component.

Anatomy and Physiology

Blood is made of cellular components, each with specialized functions, and a fluid component called *plasma,* which serves as the transport medium. The cells that comprise whole blood are categorized as *erythrocytes,* or red blood cells (RBCs); *leukocytes,* or white blood cells (WBCs); and *thrombocytes,* or platelets (Fig 39.1). Plasma is the clear yellow fluid in which proteins (e.g., albumins, globulins, fibrinogen) are the major solutes. Plasma proteins maintain intravascular volume, contribute to coagulation, and are important in acid-base balance.

The complete blood count (CBC), which provides an assessment of all cell categories, is commonly used in routine health screening. Abnormally high or low counts in any cell category can indicate or provide insight into the presence of many conditions; however, because different conditions present at different ages, values must be interpreted using age-appropriate, pediatric hematologic parameters (Table 39.1). It is also important to remember that hematologic values in neonates differ significantly from those in older children and adults—a reflection of the developmental changes during fetal hematopoiesis that correlate with gestational age (Jacob, 2016). Blood formation in the human embryo begins in the yolk sac during the first several weeks of gestation. During the second trimester, blood is formed primarily in the fetal liver, spleen, and lymph nodes. In the last half of gestation, hematopoiesis shifts from the fetal liver and spleen to the bone marrow where, by birth, most blood formation is taking place.

Erythrocytes

Erythropoietin, produced primarily by renal glomerular epithelial cells, regulates the production of erythrocytes, or RBCs. In response to a decrease in the number of circulating RBCs or a decrease in the oxygen pressure (Pao_2) of arterial blood, erythropoietin stimulates the bone marrow to convert certain stem cells to proerythroblasts. Substances essential for RBC formation include iron, vitamin B_{12}, folic acid, amino acids, and other nutrients.

The RBC matures in stages: proerythroblast, erythroblast, normoblast, reticulocyte, and erythrocyte. As cellular differentiation occurs, the nucleus present in the early forms of the cell is extruded and replaced by hemoglobin (Hgb). The RBC assumes its characteristic anucleated biconcave disk shape, which enables it to pass through small capillaries and sinuses without being destroyed. The large surface-to-volume ratio of the semipermeable membrane facilitates rapid gas exchange.

The youngest circulating RBCs are the reticulocytes (i.e., blast forms are typically seen only in the bone marrow). Once released from the bone marrow, reticulocytes are in circulation for 1 to 2 days before becoming mature RBCs. A mature RBC survives about 120 days before it is destroyed through phagocytosis in the spleen, liver, or bone marrow. The *reticulocyte count* is about 4% to 6% for the first 3 days of life, which reflects the relatively greater amount of erythropoiesis that occurs in the fetus. This increase is followed by a sudden drop, a second surge around 2 months, and a slow decline to from 0.5% to 1.5% by 1 year of age, which remains the norm for the rest of the individual's life. Although it is not routinely ordered, a reticulocyte count can be used to assess hematologic stress and/or the effectiveness of the body's early response to treatment (e.g., a tracking response to iron therapy for anemia).

Hemoglobin

Hgb is the oxygen-carrying protein molecule in the RBC. Production of Hgb requires circulating iron, the synthesis of a protoporphyrin ring, and the production of globin. Each Hgb molecule comprises two pairs of polypeptide chains. The globin portion contains protein in a precise sequence of amino acids coded by genes located on chromosomes 11 and 16. Hgb contains two alpha (α) and two beta (β) chains, which attach to heme groups; large iron-containing disks; and porphyrin, a nitrogen-containing organic compound.

Each of the four iron atoms in the Hgb molecule combines reversibly with an atom of oxygen to form oxyhemoglobin. The percentage of oxyhemoglobin is the arterial oxygen saturation (Sao_2), which is measured indirectly through pulse oximetry or directly through arterial blood gas determination. When the oxygen concentration is lower (as in the tissues), oxygen is released from Hgb to meet cellular demands.

Structural Variations

Adult Hgb contains two alpha (α) and two beta (β) chains. Equal numbers of each chain are essential for normal cell function. An imbalance of the chains damages and destroys RBCs, thereby producing anemia. At birth, approximately 70% of Hgb is made up of fetal hemoglobin (Hgb F), which is composed of two alpha

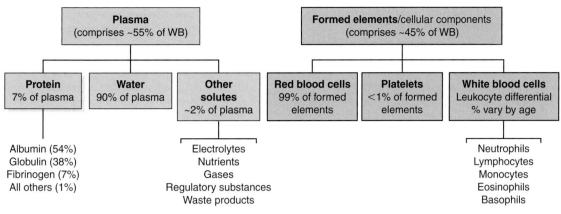

• **Fig 39.1** Composition of Whole Blood (WB).

TABLE 39.1 Age-Specific Blood Cell Indices

Age	Hgb (g/dL)[a]	HCT (%)[a]	MCV (fL)[a]	MCHC (g/dL RBC)[a]	Reticulocytes	WBCs (×10³/mL)[b]	Platelets (10³/mL)[b]
26-30 weeks gestation[c]	13.4 (11)	41.5 (34.9)	118.2 (106.7)	37.9 (30.6)	—	4.4 (2.7)	254 (180-327)
28 weeks	14.5	45	120	31.0	(5-10)	—	275
32 weeks	15.0	47	118	32.0	(3-10)	—	290
Term[d] (cord)	16.5 (13.5)	51 (42)	108 (98)	33.0 (30.0)	(3-7)	18.1 (9-30)[e]	290
1-3 days	18.5 (14.5)	56 (45)	108 (95)	33.0 (29.0)	(1.8-4.6)	18.9 (9.4-34)	192
2 week	16.6 (13.4)	53 (41)	105 (88)	31.4 (28.1)	—	11.4 (5-20)	252
1 month	13.9 (10.7)	44 (33)	101 (91)	31.8 (28.1)	(0.1-1.7)	10.8 (4-19.5)	—
2 months	11.2 (9.4)	35 (28)	95 (84)	31.8 (28.3)	—	—	—
6 months	12.6 (11.1)	36 (31)	76 (68)	35.0 (32.7)	(0.7-2.3)	11.9 (6-17.5)	—
6 months-2 years	12.0 (10.5)	36 (33)	78 (70)	33.0 (30.0)	—	10.6 (6-17)	(150-350)
2-6 years	12.5 (11.5)	37 (34)	81 (75)	34.0 (31.0)	(0.5-1.0)	8.5 (5-15.5)	(150-350)
6-12 years	13.5 (11.5)	40 (35)	86 (77)	34.0 (31.0)	(0.5-1.0)	8.1 (4.5-13.5)	(150-350)
12-18 Years							
Male	14.5 (13)	43 (36)	88 (78)	34.0 (31.0)	(0.5-1.0)	7.8 (4.5-13.5)	(150-350)
Female	14.0 (12)	41 (37)	90 (78)	34.0 (31.0)	(0.5-1.0)	7.8 (4.5-13.5)	(150-350)
Adult							
Male	15.5 (13.5)	47 (41)	90 (80)	34.0 (31.0)	(0.8-2.5)	7.4 (4.5-11)	(150-350)
Female	14.0 (12)	41 (36)	90 (80)	34.0 (31.0)	(0.8-4.1)	7.4 (4.5-11)	(150-350)

[a]Data are mean (−2 SD).
[b]Data are mean (±2 SD).
[c]Values are from fetal samplings.
[d]1 month, capillary hemoglobin exceeds venous: 1 h: 3.6-g difference; 5 day: 2.2-g difference; 3 week: 1.1-g difference.
[e]Mean (95% confidence limits).

Hgb, Hemoglobin; *HCT*, hematocrit; *MCHC*, mean cell hemoglobin concentration; *MCV*, mean corpuscular volume; *RBC*, red blood cell; *WBC*, white blood cell.
Data from Forestier F, Dattos F, Galacteros F, et al. Hematologic values of 163 normal fetuses between 18 and 30 weeks of gestation. *Pediatr Res.* 1986;20:342; Oski FA, Naiman JL. *Hematological Problems in the Newborn Infant.* Philadelphia: WB Saunders; 1982; Nathan D, Oski FA. *Hematology of Infancy and Childhood.* Philadelphia: WB Saunders; 1998; Matoth Y, Zaizor K, Varsano I, et al. Postnatal changes in some red cell parameters. *Acta Paediatr Scand.* 1971;60:317; and Wintrobe MM. *Clinical Hematology.* Baltimore: Williams & Wilkins; 1999.
From The Johns Hopkins Hospital. *Harriet Lane Handbook.* (20th ed.). Philadelphia: Elsevier; 2018.

and two gamma chains. By 12 months of age, the percent of Hgb F is less than 2%, whereas it is 95% is adult Hgb (A_1). Hgb A_2 is another adult Hgb, which consists of two α and two delta (δ) chains. Hgb A_2 normally makes up only 2.5% of the total Hgb; however, it may be increased in β thalassemia.

Among the most commonly occurring Hgb variants are Hgb S (sickle), Hgb C, Hgb E, persistence of Hgb F, and Hgb H. The incidence of these Hgbs tends to peak within certain geographic/regional populations. Atypical combinations of Hgb variants can occur, each with its own resulting condition or problems. *Hemoglobin electrophoresis,* which separates each Hgb out on a gel medium, is the diagnostic test used to differentiate the Hgb variants from Hgb A, thus aiding in the diagnosis of specific hemoglobinopathies. Other hemoglobinopathies occur because of diminished production of one of the two subunit chains, the most common being one of the *thalassemias.* Another Hgb variant is an altered state, as occurs with methemoglobin. In this condition, the ferrous form of iron oxidizes to the ferric state, causing the *heme* to be incapable of carrying oxygen. If reduced Hgb levels exceed 5 g/dL (i.e., 5 g/L not transporting oxygen), serious tissue hypoxia and cyanosis can occur. Methemoglobinemia can be congenital or caused by exposure to certain drugs and chemicals.

Normal Values

Hgb increases with increased gestational age. In the full-term newborn, Hgb levels are typically high (≥14 g/dL) as a result of increased tissue oxygenation and reduced production of erythropoietin. Hgb levels begin to drop shortly after birth, reaching a low point (11 g/dL) at about 6 to 9 weeks. This drop represents a *physiologic* anemia caused by the shortened survival of fetal RBCs and the rapid expansion of blood volume during this period. A decrease in Hgb, or anemia, can also develop secondary to a decrease in RBC production, blood loss, or increased RBC destruction. Owing to the effect of the latter processes, oxygen transport to the tissues is adversely affected, and the individual can become clinically anemic, as manifested by pallor, heart failure, or shock.

Anemias are often categorized on the basis of RBC size (e.g., normocytic, microcytic, or macrocytic), which is reflected in the mean corpuscular volume (MCV), and appearance (e.g., hypocytic or normochromic), which is reflected in the mean corpuscular hemoglobin (MCH). Examination of the peripheral smear can also reveal nuances in RBC appearance, which can, in turn, help to narrow diagnostic categories (e.g., basophilic stippling may suggest lead poisoning).

Antigenic Properties of Red Blood Cells (Blood Type)

RBCs are classified into different types according to the presence of antigens on the cell membrane. The antigenicity is genetically determined, representing contributions from both parents. The most common antigens are designated A, B, and Rh. A person inherits either A or B antigen (type A or B blood), both antigens (type AB blood, making that person a universal recipient), or neither antigen (type O blood, making that person a universal donor). The A and B antigens are sugars, whereas Rh antigens are proteins (Fig 39.2). The antigens expressed in the RBCs determine an individual's blood type. These distinctions become important either when blood transfusions are necessary or in the assessment of maternal-fetal blood incompatibilities. Individuals belong to one of eight different blood types: A Rh+, A Rh-, B Rh+, B Rh-, AB RH+, AB Rh-, 0 Rh+, or 0 Rh-, each having different combinations of *antigens* on the surface of the RBCs.

Leukocyte

Leukocytes, or WBCs, are larger and fewer in number than erythrocytes. The primary function of WBCs is to protect the body from invasion by foreign organisms (e.g., viruses, bacteria, parasites, and fungi) and to distribute antibodies and other immune response components. When the WBC count reaches a critically low level, the individual is at risk for infection. Whereas an elevated WBC count typically indicates that an infection or serious disease, such as leukemia, exists. The WBC count has two components: (1) the total number of WBCs and (2) the differential, which indicates the percentage of each type of WBC present in the same specimen. It is important to remember that an increase in the percentage of one type of WBC means a decrease in the percentage of the other, and vice versa.

There are five types of WBCs: neutrophils, lymphocytes, monocytes, eosinophils, and basophils (Table 39.2). WBCs can be grouped into two broad classifications: (1) granulocytes and (2) agranulocytes. Table 39.3 provides normal leukocyte and differential counts by age.

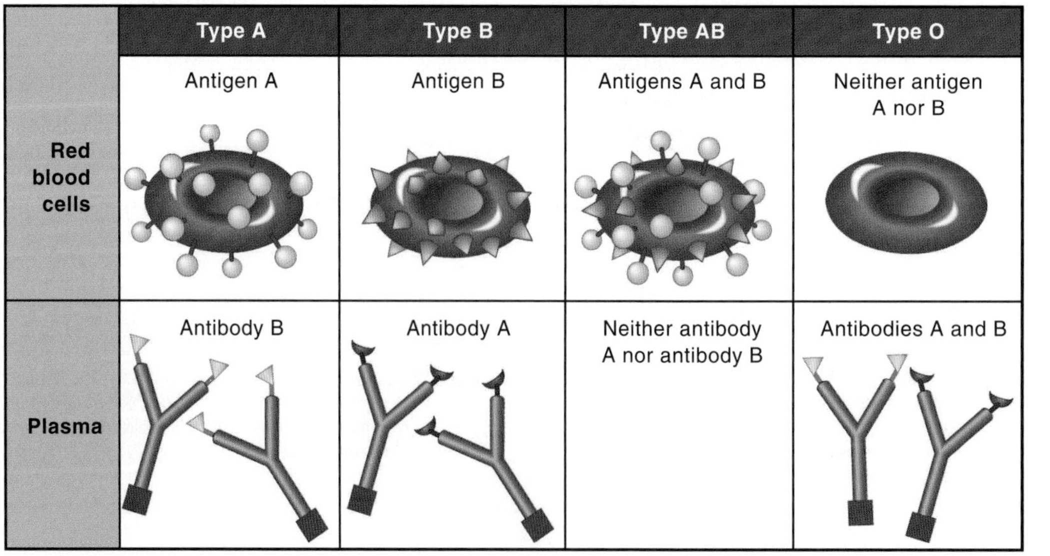

	Type A	Type B	Type AB	Type O
Red blood cells	Antigen A	Antigen B	Antigens A and B	Neither antigen A nor B
Plasma	Antibody B	Antibody A	Neither antibody A nor antibody B	Antibodies A and B

• **Fig 39.2** Red Cell Antigenicity. (From Patton K. *Anatomy & Physiology.* 7th ed. St. Louis: Mosby/Elsevier; 2010.)

TABLE 39.2   White Blood Cell Differential and Key Characteristics

Major Division of White Blood Cells	Differential	Description
Granulocytes (50%-75%)	Neutrophils	Primary defense against bacterial infection and mediating stress Elevated with bacterial or inflammatory disorders
	Bands (<1%)	Immature neutrophils put out by the bone marrow
	Eosinophils (2%-4%)	Associated with antigen-antibody response; elevated with exposure to allergens or inflammation of skin, parasites
	Basophils (1%-2%)	Phagocytes: Contain heparin, histamines, and serotonin Increased in leukemia, chronic inflammation, hypersensitivity to food, radiation therapy Mast cells
Agranulocytes (30%-40%)	Lymphocytes (25%-35%)	Primary components of the immune system Elevated with viral infections, leukemia, radiation exposure; decreased with diseases affecting the immune system
	Monocytes (<2%)	Elevated in infections and inflammation, leukemia; decreased with some bone marrow injury, leukemias

TABLE 39.3	Normal Leukocyte and Differential Counts			
	12 Months Old	**4 Years Old**	**10 Years Old**	**21 Years Old**
Leukocytes, total	11.4 (6.0-17.5)	9.1 (5.5-15.5)	8.1 (4.5-13.5)	7.4 (4.5-11.0)
Neutrophils, total	3.5 (1.5-8.5) (31%)	3.8 (1.5-8.5) (42%)	4.4 (1.8-8.0) (54%)	4.4 (1.8-7.7) (59%)
Neutrophils, band forms	0.35 (3.1%)	0.27 (0-1.0) (3.0%)	0.24 (0-1.0) (3.0%)	0.22 (0-0.7) (3.0%)
Neutrophils, segmented	3.2 (28%)	3.5 (1.5-7.5) (39%)	4.2 (1.8-7.0) (51%)	4.2 (1.8-7.0) (56%)
Eosinophils	0.30 (0.05-0.70) (2.6%)	0.25 (0.02-0.65) (2.8%)	0.20 (0-0.60) (2.4%)	0.20 (0-0.45) (2.7%)
Basophils	0.05 (0-10) (0.4%)	0.05 (0-0.20) (0.6%)	0.04 (0-0.20) (0.5%)	0.04 (0-0.20) (0.5%)
Lymphocytes	7.0 (4.0-10.5) (61%)	4.5 (2.0-8.0) (50%)	3.1 (1.5-6.5) (38%)	2.5 (1.0-4.8) (34%)
Monocytes	0.55 (0.05-1.1) (4.8%)	0.45 (0-0.8) (5.0%)	0.35 (0-0.8) (4.3%)	0.30 (0-0.8) (4.0%)

Values are expressed as cells ×10³/μL. Mean values are given; ranges are in parentheses. Percentage values are for mean values.

From Altman PL, Dittmer DS, eds. *Blood and Other Body Fluids.* Washington, DC: Federation of American Societies for Experimental Biology; 1961.

From Zitelli, BJ, McIntire SC, Nowalk AJ. *Zitelli and Davis' Atlas of Pediatric Physical Diagnosis.* 7th ed. Philadelphia: Elsevier; 2018.

Granulocytes

In children, granulocytes typically make up 40% to 70% of all WBCs. Granulocytes are further divided into neutrophils (also known as polymorphonucleocytes, or polys), eosinophils, and basophils.

Neutrophils. The major function of neutrophils is the phagocytosis or destruction of harmful particles and cells, particularly bacterial organisms. Neutrophils evolve as they mature in the bone marrow and are released into the blood from myeloblasts; they include—in the order of degree of maturity—promyelocytes, myelocytes, metamyelocytes, bands, and segmented neutrophils. A relative increase in the number of circulating immature neutrophils (bands) is referred to as a "left shift" and typically signifies the presence of an acute bacterial infection or inflammatory process.

Basophils. *Basophils*, or mast cells, typically account for less than 3% of WBCs present in blood. Although they do not respond to bacterial or viral infection, they are involved in the phagocytosis of antigen-antibody complexes. The cytoplasm of basophils contains heparin, histamine, and serotonin. A decrease in basophils (baso*penia*) can occur with acute allergic reactions and hyperthyroidism as well as stress, ovulation, and pregnancy. An increase in basophils (baso*philia*) can occur with allergic rhinitis/seasonal pollenosis, nephrosis, ulcerative colitis, and hypothyroidism.

Eosinophils. *Eosinophils*, which typically make up only 1% to 2% of WBCs, are similar to basophils in that they are involved in the phagocytosis of antigen-antibody complexes and are not responsive to bacterial or viral infections. They are also helpful in evaluating the severity of asthma. An elevation in eosinophils (eosino*philia*) can occur in allergic reactions, atopic dermatitis, asthma, and autoimmune disorders as well as parasitic infections and malignancies. A decrease in eosinophils (eosino*penia*) may occur with increased adrenosteroid production.

Agranulocytes: Lymphocytes and Monocytes

Lymphocytes. Lymphocytes (or immunocytes) make up 25% to 35% of WBCs. They originate in the bone marrow but differentiate in lymphoid tissues (e.g., spleen, liver, thymus, lymph nodes, intestines). Thymus-dependent lymphocytes (T cells) are part of the cell-mediated immune response whereby cytotoxic agents and macrophages are synthesized. There are three types of T cells: cytotoxic (killer T cells), helper T cells, and regulatory T cells. Lymphocytes that remain in the bone marrow (B cells) are precursors that can recognize antigens and transform into plasma cells, which release immunoglobulins or antibodies into the bloodstream.

Monocytes. *Monocytes* constitute 4% to 6% of WBCs. After briefly circulating in the peripheral vascular system, monocytes migrate to the tissues to mature and become part of the monocyte/histiocyte/immune cell system. Their primary function is the phagocytosis of bacteria and cellular debris; they serve as a backup system to the granulocytes, which are the body's first line of defense.

Platelet Cells and Coagulation Factors

The smallest cellular components in blood are the platelets, or thrombocytes, which are essential to hemostasis and clot formation. When a blood vessel is injured, platelets adhere to the inner surface of the vessel and form a hemostatic plug. As platelets degrade, a series of at least 13 clotting factors or proteolytic enzymes are released; these bring about the clotting process in a cascading sequence of successive reactions (Fig 39.3). Age-specific coagulation values exist for each aspect of the coagulation process and should be referenced for proper assessment and treatment management (Table 39.4).

Pathophysiology

Hematologic problems are generally classified as disorders of RBCs, WBCs, and platelets and/or coagulation function. These three broad categories of function are further divided into disorders of blood cell production, maturation, or destruction.

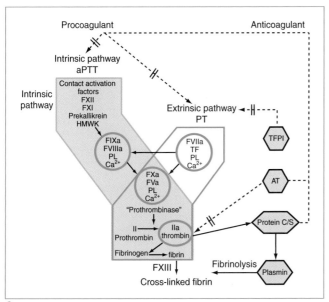

Fig 39.3 Differential Diagnosis *(DDX)* of Bleeding Disorders. *aPTT,* Activated partial thromboplastin time; *DIC,* disseminated intravascular coagulation; *PT,* prothrombin time (From The Johns Hopkins Hospital. *Harriet Lane Handbook.* 20th ed. Philadelphia: Elsevier; 2018.)

Assessment of Erythrocyte Disorders

History

A comprehensive history and physical examination are essential to unravel the mystery behind any suspected hematologic disorder, keeping in mind that many hematologic disorders have a genetic basis. In order to discern inheritable disorders, it is necessary to obtain a detailed family history. Certain disorders—such as thalassemia, sickle cell anemia (SCA), and glucose-6-phosphate dehydrogenase (G6PD) deficiency—occur with greater frequency in individuals whose ancestors came from specific geographic regions. A three-generation pedigree can provide visual clues to patterns of heritability and thus may help to narrow down the diagnostic possibilities. In particular, the primary care provider (PCP) should ask about family members with a history of anemia, jaundice, and/or splenomegaly (or history of splenectomy), as well as gallbladder disease/gallstones (or history of cholecystectomy), bleeding tendencies, and/or chronic illnesses.

A comprehensive review of each child's medical and social history as well as a thorough review of systems is fundamental. Particular attention should focus on the following:
- Birth history, including gestational age/weight, neonatal jaundice, birth/neonatal complications
- Alterations in growth and/or development
- Behavioral changes—irritability, lethargy, fatigue, school issues
- Presence of pallor, petechiae/bruising, extremity pain/swelling
- Nutritional history
- Gastrointestinal (GI) disorders/changes in output
- Bone fractures
- Recent acute infections/illness
- Drug/environmental/toxin exposures and/or history of pica
- International travel

In addition, for infants, the newborn screening panel results must be reviewed. The PCP should validate home address and phone while doing newborn rounds to make sure that there is correct information to contact the family if abnormal results are noted. The PCP must also verify and document the results in the child's medical record. In the United States, sickle cell disease is the most common genetic disease identified through the state-mandated screening programs. It exceeds the incidence of hypothyroidism and cystic fibrosis (more information about newborn screening can be found at https://www.cdc.gov/newbornscreening/).

Physical Examination

The physical examination should be comprehensive, including vital signs and growth documentation. The following positive signs are particularly important to identify owing to their association with specific problems:
- Pallor (conjunctivae, buccal mucosa, palmar creases), jaundice, petechiae/bruising, hyperpigmentation
- Retinal hemorrhages, glossitis, and/or bleeding from mucous membranes
- Lymphadenopathy, hepatosplenomegaly
- Frontal bossing and/or prominent maxilla
- Joint or extremity pain, spoon nails
- Heart murmurs, tachycardia

Erythrocyte Disorders

Anemia

Anemia is a reduction in circulating RBCs. It can occur due to a decrease in RBC production, abnormalities of the RBCs, a shortened RBC life span, RBC destruction, or an acute/ongoing loss from bleeding. RBC indices (e.g., MCV, MCH, MCHC) provide insight regarding the cell size and/or color, which, in turn, provides an organizing framework in approaching anemias. For instance, common causes of *microcytic* (↓MCV), *hypochromic* (↓MCH) anemia are iron deficiency, lead poisoning, and thalassemia trait, whereas common causes of *macrocytic* (↑MCV) anemia include exposure to certain medications (e.g., anticonvulsants), deficiencies in vitamin B12 or folate, liver disease, and hypothyroidism. RBC indices are therefore helpful in narrowing the diagnostic possibilities, especially because anemia can generally be classified on the basis of the MCV (Fig 39.4). The reticulocyte count helps to distinguish disorders resulting from hemolysis (↑retic; rapid destruction) or bleeding (loss of RBCs) from disorders resulting in the inability to produce RBCs (↓retic), as in bone marrow depression. Variations in RBC morphology (Box 39.1) can also provide clues and/or help to distinguish between disorders.

Another classification system to describe anemia reflects RBC production, maturation, or destruction (Fig 39.5). *Hypoproliferative* anemias result from a failure in RBC production and tend to be *normocytic, normochromic* anemias with a decreased reticulocyte count, making it seem that the body is not responding to the anemia. *Maturational anemias* reflect a defect in nuclear maturation, typically cause by nutritional deficiencies or a chemical/toxic exposure. The third category, *hemolytic anemias,* refers to anemias that result from increased

TABLE 39.4	Age-Specific Coagulation Values							
Coagulation Test	Preterm Infant (30-36 weeks), Day of Life 1[a]	Term Infant, Day of Life 1	Day of Life 3	1 Month-1 Year	1-5 Years	6-10 Years	11-16 Years	Adult
PT (s)	13.0 (10.6-16.2)	15.6 (14.4-16.4)	14.9 (13.5-16.4)	13.1 (11.5-15.3)	13.3 (12.1-14.5)	13.4 (11.7-15.1)	13.8 (12.7-16.1)	13.0 (11.5-14.5)
INR		1.26 (1.15-1.35)	1.20 (1.05-1.35)	1.00 (0.86-1.22)	1.03 (0.92-1.14)	1.04 (0.87-1.20)	1.08 (0.97-1.30)	1.00 (0.80-1.20)
aPTT (s)[b]	53.6 (27.5-79.4)	38.7 (34.3-44.8)	36.3 (29.5-42.2)	39.3 (35.1-46.3)	37.7 (33.6-43.8)	37.3 (31.8-43.7)	39.5 (33.9-46.1)	33.2 (28.6-38.2)
Fibrinogen (g/L)	2.43 (1.50-3.73)	2.80 (1.92-3.74)	3.30 (2.83-4.01)	2.42 (0.82-3.83)	2.82 (1.62-4.01)	3.04 (1.99-4.09)	3.15 (2.12-4.33)	3.1 (1.9-4.3)
Bleeding time (min)[a]					6 (2.5-10)	7 (2.5-13)	5 (3-8)	4 (1-7)
Thrombin time (s)	14 (11-17)	12 (10-16)[a]		17.1 (16.3-17.6)	17.5 (16.5-18.2)	17.1 (16.1-18.5)	16.9 (16.2-17.6)	16.6 (16.2-17.2)
Factor II (U/mL)	0.45 (0.20-0.77)	0.54 (0.41-0.69)	0.62 (0.50-0.73)	0.90 (0.62-1.03)	0.89 (0.70-1.09)	0.89 (0.67-1.10)	0.90 (0.61-1.07)	1.10 (0.78-1.38)
Factor V (U/mL)	0.88 (0.41-1.44)	0.81 (0.64-1.03)	1.22 (0.92-1.54)	1.13 (0.94-1.41)	0.97 (0.67-1.27)	0.99 (0.56-1.41)	0.89 (0.67-1.41)	1.18 (0.78-1.52)
Factor VII (U/mL)	0.67 (0.21-1.13)	0.70 (0.52-0.88)	0.86 (0.67-1.07)	1.28 (0.83-1.60)	1.11 (0.72-1.50)	1.13 (0.70-1.56)	1.18 (0.69-2.00)	1.29 (0.61-1.99)
Factor VIII (U/mL)	1.11 (0.50-2.13)	1.82 (1.05-3.29)	1.59 (0.83-2.74)	0.94 (0.54-1.45)	1.10 (0.36-1.85)	1.17 (0.52-1.82)	1.20 (0.59-2.00)	1.60 (0.52-2.90)
vWF (U/mL)[a]	1.36 (0.78-2.10)	1.53 (0.50-2.87)			0.82 (0.47-1.04)	0.95 (0.44-1.44)	1.00 (0.46-1.53)	0.92 (0.5-1.58)
Factor IX (U/mL)	0.35 (0.19-0.65)	0.48 (0.35-0.56)	0.72 (0.44-0.97)	0.71 (0.43-1.21)	0.85 (0.44-1.27)	0.96 (0.48-1.45)	1.11 (0.64-2.16)	1.30 (0.59-2.54)
Factor X (U/mL)	0.41 (0.11-0.71)	0.55 (0.46-0.67)	0.60 (0.46-0.75)	0.95 (0.77-1.22)	0.98 (0.72-1.25)	0.97 (0.68-1.25)	0.91 (0.53-1.22)	1.24 (0.96-1.71)
Factor XI (U/mL)	0.30 (0.08-0.52)	0.30 (0.07-0.41)	0.57 (0.24-0.79)	0.89 (0.62-1.25)	1.13 (0.65-1.62)	1.13 (0.65-1.62)	1.11 (0.65-1.39)	1.12 (0.67-1.96)
Factor XII (U/mL)	0.38 (0.10-0.66)	0.58 (0.43-0.80)	0.53 (0.14-0.80)	0.79 (0.20-1.35)	0.85 (0.36-1.35)	0.81 (0.26-1.37)	0.75 (0.14-1.17)	1.15 (0.35-2.07)
PK (U/mL)[a]	0.33 (0.09-0.57)	0.37 (0.18-0.69)			0.95 (0.65-1.30)	0.99 (0.66-1.31)	0.99 (0.53-1.45)	1.12 (0.62-1.62)
HMWK (U/mL)[a]	0.49 (0.09-0.89)	0.54 (0.06-1.02)			0.98 (0.64-1.32)	0.93 (0.60-1.30)	0.91 (0.63-1.19)	0.92 (0.50-1.36)
Factor XIIIa (U/mL)[a]	0.70 (0.32-1.08)	0.79 (0.27-1.31)			1.08 (0.72-1.43)	1.09 (0.65-1.51)	0.99 (0.57-1.40)	1.05 (0.55-1.55)
Factor XIIIs (U/mL)[a]	0.81 (0.35-1.27)	0.76 (0.30-1.22)			1.13 (0.69-1.56)	1.16 (0.77-1.54)	1.02 (0.60-1.43)	0.97 (0.57-1.37)
d-dimer		1.47 (0.41-2.47)	1.34 (0.58-2.74)	0.22 (0.11-0.42)	0.25 (0.09-0.53)	0.26 (0.10-0.56)	0.27 (0.16-0.39)	0.18 (0.05-0.42)
FDPs[a]								Borderline titer = 1:25-1:50 Positive titer < 1:50

TABLE 39.4 Age-Specific Coagulation Values—cont'd

Coagulation Test	Preterm Infant (30-36 weeks), Day of Life 1[a]	Term Infant, Day of Life 1	Day of Life 3	1 Month-1 Year	1-5 Years	6-10 Years	11-16 Years	Adult
Coagulation Inhibitors								
ATIII (U/mL)[a]	0.38 (0.14-0.62)	0.63 (0.39-0.97)			1.11 (0.82-1.39)	1.11 (0.90-1.31)	1.05 (0.77-1.32)	1.0 (0.74-1.26)
α₂-M (U/mL)[a]	1.10 (0.56-1.82)	1.39 (0.95-1.83)			1.69 (1.14-2.23)	1.69 (1.28-2.09)	1.56 (0.98-2.12)	0.86 (0.52-1.20)
C1-Inh (U/mL)[a]	0.65 (0.31-0.99)	0.72 (0.36-1.08)			1.35 (0.85-1.83)	1.14 (0.88-1.54)	1.03 (0.68-1.50)	1.0 (0.71-1.31)
α₂-AT (U/mL)[a]	0.90 (0.36-1.44)	0.93 (0.49-1.37)			0.93 (0.39-1.47)	1.00 (0.69-1.30)	1.01 (0.65-1.37)	0.93 (0.55-1.30)
Protein C (U/mL)	0.28 (0.12-0.44)	0.32 (0.24-0.40)	0.33 (0.24-0.51)	0.77 (0.28-1.24)	0.94 (0.50-1.34)	0.94 (0.64-1.25)	0.88 (0.59-1.12)	1.03 (0.54-1.66)
Protein S (U/mL)	0.26 (0.14-0.38)	0.36 (0.28-0.47)	0.49 (0.33-0.67)	1.02 (0.29-1.62)	1.01 (0.67-1.36)	1.09 (0.64-1.54)	1.03 (0.65-1.40)	0.75 (0.54-1.03)
Fibrinolytic System[a]								
Plasminogen (U/mL)	1.70 (1.12-2.48)	1.95 (1.60-2.30)			0.98 (0.78-1.18)	0.92 (0.75-1.08)	0.86 (0.68-1.03)	0.99 (0.7-1.22)
TPA (ng/mL)					2.15 (1.0-4.5)	2.42 (1.0-5.0)	2.16 (1.0-4.0)	4.90 (1.40-8.40)
α₂-AP (U/mL)	0.78 (0.4-1.16)	0.85 (0.70-1.0)			1.05 (0.93-1.17)	0.99 (0.89-1.10)	0.98 (0.78-1.18)	1.02 (0.68-1.36)
PAI (U/mL)					5.42 (1.0-10.0)	6.79 (2.0-12.0)	6.07 (2.0-10.0)	3.60 (0-11.0)

[a]Data from Andrew M, Paes B, Milner R, et al. Development of the human anticoagulant system in the healthy premature infant. *Blood.* 1988;72:1651–1657; and Andrew M, Vegh P, Johnston M, et al. Maturation of the hemostatic system during childhood. *Blood.* 1992;8:1998–2005.

[b]aPTT values may vary depending on reagent.

α2 -*AP*, α2 -Antiplasmin; *α2* -*AT*, α2 -antitrypsin; *α2* -*M*, α2 -macroglobulin; *aPTT*, activated partial thromboplastin time; *ATIII*, antithrombin III; *FDPs*, fibrin degradation products; *HMWK*, high-molecular-weight kininogen; *INR*, international normalized ratio; *PAI*, plasminogen activator inhibitor; *PK*, prekallikrein; *PT*, prothrombin time; *TPA*, tissue plasminogen activator; *VIII*, factor VIII procoagulant; *vWF*, von Willebrand factor

Adapted from Monagle P, Barnes C, Ignjatovic, V, et al. Developmental haemostasis. Impact for clinical haemostasis laboratories. *Thromb Haemost.* 2006;95;362–372.
From The Johns Hopkins Hospital. *Harriet Lane Handbook.* 20th ed. Philadelphia: Elsevier; 2018.

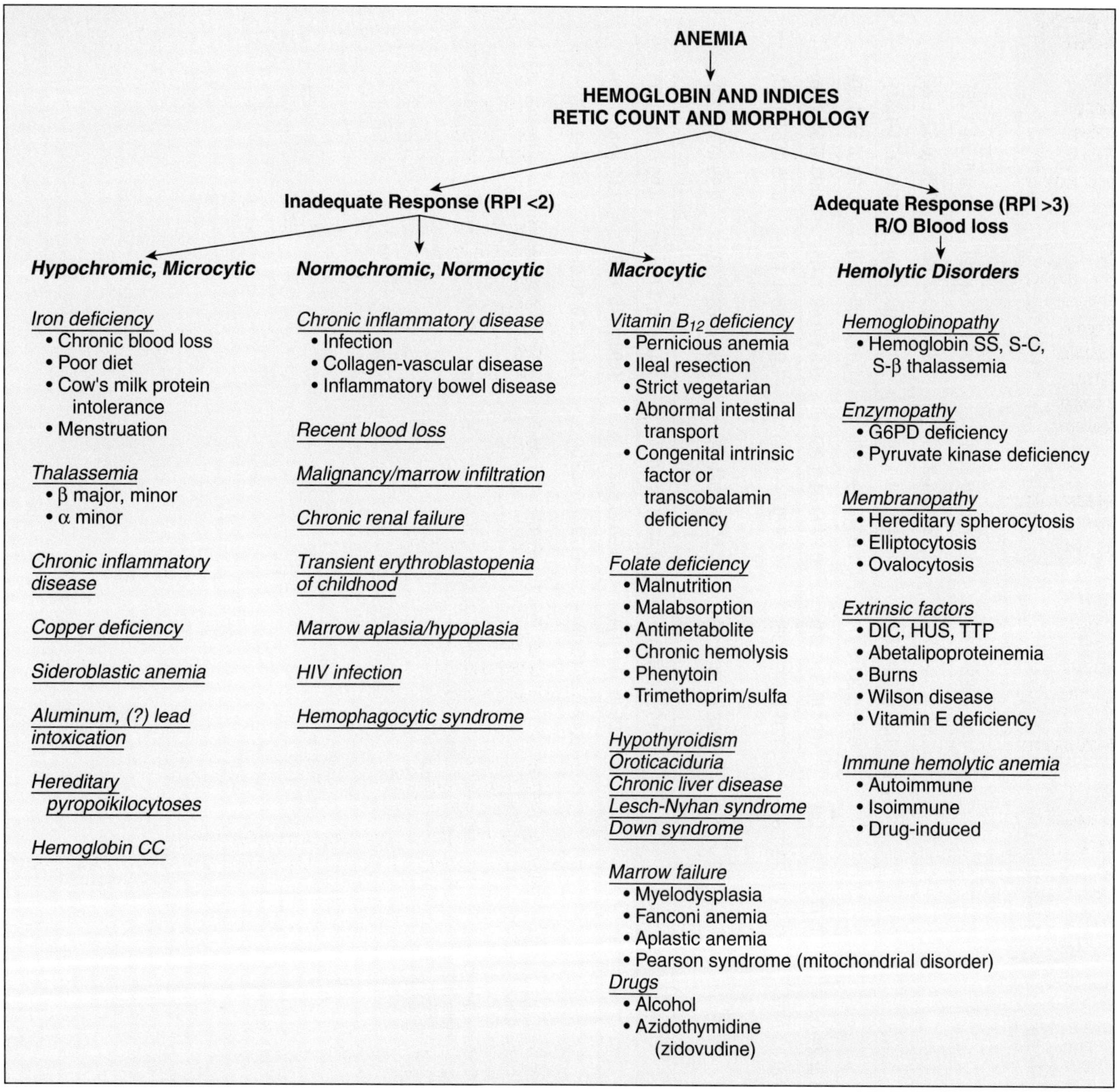

ANEMIA

↓

HEMOGLOBIN AND INDICES
RETIC COUNT AND MORPHOLOGY

Inadequate Response (RPI <2)

Adequate Response (RPI >3)
R/O Blood loss

Hypochromic, Microcytic

Iron deficiency
• Chronic blood loss
• Poor diet
• Cow's milk protein
  intolerance
• Menstruation

Thalassemia
• β major, minor
• α minor

*Chronic inflammatory
disease*

Copper deficiency

Sideroblastic anemia

*Aluminum, (?) lead
intoxication*

*Hereditary
  pyropoikilocytoses*

Hemoglobin CC

Normochromic, Normocytic

Chronic inflammatory disease
• Infection
• Collagen-vascular disease
• Inflammatory bowel disease

Recent blood loss

Malignancy/marrow infiltration

Chronic renal failure

*Transient erythroblastopenia
of childhood*

Marrow aplasia/hypoplasia

HIV infection

Hemophagocytic syndrome

Macrocytic

Vitamin B$_{12}$ deficiency
• Pernicious anemia
• Ileal resection
• Strict vegetarian
• Abnormal intestinal
  transport
• Congenital intrinsic
  factor or
  transcobalamin
  deficiency

Folate deficiency
• Malnutrition
• Malabsorption
• Antimetabolite
• Chronic hemolysis
• Phenytoin
• Trimethoprim/sulfa

Hypothyroidism
Oroticaciduria
Chronic liver disease
Lesch-Nyhan syndrome
Down syndrome

Marrow failure
• Myelodysplasia
• Fanconi anemia
• Aplastic anemia
• Pearson syndrome (mitochondrial disorder)
Drugs
• Alcohol
• Azidothymidine
  (zidovudine)

Hemolytic Disorders

Hemoglobinopathy
• Hemoglobin SS, S-C,
  S-β thalassemia

Enzymopathy
• G6PD deficiency
• Pyruvate kinase deficiency

Membranopathy
• Hereditary spherocytosis
• Elliptocytosis
• Ovalocytosis

Extrinsic factors
• DIC, HUS, TTP
• Abetalipoproteinemia
• Burns
• Wilson disease
• Vitamin E deficiency

Immune hemolytic anemia
• Autoimmune
• Isoimmune
• Drug-induced

• **Fig 39.4** Use of the complete blood count, reticulocyte count, and blood smear in the diagnosis of anemia. *DIC,* Disseminated intravascular coagulation; *G6PD,* glucose-6-phosphate dehydrogenase; *HUS,* hemolytic uremic syndrome; *R/O,* rule out; *RPI,* reticulocyte production index; *TTP,* thrombotic thrombocytopenic purpura. (From Marcdante KJ, Kliegman RM. *Nelson Essentials of Pediatrics.* 8th ed. Philadelphia: Elsevier; 2019.)

cell destruction. The hemolysis may be caused by defects in the red cell membrane, hemoglobinopathies, or congenital enzyme defects (e.g., G6PD deficiency).

Assessment

Anemia may be due to an intrinsic hematologic disorder or be a manifestation of acute or chronic disease. The workup should be directed accordingly. A knowledge of which tests to order and how to interpret laboratory data is integral to analyzing the information gleaned from the hematopoietic system. Laboratory norms vary slightly with the individual lab, so it is important to evaluate the child's results in accordance with local lab

norms and to check whether the local lab uses pediatric normal reference ranges.

The initial laboratory evaluation of suspected anemia includes a CBC with differential, including RBC indices, reticulocyte count, and review of peripheral blood smear (identifies abnormal morphology and/or staining). Following an abnormal screening for Hgb or Hct, further diagnostic studies may be indicated to delineate the type of anemia. Iron deficiency anemia is not only the most common pediatric hematologic disorder, but it is also the most frequent cause of anemia in childhood. Accordingly, the PCP may wish to consider ordering a serum ferritin, iron (Fe), total iron-binding capacity (TIBC), and/or a RBC

• BOX 39.1 Peripheral Blood Morphologic Findings in Various Anemias

Microcytes
Iron deficiency
Thalassemias
Lead toxicity
Anemia of chronic disease

Macrocytes
Newborns
Vitamin B$_{12}$ or folate deficiency
Diamond-Blackfan anemia
Fanconi anemia
Aplastic anemia
Liver disease
Down syndrome
Hypothyroidism

Spherocytes
Hereditary spherocytosis
Immune hemolytic anemia (newborn or acquired)
Hypersplenism

Sickled Cells
Sickle cell anemias (SS disease, SC disease, Sβ$^+$ thalassemia, Sβ^0 thalassemia)

Elliptocytes
Hereditary elliptocytosis
Iron deficiency
Megaloblastic anemia

Target Cells
Hemoglobinopathies (especially hemoglobin C, SC, and thalassemia)
Liver disease
Xerocytosis

Basophil Stippling
Thalassemia
Lead intoxication
Myelodysplasia

Red Blood Cell Fragments, Helmet Cells, Burr Cells
Disseminated intravascular coagulation
Hemolytic uremic syndrome
Thrombotic thrombocytopenic purpura
Kasabach-Merritt syndrome
"Waring blender syndrome"
Uremia
Liver disease

Hypersegmented Neutrophils
Vitamin B$_{12}$ or folate deficiency

Blasts
Leukemia (ALL or AML)
Severe infection (rarely)

Leukopenia/Thrombocytopenia
Fanconi anemia
Aplastic anemia
Leukemia
Hemophagocytic histiocytosis

Howell-Jolly Bodies
Asplenia, hyposplenia
Severe iron deficiency

ALL, Acute lymphocytic leukemia; *AML*, acute myeloid leukemia.

From Kliegman, RM, Lye PS, Bordini BJ, et al. *Nelson Pediatric Symptom-Based Diagnosis.* 1st ed. Philadelphia: Elsevier; 2018.

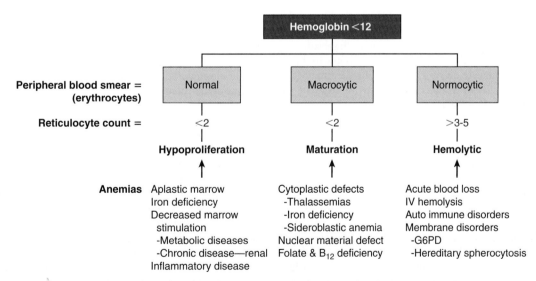

• **Fig 39.5** Classification of Anemia by Underlying Erythrocyte Disorder. *G6PD*, Glucose-6-phosphate dehydrogenase; *IV*, intravenous. (Adapted from Hillman RS, Ault KA, Rinder HM. *Hematology in Clinical Practice.* 4th ed. New York: McGraw-Hill; 2005.)

Anemia	MCV
Elevated RDW (Nonuniform Population of RBCs)	
Hemolytic anemia with elevated reticulocyte count	High
Iron deficiency anemia	Low
Anemias due to red blood cell fragmentation: DIC, HUS, TTP	Low
Megaloblastic anemias: vitamin B_{12} or folate deficiency	High
Normal RDW (Uniform Population of RBCs)	
Thalassemias	Low
Acute hemorrhage	Normal
Fanconi anemia	High
Aplastic anemia	High

DIC, *Disseminated intravascular coagulation;* HUS, *hemolytic uremic syndrome;* MCV, *mean corpuscular volume;* RBC, *red blood cell;* RDW, *red blood cell distribution width;* TTP, *thrombotic thrombocytopenic purpura.*
From Kliegman, RM, Lye PS, Bordini BJ, et al. Nelson Pediatric Symptom-Based Diagnosis. *1st ed.* Philadelphia: Elsevier; 2018.

distribution width (RDW). The RDW reflects the variability of RBC sizes (anisocytosis), which differentiates anemias (Box 39.2). Additional laboratory findings that further differentiate the microcytic anemias are presented in Table 39.5.

Microcytic Anemia: Iron Deficiency Anemia

Iron deficiency anemia (IDA) is the most common nutritional disorder and hematologic condition in the world. Some 9% of adolescent girls develop iron deficiency; 2% to 3% of such cases were due to rapid growth, heavy menses, and nutritionally inadequate diets (Abrams, 2017). The incidence of IDA among children in the United States has been declining slightly during the past four decades, although the prevalence remains high among children living at or below poverty level. Other risk factors include childhood obesity and a history of prematurity or low birth weight (Powers & Mahoney, 2019). IDA correlates with diets low in iron, as occurs with an overuse of goat's milk, cow's milk, or other milk substitutes. Deficient iron intake is also associated with prolonged bottle feeding.

Dietary iron is primarily absorbed in the duodenum. Malabsorption of iron occurs in diseases that affect this segment of the intestine, such as celiac disease, Crohn disease, giardiasis, or resection of the proximal small intestine. Disorders causing rapid transit, GI blood loss due to inflammatory bowel disease, cow's milk–induced colitis, or chronic use of aspirin or nonsteroidal anti-inflammatory drugs (NSAIDs) can also deplete iron stores and contribute to iron deficiency (Mahoney, 2017).

The minimal laboratory screening for iron deficiency is the Hgb level. Often the simplest and most cost-effective measurement is a CBC, which includes the Hgb, Hct, MCV, and RDW. A serum ferritin level is helpful because it reflects current stores of iron, but it must be interpreted carefully because ferritin is an acute-phase reactant and may be increased with inflammatory conditions (Powers & Mahoney, 2019). The American Academy of Pediatrics (AAP) Committee on Nutrition recommends universal Hgb screening for anemia at 12 months of age. This screening should include an assessment of risk factors for iron deficiency and IDA (Box 39.3).

Screening Hgb can be performed on children younger than 1 year of age when risk factors warrant it. When IDA screening

or any other routine health screening recommendation is being implemented, it is important to keep in mind that screening is not just a one-time test; the effectiveness of treatment must be determined through follow-up testing. Thus, after the routine 12-month Hgb testing, risk assessment for anemia should be performed at all preventive pediatric health care visits, with follow-up blood testing if positive. If children are at risk for IDA, a repeat Hgb should be performed as often as indicated.

Effects of Iron Deficiency

Many studies demonstrate that iron-deficient states in the first few years of life are associated with cognitive deficits that extend well into adulthood, although direct causality is difficult to prove. Children's brains reach 95% of adult size by 2 years of age; therefore any nutritional deficit, including iron, can cause lasting damage.

Lead poisoning (plumbism) is often a comorbid condition to IDA. A child at risk for lead exposure should be screened at 9 to 12 months of age and again at 24 months. An estimated 99% of lead-poisoned children are identified through screening procedures rather than clinical recognition. Additional screening should be done at 15 and 30 months of age based on at-risk status. Local health departments determine the prevalence of lead poisoning in their area and issue guidelines related to blood lead screenings for targeted children in their catchment areas (Simon et al, 2014). If the initial blood lead level is 5 mcg/dL or greater on a single visit, it is a concern for public health purposes. The United States has made great strides in reducing lead toxicity through the elimination of tetraethyl leaded gasoline, banning lead-containing solder to seal food and beverage cans, and a federal rule to limit the amount of lead allowed in paint intended for household use.

Clinical Findings

Conduct a detailed history and complete physical examination, keeping in mind children with moderate to severe anemia can be asymptomatic. Some key elements to remember are as follows:

- Infants and toddlers may be irritable and restless, but this only occurs with Hgb less than 8 g/dL and is often noticed in retrospect—after treatment.
- Pica (appetite for nonfood items such as paper, dirt, and clay) and pagophagia (the desire to ingest ice) may be present.
- Anorexia has been reported with Hgb levels less than 8 g/dL.
- Developmental delays (mental and motor areas) and social-emotional behavioral disturbances have been reported in infants and young children; adolescents may experience cognitive impairment (Powers & Mahoney, 2019).

Diagnostic Studies. IDA is frequently identified in routine screenings of Hgb level via capillary sampling. Capillary samples rely on proper technique, as excessive squeezing of the finger may produce inaccurate results. Venous sampling is the most reliable indicator. IDA is likely if there is a low Hgb level for age (in the range of 8 to 11 g/dL), a history of low iron intake, and no concern about other possible causes for the anemia or the possibility of another hemoglobinopathy. If the age of the child and the dietary patterns are consistent with IDA and there is microcytic anemia (Hgb >9 g/dL), many clinicians begin a trial of iron supplementation for 4 to 6 weeks without further diagnostic testing and then follow the child's Hgb and reticulocyte counts. The RDW is the earliest marker of iron deficiency. Serum ferritin is low with iron deficiency.

Mild to moderate IDA is characterized by Hgb levels of 7 to 10 g/dL. Levels less than 4 g/dL necessitate consultation with a

TABLE 39.5 Differentiating Features of Microcytic Anemias

Test	Iron Deficiency Anemia	Thalassemia Minor[a]	Anemia of Inflammation[b]
Serum iron	Low	Normal	Low
Serum iron-binding capacity	High	Normal	Low or normal
Serum ferritin	Low	Normal or high	Normal or high
Marrow iron stores	Low or absent	Normal or high	Normal or high
Marrow sideroblasts	Decreased or absent	Normal or increased	Normal or increased
Free erythrocyte protoporphyrin	High	Normal or slightly increased	High
Hemoglobin A_2 or F	Normal	High β-thalassemia; normal α-thalassemia	Normal
Red blood cell distribution width[c]	High	Normal	Normal/↑

[a]α-Thalassemia minor can be diagnosed by the presence of Bart hemoglobin on newborn screening.
[b]Usually normochromic; 25% of cases are microcytic.
[c]Red blood cell distribution width (RBW) quantitates the degree of anisocytosis (different sizes) of red blood cells.
See Table 150.3 for definition of microcytosis.
From Marcdante KJ, Kliegman RM. *Nelson Essentials of Pediatrics.* 8th ed. Philadelphia: Elsevier; 2019.

• BOX 39.3 Risk Factors for Iron Deficiency Anemia

- Premature and/or low-birth-weight infants
- Exclusive breastfeeding beyond 6 months without iron supplementation
- Early weaning to whole cow's milk (before 1 year)
- Excessive (>25 oz) intake of cow's, goat's, or soy milk in children 1-5 years of age
- Infants fed formula not fortified with iron
- Children with feeding problems
- Children with special health care needs/restricted diets
- Alternative diets (e.g., vegan)
- Low socioeconomic status, food insecurity
- Exposure to lead
- Eating disorders, including obesity
- Hookworm
- Adolescent female, excessive menstrual bleeding

hematologist; and levels of 7 or less should be carefully evaluated as to whether the child needs referral to hematology. If treatment with oral iron supplements is effective, follow-up Hgb in 1 month should reveal a minimal improvement of 1 to 2 g/dL; the reticulocyte count will increase to greater than 3% in 48 to 96 hours (Sills, 2016).

There is a high comorbidity between IDA and lead poisoning (Pb >5 mcg/dL) because lead molecules block iron from binding to protoporphyrin by inhibiting essential mitochondrial membrane function and interfering with enzymes. In low iron states, the lack of iron results in an accumulation of erythrocyte protoporphyrin in blood.

The typical profile for IDA is
- Microcytic, hypochromic RBCs on CBC
- Low or normal MCV; low to normal RBC number
- High RDW (>14%), low ferritin, high TIBC
- Mentzer index greater than 13 (IDA more likely)

Differential Diagnosis

Iron deficiency should be differentiated from other microcytic, hypochromic anemias, such as lead poisoning, thalassemia minor, anemia of chronic disease, and hereditary sideroblastic anemia. In lead poisoning, the free erythrocyte protoporphyrins (FEP) may be more than 200 mcg/dL, and basophilic stippling may be seen on the RBCs in the peripheral smear. β thalassemia is indicated by elevations in Hgb A_2 on electrophoresis and a Mentzer index of less than 13.

If there is no response to iron therapy within 1 month and there is confidence that the iron supplements are being given correctly, a more extensive workup should include a CBC with differential, platelet count, RBC indices, and reticulocyte count. A peripheral blood smear should also be examined to assess the number and morphology of RBCs, WBCs, and platelets. The differential diagnosis for anemia can then be determined on the basis of whether RBC production is adequate or inadequate and whether the cells are microcytic, normocytic, or macrocytic.

Other causes of anemia, such as blood loss with occult rectal bleeding, should be considered in children with a low Hgb level who eat a normal diet with adequate servings of iron-rich foods. Additional investigation is warranted in children younger than 6 months of age or older than 18 months or who demonstrate no response to treatment after 2 to 4 weeks. For those children with low Hgb/Hct who do not have a history suspicious for IDA, the investigation must expand to include less common sources for the anemia. Findings of severe anemia or atypical hematologic results require consultation and further investigation. Pairing the classification of the cells with the clinical findings, red cell indices, and additional diagnostic studies enables the provider to determine the appropriate treatment plan.

Management

For infants and children, the treatment for IDA consists of iron supplementation, typically as ferrous sulfate (3 to 6 mg/kg/day of elemental iron in two to three divided doses or 3 mg/kg/day in one or two divided doses for mild or moderate IDA) (Sills, 2016). In adolescents the daily maximum of elemental iron is 200 mg. The child's reticulocyte count should be reassessed within 1 week, as reticulocytosis may be seen within a few days of treatment. Hgb should return to a normal level within 4 to 6 weeks. If a therapeutic response is observed (Hgb increase of >1 g/dL or >3% increase

• **BOX 39.4** **Red Flags During an Anemia Workup**

Anemia Accompanied by

Abnormal vital signs (tachycardia, hypotension, hypertension)
Neutropenia and/or thrombocytopenia
High MCV with normal RDW
Blasts on the peripheral smear
Firm adenopathy
Bruising or bleeding
Weight loss, failure to thrive
Shortness of breath, fatigue
Fever
Hypoxia
Organomegaly
Edema
Oliguria-anuria
Bloody diarrhea
Red urine (hemoglobinuria)
Family history of anemia

MCV, *Mean corpuscular volume;* RDW, *red blood cell distribution width.*
From Kliegman, RM, Lye PS, Bordini BJ, et al. Nelson Pediatric Symptom-Based Diagnosis. *1st ed.* Philadelphia: Elsevier; 2018.

in Hct), iron supplementation should continue to normalize Hgb, then continue for 2 to 3 months to replete iron stores. Serum ferritin levels should be rechecked 6 months after iron supplements are stopped to determine resolution of the anemia and adequacy of iron stores (Powers & Mahoney, 2019).

Iron Requirements. Full-term infants accumulate almost 80% of their iron stores during the last trimester of pregnancy. Delayed clamping of the umbilical cord also ensures that newborns receive the maximal transfusion to begin life. Along with prematurity, maternal anemia, maternal hypertension with intrauterine growth retardation, and/or gestational diabetes can result in less iron transferred to the fetus. In the case of preterm births, the decreased iron stores are depleted rapidly and the normal physiologic nadir occurs earlier, aggravated by a smaller total blood volume at birth and poor GI absorption. The use of erythropoietin to prevent and treat anemia of prematurity also increases the risk of iron deficiency (Powers & Mahoney, 2019). In general, preterm (<37 weeks' gestation) infants require an oral supplement of elemental iron at 2 mg/kg per day from 2 weeks through 12 months of age (Powers & Mahoney, 2019).

Breast milk provides an average iron content of 1.0 to 0.3 mg/L with a high bioavailability. Because there is large variation in the iron content in human milk, the content of maternal milk may not always provide for the needs of the growing infant. It is recommended that the exclusively breastfed term infant receive elemental iron supplementation of 1 mg/kg/day (15 mg maximum) beginning at 4 months of age and continuing until iron-containing complementary foods are introduced and taken in adequate quantities (Powers & Mahoney, 2019). This same iron supplementation recommendation holds for the partially breastfed infants who receive more than half of their daily feeding as human milk. Infants fed with standard infant formulas receive a sufficient iron intake of 12 mg/dL.

The intake of iron should increase dramatically to 11 mg/day between 7 and 12 months of age based on cells sloughing and the demands of increasing body mass (Hernell et al., 2015). As the rate of growth decreases in early childhood, so does the nutritional requirement of iron, down to 7 mg/day between 1 and 3 years of age. Iron deficiency becomes more prevalent during these

ages as well, reaching 6.6% to 15.2% depending on ethnicity and socioeconomic status, although the occurrence of IDA is 0.9% to 4.4%. Despite these seemingly low levels of incidence, IDA accounts for almost half of the anemias of early childhood. Liquid supplementation for this age group is appropriate until 36 months of age. Chewable multivitamins can be used for children older than 3 years of age, but the supplement formulation must be evaluated for adequate replacement.

Complications

Adherence issues and alternative diagnoses should be explored if there is no response to iron supplementation. Dietary counseling is critical, and families may need support to make the necessary changes. Iron-deficient states can exist in the absence of anemia as a precursor to IDA and they require intervention. A more extensive determination of the child's iron status is obtained by measuring serum iron, iron-binding capacity, and the venous lead level. Stool guaiac should be checked for occult blood loss. Children with extremely low Hgb, abnormal vital signs, and/or associated red flags (Box 39.4) should immediately be attended to and/or referred to a pediatric hematologist and may need hospitalization. Laboratory results that also indicate referral are co-occurring neutropenia, thrombocytopenia, nucleated RBCs, or immature myeloid elements. When disorders of all elements—erythrocytes, platelets, and leukocytes—are found, a bone marrow disorder is probable.

Patient and Family Education

Parents or caretakers should be counseled to increase iron-rich foods in their child's diet. Exclusively breastfed term infants should be started on iron supplementation at 4 months of age and iron-fortified cereal and/or pureed meats added to the child's diet after 6 months of age. Whole cow's milk should be avoided in infants younger than 12 months of age due to its low iron content and the possibility of insensible GI blood loss. After 12 months of age, cow's milk ingestion should be limited to 24 oz/day. Goat's milk should not be the sole diet of a child, not only because of its lack of iron but also its lack of folic acid. For preterm infants, supplementation with oral iron drops should begin no later than 1 month of age. Education for older children taking iron supplements includes advising parents to avoid giving iron with meals or milk, that vitamin C juice enhances absorption, and that the child's stools will probably turn black. Foods containing soy can inhibit the absorption of iron. Any dental staining associated with taking iron can be removed with dental cleaning. Parents should also be cautioned to keep the medication safely out of reach to prevent accidental ingestion.

Thalassemias

Thalassemias are categorized into two types: alpha (α) and beta (β), based on the affected chain. In the carrier of α *thalassemia* (minor/trait), only one α chain is present, which enables the production of adequate amounts of Hgb with few or no symptoms; however in α-thalassemia disease (major), there are no α chains, so the β-globulin subunits cluster into groups of four. These β tetramers are incapable of carrying oxygen, and the affected fetuses die in utero (hydrops fetalis). In the carrier of β *thalassemia* (minor/trait), there are sufficient β chains to bind with the abundant α chains and create functional Hgb molecules; however, a resultant asymptomatic mild microcytic anemia is present (see Box 39.3).

In β thalassemia major, the α chains do not bind with each other but rather degrade in the absence of β chains; ongoing degradation results in severe anemia and the need for ongoing transfusions. The possibility of thalassemia increases if the onset of anemia and symptoms occurs prior to 3 to 6 months of age and there is a prior family history of thalassemia or a family history of anemia, miscarriage, or fetal demise or jaundice, gallstones, anemia, or splenomegaly.

Categorizing the thalassemias is less straightforward than with many anemias because although the heterozygous disease is hypochromic and microcytic, the homozygous diseases are also hemolytic. There is anemia and increased erythropoiesis. The erythropoiesis results in bone marrow expansion, but the pathogenesis of this is not fully understood. Focal osteomalacia and delayed bone maturation are at least partially explained by suboptimal blood transfusions and iron overload. Furthermore, the marrow expansion results in frontal bossing and hyperplasia of the maxillary bones, leading to typical facies (DeBaun et al., 2016).

α Thalassemias

The α thalassemias are composed of several variant Hgbs that are responsible for the various presentations. Current nomenclature often refers to the subtypes by including an indication of the number of gene deletions of α globin; the severity of symptoms increases with more deletions. Three gene deletions result in severe, even fatal, manifestations of disease. Two gene deletions present with hypochromia; the absence of gene deletions causes mild anemia and often erythrocytosis. A single globin gene deletion is clinically insignificant (DeBaun et al., 2016).

There are two manifestations of the disease expression of α thalassemia. The homozygous Hgb type, Hgb Bart (or Hgb H) with four γ-chains, results in *hydrops fetalis* and is incompatible with life because of severe anemia. Homozygous Hgb H disease can also present as a microcytic, hypochromic anemia that most often manifests as a hemolytic anemia, hepatosplenomegaly, and mild jaundice and sometimes includes thalassemia-like bone changes. During times of physiologic stress, the child may require RBC transfusion.

There are two different carrier states of α thalassemia. In α-thalassemia trait, the child exhibits microcytosis and hypochromia but has normal percentages of Hgb A₂ and Hgb F. The other trait state is referred to as a *silent carrier state* but can have either a silent hematologic phenotype or present with microcytic hypochromia and some erythropoiesis.

Management

Hgb H disease exacerbations may necessitate occasional transfusion during hemolytic or aplastic crises. No treatment is indicated for the carrier trait expressions of disease, and the microcytosis seen in these expressions require that serum iron studies should be done before starting any iron supplements. Those carrying the α-thalassemia trait alleles require careful genetic counseling, because there are complex patterns of inheritance that could affect the phenotype of such individuals' offspring (Benz, 2017).

β Thalassemia Minor/Minima

β thalassemia minor and minima disease, also known as β thalassemia *trait,* is associated with a mild hypochromic, microcytic anemia in which Hgb levels are 2 to 3 g/dL below normal and the MCV averages 65 fL. These children must be monitored for iron accumulation but are otherwise asymptomatic. The disease may be

---

> **• BOX 39.5 Mentzer Index**

Mentzer index = MCV/RBC. If the ratio is less than 13, the anemia is more likely to be thalassemia trait; if the ratio is greater than 13, the anemia is more likely to be due to iron deficiency.

---

confused with iron deficiency or lead poisoning and can be differentiated by measuring serum iron or lead levels, transferrin saturation, or serum ferritin levels. It is particularly important to diagnose this condition correctly in order to avoid unnecessary administration of iron supplements, which do not improve the Hgb level and could result in iron overload. The primary diagnostic feature is increased Hgb A₂ (>3.5%) on electrophoresis (Benz, 2017).

Clinical Findings

Clinically most individuals with thalassemia trait are asymptomatic, although mild pallor and splenomegaly may be found. A Hgb of 9.5 to 11 g/dL, Hct less than 30%, and a MCV of less than 75 fL are commonly seen in thalassemia minor. The MCV/RBC count per milliliter is less than 13 (Box 39.5). In contrast, the Mentzer index of iron deficiency is usually greater than 13; however, some sources use 13.5 as the indicator for IDA (Benz, 2017). The degree of anemia may be exacerbated in concurrent illness or pregnancy.

Management

No specific treatment is known for β thalassemia minor. Primary emphasis should be on the education of all family members and genetic testing, and counseling should be offered.

β Thalassemia Intermedia

This variant of thalassemia is the result of various mutations that cause a disorder with a clinical severity that spans from the mild symptoms of the β-thalassemia trait to the severe manifestations of β-thalassemia major. Classification is typically based on the severity of the symptoms and the type of treatment necessary rather than by the specific genotype. Diagnosis and management are clinically based with the goal of maintaining a satisfactory Hgb of at least 6 to 7 g/dL without the regular need for RBC transfusions. Transfusions alleviate thalassemic features, but there is controversy as to whether these children should receive transfusions. This decision must be balanced against the future need for chelation if there is iron overload from repeated transfusions (DeBaun et al., 2016).

β Thalassemia Major

Homozygous forms are thalassemia intermedia and thalassemia major. Homozygous β thalassemia major (or Cooley anemia) is associated with severe anemia resulting from the decreased or absent production of Hgb A and hemolysis caused by the precipitation of excess α chains in the RBCs.

Clinical Findings

Affected infants usually become symptomatic in the first year of life and have pallor, failure to thrive, hepatosplenomegaly, and a severe anemia with an average Hgb of 6 g/dL and low MCV (60 to 70 fL). RBC morphology reveals significant microcytosis, poikilocytosis, hypochromia, target cells, and nucleated RBCs. Hgb A₂ and Hgb F levels are elevated.

Management

Proper management of the child requires collaboration with a pediatric hematologist. Standards of care for thalassemia patients should be followed (Vichinsky and Levine, 2012). RBC transfusions are usually necessary every 2 to 4 weeks with the goal of maintaining a pretransfusion Hgb level between 9.5 and 10.5 g/dL. To help with future cross matching, the provider should obtain a complete typing of the patient's erythrocyte profile before the first transfusion (phenotyping). This helps to decrease difficulties with subsequent transfusions. Splenectomy may also be indicated. Hematopoietic stem cell transplantation is the only curative modality for β thalassemia major. This has been most successful in children younger than 15 years of age without excessive iron overload and hepatosplenomegaly who have sibling-matched human leukocyte antigen (HLA) allogeneic hematopoietic transplantation (Benz, 2017; DeBaun et al., 2016). Gene therapy is being investigated and holds promise for those with this major disorder.

Iron chelation is necessary to treat the hyperferric state produced by repeated transfusions and prevent complications primarily of the heart, liver, and endocrine system. Iron overload can develop even without the use of blood transfusions because of the increased iron absorption associated with high rates of erythropoiesis and red cell destruction. Monitoring for iron stores should be done on a regular basis (Benz, 2017). Chronic iron chelation therapy is necessary in order to remove the excess iron resulting from frequent transfusions.

Indications for chelation occur when the serum ferritin concentrations are excessive (variably stated as >300, >400, or >1000 mcg/L) and/or magnetic resonance imaging (MRI) T_2 suggest the presence of iron loading in critical organs such as the liver (>3 mg of iron per gram of dry weight) and the heart (Benz, 2017). Deferoxamine is administered parenterally or subcutaneously, usually via a pump overnight. It is time-consuming and associated with pain. Subcutaneously infused medications have been replaced by oral chelators. Deferasirox is an oral agent taken once daily at 20 to 30 mg/kg/day; it stabilizes the ferritin levels, thus achieving a negative iron balance (DeBaun et al., 2016). Iron excretion through chelation is further aided by the ingestion of vitamin C. Because the iron is excreted through the kidneys, hydration and monitoring of renal status are vital.

Complications

If the condition is left untreated, bone marrow expansion causes the characteristic facies, with frontal bossing and maxillary overgrowth. Other complications of disease and treatment include osteopenia, thrombolytic symptoms, cardiopulmonary problems, asplenia secondary to splenectomy, cholelithiasis, and extramedullary hematopoiesis.

The medications used to chelate iron have additional side effects. Deferasirox, the daily oral agent, commonly produces headache, nausea, vomiting, joint pain, and fatigue. It has a black box warning of GI hemorrhage as well as kidney and liver failure. Deferoxamine has risks associated with the administration of intravenous medication (infection) and vision and hearing loss. Additionally there are the inherent risks and complications of transfusion, including transfusion reaction, fever, and, although rare, hepatitis or human immunodeficiency virus (HIV) infection.

The disease as well as its complications and treatments are painful for the child and monopolize a large portion of these patients' and their and families' lives. Families need not only professional support and education but also interaction with other families affected by this disorder, such as those that can be found through the resources of the Thalassemia Support Foundation or Cooley's Anemia Foundation.

Macrocytic Anemia

Macrocytic (megaloblastic) anemias are characterized by macrocytic RBCs, hypersegmented polymorphonuclear leukocytes (PMNs) in the peripheral blood, and megaloblasts in the bone marrow. Relatively rare, macrocytic anemias are primarily due to a lack of folic acid, vitamin B_{12}, or both. These anemias may develop if the diet (e.g., goat's milk) lacks these two substances or if the gastric intrinsic factor necessary for the absorption of vitamin B_{12} is absent.

Clinical Findings

History. Suspicion should be high if there is a history of young infants being fed a diet of powdered cow's milk products and/or alternative milk sources, such as goat's milk, as these are deficient in folic acid and vitamin B_{12}. Of equal concern are older children who have strict vegetarian or vegan diets and those with signs of severe nutritional deficiencies, absorption problems, or tapeworm infestations. Children with folic acid deficiency tend to be irritable and also to have inadequate weight gain and chronic diarrhea.

Physical Examination. Physical findings relate to the severity of the anemia but commonly include weakness, pallor, and a beefy-red, smooth sore mouth and tongue.

Diagnostic Studies. The following results may be seen:
- Elevated MCV (>100 fL) and decreased reticulocyte count.
- Blood smear showing nucleated RBCs and macro-ovalocytes with anisocytosis and poikilocytosis.
- Normal WBC and platelet counts but possibly decreased in more severe cases.
- Large and hypersegmented neutrophils.
- Thrombocytopenia or possible large platelets.
- In suspected folic acid deficiency the RBC folate level is decreased whereas iron and B_{12} levels tend to be normal or elevated (Schrier, 2017).

Management

Management of folic acid deficiency and juvenile pernicious anemia (caused by a lack of vitamin B_{12}) is typically best done in consultation with a pediatric hematologist. Treatment is dietary supplementation and correction of the underlying disorder (e.g., infection) if possible.

In folic acid deficiency confirmed by measurement of the RBC folate level, folic acid may be administered in a dose of 1mg/day until complete hematologic recovery. Maintenance therapy follows with .1mg -.4 mg/day, depending on the child's age. In Vit B12 deficiency, a prompt hematologic response is usually seen after parenteral administration (either intramuscular or deep subcutaneous) of vitamin B12. Treat with 100mcg/day vitamin B12 until complete hematological recovery, followed by 60mcg/month for maintenance (Schrier, 2017).

Normocytic Anemias

Anemias that have an RBC size within the normal range are termed *normocytic*. Normocytic anemias tend to coincide with chronic illness, B_{12} deficiency, traumatic blood loss, or pregnancy. They are not common in children. Final determination of the etiology extends beyond blood cell indices and includes further chemistry laboratory tests such as blood urea nitrogen (BUN), creatinine, serum glutamic-oxaloacetic transaminase (SGOT), alkaline phosphatase, bilirubin, erythrocyte sedimentation rate, urinalysis, and thyroid profile.

Transient Erythroblastopenia of Childhood

Idiopathic or transient erythroblastopenia of childhood, or TEC, is a benign disorder of unknown cause that occurs in children during the first few years of life, usually after the first year of life. It is characterized by anemia, reticulocytopenia, and erythroid hypoplasia of the bone marrow. The cause of this transient suppression of erythropoiesis with resultant decreased RBC production is not clear, although it frequently follows a viral infection. Thus viral and immunologic mechanisms are suspected but no specific virus has been implicated. TEC is associated with a temporary failure of erythropoiesis caused by probable viral suppression or as a result of an IgG, IgM, or cell-mediated autoimmune response (van den Akker et al., 2014).

Clinical Findings

History. TEC occurs mainly in previously healthy children between 6 months and 3 years of age. The child may have a history of a preceding infection.

Physical Examination. Patients have symptoms of anemia, typically a gradually increasing pallor. Parents may report noticing decreased energy levels or fatigue in their child. Pallor and fatigue develop over a course of days or weeks and are often associated with viral symptoms, such as fever, malaise, lethargy, abdominal pain, or upper respiratory symptoms. Jaundice may be noted, especially if the child has a preexisting hemoglobinopathy.

Diagnostic Studies. The following are seen in TEC:
- Anemia (in which the Hgb content may be as low as 2.5 g/dL or only slightly decreased but generally around 6 to 8 g/dL)
- Markedly low reticulocyte count
- MCV characteristically normal for age
- WBC count usually normal but some degree of neutropenia can occur in up to 20%
- Platelet count normal or elevated
- High serum iron level reflecting decreased utilization
- Bone marrow aspiration indicating erythroid hypoplasia

Differential Diagnosis

The syndrome can be differentiated from congenital hypoplastic anemia (Diamond-Blackfan syndrome) by the normal size of the RBCs (MCV <80 fL). Approximately 50% of children with Diamond-Blackfan syndrome have dysmorphic features (e.g., short stature, congenital heart disease, and mental retardation), whereas children with TEC have a normal physical examination. The peak incidence of TEC coincides with that of IDA, but the differences in MCV should help differentiate between these diagnoses.

Management

TEC is self-limited, with recovery taking place 1 to 2 months after diagnosis. No specific treatment is indicated, although transfusions may be required for severe anemia. A referral to a hematologist may be needed.

Hemolytic Anemia

Hemolytic anemias are caused by premature destruction of RBCs and increased marrow production of reticulocytes. They can be classified as either hereditary or acquired and should be suspected in cases of an elevated reticulocyte count in the absence of bleeding or heparin therapy. In particular, the hereditary and congenital anemias manifest in infancy and early childhood. They may be due to a variety of hemoglobinopathies or defects in the red cell membrane. Determining the etiology of hemolysis necessitates careful history taking, including family medical history, child's medical history, diet, medication intake, and environmental exposures. Confirmation of the diagnosis comes from Hgb electrophoresis, Heinz body stain, and osmotic fragility test.

Sickle Cell Anemia and Trait

Sickle cell disease describes a group of complex, chronic disorders characterized by hemolysis, unpredictable acute complications that may become life-threatening, and the possible development of chronic organ damage. Children who have homozygous inheritance have sickle cell anemia (SCA) or disease (Hgb SS). Their bodies do not form the normal Hgb A molecule but rather synthesize hemoglobin S (Hgb S), which carries the amino acid valine instead of glutamic acid. Because of this change, Hgb S tends to polymerize or come out of solution at low Pao_2, low pH, low temperature, and low osmolality. This process collapses the RBC, giving it a "sickled" shape and producing a chronic hemolytic anemia. The new shape is rigid and clogs small blood vessels, producing ischemia, pain, and other vaso-occlusive problems.

Sickle cell disease has an autosomal recessive inheritance pattern. It is found most often in people of African descent but is also detected among ethnic groups from the Mediterranean, the Caribbean, Central and South America, and India. Owing to migration, it now occurs worldwide. Sickle cell trait occurs in 8% of African Americans. This incidence exceeds that of most other serious genetic disorders in children, including cystic fibrosis and hemophilia; only α thalassemia is more common. Routine neonatal screening identifies most infants with sickle cell disease born in the United States because such screening is mandated in all states and the District of Columbia. It is still important to obtain a careful family medical history because many adults do not realize that they are carriers.

Clinical Findings

The clinical findings in sickle cell disease are multisystemic, necessitating vigilant care to minimize the occurrence of crises and complications, including the following:
- Fatigue and anemia, abdominal pain, and pain crises
- Dactylitis (swelling and inflammation of the hands and/or feet) and arthritis
- Bacterial infections, leg ulcers
- Eye damage, lung and heart injury, aseptic necrosis and bone infarcts (death of portions of bone)
- Priapism, splenic sequestration (sudden pooling of blood in the spleen) and liver congestion

Children with sickle cell trait who are heterozygous (Hgb A + Hgb S) for the gene essentially have a benign clinical course. Their RBCs contain only 30% to 40% Hgb S, and sickling does not occur under most conditions. It is only in rare instances of hypoxia, such as in shock, while flying in unpressurized aircraft, or traveling to high elevations that signs of vaso-occlusion can appear. However, the presence of sickle cell trait has been implicated as a causative factor in the sudden deaths of young military recruits, college football players, and some teens. Extreme exercise, typically to exhaustion; dehydration; and relative hypoxia (altitude) are major confounding factors.

Physical Examination. SCA symptoms typically begin to emerge in the second 6 months of life as the amount of Hgb S increases and Hgb F declines. Thereafter painful vaso-occlusive crises occur. Owing to the multisystemic nature of complications these children need prompt, detailed evaluation and intervention. After 5 years of age, splenomegaly usually disappears because of autoinfarction of the organ. Rates of height and weight gain usually slow after 7 years of age, and puberty may be delayed by 3 to 4 years.

Diagnostic Studies. The following laboratory results are seen in sickle cell disease:
- Hct of 20% to 29%
- Hgb 6 to 10 g/dL (severe)
- Reticulocyte count elevated: 5% to 15%
- Normal to increased WBCs and platelets
- MCV greater than 80 fL; mean corpuscular hemoglobin concentration (MCHC) greater than 37 mg/dL
- Hgb electrophoresis (after infancy), isoelectric focusing, or high-performance liquid chromatography showing a predominance of Hgb S and no Hgb A
- Morphology: Irreversibly sickled cells or chronic elliptocytes, Howell-Jolly bodies, nucleated RBCs

Hgb electrophoresis results in a newborn with sickle cell trait will be Hgb FAS, and Hgb FS for a child with either SCA or sickle β-zero thalassemia (SBO). Normal results of Hgb electrophoresis are Hgb FA.

Differential Diagnosis

Chronic hemolytic anemia should be included in the differential diagnosis. Other syndromes characterized by hemolytic anemia and vaso-occlusion are Hgb SC disease, SCA, and a combination of Hgb S with α or β thalassemia. These diseases may be differentiated through electrophoresis and family testing if necessary. Hgb SC disease is typically less severe than Hgb SS; the course of sickle cell β thalassemia can be severe or mild depending on the amount of β globin; sickle cell α thalassemia is associated with milder anemia (Vichinsky, 2017). Prenatal genetic testing is available in instances of high suspicion; otherwise mandated newborn screening provides the diagnosis in most cases before symptoms present.

Management

Management of the child with SCA is complicated and should be done in consultation with a pediatric hematologist. Remarkable progress in the care of children with SCA can be directly attributed to the development of standards of care and anticipatory guidance. The National Heart, Lung, and Blood Institute (NHLBI) has developed evidence-based clinical practice guidelines for the management of SCA (2014).

Children with sickle cell disease need regular primary care services and coordinated consultative services and information. Growth is closely monitored, immunizations must be done on time, parents require support, and communication with specialty services should be coordinated (e.g., an annual ophthalmologic examination by a retinal specialist). Care is comprehensive, spanning normal well-child issues through acute crises and hospitalization. Some of the key aspects of care for the child with SCA are as follows:
- Hydration, illness prevention, and pain management are fundamental aspects of disease management. NSAIDs or acetaminophen may be adequate for mild to moderate pain, but narcotics should be used when these are not adequate for management. (As in the case of anyone taking narcotics, abuse and addiction issues must be considered.)
- The CBC and reticulocyte count are monitored every few months.
- All the usual immunizations of childhood are to be administered on time, including 13-valent pneumococcal conjugate (four doses at appropriate intervals) and 23-valent pneumococcal polysaccharide vaccines (first dose at or after 24 months of age), with a second dose of PPSV23 given 3 years after the first dose. The conjugate Hib and meningococcal vaccine (Hib-MenCY) is recommended for infants with sickle cell disease at 2, 4, 6, and 12 to 15 months of age and booster doses of MCV4 every 5 years thereafter. An annual flu vaccination is essential (Rogers, 2017).
- Invasive bacterial infection is the leading cause of death in young children with SCA. Penicillin V prophylaxis (125 mg PO twice daily) is initiated by 2 months of age. At 3 years of age, the dose is increased to 250 mg PO twice daily and continued at least until the fifth birthday or until the child has received two doses of PPSV23 (Rogers, 2017).
- Folic acid supplementation at 1 mg/day is typically given to adults to prevent folate deficiency due to hemolysis. This is not standard therapy for children unless a folic acid deficiency is suspected; it should be individualized for each patient (Rogers, 2017).
- Aggressive treatment of infections and maintenance of hydration and body temperature are used to prevent hypoxia and acidosis; volume replacement may be necessary to prevent circulatory collapse.
- Coexisting medical problems associated with lower oxygen saturations, such as asthma and obstructive sleep apnea, must be treated.
- In children with severe SCA, hydroxyurea is used to reduce the number of painful crises and the incidence of acute chest syndrome (a leading cause of death in adolescents with SCA). It is a preventive medication and not effective during the acute crisis. Hydroxyurea use is associated with a lower need for blood transfusions and fewer hospital visits by reducing the frequency and severity of painful events and episodes of acute chest syndrome. It increases Hgb F levels within cells, which decreases Hgb S levels, increases RBC water content, and alters the adhesion of RBCs to endothelium. There is some early evidence suggesting that it helps to improve growth and preserves organ function. The results of two studies suggest that hydroxyurea may be given safely to children as young as 8 months of age, although it is not approved for this age group (Rogers, 2017). Despite these benefits, side effects do occur, including an increased risk for serious infection. As always, the practitioner must carefully weigh all risks and benefits before integrating this medication into the treatment plan.
- Annual stroke prevention screening of major intracranial vessels with transcranial Doppler ultrasound evaluation is planned for 2- to 16-year-old children or as long as their bone windows allow meaningful waveforms to be evaluated. A reading of greater than 200 cm/s time-averaged mean maximal velocity indicates a high risk for stroke as well as the need to start a transfusion program to maintain Hgb S levels less than 30% (Rogers, 2017).

Children with sickle cell disease are usually comanaged by their PCPs and specialists in hematology. Emergency admission or referral is necessary in the presence of the following:
- Fever (to rule out sepsis) greater than 101°F (38.3°C)

- Pneumonia, chest pain, or other pulmonary symptoms (acute chest syndrome)
- Sequestration crisis (splenomegaly with decreased Hgb or Hct)
- Aplastic crisis (decreased Hct and reticulocyte count)
- Severe painful crisis, priapism
- Unusual headache, visual disturbances

Consultation is also necessary for the chronic sequelae of persistent bone pain or leg ulcers, pregnancy, and contraception. Stem cell transplantation may be a consideration in children with significant disease and is curative in some. Gene therapy is under investigation and may be available in the future. New medications are under investigation as well.

Complications

Because of functional asplenia, the greatest concern is febrile illness, indicating infection and possible sepsis. In view of the serious threat of pneumococcal sepsis in children younger than 5 years of age, all complaints of fever, poor feeding, lethargy, and irritability should be clinically evaluated. The consequences of hemolysis may include chronic anemia, jaundice, cholelithiasis, and delayed growth and sexual maturation. Vaso-occlusion and tissue ischemia may result in acute and chronic injury to virtually every organ system, with stroke being a major concern.

Patient and Family Education

The parents of children with SCA need a great deal of support in raising a child with a genetically transmitted chronic disease. Clear patterns of communication should be established between the family and the PCP using a partnership model. Initial education includes the genetics and pathophysiology of the disease and the importance of regular health maintenance visits. Discussion should emphasize the need for early evaluation and treatment of febrile illness, acute splenic sequestration, aplastic crisis, and acute chest syndrome. Parents can be taught to palpate their child's spleen. Any downward displacement or enlargement of the spleen below the left costal margin should be evaluated by a healthcare professional and the blood counts monitored for increasing anemia. As the child grows, the family should be educated about other potential clinical complications, such as stroke, enuresis, priapism, cholelithiasis, delayed puberty, retinopathy, avascular necrosis of the hip and shoulder, and leg ulcers (Rogers, 2017).

Preventive care measures also include the following:
- Timely administration of routine immunizations, including pneumococcal and meningococcal vaccines, and yearly influenza vaccine
- Prophylactic antibiotics
- Genetic counseling for those with sickle cell trait and gene therapy (under investigation)
- Support groups
- Educating adolescents with the trait about their status and the risk of disease transmission
- Hematopoietic stem cell transplant (the only intervention that can cure sickle cell disease with strict inclusion criteria identified for transplant eligibility)

Hereditary Spherocytosis

Hereditary spherocytosis (HS) is a hemolytic anemia characterized by a deficiency or abnormality of the RBC membrane protein spectrin, which reduces the RBC surface area. The RBC membranes assume a more spherical shape. Hence RBCs are more likely to be sequestered and prematurely destroyed in the spleen. HS causes mild chronic hemolysis to severe transfusion-dependent anemia. HS occurs in 1 in 5000 persons of mainly northern European ancestry.

Clinical Findings

Jaundice usually appears in the newborn period, and it may be difficult to differentiate HS from hyperbilirubinemia caused by ABO incompatibility. After 2 years of age, splenomegaly is usually present. Chronic fatigue, malaise, and abdominal pain may also be noted.

Diagnostic Studies. Laboratory findings in HS include the following:
- Chronic anemia: Hgb is 6 to 10 g/dL.
- Reticulocyte count ranges from 5% to 20%.
- On peripheral smear, a small proportion of the RBCs is spherocytic and smaller than normal and lacks the central pallor of the usual biconcave disk-shaped cell.
- Osmotic fragility of the cells is increased, as is the rate of autohemolysis of incubated blood.
- Prenatal and carrier testing for sequence analysis of the entire coding region has limited laboratory availability.

Management

The treatment of choice for children with severe HS requiring multiple transfusions is splenectomy (with removal of the gallbladder), which usually produces a clinical cure. It should be deferred until after 6 years of age because of the increased risk of encapsulated bacterial infection before that age. Risks associated with splenectomy are postsplenectomy sepsis, penicillin-resistant pneumococcal infection, pulmonary hypertension, and ischemic heart disease and stroke. Pneumococcal and meningococcal vaccines should be given before splenectomy.

After splenectomy, prophylactic penicillin therapy (in those younger than 5 years of age, 125 mg orally twice a day; in those older than 5 years of age, 250 mg orally twice a day) through adulthood is recommended; prophylaxis after 5 years of age is individualized depending on a history of prior pneumococcal disease and having recommended pneumococcal vaccine. Because of increased hemolysis, children with HS and active hemolysis should receive 1 mg of folic acid daily until splenectomy, especially if the reticulocyte count is more than 3%. Splenectomy is an effective strategy to eliminate most of the hemolysis associated with HS.

Complications

Aplastic crisis (often indicated by fever, fatigue, abdominal pain, and jaundice) associated with parvovirus and other viral infections is the most serious complication during childhood. Febrile illnesses should be vigorously treated. A child who is postsplenectomy and has a temperature greater than 101.5°F (>38.5°C) without an obvious source of infection should be hospitalized and treated with intravenous antibiotics until blood cultures are negative. Gallstone formation can occur as a result of chronic hemolysis, and an ultrasound should be performed annually, before splenectomy, and for increased abdominal symptoms (Segel and Casey, 2016).

Glucose-6-Phosphate Dehydrogenase Deficiency

A drug-induced hemolytic anemia can be caused by genetic deficiency of the G6PD enzyme in the RBC. Symptoms are generally associated with infections or exposure to oxidant metabolites of certain drugs that cause the precipitation of Hgb, injury to the red cells, and rapid hemolysis. The *G6PD* gene is found on the X chromosome. G6PD deficiency is transmitted as an X-linked recessive trait. In the United States, about 13% of African American males and 1% to 2% of African American females are affected. It may also occur in a more severe form in Greeks, Italians, Arabs, Southeast Asians, and Chinese, with the incidence ranging from 5% to 40% (Segel and Hackney, 2016).

Clinical Findings

History. Patients generally have a history of recent infection (particularly hepatitis) or oxidant drug ingestion—specifically, aspirin-containing antipyretics, sulfonamides, antimalarials, antihelmintics, naphtha quinolones—and fava beans. The degree of hemolysis is dependent on the amount of the drug ingested and the extent of enzyme deficiency.

Physical Examination. The patient may have pallor and jaundice if there is chronic hemolysis or jaundice, pallor, lethargy, irritability, headache, and red or dark clear urine after drug ingestion.

Diagnostic Studies. Several dye reduction tests provide the diagnosis. Screening tests available to measure a deficiency of G6PD should be used in high-risk groups. Only a few states include G6PD in their routine newborn screening panels. These tests measure G6PD enzyme activity in the RBC. After a hemolytic crisis, however, screening may produce a false-negative result because the younger blood cells that remain after hemolysis may show normal enzymatic activity. This is thought to be associated with higher G6PD activity taking place in reticulocytes. The enzyme assay should be obtained 2 to 3 months after an episode (Segel and Hackney, 2016).

Management

No specific treatment is available. RBC transfusion and supportive therapy may be indicated in cases of severe anemia. Keeping the child well hydrated and monitoring for renal failure are important during a hemolytic crisis.

Patient and Family Education

Patients should avoid the offending foods and drugs—the most common being fava beans, foods containing menthol and sulfites, aspirin, sulfonamide antibiotics, and antimalarials.

Platelet and Coagulation Disorders

Platelet disorders should be ruled out in children before undergoing extensive surgery and in children with petechiae, frequent nosebleeds, mucous membrane bleeding, or excessive bleeding from minor trauma. Evaluation of these complaints includes a family history of bleeding or platelet disorders and a history of drug or toxin exposure. Initial laboratory studies should include a CBC, platelet count, prothrombin time (PT), and activated partial thromboplastin time (aPTT). The diagnoses that may be differentiated with these tests are idiopathic thrombocytopenic purpura (ITP), hemophilia, von Willebrand disease, and leukemia. The coagulation cascade provides a mechanism for understanding the interconnectedness of all the factors involved in coagulation.

Overview of Diagnostic Studies

- Platelet count (normal range is 150,000 to 450,000/mm^3).
- Platelet function tests, such as platelet function analysis (PFA).
- PT (normal range is 11.5 to 14 seconds).
- aPTT is the method used to determine partial thromboplastin time (PTT) and is commonly still referred to as the PTT (normal range is 25 to 40 seconds).
- Specific coagulation factor assays determine which clotting factors are absent.

The PT and aPTT measure all of the clotting factors except factor XIII. If the platelet count is normal and either the aPTT or PT is prolonged or both, then a coagulation factor deficiency is possible. The typical laboratory findings of hemophilia are normal PT and PFA and an abnormal aPTT.

If the PT and aPTT are elevated in association with thrombocytopenia, the probable diagnosis is disseminated intravascular coagulation (DIC), which is a syndrome secondary to an underlying disorder such as sepsis, malignancy, toxins, or liver failure. In DIC, there is a systemic activation of the coagulation process. Extensive, ongoing activation of coagulation results in the depletion of platelets and coagulation factors, which then leads to bleeding and thrombosis.

Immune or Idiopathic Thrombocytopenic Purpura

Immune or ITP is the most common of the thrombocytopenic purpuras in childhood and is believed to be an autoimmune response in which circulating platelets are destroyed. It usually occurs after viral illnesses. In many cases the cause is autoimmune. Most cases occur between 1 and 4 years of age. The vast majority of cases resolve within 6 months even without treatment. If ITP lasts longer than 12 months, it is termed *chronic ITP*, and a careful reevaluation for associated disorders should be done. These disorders include leukemia, reactions to medications (e.g., quinine, heparin), lupus erythematosus, cirrhosis, HIV, hepatitis C, congenital causes (such as, X-linked thrombocytopenia), autosomal macrothrombocytopenia, Wiskott-Aldrich syndrome (WAS), and von Willebrand factor (vWF) deficiency.

Clinical Findings

ITP is essentially a clinical diagnosis and not established by a single diagnostic test, although most symptoms do not develop until the platelet count is less than 20,000/mm^3. It is characterized by the following:

- Acute onset of petechiae, purpura, and bleeding in an otherwise healthy child; the bruising or bleeding may be most prominent over the legs.
- A recent viral illness 1 to 4 weeks before onset is common.
- Hemorrhage of the mucous membranes, particularly the gums and lips.
- Nosebleeds that can be severe and difficult to control.
- Menorrhagia in an adolescent female.
- Liver, spleen, and lymph nodes are not generally enlarged.
- Bone pain and pallor are rare.

Diagnostic Studies. Laboratory findings in ITP include:

- Low platelet count (<150,000/mm^3) with an otherwise normal CBC.
- Severe thrombocytopenia with the platelet count less than 20,000/mm^3 is common and platelet size is normal or increased.
- Normal PT and aPTT and normal WBC and RBC counts.
- Megathrombocytes on the peripheral smear.
- Hgb may be decreased if there is a history of significant nose or menstrual bleeding but the MVC remains normal.

Differential Diagnosis

If the smear shows fragmented RBCs, BUN and creatinine levels should be measured to rule out hemolytic-uremic syndrome. If the PT and aPTT are elevated with thrombocytopenia, DIC is a possibility, and cultures should be taken to identify sources of infection. A prolonged PT and aPTT with a normal platelet count suggest a coagulation factor deficiency. If the syndrome is complicated by prolonged thrombocytopenia, neutropenia, anemia, bone pain, or congenital anomalies, the child should be referred to a hematologist for possible bone marrow aspiration to rule out acute lymphoblastic leukemia (ALL) and other disorders. In a *sick, febrile child* with isolated thrombocytopenia, petechiae, or purpura, the major diagnosis to consider first is meningococcemia. These children should also be referred, hospitalized, and treated for presumed sepsis.

Management

The prognosis for patients with ITP is excellent, with spontaneous recovery in the majority of pediatric cases within the first 6 months. Most cases can be managed on an outpatient basis without any specific therapy. If the platelet count is greater than 20,000/mm^3 and no bleeding is observed, children and parents should be advised to avoid contact sports, aspirin and other NSAIDs, and any other herbal or pharmacologic agents that interfere with platelet function; they should also to notify the practitioner of any excessive bleeding. Epistaxis can be treated with local measures. In severe cases (platelets <20,000/mm^3), a short course of corticosteroid therapy may reduce severity in the initial phases. Whether bone marrow evaluation is done to rule out other causes of acute thrombocytopenia, such as ALL, before initiating steroid treatment is controversial. Intravenous immunoglobulin (IVIG) is also given to children with active severe bleeding and those who have contraindications for steroid use; WinRho (Anti-D) is given intravenously with the dose depending on Hgb level; Rh(D) immune globulin is useful only in Rh-positive individuals. Splenectomy, immunosuppressives, and anti-CD20 antibody are options for those children with refractory or chronic ITP. New agents that stimulate thrombopoiesis, such as romiplostim and eltrombopag, have been approved by the FDA for use in adults with chronic ITP, but there are no data regarding their safety or efficacy in children (Scott, 2016). Guidelines for immune thrombocytopenia are available through The American Society of Hematology's evidence-based practice guideline for immune thrombocytopenia (Neunert et al., 2011).

Complications

The most serious complication is intracranial hemorrhage, which occurs in less than 1% of cases. Complaints of significant headache necessitate a careful neurologic evaluation.

Hemophilia A and B and von Willebrand Disease

Inherited coagulation deficiencies are described according to the absent coagulation factor. Most result in abnormal bleeding. Hemophilia results from a deficiency of factor VIII (hemophilia A) or factor IX (hemophilia B). In hemophilia A and B, absence or deficiency of the coagulation factor results in prolonged bleeding either spontaneously from small vessels or as a result of trauma. A rough guide to gauge the severity of hemophilia is the percentage of function of the factor levels with 100% (100 U/dL) equal to the function of factor found in 1 mL of normal plasma. The clotting factor levels with percentage of factor activity associated with severity of bleeding are as follows: less than 1 U/dL (<1%), severe; between 1 and 5 U/dL (1% to 5%), moderate; and more than 5 U/dL (>5%), mild.

In plasma, factor VIII binds with vWF, which is a specific circulatory protein and acts as a carrier protein. von Willebrand disease (also known as *vascular hemophilia*) is a heterogeneous group of hereditary bleeding disorders caused by a quantitative or qualitative abnormality of vWF protein (Table 39.4). In type I, the protein is quantitatively reduced; in type II, it is qualitatively abnormal; and it is absent in type III.

Because the genes for the coagulation factors are sex linked (carried on the X chromosome) and recessive, hemophilia A and B affect primarily males. Females are generally only carriers of the disorder. According to the CDC (https://www.cdc.gov/ncbddd/hemophilia/data.html), about 1 in 5000 males is affected with hemophilia A; each year about 400 babies are born with hemophilia A; hemophilia A is approximately four times more common than hemophilia B. von Willebrand disease occurs in both sexes with an incidence of 1 in 100 individuals. It is the most common inherited bleeding disorder and is associated with either a qualitative or quantitative defect in vWF. The primary sites of bleeding differ depending on whether the problem is hemophilia A or B or von Willebrand disease.

Clinical Findings

Table 39.6 provides comparisons of Hemophilia A, Hemophilia B, and von Willebrand Disease.

Additional findings associated with **hemophilia** include the following:
- A positive family history in the vast majority of cases.
- Excessive bruising.
- Prolonged bleeding from mucous membranes after minor lacerations, immunizations, circumcision, or during menstruation (menorrhagia).
- Hemarthrosis characterized by pain and swelling in the elbows, knees, and ankles.
- A greatly prolonged aPTT.
- A specific assay for factor VIII or IX activity confirms the diagnosis.

Additional findings associated with **von Willebrand disease** include the following:
- Mucous membrane bleeding (epistaxis, menorrhagia), easy bruising, and excessive posttraumatic or postsurgical bleeding.
- History of ecchymosis of trunk, upper arms, and thighs.
- Factor VIII clotting activity usually decreased.
- vWF antigen usually decreased and decreased vWF. Normal platelet count but isolated decreased platelet count associated with type 2B (Flood and Scott, 2016).

Management

Treatment of hemophilia consists of prevention of trauma and replacement therapy to increase factor VIII or factor IX activity in plasma. Plasma-derived and recombinant factor concentrates are available for replacement, with recombinant factor preferred. Hemarthrosis is the leading type of significant local bleeding. Local measures include the application of cold and pressure to affected painful joints. As with all bleeding disorders, aspirin and other NSAIDs should be avoided. Anticipatory guidance should be directed at avoiding high-risk behaviors and contact sports and the importance of wearing a bike helmet. Physical therapy may be needed to assist with decreased mobility caused by hemarthrosis and joint scarring. Psychosocial intervention may be needed to help families avoid overprotectiveness or permissiveness.

TABLE 39.6	Comparisons of Hemophilia A, Hemophilia B, and von Willebrand Disease		
	Hemophilia A	**Hemophilia B**	**von Willebrand Disease**
Inheritance Factor deficiency	X-linked factor VIII	X-linked factor IX	Autosomal dominant vWF and VIIIC
Bleeding site(s)	Muscle, joint, surgical	Muscle, joint, surgical	Mucous membranes, skin, surgical, menstrual
Prothrombin time (PT)	Normal	Normal	Normal
Activated partial thromboplastin time (aPTT)	Prolonged	Prolonged	Prolonged or normal
Bleeding time	Normal	Normal	Prolonged or normal
Factor VIII coagulant activity (VIIIC)	Low	Normal	Low or normal
von Willebrand factor antigen (vWF: Ag)	Normal	Normal	Low
von Willebrand factor activity (vWF: Act)	Normal	Normal	Low
Factor IX	Normal	Low	Normal
Ristocetin-induced	Normal	Normal	Normal, low, or increased at low-dose ristocetin
Platelet aggregation	Normal	Normal	Normal
Treatment	DDAVP[a] or recombinant VIII	Recombinant IX	DDAVP[a] or vWF concentrate

From Scott J. Hematology. In: Kliegman R, Marcdante K, Jenson H, et al., eds. *Nelson Essentials of Pediatrics*. 5th ed. Philadelphia: Saunders; 2006:718.

[a]Desmopressin (DDAVP) for mild to moderate hemophilia A or type I von Willebrand disease.

Ideally most children with hemophilia should be enrolled in a comprehensive hemophilia treatment center (HTC) to facilitate a collaborative, interdisciplinary approach to management. The PCP should remain central to the care of the child. Immunizations should be given either subcutaneously with a 26-gauge needle or intramuscularly with a 23-gauge needle followed by firm pressure, without rubbing, and ice at the site for several minutes. Iron replacement may also be necessary in children with severe bleeding disorders.

von Willebrand disease is treated depending on the type and severity of the bleeding. The treatment for von Willebrand disease is desmopressin (DDAVP) and factor VIII-vWF concentrates. Local measures to control bleeding may also be part of the treatment plan. Adjunctive therapy (e.g., estrogen and/or aminocaproic acid) depends on the type of von Willebrand disease (type 1, 2A, 2B, 2M, 2N, or 3), which is determined by the level of qualitative or quantitative factor deficiency. The use of aminocaproic acid, an antifibrinolytic agent, is sometimes recommended for dental extraction and nosebleeds (Flood and Scott, 2016).

Most patients are now given lifelong prophylaxis to prevent spontaneous bleeding and preserve joints. The National Hemophilia Foundation recommends that prophylaxis therapy be considered optimal treatment for children with severe hemophilia and is usually initiated with the first joint bleed. This is often in the first year of life as mobility increases. A written treatment plan tailoring replacement product dosage based on the location of the bleed should be in the electronic health record (EHR) and given to the parents to carry with them. The child should wear a medical alert bracelet or necklace.

Complications

In patients with hemophilia A and B, bleeding occurs particularly in closed areas, such as the joints, when levels of coagulation factor

decrease. Brain hemorrhage can be a serious consequence of head trauma. Continued hemorrhage results in anemia and eventually hypovolemic shock. The National Hemophilia Foundation publishes recommendations supported by the Medical and Scientific Advisory Council (MASAC); their recommendations are available through the National Hemophilia Foundation website (www.hemophilia.org). Clinical Practice Guidelines on the Evaluation and Management of von Willebrand disease are available through the National Heart, Lung, and Blood Institute.

Thrombophilia

Thrombophilia refers to the increased ability to form blood clots and may result from either acquired and/or inherited risks factors. Thrombotic events (venous thromboembolism [VTE] and stroke) are rare in healthy children, 0.07 out of 100,000, but have been increasingly recognized in tertiary pediatric centers (Raffini, 2017). Advances in treating critically ill children—coupled with increased awareness of inherited factors, improved imaging to identify thrombosis, and the prothrombotic lifestyle choices in society today—have led families to seek testing in healthy children. Screening for inherited thrombophilia in children with venous thromboembolism (VTE) is controversial, but the testing of healthy children who have a family history of thrombosis or thrombophilia is even more controversial (Raffini, 2017).

The most common inherited thrombophilias are factor V Leiden mutation, prothrombin 20210 mutation, antithrombin deficiency, and protein C or S deficiency. Also to be considered are factors that may be either inherited or acquired and are helpful in identifying patients who have multiple prothrombotic risk factors and may need testing: these would include antiphospholipid antibodies, elevated fasting homocysteine levels, and elevated factor VIII (Raffini, 2017).

Pediatric patients who have two or more inherited thrombophilia traits have been shown to be at increased risk for VTE. The most common risk factor is the presence of a central (indwelling) venous catheter (CVC), but other factors include surgery, trauma, use of oral contraceptives, immobilization, infection, systemic lupus erythematosus, structural venous anomalies, and cancer (Raffini, 2017).

Those with potential benefits from screening and testing are children with a strong family history of thrombophilia, such as a VTE in a first-degree relative younger than 40 years of age. Identifying these children has the benefit of counseling adolescent females who may be considering the use of oral contraceptives and targeted thromboprophylaxis in high-risk situations (femoral fracture in an obese teen who also has inherited thrombophilia). Educating patients about signs and symptoms of VTE, which could lead to earlier diagnosis, may also be useful. Counseling should revolve around lifestyle modifications including avoiding a sedentary lifestyle, overweight or obesity, and smoking (Raffini, 2017).

The American College of Chest Physicians has developed evidence-based guidelines and recommendations for neonates and children and recommends referral to pediatric hematologists (Monagle & Newall, 2018). Testing for children who have had a stroke is common but should be done when the child has recovered because some factor levels may be affected by acute episode-specific events (such as sepsis, asphyxia, dehydration, and central venous line infection).

Pancytopenia

Pancytopenia is marked by a decrease in all three formed elements of the blood—erythrocytes, leukocytes, and platelets. A child usually presents with clinical findings of infection or bleeding rather than anemia because of the longer life span of RBCs compared with platelets and WBCs. As such, it is not a single disease but results from a combination of disease processes. Pancytopenia is caused by one of the three following processes:
- Production failure (e.g., aplastic anemia)
- Sequestration (e.g., hypersplenism)
- Increased peripheral destruction of mature cells (e.g., certain infections/known medications)

The child should be referred to a pediatric hematologist for treatment focused at correcting the underlying mechanism, such as hematopoietic stem cell transplantation (failure of production), splenectomy, or other treatments aimed at reducing peripheral destruction of cells or sequestration.

White Blood Cell Disorders

White Blood Cell Count

The WBC count is used as an indicator of infection or illness; the percentages of the different types of cells also provide useful diagnostic information. The WBC count is automated and is a routine part of the CBC. The WBC differential is obtained on a smear of blood one cell layer thick, usually with a Wright stain procedure that contains both basic and acidic dyes. The absolute neutrophil count (ANC) is calculated from the results of the differential: If WBCs = 3600/mm^3, percentage of segmented neutrophils = 20, percentage of band neutrophils = 5, lymphocytes = 60, monocytes = 10, and eosinophils = 5, then ANC = 3600 × 0.25 (sum of % segs and bands) = 900.

White Blood Cell Dysfunction

The WBC count and differential are useful diagnostic guides in the management of a variety of childhood illnesses. The normal range of granulocyte and lymphocyte counts varies throughout childhood. Leukocytosis is an increase in the number of circulating leukocytes, primarily with a neutrophilic response particularly to bacterial infections. A relative increase in the number of circulating immature neutrophils (bands), or "left shift," is a defensive mechanism in response to an inflammatory process or acute bacterial infection. Multiple abnormalities in WBC indices should raise suspicion of a malignant disorder.

Alterations of Granulocytes

Neutropenia (measured as the ANC) is defined as a decrease in the number of circulating neutrophils and bands (ANC) in the peripheral blood to fewer than 1500/mm^3 for children older than 1 year and to fewer than 1000/mm^3 in infants between 2 weeks and 1 year of age. There are some racial differences in neutrophil counts, with some African American children having slightly lower counts than white children. Neutropenia is classified as mild (ANC of 1000 to 1500/mm^3), moderate (ANC of 500 to 1000/mm^3), or severe (ANC <500/mm^3).

Neutropenia results from decreased cellular production (as in various hematologic diseases, infections, drug-induced states, and nutritional deficiencies), increased peripheral destruction (as in autoimmune disorders), or peripheral pooling (as in bacterial infections, hemodialysis, and cardiopulmonary bypass). Most cases of neutropenia are discovered during evaluation of the WBC count in a child with an acute febrile illness, and the most common infectious causes are hepatitis A and B, respiratory syncytial virus, influenza A and B, Epstein-Barr virus, and cytomegalovirus. The general management of neutropenic patients includes careful identification and prompt treatment of any suspected or proven infections.

Neutropenia is frequently seen in preterm infants and those with intrauterine growth retardation. Because the neutrophil storage pool in newborn infants is only 20% to 30% of that of adults, it is easily depleted under stressful conditions, such as infection with resultant sepsis. Isoimmune neonatal neutropenia is a transient process resulting from the transplacental transfer of maternal antibodies to fetal neutrophil antigens. Antineutrophil antibodies can be detected in maternal and infant serum.

The largest group of neutropenic patients includes children who are receiving chemotherapy. They are at risk for developing severe, life-threatening bacterial infections depending on the degree and duration of neutropenia. Despite improvements in supportive care and treatment with granulocyte colony–stimulating factor (G-CSF), bacterial and fungal infections remain a major cause of morbidity and mortality in these patients.

Qualitative abnormalities of granulocytes are usually related to defects of phagocytosis. Although individually rare, these defects may be genetic or acquired. Malnutrition, sepsis, diabetes, and leukemia are acquired disorders related to defects in leukocyte function, particularly phagocytosis and microbicidal activity. Granulomatous diseases are relatively rare disorders of granulocytes, particularly neutrophils, in which the enzymes necessary for bactericidal activity are lacking. Such diseases result in severe, recurrent infections of the skin, lymph nodes, lungs, liver, and bone.

Lymphocytosis

Lymphocytosis is produced by viral illnesses, including mumps, measles (rubeola), rubella, varicella, mononucleosis, and hepatitis. Pertussis and chronic lymphocytic leukemia also elevate the lymphocyte count. An increase in the number of atypical lymphocytes is evident in infectious mononucleosis, cytomegalic inclusion disease, and toxoplasmosis.

Cancer

Childhood cancer is uncommon and often presents with symptoms of a benign illness. The signs and symptoms are variable and nonspecific and can include continued unexplained weight loss; headaches (typically in the early morning); swelling or persistent pain in bones, joints, back, or legs; lumps or masses; excessive bruising, bleeding, or rash; constant infections; persistent nausea or vomiting without nausea; persistent tiredness; vision changes; and/or recurrent or persistent fevers of no known etiology. Many different types of cancer can occur in young people, including cancers seen in adults as well as cancers unique to children. More than 15,000 cases of pediatric cancer are diagnosed in the United States each year, the most common being: leukemia, lymphoma, and brain cancer (Siegal et al., 2018); however, the rate of childhood cancers in the United States varies by state and region. According to the CDC,

- The Northeast had the highest rate of child/adolescent cancer, whereas the South had the lowest rate.
- Children and teens who lived in a city and/or in prosperous counties had higher rates of cancer than those living outside cities and/or in poorer counties.
- The highest incidence of leukemia is seen in the West.
- The highest incidence of lymphoma and brain tumors is seen in the Northeast.

In contrast to adult cancers, only a small percentage of all childhood cancers have a known preventable cause. Ionizing radiation is a well-recognized risk factor, and healthcare providers are encouraged to limit the use of computed tomography (CT) scans in children and pregnant women to those situations with a defined clinical indication; then the lowest possible radiation dose should be used. Numerous epidemiologic studies have investigated potential environmental causes of childhood cancer, but few strong or consistent associations have been found.

Leukemias

The leukemias are a group of malignant hematologic diseases in which normal bone marrow elements are replaced by abnormal, poorly differentiated lymphocytes known as *blast cells.* Genetic abnormalities in the hematopoietic cells take over, resulting in the unregulated clonal proliferation of malignant cells. Leukemias are classified according to cell type involvement (i.e., lymphocytic or nonlymphocytic) and by cellular differentiation. ALL is characterized by preponderantly undifferentiated WBCs.

The leukemias are the most common form of childhood cancer, accounting for up to 30% of all pediatric cancers. Although there have been dramatic improvements in survival for ALL over the past four decades, with outcomes approaching 90% in the latest studies, progress has been slower for myeloid leukemia and certain subgroups such as infant ALL, adolescent/young adult ALL,

and relapsed ALL (Madhusoodhan et al., 2016). Recent advances include the recognition of molecularly defined subgroups, which continues to inform precision medicine approaches.

ALL accounts for about 80% of childhood leukemia cases, with a peak incidence between 2 and 6 years of age, and 56% of leukemia cases in adolescents (Siegel, 2018). Acute myeloid leukemia (AML) is less common in children than ALL and accounts for about 15% of leukemia cases in children and 31% of those in adolescents.

Clinical Findings

Most of the clinical signs and symptoms of leukemia are related to leukemic replacement of the bone marrow and the absence of blood cell precursors. The child may be anemic, pale, listless, irritable, or chronically tired and may have the following:

- A history of repeated infections, fever, weight loss
- Bleeding episodes characterized by epistaxis, petechiae, and hematomas
- Lymphadenopathy and hepatosplenomegaly
- Bone and joint pain

Central nervous system (CNS) symptoms—such as headache, vomiting, or lethargy—are rare at the time of diagnosis but can present due to an intracranial or spinal mass (Horton and Steuber, 2017). All these symptoms may be vague or nonspecific; providers must maintain a high index of suspicion for cancer.

Diagnostic Studies. The following are used to diagnose leukemia:

- CBC with differential, WBCs, platelet and reticulocyte counts. Thrombocytopenia and anemia are present in most cases. The WBC count may be elevated, normal, or low with varying levels of neutropenia.
- A peripheral smear may demonstrate malignant cells.
- Bone marrow examination showing an infiltration of blast cells replacing normal elements of the marrow (Horton and Steuber, 2017).
- Chromosomal and genetic abnormalities are found in most children with ALL. The genetic alterations in their leukemic blast cells may include changes in the number of chromosomes and a structure with recurrent translocations and deletions, which provide important prognostic information (Horton and Steuber, 2017).

Further classification regarding cell type, morphologic characteristics, and cell surface markers is generally made at the cancer treatment center to which the child is referred.

Management

Approximately 90% of children diagnosed with ALL can now be cured; they are considered cured after 10 years in remission. Key genetic features are critical factors in the management plan. The treatment program for most types of acute leukemia involves 4 to 6 weeks of induction phase (usually with vincristine, prednisone, and L-asparaginase), with the goal of inducing a complete remission and restoring normal hematopoiesis. This is followed by a consolidation phase of therapy lasting several months and then a maintenance phase for 2 to 3 years. Chemotherapy, CNS therapy (cranial irradiation, which is now reserved only for a high-risk child—those with CNS disease or high WBC counts at diagnosis), or intrathecal administration of chemotherapy and systemic administration of corticosteroids are the key interventions. The use of cranial irradiation as part of therapy is decreasing. For children with ALL who relapse, the need for allogeneic stem cell transplantation is not considered until the second complete remission. However, children with certain chromosomal rearrangements or those who are not in remission by the end of the first induction phase are considered at high risk for relapse; thus transplantation must be considered sooner. The measurement of minimal residual disease is part of the current treatment protocol to determine the burden at the end of leukemic induction and the ALL outcome (Horton and Steuber, 2017).

For those with AML, treatment consists of induction chemotherapy, CNS prophylaxis, and postremission therapy. Allogeneic stem cell transplantation from an HLA-matched sibling or parent is considered in the first complete remission for children with high-risk disease.

Long-term sequelae of cancer therapy for ALL have been identified in research studies and include effects on cognition, neuropsychologic functioning, and growth deficiencies and an increased risk for second malignancies, such as AML or lymphoma. CNS irradiation has been linked to learning disabilities and impaired IQ, especially in children younger than 5 years of age who also received intrathecal therapy. As a result, cranial radiation dosages have been reduced, and earlier neuropsychologic testing is recommended. Other documented potential late effects of ALL treatment include congestive heart failure, avascular necrosis, and osteoporosis. Late effects associated with common childhood cancers are further discussed at the end of this chapter.

The role of the PCP is crucial to facilitate proper referrals and effective interdisciplinary communication and to assist the family in their coping and adaptation processes. Regular health supervision visits are also important and should not be overlooked. Immunizations should be given as appropriate depending on the stage of treatment and the child should be monitored for failed remission or metastasis (CNS and testicles are common sites) and late effects.

Lymphomas

Non-Hodgkin Lymphoma

The NHLs are a diverse group of solid tumors of the lymphatic tissues that form from malignant proliferation of T cells, B cells, or indeterminate lymphocyte cells. Different classification systems have been used to categorize these tumors. In pediatrics, the common types of NHL are small noncleaved cell lymphoma (Burkitt and non-Burkitt subtypes, B-cell origin), lymphoblastic lymphoma, and diffuse large B-cell lymphoma (Kupfer, 2015). NHLs account for 6% of all pediatric cancers.

Each year in the United States, approximately 500 children and 400 teens are diagnosed with NHL. The subtypes most common in pediatrics include Burkitt lymphoma (19%), diffuse large B-cell lymphoma (22%), lymphoblastic lymphoma (20%), and anaplastic large-cell lymphoma (10%). Incidence rates of most subtypes of NHL are higher in boys than in girls, but the incidence and subtype distribution vary throughout the world (Johnston, 2014). NHL occurs most frequently in children during the second decade of life and infrequently in children younger than 3 years of age. It is the most frequent malignancy in children with acquired immunodeficiency syndrome and is also associated with Epstein-Barr and cytomegalovirus infections.

Clinical Findings. The most common site of origin is in the lymphoid structures of the intestinal tract. The most common manifestations in children are (1) acute abdomen, including abdominal pain, distention, fullness, and constipation, and (2) nontender lymph node enlargement. Histologic differences

account for varying disease sites; lymphoblastic NHLs often present as intrathoracic tumors; in contrast, small noncleaved cell lymphomas commonly present as abdominal tumors. Other sites include the CNS and the bone marrow. Initial presentation is often with advanced disease of stage III or IV in approximately 70% of the patients (HocHgberg et al., 2016). Duration of symptoms before a diagnosis is made is typically 1 month or less, and a common presentation is enlarging, nontender lymphadenopathy or symptoms indicating compression of surrounding tissue and structures. Three clinical manifestations that may present as emergencies are superior or inferior vena cava obstruction, acute paraplegias due to spinal cord or CNS compression, and tumor lysis syndrome (Termuhlen and Gross, 2017).

Diagnostic Studies. Diagnostic studies are ordered depending on the location of the lymphoma and symptoms. They include CBC with differential, but this may be normal at diagnosis; liver function tests; lactate dehydrogenase (LDH); uric acid; and electrolyte levels. Unexplained anemia, thrombocytopenia, or leukopenia can be due to bone marrow infiltration, and elevated electrolytes and LDH may indicate rapidly proliferating tumors and tumor lysis syndromes. Imaging studies such as chest radiography, ultrasound, CT or MRI scan, or positron emission tomography (PET) of the area in question may demonstrate masses and/or lymphadenopathy in the neck, chest, or abdomen. Staging the extent of the disease is mandatory before beginning treatment and may include gallium and/or bone scans, bone marrow aspirates and biopsies, and lumbar puncture with CNS fluid analysis (Termuhlen and Gross, 2017).

Management. Optimal therapy involves a multidisciplinary approach from the time of diagnosis. Because of rapid developments in treatment and the importance of careful histologic evaluation, these children should be referred to a comprehensive pediatric oncology center for care. Lymphomas are sensitive to chemotherapy. Unlike the case in adults, radiation therapy is not commonly used in pediatric care. The prognosis has improved dramatically, with an estimated 5-year survival rate of over 85% (Termuhlen and Gross, 2017).

Hodgkin Lymphoma

Like the NHLs, Hodgkin lymphoma is a malignancy of the reticuloendothelial and lymphatic systems and involves B cells. It usually originates in a cervical lymph node and spreads to other lymph node regions; if left untreated, it will spread to organ systems including the liver, spleen, bone, bone marrow, and brain. Unlike the NHLs, involvement of the bone marrow and CNS is rare. Clinical and pathologic staging of the disease is usually done by specialists according to the Ann Arbor Staging Criteria (Termuhlen and Gross, 2017). Hodgkin lymphoma represents 6% of the childhood cancers. It is rare in children younger than 15 years of age (5.5 cases per million per year). The NIH National Cancer Institute (NCI) has estimated that the incidence of Hodgkin lymphoma in the United States in adolescents (15 to 19 years of age) is 29 cases per million per year. Clusters of cases in families suggest a genetic predisposition, but this association may include shared environments and exposure to viruses as well as inherited immunodeficiency states (McClain and Kamdar, 2017).

Clinical Findings. The most common manifestations of Hodgkin lymphoma include the following:
- Painless enlargement of the lymph nodes, usually in the cervical area; the nodes may feel rubbery and firm, are often matted together, and are nontender to palpation

- Chronic cough if the trachea is compressed by a large mediastinal mass
- Fever, decreased appetite, weight loss of 10% or more of total body weight within 6 months of diagnosis, and drenching night sweats; these systemic symptoms (B symptoms) are important for staging (McClain and Kamdar, 2017)

Diagnostic Studies. Hematologic findings are often normal but may include the following:

- Anemia and elevated or depressed leukocytes or platelets
- Elevated sedimentation rate and C-reactive protein
- Elevated serum copper and ferritin level
- Abnormal liver function test results
- Urinalysis showing proteinuria
- Imaging studies: chest radiography, ultrasound, CT, MRI, and PET

Management. The child should receive treatment at a comprehensive pediatric oncology center in collaboration with the PCP. The diagnosis is confirmed by histologic examination of an excised lymph node, followed by bone marrow studies to determine the extent of the disease. Multiple treatment agents allow different mechanisms of action to avoid overlapping toxicities. Optimal results are obtained through irradiation, chemotherapy with numerous agents, or a combination of both. Infertility is problematic for those receiving high doses of alkylators; sperm banking is discussed as an option for males before starting therapy. Approximately 75% of children who survive Hodgkin lymphoma have chronic medical conditions. They may develop a secondary malignancy 30 years later—typically a thyroid, breast, or nonmelanoma skin cancer—as well as NHL and acute leukemia. Therefore lifelong monitoring is necessary through a comprehensive pediatric oncology center where long-term complications can be anticipated, monitored, and treated (McClain and Kamdar, 2017).

Late Effects of Childhood Cancers

Adults treated for cancer during childhood can experience late effects that contribute to a high burden of morbidity after childhood, well into their adult years. For example,

- 60% to 90% will develop one or more chronic conditions
- 20% to 80% will experience a severe or life-threatening complication

According to the NCI (https://www.cancer.gov/types/childhood-cancers/late-effects-hp-pdq), the cumulative incidence of a self-reported severe, disabling, life-threatening, or fatal health condition by 50 years of age was 53.6% among survivors, compared with 19.8% among a sibling control group.

Any adverse effect or problem that does not resolve after completion of therapy is labeled a late effect of childhood cancer. Late effects can be attributed to radiation therapy, chemotherapy, or a combination of both and can occur later during puberty or with aging. Common problems have been identified, and pediatric survivors of cancer must be monitored for these issues. Problems must be identified early and addressed promptly. They can include the following:

- Short stature from cranial irradiation and intensive chemotherapy.
- Precocious puberty after cranial irradiation and hypothyroidism with neck or mantle radiation therapy.
- Avascular necrosis of the bone caused by high-dose steroid therapy—more pronounced in young children—and with local irradiation.

- Osteoporosis from cranial irradiation, glucocorticoids, and antimetabolites.
- Leukoencephalopathy resulting from cranial irradiation, methotrexate, glucocorticoids.
- Peripheral neuropathy and hearing loss from cisplatin.
- Cognitive dysfunction, stroke, and seizures from intrathecal chemotherapy, certain systemic chemotherapy agents, and radiation: cranial radiation effects are dose-dependent and more deleterious on young developing brains.
- Vision, auditory, and skeletal changes from head and neck radiation.
- Obesity and gonadal dysfunction resulting from a neuroendocrine effect.
- Potential alterations in pubertal development and gonadal function if given high-dose alkylating agents, especially in puberty and to girls.
- Cardiomyopathy and arrhythmias if given anthracyclines: Children given these drugs need to be educated just before their teen years about avoiding alcohol, which increases the likelihood of cardiotoxicity, and cautioned about cigarette smoking.
- Pericardial effusion, constrictive pericarditis, or late coronary artery disease from radiation therapy that includes all or part of the heart (e.g., used in treatment for some Hodgkin lymphoma cases).
- Pneumonitis and pulmonary fibrosis from chest and thoracic radiation and with chemotherapy agents such as bleomycin and carmustine.
- Malignant glioma associated with cranial irradiation and sarcomas associated with musculoskeletal radiation.
- Secondary leukemias (usually AML) associated with therapy with alkylating agents and epipodophyllotoxins; secondary solid tumors are associated with radiation therapy.
- Glomerular or tubular injury, renal insufficiency with heavy metals (e.g., cisplatin).
- Infertility and early menopause with alkylator therapy.
- Cystitis or bladder dysfunction with cyclophosphamide.
- Delayed recovery of normal immune function (may need readministration of immunization).
- Psychosocial effects associated with chronic illness (e.g., less likely to go to college, marry, and be employed).
- Cancer relapse.
- Possibility of hepatitis C virus infection if the individual had a blood transfusion before 1992.
- Bone marrow transplant recipients can experience unique late effects associated with treatment and require monitoring; medical insurance coverage may also be problematic in later years.

The Children's Oncology Group (COG), a NIC–supported clinical trials group, cares for more than 90% of children and adolescents diagnosed with cancer in the United States. Monitoring programs for childhood cancer survivors provides a rich source of data to guide cancer treatment and its follow-up. All survivors of childhood cancers need regular health care supervision from a provider who is aware of their prior treatment modalities and knowledgeable of late effects, aware of their risk of occurrence, and comfortable with risk-based monitoring for such problems. COG survivorship guidelines are available at http://www.survivorshipguidelines.org/. Healthy lifestyles and dietary practices and avoidance of sun, alcohol, recreational drugs, and tobacco should always be stressed.

If a neoplasm of some sort is suspected by the PCP, a phone call to the nearest comprehensive pediatric oncology/hematology center enables the child to be seen quickly and prevents a delay in diagnosis by waiting for insurance authorization. Staff in these centers can obtain authorization quickly based on clinical findings. As part of coordinated care, the PCP must maintain a relationship and follow the child for well-child care when the disease process is stabilized by: (1) securing basic information on the type of cancer, stage, location, and histology; (2) treatments (i.e., chemotherapy, radiation, surgery); (3) listing potential or at-risk late effects and monitoring needs; (4) any psychological issues; and (5) implementing preventive strategies (e.g., immunizations, exercise, diet). The NIH NIC has excellent materials for health professionals, parents, and children about childhood cancer (www.cancer.gov/types/childhood-cancers). This resource provides up-to-date information about changes in treatment and long-term effects.

Additional Resources

2011 Evidence-Based Practice Guideline for Immune Thrombocytopenia. https://www.bloodjournal.org/content/117/16/4190?sso-checked=true
American Childhood Cancer Organization.
www.acco.org/
Cooleys Anemia Foundation.
www.cooleysanemia.org
CureSearch: National Childhood Cancer Foundation.
www.curesearch.org
Leukemia and Lymphoma Society.
www.leukemia.org
National Cancer Institute: Surveillance, Epidemiology, and End Results (SEER) Program.
http://seer.cancer.gov/csr/1975_2014/
National Hemophilia Foundation.
www.hemophilia.org
National Institutes of Health: Childhood Cancer.
www.cancer.gov/types/childhood-cancers
National Institutes of Health: The Management of Sickle Cell Disease.
www.nhlbi.nih.gov/health-topics/evidenced-based-management-sickle-cell-disease(2014)
National Newborn Screening Information.
www.cdc.gov/newbornscreening/
Sickle Cell Disease Association of America (SCDAA).
www.sicklecelldisease.org

References

Abrams SA. *Iron requirements and iron deficiency in adolescents, UpToDate (website)*; 2017. Available at www.uptodate.com/contents/iron-requirements-and-iron-deficiency-in-adolescents. Accessed October 31, 2017.
Benz EJ. *Clinical manifestations and diagnosis of the thalassemia, UpToDate (website)*; 2017. Available at www.uptodate.com/contents/clinical-manifestations-and-diagnosis-of-the-thalassemias. Accessed October 31, 2017.
Benz EJ. *Management and prognosis of thalassemias, UpToDate (website)*; 2017. Available at www.uptodate.com/contents/management-and-prognosis-of-thalassemias. Accessed October 31, 2017.
DeBaun MR, Frei-Jones M, Vichinsky E. Hemoglobinopathies. In: Kliegman RM, Stanton BF, St Geme JW, et al., eds. *Nelson Textbook of Pediatrics*. 20th ed. Philadelphia: Saunders/Elsevier; 2016: Chapter 462:2336–2353.
Flood VH, Scott JP. von Willebrand disease. In: Kliegman RM, Stanton BF, St Geme JW, et al., eds. *Nelson Textbook of Pediatrics*. 20th ed. Philadelphia: Elsevier/Saunders; 2016:2390–2392.
Gillespie MA, Lyle CA, Goldberg NA. September 2015. in pediatric venous thromboembolism. *Curr Opin Hematol*. 22(5):413–419. https://doi: 10.1097/MOH.0000000000000168, PMID.
Hernell O, Fewtrell MS, Georgieff MK, Krebs NF, Lonnerdal B. Summary of current recommendations on iron provision and monitoring of iron status for breastfed and formula-fed infants in resource-rich and resource-constrained countries. *The Journal of Pediatrics*. 2015;167(4):S40–47. https://doi.org/10.1016/j.jpeds.2015.07.020.
Horton TM, Steuber CP. *Overview of the presentation and diagnosis of acute lymphoblastic leukemia in children and adolescents, UpToDate (website)*; 2017. Available at www.uptodate.com/contents/overview-of-the-presentation-and-diagnosis-of-acute-lymphoblastic-leukemia-in-children-and-adolescents. Accessed October 31, 2017.
HocHgberg J, Guidino-Roth L, Cairo MS. Lymphoma. In: Kliegman RM, Stanton BF, St Geme JW, et al., eds. *Nelson Textbook of Pediatrics*. 20th ed. Philadelphia: Saunders/Elsevier; 2016:2445–2453.
Horton TM, Steuber CP. *Overview of the Treatment of Acute Lymphoblastic Leukemia in Children and Adolescents, UpToDate (website)*; 2017. Available at www.uptodate.com/contents/overview-of-the-treatment-of-acute-lymphoblastic-leukemia-in-children-and-adolescents. Accessed October 31, 2017.
Huang LH, Portwine C, Miller R. *Transient Erythroblastopenia of Childhood*. Medscape (website); 2014. Available at http://emedicine.medscape.com/article/959644.
Johnston JM. Non-Hodgkin lymphoma. *Medscape (website)*; 2014. Available at http://emedicine.medscape.com/article/987540. Accessed June 19, 2014.
Kupfer GM. Childhood cancer epidemiology. *Medscape (website)*; 2015. Available at http://emedicine.medscape.com/article/989841. Accessed December 1, 2015.
Madhusoodhan PP, Carroll WL, Bhatla T. Progress and prospects in pediatric leukemia. *Curr Probl Pediatr Adolesc Health Care*. 2016;46(7):229–241. https://doi.org/10.1016/j.cppeds.2016.04.003.
McClain KL, Kamdar K. *Overview of Hodgkin lymphoma in children and adolescents, UpToDate (website)*; 2017. Available at www.uptodate.com/contents/overview-of-hodgkin-lymphoma-in-children-and-adolescents. Accessed October 31, 2017.
Monagle P, Newall F. Management of thrombosis in children and neonates: Practical use of anticoagulants in children. *Hematology Am Soc Hematol Educ Program*. 2018(1):399–404. https://doi.org/10.1182/asheducation-2018.1.399.
National Hemophilia Foundation. *MASAC recommendations for hepatitis A and B immunization of individuals with bleeding disorders. national hemophilia foundation (website)*; 2001. https://www.hemophilia.org/Researchers-Healthcare-Providers/Medical-and-Scientific-Advisory-Council-MASAC/MASAC-Recommendations/MASAC-Recommendations-for-Hepatitis-A-and-B-Immunization-of-Individuals-with-Bleeding-Disorders. Accessed January 14, 2017.
NHLBI (2014). Evidence-based management of SCD - Expert Panel Report (EPR) available at https://www.nhlbi.nih.gov/sites/default/files/media/docs/sickle-cell-disease-report%20020816_0.pdf.
Neunert C, Lim W, Crowther M, et al. The American Society of Hematology 2011 evidence-based practice guideline for immune thrombocytopenia. *Blood*. 2011;117(16):4190–4207.
Powers JM, Mahoney DH. Iron deficiency in infants and children < 12 years. UpToDate (website). Available at https://www.uptodate.com/contents/iron-deficiency-in-infants-and-children-less-than12-years-treatment. Accessed August 26, 2019.
Raffini L. *Screening for inherited thrombophilia in children, UpToDate (website)*; 2017. Available at www.uptodate.com/contents/screening-for-inherited-thrombophilia-in-children. Accessed October 30, 2017.
Rogers ZR. *Routine comprehensive care for children with sickle cell disease, UpToDate (website)*; 2017. Available at www.uptodate.com/contents/routine-comprehensive-care-for-children-with-sickle-cell-disease. Accessed October 31, 2017.
Schrier SL. *Diagnosis and treatment of vitamin B12 and folate deficiency, UpToDate (website)*; 2017. Available at www.uptodate.com/contents/diagnosis-and-treatment-of-vitamin-b12-and-folate-deficiency. Accessed October 31, 2017.
Scott JP. Platelet and blood vessels disorders. In: Kliegman RM, Stanton BF, St Geme JW, et al., eds. *Nelson Textbook of Pediatrics*. 20th ed. Philadelphia: Saunders/Elsevier; 2016:2400–4208.

Segel GB, Casey D. Hereditary spherocytosis. In: Kliegman RM, Stanton BF, St Geme JW, et al., eds. *Nelson Textbook of Pediatrics*. 20th ed. Philadelphia: Saunders/Elsevier; 2016:2330–2335.

Segel GB, Hackney LR. Glucose-6-phosphate dehydrogenase deficiency and related deficiencies. In: Kliegman RM, Stanton BF, St Geme JW, et al., eds. *Nelson Textbook of Pediatrics*. 20th ed. Philadelphia: Saunders/Elsevier; 2016:2353–2357.

Siegel DA, Li J, Henley SJ, et al. Geographic variation in pediatric cancer incidence—United States. 2003–2014. *MMWR*. 2018;67(25):707–713. https://www.cdc.gov/mmwr/volumes/67/wr/mm6725a2.htm.

Simon GR, Baker C, Barden GA, et al. 3rd. 2014 recommendations for pediatric preventative health care. *Pediatrics*. 2014;133(3):568–570.

Termuhlen AM, Gross TG. *Overview of non-Hodgkin lymphoma in children and adolescents, UpToDate (website)*; 2017. Available at www.uptodate.com/contents/overview-of-non-hodgkin-lymphoma-in-children-and-adolescents. Accessed October 31, 2017.

van den Akker M, Dror Y, Odame I. Transient erythroblastopenia of childhood is an underdiagnosed and self-limiting disease. *Acta Paediatr*. 2014;103(7):e288–e294.

Vichinsky EP. *Overview of variant sickle cell syndromes, UpToDate (website)*; 2017. Available at www.uptodate.com/contents/overview-of-sickle-cell-syndromes. Accessed October 31, 2017.

Vichinsky EP, Levine L. *Standards of care guidelines for thalassemia*. 2012 Available at http://thalassemia.com/documents/SOCGuidelines2012.pdf. Accessed November 30, 2015.

40

Gastrointestinal Disorders

ELIZABETH E. WILLER AND BELINDA JAMES-PETERSEN

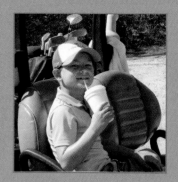

The gastrointestinal (GI) system, also known as the *digestive system,* provides the nutrients that give the body's cells the energy needed to function. Sustained operation and maintenance of this system are essential for normal growth and development and for the effective functioning of other organ systems. The pediatric primary care provider plays an integral role in the care of children with GI dysfunction. A thorough understanding of the anatomy, physiology, and common disorders of the GI system is needed to appropriately assess and treat pediatric GI problems. This chapter focuses on pathologic GI disorders commonly seen in children. Other problems of the GI system, such as obesity, anorexia, and bulimia, are discussed in Chapters 15, 17, and 18.

Anatomy and Physiology

The GI system begins to develop during the third week of gestation. The primitive gut is initially formed and then divides into the foregut, midgut, and hindgut. The structures further develop in an intricate and complex fashion to become the digestive tract and accessory organs.

The GI tract extends from the mouth to the anus. It includes the organs of digestion and accessory organs, such as the liver, pancreas, and gallbladder. The system provides the following functions: ingestion of food, movement of food from the mouth toward the rectum, mechanical and chemical dissolution of food, absorption of nutrients, and expulsion of waste products. The mouth serves as the site for ingestion, chewing, and mixing of food with saliva. The tongue senses the texture and taste of foods, which initiates salivation and the release of gastric juices in the stomach. The esophagus transports food from the mouth to the stomach by *peristalsis,* the sequential contraction and relaxation of the musculature in the esophagus. The upper esophageal sphincter prevents air from being swallowed while breathing. The lower esophageal sphincter (LES) prevents food from being regurgitated from the stomach, which is important because intraabdominal pressure exceeds intrathoracic and atmospheric pressures. The stomach serves as a reservoir for ingested foods. It secretes digestive juices, mixes food with the gastric fluids, and propels the liquid material into the small intestine. The small intestine's primary function is absorption of nutrients (carbohydrates, fats, proteins, minerals, and vitamins) into the systemic circulation. Absorption occurs through villi, which cover the mucosal folds and serve as the functional unit of the intestine. Each villus contains an artery, a vein, and a lymph vessel that transport nutrients from the intestine into

the systemic circulation. The villi are covered with enterocytes, whose major role is the digestion of carbohydrates and proteins. Enterocytes secrete proteins and enzymes known as *brush border enzymes,* which assist in digestion.

Carbohydrates must be converted to monosaccharides before their absorption is possible. This process begins in the mouth, where the salivary enzyme amylase breaks down complex starches into disaccharides. The brush border enzymes in the small intestine convert disaccharides into monosaccharides (sucrose to glucose and fructose, lactose to glucose and galactose, and maltose to glucose). When this process is hindered, disaccharides remain osmotically active and can cause diarrhea.

Fat absorption, which occurs mainly in the jejunum, is accomplished through the addition of lipases secreted by the pancreas. Lipases break down fats into particles that are easily absorbed by the villi. Fats then rely on the lymphatic system for absorption.

Proteins are converted to amino acids by pancreatic enzymes. The resulting amino acids are further divided into smaller amino acid particles that are absorbed via the brush border into the systemic circulation. After appropriate absorption of nutrients, the small intestine is left with the initial fecal liquid. This liquid is then propelled by peristalsis into the large intestine. The large intestine removes water from the fecal liquid and allows for short-term storage. The fecal mass, which consists of waste products, bacteria, intestinal secretions, and shed cells, is pushed into the sigmoid colon.

Entry of feces into the rectum stimulates the defecation reflex. This reflex stretches the rectal wall, relaxes the internal anal sphincter, and thereby creates the need to defecate. If this urge is ignored, further fluid resorption occurs as the stool is retained, resulting in an increase in stool mass and dryness. Excessive stretching of the colon from the hard, dry stool bolus can lead to decreased peristalsis, further complicating the retention of stool.

Pathophysiology

The GI tract can be affected by illness, injury, or other problems that prevent it from functioning normally. Dysfunction can be localized or systemic. Categories of dysfunction include disorders of motility; infection; malabsorption syndromes; impairment of digestion, absorption, and nutrition; congenital malformations and genetic syndromes; metabolic disorders; behavioral problems; injuries and trauma; and food intolerances, such as lactose and gluten intolerance due to absence of essential enzymes.

Assessment

History

The history assesses the following:

- How long has the symptom been present? What makes it better or worse? What have you tried or attempted to treat it? Has it impacted your activities of daily living?
- Any vomiting, belching, and flatulence?
- Nutritional patterns:
  - Feeding habits and nutrition history or current diet (what, when, how often, what tolerated)
  - Thirst level (increased or decreased)
  - Changes in appetite
  - Food intolerance or allergy (what foods, symptoms, treatment)
- Elimination patterns: Bowel habits (frequency, times per week, consistency, associated pain, the need for medications or enemas)
  - Constipation and diarrhea (definition of each, how often they occur, and treatment tried)
- Presence of pain (onset, location, type, quality, aggravating and alleviating factors)
  - *Epigastric* pain usually indicates pain from the liver, pancreas, biliary tree, stomach, and upper part of the small bowel (duodenum).
  - *Periumbilical* pain is generated from the distal end of the small intestine, cecum, appendix, and ascending colon.
  - *Colonic* visceral pain is lower abdominal pain that can be dull, diffuse, cramping, or burning.
  - *Suprapubic* discomfort indicates distal intestine, urinary tract, and pelvic organ dysfunction.
  - *Referred* pain is a diagnostic challenge. For example, because of convergent nerve pathways, inflammation of the diaphragm can generate pain that is perceived as shoulder or lower neck pain. When visceral pain is overwhelming, referred pain occurs.
  - *Acute* continuous pain is more indicative of an acute process.
- Family history of any GI disease (e.g., gallbladder disease, ulcers, or allergy to any food product)
- Past medical history related to the GI system (e.g., illnesses, surgeries, anatomic problems, such as cleft lip or palate, esophageal atresia)
- Review of systems: Apnea or asthma that may be caused by gastroesophageal reflux (GER), concerns/symptoms of cardiac insufficiency, other autoimmune symptoms (e.g., rashes)

Physical Examination

When assessing a suspected GI problem, a head-to-toe physical examination is indicated.

- Plot growth parameters, including weight for height, to establish proportionality of the patient and exclude certain growth aberrations from the diagnosis.
- Determine body mass index (BMI). The BMI is one of the first indicators used to assess body fat and is a common method of tracking weight problems and obesity in children 2 years old and older (see Chapter 17 for more details).
- Determine hydration status (skin turgor, mucous membranes, peripheral pulses, tears, capillary filling).

- Inspect the abdomen for visible peristalsis, rashes, lesions, asymmetry, masses, enlarged organs, and pulsations.
- Auscultate for frequency of bowel sounds (normal is 5 to 20 per minute).
- Percuss for density and to measure organs.
- Palpate both lightly and deeply.
- Assess peritoneal irritation:
  - Have the patient walk standing straight up or cough.
  - Have the patient stand on tiptoes and fall onto the heels or jump.
  - Palpate for rebound tenderness and a positive Rovsing sign (palpation in the left iliac fossa produces pain in the right iliac fossa).
  - Check for the obturator sign: A supine patient flexes the right thigh at the hip with the knee bent and internally rotates the hip. The sign is positive when it induces abdominal pain.
  - Check for the psoas sign: The patient lies on the left side and extends and then flexes the right leg at the hip. A positive sign is one that induces abdominal pain.
- Perform a rectal examination when intraabdominal, pelvic, or perirectal disease is suspected (the newborn examination should routinely assess for anal stenosis). Include external inspection and internal palpation for masses, stool, or irregularities. The index finger is typically used because of its increased sensitivity; however, in infants and young children, use the fifth finger. Insert a gloved, lubricated finger into the rectum. Place the other hand on the abdomen for a bimanual examination. Young pediatric patients should be supine with their feet held together and knees and hips flexed, putting their legs over their abdomen. Adolescent males can be lying on their side or standing with the hips flexed and the upper part of the body on the examination table. Adolescent females can be lying on their side or, if a concurrent pelvic examination is to be done, in the lithotomy position.
- Perform a gynecologic examination if a pathologic pelvic condition is suspected (see Chapter 42).

Common Diagnostic Studies

Laboratory tests

are performed as indicated:
- Urinalysis (UA) and urine culture
- Complete blood count (CBC) with differential
- Serum chemistry screen, liver profile, lipid profile, erythrocyte sedimentation rate (ESR), C-reactive protein (CRP), thyroid function
- Stool examination for ova and parasites (O&P), culture, blood, white blood cells (WBCs), pH, reducing substances
- Fecal fat collection for 72 hours to rule out fat malabsorption
- Pregnancy test
- Urine tests for gonorrhea or chlamydia, Papanicolaou (Pap) smear and vaginal cultures and/or smears if a pelvic or gynecologic pathologic condition is suspected

Imaging of the abdomen may include the following:

Radiography

- Abdominal x-ray, as the preliminary study; available, less expensive, with lower radiation
- Upper and lower GI with fluoroscopy and barium swallow studies to demonstrate anatomy and function. An upper gastrointestinal (UGI) series may be warranted to evaluate bowel obstruction (e.g., late presentation of malrotation, surgical

adhesions, etc.) in patients with significant vomiting (e.g., bilious, protracted); small bowel follow-through may be added if inflammatory bowel disease (IBD) (particularly Crohn disease) is suspected. An air contrast enema can diagnose and treat intussusceptions

Abdominal Ultrasonography

- No ionizing radiation, noninvasive, relatively inexpensive
- May be indicated to evaluate gallstones, extrahepatic bile ducts, pancreatic pseudocyst, hydronephrosis, or retroperitoneal mass.
- Pelvic ultrasonography may be indicated to evaluate ovarian masses or pregnancy.

Magnetic Resonance Imaging

- May be warranted if IBD is suspected, particularly Crohn disease.

Computed Tomography

- May be warranted to evaluate retroperitoneal or intraabdominal abscess (e.g., associated with IBD).
- Computed tomography (CT) usually is reserved for urgent evaluation (e.g., abscess, mass), given concerns about radiation exposure.

Specialized tests may also be considered:
- Duodenal aspirate to identify existing infection
- Esophageal pH probe to establish gastroesophageal reflux disease (GERD), with a pH of less than 4 representing a reflux episode
- Capsule endoscopy
- Breath hydrogen test if lactose intolerance is suspected
- Sweat chloride test if cystic fibrosis (CF) is suspected (see Chapter 37)

Management Strategies

Medications

Many common medications are used to treat GI disorders:
- Antibiotics, antifungals, or antihelmintics for parasitic infections
- Antiemetics for nausea or vomiting
- Antidiarrheals occasionally for persistent diarrhea or diarrhea associated with chronic disease but generally not recommended as toxins need to be excreted from the body
- Stool softeners, laxatives, and cathartics for acute treatment and long-term management of constipation and encopresis
- Medications that alter GI motility or tone to treat GERD
- Oral steroids, parenteral steroids, and other immunosuppressants in the treatment of IBD
- Pain medication and antispasmodics in selected acute and chronic GI conditions
- Medications that alter gastric acidity to treat GERD and ulcer disease
- Iron supplementation as supportive therapy for chronic disease

Probiotics and Prebiotics

Prebiotics are nondigestible dietary fibers and fructooligosaccharides (carbohydrate molecules made up of a relatively small number of simple sugars) acquired from food that are used as an energy source by certain beneficial bacteria that naturally live in the intestines. Prebiotics are sometimes known as *fermentable fiber.*

Probiotics, on the other hand, are the beneficial bacteria themselves. By acting as a food source, prebiotics give the probiotic bacteria a chance to exert their influence. The concept of prebiotics was first introduced in 1995 by Gibson and Roberfoid as an alternative approach to the modulation of the gut microbiota. The role of prebiotics in the treatment of disease is controversial, and more studies are needed to determine their usefulness. Preliminary evidence shows that prebiotics may have a role in improving antibiotic-associated diarrhea (AAD), traveler's diarrhea, and gastroenteritis; normalizing bowel function; improving colitis; reducing irritable bowel problems; aiding calcium absorption; and boosting the immune system. Some common prebiotics include oligosaccharides and inulin. Inulin is found in more than 36,000 species of plants including wheat, onions, bananas, garlic, asparagus, Jerusalem artichoke, and chicory.

Probiotics are live microbial food supplements or components of bacteria with demonstrated beneficial effects for the host. The phenomenon of eating probiotic products started 100 years ago, when the first reports showed beneficial effects of probiotic bacteria on human health. Several mechanisms have been proposed to explain the actions of probiotics. In most cases, it is likely that more than one mechanism is at work simultaneously. To be most effective, a probiotic species must be able to survive passage through the acidic environment of the stomach and grow in and colonize the intestine, even in the presence of antibiotics. Probiotics are presumed to promote healing of the intestinal mucosa by reducing gut permeability and by enhancing local intestinal immune responses, as well as by reconstituting the intestinal flora.

Probiotics are often regulated as dietary supplements rather than as pharmaceuticals or biologic products. Thus, there is usually no requirement to demonstrate safety, purity, or potency before marketing probiotics. This could lead to significant inconsistencies between the stated and actual contents of probiotic preparations. In the United States, dietary supplements generally do not require premarket review and approval by the U.S. Food and Drug Administration (FDA).

A large number of organisms are being used in clinical practice for a variety of purposes. Most of the identified benefits of probiotics relate to GI conditions, including irritable bowel syndrome (IBS), infectious diarrhea, antibiotic-related diarrhea, and traveler's diarrhea. The most widely used and thoroughly researched organisms are *Lactobacillus, Bifidobacterium,* and *Saccharomyces;* however, the mechanism of action of probiotics remains unclear. *Lactobacillus* promotes healthy bacterial flora in the digestive tract and is widely used to manage and prevent AAD, traveler's diarrhea, and infectious diarrhea. There is also some research that suggests specific strains of *Lactobacillus* may help relieve infantile colic (Szajewska et al., 2013; Chau et al., 2015). *Bifidobacterium* is widely associated with the management of abdominal bloating, flatus, and abdominal pain, which are all symptoms of IBS. *Saccharomyces* have been shown to be effective in the treatment and management of antibiotic-associated and infectious diarrhea.

Some of the most common uses of probiotics in the treatment of digestive disease include:
- IBS: A recurrent disorder of GI functioning that involves the small and large intestines with disturbances of intestinal/bowel motor function and sensation. Probiotics may improve symptoms of IBS based on systematic reviews with at least 37 randomized trials, but overall conclusions are limited by inconsistency in specific probiotics studied (World Gastroenterology Organisation, 2017).

- Infectious diarrhea: This can be caused by infectious agents, such as viruses, bacteria, and/or parasites. Rehydration is a key element in the treatment of diarrhea. Annual global mortality rates due to infectious diarrhea are about 801,000 children (CDC, n.d.) who are the most vulnerable to severe gastroenteritis with group A rotaviruses as the primary cause of disease are children. The use of probiotics and prebiotics has been related to shorter duration and severity of rotavirus diarrhea, to the prevention of infection, and reduced incidence of reinfections (Gonzalez-Ochoa, Flores-Mendoza, Icedo-Garcia, Gomez-Flores, and Tamez-Guerra, 2017).
- Antibiotic-associated diarrhea: AAD is defined as an unexplained diarrhea from other causes occurring in association with antibiotic therapy. It results when the number of healthy microorganisms in the gut decreases as a result of antibiotics given to treat infections. It occurs most frequently with the use of cephalosporins, penicillin, fluoroquinolones, and clindamycin. *Clostridium difficile* is the most serious bacteria found in AAD. Based on the most recent clinical trials, probiotics may be helpful in preventing AAD but are not commonly recommended as routine treatment as their feasibility and efficacy have not yet been fully established (Cardile et al., 2016).
- Colic: *Colic* is defined as crying for no apparent reason that lasts for 3 hours or more per day and occurs 3 days or more per week in an otherwise healthy infant younger than 3 months of age. Numerous randomized controlled trials (RCTs) over the years have demonstrated mixed results with using probiotics to decrease crying times, with differences noted between infants who are solely breastfed and those who are not (Dassow and Fox, 2016).

Upper Gastrointestinal Tract Disorders

Dysphagia

Dysphagia, or difficulty swallowing, may be caused by a variety of disorders. Younger children may be unable to swallow, and older children can have awareness that something is wrong with their swallowing ability or may complain of something stuck in their throat (globus). The physiology of swallowing is complex with oral, pharyngeal, and esophageal phases. The *oral phase* refers to ingestion, mastication, and the propulsion of food to the back of the mouth as a bolus. The *pharyngeal phase* includes the swallowing and transfer of food from the pharynx to the esophagus. Airway closure is critical during the pharyngeal phase, and the child needs to have intact motor and sensory pharyngeal protective mechanisms to prevent aspiration. The *esophageal phase* allows food to pass into the stomach.

Dysphagia may occur as a result of a structural defect, neurologic, allergic, or motor disorders, or mucosal injury. Structural defects make it more difficult to swallow solids than liquids. Common structural defects include esophageal narrowing (stricture, web, or tumor) or extrinsic obstruction (vascular ring). Nonstructural causes arise from motility disorders of the oropharynx or esophagus and are uncommon in children. Prematurity and neurologic impairment from disorders (such as cerebral palsy or muscular dystrophy) can be causes of dysphagia. Mucosal injury most commonly occurs from GERD, eosinophilic esophagitis (EoE), or gastritis, but can also be due to caustic ingestion or medication. The number of children with swallowing difficulties has escalated, because the advances in technology have increased the survival of children with special health care needs and those children with sensory motor deficits.

Clinical Findings

History
- Progressive dysfunction
- Persistent drooling or cough
- Discomfort with swallowing or a sense of food getting stuck
- Picky eating (e.g., a child who prefers liquids to solids) or food refusal
- Halitosis, chest pain

Physical Examination
- Observe the infant or child feeding, paying special attention to the adequacy of the child's oral motor skills and safety of swallowing.
- Perform a complete physical examination, paying particular attention to the mouth, throat, and neck.

Diagnostic Studies
Diagnostic tests may include:
- Lateral neck films
- Barium swallow (usually the initial procedure because it is especially effective in detecting esophageal narrowing)
- Fiberoptic endoscopy evaluation of swallowing
- Video fluoroscopy swallowing study
- Manometry (gold standard for diagnosing motor disorders)
- Magnetic resonance imaging (MRI) (for structural abnormalities)
- Electromyography

Differential Diagnosis

Obstructive and compressive lesions usually cause trouble only with solids. Physiologic dysfunction is usually associated with systemic disease, and the patient has trouble with both liquids and solids. A dysfunctional feeding relationship between child and feeder can manifest as dysphagia.

Management

Difficulty with swallowing requires evaluating associated cognitive, sensory motor, developmental, and behavioral issues. A multidisciplinary approach is recommended to provide a comprehensive, cost-effective evaluation and consistent care for the child and family. Health professionals from otolaryngology, gastroenterology, nutrition, occupational therapy, psychology, and speech-language pathology may be involved.

Vomiting

Vomiting is the forceful emptying of gastric contents coordinated by the medullary vomiting center and/or the chemoreceptor trigger zone of the brain. It is differentiated from regurgitation, which is a passive reflux of gastric contents into the oral pharynx. It can be caused by GI or extraintestinal disorders that are either acute or chronic. Vomiting can be classified as projectile (often arising from the central nervous system [CNS]) or nonprojectile (often seen in GER), and bilious, bloody, nonbilious, or nonbloody.

The age of the child helps to formulate an appropriate list of potential diagnoses:
- Newborn or young infant—infectious process, congenital GI anomaly, CNS abnormality, or inborn errors of metabolism
- Infants and young children—gastroenteritis, GERD, milk/soy protein allergies, pyloric stenosis or obstructive lesion, inborn errors of metabolism, intussusception, child abuse, intracranial mass

- Older children and adolescents—gastroenteritis, systemic illness, CNS (cyclic vomiting syndrome [CVS], abdominal migraine, meningitis, brain tumor), intussusception, rumination, superior mesenteric artery syndrome, pregnancy

Vomiting is one of the most common symptoms in childhood. Nonbilious vomit is generally caused by infection, inflammation, and metabolic, neurologic, or psychological problems. An obstructive lesion generally causes bilious vomiting. Bloody vomit accompanies active bleeding in the upper GI tract (gastritis, peptic ulcer disease [PUD]).

Following is a list of potential causes of vomiting by site of origin:

- Oropharynx: Cleft palate and laryngopharyngeal cleft
- Upper GI: Congenital stricture, foreign body (FB), gastritis and/or esophagitis, gastric web, pyloric stenosis, tracheoesophageal fistula, vascular ring, PUD
- Small intestine: Annular pancreas, choledochal cyst, intestinal atresias and stenosis, intestinal malrotation with volvulus, intestinal pseudo-obstruction
- Colon: Hirschsprung disease (HD), intussusception, meconium ileus, necrotizing enterocolitis, fecal impaction
- Hepatobiliary or pancreatic dysfunction
- Infections: Bacterial enteritis, otitis media, sepsis, urinary tract infection (UTI), viral gastroenteritis (VGE), hepatitis
- Neurologic: Congenital anatomic malformation, gray and white matter degenerative disorders, hydrocephalus, kernicterus, brain tumors, migraine headache, head trauma
- Other: Cow's-milk protein (CMP) allergy (intolerance), inborn errors of metabolism, maternal drug exposure and/or withdrawal, toxic ingestions, appendicitis, cyclic vomiting, pneumonia, drug or alcohol ingestion, eating disorders, pregnancy

Dehydration. *Dehydration* is the loss of water and extracellular fluid. *Volume depletion* or *hypovolemia* (loss of extracellular fluid) and dehydration are used interchangeably. Dehydration is classified as mild (<3% weight loss when compared with recent current weight in older children and 5% in infants), moderate (6% in older children and 10% in infants), or severe (9% or greater in older children and 15% or greater in infants) (Thomas, 2015).

Dehydration is overwhelmingly the result of an infectious process, primarily viral, that often causes diarrhea. Children are at increased risk due to their higher surface area–to-volume ratios, higher rate of insensible loss, and in younger children the inability to communicate or actively replenish losses. Depending on the cause of dehydration, water and salts (primarily sodium chloride) may be lost in physiologic proportion or disparately, producing one of three types of dehydration: isonatremic (isotonic), hypernatremic (hypertonic), or hyponatremic (hypotonic). When dehydration is caused by simple diarrhea, homeostatic mechanisms can usually maintain sodium concentrations in the serum, resulting in isonatremia. When vomiting occurs with diarrhea and water intake is less, there is greater water loss than salt loss, potentially resulting in hypernatremic dehydration. When there is massive stool loss of water and salt and only water is ingested, there is a large salt loss, potentially resulting in hyponatremia.

Clinical Findings

History. The vomiting history should assess the following:
- Symptoms with the onset of vomiting; duration of vomiting, quality and quantity, presence of blood or bile, odor, precipitating event; pain; relationship of vomiting to meals, activities, or time of day. Vomiting early in the morning is indicative of increased intracranial pressure.
- Recent exposure to illness, injury, or stress; recent travel (including camping); swimming activities; possibility of poisoning or contaminated food
- Medications currently being taken (including over-the-counter, herbal, cultural, and homeopathic remedies)
- Presence of associated symptoms: Diarrhea, fever, ear pain, UTI symptoms, vision changes, cough, headache, seizures, high-pitched cry, polydipsia, polyuria, polyphagia, anorexia
- Past history of illnesses, surgeries, or hospitalizations
- Family history of GI disease or fetal or neonatal deaths (metabolic syndrome, congenital anomaly)

The dehydration history should assess the following:
- Mental status and thirst
- Parental concern regarding decreased tearing or urination, or depressed fontanel in infants

Physical Examination
- Growth parameters and vital signs
- Neurologic examination: Nuchal rigidity, decreased level of consciousness, and behavioral changes, which can include irritability or lethargy. Sensorium remains intact until there is greater than 6% weight loss as a result of dehydration. Hypotension is a late manifestation of dehydration.
- Abdominal examination: Inspect for distention, abdominal scars from previous surgery (may be associated with obstruction and/or adhesions), or visible peristaltic waves. Auscultate bowel sounds (i.e., increased with gastroenteritis, decreased with obstruction, absent with ileus or peritonitis). Palpate the abdomen for pain and/or rebound tenderness. Assess abdominal organs (liver and spleen size, masses). Perform a rectal examination as indicated.
- Respiratory examination: Tachypnea, decreased oxygen saturation, stridor
- Assessment of dehydration (Table 40.1)
  - One of the most useful clinical signs of hydration is capillary refill time (CRT). Normal CRT is less than 2 seconds. CRT, skin turgor, and tachypnea, considered together, are most helpful in determining dehydration (Guarino et al., 2014).
  - A clinical dehydration scale (CDS) is a predictive tool regarding length of stay and need for intravenous (IV) fluids (Guarino et al., 2014). The four parameters used for assessment are general appearance, eyes (sunken or not), moistness of mucous membranes, and presence of tears.

Diagnostic Studies. Diagnostic studies are performed as indicated by the probable diagnosis:
- Laboratory studies:
  - CBC with differential, blood culture
  - Electrolytes, including blood urea nitrogen (BUN) and creatinine, glucose, and liver function tests
    - Serum sodium less than 130 (hyponatremic) or greater than 150 (hypernatremic)
  - CRP and ESR
  - Serum lactate, organic acids, ammonia for metabolic disorders (may only be abnormal during episodes of vomiting)
  - UA and urine culture
  - Toxicology screen
  - Stool for culture and occult blood, leukocytes, parasites, fat, pH, reducing substances
  - Rapid strep test and/or throat culture
  - Pregnancy test

TABLE 40.1	Stages of Dehydration		
	STAGES OF DEHYDRATION		
Symptoms	**Minimal or None (<3% Loss of Body Weight)**	**Mild to Moderate (3%-9% Loss of Body Weight)**	**Severe (>9% Loss of Body Weight)**
Mental status	Well; alert	Normal, fatigued or restless, irritable	Apathetic, lethargic, unconscious
Thirst	Drinks normally; might refuse liquids	Thirsty; eager to drink	Drinks poorly; unable to drink
Heart rate	Normal	Normal to increased	Tachycardic; bradycardic in severe cases
Quality of pulses	Normal	Normal to decreased	Weak, thready, or impalpable
Breathing	Normal	Normal; fast	Deep
Eyes	Normal	Slightly sunken	Deeply sunken
Tears	Present	Decreased	Absent
Mouth and tongue	Moist	Dry	Parched
Skinfold	Instant recoil	Recoil in <2 s	Recoil in >2 s
Capillary refill	Normal	Prolonged	Prolonged; minimal
Extremities	Warm	Cool	Cold; mottled; cyanotic
Urine output	Normal to decreased	Decreased	Minimal

From Centers for Disease Control and Prevention (CDC). *Guidelines for the Management of Acute Diarrhea After a Disaster;* 2014. http://emergency.cdc.gov/disasters/disease/diarrheaguidelines.asp. Accessed April 21, 2018.

- Imaging;
  - Abdominal radiographs (suspected obstruction or FB ingestion, organomegaly, or a palpable mass)
  - Chest radiograph (suspected pneumonia)
  - Ultrasound (abscesses, masses, stenoses, cysts, appendicitis, pyloric stenosis)
  - Barium swallow or enema (malrotation, pyloric stenosis, GER, masses)
  - CT scan or MRI to diagnose masses, inflammation, herniations, perforations, and obstructions
- Other studies
  - Endoscopy (obstruction, hemorrhage, infection, collect biopsies)
  - Esophageal pH probe analysis, scintiscan
  - Electroencephalogram (EEG)

Differential Diagnosis
See Table 40.2.

Management
Vomiting
- Identify and alleviate the cause.
- Antiemetics may at times be warranted. Off-label use of Zofran (ondansetron), a 5-HT₃ receptor antagonist, used for management of vomiting in children, has shown significant success with oral rehydration therapy (Tomasik et al., 2016).
- Refer to specialist for persistent vomiting, recurrent vomiting, or vomiting associated with significant underlying process.
Dehydration
- Determine the degree of dehydration. If minimal, mild, or moderate, oral rehydration solution (ORS) with 70 to 90 mEq/L sodium, 25 g/L glucose, 20 mEq/L potassium, 30 mEq/L

base (in the form of citrate, acetate, or lactate) with a defined osmolarity of 240 to 300 mOsm/L is recommended.
- If severe, immediate and aggressive intervention is needed (e.g., IV fluids).
- Pediatric subcutaneous rehydration using recombinant human hyaluronidase is well established as a method to aid absorption of subcutaneous fluids, reduces the risk for allergic reaction, and increases absorption (Zubairi, et al., 2017).

Initial rehydration, maintenance of fluids, and replacement of ongoing losses are stages of treatment (Table 40.3). Physiologically sodium and glucose are coupled in transport across the intestinal brush border into systemic circulation to maximize rehydration. Administration of oral fluid should be in frequent, small (5 mL or less) amounts. Larger amounts may be given as tolerated. Plain water, juices, soda, milk, and sports drinks should be avoided, because these liquids are hyperosmolar and do not provide appropriate replacement of sugars and electrolytes. Palatability of ORS does not affect the quantity consumed. Homemade solute ions can be used when premade ORS is not available (see rehydrate.org). Refeeding should resume as quickly as possible as the gut needs nutrition to facilitate mucosal repair following injury.
- Antiemetics: A single dose of an oral disintegrating tablet of ondansetron (2 mg for children 8 to 15 kg, 4 mg for children 15 to 30 kg, and 8 mg for more than 30 kg) reduces vomiting (Freedman et al., 2014).
- Treat fever over 38.2°C and monitor urine output.
- Refer if the child has a toxic appearance, severe dehydration, projectile vomiting, abnormal examination, vomiting for greater than 12 hours, or vomiting of blood, bile, or fecal matter, or decreased urine output to less than 1 mL/kg/h.

TABLE 40.2	Differential Diagnosis of Vomiting in Infants and Children		
Infant	**Child**	**Adolescent**	

Common Conditions

Infant	Child	Adolescent
Gastroenteritis	Gastroenteritis	Gastroenteritis
GERD	GERD	GERD
Overfeeding	Gastritis	Gastritis
Anatomic obstruction: Pyloric stenosis, malrotation with intermittent volvulus, intestinal duplication, Hirschsprung disease, antral/duodenal web, foreign body, or incarcerated hernia	Toxic ingestion: Lead, iron, or vitamins A and D	Toxic ingestion
Systemic infection: UTI, pneumonia, hepatitis	Systemic infection: UTI or pyelonephritis; pneumonia; hepatitis	Systemic infection
Pertussis syndrome	Pertussis syndrome	Pertussis syndrome
Otitis media	Otitis media, sinusitis	Sinusitis
	Appendicitis, small bowel obstruction Migraine Medications: (e.g., ipecac, digoxin, theophylline, etc.)	Appendicitis, small bowel obstruction, IBD Migraine Medications: (e.g., ipecac abuse/ bulimia, etc.) Pregnancy, PID

Rare Conditions

- Other gastrointestinal disorders: achalasia, gastroparesis, peptic ulcer, food allergy or pancreatitis
- Neurologic: Hydrocephalus, subdural hematoma, intracranial hemorrhage or mass, infant migraine, Chiari malformation, or meningitis
- Metabolic/endocrine: Galactosemia, hereditary fructose intolerance, urea cycle defects or amino and organic acidemias, congenital adrenal hyperplasia
- Renal: Obstructive uropathy or renal insufficiency
- Cardiac: Congestive heart failure or vascular ring
- Others: Pediatric falsification disorder (Munchausen syndrome by proxy), child neglect or abuse, CVS, or autonomic dysfunction

CVS, Cyclic vomiting syndrome; *GERD*, gastroesophageal reflux disease; *IBD*, inflammatory bowel disease; *PID*, pelvic inflammatory disease, *UTI*, urinary tract infection.

Adapted from Blanchard S, Czinn S. Peptic ulcer disease in children. In: Kliegman RM, Behrman RE, Jenson HB, et al., eds. *Nelson Textbook of Pediatrics.* 18th ed. Philadelphia: Saunders, 2011:1572–1574; Vandenplas Y, Rudolph C, Di Lorenzo C, et al. Pediatric gastroesophageal reflux clinical practice guidelines: joint recommendations of the North American Society for Pediatric Gastroenterology, Hepatology, and Nutrition (NASPGHAN) and the European Society for Pediatric Gastroenterology, Hepatology, and Nutrition (ESPGHAN). *J Pediatr Gastroenterol Nutr.* 2009;49(4):498–547. Used with permission of Lippincott Williams & Wilkins.

Complications

Dehydration, fluid and electrolyte imbalance, aspiration pneumonia, hemorrhage, or a tear of the esophagus are possible.

Patient and Family Education

Providing written information to the parent about care that is needed during all stages of oral rehydration therapy is helpful. Also include information about signs that indicate the child is worsening or not responding to treatment in the expected time frame.

Cyclic Vomiting Syndrome

Cyclic Vomiting Syndrome (CVS) is an uncommon, idiopathic disorder that, in its most classical form, is characterized by recurrent, sudden-onset attacks of repeated retching and vomiting that are separated by symptom-free intervals of weeks to months (Levinthal, 2016). Accompanying symptoms include pallor, listlessness, appetite loss, nausea, diarrhea, abdominal pain, fever, dizziness, headache, and photophobia (Kaul & and Kaul, 2015).

The etiology of CVS is unclear. It is often associated with other episodic conditions like migraine headaches and abdominal migraines. Some features of the syndrome are suggestive of a mitochondriaopathy. Triggering factors that may precipitate an episode include exposure to cold, allergies, sinus problems, emotional stress or excitement, anxiety or panic attack, intake of foods like chocolate or cheese, overeating, going to bed immediately after a meal, hot weather, physical exhaustion, menstruation, or motion sickness (Kaul & and Kaul, 2015).

Clinical Findings

History
- Red flags have been identified (Box 40.1)
- Family history positive for migraine headache is common
- A brief prodromal period (some combination of pallor, anorexia, nausea, abdominal pain, or lethargy) and/or a recovery period (from ill to playing again)
- Episodes that begin and end abruptly
- Episodes more likely to occur early in the morning (3:00 to 4:00 a.m.) or on awakening
- An identifiable trigger is commonly seen in children—physical stress (infection, lack of sleep, menstrual periods) or psychological stress (birthdays, holidays, school-related), or food products (e.g., chocolate, cheese, monosodium glutamate)

TABLE 40.3	Treatment Based on Stages and Management of Dehydration			
Degree of Dehydration	Rehydration Therapy	Maintenance	Replacement of Ongoing Losses	
Minimal or none	Not applicable	0-10 kg: 100 mL/kg/24 h 10-20 kg: 1000 mL + 50 mL/kg for each kg over 10 kg >20 kg: 1500 mL +20 mL/kg for each kg over 20 kg	<10 kg body weight: 60-120 mL ORS for each diarrheal stool or vomiting episode >10 kg body weight: 120-240 mL ORS for each diarrheal stool or vomiting episode	
Mild to moderate	ORS: 50-100 mL/kg body weight over 3-4 h or 10-20 mL/kg/h	Same	Same	
Severe	Lactated Ringer solution or normal saline[a] intravenously in boluses of 20 mL/kg body weight until perfusion and mental status improve. If after 60-80 mL/kg given then other causes of shock should be considered, then administer 100 mL/kg body weight ORS over 4 h or 5% dextrose in ½ normal saline intravenously at twice the maintenance fluid rates.	Same	Same: If unable to drink, administer through nasogastric tube or administer 5% dextrose in ¼ normal saline with 20 mEq/L potassium chloride intravenously	

Nutrition

- Continue breastfeeding.
- Lactose-containing formulas are usually well tolerated. If lactose malabsorption appears clinically substantial, lactose-free formulas can be used.
- Return to regular milk in smaller amounts more often.
- Resume age-appropriate normal diet after initial rehydration, including adequate caloric intake for maintenance.
- Complex carbohydrates, fresh fruits, lean meats, yogurt, and vegetables are all recommended.
- Avoid fatty foods and foods high in simple sugars.
- Avoid carbonated drinks or commercial juices.

[a]In severe dehydrating diarrhea, normal saline is less effective for treatment because it contains no bicarbonate or potassium. Use normal saline only if Ringer lactate solution is not available, and supplement with ORS as soon as the patient can drink. Plain glucose in water is ineffective and should not be used.

ORS, Oral rehydration solution.

Adapted from Thomas EY. Fluid and electrolytes. In: Engorn B, Flerage J, eds., eds. *The Harriet Lane Handbook: A Manual for Pediatric House Officer*. 20th ed. Philadelphia: Elsevier; 2015.

• BOX 40.1 Red Flags of Cyclic Vomiting Syndrome

- Abdominal signs (e.g., bilious vomiting, abdominal tenderness, and/or severe abdominal pain, hematemesis)
- Triggering events (e.g., fasting, high-protein meal, or intercurrent illness)
- Abnormal neurologic examination (e.g., severely altered mental status, abnormal eye movements, papilledema, motor asymmetry, and/or gait abnormality [ataxia])
- Progressively worsening episodes or conversion to a continuous or chronic pattern

- Intense nausea not relieved by vomiting
- Headache, motion sickness, photophobia, phonophobia, or vertigo may occur

Physical Examination. Physical examination is normal, although children with CVS appear substantially more ill than children with VGE. If any red flags are present, further workup is indicated.

Diagnostic Studies. *Screening labs* during a vomiting episode can help exclude other diagnoses:
- Electrolytes including HCO_3
- Upper GI radiographs (to exclude malrotation)
- Abdominal ultrasound in refractory cases (rule out transient hydronephrosis)

- If hyponatremic or hypoglycemic, rule out Addison disease and fatty acid oxidation

Differential Diagnosis

CVS is a diagnosis of exclusion. Severe GI symptoms can indicate hydronephrosis, cholelithiasis, pancreatic disease, or ureteropelvic junction. CVS precipitated by concurrent illness, fasting, or high-protein meals can indicate a metabolic disorder. An abnormal neurologic examination is suggestive of increased intracranial pressure. Approximately 10% of children with CVS-like history have a specific underlying disorder.

Management

There is no definite treatment proven to be effective in managing CVS, but some empiric treatments have shown some benefit in a case-by-case series. If there are no findings suggestive of another disorder, treatment regimens are often guided by patient and family history, physical examination, and diagnostic and laboratory test results. CVS generally occurs in three phases: the episode-prodrome, vomiting phase, and recovery phase. A trial of therapy is targeted at prophylaxis during the well phase or at acute and supportive measures during the vomiting and recovery phase. Consideration of the child's clinical course, frequency and severity of attacks, and resultant morbidity directs the treatment plan.

1. Keep a journal of potential precipitating factors in order to identify triggers (75% of children can be helped by this alone):
   • Recognize the role of excitement as a trigger (e.g., downplay big events) to avoid excessive energy output.
   • Avoid trigger foods (chocolate, cheese, monosodium glutamate, hot dogs, aspartame, antigenic foods).
2. Provide supplemental carbohydrate for fasting-induced episodes or high-energy demand times (e.g., fruit juices or other sugar-containing drinks, snacks between meals, before exertion, or at bedtime).
3. Maintain healthy lifestyle:
   • Regular aerobic exercise, avoiding overexercising.
   • Regular meal schedules; don't skip meals.
   • Maintain good sleep hygiene.
   • Maintain good hydration.
   • Avoidance or moderation in consumption of caffeine.

Children 5 Years Old or Younger
• Cyproheptadine (first choice): 0.25–0.5 mg/kg/day divided bid or tid. Maximum dosage *2–6 years:* 12 mg/24 h.

Children Older than 5 Years Old
• Amitriptyline (first choice): 0.1–0.25 mg/kg at bedtime, increase weekly by 0.1–0.25 until maximum dose of 2 mg/kg/24 h or 75 mg/24 h. For doses >1 mg/kg/24 h, divide daily dose bid and monitor electrocardiogram (ECG). Monitor ECG before starting and 10 days after peak dose. *Adult:* Initial 10–25 mg/dose qhs PO; reported range oSf 10–400 mg/24 h.
• Propranolol (second choice–see above): 0.25-1 mg/kg/day, most often 10 mg bid to tid; *<35 kg:* 10–20 mg PO tid; *≥35 kg:* 20–40 mg PO tid. Taper when discontinuing; monitor resting heart rate.

Well Phase: Prevention and Prophylaxis. Keys to successful prevention include lifestyle modifications, avoiding triggers, stress reduction, and prophylactic medications. Preventative management includes getting adequate sleep to prevent exhaustion, treating allergies and sinus problems, and instituting measures for reducing stress and anxiety. Feeding advice would include avoidance of foods with additives and those known to trigger episodes. Eating small carbohydrate-containing snacks between meals, before exercise, and at bedtime should be advised (Kaul and Kaul, 2015) (Box 40.2).
• Trial on daily prophylactic medication if abortive therapy fails consistently or episodes are frequent and/or severe (Box 40.3). Doses can be titrated every 1 to 4 weeks to achieve therapeutic dose for at least two CVS cycles. Phenobarbital and supplements (L-carnitine and coenzyme Q10) have also been used (Kaul and Kaul, 2015).

Episode: Acute Interventions
• Supportive measures include early intervention (within 2 to 4 hours of onset of symptoms), dark, quiet environment, and replacement of fluids, electrolytes, and calories. If anxiety is a trigger, relaxation exercises may be helpful.

• Pharmacologic: Administer abortive therapy as early as possible.
• Antimigraine (triptans) in children older than 12 years of age with infrequent and/or mild episodes (less than one per month); sumatriptan 20 mg intranasally at onset is contraindicated if basilar artery migraine or a migraine with at least two of the following brainstem symptoms: dysarthria, vertigo, tinnitus, hypacusis, diplopia, ataxia, or decreased level of consciousness.
• Antiemetic ondansetron (5-HT$_3$ receptor antagonist): PO. In tablet (4 mg and 8 mg), disintegrating tablet (4 mg and 8 mg), or liquid (4 mg/5 mL). Dosage is
  • 8–15 kg: 2 mg × 1
  • >15 and ≤30 kg: 4 mg × 1
  • >30 kg: 8 mg × 1
• Sedatives for unrelenting nausea and vomiting to induce sleep: Lorazepam (with ondansetron) is considered most effective, but chlorpromazine with diphenhydramine can be used.
• Treatment of specific symptoms can include histamine 2 receptor antagonists (H2RAs) or proton pump inhibitors (PPIs) for epigastric/dyspeptic pain, antidiarrheals for diarrhea, short-acting angiotensin-converting enzyme inhibitors for hypertension, and/or anxiolytic medication for anxiety (panic) triggers.
• Complementary modalities (e.g., biofeedback, massage, imagery) have also been used (see Chapter 27 under Headaches).
   Referral. Referral is recommended if red flag symptoms occur or if the child fails to respond to appropriate acute treatment and/or prophylaxis. (Response is defined as at least a 50% reduction in episode frequency and/or severity of vomiting during attacks over a 2-month period of therapy.)

Complications

Dehydration, electrolyte derangement, metabolic acidosis, hematemesis, and weight loss can be complications of an acute episode. Ongoing esophagitis may require acid suppression. Frequent or prolonged episodes may lead to growth failure. Abdominal epilepsy is an uncommon cause of cyclic vomiting; an EEG is useful in evaluation and anticonvulsants can be helpful in treatment.

Patient and Family Education

Work with families using their knowledge of the child to determine individual triggers and develop a plan of care for all stages.

Abdominal Migraine

Abdominal migraine is thought to be part of a continuum with migraine and CVS (see earlier section). It typically occurs in children rather than adults. The diagnosis is often difficult to determine during the first episode but becomes evident with cyclic episodes. The symptom-based diagnostic criteria for child and adolescent functional gastrointestinal GI disorders are called the Rome IV Criteria. The criteria for the diagnosis of an abdominal migraine must include *all* of the following occurring at least twice and for at least six 6 months prior to diagnosis (Hyams et al., 2016; Hurtado & and Li, 2017).
• Paroxysmal episodes of intense, acute periumbilical, midline, or diffuse abdominal pain lasting 1 hour or more (should be the most severe and distressing symptom).
• Episodes are separated by weeks to months.
• Intervening periods of usual health lasting weeks to months

- Stereotypical pattern and symptoms in the individual patient
- Pain associated with two or more of the following: nausea, vomiting, anorexia, headache, photophobia, or pallor
- After appropriate evaluation, the symptoms cannot be explained by another medical condition
- These criteria need to be present two or more times in the preceding 12 months

Abnormal visual-evoked responses, hypothalamic-pituitary-adrenal axis abnormalities, and autonomic dysfunction are possible mechanisms. Abdominal migraine affects 1% to 4% of children, and it is considered one of the common reasons for recurrent abdominal pain in childhood. It tends to be more common in girls than boys (3:2), with a mean onset at 7 years old and a peak at 10 to 12 years old (Dafer and Lutse, 2017).

Clinical Findings

History
- Rome IV criteria for abdominal migraine (see prior description)
- Family history of migraine or motion sickness
- History of motion sickness
- Most episodes last hours to days with a 1-hour minimum
- Aura not frequently experienced
- Headache complaints typically absent or minimal
- May have prodrome symptoms of fatigue and drowsiness

Physical Examination
- Normal physical examination; normal growth curves and BMI
- Absence of alarm signals

Diagnostic Studies. Evaluation might require excluding processes associated with severe episodic symptoms, such as intermittent small bowel or urologic obstruction, recurrent pancreatitis, biliary tract disease, familial Mediterranean fever, metabolic disorders such as porphyria, and psychiatric disorders (Hyams et al., 2016).

Differential Diagnosis

The diagnosis is often difficult to determine during the first episode. Obstructive GI and renal processes, biliary tract disease, recurrent pancreatitis, familial Mediterranean fever, and metabolic disorders, such as porphyria, should be ruled out. Cyclic vomiting is thought to be a severe variant of abdominal migraine (Dafer and Lutse, 2017).

Management

- Identify and avoid triggers: Caffeine, nitrates, and amine-containing foods; excessive emotional stress; travel; prolonged fasting; altered sleep; flickering or glaring lights.
- Sleep often relieves symptoms; antiemetics may abort an attack
- Abdominal migraine should respond to migraine prophylactic therapy (cyproheptadine, amitriptyline, topiramate). A positive response helps confirm diagnosis.

Prognosis

Complete resolution of all symptoms occurs in 61% of patients. Of those patients with abdominal migraines, 70% will ultimately develop migraine headaches later in life (Hurtado and Li, 2017).

Gastroesophageal Reflux Disease

Gastroesophageal reflux (GERD) refers to the passage of gastric contents into the esophagus from the stomach through the LES. It is a normal physiologic process that occurs several times a day in healthy infants, children, and adults. The etiology of GERD is unclear and probably multifactorial. Inappropriate relaxation of the LES with failure to prevent gastric acid reflux into the esophagus, prolonged esophageal clearance of the gastric refluxate, and impaired esophageal mucosal barrier function are the likely causes of most GERD. LES function usually is influenced by intraabdominal pressure, hormones, neurologic control, and age. Young infants have increased intraabdominal pressure because of their inability to sit upright. They can also regurgitate when they cough, cry, or strain. Daily regurgitation is more common in young infants than in older infants and children and is found in higher rates in neonates. One study of 1,447 mothers throughout the United States showed a prevalence of infant regurgitation of 26%. Regurgitation occurs more than once a day in 41% to 67% of healthy 4-month-old infants. Although regurgitation can occur at any age, the peak is around 4 months of age, with tapering beginning at 6 months and then declining in frequency until 12 to 15 months (Benninga et al., 2016).

Alterations in swallowing, pharyngeal coordination, esophageal motility, and delayed gastric emptying are also potential factors related to GERD. Increased muscle tone, chronic supine positioning, and altered GI motility exacerbate GERD. *Helicobacter pylori* is associated with GERD. Children with *H. pylori* are about six times more likely to develop GERD than non–*H. pylori*-positive children. In infants younger than 1 year old with regurgitation, approximately 10% develop significant complications (AAO-HNS, 2018). Risk factors include prematurity, neurologic impairment, obesity, CF, hiatal hernia, and family history of GERD.

Clinical Findings

Common signs and symptoms by age that should lead the clinician to suspect GERD are presented in Table 40.4. There is no symptom or symptom complex that is diagnostic of GERD or predicts response to therapy. In older children and adolescents, history and physical examination may be sufficient to diagnose GERD. The most common symptom is "heartburn," however in children this discomfort is described as chest pain or pain at the sternum. Recurrent regurgitation with or without vomiting, weight loss or poor weight gain, ruminative behavior, hematemesis, dysphagia, and respiratory disorders such as wheezing, stridor, cough, apnea, hoarseness, and recurrent pneumonia are also associated with GERD.

History. GERD history to be elicited is presented in Box 40.4. Box 40.5 presents the warning signs that merit urgent investigation of vomiting.

Physical Examination
- Review of height, weight, and head circumference
- Signs of failure to thrive (FTT)
- Torticollis: Neck arching
- Hoarseness
- Anemia
- Tooth erosion resulting from destruction of enamel by gastric acids caused by frequent vomiting
- Facial rash, recurrent diarrhea, persistent vomiting, or early-morning vomiting (symptoms of other primary disease with GERD as a secondary problem)

Diagnostic Studies. In most infants with vomiting and in older children with regurgitation and heartburn, a history and physical examination are sufficient to reliably diagnose GERD, recognize complications, and initiate treatment. An empiric trial of acid suppression with a PPI for 4 weeks may be used as a diagnostic

TABLE 40.4 Symptoms and Signs that May be Associated With Gastroesophageal Reflux

Symptoms and Signs that Vary by Age	Symptoms for All Children	Signs for All Children
Infancy: Regurgitation; signs of esophagitis (irritability, arching, choking, gagging, feeding aversion); FTT. Usually symptoms resolve between 12 and 24 months of age. Also, obstructive apnea, stridor, lower airway disease by which reflux complicates a primary airway disease (e.g., bronchopulmonary dysplasia), otitis media, sinusitis, lymphoid hyperplasia, hoarseness, vocal cord nodules, laryngeal edema. *Child and adolescent:* Regurgitation during preschool years, complaints of abdominal and chest pain, neck contortions (arching, turning of head), asthma, sinusitis, laryngitis.	Recurrent regurgitation with/without vomiting Ruminative behavior Heartburn or chest pain Hematemesis Dysphagia, odynophagia Respiratory disorders, such as wheezing, stridor, cough, hoarseness, or persistent throat clearing Halitosis	Esophagitis Esophageal stricture Barrett esophagus Laryngeal/pharyngeal inflammation Recurrent pneumonia Anemia Dental erosion Apnea spells BRUE (brief, resolved, unexplained event) Weight loss or poor weight gain

FTT, Failure to thrive.

Adapted from Vandenplas Y, Rudolph C, Di Lorenzo C, et al. Pediatric gastroesophageal reflux clinical practice guidelines: joint recommendations of the North American Society for Pediatric Gastroenterology, Hepatology, and Nutrition (NASPGHAN) and the European Society for Pediatric Gastroenterology, Hepatology, and Nutrition (ESPGHAN). *J Pediatr Gastroenterol Nutr.* 2009;49(4):498–547.

• **BOX 40.4 History for the Child with Suspected Gastroesophageal Reflux Disease**

Feeding and Dietary History
- Amount/frequency (overfeeding)
- Preparation of formula
- Observe the child during a feeding (clinician)
- Recent changes in feeding type or technique
- Position during feeding, burping technique and frequency
- Behavior during feeding
- Choking, gagging, coughing, arching, discomfort, refusal
- Other concerning behaviors
- Sandifer syndrome: torsional dystonia with arching of the back and rigid opisthotonic posturing, involving primarily the neck, back, and upper extremities
- Pattern of vomiting
- Blood or bile
- Associated fever, lethargy, diarrhea
- Medical history
- Prematurity and newborn screen results
- Growth and development, previous weight and height gain (growth charts)
- Past surgery, hospitalizations
- Recurrent illnesses, especially croup, pneumonia, asthma
- Symptoms of hoarseness, fussiness, hiccups, apnea
- Other chronic conditions
- Medications: Current, recent, prescription, nonprescription
- Family psychosocial history
- Sources of stress and/or postpartum depression
- Maternal or paternal drug use
- Family medical history
- Significant illnesses
- Family history of gastrointestinal (GI) disorders or atopy

• **BOX 40.5 Warning Signals Requiring Urgent Investigation in Infants with Regurgitation or Vomiting**

- Bilious vomiting
- Gastrointestinal (GI) bleeding, hematemesis, hematochezia
- Consistently forceful vomiting or onset of vomiting after 6 months old
- Failure to thrive (FTT)
- Recurrent respiratory infections
- Feeding problems (uncoordinated swallow, choking, or cough associated with feeding)
- Diarrhea or constipation
- Fever and/or lethargy
- Hepatosplenomegaly
- Bulging fontanelles, macrocephaly, or microcephaly
- Seizures
- Abdominal tenderness or distension
- Documented or suspected genetic/metabolic syndrome

The following specialized tests may be obtained following consultation with a physician or a pediatric gastroenterologist.
- Esophageal pH monitoring has been the gold standard to diagnose reflux. However, the presence of reflux may not correlate with the severity of illness, and some gastric contents may not be acidic. Transnasal pH placement may be uncomfortable, decrease appetite and activity, and thus underestimate the true incidence of reflux episodes. Typically, H_2 blockers are discontinued for 72 hours before the test and PPIs for 1 week before the study.
- Multichannel intraluminal impedance (MII) measures episodes of reflux independent of the pH of the fluid. It is especially useful for making a diagnosis in children with respiratory events related to reflux, because it can measure multiple indices, such as heart rate, oxygenation, sleep state, and apnea episodes. It also measures the height of refluxed material and the content and direction of the reflux (liquid, air, or both). In infants and children, pH-MII optimizes the yield of the GER-symptom association. Indications for pH-MII include: (1) evaluating the efficacy of antireflux therapy; (2) endoscopy-negative patients with symptoms concerning for reflux despite PPI therapy in whom documentation of nonacid reflux will alter clinical management; (3) evaluating tube-fed patients for reflux, because

test in older children and adolescents but is not recommended in infants and young children.

Non radiologic diagnostic tests as indicated:
- CBC with differential to rule out anemia and infection
- UA and urine culture
- Stool for occult blood
- Testing for *H. pylori*

the majority of refluxate during tube feeding is nonacidic; and (4) differentiating aerophagia from GER (Mousa and Hassan, 2017).

- Wireless pH monitoring is also available. A pH probe is placed transorally, temporarily attached to the esophageal mucosa where it is programmed to record events for 48 hours. The capsule typically sloughs in about 5 days. Failure to attach, chest pain, feeling of FB, and premature detachment are negative aspects of this technology.
- Endoscopy to obtain a biopsy can help determine severity of reflux esophagitis. It can rule out esophagitis and other pathologic conditions if deemed necessary. It may also be used to re-dilate strictures.
- Barium upper GI series should only be used if obstruction or an anatomic abnormality of the upper GI tract is suspected.
- Radionuclide scan with scintiscan and esophageal and gastric ultrasonography studies are not recommended for routine evaluation of GERD.
- Gastric emptying scan can be used to evaluate for delayed gastric motility associated with GER.
- A video swallow study may be necessary if recurrent respiratory infection, persistent cough, or feeding refusal (or difficulty) is present to evaluate for effective esophageal swallow and to rule out aspiration.

Differential Diagnosis

The clinician should also consider other causes of vomiting as found in Table 40.2.

Management

See Figs. 40.1 to 40.3, and Table 40.5.

Pharmacologic. Acid-suppression agents are the mainstays of treatment. These pharmacologic agents include H2RAs, PPIs, and buffering agents (Table 40.6). Histamine 2 receptor agonists (H2RAs) suppress gastric acid secretion by competitively inhibiting histamine at the parietal cell's H_2 receptor. Dosage requirements vary by age, but children require a relatively higher dose than adults. PPIs are the most potent acid suppressants. They work by blocking the final step in acid secretion. PPIs provide faster and increased relief of symptoms. Antacids are compounds containing different combinations, such as calcium carbonate, sodium bicarbonate, aluminum, and magnesium hydroxide. They provide rapid but short-term symptom relief by buffering gastric acid (Mousa and Hassan, 2017).

There is insufficient evidence to justify the routine use of prokinetic agents such as cisapride, metoclopramide, domperidone, bethanechol, erythromycin, or baclofen for GERD.

Nutrition. Feeding techniques, volumes, and frequency of feeding should be normalized. A trial of extensively hydrolyzed protein formula may be used for 2 to 4 weeks in formula-fed infants with vomiting. Thickened feedings have long been a recommended treatment for GERD; however, the efficacy of this approach is limited and in a review of 14 RCTs found that thickeners were only moderately effective. (Barnhart D, 2016). An increase in caloric density may be necessary in infants with FTT (poor weight gain or weight loss). In older children and adolescents, there is no evidence to support specific dietary restrictions to decrease symptoms; however, avoiding eating less than 2 hours before bedtime may be helpful. Obesity is related to GERD, so weight management is recommended as a component of a treatment program.

Lifestyle. Because prone positioning is associated with increased risk of sudden infant death syndrome (SIDS), supine

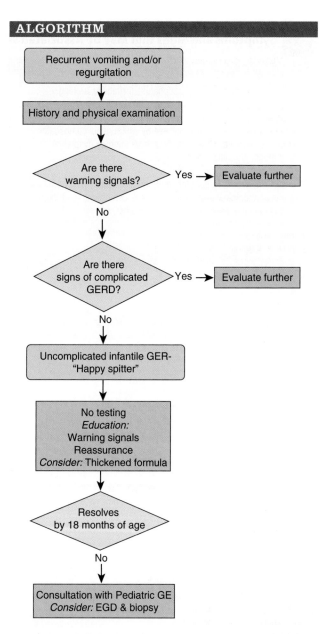

ALGORITHM

• **Fig 40.1** Approach to the Infant With Recurrent Regurgitation and Vomiting. *EGD,* Esophagogastroduodenoscopy; *GE,* gastroenterologist; *GER,* gastroesophageal reflux; *GERD,* gastroesophageal reflux disease. (From Vandenplas Y, Rudolph C, Di Lorenzo C, et al. Pediatric gastroesophageal reflux clinical practice guidelines: joint recommendations of the North American Society for Pediatric Gastroenterology, Hepatology, and Nutrition [NASPGHAN] and the European Society for Pediatric Gastroenterology, Hepatology, and Nutrition [ESPGHAN]. *J Pediatr Gastroenterol Nutr.* 2009;49[4]:498–547.)

positioning during sleep in infants is recommended. Positioning infants upright may worsen reflux. There may be some benefit in older children to left-side positioning during sleep or elevation of the head of the bed (elevate the head of the bed and do not add pillows because it may increase abdominal flexion and compression).

Surgical. Antireflux operations are among the most common procedures performed by pediatric surgeons in the United States. Antireflux surgery strategies, such as fundoplication, are used for management of cases that have not responded to less invasive

ALGORITHM

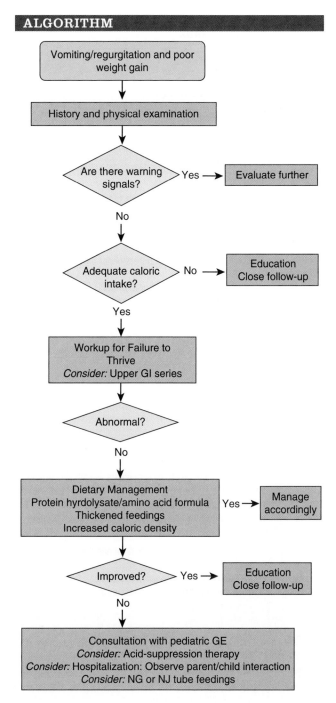

• **Fig 40.2** Approach to the Infant With Recurrent Regurgitation and Weight Loss. *GE,* Gastroenterologist; *GI,* gastrointestinal; *NG,* nasogastric; *NJ,* nasojejunal. (From Vandenplas Y, Rudolph C, Di Lorenzo C, et al. Pediatric gastroesophageal reflux clinical practice guidelines: joint recommendations of the North American Society for Pediatric Gastroenterology, Hepatology, and Nutrition [NASPGHAN] and the European Society for Pediatric Gastroenterology, Hepatology, and Nutrition [ESPGHAN]. *J Pediatr Gastroenterol Nutr.* 2009;49[4]:498–547.)

strategies, have life-threatening complications, or will have long-term dependence on medical therapy in which compliance or patient preference precludes ongoing use. A recent prospective, multicenter study showed significant reduction of reflux symptoms, total acid exposure time, and acid reflux episodes in patients after laparoscopic fundoplication (Mauritz et al., 2017).

ALGORITHM

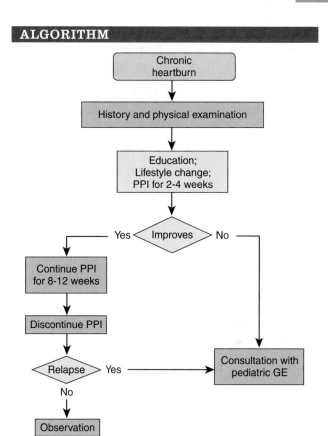

• **Fig 40.3** Approach to the Older Child or Adolescent With Heartburn. *GE,* Gastroenterologist; *PPI,* proton pump inhibitor. (From Vandenplas Y, Rudolph C, Di Lorenzo C, et al. Pediatric gastroesophageal reflux clinical practice guidelines: joint recommendations of the North American Society for Pediatric Gastroenterology, Hepatology, and Nutrition [NASPGHAN] and the European Society for Pediatric Gastroenterology, Hepatology, and Nutrition [ESPGHAN]. *J Pediatr Gastroenterol Nutr.* 2009;49[4]:498–547.)

Complications

Complications include chronic cough, FTT, irritability, and malnutrition. Esophageal injury secondary to reflux results in bleeding, stricture formation, and Barrett esophagus. GERD is circumstantially associated with significant asthma, recurrent pneumonia, or laryngeal disorders. In most infants with brief, resolved, unexplained event (BRUE), GERD is not the cause. However, in the rare case where a relationship is suspected, pH monitoring in combination with polysomnographic recording and precise, synchronous symptom recording may aid in establishing cause and effect. Red flags in infants are bilious vomiting and/or hematemesis (see Box 40.5).

Patient and Family Education

- Assure parents of infants that regurgitation is usually self-limited and symptoms improve as the child grows. Parental education and reassurance are recommended for infants with uncomplicated regurgitation. Remind parents that GERD may temporarily worsen during illness.
- Review medication information, including dosages and side effects.

Pyloric Stenosis

Pyloric stenosis is characterized by hypertrophied pyloric muscle, causing a narrowing of the pyloric sphincter. Pyloric stenosis

TABLE 40.5	Management Strategies for Infants and Children With Gastroesophageal Reflux	
Population	**Diagnostic Tests**	**Management Strategies**
Infant with uncomplicated recurrent regurgitation (GER)	None needed	Provide parental education and reassurance. In formula-fed babies, a thickened formula may reduce over-regurgitation and vomiting but does not reduce the reflux itself.
Infants with recurrent vomiting and poor weight gain (GERD)	Diet history, UA, CBC, serum electrolytes, BUN, serum creatinine Other tests as indicated	For breastfed infants, continue to breastfeed. For formula-fed babies, 2-week trial of extensively hydrolyzed formula or amino acid–based formula to exclude CMA. Increase caloric density. Thicken formula if needed. Educate regarding formula intake needed to sustain normal weight gain. Refer to pediatric gastroenterologist if management fails to improve symptoms and weight gain.
Infants with unexplained crying and/or distressed behavior	Evaluate for CMA, neurologic disorders, constipation, infection (especially UTIs)	Empiric trial with extensively hydrolyzed protein formula or amino acid–based formula. No evidence to support the empiric use of acid suppression for the treatment of irritable infants. However, if irritability persists and no condition other than GERD remains, then continued support of parents with the anticipation of improvement over time; workup to establish the relationship of reflux to feeding or to diagnose esophagitis; or trial of antisecretory therapy, although there is a potential risk for adverse effects. Clinical improvement following empiric therapy may result in spontaneous symptom resolution or placebo response.
Child older than 18 months old with chronic regurgitation or vomiting	Consider diagnosis other than GERD; testing may include upper GI endoscopy, esophageal pH/MII, and barium upper GI series	Treatment depends on diagnosis.
Heartburn in older children and adolescents	No further studies needed if problem is episodic and not severe	On-demand therapy with buffering agents, sodium alginate, or H2RA may be used for occasional symptoms. For chronic heartburn, lifestyle changes, such as diet change, weight loss, smoking avoidance, sleeping position, no late-night eating, and a 2-week trial with a PPI may help. PPI can be continued for up to 3 months if symptoms resolve. Persistent heartburn after that time should be referred to a pediatric gastroenterologist if needed.
Reflux esophagitis—endoscopically diagnosed	No further studies needed	PPI for 3 months is initial therapy. Trial of tapering the dose and then withdrawal of PPI. Chronic relapsing esophagitis may be the diagnosis if PPI cannot be withdrawn and may involve long-term therapy with PPI or antireflux surgery.

BUN, Blood urea nitrogen; *CBC*, complete blood count; *CMA*, cow's-milk allergy; *GER*, gastroesophageal reflux; *GERD*, gastroesophageal reflux disease; *GI*, gastrointestinal; *H2RA*, histamine 2 receptor antagonist; *MII*, multichannel intraluminal impedance; *PPI*, proton pump inhibitor; *UA*, urinalysis; *UTI*, urinary tract infection.

Adapted from Vandenplas Y, Rudolph C, Di Lorenzo C, et al. Pediatric gastroesophageal reflux clinical practice guidelines: joint recommendations of the North American Society for Pediatric Gastroenterology, Hepatology, and Nutrition (NASPGHAN) and the European Society for Pediatric Gastroenterology, Hepatology, and Nutrition (ESPGHAN). *J Pediatr Gastroenterol Nutr.* 2009;49(4):498–547.

occurs in 3 per 1000 live births, with a fourfold increase in males compared with females and in preterm compared to term infants (Eberly et al., 2015). It tends to be familial and is seen more commonly in Caucasian first-born males.

Clinical Findings

History. Regurgitation and nonprojectile vomiting during the first few weeks of life
- Projectile vomiting beginning at 2 to 3 weeks old
- Insatiable appetite with weight loss, dehydration, and constipation
- An association of pyloric stenosis with the administration of erythromycin in the first 2 weeks of life has been demonstrated. There is also an association with azithromycin (Eberly et al., 2015).

Physical Examination
- Weight loss
- Nonbilious vomitus that can contain blood and occur immediately after feeding
- A distinct "olive" mass may be palpated in the epigastrium to the right of midline
- Reverse peristalsis visualized across the abdomen

Diagnostic Studies. Ultrasound, with measurement of the pyloric muscle thickness, is used in most centers. An upper gastrointestinal UGI series demonstrates a "string sign," indicating a fine, elongated pyloric canal; it may be required if ultrasound is unavailable or inconclusive.

Management and Prognosis. Surgical intervention (pyloromyotomy) is indicated after correction of fluid and electrolyte imbalance. Vomiting can continue for a few days after surgery,

TABLE 40.6	Common Medications Used to Treat Gastroesophageal Reflux Disease
Medication	**Pediatric Dosage**
Histamine 2 Receptor Antagonists	
Famotidine (Pepcid)	Infants: 1-3 months old: 0.5 mg/kg/dose once daily for up to 8 weeks
	Infants >3 months old to 1 year old: 0.5 mg/kg/dose twice daily for up to 8 weeks
	Children and adolescents: Initially 0.25 mg/kg/dose every 12 h (maximum dose: 20 mg/dose)
Ranitidine (Zantac)	Infants >1 month, children, and adolescents <16 years old: 4-8 mg/kg/day divided twice daily (maximum dose: 300 mg)
	Adolescents >16 years old: 150 mg twice daily or 300 mg once HS
Proton Pump Inhibitors	
Lansoprazole (Prevacid)	Children 1-11 years old:
	<30 kg: 15 mg once daily for up to 12 weeks
	>30 kg: 30 mg once daily for up to 12 weeks
Omeprazole (Prilosec)	Children >1 year:
	5-10 kg: 5 mg once daily for up to 12 weeks
	10-20 kg: 10 mg once daily for up to 12 weeks
	>20 kg: 20 mg once daily for up to 12 weeks
Pantoprazole (Protonix)	Infants and children <5 years old: 1.2 mg/kg/day once daily for 4 weeks
	Children 5-11 years old: <40 kg 20 mg/once/day
	>40 kg = 40 mg/once/day up to 8 weeks
	Children and adolescents 12-16 years old: 20 or 40 mg once daily for up to 8 weeks
Cytoprotective Agent	
Sucralfate (Carafate)	40-80 mg/kg/day divided every 6 h
	Adult dose 250 mg divided every 6 h
	Take on an empty stomach 1 h before meal and at bedtime

Data from Engorn B, Flerage J. *The Harriet Lane Handbook: A Manual for Pediatric House Officer*. 20th ed. Philadelphia: Elsevier; 2015; Khan S, Orenstein S. Gastroesophageal reflux disease. In: Kliegman RM, Stanton BF, St. Geme JW, et al., eds. *Nelson Textbook of Pediatrics*. 19th ed. Philadelphia: Elsevier; 2011; and Lightdale JR, Gremse DA, Section on Gastroenterology, Hepatology, and Nutrition. Gastroesophageal reflux: management guidance for the pediatrician. *Pediatrics*. 2013;131(5):e1684–e1685.

although it is not as significant as it was preoperatively; feedings should be introduced gradually. The prognosis is excellent.

Eosinophilic Esophagitis

Eosinophilic esophagitis (EoE) is an emerging disease related to food ingestion. It is characterized by an isolated inflammation of the esophagus by a specific WBC, the eosinophil. Young children may present with feeding refusal or FTT. Recurrent vomiting and abdominal pain may occur in school-age children. Older children and adolescents often present with dysphagia, choking, and food impaction (Bohm, et al., 2017).

Clinical Findings

History and Physical Examination. Differentiating EoE from GERD may be difficult because both entities may present with similar clinical history and physical examination findings.

Diagnostic Studies. Currently the only way to accurately diagnose EoE is by upper endoscopy and biopsy. Esophageal mucosa

may appear normal in up to a third of patients. Esophageal edema, longitudinal furrows, mucosal fragility, whitish exudates, transient esophageal rings (feline folds), fixed esophageal rings (trachealization), diffuse esophageal narrowing, and small-caliber esophagus are typical macroscopic findings (Muir et al., 2016).

Management

Objectives of EoE therapy include improvement in histology and quality of life, reduction in clinical symptoms, and prevention of complications (such as food impactions or food stuck in the esophagus) or long-term sequelae (such as strictures or small-caliber esophagus). Current treatment modalities include dietary modification and pharmacotherapy.

Three dietary strategies include elemental diet administration, empiric dietary elimination, and targeted food elimination. Use of an elemental diet consisting of an amino acid-based formula remains the most effective and accepted dietary intervention for EoE in infants. For older children, many clinicians will recommend initially initiating the six-food (milk, soy, egg, wheat, peanut/tree nuts, and fish/shellfish) elimination diet and then an immediate referral to a pediatric allergist for identification and targeted food elimination, based on allergy testing results. Although expensive and unpalatable, the elemental diet makes the most sense, because it is devoid of all food antigens that cause eosinophil infiltration and inflammation. In children, an elemental diet produces nearly complete remission of EoE in 80%-90% of affected children (Straumann and Katzka, 2017).

Treatment of EoE usually consists of PPIs and swallowed inhaled corticosteroids (fluticasone, propionate, budesonide, and ciclesonide) for 12 weeks. However, currently there is no medication specifically FDA approved for the disease.

Peptic Ulcer Disease

PUD consists of a group of gastric and duodenal disorders ranging from gastritis to ulceration. With duodenal ulcers, mucosal defects penetrate the duodenal mucosa and submucosa. Gastric ulcers result from mucosal defects that penetrate the gastric mucosa and submucosa.

PUD is classified as primary or secondary. Most *primary ulcers* are duodenal, have no underlying cause, and tend to be chronic with resulting granulation tissue and fibrosis. They tend to recur and are more common in adolescents and rare in children. *Secondary ulcers* are more often gastric, generally more acute, and associated with known ulcerogenic events. Severe erosive gastropathy can result in bleeding ulcers or gastric perforations, more commonly in the stomach than duodenum. Head trauma, severe burns, use of corticosteroids, and nonsteroidal anti-inflammatory drugs (NSAIDs) are associated with secondary ulcers. Aspirin or NSAIDs cause mucosal injury by direct injury or inhibiting cyclooxygenase and prostaglandin formation. Chronic therapy with these medicines causes gastric mucosal damage but is not associated with ulcer formation. Stress ulceration usually occurs within 24 hours of critical illness and may occur in 25% of critically ill children in intensive care units. Preterm and term infants in neonatal intensive care units (NICUs) can also develop gastric mucosal lesions with bleeding or perforation. *Idiopathic ulcers* are found in *H. pylori*–negative children who have no history of taking NSAIDs; 20% of pediatric duodenal ulcers are of this type. A strong familial predisposition for PUD is noted, and most children with duodenal ulcers have a positive family medical history, which is a key finding.

There is no evidence that diet plays a role in the formation of ulcers.

Peptic ulcers result from an imbalance between protective and aggressive factors. *Protective factors* include the water-insoluble mucous gel lining, local production of bicarbonate, regulation of gastric acid, and adequate mucosal blood flow. *Aggressive factors* include the acid-pepsin environment, infection with *H. pylori,* and mucosal ischemia. Colonization rates with *H. pylori* in the United States and Europe are less than 10%; there are much higher rates in less-developed countries. Colonization likely occurs during the first years of life, but the infection often remains asymptomatic with low-grade inflammation or no mucosal changes. Zollinger-Ellison syndrome (ZES) is a rare syndrome involving refractory severe PUD caused by gastric hypersecretion due to the autonomous secretion of gastrin by a neuroendocrine tumor.

Clinical Findings

The most common symptom of PUD is vague, dull abdominal pain; however, presenting symptoms vary depending on the age of the child. Hematemesis or melena is reported in up to 50% of patients. Neonates can present with gastric perforation. Infants usually present with feeding difficulty, vomiting, crying episodes, hematemesis, or melena. Epigastric pain and nausea are reported more often by school-age children and adolescents. The classic adult symptom of PUD, pain alleviated by ingestion of food, is present in only a minority of children. Most children presenting with epigastric or periumbilical pain do not have PUD, but rather functional bowel disorder, IBS, or functional dyspepsia.

History
- Asymptomatic or symptoms wax and wane. Remissions may last from weeks to months.
- Pain with eating, dyspepsia; can awaken from sleep.
- GI tract bleeding may be a presenting symptom.
- Infants: Poor feeding, GI bleeding, vomiting, intestinal perforation, slow growth; history of prematurity or time in NICU.
- Toddlers and preschoolers: Poorly localized abdominal pain, vomiting, GI bleeding. May worsen after eating; irritability; anorexia.
- School-age children and adolescents: Poorly localized epigastric or right lower quadrant (RLQ) pain. Pain is often described as dull, aching, and lasting from minutes to hours. Nocturnal pain is common in older children. Relief from antacids is reported by less than 40% of children. If the pain awakens the child, worsens with food, and is relieved by fasting, this may help distinguish GI pathology from psychogenic pathology, although these symptoms are infrequently described in children. Recurrent vomiting may occur.
- GI bleeding may lead to iron deficiency anemia with symptoms of fatigue, headache, dyspnea, and malaise.
- Family history of PUD.
- Predisposing factors: Alcohol, smoking, aspirin, NSAIDs, corticosteroids, emotional stress, serious systemic disease, sepsis, hypotension, respiratory failure, multiple traumatic injuries, and extensive burns.
- ZES presents with severe peptic ulceration, kidney stones, watery diarrhea, or malabsorption (fasting serum gastrin level >200 pg/mL and baseline gastric acid hypersecretion at more than 15 mEq/h).

Physical Examination. A careful physical examination should be performed; however, there may be no physical findings. The physical examination should include the following:
- Height, weight, head circumference, BMI, and percentiles

- Vital signs
- General observation of the child's appearance
- Assessment of perfusion: Mental status, heart rate, pulses, capillary refill, pallor
- Assessment of hydration: Mucous membranes and skin turgor
- Careful mouth inspection for ulcers (associated with Crohn disease) and dental enamel erosion (associated with GERD)
- Lung examination for wheezing (associated with GERD)
- Abdominal examination for tenderness and hepatosplenomegaly
- Rectal examination (to assess perirectal disease)
- Pelvic examination in sexually active female patients with pain
- Testicular and inguinal examinations in male patients

Diagnostic Studies

Endoscopy with mucosal biopsy is the diagnostic test of choice and validates *H. pylori* infection. However, if a child has mild PUD, minimal laboratory studies are needed. Diagnostic studies to consider include the following.

Laboratory Studies
- Initially (red flags for systemic disease): CBC (anemia is associated with chronic infection with *H. pylori* or acute or chronic blood loss due to ulcer perforation into the abdominal cavity), albumin (low), and ESR (high). May also consider stool for guaiac and *H. pylori* (especially in children).
- If child is unstable, severe, or has chronic, recurrent symptoms, or serious complications also consider iron studies; *H. pylori* serology (most useful in teenagers, only helpful in children if negative due to high false-positive rate); prothrombin time and activated partial thromboplastin time (aPTT), useful to identify coagulopathy; electrolyte, BUN, creatinine levels (to assess volume depletion); arterial blood gases (acidosis); UA (hydration, infection, or stones); serum gastrin and gastrin-releasing peptide levels (in patients with refractory ulcers to exclude ZES). *Note:* PPIs must be discontinued 2 weeks before gastrin level measurement. Type and crossmatch for blood may also be done.

Imaging Studies
- Abdominal or chest x-ray for perforation
- Upper GI series helps to diagnosis about 70% of children (sensitivity higher for duodenal ulcers). A fibrinous clot in the ulcer may lead to false-negative findings. Barium studies have false-positive rates as high as 30% to 40%. Gastric outlet obstructions often due to pyloric lesions can be identified.
- Angiography is sometimes done if there is a massive bleed and endoscopy cannot be performed.

Procedures
- Esophagogastroduodenoscopy (EGD) is the procedure of choice in children for detecting PUD, because it allows direct visualization of mucosa, localization of the source of bleeding, and collection of biopsy specimens. It is also used therapeutically for acute bleeding.

Studies to Detect Helicobacter Pylori

- Histologic examination and culture biopsies obtained via endoscopy are the gold standard for detecting acute infection; however, it is an invasive procedure that requires anesthesia. It is appropriate for persistent or recurrent infection or severe symptoms.
- C-urea breath test is the noninvasive diagnostic test of choice; it can distinguish between past and present infection. It is sensitive in children older than 2 years of age, but requires special

equipment. It should be performed off acid suppression to avoid false-negative results.

- Stool monoclonal antibody test distinguishes between past and present infection. It is reliable for evaluating response to therapy if symptoms persist and should be performed off acid suppression (4 weeks) to avoid false-negative results.
- Serum immunoglobulin G (IgG) antibody titer. A positive result (>500 units) only means exposure to the disease. This test should not be the sole basis for starting therapy or used to test for eradication. It is beneficial for initial screening in the workup of epigastric pain/dyspepsia.

Differential Diagnosis

All other causes of abdominal pain, especially GERD, IBS, GI bleeding, cholelithiasis, cholecystitis, pancreatitis, lactose intolerance, hyperkalemia, and hypercalcemia, are in the differential.

Management

- The goals of treatment include ulcer healing, elimination of the primary cause, relief of symptoms, and prevention of complications.
- Medications:
  - H2RAs or PPIs are first-line therapy (see Table 40.6). PPIs are most effective if given before a meal.
  - Antacids: Any liquid preparation given between 1 and 3 hours after eating and before bed.
  - *Eradication therapy* for *H. pylori* is indicated for children with a duodenal or gastric ulcer identified by endoscopy and histopathology. *Empiric therapy* for suspected *H. pylori* is not recommended. There is increasing antibiotic resistance to *H. pylori*. Therapy is not indicated for gastritis without PUD, recurrent abdominal pain, or for children with asymptomatic PUD or with a family member with PUD. See Table 40.7 for treatment guidelines when *H. pylori* is confirmed. Compliance with the treatment regimen is the single most important determinant of eradication. Eradication rates are more than 90%. The test of cure can either be the stool antigen test or the urea breath test.
- Referral to a gastroenterologist should occur if there is:
  - Lack of improvement or inability to wean off medications
  - History of hematemesis, melena, occult blood in stools, anemia, and/or weight loss
- Idiopathic ulcers: The preferred treatment is acid suppression with either H2RAs or PPIs. Patients should be followed closely and, if symptoms recur, restart acid suppression treatment. PPIs are preferred for maintenance in children older than 1 year of age.

Complications

Acute hemorrhage, chronic blood loss, penetration of the ulcer into the abdominal cavity, or adjacent organs may produce shock, anemia, peritonitis, or pancreatitis. Obstruction can occur if inflammation and edema are extensive. Hemorrhage occurs in 15% to 20% of patients, and perforation occurs in less than 5%. Recurrence, gastric outlet obstruction, gastric adenocarcinoma, and gastric lymphoma are other possible complications.

Patient and Family Education

Treatment success depends on the child completing the drug regimen. PUD in children is being actively studied, and clinicians must be aware of ongoing changes. With the introduction of H2RAs and PPIs and the recognition that *H. pylori* can be treated, the incidence of complications has decreased dramatically.

TABLE 40.7	Recommended Eradication Therapies for *Helicobacter pylori* Disease in Children	
Medications	Dosage
Option 1 (Three Drugs)	
Amoxicillin	50 mg/kg/day up to 1 g twice daily
Clarithromycin	15 mg/kg/day up to 500 mg twice daily
Omeprazole	1 mg/kg/day up to 20 mg twice daily
Option 2 (Three Drugs)	
Amoxicillin	50 mg/kg/day up to 1 g twice daily
Metronidazole	20 mg/kg/day up to 500 mg twice daily
Omeprazole	1-2 mg/kg/day up to 20 mg twice daily
Option 3 (Three Drugs; 8 Years Old or Older)	
Bismuth sub salicylate	8-12 years old: 8 mg/kg/day times a day
Amoxicillin	50 mg/kg/day up to 1 g twice daily
Metronidazole	20 mg/kg/day divided up to 500 mg twice daily
Option 4 (Sequential Therapy)	
	Omeprazole and amoxicillin for 5 days then omeprazole, clarithromycin, and metronidazole for 5 days at dosages above

From Koletzko S, Jones NL, Goodman KJ. Evidence-based guidelines from ESPGHAN and NASPGHAN for *Helicobacter pylori* infection in children. *J Pediatr Gastroenterol Nutr.* 2011;53(2):230–243.

Lower Gastrointestinal Tract Disorders

Foreign Body Ingestion

Most foreign body (FB) ingestions are not serious; objects pass through the gut without consequence. Most swallowed items are radiopaque; coins and small toy objects are the most commonly ingested items. Food impactions are less common in children than adults. Most ingestions of foreign bodies (FBs) occur in children between 6 months and 3 years of age (80%) and more than 125,000 ingestions occur annually in patients younger than 19 years old (Sandoval, 2017). Teens may have psychiatric problems or engage in risk-taking behaviors leading to ingestion of FBs. The size and power of batteries have changed over decades. Despite warnings such as blister packs and education of families, there is often a failure to prevent accidental ingestion, and the incidence of these events is increasing (Kodituwakku, Palmer, & and Paul, 2017).

Esophageal Foreign Bodies

Esophageal FBs lodge at three spots most commonly—at the thoracic inlet where skeletal muscle changes to smooth muscle (between the clavicles at about C6) (70%), at the mid-esophagus where the aortic arch and carina overlap the esophagus (15%), or at the lower esophageal sphincter (LES) (15%). Pointed objects or small objects, such as pills or small button batteries, may lodge anywhere along the slightly moist esophageal mucosa. Common symptoms include an initial episode of choking, gagging, and coughing. Excessive salivation; dysphagia; food refusal; emesis/hematemesis; or pain in the neck, throat, or sternal notch areas may follow. Respiratory symptoms such as stridor, wheezing, cyanosis, or dyspnea may occur if the esophageal body impinges on the larynx or tracheal wall. Cervical swelling, erythema, or subcutaneous crepitations may indicate perforation of the oropharynx or proximal esophagus (Sandoval, 2017). Drooling or pooling of secretions may be related to an esophageal FB or abrasion of the esophagus as a result of swallowing the object. Disk batteries cause a liquefactive necrosis, electrical discharge leading to low-voltage burns, and pressure necrosis. Children who have swallowed lithium batteries greater than or equal to a 20 mm diameter are at greatest risk of problems due to battery ingestion Some patients have documented severe erosion or ulceration in as little as 2 hours after ingestion. Emergency endoscopic removal is essential. (Thomson and Sharma, 2015).

Abdominal Foreign Bodies. Most ingested objects that reach the stomach pass through the remainder of the GI tract without difficulty. Items greater than 5 cm in diameter or 2 cm in thickness tend to lodge in the stomach and need to be retrieved. Thin objects longer than 10 cm may not make the duodenal sweep turn and also need to be retrieved. In infants and toddlers, FBs greater than 3 cm in length or 20 mm in diameter may not pass through the pyloric sphincter. Open safety pins or other pointed objects, such as needles or thumbtacks, also should be retrieved.

Perforation after ingestion occurs in only 1% of ingestions. Perforation occurs near physiologic sphincters, areas of angulation, congenital malformations of the gut, or near areas of previous bowel surgery. Coins made with nickel have been reported to interact with gastric acid to cause stomach ulceration (Sandoval, 2017). Abdominal distention or pain, vomiting, hematochezia, and unexplained fever are symptoms related to ingestions lodging in the stomach or intestinal areas. Items that pose a greater risk include multiple small magnets that may cling together across the bowel wall, leading to pressure necrosis; items containing lead; and batteries, which usually do not cause problems but might lead to symptoms if there is leakage of alkali or mercury from battery degradation. Lithium toxicity has been reported. Nickel in coins can lead to allergic symptoms in children with a nickel allergy.

Rectal Foreign Bodies. Children sometimes put items into their rectum. Small blunt objects usually will pass spontaneously, but large or sharp objects should be retrieved after sedation to relax the anal sphincter.

Clinical Findings

History, Physical Examination, and Laboratory Studies. Specific physical findings are unusual. Abrasions, streaks of blood, or edema of the hypopharynx may occasionally indicate an FB. Laboratory studies are usually not helpful, although they may be useful to identify potential infection.

Imaging Studies. Most FBs are radiopaque. A single frontal radiograph that includes the neck, chest, and entire abdomen is usually sufficient to locate the object. Subsequent radiographs may be useful to more fully evaluate the patient. Esophageal objects should be precisely located with frontal and lateral chest radiographs and to make sure there are not two objects closely aligned. Coins in the esophagus are usually seen on the frontal view, whereas tracheal coins are more often seen from the side view (Sandoval, 2017). Having the child ingest a small amount of dilute contrast material may help locate radiolucent objects. Endoscopy may be needed and also allows removal of the object.

Management

Most children do not require special care. Patients who are drooling may require suction.

Esophageal Foreign Bodies. Objects in the esophagus should generally be considered impacted. Removal is mandatory except for blunt objects that have been in place less than 24 hours. Disk batteries and sharp objects should be removed without waiting. Endoscopy is the method of choice for removal except that experienced gastroenterology practitioners may use a Foley catheter to pull the object up or a bougienage method to push the object into the stomach. Only experienced clinicians working with healthy children who ingested an item less than 24 hours previously should try these methods. A radiograph is done immediately before the procedure to be sure the item has not moved and another radiograph follows the procedure to be sure there are no retained parts or complications, such as a pneumomediastinum.

Stomach/Lower Gastrointestinal Tract Foreign Bodies. Most FBs that reach the stomach may be left to pass through the system, usually within 2 to 3 days. Very sharp items may perforate the bowel and should be removed endoscopically from the stomach or surgically from the intestine. Button batteries in the stomach or intestine may be left to pass but should be removed if the family has not identified the battery in the stool after 2 to 3 days. It should be removed endoscopically from the stomach at that time or watched with repeat radiographs to be sure it is progressing through the tract if it is in the intestine. Items may not pass through the gut if the child has a bowel abnormality or had bowel surgery. Use of laxatives is not necessary. Inducing vomiting may lead to aspiration.

Complications

Systemic reactions from allergy or toxic response to massive ingestion can occur. Retained FBs may cause erosion, abrasion, local scarring, obstruction, abscess, FTT, perforation, pneumomediastinum, pneumonia, or other respiratory disease. Complications from the removal process can occur. Traumatic epiglottitis can occur from trauma during swallowing or a finger sweep trying to dislodge the item.

Appendicitis

Appendicitis is inflammation of the appendix that leads to distention and ischemia that can result in necrosis, perforation, and peritonitis or abscess formation. Although a classic presentation is easy to discern, appendicitis can mimic many other intraabdominal conditions, making diagnosis challenging.

Following a closed-loop obstruction of the appendiceal lumen by a fecalith, lymphoid tissue, tumor, parasite, FB, or inspissated CF secretions, the appendix becomes distended, experiences increased bacterial overgrowth, and becomes subject to ischemia and necrosis. Peritoneal inflammation around the infected appendix causes the characteristic symptoms. There is about a 36- to 72-hour maximum window from the onset of pain to the rupture of the gangrenous appendix. Rupture results in the release of inflammatory fluid and bacteria into the abdominal cavity, resulting in infection of the peritoneum with resultant generalized peritonitis. The infected fluid may be walled off by the omentum and loops of small bowel with resultant abscess formation and localized pain (Rentea, & and St. Peter, 2017).

The average age of appendicitis in children is 6 to 10 years old, with a male-to-female ratio of approximately 2:1. It is rare in infancy. The incidence is 4 cases per 1000 children. Perforation is most common in younger children (under 5 years old) and is complicated by the fact that appendicitis is less common in this age group and the ability of very young children (younger than

5 years) to communicate location and type of pain is not yet well developed (Rentea and St. Peter, 2017). It is challenging at times to make a timely diagnosis.

Clinical Findings

History
- The most reliable information is gained from the sequence of symptoms:
  - Pain: Initially poorly defined periumbilical pain (earliest sign); acute onset of severe pain is not typical of acute appendicitis. A shifting of pain to the RLQ may occur after a few hours and becomes more intense, continuous, and localized.
  - Nausea and vomiting: Typically occurs after pain; however, in retrocecal appendicitis, this may be reversed. In gastroenteritis, vomiting precedes the pain.
  - Anorexia occurs (although up to 50% of children state that they are hungry).
  - Stool is low volume with mucus; diarrhea is atypical but can occur especially after perforation (gastroenteritis has high-volume, watery stools).
  - Fever is neither sensitive nor specific for appendicitis; many children present as afebrile or with low-grade fever. High fever may be associated with perforation.
- A scoring system may be helpful (Sayed et al., 2017). A score of 4 or less is highly sensitive in the exclusion of the diagnosis of appendicitis:
  - Nausea/emesis (1 point)
  - Anorexia (1 point)
  - Migration of pain to RLQ (1 point)
  - Low-grade fever (1 point)
  - RLQ tenderness on light palpation (2 points)
  - Cough/percussion/heel tapping tenderness at RLQ (2 points)
  - Leukocytosis (>10,000/mm^3) (1 point)
  - Left shift (>75% neutrophilia) (1 point)
  Total 10 points
- The process evolves over 12 hours, with the potential for infants and young children to become ill much more quickly.
- Following perforation, symptoms lessen, with less vomiting, fever greater than 101°F (38.3°C), and the most comfortable position being on the side with the legs flexed.
- Infants demonstrate irritability, pain with movement, and flexed hips.
- The child may become quiet because crying and movement hurt.

Physical Examination. A complete physical examination is necessary. Reexamination may be needed in 4 to 6 hours.
- Presence of involuntary guarding, RLQ rebound tenderness, maximal pain over McBurney point (1.5 to 2 inches in from the right anterior superior iliac crest on a line toward the umbilicus) on abdominal examination (most reliable finding); percussion is best method for eliciting rebound tenderness.
- Heel-drop jarring test (on toes for 15 seconds, dropping down forcefully on heels); inability to stand straight or climb stairs; winces when getting off examination table or riding in a car over bumps; child most comfortable with bent knees.
- Positive psoas sign or obturator sign (or both).
- Rovsing sign or rebound tenderness (pressure deep in left lower quadrant with sudden release elicits RLQ pain) strongly suggests peritoneal irritation.

- Tenderness and possibly a mass (abscess) on the right side on rectal examination.

Diagnostic Studies. The following may be noted with appendicitis (Rentea and St. Peter, 2017):
- CBC with differential may show an increased WBC count (>10,000) with an increased neutrophil count. This occurs in 70% to 90% of those with acute appendicitis. However, an elevated WBC count may be neither sensitive nor specific in the clinical diagnosis of appendicitis; during the first 24 hours of symptoms it is often within a normal range.
- Amylase, lipase, and liver enzymes help to differentiate liver, gallbladder, or pancreatic issues.
- UA can show small numbers of WBCs (<20) and red blood cells (RBCs) (<20 per high-power field).
- Examination of stool may demonstrate blood and pus (rare finding).
- Abdominal radiographs can show a fecalith, especially if rupture has occurred.
- Ultrasound demonstrates enlargement of the appendix and changes in its wall, increased field around the appendix, or an abscess. Ultrasound has excellent specificity, but it has only fair sensitivity and is operator dependent.
- CT scan with contrast has the highest accuracy, especially in adolescents. CT scan compared with ultrasound has higher sensitivity and specificity, is not operator dependent, and may be more cost effective in preventing an unnecessary appendectomy. An appendiceal diameter of greater than 6 mm is considered diagnostic (in both ultrasound and CT scan).
- A β-human chorionic gonadotropin (β-hCG) test to rule out pregnancy or ectopic pregnancy.

Differential Diagnosis

The differential diagnosis includes vomiting and gastroenteritis (fever and crampy abdominal pain with vomiting, diarrhea, or both), constipation, UTI (fever, chills, and urinary symptoms), pregnancy, pelvic inflammatory disease (PID) or organ pathologic condition, pneumonia, duodenal ulcer (gnawing and burning pain), intestinal obstruction (crampy pain), peritonitis (worse pain when jumping or coughing), and intussusception (child younger than 2 years old with a right upper quadrant [RUQ] mass) (Fig 40.4).

Management

- A surgical consultation for an appendectomy is needed. Administering opioid narcotics for pain before surgical consultation effectively reduces acute abdominal pain, does not impede the diagnostic process, and does not lead to an inappropriate increased use of CT scanning preoperatively. IV and preoperative antibiotics are given if perforation is suspected.
- Open appendectomy (OA) or laparoscopic appendectomy (LA) is indicated in nonperforated appendicitis. The management of perforated appendicitis is controversial, including surgical intervention. Urgent appendectomy may not be indicated in cases of perforated appendicitis. Instead, surgeons may choose to perform appendectomy once fluid resuscitation and antibiotics have been administered. This nonoperative approach is utilized as long as the child's clinical condition improves with antibiotic treatment. An appendectomy may be performed 8 to 12 weeks after recovery.
- Patients should be seen for follow-up 2 to 4 weeks after surgery. If appetite, bowel function, energy, and activity level are normal; no pain or fever is present; findings on physical

Differential Diagnosis

Accidental injury	Ectopic pregnancy	Pneumonia
Accidental ingestion	Food intolerance	Renal stones
Anaphylactoid purpura	Gastroenteritis	Sickle cell anemia
Appendicitis	Hemolytic uremic syndrome	Torsion of ovary or testicle
Child abuse	Mechanical obstruction	Trauma
Constipation	Mononucleosis	Urinary tract infection
		Viral syndrome

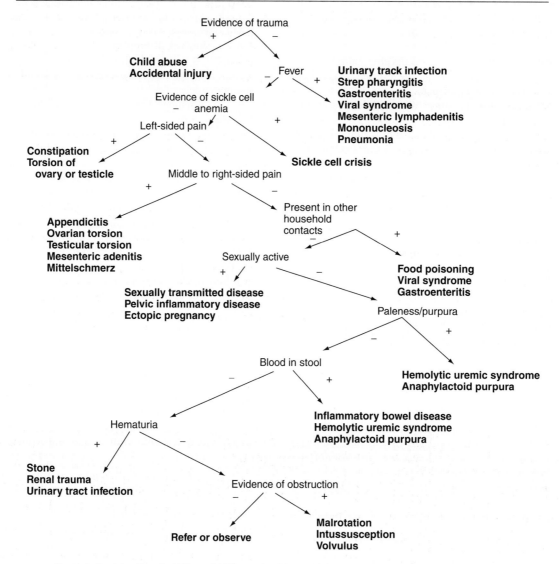

• **Fig 40.4** Decision Tree for Differential Diagnosis of Acute Abdominal Pain. (From Schwartz MW, Curry TA, Sargent J, eds. *Pediatric Primary Care: A Problem-Oriented Approach.* 3rd ed. St. Louis: Mosby; 1997.)

examination are normal; and the wound is well healed, the child can resume unrestricted activity. If at the 2- to 4-week follow-up (or earlier) the child has signs or symptoms of delayed infection, abnormal bowel function, or unexplained weight loss, refer back to the surgeon (Alder, 2017).

Complications

Perforation, peritonitis, pelvic abscess, ileus, obstruction, sepsis, shock, and death can occur.

Intussusception

Intussusception involves a section of intestine being pulled antegrade into adjacent intestine with the proximal bowel trapped in the distal segment. The invagination of bowel begins proximal to the ileocecal valve and is usually ileocolic, but it can be ileoileal or colocolic. Intussusception is thought to be the most frequent reason for intestinal obstruction in children. Intussusception most commonly occurs between 5 and 10 months of age and is also the most common cause of intestinal obstruction in children

3 months to 6 years old; 80% of the cases occur before 2 years of age. In younger infants, intussusception is generally idiopathic and responds to nonoperative approaches. In some children, there is a known medical predisposing factor, such as polyps, Meckel diverticulum, Henoch-Schönlein purpura, constipation, lymphomas, lipomas, parasites, rotavirus, adenovirus, and foreign bodies. Intussusception may also be a complication of CF. Children older than 3 years are more likely to have a lead point caused by polyps, lymphoma, Meckel diverticulum, or Henoch-Schönlein purpura; therefore, a cause must be investigated. The absolute risk of intussusception is only marginally increased by the rotavirus vaccination (Koch, Harger, von Kries et al., 2017).

Clinical Findings

History
- The classic triad for intussusception, intermittent colicky (crampy) abdominal pain, vomiting, and bloody mucous stools, are present in fewer than 25% of cases (Territo et al., 2014).
  - Paroxysmal, episodic abdominal pain with vomiting every 5 to 30 minutes. Vomiting is nonbilious initially. Some children do not have any pain.
  - Screaming with drawing up of the legs with periods of calm, sleeping, or lethargy between episodes.
  - Stool, possibly diarrhea in nature, with blood ("currant jelly").
- A history of a URI is common.
- Lethargy is a common presenting symptom.
- Fever may or may not be present; can be a late sign of transmural gangrene and infarction.
- Severe prostration is possible.

Physical Examination
- Observe the infant's appearance and behavior over a period of time; often the child appears glassy-eyed and groggy between episodes, almost as if sedated.
- A sausage-like mass may be felt in the RUQ of the abdomen with emptiness in the RLQ (Dance sign); observe the infant when quiet between spasms.

- The abdomen is often distended and tender to palpation.
- Grossly bloody or guaiac-positive stools.

Diagnostic Studies
- An abdominal flat-plate radiograph can appear normal, especially early in the course and reveal intussusceptions in only about 60% of cases (Fig 40.5). A plain radiograph may show sparse or no intestinal gas or stool in the ascending colon with air-fluid levels and distension in the small bowel only.
- Ultrasound is the diagnostic test of choice for its high sensitivity and specificity, pathology characterization, and lack of ionizing radiation (Edwards et al., 2017). The ultrasound can show the "target sign" and the "pseudo kidney" sign and can also be used to evaluate resolution following air contrast enema.
- An air contrast enema is both diagnostic and a treatment modality.

Differential Diagnosis

The differential diagnosis includes incarcerated hernia, testicular torsion, acute gastroenteritis, appendicitis, colic, and intestinal obstruction.

Management
- Emergency management and consultation with a pediatric radiologist and a pediatric surgeon is recommended.
- Rehydration and stabilization of fluid status; gastric decompression.
- Radiologic reduction using a therapeutic air contrast enema under fluoroscopy is the gold standard.
- Surgery is necessary if perforation, peritonitis, or hypovolemic shock is suspected or radiologic reduction fails.
- IV antibiotics are often administered to cover potential intestinal perforation.
- A period of observation following radiologic reduction is recommended (12 to 18 hours); clear discharge instructions to return with any recurrence of symptoms are required, and close phone follow-up for up to 72 hours is prudent.

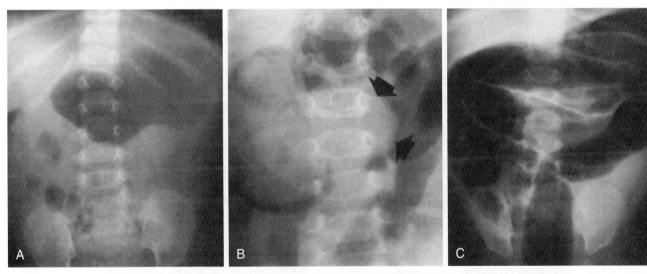

• **Fig 40.5** Intussusception. (A) Plain abdominal radiograph demonstrating a gas-filled stomach and relatively little gas in the distal end of the bowel. This baby had typical clinical features of intussusception and a palpable upper abdominal mass. Therefore, an enema with air was performed. (B) The intussusception *(arrows)* is outlined by air. (C) Reduction is proved by air refluxing into loops of small bowel. (From Burg FD, Ingelfinger JR, Wald ER, eds. *Gellis and Kagan's Current Pediatric Therapy.* 15th ed. Philadelphia: Saunders; 1999.)

Complications

Swelling, hemorrhage, incarceration, and necrosis of the bowel requiring bowel resection may occur. Perforation, sepsis, shock, and re-intussusception (reported to typically be <10%, usually within 72 hours of radiologic reduction but can occur up to 36 months later) can all occur. Recurrence is associated with the lead points described earlier.

Hirschsprung Disease (Congenital Aganglionic Megacolon)

Hirschsprung Disease (HD) is an absence of ganglion cells in the bowel wall, most often in the rectosigmoid region. This results in a portion of the colon having no motility causing functional obstruction. This disorder occurs in 1 in 5000 live births. It is the most common cause of neonatal obstruction of the colon and accounts for approximately 40% of all neonatal obstructions. The disease is familial, affects males four times more commonly than females. There is an increased risk of HD in children with trisomy 21 and several other genetic disorders.

Clinical Findings
- Failure to pass meconium within the first 48 hours of life
- FTT, poor feeding
- Chronic constipation, vomiting, abdominal obstruction
- Diarrhea, explosive bowel movements, or flatus
- Down syndrome

Diagnostic Studies
- Barium enema/unprepped (emptying intestinal contents not required) contrast study
- Anorectal manometry study—A lack of relaxation of the internal anal sphincter with balloon rectal distension suggests HD. Anorectal manometry has a 75% to 95% accuracy in diagnosing HD (Tang, 2014).

Abdominal X-ray—Radiographs indicate dilated loops of bowel. The diagnosis of HD is established by rectal suction biopsy. This will determine the absence of ganglion cells.

Differential Diagnosis. The differential diagnosis includes acquired functional megacolon, colonic inertia, chronic idiopathic constipation, obstipation, small left colon syndrome, meconium plug syndrome, and ileal atresia with microcolon.

Management. Surgical resection of the affected bowel is indicated, with or without a colostomy.

Childhood Functional Abdominal Pain and Functional Abdominal Pain Syndrome

Children who have recurrent abdominal pain with no specific organic etiology are said to have functional abdominal pain (FAP), which is also known as *recurrent abdominal pain* and is often a puzzling problem for providers. FAP is much more common than organic reasons for abdominal pain. The Rome IV criteria are used as the diagnostic standards (Zeevenhooven et al., 2017). These criteria include (Hyams, 2016):
- FAP: The following must occur at least 4 times per month for at least 2 months before diagnosis:
  - Episodic or continuous abdominal pain that does not occur solely during physiologic events (e.g., eating, menses)
  - Insufficient criteria for IBS, functional dyspepsia, or abdominal migraine
  - After appropriate evaluation, the abdominal pain cannot be fully explained by another medical condition

FAP is a fairly common pediatric complaint. The pain is genuine, but its cause remains unclear. There is no evidence of visceral hypersensitivity in the rectum as occurs with IBS. Affected children have an involuntary predisposition for the development of physiologic pain (e.g., a family history of FAP). Temperament and personality can make the child more vulnerable to environmental stressors (often minor) that precipitate the sensation of pain. Children who are perfectionists and have a tendency toward anxiety are more likely to experience FAP. Stress at school, home, with friends, or because of a novel social situation may be associated with FAP symptoms (Bishop and Ebach, 2015). Positive and negative reinforcement can modify the pain.

Approximately 15% to 35% of children worldwide have recurrent abdominal pain with about one-third of those having no specific organic disorder. FAP is the most common pain complaint of preschoolers and accounts for 2% of pediatric visits. The peak incidence of FAP occurs between 7 and 12 years old (Bishop and Ebach, 2015).

Clinical Findings
History
- A complete review of systems
- Parental history of FAP
- A careful psychosocial history (home, school, parents, friends); secondary gains from symptoms and lack of coping skills; endeavor to determine the degree of functional impairment
- Existence of associated symptoms, such as headache, joint pain, anorexia, vomiting, nausea, excessive gas, and altered bowel pattern
- Comorbidity of anxiety and/or depression, behavioral problems, a negative life event
- Identification of red flags (Box 40.6); there is an association between these symptoms and an organic cause to the chronic pain (Bishop and Ebach, 2015)
- Presence of Rome criteria for FAP (see prior description)
- Report of abdominal pain often accompanied by a dramatic reaction (clutching abdomen, doubling over, or throwing self to ground)

• BOX 40.6 Red Flags for Functional Abdominal Pain

Red Flags on History
- Localization of the pain away from the umbilicus, especially right or left upper quadrant
- Pain associated with a change in bowel habits, particularly chronic, severe diarrhea; constipation; or nocturnal bowel movements
- Pain associated with night wakening
- Repetitive, significant emesis, especially if bilious
- Constitutional symptoms, such as recurrent fever, loss of appetite or energy
- Recurrent abdominal pain occurring in a child younger than 4 years old
- Blood in stool or emesis
- Red flags on physical examination
- Unexplained fever
- Unintentional loss of weight or decline in height velocity
- Organomegaly
- Localized abdominal tenderness, particularly removed from the umbilicus
- Perirectal abnormalities (e.g., fissures, ulceration, or skin tags)
- Joint swelling, redness, heat, or discoloration
- Ventral hernias of the abdominal wall

- Determination that symptoms may be worse in the morning, preventing the child from going to school and resulting in school avoidance
- Report that pain medications do not alleviate pain
- Illicit drug use
- Sexual activity or abuse and possibility of pregnancy

Physical Examination. Following initial examination, reexamination should be done during an acute episode and with each subsequent visit. The physical examination is usually normal, but should include:

- Weight, height, and BMI plotted on growth curves
- Vital signs (temperature, heart rate, respiratory rate, blood pressure)
- Abdominal examination: Presence of pain, rebound tenderness, masses
- Perianal and rectal examination
- Complete neurologic examination
- Pelvic examination as indicated
- Examination of skin and joints
- Red flag signs and symptoms (see Box 40.6)

Diagnostic Studies. There are two different approaches the clinician can consider:

- In the move from the Rome III criteria to the new Rome IV criteria, the dictum that there was "no evidence for organic disease" in all definitions was replaced with "after appropriate medical evaluation the symptoms cannot be attributed to another medical condition." Therefore, this change allows for clinicians to opt for either no testing or selective testing as indicated (Hyams et al., 2016). In these situations, testing includes:
  - CBC, ESR, CRP, UA, and urine culture if FAPS is suspected. If indicated, a biochemical profile (liver and kidney function); stool for O&P and culture; and breath hydrogen testing may be useful.
  - Other tests to consider in addition to the above are stool for *H. pylori* antigen and serum IgA, IgG, tissue transglutaminase (TTG) antibody to rule out celiac disease (CD).
  - Ultrasound, endoscopy with or without biopsy, and esophageal pH monitoring as indicated by alarm symptoms.
- After performing a complete history and physical examination, Bishop and Ebach, (2015) suggest the following *initial* approach for ordering diagnostic studies to evaluate FAP:
  - CBC, ESR, amylase, lipase, UA, and abdominal ultrasound (liver, bile ducts, gallbladder, pancreas, kidneys, ureters).
  - A 3-day trial of a lactose-free diet.
  - If results are negative and there are no red flags, further testing is not needed.
  - Fecal calprotectin assay can also be a useful initial test in a child with recurrent abdominal pain and changes in stool habits (Pieczarkowski et al., 2016).

Follow-up evaluation with additional and more invasive GI or other testing should be considered if there are positive results noted in the initial diagnostic testing, symptoms progress, or warning signs develop. These may include such testing as CT, endoscopy, CD serology, and/or colonoscopy.

Differential Diagnosis

There is no evidence that the presence of the associated symptoms, a negative life event, or the presence of anxiety or depression can help distinguish between organic and FAP. Fig 40.6 outlines a decision tree for differential diagnosis of chronic abdominal pain. The following are included in the differential

diagnosis: all organic causes of abdominal pain, including urinary tract, GI tract (IBS, CD, intestinal malformations), and extraabdominal causes; malabsorption syndromes (usually with diarrhea, belching, flatulence, and bloating); lactose intolerance; constipation; small intestine bowel overgrowth (SIBO); abdominal pain associated with depression (usually includes social isolation, decreased activity and attention span, difficulty sleeping, and irritability); and school avoidance (usually associated with severe pain and anxiety on weekday mornings only). Consider SIBO as a diagnosis, which also has dietary interventions in addition to antibiotics.

Management

- Establish a therapeutic parent-child-practitioner relationship to improve patient satisfaction, adherence to treatment, symptom reduction, and other outcomes.
- Explain the brain-gut interaction and that biopsychosocial interventions are the most effective evidence-based treatments of FAP (Chopra et al., 2017).
- Use medications judiciously. H_2 blockers should not be used unless dyspepsia is present.
- Early in the visit, discuss the possibility with the child and parent that the pain can be functional (inorganic). Assure them that the symptoms are real and will be addressed.
- Encourage return to school and normalization of lifestyle. Limit attention given for pain episodes.
- Consider the use of complementary and alternative medicine (CAM) approaches (see Chapter 27). If certain dietary practices seem to cause pain, a blander diet may be helpful (e.g., a lactose-free diet with documented lactose intolerance). Avoiding sorbitol and fructose may be useful if malabsorption is considered a contributing factor. A Cochrane review of dietary interventions concluded that there is moderate-to low-quality evidence suggesting that probiotics may be effective in improving pain in children with recurrent abdominal pain (Newlove-Delgado et al., 2017). A mind-body approach is often useful, combining relaxation, behavioral management, stress coping training, meditation, and biofeedback. Acupuncture, massage, and hypnosis have also been shown to help with chronic abdominal pain.
- Explore psychological triggers and use management strategies for the pain. Discuss how stressful events and emotional issues might affect the pain. Suggest distraction to shift attention from abdominal pain to other activities; attending school is a good distraction. Biofeedback provides evidence to the child that he or she can change muscle tension, skin temperature, and relaxation. Relaxation and guided imagery decrease abdominal pain.
- Identify, treat, and refer for any significant psychological issues. Psychotherapy and family therapy may be of some benefit. Cognitive behavioral therapy has also been helpful for all forms of FAP (Sood and Matta, 2016). Using a biopsychosocial approach is especially helpful for FAP symptoms. Refer for psychological dysfunction (maladaptive behavior, conversion reaction, depression, anxiety).
- Discuss red flag symptoms (see Box 40.6) so that the parents and child can identify changes in status and illness.
- Establish regular follow-up.

Prognosis and Complications

If managed effectively, the prognosis is positive in most cases. Pain resolves completely for 30%-50% of patients within 2

ALGORITHM

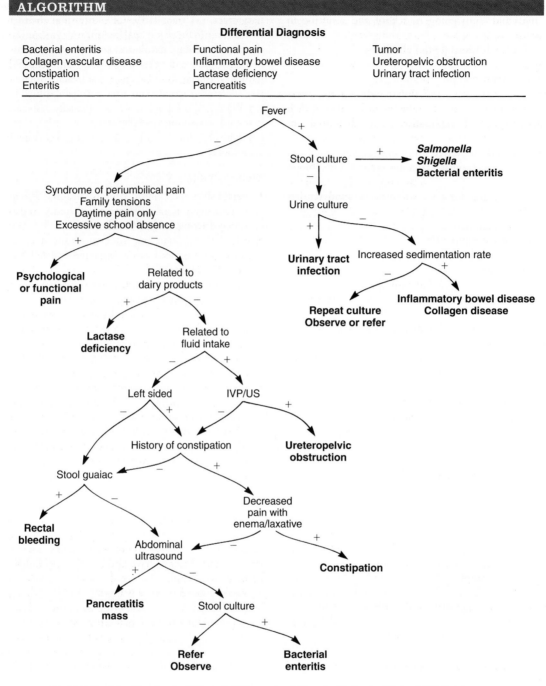

Differential Diagnosis

Bacterial enteritis	Functional pain	Tumor
Collagen vascular disease	Inflammatory bowel disease	Ureteropelvic obstruction
Constipation	Lactase deficiency	Urinary tract infection
Enteritis	Pancreatitis	

• **Fig 40.6** Decision Tree for the Differential Diagnosis of Chronic Abdominal Pain. *IVP/US,* Intravenous pyelogram/ultrasound. (From Schwartz MW, Curry TA, Sargent J, et al., eds. *Pediatric Primary Care: A Problem-Oriented Approach.* 3rd ed. St. Louis: Mosby; 1997.)

to 6 weeks of diagnosis. Parental reassurance and acceptance, and environmental modification play a significant role in this. Poor prognostic indicators include other "painful" associations among family members, male sex, school absence (more than 10 days off school in a year), anxiety disorders, onset under 6 years of age, and the presence of pain before treatment is longer than 6 months. Adults with IBS often recall having had chronic abdominal pain in childhood and are at increased risk of developing FAP, headaches, backaches, and menstrual irregularities as adults (Brown et al., 2016; Chopra et al., 2017).

Irritable Bowel Syndrome

IBS is defined as a chronic condition or FAP with altered bowel habits and bloating that is not explained by structural or biochemical abnormalities (El-Baba, 2016). It is considered a functional GI disorder. The Rome IV criteria for IBS (Hyams et al., 2016) must include *all* the following at least once per week for at least 2 months before diagnosis:

Abdominal pain at least 4 days per month associated with one or more of the following:
- Related to defecation
- A change in frequency of stool

- A change in form (appearance) of stool
- In children with constipation, the pain does not resolve with resolution of the constipation (children in whom the pain resolves have functional constipation not IBS)
- After appropriate evaluation, the symptoms cannot be fully explained by another medical condition.

IBS is the most common cause of FAP in children in the Western world. The exact etiology of IBS remains to be determined. There is some debate on whether it is caused by hereditary or environmental factors. Infection, inflammation, visceral hypersensitivity, allergy, and disordered gut motility may also be involved. There is a strong familial trend, and finding a genetic link is currently being investigated. Psychological comorbidity (somatic symptoms, anxiety, and depression) has also been reported. It is estimated that 10% to 15% of older children and adolescents suffer from IBS (El-Baba, 2016).

Clinical Findings
History
- The Rome criteria symptoms for IBS (see prior description)
- Abnormal stool frequency (four or more stools per day and two or fewer stools per week)
- Abnormal stool form (lumpy/hard or loose/watery or alternating constipation and diarrhea)
- Abnormal stool passage (straining, urgency, or feeling of incomplete evacuation)
- Passage of mucus
- Bloating or feeling of abdominal distention
- Dyspepsia (present in 30% of pediatric patients)
- Potential triggering events and psychosocial factors
- Family history of IBS
- Psychosocial history
- Nutrition history: fiber and water intake, excessive sorbitol or fructose intake

Physical Examination
- Normal physical examination; normal growth curves and BMI
- Absence of alarm signals

Diagnostic Studies. There are no specific laboratory markers for IBS.

Differential Diagnosis
See FAP for differential diagnosis. Consider SIBO.

Management
- Confirm and explain diagnosis.
- The goal is to modify severity of symptoms. Identify and develop strategies to deal with triggering events and psychosocial factors.
- Antidepressants and serotonergic agents have not been widely used in children.

Treatment goals should be to improve the quality of life. This includes ensuring pain is minimized and stool consistency and frequency is normalized. The following therapeutic interventions have been used in children with IBS:

- Dietary interventions (fiber supplement; fermentable oligo-di-monosaccharides and low FODMAP diet and polyol diet) (Schuman et al., 2018). Avoid trigger foods known to exacerbate pain episodes: caffeine; sorbitol; fatty food; large meals; gas-producing foods, such as carbonated beverages, lactose (with lactose intolerance), and cruciferous vegetables.
- Probiotics lactobacillus and bifidobacteria are commonly used.

- Drug therapy (peppermint oil, tegaserod, antispasmodic agents, antidiarrheal agents, antibiotics, and amitriptyline) or selective serotonin reuptake inhibitors (SSRIs) are sometimes used.
- Biopsychosocial therapy for IBS includes hypnotherapy, cognitive behavioral therapy, yoga, and acupuncture.

Malabsorption Syndromes: Celiac Disease, Lactose Intolerance, Cow's-Milk Protein Intolerance or Allergy, Food Protein Immunologic Enterocolitis Syndrome

Malabsorption syndromes can be caused by many different genetic, congenital, and acquired conditions and usually lead to an initial decrease in weight followed by a deceleration in height velocity. This section discusses celiac disease (CD), lactose intolerance, and cow's-milk protein intolerance (CMPI), and food protein immunologic enterocolitis syndrome (FPIES).

CD, also known as gluten-sensitivity enteropathy, is an immune-mediated systemic disorder triggered by dietary exposure to wheat gluten and related proteins in barley and rye. It is characterized by the presence of a variable combination of gluten-dependent clinical manifestations, celiac disease–specific antibodies, HLA-DQ2.5 or HLA-DQ8 haplotypes, and enteropathy. This disease frequently co-occurs with other autoimmune diseases: diabetes mellitus type 1, autoimmune thyroiditis, autoimmune liver disease, IgA nephropathy, and juvenile chronic arthritis (Hill et al., 2016; Shannahan and Leffler, 2017). Many conditions or variables may contribute to the development of CD. It is suggested that demographic changes, such as immigration from developing to developed countries, increase exposure to gluten and an increased incidence of CD follows.

CD is greater among infants born by cesarean section; the development of enteric homeostasis in the newborn period may be altered, increasing susceptibility. CD has a worldwide distribution with overall prevalence of 1%. The most typical presentation occurs between 6 months and 2 years old with a female predominance of 2:1 (Hill et al., 2016). According to Khatib and colleagues (2016), the prevalence of CD is estimated to range between 0.3% and 1.3% among Americans. This has increased during the recent years. The increased recognition of the wide distribution of CD, the low threshold for screening, and improved screening tools has led to diagnosing patients who would not have been diagnosed in the past. The classic clinical features of CD include symptoms such as diarrhea, steatorrhea, weight loss, and growth failure. Nonclassical and symptomatic patients tend to have either some gastrointestinal GI symptoms, such as abdominal pain or constipation, or may have extraintestinal symptoms (Shannahan & and Leffler, 2016).

Lactose intolerance is a clinical syndrome characterized by abdominal pain, diarrhea, nausea, flatulence, and bloating after the ingestion of lactose-containing foods. The symptoms are caused when lactose, a disaccharide (glucose and galactose) found exclusively in mammalian milk, is not absorbed in the gut. It is usually secondary to a deficiency of the lactase enzyme. Increased lactose draws fluid and electrolytes into the intestine, resulting in an osmotic diarrhea. Intestinal bacteria also metabolize excess lactose in the gut, creating methane, carbon dioxide, and hydrogen gases that lead to bloating and flatulence (National Institute of

Diabetes and Digestive and Kidney Diseases ([NIDDK],], 2018). Four types of lactase deficiency have been noted:
- Primary lactase deficiency, also known as lactase nonpersistence, is the most common cause of lactose intolerance. It develops in most children after weaning and at varying ages and is more common in various ethnic groups. The prevalence of primary lactase deficiency has not been established in the United States, although it is found more often in Hispanic, African American, Ashkenazi Jewish, Asian, and Native American populations than in Caucasian European Americans.
- Secondary lactase deficiency results from small bowel injury (e.g., gastroenteritis, chemotherapy, chronic diarrhea) and is more common in infancy.
- Congenital lactase deficiency is an extremely rare congenital absence of lactase, but if it is left untreated, it can be fatal in early infancy.
- Developmental lactase deficiency describes the lactase deficiency that occurs in preterm infants born before 34 weeks because of the immaturity of the intestinal tract.

Cow's milk allergy protein *(CMPI)* and cow's-milk allergy *(CMA)* can have similar clinical pictures; however, the body's immune response differs in each of these conditions. CMPI is a nonallergic hypersensitivity to CMP, whereas CMA is antigen mediated. Most CMA is immunoglobulin E (IgE) mediated, an expression of atopy in which eczema, allergic rhinitis, and/or asthma may also be seen. Some cases of CMA are probably cell-mediated, presenting with primarily GI symptoms (Fiocchi et al., 2018).

CMA typically develops in the neonatal period, peaks in infancy, and tends to remit during childhood. Approximately 2% to 5% of infants have CMA diagnosed by food challenge and elimination diet (Fiocchi et al., 2018). IgE-mediated CMA decreased from about 4% in 2-year-olds to less than 1% in 10-year-olds. Up to 80% of children with CMA develop tolerance within 3 to 4 years of diagnosis.

Food Protein-Induced Enterocolitis Syndrome is inflammation involving the small and large intestine. IgE is a type of antibody formed to protect the body from infections that function in allergic reactions. An IgE mediated reaction is described as one with an immediate hypersensitivity reaction, whereas non-IgE reaction is considered to be a delayed hypersensitivity reaction, which is the case in FPIES.

FPIES is classified as non-IgE–mediated GI food allergy. There are two types of FPIES: acute and chronic. The acute form presents 1 to 6 hours following ingestion of the causative food, while the chronic form (which is less common) is linked to the continuous use of the causative food.

FPIES is commonly seen in infants at the point where they are introduced to formula or solids. For those who are exclusively breast fed, it can present at a later stage. The most common FPIES triggers are cow's milk (dairy) and soy proteins. Rice and oats (grains) are also common triggers; however, other foods can also elicit FPIES reactions (Nowak-Wegrzyn et al., 2017).

The typical pattern of symptoms presents in a healthy infant usually within hours of ingestion. This is often characterized by a delay of 1 to 4 hours before onset of severe and repetitive vomiting and diarrhea (may not always be present until later stage in some cases). This subsequently leads to:
- Lethargy
- Unhealthy pale appearance
- Poor growth, FTT (in cases of recurrent acute reactions where there is prolonged use of causative food)

- Dehydration
- Hypotension
- Nutrient deficiencies

Diagnostic Studies. There is often a delayed diagnosis with FPIES, or more commonly, it is misdiagnosed, particularly because of the presenting symptoms which are nonspecific and a lack of definitive diagnostic biomarkers. It is often confused with sepsis, metabolic disease, and acute/severe gastroenteritis.

Diagnosis is based on clinical history, symptoms and timing, exclusion of other causes, and ultimately symptom improvement with avoidance of the offending food. Definitive diagnosis is often achieved through oral food challenge (OFC) done under supervision of a physician or suitable qualified clinician. In some cases, where the clinical history includes numerous episodes of typical symptoms, a food challenge is not necessary to confirm a diagnosis.

Management and Prognosis. Early recognition of FPIES is necessary to deter recurrent acute episodes, thus avoiding further complications related to the syndrome, particularly nutritional deficiencies.
- Initial management: first line of intervention is fluid replacement if profuse vomiting is present leading to dehydration. This starts with oral hydration, and if necessary IV fluids. Removal of and continuous elimination of the causative food from the diet is necessary. Introduce new food one at a time to observe for any reactions.
- Long term management: this care involves dietary monitoring, with a goal of possible resolution for the allergy. Monitor for nutritional deficiencies and provide supplements where necessary, and ultimately develop care plans on how to deal with episodes.

Prognosis is usually good, with a large percentage of the population having resolution of their reactions after many years. This is usually determined by an OFC under supervision of a physician. However, a small percentage of the population goes on to develop IgE-mediated food allergy (Michelet et al., 2017).

Clinical Findings

General History for Malabsorption Syndromes. Careful medical and family medical histories are important in the evaluation of a malabsorption syndrome and are often the key to the diagnosis. In addition, a complete dietary history is needed to distinguish between undernutrition and malabsorption. Significant historical findings include:
- Past surgical and trauma history
- Growth failure (a common symptom of nutritional deficiency and malabsorption)
- Delayed puberty can coexist with malabsorption.
- A voracious appetite or particular food avoidance is present in small children with malabsorption syndromes.
- Chronic diarrhea with frequent, large, foul-smelling, pale stools
- Excessive flatus with abdominal distention
- Pallor, fatigue, hair and dermatologic abnormalities, digital clubbing, dizziness, cheilosis, glossitis, peripheral neuropathy (symptoms of vitamin deficiency seen with malabsorption)

Disease-Specific History. In addition to the list in the earlier section, the following may stand out.

Celiac Disease
- Chronic or intermittent diarrhea, persistent or unexplained GI symptoms (e.g., nausea and vomiting), sudden or unexpected weight loss, and prolonged fatigue

Lactose Intolerance
- Abdominal pain, diarrhea, nausea, flatulence, and bloating often related to the amount of lactose ingested

Cow's-Milk Protein Intolerance and Cow's-Milk Allergy
- Family history of allergy and/or atopy

General Physical Examination
- Growth parameters and percentiles (weight, height, BMI, head circumference)
- Skinfold thickness and lean body mass
- Examination for delayed growth and puberty, including Tanner staging

Disease-Specific Physical Examination

Celiac Disease
- Impaired growth, FTT, unexplained iron deficiency anemia, abdominal distention, bloating or cramping pain
- May have no symptoms at all despite evidence of small bowel changes; maintain a high suspicion for CD in children with metabolic bone disease (such as rickets or osteomalacia), low-trauma fractures, or those with dental enamel defects. An estimated 85% to 90% of individuals with CD are undiagnosed.

Lactose Intolerance
- Abdominal distention

Cow's-Milk Protein Intolerance and Cow's-Milk Allergy. Symptoms may be immediate or late onset (Fiocchi etal,et al., 2018):
- Immediate
  - Anaphylaxis (rare) but can be life threatening
  - GI: Lip or tongue swelling, oral pruritus, nausea, vomiting
  - Skin: Urticaria, rash, flushing, angioedema
  - Respiratory: Nasal pruritus, sneezing, rhinitis, congestion, wheezing, dyspnea, chest tightness
- Late onset (1 hour to several days after ingestion of CMP)
  - Typically, non–IgE-mediated allergic reaction
  - Symptoms are mostly GI: Varied, including nausea, vomiting, abdominal pain, diarrhea, bloody stool, GERD-like symptoms, pyloric stenosis, malabsorption, FTT, IBD
  - Can see urticarial rash (with both IgE- and non–IgE-mediated allergy); eczema
  - Respiratory: Heiner syndrome is very rare

Diagnostic Studies
- Stool assessment for occult blood, WBCs, and culture; liquid stool for pH and reducing substances; 72-hour fecal fat collection or Sudan stain for stool fat
- Spot stool testing for α1-antitrypsin level to establish the diagnosis of protein-losing enteropathy
- Sweat chloride test (in the presence of steatorrhea to evaluate for CF)
- Stool for O&P: Giardiasis is a common intestinal infection causing malabsorption. See later discussion for symptoms suggestive of infestation.
- CBC with differential, mean corpuscular hemoglobin concentration (MCHC), iron, folic acid, and ferritin
- Serum calcium, phosphorus, magnesium, alkaline phosphatase, serum protein, liver function tests, vitamin D and its metabolites, vitamins A, B_{12}, E, and K
- Human immunodeficiency virus (HIV) testing (for symptoms of FTT and chronic diarrhea)
- Small bowel biopsy helps identify diseases of the small bowel mucosa and obtains material for culture and sensitivity
- Plain abdominal radiographs and barium contrast studies as indicated

- Abdominal ultrasound can detect masses and stones in the hepatobiliary system
- Retrograde studies of the pancreas and biliary tree if indicated
- Bone age

Specific Tests for Celiac Disease
- Serologic testing should be done if there is clinical suspicion of CD, the child has an associated disorder, or there is a first-degree relative with CD. Gluten should be eaten in more than one meal every day for 6 weeks prior to testing. Recommended serologic tests include IgA tissue transglutaminase antibody (tTGA) and IgA endomysial antibody (EMA) because of their high sensitivity and specificity. EMA is more expensive and less accurate in children younger than 2 years old (Leonardt et al., 2017).
- Home blood testing is not recommended.
- If serologic testing is positive, refer for endoscopy with biopsy for a definitive diagnosis, although colonoscopy may not be necessary if the tTGA level is greater than 100 units/mL (Shannahan and Leffler, 2017).
- Careful follow-up of growth parameters, tTGA testing after 6 months of gluten-free diet (GFD), and then yearly (Shannahan and Leffler, 2017).
- Bone density testing (bone problems may be first symptom of CD).

Specific Tests for Lactose Intolerance
- Lactose hydrogen breath test is the gold standard. Children should not be taking antibiotics at the time of the study, because the intestinal bacteria that act on lactose may be diminished.
- Trial of a lactose-free diet for 2 weeks, being aware of hidden sources of lactose. Symptoms should disappear with the diet and reappear when lactose is reintroduced.
- Bone density if calcium deficiency is suspected (lactose is necessary for calcium absorption into bone, and lactose-free diets can predispose to osteoporosis).
- If secondary cause of lactose intolerance is suspected, continue workup for all other causes of malabsorption.

Cow's-Milk Protein Intolerance and Cow's-Milk Allergy
- Elimination diet followed by a double-blind placebo-controlled OFC.
- Skin patch test for allergies may be performed.
- Serum IgE antibodies testing may be performed.
- Diagnosis of CMPI is made when there is clinical improvement on CMP-free diet.

Differential Diagnosis
Organic and nonorganic FTT, colic, short stature, chronic diarrhea, CF, immunodeficiency, cholestatic liver disease, GERD, SIBO, and IBD are included in the differential diagnoses.

Management

Celiac Disease
- A strict GFD for life is currently the only effective treatment for CD. The standard for being gluten-free is a limit of 10 mg of gluten (Shannahan and Leffler, 2017).
- Alternative treatments are being explored, including enzyme therapy, developing genetically engineered grains, inhibiting tTGA in the intestine, and correcting intestinal barrier defects (particularly increased permeability).

Lactose Intolerance
- Test to ensure that the individual actually has lactose intolerance.
- Reduce exposure to lactose:
  - Avoid lactose-containing milk and other dairy products, including goat's milk.
  - Use lactose-free dairy products (e.g., milk pre-hydrolyzed with lactase).
  - Use alternate milk sources (soy, rice, and so on).
- Use oral lactase supplements.
- Ensure adequate intake of calcium and vitamin D from other food products.
- Most individuals with primary lactase deficiency can ingest dairy products in small to moderate amounts, especially if taken with other foods.

Cow's-Milk Protein Intolerance and Cow's-Milk Allergy. Take the following precautions for infants and young children (Fiocchi et al., 2018):
- Breastfeed.
- Restrict milk and milk products from the diet of breastfeeding mothers.
- If formula fed, use extensively hydrolyzed formula initially. Partially hydrolyzed formula is *not* appropriate for infants with CMA.
- Use amino-acid formula for infants who demonstrate severe allergy (e.g., prior history of anaphylaxis) or who do not respond to extensively hydrolyzed formula.
- Extensively hydrolyzed soy formula is appropriate for infants after 6 months old only; before 6 months old, infants fed soy formula are at risk for nutritional deficit.
- Avoid use of other mammals' milk (e.g., sheep, goat, camel) due to risk of cross-allergic reaction.
- After 2 years old, formula is not appropriate, but ensure daily dietary intake of 600 to 800 mg of calcium.
- Probiotics may be helpful in creating tolerance, but more clinical research is needed.
- Have EpiPen if anaphylaxis is a concern.
- Monitor growth and development carefully.
- Refer to an allergist or gastroenterologist if symptoms are severe; immunotherapy is not recommended.
- Annual reevaluation of sensitivity, preferably an OFC under medical supervision.

Complications and Prognosis

Celiac Disease. Growth failure is the primary complication of CD. With delayed diagnosis or inadequate treatment, there is risk for fractures and osteoporosis (due to reduced bone mineral density), lymphoma, autoimmune diseases (e.g., type 1 diabetes, thyroid disorders), primary biliary cirrhosis, and primary sclerosing cholangitis. Sensory peripheral neuropathy may be related to gluten sensitivity (Zis et al., 2017). Celiac crisis consisting of abdominal distention, explosive watery diarrhea, dehydration with hypoproteinemia, electrolyte imbalance, hypotensive shock, and lethargy, although rare, can be the first indication of CD. Prognosis is improved with lifelong GFD.

Lactose Intolerance. Unabsorbed lactose does not cause clinical intestinal damage despite clinical symptoms. Bone density loss may occur if there is inadequate calcium and vitamin D. Other conditions misdiagnosed as lactose intolerance may worsen.

Cow's-Milk Protein Intolerance and Cow's-Milk Allergy. CMPI usually resolves by 1 to 3 years old; when there are only GI symptoms, CMPI resolves completely. CMA cannot be reversed, and there is a high likelihood of other food allergies. Complications include rickets, poor growth, and FTT.

Rectal and Intestinal Polyps

Intestinal polyps in children may be benign or present a risk for subsequent cancer or other conditions (e.g., anemia). *Solitary polyps,* often called *juvenile polyps,* are the most frequently seen (90%) polyps in children. They are most often found in preschool-age children (4 to 5 years old), are usually located in the rectosigmoid area, have an incidence of about 2% in children younger than 10 years old, and are considered to present negligible or no risk for malignancy. Polyps are also found in familial adenomatous polyposis, juvenile polyposis syndrome (JPS), phosphatase and tensin homolog (PTEN) hamartoma tumor syndrome, and Peutz-Jeghers syndrome (PJS), all of which are autosomal dominant conditions with variable penetrance.

Clinical Findings

History
- May be asymptomatic. A careful family history is imperative to identify children at risk for polyposis.
- Painless, bright red rectal bleeding (hematochezia). Usually the blood coats or is mixed in with the stool. Bleeding can be daily, intermittent, or infrequent. Large volume blood loss is extremely rare.
- Familial adenomatous polyposis: Nonspecific complaints, diarrhea, constipation, or changes in bowel habits.

Physical Examination
- Anorectal examination to find polyp or other source of rectal bleeding
- Pallor and edema caused by anemia and hypoproteinemia from GI hemorrhage and protein-losing enteropathy indicate a heavy polyp burden
- Extraintestinal symptoms of familial adenomatous polyposis include ophthalmologic changes (may see hypertrophy of retinal pigment); dental anomalies (supernumerary or unerupted teeth); osteomas of skull, jaw, or extremities; and multiple lipomas

Diagnostic Studies
- CBC with differential and ESR, CRP, prothrombin time, and partial thromboplastin time
- Fecal occult blood test, even if blood appears to be present
- Stool culture for bacterial pathogens and O&P
- Colonoscopy to the terminal ileum with biopsy evaluation is the diagnostic test of choice
- Upper endoscopy if there is concern for gastric or duodenal polyps; small-bowel video capsule endoscopy may be used
- Barium contrast of upper intestine

Management
- Refer to a pediatric gastroenterologist for management and follow-up screening.
- Treatment involves resection of the polyp(s), usually with diagnostic or surveillance screening. If multiple polyps are present, bowel resection (colectomy) is common. For familial adenomatous polyposis, colectomy is standard therapy.
- Children with one or two juvenile colonic polyps at diagnosis usually need no further follow-up.
- Follow-up is required if:
  - There is a family history of polyps (i.e., all children are at risk for polyposis).
  - The child has three or more polyps on colonoscopy.

- Polyps are found outside the colon.
- Extraintestinal symptoms are present.
- Follow-up varies by condition, severity, and pediatric specialist provider. Genetic testing to determine presence of gene mutation is usually done at 8 to 10 years old.
- Ophthalmologic evaluation may be recommended.
- Genetic counseling may be recommended.

Complications

Children with polyps are at risk for colorectal, gastric, duodenal, pancreatic, and extraintestinal cancer as adults (usually appearing in the fourth decade of life or later). Psychological issues related to having a hereditary condition with uncertain long-term outcomes (i.e., high risk for malignancies) can cause family problems.

Anal Fissure

Anal fissures are small tears in the anal mucosa. The usual cause of an anal fissure is passage of frequent or hard stools. Anal stenosis and other trauma can also be causative factors. Anal fissures are the most common cause of rectal bleeding in all pediatric groups.

Clinical Findings

History
- Crying with bowel movement
- Bright red streaks of blood in the stool or diaper
- Withholding of stool

Physical Examination. With the patient in the knee-chest position and the anus slightly everted, small tears in the anal mucosa can be visible. An otoscope with a large speculum is needed if the external fissures are not readily visible. A digital anal examination with the fifth finger rules out anal stenosis.

Differential Diagnosis

Other sources of lower intestinal hemorrhage, such as infection, formula intolerance, necrotizing enterocolitis, intussusception, juvenile polyps, hemolytic-uremic syndrome, Henoch-Schönlein purpura, irritable bowel disease, and vascular lesions are included in the differential diagnosis. Sexual abuse should be considered in children with large, irregular, or multiple fissures.

Management
- Treat the constipation.
- Local wound care should include sitz baths twice a day and application of 0.5% hydrocortisone cream or K-Y jelly to the anus.

Complications

Recurrence is common. Constipation causes a fissure, which leads to a stool withholding-encopresis–painful stooling cycle.

Patient and Family Education

Preventive measures include avoiding constipation, encouraging regular toileting habits, and avoiding the use of laxatives and enemas.

Inflammatory Bowel Disease

IBD is thought to be a dysregulated immune response of intestinal mucosa to microbes in genetically susceptible individuals. Defects may be present in both the barrier function of intestinal epithelium and the immune system. Three primary types of IBD are recognized: (1) (CDC, 2017) Crohn disease, (2) ulcerative colitis, and (3) unclassified IBD. See Table 40.8 for features contrasting Crohn disease and ulcerative colitis. Symptoms of IBD in children can be difficult to interpret and a definitive diagnosis between Crohn disease and ulcerative

TABLE 40.8 Features of Crohn Disease and Ulcerative Colitis

Feature	Crohn Disease	Ulcerative Colitis
Age at onset	10-20 years old	10-20 years old
Area of bowel affected	Can affect any part of the GI system; often in terminal ileum or colon; may be small bowel only; small bowel and cecum; small bowel and colon; or colon only; occasionally isolated perianal disease	Affects colon and rectum; entire colon may be inflamed (pancolitis); may have subtotal colitis or "ileal backwash" (i.e., superficial inflammation of ileum proximal to splenic flexure); may be left-sided (distal to splenic flexure); may have proctitis (limited to rectum or distal 15 cm)
Distribution	Segmental; disease-free "skip" areas common	Continuous distal to proximal
Endoscopic, radiographic, or biopsy findings	Noncaseating granulomas located in the inflamed mucosa; cobblestone appearance of bowel wall; linear/serpiginous ulcers and transverse fissures; fixation and separation of loops; small bowel strictures/stenoses; bowel or perianal fistulas; perianal abscesses or large (>5 mm) skin tags	Superficial inflammation of mucosa; friable tissue with exudates and granularity; loss of vascular pattern; small perianal skin tags (<5 mm)
Intestinal symptoms	Abdominal pain, diarrhea, anorexia, weight loss	Abdominal pain with or around time of stooling, bloody diarrhea, urgency, and tenesmus
Extraintestinal manifestations: Seen more often in Crohn disease than ulcerative colitis; similar types for both conditions	Ophthalmologic conditions (uveitis, iritis, conjunctivitis) more likely in Crohn disease	Primary sclerosing cholangitis more likely in ulcerative colitis

GI, Gastrointestinal.

Data from da Silva B, Lyra A, Rocha R, et al. Epidemiology, demographic characteristics and prognostic predictors of ulcerative colitis. *World J Gastroenterol.* 2014;20(28):9458–9467; Day AS, Ledder O, Leach ST, et al. Crohn and colitis in children and adolescents. *World J Gastroenterol.* 2012;18(41):5862–5869; and Dotson JL, Hyams JS, Markowitz J, et al. Extraintestinal manifestations of pediatric inflammatory bowel disease and their relation to disease type and severity. *J Pediatr Gastroenterol Nutr.* 2010;51(2):140–145.

colitis may be elusive, especially in early, active disease. Numerous contacts with healthcare providers may be necessary to establish a diagnosis, and the initial diagnosis may change as the disease progresses (da Silva et al., 2014). Several indices are used to assess and classify IBD. The Pediatric Ulcerative Colitis Activity Index (PUCAI) is widely used for children. The scoring index defines severe disease with a score of at least 65 points. The PUCAI yields a range of scores that can also be used to monitor disease severity and treatment progress (Siow, Bhat, and Mollen, 2017). The Montreal classification of IBD was developed to accurately classify the phenotype (physical characteristics) of all subtypes of IBD, including disease location or extent, behavior, and age of onset. This classification includes features at diagnosis and during disease evolution over time not covered in the previous Vienna classification (Wilson and Russell, 2017).

The incidence of IBD appears to be increasing worldwide, especially the incidence of Crohn disease and pediatric-onset IBD (Wilson and Russell, 2017). IBD can occur at any age, with a peak onset between 15 and 30 years. Up to 25% of cases are in children and adolescents, and 4% are found in children younger than 5 years old. IBD in infants is extremely rare. In contrast to adults, children diagnosed with IBD are more likely to have Crohn disease than ulcerative colitis, to have more severe or extensive disease (both Crohn disease and ulcerative colitis), more vague symptoms, more extraintestinal symptoms (e.g., arthralgia), and more relapses (Sairenji et al., 2017).

Crohn Disease

Crohn disease is a chronic disease with dysregulated inflammation and cytokine production in the intestinal tract. Any part of the GI tract can be involved, although the terminal ileum and colon are most commonly affected. Inflammation is usually transmural, affecting the entire wall of the intestine, creating fissures and fistulas. Unaffected areas of intestine are called *skip areas.*

The exact cause is unknown, although it is likely due to environmental exposure that triggers an abnormal immune reaction in a genetically susceptible individual. Crohn disease peaks in late adolescence and early adulthood, then again in middle adulthood (50 to 70 years); 25% to 40% of cases are diagnosed in childhood and adolescence. The incidence and prevalence of esophageal Crohn disease in children ranges from 7.6% to 17.6%. It is more common in Caucasians, and males and females are affected about equally. Siblings are more likely to have Crohn disease than is the general population. Approximately 10% to 15% of cases are re-diagnosed as ulcerative colitis within the first year of illness (da Silva et al., 2014).

Clinical Findings

History
- Fever, usually low grade, of unknown etiology
- Weight loss (average of 5 to 7 kg)
- Delayed growth velocity, short stature, delayed bone age
- Arthralgias and/or arthritis in large joints, occasional joint destruction
- Obstructive symptoms associated with meals, bloating, early satiety
- Pain in the umbilical region and RLQ; may awaken at night
- Anorexia
- Malabsorption and lactose intolerance

- Diarrhea (with or without blood or mucus) and pain with stooling
- Jaundice
- Oral aphthous ulcers, especially during exacerbations of the illness
- Use of tobacco
- Positive family history

Physical Examination
- Carefully measure growth parameters (height, weight, and BMI).
- Perform an abdominal examination while observing for RLQ tenderness and a mass.
- Perianal skin tags, deep anal fissures, and perianal fistulas strongly suggest Crohn disease.
- Clubbing of digits (due to mucosal inflammatory change and fibrosis and/or platelets are sensitive in the microvasculature and release platelet-released growth factor).
- Erythema nodosum is common.

Diagnostic Studies. The following are ordered as needed:
- Inflammatory markers: ESR, CRP
- Nutritional labs: Albumin, total protein (consider iron panel, calcium, zinc, alkaline phosphatase, folate, vitamin B_{12})
- Other blood tests: CBC with differential (consider liver enzymes—aspartate aminotransferase [AST], alanine amino transferase [ALT], total bilirubin, γ-glutamyltransferase [GGT]; amylase; lipase)
- Stool: Routine culture, O&P, *C. difficile* (with recent antibiotic use), blood, WBCs, and fecal α1-antitrypsin; fecal calprotectin assay (appropriate initial test in a child with recurrent abdominal pain and changes in stool habits) (Hejl et al., 2017).
- Radiologic studies: Bone age (usually delayed by 2 years), bone density, abdominal plain films, upper GI series with small bowel follow-through, abdominal CT with contrast
- Ileocolonoscopy is a first step to assess for Crohn disease. Other endoscopic studies include small bowel capsule endoscopy (SBCE), push enteroscopy, single- or double-balloon enteroscopy, inter-operative enteroscopy or spiral enteroscopy. Esophageal endoscopy is recommended in children diagnosed with Crohn disease who have perianal disease. (De Felice et al., 2016).
- Screen for tuberculosis (TB) if child is at risk (see Chapter 31 for risk criteria). Biologic agents used in Crohn disease therapy can activate latent TB.

Differential Diagnosis

Rheumatoid arthritis, systemic lupus erythematosus, hypopituitarism, acute appendicitis, peptic ulcer, intestinal obstruction, intestinal lymphoma, anorexia, chronic granulomatous disease, sarcoidosis, and growth failure are included in the differential diagnosis.

Management

The goals of therapy are to (1) control the disease; (2) prevent relapses; and (3) achieve normal nutrition, growth, and lifestyle. Treatment is pharmacologic, nutritional, surgical, and psychosocial. The following management steps are taken:
- Refer to a pediatric gastroenterologist for colonoscopy, endoscopy, more definitive diagnosis, consultation, and follow-up care.
- In the United States, corticosteroid management is most common. In Europe, exclusive enteral nutrition (EEN) had been

used as first-line therapy. Currently, it is indicated for patients who are malnourished or at risk of becoming malnourished and who have an inadequate or limited oral intake (Lane, Lee, and Suskind, 2017).

- Medications:
  - Corticosteroids (e.g., prednisone, budesonide) are used orally, rectally, or intravenously for acute inflammation of mild to moderate disease. They are not intended for use in remission.
  - 5-aminosalicylates (balsalazide, sulfasalazine, olsalazine, and mesalamine) are used orally or rectally for mild disease to control inflammation.
  - Immunomodulator agents are used (azathioprine, 6-mercaptopurine, methotrexate, and cyclosporine) for severe small or large bowel disease, steroid-dependent or refractory disease, severe fistula, and growth failure.
  - Biologic agents (e.g., infliximab, a chimeric, anti-tumor necrosis factor α [anti-TNF-α] antibody) for steroid-dependent or refractory disease, perirectal fistula, and maintenance of remission, can be given alone or in combination with immunomodulators. One IV infusion of infliximab has been shown to induce remission in Crohn disease. Greater mucosal healing follows treatment with immunomodulators and biologic agents than with corticosteroids and improved growth is seen with early anti-TNF-α treatment (Jeuring et al., 2016).
  - Antibiotics are used for acute infections (ampicillin, gentamicin, clindamycin, ciprofloxacin, or metronidazole).
  - Adjunctive therapy, including growth hormone prior to or at the time of puberty, enhances optimal growth (Altowati et al., 2016).
- Severe disease can require hospitalization, total parenteral nutrition, a nasogastric tube for decompression, or surgery. Despite the availability of new therapeutic agents, surgery may still be required for patients with refractory disease, or for those who are intolerant of medication side effects. With pediatric patients, poor growth, unresponsive to medical therapy, may also be an indication for surgery. A recent systematic review determined that cumulative rates of surgery among pediatric Crohn disease ranged from 10% to 72% (Stokes et al., 2017; Rinawi et al., 2016).
- Monitor growth and pubertal changes.
- An ophthalmologic examination is needed to rule out underlying ophthalmologic manifestations of the disease.
- Refer for nutritional counseling during remission, to prevent or correct malnutrition, and to maintain and promote growth. See Chapter 17 for specific nutritional recommendations.
- Encourage participation in social activities, such as support and fitness groups (e.g., Team Challenge, a fund-raising running event for Crohn disease and colitis), and Crohn disease camps. Refer for psychosocial and family therapy as indicated.

Complications

Intestinal obstruction with scarring and strictures is the major complication of Crohn disease. Growth failure (especially linear growth) is extremely common. Fistula and abscesses can occur; however, perforation and hemorrhage are rare. Primary sclerosing cholangitis, pancreatitis, pericarditis, arthritis, and peripheral neuropathy are other complications of Crohn disease (Martin-de-Carpi et al., 2017; Stenke et al., 2017). Treatment with corticosteroids or immunosuppressive drugs increases the risk for opportunistic infections and inadequate response to immunizations (Nguyen

et al., 2017). Care must be taken with long-term use of biologics in children because of the risk of infection or malignancy. The child and family are at risk for social functioning difficulties, anxiety, depression, somatization disorders, and school difficulties.

Prevention and Prognosis

Follow recommended therapy to prevent sequelae. Crohn disease is progressive and without cure, although about 55% of individuals are in remission at any one time and only about 1% of individuals experience continuous active disease. Child-onset disease tends to be more severe and requires more immunosuppressive treatment than adult-onset disease (Rinawi et al., 2016).

Ulcerative Colitis

Ulcerative colitis is a chronic disease that is characterized by diffuse inflammation of the rectal and colonic mucosa. Ulcerative colitis involves the rectum in 95% of cases and may be extended continuously and circumferentially to more proximal parts of the large intestine (da Silva et al., 2014). Pediatric patients, especially those younger than 10 years old, may appear to have no lesions in the rectum, and can lead to a misdiagnosis of Crohn disease.

The cause is unknown, but the disease has a multifactorial basis (i.e., heredity, diet, environment, immunologic alterations, and ineffective mucosal integrity). The annual incidence rate in the United States is 10 to 12 cases per 100,000, and the overall prevalence rate is 37 to 238 cases per 100,000 individuals. The incidence of ulcerative colitis has increased worldwide over recent decades, especially in developing nations. Although ulcerative colitis is less common in children, recent studies have shown that the number of cases has increased in children and adolescents (da Silva et al., 2014).

Clinical Findings

History
- Fever
- Weight loss (average of 4 kg)
- Delayed growth and sexual maturation
- Arthritis and/or arthralgias of the large joints
- Anorexia
- Diarrhea
- Lower abdominal cramping, left lower quadrant pain
- Pain increased before stooling and passing flatus
- Stool with bright red blood and mucus
- Nocturnal stooling
- Oral aphthous ulcers
- Skin lesions (erythema nodosum, pyoderma gangrenosum, and diffuse papulonecrotic eruptions)

Physical Examination
- Carefully measure growth parameters (weight, height, and BMI) and perform a complete physical examination. Abdominal examination can reveal rebound tenderness if the disease is severe.

Diagnostic Studies
- CBC with differential, iron-binding capacity, total protein, albumin, ESR, and CRP
- Stool for WBCs, blood, and culture (bloody diarrhea with negative stool culture characteristic of ulcerative colitis)
- Bone age (usually delayed up to 2 years)
- Colonoscopy (diffuse mucosal inflammation)
- Perinuclear neutrophil cytoplasmic antigen (positive in 60% to 70% of cases)
- Fecal calprotectin assay (Moen et al., 2017)

Differential Diagnosis

Shigella, Salmonella, Yersinia, Campylobacter, E. coli, C. difficile, IBS, self-limited colitis, and Crohn disease are in the differential diagnosis.

Management

The goals of therapy are to (1) control the disease; (2) prevent relapses; and (3) achieve normal nutrition, growth, and lifestyle. Treatment is pharmacologic, nutritional, surgical, and psychosocial. Management involves the following:

- Refer for colonoscopy, biopsy, definitive diagnosis, consultation, and close follow-up care.
- Pharmacologic treatment options: Treatment for ulcerative colitis can become quite complex and requires an individualized approach. Patients with mild-to-moderate disease can usually be managed in the outpatient setting, whereas severe ulcerative colitis warrants inpatient care.
  - Mild to moderate ulcerative colitis: Topical mesalamine, oral 5-aminosalicylates, or topical steroids with topical mesalamine as a superior first-line agent.
  - Moderate-to-severe ulcerative colitis: Systemic steroids, Systemic steroids for 1 to 2 weeks until clinical response is established followed by a slow taper off of the steroid.
  - Thiopurines: Azathioprine and 6-mercaptopurine have limited utility in the acute setting. Adverse effects include fever, rash, nausea, diarrhea, arthralgia, thrombocytopenia, leukopenia, infection, pancreatitis, hepatitis, non-Hodgkin lymphoma, and hepatosplenic T-cell lymphoma.
  - Biologic agents (infliximab, adalimumab, golimumab) for induction of remission and maintenance in steroid-refractory and moderate to severe disease
  - Hydrocortisone rectal preparation for tenesmus.
  - Cyclosporine monotherapy is as effective as or more effective than corticosteroids for initial treatment of fulminating disease.
  - Probiotics (e.g., VSL#3, *Saccharomyces boulardii*) may provide benefits when used with other therapies in mild to moderately active disease.
  - Curcumin (active ingredient in turmeric) may assist in maintaining inactive disease.
  - Iron supplementation to correct anemia; multivitamin.
- Nutrition (see Chapter 17 for nutritional recommendations):
  - Diet: High in protein and carbohydrates, normal amount of fat, and decreased roughage. Omega-3 fatty acids (in contrast to omega-6 fatty acids) have an anti-inflammatory effect on the bowel, though there is not enough evidence currently to recommend their use for treatment of ulcerative colitis (Lewis and Abreu, 2017).
  - Lactose is poorly tolerated.
  - Parenteral or enteral nutritional supplements (60 to 70 cal/kg/day) may be used.
  - Refer for nutritional therapy to prevent or correct malnutrition and maintain and promote growth.
- Monitor growth.
- Surgery may be indicated (complete proctocolectomy with permanent ileostomy is curative).
- Refer for ophthalmologic examination to rule out ophthalmologic manifestations of the disease.
- Refer for psychosocial therapy as indicated. Depressive disorders are common.

- Assess immunization status and ensure child is up to date; there is controversy regarding immunizing with live vaccines (e.g., varicella) (Nguyen et al., 2017; Reich et al., 2017).

Complications

Complications can include growth failure, toxic megacolon, intestinal perforation, liver disease, sepsis, cancer of the colon (a long-term sequela—1% to 2% per year after 10 years of disease), arthritis, uveitis, malnutrition, as well as behavioral and emotional problems similar to those of children with CD.

Prevention and Prognosis

Follow the recommended therapy to optimize remission, maintain inactive disease state, and prevent complications. Prognosis is good for patients with mild disease and those who respond quickly to initial therapy. Those with untreated or poorly treated disease are at increased risk for colectomy and colon cancer. In one study of children who had colectomy, 73% reported pouchitis (inflammation of the ileal pouch), and 56% required a second surgery, but overall quality of life, BMI, and number of offspring were equal to that of control subjects (da Silva et al., 2014).

Failure to Thrive

FTT is a broad term referring to a symptom of a lack of weight gain proportional to age as determined by standardized growth charts. The diagnosis is based on a child's weight but the definition varies in the literature. It is also called *growth deficiency, growth delay, protein energy malnutrition, faltering weight,* and *faltering growth.* FTT should be considered if any of the criteria in Box 40.7 are found. The pathway to FTT is based on interventions needed to impact the complex system of biological, psychosocial, and environmental factors contributing to a child's growth and development. FTT has three basic causes: (1) inadequate caloric intake, (2) inadequate caloric absorption, and (3) excessive caloric expenditure. The most common cause is nutritional deficiency without an underlying medical condition (greater than 80%). Generally, the prevalence rates are thought to be around 5% to 10% in the United States. Children living in poverty and/or from developing countries with higher rates of malnutrition and/or HIV infection are more likely to have FTT. Rates may be increasing, because more preterm infants are surviving (Larson-Nath et al., 2016).

Onset between 2 weeks and 4 months is more often associated with congenital disorders, serious somatic illness, and with deviant mother-infant interactions. Onset between 4 and 8 months in otherwise healthy children is more clearly associated with feeding

---

• BOX 40.7 Criteria that Define Failure to Thrive

- Weight less than 80% of median weight for length
- Weight for length less than 80% of ideal weight
- Weight for length less than the 10th percentile
- Body mass index (BMI) for chronologic age less than 5th percentile
- Weight for chronologic age and sex less than 5th percentile or more than two standard deviations below the mean
- Length for chronologic age and sex less than 5th percentile
- Weight deceleration crossing more than two major percentile lines on age and population appropriate growth chart
- Height, head circumference, and developmental skills may be affected

problems. In chronic cases, weight for height may appear to be normal because of concurrent reductions in velocity.

Clinical Findings and Risk Factors

Clinical findings include poor weight gain associated with poor intake, vomiting, food refusal, food fixation, abnormal feeding practices, presence of anticipatory gagging, irritability, chronic physical problems in any body system, or psychosocial problems. Inborn errors of metabolism should be suspected with history of acute, severe, and potentially life-threatening symptoms, liver dysfunction, recurrent vomiting, neurologic symptoms, cardiomyopathy, impairment of vision or hearing, renal symptoms, dysmorphic features, organomegaly, and/or high anion gap acidosis, lactic acidosis, or hypoketotic hypoglycemia. In more severe cases, height, head circumference, and developmental progress may also be affected.

Yoo and colleagues (2013) studied the predictive value of a set of predefined symptoms and signs that might point toward "nonorganic" versus "organic" etiologies for FTT. They found that the presence of vivacity, food restriction, and/or feeding rituals and poor appetite were more predictive of nonorganic (or inadequate caloric intake) and that vomiting, diarrhea, irregular bowel movements, and abdominal distention were more typical symptoms of organic (or malabsorption/excessive expenditure of calories). Vomiting and abdominal distention were noted to be of particular significance. Yoo and colleagues' review (2013) also noted that infants hospitalized for FTT predictably related to social encounters and objects differently, depending on what their eventual causative deficiency proved to be. Infants with organic causes were more likely to prefer close, personal interactions (i.e., with touching/holding) than those later diagnosed as having a nonorganic deficiency due to psychosocial factors (preferred distant social encounters and relating to inanimate objects).

Therefore, a thoughtful approach to the history (medical, developmental-behavioral, nutritional, and social), physical examination, and limited laboratory evaluation of children with FTT can be more predictive than relying on a battery of laboratory tests or empiric hospitalization. The following should be included in the assessment.

History. General parental concerns about the child's weight and growth need to be addressed. Look for conditions that would negatively affect the child's growth potential, increase the caloric needs, decrease the availability or use of calories, or affect the child's ability to feed or willingness to feed or factors that might affect the parent's ability or interest in feeding the child.

Prenatal
- Maternal health including chronic illness, such as diabetes mellitus, HIV, cytomegalovirus (CMV), infection; maternal habits, such as nutrition, alcohol, cigarette use
- Obstetric complications, such as toxemia, hemorrhage, multiple pregnancies

Perinatal
- Birthweight, Apgar scores, complications, length of stay in the hospital, congenital anomalies, neurologic insults, newborn screening results, weight for gestational age

Neonatal
- Intraventricular hemorrhage, seizures, hypoxia, extreme hyperbilirubinemia, infection

Postnatal Health
- Hospitalizations, medications, surgeries, accidents, illnesses
- Serious or recurrent infections

- Recurrent symptoms, such as vomiting, diarrhea, wheezing, snoring
- Chronic health conditions (Table 40.9)
- Collection and interpretation of growth data, percentiles, BMI, height for weight over time
- Stooling and voiding history: Diarrhea, constipation, vomiting, poor urine stream
- Careful review of systems

Developmental Trajectory and Temperamental Style
- Developmental and behavioral history

Family and Psychosocial History
- Social and family factors: Family composition, caregiving environment, day care, family support, poverty, parent-child relationship, parenting attitudes, typical day
- Family health history: Size and growth, developmental disabilities, inherited diseases that may affect growth and development

TABLE 40.9 Major Causes of Failure to Thrive

System	Cause
Gastrointestinal	GER, Crohn disease, pyloric stenosis, cleft palate or cleft lip, lactose intolerance, Hirschsprung disease, CMPI, hepatitis, cirrhosis, pancreatic insufficiency, biliary disease, IBD, malabsorption, alkaline foods
Cardiac	Cardiac diseases leading to congestive heart failure
Renal	UTI, renal tubular acidosis, diabetes insipidus, chronic kidney disease
Pulmonary	Asthma, bronchopulmonary dysplasia, CF, anatomic abnormalities of the upper airway; obstructive sleep apnea; recurrently infected adenoids and tonsils
Endocrine and metabolic	Hypothyroidism, diabetes mellitus, adrenal insufficiency or excess, parathyroid disorders, pituitary disorders, growth hormone deficiency; inborn errors of metabolism
Neurologic	Mental retardation, cerebral hemorrhage, degenerative disorders, cerebral palsy
Infectious	Parasitic or bacterial infections of the GI tract, TB, HIV
Congenital	Many genetic abnormalities
Malignancy and autoimmune disorders	Many cancers of childhood, collagen-vascular disease, juvenile idiopathic rheumatoid arthritis
Nutritional	Lack of calories, lack of micronutrients including vitamin A, zinc, iron
Hematologic	Sickle cell disease and others
Prenatal	Small for gestational age, perinatal infection
Psychosocial	Depression, anorexia nervosa, bulimia, maternal depression, child abuse or neglect, ADHD, autism, chronic pain
Environmental toxins	Heavy metal poisoning; other toxins

ADHD, Attention-deficit/hyperactivity disorder; *CF*, cystic fibrosis; *CMPI*, cow's-milk protein intolerance; *GER*, gastroesophageal reflux; *GI*, gastrointestinal; *HIV*, human immunodeficiency virus; *TB*, tuberculosis; *UTI*, urinary tract infection.

Physical Examination

- Weight, height, BMI, and head circumference (in those younger than 2 years old) plotted on standardized growth curves and percentiles, including weight-for-height graphs (include past and present growth parameters)
- Skinfold measurements: Loss of subcutaneous fat; general wasting (more common in developing countries; seen with malignancy, HIV, cerebral palsy, inflammatory diseases)
- Vital signs (temperature, pulse, respiratory rate, blood pressure)
- Hydration status
- Presence of dysmorphic features
- Skin, hair, nails, and mucous membranes: Scaling skin (seen with zinc deficiency); rough or hard skin (with hypothyroidism); edema (with protein deficiency); alopecia (with hypervitaminosis, kwashiorkor, or syphilis); hair color/texture changes (with zinc deficiency, Menkes kinky hair disease); spoon-shaped nails (with iron deficiency or GI diseases); cyanosis (with heart disease); and labial fissures (with vitamin deficiency)
- Evidence of abuse or neglect: Unexplained burns or skin lesions; fractures; retinal hemorrhages; unwashed skin; diaper rash; untreated impetigo; uncut and dirty fingernails; unwashed clothing
- Oral findings: Dental caries, tonsillar hypertrophy, submucous cleft palate, or tongue enlargement (may require oral-motor function studies, including lip/tongue/swallowing assessment)
- Respiratory compromise (with CF, bronchopulmonary dysplasia)

- Cardiovascular examination for congenital heart disease
- Abdominal: Lymphadenopathy, hepatosplenomegaly, masses, distention (with malignancy, inborn errors of metabolism, and immunodeficiency)
- Endocrine: Thyroid enlargement, precocious or ambiguous sexual development
- Neuromuscular tone and strength, cranial nerves for swallowing (cerebral palsy)
- Hypertonicity/hyperreflexia for cerebral palsy

Diagnostic Studies

- Feeding assessment: Nutritional and feeding history for calorie, protein, micronutrient intake.
  - Quality of food for age and ability to suck, chew, and swallow
  - Social nature of the feeding event and family eating patterns (meals and child feeding)
  - Feeding history: Caloric intake; feeding behavior; feeding cues; cues to hunger and satiety; progression to solids; frequency of feedings; amount taken per feeding; preparation of formula (over dilution)
  - Twenty-four-hour diet recall for infants, 3-day diet history for older children eating solid foods
  - Parental understanding of nutrition and feeding of children
- Developmental assessment
- Laboratory and imaging studies as delineated in Table 40.10

TABLE 40.10 Evaluation Studies for Failure to Thrive

Generic Cause	Associated Conditions	Physical Findings	Diagnostic Evaluation
Inadequate caloric intake	Poor food intake Chronic illness Inappropriate type/volume of feeding Anorexia, bulimia Food not available, parental withholding Poverty, neglect	Signs of neglect or abuse Minimal subcutaneous fat Protuberant abdomen	Complete dietary history Complete psychosocial evaluation Basic metabolic profile, vitamin D (calcidiol), lead, zinc, iron screening, albumin for protein status in severe FTT
Inadequate caloric absorption	GI causes (malabsorption, chronic vomiting, pancreatic insufficiency, celiac disease, chronic reflux, IBD) Chronic renal disease, CF, inborn errors of metabolism, infestations	Dysmorphism suggestive of chronic disease, organomegaly, skin/mucosal changes	CBC/ESR, basic metabolic profile, serum electrolytes (include total CO_2 to rule out renal tubular acidosis), UA and urine culture, sweat test, stool studies for fat, reducing substances, O&P, and culture Review of newborn metabolic screening tests Extremity radiographs if indicated (e.g., rickets)
Excessive caloric expenditure	Hyperthyroidism, chronic disease (cardiac, renal, endocrine, hepatic), malignancy	Dysmorphisms, skin dysmorphology, cardiac findings, abdominal mass or lymphadenopathy, hepatosplenomegaly	TSH, CBC/ESR, serum protein, albumin, alkaline phosphatase, BUN, creatinine, liver function tests Chest radiograph Renal ultrasound and voiding cystourethrography
Growth failure	Genetic, familial short stature, small for gestational age, hypothyroidism	Short stature, dysmorphisms, decreasing height growth with symmetric weight to height	Thyroid studies, HIV screening Karyotype (especially in small girls for Turner syndrome) Bone age Developmental testing Growth hormone (expensive, often done later in workup)

BUN, Blood urea nitrogen; *CBC*, complete blood count; *CF*, cystic fibrosis; *ESR*, erythrocyte sedimentation rate; *FTT*, failure to thrive; *GI*, gastrointestinal; *HIV*, human immunodeficiency virus; *IBD*, inflammatory bowel disease; *O&P*, ova and parasites; *TSH*, thyroid-stimulating hormone; *UA*, urinalysis.

Data from Goh L, How C, Ng KH. Failure to thrive in babies and toddlers. *Singapore Med J.* 2016;57(6):287–291; and Dobowitz H, Black M. Failure to thrive. *BMJ Best Practice (Online).* http://bestpractice.bmj.com/best-practice/monograph/747.html. Accessed April 13, 2018.

Differential Diagnosis

See Tables 40.9 and 40.10.

Management

Management is often best addressed by an interdisciplinary team that includes pediatrics (with specialty consultants for specific medical conditions), nutrition (may include lactation specialist), mental health, other community resources (e.g., Women, Infants, and Children [WIC] program, food stamps, Medicaid, housing authorities), and social work personnel. Community nurse home visits can aid in observations (mealtime behaviors, such as food refusal, spitting, food throwing, oral retention), assessment, and support.

- Manage treatable causes with prompt attention to urgent, life-threatening medical conditions.
- Restore nutritional intake and appropriate intake patterns.
- Provide nutritional rehabilitation: Vitamin supplementation with iron, zinc, and minerals; calorically enriched formula and foods (up to 150 cal/kg/day for infants <6 months old). In older infants and toddlers, solids should be offered before liquids, and they should not be force fed. See Chapter 17 for further information related to nutrition for FTT. The expected normal weight gain by age should be:
  - Birth to 3 months old: 25 to 30 g/day
  - 3 to 6 months old: 15 to 20 g/day
  - 6 to 12 months old: 10 to 15 g/day
  - 12 months old and older: 5 to 10 g/day
- Provide parent education and support and improve parent-child interaction.
- Treat underlying chronic condition.
- Make referrals as needed including feeding clinics.
- Evaluate for normal weight gain every 1 to 3 weeks. Catch-up growth can occur rapidly but can take up to 2 weeks before growth occurs with more involved cases. One must be careful to not overshoot the mark, resulting in overweight.
- Hospitalize for evaluation and intervention to protect from abuse when intentional etiology is suspected, to avoid further starvation and sequelae, to manage extreme child-parent interaction problems, to provide care when outpatient management is not feasible or practical, and to provide more intensive care after failure of outpatient management.

Prognosis

The goal of nutrition management is to achieve symmetry of weight and height and genetic growth potential. Nutritional effects of chronic conditions may persist if not treated with the primary condition. Outcomes are variable depending on the underlying condition and severity.

Most children achieve expected growth and development. However, because brain growth occurs maximally in the first 6 months of life, nutritional insufficiency in an infant can severely affect long-term development and social/emotional health. Subtle neurodevelopmental abnormalities, the home environment, and the quality of nurturing by caregivers can affect outcomes. Many studies document that FTT can result in long-term detrimental effects—short stature, lower cognitive functioning, poorer academic functioning, and increased risk for adult diseases, such as cardiovascular disease, obesity, hypertension, and diabetes (Larson-Nath and Biank, 2016; Goh, How, and Ng, 2016).

Encopresis/Constipation

The North American and European Societies for Pediatric Gastroenterology, Hepatology and Nutrition (NASPGHAN and ESPGHAN) reviewed evidence-based data on constipation and encopresis in children to include definition, epidemiology, assessment, and management. This discussion draws on that review (Tabbers et al., 2014).

Constipation is a common condition in childhood that accounts for 3% to 5% of primary care office visits and 25% of gastroenterology consultations (Philichi, 2018). It is an acute or chronic condition in which stool is retained, hard, infrequent, and can become impacted in the colon. Box 40.8 outlines the Rome IV criteria defining functional constipation in infants and children; Fig 40.7 presents the Bristol Stool Form Scale with qualitative stool characteristics.

Encopresis, also known as fecal soiling or fecal incontinence, is most often defined as repetitive, voluntary, or involuntary passage of stool in the underwear or inappropriate places after an age when the child should be able to control bowel movements, usually 4 years old. Fecal soiling or incontinence occurs at least once per month for at least 2 months prior to diagnosis. It is associated most often with or probably caused from underlying constipation. (Benninga et al., 2016; Hyams et al., 2016). It is important to determine if there is underlying constipation as a cause for fecal incontinence to appropriately direct a treatment plan. Primary, or continuous, encopresis is present in children who have never been toilet trained. Secondary, or discontinuous, encopresis is seen in those who were previously trained but who begin to soil. There are two subtypes of encopresis: (1) encopresis with constipation, associated with stool retention, constipation, and incontinence overflow (functional retentive fecal incontinence); and (2) encopresis without constipation, or functional non-retentive fecal incontinence, which is less common. The child with non-retentive fecal incontinence has a normal physical exam with no stool retention on exam or radiographic study and no evidence of anorectal sensorimotor function or motility disorder (Hyams, 2016).

Encopresis may be more common than believed because many families hesitate to inform their healthcare provider about it due to social perceptions that the issue is related to either their parenting skills or abuse. The cause of encopresis is unclear, is usually

---

• BOX 40.8 Rome IV Criteria for Functional Constipation in Infants and Children

Must include 2 or more of the following occurring at least once per week for a minimum of 1 month with insufficient criteria for a diagnosis of irritable bowel syndrome:

1. Two or fewer defecations in the toilet per week in a child of a developmental age of at least 4 years
2. At least 1 episode of fecal incontinence per week
3. History of retentive posturing or excessive volitional stool retention
4. History of painful or hard bowel movements
5. Presence of a large fecal mass in the rectum
6. History of large diameter stools that can obstruct the toilet
7. After appropriate evaluation, the symptoms cannot be fully explained by another medical condition.

From Hyams J, Di Lorenzo C, Saps M, et al. Functional disorders: child/adolescent. *Gastroenterology.* 2016;150[6]:1456–1470.

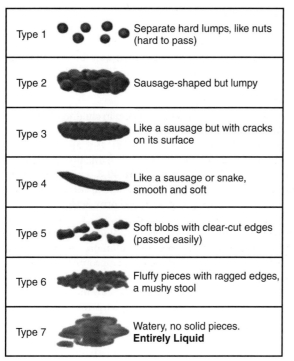

Type 1		Separate hard lumps, like nuts (hard to pass)
Type 2		Sausage-shaped but lumpy
Type 3		Like a sausage but with cracks on its surface
Type 4		Like a sausage or snake, smooth and soft
Type 5		Soft blobs with clear-cut edges (passed easily)
Type 6		Fluffy pieces with ragged edges, a mushy stool
Type 7		Watery, no solid pieces. **Entirely Liquid**

• **Fig 40.7** Bristol Stool Chart. (From Kliegman RM, Stanton BF, Geme JW, Schor NF, Behrman RE. *Nelson Textbook of Pediatrics.* 20th ed. Philadelphia: Elsevier; 2016.)

multifactorial, and appears to differ among children. Both physiologic and psychosocial factors can be involved.

Children with encopresis with constipation often have a history of an acute stool problem that was not adequately managed (e.g., the child had an illness that caused dehydration and constipation), leading to a cycle of constipation, painful defecation, stool retention, more severe constipation, more painful defecation, more stool retention, and so on. In encopresis with constipation, stool retention over time leads to distention of the colon and stretching of the rectum, ineffective peristalsis, decreased sensory threshold in the rectum, and weakened rectal and sphincter muscles (see Fig 40.8). Soft, semi-formed, or liquid stool from higher in the colon leaks around retained stool and passes uncontrollably through the rectum, causing soiling. The child is almost always unaware of the actual incontinence. Children with encopresis with constipation may either refuse or be willing to use the toilet.

Children with encopresis without constipation (functional non-retentive fecal incontinence) are not constipated, but have overflow incontinence or voluntary bowel movements in their clothing or other inappropriate places. Children with non-retentive encopresis appear to have more behavioral problems and externalizing behavior than children with retentive encopresis or those without stooling problems, although it is unclear which causes which. Some of these children may also have a developmentally delayed or faulty perception of the need to stool and will soil as a result (Tabbers et al., 2014).

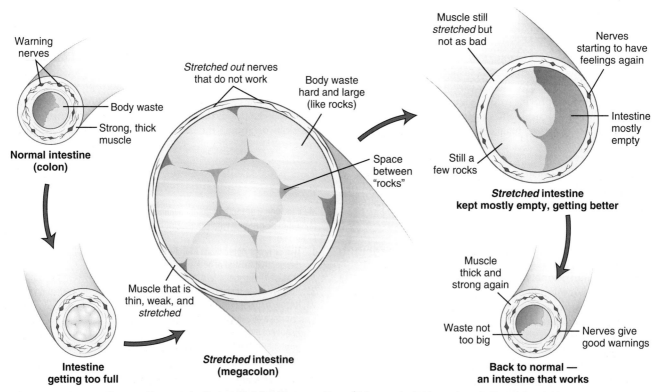

• **Fig 40.8** Encopresis: Patient Training Diagram. (From Weissman L, Bridgemohan C. Bowel function, toileting, and encopresis. In: Carey WB, Croker AC, Coleman WL, et al., eds. *Developmental-Behavioral Pediatrics.* 4th ed. Philadelphia: Saunders; 2009.)

Physiologic

Possible physiologic factors related to encopresis with constipation may include the following:
- Inadequate fluid intake
- Dehydration caused by illness and fever or during active play in hot weather
- A change in diet, such as the introduction of solids or increased carbohydrates; there is conflicting information on the role of fiber intake pre- and post-constipation diagnosis (Tabbers et al., 2014)
- Secondary stool retention and constipation due to:
  - Painful bowel movements
  - Anal fissures
  - Paradoxic constriction of the external anal sphincter muscle during attempted defecation
  - Neurogenic conditions (e.g., aganglionic colon [HD], cerebral palsy, myelomeningocele)
  - Endocrine and metabolic conditions (e.g., hypothyroidism)
  - Medications (e.g., opioids, iron supplements, anticholinergics)

Psychosocial

Psychosocial treatment, which may include health education in the office setting or more formal counseling therapy, is indicated if these types of factors are present:
- Major family or life adjustments, such as loss of a parent, sibling, or other significant person
- Inappropriate toilet-training techniques leading to a power struggle; children who are pushed might rebel in the only way they can, by refusing to cooperate
- Irregular toileting patterns, often caused by travel, unfamiliar or unpleasant bathrooms ,or lack of regular routine
- Physical abuse and sexual abuse
- Children absorbed in play or an activity who do not want to stop to defecate
- Behavioral and attention problems as well as anxiety and depressive symptoms
- Social structure: toilet habits at school. School often regulates bathroom use therefore the child will withhold

Clinical Findings

History. Early detection and treatment are important, so specific and directed questions need to be asked in well-child visits. "Is pooping and peeing going okay?" is not a sufficient question to ask while obtaining history. The history can include the following:
- Is there a significant family or child history related to stooling (e.g., Hirschsprung? Constipation in infancy? Late meconium passage?)
- Does the child complain of abdominal pain, bloating, loss of appetite?
- How often does the child have a bowel movement?
- Are there situations when the child refuses to defecate or urinate (e.g., at school, in public bathrooms, when playing)?
- Describe the process of when the child defecates (e.g., painful? Child resists using toilet? Child hides, defecates outside toilet?).
- What is the quality of stool (e.g., ribbon, hard, large-caliber)?
- Describe any issues with hygiene (e.g., stained underwear, odor, leakage of stool).
- Does the child have enuresis? A history of UTIs?

Box 40.9 outlines specific findings that are red flags for constipation and require further investigation.

Physical Examination. The NASPGHAN and ESPGHAN state that a digital examination is not supported by evidence (Benninga et al., 2016). The physical examination should assess for the following:

- Overflow soiling
- Abdominal distention
- Abdominal tenderness on palpation
- Mass felt at the midline in the suprapubic area (descending colon)
- Anal fissures
- Sacral dimple or hair tuft
- Neurologic signs: absent or diminished abdominal, cremasteric, anal wink reflexes, and deep tendon reflexes (DTRs) in lower extremities

Diagnostic Studies. X-rays and laboratory tests to identify structural or organic causes of constipation are not recommended by NASPGHAN and ESPGHAN unless there are alarming signs that indicate an underlying condition for constipation is present. However, an abdominal flat plate radiograph can be indicated when fecal impaction is suspected, abdominal exam cannot be performed or unreliable. The abdominal film can show accumulation of stool in the sigmoid colon and can help parents who may deny their child is constipated to better understand their child's problem. Laboratory studies can be done when suspicion for thyroid disease, CD, or hypercalcemia is present (Benninga et al., 2016; Philichi, 2018).

Differential Diagnosis

The differential diagnoses for encopresis with constipation are anorectal stenosis, spina bifida occulta, spinal cord dysplasia, HD, mental retardation, hypothyroidism, hypercalcemia, cerebral palsy, and CF. The infant exhibiting normal red-faced grunting and straining with defecation is not constipated.

Management

In all cases, the goals of treatment are to establish a regular bowel routine, "demystify" the problem, alleviate blame, and gain cooperation for treatment plans. Treatment approaches for children with constipation have followed a pattern of:
- Bowel evacuation using oral polyethylene glycol (PEG) solutions are as effective as enemas but much less traumatizing to children and families (Tabbers et al., 2014)
- Bowel retraining to establish a regular pattern of stooling
- Ongoing maintenance with medications as needed, normal physical activity as per AAP recommendations, and regular toileting hygiene to prevent recurring constipation.

Additional treatment may include:

Biofeedback—sensory retraining and relaxation of the sphincter muscle during defecation. This is used in children with confirmed abnormal sensory threshold and defecation mechanics on anorectal manometry. Surgical treatment is used but rare; this includes a cecostomy button for anterograde colonic enemas.

The emphasis in treating nonretentive fecal soiling is on behavioral therapy, educating the child and parent about normal stooling, and establishing a structured pattern of toileting. Box 40.10 outlines approaches to treating a child with encopresis without constipation (also see the Management subsection in the Toilet Refusal Syndrome section below). Active pre-toilet training education can be used as a preventive option.

Children who have encopresis with constipation present a greater challenge. Education of parents and children is equally vital to successful treatment. A clear message to children and parents should be that the dynamics of encopresis (retention, colon stretching, decreased peristalsis, impaction, leaking) are not voluntary—no one is to blame; they can, however, be reversed through bowel rehabilitation. Correcting them takes hard work, cooperation, and time, and the provider will work with the family to ensure success. Fig 40.8 can be used to educate parents and children about the bowel rehabilitation process involved in the treatment plan. Timed urination may also be helpful, because children who struggle to hold their urine activate the pelvic floor and, as a result, hold their stool as well.

In some cases, child mental health referral may be indicated but should not be the first referral and alone cannot cure the problem. This referral should be reserved for situations in which there are other indications that mental health interventions may be helpful to the child and/or family.

Figs 40.9 and 40.10 present algorithms for constipation in infants 6 months and younger and those infants and children older than 6 months. Table 40.11 provides guidelines to treating a child with encopresis with constipation, including appropriate medications. According to the ESPGHAN and NASPGHAN, although not U.S. FDA-approved for use in children, PEG is the first-line therapy for children presenting with functional constipation and/or fecal impaction. Further research is being conducted to determine the safety of its long-term use in children (Tabbers et al., 2014; NASPGHAN Neurogastroenterology and Motility Committee, 2015). Enemas are recommended *only* if PEG is not available.

For maintenance, PEG is recommended as first-line therapy, although lactulose may be given if PEG is not available. Milk of magnesia, mineral oil, and stimulant laxatives may also be considered for maintenance or as second-line treatment. Enemas are not recommended for maintenance therapy. Maintenance medications need to be continued for a minimum of 2 months and should not be stopped until 1 month after resolution of the problem. At this time, medications should be decreased gradually and if any problems recur, the medication should be adjusted back to the last successful dose and given an additional 2 weeks before attempting to decrease again. Throughout the treatment, medications must be adjusted according to the clinical response, so the provider must be readily available for the family to ask questions and make modifications.

Because this problem often occurs in school-age children and the nature of the school setting can discourage children from using the restroom, providers should consult with the school nurse to ensure that children are allowed to use the toilet without going through extra steps and without having to draw attention to themselves. Hygiene management (e.g., may include access to a more private toilet and extra underwear) and psychological and emotional support in the school setting are important to a child's success in overcoming encopresis.

Complications

Persistent encopresis is an unpleasant condition, and children with encopresis often experience ridicule and shame. Age-group peers frequently treat children with scorn, hostility, and rejection. Teachers and other adults might be disgusted by children with encopresis, and parents, dealing with anger, guilt, embarrassment, and helplessness, find their children and the condition extremely difficult to manage. Social, interpersonal, and family relations are at grave risk.

Intractable constipation, and even megacolon, can be seen in children with Down syndrome, cerebral palsy, or neurologic conditions. When medical management is unsuccessful, an antegrade continence enema procedure may be necessary.

Patient and Family Education

The best treatment of encopresis is prevention. If constipation or encopresis is caused by an underlying anatomic or organic cause (e.g., HD, occult spina bifida, hypothyroidism), early diagnosis and referral is essential. The pediatric provider must understand the relationship between constipation and encopresis and/or diarrhea, recognize conditions that may contribute to each, and provide parents with anticipatory guidance related to toilet training and normal elimination habits in order to prevent problems. It is equally important to promote consistent, positive, and supportive attitudes during treatment and remove negative attributions to soiling. Although parents should be informed that treatment may be required for months or years, providers should emphasize that by following a clear, consistent, aggressive treatment protocol the condition can be managed. Finally, providers, parents, and the child must work together to prevent recurrence of symptoms after successful treatment.

Toilet Refusal Syndrome

Toilet refusal syndrome (TRS) is present when a child demonstrates a pattern of successfully using the toilet to urinate, but refuses to use the toilet for bowel movements. These children usually defecate in a diaper, training pants, or "pull-ups." In some cases, children retain stool or defecate outside the toilet. Encopresis without constipation also fits this description; the child defecates outside the toilet when beyond the age of expected training.

Many young healthy children experience TRS for a short period of time. In a study of children who were trained at early ages (some as early as the first 6 months of life), there was a nearly 12% incidence of TRS. The cause of TRS is unknown, but the presence of younger siblings in the household and the parents' inability to set limits for the child may be related. TRS can persist in preschool and school- age children and may be associated with comorbid conditions. Constipation and painful bowel movements appear to precede rather than follow the problem.

Clinical Findings

History
Parents or caregivers report that the child demonstrates the following:
- Bladder control but refusal to defecate on the toilet
- A regular or irregular pattern of bowel movements
- Consistent signs from child that a bowel movement is imminent
- May have a history of hiding when defecating, either before or after toilet training begins

Physical Examination
- The physical examination is unremarkable.
- Examine the anus for fissures or irritation that may cause a child to refuse to defecate and the presence of an anal wink. A digital examination is not indicated.
- Check for signs of stool retention:
  - Abdominal distention
  - Abdominal tenderness on palpation
- Palpate for a mass in the sigmoid colon or at the midline in the suprapubic area (impaction).

Differential Diagnosis

The differential diagnosis includes stool withholding, constipation, and encopresis.

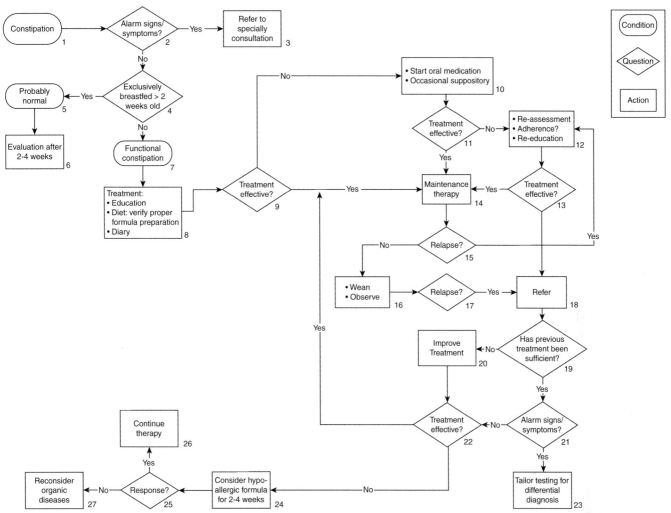

• **Fig 40.9** An Algorithm for the Evaluation and Treatment of Constipated Infants Less Than 6 Months Old. *Ca,* Calcium; *MRI,* magnetic resonance imaging; *Pb,* lead; *PEG,* polyethylene glycol; *Rx,* medication; *T₄,* thyroxine; *TSH,* thyroid-stimulating hormone. (From Tabbers MM, DiLorenzo C, Berger MY, et al. Evaluation and treatment of functional constipation in infants and children: evidence-based recommendations from ESPGHAN and NASPGHAN. *J Pediatr Gastroenterol Nutr.* 2014;58[2]:258–274.)

Management

Return the child to diapers and reintroduce toilet training in about a month or when the child indicates interest. Some children prefer not to wear diapers all the time, but ask to have one put on when they feel the urge to defecate. If possible, have parents encourage the child to go into the bathroom for these diaper defecations. After having a bowel movement, the child asks to be changed and returns to wearing training pants. This pattern may continue for several weeks or months. When parents refrain from expressing negative messages about stooling or fecal matter and matter-of-factly clean up the child after defecating in the diaper, the duration of TRS appears to shorten. For older children, schedule a daily time for the child to sit on the toilet for 5 to 10 minutes when the child typically has a bowel movement; have these times be positive, never punitive or forced. Never flush the toilet while the child is sitting on it. If in a public restroom, have parents keep sticky notes with them to cover automatic flush sensors. Incentives and positive feedback when the child successfully uses the toilet for bowel movements may be effective (e.g., the parent can

use star charts or cards on the wall and the child can remove them and turn them in for a prize), but excessive praise is not recommended, because the child is simply doing what is to be expected. If the child has constipation, fecal impaction, or both, initial bowel clean-out is necessary using PEG. Then a daily dose adjusted to clinical response is recommended until toilet training is complete.

Complications

Refusal to use the toilet for bowel movements may lead to stool withholding, constipation, and impaction, which are conditions that result in primary encopresis. Psychological complications include embarrassment, shame, conflict, and stress between children and parents, especially as the child becomes older. Child maltreatment can be a significant complication.

Patient and Family Education

Prevention through appropriate toilet training is key (see Elimination: Chapter 18). If a child refuses to defecate on the toilet, use of punishment or force can complicate the problem. Parents

• BOX 40.9 Alarm Signs and Symptoms in
Constipation

- Constipation starting extremely early in life (<1 month)
- Passage of meconium >48 h
- Family history of Hirschsprung disease
- Ribbon stools
- Blood in stools in the absence of anal fissures
- Failure to thrive
- Fever
- Bilious vomiting
- Abnormal thyroid function
- Severe abdominal distension
- Decreased lower extremity strength/tone/reflex
- Perianal fistula
- Abnormal position of anus
- Absent anal or cremasteric reflex
- Tuft of hair on spine
- Sacral dimple
- Gluteal cleft deviation
- Extreme resistance or fear during anal inspection
- Anal scars

Tabbers M, DiLorenzo C, Berger M, et al. Evaluation and treatment of functional constipation in infants and children: evidence-based recommendations from ESPGHAN and NASPGHAN. *J Pediatr Gastroenterol Nutr.* 2014;58[2]:258–274; and Philichi, L. Management of childhood functional constipation. *J Pediatr Health.* 2018;32[1]:103–111.

• BOX 40.10 Management of Children With Mild Encopresis Without Constipation

- Monitor diet:
  - Ensure adequate fiber and water intake for age:
    - Recommended water intake is about 1 oz/kg/day.
    - Fiber recommendations: 4- to 8-year-olds: about 25 g of fiber each day; 9- to 13-year-old girls: about 26 g of fiber each day; 9- to 13-year-old boys: about 31 g of fiber each day; 14- to 18-year-old girls: about 26 g of fiber each day; and 14- to 18-year-old boys: about 38 g of fiber each day. Legumes, vegetables, and some fruits are good sources of fiber.
  - Decrease milk to 16 oz/day.
  - Do not allow excessive dairy, rice, applesauce, bananas, white flour, or potatoes.
- Give child all responsibility for own toilet habits. Stop parental reminders to use toilet. Stop all encouragement and criticisms.
- Establish a regular toileting routine.
- Avoid use of stool softeners or laxatives.
- Encourage daily physical activity per American Academy of Pediatrics (AAP) recommendations.
- May use incentives or rewards to reinforce positive behavior. Have parent and child agree on reward beforehand so that it can be discussed as a positive, subtle reminder.

should be alert for signs of constipation and should be encouraged to contact the pediatric provider sooner rather than later if there is any concern.

Diarrhea

Acute and chronic diarrhea results from alterations in the normal functioning of the intestinal system. The altered intestinal mechanisms that result in diarrhea vary; briefly, diarrhea can occur as a result of:

- Nonabsorbable solutes in the GI tract, when fluids exceed the transport capacity, or when water-soluble nutrients are not absorbed (osmotic diarrhea). Such nutrient malabsorption and/or excessive fluid intake account for most chronic diarrhea; dumping syndrome, lactase deficiency, overfeeding, and malabsorption syndromes are causative conditions (Giannattasio et al., 2016).
- Invasion, inflammation, and/or release of toxins by bacteria or viruses (such as in traveler's diarrhea) that decrease absorption and increase secretion and transportation of electrolytes and water from mucosal crypt cells in the small intestine into the bowel lumen (secretory diarrhea). As an example, viruses injure the absorptive mature mucosal surface cells, thereby altering the release of disaccharides and preventing the conversion of carbohydrates to monosaccharides necessary for normal absorption. Congenital disorders, mucosal disorders, and tumors can also lead to secretory diarrhea.
- Mutations in the ion transport proteins, such as chloride-bicarbonate exchange.
- Alterations in the anatomy of the intestinal surface or functional ability due to inflammation or surgical procedures (e.g., short bowel syndrome, CD, IBS) with a subsequent loss of fluids, electrolytes, macronutrients and micronutrients, and normal peristalsis.
- A change in intestinal motility, either increased or decreased (e.g., irritable bowel, bacterial overgrowth due to stasis [pseudo obstruction], toddler's diarrhea).
- Altered immune function.

Acute Diarrhea

The term *acute gastroenteritis* was formerly used to describe acute diarrhea, but this term is technically a misnomer because the etiology of diarrhea does not technically involve the stomach (Guandalini, 2017). With acute diarrhea, there is a disruption of the normal intestinal net absorptive versus secretory mechanisms of fluids and electrolytes, resulting in excessive loss of fluid into the intestinal lumen. This can lead to dehydration, electrolyte imbalance, and in severe cases, death in those also malnourished. In children younger than 2 years old, this translates to a daily stool volume of more than 10 mL/kg (this definition excludes the normal breastfeeding stooling of five or six stools per day). In children older than 2 years old, diarrheal stooling is described as occurring four or more times in 24 hours. The duration can last up to 14 days.

Viruses can injure the absorptive surface of mature villous cells, which reduces the amount of fluid absorbed. Some can release a viral enterotoxin (e.g., rotavirus). A loss of water and electrolytes ensues, and there can be volumes of watery diarrhea, even if the child is not being fed. Bacterial and parasitic agents can adhere and/or translocate, causing noninflammatory diarrhea. Bacteria can also damage the anatomy and functional ability of the intestinal mucosa by direct invasion. Some bacteria release endotoxins, whereas others release cytotoxins that result in the excretion of fluid, protein, and cells into the intestinal lumen and an inflammatory response in some cases. Abnormal peristalsis for any reason can result in acute diarrhea. The enteric pathogens are spread through the fecal-oral route and by ingestion of contaminated food or water.

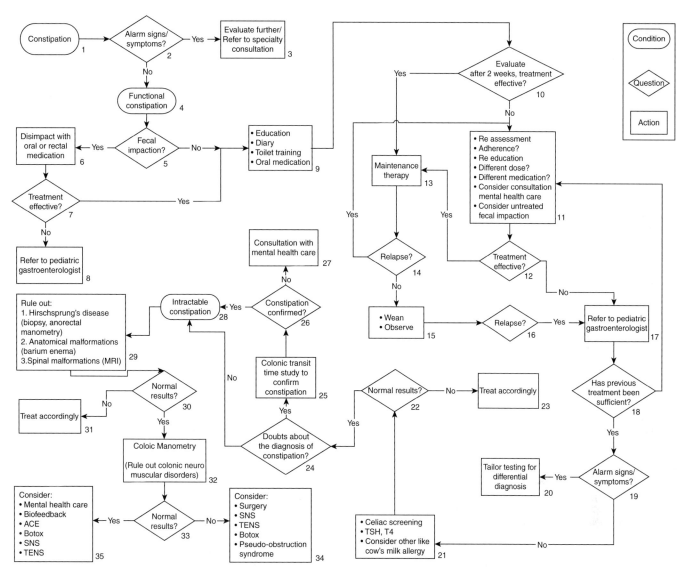

- **Fig 40.10** An algorithm for the evaluation and treatment of constipated infants and children 6 months old or older. *Ca,* Calcium; *MRI,* magnetic resonance imaging; *Pb,* lead; *T₄,* thyroxine; *TSH,* thyroid-stimulating hormone. (From Tabbers MM, DiLorenzo C, Berger MY, et al. Evaluation and treatment of functional constipation in infants and children: evidence-based recommendations from ESPGHAN and NASPGHAN. *J Pediatr Gastroenterol Nutr.* 2014;58[2]:258–274.)

Worldwide, the burden of acute diarrhea is huge, resulting in 3 to 5 billion cases and nearly 2 billion deaths (20% of total child deaths) in children younger than 5 years old (particularly vulnerable). Developing countries also see their share of the burden of this disease (approximately 10%), attributable to poor water, sanitation, and hygiene (Guandalini, 2017; Pavlinac et al., 2018). Globally, females have higher rates of *Campylobacter* species infections and hemolytic uremic syndrome; otherwise the incidence of cases shows no gender preference. Nontyphoidal *Salmonella, Shigella, Campylobacter, E. coli* organisms (bacteria); rotavirus, norovirus, enteric adenovirus (viruses); and *Giardia, Cryptosporidium,* and *Strongyloides* (parasites) cause most disease. *Shigella, E. coli, Giardia lamblia, Cryptosporidium parvum,* and *Entamoeba histolytica* are particularly infectious in small amounts. The term "dysentery" is used to indicate infection with specific species of *Shigella* and *Salmonella* (e.g., *Shigella dysenteriae*) (Tian et al., 2016).

In the United States, those most vulnerable include Native Americans and Native Alaskans, where remote residential locations or living on reservations compromises sanitation and safe water supplies, and where severe rotavirus diarrhea occurs. About 200,000 hospitalizations in the United States occur annually due to diarrheal illness with 300 deaths. The most common viral pathogens are noroviruses and rotavirus, followed by adenoviruses and astroviruses. Food-borne bacterial or parasitic diarrheal diseases are most commonly due to *Salmonella* and *Campylobacter* species, followed by *Shigella, Cryptosporidium, E. coli* O157:H7, *Yersinia, Listeria, Vibrio (Vibrio cholerae* and other species), and *Cyclospora* species. *C. difficile* has been associated with pseudomembranous colitis and diarrhea after the use of antibiotics; it is not the causative agent in most antibiotic associated diarrhea (AAD) in children in the United States (Tian et al., 2016).

Tables 40.12 and 40.14 discuss the characteristics of diarrheal diseases caused by bacteria, viruses, and parasites that a primary care provider is more likely to encounter and needs to differentiate. Infections due to *Cryptosporidium, E. coli* O157:H7, *Giardia, Listeria, Salmonella, Shigella,* and *V. cholerae* must be reported to the CDC. The enteric pathogens encountered more in day care settings include rotavirus, astrovirus, calicivirus, *Campylobacter, Shigella, Giardia,* and *Cryptosporidium* species (Guandalini, 2017).

Nausea and vomiting are not good indicators of the severity of a condition; however, the absence of or low-grade fever, mild to moderate periumbilical pain, and watery diarrhea are more typically associated with less serious bacterial infection and suggest small intestine involvement (Camilleri et al., 2017). The following are more indicative of potentially serious infection in the upper intestine:

- Food-borne illness suspected
- Bloody diarrhea, weight loss, dehydration, severe abdominal pain, and fever
- Diarrhea lasting several days with more than three stools per day
- Neurologic involvement on physical examination

Clinical Findings

History
- Pattern of diarrhea: Onset, number of stools, volume, frequency
- Appearance of stool: Odor, mucoid, and/or bloody
- Associated symptoms: Abdominal pain, nausea, vomiting, or fever
- Number of wet diapers in the past 24 hours and approximate time of last void
- Dietary consumption: Changes in diet that might correlate with increased stooling; ingestion (and when) of raw or poorly cooked foods (e.g., raw or undercooked eggs, meat, shellfish, fish, poultry), unpasteurized or under-pasteurized milk or juices, home-canned foods, fresh produce (fruits/vegetables), soft cheeses, deli meats
- If given, response to oral rehydration therapy
- Food allergies
- Family members or close friends with similar illness or other GI diseases
- Day care, school attendance, recreational swimming exposure (even if chlorinated): Illness patterns and contacts at these locations; walking in soil without shoes
- Travel history: Foreign or coastal areas; camping or travel where untreated water might have been consumed
- Attendance at picnics or other outings where food was consumed
- Most recent weight and previous growth pattern
- Medications: Antibiotics, laxatives, antacids, opiates (withdrawal), vitamins (toxicity)
- Pica (metals, plants)
- Chemotherapy
- Recent surgeries (abdominal)

Physical Examination
- Complete physical examination including vital signs and assessment of behavior/mental status changes
- Assess for dehydration (see Table 40.1)

Diagnostic Studies. Diagnostic studies are ordered if the symptoms (discussed earlier) of more serious infection are present. Some specific diagnostic findings associated with the more common infectious diarrheal illness are found in Table 40.12. Molecular diagnostic tests (e.g., polymerase chain reaction [PCR]) have greatly improved the ability to diagnose diarrheal illness due to bacteria. The following tests may be ordered:

- Stool examination (color, consistency, blood, mucus, pus, odor, volume): In endemic areas, microscopy examination for parasites (e.g., *G. lamblia* and *E. histolytica*).
- Stool: pH (<5.5 suggests carbohydrate intolerance typically seen in viral infections), leukocytes (suggest bacterial invasion), reducing substances (viral infections), and occult blood. Normal stool: pH greater than 5.5, carbohydrate negative.
- Stool cultures should be considered early in the course of illness for bloody or prolonged diarrhea; in the presence of leukocytes; if clinical signs of colitis are present; for suspected food-borne illness outbreaks (especially with *E. coli* O157:H7); in the immunocompromised; or after recent travel abroad.
- Electrolytes, if indicated, to evaluate degree of dehydration and for more serious signs and symptoms of infectious disease.
- CBC, as indicated for serious infectious disease.

Differential Diagnosis

Diarrhea from viral etiology and antibiotic use are the most common causes of diarrhea in all age groups. Systemic infection is a common cause in infants and children, and food poisoning is a common cause in children and adolescents. Overfeeding should also be considered in infants. Rare causes of acute diarrhea in infants include primary disaccharidase deficiency, Hirschsprung toxic colitis, adrenogenital syndrome, and neonate opiate withdrawal; toxic ingestion in children; and hyperthyroidism in adolescents.

Management

The foundation of all treatment of acute diarrhea is fourfold:
- Restore and maintain hydration and correct/maintain electrolyte and acid-base balance. Oral rehydration with an oral electrolyte solution should be attempted when dehydration is assessed between 3% and 9%. Administer parenteral hydration if necessary for the following: impaired circulation and possible shock, weight less than 4 to 5 kg or a child younger than 3 months old, intractable diarrhea, lethargy, anatomic anomalies, or failure to gain weight or continued weight loss despite oral fluids (see Table 40.3).
- Maintain nutrition. Resume early refeeding because contents of the bowel stimulate the growth of enterocytes and help facilitate mucosal repair following injury (see Table 40.3).
- Prescribe antibiotics prudently. Antibiotics are recommended for acute diarrhea caused by *G. lamblia, V. cholerae,* and *Shigella* species and can be considered for infections caused by enteropathogenic *E. coli* (if infection prolonged), enteroinvasive *E. coli, Yersinia* for those with sickle cell disease, and *Salmonella* in young infants with fever or positive blood culture findings (Guandalini, 2017) (see Table 40.12). Children with HIV at risk for acute diarrhea may benefit from cotrimoxazole and vitamin A (Polyak et al., 2016).
- Treat any related conditions, such as sepsis and cardiovascular collapse.

Some adjunct medications and treatments have received wider use in countries outside of the United States and show efficacy in some studies. Some of these include:
- Antidiarrheals (antimotility agents or adsorbents) are not generally recommended. However, a review of literature demonstrated that loperamide in children older than 3 years old is safe and decreases the duration and frequency of diarrhea compared with placebo. Children younger than 3 years old and those who are malnourished, those with moderate or severe dehydration, those who are systemically ill, or those who have

TABLE 40.11 Management of Children with Encopresis With Constipation		
Treatment Phase	**Treatment Program**	**Comments**

Phase I: Catharsis (bowel clean-out over 3-5 days; maximum of 6 consecutive days)	Oral clean-out if >3 years administered at home (preferred):
	• PEG 4050: 1-1.5 g/kg/day in 2-4 divided doses (preferred method)
	• Enema (only if PEG is not available; infrequently used)
	• Sodium phosphate (Fleet) enema:
	  • 2-11 years: 6 mL/kg/day per rectum; may give up to 135 mL once a day in older children
	  • >11 years: An adult enema or 135 mL per rectum once a day
	Pediatric enema is 67.5 mL; adult enema is 135 mL.
		Home treatment is preferred, should take 3-5 days or until stool output is runny diarrhea.
		PEG can be premixed and stored in refrigerator for 48 h.
		Catharsis may need to occur in the hospital if:
		• Retention is severe
		• Home compliance is poor
		• Parents prefer admission
		• Child needs enema for clean-out and parent should not administer
		The child may have watery or soft stools for several days after clean-out. Child and parents should be informed that this does not indicate cure, but that ongoing maintenance and bowel retraining is essential for the bowel to return to normal functioning (see Fig 40.8).

Phase II: Maintenance (regular bowel movements over 4-12 months)	Oral laxatives
	• PEG 4050 starting at 0.4 and up to 0.8 g/kg/day PO in two divided doses
	• Lactulose 1 to 2 mL/kg/24 hours in two divided doses. Max dose 60 mL/24 hours
	• Magnesium hydroxide
	  • 2-5 years: 0.4-1.2 g/day, PO once or divided
	  • 6-11 years: 1.2-2.4 g/day, PO once or divided
	  • 12-18 years: 2.4-4.8 g/day, PO once or divided
	• Mineral oil 1-3 mL/kg/day PO once or divided, maximum 90 mL/day
	• Stimulant laxative Bisacodyl: 3-10 years: 5 mg/day; >10 years: 5-10 mg/day
	Behavioral training
	• Establish daily toilet sitting 15-20 min after meals 2-3 times a day for 5-10 min
	• Provide positive reinforcement for toilet sitting and stooling
	• Keep a diary of bowel movements, recording time and amount
	• Ensure child has at least 1 h of physical exercise per day; have child be active in the 15-20 min between mealtime and sitting on toilet
	Dietary treatment
	• Ensure adequate dietary fiber intake
	• Ensure adequate fluid intake
		• Adjust daily medications to achieve one to three soft, mushy stools per day.
		• PEG has been shown to be safe and effective when used alone and more effective than lactulose (Gordon et al., 2016).
		• Adding enemas to the chronic use of PEG is not supported by evidence (Tabbers et al., 2014).
		• Use of senna is not recommended.
		• Plan on 6 months of treatment before bowel regains normal function.
		• Stimulant laxatives used as second- or third-line treatment.

Phase III: Weaning: Follow-up	Continued treatment for at least 1 month after all symptoms are resolved. Gradual tapering of laxative Regular visits (about every 4-10 weeks) depending on severity and need of family Telephone availability to discuss progress and adjust doses Counseling or referral as appropriate for psychosocial and developmental issues Continued education regarding normal bowel function	Goals of follow-up visits: • Monitor compliance. • Provide encouragement and support. • Detect and treat relapse early if it occurs.

PEG, Polyethylene glycol; *PO*, per os (by mouth, orally).

Adapted from Kehoe TD. The constipated 8-year-old. In: Burns CE, Richardson B, Brady MA, eds. *Pediatric Primary Care Case Studies*. Sudbury, MA: Jones and Bartlett; 2010.

bloody diarrhea should not be treated with this drug. Some over-the-counter products intended for diarrhea contain salicylates (e.g., Pepto-Bismol), and there is concern for Reye syndrome.

• Probiotics: *Lactobacillus casei* strain GG or *S. boulardii* (a yeast) given early in a viral diarrheal illness or AAD can both treat diarrhea (decrease duration by about 25 hours) and ameliorate the risk of AAD (Hojsak, 2017).

TABLE 40.12   Diarrheal Illnesses Due to Common Bacterial or Viral Pathogens

Etiology	Incubation Period	Signs and Symptoms	Duration of Illness	Route of Transmission	Laboratory Testing	Treatment and Complications*
Campylobacter jejuni	2-5 days, but can be longer	Diarrhea (foul smelling), cramps, fever, nausea and vomiting; diarrhea may be bloody in neonates Occurs in warm weather months	2-10 days	Raw and undercooked poultry, unpasteurized milk, contaminated water; low inoculum dose produces infection	Routine stool culture; *Campylobacter* requires special media and incubation temperature; positive gross blood, leukocytes; CBC: ↑WBCs	Rehydration is the mainstay. **Azithromycin, erythromycin, and metronidazole** shorten the duration of the illness when given early, and usually eradicates the organism from stool within 2-3 days. **Ciprofloxacin** (not routinely first-line therapy)
Clostridium difficile	Unknown	Variety of symptoms and severity are seen: mild to explosive diarrhea, bloody stools, abdominal pain, fever, nausea, vomiting Mild to moderate illness is characterized by watery diarrhea, low-grade fever, and mild abdominal pain	During or after several weeks of antibiotic use; can occur without being associated with such treatment	Acquired from the environment or from stool of other colonized or infected people by the fecal-oral route	Stool cultures; enzyme immunoassay for toxin A, or A and B; positive gross blood, leukocytes; CBC: ↑WBCs; ESR normal	Discontinue current antibiotic (any antibiotic, but notably ampicillin, clindamycin, second- and third-generation cephalosporins). Fluids and electrolyte replacement are usually sufficient. If antibiotic is still needed or illness is severe, treat with oral **metronidazole** (drug of choice in children) or **vancomycin** for 7 to 10 days. Supplement with probiotics. Lactobacillus GG, *Saccharomyces boulardii* are recommended. Complications include pseudomembranous colitis, toxic megacolon, colonic perforation, relapse, intractable proctitis, death in debilitated children.
Enterohemorrhagic *Escherichia coli* (EHEC) including *E. coli* O157:H7 and other Shiga toxin–producing *E. coli* (STEC)	1-8 days	Severe diarrhea that is often bloody, abdominal pain, and vomiting Usually little or no fever More common in children <4 years old	5-10 days	Undercooked beef, especially hamburger, unpasteurized milk and juice, raw fruits, vegetables (e.g., sprouts, spinach, lettuce), salami (rarely) Contaminated water; petting zoos	Stool culture; *E. coli* O157:H7 requires special media to grow. If *E. coli* O157:H7 is suspected, specific testing must be requested. Shiga toxin testing may be done using commercial kits; positive isolates should be forwarded to public health laboratories for confirmation and serotyping. Stool grossly positive for blood.	Supportive care: Monitor CBC, platelets, and kidney function closely. *E. coli* O157:H7 infection is also associated with HUS, which can cause lifelong complications. Studies indicate that antibiotics may promote the development of HUS.

TABLE 40.12   Diarrheal Illnesses Due to Common Bacterial or Viral Pathogens—cont'd

Etiology	Incubation Period	Signs and Symptoms	Duration of Illness	Route of Transmission	Laboratory Testing	Treatment and Complications*
Enterotoxigenic E. coli (ETEC) and enteroadherent E. coli (frequent cause of traveler's diarrhea)	1-3 days	Watery diarrhea, abdominal cramps, some vomiting; often cause of mild traveler's diarrhea	3 to >7 days	Water or food contaminated with human feces	Stool culture. ETEC requires special laboratory techniques for identification. If suspected, must request specific testing.	Supportive care: Antibiotics are rarely needed except in severe cases. Recommended antibiotics include **TMP-SMX, azithromycin, ciprofloxacin,** and **metronidazole.** See www.cdc.gov/travel.
Listeria monocytogenes	Variable, ranging from 1 day to more than 3 weeks	Rare, but serious Fever, muscle aches, and nausea or diarrhea Pregnant women may have mild flulike illness, and infection can lead to premature delivery or stillbirth Older adults or immunocompromised patients may have bacteremia or meningitis Infants infected from mother at risk for sepsis or meningitis	Variable	Thrives in salty and acidic conditions, such as fresh soft cheeses, ready-to-eat deli meats, hot dogs; also unpasteurized milk, inadequately pasteurized milk; multiplies at low temperatures, even in properly refrigerated foods	Blood or cerebrospinal fluid cultures. Asymptomatic fecal carriage occurs; therefore, stool culture usually not helpful. Antibody to listeriolysin O may be helpful to identify outbreak retrospectively.	Initial therapy with IV **ampicillin** and an **aminoglycoside** usually **gentamicin,** recommended for severe infections.
Adenovirus, enteric	3-10 days	Children >4 years old	Variable	Fecal-oral, throughout year; can remain viable on inanimate objects	Stool specimen for adenovirus antigen via rapid commercial immunoassay techniques or per electron microscopy.	Supportive care: Monitor intake and hydration status. Preventive care: Good hand washing and diapering precaution.
Norovirus	12-48 h	Abrupt-onset watery diarrhea, nausea, vomiting, abdominal cramps	24-60 h Often associated with closed venues (child care centers, cruise ships)	Fecal-oral; contaminated food (ice, shellfish, ready-to-eat foods [e.g., salads, bakery products], or water)	No commercial assay available; CDC can support laboratory evaluation or state and local health department laboratories can perform RT-PCR assays.	Supportive care: May need to treat dehydration and/or electrolyte imbalance. Preventive care: Hand hygiene, clean surfaces and food preparation areas; no swimming in recreational venues for 2 weeks after symptoms resolve.
Rotavirus	1-3 days; prevalent during cooler months in temperate climates	Acute-onset fever, vomiting, and watery diarrhea occur 2-4 days later in children <5 years old, especially those between 3 and 24 months old	3-8 days	Fecal-oral; viable on inanimate objects; rarely contaminated water or food	Enzyme immunoassay and latex agglutination assays for group A rotavirus antigen; virus can be found by electron microscopy and specific nucleic acid amplification methods.	Supportive care: May need to correct dehydration and electrolyte imbalances. Oral IG has been used in those immunocompromised. Preventive care: Rotavirus vaccine; hygiene and diapering precautions in day care facilities.

Continued

TABLE 40.12 Diarrheal Illnesses Due to Common Bacterial or Viral Pathogens—cont'd

Etiology	Incubation Period	Signs and Symptoms	Duration of Illness	Route of Transmission	Laboratory Testing	Treatment and Complications*
Salmonella spp.	1–3 days	Diarrhea, fever, abdominal cramps, rebound tenderness, vomiting. *Salmonella typhi* and *Salmonella paratyphi* produce typhoid with insidious onset characterized by fever, headache, constipation, malaise, chills, and myalgia; diarrhea is uncommon, and vomiting is not usually severe	4–7 days	Contaminated eggs, poultry, unpasteurized milk or juice, cheese, contaminated raw fruits and vegetables (alfalfa sprouts, melons) *S. typhi* epidemics are often related to fecal contamination of water supplies or street-vended foods	Routine stool cultures; positive leukocytes and gross blood. CBC: WBC can be slightly ↑ with left shift, ↓, or normal.	Supportive care: *Only consider antibiotics (other than for S. typhi or S. paratyphi)* for infants <3 months old, those with chronic GI disease, malignant neoplasm, hemoglobinopathies, HIV, other immunosuppressive illnesses or therapies. If indicated, consider **ampicillin or amoxicillin, azithromycin,** or **TMP-SMX**; if resistance shown to any of those, use IM **ceftriaxone, cefotaxime;** or **azithromycin** or **quinolones.** A vaccine exists for *S. typhi* in certain cases.
Shigella spp.	Varies from 1–7 days, but typically is 1–3 days	Abdominal cramps, fever, and diarrhea; Stools may contain blood and mucus. Seen most commonly in those 6 months old to 3 years old	4–7 days	Food or water contaminated with human fecal material. Usually person-to-person spread, fecal-oral transmission. Ready-to-eat foods touched by infected food workers (e.g., raw vegetables, salads, sandwiches)	Routine stool cultures; gross blood, leukocytes. CBC: normal or slightly ↑ WBCs with left shift.	Supportive care: If antibiotics indicated (severe disease, dysentery, immunocompromised), test first for susceptibility. Oral **ampicillin (amoxicillin** less so) or **TMP-SMX** recommended in the United States; for organism resistance, use IM **ceftriaxone** for 2–5 days; PO **ciprofloxacin; azithromycin** (oral cephalosporins not useful). If child is at risk of malnutrition, supplement with vitamin A (200,000 international units). No swimming in recreational pools/slides for 1 week after symptoms resolve.
Yersinia enterocolitica and *Y. pseudotuberculosis*	Typically 4–6 days with a range of 1–14 days	Appendicitis-like symptoms (diarrhea and vomiting, fever, and RLQ pain) occur primarily in older children and young adults. May have a scarlatiniform rash or erythema nodosum with *Y. pseudotuberculosis*. Seen in all ages	1–3 weeks, usually self-limiting	Undercooked pork, unpasteurized milk, tofu, contaminated water. Infection has occurred in infants whose caregivers handled chitterlings	Stool, vomitus, or blood culture. *Yersinia* requires special medium to grow. If suspected, must request specific testing. Serology is available in research and reference laboratories.	Supportive care: If septicemia or other invasive disease occurs, antibiotic therapy with **gentamicin** or **cefotaxime (doxycycline** and **ciprofloxacin** also effective) after susceptibility testing is done.

CBC, Complete blood count; *CDC*, Centers for Disease Control and Prevention; *ESR*, erythrocyte sedimentation rate; *GI*, gastrointestinal; *HIV*, human immunodeficiency virus; *HUS*, hemolytic uremic syndrome; *IG*, immunoglobulin; *IM*, intramuscular; *IV*, intravenous; *RLQ*, right lower quadrant; *RT-PCR*, reverse transcription-polymerase chain reaction; *TMP-SMX*, trimethoprim-sulfamethoxazole; *WBC*, white blood cell.

Adapted from Department of Health and Human Services, Centers for Disease Control and Prevention (CDC). Diagnosis and management of food borne illnesses: a primer for physicians and other health professionals. *MMWR Morb Mortal Wkly Rep.* 2004;53(RR04):7–9. Additional information from Mezoff EA, Cohen MB. *Clostridium difficile* infection. In: Kliegman RM, Behrman RE, Jenson HB, et al., eds. *Nelson Textbook of Pediatrics.* 19th ed. Philadelphia: Elsevier; 2011:994; and Red book. *2012 Report of the Committee on Infectious Diseases.* 29th ed. Elk Grove Village: American Academy of Pediatrics; 2012.

TABLE 40.13 Common Causes of Chronic Diarrhea Seen in Children

Age	Conditions
0-6 months old	• Carbohydrate malabsorption (acquired, congenital) (e.g., CMPI) • Protein hypersensitivity • Excessive intake of formula or other fluid (water, juice [especially those containing sorbitol/fructose], high-carbohydrate liquids) • Postenteritis • Infections • CF or other fat absorption conditions • Neuroblastoma (rare) • Immunodeficiency (e.g., HIV/AIDS and others) • Lymphangiectasia (rare) • Hirschsprung disease • Neonatal or infant enteropathies (rare) • Radiation treatments
7-24 months old	First eight bulleted conditions listed above plus: • Chronic nonspecific diarrhea • Small-bowel overgrowth • Celiac disease • Graft-versus-host enteropathy • Autoimmune enteropathy • Radiation treatments
>24 months old	• Excessive intake of fruit juice/high-carbohydrate drinks • Infections • Small-bowel bacterial overgrowth • Celiac disease • Munchausen syndrome by proxy • Grant-versus-host enteropathy • Carbohydrate malabsorption • IBS • Adult-type hypolactasia • Encopresis • IBD (e.g., Crohn disease) • Excessive use of laxatives • Radiation treatments • Acquired lactase deficiency in older children, primarily of African, Asian, or Middle Eastern descent • Perforated appendix

AIDS, Acquired immune deficiency syndrome; *CF*, cystic fibrosis; *CMPI*, cow's-milk protein intolerance; *HIV*, human immunodeficiency virus; *IBD*, inflammatory bowel disease; *IBS*, irritable bowel syndrome.

Data from Guarino A, LoVecchio A, Berni Canani R. Chronic diarrhea in children. *Best Pract Res Clin Gastroenterol.* 2012;26(5):649–661; Lee KS, Kang DS, Yu J, et al. How to do in persistent diarrhea of children? Concepts and treatments of chronic diarrhea. *Pediatr Gastroenterol Hepatol Nutr.* 2012;15(4):229–236.

• Dioctahedral smectite, adsorbent clay, is used in many countries to protect the intestinal mucosa by absorbing viruses, bacteria, and bacterial toxins; there are few reported side effects. Studies have shown that smectite can reduce the duration of diarrhea (Piescik-Lech et al., 2013).
• Oral enteric peppermint oil capsules have been studied for use with diarrhea, cramping, and bloating, especially when related to IBS. It may produce smooth muscle relaxation, slow food transit through the intestines, and help with general symptom relief; its efficacy is still debated. Essential peppermint oil *(Mentha piperita)* aromatherapy can be used for abdominal pain and relaxation. See Chapter 27 for complementary medicine therapies for diarrhea.
• Zinc is commonly prescribed to shorten the duration of acute diarrhea in children >6 months from developing countries. Zinc was efficacious for diarrhea caused by *Klebsiella,* not necessarily for *E. coli* or parasitic infections, and was detrimental when used in infections caused by rotavirus. The administration of zinc was shown to reduce the duration of the diarrhea as well as frequency and amount of stool. The World Health Organization (WHO) recommends routine use of zinc supplementation, at a dosage of 20 mg per day for children older than 6 months. In the study by Yazar et al. (2016), they used a standard dose of 15 mg per day.

Complications

See Table 40.12 for complications associated with some common pathogens.

Prevention

Preventive measures include the following:
• Good hand washing by all individuals (including children and all care providers), especially when handling food: Liquid soap and paper towels are recommended at day care centers. Use of non-water alcohol hand sanitizers with an ethanol content of at least 60% has also shown efficacy to reduce GI illnesses (CDC, 2011).
• Good sanitation and appropriate removal of soiled clothing and diapers: The diapering area should be cleaned after changing each child at day care centers.
• Avoid contaminated sources; meat should be properly cooked.
• Promote exclusive breastfeeding for the first 6 months of life to promote passive immunity and guard against exposure to contaminated food and water.
• Promote appropriate supplemental nutrition starting at 6 months (breastfeeding should continue through the first year or longer in developing countries), food handling, and storage.
• In developing countries, consider addition of vitamin A and zinc in cases of malnutrition.
• With *Shigella,* culture all symptomatic contacts and treat those with positive stool cultures.
• Avoid unnecessary antibiotic usage.
• Promote well-functioning sewage system in developing countries (including latrines, septic tanks, dry-composting toilets), which can cut diarrheal illness by up to 30%.
• Promote rotavirus vaccine for all children worldwide.

Chronic Diarrhea

Chronic diarrhea is defined as loose stools of less than 10 mL/kg/day in infants and less than 200 g/24 hours in older children. The terms *persistent* or *prolonged diarrhea* have also been used when describing a state of chronic diarrhea; these generally refer to a continuing diarrheal illness that started as acute diarrhea and is affecting growth. Diarrhea that is chronic is the result of intraluminal factors (that influence digestion) or mucosal factors (that influence digestion and transport of nutrients across the mucosa); either factor affects the normal cellular mechanisms of the GI tract. Because "persistent" diarrhea is generally associated with an acute diarrheal onset, it is surmised that there is either persistent infectious colonization with an enteric pathogen or impaired healing and return to the normal intestinal processes/structure. Table 40.13 lists the most common causes of chronic diarrhea by age group. Infants and children have difficulty absorbing volumes of liquid larger than 200 mL/kg/day; an excess can cause diarrhea, which is not an uncommon finding in early childhood ("toddler's diarrhea").

Clinical Findings
History
- Occurrence of three or more watery stools per day for more than 2 weeks; 10 watery/runny stools per day that often contain undigested food particles is more typical of "toddler's diarrhea"
- Presence of red flags:
  - Hematochezia or melena
  - Persistent fever
  - Weight loss or growth arrest
  - Anemia
- Dietary history (including amount of fruit juices or high-carbohydrate fluids ingested per day)
- Stool consistency, blood, mucus, pus, particles of food
- Stool incontinence
- Exposure to illness (including day care; contact with pets/other animals)
- Teething
- Prior treatments for diarrhea (any dietary manipulation, drug, or home treatments)
- Recent travel

Physical Examination. Look for physical findings associated with the underlying pathologic condition:
- Assessment of hydration status
- Weight and height measurements; any weight loss
- Growth retardation
- Skin and hair condition, color of skin and conjunctivae
- Vital signs (heart rate and blood pressure)
- Palpation of the thyroid for enlargement
- Increased heart rate
- Respiratory symptoms
- Clubbing of fingers
- Abdominal examination
- Rectal examination (skin tags, impaction, tenderness)

Diagnostic Studies
- Stool: Culture, O&P (best done on three specimens collected on separate days), pH (Normal stool pH greater than 5.5 indicates negative carbohydrate.), reducing substances, occult blood, leukocytes, fat and fecal elastase (to evaluate for pancreatic insufficiency)
- CBC with differential, electrolytes, and albumin
- UA and culture in young children

The following are ordered as indicated by the history, physical examination, and consideration of differential diagnoses:
- ESR, CRP
- Hormonal studies to assess for secretory tumors (vasoactive intestinal peptide, gastrin, secretin, urine assay for 5-hydroxytryptamine [5-HT])
- Breath hydrogen test for lactose or sucrose intolerance (difficult to assess in infants)
- Viral serologies, such as HIV or CMV
- Sweat chloride test
- Endoscopy, barium studies

Differential Diagnosis
See Table 40.13.

Management
- Treat the underlying cause.
- Chronic nonspecific diarrhea (toddler's diarrhea): Normalize the diet; remove offending foods and fluids; eliminate sorbitol and fructose-containing fluids; reduce fluid intake to no greater than 90 mL/kg/24 hours (give half of fluid as milk [whole or 2%]); increase fat intake to 35% up to 40% of the diet; and increase fiber to bulk up stools.
- Treat carbohydrate malabsorption by decreasing lactose or sucrose; add lactase or sacrosidase as indicated by particular carbohydrate intolerance.
- Post-gastroenteritis malabsorption syndrome (evidenced in infants with weight loss and fat globules in the stool) can be given a predigested formula (e.g., Pregestimil or Alimentum), if tolerated, for 3 to 4 weeks (elemental formula can be used if those are not tolerated). Refer the following patients to a gastroenterologist: Newborns with diarrhea in first hours of life; patients with growth delay or failure or abnormal physical findings (anorexia, abdominal pain, chronic bloating, vomiting, or weakness); or those with severe illness.

Complications
Malnutrition, growth failure, and cognitive/developmental impairments (found more in developing countries) can occur.

Intestinal Parasites

Various protozoa and helminths can invade the GI tract and cause disease. In developed countries, such infestations are usually by protozoa. Endemic areas of developing countries are subject to more significant morbidity and mortality from parasitic infestations. All can multiply within the human body, are associated with diarrheal symptoms, and are spread by fecal contamination due to poor water and sewage disposal practices. Cysts of these parasites are often resistant to chlorine.

Helminths are worm: nematodes (roundworms), cestodes (tapeworms), and trematodes (flatworms) that most commonly reside in the human intestines but do not multiply there. Fecal-oral contact with eggs or cysts excreted from the initial vector via ingestion of contaminated food or water is one route of infestation. Some helminths (hookworms and whipworms) release larvae into the soil; humans become infected when they walk barefoot on contaminated soil and the skin is penetrated by the larvae. These larvae then travel to the lungs and intestines. Eggs can also be excreted in the stool; poor sanitary disposal of human waste into soils affords the further potential for ingestion via contamination of food and water. They are found worldwide, principally in tropical and subtropical developing countries. In industrialized countries, infestation is found in those who travel to endemic areas, in the immunocompromised, and immigrants from endemic areas. Their insidious nature causes chronic health and nutritional problems that can impair physical and mental growth of children. *Enterobius vermicularis* (pinworm), *Ascaris lumbricoides* (roundworm), and *Taenia* (tapeworm) are some of the more common intestinal parasites that affect the pediatric population (CDC, 2015).

Clinical Findings, Management, and Differential Diagnosis
See Tables 40.14 and 40.15 for clinical findings and management. The differential diagnosis includes all other causes of infectious and noninfectious diarrhea.

TABLE 40.14 Intestinal Illnesses Due to More Common Parasites (Protozoa and Helminths)

Etiology	Incubation Period	Signs and Symptoms	Duration of Illness	Route of Transmission	Laboratory Testing	Treatment[a]
Cryptosporidium parvum	3–14 days	Diarrhea (usually watery), stomach cramps, upset stomach, bloating, slight fever, anorexia, weight loss, flatulence, nausea, vomiting, fatigue	Self-limiting, usually lasts 6–14 days	Fecal–oral route; from uncooked food or food contaminated by an ill food handler after cooking; drinking water (collects on water filters and membranes that cannot be disinfected); reservoirs include cattle, sheep, goats, birds, reptiles, young animals	Request specific testing of the stool for Cryptosporidium using antigen-detection tests. May need to examine water or food.	Supportive care, self-limited. If severe, or individual immunocompromised consider **paromomycin** for 7 days. For children 1–11 years old, consider **nitazoxanide** for 3 days.
Cyclospora cayetanensis	Usually 7 days, but can range from 2 to 14 days	Diarrhea (usually watery), loss of appetite, substantial loss of weight, stomach cramps, nausea, vomiting, fatigue, myalgia, low-grade fevers	May remit and relapse over weeks to months	Fecal–oral from sewage or nontreated water; food (various types of fresh produce [imported berries, lettuce])	Request specific examination of the stool for Cyclospora. May need to examine water or food.	**TMP-SMX** for 7–10 days.
Entamoeba histolytica	Commonly 2–4 weeks (known to also range from days, months, to years); fecal–oral transmission	Can be asymptomatic with nonspecific complaints of diarrhea, lower abdominal pain In invasive disease (amebic colitis) symptoms of increasing diarrhea, bloody diarrhea, lower abdominal pain, tenesmus, weight loss progress over a 1- to 3-week period; occasional fever Advanced disease hepatomegaly, liver tenderness	Weeks to years, depending on response to treatment; no drug is completely effective	Spread by fecal–oral route	Stool examination for trophozoites or cysts; PCR, isoenzyme analysis, monoclonal antibody–based antigen; enzyme immunoassay; ultrasounds and CT scans to identify suspected liver abscess or other extraintestinal infection.	Asymptomatic cyst excreters: Luminal amebicide (**iodoquinol, paromomycin, diloxanide**). Mild to moderate or severe involvement/liver abscesses: **metronidazole** or **tinidazole** followed by luminal amebicide. Follow-up stool examination after treatment. Perform stool examinations on household members or other suspected contacts. Do not treat with corticosteroids or antimotility drugs. Complications include liver abscess, ameboma.
Giardia intestinalis	3 weeks	Can include bouts of watery diarrhea; abdominal pain, greasy, foul-smelling stools; bloody diarrhea (rare); flatulence; abdominal distention; anorexia; weight loss; FTT; anemia; asymptomatic infection common	Pending effective treatment	Fecal–oral or contaminated food or water. Water can be contaminated by *Giardia* from dogs, cats, beavers, and other animals.	Stool specimens for trophozoites or cysts using staining methods; antigens using enzyme immunoassay; PCR techniques. Increased sensitivity by obtaining three or more specimens every other day and by rapid examination of stool (can be placed in a fixative).	Correct for any dehydration or electrolyte imbalance. **Tinidazole, metronidazole, nitazoxanide** drugs of choice. **Albendazole, mebendazole** effective also in children with fewer side effects. Consult for those immunocompromised. Contact local health departments in cases of outbreaks. Infected individuals should not use recreational water sources for swimming until 2 weeks after symptoms resolve. Filtration, boiling, chemical disinfection may be required for drinking water. Some infections are self-limited and treatment is not required. Dehydration and electrolyte abnormalities can occur and should be corrected. Complications: Debilitating disease leading to malabsorption; anorexia; weight loss; FTT.

Continued

TABLE 40.14 Intestinal Illnesses Due to More Common Parasites (Protozoa and Helminths)—cont'd

Etiology	Incubation Period	Signs and Symptoms	Duration of Illness	Route of Transmission	Laboratory Testing	Treatment[a]
Ancylostoma duodenale (hookworm)	5–8 weeks for eggs to appear in feces; 4–12 weeks for onset of symptoms	Often asymptomatic or stinging/burning sensation in feet followed by pruritus, papulovesicular rash (lasting up to 2 weeks), pharyngeal itching, hoarseness, nausea, vomiting. As migrates through lungs: Mild cough, pneumonitis. Chronic infestation: Anemia, edema, growth delays, slowed development and cognition in children	5 years unless treated	Larvae in feces-contaminated soil penetrate skin (travel to lungs and settle in the intestines) or are directly ingested from contaminated food or water, including human milk.	CBC shows hypochromic microcytic anemia, eosinophilia; hypoproteinemia. Stool microscopic examination for ova.	**Albendazole, pyrantel pamoate**; repeat stool examination in 2 weeks recommended. Iron and nutritional supplementation if indicated; severe cases require blood transfusions. Complications: Delayed growth, developmental/mental status delays in children.
Enterobius vermicularis (pinworm)	1–2 months, or longer from ingestion to migration to perianal area	Perirectal and/or vaginal pruritus; nervous irritability, hyperactivity, insomnia; urethritis, vaginitis, salpingitis, and pelvic peritonitis have been reported	Reinfection common in children	Ingested eggs from soil, water contamination, or direct fecal-oral route from fomites on bedding, clothing, toys, baths; person-to-person. Female lays eggs in perianal area and dies; ingested eggs hatch, become larvae in small intestine, and migrate to rectum.	1 cm long white, thread-like worms can be visualized at anus during night after child has been asleep for 2–3 h. Microscopic examination: Use transparent adhesive tape applied to anus to collect any eggs or pinworms present on three consecutive nights or mornings before child arises. Direct stool examination usually not productive.	**Mebendazole, pyrantel pamoate, or albendazole** and repeated in 2 weeks; also treat family members; vaginitis is self-limiting. Easily spread among family members, in day care settings, and institutions (up to 50% infestation rates in these populations). Preventive: Morning baths, change bedding, hand hygiene, clip fingernails, avoid scratching perianal region, avoid nail biting. Day care precautions include hand hygiene, proper handling of underwear and diapers.
Ascaris lumbricoides (roundworm)	8 weeks from egg ingestion to adult egg-laying capacity	Weight loss, malnutrition; worms can be seen in vomitus and stools; can cause cough, fever, chest discomfort if pass through lungs (not a common occurrence). Children can have large worm burdens. Stressful conditions (fever, illness) and some anthelmintic drugs can cause adults to migrate	12–18 months without treatment	Fecal-oral from ingestion of eggs from contaminated food (fruit, vegetables) or soil (where incubation occurs; adult worms live in small intestine and eggs are excreted in feces). Larvae migrate from intestines via portal blood to liver and lungs, ascend through tracheobronchial tree to pharynx, to intestines again to develop into adults. Found in areas where human feces are used for fertilizer.	Stool/vomitus/nares: Worms seen via microscopy. CBC: Marked eosinophilia. Have laboratory check for all concurrent worm infestations in order to treat all worms appropriately.	**Albendazole, mebendazole, ivermectin**; surgical intervention if necessary. Complications: Impaired nutritional status of children and growth; bowel or biliary obstruction, peritonitis, obstruction of common bile duct (biliary colic, cholangitis, pancreatitis); Löffler syndrome due to allergic response as larvae migrate to the lungs. Reinfection common. Globally, most common human intestinal nematode.

TABLE 40.14   Intestinal Illnesses Due to More Common Parasites (Protozoa and Helminths)—cont'd

Etiology	Incubation Period	Signs and Symptoms	Duration of Illness	Route of Transmission	Laboratory Testing	Treatment[a]
Taenia (tape-worm) (*T. saginata* [beef]; *T. solium* [pork])	2-3 months after larvae ingested to feces excretion	Worm(s) may be seen in peri-anal region. May be asymptomatic or have abdominal pain, nausea, diar-rhea, excessive appetite	Several years before cysticercosis symptoms evident	Fecal-oral from ingestion of water or food contami-nated with eggs or from ingested cysts or larvae in inadequately cooked pork or beef.	Stool microscopy: ova seen.	**Praziquantel, niclosamide, nitazoxanide.** Complications: Systemic cysticercosis from *T. solium* (viscera, brain, muscle invasion with possible seizures).
Trichuris trichiura (whip-worm)	12 weeks	Asymptomatic unless infestation is heavy; abdominal pain, tenesmus, bloody diarrhea with mucus; can mimic IBD; growth retardation		Fecal-oral from contaminated soil (where eggs incubate), water, and/or food (embeds in mucosal lining of large intestines). Not spread person to person.	Stool microscopy or con-centration techniques.	**Mebendazole, albendazole, ivermectin** for 3 days; can reexamine stools after 2 weeks to ensure resolution. Complications: Chronic colitis, rectal prolapse, com-promised nutritional status, growth retardation.

CBC, Complete blood count; *CT,* computed tomography; *FTT,* failure to thrive; *IBD,* inflammatory bowel disease; *PCR,* polymerase chain reaction; *TMP-SMX,* trimethoprim-sulfamethoxazole.
[a]See Table 40.15 for dosages.

TABLE 40.15	Medications for Treatment of Parasite Infestations
Drug	**Dosage**
Albendazole (Albenza): Take with food. The tablet may be crushed or chewed and swallowed with a drink of water.	*Ascariasis:* 1 year old: 200 mg once; >2 years old: 400 mg once *Taenia solium:* 15 mg/kg/day in 2 doses × 8-30 days; can be repeated as necessary (maximum 400 mg per dose)
Mebendazole (Vermox): Tablet may be crushed, mixed with food, swallowed whole, or chewed.	*Pinworms:* 100 mg once; may need to repeat in 2 weeks Whipworms, roundworms, and hookworms: 100 mg twice daily for 3 days *Toxocariasis:* 100-200 mg twice daily for 5 days
Diloxanide furoate (Furamide): Give with meals.	20 mg/kg/day in 3 doses × 10 days (maximum 500 mg per dose)
Ivermectin (Stromectol): Take on an empty stomach.	All ages: 150-200 mcg/kg/dose once
Iodoquinol (Yodoxin): Administer after meals, tablets may be crushed and mixed with applesauce or chocolate syrup.	30-40 mg/kg/day in 3 doses × 20 days (maximum 2 g) Adults: 650 mg 3 times daily × 20 days
Metronidazole (Flagyl)	35-50 mg/kg/day in 3 doses × 7 to 10 days (maximum 500-750 mg per dose) *Giardia lamblia:* 15 mg/kg/day in 3 doses × 5 days (maximum 250 mg per dose)
Nitazoxanide (Alinia): Administer with food, shake suspension well prior to use.	1-3 years old: 100 mg in 2 doses × 3 days 4-11 years old: 200 mg in 2 doses × 3 days 11 years old to adult: 500 mg twice daily × 3 days
Paromomycin (Humatin): Administer with or without meals, protect from moisture.	25-35 mg/kg/day in 3 doses × 7 days
Praziquantel (Biltricide): Administer tablets with water during meals; do not chew due to bitter taste.	*Tapeworm:* 5-10 mg/kg once *Liver Fluke:* Up to 75 mg/kg in 3 doses in 1 day
Pyrantel pamoate (Pamix, Pin-X): Over the counter. May be mixed with milk or fruit juice. Shake suspension well.	11 mg/kg daily (maximum 1 g) × 3 days Use with caution in children <2 years old
Tinidazole (Tindamax)	*Giardia lamblia:* 50 mg/kg once (maximum 2 g)

Medication choices and dosages are dependent upon child's condition at diagnosis and parasite. Consult CDC or latest recommendations for treatment regimens.

Data from Schleiss MR, Chen SF. Principles of antiparasitic therapy. In: Kliegman RM, Behrman RE, Jenson HB, et al., eds. *Nelson Textbook of Pediatrics.* 19th ed. Philadelphia: Elsevier; 2011.

Patient and Family Education

Most parasitic infestations can be prevented by good hand washing and good sanitation. The following preventive measures are recommended:

- Travelers to developing countries need to eat only foods that can be peeled or have been cooked. Ice, "washed" foods, and tap water can be contaminated. Bottled or treated water is advised for drinking and brushing teeth. Shoes should be worn when walking on potentially contaminated soil.
- *G. lamblia:* Encourage good hand hygiene. Prevent contamination of water sources. Treat questionable water with iodine, boiling for 20 minutes, or use commercial filters to filter contaminated water. Exclude symptomatic children and staff from school and day care until asymptomatic.
- *E. vermicularis:* Avoid scratching. Wash sheets and clothing in hot water and detergent.
- *A. lumbricoides:* Appropriate food preparation is necessary to prevent infection. When human feces are used for fertilizer, thoroughly cook or soak fruits and vegetables in diluted iodine solution before consuming. Periodic, empiric treatment of children may prevent nutritional and cognitive deficits in endemic areas.
- *Taenia:* Avoid raw or undercooked beef or pork.

Congenital Gastrointestinal Conditions

These are discussed in Chapter 29 with other perinatal concerns.

Additional Resources

American Gastroenterological Association.
    www.gastro.org
Canadian Celiac Association.
    www.celiac.ca
Celiac Disease Foundation.
    http://celiac.org
Celiac Support Association.
    www.csaceliacs.org
Crohn's and Colitis Foundation of America (CCFA).
    www.ccfa.org
Cyclic Vomiting Syndrome Association.
    www.cvsaonline.org
Gastroparesis and Dysmotilities Association.
    www.digestivedistress.com/
Improve Care Now.
    www.improvecarenow.org
International Foundation for Functional Gastrointestinal Disorders (IFFGD).
    www.iffgd.org
National Institute of Diabetes and Digestive and Kidney Diseases.
    www.niddk.nih.gov
North American Society for Pediatric Gastroenterology, Hepatology, and Nutrition (NASPGHAN).
    www.naspghan.org
Rehydration Project.
    http://rehydrate.org/solutions/homemade.htm
Rome Foundation: Functional Gastrointestinal Disorders.
    www.romecriteria.org

References

Alder AC. *Pediatric Appendicitis. Medscape (Website)*; 2017. Available at http://emedicine.medscape.com/article/926795. Accessed April 13, 2018.
Altowati M, Jones A, Hickey H, et al. Assessing the feasibility of injectable growth-promoting therapy in Crohn's disease. *Pilot Feasibility Studies.* 2016;2(71):1–9.

American Academy of Otolaryngology—Head and Neck Surgery (AAO-HNS). *Pediatric GERD (gastroesophageal reflux disease)*; 2018. Available at www.entnet.org/HealthInformation/pediatricGERD.cfm Accessed April 13, 2018.

Barnhart DC. Gastroesophageal reflux disease in children. *Semi Pediatr Surg.* 2016;25(4):212–218.

Benninga M, Faure C, Hyman P, St James Roberts I, Scvhecter N, Nurko S. Childhood functional gastrointestinal disorders: Neonate/Toddler. *Gastroenterology.* 2016;150:14443–14457.

Bishop WP, Ebach D. The digestive system. In: Marcdante KJ, Kliegman RM, eds. *Nelson Essentials of Pediatrics.* 7th ed. Philadelphia: Elsevier; 2015.

Bohm M, Jacobs JW, Gupta A, Gupta S, Wo JM. Most children with eosinophilic esophagitis have a favorable outcome as young adults. *Dis Esophagus.* 2017;30(1):1–6.

Brown L, Beattie R, Tighe M. Practical management of functional abdominal pain in children. *Arch Dis Child.* 2016;101(7):677–683.

Camilleri M, Sellin J, Barrett K. Pathophysiology, evaluation, and management of chronic watery diarrhea. *Gastroenterology.* 2017;152(3):515–532.

Cardile S, Alterio T, Arrigo T, Salpietro C. Role of prebiotics and probiotics in pediatric diseases. *Minerva Pediatrica.* 2016;68(6):487–497.

Centers for Disease Control and Prevention (CDC). *Diarrhea: Common illness, global killer.* CDC (website); N.D. Available at https://www.cdc.gov/healthywater/pdf/global/programs/globaldiarrhea508c.pdf. Accessed October 31, 2018.

Centers for Disease Control and Prevention (CDC). *Guideline for the Prevention and Control of Norovirus Gastroenteritis Outbreaks in Healthcare Settings: Summary of Guidelines.* CDC (Website); 2015. Available at https://www.cdc.gov/infectioncontrol/guidelines/norovirus/index.html. Accessed April 14, 2018.

Centers for Disease Control and Prevention (CDC). *Inflammatory Bowel Disease.* CDC (Website); 2017. Available at www.cdc.gov/ibd/. Accessed April 14, 2018.

Centers for Disease Control and Prevention (CDC). *Parasites: Children.* CDC (Website); 2015. Available at https://www.cdc.gov/parasites/children.html. Accessed April 14, 2018.

Chau K, Lau E, Greenberg S, et al. Probiotics for infantile colic: a randomized, double-blind, placebo-controlled trial. *J Pediatr.* 2015;166(1):74–78.

Chopra J, Patel N, Basude D, Gil-Zargozano E, Paul S. Abdominal pain-related functional gastrointestinal disorders in children. *British J Nurs.* 2017;26(11):624–631.

Dafer RM, Lutse HL. Migraine variants; 2017. Available at https://emedicine.medscape.com/article/1142731-overview. Accessed April 14, 2018.

da Silva B, Lyra A, Rocha R, Santana G. Epidemiology, demographic characteristics and prognostic predictors of ulcerative colitis. *World J Gastroenterol.* 2014;20(28):9458–9467.

Dassow P, Fox S. When infants and children benefit from probiotics? *J Fam Pract.* 2016;65(11):789–794.

De Felice K, Katzka D, Raffals L. Crohn's disease of the Esophagus: clinical features and treatment outcomes in the biologic era. *Inflamm Bowel Dis.* 2016;21(9):2106–2113.

Dobowitz H, Black M. *Failure to thrive, BMJ Best Practice* (Online). 2018. Available at: http://bestpractice.bmj.com/best-practice/monograph/747.html. Accessed April 14, 2018.

Eberly MD, Eide MB, Thompson JL, Nylund CM. Azithromycin in early infancy and pyloric stenosis. *Pediatrics.* 2015;135(3):483–488.

Edwards A, Pigg N, Courtier J, Zapala M, MacKenzie J, Phelps A. Intussusception: past, present and future. *Pediatric Ultrasound.* 2017;47(9):1101–1108.

El-Baba MF, Cuffari C. *Pediatric Irritable Bowel Syndrome.* Medscape (Website); 2016. Available at https://emedicine.medscape.com/article/930844. Accessed April 13, 2018.

Fiocchi A, et al. The global impact of the DRACMA guidelines cow's milk allergy clinical practice. *World Allergy Organ J.* 2018;11(1).

Freedman S, Hall M, Shah S, et al. Impact of increasing ondansetron use on clinical outcomes in children with gastroenteritis. *JAMA Pediatr.* 2014;168(4):321–329.

Giannattasio A, Guarino A, Lo Vecchio A. Management of children with prolonged diarrhea. *F1000 Faculty Reviews.* 2016;206:1–11.

Gibson G, Roberfroid M. Dietary modulation of the human colonic microbiota: introducing the concept of prebiotics. *J Nutr.* 1995;125(6):1401–1412.

Goh L, How C, Ng K. Failure to thrive in babies and toddlers. *Singapore Med J.* 2016;57(6):287–291.

Gonzalez-Ochoa G, Flores-Mendoza L, Icedo-Garcia R Gomez-Flores R, Tamez-Guerra P. Modulation of rotavirus severe gastroenteritis by the combination of probiotics and prebiotics. *Arch Microbiol.* 2017;6:953–961.

Gordon M, MacDonald J, Parker C, Akobeng A, Thomas A. Osmotic and stimulant laxatives for the management of childhood constipation. *Cochrane Database Syst Rev.* 2016;8:CD009118. https://doi.org/10.1002/14651858.CD009118.pub3.

Guandalini S. *Diarrhea.* Medscape (Website); 2017. Available at http://emedicine.medscape.com/article/928598. Accessed April 14, 2018.

Guarino A, Ashkenazi S, Gendrel D, LoVecchio A, Shamir R, Szajewska H. European society for pediatric gastroenterology, hepatology, and Nutrition/European society for pediatric infectious diseases evidence-based guidelines for the management of acute gastroenteritis in children in Europe: updated 2014. *J Pediatr Gastroenterol Nutr.* 2014;59(1):132–152.

Hejl J, Theede K, Mollgren B, et al. Point of care testing of fecal calprotectin as a substitute for routine laboratory analysis. *Practical Laboratory Medicine.* 2017;10:10–14.

Hill HD, Fasano A, Guandalini S, et al. NASPGHAN Clinical report on the diagnosis and treatment of gluten-related disorders. *J Pediatr Gastroenterol Nutr.* 2016;63(1):156–165.

Hojsak I. Probiotics in children: what is the evidence? *Pediatr Gastroenterol Hepatol Nutr.* 2017;20(3):139–146.

Hurtado C, Li BU. *The NASPGHAN Fellows Concise Review of Pediatric Gastroenterology, Hepatology and Nutrition.* 2nd ed; 2017.

Hyams J, Di Lorenzo C, Saps M, Shulman R, Staiano A, Van Tilburg M. Functional disorders: Child/Adolescent. *Gastroenterology.* 2016;150(6):1456–1470.

Jeuring S, van den Heuvel T, Liu L, et al. Improvements in the long-term outcome of Crohn's disease over the past two decades and the relation to changes in medical management: results from the population-based IBDSL cohort. *Am J Gastroenterol.* 2016;112:325–406.

Kaul A, Kaul K. Cyclic vomiting syndrome: a functional disorder. *Pediatr Gastroenterol Hepatol Nutr.* 2015;18(4):224–229.

Khatib M, Baker R, Ly E, Kozielski, Baker S. Presenting pattern of pediatric celiac disease. *JPGN.* 2016;62(1):60–63.

Koch J, Harger T, von Kries R, Wichmann O. Risk of intussusception after rotavirus vaccination- a systematic literature review and meta-analysis. *Deutsches Arzteblatt International.* 2017;114:255–262.

Kodituwakku R, Palmer S, Paul S. Management of foreign body ingestions in children: button batteries and magnets. *Br J Nurs.* 2017;26(8):456–461.

Lane E, Lee D, Suskind D. Dietary therapies in pediatric inflammatory bowel disease. *Gastroenterol Clin N Am.* 2017;46:731–744.

Larson-Nath C, Biank V. Clinical review of failure to thrive in pediatric patients. *Pediatric Annals.* 2016;45(2):46–49.

Leonard MM, Sapone A, Catassi C, Fasano A. Celiac disease and nonceliac gluten sensitivity, a review. *JAMA.* 2017;318(7):647–656.

Levinthal D. The cyclic vomiting syndrome threshold: a framework for understanding pathogenesis and predicting successful treatments, clinical and translational. *Gastroenterology.* 2016;7(10):1–8.

Lewis J, Abreu M. Diet as a trigger for inflammatory bowel diseases. *Gastroenterology.* 2017;152:398–414.

Martin-de-Carpi J, Moriczi M, Pujol-Muncunill G, Navas-Lopez V. Pancreatic involvement in pediatric inflammatory bowel disease. *Front Pediatr.* 2017;5(218):1–5.

Mauritz F, Conchillo J, van Heurn, et al. Effects and efficacy of laparoscopic fundoplication in children with GERD: a prospective multicenter study. *Surg Endosc*. 2017;31(3):1101–1110.

Michelet M, Schluckebier D, Petit L, Caubet J. Food protein-induced Enterocolitis syndrome- a review of the literature with focus on clinical management. *J Asthma Allergy*. 2017;10:197–207.

Moen S, Qujeq D, Tabarti M, Kashifard M, Hajian-Tilaki K. Diagnostic accuracy of fecal calprotectin in assessing the severity of inflammatory bowel disease: from laboratory to clinic. *Caspian J Intern Med*. 2017;8(3):178–182.

Mousa H, Hassan M. Gastroesophageal reflux. *Pediatr Clin N Am*. 2017;64:487–505.

Muir A, Merves J, Liacouras C. Role of endoscopy in diagnosis and management of pediatric eosinophilic esophagitis. *Gastrointest Endosc Clin N Am*. 2016;26(1):187–200.

NASPGHAN Neurogastroenterology and Motility Committee. *Polyethylene Glycol 4050 (PEG 4050) Frequently Asked Questions*; 2015. https://www.gikids.org/files/PEG_4050_FAQ_formatted.pdf. Accessed January 22, 2018.

National Institute of Diabetes and Digestive and Kidney Diseases (NIDDK). *Lactose Intolerance*; 2018. https://www.niddk.nih.gov/health-information/digestive-diseases/lactose-intolerance. Accessed on April 13, 2018.

Newlove-Delgado T, Martin A, Abbott R, et al. Dietary interventions for recurrent abdominal pain in childhood. *Cochrane Database Syst Rev*. 2017;3.

Nguyen H, Minar P, Jackson K, Fulkerson P. Vaccinations in immunosuppressive-dependent pediatric inflammatory bowel disease. *World J Gastroenterol*. 2017;23(42):7644–7652.

Nowak-Węgrzyn A, Chehade M, Groetch M. International consensus guidelines for the diagnosis and management of food protein-induced enterocolitis syndrome: executive summary-workgroup report of the adverse reactions to foods committee, American Academy of Allergy, Asthma & Immunology. *J Allergy Cin Immunol*. 2017:139–1111.

Pavlinac P, Brander R, Atlas H, John-Stewart G, Dennu D, Watson J. Interventions to reduce post-acute consequences of diarrheal disease in children: a systematic review. *BMC Public Health*. 2018;18:208. 1–27.

Philichi L. Management of childhood functional constipation. *J Pediatr Health*. 2018;32(1):103–111.

Pieczarkowski S, Kowalska-Duplaga K, Kwinta P, Tomasik P, Wedrychowicz A, Fyderek K. Diagnostic value of fecal calprotectin test in children with chronic abdominal pain. *Gastroenterol Res Pract*. 2016:1–7.

Piescik-Lech M, Urbanska M, Szajewska H. Lactobacillus GG (LGG) and smectite versus LGG alone for acute gastroenteritis: a double-blind, randomized controlled trial. *Eur J Pediatr*. 2013;172(2):247–253.

Polyak C, Yuhas K, Singa B, et al. Cotrimoxazole prophylaxis discontinuation among antiretroviral-treated HIV-1infected adults in Kenya: a randomized non-infertility trial. *PLOS Medicine*. 2016;13(1):1–16.

Reich J, Wasan S, Farraye F. Vaccination and health maintenance issues to consider in patients with inflammatory bowel disease. *Gastroenterol Hepatol*. 2017;13(12):717–750.

Rentea RM, St. Peter SD. Contemporary management of appendicitis in children. *Adv Pediatrics*. 2017;64:225–251.

Rinawi F, Assa A, Hartman C, et al. Incidence of bowel surgery and associated risk factors in pediatric-onset Crohn's disease. *Inflamm Bowel Dis*. 2016;22(12):2917–2923.

Sairenji T, Collins K, Evans D. An update on inflammatory bowel disease. *Prim Care Clin Office Pract*. 2017;44:673–692.

Sandoval J. *Pediatric Foreign Body Ingestion*. Medscape (Website); 2017. Available at http://emedicine.medscape.com/article/940015-overview. Accessed April 15, 2018.

Sayed A, Zeidan A, Fahmy D, Ibrahim H. Diagnostic reliability of pediatric appendicitis score, ultrasound and low-dose computed tomography scan in children with suspected acute appendicitis. *Ther Clin Risk Manag*. 2017;13:847–854.

Shannahan S, Leffler D. Diagnosis and updates in celiac disease. *Gastrointest Endoscopy*. 2017;27:79–92.

Siow A, Bhat R, Mollen K. Management of acute severe ulcerative colitis in children. *Semi Pediatr Surg*. 2017;26:367–372.

Sood M, Matta S. Approach to a child with functional abdominal pain. *Indian J Pediatr*. 2016;83(12):1452–1458.

Stenke E, Bourke B, Knaus U. Crohn's strictures-moving away from the knife. *Front Pediatr*. 2017;5(141):1–8.

Stokes A, Kulaylat A, Rocourt D, Hollenbeak C, Koltun W, Falaiye T. Rates and trends for inpatient surgeries in pediatric Crohn's disease in the United States from 2003 to 2012. *J Pediatr Surg*. 2017:1–5.

Straumann A, Katzka D. Diagnosis and treatment of eosinophilic esophagitis. *Gastroenterology*. 2017.

Szajewska H, Gyrczuk E, Horvath A. Lactobacillus reuteri DSM 17938 for the management of infantile colic in breastfed infants: a randomized, double-blind, placebo-controlled trial. *J Pediatr*. 2013;162(2):257–262. 20.

Tabbers M, DiLorenzo C, Berger M, et al. Evaluation and treatment of functional constipation in infants and children: evidence-based recommendations from ESPGHAN and NASPGHAN. *J Pediatr Gastroenterol Nutr*. 2014;58(2):258–274.

Tang Y, Chen J, An H, et al. High-resolution anorectal manometry in newborns: normative values and diagnostic utility in Hirschsprung disease. *Neurogastroenterol Motil*. 2014;26(11):1565–1572.

Territo H, Wrotniak B, Qiao H, Lillis K. Clinical signs and symptoms associated with intussusception in young children undergoing ultrasound in the emergency room. *Pediatr Emerg Care*. 2014;30(10):718–722.

Thomas E. Fluid and electrolytes. In: Engorn B, Flerage J, eds. *The Harriet Lane Handbook: A Manual for Pediatric House Officer*. 20th ed. Philadelphia: Elsevier; 2015.

Tian L, Zhu X, Chen Z, et al. Characteristics of bacterial pathogens associated with acute diarrhea in children under 5 years of age: a hospital based cross-sectional study. *BMC Infectious Diseases*. 2016;16(253):1–8.

Tomasik E, Ziotkowska E, Kotodziej, Szajewska H. Systematic review with meta-analysis: ondansetron for vomiting in children with acute gastroenteritis. *Aliment Pharmacol Ther*. 2016;44:438–446.

Vandenplas Y, Rudolph C, Di Lorenzo C, et al. Pediatric gastroesophageal reflux clinical practice guidelines: joint recommendations of the North American Society for Pediatric Gastroenterology, Hepatology, and Nutrition (NASPGHAN) and the European Society for Pediatric Gastroenterology, Hepatology, and Nutrition (ESPGHAN). *J Pediatr Gastroenterol Nutr*. 2009;49(4):498–547.

Wilson D, Russell R. Overview of pediatric IBD. *Semi Pediatr Surg*. 2017;26:344–348.

World Gastroenterology Organisation (WGO) Global Guideline. *Probiotics and Prebiotics*; 2017. Retrieved from http://www.worldgastroenterology.org/guidelines/global-guidelines/probiotics-and-prebiotics/probiotics-and-prebiotics-english.

Yazar A, Guven S, Dinelyici E. Effects of zinc or symbiotic on the duration of diarrhea in children with acute infectious diarrhea. *Turk J Gastroenterol*. 2016;27:537–540.

Yoo S, Hwang E, Lee Y, Park J. Clinical characteristics of failure to thrive in infant and toddler: organic vs. nonorganic. *Pediatr Gastroenterol Hepatol Nutr*. 2013;16(4):261–268.

Zis P, Rao D, Sarrigiannis P, et al. Transglutaminase 6 antibodies in gluten neuropathy. *Dig Liver Dis*. 2017;49(11):1196–1200.

Zubairi H, Nelson B, Tulshian P, et al. Hyaluronidase resuscitation in Kenya for severely dehydrated children. *Pediatr Emerg Care*. 2017;00(00).

Zeevenhooven J, Ilan J, Koppen N, Benninga MA. The New Rome IV Criteria for functional gastrointestinal disorders in infants and toddlers. *Pediatr Gastroenterol Hepatol Nutr*. 2017;1:1–13.

41

Genitourinary Disorders

AMBER WETHERINGTON

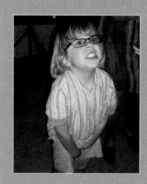

The genitourinary (GU) system maintains an optimal environment for metabolism by regulating water and electrolytes (sodium, potassium, chloride, calcium, phosphate, and magnesium); excreting waste products (urea, creatinine, poisons, and drugs); and regulating acid-base and hormone secretion (vitamin D, renin, erythropoietin, and prostaglandins). The male GU system system has both reproductive and excretory functions. GU problems in children and adolescents range from commonly occurring, easily treated diseases to significant congenital or acquired conditions. Pediatric primary care providers (PCPs) play a significant role in working with children, adolescents, and families to identify problems, manage disorders, maintain optimal function, and provide education and support related to GU function. First-line assessment and management, provision of continuity of care, and referral to and collaboration with pediatric urologists and nephrologists are important components of patient management.

Standards of Care

The American Academy of Pediatrics (AAP) and the *Bright Futures Practice Guidelines* do not recommend screening for asymptomatic bacteremia or chronic kidney disease with a urine dipstick or complete urinalysis (UA) at any age (Hagan et al., 2017).

Hypertension in infants and young children is usually secondary to another disease process and is most commonly renal in origin. Older school-age children and adolescents may present with primary hypertension due to increased obesity rates; however, the GU system must be considered. Routine blood pressure (BP) screening is recommended at every preventive health care visit beginning at 3 years old (Hagan et al., 2017). The management and treatment of hypertension is discussed in Chapter 38.

Anatomy and Physiology

The renal system is composed of two kidneys, two ureters, a bladder, and a urethra. The kidneys are positioned posteriorly on the abdominal wall. The main structures of the kidney are the cortex, the medulla, and the collecting system. The renal medulla and nephrons are present at birth, but the peripheral tubules are small and immature. By adolescence, the kidneys are adult size and weight. The ureters are muscular tubes that move urine from the kidneys to the bladder by peristaltic contractions. The bladder is a muscular reservoir that collects urine, lies close to the anterior abdominal wall in early childhood, and descends with growth into the pelvis changing shape from cylindrical to pyramidal. As the bladder fills

to capacity, nerve signals transmit to the brain that urination is required. When urination occurs, the sphincter between the bladder and urethra opens and contractions of the bladder create pressure to force urine out the urethral meatus. The male urethra is significantly longer than the female urethra because it leaves the bladder in the lower pelvis, passes through the prostate with openings for the release of bulbourethral gland fluids and semen during sexual activity, and extends the full length of the penile shaft. The urethral meatus is normally located on the tip of the glans in the male. The female urethra descends from the bladder and exits the body inside the labia minora, midline, just posterior to the clitoris.

Physiologically the kidneys serve to filter, clear, reabsorb, and secrete substances essential to metabolism. The urinary system begins forming and excreting urine at 3 months of gestational age. Glomerular filtration and renal blood flow increase at birth and become stable by 1 to 2 years old. In infants, total extracellular fluid volume is significantly greater than that of adults, and fluid composition tends to have a lower bicarbonate concentration. Normal urine excretion is 1 to 2 mL/kg/h. The kidneys mature throughout infancy, and kidney function approaches adult values between 6 and 12 months old.

Pathophysiology and Defense Mechanisms

Disorders in the urinary system can occur anywhere in the system from the kidneys to the urethral meatus. Upper tract disorders involve the kidneys and ureters, while lower tract disorders involve the bladder, urethra, or meatus. This differentiation can be difficult because frequently disorders in one part of the system affect the entire system, and can present silently or symptomatically. The main mechanisms of GU disorders are infection, inflammatory response, congenital malformation, or injury.

The urinary tract is normally sterile. The mucosal lining of the bladder serves as the first line of defense and inhibits bacterial growth and adherence. The acid pH of the urine also protects the urinary system by inhibiting bacterial growth. Finally, the urine flow out of the bladder provides mechanical defense by its flushing action.

Assessment of the Genitourinary System
History and Clinical Findings

- History of the present illness
  - Symptom onset and pattern (e.g., acute, chronic, cyclic)
  - Fever

- Abdominal pain
- Flank pain
- Preceding injury or illness, especially streptococcal infection
- Vomiting
- Voiding pattern: Stream force and direction, dribbling or discharge, enuresis or incontinence, dysuria, or urinary urgency or hesitancy
- Color, odor, frequency, and volume of urine
- Bowel patterns or chronic constipation
- Sexual activity or abuse
- Family history
  - Renal disease, deafness, hypertension, structural abnormalities, or syndromes involving the GU system
  - Past history of urinary tract infection (UTI), hematuria, proteinuria, syndromes associated with GU abnormality

Physical Examination

- Growth parameters: Failure to thrive (FTT) can be associated with UTI, renal tubular acidosis (RTA), and chronic renal failure in infants. Unusual weight gain can be associated with nephrotic syndrome or acute renal failure
- BP: Often elevated with nephritis and nephrotic syndrome
- Edema or pallor
- Ear position and formation: If low-set or abnormal, may have concurrent renal involvement
- Abdominal masses, ascites, flank (including costovertebral) or suprapubic tenderness
- External genitalia abnormalities
- Unusual facial features associated with syndromes that include renal disease

Diagnostic Studies

Diagnostic studies are ordered as indicated. The proper collection, transport, and storage of urine is essential to obtain accurate results. The normal composition of urine varies considerably during a 24-hour period. Most reference values are based on analysis of the first morning voided urine. This specimen is preferred because it has a uniform volume and concentration and lower pH which preserves the formed elements. Urine should be evaluated within 30 minutes and kept refrigerated (below 39.2°F or 4°C) if stored. Specimens that require extended storage (i.e., overnight) require preservative containing containers (Quest Diagnostics, 2017).

The following should be noted on the UA:

- Physical characteristics: Color, clarity, odor, specific gravity, and osmolality.
- Specific gravity is a measure of hydration and renal concentration ability and varies from 1.003 to 1.030. A first-voided urine specimen specific gravity of 1.010 or more indicates intact renal concentrating ability. Urine with a specific gravity greater than 1.030 is considered concentrated.
- Chemical characteristics: Urine dipsticks are Clinical Laboratory and Improvement Amendments of 1988 (CLIA) waived and are widely used to determine pH, specific gravity, glucose, ketones, protein, bile pigments, hemoglobin, nitrites, and leukocyte esterase. For correct results, strips must remain in their original containers and not be exposed to moisture, light, cold, or heat until used. Urine must be fresh, warmed to room temperature if refrigerated, and read at correct time intervals for each test strip (Table 41.1). Urine pH varies from 4.6 to 8 and reflects the ability to maintain acid-base balance. Blood

indicates the presence of hemoglobin. Intact erythrocytes cause spotty changes on the dipstick, whereas free hemoglobin or myoglobin cause uniform color change. Leukocyte esterase indicates white blood cells (WBCs) in the urine (pyuria) and warrant further investigation. Nitrites are an indirect measure of bacteria in the urine and the most specific marker for infection. Common urinary pathogens contain enzymes that reduce nitrate in urine to nitrite. There is an increased risk of false negative results for leukocyte esterase and nitrite in children younger than 3 years; however, new research supports UA dipstick testing alone as statistically reliable given the ease and speed of results (Schroeder, et al., 2015).

A urine culture should be done on any urine sample positive for nitrites or leukocyte esterase if the child has symptoms of UTI, the risk criteria for UTIs are met, or the child has a high fever without a source. The combination of leukocyte esterase and nitrites is highly predictive of a positive urine culture. Negative leukocyte esterase and nitrites reasonably rule out a UTI; however, a culture is still indicated for both negative and positive urine dipstick findings, especially if the urine was not in the bladder at least 4 hours (Mambatta, et al., 2015).

Microscopic urine examination: This can be accomplished on centrifuge-spun and unspun urine and consideration must be given to which method of collection was used. Urine that is positive for blood or protein on dipstick should be sent to lab for a UA with reflexive microscopy.

- RBCs: In general, more than 2 to 5 per HPF (×40) in unspun urine or more than 2 to 10 per HPF in spun urine is thought to be abnormal. If cells are dysmorphic, the origin of the blood is most likely the kidney.
- WBCs: Normal findings include fewer than two WBCs per HPF. More than 10 WBCs often indicates an infection.
- Bacteria: Leukocytes seen in unspun urine are associated with bacterial colony counts of greater than 100,000.
- Casts: RBCs, hyaline, waxy, epithelial, leukocyte, or fatty casts are seen in various disease states.
- Crystals, if amorphous, are not unusual.

Depending on the results of the UA and/or clinical symptoms, other tests may be indicated, including:

- Gram stain: Bacteria on the Gram stain are highly predictive of a UTI and if present, a urine culture should be performed.
- Urine culture and sensitivities: Culture remains the gold standard for diagnosing and treating UTIs. Urine should be cultured immediately but may be refrigerated for up to 24 hours before plating. Urine specimens unrefrigerated for 2 hours or more are subject to bacterial overgrowth, change in pH, and dissolution of RBC and WBC casts. Bacterial identification and sensitivities are recommended.
- A 24-hour urine collection: A 24-hour urine sample determines calcium excretion, the calcium-creatinine ratio, and protein quantification.
- Blood urea nitrogen (BUN) estimates the urea concentration in blood and measures toxic metabolites that can cause uremic syndrome.
- Serum creatinine and creatinine clearance estimate the glomerular filtration rate (GFR), a measure of kidney function.
- Serum electrolytes and acid-base status help detect renal tubular abnormalities.
- Ultrasonography provides noninvasive structural information.
- Dimercaptosuccinic acid (DMSA) scanning is the most sensitive tool for detecting acute pyelonephritis and renal scarring. DMSA is most appropriate when there is concern for scarring

TABLE 41.1 Chemical Characteristics of Urine

Constituent	Positives Indicate	Cause of False Positive	Cause of False Negative
Glucose	Metabolic problem (e.g., diabetes), recent high glucose intake, oral corticosteroids, galactosemia	Antibiotics, delay in reading, myoglobin, oxidizing contaminants	Ascorbic acid intake, ketones, high specific gravity
Ketones	Dehydration, starvation, missed breakfast, strenuous exercise, stress, fever, metabolic problems (e.g., diabetes)	Irrigating solution, highly pigmented urine	If urine left standing, acetone evaporates
Protein	Renal disease, orthostatic proteinuria	Exercise, fever, dehydration, alkaline or concentrated urine (specific gravity >1.02), semisynthetic penicillin, oxidizing, cleansing agents	Dilute or acidic urine
Blood (hemoglobin)	If concurrent microscopic examination is negative for RBCs: Free hemoglobin secondary to chemicals, illness, or drugs; myoglobin secondary to burns, muscle trauma, physical child abuse, myositis, strenuous exercise. If concurrent microscopic examination is positive for RBCs: External excoriation, renal problems	Menses, oxidizing cleansing agents, dilute urine, myoglobinuria, strenuous exercise	Ascorbic acid, dipstick exposed to air, pH of urine <5.1
Nitrite	Bacteria causing urinary tract infection	Rare	Common; urine should be in bladder at least 4 h, dilution of nitrate in urine
Leukocyte esterase	Pyuria (white blood cells in urine); inflammation from irritation or infection of vulva, vagina, or urethra; bladder or kidney inflammation with or without infection	Oxidizing agents	Immunocompromised, proteinuria, vitamin C in the urine, technical error related to time at reading dipstick
Urobilinogen	Hemolytic disease; hepatic disease	Sulfonamides, presence of phenazopyridine	Exposure to light, urine remains at room temperature too long
Bilirubin	Hepatic disease; biliary obstruction	Presence of phenazopyridine	Urine remains at room temperature too long

RBC, Red blood cell.

Mambatta AK, Jayarajan J, Rashme VL, et al. Reliability of dipstick assay in predicting urinary tract infection. *J Fam Med Prim Care.* 2015;4(2):265–268.

or when serum creatinine is elevated (American Urological Association guideline 2010, revised and confirmed 2017).
- Voiding cystourethrogram (VCUG) is the most reliable method for detection of vesicoureteral reflux (VUR). Indications for VCUG in a child with a UTI are limited to febrile UTIs after an abnormal ultrasound or DMSA scan, or when there is a second febrile UTI (AAP Subcommittee on Urinary Tract Infection, 2016).

Management Strategies

Education and Counseling

Education and counseling are essential components in the management of GU tract disorders. Parents and children must be informed about the pathologic condition, etiology, treatment, prevention strategies, and prognosis with and without treatment. The PCP and family must decide on an agreeable plan of care. Urinary problems can occur any time during infancy, childhood, or adolescence and vary in severity, chronicity, and disability.

Referral

Referral to a pediatric urologist, nephrologist, or surgeon may be required. When a referral is made, the PCP retains the essential role of case manager for the child and providing care continuity. The PCP is often the person the family knows best and is most comfortable with when discussing concerns, potential plans, and long-term management.

Dysfunctional Voiding

Dysfunctional voiding is defined as a problem of bladder emptying. During voiding, the child contracts the external urethra in either a "staccato pattern," resulting in intermittent flow, prolonged micturition time, and often, incomplete bladder emptying, or there is a "plateau pattern" related to continuous, tonic sphincter contraction that results in a dynamic bladder outlet obstruction. Either detrusor overactivity or underactivity may be present. A long-standing pattern of incomplete emptying can lead to overextension of the bladder and subsequent underactive detrusor function. As a result, UTI, symptoms of urgency, frequency, and overflow incontinence can occur (Austin et al., 2015).

The cause of dysfunctional voiding is unknown, but it is believed to be multifactorial and is often accompanied by constipation. UTI, structural abnormalities, stress, and abuse must also be considered.

History and Clinical Findings

Because of the varied problems associated with dysfunctional void-ing, this history of a child includes differing symptoms, including:

- Infrequent voiding
- Cluster voiding where they void a lot after a period of not void-ing during each day (e.g., not voiding at school)
- Holding maneuvers
- Sudden daytime incontinence after having been dry
- Urgency
- Frequency
- Inability to stop the voiding stream
- Occasional nocturnal enuresis, but usually daytime wetting
- Urine pooling in the vagina during voiding that results in later leakage (e.g., vaginal voiding)
- Constipation
- UTI

Include information about the child's general development, developmental milestones, pattern of toilet training and elimi-nation (i.e., frequency and volume of voiding and stooling as well as timing of episodes of any incontinence), stressors experi-enced following toilet training, family history of voiding prob-lems, and the child's behavioral patterns including the child's and family's emotional response to the condition. It is impor-tant to get direct information from the child because parents are often unaware of elimination patterns of their older, toilet-trained child.

Physical Examination

Genital and abdominal examinations should be completed, including checking for labial adhesions in females. Males should be checked for meatal stenosis, which can lead to a deflected stream that sprays upward. Consider, particularly, the possibil-ity of constipation and check for abdominal masses indicating retained stool.

Diagnostic Studies

Urodynamic diagnostic procedures are not routinely done. The following tests may be indicated:

- UA
- Urine culture and sensitivity
- Bladder ultrasound done by a urologic provider to measure post-void residual urine volume
- Renal and bladder ultrasound if structural abnormalities are suspected which may show a normal upper renal system and a thick-walled bladder
- VCUG ordered by a pediatric urology provider if VUR sus-pected.

Differential Diagnosis

The differential diagnoses for dysfunctional voiding are as follows:

- UTI
- Structural abnormality, such as abnormal sphincters, ectopic ureter, duplicated urethra, or urethral valves
- Neurogenic bladder
- Non-neurogenic dysfunctional voiding (Hinman-Allen syn-drome), in which the child holds urine, which leads to over-activity of the detrusor muscle, high voiding pressure, bladder decompensation, and a predisposition for infection and renal damage (Clothier and Wright, 2018).

- Asymptomatic VUR that does not cause voiding symptoms
- Trauma or abuse
- Urethritis (which may be caused by chemicals in soaps, bubble baths)

Management

The management goal is to prevent or break the cycle of urinary dysfunction and its complications. Intervention includes the following:

- Treat UTI if present.
- Treat constipation if present. This may eliminate the entire problem but can take months to correct (see Encopresis/Con-stipation in Chapter 40). Parents must be aware of the possible need for long-term treatment.
- First-line treatment should involve urotherapy (Box 41.1). At the start of the program, the family should focus on children doing the "jobs" given to them and not on successful resolution of the issue (Austin et al., 2015). There is conflicting evidence on the addition of biofeedback to urotherapy. Implementing biofeedback also has the drawback of needing multiple visits, which families may find difficult to attend and can be very costly.
- Second-line treatment combines urotherapy with pharmaco-therapeutics. The International Children's Continence Society (ICCS) notes that medication use is "an off-label method"

• BOX 41.1 Urotherapy for Dysfunctional Voiding and Enuresis

- Educate parents and child on how the bladder works: Describe filling and emptying process, especially as it is related to problem of external sphincter contraction during voiding.
- Explain the relationship between abdominal, pelvic floor, and external sphincter muscles; how to be aware of and to relax muscles to allow complete voiding.
- Explain the relationship of bladder and bowel function as they are connected by the pelvic floor.
- Implement bladder retraining:
  - Establish a consistent, structured regimen of toileting: Set a timed-voiding schedule, usually every 2 h, 1½ if actively treating, because the goal is to void before bladder contractions activate the pelvic floor; void before going to bed and immediately upon rising in morning.
  - Use correct toilet posture: Sit comfortably with hips abducted, knees wide, and feet and buttocks well supported with a pelvic tilt.
  - Void with relaxation: Have child take a deep breath and relax the sphincter when exhaling; use a straw to breathe through.
  - Void to completion: If not accomplished on the first voiding, double void by having child void and count to five and void again and repeat until no further urine is produced.
  - Avoid Credé maneuver or injury can result from external pressure on the bladder.
  - Give lifestyle advice related to diet and fluid intake.
  - Encourage 1 oz/kg/day of water to be consumed at regular intervals between breakfast and dinner (this most often eliminates evening thirst).
- Monitor progress:
  - Keep frequency, volume charts, or a voiding diary.
  - Actively manage bowel dysfunction.
  - Implement behavioral interventions as indicated, based on child and family history.
  - Neuromodulation and catheterization may be appropriate in resistant cases.

(Austin et al., 2015) and a pediatric urology referral is indicated before using medications. Anticholinergics may be used, but their side effects can be significant (e.g., constipation).
- Treat skin breakdown if present. Vinegar sitz baths can be very effective.

Patient and Family Education

Effective toilet training can prevent bowel and bladder dysfunction (BBD), especially if children learn to be responsive to cues to urinate and defecate. Instruct parents that holding urine is not the goal; because, paradoxically, if a person activates the pelvic floor to hold urine, often a feedback loop to the brain is activated and one feels a decreased need to go. Parents need to be alert to signs of dysuria as this may cause children to struggle to retain urine or void incompletely. Early treatment for UTIs is essential to prevent renal dysfunction. Teach elimination norms at every well-child check.

Enuresis

Enuresis is the voluntary or involuntary urination at an age when toilet training should be complete. Children who never established control have primary enuresis. Secondary enuresis is present when children have been dry for more than 6 to 12 months and then begin wetting. Nocturnal enuresis is incontinence during sleep. If a child has normal daytime elimination with no concerns, then nighttime wetting is called *monosymptomatic nocturnal enuresis (MNE)*. More commonly, children with nocturnal enuresis have BBD symptoms during the day; this type of nocturnal enuresis is *non-monosymptomatic nocturnal enuresis (NMNE)*. Diurnal enuresis, daytime wetting, occurs during waking hours.

Diagnosing enuresis can be a challenge. According to the ICCS a diagnosis of enuresis requires a minimum age of 5 years old, and one episode a month for a duration of 3 months. Enuresis is frequent if it occurs four or more times a week and infrequent if it occurs four or less times a month (Austin et al., 2015). It is important to remember that the age at which urinary continence is normally achieved varies greatly, and children should be evaluated on a case-by-case basis, considering the child and family dynamics, developmental stages, and the amount of duress the issue causes. If the parent or child asks for help, they should receive it.

The cause of enuresis varies among children and can be difficult to determine. A number of factors are associated with enuresis, including the following:
- Constipation: It cannot be overemphasized how important it is to determine if constipation or impaction exists before treating nocturnal enuresis.
- Familial disposition: Even if there is a presumed genetic predisposition based on parental history, many of these children have constipation that if treated causes improvement.
- Neurologic developmental delay.
- Behavioral comorbidities (e.g., externalizing behaviors): There is an association between enuresis (especially daytime enuresis) and attention-deficit/hyperactivity disorder (ADHD) (Kovacevic et al., 2017), obsessive-compulsive disorder (Yousefichaijan, 2016), and other mental health concerns.
- Functional small bladder capacity: In some children, bladder capacity is normal during the day but is functionally reduced at night (Kuwertz-Bröking and von Gontard, 2017).

- Sleep disorders: Obstructive sleep apnea and disordered sleep patterns result in increased nocturnal enuresis incidence (Kuwertz-Bröking and von Gontard, 2017).
- Stress and family disruptions: Examples include divorce, move, or a new family member.
- Polyuria: This can be caused by nocturnal drinking as well as caffeine intake (Kuwertz-Bröking and von Gontard, 2017).
- Inappropriate toilet training: This is especially common when parents are overly demanding or punitive of the child.

History and Clinical Findings

The goals of assessment are to (1) determine if there are comorbid or underlying conditions that require pediatric urology referral and (2) establish the best approach to treating this particular child's condition.

It is essential to gather the most honest nighttime *and* daytime history of bowel and bladder elimination habits. Ask parents about the following:
- Voiding characteristics:
  - Urgency, dysuria, or dribbling
  - Are there voiding or stooling postponement behaviors?
  - Number of voids per day: is nocturia present?
  - Cluster voiding: for example, is the child waiting until after school?
  - Frequency of wetting—day and night
  - Type of urinary stream
- These findings warrant referral to a pediatric urologist:
  - Weak or interrupted urinary stream
  - Need to use abdominal pressure to urinate
  - Combined daytime incontinence and nocturnal enuresis
- Fluid intake, including timing, type, and volume
- UTI
- Family history of enuresis, treatment, and age of resolution, including parents
- Toilet training history: What age was toilet training begun? How was it handled? Was the child ever dry? For how long?
- Effect of enuresis on child and parents
- Manner in which family deals with the enuresis: For example, is the child punished? Who changes the bed? Any previous medical treatment?
- Bowel patterns: What is the frequency? Is there constipation? Is there fecal incontinence? What is the quality of stool? (see Chapter 40).
- Sleep patterns: Assess for symptoms of obstructive sleep-disordered breathing or apnea. Reassure parents that deep sleep is not a cause for nocturnal enuresis.
- General health:
  - Prenatal and perinatal history
  - Is child tired? Has child lost weight? Does child have excessive thirst or hunger (e.g., diabetes)?
  - Does the child have a neuropsychological condition (e.g., ADHD) or other behavioral problem?
  - Changes in the home, family, or school environment: Be sure to determine if the enuresis was present before disruptive changes occurred.

Physical Examination

- The physical examination includes the following:
  - Assess the external genitalia for signs of irritation, infection, labial fusion, and/or meatal stenosis.

- Examine the abdomen for masses, especially at the suprapubic midline and in the left lower quadrant.
- Examine the lower back for dimples and hair tufts.
- Assess for neurologic function and deep tendon reflexes.

Diagnostic Studies

A UA is recommended in all children with enuresis. A culture should be done if there are clinical symptoms to warrant it. More sophisticated testing is usually not necessary.

Differential Diagnosis

The differential diagnosis includes benign idiopathic urinary frequency (pollakiuria), a condition of excessive urination (more than 8 to 12 times/day, often as frequent as every 15 to 30 minutes) seen in previously toilet-trained children who do not need to void at night. Pollakiuria has no known cause, but may be associated with viral cystitis or urethritis, stress, tic disorders, and hypercalciuria. Although considered self-limited because it does not typically respond to medication, pollakiuria can persist for months or even years; however, it typically lasts about 6 months (Elder, 2016e).

Organic causes of enuresis must be identified. The most common organic cause is UTI that may be related to BBD. Worsening incontinence, development of neurologic signs (e.g., weakness in legs), and increased urine volumes or dilution warrant referral to specialists for further evaluation. Other organic causes of enuresis include:

- Diabetes mellitus
- Diabetes insipidus
- Sickle cell disease due to forced fluids leading to increased urine output
- Chronic renal failure secondary to kidneys' inability to concentrate urine
- Structural anomalies, such as ectopic ureter (constant leakage is noted) or a vesicovaginal fistula
- Neurologic abnormalities, including neurogenic bladder
- Hypercalciuria
- Obstructive uropathy other than that due to ⚫ BBD
- Eosinophilic cystitis
- Vaginitis
- Sleep apnea
- Pinworms

Management

The treatment goals are to establish normal bladder function and prevent both physical and emotional complications. A thorough examination to distinguish between organic and nonorganic causes is the first crucial step. Intervention is based on the underlying cause and involves behavioral modification, medication, treatment of comorbid or organic conditions, or a combination of these modalities. Treatment of daytime urinary dysfunction and constipation should be done before treating nocturnal enuresis. Referral to a pediatric urology specialist may be necessary. Outcomes of treatment are categorized as:

- No response: Less than 50% decrease in enuresis
- Partial response: 50% to 99% reduction
- Complete response: 100% reduction
  Over the long term, outcomes include:
- Relapse: More than one symptom relapse per month

- Continued success: No return of symptoms in 6 months
- Complete success: No return of symptoms after 2 years

Because functional enuresis is largely self-limited, there is consensus to delay aggressive treatment until the child is 6 to 8 years old. Treatment strategies for children 6 years old or older include the following:

- *Urotherapy:* A non-pharmacologic, nonsurgical intervention, urotherapy is basic to enuresis treatment (see Box 41.1). Urotherapy increases daytime urination by establishing a regular voiding schedule—not waiting until the micturition urge is felt. It also limits nighttime urine production by regulating fluid intake. The goal is for the bladder to hold urine produced overnight. Children should void before going to bed and again immediately upon waking in the morning. Proper posture while urinating is important to help the child be more sensitive to cues of a full bladder and to control urination. This approach is effective for children with hyperactive bladders and may make medication unnecessary for many children. Urotherapy also involves aggressive treatment of constipation.
- *Enuresis alarms:* The decision to use an alarm should be made after discussion with the child and family and be based on their preference. Alarm therapy is more effective in children with "decreased maximal voided volumes." A review of the literature indicates that long-term alarm therapy is more effective than desmopressin for treatment of primary nocturnal enuresis (Apos et al., 2018) and an enuresis alarm should be first-line treatment when conditions such as diabetes, kidney disease, or urogenital malformations have been ruled out. Use of an alarm requires commitment and effort on the part of children and parents and support from the PCP.
- *Drug therapy:* Drug therapy (see Table 41.2 for dosing and comments) can be combined with urotherapy and/or alarm therapy, but it is not curative. It usually has high initial success rates. Unfortunately, drug therapy can be expensive, and high relapse rates occur when the drug is discontinued. When the wetting recurs, it can be very upsetting to the child, which is a factor that needs to be considered when prescribing. However, it can be very useful for overnight stays (e.g., camp) when staying dry is important to the child.

Desmopressin has an antidiuretic effect and appears to be most effective in children with large nocturnal urine production and normal nocturnal bladder capacity. Its effect is immediate and it can be taken only on nights that the child wants to be sure to stay dry. Desmopressin is available in three forms: nasal spray, oral tablets, or oral lyophilisate preparation (MELT) (sublingual administration). Nasal spray has led to hyponatremia, has a black box warning from the FDA, and is not recommended for routine use (Kamperis et al., 2017).

Caution patients to avoid high fluid intake with the oral medication, to give the correct dosage, and to discontinue the medication if headache, nausea, or vomiting occurs (Kamperis et al., 2017). Desmopressin may be more effective when combined with urotherapy and long-term success is best when desmopressin is tapered slowly over time (Chua, 2016).

Other drugs are not recommended as first-line treatment. These include anticholinergics (antimuscarinic drugs [also used for treatment of overactive bladder]: oxybutynin, tolterodine, and solifenacin), which cause constipation and could complicate the problem; botulinum toxin type A (BtA), and imipramine, which should only be used by specialists, if at all, due to its cardiotoxic side effects.

TABLE 41.2	Drug Therapy for Children 6 Years or Older With Monosymptomatic Nocturnal Enuresis	
Medication	**Dosing**	**Comments**
Desmopressin acetate (DDAVP)	Oral: 0.2 mg tablet once daily at bedtime; can be adjusted up to maximum of 0.6 mg/day Oral: 120 mcg Melt (dissolves sublingually) once daily at bedtime; this is the bioequivalent of 0.2 mg tablet; can be adjusted up to 240 mcg/day	Effective in children with nocturnal polyuria and normal bladder volume. Short-term treatment only (4-8 weeks). Not recommended in children younger than 6 years. Not recommended to use nasal spray. Caution must be used with patients who are hypertensive or have a potential for fluid-electrolyte imbalance (e.g., children with cystic fibrosis susceptible to hyponatremia). Use least amount effective. Take on empty stomach; avoid caffeine, chocolate, NutraSweet, and carbonated beverages. Wake children to urinate within 10 h of taking the medication.
Oxybutynin chloride, immediate release Oxybutynin chloride, extended release	5 mg once daily at bedtime; increase as tolerated in 5 mg increments to maximum of 20 mg daily	Effective in children with daytime enuresis. Not recommended in children 5 years old or younger.

Sacral nerve stimulation for children with severe voiding dysfunction that has not responded to aggressive urotherapy and medical interventions is currently being studied.

Patient and Family Education

Supportive, proactive education of parents and positive reinforcement of the child's efforts help prevent enuresis. For 3- to 5-year-old children, a nonjudgmental attitude of "benign neglect" in the face of accidents is the best approach. For older children with enuresis, aggressive, long-term interventions are appropriate; wetting is a common phenomenon, and parents should be reassured that it rarely indicates disease. Dealing with a child who wets frequently can be frustrating, however, and parents need to know that the PCP is committed to working closely with them until the child is dry.

Genitourinary Tract Disorders

Urinary Tract Infection and Pyelonephritis

There are three kinds of UTI in children: (1) asymptomatic bacteriuria, (2) cystitis, and (3) pyelonephritis. Young children may have limited or unusual symptoms; therefore, a high degree of suspicion must be maintained to diagnose UTI. Inflammation and infection can occur at any point in the urinary tract, so a UTI must be identified according to location. *Asymptomatic bacteriuria* is bacteria in the urine without other symptoms, is benign, and does not cause renal injury. *Cystitis* is an infection of the bladder that produces lower tract symptoms but does not cause fever or renal injury. *Pyelonephritis* is the most severe type of UTI involving the renal parenchyma or kidneys and must be readily identified and treated because of the potential irreversible renal damage. Clinical signs thought to be consistent with pyelonephritis include fever, irritability, and vomiting in an infant, and urinary symptoms associated with fever, bacteriuria, vomiting, and renal tenderness in older children. UTIs are the most common cause of serious bacterial infection in infants younger than 24 months old with fever without a focus (Elder, 2016d). A *complicated UTI* is defined as a UTI with fever, toxicity, and dehydration, or a UTI occurring in a child younger than 3 to 6 months old. UTIs may be classified based on their association with other structural or functional abnormality such as VUR, obstruction, dysfunctional voiding, or pregnancy. Additionally, a UTI must be identified as a first occurrence, recurrent (within 2 weeks with the same organism or any reinfection with a different organism), or chronic (ongoing, unresolved, often caused by a structural abnormality or resistant organism). Age and gender of the pediatric patient are important factors in determining the evaluation method and the course of treatment.

The organism most commonly associated with UTI is *Escherichia coli* (70%), although other organisms (such as *Enterobacter, Klebsiella, Pseudomonas*, and *Proteus*) can cause infection. UTI secondary to group B streptococcus is more common in neonates. Several factors contribute to the etiology of UTIs. Most UTIs are thought to be ascending (i.e., the infection begins with colonization of the urethral area and ascends the urinary tract). If the infection progresses to the kidney, intrarenal reflux deep into the kidneys can lead to scarring. However, the most important risk factor for the development of pyelonephritis in children is VUR, which can be detected in 10% to 45% of young children who have symptomatic UTIs. Furthermore, reflux of infected urine from the bladder increases the risk of pyelonephritis. This kidney damage occurs in the compound papillae, which have wide and gaping openings allowing intrarenal reflux. The compound papillae are located in the upper and lower poles of the kidney, the usual site of scarring.

Host resistance factors and bacterial virulence factors are also important in the etiology of UTIs. These include the presence of a structural abnormality or dysplasia (such as VUR, obstruction, or other anatomic defect), or the presence of functional abnormalities (such as dysfunctional voiding or constipation). Other host factors affecting risk include female gender (having a short urethra), poor hygiene, irritation, sexual activity or sexual abuse, and pinworms. Several bacterial factors are known, but the two most important ones are adherence and bacterial virulence. Bacteria that have fimbriae or pili are able to adhere to the surface of the bladder mucosa; this allows the bacteria to resist the bladder's defensive cleansing flow of urine and causes tissue inflammation and cell damage. Adherence may also play a role in bacteria ascending the urinary tract. Virulence refers to the toxicity of substances released by bacteria. The greater the virulence, the greater the damage to the urinary tract. Both of these factors enhance colonization of the urinary tract and aid in the persistence and effect of the bacteria.

TABLE 41.3	Clinical Findings of Urinary Tract Infection in Children of Various Ages		
Neonates	**Infants**	**Toddlers and Preschoolers**	**School-Age Children and Adolescents**
Jaundice	Malaise, irritability	Altered voiding pattern	"Classic dysuria" with frequency, urgency, and discomfort
Hypothermia	Difficulty feeding	Malodor	
Failure to thrive (FTT)	Poor weight gain	Abdominal/flank pain[a]	Malodor
Sepsis	Fever[a]	Enuresis	Enuresis
Vomiting or diarrhea	Vomiting or diarrhea	Vomiting or diarrhea[a]	Abdominal/flank pain[a]
Cyanosis	Malodor	Malaise	Fever/chills[a]
Abdominal distention	Dribbling	Fever[a]	Vomiting or diarrhea[a]
Lethargy	Abdominal pain/colic	Diaper rash	Malaise

[a]Findings increase likelihood of pyelonephritis.

The risk of UTI in infants 2 to 24 months old is about 5%. The incidence in females is more than twice that of males (2.27%); uncircumcised boys have a rate 4 to 20 times greater than circumcised boys (AAP Subcommittee on Urinary Tract Infection, 2016). There is a greater frequency in premature and low-birth-weight infants. Females older than 12 months old have 2.1% prevalence; after the first year of life, it is also more common to find a UTI in females than in males with an overall incidence of 1% to 3% in girls and 1% in boys (Elder, 2016d). The incidence of UTI is often increased in sexually active adolescent girls. The risk of recurrence within the first year after an initial infection iscommon.

History and Clinical Findings

The following information should be obtained:
- Family history of VUR, recurrent UTI, or other kidney problems
- Prenatally diagnosed renal abnormality
- Previous infection: Request records from the past infection evaluation and diagnostic studies
- Circumcision
- Risk factors for infants 2 to 24 months old with no other source of infection (AAP Subcommittee on Urinary Tract Infection, 2016)
- Female—white race, age younger than 12 months old, temperature 39°C or higher, fever for 2 days or more
- Male—nonblack race, temperature 39°C or higher, fever for more than 24 hours
- Hygiene habits: Wiping front to back
- Voiding patterns: Frequency, abnormal stream, complete emptying, dribbling, enuresis, holding urine, incomplete emptying, and bathroom avoidance
- Constipation, perianal itching (pinworms)
- Irritants, such as nylon underwear or clothing (spandex, tight pants or shorts that rub); bubble bath or sitting in soapy bath water
- Hypertension
- Sexual activity, masturbation, or sexual abuse
- Other infection: Pinworms, diaper rash

Physical Examination

See Table 41.3 for age-related symptoms.
- General appearance (toxic appearing?)
- Vital signs: Temperature, BP
- Growth parameters: Growth may be decreased with chronic UTI or renal insufficiency, especially in infants
- Flank pain or costovertebral angle tenderness
- Abdominal examination: Suprapubic tenderness, bladder distention or a flank mass (obstructive signs), mass from fecal impaction
- Genitalia: Vaginal erythema, edema, irritation, or discharge; labial adhesions; uncircumcised male, urethral ballooning; weak, dribbling, threadlike stream
- Neurologic examination (if voiding is dysfunctional): Perineal sensation, lower extremity reflexes, sacral dimpling, or cutaneous abnormality

Diagnostic Studies

The method used to collect urine has an effect on the interpretation of results. Bagged urine specimens, even after cleaning the external genitalia prior to placement, produce a high incidence of false positive UA results due to contamination and thus must not be used to determine UTI. If antimicrobial therapy must be initiated due to an ill-appearing child, catheterization and urine culture must be obtained prior to administering antibiotics (AAP Subcommittee on Urinary Tract Infection, 2016). Older children who can void on command should be able to obtain a clean-catch void. Having the female child sit with knees apart, feet supported, and torso leaned forward while on the toilet separates the labia and decreases contamination.

Urine culture is essential to confirm the diagnosis. UTIs cause cultures with greater than 100,000 colonies of a single pathogen in a clean catch urine specimen, greater than 50,000 in a catheterized or suprapubic specimen, or 10,000 colonies of a single pathogen in the symptomatic (Elder, 2016d; Desai, 2018).

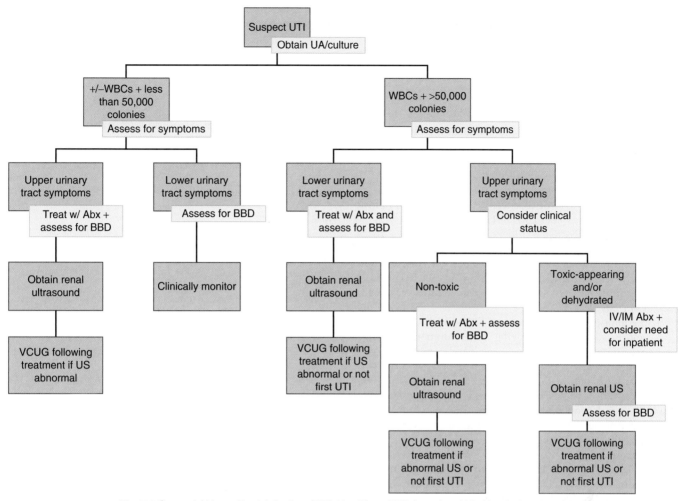

• **Fig 41.1** Suspect Urinary Tract Infection *(UTI)* Algorithm. *BBD*, bowel and bladder dysfunction; *IM*, intramuscular; *IV*, intravenous; *UA*, urinalysis; *US*, ultrasound; *VCUG*, Voiding cystourethrogram; *WBCs*, white blood cells. Lower urinary tract symptoms include bladder symptoms (urinary frequency/urgency/incontinence/dysuria); upper urinary tract symptoms include fever, flank pain, gross hematuria, vomiting, malaise), abnormal renal ultrasound includes findings such as hydronephrosis, renal scarring, abnormal renal size (AAP Subcommittee on UTI, 2016; AUA, 2010/2017).

- UA should be used only to raise or lower suspicion. Suspicious findings include foul odor, cloudiness, nitrites, leukocytes, alkaline pH, proteinuria, hematuria, pyuria, and bacteriuria.
- Leukocyte esterase chemical tests detect pyuria, but pyuria may arise from causes other than UTI.
- Consider obtaining a lab UA with reflexive gram stain and microscopy if dipstick findings are positive.
- Bacterial identification and determination of sensitivities are necessary in patients who appear toxic or could have pyelonephritis, have relapses or recurrent UTI, or are nonresponsive to medication.
- Complete blood count (CBC) (elevated WBC count), erythrocyte sedimentation rate (ESR), C-reactive protein (CRP), BUN, and creatinine should be done if the child is younger than 1 year old, appears ill, or if pyelonephritis is suspected.
- Blood culture should be done if sepsis is suspected (see Chapter 28).

Differential Diagnosis

The differential diagnosis includes urethritis, vaginitis, viral cystitis, foreign body, sexual abuse, dysfunctional voiding, appendicitis, pelvic abscess, and pelvic inflammatory disease. Any child who has acute fever without a focus, FTT, chronic diarrhea, or recurrent abdominal pain should be evaluated for UTI.

Management

Goals of treatment are to quickly identify the extent and level of infection; to eradicate infection; to provide symptomatic relief; to find and correct anatomic or functional abnormalities; and to prevent recurrence and renal damage (AAP Subcommittee on Urinary Tract Infection, 2016). When deciding on a treatment plan, the child's age, gender, symptoms, the suspected location of the UTI, and antibiotic resistance patterns in the community must be considered. Fig 41.1 outlines treatment of UTIs in the child.

Infants 2 to 24 Months Old

To diagnose UTI, the child should have both a UA suggesting infection (positive leukocyte and/or nitrite tests) and urine culture from a sterile catheterization or suprapubic aspiration (SPA) with at least 50,000 cfu/mL. Risk factors have been identified to help steer management as judged by the clinician. Higher risk for girls is white race, age younger than 12 months, temperature of at least 102.2°F (39°C), fever lasting at least 2 days, and absence of another source of infection. Higher risk for boys is nonblack race, temperature of at least 102.2°F (39°C), fever lasting more than 24 hours, and absence of another source of infection (Roberts, 2012; AAP, 2016).

Asymptomatic Bacteriuria

If there are no leukocytes on UA, no treatment is indicated.

Uncomplicated Cystitis

Use regional antibiotic resistance patterns and culture and sensitivity results when choosing antibiotics. Short-term (3 to 5 days) antibiotics may be as effective in treating non-febrile bladder infections as standard 7- to 10-day dosing with no increased risk of recurrence (Elder, 2016d). Children 2 to 24 months old and febrile children should have 7 to 14 days of antibiotics. Additional specific recommendations for the febrile child less than 24 months can be found in the AAP Guidelines. Recommended oral medications include the following (Lee et al., 2018):

- Trimethoprim-sulfamethoxazole (TMP-SMX): More than 2 months old—8 to 12 mg/kg TMP component in two divided doses; adolescents, 160 mg TMP component every 12 hours.
- Amoxicillin: Younger than 3 months old—20 to 30 mg/kg/day in two divided doses every 12 hours; older than 3 months old—25 to 50 mg/kg/day in two divided doses; adolescents, 250 to 500 mg every 8 hours or 875 mg every 12 hours.
- Amoxicillin clavulanate (doses for amoxicillin component): Younger than 3 months old—30 mg/kg/day in two divided doses; older than 3 months old—20 to 45 mg/kg/day in two or three divided doses; adolescents—250 to 500 mg every 8 hours or 875 mg every 12 hours.
- Cephalexin: 50 to 100 mg/kg/day divided in four doses and given every 6 hours (maximum dose of 4 g/day).
- Cefixime: Older than 6 months old—16 mg/kg/day divided every 12 hours for first day, then 8 mg/kg/day divided every 12 hours to complete 13-day treatment; adolescents—400 mg every 12 to 24 hours.
- Nitrofurantoin: Older than 1 month old—5 to 7 mg/kg/day divided every 6 hours (maximum 400 mg/24 hours); adolescents—50 to 100 mg/dose every 6 hours (macrocrystals) or 100 mg twice a day (dual release).
- Recurrent UTI: Further evaluation required. Prophylactic antibiotic use (Box 41.2) is controversial and not routinely recommended.
- Acute pyelonephritis: Oral therapy is equally as effective as parenteral therapy in treating pyelonephritis and preventing kidney damage.
- Hospitalization is required if severity of symptoms warrants—dehydrated, vomiting, or not drinking. Children 1 month old and younger should be admitted and provided a parenteral regimen.
- Infants over 1 month and children with uncomplicated pyelonephritis (well hydrated, no vomiting, no abdominal pain) can be effectively treated with cefixime, cephalexin, or amoxicillin clavulanate.
- Adolescents with uncomplicated pyelonephritis can be treated with either amoxicillin clavulanate (875/125 mg twice a day) or ciprofloxacin (500 mg twice a day or extended release 1000 mg once a day).

• BOX 41.2 Radiologic Workup and Prophylaxis for Urinary Tract Infections

Why Do a Radiologic Workup?
- To identify any structural or functional abnormality of the urinary tract
- To identify any renal scarring or damage

Who Requires a Workup?
- Order a renal and bladder ultrasound on children with the first positive urine culture and with fever and systemic illness. In children with one or more infections of the lower urinary tract (dysuria, urgency, frequency, suprapubic pain), renal and bladder ultrasound may be considered; however, assessment and treatment of bladder and bowel dysfunction is most important.
- If the renal ultrasound is abnormal, voiding cystourethrogram is indicated.

What about Prophylaxis?
- There is controversy about if and when prophylaxis should be used (AAP Subcommittee on Urinary Tract Infection, 2016). If a decision to use prophylaxis is made and depending on the source, between one-quarter to one-half of the treatment dose of antibiotic may be given at bedtime.
- Nitrofurantoin: Older than 2 months old: 1-2 mg/kg as a single daily dose; expensive; liquid form poorly tolerated; consider sprinkling capsules over applesauce, yogurt, pudding
- TMP-SMX: TMP 2 mg/kg as a single daily dose or 5 mg/kg twice per week (based on TMP component) if older than 1 month
- Cephalexin: 10 mg/kg as a single daily dose
- Amoxicillin: 10 mg/kg as a single daily dose; can be used for a newborn or premature infant; not used past the first 2 postnatal months; shelf life for liquid is 14 days

AAP, American Academy of Pediatrics; TMP-SMX, trimethoprim-sulfamethoxazole.

- Follow-up cultures are not routinely needed. However, follow-up urine culture should be done 48 to 72 hours after initiating treatment if symptoms persist or organism resistance is found in the community.
- If the culture is not sterile or if no clinical improvement is seen, antibiotic change should be based on sensitivity report. Urine should be sent for bacterial identification and sensitivity studies if not performed initially, and an alternative broad-spectrum antibiotic should be used pending those results. Culture should again be repeated after 48 to 72 hours if response to therapy limited.
- Phenazopyridine may be given at 12 mg/kg/day for 6- to 12-year-olds and 200 mg for those older than 12 years old, three times a day for dysuria.
- Radiologic workup (Table 41.4) is recommended to identify any structural or functional abnormality of the urinary tract and any renal scarring or damage.
- Children younger than 2 years old with the first UTI should have a renal and bladder ultrasound as soon as the urine is sterile or when the prescribed antibiotic has been completed. Additionally, all children with fever, diagnosed with pyelonephritis, or with recurrent UTIs should have a renal and bladder ultrasound. VCUG does not need to be done routinely with first febrile UTI. However, if ultrasound reveals hydronephrosis, scarring, or other atypical or concerning findings, VCUG should be utilized (American Urological Association [AUA], 2010/2017).
- DMSA scan ordered by the urological specialist may be obtained when renal scarring is suspected or when diagnosis of pyelonephritis is uncertain (AUA, 2010/2017).

TABLE 41.4 Radiologic Studies Done for Evaluation of Urinary Tract Conditions

Study	Cost	Advantages	Disadvantages	Use
Ultrasound	Least expensive	Shows structure, shape, and growth Detects structural abnormality, obstruction, pyelonephritis, large scars Painless, low risk, no radiation, noninvasive, available	Does not detect small scars of VUR Poor visualization of ureters Does not measure renal function or transient injury to kidney	Initial evaluation with first UTI and follow-up
Voiding cysto-urethrogram (VCUG) (radiographic)	Least expensive	Detects and grades VUR if high or low pressure, high or low bladder volumes, during voiding, during early or late bladder filling Visualizes bladder and urethra (especially in males) and diverticula	Does not detect obstruction, pyelonephritis, scars Greater radiation than with scan Requires intravesical administration of contrast	Indicated in infants and children with abnormal ultrasound
Dimercaptosuccinic acid (DMSA) renal scan (nuclear)	Most expensive	Detects acute inflammation, scars, and obstruction Earlier detection of parenchymal damage—large or small scars, permanent or focal—than with IVP (1-3 years old)	Does not detect VUR or measure renal function Does not evaluate calyces, ureters, bladder, or urethra	Follow-up for fever of unknown origin and negative ultrasound in neonates To diagnose acute pyelonephritis To detect renal scars
Computed tomography (CT) (contrast)	Expensive	Detects obstruction, pyelonephritis, large scars	Does not detect small scars or VUR Risk of allergic reaction, acute renal failure	Trauma

IVP, Intravenous pyelogram; *UTI,* urinary tract infection; *VUR,* vesicoureteral reflux.

Patient and Family Education, Prevention, and Prognosis

Discuss the following with parents and/or patients:
- Clear explanation of the cause, potential complications, and overall treatment plan, including short- and long-term plans.
- Frequent and complete voiding and increased fluid intake, especially water. Scheduled voiding times, voiding with knees spread apart, or double voiding (voiding and then immediately attempting to void again) is helpful.
- Proper hygiene and avoiding irritants, such as bubble baths, sitting in soapy water, and perfumed soaps. Avoid wearing tight pants, especially spandex pants. Wear cotton underwear. Treat perineal inflammation to help prevent UTI.
- Treat constipation, pinworms.
- Encourage sexually active females to drink water before intercourse and void immediately afterward.
- Decrease intake of bladder irritants, such as the "four Cs" (caffeine, carbonated beverages, chocolate, citrus), aspartame (NutraSweet), alcohol, and spicy foods.
- Seek prompt medical attention with recurrence of fever and/or duration of fever for more than 48 hours, especially if younger than 24 months old.

Vesicoureteral Reflux

VUR is retrograde regurgitation of urine from the bladder into the ureters, and potentially the kidney. The major concern with VUR is the exposure of the kidney to infected urine which may cause pyelonephritis. Primary VUR is the most common type and typically involves an abnormally short ureter and ineffective valve. Secondary VUR is due to either functional or structural bladder outlet obstruction. It is graded according to an international classification (Fig 41.2). Grade I does not reach the renal pelvis; grade II extends up to the renal pelvis without dilation; grade III describes reflux to the renal pelvis with mild to moderate dilation of the ureter and the renal pelvis; grades IV and V (high grade) include definite distention of the ureters and renal pelvis and can include hydronephrosis or reflux into the intrarenal collecting system (Elder, 2016f).

VUR is the most common anatomic abnormality found in young infants and children with UTI. Approximately 30% to 40% of children with affected siblings have reflux, and 50% of children with affected mothers have reflux (Elder, 2016f). A meta-analysis identified a positive correlation with recurrent UTIs, BBD and renal scarring (AUA 2010/2017).

History and Clinical Findings

The history may be positive for a previous UTI, abnormal voiding pattern or dysfunction, unexplained febrile illness, chronic constipation, prenatal high-grade hydronephrosis, and/or UTI symptoms. The family history may be positive for VUR.

Diagnostic Studies

- Ultrasonography (may be normal even in the presence of reflux)
- VCUG establishes the presence of reflux and determines the grade.
- DMSA scan to assess for renal scarring if renal ultrasound is abnormal.
- BP and serum creatinine if bilateral renal abnormalities are found.
- UA, and subsequent urine culture if UA suggests UTI.

Management

The goal of treatment is the prevention of infection and subsequent scarring. Early identification and appropriate treatment of infection achieve this goal (Table 41.5).

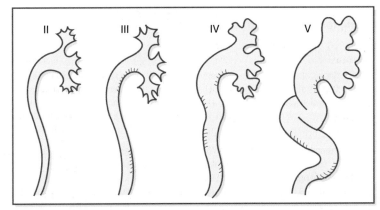

• **Fig 41.2** Grading of Vesicoureteral Reflux. Grade I: Vesicoureteral reflux (VUR) into a nondilated ureter. Grade II: VUR into the upper collecting system without dilation. Grade III: VUR into dilated ureter and/or blunting of calyceal fornices. Grade IV: VUR into a grossly dilated ureter. Grade V: massive VUR, with significant ureteral dilation and tortuosity and loss of the papillary impression. (From Elder JS. Vesicoureteral reflux. In Kliegman RM, Stanton BF, St Geme JW, et al., eds. *Nelson Textbook of Pediatrics*. 20th ed. Elsevier; 2016:2562–2567.e. Fig 539.2.)

TABLE 41.5 Management of Primary Vesicoureteral Reflux in Children

	Monitor Clinically	Treat BBD	CAP	Yearly renal ultrasound +VCUG	Surgical Correction
Grade I	Yes	Yes	Avoid	Avoid	Avoid
Grade II	Yes	Yes	Consider	Consider	Consider
Grade III	Not alone	Yes	Yes	Yes	Consider
Grade IV-V	Not alone	Yes	Yes	Yes	Consider

BBD, Bowel bladder dysfunction; *CAP*, continuous antibiotic prophylaxis; *VCUG*, voiding cystourethrogram.

• Most children outgrow their reflux secondary to an increase in the ureter intramural length. Grades I and II reflux resolve spontaneously in up to 85% of children, grade III reflux resolves spontaneously in 50%. Factors associated with decreased chance for resolution include grades IV and V reflux, bilateral reflux, and older children who present with reflux. Very few children with low-grade VUR require surgery (Elder, 2016f).
• Providers should treat underlying comorbidities, such as constipation and dysfunctional voiding.
• Prophylactic antibiotics to prevent UTI, pyelonephritis, renal injury, and other sequelae may be used when a child has VUR. Prophylaxis is recommended for children with history of a febrile UTI, VUR grades III-V, or for children younger than 1 year old (AUA 2016/2017). Recently, a number of other studies questioned the efficacy of prophylactic antibiotics for both VUR and recurrent UTI. There are no set guidelines for prophylaxis in children over 1 year of age, and management should consider the presence of BBD, VUR grade, renal scarring, and parental choice (AUA 2016, 2017). Untreated BBD can increase incidence of breakthrough UTIs while on continuous antibiotic prophylaxis (AUA 2016/2017).
• Interval urine cultures are performed with symptoms of unexplained illness.
• Repeat VCUG once every 12 to 24 months after diagnosis, with the 24-month intervals in patients with less chance for spontaneous resolution, such as high-grade or bilateral VUR or presence of BBD. Annual BP and growth measurement.

VCUG is optional if parents choose an observation-only approach, which is appropriate in the absence of UTIs or BBD.
• Surgical correction includes endoscopic injection of a bulking agent at the ureteral orifice and open surgical correction (ureteral reimplantation) (AUA 2010/2017).

Patient and Family Education, Prevention, and Prognosis

• VUR does not cause scarring, infection does; but VUR is a risk factor for pyelonephritis and subsequent scarring. Ensure prompt treatment of UTI. Emphasize the necessity of urine culture with any suspicious symptoms. The potential for untreated, chronic UTI leading to chronic renal disease must be explained. BP and growth should be monitored.
• Treating of BBD improves surgical outcomes.
• Siblings are no longer routinely screened for presence of VUR (AUA 2010/2017).
• Prophylactic medicines are best given at night because of urinary stasis while asleep. Recommended medications used for prophylaxis are listed in Box 41.2.
• Review the education discussed in the UTI section.

Hematuria

Hematuria is the presence of five or more RBCs per HPF in three consecutive fresh, centrifuged specimens obtained over several weeks (Pan and Avner, 2016b). The number of RBCs per HPF considered to be abnormal ranges from 1 to more than 5 per HPF in unspun urine, and more than 5 to 10 per HPF in spun urine. In this text, *hematuria* is defined as more than two RBCs per HPF in unspun urine or five per HPF in spun urine. The term *gross hematuria* is blood seen in the urine and the color is significant in the location of the disorder. Brownish, tea-colored urine with casts or protein is usually glomerular in origin. Blood clots and red-to-pink urine with isomorphic RBCs but no protein usually originates from the lower tract. Factors causing hematuria can arise anywhere in the urinary system, from the urinary meatus to the kidneys. Urine can be discolored with a positive urine dipstick when there is myoglobinuria or hemoglobinuria, in which case no RBCs are seen on microscopic examination, so dipstick hematuria should be confirmed via UA. Hematuria can be microscopic or macroscopic. Microscopic hematuria may be either persistent or transient.

The causes of macroscopic hematuria include hypercalciuria, immunoglobulin A (IgA) nephropathy, glomerulonephritis (GN), UTI, hydronephrosis, tumor, cystitis cystica, polyps, or epididymitis. The incidence of hematuria is 0.5% to 2% when confirmed with repeat UA (Pan and Avner, 2016b). However, 50% of children with gross hematuria have UTIs.

History and Clinical Findings

- Previous medical history of cystic kidney disease, sickle cell disease, systemic lupus erythematosus (SLE), malignancy
- Family or previous history of hematuria, nephrolithiasis, cystic kidney, hemoglobinopathy, sickle cell disease or trait, SLE, hypertension, congestive heart disease, malignancy, deafness, renal failure
- Preceding illness: Viral or streptococcal pharyngitis, impetigo
- Onset, duration, pattern, and timing of hematuria; color of urine
- Dysuria, urgency, frequency, or enuresis
- Presence of pain (back, abdominal, or flank) with voiding
- Straining or squatting with urination (tumor)
- Strenuous exercise or trauma (including bladder catheterization)
- Trauma, foreign body
- Sexual activity or abuse
- Current menstruation
- Edema, rash, pallor, or arthralgias
- Certain drugs (sulfonamides, nitrofurantoin, salicylates, phenazopyridine, toxins [lead, benzenes]), and foods (food color, beets, blackberries, rhubarb, and paprika) can discolor the urine but will not result in RBCs in the urine (Pan and Avner, 2016b)
- Symptoms related to chronic renal disease (Box 41.3)

Physical Examination

- Growth parameters: FTT or falling growth curves (chronic renal insufficiency or long-standing acidosis)
- Vital signs, especially BP
- Malformed ears (congenital renal disease)
- Oliguria or anuria
- Edema, hypertension, and proteinuria, which are suggestive of glomerular disease
- Flank pain, which is suggestive of an upper tract disorder

> • **BOX 41.3** **Seven "Red Flags" for Chronic Renal Failure**
>
> 1. Failure to thrive (poor growth, fatigue, anorexia, nausea, gastroesophageal reflux, vomiting)
> 2. Chronic anemia (normochromic, normocytic, nonresponsive to medication)
> 3. Complicated enuresis (daytime frequency, urgency, incontinence, chronic constipation, encopresis, infrequent voiding, straining to void, recurrent urinary tract infection)
> 4. Prolonged, unexplained vomiting or nausea (especially in the morning), anorexia, weight loss without diarrhea
> 5. Hypotension
> 6. Unusual bone disease (e.g., rickets, valgus deformity, fracture with minor trauma)
> 7. Poor school performance (e.g., headache, fatigue, inattention, withdrawal from activities)

- Abdominal or flank mass, which suggests an obstruction, such as Wilms tumor, cystic disease, or posterior valves
- External genitalia: Excoriation, bleeding, foreign body, abuse

Diagnostic Studies

- Urine dipstick analysis for pyuria, proteinuria, hematuria, and concentration
- If greater than 1+ hematuria by dipstick (which equals three RBCs/HPF or 0.02 mg/dL hemoglobin), microscopic examination for RBCs is needed to differentiate RBCs from hemoglobinuria or myoglobinuria.
- The most significant differentiating factor is the presence of proteinuria. If present, rapid evaluation and early referral to a nephrologist are essential. See section on "Nephrotic Syndrome."
- Microscopic examination of the urine includes RBCs, size and shape of the cells, casts, crystals, and WBCs
- Distorted, misshapen RBCs of different sizes suggest glomerular disease.
- Crystalluria is most commonly caused by hypercalciuria.
- Urine culture
- 24-hour urine collection
- First morning UA on first-degree relatives
- Renal ultrasound if Wilms tumor or nephrolithiasis is suspected. Spiral helical computed tomography (CT) scan is the most sensitive modality for diagnosing nephrolithiasis, but there is a large radiation exposure (Pan and Avner, 2016b).
- If there are systemic symptoms (e.g., edema, hypertension, changes in urine output), consider further evaluation as described in the "Nephritis and Glomerulonephritis" section (Pan and Avner, 2016a).
- Renal biopsy is recommended for recurrent gross hematuria and coexisting nephritic syndrome, hypertension, renal insufficiency, systemic illness, and parent anxiety (Pan and Avner, 2016b).
- Cystoscopy, which is invasive and costly, rarely used, and done if other results are inconclusive and symptoms persist.

Differential Diagnosis

Categories of hematuria to be considered in the diagnostic workup of hematuria are (Pan and Avner, 2016b):
- Gross hematuria
- Urine color is red or tea-colored; microscopic examination shows RBCs.

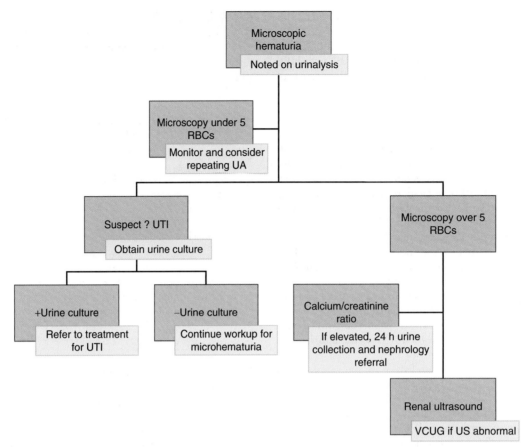

• **Fig 41.3** Management of Asymptomatic Microscopic Hematuria. *RBC, Red blood cells; UA,* urinalysis; *US,* ultrasound; *UTI,* urinary tract infection; *VCUG,* voiding cystourethrogram.

• Common causes are poststreptococcal glomerulonephritis (PSGN), renal disease, UTI, trauma, coagulopathy, crystalluria, and nephrolithiasis. Recurrent episodes of gross hematuria are rare.
• Consider Henoch-Schönlein purpura (HSP) when there is gross hematuria in the presence of abdominal pain, with or without bloody stools, arthralgias, and purpuric rash (see Chapter 25).
• Consider IgA nephropathy with gross hematuria in the presence of acute illness or strenuous exercise.
• Sickle cell disease and trait can cause recurrent gross hematuria (mostly males, unilateral kidney).
• Rhabdomyosarcoma causes gross hematuria and voiding dysfunction (Pan and Avner 2016b).
• Attention and methodic approach are required as history and physical examination guide the workup.
• Renal disease is more likely if microscopic hematuria is accompanied by proteinuria on a first morning sample.
• Other nonspecific symptoms (fever, malaise, weight change), extra renal symptoms (malar rash, purpura, arthritis, headache, dysuria, abdominal or flank pain, edema, oliguria) may be present.
• Asymptomatic microscopic hematuria rarely indicates significant renal disease.
• Family history is important to assess for benign familial hematuria.
• Hypercalciuria is commonly associated with asymptomatic microscopic hematuria, which leaves patients prone to symptomatic urolithiasis. The diagnosis is made by urine laboratory examination if the spot calcium-creatinine ratio done on the first morning specimen is elevated to more than

0.2, or the 24-hours urinary calcium to more than 4 mg/kg/day. Hypercalciuria is associated with immobilization, diuretics, vitamin D intoxication, hyperparathyroidism, and sarcoidosis (Pan and Avner, 2016b).
• Regularly monitor for hypertension and proteinuria.
• Asymptomatic hematuria with proteinuria is worrisome for renal disease and further evaluation for renal problems is required.
• Consider evaluating for orthostatic proteinuria (see "Proteinuria" section). Persistent proteinuria is more indicative of a glomerular process.
• Hematuria caused by external irritation of the urinary meatus will resolve with healing and removal of the offending irritant (diaper rash, soaps, bubble bath, lotions) or avoidance of the offending behavior (e.g., scratching, masturbation, sexual activity).

Management

A progressive approach to evaluating hematuria should be undertaken with the goal of not overlooking serious, treatable, progressive conditions while at the same time avoiding unnecessary studies (Fig 41.3). Referral is indicated for gross hematuria with unclear cause, symptomatic microscopic hematuria, or persistent asymptomatic hematuria and proteinuria as renal biopsy may be indicated (Pan and Avner, 2016b). Asymptomatic hematuria requires periodic evaluation every 1 to 2 years to reevaluate for coexisting conditions or proteinuria, and to revisit family history of hematuria or hearing deficits.

Patient and Family Education, Prevention, and Prognosis

Patient education should stress the importance of follow-up for evaluation of the hematuria. Prognosis depends on the cause of the hematuria.

Proteinuria

Protein in the urine is commonly detected by dipstick tests. It may be transient, recurrent, or fixed. Proteinuria can be a symptom of disease, or it can reflect a benign, self-limited condition. The quantity of protein and the timing of its presence determine its significance. Qualitative protein in urine, as tested by dipstick, is considered a positive result if it registers 1+ (30 mg/dL) or more in urine with a specific gravity of less than 1.015. Quantitative protein is tested by measuring a volume of urine over a set period. A level of less than 4 $mg/m^2/h$ is considered normal, 4 to 40 $mg/m^2/h$ is abnormal, and greater than 40 $mg/m^2/h$ indicates nephritic disease.

Four groups of proteinuria exist: (1) isolated, (2) transient or functional, (3) glomerular, and (4) tubulointerstitial.

- Isolated proteinuria includes orthostatic proteinuria and persistent asymptomatic proteinuria, which are the most common.
- Orthostatic proteinuria accounts for up to 60% (75% in adolescents) of cases of proteinuria (Pais and Avner, 2016a). In this condition, the child excretes abnormal amounts of protein when upright but normal amounts when lying down. Orthostatic proteinuria is demonstrated by collecting urine as described in the "Diagnostic Studies" section.
- Persistent asymptomatic proteinuria is a common, transient phenomenon in which an otherwise healthy child, with normal clinical and laboratory workup, has an abnormally high level of protein in the urine.
- Transient or functional proteinuria is usually caused by some type of stress.
- Exercised-induced proteinuria is documented by collecting a urine sample, having the patient exercise vigorously for several minutes, and then collecting another sample. The post exercise sample is usually strongly positive.
- Fever-induced proteinuria can accompany any febrile state and usually subsides with resolution of the fever. Other stress-related causes include cold exposure, infection, congestive heart failure, and seizures. This type of proteinuria usually resolves in 1 to 2 weeks, and if resolution has been verified, no further workup is required.
- Glomerular proteinuria and tubulointerstitial proteinuria are the least common types characterized by high proteinuria levels. Some authorities believe that children with persistent proteinuria, even at low levels, should be followed with a high index of suspicion for an underlying, progressive renal disorder.

Proteinuria originates from problems with glomerular filtration, tubular reabsorption or secretion, or both. The child is often asymptomatic. If proteinuria is significant enough to cause hypoproteinemia, edema is present. The incidence of proteinuria is cited at 30% to 55% in school-age children. It persists, however, in up to 6% of children when four consecutive urine specimens are tested (Pais and Avner, 2016a).

History and Clinical Findings

- Family history of deafness, visual problems, and renal disease
- Recent strenuous exercise or febrile illness
- Polydipsia or polyuria
- Vague symptoms, such as malaise, fatigue, or pallor
- Symptoms related to chronic renal disease (see Box 41.3)

Physical Examination

- Growth and development parameters (poor weight gain or FTT with chronic disease; weight gain with nephrotic syndrome)
- BP (hypertension), pulse, respiratory rate
- Edema, especially periorbital edema, or symptoms of fluid retention
- Abdominal examination for a mass, enlarged kidney, fluid, tenderness

Diagnostic Studies

- UA (repeated three times over 1 to 2 weeks), preferably done on a first-voided specimen.
- 1+ protein (30 mg/dL) is significant if the specific gravity is less than 1.015; 2+ protein (100 mg/dL) is significant if the specific gravity is greater than 1.015.
- False-positive results occur in highly concentrated or alkaline (pH greater than 5.5) urine. False-negative results occur in dilute or acidic urine.
- At least 75% of asymptomatic patients with proteinuria in a single urine specimen have normal urine on repeated testing.
- A first void urine sample collected immediately after arising can be compared with a specimen collected after several hours of activity to rule out orthostatic etiology. Have the child void before sleep to obtain accurate results. A typical result yields negative to trace amounts on the first morning specimen, but 1+ or greater on the second specimen. If the result is equivocal, back-to-back urine samples (from arising to bedtime and bedtime to arising) can be evaluated for quantitative protein.
- Microscopic urine: RBCs or WBCs (or both), casts, bacteria, oval fat bodies, or other abnormalities are present in most pathologic conditions.
- A urine protein-to-creatinine ratio on a first morning voided sample. Normal values are less than 0.5 mg/dL in children younger than 2 years old and less than 0.2 mg/dL in children older than 2 years; greater than 2 mg/dL is considered nephritic (Pais and Avner, 2016a). An abnormal urine protein-to-creatinine ratio requires further testing.
- A 12- or 24-hour timed urine collection for creatinine (normal: 14 to 20 mg/kg/24 hours) and protein excretion (normal: less than 4 $mg/m^2/h$) is elevated with proteinuria. A back-to-back sample collection (see earlier) is done to compare active or upright and resting levels.
- If protein in urine is greater than 4 $mg/m^2/h$, check the CBC, electrolytes, BUN, creatinine, albumin/total protein, C3, C4, cholesterol, liver functions, and urine culture and refer to nephrology. Other studies that may be considered by specialist include ultrasonogram, VCUG, and radionuclide scans with evaluation for systemic disease as indicated (e.g., antinuclear antibody [ANA], anti-streptolysin O [ASO], streptozyme, hepatitis B, human immunodeficiency virus [HIV], tuberculosis).

Differential Diagnosis

Pseudoproteinuria can be caused by semisynthetic penicillins or anti-inflammatory agents.

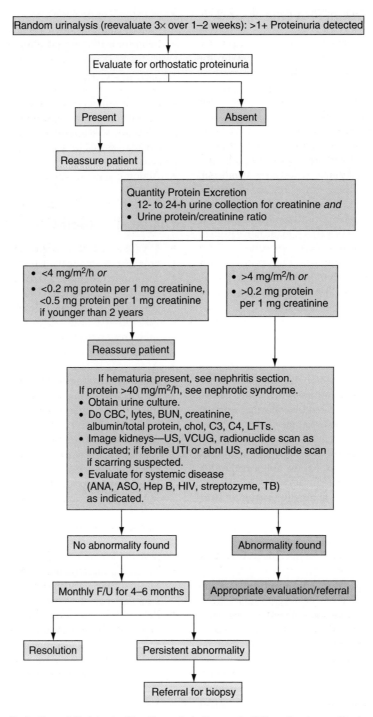

• **Fig 41.4** Evaluation of Proteinuria Algorithm. *abnl,* Abnormal; *ANA,* antinuclear antibody; *ASO,* anti-streptolysin O; *BUN,* blood urea nitrogen; *C3,* complement 3; *C4,* complement 4; *CBC,* complete blood count; *chol,* cholesterol; *F/U,* follow-up; *Hep B,* hepatitis B; *HIV,* human immunodeficiency virus; *LFT,* liver function test; *lytes,* electrolytes; *TB,* tuberculosis; *US,* ultrasound; *UTI,* urinary tract infection; *VCUG,* voiding cystourethrogram. (Adapted from Norwood VF, Peters CA. Disorders of renal functional development in children. In: Wein AJ, Kavoussi LR, Partin AW, et al., eds. *Campbell-Walsh Urology.* Elsevier; Vol. 123. 2016:2849–2872.e2.)

Management

The persistence, quantity, and presence of other abnormalities (e.g., hematuria) are key in evaluating proteinuria (see Fig 41.4).

• If protein by dipstick is trace or 1+ and specific gravity is greater than 1.015, offer reassurance; do monthly recheck of urine for

4 to 6 months. If protein is persistent, refer the patient to a nephrologist.

• If protein by dipstick is greater than 1+, evaluate the child for orthostatic proteinuria (see Diagnostic Studies mentioned previously).

• If first morning urine protein is 1+ or 2+, perform either a quantitative 12- to 24-hour urine protein excretion test or

a random urine total protein-creatinine ratio and UA with microscope. Proceed as shown in Fig 41.4.
- If protein by dipstick is greater than 2+, evaluate for nephrotic syndrome (see later section).
- If hematuria is present, evaluate for nephritis (see later section).
- Follow-up is important to monitor for any change in status.
- Refer to a nephrologist if persistent unexplained nonorthostatic proteinuria, any hematuria or RBC or WBC casts, polyuria or oliguria, nephrotic levels of protein, elevated BUN or creatinine, elevated BP, systemic complaints (e.g., joint pain, rashes, or arthralgias), or a child with a family history of renal failure, GN, sensorineural hearing loss, or kidney transplantation.

Patient and Family Education, Prevention, and Prognosis

Patient education should stress the importance of follow-up to evaluate the cause of proteinuria. Children with mild asymptomatic proteinuria who have a normal first morning specimen do not require extensive testing for kidney disease but should be monitored annually.

Nephrotic Syndrome

Nephrotic syndrome is due to excessive excretion of protein in urine as a result of alterations in the integrity of the glomerular filtration barrier. The main mechanism of the massive protein loss is increased glomerular permeability. The loss can be selective (albumin only) or nonselective (including most serum proteins), and such selectivity is an important distinction in diagnosis. The classic definition of nephrotic syndrome is massive proteinuria (3 to 4+ protein with UA, greater than 40 mg/m^2/h or a protein:creatinine ratio on a first morning void of greater than 2 to 3:1), hypoalbuminemia (less than 2.5 g/dL), edema, and hyperlipidemia. Edema formation results from a decrease in the plasma oncotic pressure due to a loss of serum albumin, which causes water to extravasate into the interstitial space. This then leads to decreased intravascular volume with decreased renal perfusion and activation of the renin-angiotensin system (Pais and Avner, 2016b). With protein loss, the liver increases its synthesis of protein and thereby causes concurrent hyperlipidemia and lipiduria. In addition, the reduced intravascular volume stimulates antidiuretic hormone, which enhances the reabsorption of water.

Nephrotic syndrome is a chronic disease characterized by periods of remission (when both the urinary protein excretion and serum albumin normalize) and relapses (recurrence of proteinuria and hypoalbuminemia after complete remission). Ninety-five percent of the children with minimum change nephrotic syndrome (MCNS) are "steroid responders," having remission with steroid treatment. Steroid responsiveness is the best prognostic indicator for nephrotic syndrome (Pais and Avner, 2016b). Of the remaining children, most are steroid resistant and show no response to steroid treatment. A small number of cases are either partial responders, with minimal response to steroids, or are steroid dependent and require high doses of prednisone with frequent relapses.

Nephrotic syndrome occurs as a result of genetic, immune, systemic, nephrotoxic, allergic, infectious, malignant, vascular, or idiopathic processes. Despite significant research, the understanding of its histopathology is better than the understanding of its pathogenesis. The primary mechanism is believed to be immunologic. The incidence of idiopathic nephrotic syndrome in the United States is 2 to 3/100,000 per year, with a 15 times greater incidence in children than in adults (Pais and Avner, 2016b).

History and Clinical Findings

- History of allergy in up to 50% of children with MCNS
- Edema is the cardinal clinical feature, especially periorbital edema, dependent areas (tight shoes or underwear), and lax tissues (puffy eyes)
- Low urine production
- Gastrointestinal symptoms: Anorexia, paleness, listlessness, diarrhea, vomiting, abdominal pain (right upper quadrant)
- Respiratory difficulties secondary to ascites, effusion, pneumonia in advanced disease

Physical Examination

- Edema initially in tissues of low resistance and dependent areas: Periorbital, scrotal, and labial. If generalized, can become massive (anasarca)
- Anorexia, irritability, fatigue, abdominal discomfort, and diarrhea
- Muscle wasting, malnourishment, growth failure if prolonged
- If the disease is progressive, hydrothorax with respiratory difficulty
- Hypertension; normal BP if hypovolemic
- Chronically ill-appearing

Diagnostic Studies

- UA and microscopic examination (protein of 2+ or greater, hyaline and fine granular casts, microhematuria [in 33%], elevated specific gravity, fat bodies, and casts in urine).
- Quantitative urine protein excretion (24-hour collection or protein-creatinine ratio on a random first morning urine).
- CBC; electrolytes, BUN, creatinine (normal); calcium; serum albumin (less than 2 g/dL), total protein; liver enzymes; triglycerides, lipoproteins, cholesterol (elevated); C3 and C4 (normal); ANA; varicella antibody test in case of exposure while on corticosteroids.
- Consideration of Venereal Disease Research Laboratory (VDRL), hepatitis B surface antigen, HIV, malaria, purified protein derivative (PPD) as indicated by history.
- Neonatal or infant nephrotic syndrome requires a karyotype because male pseudohermaphroditism can be associated with Denys-Drash syndrome.
- Referral with possible kidney biopsy is recommended if criteria for MCNS are not met, systemic disease is present, hypertension and hematuria are present, hypocomplementemia or nonselective proteinemia is present, patient is older than 7 years, patient is nonresponsive to steroids, or if relapses are frequent.

Differential Diagnosis

Infants (newborn to 1 year old) usually have congenital renal problems, children 7 years old and older are likely to have focal glomerulosclerosis or mesangial proliferative GN, and teens have membranous nephropathy. The differential diagnosis includes hypoproteinemia from starvation, liver disease, and protein-losing enteropathy; none of these conditions has associated proteinuria. GN should also be considered in the differential diagnosis.

Management

Nephrotic syndrome is a complex, often chronic disorder that responds to careful management with a gratifying long-term positive outcome. The diagnosis is made with 95% certainty on clinical impressions. A major goal is to control edema while awaiting definitive remission.

- Consultation with and/or referral to a nephrologist should occur because of the constantly changing strategies for managing these children.
- Hospitalization may be necessary initially if disease is severe.
- Prednisone (2 mg/kg/day; maximum 60 mg) to induce remission, which can occur as early as 14 days as evidenced by diuresis. Steroids are continued for at least 4 to 6 weeks (Pais and Avner, 2016b). Relapses are treated with a short course of steroids and the patient is weaned as soon as the proteinuria resolves.
- Non-corticosteroid medications (cyclophosphamide and cyclosporine) are used by nephrologists if the child is steroid-dependent, steroid-resistant, or relapses frequently (Pais and Avner, 2016b).
- Activity and diet recommendations: No limitation is placed on activity. During active disease, salt may be restricted by the nephrologist. At other times, a diet appropriate for age is recommended.
- Diuretics and albumin replacement are sometimes used in the acute phase. Home BP monitoring may be recommended.
- Daily home proteinuria testing may be recommended to monitor the child and promptly identify exacerbations. Relapses are persistent proteinuria greater than 2+ every day for 3 days.

Complications

Children with nephrotic syndrome are susceptible to pneumococcal, *E. coli, Pseudomonas,* and *Haemophilus influenzae* infection because of fluid stasis; such infection is seen as peritonitis, pneumonia, cellulitis, or septicemia. Hypertension or hypotension is a possibility. Because the child is in a hypercoagulable state, thromboembolism is possible. Protein losses and compromising edema are also potential complications.

Patient and Family Education, Prevention, and Prognosis

Patient education should stress the importance of continued, regular care to monitor renal function and the early treatment of the disease or concurrent infections. Families must know that relapses are the rule. An understanding of the disease process, side effects of steroids, recognition of infection, and the importance of monitoring proteinuria for relapses is crucial. If chronic steroid treatment is needed, the child and family must understand the side effects of the medication. The prognosis is good in steroid responders, with relapses that decrease in frequency as the child grows older, typically without any residual renal dysfunction. However, recent research hypothesizes that relapse and long-term implications of Nephrotic Syndrome may be misunderstood due to a lack of studies and follow-up through adulthood. In fact, newer studies suggest anywhere from 5% to 30% of individuals relapse into adulthood. Long-term complications range from hypertension and osteoporosis to end-stage renal disease (ESRD) (Hjorten, Anwar, and Reidy, 2016).

Nephritis and Glomerulonephritis

Nephritis is a noninfectious, inflammatory kidney response characterized by varied degrees of hypertension, edema, proteinuria, and hematuria that is either microscopic or macroscopic with dysmorphic RBCs and casts. Nephritis is classified as acute, intermittent, or chronic. Primary GN occurs when the glomerulus is the original and predominant structure impaired. Secondary GN occurs when renal involvement is secondary to systemic disease (e.g., SLE, HSP, primary vasculitis, Goodpasture syndrome, or drug hypersensitivity reactions). Involvement can be in the glomerulus, the interstitium, localized in one part of the kidney, or generalized throughout. GN refers to inflammation primarily in the glomeruli; interstitial nephritis refers to inflammation in the interstitium primarily caused by drug reactions. PSGN is the classic form of GN.

Acute nephritis most commonly occurs as PSGN, which is characterized by a history of streptococcal infection within the prior 2 weeks and an acute onset of edema, oliguria, hypertension, and gross hematuria. Consider an alternative diagnosis if the following findings are present: nephrotic levels of protein, lack of evidence for a post-infection mechanism, rapidly deteriorating renal function, or clinical or laboratory findings suggesting other forms of GN (e.g., rash, positive ANA).

Intermittent gross hematuria and proteinuria syndromes include the following:

- IgA nephropathy, or Berger disease, is the most common chronic GN in children of European or Asian descent and is uncommon in African Americans; it is more common in males than females (2:1). This condition is immunologic and causes recurrent gross and microscopic hematuria, and often proteinuria. It is present in about one-third of persons biopsied for persistent microscopic hematuria. It is often precipitated by viral infections or strenuous exercise, and each episode lasts less than 72 hours. BP is normal, no edema is present, and C3 is normal. Definitive diagnosis is made by biopsy. The prognosis is good in the absence of elevated serum creatinine or nephrotic-range proteinuria, although progression to chronic renal insufficiency can occur.
- Hereditary or familial nephritis involves many disorders, but the best known is Alport syndrome. More common and severe in males, with onset before 15 years old, this condition is inherited as an X-linked dominant trait 75% of the time. The initial manifestation is isolated, persistent, microscopic hematuria with intermittent macrohematuria and variable proteinuria, occurring with an upper respiratory infection or exercise. Laboratory abnormalities are variable; biopsy verifies the diagnosis. Extra renal abnormalities, including neurogenic deafness, ocular abnormalities, and macrothrombocytopenia are common. Vision and hearing screening are essential, and PCPs should refer if abnormalities are noted. Severe forms of the disease can lead to end-stage renal disease, which is often heralded by hypotension.
- Familial or benign recurrent nephritis, also known as *thin-basement-membrane disease,* is a disorder inherited as an autosomal dominant trait with unknown etiology. Episodes are characterized by macroscopic and microscopic hematuria and mild proteinuria, often precipitated by upper respiratory tract infection. Laboratory values other than UA are normal. The diagnosis is confirmed by biopsy, which may not be needed if the disease is mild and confirmed in relatives. In the absence of notable proteinuria, deafness, ocular defects, renal failure, and with normal biopsy findings, the prognosis is excellent.

Chronic nephritis is most commonly known as *membranoproliferative GN* and is distinguished by four types based on biopsy.

Chronic nephritis occurs after acute nephritis or in individuals with nonspecific complaints, such as anorexia, intermittent vomiting, and malaise. It is manifested by diminished renal function that ultimately has detrimental effects on other organ systems. Types I and II may respond to steroids, but the overall prognosis is guarded.

The inflammatory kidney response results from various causes such as infection, an immunologic response, drugs, toxins, and vascular or systemic disorders. PSGN is an immune response by the host to a group A beta-hemolytic skin or pharyngeal streptococcal infection, whereas acute postinfectious glomerulonephritis (APGN) can be caused by bacterial, fungal, viral, parasitic, or rickettsial agents.

PSGN is the most common form of nephritis in childhood, occurs most often between 5 and 12 years old, occurs more often in males (2:1), and is unusual in children younger than 3 years old. The incidence of APGN is difficult to determine because of the large number of patients with subclinical cases (Pan and Avner, 2016a).

History and Clinical Findings

- Streptococcal skin (more likely) or pharyngeal infection within the past 2 to 3 weeks (PSGN). A latent period of 7 to 10 days elapses between infection and the onset of symptoms; if fewer than 5 days or more than 14 days, consider other causes.
- Abrupt onset of gross hematuria.
- Reduced urine output (with diuresis in 5 to 7 days).
- Lethargy, anorexia, nausea, vomiting, abdominal pain.
- Chills, fever, backache (pyelonephritis).
- Medication taken in the past few weeks.

Physical Examination

- Hypertension that is transient and resolves in 1 to 2 weeks
- Edema, especially periorbital edema, or abrupt onset with weight gain
- Circulatory congestion—dyspnea, cough, pallor, pulmonary edema if severe
- Ear malformations
- Flank or abdominal pain or a mass (in polycystic kidney or malignancy [e.g., Wilms tumor])
- Costovertebral angle tenderness (in pyelonephritis)
- Rashes or arthralgias (with SLE, HSP, or impetigo)
- Evidence of trauma or abuse

Diagnostic Studies

- UA with microscopic examination—tea color; elevated specific gravity; macrohematuria and microhematuria; proteinuria not exceeding the amount of hematuria; pyuria in PSGN; granular, hyaline, WBC, or RBC casts; and dysmorphic RBCs
- Serum C3 or C4 (low early in disease, returning to normal in 6 to 8 weeks), total protein and albumin (elevated)
- CBC, ESR, ASO titer (elevated), streptozyme test (positive), anti–deoxyribonucleic acid (DNA) antibody titer
- Electrolytes, BUN, creatinine, and cholesterol
- Fluorescent antinuclear antibody (SLE), hepatitis titers, sickle cell or hemoglobin electrophoresis, tuberculin PPD, and fluorescent treponemal antibody absorption (syphilis)

Differential Diagnosis

Acute nephritis also occurs as part of systemic illnesses, such as SLE, HSP, hemolytic-uremic syndrome, vasculitis, or as a reaction to drugs or irradiation.

Management

Consultation with a nephrologist is recommended in all cases (Fig 41.5).

PSGN treatment is supportive because resolution occurs spontaneously 95% of the time. The course is not affected by corticosteroids, immunosuppression, or other treatment modalities. During the peak of oliguria and hypertension, in the first few days of illness, hospitalization may be required with fluid and sodium limitation and diuretic, antihypertensive, and antibiotic treatment if cultures are positive. Resolution occurs once diuresis begins. Gross hematuria persists for 1 to 2 weeks, urine can be abnormal for 6 to 12 weeks, and microscopic hematuria can persist for up to 2 years. Complement levels return to normal in 6 to 8 weeks (Pan and Avner, 2016a).

- Acute nephritis—possible hospitalization with treatment as described previously.
- IgA nephropathy—annual follow-up with BP, UA, and determination of renal function.
- Benign familial or hereditary nephritis—perform audiometry and review family medical history. Hereditary markers are being developed for this disease.
- Benign recurrent nephritis—monitor UA and renal function every 1 to 2 years.
- Chronic nephritis—a team approach is required to adequately provide care.

Complications

Prolonged oliguria and renal failure can occur if acute nephritis progresses. Hypertensive encephalopathy or congestive heart failure can occur secondary to PSGN. Irreversible parenchymal damage causes hypertension and renal insufficiency.

Patient and Family Education, Prevention, and Prognosis

Patients with PSGN may have macrohematuria or microhematuria for up to 6 to 12 months, but the long-range outcome is excellent. Thin-basement-membrane disease has a good outcome. IgA nephropathy with severe histologic findings has a poor outcome, especially if the child is African American. Patient education should stress the importance of continued, regular care to monitor renal function.

Myoglobinuria

Myoglobin in the urine is associated with acute tissue injury, or rhabdomyolysis. Myoglobinuria is often confused with hematuria as it is associated with a red- or rust-colored pigment in the urine and causes a positive blood test on a urine dipstick. Myoglobin is released into the bloodstream with muscle damage. Myoglobin breaks down into byproducts that are harmful to the kidneys, resulting in acute renal injury. As long as renal injury is prevented and rhabdomyolysis does not occur, myoglobinuria is not associated with long-term effects or high mortality (Chavez, Leon, Einav, and Varon, 2016).

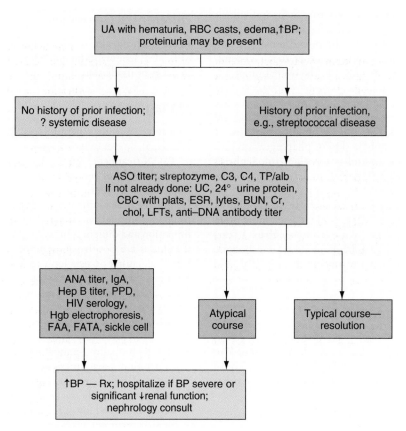

• **Fig 41.5** Evaluation of Nephritis Algorithm. *ANA*, Antinuclear antibody; *ASO*, antistreptolysin O; *BP,* blood pressure; *BUN*, blood urea nitrogen; *C3*, complement 3; *C4*, complement 4; *CBC*, complete blood count; *chol*, cholesterol; *Cr*, creatinine; *DNA*, deoxyribonucleic acid; *ESR*, erythrocyte sedimentation rate; *FAA*, fluorescent antinuclear antibody; *FATA*, fluorescent treponemal antibody absorption; *Hep B*, hepatitis B; *Hgb*, hemoglobin; *HIV*, human immunodeficiency virus; *IgA*, immunoglobulin A; *LFT*, liver function test; *lytes*, electrolytes; *plats*, platelets; *PPD*, purified protein derivative; *RBC*, red blood cell; *Rx*, prescribe; *TP/ alb*, total protein/albumin; *UA*, urinalysis; *UC*, urine culture.

History and Clinical Findings

- Crushing injury to the muscle, such as with traumatic injury
- Red or dark-colored urine
- Myalgias or weakness
- Drug abuse, toxins, or exposure to snake venom
- Strenuous exercise
- Metabolic disorder such as severe hyperkalemia or diabetic ketoacidosis

Physical Examination

- Thorough examination of body surface area to assess for muscle injury
- Areas of pressure necrosis or ischemia

Diagnostic Studies

- UA.
- Microscopic urine analysis showing few or no red blood cells. Centrifuged urine that remains pigmented.
- Markedly elevated serum creatinine kinase level. Serum CK of over 1000 is usually seen in patients with rhabdomyolysis.
- Serum complete metabolic panel. Acute renal insufficiency elevates BUN and creatinine. Creatinine elevation occurs

due to the leakage of creatinine from damaged muscles. CMP that reveals hyperkalemia, hyperphosphatemia, or hypocalcemia
- Increased levels of other muscle enzymes (aldolase, lactic acid dehydrogenase [LDH], aspartate aminotransferase [AST]).

Differential Diagnosis

Myoglobinuria must be differentiated from gross hematuria and other metabolic disorders, or other local causes of muscle pain and weakness.

Management

The primary goal of management is to prevent acute renal insufficiency, requires nephrology consultation and possible inpatient management, and treats underlying fluid and electrolyte abnormalities. Normal saline administration and induction of diuresis are mainstays of therapy. Urine alkalinization with sodium bicarbonate reduces the breakdown of myoglobin in the bloodstream. In patients with crush injuries, treatment of soft tissue injury and prevention of compartment syndrome are essential. Discontinuation or reversal of drugs, venoms, or other toxins in the system may be necessary.

Patient and Family Education, Prevention and Prognosis

Families must understand that long-term therapy may include hemodialysis or peritoneal dialysis in severe cases resulting in acute renal disease. Myoglobinuria generally clears or improves in 10 to 14 days (Chavez, Leon, Einav, and Varon, 2016).

Renal Tubular Acidosis

Dysfunction of renal tubule transport capability results in a condition known as *renal tubular acidosis (RTA)*. There are several types. Type I, classic or distal RTA (dRTA), occurs with distal tubule defects. Defects in the proximal tubules are the most common type and result in proximal RTA (pRTA), type II, or *bicarbonate-wasting RTA*. Type III is a subtype of type I that occurs primarily in preterm infants. Type IV, also known as hyperkalemic RTA, occurs with problems in the functioning of aldosterone most commonly following relief of obstructive uropathy (Sreedharan and Avner, 2016).

RTA is often an isolated, idiopathic, and primary problem. It is usually found in children evaluated for growth failure and when illness, dehydration, or starvation stresses a child. RTA is more common in males than females.

History and Clinical Findings

- Failure to gain weight (especially) and height—the most common symptoms
- Polyuria and polydipsia
- Muscle weakness (caused by hypokalemia)
- Irritability before eating, satiation after eating, vomiting, diarrhea, or constipation in dRTA
- Preference for liquids over solid foods, poor appetite, or anorexia, especially with type IV

Physical Examination

- Arrested growth curve toward the end of the first year with prior consistent growth
- Normal physical examination and development

Diagnostic Studies

Studies include serum electrolytes, including carbon dioxide (CO_2) (hypokalemia, hyperchloremic metabolic acidosis), renal function tests (BUN, creatinine), calcium, phosphorus, alkaline phosphatase, and UA (first morning void) for glucose and pH.

If any of the laboratory findings are abnormal, consider the following:
- A 24-hour creatinine clearance to establish the normal GFR, calcium (normal less than 4 mg/kg/24 hours), and calcium-creatinine ratio
- Renal ultrasonography to determine the anatomy and rule out nephrocalcinosis, nephrolithiasis, hydronephrosis, obstructive uropathy, and parenchymal damage

Differential Diagnosis

Primary RTA must be differentiated from secondary RTA, which can be due to many disease states or conditions, such as other causes of growth failure (e.g., FTT), hypothyroidism, and systemic acidosis.

Management

Goals of management include correcting the acidosis and maintaining normal bicarbonate (greater than 20 mEq/L), thereby restoring growth and minimizing complications.
- Oral alkalizing medications are given to achieve these goals. Common agents include Bicitra (sodium citrate and citric acid), Polycitra (sodium, potassium citrate, and citric acid), sodium bicarbonate, and baking soda. The dose must be titrated to the child's response as determined by weight and laboratory results (CO_2 and electrolytes). Initiate medication at 3 mEq/kg/day, and check laboratory results in a few days. Titrate the dose until a serum bicarbonate level of 20 to 22 mEq/L is achieved (Desai, 2018). Doses should be given frequently throughout the day (with meals) and as late as possible at night (at bedtime).
- The response to medication helps confirm the diagnosis and type of RTA. dRTA has a rapid response to treatment, and normal bicarbonate levels are maintained with little difficulty. pRTA requires higher doses to normalize bicarbonate and is less easily maintained. Type IV RTA requires mineralocorticoid treatment if aldosterone is deficient.
- Maximizing caloric intake to enhance growth can be accomplished by emphasizing solid foods for all meals and snacks, and avoiding water and non-caloric foods. Providing nutritional supplements is also ideal.
- Meticulous follow-up is imperative. Weight and laboratory results should be monitored biweekly to monthly until weight gain is established and CO_2 is stabilized. Weight should be measured on the same scale.
- Pseudoephedrine should be avoided because it is minimally excreted in alkalinized urine and may cause toxicity.
- Referral to a pediatric nephrologist is necessary for any child who is not growing well despite treatment, whose laboratory values are not normalizing with treatment, has unusual laboratory results, has type IV RTA, or has any RTA complications.

Complications

It is rare to have complications with pRTA. Hypercalciuria can occur with dRTA, leading to nephrocalcinosis, nephrolithiasis, renal parenchymal destruction, and occasionally renal failure. Rickets sometimes occurs in type IV RTA.

Patient and Family Education, Prevention, and Prognosis

Patient education should stress the importance of continued, regular care to monitor renal function and growth. Isolated pRTA responds quickly to treatment, with children "catching-up" growth and reaching normal maximum height. pRTA resolves spontaneously without symptom recurrence, often within 1 to 2 years, but may take up to a decade (Sreedharan and Avner, 2016). dRTA usually lasts a lifetime; type IV resolves with underlying problem correction.

Nephrolithiasis and Urolithiasis

Urinary stones (nephrolithiasis) happen anywhere in the urinary tract. In North America, most children have stones in the kidneys; bladder stones occur in less than 10% of the pediatric cases and are most often related to urologic abnormalities. Bladder stones are endemic to other parts of the world and are likely related to diet.

The prevalence of urinary stones varies by region, with a higher incidence in the Southeast United States and in Caucasians, and slightly more often in males than females. Seventy-five percent of children who have nephrolithiasis are predisposed to stone formation. Metabolic risk factors account for more than 50% of cases, structural abnormalities account for 32%, and infections account for 4%. Hypercalciuria is the most common metabolic cause (accounts for 30% to 60%) of urinary calculi and is a condition with many causes including renal tubular dysfunction, endocrine disturbances, bone metabolic disorders, UTI, familial idiopathic hypercalcemia, and medications (Elder, 2016c). Hyperoxaluria is found in up to 20% of children with nephrolithiasis. Hyperuricosuria has been documented in 2% to 10% of children with stone formation.

History and Clinical Findings

- Family history of nephrolithiasis, arthritis, gout, or renal disease
- Stones or fragments passed in urine
- Dietary history high in protein, sodium, calcium, and oxalate intake
- Infant colic
- History or symptoms suggestive of a UTI in a preschooler

Physical Examination

- Abdominal, flank, or pelvic pain (occurs at all ages, but present in 94% of adolescents)

Diagnostic Studies

- UA shows gross or microscopic hematuria (90%) and 20% of children also have a UTI (Desai, 2018).
- Hypercalciuria is diagnosed by a 24-hour urinary calcium excretion greater than 4 mg/kg. Screening may be performed on a random urine specimen by measuring the calcium:creatinine ratio (mg/dL:g/dL). Greater than 0.2 suggests hypercalciuria in an older child; normal ratios may be as high as 0.8 in infants younger than 7 months old (Porter and Avner, 2016).
- Abdominal radiography, abdominal ultrasound, and/or CT scan. Although CT scan is the most highly specific, ultrasonography is the standard of care for those under 14 years of age (Brisbane, Bailey, and Sorensen, 2016).
- Analyze stone composition to aid in the diagnosis of the metabolic abnormality, which presents in up to 75% of children (Desai, 2018).

Differential Diagnosis

Other diagnoses causing flank pain should be considered (e.g., UTI, pyelonephritis, or trauma). Slightly more than half of preschool children with nephrolithiasis have flank pain or other afebrile illnesses, including gastrointestinal viral syndromes and early appendicitis, chronic recurrent abdominal pain of no known cause, and emotional stress.

Management

Management is through urology. Increased fluid intake is the first line of therapy regardless of the cause. In adolescents, a goal of 2 L of urine output per day is helpful. Stone removal may be required if the stone is not passed and severe symptoms continue for more than 24 to 48 hours or pain is intolerable. Extracorporeal shockwave lithotripsy (ESWL) is safe in children; follow-up studies show it does not cause long-term kidney damage. Skin bruising and hematuria are almost universal side effects of ESWL. Stones may also be removed by using rigid or flexible endoscopes passed through the urethra into the bladder or ureter. Percutaneous removal and open surgical lithotomy is still an option if other techniques fail.

Refer to a dietician. Dietary restrictions control stone formation and renal injury in most metabolic disorders contributing to stone formation.

Patient and Family Education, Prevention, and Prognosis

Recurrence rates are high if left untreated, and patients with hyperuricosuria may have symptomatic or asymptomatic calculi. Despite an excellent response to therapy, children with nephrolithiasis require long-term follow-up with a nephrologist because of the potential for renal insufficiency and end-stage renal disease.

Wilms Tumor

Wilms tumor, the most common malignancy of the GU tract, is typically found as a firm, smooth mass in the abdomen or flank. It is staged as follows:
- Stage I: The tumor is limited to the kidney and can be completely excised with the capsular surface intact.
- Stage II: The tumor extends beyond the kidney but can still be completely excised.
- Stage III: There is postsurgical residual nonhematogenous extension confined to the abdomen.
- Stage IV: There is hematogenous metastasis, most frequently to the lung.
- Stage V: There is bilateral kidney involvement.

This malignancy manifests as a solitary growth in any part of either or both kidneys. There are approximately 8 cases of Wilms tumor per million in children younger than 15 years old with 500 new cases every year. Most Wilms tumors occur in children between 2 and 5 years old. The peak incidence and median age at diagnosis is 3.5 years old (Densmore and Densmore, 2018). About 1% to 2% of children with Wilms tumor have a family history of Wilms, and the tumor is inherited in an autosomal dominant manner. An important feature of Wilms tumor is the occurrence of associated congenital anomalies including renal abnormalities, cryptorchidism, hypospadias, duplication of the collecting system, ambiguous genitalia, hemihypertrophy, aniridia, cardiac abnormalities, and Beckwith-Wiedemann, Denys-Drash, and Perlman syndromes. Wilms tumor occurs with equal frequency in both sexes although males are usually diagnosed younger. There is a higher frequency in African Americans and a lower frequency in Asians.

History and Clinical Findings

- The most frequent finding is increasing abdominal size or an actual palpable mass.
- Pain is reported if the mass has undergone rapid growth or hemorrhage.
- Fever, dyspnea, diarrhea, vomiting, weight loss, or malaise may be reported.

Physical Examination

- A firm, smooth abdominal or flank mass that does not cross the midline may be noted.
- BP is elevated if renal ischemia is present (rare).
- A left varicocele is found in males if the spermatic vein is obstructed.
- A careful examination is needed to rule out congenital anomalies.

Diagnostic Studies

- Chest and abdominal radiography are performed to differentiate neuroblastoma, which is usually calcified.
- Abdominal ultrasonography is used to differentiate a solid from a cystic mass or hydronephrosis and multicystic kidney.
- UA demonstrates hematuria in 25% to 33% of children.
- Obtain a CBC, reticulocyte count, and liver and renal chemistry studies.
- A CT scan of the chest, abdomen, and pelvis to stage the disease and bone marrow is done by the oncology team.

Differential Diagnosis

Neuroblastoma is the main differential diagnosis (the mass often crosses the midline). Multicystic kidney, hydronephrosis, renal cyst, or other renal malignancies are additional conditions to consider.

Management

Diagnostic workup is the initial urgent priority, with concurrent referral to a pediatric cancer center for treatment. Surgery removes the affected kidney and possibly the ureter and adrenal gland, and combined chemotherapy and radiotherapy are instituted if the disease is advanced or has unfavorable histologic findings. Coordinate close follow-up with the cancer team.

Complications

The lungs and liver are the most common sites of metastasis. Hypertension is possible because of renal ischemia and occasionally leads to cardiac failure.

Patient and Family Education, Prevention, and Prognosis

The prognosis is determined by the histology of the neoplasm, the patient's age (the younger the better), the size of the tumor, positive nodes, and, most significantly, the extent or stage of the disease. The cure rate is about 80% to 90% for infants with stage 4S; reoccurrence of the disease has a less than 50% response to alternative chemotherapeutic agents (Shohet and Foster, 2017). A pediatric urologist should determine if a child should be allowed to participate in sports on an individual basis. Kidney protector use is highly recommended during sports. The National Wilms Tumor Study is a good reference for information about management, sequela, and prognosis.

Chronic Genitourinary Conditions in Males
Hypospadias

Hypospadias is a common congenital abnormality in which the urethral meatus is located anywhere from the proximal glans to the perineum on the ventral surface (underside) of the penis. Chordee, a ventral bowing of the penis, occurs when a tight band of fibrous tissue pulls on the penis. *Torsion* refers to rotation of the penis to the right or left.

The etiology of hypospadias is unknown. It is believed that the endocrine system probably has an important role, but what that role is remains unclear. The primitive gonad in the eighth week of embryonic development differentiates into male or female. As the genital tubercle enlarges, developmental arrest occurs along the line of urethral fusion and causes hypospadias.

Hypospadias occurs in 1 in 250 male infants with an increased risk if family members have hypospadias. Ten percent of affected boys also have undescended testicles, inguinal hernia, or hydrocele (Elder, 2016a).

History and Clinical Findings

- A family history of a male relative with GU problems may be reported.
- There is report of an unusual direction, particularly downward, to the urine stream.
- Other findings include inguinal hernia or undescended testicles (10%), and/or chordee (Elder, 2016a).

Physical Examination

In a newborn, the classic finding is a dorsally hooded foreskin. It is essential to visualize the urethral meatus, which is facilitated by pulling the ventral shaft skin in a downward and outward direction. The deformity is described by location—glanular, coronal, subcoronal, penoscrotal, scrotal, and as distal (60%), mid-penile (25%), or proximal (15%).

Differential Diagnosis

The differential diagnosis includes intersex abnormalities.

Management

The goal of surgical repair is to have a functional penis that appears normal. Historically, circumcision was avoided because the foreskin may be used in the surgical repair. However, newer surgical techniques that do not require the use of skin flaps change this standard of care. Physiologic phimosis may prevent visualization of a urethral anomaly during a well-child exam, especially with a mild form of hypospadias. Surgical success is not compromised in these cases. Referral should be made to a pediatric urologist at birth or at detection of the anomaly. Surgery to correct hypospadias is best done around 6 to 12 months old. Repair is usually accomplished in a one-stage outpatient procedure unless it is a complex defect.

Complications

With unrepaired hypospadias, peer taunting, problems with erections, abnormal urine stream, and ultimately potential for ineffective delivery of sperm are possible complications. Intersex abnormalities are possible if associated with cryptorchidism.

Patient and Family Education, Prevention, and Prognosis

Education and reassurance regarding the etiology, repair, and outcome should be provided. Carefully assess newborns when hypospadias is reported in a family member. Hypospadias is usually an isolated anomaly, but it does require further workup to assess the anatomy of the urinary system for other anomalies.

Cryptorchidism (Undescended Testes)

Cryptorchidism is a testis that does not reside in and cannot be manipulated into the scrotum. A retractile testis is out of the scrotum, but can be brought into the scrotum and remains there. A gliding testis can be brought into the scrotum, but returns to a high position in the scrotum once released. An ectopic testis lies outside the normal path of descent. An ascended testis is one that has fully descended, but has spontaneously re-ascended and lies outside the scrotum. A trapped testis is one dislocated after herniorrhaphy. Any testis that is not in the scrotum is subject to progressive deterioration. Undescended testes is a common disorder that often causes great anxiety for parents.

Testes develop in the abdomen and descend in the seventh fetal month to the upper part of the groin, subsequently progressing through the inguinal canal into the scrotum. Failure of the testes to descend can be caused by mechanical lesions or can be secondary to hormonal, chromosomal, enzymatic, or anatomic disorders.

This condition is the most common GU disorder in boys, occurring in 3.4% of term newborns. Testicular descent occurs at 7 to 8 months gestation, so it is therefore more common in preterm (30%), low-birth-weight, and twin infants. A great majority of undescended testes descend spontaneously during the first 3 months of life but after 6 months old it is rare (0.8%) for them to descend. Cryptorchidism is bilateral in 10% of cases. Retractile testes are bilateral and most common in boys 5 to 6 years old (Elder, 2016b).

History and Clinical Findings

- Family history of undescended testes or testicular malignancy
- Testes not consistently descended during the infant's bath/warm environments
- Risk factors include prematurity, hypospadias, congenital hip subluxation, low birth weight, Down syndrome, Klinefelter syndrome
- Other congenital, endocrine, chromosomal, or intersex disorders

Physical Examination

Having the child sit cross-legged, frog-legged, squat, or stand can facilitate testicle descent and palpation.
- Scrotal rugae less fully developed
- Bilateral or unilateral absence of a testicle
- Retractile testes, which move between the scrotum and external ring, but can be manipulated to the lower part of the scrotum and remain there; in children 3 months to 7 years old, retraction is especially common with tactile stimulation of the area or cold

- Gliding testes that lie between the scrotum and external ring and can be manipulated to the lower part of the scrotum, but return to the high position
- Location of the testis is described as prescrotal (at the external inguinal ring); canalicular, high or low (between the external and internal rings), the most common type; ectopic (superficial inguinal, femoral, or perineal); or intraabdominal (above the internal inguinal ring), not palpable, occurring in less than 15% of males with undescended testes.

Diagnostic Studies

None are indicated except in newborns with potential sex abnormalities, hypopituitarism, Down syndrome, or congenital adrenal hyperplasia. The risk of intersex abnormality is 27% if hypospadias and unilateral or bilateral cryptorchidism are present.

Differential Diagnosis

Anorchism and chromosomal abnormalities are the differential diagnoses.

Management

The goals of treating undescended testes are to improve fertility outcome, decrease malignancy risk, and minimize the psychological stress associated with an empty scrotum. Management is surgical intervention between 9 and 15 months old. Hormonal therapy is not effective in stimulating testicular descent. Surgery at 6 months old is appropriate if orchiopexy is performed by a skilled pediatric urologist or surgeon with an attendant and skilled pediatric anesthesiologist. In a child younger than 1 year old, regular examination to assess the position of the testes should be performed at every well-child care visit. If the testes remain undescended, referral to a pediatric urologist or surgeon should occur by 6 months old. Referral should also occur if a retractile testis does not retain scrotal residence. If undescended testes are found after 1 year old, the child should be immediately referred to a pediatric urologist or surgeon for treatment.

Complications

Poor testicular development, infertility, malignancy, vulnerability to trauma, testicular torsion, and inguinal hernia are possible complications of undescended testicles.

Patient and Family Education, Prevention, and Prognosis

Histologic changes occur in an undescended testis as early as 6 months old, with irreversible changes shown by 2 years old that contribute to infertility and are associated with malignancy. Infertility as a complication of cryptorchidism has been reported in as many as 15% of men with unilateral undescended testes and 35% to 50% if bilateral (Elder, 2016b). Testicular malignancy in males with cryptorchidism is two to four times higher than the general population. Correction of undescended testes does not diminish the incidence of testicular cancer, although an increased incidence in testicular tumors has been observed if orchiopexy is done at later ages. Malignancy is more common with an intraabdominal testis. A testicular neoplasm in one child mandates examination of his male siblings (Elder, 2016b). Testicular self-examination should be taught to these select young men.

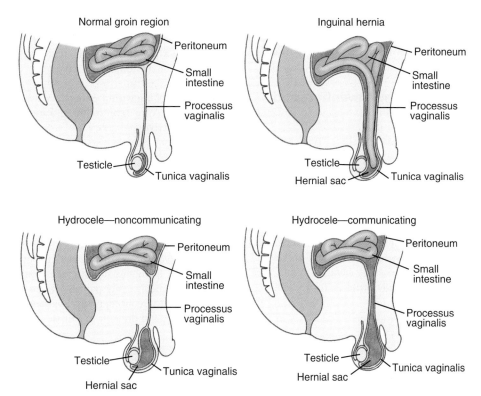

Fig 41.6 Hydroceles and Hernias. (From Katz A, Richardson W. Surgery. In: Zitelli BJ, McIntire SC, Nowalk AJ, eds. Zitelli and Davis' Atlas of Pediatric Physical Diagnosis. 2018:616–657, Figure 18–90.)

Undescended testes do not resolve with puberty; retractile testes generally settle into the scrotum by puberty. Open discussion of the problem, management, and potential complications is essential. The AAP Council on Sports Medicine and Fitness does not include an absent testicle as a condition to discourage sports participation (Mirabelli, et al., 2015).

Hydrocele

A common cause of painless scrotal swelling is a hydrocele, a collection of serous fluid in the scrotal sac. A noncommunicating hydrocele has a collection of fluid only in the scrotum. If the processus vaginalis remains patent so that fluid moves from the abdomen to the scrotum, it is called a *communicating hydrocele* and is more likely to be associated with a hernia (Fig 41.6).

Incomplete closure of the processus vaginalis through which the testes descend into the scrotum allows a hydrocele to develop. Incidence is 0.5% to 2% in neonates (Elder, 2016b).

History and Clinical Findings

Hydroceles that persist beyond 1 year old are assumed to be in conjunction with a hernia. In older children, they also occur after trauma, with an inflammatory illness, or neoplasm.
- Intermittent or constant bulge or lump in the scrotum, often more distally placed. Scrotal size increases with activity and decreases with rest.
- Overlying skin may be tense.
- Bluish discoloration in the area of bulge.
- No distress or vomiting.

Physical Examination

- Asymmetry or a scrotal mass present; if swelling is present in the inguinal area, a hernia is probable; swelling is usually unilateral
- Testes descended
- Cremasteric reflex present
- Noncommunicating hydrocele—scrotal sac tense, slightly blue tinged, fluctuant, and does not reduce; no swelling in the inguinal region
- Communicating hydrocele—fluid in the scrotal sac comes and goes (probably flat in the morning, swollen later in the day)

Differential Diagnosis

Hernia, undescended testicle, retractile testicle, and inguinal lymphadenopathy are the differential diagnoses.

Management

- Noncommunicating hydrocele: Fluid is generally absorbed spontaneously; no treatment is indicated unless the hydrocele is so large that it is uncomfortable or persists longer than 1 year.
- Communicating hydrocele: Many communicating hydroceles will resolve without surgery and deserve observation (Guerra and Leonard, 2017). If the hydrocele persists for more than 1 year, referral for surgical intervention is recommended.

For children over 12 months old, a diagnostic evaluation by the urologist is warranted if the congenital hydrocele has not resolved or with the initial onset of clinical findings. Surgery is usually done on an outpatient basis.

Patient and Family Education, Prevention, and Prognosis

Reassure parent that the increased size of the scrotal sac will resolve, usually by 1 year old, and involves no danger. Signs of hernia must be explained, and parents must be alerted to observe and report any abnormal findings.

Spermatocele

A benign, painless scrotal mass or cyst on the head of the epididymis or testicular adnexa containing sperm is called a *spermatocele.* A spermatocele is an uncommon, generally benign finding and occurs in the mature male or older adolescents.

History and Clinical Findings

- Scrotal swelling but otherwise asymptomatic
- Painless, mobile cystic nodule usually less than 1 cm in size, superior and posterior to the testicle
- No change in size with the Valsalva maneuver
- An ultrasound may be ordered if large and bothersome or painful

Differential Diagnosis

A varicocele, mass, and an epididymal cyst (identical in appearance but not containing sperm) are the differential diagnoses.

Management

No treatment is required unless the cyst is large and bothersome or painful in which case referral to a urologist is recommended.

Patient and Family Education, Prevention, and Prognosis

Any pain or discomfort should be reported. Testicular self-examination assists in early detection of this disorder in later adolescence.

Varicocele

A varicocele is a benign enlargement or dilation of testicular veins causing a painless scrotal mass of varying size that may feel like a "bag of worms." It is usually found on the left side.

The etiology of varicoceles is probably multifactorial, with the physiologic changes associated with puberty playing some role. A varicocele is caused by valvular incompetence of the spermatic vein resulting in dilated or varicose veins. Varicoceles are rare before 10 years old and may be indicative of malignancy. They occur in 5% of adolescent males and 15% of adult males. Up to 85% to 95% arise on the left side because the left spermatic vein drains into the left renal vein and arterial compression of the renal vein obstructs blood flow from the vein. In contrast, the right spermatic vein drains into the vena cava. Only 2% of varicoceles occur bilaterally (Elder, 2016b).

History and Clinical Findings

- Usually, a painless swelling is noted in the left side of the scrotum, occasionally a "dull ache" or "heavy" feeling if large.
- Scrotal swelling with prolonged standing causes pain; swelling and pain resolve upon reclining. Pain can occur with strenuous physical activity.

Physical Examination

- In the standing position, a "bag of worms" can be felt posterior and superior to the testis that collapses on lying and enlarges with the Valsalva maneuver.
- Measure and compare the size of both testes (length, width, and depth) using a standard orchidometer.
- Grade 3 varicocele, the classic "bag of worms," is larger than 2 cm and easily visualized; grade 2 varicocele is 1 to 2 cm in diameter and is easily palpable when the adolescent is standing but not visualized; grade 1 varicocele is the most common, very small, and difficult to palpate (the Valsalva maneuver may help).
- Cremasteric reflex is present.

Diagnostic Studies

- Ultrasonography to rule out malignancy in children younger than 10 years old
- Serial ultrasonography to measure testicular size every 6 to 12 months of age

Differential Diagnosis

Varicoceles must be differentiated from other testicular masses, such as lipoma, hernia, hydrocele, spermatocele, and tumors.

Management

Asymptomatic grade 1 varicocele with normal testicular volumes usually does not require intervention in adolescence but involves ultrasonographic monitoring of testicular size every 12 months (AUA, 2010/2017). Any change in comfort level should be reported. Referral to a surgeon or urologist should be made if the varicocele is grade 2 or 3, if the varicocele is painful, if the difference in testicular volume is marked (greater than 2 mm by ultrasound), if the varicocele is right sided or bilateral, or if testicular growth becomes retarded over a 6- to 12-month period (Elder, 2016b). Ligation is the usual procedure, completed on an outpatient basis with few complications.

Complications

Atrophy or testicular growth arrest, as noted by a discrepancy in testicular size, can occur. Lower fertility rates with decreased sperm concentration and motility occur and are factors in an aggressive surgical approach for the adolescent male with grade 2 or 3 varicocele. Hydrocele may be an insignificant, self-limiting complication following surgery.

Patient and Family Education, Prevention, and Prognosis

A varicocele is the most common cause of infertility. Because of this, early identification is essential. All patients should be counseled about the long-term risks to fertility. Correction of testicular atrophy and an improved sperm count and fertility have been noted in 80% to 90% of those undergoing surgery early in adolescence (Elder, 2016b). Testicular self-examination assists in early detection of this disorder.

Inguinal Hernia

A scrotal or inguinal swelling (or both) that results in bulging of abdominal contents through a weakness in the abdominal wall is an inguinal hernia (see Fig 41.6). In females, inguinal hernias cause swelling in the inguinal area and labia majora.

Incomplete closure of the processus vaginalis through which the testes descend into the scrotum allows the presence of abdominal contents in the inguinal canal or scrotum and thus the development of a hernia. Males who are obese, weight lifters, or have a family history of undescended testes are at high risk for hernias. Having a sibling with an inguinal hernia increases one's risk, and 11.5% of patients have a family member with a history of inguinal hernia (Aiken and Oldham, 2016).

Inguinal hernias are much more common in males than in females (8 to 10:1), occurring in 1% to 5% of boys. Premature infants are at increased risk (7% to 30% of males, 2% of females). More than 50% of hernias are diagnosed during the first year of life, with the peak incidence in the first 3 months of life. Bilateral hernias are common (10% to 20%). Unilateral hernias are more likely to occur on the right side (50% to 60%) than the left (30%) (Aiken and Oldham, 2016). Indirect hernias are a congenital condition and are the most common type in children. Direct hernias are rare in childhood and normally are the result of straining and weakened abdominal muscles.

History and Clinical Findings

- Family or personal history of undescended testes
- Swelling in the inguinal area, scrotum, or both that comes and goes and increases with crying or straining
- Prematurity, weight lifting, or obesity

Physical Examination

- Swelling is found in the inguinal area, scrotal area (labia majora in females), or both.
- The hernia is reducible with pressure on the distal end.
- Direct hernias push outward through the weakest point in the abdominal wall.
- Indirect hernias push downward at an angle into the inguinal canal.
- The child is fussy and has a distended abdomen if the hernia is incarcerated.
- Silk glove sign: A sensation of two surfaces rubbing against each other while one palpates the spermatic cord as it crosses the pubic tubercle.

Diagnostic Studies

An abdominal radiograph is helpful if air is present below the inguinal ligament. Ultrasonography differentiates a hernia from a hydrocele and is especially helpful if an incarcerated hernia is suspected.

Differential Diagnosis

Hydrocele, undescended testes, and inguinal lymphadenopathy are included in the differential diagnosis.

Management

If a child is seen with a hernia, an attempt should be made to reduce it, and the child should be referred to a surgeon or urologist for repair within 1 to 2 weeks. Even if no swelling is seen at the visit but is elicited by the history, the child should be referred to a surgeon or urologist. Inguinal hernias do not resolve spontaneously. Premature infants should have the hernia repaired prior to discharge. If the hernia is not easily reduced; if it is painful; or if a hard, tender, or red mass is present, refer immediately. If reduction is difficult and ischemia is ongoing, hospitalization and surgical repair within 24 to 48 hours are indicated.

Complications

Incarceration and strangulation of a hernia cause pain, irritability, erythema, vomiting, and abdominal distention. The overall incidence of incarceration is 12% to 17%, and two-thirds of incarcerated hernias occur during the first year of life (Aiken and Oldham, 2016). Both of these conditions are surgical emergencies. Bowel ischemia is of immediate concern, and testicular injury occurs from torsion as a result of the direct pressure of the incarcerated hernia or as a result of ischemia from cord compression. Because of the 40% to 60% contralateral occurrence of hernias in children, bilateral exploration is usually done at the time of surgery in infants younger than 1 year old.

Patient and Family Education, Prevention, and Prognosis

If surgery is deferred, parents must be aware of the signs and symptoms of incarceration (tenderness, redness, crying, nausea, vomiting, abdominal distention) and be cautioned to seek immediate evaluation by a health care provider should they occur.

Testicular Masses

A mass located on the testicle is most often a malignancy. Testicular tumors can occur at any age; 35% of prepubertal testicular tumors are malignant. Most of the tumors are yolk sac tumors; however, rhabdomyosarcoma and leukemia can appear in this age group; 98% of painless testicular tumors in adolescents are malignant (Elder, 2016b).

History and Clinical Findings

- Family history of testicular cancer

- Sensation of fullness or heaviness
- Possibly no complaints because testicular masses cause little or no pain and are often small
- Cryptorchidism, trauma, and atrophy

Physical Examination

- A hard, painless testicular mass.
- There may be an associated hydrocele.
- The abdomen and supraclavicular areas should be assessed for any palpable nodes.

Diagnostic Studies

- Serum levels of alpha-fetoprotein, β-human chorionic gonadotropin (β-hCG), and lactate dehydrogenase if tumor is suspected.
- Scrotal sonography establishes the location of the mass and differentiates a cystic from a solid mass.
- CT scan is indicated to evaluate for metastasis and ordered by specialists.

Differential Diagnosis

Intratesticular masses, which are almost always malignant, must be differentiated from extratesticular masses, such as hernia, varicocele, hydrocele, or spermatocele.

Management

Any child or adolescent with a testicular mass must be referred immediately for further evaluation. Treatment is dependent on the stage and type of tumor and includes orchiectomy, irradiation, and/or chemotherapy.

Patient and Family Education, Prevention, and Prognosis

Metastasis may occur before the initial tumor is noticed. Pay attention to complaints about back or abdominal pain, unexplained weight loss, dyspnea (pulmonary metastases), gynecomastia, supraclavicular adenopathy, urinary obstruction, or a "heavy" or "dragging" sensation. Early detection and therapeutic intervention can lead to a 90% survival rate; 90% of relapses occur in the first 12 months after treatment. Testicular examination should be routinely done during physical examinations.

Acute Male Genitourinary Conditions

Scrotal Trauma

Trauma to the scrotum most often occurs as a result of sports participation or play, usually from direct blows to the scrotum and straddle injuries. In a prepubertal child, the testicle is often spared damage because of the small size and mobility of the testes. Damage occurs when the testicle is forcibly compressed against the pubic bones. Significant symptoms (swelling, discoloration, and tenderness) from minor trauma suggest an underlying tumor.

Clinical Findings

- Pain after injury; older children and adolescents usually report a specific mechanism of injury, time, and place.

- Swelling, discoloration, ecchymosis, and tenderness of the scrotum are common.
- Clear transillumination is compromised if a hematoma is present.
- Ultrasound differentiates the degree and type of injury and assesses for testicular rupture.

Differential Diagnosis

Urethritis, epididymitis, orchitis, and prostatitis should all be included in the differential diagnosis. Degrees of injury include the following:
- Traumatic epididymitis: Inflammation, but no infection. Pain and tenderness with scrotal erythema and edema and a tender indurated epididymis develop within a few days after injury. UA and Doppler ultrasonographic findings are normal. The course is usually acute but short-lived.
- Intratesticular hematoma
- Hematocele with contusion and ecchymosis of the scrotal wall with severe scrotal injury
- Testicular torsion

Management

NSAIDs, cool compresses, scrotal support or elevation, and bed rest are modalities used to help relieve pain. An enlarging scrotum merits immediate surgical exploration, as does hematocele.

Patient and Family Education, Prevention, and Prognosis

On rare occasion, testicular rupture can occur and be manifested by massive swelling and ecchymosis. Prevention is the best approach to this disorder; an athletic cup should be worn when participating in sports where injury could occur. A testicular mass should be considered cancer until proven otherwise.

Testicular Torsion

Testicular torsion is the result of twisting of the spermatic cord, which subsequently compromises the blood supply to the testicle. Generally, there is a 6-hour window before significant ischemic damage and alteration in spermatic morphology and formation occurs (Elder, 2016b).

Normal fixation of the testis is absent, so the testis rotates and blocks blood and lymphatic flow. Torsion can occur after physical exertion, trauma, or on arising, and at any age but is most common in adolescence and is uncommon before 10 years old. The left side is twice as likely to be involved because of the longer spermatic cord.

History and Clinical Findings

- Sudden onset of unilateral, unrelenting scrotal pain, often associated with nausea and vomiting.
- History of intermittent testicular pain. Prior episodes of transient pain are reported in about half of patients.
- Minor trauma, physical exertion, or onset of acute pain on arising is possible.
- May be described as abdominal or inguinal pain by the embarrassed child.
- Fever is minimal or absent.

Physical Examination

- Ill-appearing and anxious male, resisting movement
- Gradual, progressive swelling of involved scrotum with redness, warmth, and tenderness
- The ipsilateral scrotum can be edematous, erythematous, and warm
- "Blue dot" sign, which is a subtle blue mass visible through the scrotal skin
- Testis larger than opposite side, elevated, lying transversely, exquisitely painful
- Spermatic cord thickened, twisted, and tender
- Slight elevation of the testis increases pain (in epididymitis it relieves pain)
- The cremasteric reflex is absent on the side with torsion
- Neonate—hard, painless, mass with edema or discolored scrotal skin

Diagnostic Studies

- UA is usually normal; pyuria and bacteriuria indicate UTI, epididymitis, or orchitis.
- Doppler ultrasound or testicular flow scan considered if Doppler ultrasound within normal and time allows.

Differential Diagnosis

Epididymal appendage torsion, acute epididymitis (mild to moderate pain of gradual onset), orchitis, trauma (pain is better within an hour), hernia, hydrocele, and varicocele are included in the differential diagnosis.

Management

Testicular torsion is a surgical emergency, and identification with prompt surgical referral critical. Occasionally manual reduction can be performed, but surgery should follow within 6 to 12 hours to prevent retorsion, preserve fertility, and prevent abscess and atrophy. Contralateral orchiopexy may be done because of a 50% occurrence of torsion in nonfixed testes. Rest and scrotal support do not provide relief.

Patient and Family Education, Prevention, and Prognosis

Testicular atrophy, abscess, or decreased fertility and loss of the testis as a result of necrosis can occur if the torsion persists more than 24 hours.

Torsion of the Appendix Testis

Torsion of the appendix testis is a common cause of acute scrotal pain and is often misdiagnosed. It most commonly occurs in the prepubertal age group and may be a response to hormonal stimulation. Once the appendix torses, it falls off and is resorbed by the body. Recurrence in another appendix, such as the appendix epididymis, can occur but is not associated with prior appendix testis torsion. This condition is the most common cause of testicular pain in boys 2 to 10 years old (Elder, 2016b).

History and Clinical Findings

- Gradual onset of scrotal pain.

- "Blue dot" sign, which is a subtle blue mass visible through the scrotal skin: Early in the process there may be a 3- to 5-mm tender indurated mass on the upper pole (Elder, 2016b).
- Doppler ultrasonography or testicular flow scan considered if Doppler ultrasound within normal and time allows.
- Cremasteric reflex present.

Differential Diagnosis

Testicular torsion, acute epididymitis, orchitis, trauma, hernia, hydrocele, and varicocele are included in the differential diagnosis.

Management

Appendix testis torsion is a self-limited condition; inflammation resolves in 3 to 5 days. Management includes NSAIDs, limited activities or bed rest until pain is gone, and warm compresses. Surgery is rarely indicated but might be necessary if testicular torsion cannot be ruled out or if symptoms do not resolve spontaneously in a few days.

Epididymitis

Epididymitis is an inflammation of the epididymis that is painful, acute, and commonly caused by *Neisseria gonorrhoeae* or *Chlamydia trachomatis* in the sexually active adolescent, often with infection in the urethra or bladder. However, it can be caused by a viral, coliform bacterial, or tubercular infection; by chemical irritation; by anomalies of the GU tract; or by dysfunctional voiding. It is rare before puberty, but it occurs in younger boys from *E. coli* infection. It may occur in children younger than 2 years old with GU tract abnormalities (Elder, 2016b).

History and Clinical Findings

- Trauma or sexual encounters within past 45 days
- Painful scrotal swelling, usually gradual but may be acute
- Dysuria and frequency, or obstructive voiding
- Fever, nausea, vomiting

Physical Examination

- Scrotal edema and erythema are noted.
- The epididymis is hard, indurated, enlarged, and tender; the spermatic cord is tender.
- The testis has normal position and consistency.
- The cremasteric reflex is normal (not present in older adolescents).
- Elevation of testis may relieve pain (in torsion it increases pain).
- Hydrocele may be present due to inflammation.
- Urethral discharge may be present: purulent in gonorrhea, and scant and watery in chlamydial infection.
- Rectal examination reveals prostate tenderness and can produce a urethral discharge.

Diagnostic Studies

- UA: Pyuria and occasional bacteria may be present
- CBC: Elevated WBC count

- Urethral culture and Gram stain: Urine nucleic acid amplification tests for gonococci and *Chlamydia*
- Testing for other STIs and HIV if there is a history of sexual activity
- Doppler ultrasonography to differentiate torsion of the testis
- If the above tests are not diagnostic, refer to urology to identify urogenital problems with evaluation by VCUG, ultrasonography, or both in prepubertal children and in those who deny sexual activity.

Differential Diagnosis

The differential diagnosis includes testicular torsion, hernia, hydrocele, varicocele, spermatocele, trauma, tumor, or concomitant urethritis. Testicular cancer has been confused with epididymitis.

Management

Management involves symptom relief and treatment of a causative organism, if found. Bed rest, scrotal support, and elevation are indicated. Apply ice packs as tolerated. Sitz baths and analgesics or NSAIDs relieve pain. Antibiotic treatment includes the following (Centers for Disease Control and Prevention [CDC], 2015):

- First line: Ceftriaxone (250 mg intramuscularly one time) plus doxycycline (100 mg twice a day for 10 days).
- Alternative treatments: Ofloxacin (300 mg twice a day for 10 days) or levofloxacin (500 mg once a day for 10 days).
- Referral to a urologist is indicated if a solitary testicle is involved, if a prompt response to treatment does not occur, or if a question about the diagnosis remains. Treatment of sexual partner(s) from the past 60 days is indicated if caused by an STI. Intercourse should be avoided until cured. Follow-up is needed within 3 days if no improvement or if symptoms recur after treatment. Follow-up after antibiotics is recommended to ensure that no palpable mass remains.

Patient and Family Education, Prevention, and Prognosis

Infertility, abscess formation, testicular infarction, and late atrophy are possible but rare complications. Because epididymitis is usually caused by an STI, partners must be evaluated and treated. Patients must understand the sexually transmitted etiology of this disease. Pain and edema usually resolve within 1 week.

Phimosis and Paraphimosis

Phimosis refers to a foreskin that is too tight to be retracted over the glans penis. Physiologic or primary phimosis occurs over the first 6 years of life when the glans does not completely separate from the epithelium. Pathologic or secondary phimosis occurs after puberty or when the foreskin cannot be retracted after previously being retracted. Paraphimosis is a retracted foreskin that cannot be reduced to the normal position.

Phimosis can be congenital or acquired from infection and foreskin inflammation. Paraphimosis causes penis constriction and results in pain, glans edema, and possible necrosis. Paraphimosis is most common in adolescents and can follow masturbation, sexual activity, or forceful retraction.

History and Clinical Findings

- May be a history of infection or inflammation of the penis
- Retraction of the foreskin with an inability to reduce it (paraphimosis)
- Pain and dysuria
- Signs of urinary obstruction—ballooning of the foreskin with urination and/or abnormal intermittent urinary stream

Physical Examination

- Phimosis—a tight, pinpoint opening of the foreskin with minimal ability to retract the foreskin; foreskin flat and effaced
- Pathologic phimosis—thickened rolled foreskin
- Paraphimosis—edema and bluish discoloration of the glans and foreskin

Management

- Phimosis: Normal cleansing with gentle stretching of the foreskin until resistance is felt. Most foreskins are retractable by 5 or 6 years old. Never forcefully retract the foreskin. Circumcision is indicated if urinary obstruction or infection is present. Persistent phimosis can be treated with 0.05% betamethasone cream twice daily for 2 to 4 weeks. This frequently allows successful retraction of the foreskin, promotes awareness of improved hygiene, and offers an alternative to circumcision. (Elder, 2016a).
- Paraphimosis: Reduction may be accomplished by lubricating the foreskin and glans, simultaneously compressing the glans, and placing distal foreskin traction. If this technique is not successful, surgical release of the constricting band must be done to prevent necrosis of the glans. Paraphimosis is a surgical emergency (Elder, 2016a). Investigation of events leading to the paraphimosis is needed to rule out sexual abuse.

Patient and Family Education, Prevention, and Prognosis

Infection and urinary obstruction can occur with phimosis; however, a tight foreskin in uncircumcised males is normal and usually resolves by 6 years old. It is not an indication for circumcision. Necrosis of the penis is possible with paraphimosis. The foreskin of infants and children should never be forcibly retracted.

Balanitis and Balanoposthitis

Balanitis is an inflammation of the glans; *balanoposthitis* is an inflammation of the foreskin and glans penis occurring in uncircumcised males or those with phimosis. Debris accumulation under the foreskin, probably resulting from poor hygiene, irritates the foreskin and glans and leads to infection. If purulent discharge with fiery-red erythema and moist translucent exudates are present, consider streptococcal etiology. Normal skin flora is the usual cause of infection, but gram-negative bacteria are possible. If a urethral discharge is present, a sexually transmitted infection (STI) must be considered. Occasionally trauma or allergy can be the cause.

History and Clinical Findings

- A fussy infant or pain and dysuria in an older child. Edema and inflammation are noted on the foreskin and glans.
- Cultures may help determine infectious causes

Management

Prescribe oral and topical antibiotics as directed by the cultures, along with warm bathtub soaks. Depending on the swelling, topical steroids might also be prescribed.

Patient and Family Education, Prevention, and Prognosis

Paraphimosis can occur with severe infections; however, avoid forcible foreskin retraction. A review of proper hygiene and the removal of irritants is needed. Occurrence is not an indication for circumcision.

Additional Resources

American Association of Kidney Patients. www.aakp.org
Fred Hutch: National Wilms Tumor Study. www.fredhutch.org/en/diseases/wilms-tumor.html
IgA Nephropathy Support Network. www.igansupport.org
National Cancer Institute: Wilms Tumor and Other Childhood Kidney Tumors Treatment. www.cancer.gov/types/kidney/patient/wilms-treatment-pdq
National Institute of Diabetes and Digestive and Kidney Diseases. www.niddk.nih.gov/health-information/health-topics/kidney-disease/Pages/default.aspx
National Kidney Foundation. www.kidney.org
Testicular Cancer Awareness Week. www.tcaw.org
Urology Care Foundation: The Official Foundation of the American Urologic Association. www.urologyhealth.org

Enuresis
Bedwetting Store. www.bedwettingstore.com
Education and Resources for Improving Childhood Continence (ERIC). www.eric.org.uk
International Children's Continence Society (ICCS). www.i-c-c-s.org
National Association for Continence. www.nafc.org
National Institute of Diabetes and Digestive and Kidney Diseases. www.niddk.nih.gov/health-information/health-topics/urologic-disease/urinary-incontinence-in-children/Pages/facts.aspx
National Kidney Foundation. www.kidney.org/patients/bw/
Potty MD. www.pottymd.com
Society of Urologic Nurses and Associates. www.suna.org
Urology Care Foundation. www.urologyhealth.org

General
General information for parents, children, and adolescents, including encopresis and enuresis can be found at the following websites:
Nemours Foundation. www.kidshealth.org
National Institute of Diabetes and Digestive and Kidney Diseases, Digestive Diseases A-Z. www.niddk.nih.gov/health-information/health-topics/digestive-diseases/Pages/default.aspx

References

Aiken JJ, Oldham KT. Inguinal hernias. In: Kliegman RM, Stanton BF, St Geme JW, Schor NF, eds. *Nelson Textbook of Pediatrics*. 20th ed. Philadelphia: Elsevier; 2016. 1903–1909.e1.
Bright Futures/American Academy of Pediatrics (AAP) Committee on Practice and Ambulatory Care. *Recommendations for Preventive Pediatric Health Care*. 2017. Retrieved from: https://www.aap.org/en-us/Documents/periodicity_schedule.pdf.
American Academy of Pediatrics (AAP). *Subcommittee on Urinary Tract Infection. Steering*. 2016.
Committee on Quality Improvement and Management. *Reaffirmation of the AAP Clinical Practice Guideline: The Diagnosis and Management of the initial UTI in febrile infants and children 2 to 24 Months of Age*. 2016. Retrieved from: http://pediatrics.aappublications.org/content/138/6/e20163026.
American Urological Association (AUA). *Management and Screening of Primary Vesicoureteral Reflux in Children: Aua 2010 Guideline*. Originally published 2010. Reviewed and validity confirmed 2017. Retrieved from: https://www.auanet.org/education/guidelines/vesicoureteral-reflux-a.cfm.
Apos E, Schuster S, Reece J, Whitaker S, Murphy K, Golder J, et al. Enuresis management in children: retrospective clinical audit of 2861 cases treated with practitioner-assisted bell-and-pad alarm. *J Pediatr*. 2018;193. https://doi.org/10.1016/j.jpeds.2017.09.086.
Austin PF, Bauer SB, Bower W, Chase J, Franco I, Hoebeke P, et al. The standardization of terminology of lower urinary tract function in children and adolescents: update report from the standardization committee of the international children's continence society. *Neurourol Urodyn*. 2015;9999:1–11. https://doi.org/10.1002/nau.22751.
Brisbane W, Bailey MR, Sorensen MD. An overview of kidney stone imaging techniques. *Nat Rev Urol*. 2016;13(11):654–662.
Centers for Disease Control and Prevention (CDC). Sexually transmitted diseases treatment guidelines. *MMWR*. 2015;64(3):1–140.
Chavez LO, Leon M, Einav S, Varon J. Beyond muscle destruction: a systematic review of rhabdomyolysis for clinical practice. *Critical Care*. 2016;20:135.
Chua ME, Silangcruz JM, Chang SJ, et al. Desmopressin withdrawal strategy for pediatric enuresis: a meta-analysis. *Pediatrics*. 2016;138(1).
Clothier C, Wright AJ. Dysfunctional voiding: the importance of noninvasive urodynamics in diagnosis and treatment. *Pediatr Nephrol*. 2018;33:381–394. https://doi.org/10.1007/s00467-017-3679-3.
Desai R. Nephrology. In: Hughes HK, Kahl LK, eds. *The Harriet Lane Handbook: A Manual for Pediatric House Officers*. 21st ed. Philadelphia: Elsevier; 2018:516–547.
Elder JS. Anomalies of the penis and urethra. In: Kliegman RM, Stanton BF, Geme St JW, Schor NF, eds. *Nelson Textbook of Pediatrics*. 20th ed. Philadelphia: Elsevier/Saunders; 2016a:2586–2592.e1.
Elder JS. Disorders and anomalies of the scrotal contents. In: Kliegman RM, Stanton BF, Geme St JW, Schor NF, eds. *Nelson Textbook of Pediatrics*. 20th ed. Philadelphia: Elsevier/Saunders; 2016b:2592–2598.e1.
Elder JS. Urinary lithiasis. In: Kliegman RM, Stanton BF, Geme JW, Schor NF, eds. *Nelson Textbook of Pediatrics*. 20th ed. Philadelphia: Elsevier/Saunders; 2016c:2600–2604.e1.
Elder JS. Urinary tract infections. In: Kliegman RM, Stanton BF, St. Geme JW, Schor NF, eds. *Nelson Textbook of Pediatrics*. 20th ed. Philadelphia: Elsevier; 2016d:2556–2562.e1.
Elder JS. Voiding disorders. In: Kliegman RM, Stanton BF, Geme JW, Schor NF, eds. *Nelson Textbook of Pediatrics*. 20th ed. Philadelphia: Elsevier/Saunders; 2016e:2562–2567.e1.
Elder JS. Vesicoureteral reflux. In: Kliegman RM, Stanton BF, Geme JW, Schor NF, eds. *Nelson Textbook of Pediatrics*. 20th ed. Philadelphia: Elsevier/Saunders; 2016f:2562–2567.e1.
Guerra L, Leonard M. Inguinoscrotal pathology review. *Can Urol Assoc J*. 2017;11(1–2 suppl1):S41–S46. Retrieved from: https://doi.org/10.5489/cuaj.4336.
Hagan JF, Shaw JS, Duncan PM, eds. *Bright Futures: Guidelines for Health Supervision of Infants, Children and Adolescents*. 4th ed. Elk Grove Village, IL: American Academy of Pediatrics; 2017.
Hjorten R, Anwar Z, Reidy KJ. Long term outcomes of childhood onset nephrotic syndrome. *Front Pediatr*. 2016;53(4):1–7.
Kamperis K, Van Herzeele C, Rittig S, Vande Walle J. Optimizing response to desmopressin in patients with monosymptomatic nocturnal enuresis. *Pediatr Nephrol*. 2017;32(2):217–226.

Kovacevic L, Wolfe-Christensen C, Rizwan A, Lu H, Lakshmanan Y. Children with nocturnal enuresis and attention deficit hyperactivity disorder: a separate entity? *J Pediatr Urology*. 2017. https://doi.org/10.1016/j.jpurol.2017.07.002.

Kuwertz-Bröking E, von Gontard A. Clinical management of nocturnal enuresis. *Pediatric Nephrology*. 2017. https://doi.org/10.1007/s00467-017-3778-1.

Lee CKK. Drug dosages. In: Hughes HK, Kahl LK, eds. *The Harriet Lane Handbook: Handbook for Pediatric House Officers*. 21st ed. Philadelphia: Elsevier; 2018:732–1109.

Mambatta AK, Jayarajan J, Rashme VL, Harini S, Menon S, Kuppusamy J. Reliability of dipstick assay in predicting urinary tract infection. *J Family Med Prim Care*. 2015;4(2):265–268.

Mirabelli MH, Devine MJ, Singh J, Mendoza M. The preparticipation sports evaluation. *Am Fam Physician*. 2015;92(5):371–381.

Pais P, Avner ED. Introduction to the child with proteinuria. In: Kliegman RM, Stanton BF, Geme JW, Schor NF, eds. *Nelson Textbook of Pediatrics*. 20th ed. Philadelphia: Elsevier/Saunders; 2016a:2517–2518.e1.

Pais P, Avner ED. Nephrotic syndrome. In: Kliegman RM, Stanton BF, Geme JW, Schor NF, eds. *Nelson Textbook of Pediatrics*. 20th ed. Philadelphia: Elsevier; 2016b:2521–2528.e1.

Pan CG, Avner ED. Glomerulonephritis Associated with Infections. In: Kliegman RM, Stanton BF, Geme JW, Schor NF, eds. *Nelson textbook of pediatrics*. 20th ed. Philadelphia: Elsevier; 2016a. 2498–2501.e2.

Pan CG, Avner ED. Clinical evaluation of the child with hematuria. In: Kliegman RM, Stanton BF, St. Geme JW, Schor NF, eds. *Nelson Textbook of Pediatrics*. 20th ed. Philadelphia: Elsevier; 2016b:2494–2496.e1.

Porter CC, Avner ED. Upper Urinary Tract Causes of Hematuria. In: Kliegman RM, Stanton BF, St. Geme JW, Schor NF, eds. *Nelson Textbook of Pediatrics*. 20th ed. Philadelphia: Elsevier; 2016:2510–2512.e1.

Roberts KB. Revised AAP Guideline on UTI in febrile infants and young children. *Am Fam Physician*. 2012;86(10):940–946.

Quest Diagnostics. *Urine Collection*. 2017. Retrieved from: www.questdiagnostics.com/home/physicians/testing-services/specialists/hospitals-labstaff/specimen-handling/urine.html.

Schroeder AR, Chang PW, Shen MW, Biondi EA, Greenhow TL. Diagnostic accuracy of the urinalysis for urinary tract infections under three months of age. *Pediatrics*. 2015;135(6):0031–4005.

Shohet Foster J. Neuroblastoma. *BMJ*. 2017:357. https://doi.org/10.1136/bmj.j1863.

Sreedharan R, Avner ED. Tubular function. In: Kliegman RM, Stanton BF, Geme JW, Schor NF, eds. *Nelson Textbook of Pediatrics*. 20th ed. Philadelphia: Elsevier; 2016. 2528–2528.e2.

Yousefichaijan P, Khosrobeigi A, Salehi B, Taherahmadi H, Shariatmadari F, Ghandi Y, et al. Incidence of obsessive–compulsive disorder in children with nonmonosymptomatic primary nocturnal enuresis. *J Pediatr Neurosci*. 2016;11(3):197–199, 2016. https://doi.org/10.4103/1817-1745.193371.

42

Pediatric and Adolescent Gynecology

ELIZA BUYERS AND ELIZABETH ROMER

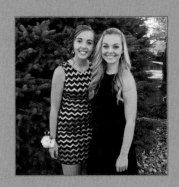

Pediatric and adolescent gynecology provides the primary care provider (PCP) with varied and interesting challenges. Knowledge, sensitivity, and comfort with this topic gives the PCP the ability to work with the child and parent or adolescent, providing education about children's bodies as they mature and approaching issues that may be considered personal or embarrassing. Establishing and maintaining an open relationship with parents and children helps ease the transition as adolescents take an increasingly larger role in determining their own care. Gynecologic issues include concerns about vulvar, vaginal, menstrual, and breast health and development as well as sexual health. PCPs who understand the anatomy and physiology of the female reproductive system provide guidance and support that can empower girls and adolescents throughout their entire life.

The most common gynecologic concerns for children are vulvovaginal issues, which overwhelmingly respond to general measures that reduce irritation. The onset of puberty introduces the presence of endogenous estrogen and dramatically changes the anatomy and physiology of the reproductive system. The menstrual cycle is the hallmark of female puberty and can be understood as an additional vital sign reflecting overall pubertal status and insight into other factors affecting health and well-being. Concerns about the menstrual cycle should be discussed, evaluated, and treated when indicated. Sexual health, including discussions of healthy relationships, family planning, contraception, and counseling for the prevention of sexually transmitted infections (STIs) is another fundamental aspect of primary care for adolescents.

Anatomy, Physiology, and Assessment of the Female Reproductive System

The fetus is sexually undifferentiated for the first 6 weeks of gestation, having two bipotential gonads and bipotential paramesonephric (müllerian) and mesonephric (wolffian) ducts. Testes-determining factor on the Y chromosome causes testicular differentiation. The production of anti–müllerian hormone (AMH) by the Sertoli cells in the male gonad inhibits müllerian duct development, and the wolffian duct differentiates into the epididymis, vas deferens, and seminal vesicle. Without the influence of the Y chromosome, the gonads develop into ovaries by about 8 weeks' gestation and reach maturity by 20 weeks' gestation. The müllerian ducts develop into

the fallopian tubes, uterus, cervix, and the superior portion of the vagina. Differentiation of the external genitalia and the lower third of the vagina, including the hymen, occurs with the development of external urologic structures.

In utero, maternal estrogen thickens and enlarges the female genital structures and also stimulates the lining of the uterus. Mucus produced by the cervix results in physiologic leukorrhea of the newborn period. After birth, maternal hormones are withdrawn, resulting in endometrial shedding; this may cause a small amount of vaginal bleeding.

The External Genitalia and Vagina Before Puberty

By 8 weeks after birth, without the influence of maternal or endogenous estrogen, the labia majora flattens and the labia minora thins. Because of the absence of estrogen, the genital epithelium of the vaginal opening is atrophic, erythematous, and easily traumatized (Fig 42.1 and Table 42.1). There are several different normal hymenal configurations, with annular and crescent being the most common (Fig 42.2).

The microbiology of the prepubertal vagina reflects the hypoestrogenic atrophic epithelium with a pH of 6.5 to 7.5. Normal flora includes lactobacilli, common aerobic, anaerobic, and enteric organisms. If done, a routine bacterial culture of the prepubertal vagina will demonstrate a broad variety of organisms, including skin and fecal flora. The presence of these organisms does not in itself signal disease or infection and must be correlated with clinical concerns.

When the prepubertal child is in a squatting position, the labia are open and allow for a visual exam of the vulva and lower vagina. Although special attention will be paid to the external genitalia when the child or parent has a specific concern, inspection of the genitals should be a part of all complete physical exams. There are a variety of positions in which to examine the external genitalia: the "frog-leg" position is usually comfortable and easily incorporated into part of a complete physical exam (Fig 42.3).

A brief and routine genital exam demonstrates to the child and her parents that the external portion of her urinary, gastrointestinal, and reproductive systems are important and normal parts of her body. It can be tempting to skip over the genital exam, especially if a child or parent is anxious or uncooperative. However, it is important to be able to attest to the normal appearance (vs. a postpubertal or diseased state) of the vulva and vaginal opening in the prepubertal child. The exam also provides context for any questions or concerns and allows for the discussion of topics that may not otherwise be brought up, such as:

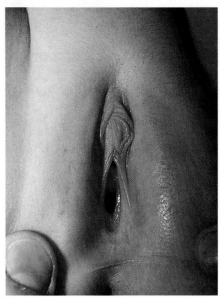

• **Fig 42.1** Prepubertal Vulva. (From Zitelli BJ, McIntire SC, Nowalk AJ. *Zitelli & Davis' Atlas of Pediatric Physical Diagnosis*. 7th ed. Philadelphia: Elsevier; 2018.)

TABLE 42.1	Prepubertal External Genitalia, Normal Findings	
Finding	**Typical Appearance/Description**
Pubic hair	Absent (Tanner 1)
Labia majora	Flat, no fat pads
Labia minora	Thin
Clitoris	Not enlarged (<3 mm length or width)
Hymen and vaginal epithelium	Tissue hypoestrogenic: thin, erythematous, fragile
Anus and perianal region	Without lesions or skin changes

• Explain that an exam of the genitalia is an important part of a full health exam, just like checking the heart, lungs, throat, etc.
• Explain that the exam is visual only and looks at the outside of the body.
• Explain that the parent/guardian gives permission for exam and is present with the child (unless sexual abuse is a consideration).
• The exam gives an opportunity to label body parts with correct anatomic terms such as vulva, vaginal opening, and labia and discuss socially appropriate language and behaviors when in public.
• Discuss basic hygiene.
• Discuss safety, privacy, and body boundaries.
• Encourage questions and discussion with child and parent, acknowledging the medical office as the appropriate place for such discussions.

Additionally, a complete external exam is needed to accomplish pubertal staging, which allows for anticipatory guidance regarding the physical changes of puberty and also to assess for premature or delayed development.

External Genitalia and Vagina After the Onset of Puberty

The sexual maturity rating (SMR) is discussed in Chapter 13. The vulva and vagina of the postpubertal female vary significantly from the prepubertal state (Fig 42.4 and Table 42.2). Some adolescents choose to remove some or all of their pubic hair, which can make this staging more difficult. As pubic hair grows on the mons pubis and labia majora, so do the fat pads in these areas, which serve to protect the vulva and vaginal opening. At the time of puberty, the labia minora also enlarge and grow to adult size. Normal labia minora are varied in size, shape, color, and appearance. Asymmetry in the size of the labia minora is very common and considered a normal variant. The minora may or may not extend past the labia majora.

Inspection of the vaginal opening will now reveal that the tissue, including the hymen, is estrogenized and thickened. The vaginal tissue is stretchy, and most girls can comfortably place and use internal feminine hygiene products (e.g., tampons, diva cup) without difficulty. Postpubertal vaginal secretions occur daily; small amounts of clear or cloudy fluid are produced, the amount and color of the discharge changing normally throughout the menstrual cycle or due to other factors such as clothing, bathing,

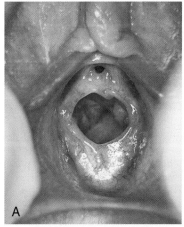 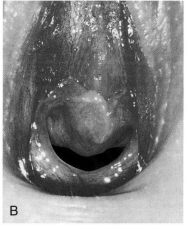

• **Fig 42.2** Normal Hymenal Configurations. A, Annular. B, Crescent. (From Zitelli BJ, McIntire SC, Nowalk AJ. *Zitelli & Davis' Atlas of Pediatric Physical Diagnosis*. 7th ed. Philadelphia: Elsevier; 2018.

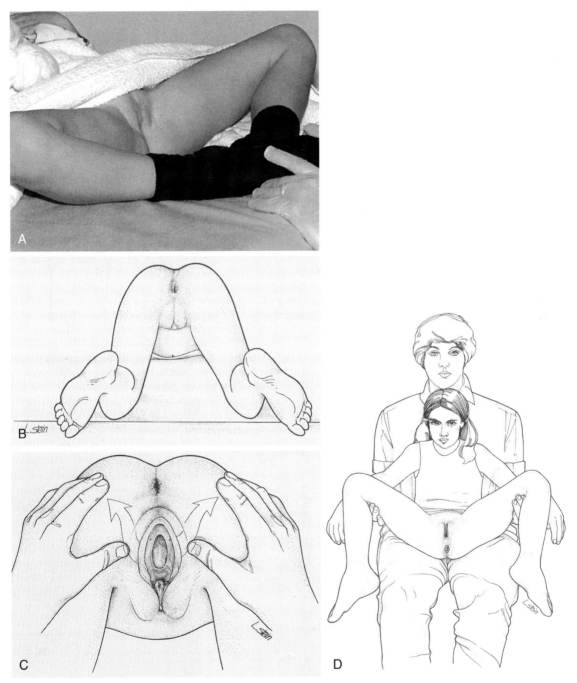

• **Fig 42.3** Different exam positions for performing a gynecologic exam on a child. A. Frog leg position. B. Knee chest position. C. Prone position. D. Sitting on parent's lap. From Lara-Torre E, Valea FA. Pediatric and adolescent gynecology: gynecologic examination, infections, trauma, pelvic, mass, precocious puberty ([A] From McCann JJ, Kerns DL. *The Anatomy of Child and Adolescent Sexual Abuse: A CD-ROM Atlas/ Reference*. St. Louis: InterCorp; 1999; [B–D] From Finkel MA, Giardino AP, eds. *Medical Examination of Child Sexual Abuse: A Practical Guide*. 2nd ed. Thousand Oaks, CA: Sage, 2002:46–64. In Lobo, RA, Gershenson DM, Lentz GM, Valea FA. *Comprehensive Gynecology*. Philadelphia: Elsevier; 2017,12:219–236.)

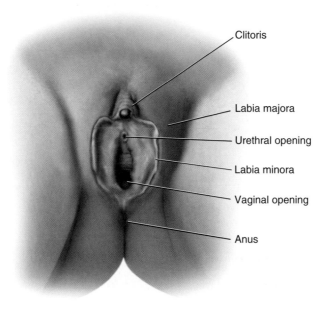

Normal

● **Fig 42.4** Postpubertal Vulva. (From Zitelli BJ, McIntire SC, Nowalk AJ. *Zitelli & Davis' Atlas of Pediatric Physical Diagnosis*. 7th ed. Philadelphia: Elsevier; 2018.)

TABLE 42.2	Postpubertal External Genitalia, Normal Findings	
Finding	**Typical Appearance/Description**	
Pubic hair and labia majora	Mons pubis and labia majora develop fat pads. Tanner stage 4-5, but hair may be partially or completely removed.	
Labia minora	May or may not be symmetric. Size and shape different for every woman. Normal variant may extend past labia majora.	
Hymen, vaginal epithelium	Tissue is estrogenized, moist. Discharge may be clear, white, thin or thick. Mild to no odor with adequate hygiene.	
Anus and perianal region	Normal exam without lesions or skin changes.	

and dietary habits. Education about the normalcy of vaginal discharge even before the onset of menarche helps reassure girls and parents who are bothered or alarmed by its presence.

Estrogen increases the glycogen content in vaginal epithelial cells, encouraging the colonization of lactobacilli, production of lactic acid, and a decrease in vaginal pH to less than 4.7. The normal vaginal flora in the postpubertal girl remains heterogeneous, including lactobacillus and other components of the vaginal flora, such as *Gardnerella vaginalis, Escherichia coli,* group B streptococci (GBS), genital mycoplasma, and *Candida albicans* (ACOG Practice Bulletin, Vaginitis, 2017). Detection of these organisms on culture or on DNA testing does not signal infection and must be correlated with clinical concerns.

When a formal inspection of the vulva is indicated in the adolescent, many recommend that the patient be given a handheld mirror while the PCP, using a moistened cotton swab, points out the major anatomic structures. Often girls have questions about the vulva, and this offers a perfect opportunity to educate them and reassure of their normalcy.

General principles of vulvar and vaginal self-care that are helpful for girls and women of all ages are included in Box 42.2. When needed, plain warm-water baths are best, with the avoidance of baking soda or any other additives. Products labeled and marketed for "feminine hygiene" are unnecessary and in some cases can be harmful.

Internal Reproductive Organs

The size and growth of the internal reproductive organs correlate with the stage of pubertal development. The prepubertal cervix and uterus are small and approximately of equal size; the endometrium is atrophic owing to the absence of estrogen-induced stimulation; the ovaries are small (1 to 3 cm^3) With exposure to endogenous estrogen, the internal reproductive structures grow significantly and reach adult size once menarche has occurred (Fig 42.5).

An internal pelvic exam is not indicated as part of routine health screening in adolescents. At age 21, women should have a Papanicolaou test (i.e., pap test, pap smear, cervical screening) done via pelvic exam, to screen for cervical cancer. If the pap test is negative, it should be repeated every 3 years (ACOG, 2017). Routine recommended screening for STIs can be done via urine sample or a self-collected vaginal swab.

When an internal pelvic exam is indicated in a postpubertal adolescent (indications discussed later), it is usually well tolerated as long as the teen understands the reasons for the exam and how it will be performed. A moistened cotton swab can be used to explore the vaginal opening, hymenal configuration, and confirm

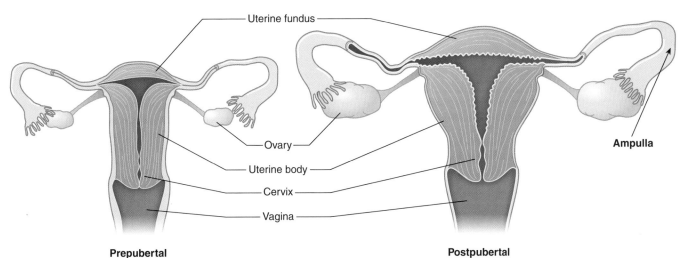

• Fig 42.5 Prepubertal and Postpubertal Cervix, Uterus, and Ovaries. Note 1:1 ratio of cervix to uterus, atrophic endometrium, and small ovaries in prepuberty. Estrogen induces growth of the uterus in proportion to the cervix (1:3), thickens endometrium, and reproductive-age ovarian size.

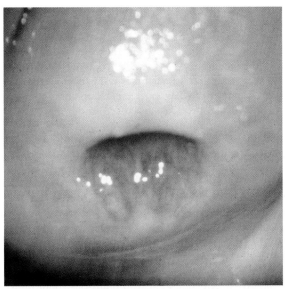

• Fig 42.6 Normal-Appearing Cervix of an Adolescent Female During Speculum Examination. (From Zitelli BJ, McIntire SC, Nowalk AJ. *Zitelli & Davis' Atlas of Pediatric Physical Diagnosis*. 7th ed. Philadelphia: Elsevier; 2018.)

vaginal patency when needed. A small lubricated gloved finger can palpate the vagina and cervix. When needed, a small, lubricated speculum can be used to visualize the cervix and upper vagina (Fig 42.6).

Female Pubertal Development and the Menstrual Cycle

Ovarian estrogen production initiates pubertal changes. The menstrual cycle is the hallmark of female puberty. Educating girls and their families reduces anxiety and encourages communication with the PCP. Based on pubertal staging, providers can offer anticipatory guidance on the timing of the first menstrual period, or menarche, as well as practical education about how to record the frequency, duration, and amount of menstruation, encouraging

girls to bring their data to each appointment. Smartphone apps offer an accurate and appropriate way of collecting this information (Box 42.1).

Physiology of Menstrual Bleeding

Menstrual bleeding occurs due to a complex interaction between the hypothalamus, anterior pituitary gland, ovary, and endometrium. Table 42.3 and Fig 42.7 describe and illustrate the physiology of a normal ovulatory cycle at the level of the brain, ovaries, and uterus.

Ovulatory and Anovulatory Menstrual Cycles

Ovulatory menstrual cycles are regular in frequency, duration, and blood loss. In anovulatory cycles, the absence of progesterone produced by the corpus luteum, the endometrium is stimulated by unopposed estrogen and becomes fragile, resulting in unpredictable bleeding. Immaturity of the hypothalamic-pituitary-ovarian (HPO) axis is the most common cause of anovulation in early adolescence, although other causes must be considered and are discussed in the sections on amenorrhea and abnormal uterine bleeding (AUB). Despite the frequency of anovulation among adolescents, most cycles still align with the norms listed in Table 42.4. Further evaluation is needed in individuals with repeated erratic menstrual cycles or the absence of periods for longer than 90 days.

TABLE 42.3	Physiology of an Ovulatory Cycle in Brain, Ovaries, and Endometrium

Brain

- Early in follicular phase, increasing gonadotropin-releasing hormone (GnRH) pulsations from the hypothalamus signal the anterior pituitary to secrete follicle stimulating hormone (FSH). FSH also stimulated by lower levels of estrogen noted at the end of the menstrual cycle.
- Later in follicular phase, increasing levels of estrogen produced by ovary causes FSH suppression and luteinizing hormone (LH) secretion and surge.
- During luteal phase, LH production continues.
- During menstrual phase, FSH levels increase again.

Ovaries

- Early in follicular phase, ovarian follicles are stimulated by FSH to develop a dominant follicle.
- FSH stimulates granulosa cells to increase production of estrogen. Increasing estrogen production feeds back to anterior pituitary to cause LH surge in the later follicular phase.
- LH surge stimulates rupture of the dominant follicle, also called ovulation.
- During the luteal phase, the remains of the follicle become the corpus luteum. Its theca lutein cells secrete progesterone.
- If pregnancy does not occur, the corpus luteum decays and stops secreting progesterone after 10 days.

Endometrium

- During the first part of an ovulatory cycle, the endometrium is exposed to estrogen alone. This causes proliferation of the glands and arteries of the endometrium (proliferative phase).
- After ovulation, the endometrium is exposed to a combination of estrogen and progesterone. The progesterone stops endometrial proliferation and causes the lining to change to a secretory phase (secretory phase).
- With the demise of the corpus luteum, progesterone levels drop. The endometrium sheds, which results in menstrual bleeding (menstrual phase).
- Menstrual fluid leaves the uterus through the cervix and then exits the body through the vagina.

Coagulation Pathway and the Menstrual Cycle

During the menstrual phase, blood vessels within the endometrium are rapidly repaired due to interactions of platelets and clotting factors. Inherited or acquired conditions (e.g., von Willebrand, Fe deficiency anemia, endometriosis, STI) that affect the coagulation system may result in heavy, prolonged bleeding and associated blood loss. Further evaluation is needed when cycles are outside of the norms given in Table 42.4.

Early Pregnancy: Key Concepts for Adolescent Providers

For adolescents, a prerequisite to making responsible and informed decisions about their pregnancy is medically accurate information on sexual health and human reproduction. PCPs play a critical role in teaching and discussing these issues. Clinicians can educate adolescent patients and their families in the clinic setting and advocate for scientifically accurate information to be taught in school as well as at home (Cora, Breuner, Mattson, 2016).

Physiology of Early Pregnancy

In educating adolescents who are considering withdrawal as a contraceptive method, it is important for them to know that precum (pre-ejaculate) and other secretions from the penis may contain active sperm and be able to travel through the cervix, uterus, and fallopian tubes to the ampulla, where they remain active and capable of fertilization for 5 days following intercourse (Fig 42.8). Ovulation is unpredictable in women of all ages, especially in adolescents, so fertility awareness is also considered a less effective method of contraception. Implantation occurs 5 to 6 days after fertilization when the fertilized egg, now called a blastocyst, implants inside the uterine wall. Some women will have bleeding with implantation, which can be mistaken for a short menstrual period. Due to a wide range of genetic, environmental, and other factors, over half of fertilized eggs in normal, healthy couples fail to implant inside the uterus and therefore pregnancy does not occur. When implantation does occur, the placenta is formed and begins to produce human chorionic gonadotropic (hCG), which can be detected in the blood and urine as soon as a few days after implantation. Urine hCG testing is considered a highly accurate confirmation of pregnancy, although home test instructions can be confusing and a repeat test in the clinic is always warranted. However, it may take 2 to 3 weeks from intercourse for a pregnancy test to become positive.

During pregnancy, hCG, estrogen, and progesterone levels increase. Box 42.3 lists common symptoms of early pregnancy. It is appropriate to screen for pregnancy when adolescents present with these concerns even if sexual contact is not reported. It may be necessary to reassure families and patients that pregnancy screening is part of the diagnostic evaluation and does not mean that the provider suspects sexual activity.

Addressing Common Misperceptions About Pregnancy

When PCPs address common misperceptions and provide accurate information on sexual health, they empower young people to make intentional and informed decisions. Key misperceptions that put young people at risk for unplanned pregnancy are listed in Box 42.4. Interestingly, most teens overestimate the risk of pregnancy with a single act of unprotected intercourse and may believe that they are infertile when pregnancy does not occur. In fact, a single act of sex without knowledge of where a woman is in her cycle confers a 5% chance of resulting in pregnancy (Li et al., 2015). An adolescent who is anxious about unplanned pregnancy needs support, education, and testing; as a result, she may be highly motivated to initiate a contraceptive method.

Vulvar and Vaginal Concerns

Vulvar and vaginal concerns are common among girls and adolescents. Vaginitis is the spectrum of conditions that cause vulvovaginal symptoms such as a change in vaginal discharge, pruritus, burning, irritation, erythema, dysuria, and spotting. Vulvar skin conditions cause similar symptoms and must be considered.

Evaluation

Evaluation of vulvar and vaginal concerns includes a focused history with special attention to the quality, location, and duration of symptoms. Ask patients about hygiene practices and materials and products that come in contact with the vulva. The physical exam assesses the external genitalia for the presence or absence of clinical findings, including patient identification of the area that is causing discomfort. An internal pelvic exam may be indicated

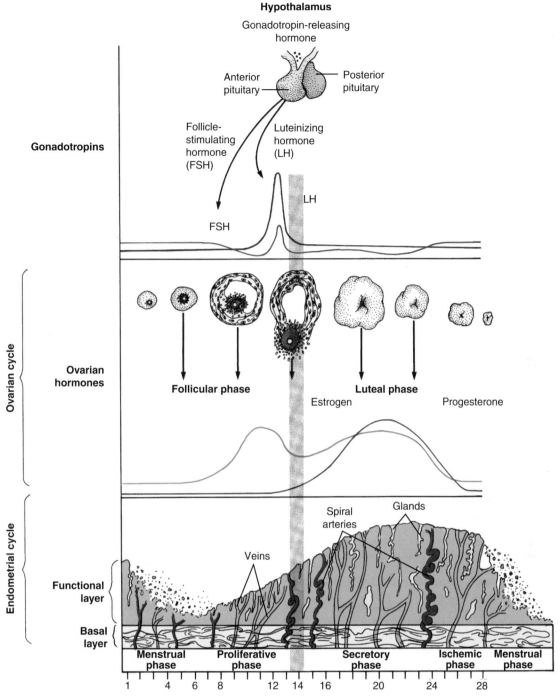

• **Fig 42.7** Female Reproductive Cycle Showing Changes in Hormone Secretion, the Ovary, and the Uterine Endometrium.

TABLE 42.4	**Norms for the Menstrual Cycle in Adolescent Girls.**
Median age at menarche	Between 12 and 13 years
Normal interval range	21-45 days (mean: 34 days)
Flow length	7 days or less
Product use	3-6 pads or tampons per day

in certain adolescents who have concerns about vaginal discharge and are agreeable to a pelvic exam. Testing for STIs can be done via urine or self-collected vaginal swab if preferred (ACOG practice Bulletin, Vaginitis, 2017).

A saline-moistened swab can be used to collect vaginal discharge for culture in the prepubertal child with a suspected acute bacterial infection. When nonspecific causes are suspected, a bacterial culture may not be helpful because of the broad range of organisms, including skin and fecal flora, found in the hypoestrogenic and alkaline prepubertal vagina. Common causes of vaginitis in women, such as yeast, are very uncommon in prepubescent girls.

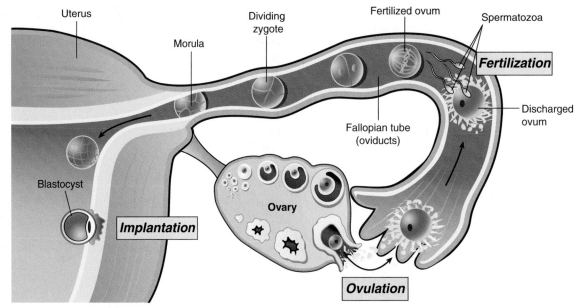

• **Fig 42.8** Ovulation, Fertilization, and Implantation. (From Salvo SG. *Massage Therapy*. 3rd ed. St. Louis: Saunders; 2007.)

• **BOX 42.2** **General Recommendations for Hygiene and Self-Care for the Vulva and Vagina**

- Cool compresses can be used if needed to soothe itching or irritation.
- In general, gently wash with plain warm water. Avoid bubble baths and sitting in water with soap or shampoo, as this removes moisture and causes dryness and itching.
- When bathing, gently wipe away any debris from the labial folds if needed. Avoid scrubbing with washcloth or scrubby brush.
- Gently dry off the vulva after washing. If desired, a hair dryer on the cool setting may be used for drying.
- Always wipe from front to back after a bowel movement.
- Limit the use of "commercial" wipes only to remove visible debris. All wipes contain chemicals that cause dryness and possible irritation.
- Wear white cotton underwear. Certain colors contain dyes that cause irritation and noncotton materials are less breathable.
- Wear loose-fitting and breathable clothing. Thong underwear, spandex, Lycra, and tight pants can cause irritation.
- Change promptly out of wet swimsuits and sweaty exercise clothes.
- Sleep without underwear or wear only very loose pajama pants. Avoid tight sleepers or "onesies" that do not allow air to circulate.
- Avoid scented pads and tampons.
- Some girls wear a pad or panty liner every day to deal with normal vaginal discharge. Educate girls about the physiologic and protective role of discharge and offer the option of changing underwear more often if the moisture is bothersome.
- Avoid sprays, washes, vaginal douches, and other products marketed for "feminine hygiene."
- If irritation occurs, soak in plain water a few times each day; also wear looser clothes and no underwear when possible.
- If irritation occurs, wash underwear separately from other clothes. Use a small amount of laundry soap and double rinse. Do not use fabric softeners.

• **BOX 42.3** **Common Symptoms in Early Pregnancy**

- Late or skipped menstrual period
- Abnormal bleeding
- Painful or swollen breasts
- Nausea with or without vomiting
- Fatigue

• **BOX 42.4** **Key Findings of the Fog Zone: How Misperceptions, Magical Thinking, and Ambivalence Put Young Adults at Risk for Unplanned Pregnancy**

A survey of 1800 unmarried young people aged 18 to 29 found the following:
- 18% Believe that douching after sex can prevent pregnancy.
- 25% Believe that after giving birth, a woman cannot get pregnant before her first period.
- 22% Believe that there is an almost certain chance of pregnancy after a single act of unprotected sex.
- 16% Believe it is quite or extremely likely that they are infertile.
- 40% Agree with the statement "It doesn't matter whether you use birth control or not, when it's your time to get pregnant, it will happen."

From Kaye K, Suellentrop K, Sloup C. The Fog Zone: How Misperceptions, Magical Thinking, and Ambivalence Put Young Adults at Risk for Unplanned Pregnancy. Washington, DC: The National Campaign to Prevent Teen and Unplanned Pregnancy; 2009.

In postpubertal adolescents, vaginal discharge can be collected by inserting a cotton-tipped swab inside the vagina or collected at the time of a speculum exam. Measurement of vaginal pH is helpful in the diagnosis of vaginal discharge in reproductive-age women. An elevated pH suggests bacterial vaginosis (pH >4.5) or trichomoniasis (pH 5 to 6) and helps to exclude candidal vulvovaginitis (pH remains normal at 4 to 4.5). Narrow-range pH paper (4 to 5.5) should be applied directly to the vaginal secretions; false elevation in pH can occur due to cervical mucus, blood, and semen. Microscopy can be performed by mixing the swab with 1 to 2 drops of saline on one slide and adding one drop of 10% KOH to a smear on a second slide. A bacterial culture is typically not helpful in adolescents given the heterogeneity of the normal vaginal flora. When microscopy is not available, commercial diagnostic testing methods (rapid antigen and nucleic acid amplification tests [NAATs]) are available for identifying bacterial vaginosis, candidiasis, and trichomoniasis. In sexually active females or when sexual abuse may be suspected, a NAAT may be used to check for gonorrhea and chlamydia. Yeast culture is helpful if clinical suspicion is high for candidal infection but microscopy is negative.

Prepubertal Vulvar and Vaginal Concerns

Prepubertal vulvovaginitis is one of the most common gynecologic concerns. Atrophic vaginal epithelium and absence of labial fat pads and pubic hair predispose to vulvar trauma and irritation. "Nonspecific" vaginitis causes as many as 75% of vulvovaginal symptoms and occurs as a result of poor hygiene—especially noted around the time of toilet training—or the use of soap, detergent, or cream. Symptoms due to nonspecific causes tend to be bothersome but are usually not severe and may come and go over weeks or months.

Vulvovaginal infections due to specific bacterial causes are less common than nonspecific causes and usually have an acute onset with visible discharge. Infectious causes include group A streptococci and *Haemophilus influenzae* as well as enteric organisms. STIs must be considered. Yeast infections are rare in prepubertal girls, as a high vaginal pH does not allow for growth of *Candida* species. Other causes of vulvar and perianal itching include pinworms and lichen sclerosis. A foreign body usually causes odor, discharge, and possibly bleeding but is less likely to cause vulvar symptoms. Consider sexual abuse with all vulvovaginal concerns. Ask patients about other systems and screen for urinary tract infection, constipation, and bowel and bladder dysfunction.

Advise all patients with vulvovaginal symptoms to stop the use of irritating products and follow the hygiene measures outlined in Box 42.2. For nonspecific causes and dermatitis, symptoms should improve greatly or resolve within 2 to 3 weeks. When patients have persistent complaints in spite of treatment or the provider is unsure about the diagnosis, referral to a specialist with expertise in the diagnosis and treatment of prepubertal vaginitis is indicated. Exam under anesthesia along with vaginoscopy may be indicated to assess for a foreign body (most commonly tissue paper) or a cervical or vaginal lesion as the cause (Table 42.5).

TABLE 42.5 **Characteristics, Evaluation, and Treatment of Prepubertal Vulvovaginitis**

Cause and Characteristics	Evaluation	Treatment
Nonspecific Vulvovaginitis • Discharge may be clear, yellow, green, malodorous • With or without itching; less commonly, dysuria • Vulvar erythema, may extend to anus and there may be excoriations • May have contact dermatitis concurrently	Careful history and exam with attention to hygiene practices. If vaginal culture is done, it will likely reveal diverse flora.	See Box 42.2
Irritant or Contact Dermatitis • Vulvar soreness and itching • History of bubble bath, sandbox, prolonged contact with urine/feces • May develop after prolonged exposure to commercial products (e.g., perfumes, clothing dyes) • May occur after use of topical agent to treat vulvovaginal symptoms	Careful history and exam with attention to hygiene practices. Attention to products used in vulvar area (e.g., soaps/detergents, underwear).	
Specific Bacterial Infections • Acute onset, with pain, possible itching and bleeding • "Beefy red" appearance with group A strep infection • Respiratory pathogens may be associated with current or recent respiratory infection • Enteric pathogens may be associated with recent or current diarrhea	Culture confirms pathogen. Respiratory: *Streptococcus pyogenes* (group A β-hemolytic streptococcus), *Staphylococcus aureus, Haemophilus influenzae, Streptococcus pneumoniae*, other flora. Enteric: *Shigella, Yersinia*, other flora.	Specific to pathogen For example, *S. pyogenes*: penicillin V, amoxicillin *Shigella*: Trimethoprim-sulfamethoxazole, ampicillin
Pinworms (enterobius vermicularis) • Itching including perianal areas, especially at night • Excoriations and erythema but no discharge	Tape test reveals eggs. Treatment is indicated if other family members infected or symptoms suggestive of infection.	Single does of mebendazole or albendazole, repeated in 2 weeks
Candidal Diaper Dermatitis • Itching and erythema in groin and labial skin folds • Beefy red areas, vesicles and pustules at periphery • Vaginal involvement unlikely before puberty	KOH prep shows budding yeast and pseudohyphae.	Topical nystatin or miconazole; fluconazole orally Dryness and frequent diaper changes must be maintained
Infections Due to Sexual Abuse • Gonorrhea, chlamydia, trichomoniasis, herpes simplex, human papillomavirus	Teat for STI if sexual abuse suspected and/or there are suspicious clinical findings.	See CDC treatment guidelines for sexually transmitted infections Report to child protection services (CPS); exam as indicated
Foreign Body • Malodorous discharge, minimal vulvar symptoms, possible bleeding • Tissue paper most common • Patient/parent may report item inserted into vagina	Can attempt removal with warm irrigation fluid after introitus is treated with a topical anesthetic. Exam under anesthesia and vaginoscopy may be needed.	Try general self-care measures if symptoms mild Refer if symptoms increased

CDC, Centers for Disease Control.

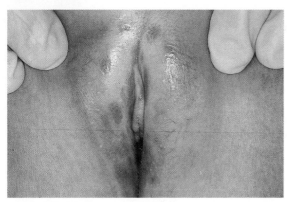

• **Fig 42.9** Lichen Sclerosis. (From Zitelli BJ, McIntire SC, Nowalk AJ. *Zitelli & Davis' Atlas of Pediatric Physical Diagnosis*. 7th ed. Philadelphia: Elsevier; 2018.)

Lichen Sclerosis

Patients who have lichen sclerosis report intense itching and soreness; they may also report bleeding. Diagnosis is made clinically by visualizing white, atrophic skin along with ulcerations and subepithelial hemorrhages on the genitalia, perineum, or perianal area. The clitoris has a normal appearance but the labia minora are flattened and may be scarred (Fig 42.9). Left untreated on or near the vulva, the labia shrink and the opening to the vagina may be scarred. Treatment is with clobetasol propionate 0.05% to the affected area once to twice each day for 2 weeks. Treatment continues until the child is asymptomatic and the disease is not visible, followed by careful tapering of the medication. Referral to a specialist such as a pediatric gynecologist or dermatologist should be made if there is any uncertainty about diagnosis and/or treatment.

Prepubertal Vaginal Bleeding

Bleeding in the first week of life secondary to withdrawal from maternal hormones is physiologic. Other prepubertal vaginal bleeding is not normal and should be promptly evaluated with a careful history and physical exam. Local causes of vaginal bleeding include vaginitis, lichen sclerosis, retained foreign body, condyloma, trauma (including sexual abuse), urethral prolapse, and other benign or rare growths. Endometrial causes include precocious puberty, other endocrine abnormalities, and functional estrogen-producing ovarian cysts or tumors. Patients with thrombocytopenia or bleeding disorders may have other signs such as epistaxis, petechiae, and hematomas. Referral to a specialist in pediatric gynecology should be made if the cause of bleeding is not identified.

Labial Adhesions

This common finding occurs primarily in girls 3 months to 6 years of age due to the hypoestrogenic state of the vulva. The labia minora adhesions are usually found on routine exam; they may be partial or appear to completely occlude the vaginal opening and usually do not cause symptoms but may cause postvoid dripping of urine, frequent urinary tract infections, or nonspecific complaints (Fig 42.10). A careful history should be obtained for functional concerns with voiding, trauma, and inadequate hygiene. Treatment in asymptomatic patients is conservative, with careful attention to vulvar hygiene and reassurance. In symptomatic patients, topical estrogen and/or steroid cream applied to the adhesion with gentle pressure is curative, but recurrence is common until the girl goes through puberty.

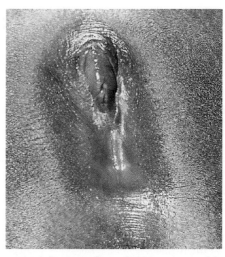

• **Fig 42.10** Labial Adhesions. (From Zitelli BJ, McIntire SC, Nowalk AJ. *Zitelli & Davis' Atlas of Pediatric Physical Diagnosis*. 7th ed. Philadelphia: Elsevier; 2018.)

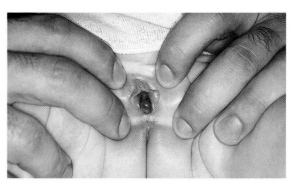

• **Fig 42.11** Imperforate Hymen (Bulging). (From Zitelli BJ, McIntire SC, Nowalk AJ. *Zitelli & Davis' Atlas of Pediatric Physical Diagnosis*. 7th ed. Philadelphia: Elsevier; 2018.)

Imperforate Hymen

Occasionally imperforate hymen is diagnosed in the newborn when uterovaginal secretions due to maternal estrogen accumulate in the vagina (i.e., hydrocolpos) (Fig 42.11). A careful history and exam will differentiate imperforate hymen from labial adhesions.

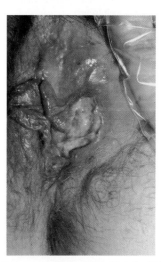

• **Fig 42.12** Vulvar Uclers. (From Zitelli BJ, McIntire SC, Nowalk AJ. *Zitelli & Davis' Atlas of Pediatric Physical Diagnosis*. 7th ed. Philadelphia: Elsevier; 2018.)

TABLE 42.6   Common Causes of Vaginitis and Vulvar Complaints in Post-Pubertal Adolescents

	Discharge	Cause and Diagnosis	Acuity, Additional Symptoms/History	Treatment[a]
Physiologic Discharge	White or transparent. Thick or thin. Usually no odor, but may have slight odor. Gradual onset as occurs due to estrogen and then changes in hormones during menstrual cycle. Patient reports discharge on and off for weeks, months, or years.	Endocervical secretions and vaginal cells sloughing. Mediated by normal, healthy production of estrogen, and may change in mid–menstrual cycle with ovulation. Diagnostic testing negative. Wet prep reveals numerous epithelial cells without inflammation.	Weeks to months of concern, may get heavier and lighter. No vulvar symptoms or minimal pain and itching. Patient has concerns about wetness of underwear and feels the need to wear panty liners, which may cause irritation.	Reassure and educate about protective functions of physiologic discharge. Review best practices for hygiene and self-care (Box 42.2).
Contact Dermatitis	Normal to increased discharge. Thick or thin. Usually no odor: may have slight odor.	Soaps, perfumes/sprays, pads, panty liners, laundry detergents and fabric softeners, OTC creams marketed to treat vaginal itching and/or yeast, baby wipes. Due to excessive cleaning or poor hygiene. Diagnostic testing negative.	Usually chronic symptoms; can have acute flares. Obtain careful history about all habits.	Stop using all possible irritants. Soak in plain water bath 1-3 times a day, use cool compresses as needed. Wear loose-fitting and breathable clothes, avoid Lycra and thongs. Skip underwear when not needed (as when sleeping at night).
Candidiasis	Discharge scant or thick, white, and curd-like. Usually no odor. Itching, pain, and swelling dominant concern, not discharge itself.	80% of infections due to *Candida albicans*. Vaginal pH is normal (4-4.5). Wet prep KOH slide reveals budding pseudohyphae and yeast forms. DNA probe test available. Consider yeast culture if no response to treatment.	Acute inflammatory symptoms of itching and soreness, redness, external dysuria, and swelling of vulva. Candida part of normal, vaginal flora. Correlate with findings/symptoms if detected on lab test.	OTC intravaginal agents in creams and suppositories: clotrimazole, miconazole, tioconzazole. Prescription intravaginal: butoconazole 2% cream, 5 g in one application Or teroconazole 0.4% cream 5 g for 7 days Prescription oral: fluconazole 150 mg PO once
Bacterial Vaginitis	Thin, gray, or yellow; malodorous; "fishy smelling." Fishy odor may increase after intercourse when semen mixes with discharge.	Vaginal pH is elevated (>4.5). Wet prep shows "clue cells," epithelial cells studded with coccobacilli and rare leukocytes. Fishy, amine odor after applying KOH to wet mount. DNA probe test available for *G. vaginalis* and vaginal fluid sialidase activity.	Minimal irritation or inflammation. No vulvar symptoms. *Gardnerella vaginalis* is part of normal, vaginal flora. Correlate with findings/symptoms if detected on test results.	metronidazole 500 mg PO bid for 7 days Or metronidazole gel 0.75%, 5 g intravaginally daily for 5 days Or clindamycin cream 2%, 5 g intravaginally at bedtime for 7 days
Trichomoniasis	Thin, frothy, green-yellow, purulent, malodorous.	Vaginal pH is elevated (5-6). Motile trichomonads on wet prep (but only in 60% of patients). Strongly consider DNA probe test or other diagnostic test if patient is sexually active or infection is suspected.	May have burning, itching, dysuria.	Metronidazole 2 g PO once Or metronidazole 500 mg PO bid for 7 days Or tinidazole 2 g PO once
Acute Cervicitis (due to chlamydia or gonorrhea)	May be yellow. May cause no symptoms or minimal symptoms.	Numerous white cells (>10 per high power field) on wet prep. NAAT testing is diagnostic. Can be done via urine, self-collected vaginal swab, or endocervical swab.	May have dysuria, increased discharge, spotting, pelvic pain.	*See the CDC's STI treatment guidelines for updated recommendations.*

[a]Treatments are recommended by the Centers for Disease Control at www.cdc.gov.

NAAT, Nucleic acid amplification test; *OTC*, over-the-counter; *STI*, sexually transmitted infection.

Associated complications are rare and treatment is usually delayed until the onset of puberty, but findings of an imperforate hymen warrant consultation with a pediatric gynecologist.

Adolescent Vulvar and Vaginal Concerns

The vulva and vagina of the postpubertal female vary significantly from the prepubertal state, primarily due to the presence of endogenous estrogen. Physiologic discharge can cause concern and warrants evaluation and then reassurance when indicated. Vulvovaginitis is more likely to be caused by a specific infection in adolescents than in prepubescent girls, but it can still be exacerbated or entirely due to noninfectious processes.

Vulvovaginitis in Adolescents

Initial diagnostic evaluation of acute symptoms should include testing for candidiasis, bacterial vaginitis, and trichomoniasis, which account for over 90% of infection-related vaginitis episodes. Table 42.6 lists common causes and characteristics of vaginitis and vulvar complaints in post-pubertal girls.

Nonsexual Genital Ulcers

The condition of nonsexual genital ulcers (NSGUs), or vaginal aphthosis, is poorly understood. Vulvar ulcers are unusual, painful, and distressing, particularly in young teens who have never been sexually active. Patients report intense vulvar pain and extreme external dysuria and have significant ulcerated vulvar lesions (Fig 42.12). The vast majority of patients recall systemic signs and symptoms of a viral illness (fever, malaise, headache, gastrointestinal symptoms) preceding the symptom onset. Diagnosis is made by a careful history excluding sexual abuse or sexual contact, a complete exam (including inspection of the mouth for additional ulcers), and polymerase chain reaction (PCR) testing of the lesion to rule out herpes simplex. Other causes of ulcers—such as syphilis, Crohn's disease, systemic lupus erythematosus (SLE), and other immune diseases—should be considered. The primary goal of treatment is pain relief and the prevention of superimposed infection. Comfort measures include plain water baths, topical anesthetics (viscous xylocaine), voiding in the tub to reduce external dysuria, and acetaminophen or ibuprofen for pain. Significant pain may be present for 10 to 14 days, with complete resolution in 3 weeks. Recurrence is not unusual, but symptoms are usually less severe. PCPs not familiar with this condition should consult with a specialist in adolescent gynecology.

Concerns About Labial Appearance

The trend to remove pubic hair and increased access to idealized images are likely contributing factors to concerns about labial appearance. At the time of puberty, the labia minora enlarge and grow to adult size. Despite conventional images and diagrams of female genitalia, normal labia minora are endlessly varied in size, shape, color, and appearance. Asymmetry in the size of the labia minora is common and considered a normal variant. If there is irritation, the PCP can offer solutions such as the application of emollients and changing the type of clothing worn so as to stop irritation. Many are unaware of normal variations in the labia minora and may need additional education and reassurance. Labiaplasty is not recommended for adolescents (ACOG Committee Opinion 686, January 2017).

Menstrual Concerns

Amenorrhea

Amenorrhea is the absence of menstrual periods and can be temporary or permanent due to central, gonadal, or peripheral dysfunction. PCPs should use their understanding of the normal physiology of the menstrual cycle (see Table 42.3 and Fig 13.2) to evaluate amenorrhea and oligomenorrhea in a stepwise fashion that avoids unnecessary testing and reduces anxiety for the patient and her family. An adolescent who has not entered puberty by 13 years of age warrants evaluation. Causes of pubertal delay are discussed in Chapter 45, although there is significant overlap between the causes of pubertal delay and amenorrhea. *Primary amenorrhea* describes the failure to have a period within 3 years of breast development or by age 15. *Secondary amenorrhea* is no menstrual period for three menstrual cycles (~90 days) or the absence of menstrual periods for at least 6 months in women who have had at least one period but do not have regular cycles. *Oligomenorrhea* describes infrequent menstrual periods (fewer than 6-8 per year).

History and Physical

A careful history, physical exam, and pregnancy testing are the first steps in the evaluation of all cases of amenorrhea. Historical items to discuss with patients and families are listed in Table 42.7. Physical finding to note include:

- External genital exam to confirm that vagina is present; confirm that hymen is patent.
- Sexual maturity rating (SMR) of breasts given that menstrual periods usually occur when breast at SMR IV and rare before SMR III.
- Physical signs of an eating disorder. Anorexia/dehydrated; low pulse, blood pressure, and temperature; dry skin; lanugo. Bulimia-swollen cheeks (parotid glands), calluses on hands/fingers, enamel erosion and/or stains on teeth (see Chapter 30).
- Signs of androgen excess: cystic or severe acne, excess hair on face or body, male pattern (temporal) baldness.
- Body changes suggestive of hyperinsulinemia: central adiposity, acanthosis nigricans, striae.

Women with primary amenorrhea who have an abnormal genital exam, such as imperforate hymen or absence of a vaginal opening with otherwise normal labia and hymenal tissue (e.g., müllerian agenesis and androgen insensitivity syndrome), should have an internal pelvic exam, and/or a pelvic ultrasound done to confirm the presence of an upper vagina, cervix, uterus, and ovaries as well as to assess for any obstruction of menstrual flow. Any abnormalities warrant consultation with a gynecologist, endocrinologist, or other provider experienced at diagnosing and treating primary amenorrhea.

Additional Testing

Laboratory testing for causes of amenorrhea can be expensive and confusing (Box 42.5). After performing a pregnancy test, the tests that are most helpful initially include follicle stimulating hormone (FSH), estradiol, TSH, T4 and prolactin. PCPs who are not comfortable with the interpretation of these labs should refer patients to a gynecologist, endocrinologist, or adolescent medicine provider. Additional follow-up testing such as chromosomal analysis and brain magnetic resonance imaging (MRI) may be indicated after evaluation by the specialist.

TABLE 42.7	Patient History for Evaluating the Cause of Amenorrhea

History	Significance of Positive Finding
Age of thelarche (onset of puberty in girls, noted as breast budding)	Normal age of thelarche 8-13 years, average age 10. Menarche (first period) usually 2-3 years after thelarche.
Menstrual history: age of first period, length between cycles, and days of bleeding	Need to distinguish between primary and secondary amenorrhea, given 15% of primary cases have abnormal findings on pelvic exam/ultrasound. Menstrual history can suggest previously ovulatory (regular) or anovulatory (chaotic) cycles.
Pubertal and menstrual timing for for both parents and all siblings	Familial or constitutional delay is the most common reason for delayed onset of puberty; menarche still should occur 2-3 years after thelarche.
Height and weight growth curves	Menarche typically occurs after the most rapid pubertal growth spurt, with growth slowing after menarche. Obesity and/or rapid weight gain can cause anovulation; it may be associated with polycystic ovarian syndrome (PCOS) and/or eating disorders or other conditions. Weight loss or being underweight can cause hypothalamic amenorrhea/anovulation or suggest restrictive eating and/or eating disorders.
Patient involvement in competitive athletics Screening for female athlete triad, usually characterized by frequent exercise, high stress and perfectionism, restrictive or "very healthy" eating habits	Intense activity can cause pubertal delay and amenorrhea. Female athlete triad can cause functional hypothalamic amenorrhea/anovulation due to inadequate energy intake.
Anxiety, depression, self-harm, obsessive thoughts about diet, exercise, and/or body image Consultation with parent and during one-on one interview	Stress can induce hypothalamic amenorrhea. Mental health concerns associated with eating disorder or poor energy intake.
Concerns about severe acne, excess facial hair, male-pattern baldness	Androgen excess conditions such as PCOS can cause anovulation.
Autoimmune disorders (e.g., Graves disease, celiac disease)	Certain autoimmune conditions associated with primary ovarian insufficiency.
Previous surgeries	Previous dilation and curettage (D&C) can cause scarring of uterine lining.
Congenital anomalies and/or syndromes	Renal, skeletal, abdominal wall, and anorectal anomalies associated with müllerian anomalies. Turner syndrome (XO) associated with ovarian hypofunction or premature ovarian failure.
Previous malignancy treated with radiation, chemotherapy, surgery	May cause damage to reproductive system.
Family history of Fragile X syndrome (FXS)	Female carriers of fragile X premutation have increased risk of primary ovarian insufficiency (FX-POI).
Current use of hormonal contraception *During one-on-one interview, ask about all medications used, and specifically contraceptive use. Teens may initiate and use contraception confidentially.*	Hormonal methods may induce amenorrhea. After negative pregnancy test, reassure this is an expected side effect and benefit of many hormonal methods.
History of sexual contact *During one-on-one interview, ask about any type of intimate contact. Do not use the term "sexually active."*	Hormonal methods may induce amenorrhea. After negative pregnancy test, reassure this is an expected side effect and benefit of many hormonal methods.

Causes of Amenorrhea

There are four major causes of amenorrhea: pregnancy, hypogonadotropic conditions, ovarian dysfunction, and structural causes. The most common cause of amenorrhea in reproductive-age females is pregnancy, which can occur even before the onset of the first menstrual period. Parents and patients may have to be reassured that pregnancy testing, usually via urine hCG, is part of the standard, evidence-based protocol for the evaluation of amenorrhea. Further testing should be delayed until a negative pregnancy test has been documented.

Central causes of amenorrhea include hypothalamic or pituitary gland dysfunction; depressed production of gonadotropins (FSH and luteinizing hormone [LH]) resulting in inadequate stimulation of the ovary, low estrogen levels, and anovulation. The history often suggests these conditions, and lab testing confirms low estrogen levels and normal or low FSH levels. Functional causes include chronic diseases and illnesses, stress, competitive athletics, and eating disorders. Structural causes of dysfunction include prolactinomas and other pituitary tumors, pituitary infarction, and previous irradiation.

Pregnancy Test: Done via urine sample. Explain to patient and family that this must be done in all cases of amenorrhea, even when earlier sexual contact seems very unlikely.

Follicle Stimulating Hormone (FSH): An elevated FSH suggests premature, primary ovarian insufficiency, which warrants referral to endocrinology and/or gynecology for additional testing for a chromosomal abnormality, possible associated conditions, counseling about future fertility, and hormonal replacement therapy when indicated.

Thyroid Studies (TSH and T4): Hypothyroidism and hyperthyroidism can cause amenorrhea as well as other medical complications. Detection of central hypothyroidism warrants evaluation for deficiency of other pituitary hormones.

Prolactin: An elevated prolactin should be repeated fasting and before 8 a.m. when possible. Hyperprolactinemia, due to a tumor or other causes, can cause hypothalamic dysfunction leading to amenorrhea. A slight elevation in prolactin can be associated with the use of certain medications and can also occur when a patient has PCOS. Hyperprolactinemia warrants consultation with an endocrinologist or another provider (gynecologist, adolescent medicine) who is familiar with causes and treatment.

Estradiol: This test can be helpful when a patient is being assessed for hypothalamic causes of amenorrhea. A normal level of estradiol is reassuring that the ovary is producing adequate levels of estrogen. A low level of estradiol is seen when there is primary ovarian insufficiency or when hypothalamic suppression of the ovaries is significant, as seen in girls with anorexia.

Luteinizing Hormone (LH): May sometimes be included in the initial evaluation of amenorrhea but is more useful when central causes are being considered. A low LH is consistent with a hypogonadotropic process.

Total and Free Testosterone: Total serum testosterone is useful in assessing for an androgen-secreting tumor when a patient presents with hirsutism in addition to amenorrhea. Free testosterone is needed to assess for biochemical hyperandrogenism in evaluation of PCOS (Chapter 26). Serum testosterone is also useful in assessing patients with primary amenorrhea who are found to have absent reproductive organs. It will be at male levels when androgen-insensitivity is the cause but at normal female levels with mullerian agenesis.

DHEA-S and Androstenedione: These are androgens that may be assessed when considering causes of amenorrhea that also cause hirsutism and may be elevated in PCOS.

17-OH Progesterone (17-OHP): Used to evaluate for non-classic congenital adrenal hyperplasia, which needs to be ruled out before diagnosing PCOS.

Pelvic Ultrasound: Assesses for the presence or absence of internal reproductive organs and obstruction of menstrual blood flow if this cannot be done adequately by pelvic exam. In cases of secondary amenorrhea, a pelvic ultrasound is usually not indicated.

Chromosomal Analysis: Some patients with amenorrhea should have this testing—for example, those who are found to have primary ovarian insufficiency (elevated FSH, low estradiol) and when androgen-insensitivity syndrome is possible.

Pituitary MRI: Imaging of the pituitary to assess for tumor or mass effect is indicated when there are concerns about a central cause of amenorrhea. Examples include significantly elevated prolactin, central hypothyroidism, low FSH and LH suggestive of pituitary hormone deficiency.

MRI, Magnetic resonance imaging; PCOS, polycystic ovarian syndrome.

Ovulatory dysfunction in adolescence is common and is usually due to immaturity of the HPO axis. Many adolescents experience anovulation for several years following their first period; this may result in erratic bleeding or no bleeding at all. This condition generally accompanies a normal history, physical exam, and lab testing. Treatment is based on the individual needs of the patient and at a minimum should involve close monitoring of the patient

- Bleeding more frequently than every 21 days or going longer than 90 days without a period.
- Soaking more than one or two menstrual pads or products every hour.
- Menstrual flow lasting longer than 7 to 8 days in a row.

and her menstrual periods, which should return to a normal frequency of at least every 45 days.

Ovarian insufficiency is marked by a low serum estradiol and elevated FSH (typically above 40 mIU/mL). In these cases, chromosomal analysis should be obtained and management coordinated with a genetics specialist. The most common cause of gonadal failure is Turner syndrome (XO, or mosaic with XO). Polycystic ovarian syndrome (PCOS) is one of the most common causes of secondary amenorrhea and oligomenorrhea. This complex condition involves ovulatory dysfunction, hyperandrogenism, and insulin resistance (Chapter 45).

Congenital anomalies of the reproductive system causing primary amenorrhea include imperforate hymen, transverse vaginal septum, and partial or complete absence of the vagina and uterus. Girls with an imperforate hymen may have cyclic abdominal pain due to the buildup of trapped menstrual blood. Referral to a gynecologist is needed for surgical correction of this condition. Patients with müllerian agenesis have an abnormal external genital exam or pelvic ultrasound, otherwise normal growth and development, normal 46,XX karyotype, and a normal female hormonal profile (ACOG Committee Opinion, 2016). When a congenital anomaly is discovered, referral to an adolescent gynecologist or other specialist familiar with this condition is essential.

In postmenarchal adolescents, anatomic causes of amenorrhea are unlikely. However, if a uterine procedure such as curettage has been done, there may be scarring of the uterine lining, which would prevent normal growth of the endometrium.

Abnormal Uterine Bleeding

Menstrual flow outside of normal volume, duration, regularity, or frequency of the cycle is called AUB. Irregularity in menstrual cycles is common and expected during adolescence but may warrant further evaluation (Box 42.6). AUB can be a presenting symptom of anovulation or of a bleeding disorder. The evaluation and management of vaginal bleeding due to trauma or pregnancy is discussed elsewhere.

Heavy Menstrual Bleeding

History alone is not a reliable measure of blood loss; without objective assessment, significant conditions may be overlooked. The following require further workup:

- Heavy or prolonged menstrual bleeding that causes anemia or has been ongoing since menarche.
- History of surgery-related bleeding or bleeding associated with dental work.
- Two or more of the following: bruising one to two times per month, epistaxis one to two times per month, frequent gum bleeding, or a family history of excessive bleeding.
- Family history of a known bleeding disorder.

Adolescents with heavy and/or prolonged bleeding patterns should have a pregnancy test, complete blood count (CBC)

TABLE 42.8	Causes of Abnormal Uterine Bleeding in Adolescent Girls	
Cause	**Clinical Considerations**	
Pregnancy	Test all patients with abnormal uterine bleeding (AUB) even when sexual contact has not been reported.	
Bleeding disorders (von Willebrand disease, platelet function disorders, acquired disorders)	Screen if there is anemia or other concerning symptoms or signs.	
Anovulation • Immaturity of hypothalamic-pituitary-ovarian (HPO) axis • Hyperandrogenic anovulation [PCOS]) • Anovulation due to thyroid disease, or primary pituitary disease. • Primary ovarian insufficiency (will usually present with oligomenorrhea or amenorrhea)	Anovulation allows for a disordered endometrium, which can result in chaotic and heavy bleeding. Consider lab testing for TSH, FSH, and androgens when indicated.	
Medications Hormonal therapy, contraception, anticoagulation therapy.		
Cervicitis due to sexually transmitted infections (STIs)	Test for chlamydia, gonorrhea.	
Benign structural causes (fibroids, polyps)	Uncommon in adolescents	
Rare tumors (estrogen- and/or androgen-secreting tumors, rhabdomyosarcoma)	Uncommon, rare cause.	

FSH, Follicle stimulating hormone.

TABLE 42.9	Overview of Hormonal Therapy

Common Indications for Hormonal Therapy
- Abnormal uterine bleeding
- Dysmenorrhea
- Chronic pelvic pain
- Endometriosis
- Premenstrual syndrome
- Menstrual migraines
- Seizures associated with the menstrual cycle
- Acne
- Hirsutism
- Menstrual suppression
- Patient preference

Mechanism of Action
- All methods contain progestin, which induces endometrial atrophy and results in less bleeding and cramping. Progestin effect on endometrium allows for a safe way to reduce or eliminate periods.
- Combined hormonal methods (oral contraceptive pill [OCP], skin patch, vaginal ring) contain progestin and estrogen. Estrogen increases sex-hormone binding globulin (SHBG), which results in lower free testosterone and therefore fewer androgenic concerns like acne and hirsutism. Takes 3-6 months or longer of use for full effects.
- Systemic methods (OCP, skin patch, vaginal ring, depot medroxyprogesterone acetate [DMPA], implant) prevent ovulation, which may be a trigger for pain, premenstrual syndrome (PMS), and other concerns in some adolescents.

Key Counseling Points
- Methods are labeled as "birth control," but this should not be a barrier to use in preteens or adolescents who would greatly benefit from these medications. Can reassure patients and families that there is no change in sexual behavior/interest when adolescents initiate these methods for medical reasons.
- Do not negatively affect future fertility and do not cause cancer.
- There are many different kinds of hormonal therapy. If one option does not meet a patient's/family's needs, another option can be tried.
- During the first 3-6 months of hormonal therapy, breakthrough bleeding is common and should be expected. Unplanned bleeding can be minimized by using the method correctly (e.g., pill must be taken at the same time each day; expect breakthrough bleeding if a pill is missed.)

with platelets and ferritin (iron deficiency). Patients who are actively bleeding and found to have significant anemia, or who exhibit symptoms of hemodynamic instability such as hypotension and tachycardia should be sent to an emergency department (ED) for evaluation and management, including assessment for a bleeding disorder, blood type, screen and crossmatch with potential blood administration and estrogen therapy. 🔵 Those with significant anemia, who require hospitalization, or who have a compelling history of a bleeding disorder should be screened for a coagulopathy (see Chapter 39). As many as 20% of this population will be found to have a coagulopathy, and consultation with hematology and gynecology and close follow-up as an outpatient is warranted. Ongoing concerns about anemia or excessive bleeding also warrant referral to a hematologist for further evaluation and treatment.

Causes of Abnormal Uterine Bleeding

Most adolescents with AUB do not have a bleeding disorder; they have AUB due to anovulation. Anovulation causes the lining of the endometrium to become disordered and fragile, resulting in chaotic bleeding patterns. Table 42.8 lists causes of AUB in

adolescents and should be considered and evaluated by lab testing when indicated. Given that structural causes are very rare in this population, a pelvic ultrasound is not typically indicated in the initial evaluation for bleeding in adolescence.

Treatment of Abnormal Uterine Bleeding

The treatment of AUB depends on the severity of the condition, its cause, and the preference of the patient and her family. Hormonal therapy (Table 42.9 and Box 42.7) is the mainstay of treatment. Iron supplementation (3 to 6 mg/kg per day of elemental iron divided into thrice daily dosing) is indicated for anemia or low iron stores. Treatment should be continued until abnormal bleeding patterns have resolved for for 3 months and lab values have normalized.

Mild Symptoms. For patients who have only mild symptoms, nonsteroidal antiinflammatory drugs (NSAIDs) such as ibuprofen or naproxen are recommended. In addition to reducing pain, these medications decrease associated menstrual blood loss. If iron stores are depleted, iron supplementation is indicated. Patients should track their menstrual bleeding and alert their PCP about any concerns. Bleeding patterns should be reviewed periodically and the evaluation repeated when indicated. Patients with mild symptoms should be educated that hormonal therapy is an option if medical or functional concerns increase.

Moderate Symptoms and/or Anemia. Patients with moderate symptoms need iron supplementation and hormonal therapy to reduce further blood loss. Patients should have a repeat CBC and ferritin in 3 months to ensure that anemia and iron deficiency are improved or resolved. Iron supplementation should continue for 3 months after hemoglobin and ferritin levels have normalized. Hormonal therapy should continue for a minimum of 3 to 6 months and possibly longer based on patient and family preference.

Severe Anemia and/or Bleeding Disorder. Patients with severe anemia require immediate treatment for their bleeding in an ED setting. Iron supplementation and hormonal therapy will control and prevent further bleeding. Patients should be seen within 5 to 7 days after leaving the hospital to assess hemoglobin status. Increased bleeding as an outpatient should prompt the patient or family to call their PCP and return to the ED if necessary. Hormonal therapy should be continued for a minimum of 6 to 9 months. Consultation with gynecology or adolescent medicine is indicated to ensure appropriate evaluation, management, and follow-up. Patients with a suspected or diagnosed bleeding disorder should be referred to hematology.

Treating the Underlying Cause of Abnormal Uterine Bleeding

Most commonly, AUB in adolescents is due to anovulation caused by immaturity of the HPO axis. AUB due to this cause may warrant treatment; however, the underlying condition will resolve as the endocrine system matures. For adolescents found to have medical conditions (e.g., PCOS, thyroid dysfunction), treatment of the underlying condition results in a return to regular ovulatory cycles; however, hormonal therapy may be needed in the interim.

Pelvic Pain

There are many causes of pelvic pain in female adolescents. Pain is a response to distention, stretching, compression, irritation, and ischemia and can be referred from another site. The clinical neuroanatomy of the female pelvis is complex, with several organ systems sharing visceral and somatic innervation. Stress and overall sense of health and well-being greatly affect an individual's response to pain and her ability to cope with it.

TABLE 42.10 Gynecologic Causes of Pelvic Pain in Adolescents

Serious, requiring urgent intervention
- Ectopic pregnancy
- Rare obstetric emergencies (abruption, uterine rupture)
- Ovarian or fallopian tube torsion

Common
- Dysmenorrhea
- Mittelschmerz
- Pelvic inflammatory disease with or without tubo-ovarian abscess
- Ovarian and paratubal cysts
- Vulvovaginitis

Other
- Pregnancy
- Endometriosis
- Vaginal foreign body
- Müllerian anomalies causing obstruction
- Leiomyoma (fibroids)
- Vaginismus
- Pelvic floor dysfunction

Acute Pelvic Pain

Common gynecologic causes of acute pain in adolescent females include pelvic inflammatory disease (PID), ovarian cysts, ovarian torsion, and ectopic pregnancy (Table 42.10). Nongynecologic causes of acute, severe pelvic pain include appendicitis, kidney stones, and urinary tract infection. Evaluation of acute pain must include a careful history, physical exam, and pregnancy testing. Other testing includes pelvic ultrasound to assess for ovarian causes, imaging for appendicitis, urinalysis, and testing for STIs. The adolescent girl with acute pelvic pain should receive immediate attention at a medical center that can provide aggressive evaluation and treatment for gynecologic and nongynecologic causes (Table 42.11). 🔊 *Ovarian or fallopian tube torsion* describes the twisting of the adnexa, resulting in partial or complete tissue ischemia. The onset of pain is acute, sharp, and associated with nausea and vomiting. Surgical intervention is necessary to detorse the adnexa and prevent necrosis and loss of the ovary. Patients with suspected torsion should be sent to an ED and surgical consultation obtained. 🔊

Chronic and Recurrent Pelvic Pain

The initial evaluation of mild to moderate, recurrent, or chronic pelvic pain is best done with a comprehensive approach to the patient and her symptoms. In additional to the gynecologic causes of pain listed in Table 42.10, there are gastrointestinal, urinary, musculoskeletal, neurogenic, and psychologic causes that must be considered (Table 42.11). History, including a confidential interview to screen for social and emotional concerns and a physical exam are the first steps in evaluation. Common causes of chronic or recurring gynecologic pain are discussed next.

Dysmenorrhea

Dysmenorrhea is painful menstruation. Pain usually begins with the onset of menses but can occur 1 to 2 days before the onset of bleeding in some adolescents. There may be associated nausea, vomiting, diarrhea, headaches, dizziness and back pain. *Primary*

TABLE 42.11 Differential Diagnosis of Pelvic Pain in Adolescents, Nongynecologic Causes

Gastrointestinal
- Constipation
- Appendicitis
- Irritable bowel syndrome
- Celiac disease
- Lactose Intolerance
- Gastroenteritis
- Hernia
- Inflammatory bowel disease
- Intestinal obstruction

Urinary
- Urinary tract infection (UTI), pyelonephritis
- Renal calculi
- Urethral syndrome
- Interstitial cystitis

Musculoskeletal
- Trauma
- Joint pain or injury
- Inflammation of muscles and ligaments

Neurogenic
- Nerve compression due to injury
- Neuropathic pain

Psychologic
- Physical and/or sexual abuse (current or previous)
- Depression and/or anxiety
- Eating disorder
- School avoidance
- Substance use/abuse
- Fear of pregnancy

• BOX 42.8 Characteristics of Primary Dysmenorrhea in Adolescents

- Onset of severe cramps usually 1 to 2 years after the onset of menses, but can be anytime, especially if bleeding is heavy.
- Pain is in the lower or midabdomen. May radiate to back or thighs.
- Character is crampy and stabbing at times. May be severe.
- NSAIDs and heat usually helpful but may not alleviate pain.
- Missing of school and activities not uncommon if pain is severe.
- Absence of pain outside menstruation.
- Physical exam is normal.

NSAIDs, Nonsteroidal anti-inflammatory drugs.

---

dysmenorrhea refers to recurrent, menstrual-related pain in the absence of pelvic pathology and is thought to be due to the release of prostaglandins from the endometrium. *Secondary dysmenorrhea* describes painful menstruation in the presence of pelvic pathology such as endometriosis, ovarian cysts, or infection. The evaluation of dysmenorrhea in adolescents starts with a detailed medical and menstrual history. Typical characteristics of dysmenorrhea are listed in Box 42.8. The physical exam should be normal, and pelvic ultrasound is not routinely indicated.

Treatment for dysmenorrhea starts with education about the condition, tracking the menstrual cycle, and basic self-care before and during menstrual periods. Over-the-counter and prescription

NSAIDs are effective in many cases due to their antiprostaglandin effect. The patient should take the medication as soon as she knows her menses is coming so as to block prostaglandin production before the onset of severe pain. Ibuprofen 400 to 800 mg every 8 hours or naproxen 550 mg every 12 hours are commonly used. Acetaminophen is unlikely to be helpful in relieving dysmenorrhea. Hormonal therapy, which causes the endometrial lining to become more atrophic, therefore releasing less prostaglandin, is another treatment option for adolescents who fail initial treatment and includes combined hormonal methods (oral contraceptive pills [OCPs], skin ptch, vaginal ring). For adolescents who still have cramps with their periods or who prefer fewer periods, these methods can be given in extended or continuous fashion. Progesterone-only treatments for dysmenorrhea include the levonorgestrel IUD, etonogestrel subdermal implant, depot medroxyprogesterone acetate (DMPA), and norethindrone acetate. Patients who continue to have pain after several months of treatment should be referred to a gynecologist for additional evaluation.

Mittelschmerz

The term mittelschmerz refers to the pain causes by normal ovarian function at the time of ovulation. It occurs during the middle of the menstrual cycle, is typically unilateral and mild to moderate in severity, and lasts for a few hours to several days. If needed, treatment is with an over-the-counter (OTC) pain medication; hormonal therapies that block ovulation are another option.

Ovarian Cysts

Ovarian cysts in women of reproductive age are common and cause pain of wide-ranging severity. Ultrasound is the preferred method of imaging for ovarian cysts and describes location, size, and cyst complexity. Severe pain caused by an ovarian cyst occurs when it ruptures or leaks fluid onto the peritoneum. Severe pain associated with nausea and vomiting should be addressed immediately given the risk of ovarian torsion.

Ovarian cysts in adolescents are often due to normal physiologic functions and resolve on their own. Supportive care with OTC pain medications, heat, and rest may be helpful. Pain from an ovarian cyst should gradually improve over the days to weeks following its onset, with complete resolution of symptoms within 1 to 3 months. A repeat ultrasound done 3 months following initial imaging is recommended to confirm that the cyst has resolved. Cysts that do not resolve in 3 months are less likely to be functional and may represent a neoplasm, such as teratoma, cystadenoma, or paratubal cyst. Ovarian cancer is rare in adolescents but must be considered. Patients who have ovarian or adnexal findings that do not resolve within 3 months should be referred to a gynecologist for consultation for possible removal. Patients with increasing pain should be referred sooner.

Endometriosis

Endometriosis is the presence of endometrial glands and stroma outside their normal location within the lining of the uterus. Historically endometriosis was considered a disease of adult women only. However, current studies show endometriosis in about 5% of adolescents 15 to 19 years of age, and nearly half of those adolescents have chronic pain (de Sanctis et al., 2018). The most common symptoms are cyclic as well as noncyclic pelvic pain, gastrointestinal pain, and urinary symptoms. The cause of endometriosis is multifactorial, with several theories about its origins. A family history of endometriosis is correlated with a higher risk of

Symptoms attributable to PMS are as follows:
- Present during the 5 days before the period
- Occur for at least 2 menstrual cycles in a row
- End within 4 days after period starts
- Interfere with some normal activities
  Exclude depression, anxiety, and social-emotional stressors, which can mimic premenstrual syndrome but will not occur in a cyclic pattern that align with the menstrual cycle.

the condition. NSAIDs and hormonal therapy may help to resolve symptoms, but if there is no response to therapy within 3 months, referral to a gynecologist is warranted.

Premenstrual Syndrome

Premenstrual syndrome (PMS) includes a cluster of emotional and physical symptoms that occur in cyclic fashion about 1 to 2 weeks prior to the menstrual period and resolve with menses onset. Common PMS symptoms include bloating, breast pain, headache, food cravings, anxiety, fatigue, irritability, and depression. Premenstrual dysphoric disorder (PMDD) is a severe form of PMS defined in the American Psychological Association's *Diagnostic and Statistical Manual of Mental Disorders,* fifth edition (DSM-5). The diagnosis of PMS is made with the patient's prospective recording of her symptoms for 2 to 3 months (Box 42.9). Depression and anxiety can overlap or mimic PMS, so screening for underlying mental health concerns due to PMS or PMDD is important. Mild and moderate PMS symptoms often improve with lifestyle changes, such as increased aerobic exercise, relaxation techniques, adequate sleep, and avoidance of foods high in fat, salt, sugar, and caffeine. Hormonal therapy used to prevent ovulation and the subsequent fluctuations in hormone levels can also be used to to treat PMS, along with other evidence-based treatments (Yonkers & Simoni, 2017).

Breast Concerns

Breast development (thelarche) begins in most girls between the ages of 8 and 13 years and is often the first sign of puberty. Breast concerns are not uncommon among adolescents; PCPs can offer reassurance following a normal exam as well as educate patients on basic breast anatomy (ACOG practice Bulletin, June 2016a).

Asymmetric Breasts

Significant differences in breast size can cause distress for patients and their parents. A breast exam should be done to confirm normal findings and verify that the size difference is not due to a cyst or mass in the larger breast. Young adolescents with this concern can be reassured that asymmetry will often improve over time and that surgical intervention is not usually needed.

Mastalgia

Mild breast pain is common among young women. Many fear that this symptom is due to breast cancer. Reassure patients and families that breast cancer is extremely uncommon in adolescents; it can also be helpful to explain that this condition usually does not cause pain. History elucidates whether breast pain is cyclic or noncyclic, as well as other possible factors including new medications, trauma, type of bra, and breast growth. Examine the patient

for fibrocystic changes, mastitis, cysts, and chest wall pain. Pregnancy testing should also be done.

Breast Cyst or Mass

Due to increased awareness of breast cancer, a palpable breast cyst or mass in an adolescent can be very alarming to the patient and her family. Breast cancer is extremely rare in the adolescent population, but all findings require evaluation and appropriate clinical follow-up. The first step is a careful history, assessing for history of trauma, previous thoracic (chest/back) irradiation, associated symptoms, and family history of breast cancer. The breast exam in many cases reveals normal physiologic tissue or fibrocystic changes. Breast ultrasound is indicated for masses that are persistent or worrisome due to physical findings such as large size (>5 cm), skin changes, solid, or fixed on the underlying tissue. If a discrete but nonsuspicious mass is found, it is reasonable to observe it for 1 to 2 months and have the patient return for a repeat breast exam.

Nipple Discharge

Adolescents can express a small amount of clear discharge from their nipples; however, spontaneous nipple discharge needs further evaluation. Common causes include mechanical stimulation and irritation from clothing. Galactorrhea, which is a milky white discharge from both nipples, can be caused by hormonal medication, certain tranquilizers, antidepressants, and antihypertensives, as well as hypothryoidam or a prolactin-secreting pituitary adenoma. When nipple discharge persists, consultation with an adolescent gynecologist or pediatric endocrinologist should be obtained, depending on the rest of the exam.

Gynecologic Concerns in Adolescents With Physical and Developmental Disabilities

Similar to their peers, adolescents with physical and developmental disabilities need reproductive health care (ACOG Committee Opinion 668, August 2016b). Menstrual suppression or reduction is a common request from adolescents and their families due to concerns about hygiene, mood changes before or during the menstrual cycle, exacerbation of conditions such as seizures, as well as other concerns. Many disabled teens can consent to sexual activity and desire contraception. Furthermore, caregivers may request contraception because of concerns that sexual abuse might occur. Safety of the teen's environment and abuse prevention should be discussed with all teens and their families. Studies show that rates of all types of abuse among children with disabilities is 31%, compared with 9% for nondisabled children (deAlwis and Horrideg, 2016) with the risk of sexual abuse 4.62 times as likely and emotional abuse 4.31 times as likely (Sobsey, 2014). Disabled teens in romantic relationships are at greater risk for dating violence than are their nondisabled peers (Mitra, 2013).

PCPs who care for adolescents with disabilities are well equipped to provide appropriate counseling for menstrual management and contraception. The U.S. Medical Eligibility Criteria (USMEC), described later, help guide providers as to relative and absolute contraindication for contraception for individuals with medical conditions. Combined OCP, skin patches, and vaginal rings can be used in extended or continuous dosing to reduce or eliminate menstrual periods. Amenorrhea will occur in 50% of patients after 1 year using continuous dosing. Breakthrough bleeding occurs most often in the first 3 months of use. When bleeding occurs with prolonged use, it can be managed with a 5-day break to allow for a withdrawal bleed and then restart. DMPA and amenorrhea will occur in 50% to 80% of patients after 1 year of use, but initial bleeding is very common. Concerns about weight gain and bone mineral density may limit its use. The levonorgestrel IUD 52 mg (Mirena, Liletta) is an excellent option for menstrual suppression as well as long-acting, highly effective contraception. There are very few medical contraindications to this IUD, and amenorrhea rates are 50% or higher at 1 year of use, with decreased flow in almost all users. Initial bleeding and spotting should be expected for first 3 to 6 months after IUD placement. The procedure for IUD insertion may require anesthesia but can be coordinated with other procedures such as dental work. Oral progesterone (norethindrone acetate) is another option for menstrual suppression.

Sexual Health

PCPs who provide health care to children, adolescents, and young adults should understand sexuality in a developmental context (Chapter 21). PCPs are instrumental in fostering the sexual well-being of their patients, with the potential for self-efficacy, positive relationships, and responsible, healthy choices. There are many key elements of sexual health; the following section addresses those aspects directly related to the gynecologic health of adolescents, specifically contraception to avoid unintended pregnancy, access to prenatal care and abortion, and STI education, prevention, testing, and treatment.

Best Practices in Contraceptive Counseling

An overwhelming 82% of all teen pregnancies are unintended, and the majority are preventable with effective contraception. Long-acting, reversible contraception (LARC) is the first-line option for teens and young women who want birth control (ACOG, 2018). This section reviews best practices in contraceptive counseling and then provides an overview of available methods.

PCPs seeing adolescents are uniquely positioned to provide sexual health education including counseling on contraceptive options. High-quality counseling has a significant impact on reproductive health outcomes, and with regards to contraception, results in higher rates of satisfaction and continuation of a method, which then results in more effective pregnancy prevention. Creating the time and space for a one-on-one interview, listening to what teen patients have to say, and demonstrating empathy on difficult issues will allow for productive discussions between PCPs and adolescents about sensitive health topics such as sexuality and family planning. Additional information on the sexual health interview is covered in Chapter 21, but central issues when contraception is discussed are highlighted here. Box 42.10 provides a summary of best practices in adolescent contraceptive counseling, with a more in-depth discussion of several of these issues in the following paragraphs.

Address Confidentiality Concerns
Confidentiality is an essential component of adolescent health care and teens often forgo needed medical care unless confidentiality can be assured. Twenty-one states explicitly allow minors to consent to contraceptive services on their own, without the approval or consent of their parents. Other states allow minors to consent in certain circumstances, and four states have no explicit policy. Clinicians who provide health services to adolescents must be aware of the regulations in their state. The Guttmacher Institute is a valuable resource to learn about state laws and policies related to minors' access to contraception (www.guttmacher.org). When necessary, providers should be aware of local resources for free and

• BOX 42.10 Summary of Best Practices in Adolescent Contraceptive Counseling

- Address confidentiality concerns:
  - Take the time to do a one-on-one interview, even when the teen presents with her parent or partner.
  - Discuss confidentiality, privacy, limitations, and support conversations with family and friends.
  - Know your state laws and policies.
  - Develop and identify local resources for free and confidential reproductive health care.
- Use tools and techniques that reflect best practices:
  - Designed for young adults, with content and format for them.
  - Reflects best practices and current recommendations.
  - Ensure that teen knows about LARC, how and where to get it.
  - Address common myths and misperceptions about contraception.
  - Ask about opinions of friends and family members.
  - Educate teen on noncontraceptive benefits as well as possible common side effects.
  - Discuss the prevention of STIs: risk reduction strategies including condom use and all other methods.
  - Invest time in phone calls and return visits when needed to listen to concerns and provide reassurance.
- Follow updated clinical recommendations:
  - Use same-day start or "quick start" for all methods when possible.
  - Pelvic exam and testing not required before starting any method.
  - Multiple visits before or after starting a method are not required.
  - Do not unnecessarily restrict the use of contraception in teens with medical conditions. Instead, refer to USMEC.

LARC, Long-acting, reversible contraception; *STIs*, sexually transmitted infections; *USMEC*, US Medical Eligibility Criteria.

confidential reproductive health care. Examples may include Title X family planning clinics, community health centers, state and county public health clinics, school-based clinics, and private and/or nonprofit providers and organizations.

Use Tools and Techniques That Reflect Best Practices
One of the most significant changes over the last decade is the recommendation that LARC be offered as the first-line option for teens requesting birth control. This evidence-based guideline (ACOG, 2018) was based on findings from a meta-analysis of 12 studies on the LARC method in adolescents and women under 25 years of age. Overall, an 84% continuation rate was found for LARC. Within the studies the Contraceptive Choice project (Secura et al., 2010), which included almost 10,000 women and demonstrated that two-thirds of them choose a long-acting method when financial and knowledge barriers were removed, over 50% of young women ages 14 to 17 chose the contraceptive implant, and over 40% of young women ages 18 to 20 choose the IUD. Adolescents using LARC were significantly less likely to experience a pregnancy, live birth, or abortion compared with their peers. These positive outcomes, including safety and efficacy in the adolescent population, were reproduced in numerous subsequent studies (Diedrich et al., 2017; ACOG, 2018).

When clinicians discuss options for birth control, it is important to use updated tools that reflect best practices. For example, outdated patient handouts may contain inaccurate information about the safety of IUDs in teens. Fig 42.13 is an example of a visual aid that reflects best practices by depicting LARC as the most effective option. Other visual tools and models are helpful for explaining the various methods and how they work. When requested, the manufacturers of LARC supply clinics with models

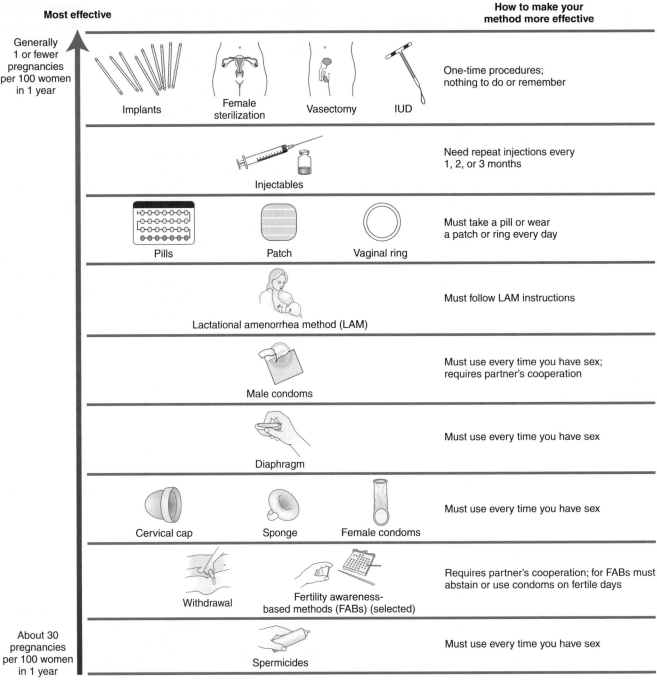

Most effective

Generally 1 or fewer pregnancies per 100 women in 1 year

How to make your method more effective

Implants · Female sterilization · Vasectomy · IUD — One-time procedures; nothing to do or remember

Injectables — Need repeat injections every 1, 2, or 3 months

Pills · Patch · Vaginal ring — Must take a pill or wear a patch or ring every day

Lactational amenorrhea method (LAM) — Must follow LAM instructions

Male condoms — Must use every time you have sex; requires partner's cooperation

Diaphragm — Must use every time you have sex

Cervical cap · Sponge · Female condoms — Must use every time you have sex

Withdrawal · Fertility awareness-based methods (FABs) (selected) — Requires partner's cooperation; for FABs must abstain or use condoms on fertile days

About 30 pregnancies per 100 women in 1 year

Spermicides — Must use every time you have sex

Least effective

• **Fig 42.13** How Well Does Birth Control Work? (Redrawn from Association of Reproductive Health Professionals [ARHP]: You decide tool kit: contraceptive efficacy tools. Adapted from World Health Organization. Comparing typical effectiveness of contraceptive methods. [Job Aid]. Geneva, Switzerland, WHO, 2006). In Lobo RA: Gershenson DM, Lentz GM, Valea FA: Comprehensive Gynecology, ed 7, Philadelphia, 2017, Elsevier.)

of devices that allow teens to see and feel their size and shape. Patients are often surprised to see that the IUD is much smaller than they expected or that the implant is very thin, flexible, and will go unnoticed beneath their skin.

Many adolescents seek online resources. Table 42.12 lists websites that present medically accurate, nonjudgmental health content in a format that is likely to appeal to teens and young adults. Given the volume of inaccurate information on the Internet, it is important for providers to highlight that these websites provide material that is written and reviewed by sexual health experts. This

type of supplement to in-clinic conversations can allow teens and families to research options before and after their visits as well as provide ongoing support once a method is initiated.

Dual use of a contraceptive method along with condoms to prevent STIs is important and should be reaffirmed in counseling visits and education tools. Key elements in a discussion on contraceptive options should include information on their effectiveness and potential side effects (Dehlendorf, Krajewski, and Borrero, 2018). Ask about the opinions and experiences of friends and families, and address common myths and misperceptions that

TABLE 42.12   Medically Accurate Websites on Sexual Health[a]

http://www.bedsider.org

An online birth control support network. No funding from pharmaceutical companies. Medical partners include the American College of Obstetricians and Gynecologists.
- Information and comparison of all contraceptive methods.
- Health clinic finder (enter zip code).
- Can set up daily, weekly, monthly text message reminders (for short-acting methods).
- Can set up text and email reminders for next clinic appointment:

www.itsyoursexlife.org

MTV's public health campaign to support young people to make responsible decisions about their sexual health. Also supported by the Kaiser Family Foundation, Advocates for Youth and others.
- Information and about sexually transmitted infections (STIs) and tips for their prevention.
- Talking to partner about STIs.
- Links to other trusted sexual health resources including live chat features.

www.goaskalice.org

Written and run by a team of health professionals and researchers at Columbia University.
- Sexual and reproductive health in questions and answer format.
- General health including alcohol and drugs, nutrition, relationships and more.

[a]These sites are directed to college-age teens and young adults.

TABLE 42.13   Quick-Start Contraception

All methods of contraception can be quick started at any time during the menstrual cycle as long as the provider is reasonably certain that the woman is not pregnant.
Criteria include any of the following:
- Has never had sexual intercourse before
- Is currently using another effective method of contraception
- Has regular monthly periods and is less than 7 days from the start of a normal period
- Is less than 4 weeks postpartum or less than 7 days after spontaneous or induced abortion
- Has not had unprotected sexual intercourse in more than 3 weeks and has a negative pregnancy test today

If the woman has had unprotected sex in the previous 3 weeks but has a negative pregnancy test today, all methods except intrauterine devices can be quick-started.
- Advise teen that the pregnancy test is not conclusive but contraceptive hormones do not cause harm to the pregnancy or fetus so it is OK to start the method today.
- Use backup method or no sex for 1 week.
- Return for repeat pregnancy test in 2 weeks.

might otherwise prevent the adolescent from considering a given method.

Finally, contraceptive counseling also includes ongoing support, education, and reassurance. When adolescents leave the clinic with a new contraceptive method, they must know how to contact the clinic with questions and concerns. Phone calls and follow-up visits should be encouraged and viewed as valued opportunities to provide

additional support and education. Teens may need reassurance that an expected side effect, like breakthrough bleeding, is common and does not mean that the method is not working. For most women, contraceptive choice is an issue they address throughout most of their adult lives. Using a patient-centered approach to contraceptive counseling allows adolescents to make decisions about which method best suits their needs at this time and empowers them to make decisions about family planning for the future.

Follow Updated Clinical Recommendations

There are several updated clinical recommendations for providing contraception that remove traditional barriers to initiating birth control. Published by the CDC, *U.S. Selected Practice Recommendations for Contraceptive Use* addresses common issues and offers evidence-based clinical guidance (Curtis et al., 2016). All methods can be started on the same day as long as the provider can be reasonably sure a patient is not pregnant. "Quick Start" (Table 42.13) refers to the practice of initiating a contraceptive method on the same day of the contraceptive visit, or on any day during the menstrual cycle as continuation rates are higher. Multiple visits before or after starting a method should never be required. Tests and exams required before initiation of a method are minimal to none. Most providers obtain a urine pregnancy test before starting contraception, even when the chance of pregnancy is extremely low. If the adolescent had unprotected sexual intercourse in the previous 3 weeks before starting a method, she should return for another pregnancy test in 2 weeks to make sure she is not pregnant. The use of emergency contraception (EC) may be indicated if pregnancy is a risk. All women should be instructed to abstain or use a backup method for 7 days after starting a new method. Blood pressure should be assessed before initiating combined hormonal methods (OCPs, patch, ring), and initiation of an IUD requires a pelvic exam that, along with STI testing, if indicated, can be done at the time of insertion. There are no evidenced-based recommendations for follow-up testing or exams once a method has been initiated.

The concept of bridging methods is helpful for women who prefer to have no gaps in their contraceptive coverage. For example, an adolescent who is interested in LARC but cannot receive it that day should be started on a shorter-acting method she can use until LARC is obtained; a teen who is switching from birth control pills to an implant can continue to use her pills for 7 days after the implant is placed. Sometimes concern about the safety of birth control creates a barrier to its initiation.

The US Medical Eligibility Criteria for Contraceptive Use was developed by the Centers for Disease Control (CDC) and World Health Organization (WHO); it provides evidence-based guidance for safe contraceptive use in adolescents and women with medical conditions. The USMEC, available free online and with a free smartphone application, is an evidence-based tool that is easy to use and can provide an immediate, direct answers to common clinical questions (https://www.cdc.gov/reproductive-health/contraception/pdf/summary-chart-us-medical-eligibility-criteria_508tagged.pdf). Table 42.14 describes common clinical scenarios where providers may have questions about contraceptive safety. USMEC presents evidence-based recommendations for safe use in these conditions as well as many others.

Contraceptive Methods

It is important for providers to have a working knowledge of contraceptive methods. Given that LARC is recommended as the first-line approach, PCPs must be familiar with these options even if they are not provided in their practice. A brief overview

TABLE 42.14	Common Clinical Scenarios in Providing Contraception and US Medical Eligibility Criteria for Contraceptive Use

Sixteen-year-old with a family history of breast cancer. Both grandmother and mother of patient were diagnosed in their 40s, and mother of patient is worried that "hormones will cause cancer." *USMEC: All contraceptive methods, including OCPs, are safe to use and do not increase the risk of cancer. Of note, OCPs are known to decrease the risk of ovarian cancer.*

Fifteen-year-old with previous pelvic inflammatory disease due to gonorrhea infection *requests an intrauterine device (IUD) for contraception. USMEC: There are no restrictions for IUD use based on age, parity, history of sexually transmitted diseases (STDs), history of pelvic inflammatory disease (PID), or prior ectopic pregnancy.*

Seventeen-year-old who is morbidly obese and has major depression. *USMEC: All contraceptive methods are safe to use in women with obesity and depressive disorders.*

Fourteen-year-old with migraine headaches without aura. *USMEC: All contraceptive methods are safe to use. Combined hormonal contraception (methods that contain estrogen) should be avoided in patients who have migraine WITH aura.*

Seventeen-year-old with epilepsy, currently on the anticonvulsant topiramate. *USMEC: All contraceptive methods are safe to use in women with epilepsy. However, combined hormonal contraception (CHC) should not be used in women on certain anticonvulsants like topiramate due to decreased contraceptive efficacy. (Medications to avoid with CHCs are listed at USMEC.)*

OCP, Oral contraceptive pill; *USMEC*, US Medical Eligibility Criteria for Contraceptive Use.

TABLE 42.15	Advantages and Potential Challenges of Common Birth Control Methods	
	Advantages	**Potential Challenges**

Implant

Advantages	Potential Challenges
• Highest efficacy • High satisfaction and continuation. • Simple and quick insertion • Discreet, immediate reversibility • Relief of dysmenorrhea	• Uterine bleeding, although not dangerous, may be frequent, unpredictable, and prolonged.

Intrauterine Device (IUD)

Advantages	Potential Challenges
• Very high efficacy • Highest satisfaction and continuation of any method • Discreet, immediate reversibility • Levonorgestrel IUDs, treatment for bleeding, dysmenorrhea, anemia due to heavy bleeding • Safe for almost all teens, including those with complex medical conditions; no medication interactions	• Pelvic exam required for insertion.

Depot Medroxyprogesterone Acetate ([DMPA], aka "Depo")

Advantages	Potential Challenges
• High efficacy • Simple and quick injection • Discreet • Relief of dysmenorrhea and heavy bleeding • No medication interactions	• Possible increased appetite and associated weight gain not uncommon. • Irregular bleeding common in first 3-9 months. • Visit every 11-13 weeks.

Combined Hormonal Contraception: Oral Contraceptive Pills (OCPs), Skin Patch, Vaginal Ring

Advantages	Potential Challenges
• Good efficacy when used correctly and consistently • Widespread familiarity • Many noncontraceptive benefits • User can start or stop at anytime • Immediate reversibility	• Remember each day (pills), week (patch), month (ring). • Visits to pharmacy for refills. • Requires medication storage. • Contain estrogen that may limit use in select medical conditions.

of the advantages and potential challenges of the most effective and commonly prescribed methods is given in Table 42.15. In the following section, each contraceptive method is reviewed, including a description of the method and its mechanism of action, its advantages, counseling about what to expect with its use, and how to address common side effects.

The Implant

The contraceptive implant is a single rod 4 cm in length and 2 mm in diameter; it is placed into the subdermal space of the upper inner nondominant arm. It consists of an ethylene vinyl acetate copolymer (latex-free) that allows for the controlled release of etonogestrel (68 mg) over a period of 3 years, with contraceptive efficacy documented at 4 years. Etonogestrel is the main active metabolite of desogestrel, a progestin used in many OCPs. The implant is a progestin-only method. The currently available etonogestrel implant (Nexplanon) contains barium sulfate and is radiopaque.

The primary mechanism of action is ovulation suppression, which may prevent conception by thickening the cervical mucus and altering the endometrial lining. It is the most effective of any contraceptive option and the method of choice for many teens, particularly those ages 14 to 17. Insertion is quick and easy, and does not require a pelvic exam. A teen can easily palpate her implant and be confident about its presence. Many teens as well as women of all ages prefer a method that requires no action on their part and is highly effective. The implant can be inserted at any time during the menstrual cycle using a quick start protocol. Users should be instructed to avoid sexual intercourse or use an alternative method

for the first week. The implant can be placed immediately postpartum or following a spontaneous or induced abortion.

All PCPs who perform insertions and removals are required by the US Food and Drug Administration (FDA) to receive training from the manufacturer. The procedure takes an average of 30 seconds and starts with the injection of a local anesthetic followed by device insertion. The application site is then dressed with a bandage and the patient can return immediately to her usual activities. Infection site complications are rare and most commonly include local redness and bruising. The implant is palpable by the user but is very discreet, given its location in the upper inner arm as well as its subdermal placement. It is helpful to reassure teens that the implant will not migrate and will not break. The procedure to remove the implant involves injection of a local anesthetic followed by a small incision for removal. If a woman wants to continue to use an implant at the end of 3 years, it is best practice to remove the current implant and replace with a new device at the same visit.

Managing Common Expected Side Effects of the Implant. The contraceptive implant causes bleeding pattern changes that are unpredictable for the duration of use. Episodes of frequent bleeding are more common in the first 3 months but may continue. The bleeding pattern that a user experiences in the first 3 months is broadly predictive of future bleeding. There is no way to predict the type of bleeding pattern that a woman will have with implant use, but women with lower body weight tend to have less bleeding than those with higher weights. Counseling and education about changes in bleeding patterns *prior* to receiving the implant increase satisfaction and continuation of the method.

When irregular or prolonged bleeding occurs, reassurance from the PCP is crucial and is usually all that is necessary. With prolonged progestin exposure, the endometrium becomes atrophic, which can result in amenorrhea or spotting or frequent bleeding due to endometrial instability. Most patients who are concerned about their bleeding respond to reassurance alone. When continued bleeding is being evaluated, it is usually not necessary to obtain lab testing, although some patients or providers feel more comfortable after the assessment of hemoglobin. It is reasonable to consider STI testing and any other clinically indicated tests. The CDC recommends NSAIDs for 5 to 7 days or (if medically eligible) combined an OCP or estrogen for 10 to 20 days. Many providers offer hormonal treatment to manage bleeding for longer periods if necessary, given the benefit of continuing this highly effective method.

Intrauterine Devices

Five different IUDs are now available in the United States, all of which are safe and effective for teens and women who have not yet had children.

The copper-containing IUD is marketed under the name Para-Gard and has been approved by the FDA for 10 years, although contraceptive efficacy has been documented for 12 years. It is made of polyethylene with barium sulfate added to create x-ray visibility. Copper wire is wound around the vertical stem of the T-shaped device. Four IUDs contain the hormone levonorgestrel and include Liletta, Mirena, Kyleena, and Skyla. Mirena has been available in the United States since 2001 and in Europe a decade prior to that. The product consists of a T-shaped polyethylene frame with a vertical cylinder that slowly releases levonorgestrel directly into the endometrial cavity. Mirena is FDA-approved to use for 5 years, although its contraceptive efficacy has been documented for 7 years of use. Liletta, a generic levonorgestrel IUD, is identical to Mirena. Skyla and Kyleena are levonorgestrel IUDs that contain a lower dose of levonorgestrel and therefore are less likely to induce amenorrhea.

All IUDs produce a sterile foreign body reaction within the uterine cavity, which creates a hostile environment for sperm. The contraceptive effects of continuous IUD use occur prior to fertilization; therefore IUDs are not abortifacients. The copper IUD causes an increase in copper ions, enzymes, white blood cells, and prostaglandins in uterine and tubal fluids, which impair sperm function and prevent fertilization. Levonorgestrel IUDs have a local effect on the endometrium, causing the release of foreign body mediators, inhibiting sperm capacitation and survival, thickening cervical mucus, and suppressing the endometrium. Systemic absorption of levonorgestrel is low and most cycles are ovulatory. IUDs are very effective, with failure rates of less than 1%. The levonorgestrel IUDs have slightly lower failure rates than the copper IUD.

Advantages and Method Counseling. IUD users report higher satisfaction and continuation than users of any other contraceptive method. Satisfaction and continuation of the levonorgestrel IUD is higher than with the copper IUD. An IUD can be inserted at any time in a woman's menstrual cycle as long as the provider is reasonably sure she is not pregnant. Screening for chlamydia and gonorrhea is indicated at least annually for all sexually active teens and can be done at the same visit as insertion. If an STI is detected, treatment should occur with the IUD in place. An IUD can be inserted immediately following vaginal delivery or cesarean section. The procedure for IUD insertion includes a bimanual exam, speculum exam, measuring for uterine size, and placement of the IUD using a sterile, prepackaged applicator. IUD strings are cut to 3 cm in length, which allows them to curl up around the cervix so that they cannot be felt during intercourse. The pain experienced with IUD insertion is rated as tolerable by most women, including young women and those who have not had children. After a detailed explanation of the insertion procedure, most women clearly express their interest or noninterest in this method and the procedure required for insertion.

Managing Common Expected Side Effects. In the first days and weeks after IUD insertion, there may be bleeding and cramping related to the procedure itself. NSAIDs decrease bleeding and pain following insertion. Heavy bleeding, severe pain, nausea, vomiting, or fevers should be evaluated with a complete history and exam including a speculum exam to look for IUD strings and a bimanual exam to assess uterine tenderness. The risk of complications such as uterine perforation and infection is low but should be considered. There is a 5% risk of IUD expulsion, which is usually accompanied by increased cramping and bleeding. If the IUD strings are not visible, a pelvic ultrasound will confirm the intrauterine location. The patient must refrain from sex or use another effective method until the IUD location has been confirmed.

Users of the levonorgestrel IUD should expect unscheduled bleeding or spotting in the first 3 to 6 months of use; this bleeding is not harmful and decreases with continued use. Over time, many women experience only light menstrual bleeding or amenorrhea. Patients may need reassurance that amenorrhea is a safe, expected benefit of this IUD and that no treatment is needed. A pregnancy test can be done at any time if reassurance is needed, and some patients may request a pelvic exam to confirm that the IUD strings are present if they are unable to feel them on their own.

Missing Strings. There is no evidence-based recommendation to have patients "check their strings" during IUD use. However, PCPs should be able to palpate and visualize IUD strings on pelvic exam. If strings are not visible, a pregnancy test should be done, followed by a pelvic ultrasound to confirm the intrauterine location of the IUD. Encourage patients to use another contraceptive method until the IUD location is confirmed. If the IUD is confirmed to be inside the uterus, no other treatment is needed.

Depot Medroxyprogesterone Acetate

DMPA (or *Depo-Provera*) is a progestin-only contraceptive. The most commonly used form is a 150-mg dose injected intramuscularly (deltoid or gluteus maximus) every 3 months. Another formulation of DMPA allows for a self-administered subcutaneous dose of 104 mg every 3 months. DMPA increases the circulating levels of progestin, which acts on the HPA axis to suppress ovulation. Progestin thins the lining of the endometrium and, over time, induces significant endometrial atrophy.

DMPA can be initiated in quick-start fashion. Patients who are at risk for an interval pregnancy due to recent unprotected intercourse

TABLE 42.16   Key Differences in Oral Contraceptive Pills

Variation	Detail	COMMENT
Amount of estrogen (EE = ethinyl estradiol)	Most OCPs contain 35 µg or less, (low dose). "Very" low-dose pills contain 20 µg or less.	No difference in safety or efficacy among OCPs with <35 µg EE. Reasonable to try lower EE dose to manage side effects such as nausea or breast tenderness.
Type of progestin	Several generations of progestins: First: norethindrone Second: levonorgestrel Third: desogestrel, norgestimate Fourth: drosperinone	Third- and fourth-generation progestin considered less androgenic. Certain progestins may confer an increased risk of venous thromboembolism (VTE)/stroke than others; counsel users about the increased risk of VTE/stroke with CHC use. Medical contraindications to CHC use apply to all types in this method category.
Formulation	Monophasic: all active pills contain the same dose of estrogen and progestin. Triphasic: dose of estrogen and progestin changes each week.	Data do not support any advantage to triphasic formulations.
Regimen	Traditional 21/7 (most common): 21 days of active pills + 7 days of placebo. Extended 84/7 or other: With traditionally packaged pills write SIG: Take 1 active pill for 84 (4 packs) in a row then 7 days off. Continuous: all pills active (no placebo breaks) With traditionally packaged pills write SIG: Take 1 active pill every day.	Bleeding occurs monthly due to hormonal withdrawal while placebo pills are being taken. Bleeding occurs during placebo break every few months with extended use. No scheduled bleeding with continuous use. More likely to have unscheduled or "breakthrough bleeding," which will decrease with consistent use. Breakthrough bleeding can be managed with a 5-day break from OCPs. Any OCP can be used in extended or continuous fashion.

CHC, Combined hormonal contraception; *OCP*, oral contraceptive pill.

should return in 2 to 4 weeks for a repeat pregnancy test. Repeat injections should be given at 11- to 13-week intervals. An injection can be given early when necessary (e.g., a patient is in clinic and this timing is more convenient than a return visit). The repeat injection can be given up to 2 weeks late (15 weeks from the last injection) without additional contraceptive protection or pregnancy testing (Curtis et al., 2016). If a woman is more than 2 weeks late (that is, more than 15 weeks from her last injection) and she wishes to continue the method, the PCP should follow the quick-start protocol.

DMPA is safe in women with medical contraindications to estrogen. Noncontraceptive benefits include improvements in dysmenorrhea and pain related to endometriosis, reduction of bleeding, and high rates of menstrual suppression with continued use. DMPA levels are not decreased by antiepileptics and there may be reduced seizure activity in certain women with epilepsy as well as reduced pain crises in women with sickle cell disease.

Side Effects. The main side effect of DMPA is irregular menstrual bleeding, which most women experience. Irregular bleeding is common in the first 6 months of use and likely improves with method continuation. Amenorrhea occurs in most women after 1 to 2 years of use and sooner for some. If bleeding becomes bothersome, a 5- to 7-day short-term treatment with NSAIDs or hormonal treatment with a combined hormonal contraceptive can be offered. Weight gain on DMPA is unpredictable and varies widely among users. Women should be counseled about the possibility of increased appetite, which is thought to be the mechanism of weight gain. The package insert reports an average weight gain of 5 lb in the first year, although some women may gain more and may do so quickly. Nutrition and counseling about lifestyle changes can be offered, but obesity and weight gain should never preclude use in an adolescent who feels that DMPA is her best contraceptive option. DMPA may have an effect on bone density that is reversible once the method is discontinued and may not be of clinical significance (ACOG Opinion 602, 2014a). Experts do not recommend limiting its use in women who choose DMPA as their contraceptive method due to this risk.

Combined Hormonal Contraception

Combined hormonal contraception (CHC) contains both estrogen and progestin. This includes OCPs, the contraceptive patch, and the contraceptive ring. OCPs have been available in the United States since the 1960s and have been extensively studied. The levels of hormones contained in OCPs have decreased dramatically over the past 50 years as lower doses have been found to be efficacious, safer, and better tolerated. Although there are approximately 70 different combined OCPs available in the United States, differences in side effects are minimal. Furthermore, medical eligibility and counseling regarding risk should remain constant among all combined hormonal methods, including those labeled as containing very low doses. Examples of how pills differ are listed in Table 42.16. The major differences are in estrogen dose, progestin type, and packaging regimen of active and placebo pills. Best practices in prescribing CHC are listed in Table 42.17.

The transdermal contraceptive patch (Xulane) is a thin, beige adhesive patch that contains progestin norelgestromin and ethyl estradiol.

TABLE 42.17	Best Practice for Prescribing Combined Hormonal Contraception
Dispense	Provider writes to dispense a 3-month supply. Most insurance companies will dispense a 3-month supply. Dispensing 13 months is ideal and the best option if insurance barriers can be overcome.
Refills	Provide enough refills for at least 1 year.
Quick Start	Teen should start combined hormonal contraception as soon as she obtains it. No requirement for pelvic exam or pregnancy test. Can return for a pregnancy test in 2 weeks if any possibility of interval pregnancy.

BOX 42.11 Approach to Counseling About Risk for Venous Thromboembolism/Stroke Before Initiating Combined Hormonal Contraception

1. Discuss that nonusers and users both risk VTE.
   - Healthy, non-OCP users: 1-4/10,000 women years
   - OCP users: 3-9/10,000 women years
   - Pregnancy: 5-20/10,000 women years
   - Postpartum: 40-65/10,000 women years
2. Do not use CHC if USMEC Category 3 and 4.
3. Overall risk very, low, especially in healthy teens.
4. As with any treatment, benefits need to outweigh risks.

CHC, Combined hormonal contraception; *OCP*, oral contraceptive pill; *USMEC*, US Medical Eligibility Criteria; *VTE*, venous thromboembolism.

Committee on Gynecologic Practice. ACOG Committee Opinion Number 540: Risk of venous thromboembolism among users of drospirenone-containing oral contraceptive pills. Obstet Gynecol. 2012;120:1239–42.

It can be applied to the torso, buttocks, or upper arms and must be changed each week. The vaginal contraceptive ring (NuvaRing) is a soft, clear, flexible 54-mm-diameter ring that releases the progestins etonogestrel and ethinyl estradiol (EE). The ring is inserted by the user into the vagina and must be replaced monthly.

Mechanism of Action. The progestin component of combined hormonal methods provides the majority of its contraceptive efficacy by preventing ovulation via negative feedback on the HPO axis. The estrogen component is added to stabilize the endometrium and allow for better cycle control.

Managing Common Expected Side Effects

Missed Pills. OCP users who forget to take their pill should be advised to take it as soon as they remember. If a single pill is missed in a pill pack but taken within 24 hours of its usually scheduled time, contraceptive efficacy should not be affected. For the sake of simplicity and to avoid contraceptive failure, women who miss more than 1 pill in any given cycle should be advised to use another form of contraception (such as condoms) or avoid sex until they have had at least 7 days of consistent pill use. Women who have missed pills may have unscheduled bleeding. Finally, OCP users who are missing pills should always be counseled about other options, specifically LARC, which has a level of efficacy 20 to 30 times higher than that of OCPs in the teen population.

Unexpected Bleeding. In the first 3 months of CHC use, unexpected bleeding is not uncommon and no treatment is needed. Providers should confirm that the user is taking the pill at the same time each day (or changing the patch or ring as directed) and reassure the user that bleeding resolves with continued and consistent use. Users with unexpected bleeding due to missed or late pills will benefit from a review of all contraceptive options, specifically LARC, which makes no demands on the user. Users of extended or continuous CHC should expect unscheduled bleeding especially in the first 4 months of use. Prolonged progestin exposure causes the endometrium lining to become thin and instability may result in bleeding. Users can either continue on the method, take a 5-day break to allow for a withdrawal bleed and enable the endometrium to stabilize, or try a 5-day course of NSAIDs.

Pill-Induced Amenorrhea. Some users of CHC experience amenorrhea during the hormone-free interval (that is, the placebo pills of OCPs or the hormone-free week of patch or ring use). It is reasonable to obtain a urine pregnancy test to make sure that

pregnancy has not occurred. Otherwise no treatment is needed and the patient can be reassured that this is due to the progestin causing the endometrium to become atrophic. OCP users who prefer to have a monthly period can try switching to a different brand of pill.

Other Side Effects. CHC is well tolerated and causes minimal side effects. Breast pain and nausea may occur initially but usually resolve within the first few weeks of use. Switching to a different brand of OCP is always an option; trying a lower dose of estrogen (e.g., a pill that contains 20 µg of EE or less) or a different progestin is reasonable. Some women experience side effects that continue with use or are not attributable to the OCP. These include new-onset headaches, mood changes, and weight gain. Providers should evaluate patients for other causes of these symptoms as well as discuss different options for CHC or other methods.

Deep venous thrombosis (DVT) and stroke are rare with the use of CHC and can occur in healthy teens who are not on hormones. Patients who call with symptoms that are concerning for any serious medical condition should be evaluated immediately. Box 42.11 outlines the risk of venous thromboembolism (VTE) and/or stroke with use of CHC, which should be discussed with all users of these methods prior to initiation. Women with USMEC category 3 or 4 CHC contraindications should not use these methods.

Progestin-Only Pills

The progestin-only pill (POP), also referred to as the "minipill," contains 0.35 mg of norethindrone acetate. The primary contraceptive mechanism of POPs is progestin-induced thickening of cervical mucus, which blocks sperm from entering the uterus. POPs do not consistently suppress ovulation. Failure rates with POPs are found to be higher than those with combined OCPs. For effective use, POPs must be taken at the same time each day and must be taken continuously to be effective. Patient should be counseled that there should be no placebo breaks. Women who use POPs may have regular ovulatory cycles, irregular bleeding, or amenorrhea.

Emergency Contraception

Emergency contraception (EC) comprises methods of birth control used after unprotected intercourse or if there are concerns about method failure, such as missed pills or a broken condom. The use of EC is highly time-sensitive, with better efficacy the sooner it is used after intercourse. For this reason clinicians are strongly encouraged to discuss EC with their patients as part of

TABLE 42.18	Types of Emergency Contraceptive Pills Available in the United States

Progestin-only emergency contraceptive (EC): levonorgestrel 1.5 mg in one dose

- Brand names: *Plan B One-Step, Take Action, Next Choice One Dose, My Way*
- Over-the-counter with unrestricted sale to any gender, any age

Ulipristal acetate 30-mg tablet

- Brand name: *Ella*
- Sold by prescription only regardless of age
- More effective than levonorgestrel ECPs; preferred option when possible

Yuzpe regimen (combined OCPs)

- For options: http://ec.princeton.edu/questions/dose.html#dose
- Unlike other ECPs, may cause nausea

ECPs, Emergency contraceptive pills.

• BOX 42.12 Male Condom Information

- There are no age or other restrictions on who can buy condoms.
- Carry a condom with you if sex is a possibility.
- Check the expiration date and make sure that the package is not damaged.
- Use a water-based lubricant (like KY jelly) and not petroleum jelly or oils.
- Unroll the condom on an erect penis.
- Withdraw when the penis is still erect, holding onto the base.

---

routine sexual health counseling. Some adolescents choose to obtain EC pills in advance to have them available for immediate use. When adolescents are being counseled on the use of EC, PCPs should explain that it works best when taken right away and there is no reason to wait until "the morning after."

Three types of EC pills are available in the Unites States (Table 42.18). Their mechanism of action is to delay or inhibit ovulation. Ulipristal acetate is a progesterone-receptor modulator that can be taken up to 5 days after the unprotected encounter with an effectiveness that ranges from 62% to 85%. Levonorgestrel is available over the counter, providing 74% effectiveness, and can be taken up to 72 hours (3 days) after unprotected intercourse.

The copper IUD when used for EC prevents sperm from fertilizing an egg and may prevent implantation. It is 99% effective if inserted within 5 days of the unprotected encounter. Continued use of the copper IUD provides ongoing contraception by creating a hostile environment for sperm so that they do not travel into the tubes, where fertilization occurs.

There are no medical contraindications to oral EC and few contraindications to the copper IUD. Women who use oral EC may experience irregular bleeding and should be counseled to do a pregnancy test if she does not have a period in the following weeks after use. Visits for EC are optimal times to counsel patients and initiate more effective methods of contraception. If ulipristal acetate is used for EC, hormonal methods should not be initiated for 2 weeks to ensure the highest efficacy possible.

Condoms

Male and female condoms are the only methods of contraception that also provide protection against STIs. Male condoms are the most common form of contraception used. Condoms must be used consistently and correctly to be effective; most failures are due to incorrect and inconsistent use, resulting in a 15% or higher failure rate per year in most users. Adolescents benefit from learning how to obtain condoms and how to negotiate for their use as well as from a demonstration of correct condom use (Box 42.12). Condom use should be strongly encouraged and continued for STI prevention even if a more effective contraceptive method is started. Female condoms have not been studied as extensively but do offer protection from pregnancy and STIs and should be offered as an alternative if male condoms are not an option.

Coitus Interruptus and Other Less Effective Methods

Withdrawal (coitus interruptus) is not an effective method of contraception, with a failure rate of 27% each year with typical use. This method often fails because precum can contain active sperm and the male partner may not be able to withdrawal prior to ejaculation. Other less effective methods include spermicides or a sponge, diaphragm, cervical cap; these have fertility failure rates of 25% or higher per year. Patients who use any of these methods as their primary contraception should be counseled on their efficacy compared to other methods and supported to make changes if requested.

Teen pregnancy

Understanding Teen Pregnancy

The American Academy of Pediatrics Policy Statement on Adolescent Pregnancy (2014) provides some perspective on this subject. Unintended pregnancy results from not using contraception or using a method incorrectly or inconsistently; a small percentage of unintended pregnancies are due to contraceptive failure. Teen pregnancy and unintended pregnancy in women of all ages is more likely to occur among those who are less educated and have a lower income. This disparity is primarily due to lack of access and less use of contraception. *Healthy People 2020* aims at improving pregnancy planning, spacing, and the prevention of unintended pregnancy.

Over the last several decades there has been a significant and continued decline in the US teen pregnancy rate, with data from 2015 at 22.3/1000 women aged 15 to 19—an 8% drop from 2014 (CDC, 2018). Data on age, race, ethnicity, and by state can be found at https://www.cdc.gov/teenpregnancy or https://data.guttmacher.org. The decreased in adolescent pregnancy is primarily attributable to the increased use of contraception (Lindberg, Santelli, and Desai, 2016). The United States maintains the highest teen birth rate of all developed countries, with a teen pregnancy rate of 57 pregnancies per every 1000 women age 15 to 19 in the United States compared with just 8/1000 in Switzerland (Sedgh et al., 2015). Much lower teen pregnancy rates in other developed nations reflect long-established and universal sex education programs, increased acceptance of adolescent sexuality, social expectations regarding the use of contraception, free family planning services, and low-cost EC. Adolescents in other developed nations do not have lower pregnancy rates because they are less sexually active than teens in the United States; they are, however, more likely to use an effective contraceptive method when they engage in sex.

The geographic teen pregnancy disparities in the Unites States are striking. The teen pregnancy rate low is 9.4/1000 in Massachusetts compared with 38/1000 in Arkansas (CDC, 2018). Birth rates are higher in rural counties and in lower socioeconomic groups. These differences reflect racial and ethnic disparities in income and education as well as access to sex education, contraceptive services, and health care in general. PCPs play a central role in implementing practices and policies that improve health outcomes for all teens.

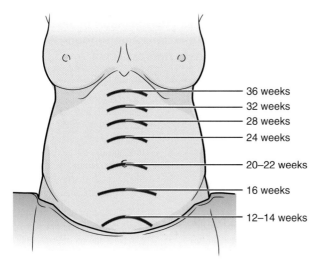

• **Fig 42.14** Assessment of Gestation in Pregnancy by Uterine Size. (From Niedzwwiecki B, Pepper J, Weaver PA. *Kinn's Medical Assisting Fundamentals*. 1st ed. St. Louis: Elsevier; 2019.)

Labels on figure:
- 36 weeks
- 32 weeks
- 28 weeks
- 24 weeks
- 20–22 weeks
- 16 weeks
- 12–14 weeks

Diagnosis of Teen Pregnancy

Pregnancy testing should be done in any adolescent who is menarchal and has missed one or more periods. Though rare, pregnancies have been reported in pubertal girls who have not yet had their first period. Concerns about breast pain, nausea, vaginal bleeding, and pelvic pain all warrant pregnancy testing. Pregnancy can also present with fatigue, weight gain, and urinary frequency.

Urine hCG tests are sensitive and specific; they will detect pregnancy 14 to 21 days from sexual intercourse or at the time of the missed period in women with regular ovulatory cycles. False negatives occur with dilute urine or if testing is done too soon and hCG levels have not reached 100 mIU/mL. Serum hCG testing is not usually necessary but detects very low levels of hCG. In general, serum hCG results below 5 mIU/mg are considered negative.

When an adolescent presents with reports of a positive urine pregnancy test done at home, it is best to perform a urine pregnancy test in the clinic. Urine pregnancy kits can be misread, often because the control indicator is interpreted as a positive result. Teens who express concerns that they may be pregnant should be seen quickly for pregnancy confirmation and counseling. If negative pregnancy results are obtained, the PCP should provide sexual health counseling, offer EC if it has been less than 5 days since the most recent unprotected intercourse, and initiate contraception with a quick-start protocol if the teen is motivated to avoid similar concerns in the future.

When pregnancy is diagnosed, an abdominal exam should be performed. The 12-week uterus is about the size of a grapefruit and can be palpated just above the pubic bone. The top of the uterus in a 20- to 22-week pregnancy is palpable at the umbilicus (Fig 42.14). A pelvic exam is needed to assess uterine size before 12 weeks.

After Diagnosing Pregnancy

The overwhelming majority of teen pregnancies are unintended; therefore the diagnosis of pregnancy may be unexpected and can be devastating for the teen, her partner, and her family. Disclosure of the result should occur with the adolescent alone. Sometimes the teen may insist that her partner or family member remain in the room. The provider then must balance respect for the teen's autonomy with concerns for her privacy, safety, and any other factors known about the clinical situation. It is not necessary for the adolescent to make any decision about her intentions regarding the pregnancy at the time of diagnosis. The PCP and staff must remain supportive and unbiased. The teen should be allowed as much time as she needs to understand the results. Most teens want to inform their parents or guardians; clinicians can play an instrumental role in facilitating this communication. *Options counseling* refers to the choices that women make regarding pregnancy: continue the pregnancy and raise the child, continue the pregnancy and make an adoption or kinship care plan, or end the pregnancy. Clinicians who do this work must be well versed in nonjudgmental, nondirective options counseling and respect the teen's personal, family, and spiritual beliefs as well as her and cultural practices.

If the adolescent is certain that she wants to continue the pregnancy, she should be seen by a prenatal provider within 1 to 2 weeks from diagnosis. Adolescent pregnancies are at higher risk for preterm delivery, a low-birth-weight infant, and social and emotional concerns such as depression and partner violence. The teen should be strongly advised to avoid all alcohol, tobacco, marijuana, and other recreational drugs. Prescription medication should be reviewed and any category X medications (for example, isotretinoin and warfarin) should be stopped immediately. If the patient was using hormonal contraception, she should stop this medication and be reassured that it has not caused any harm. Additional referral to social services can provide help with food stamps, living arrangements, and adoption possibilities.

If the adolescent is certain that she wants to end the pregnancy, referral to a provider who performs abortions is made. Relevant information on consent, cost, timing, and rules regarding parental notification, when applicable, as well as additional counseling, education, and resources for assistance should be provided. When an adolescent expresses the desire to have an abortion, it is not appropriate for her to be referred to a crisis pregnancy center or pregnancy resource center that will not provide balanced counseling regarding options.

Preconceptual Counseling

Some adolescents seek to become pregnant, and some may be ambivalent about pregnancy and therefore do not use contraception. Ninety percent of adolescent become pregnant during a single year of sexual activity when no birth control method is used. Preconceptual counseling is recommended for reproductive-age women and focuses on factors that result in better outcomes (Box 42.13). Once rapport is well established, the PCP should inquire about goals for education and career as well as the social, emotional, and financial supports available.

Ectopic Pregnancy

An ectopic pregnancy is one that occurs when the fertilized egg implants outside of the uterine cavity, most commonly in the fallopian tube. Symptoms usually occur during the first few weeks of pregnancy when a teen may not even know she is pregnant; they can include vaginal bleeding, pelvic and abdominal pain, nausea and vomiting. If the ectopic pregnancy starts to rupture, there may be dizziness, fatigue, bloating, and referred pain in the shoulder, neck, or back. Adolescents who present with vaginal bleeding and abdominal pain should be assessed for pregnancy. If they are pregnant and having worrisome symptoms, a transvaginal ultrasound should be performed to determine the location of the pregnancy; referral to the ED may be appropriate. Serial hCG levels that do not rise appropriately can be helpful in confirming the diagnosis. Women who use an IUD for contraception have a lower risk for ectopic pregnancy than women not using effective contraception because the risk of pregnancy overall is much decreased. However, when a pregnancy does occur with an IUD in place, close to half of them are ectopic. Tubal pregnancy in an unstable patient is a medical emergency. ● Ruptured ectopic pregnancy is a significant cause of pregnancy-related mortality (ACOG, 2018).

Sexually Transmitted Infections

STIs pass from one person to another during intimate physical contact and sexual behaviors such as vaginal, oral, and anal sex. The most common and reportable STIs include chlamydia and gonorrhea. *STI* is a broader term that includes conditions that can cause infection but do not necessarily result in a disease process.

STI: Adolescent Health Disparity

Compared with other age groups, adolescents and young adults have disproportionately high rates of STIs. The CDC (2018) estimates that adolescents ages 15 to 24 account for over half of the 20 million new STIs in the United States each year. One in every four sexually active adolescent females has an STI such as chlamydia or human papillomavirus (HPV). Table 42.19 lists many of the factors that contribute to the high prevalence of STIs among young people and corresponding strategies that providers can adopt to address this health disparity. Discussing common myths about STIs (Table 42.20) with adolescent patients is an effective way for clinicians to establish rapport on the topic. This also provides accurate information, which may guide the teen to healthier decisions.

STI: Prevention and Screening

The CDC's STI Treatment Guidelines are continually updated based on disease surveillance and should be consulted for up-to-date recommendations for prevention, screening, and treatment. The CDC website (www.cdc.gov) and the CDC's free smartphone app (CDC STD TX Guide) are convenient ways for providers to access this information when needed. Avoid referring to outdated textbooks or handbooks that may contain older information.

PCPs are central to the prevention of STIs in the adolescent population (Box 42.14). STI prevention starts with appropriate vaccination, which is greatly influenced by the strength of the health provider's recommendation (Ventola, 2016). Appropriate STI screening founded on evidence-based recommendations is a key strategy for prevention, as early treatment and risk reduction counseling results in improved outcomes. Table 42.21 outlines the screening recommendations for sexually active adolescents.

TABLE 42.19	Factors That Lead to High Rates of Sexually Transmitted Infections Among Young People and Strategies to Address Them	
Factors	**Provider Strategy**
Young women have increased biologic susceptibility to infection	• Follow age-based screening recommendations for annual GC/Chlamydia testing: test all sexually active females annually until age 25. • Teach how to use and to negotiate for condom use with every partner for oral, anal and vaginal sex.
Adolescent concerns about confidentiality and privacy	• Make it your regular practice to have a one-on-one interview with teens at each visit. • Know the laws in your state. All states allow minors to consent to sexually transmitted infection (STI) services. Go to www.guttmacher.org and learn about your state's laws and then share with your clinic team. • Work with clinic schedulers, business managers to develop policies that follow state laws and allow for teen confidentiality. • Understand how tests will be billed in your clinic and develop options to manage situations when confidentiality must be assured. • Know and/or develop local resources for free and confidential testing when needed.
Embarrassment about STIs	• Get comfortable talking about STIs and STI testing in a way that allows for questions and discussion. For example, talk about age-based screening in general, and common myths about STIs. • During your confidential interview, establish rapport before taking a sexual history on all patients, not just those who ask for STI testing.
Fear of testing method	• Urine testing for STIs is not painful or invasive. • Pelvic exam (females) or urethral swab (males) is not needed for testing.
Insurance coverage	• Help families and adolescents obtain coverage. • Know local resources and/or offer free screening.
Myths about STIs	• Address common myths and misperceptions when discussing STI testing and prevention (see Table 42.20).

TABLE 42.20 Common Sexually Transmitted Infections: Myths and Facts

Myth	Fact
"I can't have an STI if I've only had 1 partner," or "Only people that sleep around get STIs."	All sexually active adolescents should have testing for STIs based on screening recommendations and/or symptoms. It only take one partner to get an STI.
"You can tell if someone has a STI."	Over 70% of chlamydial and gonorrheal infections have no symptoms.
"You can get a STI from a toilet seat."	No you can't. Intimate skin-to-skin contact is necessary for infection to occur.
"You can't get a STI from oral sex."	Yes you can. Chlamydia, gonorrhea, HPV, and herpes are transmitted by oral sex.
"Using 2 condoms at once will prevent STIs better than using just 1."	One condom, used correctly, is best to prevent STIs. Two condoms may increase friction and cause them to break or tear.
"If the guy pulls out, this will prevent the spread of STIs."	Precum contains fluids that can spread infection. Some STIs can be spread via skin-to-skin contact alone.
"HIV is a death sentence, so why bother getting tested?"	With regular treatment, HIV-infected people can live normal, healthy lives and have children that are HIV-negative. Knowing your HIV status is the only way to prevent spread of disease to people you care about.
"I'm not gay so I don't need an HIV test."	HIV infection is also spread through heterosexual sex.
"I've already had PID and STIs. I can't get them again, and it doesn't matter anyway."	Repeat gonorrhea and chlamydia infections are common. You are not immune after having an infection. With each infection, there is a risk of serious complications.
"My birth control will also protect me from STIs."	Except for condoms, birth control methods do not protect from STIs.
"I hate condoms and never have one to use. There is nothing that works for me to prevent STIs."	Risk reduction makes a difference. Start using condoms some of the time. Bring condoms with you when going out. Get frequent STI testing so any infection is treated quickly. If at significant risk for HIV, start taking PrEP.

HPV, Human papillomavirus; *PID,* pelvic inflammatory disease; *PrEP,* preexposure prevention; *STI,* sexually transmitted infection.

BOX 42.14 The Five Major Strategies to Prevent and Control Sexually Transmitted Infections

1. Preexposure vaccination for HPV, hepatitis B, hepatitis A
2. Identification of asymptomatic infected persons by following screening guidelines and testing of persons with STI symptoms
3. Education and counseling on ways to avoid STIs through reducing number or sexual partners, sexual abstinence, and consistent use of condoms
4. Effective diagnosis, treatment, counseling, and follow-up of infected persons
5. Evaluation, treatment, and counseling of sex partners, including expedited partner therapy

HPV, Human papilloma virus.

From Center for Disease Control and Prevention. Sexually Transmitted Disease Treatment Guidelines, 2015. MMWR Recomm Rep.2015;64(3):1–137.

TABLE 42.21 Routine Sexually Transmitted Infection Screening Recommendations for Sexually Active Populations

Adolescent females	• Annual testing for chlamydia and gonorrhea until age 25 and/or when presenting for STI evaluation and/or GU/GYN symptoms • HIV test at least once; *Tests that are not routinely indicated unless there are symptoms or other risk factors: bacterial vaginosis, trichomoniasis, herpes, syphilis, hepatitis A/B/C*
Adolescent males	• Test for chlamydia and gonorrhea if: high prevalence community, seen at teen clinic, STI clinic, or correctional facility; and/or presenting for STI evaluation and/or GU symptoms • HIV test at least once
Pregnant women	• HIV, syphilis (RPR), Hepatitis B (HBsAg); chlamydia and gonorrhea if less than age 25, hepatitis C if high risk for infection
MSM (men who have sex with men)	• Annual testing for HIV, syphilis (RPR), chlamydia, and gonorrhea (pharyngeal, rectal, and/or urethral, depending on site of sexual contact)
WSW (women who have sex with women)	*Same as adolescent female*
Transgender men and women	*Follow screening guidelines based on current anatomy and sexual behaviors*

GU/GYN, Genitourinary/gynecologic.

From Center for Disease Control and Prevention. Sexually Transmitted Disease Treatment Guidelines, 2015. *MMWR Recomm Rep.* 2015:64(3);1–137.

Everyone should be tested for HIV at least once between ages 13 and 64. Females should be screened at least annually for gonorrhea and chlamydia. Additional STI testing is recommended if a teen is pregnant, symptoms are present, or if the PCP is dealing with a high-risk group like men having sex with men (MSM).

Common Sexually Transmitted Infections

Although many people with STIs are asymptomatic, it is important for providers to recognize the symptoms of common STIs and test when indicated. Chlamydia and gonorrhea are the most common reportable STIs, and annual screening for them is indicated. Testing is also recommended in patients who present with genitourinary or gynecologic symptoms and report sexual activity, or when sexual abuse or sexual activity is suspected. Concerns about vaginal discharge and appropriate testing are discussed earlier in the chapter (refer to Table 42.6).

Genital herpes causes a small, painful herpetic ulcer (Fig 42.15). Primary HSV infection, when recognized, is often preceded by flu-like symptoms as well as multiple painful lesions that cause intense external dysuria and swelling. A single small painful lesion may be due to a recurrent HSV outbreak. Test lesions for HSV with a type-specific PCR test; serology can be done later if helpful but may not reveal antibodies to HSV until several weeks following infection. NSGUs, discussed earlier, also cause exquisitely painful vulvar ulcers, but the lesions are often larger than those due to herpes and PCR testing of the NSGU lesion will be negative for HSV.

Treatment and Counseling

Treatment for common STIs is generally straightforward and effective (Table 42.22). When possible, onsite and directly observed single-dose therapy allows for maximum adherence and increases the opportunity for counseling. Ongoing care must be supportive of the teen with regard to their medical, emotional, and social situation. Once trust is established, adolescents may ask the PCP or clinic staff to help them discuss related issues with their partners and their families. General counseling topics that should be reviewed with adolescents who are receiving treatment for an STI are listed in Box 42.15.

Partner notification and treatment is a necessary step when a reportable infection is diagnosed. Time spent counseling on the importance of notification and providing patients with written information about the infection increases the rate of partner notification and treatment. Ideally, sexual partners will see their own PCP for counseling and treatment. In the case of chlamydia and gonorrhea infection, the partner of the infected individual should be presumptively treated without retesting given the high rates of coinfection among partners.

Expedited partner therapy is an effective strategy to prevent reinfection, transmission of new infections, and prevention of PID and other complications. It should be routinely offered to heterosexual patients with chlamydia or gonorrhea infection when the provider cannot confidently ensure that the patient's sex partners will be treated (Box 42.16).

Pelvic Inflammatory Disease

PID is an infection of a woman's reproductive organs. It is most commonly caused by chlamydia and gonorrhea but can be caused by other infections. There is no simple test for PID and many episodes are subclinical and go unrecognized. The CDC recommends presumptive treatment for sexually active young women if they experience pelvic or lower abdominal pain when no other cause of pain can be identified (CDC, 2015). Table 42.23 outlines clinical criteria for the diagnosis of PID and treatment guidelines. Women with PID should also be tested for HIV. A young woman with an IUD and diagnosis of PID should be reassured that the IUD does not have to be removed. There may be an increased risk of PID in the first weeks after IUD placement because bacteria from the cervix are introduced into the uterus with the insertion procedure (Hubacher, 2014); however, following this initial time period, IUD users are no more likely to contract STIs than nonusers.

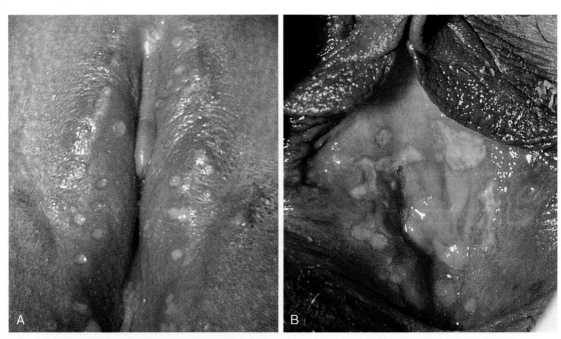

• **Fig 42.15** Primary Herpes Simplex Virus With Vulvar Lesions. A. Prepubertal child with numerous vesicular lesions, a few of which have ulcerated over perineum. B, Full-blown ulcerative phase of herpetic Vulvovaginitis in an adolescent. (From Zitelli BJ, McIntire SC, Nowalk AJ. *Zitelli & Davis' Atlas of Pediatric Physical Diagnosis.* 7th ed. Philadelphia: Elsevier; 2018.)

TABLE 42.22   Overview of Common Sexually Transmitted Infections

Infection	Test	Symptoms/Sequelae	Treatment and Specific Follow-up
Chlamydia Most common reportable infection in the United States. Largest burden of infection is in women below age 25.	Nucleic acid amplification test (NAAT) via urine sample, vaginal, endocervical, rectal, or oropharyngeal swab. Vaginal and rectal swabs can be self-collected. High specificity and high sensitivity.	The majority of infections (75%) cause no symptoms. In males, may cause dysuria, urethritis, proctitis, pharyngitis. In women, may cause dysuria, vaginal discharge, vaginitis, cervicitis, post-coital bleeding, breakthrough bleeding, painful intercourse, and pelvic pain. Sequelae of infection in women include PID, ectopic pregnancy, and infertility due to tubal disease.	Azithromycin 1 g orally single dose or Doxycycline 100 mg orally bid for 7 days Treat all sex partners in previous 60 days. If no sexual contact in >60 days, treat the most recent partner. Retesting at <3 weeks can lead to false positive result; re-treat if concerns about med compliance or reinfection. Men and women treated for chlamydia should be retested at 3 months (due to risk of reinfection).
Gonorrhea Second most common reported infection in the United States. Infections often concentrate in specific geographic locations and communities.			Use dual therapy due to concerns about antibiotic resistance: Ceftriaxone 250 mg IM in single dose *plus* 1 g azithromycin in a single dose. Administer both meds on same day, same time if possible. Treat all sex partners in previous 60 days. If no sexual contact in >60 days, treat the most recent partner. Symptoms that persist after treatment should be evaluated by NAAT and culture with antimicrobial susceptibility due to concerns about resistant organisms. Contact local public health department for guidance when needed. Men and women who have been treated for gonorrhea should be retested at 3 months (due to risk of reinfection).
Trichomoniasis Most common nonviral STI, but infection not reportable in the United States. Untreated infections may last months to years.	Testing should be done when sexually active women seek care for vaginal discharge. Screening in asymptomatic patients may be considered in high-prevalence settings and is recommended in women with HIV. NAAT testing (or microscopy when not available) of vaginal/urethral secretions. NAAT tests are 3-5 times more sensitive than microscopy. Testing of rectal and oral sites not recommended.	The majority of infections (70%-85%) cause no or minimal symptoms. In women, may cause diffuse, malodorous, or yellow-green discharge with or without vulvar irritation. In men, may cause urethritis, epididymitis, or prostatitis. Infection with trich is associated with an increased risk for PID and HIV acquisition.	Metronidazole 2 g in one dose. Current partners should be referred for treatment. Testing for chlamydia, gonorrhea and HIV should be performed when trich is detected. Women who have been treated for trich should be retested at 3 months (due to risk of reinfection).
Syphilis Systemic disease caused by *Treponema pallidum*.	Screening recommended in pregnant women, MSM, and HIV-infected individuals. Diagnostic testing when patients have signs and symptoms of infection. Serologic nontreponemal (RPR) and treponemal tests (FTA-ABS) can be used for initial screening.	Primary infection: painless ulcer or chancre Secondary: skin rash, lymphadenopathy Latent infection are those lacking clinical manifestations.	Penicillin G, administered parentally, is the preferred drug for treatment in all stages of disease. See CDC STI treatment guidelines[a] and consult infection disease experts as needed. All persons with infection should be screened for HIV. Partners in previous 90 days preceding diagnosis should be treated presumptively. Partners previous to last 90 days should be screened for infection.

Continued

TABLE 42.22 Overview of Common Sexually Transmitted Infections—cont'd

Infection	Test	Symptoms/Sequelae	Treatment and Specific Follow-up
Genital herpes Lifelong viral infection. Most people with infection are unaware of it. Most cases of recurrent genital herpes are due to HSV-2, but HSV-1 can cause genital lesions.	Testing should be type-specific to differentiate between HSV-1 and HSV-2 infection given different prognoses for recurrent disease and viral shedding. Polymerase chain reaction (PCR) test of the herpetic lesion is the test of choice in the acute setting. Serologic testing weeks after infection can be helpful to guide counseling. Presence of HSV-2 antibodies strongly suggests anogenital infection. Presence of HSV-1 antibodies alone may reflect oral HSV infection acquired in childhood, or genital HSV-1. General screening not recommended.	Primary infection can present as flu-like illness in addition to multiple, extremely painful vesicles on the genital area. Presenting complaint may be dysuria, tingling, burning, or itching: physical exam crucial for diagnosis. Recurrent infections produce a single lesion and may have a prodrome.	Many options: First clinical episode: Acyclovir 400 mg PO tid for 7-10 days or Valacyclovir 1 g PO bid for 7-10 days Recurrent episode: Acyclovir 800 mg bid for 5 days or Valacyclovir 1 g PO qd for 5 days Suppressive therapy: Acyclovir 400 mg bid daily or Valacyclovir 1 g PO daily Many patients with HSV-2 opt for suppressive therapy to reduce shedding and transmission of infection as well as to reduce recurrences by 70%-80%. Safety and efficacy of therapy are well established. Asymptomatic sex partners should be offered serologic testing.
HIV 1.2 million people in the United States have HIV; 16% are unaware of the infection.	All persons who seek evaluation and treatment for STIs should be screened for HIV. All persons aged 13-64 should be screened for HIV at least once. Additional consent forms for testing is not recommended. Serologic testing for HIV-1 and HIV-2. Rapid tests are also available.	Begins as brief, acute viral syndrome and transitions into chronic illnesses and immunodeficiency (AIDS).	Treatment is lifesaving and prevents spread of infection. Partners need counseling and should be offered preexposure prevention (PrEP) to prevent infection. Refer to Chapter 31 for a complete discussion of HIV infection.

aCheck www.CDC.gov for updates.

CDC, Centers for Disease Control; *HSV,* herpes simplex virus; *PID,* pelvic inflammatory disease; *STI,* sexually transmitted infection.

• BOX 42.15 Things to Consider When an Adolescent Is Being Treated for a Sexually Transmitted Infection

- Check www.cdc.gov when needed to confirm current treatment guidelines.
- Discuss how medications will be obtained as well as detailed instructions for use.
- Discuss the need for partner treatment and notification when appropriate. Offer expedited partner therapy (EPT) if there is infection with gonorrhea/chlamydia.
- No sexual contact until 7 days after patient *and* partner have been treated.
- Review consistent and correct condom use to prevent future infections.
- Review current contraceptive method when appropriate.
- Screen for other HIV and other STIs when indicated.
- Schedule a follow-up visit in 3 months to test for reinfection.

STIs, Sexually transmitted infections.

• BOX 42.16 Expedited Partner Therapy and the Reduction of Sexually Transmitted Infections in Adolescents

- Effective treatment of chlamydia and gonorrhea includes treatment of sex partners to prevent reinfection, transmission of new infections, and prevention of PID and other complications.
- EPT allows the clinician to provide a prescription for the sex partner or partners of the infected patients without an exam or visit.
- Encouraged by most state public health departments, visit www.cdc.gov/STI/ept to check for updated information on your state.

EPT, Expedited partner therapy; PID, pelvic inflammatory disease.

TABLE 42.23 Pelvic Inflammatory Disease Overview

Diagnosis

- Presumptive PID if one or more present on pelvic exam in sexually active adolescent without other explanation for pain:
  - Cervical motion tenderness
  - Uterine tenderness
  - Adnexal tenderness
- Increased specificity of PID diagnosis if one or more present:
  - Oral temperature >101°F (38.3°C)
  - Mucopurulent cervical discharge or cervical friability
  - Abundant white blood cells in vaginal discharge microscopy
  - Elevated erythrocyte sedimentation rate, elevated C-reactive protein
  - Positive gonorrhea and/or chlamydia

Management

- Test for pregnancy, gonorrhea and chlamydia, HIV; other STIs if additional symptoms
- Treat partner(s) if gonorrhea/chlamydia detected
- Counsel to avoid sexual contact until patient and partner have completed treatment
- See patients within 72 h (3 days) to confirm response to treatment
- If gonorrhea/chlamydia detected, test for reinfection in 3 months
- Most patients can be treated on an outpatient basis. Decision to hospitalize for treatment is based on clinical judgment and often advised if any of the following:
  - Surgical emergency (i.e., appendicitis) cannot be reasonably excluded
  - Presence of tubo-ovarian abscess
  - Pregnancy
  - Severe illness, nausea, vomiting, high fever
  - Unable to tolerate or follow outpatient regimen
  - No response to oral therapy
- Antimicrobial treatment (always check for updates at www.cdc.gov)
  - Inpatient: Cefotetan 2 g IV q 12 h, PLUS doxycycline 100 mg PO or IV q 12 h. See www.cdc.gov for alternative parental options.
  - Outpatient: Ceftriaxone 250 mg IM in a single dose, PLUS doxycycline 100 mg PO bid for 14 days with or without metronidazole 500 mg PO bid for 14 days. See www.cdc.gov for alternative parenteral options.

PID, Pelvic inflammatory disease; *STI,* sexually transmitted infection.

References

ACOG. *Cervical Cancer Screening;* 2017. Available at: https://www.acog.org/-/media/For-Patients/faq085.pdf?dmc=1&ts=20180831T1947142721. Accessed August 31, 2018.

ACOG. *Committee Opinion on Adolescent Health Care 735: Adolescents and Long-Acting Reversible Contraception: Implants and Intrauterine Devices;* 2018. Available at: https://www.acog.org/Clinical-Guidance-and-Publications/Committee-Opinions/Committee-on-Adolescent-Health-Care/Adolescents-and-Long-Acting-Reversible-Contraception. Accessed September 1, 2018.

ACOG. *Committee Opinion on Adolescent Health Care 602: Depot medroxyprogesterone acetate and bone effects;* 2014a. Available at: https://www.acog.org/Clinical-Guidance-and-Publications/Committee-Opinions/Committee-on-Adolescent-Health-Care/Depot-Medroxyprogesterone-Acetate-and-Bone-Effects. Accessed March 13, 2018.

ACOG. *Committee Opinion on Adolescent Health Care: 605, Primary Ovarian Insufficiency in Adolescents and Young Women;* 2014. Available at: https://www.acog.org/Clinical–Guidance–and– Publications/Committee–Opinions/Committee–on–Adolescent–Health–Care/Primary–Ovarian–Insufficiencyin–Adolescents–and–Young–Women. Accessed March 13, 2018.

ACOG. *Committee Opinion on Adolescent Health Care 668: Menstrual Manipulation for Adolescents With Physical and Developmental Disabilities;* 2016. Available at: https://www.acog.org/-/media/Committee-Opinions/Committee-on-Adolescent-Health-Care/co668.pdf?dmc=1&ts=20170217T1426048189. Accessed March 13, 2018.

ACOG. *Committee Opinion on Adolescent Health Care 686: Breast and Labial Surgery in Adolescents;* 2017. Available at: https://www.acog.org/–/media/Committee–Opinions/Committee–on–Adolescent–Health–Care/co686.pdf?dmc=1&ts=20170217T0416002970. Accessed March 13, 2018.

ACOG. *Committee Opinion on Adolescent Health Care 728: Müllerian Agenesis: Diagnosis. Management, and Treatment;* 2018. Available at https://www.acog.org/Clinical–Guidance–and–Publications/Committee–Opinions/Committee–on–Adolescent–Health–Care/Mullerian–Agenesis–Diagnosis– Management–and–Treatment. Accessed March 13, 2018.

ACOG. *Practice Bulletin 108: Polycystic Ovarian Syndrome;* 2009. Available at https://www.ncbi.nlm.nih.gov/pubmed/19888063. Accessed March 13, 2018.

ACOG. *Practice Bulletin 136: Management of Abnormal Uterine Bleeding Associated With Ovulatory Dysfunction;* 2013. Available at: https://www.ncbi.nlm.nih.gov/pubmed/23787936. Accessed March 13, 2018.

ACOG. *Practice Bulletin 164: Diagnosis and Management of Benign Breast Disorders;* 2016. Available at: https://www.ncbi.nlm.nih.gov/pubmed/27214189. Accessed March 13, 2018.

ACOG. *Practice Bulletin 191: Tubal ectopic pregnancy;* 2018. Available at: https://www.ncbi.nlm.nih.gov/pubmed/29232273. Accessed March 13, 2018.

American Academy of Pediatrics Committee on Adolescence Policy Statement. Addendum—adolescent pregnancy: current trends and issues. *Pediatrics.* 2014;133(5):954–957.

Bacon JL, Romano ME, Quint EH. Clinical recommendation: labial adhesions. *J Ped Adol Gyn.* 2015;28(5):405–409.

Bercaw-Pratt JL, Boardamn LA, Simms-Cendan JS. *Clinical Recommendation: Pediatric Lichen Sclerosis;* 2014. Available at: https://pdfs.semanticscholar.org/b0b6/ae3dc6d3e0426d01e01fda7ff69178f9f57e.pdf. Accessed September 1, 2018.

Breuner C, Mattson G. Committee on Adolescence, Committee on psychosocial aspects of child and family health: sexuality education for children and adolescents. *Pediatrics.* 2016;138(2):e20161348.

Centers for Disease Control. Reproductive Health: *Teen Pregnancy.* Available at https://www.cdc.gov/teenpregnancy/about/social-determinants-disparities-teen-pregnancy.htm, Accessed September 1, 2018.

Centers for Disease Control. *STDs in adolescents and young adults: Public Health Impact.* Available at https://www.cdc.gov/std/stats16/adolescents.htm, Accessed September 1, 2018.

Centers for Disease Control. *STI Treatment Guidelines;* 2015. Available at: https://www.cdc.gov/STI/default.htm. Accessed March 14, 2018.

Curtis KM, Jatlaoui TC, Tepper NK, et al. U.S. Selected practice recommendations for contraceptive use. *MMWR Recomm Rep.* 2016;65(No. RR-4):1–66.

de la Rosa FG, Zakzuk J, Guzman NA, et al. Efficiency of the use of long-acting reversible contraception: a systematic review of the literature. *Value in Health.* 2018;21:S164.

de Sanctis V, Matallioticis M, Soliman AT, et al. A focus on the distinctions and current evidence of endometriosis in adolescents. *Best Pract Res Clin Obstetric Gynecol.* 2018. [in press].

Dehlendorf C, Krajewski C, Borrero S. Contraceptive counseling: best practices to ensure quality communication and enable effective contraceptive use. *Clin Obstetr Gynecol.* 2014;57(4):659–673.

Diedrich JT, Klein DA, Peipert JF. Long-acting reversible contraception in adolescents: a systematic review and meta-analysis. *Am J Obstet Gynecol.* 2017;216(4). 364.e1–e364.

Emans SJ, Laufer MR. *Pediatric and Adolescent gynecology.* Lippincott Williams & Williams; 2012.

Hillard PJ. Menstruation in Adolescents: what do we know? And what do we do with the information? *J Ped Adol Gyn*. 2014;27(6):309–319.

Hubabcher D. Intrauterine device & infection: review of the literature. *Indian J Med Res*. 2014;140:S53–S57.

Lindberg L, Santelli J, Desai S. Understanding the decline in adolescent fertility in the US, 2007–2012. *J Adolesc Health*. 2016;59(5):577–583.

Mitra M, Mouradian V, McKenna. Dating violence and associated health risks among high schools students with disabilities. *Matern Child Health J*. 2013;17(6):1088–1094.

Ott MA, Sucato GS. Contraception for Adolescents. *Pediatrics*. 2014;134(4):e1244–1256.

Reindollar RH, Byrd JR, McDonough PG. Delayed sexual development: a study of 252 patients. *Am J Obstet Gynecol*. 1981;140:371.

Rietmeijer CA. Risk reduction counseling for prevention of sexually transmitted infections: how it works and how to make it work. *Sexually Transmitted Infections*. 2007;83(1):2–9. https://doi.org/10.1136/sti.2006.017319.

Secura GM, Allsworth JE, Madden t, et al. The Contraceptive CHOICE Project: reducing barriers to long-acting reversible contraception. *Am J Obstetr Gynecol*. 2010;203(2):115.e1–115.e7.

Sedgh G, Finer LB, Bankole A, et al. Adolescent pregnancy, birth, and abortion rates across countries: levels and recent trends. *J Adolescent Health*. 2015;56(2):223T–230T. Available at: http://www.jahonline.org/article/S1054-139X(14)00387-5/abstract. Accessed March 14, 2018.

Sobsey D. *Violence and Disability*; 2014. Available at http://eugenic-sarchive.ca/discover/encyclopedia/535eee9d7095aa0000000262. Accessed August 31, 2018.

Ventola CL. Immunization in the US. Recommendations, barriers, and measures to improve compliance: part 1: childhood vaccinations. *Pharm Ther*. 2016;41(7):426–436.

Yonkers KA, Simoni MK. Evidenced-based treatments for premenstrual disorders. *Am J Obs Gyn*. 2017;218(1):68–74.

43

Musculoskeletal Disorders

CYNTHIA MARIE CLAYTOR

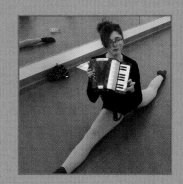

Primary care providers (PCPs) play a vital role in the early detection and appropriate management of musculoskeletal conditions in children and adolescents. Common musculoskeletal disorders include athletic injuries, back pain, foot injuries, knee disorders, shin splints, and stress fractures. Congenital problems include spinal deformities, hip and foot anomalies, growth disorders and developmental delay, metabolic disorders, and neuromuscular disorders ranging from cerebral palsy to muscular dystrophy. A variety of other conditions can cause musculoskeletal findings, including intentional and unintentional injury, cancer, and juvenile idiopathic arthritis. Iatrogenic deformities that result from cultural practices, such as using a cradleboard, or from fetal position and intrauterine compression can also cause deformities. Disorders of the musculoskeletal system present unique problems because growth and development of this system contribute to the evolution of pathologic conditions over time. Limited mobility, pain, and deformity can interfere with the child's lifestyle. Children with functional disabilities may not be able to fully participate in all activities with peers and family or meet the physical requirements of various occupations. They may also face challenges related to self-esteem. PCPs must be vigilant and seek to help children and their families prevent these problems.

PCPs assess development of the musculoskeletal system, identify problems requiring early intervention, focus on lifestyle assessment and injury prevention, and monitor the long-term outcomes of orthopedic care. They are often the first to refer to specialists as needed for early diagnosis and treatment. When necessary, they help families integrate orthopedic care within the daily living activities at home and school and help families to cope with the issues of disability, deformity, and long-term care.

Anatomy and Physiology

Limb formation occurs early in embryogenesis (4 to 8 weeks of gestation); primary ossification centers are present in all the long bones of the limbs by the 12th week of gestation. Development of the skeletal system begins around the 4th week of gestation, with ossification of the fetal skeleton beginning during the 5th month of gestation. The clavicles and skull bones are the first to ossify, followed by the long bones and spine. The epiphyses of the newborn's long bones are composed of hyaline cartilage. Soon after birth, the cartilage along the epiphyseal plate begins secondary ossification. The shape of the spine also changes from a C shape at birth to an S curve by late adolescence. As the child starts to walk, the lumbar curve develops. The sacrum starts out as five separate bones at birth, only to become fused as one large bone by 18 to 20 years of age (Duderstadt and Schapiro, 2019).

Bone age, measured by radiographs of the left hand and wrist, can be used to quantitatively determine somatic maturation and serves as a mirror that reflects the tempo of growth. In adolescents, the skeletal growth spurt begins at about Tanner stage 2 in girls and Tanner stage 3 in boys. Growth peaks around stage 4 and then ends with stage 5. The growth spurt lasts longer in boys than in girls. The pelvis widens early in pubescent girls. In both sexes, the legs usually lengthen before the thighs broaden. Next the shoulders widen and the trunk completes its linear growth. Bone growth ends when the epiphyses close.

Long bones have a growth plate, or physis, at each end that separates the epiphysis from the diaphysis or shaft. Openings through this plate allow blood vessels to penetrate from the epiphysis. In the growth plate, chondrocytes produce cartilage cells, dead cells are absorbed, and the calcified cartilage matrix is converted into bone. The entire growth plate area is weaker than the remaining bone because it is less calcified. Because blood supply to the growth plate comes primarily through the epiphysis, damage to epiphyseal circulation can jeopardize the survival of the chondrocytes. If chondrocytes stop producing, growth of the bone in that area stops (Fig 43.1).

There are two ways that children's bones grow. Longitudinal growth occurs in the ossification centers; changes in bone width and strength take place via intramembranous ossification. The length of long bones comes from growth at the epiphyseal plates, whereas their diameter increases as a result of deposition of new bone on the periosteal surface and resorption on the surface of the medullary cavity. Growth of the small bones, hip, and spine comes from one or more primary ossification centers in each bone. Apophyses are the sites for connection of tendons to bone. In children, these sites, which are similar to epiphyses, allow for growth and are weaker than bone. These sites can become inflamed with overuse, as occurs in Osgood-Schlatter disease.

The development of bones and muscles is influenced by use. In infants and toddlers, the legs straighten and lengthen with the stimulus of weight bearing and independent walking. The infant is born with the full complement of muscle fibers. Growth in muscle length results from lengthening of the fibers, and growth in bulk comes from hypertrophy. Length of muscles is related to growth in length of the underlying bone. If a limb is not used, it grows minimally. If muscles and bones are not used in their intended normal manner, as occurs with spastic diplegia, the forces for development tend to stimulate growth in abnormal patterns. Thus scoliosis can

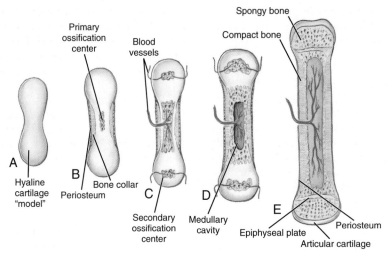

• **Fig 43.1** Growth Plates and the Transition From Cartilage to Bone at the Epiphyseal Plate. (A) Hyaline cartilage "model." (B) Periosteum and bone collar form. (C) Blood vessels and osteoblasts infiltrate primary ossification centers. (D) Osteoclasts form the medullary cavity. (E) Ossification is complete. Hyaline cartilage remains as articular cartilage and in the epiphyseal plate. (From Duderstadt KG, Schapiro NA. Musculoskeletal system. In: Duderstadt KG, ed. *Pediatric Physical Examination: An Illustrated Handbook.* Philadelphia: Elsevier; 2014:260, fig 18-1.)

develop or bowlegs may increase in severity. Muscle contractures occur if muscles are not used regularly and put through their full range of motion. The growth of fibrous tissue, tendons, and ligaments is also dependent on mechanical demands.

Nutritional, mechanical, and hormonal factors during the growth process influence the thickness of bones and the health of the marrow. Adequate protein, calcium, and vitamin D in the diet are key nutritional elements that affect the growth and development of a child's musculoskeletal system.

The muscle structures originate from the embryonic mesoderm. Muscle fibers are developed by the fourth or fifth month of gestation and grow in tangent with their respective bones. The rate of muscle growth (muscle mass and cell sizes) speeds up dramatically around 2 years of age, with girls exhibiting a greater rate of growth than boys until this gender trend is reversed at puberty (Duderstadt and Schapiro, 2019). Tendons are associated connective tissues; they are tough, flexible fibrous bands connecting muscles to bones. Ligaments are composed of fibrous connective tissue that joins bones to each other.

Pathophysiology and Defense Mechanisms

Pathophysiology

Muscles and bones can be affected by localized or systemic problems. An initial orthopedic problem can be symptomatic of a larger problem (e.g., juvenile arthritis). Tendon and ligament injuries that result in sprains and strains or apophysitis are the result of traumatic injury or overuse.

Systemic Problems

Musculoskeletal presentation in children and adolescents can be a feature of potentially life-threatening conditions (such as sepsis, malignancy, or nonaccidental injury) and chronic pediatric conditions (such as inflammatory bowel disease, cystic fibrosis, and juvenile idiopathic arthritis).

Systemic problems can include chronic conditions such as hemophilia, sickle cell disease, and arthritic diseases; neurologic problems, such as cerebral palsy; and various cancers, including osteosarcoma and leukemia. Children with metabolic problems, such as vitamin D–resistant rickets, have bony deformities. Acute systemic disorders can also affect the musculoskeletal system. For example, viruses and bacteria can infect joints and bones. In developing countries, tubercular infections of bones are common and devastating. PCPs must assess patients from a broad perspective, obtain a thorough history to include other body systems, and order appropriate laboratory studies that might identify systemic problems.

Genetic Disorders

Many genetic problems have an orthopedic component. Osteogenesis imperfecta (OI) is a genetic disorder characterized by decreased levels of collagen, the major protein of the body's connective tissue. Mutations in genes encoding type 1 collagen (*COL1A1* or COL1A2 genes) account for approximately 80% of OI cases (Abdelgawad and Naga, 2014). Children with OI have bones that break easily, even from minor trauma. Down syndrome is a consequence of a trisomy 21 chromosome. The main orthopedic pathology is hypotonia and the possibility of loose joint capsules and ligaments. Children with Down syndrome have a higher incidence of scoliosis, dislocation of the hip, Legg-Calvé-Perthes disease (LCPD), instability of the patella, and pes planus (flat feet). Children with Marfan syndrome may have longer than normal fingers, low muscle tone, and lax joints that are prone to dislocate. Severe scoliosis may develop in children with neurofibromatosis, Turner syndrome, and Noonan syndrome. Girls with Turner syndrome may present with webbed neck, short stature, valgus deformity of the elbow, and short fourth metacarpal deformity. Children with Noonan syndrome can present with webbed neck, pectus carinatum or excavatum, clumsiness, poor coordination, and motor delay. (See Chapter 32 for a discussion of various genetic conditions.)

Many orthopedic problems have a multifactorial inheritance pattern. If one child in a family has a dislocated hip or scoliosis, the risk for these conditions increases for the other siblings. The pediatric provider must understand the genetic disorder to monitor related orthopedic problems, consider the genetic implications, and provide families with appropriate genetic information or refer them for genetic counseling.

Intrauterine Compression Deformations

The developing fetus moves its body parts frequently, which influences musculoskeletal development. When the fetus fills the uterine space, movements are restricted and body parts begin to assume the shape in which they are fixed. Because of in utero positioning, joint and muscle contractions can develop and are generally considered physiologic in nature. Fetal movement is required for proper development of the musculoskeletal system, and anything that restricts fetal movement can cause deformation from intrauterine molding. Two major intrinsic causes of deformations are neuromuscular disorders and maternal oligohydramnios. Extrinsic causes are related to fetal crowding that restricts fetal movement. Infants with deformations caused by extrinsic causes (e.g., breech position) have an excellent prognosis with corrections occurring spontaneously. Because much of the bony structure is cartilaginous, molding occurs with relative ease. Intrauterine positioning issues can result in tibial bowing and 20 to 30 degrees of hip flexion. Occasionally a foot may be turned awkwardly, legs might be fixed straight up with the feet near the ears, or the neck may be tipped to one side. Such positioning issues are outside the range of normal and the outcomes are deformities in various degrees. The longer the position is maintained, the more severe the problems will be. In general there is a tendency for bowing and late deformations to straighten; however, the effects related to in utero positioning may not fully abate until the child is 3 to 4 years of age. More severe deformities (i.e., rigid metatarsus adductus [MA]) must be referred to orthopedists for treatment as soon as they are identified. A softer skeleton is easier to realign in a positive direction.

Injuries

Unique differences in the pediatric skeletal system predispose children to injuries unlike those seen in adults. The important differences are the presence of periosseous cartilage, physes, and a thicker, stronger, more osteogenic periosteum that produces new bone, called *callus*, more rapidly and in great amounts. Sports- and recreation-related injuries account for a significant number of emergency department visits each year for children ranging in age from 5 to 14 years. Physeal fractures in preadolescent children are the most common musculoskeletal injuries seen. Clavicular fractures are seen at all ages ranging from a newborn birth injury to trauma in adolescence. Injury to the clavicle is usually sustained by a fall on an outstretched hand or by direct force; approximately 80% of fractures occur in the middle third of the clavicle (Murphy and Karlin, 2016). Fractures of the wrist and forearm account for nearly half of all fractures in children. Tendinosis may occur in the young athlete in the rotator cuff from throwing motions and swimming, in the iliopsoas in dancers, and in the ankle of dancers, gymnasts, and figure skaters. Shoulder injuries can be acute or may result from chronic overuse. Overuse injuries are common chronic injuries in children; they are related to repetitive stress on the musculoskeletal system without sufficient time to recover. Apophysitis is an overuse injury unique to the skeletally immature active child or athlete. Tensile loading and stress to the apophysis—which is a secondary growth center at the insertion of the tendon—cause irritation, inflammation, and microtrauma affecting muscles, ligaments, tendons, bones, and growth plates (Winell and Davidson, 2016).

The possibility of nonaccidental trauma should always be considered when orthopedic injuries, especially fractures, are present. PCPs should have a high index of suspicion if an injury is unexplained, if the severity of injury is incompatible with the history, or if the injury is inconsistent with the child's developmental capabilities. Rib fractures and any unexplained fracture in a child younger than 3 years of age, metaphyseal fractures, multiple fractures in various stages of healing, and complex skull fractures should be carefully evaluated (Flaherty et al., 2014). The management of traumatic injuries is discussed in Chapter 44. Assessment of nonaccidental trauma is also discussed in Chapter 24.

Defense Mechanisms

Fracture Healing

One of the major differences between adult and pediatric bones is that the periosteum in children is very thick. The major reason for increased healing speed of children's fractures is the periosteum, which contributes to the largest part of new bone formation around a fracture. Children have significantly greater osteoblastic activity in this area because bone is already being formed beneath the periosteum as part of normal growth. This already active process is readily accelerated after a fracture. Periosteal callus bridges a fracture in children long before the underlying hematoma forms cartilage anlagen that go on to ossify. Once cellular organization from the hematoma has passed through the inflammatory process, repair of the bone begins in the area of the fracture. In most children, by 10 days to 2 weeks after a fracture, a rubber-like bone forms around the fracture and makes it difficult to manipulate. As part of the reparative phase, cartilage formed as the hematoma organizes; it is eventually replaced by bone through the process of endochondral bone formation. The more growth potential the child has, the more remodeling will occur. Remodeling power is highest near the physis and across the coronal and sagittal planes (Abdelgawad and Naga, 2014).

Growth Plate Fractures

Fractures of the long bones can produce permanent deformities in children if the fracture occurs through the growth plate. The outcome depends on the fracture location and type, age of the child, status of the blood supply to the physis, and treatment. The Salter-Harris classification is based on the mechanism of injury, relationship of the fracture line to the layers of physis, and prognosis with respect to subsequent growth disturbance. There are five classifications (Fig 43.2). Type I involves a fracture through the zone of hypertrophic cells of the physis with no fracture of the surrounding bone. Type II fractures, the most common type of growth plate fracture, are similar to type I except that a metaphyseal fragment is present on the compression side of the fracture. Growth disturbance in types I and II is rare.

Type III fracture involves physeal separation with fracture through the epiphysis into the joint and requires anatomic reduction, occasionally through an open approach. Type IV fracture involves the metaphysis, physis, and epiphysis. Type V fracture involves a compression or crushing injury to the physis. Type V fractures are rare and are difficult to diagnose initially due to the lack of radiologic signs. Types IV and V require anatomic reduction to prevent articular incongruity and osseous bridging across the physis. Certain growth plates are more prone to growth disturbances. Children should be reevaluated intermittently for 1 year after healing to assess possible growth or functional disturbances.

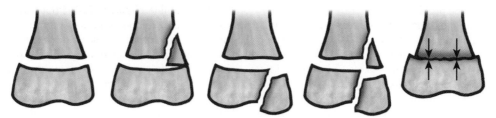

● **Fig 43.2** Salter-Harris Classification of Physical Fractures, Types I to V. (From Wells L, Sehgal K, Dormans JP. Pediatric fracture patterns. In: Kliegman RM, Stanton BF, St. Geme JW, et al., eds. *Nelson Textbook of Pediatrics*. 19th ed. Philadelphia: Saunders/Elsevier; 2011:2389–2391.)

Shaft Fractures

The mechanism of injury is an important part of the history in evaluating a child for a traumatic injury. Closed pediatric fractures are largely caused by low-energy activities and play; open fractures are generally caused by more force.

There are a variety of shaft fractures. In children between 9 months and 6 years of age, torsion of the foot may produce an oblique fracture of the distal aspect of the tibial shaft without a fibular fracture. These fractures are usually the result of tripping while walking or running, stepping on a ball or toy, or falling from a modest height. The child is typically seen due to failure to bear weight, a limp, or pain when asked to stand on the involved extremity. Physical findings may be minimal, and radiographs may show the characteristic faint oblique fracture line crossing the distal tibial diaphysis and terminating medially. Treatment is immobilization. Fractures of the forearm in children most often result from a fall on an outstretched hand. This results in forceful axial loading with resultant bony failure in compression and bending of the arm. These forces generally cause torus or greenstick fractures. The rotational malalignment may not be identified and may be undertreated. During physical examination, PCPs should observe for soft tissue injury, subtle rotational deformities, and neurovascular involvement and compare the injured limb with the contralateral one. Anteroposterior (AP) and lateral radiographs as well as oblique views of the wrist and forearm should be obtained if the physical examination suggests a fracture or dislocation. It is important to examine the entire arm and consider radiographic views of the joints above and below suspected fractures. Failure to diagnose and treat rotational malalignment is the most common cause of loss of forearm rotation in children.

Assessment of the Orthopedic System

History

- History of present illness or complaint
  - Onset: Appearance of first symptoms,; insidious or sudden, association with injury or strain, accompanied by any constitutional symptoms or signs (e.g., fever, malaise, swelling, ecchymosis)
  - Pain: Location and character, course of radiation, severity, extent of disability produced, effect of various activities including weight bearing, relief measures, changes from day to night or from day to day, child's refusing to move the painful part or assuming a pain-relieving position, effects of previous treatment, presence of pain or discomfort in other parts of the body

- Deformity: Character (swelling, inflammation, contracture, joint stiffness, unusual positioning, appearance), first appearance and who noted it, association with injury or disease, rate of change, extent of disability, a cosmetic problem or a cause of embarrassment
- Injury: How, when (time and date), and where; mechanism or manner in which injury was produced; involvement in organized or competitive sports
- Altered function: Weakness, limp, decreased range of motion, loss or decrease sensation, or alteration in perfusion that may be associated with circumferential swelling
- Altered gait patterns: Toe walking, in-toeing or out-toeing, limping, shortened single-limb stance phase, Trendelenburg gait, steppage gait (associated with footdrop), or Gower sign
- Other factors or constraints: Type of shoe worn; use of backpack and amount of weight in backpack, amount of time spent at repetitive tasks or at computer station; sitting in TV squat or "W" position; aggravating factors: dominant hand; use of complementary or alternative modalities
- Medication use: Steroids, anti-inflammatories, analgesics
- Family history
  - Any family members with musculoskeletal problems; many orthopedic problems have a genetic component
- Medical history
  - Pregnancy history and birth history: Breech delivery, shoulder presentation, multiple births, oligohydramnios, asphyxia at birth; maternal alcohol or substance abuse
  - Development history: Milestones met at appropriate age, such as first walking and sitting; delays in achieving gross or fine motor developmental milestones
  - Illnesses, accidents, or surgeries: Trauma, meningitis, juvenile arthritis, chronic diseases; especially those affecting nutritional status (i.e., inflammatory bowel disease, sickle cell disease)
- Review of systems
  - Any infections, constitutional diseases, or congenital problems that might have an orthopedic component? Any history of fractures, joint pains, strains or sprains? Any limitation is physical activity or sports participation?

Physical Examination

Special orthopedic examination techniques specific to children are described in the following sections and should be completed in addition to the normal orthopedic examination maneuvers.

Inspection and Palpation

Inspection of the skin—noting the skin color, presence of swelling or atrophy, erythema, ecchymosis, scars, or unusual pigmentation—is essential. Palpate skin for differences or inconsistencies in temperature and perfusion and palpate bone and joints to ascertain tenderness, prominence, indentations, and crepitus.

Range-of-Motion Examination

Observe the child's posture while sitting, standing, and walking as well as assess and evaluate the proportion of upper extremities to lower extremities. Evaluation of symmetry as well as range of motion, muscle size, strength, and tone should be a part of a musculoskeletal examination. Range of motion is the normal range, flexion, extension, and rotation of a joint. Joint hypermobility is the ability of the joint to move beyond its normal range. Hypermobility of joints generally does not cause problems, although there is a slight increase in dislocation and sprain of the involved joint. Normal joint motion is age related (e.g., external hip rotation is greatest in early infancy). Passive range of motion, in which the examiner moves the joint, provides information about joint mobility and stability. It can also provide information about the limits of contracted tendons and muscles. Active range of motion, in which the child moves the joint, provides information about both muscle and bony structures working together for functional movement.

Limited range of motion can be the result of mechanical problems, swelling, muscle spasticity, pain, infection, injury, or arthritis. Note pain, stiffness, limitations or deviations, and rigidity.

Gait Examination

Ambulation typically begins between 8 and 16 months of age. The development of a normal gait is dependent on progressive neurologic maturation. Initially a child's gait is characterized by a short stride length, a fast cadence, and slow velocity with a wide-based stance. The gait undergoes developmental changes. Walking velocity, step length, and duration of the single-limb stance increase with age, whereas the number of steps taken per minute decreases. A mature gait pattern is well established by 3 years of age. Normal neurologic maturation results in efficiency and smoothness of gait; by 7 years of age, the gait characteristics are similar to those of an adult (Baldwin et al., 2016). A normal gait cycle consists of the stance phase, during which the foot is in contact with the ground, and the swing phase, during which the foot is in the air. The stance phase is further divided into three major periods: the initial double-limb support, followed by the single-limb stance, and then another period of double-limb support.

Observe the child walking without shoes and with minimal covering. Compare stance and swing phases in both legs, and the range of motion of each joint should be evaluated. Inspect from the front, side, and back as the child walks normally, on his or her toes, and then on the heels. The gait should be smooth, rhythmic, and efficient. Ankle, knee, and hip movements should be symmetric and full with little side-to-side movement of the trunk.

Limping is a disturbance in the normal pattern of gait. Abnormal gait can be antalgic or nonantalgic. An antalgic gait is characterized by a shortening of the single-limb stance phase to prevent pain in the affected leg. Painful or antalgic gaits serve to reduce stress or pain at the affected area. The trunk shifts to the opposite side to keep balance and reduce stress; the stance phase and stride length are shortened as compensatory mechanisms.

Causes of a painful gait include infection, trauma, or acquired disorders. A nonantalgic gait may be caused by general weakness, spasticity, muscular disorders, or leg-length discrepancies. Gait disturbances may become more apparent with fatigue. When there is a concern regarding sensory or motor deficits, the provider should assess and evaluate the child's spinal nerves and deep tendon reflexes.

Posture

To assess posture adequately, the child should be examined undressed to his or her underwear. The examiner must look at the child from the front, side, and back.
- Pelvis and hips should be level. Place hands on the iliac crest to test for a pelvic tilt caused by limb-length discrepancy.
- Legs should be symmetric in shape and size. Patellas should be straight ahead.
- The feet should point straight ahead, with an imaginary line from the center of the heel through the second toe. There should be an arch (except in babies, in whom a fat pad obscures the arch) and straight heel cords.
- The spine should be straight, and the back should look symmetric, with shoulder and scapular heights and waist angles equal. There should be slight lordotic curves at the cervical and lumbar areas.

Hip Examinations

Galeazzi Maneuver

The Galeazzi sign can signal conditions that cause leg-length discrepancies. The Galeazzi maneuver includes flexing the hips and knees while the infant or child lies supine, placing the soles of the feet on the table near the buttocks, and then looking at the knee heights for equality (Fig 43.3A). The Galeazzi sign is positive if the knee heights are unequal. However, it is not reliable in children with dislocatable but not dislocated hips or in children with bilateral dislocation.

Barlow Maneuver

The Barlow maneuver assesses the potential for dislocation of a nondisplaced hip in an infant during the first month of life (Fig 43.4A), looking for laxity and instability. The infant should be unclothed and placed in the supine position with knees flexed. The hip is flexed and the thigh is brought into an adducted position while applying gentle downward pressure. With hip instability, the femoral head slips/drops out of the acetabulum or can be gently pushed out of the socket; this is termed a *positive Barlow*. The dislocation is palpable as this maneuver is performed. The maneuver must be performed gently in a noncrying neonate/infant to keep from damaging the femoral head. Examine the hips one at a time. The hip generally relocates spontaneously after release of the downward (posterior) force. (See resource for Barlow maneuver video https://www.youtube.com/watch?v=lqtLIhNnJUw).

Ortolani Maneuver

The Ortolani maneuver is the reverse of the Barlow maneuver (see Fig 43.4B). It reduces a posteriorly dislocated hip and is performed gently to reduce a recently dislocated hip. The infant is in the supine position with both knees flexed. The provider' thumb is placed near the lesser trochanter and the pad of the second finger is positioned on the bony prominence of the greater trochanter.

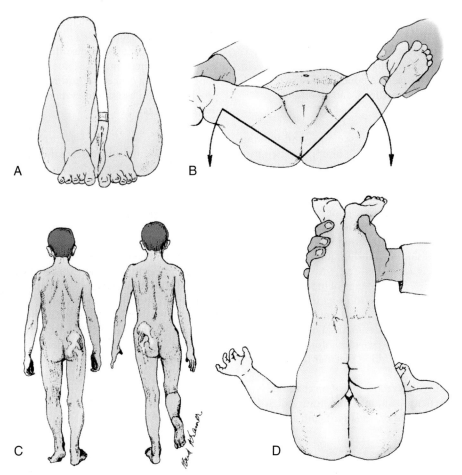

• **Fig 43.3** Physical Findings in Congenital Hip Dislocation. (A) Leg-length inequality is a sign of unilateral hip dislocation (Galeazzi sign). (B) Limitation of hip abduction is often present in older infants with hip dislocation. Abduction of greater than 60 degrees is usually possible in infants. Restriction or asymmetry indicates the need for careful radiologic examination. (C) Trendelenburg sign. In single-leg stance, the abductor muscles of the normal hip support the pelvis. Dislocation of the hip functionally shortens and weakens these muscles. When the child attempts to stand on the dislocated hip, the opposite side of the pelvis drops. (D) Thigh-fold asymmetry is often present in infants with unilateral hip dislocation. An extra fold can be seen on the abnormal side. However, the finding is not diagnostic. It may be found in normal infants and may be absent in children with hip dislocation or dislocatability. (From Scoles P. *Pediatric Orthopedics in Clinical Practice*. 2nd ed. St. Louis: Mosby; 1988.)

The leg is flexed at the hip and then abducted while pushing up with the fingers located over the trochanter posteriorly. The femoral head is lifted anteriorly into the acetabulum. A palpable *clunk* as the femoral head is relocated is considered a positive Ortolani sign. A high-pitched hip *click* may be audible or felt at the very end of abduction (Sankar et al., 2016). A click is a common sound and is not considered a positive Ortolani sign. Positive Barlow and Ortolani maneuvers may be achieved only during the first few months of life. Dislocations can occur later in infancy; PCPs must test the hips using other strategies and note limited abduction in older infants until they are walking independently (Fig 43.5). See resource for Ortolani test video (https://www.aap.org/en-us/about-the-aap/Committees-Councils-Sections/Section-on-Orthopaedics/Pages/Barlow-Ortolani-Maneuvers.aspx/).

Klisic Test

The Klisic test provides an observational sign of hip placement. The PCP places the tip of the third finger of one hand over the greater trochanter and the index finger of the same hand on the anterosuperior iliac spine. An imaginary line is drawn between the index and third fingers. Normally the imaginary line points to the umbilicus. If the hip is dislocated, the trochanter is elevated and the imaginary line points halfway between the umbilicus and the pubis (i.e., the line points below the umbilicus). This sign is another physical assessment marker of hip dislocation (Sankar et al., 2016) (Fig 43.6).

Trendelenburg Sign

The Trendelenburg test can be used to identify conditions that cause weakness in the hip abductors. It is elicited by having the child stand and then raise one leg off the ground. If the pelvis (iliac crest) drops on the side of the raised leg, the sign is positive and indicates weak hip abductor muscles on the side that is bearing the weight. It may or may not be painful as it involves muscle weakness around the hip joint. Normally the muscles around a stable hip are strong enough to maintain a level pelvis if one leg is raised (see Fig 43.3C). With bilaterally dislocated hips, a wide-based Trendelenburg limp is noted.

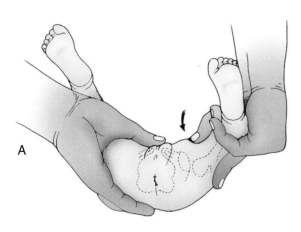

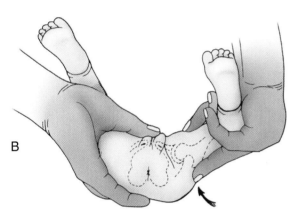

• **Fig 43.4** (A) Barlow (dislocation) test. The "stabilizing hand" is positioned with the thumb on the symphysis and the fingers on the sacrum. The thumb of the abducting hand is placed on the inner aspect of the thigh and gives lateral pressure to the adductor region, while the hand (wrapped around the knee with the index finger on the lateral side of the thigh) provides gentle downward pressure. If there is hip instability, dislocation is palpable as the femoral head slips out of the acetabulum. Diagnosis is confirmed with the Ortolani test. (B) Ortolani (reduction) test. With the infant relaxed on a firm surface, the hips and knees are flexed to 90 degrees. The hips are examined one at a time. The infant's thigh is grasped with the middle finger over the greater trochanter and the thigh is lifted to bring the femoral head from its dislocated posterior position to opposite the acetabulum. Simultaneously the thigh is gently abducted, reducing the femoral head in the acetabulum. In a positive finding, the examiner senses reduction by a palpable, nearly audible "clunk." Test one hip at a time for both of these tests. (From Marcdante KJ, Kliegman RM, Jenson HB, et al., eds. *Nelson Essentials of Pediatrics*. 6th ed. Philadelphia: Saunders/Elsevier; 2011.)

Medial (Internal) and Lateral (External) Rotation

The child is placed prone and the knees are flexed 90 degrees. Medial rotation is measured as the legs are allowed to fall apart as far as possible, using gravity alone or with light pressure. The angle between vertical (0 degree) and the leg position is the medial rotation. It is measured for each leg (Fig 43.7A). Asymmetric hip rotation is abnormal. Lateral rotation is measured by allowing the legs to cross while the child is still prone. The angle between vertical and the leg position is measured for each leg (see Fig 43.7B). Again, asymmetric hip rotation is abnormal. By 1 year of age, a normal child has approximately 45 degrees of internal and external hip rotation.

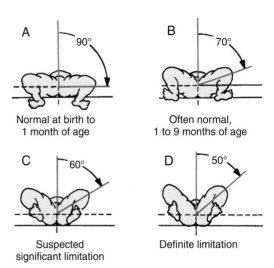

• **Fig 43.5** Hip Abduction Test. The child is placed supine and the hips are flexed 90 degrees and fully abducted. Although the normal abduction range is quite broad (A and B), one can suspect hip disease in any patient who lacks more than 35 to 45 degrees of abduction (C suspicious and D abnormal). (From Chung SMK. *Hip Disorders in Infants and Children*. Philadelphia: Lea and Febiger; 1981.)

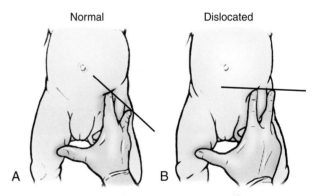

• **Fig 43.6** The Klisic Test. (A) Normal position of imaginary line when hip in socket. (B) Imaginary line position when hip is dislocated. (From Kliegman RM, Stanton BF, St. Geme JW, et al., eds. *Nelson Textbook of Pediatrics*. 19th ed. Philadelphia: Saunders/Elsevier; 2011.)

Back Examination

Adams Test or the Adams Forward Bend Test

The Adams forward bend test (Adams test) looks for asymmetry of the posterior chest wall on forward bending and allows for the evaluation of structural scoliosis. The child bends at the waist to a position of 90 degrees back flexion with straight legs, ankles together, and arms hanging freely or with palms together (in a diving position) but not touching the toes or floor (Fig 43.8). The back is then inspected for asymmetry of the height of the curves on the two sides or rib hump; the provider inspects the child's back by looking at it from the rear and side positions. The examiner should be seated or standing in front of the child to best scan each level of the spine visually. If a rib hump is present, a scoliometer, if available, can be used to measure the angular tilt of the trunk. A spinal rotation greater than 5 to 7 degrees measured by placing the scoliometer at the peak of the curvature indicates the need for further evaluation (Duderstadt and Schapiro, 2019).

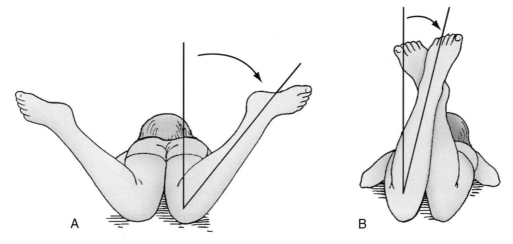

• **Fig 43.7** Hip Rotation in Extension. This is measured with the child in prone position and the knee flexed 90 degrees. The lower leg is vertically oriented. This is considered the neutral position. On outward rotation (A), the leg produces internal hip rotation, and on inward rotation (B), the leg produces external hip rotation. (From Thompson GH. Gait disturbances. In: Kliegman RM, ed. *Practical Strategies in Pediatric Diagnosis and Therapy*. Philadelphia: Saunders; 1996.)

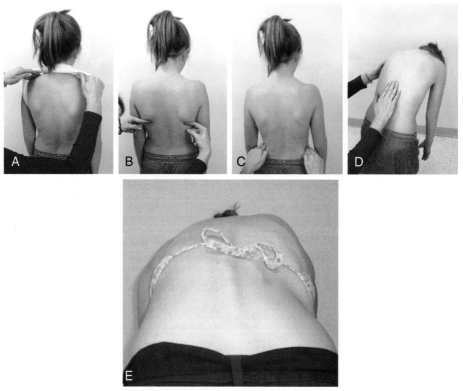

• **Fig 43.8** Assessment of the Spine. (A) Testing shoulder symmetry. (B) Scapular symmetry. (C) Iliac crest symmetry. (D) Beginning Adams forward bend test. (E) Positive rib hump. (From Skirven T, Osterman A, Dedorczk J, et al. *Rehabilitation of the Hand and Upper Extremity*. 6th ed. Philadelphia: Mosby; 2012; and Duderstadt KG, ed. *Pediatric Physical Examination: An Illustrated Handbook*. Philadelphia: Elsevier; 2014:277.)

Diagnostic Studies

Radiographs are an important diagnostic tool for the musculoskeletal system. Imaging should begin with standard radiographs of the area of concern. AP and lateral views of the affected area, bone, or joint are typically ordered to analyze the anatomic structures. Views of both extremities may be ordered so that comparisons can be made. Computed tomography (CT) scans augment radiographs to detail specific areas of the body. CT is useful in detailing the relationship of bones to their contiguous structures. Magnetic resonance imaging (MRI) provides excellent visualization of joints, soft tissues, cartilage, and medullary bone. It can distinguish between various physiologic changes that occur in bone marrow related to age and disease process. Ultrasonography can provide information about cartilaginous areas or tissues not visible on radiograph and is highly sensitive for detecting effusion of the hip joint. Bone scans (scintigraphy) are more sensitive than radiographs, demonstrate abnormal uptake earlier than conventional radiographs, and are useful in detecting causes of obscure skeletal pain. Although CT scanning and radiographs offer tremendous benefits in diagnosing and guiding care for children with musculoskeletal problems, PCPs must be mindful of the cost and amount of radiation a child is exposed to and weigh the risks versus benefits of their use.

Laboratory studies can help to identify systemic disease, infection, or inflammation. Erythrocyte sedimentation rate (ESR), C-reactive protein (CRP), complete blood count (CBC), blood cultures, rheumatoid factor, and antinuclear antibodies are hematologic tests that can assist in the diagnosis and management of bone disorders. Other laboratory tests also provide an understanding of muscle metabolism (e.g., carnitine, lactic acid, leptin, pyruvates). Some bony lesions and joint effusions of muscle tissue may have to be biopsied.

Management Strategies

Counseling

Counseling for orthopedic problems involves several components. The family should understand and have time to ask questions about all of the following issues: the pathologic condition, including possible etiologies; treatment plan; prognosis with and without treatment; any genetic implications of the diagnosis; and long-term-care issues. Counseling helps families cope with a poor, chronic, or challenging diagnosis and its short- and long-term implications. Congenital problems are often identified prenatally, at birth, or shortly thereafter. Families must be given the diagnosis truthfully, humanely, and as soon as possible. Issues of etiology must be discussed to address parents' feelings of guilt for causing the problem and to discuss genetic implications if any. A plan of care that is mutually agreed on by the family and the provider must be developed before the infant is discharged from the hospital or clinic.

Anticipatory Guidance: Musculoskeletal Development

Families are sometimes concerned about problems that providers believe are within normal limits and do not require an orthopedic referral. PCPs should provide the child's family with a description of the child's predicted musculoskeletal development. Timelines and markers that parents can use to monitor their child's development are particularly helpful in allowing families to understand their child's pattern of growth. Misperceptions about the implications of minor variations must be clarified, and the family should always be given the opportunity to return for further assessment or discussion if concerns remain. Examples of common developmental concerns are flat feet in infants and toddlers, "bowed" legs in toddlers, and "knock knees" in preschool children.

Shoes

The use of therapeutic shoes to correct orthopedic problems is controversial. Studies confirm that therapeutic shoes do little to correct deformities. Shoes for the average child should keep the feet warm and protected from injury. Shoes should be selected to fit properly and comfortably with room for growth. High-top shoes for toddlers may have the advantage of staying on little feet with fat pads better, but they do not provide additional support. Toddlers' feet do not need extra support. Features of a good shoe are as follows:

- Flexible sole—to allow as much free motion as possible; for young children, test to see if the shoe can be flexed in the parent's hand.
- Flat—do not allow high heels.
- Foot shaped—avoid pointed toes or other shapes that do not conform to the normal configuration of the foot.
- Fitted generously—better to be too large than too small.
- Friction similar to skin—the soles should have the same friction as skin so that they are not slippery.

Well-cushioned, shock-absorbing shoes are helpful in the child or adolescent athlete in order to decrease the chances of developing overuse syndrome. Shoe modifications may be needed in certain conditions. Shoe lifts are needed if limb-length differences exceed 2.5 cm. Orthotics can also be used in certain orthopedic situations to distribute pressure on the sole of the foot more evenly and facilitate function. Orthopedists recommend using Superfeet insoles as a first-line treatment.

Care of Children in Casts and Splints

Casts and splints are applied in order to immobilize a limb, promote healing, maintain bone alignment, diminish pain, protect the injury, and help compensate for surrounding muscular weakness. Splints are noncircumferential immobilizers that accommodate swelling. Splints are used in orthopedic conditions where swelling is anticipated— that is, in acute fractures or sprains and for initial stabilization of reduced, displaced, or unstable fractures before orthopedic intervention. Casts are circumferential immobilizers. They provide superior immobilization but are less forgiving than splints and have a higher rate of complications. The use of casts and splints is generally limited to a short period of time. If prolonged immobilization is required, joint stiffness and muscle atrophy may occur, generally warranting physical or occupational therapy to regain function.

The child's cast should be kept cool, clean, and dry. Cover it with plastic wrap or a plastic bag when the child bathes or is in a situation where the cast may get wet. If the cast becomes wet, a hair dryer set on cool setting can be used for drying small areas. If the cast becomes soiled, clean it with a slightly damp washcloth and cleanser.

Teach the family how to do a circulatory inspection to check the function of nerves and blood vessels. Casts can be perceived by children to be itchy, and they may insert small toys or long thin objects that cannot be seen externally in attempt to relieve the itching. These objects or an area of swelling may impede the blood flow or neurologic innervation. The child's toes or fingers below the cast should be pink and warm to the touch. The child should be able to feel all sides of his or her fingers or toes when touched and be able to wiggle all of the fingers or toes. Skin care following cast and splint removal is imperative. For the first few days following splint and cast removal, the skin will be delicate and sensitive.

It may appear pale yellow and will be flaky. The family should be instructed to soak and gently cleanse the skin, pat it dry, and avoid rubbing or peeling excess skin.

The family must know when to call the provider—that is, if the toes or fingers are cold to the touch and appear pale or blue, complaints of tingling or numbness, inability to move fingers or toes, and excessive swelling. Additional problems with casts (i.e., foul smell, breakage, or loosening) and/or alteration in skin integrity following the removal of a cast or splint must be reported.

Physical and Occupational Therapy

Children with developmental delays, cerebral palsy, spinal disorders, and torticollis should be referred for physical and/or occupational therapy. Treatments focus on improving gross and fine motor skills, balance and coordination, strength and endurance, as well as cognitive and sensory processing. Structured physical therapy after orthopedic injury can be helpful.

Orthopedic Conditions Specific to Children

Annular Ligament Displacement

Annular ligament displacement, previously described as a subluxation of the radial head and frequently called *nursemaid's elbow*, is a frequent injury that occurs in children 6 months to 5 years of age. The injury typically occurs when traction is applied to the arm of a young child, which is most often the result of pulling a child by the hand or grasping a child's hand to prevent a fall. This motion causes the annular ligament to slide over the head of the radius, where it becomes entrapped in the radiohumeral joint when the distal traction is released (Bexkens et al., 2016) (Fig 43.9A).

Clinical Findings

History. Often the history is nonspecific as to a report of an injury, and the parent may not have been aware of when the injury occurred. Alternatively, a caregiver will commonly report that the child cried, complaining of arm pain after being pulled up by his or her arm or swung by the arms. The caregiver typically reports that since the incident, the child has refused to use the affected arm, crying out in pain if the arm is moved, particularly the elbow.

The injury produces immediate pain and limited supination. Swelling and ecchymosis are not always present. Pain may be present with movement but not on palpation. Following the injury a toddler typically will resist moving his or her arm and can be observed holding the affected arm in pronation and slight flexion against their body (Bexkens et al., 2016).

Diagnostic Studies. Radiographs are not routinely recommended when the history and clinical presentation are classic. If obtained, radiography of the elbow is normal. If the history of the injury is not consistent with a mechanism expected to cause angular ligament displacement or if the physical examination leads to the possibility of additional injury, radiographs are indicated.

Differential Diagnosis. Subluxation has a classic history and presentation. If the child does not improve after the reduction procedure (see next section), a fracture of the elbow or clavicle should be considered. The clinical presentation of a fracture may be similar to that of an angular ligament displacement injury and therefore must be ruled out. Consider maltreatment if recurrent dislocations or other symptoms or signs are present.

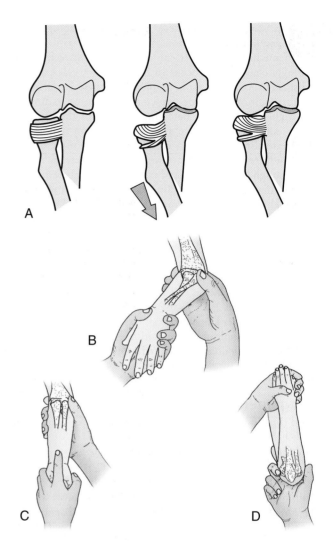

• **Fig 43.9** (A) Annular ligament displacement, formerly known as *subluxation of the radial head*. The pathology of nursemaid's elbow, or pulled elbow. The anterior ligament is partially torn when the arm is pulled. The radial head moves distally, and when traction is discontinued, the ligament is carried into the joint. (B and D) Reduction of radial head subluxation by supination and flexion technique. (B) The palm of the child's hand is grasped as if to shake it. Axial traction is applied to the forearm with the wrist adducted to the ulnar side. Pressure is also applied directly over the radial head of the elbow. (C) The forearm is supinated while axial traction and pressure are maintained over the forearm and radial head. (D) The elbow is flexed to the shoulder while supination and pressure are maintained over the radial head. (A, From Rang M. *Children's Fractures*. 2nd ed. Philadelphia: JB Lippincott; 1983:193. Found in Kliegman RM, Stanton BF, St. Geme JW, et al., eds. *Nelson Textbook of Pediatrics*. 19th ed. Philadelphia: Saunders/Elsevier; 2011. B–D, From Shah B. Reduction of radial head subluxation. In: Finberg L, Kleinman RE, eds. *Saunders Manual of Pediatric Practice*. 2nd ed. Philadelphia: Saunders; 2002:1162.)

Management. Two techniques can be used to reduce the radial head: supination and flexion or pronation. Do not attempt either procedure if epitrochlear tenderness is present because this may be indicative of a more serious injury (e.g., fracture).

The steps to correct the angular ligament displacement are as follows:

• Approach the child in a slow, nonthreatening way and distract him or her by talking or other diversionary tactics.

TABLE 43.1 Brachial Plexus Injury Using the Narakas Classification

Name	Nerves and Muscles Involved	Prognosis
Narakas type I	C5 and C6; shoulder and biceps	Recovery is usually complete.
Narakas type II	C5–C7; shoulder, biceps, and forearm extensors	Recovery is usually complete.
Narakas type III	C5–T1	Variable with complete paralysis of limb; shoulder and biceps recovery is fair to poor with hand recovery variable.
Narakas type IV	C5–T1	Complete paralysis of the limb and Horner syndrome; shoulder and biceps recovery is fair to poor with hand recovery variable.

- Use either the supination and flexion technique as illustrated in Fig 43.9B, or the hyperpronation technique. With the pronation maneuver, the provider gently extends the elbow in order to pronate (palm down) the child's forearm and continues to gently rotate the child's forearm (hyperpronate) until thumb faces downward (Bexkens et al., 2016). Once hyperpronation and extension are achieved, the provider then releases the forearm and elbow and evaluates if the attempt at reduction was successful.
- A palpable or audible "pop" or "click" usually signals successful reduction. Typically the child begins reaching for objects again with the affected arm within 15 minutes of reduction. If reduction is successful, no further treatment is necessary.

Complications. Several attempts (up to three at reduction) may be necessary before the patient resumes normal use of the arm. If normal use does not follow reduction attempts, immobilization using a sling with prompt orthopedic follow-up is indicated. Recurrence of angular displacement is seen in approximately one-third of patients. Education and anticipatory guidance should be provided to caregivers in an effort to prevent reinjury (Carrigan, 2016).

Patient and Parent Education. Key points to cover include instructing caregivers not to lift or pull the child by the hand or elbow and to lift the child from the axillae.

Brachial Plexus Injuries

The brachial plexus is a network of nerves in the shoulder arising from the spinal cord; it enables movement and sensation in the shoulders, arms, and hands. Injury to the shoulder and brachial plexus during the birthing process is known as *obstetric brachial plexus palsy* or *neonatal brachial plexus palsy*. Brachial plexus injuries types I through IV are typically classified using the Narakas criteria (Table 43.1). Most injuries affect the upper brachial plexus (C5 and C6 nerve roots), resulting in weakness or paralysis of the shoulder and upper arm; they are known as *Erb-Duchenne (or Erb) palsy*. More severe injuries involving the lower plexus (C7, C8, and T1 nerve roots) impair hand function and cause ipsilateral ptosis and miosis; they are known as *Dejerine-Klumpke (or Klumpke) palsy* (Somashekar et al., 2016).

Risk factors for neonatal brachial plexus palsies may be divided into three categories: neonatal, maternal, and labor-related factors. Breech presentation and macrosomic infants are at increased risk for brachial plexus injuries. Maternal characteristics include diabetes, obesity, maternal age (>35 years), and maternal pelvic anatomy. Labor-related factors (such as shoulder dystocia) account for approximately 45% of brachial plexus injuries. Vacuum extraction, direct compression of the fetal neck during delivery by forceps, or application of lateral traction on the head during delivery of the shoulder can cause stretching of the cervical nerve roots and eventually brachial plexus injury (Russman, 2018).

Clinical Findings

History. History should include obstetric history, mode of delivery, and postnatal health of the infant.

Physical Examination. A thorough head-to-toe examination is required to identify any deformations or other injuries that may have occurred in utero or during delivery. Assess passive range of motion, and newborn reflexes should be tested in order to identify neurologic deficits. Findings may include:

- Erb palsy, presenting with an adducted arm, which is internally rotated at the shoulder: The wrist is flexed, and fingers are extended, resulting in a characteristic "waiter's tip" posture.
- Absent bicep reflex with asymmetric Moro and tonic neck reflex on the affected side
- Limp wrist and hand with absent grasp reflex (lower plexus involvement)
- Horner syndrome (ipsilateral ptosis, miosis, enophthalmos, anhidrosis) if the sympathetic fibers of the T1 nerve root are involved
- Occasionally hand paralysis with normal shoulder movement, which is a rare occurrence of an isolated C8 through T1 injury
- Limited neck movement due to damage to the sternocleidomastoid muscle; skull fracture
- Impaired respiratory effort as a result of diaphragmatic paralysis and flaccidity
- Ruptured intra-abdominal structures, especially the liver and spleen, which require careful abdominal examination

Diagnostic Studies. Radiologic examination, electrophysiologic studies, and MRI are useful to confirm a clinical diagnosis and the extent of injury. Radiographs of the chest and upper limbs are important because they reveal associated injuries, such as rib, transverse process, and clavicular/humeral fractures. A chest radiograph is necessary to rule out phrenic nerve injury. Electrodiagnostic studies with electromyography and nerve conduction velocities are used to determine the severity of the neural lesion.

Differential Diagnosis. The differential diagnosis of upper extremity paralysis in a newborn includes epiphyseal separation of the humeral head, fracture of the clavicle or humerus, septic arthritis, acute osteomyelitis of the upper extremity, spinal cord injury, cervical cord lesions, and congenital malformations of the plexus and upper limb (Herring and Ho, 2014).

Management. An interprofessional team approach is ideal, with referral to providers who specialize in treating brachial plexus injuries. Referral should be made in the first week of life. The initial goal of therapy is to maintain passive range of motion, supple joints, and muscle strength. Indications for surgical exploration and reconstruction of the brachial plexus include failure of recovery of elbow flexion and shoulder abduction from the third to the sixth months of life. The spectrum of nerve surgery includes neurolysis, neuroma resection, nerve grafting, and nerve transfers.

Complications. Late sequelae include internal rotation contractures, hypoplasia of the arm, altered sensibility, flexion contractures of the elbow, dislocation of the radial head, and psychologic and social consequences.

Prognosis. Recovery can occur spontaneously and is highly dependent on the level and extent of nerve injury. Paralysis of the upper portion of the arm generally has a better prognosis than does paralysis of the lower part. If the paralysis is due to edema surrounding the nerve fibers (neurapraxia), spontaneous full recovery within a few weeks is likely; if it is due to disruption of the nerve fibers (axonotmesis), function generally returns in a few months. More severe injuries, total disruption of the nerves (neurotmesis), and root avulsion require surgery with partial or complete recovery observed over several years. Fortunately 50% of plexus injuries occur at the upper nerve roots (C5 to C6), involve neurapraxia and axonotmesis, and heal spontaneously (Russman, 2018).

Clavicular Fracture

Clavicular fractures seen in newborns result from birth trauma. In young children they can result from accidental or nonaccidental trauma, can occur as a result of a direct hit or indirect trauma and are most commonly associated with a fall. Approximately 80% to 85% of these fractures occur in the middle third of the clavicle and 12% to 15% in the distal third. The clavicle is the first bone to ossify and the last physis in the body to close, usually not until age 25 to 30 years (Herring and Ho, 2014).

Clinical Findings

History. History varies depending on the age of the child. In the neonate, it may include:
- Difficult delivery, high birth weight, midforceps delivery, and shoulder dystocia
- Irritability when infant is moved or lifted
In the older child, it may include:
- History of fall or trauma with focus on mechanism of injury; typically the fall is on an outstretched hand (Apel, 2014)

Physical Examination. In all children, look for the following:
- Pain with shoulder movement
- Decreased arm movement on affected side (asymmetric spontaneous arm movements) or absent Moro reflex
- Swelling, bony abnormality, discoloration, and/or crepitus elicited over the fracture site
- Callus felt over the fracture site within a few days
- Spasm of the sternocleidomastoid muscle on the affected side
- An associated Erb palsy

Diagnostic Studies. Imaging studies are recommended. Radiography with routine clavicular views is sufficient.

Differential Diagnosis. Brachial palsy, shoulder dislocation, or other bony problems should be considered.

Management. Management involves the following:
Neonate
- Incomplete fractures that do not cause pain need no treatment.
- Immobilization of the shoulder is an option when movement results in a painful arm (usually with a complete fracture). Pin the sleeve of the infant's arm to the front of the shirt for 1 to 2 weeks (Apel, 2014).

Older child
- Sling immobilization for comfort to support the affected extremity is often sufficient. Generally sling immobilization can be discontinued at 3 to 4 weeks.
- A figure-eight clavicular brace can be used if displacement results in a decreased shaft length. However, it is uncomfortable to wear and its effectiveness is questionable.
- Protection for 4 to 5 weeks is generally sufficient because union requires about 4 weeks of healing.

- An older child may need analgesics or a nonsteroidal anti-inflammatory drug (NSAID) for pain.
- The need for surgical intervention is uncommon with clavicular fractures. Surgery may be needed in the case of open fractures, neurovascular compromise, multiple trauma, rib cage fractures, and fractures with greater than 100% displacement with severe skin tenting.

Prognosis. The prognosis is excellent. Often the injury in neonates is identified only at later primary care visits when the callus lump is palpated, although the child may be irritable until the fracture is stable. The infant is usually asymptomatic within 7 to 10 days. Parents need information and emotional support. In older children, general healing time is 6 to 8 weeks with average return to noncontact sports in 4 to 6 weeks and contact sports in 8 to 12 weeks. Bony callus appears approximately 10 days after injury as a painless firm "lump."

Costochondritis and Sternochondritis

Costochondritis is a common cause of chest pain in children and adolescents. The condition is characterized as an inflammatory process of one or more of the costochondral cartilages that causes localized tenderness and pain in the anterior chest wall. Trauma to the area and unaccustomed physical effort (lifting heavy objects or coughing) are factors known to cause costochondritis; however, most cases are idiopathic (Garry, 2018). Inflammation is the underlying problem.

Clinical Findings

History. Pain localized to the costosternal or costochondral junction is the major symptom. It often presents with tenderness over more than one rib as a result of referred pain. The primary rib that is inflamed and usually responsible for the symptoms is most often the one that exhibits the greatest sensitivity to palpation. Characteristics of the pain include the following:
- Acute or gradual onset; typically insidious, occurring over several days or weeks
- Sharp, darting, or dull quality
- Radiation from chest to upper abdomen or back
- Occasional complaints of a feeling of tightness caused by muscle spasm
- Exacerbating factors may include coughing, sneezing, deep inspiration, movement of the upper torso and upper extremities

Physical Examination. Palpation reveals tenderness over the costochondral junction. The tenderness is localized and most common at the sternocostal cartilage of the second through seventh ribs. The presence of pain, swelling (a unique bulbous enlargement of the joint commonly noted over a single upper costochondrial junction) with or without redness, and tenderness at the costal cartilage are referred to as the *Tietze syndrome*. Ecchymosis may be seen in cases of trauma. Respiratory effort is normal. Auscultation of the lungs, heart, and abdomen is normal.

Diagnostic Studies. No diagnostic studies are needed because history and physical findings are diagnostic. Chest radiography may exclude other possible causes but offers no diagnostic value. A CT scan can demonstrate swelling of the costal cartilage.

Differential Diagnosis. Rib fractures are the key differential diagnosis if pain is associated with an injury. Childhood rheumatic diseases can also produce complaints similar to those of costochondritis but generally have other characteristic physical findings. Costochondritis is one of the differential diagnoses of pediatric chest pain (see Chapter 38).

Management. Treatment consists of using mild analgesia and NSAIDs to relieve discomfort and avoiding strenuous activity. Cough suppressants may be beneficial if cough is an aggravating factor. Stretching exercises and the application of ice to the area are useful. Parents and children must be reassured that this is a benign, self-limited condition and is not related to cardiac disease.

Back Pain

Young children do not commonly complain of severe back pain. Most episodes of back pain in pediatric patients are brief, with nonspecific findings and history. Back pain that warrants immediate attention includes complaints from children younger than 4 years of age, persistent symptoms, self-imposed activity limitations, systemic symptoms, increasing discomfort, persistent nighttime pain, neurologic symptoms, history of tuberculosis or cancer, and back pain accompanied by unexplained weight loss (Mistovich and Spiegel, 2016). Younger children who have such complaints should be carefully evaluated for occult pathologic conditions, and the provider's index of suspicion about underlying pathologic conditions should be raised.

The older the child or adolescent, the more likely it is that the back pain is musculoskeletal in origin. The young athlete is especially susceptible to back injury. Intense training can cause repetitive microtrauma. Back pain can result from sprains of the ligaments or muscles (or both) of the back due to injury.

Clinical Findings

History. Onset, duration, location, frequency, and intensity of the pain are key questions to ask in forming an initial impression. In addition, it is important that PCPs differentiate between mechanical and inflammatory causes. The history should include questions related to the timing of back pain and aggravating or relieving factors. Specifically the back pain reported with morning stiffness or prolonged rest is associated with inflammatory causes, whereas back pain reported with activity is associated with mechanical causes.

The following findings should alert the pediatric provider to possible pathologic conditions:

- Pain that prohibits play or activities, persists or worsens, or occurs at night
- History of trauma (vertebral fracture)
- Positive neurologic or musculoskeletal signs on examination
- Systemic signs, such as fever, chills, weight loss, and malaise
- Presence of any radicular symptoms, gait disturbances, muscle weakness, altered sensation, and changes in bowel and/or bladder function

In school-age children and adolescents, back pain can be associated with a history of the following:

- Muscle strain as a result of "overuse syndrome" from excessive muscular exertion, usually related to sports, commonly in sedentary children who have recently increased their activity level
- Wearing high heels (females)
- Neck/shoulder, low back, and arm pain in relation to computer or video game use; excessive TV watching

Physical Examination. The examination should include a complete musculoskeletal and neurologic assessment with the child adequately exposed for the clinical examination. Inspect for any changes in alignment in the frontal or sagittal plane; range of motion should be assessed in flexion, extension, and lateral bending. Younger children may be asked to pick an object up off the floor to assess spinal flexion. Palpation reveals any areas of tenderness and/or muscle spasm. Palpate the top of the iliac crests while the child is standing to assess leg lengths. A careful neurologic examination should be performed.

Diagnostic Studies. A CBC with differential, ESR, and CRP are useful tests for infectious conditions; rheumatoid factor and antinuclear antibodies are useful tests for suspected rheumatologic disorders. Initially AP and lateral radiographs of the involved region of the spine are recommended. With lumbar back pain, right and left oblique views are also recommended. MRI is most helpful for viewing soft tissue and intraspinal detail, and CT is superior for assessing bone involvement.

Differential Diagnosis. Occult pathologic conditions should be ruled out. Discitis, vertebral osteomyelitis, vertebral fracture, or tumor can cause significant back pain in toddlers. Older children can experience these same problems in addition to intervertebral disc herniation, vertebral endplate fractures, low back stress fracture, and spondylosis. Back pain is a commonly reported symptom in somatizing children. Athletes with a history of low back pain lasting more than 1 month deserve careful evaluation. A low back stress fracture or spondylosis must be included in the differential diagnoses.

Management. Treatment is determined by findings on history and physical examination and can include referral for radiographs (AP and lateral views) and imaging studies or referral to a pediatric orthopedist. If the back pain is due to injury, pain management and physical therapy may be part of the treatment plan.

Scoliosis

Scoliosis is a three-dimensional deformity most commonly described as a lateral curvature of the spine in the frontal plane. There are two types of scoliosis: nonstructural and structural. Nonstructural, also known as *functional scoliosis,* involves a curve in the spine without rotation of the vertebrae. The curve is reversible, because it is caused by conditions such as poor posture, muscle spasms, pain, or leg-length discrepancy. Structural scoliosis involves a rotational element of the spine and has various classifications depending on the cause. The remaining discussion pertains to structural scoliosis.

The diagnosis is based on a curvature of more than 10 degrees using the Cobb method, in which the angle between the superior and inferior end vertebrae (tilted into the curve) is measured by a radiologist (see Diagnostic Studies). In most pediatric cases, the etiology is unknown and is termed and classified as idiopathic. Other classifications include congenital, in which vertebrae fail to form (e.g., hemivertebrae), and neuromuscular (e.g., cerebral palsy, neurofibromatosis, Marfan syndrome). Kyphosis, which results from disorders of sagittal alignment (such as postural kyphosis and Scheuermann disease) is another classification of structural scoliosis. Kyphosis, commonly termed *round back,* is discussed following scoliosis.

- Idiopathic: Etiology is unknown and is likely multifactorial. It is the most common type of scoliosis. There are three types classified by age at onset:
  - Infantile (0 to 3 years of age)
  - Juvenile (3 to 10 years of age)
  - Adolescent (11 years of age and older)
- Congenital: A structural anomaly present at birth (e.g., hemivertebrae) often associated with other congenital abnormalities, such as renal and cardiac anomalies; progression of curvature can worsen rapidly, particularly during periods of rapid growth (e.g., first 2 to 3 years of life and adolescence).

TABLE 43.2 Scoliosis, Kyphosis, and Lordosis

	Curve	Etiology	Clinical Findings	Radiographs	Management
Scoliosis	Lateral	Classifications: Idiopathic (most common); neuro-muscular; constitutional; secondary; congenital; miscellaneous; functional (leg-length discrepancy—not scoliosis)	History: Positive family history; related to etiologies (classifications); painless curvature; typically have right thoracic curve	AP and lateral standing views to identify degree of curve; >10 degrees abnormal; may have one curve (C) or two curves (S); vertebrae show lateral deviation and rotation	Referral to orthopedic surgeon; brace or surgery; need to monitor progression of curve. Most curves do not increase after growth is complete; females with idiopathic scoliosis more likely to have curve progression and need close monitoring.
Kyphosis	AP curve of thoracic spine	Familial (Scheuermann disease); secondary to tumor, trauma, and so on; congenital; postural, not true kyphosis	Postural round back	Narrow disc space and loss of normal anterior height of vertebrae	Postural: PT, dancing, and swimming can be helpful. If structural, refer to an orthopedic surgeon for observation, bracing, or surgery.
Lordosis	AP curve of lumbar spine	As a result of hip contractures; physiologic; family and racial groups; before puberty	Abdomen and buttock protuberant; if result of hip contractures, lordosis disappears when sitting	Standing lateral views	If lumbar spine flattens and lordosis disappears when child bends forward, it is physiologic and no treatment is needed; if fixed, refer to an orthopedist.

AP, Anteroposterior; *PT,* physical therapy.

- Neuromuscular: Most common in nonambulatory patients. Secondary to weakness/imbalance/spasticity of the muscles of the trunk caused by primary neuromuscular problems (e.g., cerebral palsy or muscular dystrophy). In contrast to idiopathic and congenital scoliosis, curves caused by neuromuscular disorders can continue to progress after skeletal maturity.

Idiopathic scoliosis is the most common type. Its etiology is unknown, but it often has a familial or genetic pattern. The overall incidence of idiopathic scoliosis is approximately 2% to 3% with between 0.3% and 0.5% of children with scoliosis having curves greater than 20 degrees on radiography and less than 0.1% demonstrating curves greater than a 40-degree Cobb angle.

Hormonal changes and sexual maturity play a role in the disease process, and a rapid growth period is believed to be a significant factor in the progression of the curvature associated with idiopathic scoliosis. In addition, the risk of curve progression depends on the amount of growth remaining, the magnitude of the curve, and gender. Although the incidence of idiopathic scoliosis is nearly equal in girls and boys, females have a much higher risk of developing curves greater than 30 degrees (Mistovich and Spiegel, 2016). The most common type of idiopathic scoliosis is found in adolescents, and it is the major focus of the remaining discussion.

Small to moderate scoliotic curves (10% to 30%) usually do not increase significantly after skeletal growth is complete but they bear watching, particularly during periods of rapid growth. Double-S and more severe curves are more likely to progress during the growth years. For a given child, however, it is difficult to predict progression because even small curves (10% to 25%) can progress to severe deformity. Regular monitoring of any curve in a skeletally immature child by the provider is important (Table 43.2).

The female:male ratio increases with increasing curve magnitude. For curves less than 20 degrees, the risk for progression is low; these curves generally need only to be observed. However, for curves between 20 and 45 degrees, the risk for progression is high during growth, and early intervention is of paramount importance. In children with curves greater than 50 degrees, the spine loses its ability to compensate and progression is expected. Young premenarchal females with large curves are a vulnerable group because their spines are skeletally immature, with growth remaining. The majority of adolescents with idiopathic scoliosis have a right thoracic curve. Juvenile manifestation is uncommon, and infantile scoliosis is rare in the United States.

Clinical Findings

History. Scoliosis is generally painless and insidious onset is typical. Generally there is no significant history. The provider should assess the following:
- Family history of scoliosis
- Age of menarche
- Etiologic factors related to the various causes of structural scoliosis

The presence of pain with a lateral curvature of the spine suggests an inflammatory or neoplastic lesion as the cause of the scoliosis. Some children with idiopathic scoliosis complain of mild pain that is activity-related. Severe, constant, or night pain and point tenderness can be indicative of other pathologic conditions (e.g., metastatic tumor or stenosis) and warrants further investigation.

Physical Examination. Children of all ages should be evaluated in the standing position, from both the front and the side, to identify any asymmetry. Looking primarily at the straightness of the spine can be misleading because scoliosis involves both rotation and misalignment of the vertebrae. The Adams forward bend position accentuates the rotational deformity of scoliosis. Asymmetries to look for include:
- Unequal shoulder height.
- Unequal scapular prominences and heights: Note that the muscle masses may be somewhat unequal, especially if the

child uses one shoulder more than the other, as in carrying books. Look for bony, not muscular, prominence.

- Unequal waist angles: The hip touches one arm and the contralateral arm hangs free.
- Unequal rib prominences and chest asymmetry.
- Asymmetry of the elbow-to-flank distance and some deviation of the spine from a straight head-to-toe line.
- Unequal rib heights when the child stands in the Adams forward bend position (see Fig 43.8).

During the Adams test the examiner looks for asymmetry of the posterior chest wall on forward bending, the earliest abnormality seen. Rotation of the vertebral bodies toward the convexity results in outward rotation and prominence of the attached ribs posteriorly. The anterior chest wall may be flattened on the concavity due to inward rotation of the chest wall and ribs. Associated findings may include elevation of the shoulder, lateral shift of the trunk, and an apparent leg-length discrepancy.

Congenital scoliosis may be visible in the infant lying prone; it is sometimes more prominent if the infant is suspended prone. Inspect for skin abnormalities, sacral dimple, and hairy patches.

The physical examination should also include the following:

- Observation for equal leg lengths
- Examination of the skin for hairy patches, nevi, café-au-lait spots, lipomas, dimples
- Neurologic examination checking for weakness or sensory disturbance
- Cardiac examination with diagnosis of Marfan syndrome

Diagnostic Studies. Standing AP and lateral radiographs of the entire spine are recommended at the initial evaluation of patients with clinical findings suggestive of a spinal deformity. On the PA radiographs, the degree of curvature is determined by the Cobb method. An MRI is helpful when an underlying cause of the scoliosis is suspected based on age (infantile and juvenile curves), abnormal findings in the history and on physical examination, and atypical radiographic features. The latter include uncommon curve patterns, such as the left thoracic curve, double thoracic curves, high thoracic curves, widening of the spinal canal, and erosive or dysplastic changes in the vertebral body or ribs. On the lateral radiograph, an increase in thoracic kyphosis or absence of segmental lordosis may be suggestive of an underlying neurologic abnormality (Mistovich and Spiegel, 2016).

Differential Diagnosis. Structural scoliosis must be differentiated from functional scoliosis. The latter disappears when the child is placed in the Adams forward bend position, whereas the former is enhanced in this position. Persistent functional scoliosis to one side in a child with a neuromotor problem can eventually become structural and must be managed with physical therapy or other means to prevent progression. Consider systemic problems (e.g., neurofibromatosis, cerebral palsy, multiple sclerosis, Rett syndrome, rickets, tuberculosis, and tumor).

Management. The primary aim of scoliosis management is to stop the progression of curvature and improve pulmonary function. Treatment options include observation, bracing, and surgery. The management presented in this text addresses idiopathic scoliosis. Of note, genetic testing is available to provide a personalized treatment approach for selected patients diagnosed with adolescent idiopathic scoliosis. The ScoliScore is a genetic test that screens for more than 50 genetic markers (53 single nucleotide polymorphisms [SNPs]) linked to the progression of spinal curves and assigns a quantitative score to a patient's deoxyribonucleic acid (DNA) saliva sample. (See discussion of SNPs in Chapter 3.) The score identifies the patient as having a low, medium, or high risk for curve progression (Bohl et al., 2016). For children in the low-risk group, these prognostic data may lead to less frequent follow-up visits to specialists, avoiding or discontinuing bracing, and fewer radiologic tests. Combined with diagnostic information and clinical judgment, the results of the ScoliScore test can serve as a guide for healthcare providers to optimize the treatment of scoliosis.

Idiopathic Scoliosis

Adolescent scoliosis can resolve, remain static, or increase. Treatment decisions are based on the natural history of each curvature. Infantile scoliosis can resolve spontaneously; however, progressive curves require bracing and surgery in an attempt to slow the curve progression and prevent complications (e.g., thoracic insufficiency syndrome). Juvenile scoliosis is found more frequently in girls; such curves are at high risk for progression and often require surgical intervention. The treatment goal is to delay spinal fusion, allowing time for the pulmonary system and thoracic cage to have matured and maximal trunk height to be achieved. (See the various surgical procedures described in the following section.) The natural history includes the degree of skeletal maturity or growth remaining, the magnitude of the curve, and any associated diagnoses or medical conditions.

Observation is always indicated for curves less than 20 degrees. Bracing or surgery may be indicated for larger curves. Brace treatment may reduce the need for surgery, restore the sagittal profile, and change vertebral rotation. Indications for bracing are a curve of more than 30 degrees. Additional indications for brace therapy include skeletally immature patients with curves of 20 to 25 degrees that have shown more than 5 degrees of progression. The efficacy of bracing for adolescent idiopathic scoliosis remains controversial. Some studies show brace treatment to be effective in preventing progression; however, it has been found that the success of treatment is proportional to the amount of time that the patient wears the brace. Various brace treatment protocols suggest wearing a brace as much as 23 hours per day; therefore compliance is a significant factor for this treatment modality (Gomez et al., 2016).

Surgical treatment is indicated for children and adolescents who do not respond to bracing and for those with curvature exceeding 45 to 50 degrees (Richards et al., 2014). There are various surgical procedures; all aim to control progressive curvatures. In the past, surgery was limited to arthrodesis (surgical fusion) of the spine.

In recent years several procedures have been developed that are designed to postpone and, in some cases, eliminate the need for early spinal fusion and allow for growth. These include the vertical expandable prosthetic titanium rib (VEPTR). This procedure is indicated for children with restricted pulmonary function due to the curvature of the thoracic spine. The surgery involves implanting a prosthesis that serves to enlarge the constricted thorax. The prosthesis can be adjusted approximately every 4 to 6 months, thereby allowing for growth. The "growing rod" is another surgical procedure that has shown success in patients with adolescent idiopathic scoliosis and involves inserting spinal rods that are used to exert distraction forces that are adjusted approximately every 6 months. The rods serve as an internal brace to control the curvature of the spine while allowing skeletal growth. A more recent procedure involves intervertebral spinal stapling or tethering. Unlike the VEPTR and rod procedures, intervertebral spinal stapling does not require repeat adjustments and therefore eliminates the need for repeat surgical procedures. Research on this technique is limited, and clinical indications have not been universally agreed upon. Further research is necessary and long-term results are yet to be determined.

Referral to an orthopedist or a center that specializes in working with infants and children with scoliosis is essential. Support must be given to the child and family through the diagnostic and treatment phases, considering school and peer factors. PCPs must help the child with psychologic adjustment issues that arise if bracing or surgery is recommended and instituted. Some specific concerns of the child can include self-esteem problems, managing hostility and anger, learning about the disease and its care, wondering about the long-term prognosis, and concerns about clothing and participation in sports and other activities.

Complications. Progressive scoliosis can result in a severe deformity of the spinal column and cause deformities so severe that they impair both respiratory and cardiovascular function, limit physical activities, and impair comfort. The psychologic consequences of an untreated scoliosis deformity can be immense.

Prevention. Prevention is not possible; however, screening and early identification of children with scoliosis may help avoid more expensive, invasive care and prevent the potential long-term consequences of the disorder. However, screening is effective only if the identified children are referred for care. Parents must be notified, a referral arranged, and follow-up ensured.

Kyphosis

The thoracic spine normally has between 20 and 45 degrees of posterior curvature, which is considered physiologic. *Kyphosis* describes the condition when the normal posterior curvature of the thoracic spine becomes excessive or exaggerated and is outside the physiologic range of normal. With kyphosis there is an AP forward curve of the thoracic spine with the apex posterior (i.e., the back is prominent). The most common clinical type of kyphosis is postural (postural round back). The curvature of the spinal column points backward and, when viewed from the side, gives the appearance of a humpback. In postural kyphosis, the Adams forward bend test demonstrates normalization of the lateral spine profile when viewed from the side (see Table 43.2) and the child can reverse the round-back appearance with active extension. Postural kyphosis is the most common type and is more often seen in girls than in boys. It rarely causes pain and the curvature is flexible.

Scheuermann kyphosis is an osteochondrosis that presents as an abnormality of the vertebral epiphyseal growth plates. Onset generally occurs in adolescence. The kyphosis is rigid; the pain is located over the deformity and is worse at the end of the day. Scheuermann kyphosis is defined by vertebral wedging of 5 degrees or more on three adjacent vertebral bodies visualized on a standing lateral radiograph of the thoracic and lumbar spine. Associated radiographic findings include irregularities of the vertebral end plates, disk-space narrowing, and herniation of the intervertebral disk penetrating into the vertebral body (Mistovich and Spiegel, 2016).

Management. Depending on the cause and severity of the kyphosis, there are a variety of treatment options. Postural kyphosis may be improved with an exercise and physical therapy program that strengthens the supporting muscles. Activities (such as, dancing or swimming) that require a full range of motion of the shoulders, back, and arms can be helpful. Adolescent kyphosis may be treated with a combination of a back brace, exercise, and physical therapy. Surgery may be required in children with

structural problems that cause kyphosis and in adolescents with curvature of the back that exceeds 50 to 60 degrees. Kyphosis caused by infections or tumors may also require surgery.

Lumbar Lordosis

Lumbar lordosis, or hyperlordosis, is an AP curve of the lumbar area of the spine (i.e., the child stands with the abdomen and buttocks protuberant). It is the least common of the congenital spinal deformities and is often associated with kyphosis or scoliosis. Congenital lordosis deformity is usually progressive. Lordosis can be a secondary result of a hip problem in which full extension is limited by hip flexion contractures or from lumbosacral deformities.

Management. If the PCP suspects lumbar lordosis, have the child bend forward. If the lumbar spine flattens and the lordosis disappears in the forward bending position, it indicates that the spine is flexible and the lordosis is only physiologic. This child should be seen for follow-up in 6 to 12 months, and the examination should be repeated to make sure that continued physiologic findings are obtained. If the lordosis persists in the forward bending position, this indicates a fixed structural deformity and needs referral to an orthopedist. Lordosis resulting from hip flexion contractures is absent while sitting; it is commonly seen in children with cerebral palsy, spina bifida, and developmental dysplasia of the hip (see Table 43.2).

Developmental Dysplasia of the Hip

Developmental dysplasia of the hip (DDH) represents a spectrum of anatomic abnormalities in which the femoral head and acetabulum are in improper alignment and/or grow abnormally. This includes dysplastic, subluxated, dislocatable, and dislocated hips. Dysplasia is characterized by a shallow, more vertical acetabular socket with an immature hip/acetabulum. In subluxation, the hip is unstable and the head of the femur can slide in and out of the acetabulum. DDH occurs congenitally or develops in infancy or childhood. Dysplasia may be diagnosed many years after the newborn period.

The incidence of DDH is estimated to range from 1.5 to 20 per 1000 live births in the United States. It is found more commonly with breech births and is four times more common in girls than in boys. A positive family history (genetic risk factors) increases the risk for having a child with this problem. Other risk factors associated with DDH that are seen in infants include oligohydramnios, torticollis, and lower limb deformities (e.g., clubfoot, MA, and dislocated knee) (Tamai, 2018).

Physiologic, mechanical, and genetic factors are implicated in DDH. Physiologic factors include the hormonal effect of maternal estrogen and relaxin, which are released near delivery and produce a temporary laxity of the hip joint. Mechanical factors include constant compression in utero with restriction of movement late in gestation if the fetal pelvis becomes locked in the maternal pelvis. This is seen with first pregnancy, oligohydramnios, and breech presentation.

In the unstable hip, the femoral head and acetabulum may not have a normal tight, concentric anatomic relationship, which can lead to abnormal growth of the hip joint and result in permanent disability. In the newborn, the left hip is most often involved because this hip typically is the one in a forced adduction position against the mother's sacrum.

The hip can dislocate noncongenitally or in utero in children with certain muscular or neurologic disorders that affect the use of the lower extremities, such as cerebral palsy, arthrogryposis, or myelomeningocele. Dislocation results from the abnormal use of the extremity over time.

Clinical Findings

History. Risk factors for DDH include female gender, family history, high birth weight, breech positioning, and in utero postural deformities (Tamai, 2018).

Physical Examination. A hip examination should be performed on children as part of their well-child supervision until the child begins to walk (Krader, 2017). Findings of DDH include the following:

- Routine examinations of the hips and lower extremities until the infant is walking. The Barlow and Ortolani tests are used to screen for DDH in neonates. Once an infant reaches the second and third months of life, the soft tissue surrounding the hips begins to tighten and the Barlow and Ortolani tests are less reliable. The Klisic and Galeazzi tests are used to screen older infants. Routine ultrasonography is not recommended; however, an ultrasound should be obtained if there is a high index of suspicion of dysplasia based on a positive clinical examination.
- Some 60% to 80% of abnormal hips of newborns identified by physical examination resolve by 2 to 8 weeks.
- In the older infant 6 to 18 months of age,
  - Limited abduction of the affected hip and shortening of the thigh (unequal leg lengths) are reliable signs (see Figs 43.3B and 43.5).
  - Normal abduction with comfort is 70 to 80 degrees bilaterally. Limited abduction includes those cases with less than 60 degrees of abduction or unequal abduction from one side to the other (see Fig 43.5).
  - There should be a positive Galeazzi sign (see Fig 43.3A).
- Other findings include asymmetry of inguinal or gluteal folds (thigh fold asymmetry is not related to the disorder [see Fig 43.3D]) and unequal leg lengths, shorter on the affected side.

In the ambulatory child who was not diagnosed earlier or was not corrected, the following might also be noted:

- Short leg with toe walking on the affected side
- Positive Trendelenburg sign (see Fig 43.3C)
- Marked lordosis or toe walking
- Painless limping or waddling gait with child leaning to the affected side

If the hips are dislocated bilaterally, asymmetries are not observed. Limited abduction is the primary finding on examination (see Fig 43.5). Also in subluxation of the hip (not frankly dislocated), limited abduction again is the primary indicator. A waddling gait may also be noted.

Diagnostic Studies. Ultrasound is superior to radiographs for evaluating cartilaginous structures and is recommended when the infant reaches 6 weeks of age. Use of ultrasonography prior to 6 weeks has a high incidence of false-positive results (Krader, 2017). Ultrasound is used to assess the relationship of the femur to the acetabulum and provides dynamic information about acetabular development and stability of the hip. Radiologic evaluation of the newborn to detect and evaluate DDH is recommended once the proximal epiphysis ossifies, usually by 4 to 6 months (Hryhorczuk et al., 2016). Radiography prior to this is unreliable, because so much of the hip joint is cartilaginous in the young infant. AP and lateral Lauenstein (frog-leg) position radiographs of the pelvis are indicated.

Management. The goal of management is to restore the articulation of the femur within the acetabulum. Most neonatal hip instability findings resolve spontaneously by 6 to 8 weeks.

However, close observations of these infants is recommended. Any infant with persistently abnormal findings on physical examination requires prompt referral to an orthopedist.

- Refer infant to an orthopedist if the newborn exam is positive. Follow up the newborn exam again at 2 weeks of age with a thorough hip examination to check for DDH. If the exam is positive or inconclusive, refer the infant to an orthopedist (Krader, 2017).
- Refer infant if limited or asymmetric hip abduction is noted at 4 weeks or older.
- For infants less than 6 months of age with a normal DDH examination and a history of breech presentation in the third trimester, previous clinical hip instability, improper swaddling, or a positive family history (including a close relative with hip replacement for dysplasia at <40 years of age), or parental concern, imaging is an option (Krader, 2017).
- Most neonatal hip instability resolves spontaneously by 6 to 8 weeks of age. Close observation of these children is recommended.
- The treatment of choice for persistent subluxation and reducible dislocations identified in the early phase is a Pavlik harness. The harness is applied with hips having greater than 90 degrees of flexion and with adduction of the hip limited to a neutral position. Radiographic or ultrasound documentation can be used during treatment to verify the position of the hip. If the infant does not respond to treatment with the harness, surgical treatment may be needed.
- The earlier treatment is started with the Pavlik harness, the better the prognosis for a successful outcome. The harness is worn 24 hours a day except for bathing. The infant with a Pavlik harness should be seen weekly to make sure that it fits properly, to identify complications associated with the use of the harness (e.g., avascular necrosis and femoral nerve palsy), and to ensure that the femur is properly seated in the socket. Ultrasonography can be performed while the Pavlik harness is worn to assess hip reduction and acetabular development. The length of time the harness is worn depends on the age of the infant, when it was applied, and whether reduction is successful. Generally the harness is worn full time for 3 to 6 weeks and then may be required only during waking hours for decreasing periods of time.
- For a child in a Pavlik harness or spica cast, cast care, skin care, and car safety when the child cannot easily be placed in a car seat are issues to be addressed. The child needs special attention to maintain developmental stimulation while immobilized. An orthopedist should be immediately consulted for any infant seen in a primary care setting who is in a Pavlik harness and exhibits excessive hip flexion (beyond 100 degrees) or abduction (beyond 60 degrees).
- The 6- to 18-month-old infant with a dislocated hip is likely to require either closed manipulation or open reduction. Preoperative traction, adductor tenotomy, and gentle reduction are especially helpful in preventing osteonecrosis of the femoral head. After the closed or open reduction, a hip spica cast is applied in order to maintain the hip in more than 90 degrees of flexion and avoid excessive internal or external rotation. Triple diapering is no longer recommended as musculoskeletal forces far outweigh the force that can be exerted by the diaper material.
- Annual or biennial follow-up including radiographs to the point of skeletal maturity is recommended to evaluate for the possibility of late asymmetric epiphyseal closure (Tamai, 2018). Support the child and family through the treatment phases and explain management goals clearly.

Complications. The Pavlik harness and other positional devices may cause skin irritation, and a difference in leg length may remain. There may be delay in walking if the child is put in a body cast. The long-term outcomes depend on the age at diagnosis, severity of the joint deformity, and effectiveness of therapy. Untreated cases may result in a permanent dislocation of the femoral head so that it lies just under the iliac crest posteriorly. Clinically the child has limited mobility of this pseudojoint and related short leg. Forceful reduction can result in avascular necrosis of the femoral head with permanent hip deformity. Redislocation or persistent dysplasia can occur. Adult degenerative arthritis is associated with acetabular dysplasia. Charting should always include notation about hip findings, because these can change during growth and development in infants and children.

Prevention. The condition cannot be prevented, but early identification resulting in early treatment significantly reduces its long-term consequences. Screening of all neonates and infants should include full hip abduction; examination for unequal inguinal and gluteal folds and unequal leg lengths; and Barlow, Ortolani, and Galeazzi maneuvers at every examination. The hip can dislocate at any point in early development, even up to the point of first ambulation. In older children, limited abduction, gait, and standing position, including the Trendelenburg position, add important information.

Legg-Calvé-Perthes Disease

LCPD is a childhood hip disorder that results in infarction of the bony epiphysis of the femoral head. It presents as avascular necrosis of the femoral head. The basic underlying cause is insufficient blood supply to the femoral head. There is an initial ischemic episode of unknown etiology that interrupts vascular circulation to the capital femoral epiphysis. The articular cartilage hypertrophies, and the epiphyseal marrow becomes necrotic. The area revascularizes, and the necrotic bone is replaced by new bone. This process can take 18 to 24 months. There is a critical point in these dual processes when the subchondral area becomes weak enough that fracture of the epiphysis occurs. At this time the child becomes symptomatic. With fracturing, further reabsorption and replacement by fibrous bone occurs, and the shape of the femoral head is altered. Articulation of the head in the hip joint is interrupted. The bone reossifies with or without treatment; without treatment, the femoral head flattens and enlarges, causing joint deformity. Lateral subluxation of the femoral head is associated with poor outcomes.

Etiology is unclear, but certain risk factors have been identified in children. These include gender, socioeconomic group, and the presence of an inguinal hernia and genitourinary tract anomalies. Boys are affected three to five times more often than girls; incidence increases in lower socioeconomic groups and in children with low birth weights. The disease is bilateral in 10% to 20% of children. It affects children 4 to 8 years of age.

Clinical Findings

History. There can be an acute or chronic onset with or without a history of trauma to the hip, such as jumping from a high place.

- The most common presenting sign is an intermittent limp (abductor lurch), especially after exertion, with mild or intermittent pain.
- The most frequent complaint is persistent pain in the groin, anterior hip region, or laterally around the greater trochanter.

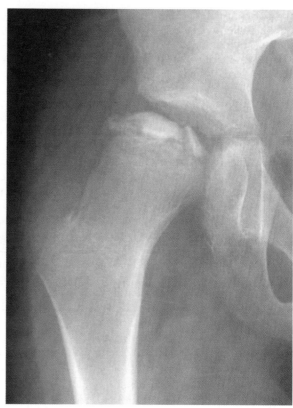

● **Fig 43.10** Anteroposterior (AP) radiograph of the right hip of an 8-year-old boy with Legg-Calvé-Perthes disease (LCPD). There is a collapsed yet dense capital femoral epiphysis with early fragmentation. The small medial triangle of the capital femoral epiphysis is uninvolved in the disease process. (From Behrman RE, Kliegman RM, Jenson HB, eds. *Nelson Textbook of Pediatrics*. 17th ed. Philadelphia: Saunders; 2004.)

- Pain may be referred to the medial aspect of the ipsilateral knee or to the anterior thigh.
- Some children may report limited range of motion of the affected extremity.

Physical Examination. Findings may include:

- Antalgic gait with limited hip movement
- Trendelenburg gait resulting from pain in the gluteus medius muscle
- Muscle spasm
- Atrophy of gluteus, quadriceps, and hamstring muscles
- Decreased abduction, internal rotation, and extension of the hip
- Adduction flexion contracture
- Pain on rolling the leg internally

Diagnostic Studies. Routine AP pelvis and frog-leg lateral views are used to confirm the diagnosis, stage the disease, and follow disease progression and response to treatment. Radiographic findings can include smaller epiphyses, increased epiphyseal density, a subchondral fracture line, lateralization of the femoral head, and other features. Changes in the epiphyseal margin are discerned by the orthopedist and radiologist (Fig 43.10). There may be no radiographic findings early in LCPD. Ultrasonography is useful in the preliminary diagnosis; capsular distention can be seen on sonographic images. Bone scans and MRI allow for precise localization of the bone involvement, but changes seen as bone marrow edema and joint effusions are nonspecific. CT is not typically used on a routine basis to evaluate patients with LCPD (Kim and Herring, 2014).

Differential Diagnosis. Acute and chronic infections, sickle cell disease, toxic synovitis, Gaucher disease, slipped capital femoral epiphysis (SCFE), osteomyelitis, juvenile idiopathic arthritis, hemophilia, and neoplasm are included in the differential diagnosis.

Management.
- Referral to an orthopedist is required for the management of LCPD. There are various approaches to the management, and treatment remains controversial. The general approach is guided by the principle of containment of the femoral head within the acetabulum. To be successful, containment must be instituted while the femoral head is still moldable. Nonoperative containment can be achieved in a variety of ways including activity limitation, protected weight-bearing, use of NSAIDs and physical therapy to maintain hip motion, and bed rest with traction, or casting to maintain hip abduction. Surgical approaches involve pelvic and femoral osteotomies of the proximal femur or pelvis.
- Support and monitor the child throughout treatment and recovery, including during interruption of school or other activities. Treatment and monitoring of LCPD requires long-term follow-up.

Complications. The condition is not preventable; however, early identification and treatment reduce its long-term complications, such as premature degenerative osteoarthritis related to femoral head deformity in early adult life. Decreased use of the hip joint may occur, depending on the femoral head's remodeling status. Older children have a poorer prognosis owing to the decreased opportunity for femoral head remodeling in the remaining growth period. Females with LCPD also have a poorer prognosis.

Slipped Capital Femoral Epiphysis

SCFE is a Salter-Harris type I fracture through the proximal femoral physis. Stress around the hip causes a shear force to be applied at the growth plate. Although trauma may play a role in the fracture, there is an intrinsic weakness in the physeal cartilage. The fracture occurs at the hypertrophic zone of the physeal cartilage. Stress on the hip causes the epiphysis to displace posteriorly and inferiorly to the metaphysis. Because the blood supply to the epiphysis crosses the weakened area, the epiphysis is at risk for avascular necrosis. The slippage is generally gradual, and the condition is categorized as stable or unstable based on the child's ability to bear weight (POSNA, 2018).

SCFE typically occurs just after the onset of puberty, often in overweight and slightly skeletally immature boys. Obesity alters the level of circulating hormones and affects the mechanical load on the physis. SCFE is also seen in children in whom puberty is delayed. African American children are affected slightly more than others. The incidence is slightly greater in boys than in girls. In children younger than 10 years of age, SCFE is associated with hypothyroidism, panhypopituitarism, hypogonadism, renal osteodystrophy, and growth hormone abnormalities (Sankar et al., 2016).

Clinical Findings. Clinical presentation is often misleading, in which case it can result in delay of diagnosis and treatment.

History
- A vague history of antecedent trauma.
- Pain in affected hip, groin, thigh, or knee.
- Some have complaints of limping or gait abnormalities.

Physical Examination

- Overweight or obesity is a major characteristic for boys and to a lesser extent for girls (Herngren, Stenmarker, Vavruch, Hagglund, 2017).
- Delayed puberty.
- Pain in the groin or diffusely over the knee or anterior thigh
- Pain and decreased internal rotation.
- Antalgic limp with a short leg component (50% are up to 1 inch shorter on the affected side).
- As the epiphysis continues to slip, there may be a more pronounced limping and external rotation of the toes when the patient is walking.
- External rotation of the thigh when the hip is flexed; lack of internal rotation of the hip with range of motion.
- Mild atrophy of the thigh and gluteal muscles.
- Limited abduction and extension.
- With unstable SCFE, the child is unable to bear weight.

Diagnostic Studies. Plain radiography is often the only imaging modality needed to diagnose and evaluate SCFE (Herring, 2014b). AP pelvis, frog-leg lateral, and true lateral views of the pelvis are obtained. Radiographic findings include flattening of the epiphyseal prominence, widening or irregularity of the growth plate, and narrowing of the area if the epiphysis has slipped posteriorly (Fig 43.11). Radiographically, the slippage is measured using the Southwick method and can be classified as mild (<33% slippage of the epiphysis or less than a 30-degree slip angle), moderate (30% to 50% slippage of the epiphysis or 30- to 50-degree slip angle), or severe (>50% slippage of the epiphysis or >50-degree slip angle).

Differential Diagnosis. LCPD, sepsis of the hip joint, and osteoarthritis should be considered.

Management. Treatment modalities aim to prevent further slippage by stabilizing the epiphysis and avoiding complications, such as osteonecrosis and chondrolysis (Peck and Herrera-Soto, 2014).
- Refer immediately to an orthopedic surgeon.
- Place child on crutches or in a wheelchair. Non–weight bearing must be emphasized to prevent further slippage. Once the diagnosis has been made, the child should immediately be admitted to the hospital and placed on bed rest.
  Standard treatment for a stable SCFE involves percutaneous pinning and placement of a single cannulated screw through the femoral neck into the central aspect of the proximal femoral epiphysis (Sankar et al., 2016).
- There is a high incidence of contralateral SCFE within 6 to 12 months. The hip or hips must be monitored until skeletal maturity has been achieved.
- Support and monitor the child throughout the treatment phase, which includes adherence to partial weight bearing with the use of crutches for approximately 4 to 6 weeks and a gradual return to normal activities. Contact sports are usually restricted by the orthopedist until growth is complete.

Complications. The two most severe complications of SCFE are avascular necrosis and chondrolysis. Avascular necrosis is loss of blood supply to the proximal femoral physis, resulting in death of a portion of the bone. It is the most serious complication and has a higher incidence if the slip is severe or unstable. Chondrolysis is acute cartilage necrosis and represents a loss of articular cartilage.

Prevention. SCFE is not a preventable condition. However, identification of the condition during the period preceding the slip allows early intervention to prevent deformity and long-term sequelae (e.g., premature degenerative arthritis). If the child is overweight, advise about the need for weight reduction.

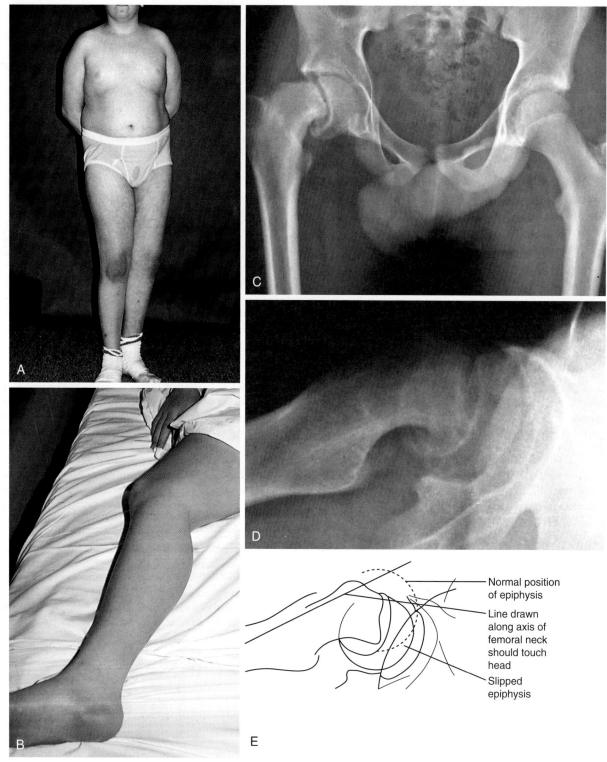

• **Fig 43.11** Slipped Capital Femoral Epiphysis. (A) Obese boy with a painful limp and reluctance to bear weight on his right leg. (B) In supine position, right leg is in external rotation to minimize discomfort. (C) An anteroposterior radiograph shows the right femoral head displaced medially to the femoral neck. (D) Lateral view shows the femoral head displaced posteriorly to the femoral neck. (E) A line drawn along the axis of the femoral neck normally touches the head. (From Basil Z, McIntire S. *Zitelli and Davis' Atlas of Pediatric Physical Diagnosis.* 6th ed. Philadelphia: Saunders/Elsevier; 2013.)

Femoral Anteversion

Femoral anteversion is a condition in which the head and neck of the femur are rotated at an increased angle anteriorly in relation to the femoral shaft, resulting in an in-toeing gait. Younger children have a somewhat wider angle. During infancy, the degree of anteversion is approximately 40 degrees; it decreases with skeletal maturity (Herring, 2014a). An in-toeing gait is most noticeable in children 3 to 6 years of age and is considered normal. By 10 to 12 years of age, the normal angle (10 to 15 degrees) of anteversion is seen. Femoral anteversion is also called *internal femoral torsion,* the etiology of which is unknown and controversial. Some attribute a worsening of the condition to sitting in a "W" position, whereas others believe the anteversion is congenital and is not altered by position. A family history is often identified, and it occurs more commonly in girls than boys (2:1).

Clinical Findings

History
- In-toeing gait, most noticeable with running
- Runs awkwardly; may actually trip or fall as a result of crossing the feet while walking or running
- Possible family history
- History of "W" sitting

Physical Examination
- In-toeing gait with patellas medial
- Internal (medial) rotation normally less than 70 degrees (mild deformity, 70 to 80 degrees; moderate, 80 to 90 degrees; severe, >90 degrees [see Fig 43.7])
- External (lateral) rotation decreased (limited to 0 to 10 degrees)
- Knees medially rotated ("kissing patella") when standing

Diagnostic Studies. Radiographs are not merited unless surgery is contemplated.

Differential Diagnosis. Consider other rotational deformities, such as internal tibial torsion or MA. Cerebral palsy with a "scissoring gait" might be mistaken for severe femoral anteversion.

Management. Inform the family that femoral anteversion is not harmful and there are no known serious consequences to the condition. Management includes observation of the child and referral to an orthopedist if medial rotations are significant (no external rotation of the hip in extension) or the child or family has significant concerns. Nonoperative management strategies (such as shoe modifications, twister cables, and night splints) are ineffective. Operative correction is successful but carries the risk of complications. Osteotomy is rarely performed and is done only in the child older than 8 years of age with significant cosmetic and functional deformity. The natural history of the condition is for the medial, or internal, rotation to decrease, providing some improvement.

Complications. Studies have shown that the condition does not cause flatfoot, bunions, knee problems, back difficulties, difficulties in running, or degenerative arthritis of the hip in adults. It is primarily a cosmetic problem unless it is severe enough to interfere with activities. Self-esteem can be affected in severe cases.

Prevention. Excessive femoral anteversion cannot be prevented. Studies have shown that in-toeing is usually but not always self-correcting and is not prevented or improved with special shoes, braces, or exercises (Herring, 2014a).

Genu Varum

Genu varum, or bowing of the legs, can be a physiologic or developmental variation of normal or a pathologic condition that involves

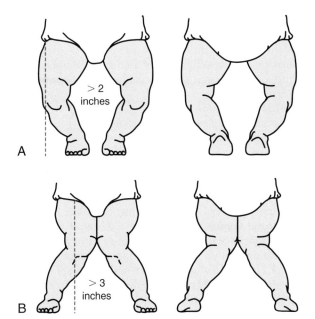

• **Fig 43.12** Genu Varum and Genu Valgum. In genu varum (A), the knees are tilted away from the midline; the intercondylar (knee) distance with the ankles together is then measured. In genu valgum (B), the knees are tilted toward the midline; the intermalleolar distance with the knees approximated is then measured.

a rotational deformity (Fig 43.12). The term *bowlegs* is used to describe physiologic variations of the normal knee angle, resulting in bowing of legs that is typically seen in children up to 2 years of age, but it can be considered normal until 3 years of age. The typical pattern of normal bowing seen in children is a symmetric lateral bowing of both tibias in the first year followed by bowlegs in the second year. Most bowing resolves spontaneously but can also progress to persistent or pathologic varus. The angle between the tibia and femur is pronounced in varus (up to 15 degrees) in normal children before 1 year of age. This is considered an in utero positioning effect. The angle approaches neutral by 18 months of age and then proceeds to a valgus angle, with an average angle of 12 degrees from 2 to 3 years of age. The angle then gradually decreases to 8 degrees in females and 7 degrees in males by adulthood. If the varus angle is greater than 15 degrees in infants, does not begin to decrease in the second year, is asymmetric, is associated with short stature, or is rapidly progressing, the condition is considered pathologic.

If the varus persists after 30 months of age or increases, it may represent Blount disease, rickets, tumor, neurologic problems, infection, or other conditions. A Salter fracture through the tibial growth plate can result in later genu varum as growth across the plate progresses unevenly.

With Blount disease (idiopathic tibia vara that affects the proximal tibia), there is abnormal growth of the medial aspect of the proximal tibial epiphysis that results in progressive varus angulation of the tibia. Blount disease is rare, but it can occur in infancy (18 months to 3 years of age), during the school years (4 to 10 years of age), and during adolescence (11 years of age and older). It is seen more frequently in African American, Hispanic, and Scandinavian populations, is associated with obesity and early walkers, and commonly has a positive family history. Onset in infancy presents the highest risk for greatest deformity (Stevens, 2017).

Clinical Findings

History. Family history is important because certain heritable conditions—Marfan syndrome, OI, or vitamin D–resistant rickets—may predispose a child to this condition. Additional history may include progression since birth. Increasing deformation is problematic.

Physical Examination

- Tibial-femoral angle greater than 15 degrees.
- Associated internal tibial torsion.
- Lower extremity length discrepancy.
- Intercondylar (knees) distance with the ankles together—measurement greater than 4 to 5 inches suggests the need for additional evaluation.
- Joint laxity of lateral collateral ligaments in older children.

Diagnostic Studies. The standard radiograph for the older child is a weight-bearing AP of the lower extremities with the patellas facing forward and a lateral radiograph of the involved extremity. Note the femur and tibia length and diaphyseal deformities. The mechanical axis is a line drawn from the center of the head of the femur to the center of the ankle; this line should bisect the knee (Stevens, 2017). In physiologic bowing, the deformity is gentle and symmetric, with a metaphyseal-diaphyseal angle less than 11 degrees and normal appearance of the proximal tibial growth plate. In Blount disease the bowing is asymmetric, abrupt, and with sharp angulation; the metaphyseal-diaphyseal angle is greater than 11 degrees; and there is medial sloping of the epiphysis and widening of the physis (Baldwin and Wells, 2016).

Differential Diagnosis. Physiologic, persistent, and pathologic genu varum, metabolic (rickets), neurologic problems, Blount disease, infections, tumor, osteochondrodysplasias, and internal tibial torsion should be ruled out.

Management

In physiologic genu varum (no increasing deformity), the following apply:

- No active treatment; spontaneous resolution is expected. Corrective shoes and splinting are unnecessary.
- Reassure parents; provide information about the natural progression of the problem.
- Observe the child's condition over time (in 3 to 6 months) to be sure the problem is resolving, especially during the second year of life. Serial photographs of the legs can be helpful.

Indications for orthopedic evaluation of genu varum include the following:

- Family history of pathologic bowing
- Asymmetric deformity: unilateral bowing, gait abnormalities, leg-length discrepancy
- Short stature (height <25th percentile)
- Late walking (>18 months of age)
- Blount varus angulation/increasing deformity
- Progressive varus deformity after 18 months of age
- Presentation at 24 months or later (Dettling and Weiner, 2017)

In pathologic genu varum (increasing deformity), the following apply:

- Blount disease may be treated with bracing in children younger than 3 years of age. Bracing is effective and can prevent progression in 50% of these children. In children older than 4 years of age, a proximal tibial valgus osteotomy and associated fibular diaphyseal osteotomy are the procedures of choice.

- Monitor to be sure braces are used consistently, with good fit.
- Observe to be sure the problem is not worsening.

Complications. Knee degeneration and deformity result if pathologic genu varum is not treated. Early identification and referral reduce the complexity and expense of treatment and residual deformities.

Genu Valgum

Genu valgum also referred to as *knock knees* (see Fig 43.12), is a common orthopedic condition in children. Lower extremity alignment goes through a predictable progression from varus to valgus over the first 6 years of life. Causes of genu valgum include physiologic and pathologic processes. Physiologic genu valgum improves spontaneously between 4 and 6 years of age. Pathologic conditions leading to valgus are rickets, renal osteodystrophy, skeletal dysplasia, posttraumatic physeal arrest, tumors, and infection (Baldwin and Wells, 2016).

Clinical Findings

History

- Progression of the deformity.
- Joint pains or stiff gait.
- Older child may report knee pain due to the stretching of the medial aspect of the knee.

Physical Examination

- Bilateral tibial-femoral angle less than 15 degrees of valgus in the child up to 6 years of age is considered normal; a valgus angle greater than 15 degrees is outside the range of normal.
- Unilateral deformity.
- Awkwardness of gait.
- Sublaxating patella.
- Intermalleolar (ankles) distance with knees together: Measurement greater than 4 to 5 inches suggests the need for additional evaluation.
- Short stature: genu valgum associated with short stature should be referred.

Diagnostic Studies. No radiographic studies are needed unless a pathologic condition is suspected. Long-length AP radiographs of the leg in a weight-bearing stance are used for preoperative planning.

Differential Diagnosis. Rule out pathologic conditions of genu valgum.

Management. Deformities greater than 15 degrees and occurring after 6 years of age are unlikely to correct with growth and require surgical intervention. In the skeletally immature, medial tibial epiphyseal hemiepiphysiodesis or stapling are common surgical approaches. In the skeletally mature, osteotomy is often necessary (Neral and Liu, 2019). Early identification and referral reduce the complexity and expense of treatment and residual deformities.

Tibial Torsion

Tibial torsion is a common problem in children that involves twisting of the long bone along its long axis. *Tibial version* describes the normal variation in tibial rotation. At birth, the tibias have a mean lateral rotation of 2.2 degrees and rotate laterally over time, with an adult mean lateral tibial rotation of about 23 degrees. Tibial torsion describes rotations that are outside the range of normal. Medial tibial torsion (MTT), also known as *internal tibial torsion*, consists of abnormal medial rotation or twisting, resulting in in-toeing of the feet; lateral tibial torsion (LTT) consists of abnormal lateral rotation resulting in out-toeing (Baldwin and Wells, 2016).

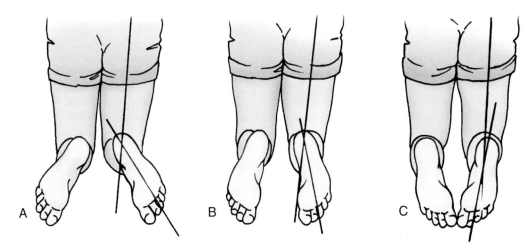

• Fig 43.13 Thigh-Foot Angle (TFA). With the child in the prone position and the knees flexed and approximated, the long axis of the foot can be compared with the long axis of the thigh. The long axis of the foot bisects the heel and the second toe or lies between the second and third toes. (A) External tibial torsion produces excessive outward rotation. (B) Normal alignment is characterized by slight external rotation. (C) Internal tibial torsion produces inward rotation of the foot and a negative angle. (From Thompson GH. Gait disturbances. In: Kliegman RM, Nieder ML, Super DM, eds. *Practical Strategies in Pediatric Diagnosis and Therapy*. Philadelphia: Saunders; 1996.)

Tibial torsion may be congenital, developmental, or acquired. MTT is the most common cause of in-toeing during the second year of life and is often noted around 6 to 12 months of age. In most cases it is a physiologic condition resulting from in utero positioning. In 90% of cases, internal tibial torsion gradually resolves on its own by the time the child reaches 8 years of age. LTT is a cause of out-toeing in late childhood and is usually an acquired deformity. Contracture of the iliotibial band is the underlying problem.

Clinical Findings

Physical Examination. Observe the child's gait for in-toeing. The thigh-foot angle (TFA) is used to assess tibial rotation. With the child prone and the knees flexed 90 degrees, the foot and thigh are viewed from directly above (looking downward at the angle of the thigh and foot). The foot should be relaxed. MTT exists if the TFA is negative by more than 10 to 20 degrees (–10 to –20 degrees), bearing in mind the child's age. In-toeing is expressed in negative values (Fig 43.13). The normal range at 13 years of age is –5 to +30 degrees. Abnormal lateral torsion is associated with forward-pointing patellas and outward-pointing feet. A TFA measurement of greater than 30 degrees indicates abnormal LTT (Baldwin and Wells 2016).

Diagnostic Studies. Radiographs are usually not necessary.

Differential Diagnosis. Differential diagnoses include genu varum (the knee has an abnormal tibial-femoral angle), femoral torsion (femoral anteversion), adducted great toe, and MA. All of these produce in-toeing gaits. Adducted great toe (the searching toe) is a benign condition that resolves spontaneously. Lateral femoral torsion also causes an out-toeing gait. Screening for associated hip dysplasia and neuromuscular problems (cerebral palsy) is recommended.

Management

- Treatment of tibial version (the normal variation in tibial rotation) is observation and monitoring.
- MTT should be referred to an orthopedist if the problem is significant (TFA >–20 degrees by 3 years of age). Stretching exercises or external rotational splints may be recommended.

Surgical intervention may be needed for severe cases that persist into late childhood and cause significant functional problems.

- Special shoes are ineffective for the treatment of MTT. Avoidance of certain postures that are thought to exacerbate MTT is controversial (e.g., sleeping in the knee-chest position and sitting with the feet tucked under the buttocks).
- LTT with TFA greater than +30 degrees should be referred to an orthopedist because it usually worsens with growth and does not correct spontaneously. Medial femoral torsion with pain also should be referred.

Complications. There are no complications with normal tibial version and no interference with activities. Tibial torsion (the TFA is outside the acceptable range of normal) can lead to significant functional problems in severe cases.

Popliteal Cysts

Popliteal cysts, or Baker cysts, are due to the egress of fluid through a normal communication of a bursa or may be caused by herniation of the synovial membrane through the joint capsule. Baker cysts appear much less frequently in children than in adults.

Clinical Findings. Findings include swelling behind the knee with or without discomfort. Cysts are generally located at or below the joint line.

Diagnostic Studies. Ultrasonography can distinguish between a fluid-filled cyst and solid tumor. Radiographs will show if there is soft calcification in the mass.

Differential Diagnosis. Lipomas, xanthomas, vascular tumors, and fibrosarcomas must be ruled out.

Management. Observation is the treatment of choice. The cyst usually resolves in 10 to 20 months. Ice and NSAIDs are used to promote comfort and relieve pain. Surgical incision is indicated only when symptoms are severe and limiting.

Sports-Related Injuries

Osgood-Schlatter Disease. Osgood-Schlatter disease is caused by microtrauma in the deep fibers of the patellar tendon at its insertion on the tibial tuberosity. The diagnosis is usually based on history and physical examination. The quadriceps femoris muscle inserts on a relatively small area of the tibial tuberosity and naturally high tension exists at the insertion site. In children additional stress is placed on the cartilaginous site with vigorous physical activity (overuse), leading to traumatic changes at insertion (Patel and Villalobos, 2017). Osgood-Schlatter disease is often seen in the adolescent years after the patient has undergone a rapid growth spurt the previous year. It occurs more frequently in boys than in girls, typically between 10 to 15 years in boys and 8 to 12 years in girls. This difference is probably related to a greater participation in specific risk activities by boys than by girls (Vaishya, Azizi, Agarwal, Vijaym 2016).

Clinical Findings

History

- Recent physical activity (such as, running track, playing soccer or football, or surfboarding) commonly produces the condition.
- Pain increases during and immediately after the activity and decreases when the activity is stopped for a while.
- Running, jumping, kneeling, squatting, and ascending/descending stairs exacerbate the pain.
- Pain is bilateral in 20% to 50% of cases.
- Approximately 25% of patients give a history of precipitating trauma.

Physical Examination. Characteristic findings include the following:

- Pain may be reproduced by extending the knee against resistance, stressing the quadriceps, or squatting with the knee in full flexion.
- Focal swelling, heat, and point tenderness found at the tibial tuberosity.
- May palpate a bony prominence over the tibial tuberosity.
- Full range of motion of knee.

Diagnostic Studies. The diagnosis is based on history and physical examination. Radiographs are not needed unless another pathologic condition is suspected.

Differential Diagnosis. Other knee derangements, tumors (osteosarcoma), and hip problems with referred pain should be considered. The referred pain of hip problems is diffuse across the distal femur without point tenderness at the tibial tubercle.

Management. Osgood-Schlatter disease is a self-limiting condition, with symptom management the key consideration. The following steps are taken:

- Avoid or modify activities that cause pain until the inflammation subsides.
- Use ice or other cold therapy to reduce pain and inflammation.
- Once the acute symptoms have subsided, quadriceps stretching exercises, including hip extension for complete stretch of the extensor mechanism, may be performed to reduce tension on the tibial tubercle. Stretching of the hamstrings may also be useful.
- Use of NSAIDs is recommended by some but thought ineffective by others. Because this condition may last up to 2 years, the chronic use of NSAIDs may be problematic.
- A neoprene sleeve over the knee may help to stabilize the patella.
- A patellar tendon strap that wraps around the joint just below the knee reduces strain on the tibial tuberosity.
- Cylinder casting or bracing with limited weight bearing for 2 to 3 weeks may be used in severe cases.

- Overuse is to be avoided and balanced training and adequate warm-up before exercise or sports participation should be encouraged.
- Use of knee pads may help protect the tibial tuberosity from direct injury for those who engage in sports that result in knee contact.

Complications. In the postpubertal child, a residual ossicle in the tendon next to the bone may cause persistent pain. Surgical removal is indicated and relieves the pain.

Knee Injuries

Chapter 19 presents a further discussion of sport-related injuries and issues related to the musculoskeletal examination and common sports. Table 43.3 outlines the etiology, assessment, management, and differential diagnosis of common knee injuries seen in children and young adults.

Pes Planus

Physiologic or flexible pes planus (flatfoot) is normal in neonates and toddlers and is due to a fat pad in the arch that makes the appearance of the arch seem flat. This generally resolves by 3 years of age. Flexible flatfoot is often familial, common, and benign. The arch is seen when the foot is suspended but flattens with weight bearing. Rigid flatfoot is pathologic.

There are three types of flat feet: a flexible flatfoot, a flexible flatfoot with a tendo-Achilles contracture, and a rigid flatfoot. Flat feet in neonates and toddlers are associated with physiologic ligamentous laxity. Flexible flat feet persisting into adolescence are usually associated with familial ligamentous laxity, as it is hereditary. Flatfoot also is associated with certain syndromes (Marfan and Down syndromes), myelodysplasia, cerebral palsy, and obesity. Flat feet may be secondary to muscle imbalance or weakness, a bony abnormality, or shortened heel cords.

History. Onset is noticed with weight bearing. The flexible flatfoot is painless and asymptomatic. Examine the shoes to see if there is abnormal wear on the inner side.

Physical Examination. Clinical manifestations include the following (Winell and Davidson, 2016):

- There is a normal longitudinal arch when examined in a non–weight-bearing position, but the arch disappears when standing.
- On standing, the hindfoot collapses into valgus and midfoot sag becomes evident.
- Generalized ligamentous laxity is commonly observed.
- Range of motion should be normal in flexible flatfoot.

Differential Diagnosis. Congenital vertical talus should be considered if the foot is rigid and no arch can be molded or if the foot has a rocker-bottom appearance. Calcaneovalgus foot might also be considered.

Management. Management involves the following:

- Symptomatic feet and rigid flatfoot should be treated; refer to a podiatrist.
- For painful, flexible flatfoot, a removable longitudinal arch support (e.g., Superfeet) may be recommended by the podiatrist.
- If the Achilles tendon is tight, passive stretching may be helpful.
- Routine radiographs are not indicated unless pathologic flatfoot is suspected.

Complications. Some cases of flatfoot are symptomatic in adulthood; in severe cases, the bones of the feet adapt to their abnormal position with pronation and the possible development

TABLE 43.3   Characteristics of Various Types of Knee Injuries and Conditions

Condition	History, Mechanism of Injury	Clinical Findings	Management	Differential Diagnosis, Prognosis, and Comments
Quadriceps contusion	Typically a sports injury that results in bruising/contusion of the quadriceps muscle. Injury can sometimes result from minor trauma or indirectly from tensile overload.	Acute pain, swelling, and restriction of active and passive range of motion of hip and knee; tenderness over quadriceps.	RICE: not to exceed 48 hours. Progressive leg and gravity-assisted ROM after rest. Flexion of the knee is the last function to return to normal, so it is a good indicator for return to sport. NSAID for pain relief.	In teens, rule out rhabdomyosarcoma of the quadriceps, Ewing sarcoma, and osteosarcoma if there is swelling and pain in the thigh without a clear history of trauma.
Meniscal tear (torn cartilage)	Associated with a significant injury in a youth; results from axial loading with rotation. Tear of a normal meniscus is rarely seen in children <12 years of age. Congenitally abnormal cartilage (discoid) can tear at any age.	Pain, swelling, and limping. Joint-line tenderness and positive McMurray sign. Patient may report a sensation of clicking or catching in the knee or locking of the knee. Can be isolated or may occur in combination with ACL or MCL injuries.	RICE initially; MRI if suspected tear; arthrography with MRI to rule out nerve injury with a prior tear; pain management. Surgical intervention: meniscectomy generally relieves symptoms.	Some 75% of patients develop degenerative articular changes on x-ray by 30 years of age. A small percentage of youths develop degenerative changes 3–5 years after injury. Chondral fractures and injuries to articular cartilage have similar histories and physical findings.
Sprain of the ACL	Acute injury; typically there is a twisting or hyperextension while the foot is planted and knee extended. Report of a "popping" feeling and knee shifting or pulling apart.	Swelling/effusion and pain. Instability with lateral movement. Positive Lachman test.	Following the injury, a knee brace or immobilizer is used until swelling and pain subside. ACL reconstruction. Pain management. Neuromuscular training to prevent injury.	Associated with MCL and meniscal tears.
Sprains of the MCL	Most commonly injured ligament of the knee due to valgus stress to an extended knee. Patient reports tearing sensation with medial pain, swelling, stiffness.	Instability with lateral movement and medial knee pain. Tenderness over the MCL. If tenderness extends along the distal femoral physis, suspect physeal fracture.	RICE, splint, or hinged knee brace to protect against valgus stress. Pain management. Plain radiographs to look for physeal and epiphyseal fractures in skeletally immature children. Surgical repair on an isolated collateral ligament is not beneficial; nonoperative treatment is the standard of care.	Combined ACL and MCL injuries are common. Physeal fractures are more common than MCL sprains in youths.
Osteochondritis dissecans	Juvenile and adolescent types common in 10- to 15-year-olds; boys more common than girls. Isolation and sometimes sequestration of an osteochondral fragment without significant trauma. May be caused by microtrauma or trauma or may involve metabolic or genetic factors. Pain increased with activity and diminished with rest and intermittent effusions. Locking and catching are unusual findings but may be present if bone fragments are detached.	Activity-related pain and swelling. Tenderness of the femoral condyle.	Plain radiographs or MRI; 4–6 weeks of immobilization and non–weight bearing if <12 years of age. Youths >12 years of age: Arthroscopic surgery. Eliminate high-impact activities; non–weight bearing for several weeks until symptoms abate. About 50% heal spontaneously with rest and protected weight bearing. Surgical intervention if still symptomatic despite 6–12 months of conservative treatment, symptomatic loose body, or nonunion.	Mimics symptoms of a torn meniscus. Articular cartilage transplantation for selected patients.

Continued

TABLE 43.3	Characteristics of Various Types of Knee Injuries and Conditions—cont'd			
Condition	History, Mechanism of Injury	Clinical Findings	Management	Differential Diagnosis, Prognosis, and Comments
Dislocation of the patella	Associated with patellar malalignment. Most cases involve lateral dislocation with pain and swelling. Most occur in youths <20 years of age. Family history in 20%–30%. More frequently seen in girls than in boys.	Massive and tense effusion. Tenderness at the medial border of the patella and medial retinaculum. Guarding with gentle pressure on the medial patella with lateral displacement.	Nonoperative management: 2–3 weeks of joint rest with splint or knee immobilizer (patella-stabilizing sleeve), then intensive rehabilitation. Isometric exercises, especially of quadriceps. Some 80%–85% of cases are successfully managed with nonoperative treatment. Surgical correction for recurrent dislocations or chronic instability.	Outcomes with nonoperative therapy vs. acute surgery are similar. Patellar dislocation tends to recur (recurrence is more frequent in a younger child) but decreases over time. Degenerative arthritis with recurrent dislocations is common with or without surgery.

ACL, Anterior cruciate ligament; *MCL,* medial collateral ligament; *MRI,* magnetic resonance imaging; *NSAID,* nonsteroidal anti-inflammatory drug; *RICE,* rest, ice, compression, and elevation; *ROM,* range of motion.

Data from Anderson SJ. Lower extremity injuries in youth sports. *Pediatr Clin North Am.* 2002;49:627–641; Hosalkar HS, Wells L. The knee. In: Kliegman RM, Behrman RE, Jenson HB, et al., eds. *Nelson Textbook of Pediatrics.* 18th ed. Philadelphia: Saunders/Elsevier; 2007; Landry GL. Management of musculoskeletal injury. In: Kliegman RM, Behrman RE, Jenson HB, et al., eds. *Nelson Textbook of Pediatrics.* 18th ed. Philadelphia: Saunders/Elsevier; 2007; McMahon P, ed. *Current Diagnosis and Treatment: Sports Medicine.* New York: Lange Medical Books/McGraw-Hill; 2007; Staheli LT, ed. *Pediatric Orthopaedic Secrets.* 2nd ed. Philadelphia: Hanley and Belfus; 2003.

of bunions, which may require surgery. Congenital vertical talus is a complication in childhood and should be identified early and referred for treatment.

Patient Education. Parents must understand that arch supports may relieve pain but do not help the foot to "grow" an arch.

Metatarsus Adductus

MA involves adduction of the forefoot relative to the hindfoot. When the forefoot is supinated and adducted, the deformity is termed *metatarsus varus.* The most common cause is intrauterine molding; the deformity is bilateral in 50% of cases (Winell and Davidson, 2016). A nonflexible foot, especially with heel valgus, or persistence may indicate a more serious problem.

Clinical Findings
History. There can be a family history.

Physical Examination
- The forefoot is adducted, whereas the midfoot and hindfoot are normal.
- The lateral border of the foot has a convex shape, with the base of the fifth metatarsal appearing prominent. Normally this border should look straight. Sometimes spreading of the toes is noted with a wider space between the first and second toes.
- The foot should normally be straight. If one draws a line from the middle of the heel, it should pass through the second toe or between the second and third toes. In MA, the forefoot has an increased angle (>15 degrees) or resists stretching (Fig 43.14).
- To determine whether the foot is flexible or rigid, the heel is grasped with one hand while the forefoot is abducted with the other. In flexible MA, the forefoot can be abducted past midline.
- A careful hip examination should be performed to rule out associated DDH.

Diagnostic Studies. Radiographs are not performed routinely. AP and lateral weight bearing are indicated in toddlers or older

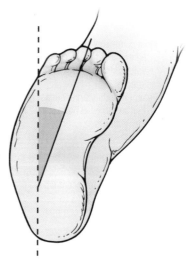

● **Fig 43.14** Metatarsus Adductus (MA) Angle. An angle (created by the intersecting lines) that is greater than 15 degrees indicates MA.

children with residual deformities. The AP radiographs demonstrate adduction of the metatarsals at the tarsometatarsal articulation and an increased intermetatarsal angle between the first and second metatarsals.

Differential Diagnosis. Consider congenital vertical talus, which will be rigid, or clubfoot, in which the foot is inverted and in the pointed-toe position.

Management. Management is based on the rigidity of the deformity; most children respond to nonoperative treatment.
- For the flexible foot that can be brought past midline, the soft tissues can be stretched by the parents with each diaper change. Instruct parents to hold the hindfoot in one hand and stretch the midfoot to overcorrect the deformity to the count of five and repeat five times. The soft tissues should blanch

with each stretch. Be sure that the parent is not just pushing on the great toe. Feet that correct just to the neutral position may benefit from stretching exercises and retention in a slightly overcorrected position by a splint or reverse shoe. If there is no improvement in 4 to 6 weeks, serial plaster casts should be considered. Once flexibility and alignment are restored, orthoses or corrective shoes are generally recommended. Surgical treatment may be considered in the small subset of children with symptomatic residual deformities that have not responded to conservative treatment. Surgery is generally delayed until 4 to 6 years of age (Winell and Davidson, 2016).

- For the nonflexible foot:
  - Refer to an orthopedist.
  - Educate the family that the treatment for infants may include serial short-leg casts or braces to stretch the foot (two or three casts for 2 weeks per cast) or other management if the bones of the foot are more severely affected. If the child is older than 2 to 3 years of age, surgery may be needed to correct the problem.
  - Surgical treatment may be considered in patients with symptomatic residual deformities that have not responded to conservative treatment. Surgery is generally delayed until the child is 4 to 6 years of age.

Talipes Equinovarus

Talipes equinovarus (clubfoot) has three elements: the ankle is in equinus (the foot is in a pointed-toe position), the sole of the foot is inverted as a result of hindfoot varus or inversion deformity of the heel, and the forefoot has the convex shape of MA (forefoot adduction). At birth, the foot cannot be manually corrected to a neutral position with the heel down.

The etiology is thought to be multifactorial and likely involves the effects of environmental factors in a genetically susceptible host. Clubfoot may be idiopathic or hereditary, neurogenic (as seen with myelomeningocele), or associated with syndromes (e.g., arthrogryposis and Larsen syndrome). It varies in severity, with uterine positioning a factor in mild clubfoot. The incidence is 1:1000 live births, with approximately 50% of cases being bilateral, and it is more common in male infants (Winell and Davidson, 2016). The problem is congenital and can be identified in neonates.

Clinical Findings

History. Clubfoot is present at birth but the parents may not note curvature.

Physical Examination. Note the inflexibility of sole of the foot. It is inverted as a result of hindfoot varus or inversion deformity of the heel, and the forefoot has a convex shape with forefoot adduction. It can be bilateral. A complete physical examination should be performed to rule out coexisting musculoskeletal and neuromuscular problems.

Diagnostic Studies. AP and lateral radiographs are recommended, often with the foot held in a maximally corrected position. Radiographic measurements can be made to describe malalignment between the tarsal bones. A common radiographic finding is "parallelism" between lines drawn through the axis of the talus and the calcaneus on the lateral radiograph, indicating hindfoot varus. Radiographs are not required in an infant to diagnosis the anomaly.

Management. The following steps are taken:
- Refer to an orthopedist upon diagnosis, ideally shortly after the infant is born, because the joints are most flexible in the first hours and days of life. Nonoperative treatment should be

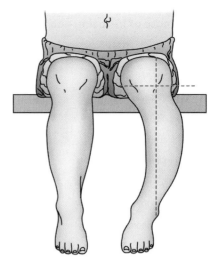

- **Fig 43.15** In-Toeing From Internal (Medial) Tibial Torsion.

initiated as soon as possible after birth. Treatments include taping and strapping, manipulation, and serial casting. The Ponseti method of clubfoot treatment involves a specific technique for manipulation and serial casting. Weekly cast changes are performed; 5 to 10 casts are usually required. Up to 90% of children will need a percutaneous tenotomy of the heel cord as an outpatient followed by a long leg cast with the foot in maximal abduction and dorsiflexion. This is followed by a full-time bracing program for 3 months and then nightly bracing for 3 to 5 years. For older children with untreated club feet or for those who have residual deformity, osteotomies may be required in addition to the soft tissue surgery (Winell and Davidson, 2016).

- Stiffness remains a concern at long-term follow-up. Although pain is uncommon in childhood and adolescence, symptoms may appear during adulthood.

Complications. With growth, the abnormality can become increasingly distorted, making correction more difficult. Calf hypoplasia and a shorter than normal foot can occur even with correction.

Overriding Toes

Overriding toes are generally identified at birth. Efforts to tape them into a correct position or otherwise modify their position are usually futile. Overriding of the second, third, and fourth toes generally resolves with time. Occasionally, if severe, they can be surgically improved. Shoe fit can be a problem.

In-Toeing and Out-Toeing Rotational Problems

When a child has an in-toeing or out-toeing gait, the degree of rotation and source of the rotational deformity must be assessed (Fig 43.15). These conditions include internal femoral torsion (femoral anteversion), internal tibial torsion, and MA. The causes of in-toeing usually are physiologic, are related to age, and resolve as the child grows (Table 43.4). In addition, in-toeing in children can vary with activities and from step to step.

Clinical Findings
History
- This should include onset, progression, functional limitations, previous treatment, evidence of neuromuscular disorder, and significant family history.

TABLE 43.4	Typical Cause of In-Toeing and Out-Toeing Rotational Problem		
Cause	Possible Diagnoses	Typical Finding	Age at Manifestation
In-toeing	Equinovarus	Plantar foot flexion, forefoot adduction, and hindfoot varus	At birth
	Metatarsal adductus	Curved foot: refer if not flexible	Birth to 6 months of age
	Abducted great toe	Searching toe: resolves spontaneously	Toddler period
	Medial tibial torsion	Refer if thigh-foot angle more than −10 to −20 degrees	12–18 months old
	Internal femoral torsion	Refer if >70 degrees medial and <10 degrees lateral hip rotation	2–5 years of age
Out-toeing	Physiologic infantile out-toeing	Feet may turn out when infant is positioned upright: resolves spontaneously	Early infancy
	Lateral tibial torsion	Refer if TFA ≥30 degrees	Late childhood
	Lateral femoral torsion	Refer if >2 standard deviations of the mean	Late childhood

Physical Examination

- Observe the gait. Note that the slightly older child may consciously or unconsciously improve or worsen the gait for the examiner. Asking the child to run may also be helpful.
- Lay the child prone on the examining table.
- Examine for femoral anteversion (medial and lateral rotations).
- Examine for internal or external tibial torsion (TFA).
- Examine for MA or other deformity.

The child may have a combination of any or all of the aforementioned problems.

Management. See the individual diagnoses for management strategies.

Toe Walking

Some young children initially stand on their toes until they establish the heel-toe pattern, usually within the first 6 months of walking. Consistent toe walking is frequently associated with neurologic problems, such as cerebral palsy. Autistic children or those with early muscular dystrophy may toe walk. Children with tight heel cords may toe walk. Unilateral toe walking can be associated with a short leg, as found with a dislocated hip. Toe walking also can be a habit, especially in children who used walkers or jumpers. In these children, toe walking generally resolves before 3 years of age and is not associated with musculoskeletal deformity. It is important to differentiate between the idiopathic toe walker and the child who toe walks because of a neuromusculoskeletal condition associated with tight heel cords and contractures.

Clinical Findings

History. The PCP should assess onset of walking, use of walker or jumper, severity of toe walking, any other developmental delays, or associated neurologic conditions.

Physical Examination. The examination should include the following:

- Looking at shoe wear and heel wear to assess extent of toe walking.
- Assessing for tight heel cords. The foot should be brought beyond a 90-degree angle.
- Conducting a neurologic assessment.
- Measuring leg lengths and examining hips.

Management

Management depends on the etiology. Orthopedic management is needed for tight heel cords, unequal leg lengths, and hip problems.

Leg Aches of Childhood

Extremity pain, often referred to as *growing pains* by the layperson, is a frequent clinical presentation. The pain is usually nonarticular; in two-thirds of children, it is described as being located in the shins, calves, thighs, or popliteal fossa. It is almost always bilateral. The pain appears late in the day or is nocturnal, often waking the child. The pain lasts from minutes to hours. By morning, the child is almost always pain-free. Because it occurs late in the day and is often reported on days of increased activity, it may represent a local overuse syndrome; it may also be associated with low vitamin D levels and decreased bone strength. Leg aches of childhood are generally not associated with serious organic disease, have a peak incidence between 4 and 8 years of age, and usually resolve by late childhood; 10% to 20% of school-age children experience intermittent leg aches (Vehapoglu et al., 2015). However, it is important to differentiate these pains from more serious pathologic conditions. Restless legs syndrome, also known as periodic limb movement disorder, is a more recently recognized common source of nocturnal leg pains in children.

Clinical Findings

History. Pain or leg aches are typically described as:

- Occurring characteristically in the evening or late in the day; may wake the child up from sleep
- Pain gone in the morning with no limitation of activity
- Poorly localized and bilateral
- Occurring commonly in the front of the thighs, in the calves, and behind the knees
- Transient and occurring over a period of time as long as several years
- Not associated with a limp or disability
- Without reported fevers or swelling
- Without report of recent or remote trauma

Physical Examination

- Have the child stand on tiptoes and heels.
- Measure leg lengths.

TABLE 43.5	Types of Limp			
Type of Limp	Cause	Characteristics	Examples
Antalgic	Pain: typically due to infection, fracture, or trauma.	Walking on a painful extremity results in an attempt to get weight quickly off affected side; gait has shortened stance phase.[a]	Sore knee: patient walks with fixed knee. Sore toe: Patient tries not to roll off toe at toe-off phase of the stride. Appendicitis causes slight slumping posture and shortened stride on the right side due to psoas muscle irritation.
Trendelenburg gait/abductor lurch	Hip problems: typically developmental, congenital, or muscular disorders.	Tilts over affected hip to decrease mechanical stresses; unaffected leg is off the ground during swing-through phase of gait.	Hip dysplasia.
Equinus/toe-to-heel gait	Neurologic incoordination.	Unsteady wide-based gait.	Cerebral palsy: toe-to-heel sequence to gait during stance phase due to heel-cord contractures.
Circumduction	Functionally longer leg; knee or ankle stiffness.	Longer leg progresses forward in swing motion.	Leg-length inequality/knee injury with hyperextension/ankle problems.

[a]Stance phase: Represents 60% of the gait cycle; swing about 40%.

- Evaluate range of motion. (Consider using the Pediatric Gait, Arms, Legs, and Spine [pGALS]. See Resources.)
- Assess for swelling, erythema, and tenderness.
- Observe for limping.

Findings include normal physical examination with no joint pain or tenderness, guarding, swelling, erythema, or reduced range of motion.

Diagnostic Studies. There is no single diagnostic test. It is a diagnosis of exclusion.

Differential Diagnosis

Restless legs syndrome, neoplastic lesions, leukemia, sickle cell anemia, juvenile arthritis, and subacute osteomyelitis apophysitis must be ruled out (Lehman and Carl, 2017).

Management

Reassure parents that these common complaints have a benign etiology and generally resolve spontaneously. Symptomatic treatment with heat and analgesia may be of benefit. Stress the need for parents to bring the child in for reevaluation if there is a change in symptoms or other signs emerge. Refer the child if the pain is localized to one region, is associated with swelling or other constitutional symptoms, is increasing in severity, or alters gait.

Limps

Deviations from the normal age-appropriate gait pattern can be caused by a wide variety of conditions. A limp is usually mild and self-limited and caused by contusion, strain, or sprain. In some cases the cause can be a sign of a serious inflammatory or infectious process. Age is an important factor in diagnosing the many causes of limping. Table 43.5 describes the various types of limps commonly seen in children.

Clinical Findings

History. A careful history is needed, including:
- Presence of pain
- History of trauma, past medical history
- Presence of fever, night sweats
- Weight loss or anorexia

- Type of limp (Table 43.6)
- Interference with activities
- Review of systems

Physical Examination
- The child should be in a diaper or underwear during examination.
- Observe for areas of erythema, swelling, atrophy, and deformity.
- Observe each limb segment.
- Identify limp type: Have the child walk and run while distracted.
- Stance and swing phase should be compared in both legs.
- Range of motion of each joint should be evaluated, especially the hip.
- Complete a neurologic examination, including strength, reflexes, balance, and coordination.
- Assess Trendelenburg sign for hip stability.

Diagnostic Studies. A CBC with differential and measurement of ESR and CRP levels should be obtained to rule out infection, inflammatory arthritis, or malignancy. Imaging should include radiographs of the area of concern. When imaging the hip, frog-leg lateral views should be obtained. Ultrasound may be used to detect effusion of the hip joint. If radiographs and ultrasound are positive, a CT scan may be indicated.

Differential Diagnosis

Fracture, DDH, LCPD, SCFE, tumor, infection, juvenile arthritis, and others should be considered (see Table 43.6).

Management

Refer the patient to an orthopedist immediately unless the etiology is a mild strain or a local lesion that can be managed conservatively by the PCP.

Overuse Syndromes of Childhood and Adolescence

Overuse injuries, overtraining, and burnout among child and adolescent athletes are growing problems. It is estimated that 60 million children and youth, ages 6 to 18 years of age, participate is some form of sport activity (Magrini, 2016). An

TABLE 43.6	Differential Diagnosis of Limping					
Condition	Age	Pain (±)	Historical Findings	Clinical Findings	Causative Factors	Management
Developmental dysplasia of the hip	Infant, toddler, child, adolescent	−	Breech delivery; MA; torticollis; poor treatment outcomes if not diagnosed at birth or shortly thereafter.	Limited abduction; Trendelenburg; radiography at 2–3 months old; shortening of leg; acetabular dysplasia	Familial; joint laxity, positioning, maternal hormones.	Newborn: no triple diapers. Pavlik harness to hold hips in flexion—see weekly; after 6 months of age, traction or open reduction; after 18 months of age, osteotomy.
Leg-length inequality	Toddler, child, adolescent	−	None.	Circumduction gait; joint contracture; >1 cm discrepancy in leg lengths	Congenital; neurogenic; vascular; tumor; trauma; infection.	Shoe lifts; epiphysiodesis (fusion of growth plate to arrest growth of the opposite side) if discrepancy 2–6 cm.
Neuromuscular (NM) disease	Toddler, child, adolescent	−	Depends on cause.	Depends on cause; equinus or abductor gait	Cerebral palsy, muscular dystrophy, and other NM diseases.	Referral to appropriate specialists.
Discitis	Toddler, child, adolescent	+	Varied: fever, malaise, unwilling to walk, backache.	Stiff back, ↑ ESR; positive x-ray within 2–3 weeks—narrow disk space, irregular vertebral body endplate; bone scan, CT, MRI show early findings; early bone scan has typical findings.	Bacterial infection in disc space (Staphylococcus aureus) or inflammatory response.	Immobilization and antistaphylococcal antibiotic therapy.
Septic arthritis	Toddler, child, adolescent	++	Moderate to high fever, malaise, arthralgias; irritability; progressive course.	Redness, warmth, and swelling of joint— knee or hip; limited hip motion; ESR >25 mm/h.	S. aureus likely organism.	Appropriate antibiotic coverage (7 days, IV; 3–4 weeks total).
Acute hematogenous osteomyelitis	Toddler, child, adolescent	+	Varied: malaise, low-grade to high fever; may have severe constitutional symptoms; toxicity.	Refusal to walk or move limb; point tenderness; limp; 7–10 days to see radiographic bony changes; 25% ↑ WBCs; ↑ CRP.	S. aureus likely organism.	Appropriate antibiotic coverage (generally 7 days, IV; 4–6 weeks total or until ESR is normal).
Neoplasm	Toddler, child, adolescent	+	Depends on type of neoplasm.	Varied.	Neoplasm—benign or malignant.	Referral to oncologist.
Trauma	Toddler, child, adolescent	+	Depends on type (fractures, strains, sprains).	Varied.	Varied.	Rule out physical abuse if discrepancy related to developmental capabilities, injury history, and type of injury.
Occult trauma: toddler fracture	Toddler	+	Well child.	Commonly radiograph (oblique view) shows spiral fracture of tibia; refusal to walk, mild soft tissue swelling.	Trauma.	See Trauma, earlier.
Transient synovitis	3–8 years of age	+	Mild to moderate fever, mild irritability; resolves within 1 week.	Limited hip motion; ESR <25 mm/h.	Inflammatory reaction; unknown etiology; often URI (50%) prior.	Rest.

		TABLE 43.6	Differential Diagnosis of Limping—cont'd			

Condition	Age	Pain (±)	Historical Findings	Clinical Findings	Causative Factors	Management
Juvenile arthritis (JA)	Childhood until 16 years of age	+	Fever, rashes, ↑ WBCs; some iritis; joint stiffness and swelling; S and S >3 months.	Mono-/polyarticular arthropathy; + ANA (25% to 88%); ↑ ESR in moderate/severe JA.	Unknown; genetic (HLA) or environmental.	Treat with NSAIDs initially; may need sulfasalazine, methotrexate, corticosteroids; joint replacements when older.
Slipped capital femoral epiphysis (SCFE)	9–15 years of age	+	>90th percentile weight; African American; male.	Limited abduction and extension; external rotation of thigh if hip flexed.	Multifactorial: mechanical; endocrine; trauma; familial.	Needs immediate surgery; non–weight-bearing with crutches until admitted; bilateral involvement does occur.
Legg-Calvé-Perthes disease (LCPD)	4–8 years of age	+	Acute or chronic onset; pain in hip, groin, knee; stiffness; male.	+ Trendelenburg, shortening; ↓ abduction, internal rotation, hip extension; + radiographs but not early.	Familial; breech birth; prior trauma (17%).	In female, tends to be more serious problem; bed rest, traction, then PT; bracing and surgery may be needed; bilateral involvement does occur.

ANA, Antinuclear antibody; *CRP,* C-reactive protein; *CT,* computed tomography; *ESR,* erythrocyte sedimentation rate; *HLA,* human leukocyte antigen; *IV,* intravenous; *MA,* metatarsus adductus; *MRI,* magnetic resonance imaging; *NSAID,* nonsteroidal anti-inflammatory drug; *PT,* physical therapy; *S and S,* signs and symptoms; *URI,* upper respiratory infection; *WBC,* white blood cell

overuse injury is microtraumatic damage to a bone, muscle, or tendon that has been subjected to repetitive stress without sufficient time to heal or undergo the natural reparative process. *Apophysitis* refers to the irritation, inflammation, and microtrauma of the apophysis. The risk of overuse injuries is more serious in the pediatric population because the growing bones cannot handle as much stress as the mature adult bone. Typical overuse injuries of childhood are varus overload of the elbow ("Little League elbow"), Osgood-Schlatter disease, calcaneal apophysitis, Sever disease, proximal humeral epiphysiolysis ("Little League shoulder"), patellofemoral pain syndrome, shin splints, and stress fractures (Table 43.7).

Clinical Findings

History. An in-depth history about the sport played, activities performed (e.g., pitching, kicking, swinging), and hours played per week, including games and practice, must be determined. The PCP must ask specific questions related to the child's pain. For example, what makes the pain better or worse? Further history and discussion with the child and adolescent should include questions such as the following related to the timing of the pain as it relates to the child's activity:

- Is there pain in the affected area after physical activity?
- Is there pain during the activity without restricting performance?
- Is there pain during the activity that restricts activity?
- Is there chronic, unremitting pain even at rest?

Physical Examination. The examination is dependent on the joint or limb involved. Check for deformity, warmth, swelling, range of motion, and ecchymosis. Observe for guarding of an extremity or limping.

Differential Diagnosis

Depending on the presenting symptoms, a plain film, CT, MRI, or bone scan may be indicated.

Management

Most of the injuries can be managed conservatively with proper and timely diagnosis. Treatment often involves resting and icing the extremity or joint, doing retraining and strengthening exercises, gradually reintroducing activities, and using analgesics. NSAIDs help reduce the inflammatory component of the trauma. Patient and parent education is important to prevent further injury and disability and to allow the child to return to safe sport participation. If not managed properly and effectively, overuse injuries can affect normal physical growth and maturation. PCPs can be instrumental in educating the active child, parents, and coaches in developing strategies to prevent overuse injuries. These include careful monitoring of training workload, especially during growth spurts; providing time for prepractice neuromuscular training to enhance strength and conditioning; and frequent evaluation of proper use and sizing of sporting equipment (DiFiori et al., 2014).

Muscle Diseases

The muscular dystrophies are a group of hereditary disorders of skeletal muscle that produce progressive degeneration of skeletal muscle, leading to weakness. The muscular dystrophies are autosomal-dominant, sex-linked, and can appear in several children in a family. The X-linked dystrophies are the most common, with the most common dystrophy being Duchenne muscular dystrophy. The prevalence of Duchenne and Becker muscular dystrophy in the United States is estimated at 1 in every 7250 males aged 5 to 24 years (CDC, 2018).

TABLE 43.7 Overuse Injuries of Childhood: Characteristic Features and Their Treatment

Condition	Clinical Findings	Treatment	Comments
Osgood-Schlatter disease	Swelling and tenderness/pain over tibial tubercle.	NSAIDs, knee pad, knee immobilizer if severe pain for 1–2 weeks.	Most resolve with time (12–18 months); x-ray only if pain persists (shows soft tissue swelling and possible residual ossicle); if pain persists, consider surgical incision of ossicle.
Patellofemoral pain syndrome	Anterior knee pain.	Rest, NSAIDs, retraining, and strengthening of quadriceps muscles.	Arthroscopic surgery only if recurring problems.
Proximal humeral epiphysiolysis ("Little League shoulder")	Shoulder pain—gradual onset; pain ↑ with throwing, especially curve ball.	Modify activity; gradual restart, but limit intensity and frequency of throwing. with retraining and muscle strengthening.	Seen in skeletally immature children; radiographs show widening proximal humeral physis.
Sever disease, calcaneal apophysitis	Swelling/tenderness/pain posterior aspect of the heel. Pain with forced dorsiflexion of the ankle.	Activity modification; limit running, jumping, and specific sport that causes pain, Heel cushions, arch supports. Pre/post sport icing. Gentle heel cord stretching exercises.	Most resolve with rest and return to previous level of activity/sport within 2 months. Radiograph evaluation is not diagnostic or prognostic. Radiographic evaluation should be used for exclusion of other causes of heel pain.
Shin splints	Pain along medial border of tibia; child has a history of prolonged running.	NSAIDs; ice after running; retraining and muscle strengthening after inflammation ↓; gradual return to running.	Associated with poor running technique, hard running surface, muscle weakness; inadequate running shoes; sudden increase in running; is an inflammatory response; may need to consider exertional compartment syndrome.
Stress fractures	Tenderness and swelling at site.	Reduce or eliminate activity that caused injury for 10–14 days; may need to cast.	Caused by microtrauma; most commonly seen in active teens but can occur during childhood; proximal tibia most common site.
Varus overload of the elbow ("Little League elbow")	Elbow pain with activity; locking and ↓ extension of elbow; medial humeral epicondylar tenderness.	Rest; NSAIDs; ice; when pain-free, gradual return to activity with retraining; surgery if elbow instability. Enforce pitch count restrictions.	Leads to osteochondral lesions and stress fractures if severe; radiographs reveal widening proximal physis; also seen in gymnasts.

NSAID, Nonsteroidal anti-inflammatory drug.

Clinical Findings

History
- Disease becomes evident between 3 and 6 years of age.
- There is usually a family history of muscle disease.
- Failure to achieve motor milestones, especially independent ambulation, is noted.
- Toe walking is commonly seen.
- Loss of motor skills, such as the ability to climb stairs easily, is typical
- Easy fatigue with physical activity is reported.
- A history of good days and bad days in relation to ability to accomplish physical activities is common.
- There is increasing difficulties with motor activities.

Physical Examination
- Toe walking
- Large firm calf muscles
- Fibrotic or "doughy" feel to the muscles
- Widely based lordotic stance
- Waddling Trendelenburg gait
- Lower extremities showing early weakness of gluteal muscle strength
- Positive Gower sign: this sign is obtained by asking the child to get up off the floor without help. The sign is positive if the child uses his or her arms to push off from the legs, gradually standing in a segmented fashion.

Management

Referral to an interprofessional team providing orthopedic, metabolic, and physical therapy as well as social services and nursing care. Genetic counseling may be necessary depending on the diagnosis.

The use of corticosteroids and deflazacort, which is approved for use in children 2 years of age and older by the US Food and Drug Administration and is not available in the United States, has been shown to preserve or improve strength, but these drugs have significant side effects, including weight gain, osteopenia, and myopathy. Dexamethasone and triamcinolone should not be used because they induce myopathy. Physical therapy is used to promote mobility and prevent contractures. Surgery may be needed for severe contractures and scoliosis.

Patient and family support is needed. Muscle diseases are chronic and debilitating; some are fatal conditions. Helping the child to lead as normal a life as possible while coping with his or her condition is a major task for parents and caregivers.

Ganglions of the Hands

Ganglions are the most common benign lesions of soft tissue in children (see Popliteal Cysts). A ganglionic cyst is an acquired, mucinous, fluid-filled painless lesion that originates from the synovial-lined space. A ganglion grows out of a joint. It rises out of the connective tissues between bones and muscles.

Clinical Findings

Ganglions of the hand are hard, fixed masses commonly found on the wrist (commonly dorsal) and flexor aspects of the finger. The etiology of these cysts is unknown. Transillumination of the cyst with an otoscope or examination by ultrasonography plus findings on physical examination are keys to the diagnosis.

Management

Ganglionic cysts in children are rarely symptomatic and usually regress spontaneously. The likelihood of recurrence with any form of treatment is higher in children than in adults with such lesions. Conservative care with rest and splinting can be tried. If conservative care fails to result in partial or complete resolution, refer for needle aspiration or surgical excision, which is the most reliable method to eliminate a ganglion because the tract that extends into the joint is removed. Steroid injections are not advised.

Additional Resources

American Academy of Orthopaedic Surgeons (AAOS).
www.aaos.org
Arthritis Research UK: Pediatric Gait, Arms, Legs, and Spine (pGALS) Video.
www.arthritisresearchuk.org/system/search-results.aspx?keywords=pGALS
Backpack Safety Tips.
http://orthoinfo.aaos.org/topic.cfm?topic=A00043
Muscular Dystrophy Association (MDA).
www.mdausa.org
National Scoliosis Foundation: The Spinal Connection.
www.scoliosis.org/resources/spinalconnection.php
Pediatric Orthopaedic Society of North America (POSNA) - Physician education study guides.
https://posna.org/Physician-Education/Study-Guide
Ortho Info (AAOS sponsored expert orthopedic information).
http://orthoinfo.aaos.org
Ortho Bullets Pediatrics High-Yield Topics.
http://www.orthobullets.com
Scoliosis Research Society (SRS).
www.srs.org
STEPS:
National charity in the United Kingdom for those affected by a lower limb condition.
www.steps-charity.org.uk
United Brachial Plexus Network, Inc.: Erb Palsy Support and Information Network.
www.ubpn.org

References

Abdelgawad A, Naga O. *Pediatric Orthopedics a Handbook for Primary Care Physicians.* New York: Springer; 2014.
Apel PJ. Evaluation and treatment of childhood musculoskeletal injury in the office. *Pediatr Clin N Am.* 2014;61:1207–1222.
Baldwin KD, Wells L. Torsional and angular deformities. In: 20th ed. Kliegman RM, Stanton BF, St Geme JW, et al., eds. *Nelson Textbook of Pediatrics.* vol. 2. Philadelphia: Elsevier; 2016:3257–3263.
Baldwin KD, Wells L, Dormans JP. Evaluation of the child. In: 20th ed. Kliegman RM, Stanton BF, St Geme JW, et al., eds. *Nelson Textbook of Pediatrics.* vol. 2. Philadelphia: Elsevier; 2016:3242–3259.
Bexkens R, Washburn FJ, Eygendaal D, et al. Effectiveness of reduction maneuvers in the treatment of nursemaid's elbow: a systematic review and meta-analysis. *Am J Emerg Med.* 2016;35(1):159–163.
Bohl DD, Telles CJ, Ruiz FK, et al. A genetic test predicts providence Brace success for adolescent idiopathic scoliosis when failure is defined as progression to greater than 45 degrees. *Clin Spine Surg.* 2016;29(3):E146–E150. https://doi.org/10.1097/BSD.0b013e3182aa4ce1.
Carrigan RB. Upper limb. In: Kliegman RM, Stanton BF, St Geme JW, et al., eds. *Nelson Textbook of Pediatrics.* 20th ed. Philadelphia: Elsevier; 2016:3302–3309.
Centers for Disease Control and Prevention (CDC). *MD STARnet Data and Statistics;* 2018. https://www.cdc.gov/ncbddd/musculardystrophy/data.html.
Dettling S, Weiner DS. Management of bow legs in children: A primary care protocol. *J Fam Pract.* 2017;66(5). E1-E-6.
DiFiori JP, Benjamin HJ, Brenner JS, et al. Overuse injuries and burnout in youth sports: a position statement from the American Medical Society for Sports Medicine. *Br J Sports Med.* 2014;48(4):287–288.
Duderstadt KG, Schapiro NA. Musculoskeletal system. In: Duderstadt KG, ed. *Pediatric Physical Examination: An Illustrated Handbook.* Philadelphia: Elsevier; 2019.
Flaherty EG, Perez-Rossello JM, Levine MA, et al. Evaluating children with fractures for child physical abuse. *Pediatrics.* 2014;133(2):e477–e489.
Garry JP. Pediatric costochondritis, *Medscape* (website). 2018. Available at http://emedicine.medscape.com/article/1006486. Accessed July 30, 2019.
Gomez JA, Hresko MT, Glotzbecker MP. Nonsurgical management of adolescent idiopathic scoliosis. *J Am Acad Orthop Surg.* 2016;24(8):555–564. https://doi.org/10.5435/JAAOS-D-14-00416.
Herngren B, Stenmarker M, Vavruch L, Hagglund G. Slipped capital femoral epiphysis: a population-based study. *BMC Musculoskelet Disord.* 2017;18(1):304. https://doi.org/10.1186/s12891-017-1665-3.
Herring JA. Disorders of the femur. In: 5th ed. Herring JA, ed. *Tachdjian's Pediatric Orthopedics from the Texas Scottish Rite Hospital for Children.* vol. 1. Philadelphia: Elsevier/Saunders; 2014a:678–681.
Herring JA. Slipped capital femoral epiphysis. In: 5th ed. Herring JA, ed. *Tachdjian's Pediatric Orthopedics from the Texas Scottish Rite Hospital for Children.* vol. 1. Philadelphia: Elsevier/Saunders; 2014b:630–665.
Herring JA, Ho C. Upper extremity injuries. In Herring JA, ed. *Tachdjian's Pediatric Orthopedics from the Texas Scottish Rite Hospital for Children.* 5th ed, Philadelphia: Elsevier/Saunders; 2014(2):356–482.
Hryhorczuk AL, Restrepo R, Lee EY. Pediatric musculoskeletal ultrasound. Practical imaging approach. *Am J Roentgenol.* 2016;206(5). https://doi.org/10.2214/AJR.15.15858.
Kim HKW, Herring JA. Legg-Calvé-Perthes disease. In: 5th ed. Herring JA, ed. *Tachdjian's Pediatric Orthopedics from the Texas Scottish Rite Hospital for Children.* vol. 1. Philadelphia: Elsevier/Saunders; 2014:580–629.
Krader CG. Developmental dysplasia of the hip. *Contemporary Pediatrics.* 2017.
Lehman PJ, Carl RL. Growing pains: when to be concerned. *Sports Health.* 2017;9(2):132–138. https://doi.org/10.1177/1941738117692533.
Magrini D. Musculoskeletal overuse injuries in the pediatric population. *Curr Sports Med Rep.* 2016;15(6):392–399.
Mistovich RJ, Spiegel DA. The spine. In: 20th ed. Kliegman RM, Stanton BF, St Geme JW, et al., eds. *Nelson Textbook of Pediatrics.* vol. 2. Philadelphia: Elsevier; 2016:3283–3293.
Murphy KP, Karlin AM. Shoulder injuries. In: 20th ed. Kliegman RM, Stanton BF, St Geme JW, et al., eds. *Nelson Textbook of Pediatrics.* vol. 2. Philadelphia: Elsevier; 2016:3339–3341.
Neral M, Liu RW. Genu valgum: Study guide: Pediatric Orthopedic Society of North America, (POSNA). 2019. https://posna.org/Physician-Education/Study-Guide/Genu-Valgum. Accessed July 30, 2019.
Patel DR, Villalobos A. Evaluation and management of knee pain in young athletes: overuse injuries of the knee. *Transl Pediatr.* 2017;6(3):190–198. https://doi.org/10.21037/tp.2017.04.05.
Peck K, Herrera-Soto J. Slipped capital femoral epiphysis: what's new? *Orthop Clin North Am.* 2014;45(1):77–86.
Pediatric Orthopedic Society of North America (POSNA). Slipped capital femoral epiphysis. *OrthoInfo.* 2016. (website). Available at: http://www.orthoinfo.org/topic.cfm?topic=A00052. Accessed July 30, 2019.

Richards B, Sucato D, Johnston C. Scoliosis. In: 5th ed. Herring JA, ed. *Tachdjian's Pediatric Orthopedics from the Texas Scottish Rite Hospital for Children.* vol. 1. Philadelphia: Elsevier/Saunders; 2014:206–290.

Russman B. *Neonatal Braxial Plexus Palsy. UpToDate* (website); 2018. Available at http://0-www.uptodate.com.patris.apu.edu/contents/neonatal-brachial-plexus-palsy?source=search_result&search=Brachial+Plexus+Injuries&selectedTitle=2~100.

Sankar WN, Horn BD, Wells L, et al. The hip. In: 20th ed. Kliegman RM, Stanton BF, St Geme JW, et al., eds. *Nelson Textbook of Pediatrics.* vol. 2. Philadelphia: Elsevier; 2016:3274–3283.

Somashekar DK, Di Pietro MA, Joseph JR, et al. Utility of ultrasound in noninvasive preoperative workup of neonatal brachial plexus palsy. *Pediatr Radiol.* 2016;46:695–703.

Stevens PM. *Pediatric Genu Varum. Medscape* (website): 2017. https://emedicine.medscape.com/article/1355974-overview. Accessed July 30, 2019.

Tamai J. Developmental dysplasia of the hip treatment & management. *Medscape* (website). 2018. https://emedicine.medscape.com/article/1248135-overview. Accessed July 30, 2019.

Vehapoglu A, Turel O, Turkman S, et al. Are growing pains related to vitamin D deficiency? Efficacy of vitamin D therapy for resolution of symptoms. *Med Princ Pract.* 2015;(24):332–338. https://doi.org/10.1159/000431035.

Vaishya R, Azizi AT, Agarwal AK, Vijay V. Apophysitis of the tibial tuberosity (Osgood-Schlatter Disease): a review. *Cureus.* 2016;8(9):e780. https://doi.org/10.7759/cureus.780.

Winell JJ, Davidson RS. The foot and toes. In: 20th ed. Kliegman RM, Stanton BF, St Geme JW, et al., eds. *Nelson Textbook of Pediatrics.* vol. 2. Philadelphia: Elsevier; 2016:3247–3254.

44

Common Pediatric Injuries and Toxic Exposures

SARA D. DEGOLIER AND JENNY BEVACQUA

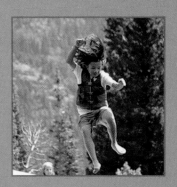

According to the Centers for Disease Control and Prevention, more than 9.2 million children ages 0 to 19 years are treated for nonfatal injuries annually in the emergency department (ED) setting (CDC, 2016). Injuries can be either intentional or unintentional. Physical injury to the body occurs in many ways, ranging from burns to toxic ingestions including environmental heavy metals. The abnormal transfer of energy by mechanical, thermal electric, chemical, or radiation between a moving and stationary object is now recognized as the underlying etiology of most injuries. Mechanical energy transfer (e.g., rough/hard surfaced object lacerates/scrapes the skin) is the most common type of injury. Environmental toxins can lead to cellular damage of organ systems.

Three main components essential to the management of an injured child include: obtaining an appropriate history, identifying the mechanism of the injury, and performing a thorough physical examination. If the injury is life threatening or there is deterioration in the child's condition, a trauma severity assessment must be performed immediately (see Chapter 46 for assessment of head injuries). Assessment should occur within the first 5 minutes of initial contact and include:

- Respiratory status, airway, circulation, and vital signs
- A brief history (allergies, medications, past medical history, and events surrounding the injury)
- Rapid assessment of essential organ status; cardiopulmonary resuscitation must be initiated if indicated

Once the patient is stabilized, a secondary assessment can be completed, to include:

- A complete physical examination with vital signs
- Laboratory and radiographic studies, as indicated

The definitive care phase includes stabilization of local injuries and preparation of the patient and family for transport to the ED if necessary.

The primary care provider (PCP) should always consider nonaccidental trauma (physical abuse) when a child presents with an injury and the caregiver's explanation for the injury is not consistent with the injury itself. According to Chiesa and Sirotnak (2016), red flags include an absent history, a history that changes each time the caregiver gives the history, or a history with significant detail lapses. Improbable or illogical explanations of the injury from the caregiver are also concerning (see Chapter 24).

Trauma to the Skin and Soft Tissue

Abrasions

Abrasions are superficial skin injuries, often the result of falls or friction that involve epidermal trauma. The depth of skin tissue involvement varies depending on the amount of force and friction. The most serious form of abrasion is an avulsion, which results in the loss of epidermal, dermal, and subcutaneous layers.

Clinical Findings

History and Physical Examination. Determine the extent of the abrasion and the presence of dirt, grime, or other foreign objects (e.g., tar at the injury site). Findings include skin that appears scraped off, as well as oozing of serous fluid and/or blood. Increasing pain, swelling, warmth, erythema, and red streaking of the injured area suggest ongoing or deeper injury or secondary infection. Assess the surrounding tissue for circulation, sensation, motion, and function.

Management

Most abrasions can be managed at home unless the abrasion is deep, involves a large area, is associated with severe pain, or has a significant amount of dirt, grime, tar, or a foreign object in the wound. Because the primary focus is prevention of infection, parents of a child who is immunocompromised should contact the child's PCP either by phone and/or office visit. Abrasion management includes:

- Cleansing the wound by scrubbing with soap or an antibacterial cleanser using a wet gauze or soft surgical nail brush, although the preferred method is gentle irrigation with copious amounts of water or normal saline (300 to 1000 mL depending on the surface area of the wound). Povidone-iodine, alcohol, and hydrogen peroxide should not be used on open wounds. If dirt or dark-colored matter is not adequately removed, new skin may grow over the particles, resulting in a permanent tattoo. A secondary infection may occur if all debris is not removed. Pieces of loose skin can be removed with sterile scissors and foreign objects with tweezers. If tar is present, rub the wound area with petrolatum, and then repeat the normal saline or water irrigation.

- Small abrasions can be left open to the air or may require a small bandage. Larger abrasions heal quicker if kept moist.
- Cover larger abrasions and abrasions of the hands, feet, and areas overlying joints with a sterile nonadherent dressing. Antibiotic ointment such as bacitracin/polymyxin B may be applied, especially to the elbows or knees to prevent cracking or reopening of the wound because of constant movement and stretching of the joints.
- Instruct the caregiver to wash the abrasion at least every 24 hours and reapply the dressing and antibiotic ointments until a protective dry scab forms.
- Provide instructions regarding the signs and symptoms of infection.
- Tetanus prophylaxis should be administered if the wound is significant or if the child has not received a tetanus immunization within the previous 5 years.

Puncture Wounds

Puncture wounds are typically classified as superficial or deep. Glass, wood splinters, toothpicks, needles, nails, metal, staples, thumbtacks, and bites are common sources of injury. Although the majority of puncture wounds heal without problems, a sizable minority are complicated by infection that can lead to cellulitis, fasciitis, septic arthritis, or soft-tissue abscesses.

Staphylococcus aureus and *β-hemolytic streptococci* are normal flora of the skin and are common causes of secondary infections in puncture wounds. *Pseudomonas aeruginosa* colonizes on the rubber soles of tennis shoes and is a common pathogen for plantar puncture wounds when the puncture occurs through the sole of a tennis shoe. Osteomyelitis can occur if the puncture wound penetrates a bone or joint, commonly *P. aeruginosa* in non-diabetic patients and *S. aureus* in diabetic patients (Baddour and Brown, 2017). Cat and dog bites can cause *Pasteurella multocida* wound infections.

Infection risk varies with the wound location and depth and the presence of a foreign object. Deep penetrating injuries to the forefoot with a dirty object, especially those involving the plantar fascia, have a higher infection risk than wounds to the arch or heel area. The forefoot has less overlying soft tissue than other plantar surfaces and is the major weight-bearing area of the foot; therefore, cartilage and bone can be involved. The metatarsophalangeal joint region is also at high risk for the same reasons.

Clinical Findings

History. The assessment of a child with a minor puncture wound begins by excluding more serious and/or occult injuries. Important information includes:

- Date/time of injury and history of wound care provided at time of injury and thereafter.
- Identification of the penetrating object and estimated depth of penetration.
- Location and condition (rusty, jagged, smooth) of the penetrating object and whether all or part of the foreign object was removed.
- Type and condition of footwear worn or if the child was barefoot.
- Tetanus immunization status
- Presence of any medical condition that increases the risk for infectious complications.

Physical Examination. A good light source is recommended. Note circulation, movement, and sensation of the surrounding area. Determine the amount of involvement of underlying tissue or bone structures. Evaluate neurologic status, as well as vascular and tendon injury (Baddour and Brown, 2017). Plantar wounds should be examined while the patient is prone and a tourniquet applied if the wound is bleeding (Chorley, 2018). Assess the wound for length and depth, presence of debris or penetrating object, and signs of infection.

Examination findings consistent with *cellulitis* include the following:

- Localized pain or tenderness, swelling, and erythema at the puncture site (may be more obvious at dorsum of the foot for plantar puncture wounds)
- Fever
- Pain with flexion or extension of the involved extremity. For plantar puncture wounds, pain along the plantar aspect of the foot during extension or flexion of the toes may indicate deep tissue injury with a higher infection risk.
- Decreased ability to bear weight

Examination findings consistent with *osteomyelitis-osteochondritis* include the following:

- Extension of pain and swelling around the puncture wound and the adjacent bony structures
- Point tenderness over the bone
- Fever and/or increasing erythema
- Decreased use of the affected extremity

Examination findings consistent with *pyarthrosis* (septic arthritis) include:

- Pain, swelling, warmth, and erythema over the affected joint
- Decreased range of motion and weight bearing of the affected joint
- Fever

Diagnostic Studies. Obtain plain film radiograph if there is suspicion of a retained foreign object; the wound is caused by a piece of glass, a nail, or something breakable, small, or thin; or if there was penetration of a joint space, bone, growth cartilage, or the plantar fascia. Radiographs are helpful if there is a concern for deep infection with the patient exhibiting fever, pain with passive movement, progressive pain over time, joint swelling, crepitus, or disproportionate pain at the wound site (Baddour and Brown, 2017). Most metal, glass, and radiopaque foreign objects are visible on a plain radiograph. Ultrasound is best for evaluation of radiolucent foreign objects including wood and plastic. Computed tomography (CT) and magnetic resonance imaging (MRI) identify foreign objects when radiograph and ultrasound fail (Baddour and Brown, 2017). Bone scans are sensitive, but not specific, for osteomyelitis while radiographs are specific, but don't show early osteomyelitis. MRI identifies subperiosteal abscess and early edema before radiographic changes occur. Clinical examination and laboratory studies and imaging should be considered early if osteomyelitis is suspected (Erickson, Rhodes and Niswander, 2016).

- A complete blood count (CBC) shows a white blood cell elevation which might indicate infection.
- Erythrocyte sedimentation rate (ESR) and C-reactive protein (CRP) are nonspecific inflammatory markers and help diagnose bony inflammation and infection.
- A wound and/or blood culture is typically indicated prior to starting antibiotics, especially if the wound appears infected.

Management

The circumstance surrounding the penetrating injury and the presenting symptoms are the best indicators of whether the injury is superficial and will heal uneventfully, or if it will result in infectious complications.

- Ensure the patient has adequate pain control prior to cleaning the wound.
- Cleanse the skin surface surrounding the wound with iodine-containing or antiseptic solution such as chlorhexidine (Baddour and Brown, 2017). After cleansing, irrigate the wound with either tap water or normal saline (Harper, 2017).
- Ensure that there are no foreign objects present.
- For animal and human bites, trim any superficial devitalized epidermal tissue (Harper M, 2017).
- Obtain imaging studies as indicated. 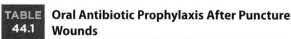 Refer a child to orthopedic surgery immediately if imaging studies demonstrate that the foreign object invaded bone, growth cartilage, or a joint space. Always suspect a retained foreign object if the puncture wound is infected, the infection is not responding to antibiotic therapy, or if pain is still present weeks after the injury. Surgical débridement/removal should be used where there is presence or concern of a deep infection, infection with a foreign object, or a rapidly progressing infection (Baddour and Brown, 2017).
- Following cleansing, cover the wound with a simple bandage and let heal by secondary intention without any repair. Deeper wounds that require exploration should have a small, sterile, damp saline gauze placed to keep the edges open to prevent superficial skin closure and promote healing. Remove the gauze 2 to 3 days after placement. Some larger or facial dog bite wounds may be repaired for cosmesis by an experienced clinician (Harper, 2017).
- Children with simple, uncomplicated puncture wounds do not need antibiotics. Exceptions include: signs of infection; cat bites; hand, foot, or genitalia wounds; the puncture is near a joint or bone; or the wound is deep or contains debris (Table 44.1). A recheck appointment should be scheduled 48 hours from the start of antibiotics for the patient receiving outpatient therapy.
- Consider surgical debridement for removal of a foreign object and/or abscess drainage with infected puncture wounds.
- Treatment for severe infections, such as septic arthritis and osteomyelitis, includes surgical debridement and parenteral antibiotics.
- Tetanus prophylaxis if indicated (see Chapter 22).

Patient and Parent Education

Home care management for a puncture wound includes:
- Cleanse the wound twice daily and when wound soiling occurs. Use warm water and soap, and then apply bacitracin or triple antibiotic ointment to the wound.
- Cover the wound with a dressing, such as an adhesive bandage.
- Observe closely for signs and symptoms of infection and if infection is suspected, notify the provider immediately; rapid re-evaluation is necessary. Further evaluation is required if a puncture wound continues to cause localized or spreading pain or discomfort.

Ingrown Toenail (Onychocryptosis) and Nail Hematoma

Ingrown toenails are caused by several factors, including abnormal position of the toenail on the nailbed, tight and improperly fitting shoes, trauma to the nail, and improper toenail trimming. The great toe is the most commonly affected. An ingrown toenail occurs when the lateral edge of the toenail pierces the lateral nail fold of the skin, entering the skin causing an inflammatory (foreign object) reaction and secondary infection.

TABLE 44.1	Oral Antibiotic Prophylaxis After Puncture Wounds	
Type	**First Line**	**Alternative**
Human bites	Amoxicillin clavulanate for 7-10 days	Cephalexin Clindamycin
Animal bites Cover for *Pasturella multocida* (dog and cat bites)	Amoxicillin clavulanate for 7-10 days	Cefuroxime, fluoroquinolone, or trimethoprim-sulfamethoxazole (TMP-SMX) plus clindamycin or metronidazole
Plantar wounds Cover for *Pseudomonas aeruginosa*	Ciprofloxacin for 7-20 days	Consult with infectious disease as may require IV therapy

From Harper (2017) and Baddour and Brown (2017).

Subungual hematomas are blood accumulations under an intact nail and may occur with Tuft fractures or lacerations. Tuft fractures are common following crush injuries and involve the distal phalanx. Another a crush injury, called a Seymore fracture, is a proximal nail fold incarceration with an open distal phalanx physeal fracture. The Seymour fracture usually causes blood at the nailfold and the nail to look longer than others.

Management

Ingrown toenail
- Pack cotton under the nail edge to elevate the nail and educate the patient to repack the cotton daily to prevent infection.
- Soak the affected foot in warm water mixed with Epsom salts for 20 minutes, three times a day. Keep the foot or affected toenail clean and dry.
- Encourage frequent elevation of the affected toe.
- Educate about the importance of clipping nails straight across with extension of toenail just over the edge of the nailbed.
- Properly fitting shoes (no toe crowding) are important.
- For persistent ingrown toenails with or without infection, consider a referral to a podiatrist.

Subungual hematoma
- May require digital or regional nerve block.
- Irrigate nail surface with saline solution, then clean with chlorhexidine or isopropyl alcohol.
- Uncomplicated nail hematomas can be drained (trephination) by PCPs. Make one or more holes above the hematoma with either a portable heat cautery device or the end of an untwisted heated-to-red paperclip (heated to melt the nail). Remove the cautery device immediately after creating a hole to ensure that the underlying tissue is not cauterized, subsequently blocking the drainage of fluid. Ensure the holes are large enough to drain the hematoma.
- Tuft fractures are often managed by PCPs with orthopedic consult if needed. Use an aluminum splint to immobilize the fracture for 2 to 3 weeks. For open Tuft fractures, an oral antibiotic (typically a first-generation cephalosporin) is used to prevent infection, such as cellulitis or osteomyelitis.

- Seymour fractures require orthopedic surgical repair, irrigation, débridement, and antibiotics due to risk of infection and permanent mallet deformity of the finger. Lateral view radiographs help identify a Seymour fracture.
- Nail injuries that involve lacerations or a crushing fracture of the distal phalanx necessitate orthopedic referral.
- Home care includes soaking the affected nailbed three times per day with antibacterial soap until the drainage stops and the underlying skin heals. Educate the patient and parent to monitor for signs of infection (increased erythema, swelling, pain, or purulent drainage) with return for further care if infection is suspected.

Lacerations

Lacerations are one of the leading causes of ED visits. They are associated with occult injuries to the deeper tissues and require careful exploration.

The most common lacerations result from shear, tension, and compression injuries. Shear injuries are caused by sharp objects and tend to cause minimal, if any, damage to the tissues surrounding the injury. These heal quickly and have the lowest potential for wound infection. The greatest danger of shear injuries is the potential for damage to nerve, tendon, and vascular structures that may require more complicated repair that should only be attempted in the ED or operating room by a skilled surgeon.

Tension lacerations are caused from stresses on the skin, usually secondary to blunt force of an object at less than a 90-degree angle. The skin tears due to the stress and causes an irregularly shaped injury edge. These are accompanied by damage to surrounding tissues. A classic example is when a child falls and bumps his or her head on the dull edge of a piece of furniture, causing the skin to break open.

Compression lacerations are caused by a crush injury, usually involving blunt force of an object at a 90-degree angle. This type of laceration usually has irregular, often stellate wound edges. Compression injuries can cause significant injury to adjacent tissues and have the highest incidence of wound infections.

Clinical Findings

History. Key questions to ask when assessing a laceration include:

- How long ago (number of hours) did the injury occur? Length of time since injury can influence the treatment plan for the patient.
- Does the child have allergies to antibiotics or anesthetics?
- What is the child's tetanus immunization status? Is there a need for further immunization?

Physical Examination. Key points in the examination of a laceration include:

- Perform a neurovascular examination, including evaluation of pulses, motor function, and sensation distal to the laceration.
- Evaluate the range of motion, especially with wounds involving the distal forearm, wrist, and hand due to the high potential for tendon injury.
- Determine whether the wound edges approximate and note the degree of tension at the wound site.

Management

Providers may repair the wound using sutures, staples, glue, or tape. Minor lacerations to the scalp, arms, and legs are commonly managed by PCPs. Significant wounds to the face, hands, or genital areas should be referred to a specialist, such as an orthopedic surgeon who specializes in hand repair, or a plastic surgeon for plastic and reconstructive surgery (particularly for the face).

The steps in wound management are summarized as follows (Attia et al, 2016):

1. *Decision to close the wound:* Most wounds are closed using a primary wound closure as soon as possible after the injury. This speeds healing, prevents infection, and improves the cosmetic result. Delayed closure increases the risk of infection. Some researchers suggest a "golden period" for wound closure of 6 hours. However, wounds considered low risk for infection, such as a clean knife wound to an extremity, can be closed even 12 to 24 hours after the injury. Children are less likely than adults to get wound infections and rates are generally believed to be less than 5%. Other guidelines to consider in wound closure include the following:
   - Most facial wounds may be closed up to 24 hours after initial injury to provide the child with the optimal cosmetic outcomes. Depending on the severity of the laceration or potential for infection (such as a dog bite), repair and management may require anesthesia.
   - Infection risk is inversely related to the area's blood flow. The lower the blood flow, the higher is the infection risk. For example, a hand or foot laceration is more likely to become infected than a scalp laceration because the extremities have lower blood perfusion.
   - Contaminated wounds, crush wounds, and lacerations in children who are immunocompromised are at high risk for infection, and should be closed within 6 hours of injury.
   - Leave animal and human bites open for healing by granulation and re-epithelialization (e.g., secondary intention). Scarring increases with this method, but the benefits of improved healing and decreased infection outweigh this.
   - Delayed primary closure involves closing a wound 3 to 5 days after initial injury when the risk of infection decreases. This is recommended for heavily contaminated wounds and those associated with extensive damage, such as high-velocity missile injuries, crush injuries, and explosion injuries. Initial management of such injuries includes wound cleansing, debridement, and a sterile dressing. Close follow-up is recommended to check for infection and for wound closure.
2. *Anesthesia:* Appropriate use of local anesthetic and conscious sedation is essential for successful repair of lacerations in children. Consider intranasal versed or conscious sedation with more complicated wound closures and patients with high anxiety levels. Wound exploration and cleansing are both painful procedures made worse by fear and anxiety. Infiltration of the wound with local anesthetic, such as 1% lidocaine with or without epinephrine (depending on location of laceration), can help control bleeding. There are a number of anesthetic and epinephrine/adrenaline topical solutions that can be placed on minor wounds 20 to 30 minutes prior to cleansing or repair procedures, but these cannot be used on eyes, ears, nose, fingers, genitals, or toes.
3. *Hair:* Hair near the wound usually creates minimal difficulty during repair. Do not shave hair because it increases the risk of infection. Instead, clip the hair with scissors, if needed, to visualize the wound during closure. Alternatively, petroleum jelly can be used to keep unwanted scalp hair away from the wound while suturing. Eyebrow hair should not be removed because this may lead to abnormal or slow regrowth.

4. *Wound cleansing:* Irrigation is the preferred method of wound cleansing as it reduces bacterial contamination and prevents subsequent infection. Tap water and sterile normal saline are equally safe to use for irrigation of the wound. A general rule for the saline irrigation volume is to use 50 to 100 mL of normal saline per centimeter of the wound. More solution may be needed if the wound is unusually large or contaminated. Use a large irrigating syringe (20 to 50 mL) to provide enough force to cleanse the wound. A splash guard attached to the syringe is recommended to reduce splatter during irrigation. It is important to remove all foreign debris to decrease infection risk and prevent skin tattooing. Chlorhexidine or povidone-iodine surgical scrub preparations may be used to clean the skin *surrounding* the wound but are not recommended for use in the wound itself. Hydrogen peroxide and alcohol are not recommended.

5. *Wound exploration:* Explore wounds for the presence of foreign objects, deep tissue layer damage, injury to nerve or blood vessel, or joint involvement. It is imperative to determine the wound depth. Probe the wound with a cotton-tipped swab, a hemostat, or a needle holder. Deep lacerations should be closed in an ED by layered closure. If tendon injury is suspected or if bone is exposed, refer to an orthopedist.

6. *Wound debridement:* Unattached loose tissues may be gently removed with sterile instruments. Debridement is advantageous because it removes wound contaminants and approximates wound edges. This allows for easier wound repair and cosmetic acceptability after the wound heals. Although it is helpful to excise necrotic skin, excessive trimming of irregular lacerations should not be attempted as it can create a defect that is difficult to close or that increases tension at the wound margin, making scarring more likely.

7. *Wound closure:* Several methods are available for wound closure.
   - *Traditional sutures* (or stitches) involve "sewing" the skin together with a needle and surgical thread. This procedure usually requires an injection and/or topical use of an anesthetic and bandaging the wound afterward. Simple, uncomplicated lacerations to the scalp, trunk, arms, or legs may be closed with sutures (called *primary closure*). In general, an absorbable suture material is used for closure of structures deeper than the epidermis, and nonabsorbable sutures are used to close the outermost layer of a laceration. See Table 44.2 for suture material, size, and removal guidelines.
   - *Staples* can be used for the scalp, trunk, and extremities (not including the hands and feet) and provide a more rapid closure time than with sutures. Laceration repair with staples is associated with a lower infection rate but can be more painful to remove and also may not be as cosmetically appealing when healed. Staples should not be used if MRI or CT is necessary.
   - *Surgical tape,* such as Steri-Strips, is used for small superficial wounds. Surgical tape cannot be used on wounds in moist areas or in areas of tension, such as flexor or extensor surfaces. Surgical tape should also be avoided in wounds on small children, who will most likely remove the tape prematurely.
   - *Topical skin adhesive,* also known as *skin glue,* is used for simple lacerations with clean edges. The adhesive is applied on top of the skin while the edges of the wound

TABLE 44.2 Suture Material, Size, and Removal Guidelines

Body Region	Monofilament[a] (for Superficial Lacerations)	Absorbable[b] (for Deep Lacerations)	Duration (Days)
Scalp	5-0 or 4-0	4-0	5-7
Face	6-0	5-0	3-5
Eyelid	7-0 or 6-0	—	3-5
Eyebrow	6-0 or 5-0	5-0	3-5
Trunk	5-0 or 4-0	3-0	5-7
Extremities	5-0 or 4-0	4-0	7-10
Joint surface	4-0	—	10-14
Hand	5-0	5-0	7
Foot sole	4-0 or 3-0	4-0	7-10

[a]Examples of monofilament nonabsorbable sutures: Nylon, polypropylene. Good for the outermost layer of skin. Polypropylene is good for scalp, eyebrows.

[b]Examples of absorbable sutures: Polyglycolic acid and polyglactin 910 (Vicryl). Good for deeper, subcuticular layers.

From The Johns Hopkins Hospital. *Harriet Lane Handbook.* 20th ed. Philadelphia: Elsevier; 2018.

are held together. Usually two or three applications of the adhesive are applied to ensure adequate closure. Adhesive in the wound or between wound margins should be avoided. Skin glue takes less time to apply than stitches and forms a strong, flexible bond over the top of the wound. Topical skin adhesive should not be used on areas of skin where there is tension, such as over a joint, due to the high probability of the wound reopening and thus requiring healing by secondary closure, causing increased risk of scarring. A bandage is not required for cover after tissue repair with skin glue. The topical skin adhesive sloughs off the wound as it heals, usually in 7 to 10 days, and does not require a return visit for removal. Infection risk is minimal due to antimicrobial properties of the adhesive. Minimal scarring is associated with this method of laceration repair.

8. *Dressing:* The purpose of dressings is to protect, compress, absorb, and immobilize, and to improve healing and affect cosmetic outcomes. A simple repaired laceration may be covered with an adhesive bandage. For more complex repaired injuries, dress the wound with nonadherent gauze for the first layer followed by a second layer of plain gauze (if needed), and secured in place with adhesive tape or elasticized gauze (tubular net bandage).

9. *Immunization:* Give tetanus booster or tetanus immunoglobulin as indicated.

10. *Antibiotics:* Antibiotic prophylaxis of clean wounds is not indicated. Its use in contaminated wounds may be helpful, but careful wound cleaning with extensive irrigation followed by prompt wound closure (when indicated) are the most effective safeguards in preventing infection.

11. *Suture and staple removal:* The timing for removal of staples and sutures depends on their location (see Table 44.2).

Patient and Parent Education

Instructions for wound care at home are best given in writing and should include the following:

- Patients can shower 24 hours after suture placement without worrying about the infection risk. However, the area should be dried well and kept dry after showering.
- Note signs and symptoms of infection that warrant an early recheck (redness, swelling, discharge, increased pain).
- Give instructions about cleansing and bandaging the wound. For surgical tape and topical skin adhesive, do not use topical antibiotic ointment or lotions because they will remove the adhesive.
- List any activity restrictions.
- Identify a date for a return appointment.

Burns

Every day in the United States more than 300 children from birth to 19 years old require burn treatment in an emergency room, and two children die from their burns (CDC, 2016). Intentionally burning a child is, unfortunately, a common form of abuse, and every child burn injury should be evaluated for potential abuse or neglect.

Common causes of burn injuries include grills, hot soups, hot water, curling irons, house fires, and appliances, such as hot stoves or coffee pots. Residential fires cause serious injury or death. Younger children tend to sustain more scald injuries from steam or hot liquid, and older children tend to incur burns from flame and direct fire contact. Scald burns may cause deeper injuries, depending on how long the skin is in contact with the substance. The longer the contact, the deeper the scald burn is. Thermal burns are deeper and involve more skin layers in children than adults due to children having thinner skin.

Burns are classified by depth of injury, percentage of body surface area (BSA) involved, location of the burn, and association with other injuries. The classification system for burns includes superficial, superficial (partial or deep), and full thicknesses. The term *fourth-degree burn* identifies burns that extend into the muscle, fascia, and/or bone and are potentially life threatening (Rice and Orgill, 2017).

- Superficial burns involve only the epidermis. The skin is erythematous, inflamed, and painful, but there are no blisters. Superficial burns typically heal in 3 to 7 days, have little risk of scarring, and require only symptomatic treatment. Sunburn is a common example of a superficial burn.
- Partial-thickness burns involve the epidermis and the dermis to a variable degree. The dermal appendages are always preserved and provide a source for regeneration.
- Superficial partial-thickness burns are erythemic, very painful, mottled, moist, and blistered. They usually heal in 7 to 14 days; scarring may occur.
- Deep partial-thickness burns appear pale and yellow and are less painful and weepy than superficial partial-thickness burns. Deep partial-thickness burns take longer to heal (3 weeks), and are more likely to scar.
- Full-thickness burns destroy the epidermis and dermis completely. The skin appears whitish (a waxy white appearance) or leathery. The surface is dry and nontender. Fluid losses can be profound with this burn. These usually require skin grafting, cause permanent scarring, and take several weeks to heal.
- Full-thickness burns with extension into deep tissue involve destruction and/or extensive injury of muscle, fascia, nerves,

tendons, vessels, and bone. They typically require surgical intervention and skin grafting.

Burns involving large body surfaces generally vary in depth. Burn wounds are dynamic, and the effect of dermal ischemia (affected by infection, exposure, and dehydration) may not be initially apparent. Their depth can change from day to day. The percentage of BSA and the part(s) of the body affected are also key factors to determine treatment, disposition, and prognosis (Table 44.3). Multiple methods estimate the burn BSA. For example, the area covered by a child's palm (from wrist crease to finger crease), also called the "rule of the palm," represents 1% of total BSA (TBSA) and may be used for estimating the extent of small burns covering less than 10% of BSA (Antoon and Donovan, 2016). Free software to calculate BSA in pediatric burn victims is available at www.sagediagram.com/.

Clinical Findings

History. The following information should be obtained:

- Description of how the burn occurred, including injury agent and length of time agent was in contact with the skin, circumstances surrounding the injury, when it occurred, and likelihood of other injuries, such as trauma or smoke inhalation
- Initial and subsequent treatment of the burn
- Previous history of burn injuries
- Other current medical problems, medications, allergies, and tetanus status
- Suspicion of child abuse if the injury does not match the history and mechanism described.

Physical Examination. The physical examination should begin with primary airway assessment. The most common cause of death during the first hour after a burn injury is respiratory impairment. Children with any sign of airway compromise should immediately be placed on 100% oxygen via a nonrebreather mask and transported to the hospital via ambulance and emergency medical services (EMS) for further care and management. Airway complications should be suspected if there is history of exposure to flame, smoke, or chemicals; the exposure was in an enclosed place; there are facial or neck burns; burns or soot over the nares or oral cavity; hoarseness; or cough, or auscultated wheezes or crackles (Micak, 2018). Once the patient is stable, a thorough physical examination requires the following determinations:

- Percentage of BSA affected (see Table 44.3)
- Mechanism of burn and associated injuries
- Burn distribution and pattern with particular concern for circumferential burns to the thorax that may cause poor chest expansion and declining oxygen saturation
- Burn depth—classified as superficial, partial thickness, or full thickness
- Assessment of the extremity vascular status
- Presence of any complicating medical condition

Diagnostic Studies

- A CBC may include elevated hematocrit secondary to fluid loss. Initial white blood cell elevation is always secondary to an acute phase reaction, but may later indicate infection.
- A basic metabolic panel may reveal elevated potassium due to cell breakdown. Blood urea nitrogen (BUN) and creatine kinase assess renal function, rhabdomyolysis, and tissue perfusion.
- A urinalysis and specific gravity help determine hydration status, and the presence of myoglobin may suggest acute tubular necrosis secondary to muscle tissue destruction and breakdown.

TABLE 44.3	Estimation of Surface Area Burned Based on Age					
	AGE (YEARS)					
Area	Birth to 1	1-4	5-9	10-14	15	Adult
Head	19	17	13	11	9	7
Neck	2	2	2	2	2	2
Anterior trunk	13	13	13	13	13	13
Posterior trunk	13	13	13	13	13	13
Right buttock	2.5	2.5	2.5	2.5	2.5	2.5
Left buttock	2.5	2.5	2.5	2.5	2.5	2.5
Genitalia	1	1	1	1	1	1
Right upper arm	4	4	4	4	4	4
Left upper arm	4	4	4	4	4	4
Right lower arm	3	3	3	3	3	3
Left lower arm	3	3	3	3	3	3
Right hand	2.5	2.5	2.5	2.5	2.5	2.5
Left hand	2.5	2.5	2.5	2.5	2.5	2.5
Right thigh	5.5	6.5	8	8.5	9	9.5
Left thigh	5.5	6.5	8	8.5	9	9.5
Right leg	5	5	5.5	6	6.5	7
Left leg	5	5	5.5	6	6.5	7
Right foot	3.5	3.5	3.5	3.5	3.5	3.5
Left foot	3.5	3.5	3.5	3.5	3.5	3.5

This modification by O'Neill of the Brooke Army Burn Center Diagram shows the change in surface area of the head from 19% in an infant to 7% in an adult. Proper use of this chart provides an accurate basis for subsequent management of the burned child.

From Joffe MD. Burns. In: Fleisher GR, Ludwig S, Henretig FM, et al. eds. *Textbook of Pediatric Emergency Medicine*. 6th ed. Philadelphia: Lippincott Williams & Wilkins; 2010:1285.

Differential Diagnosis

Chapter 24 discusses intentional burn injuries resulting from child abuse. Scalded skin syndrome caused by staphylococcal infection can cause skin exfoliation, but the clinical presentation clearly differentiates it from an accidental burn injury. Management is similar to that used for burn management.

Management. Determining the need for admission to a hospital or burn center involves many factors, including burn depth, percentage of BSA injured, and mechanism of the burn injury. Other factors that influence hospital admission include risk of infection, pain control, functional and cosmetic outcomes, and social considerations. ●Children with burn injuries who meet the following criteria should be admitted to the hospital or burn center for further management (O'Halloran, 2018; Carney and Roswell, 2016):

- Burns involving more than 20% TBSA
- Partial-thickness burns involving more than 10% TBSA
- Full-thickness burns involving more than 2% TBSA
- Circumferential burns
- Burns overlying joints and/or involving critical areas, such as the hands and feet, genitalia, and perineum
- Full-thickness burns
- Chemical burns, electrical burns (including lightning injury), inhalation injury
- Suspicion of child abuse or unsafe home environment
- Presence of an underlying chronic illness

The outpatient treatment of minor burns is an option only for superficial burns and partial-thickness burns to less than 10% of BSA. Referral and consultation with a burn specialist depends on the severity and location of the burn. Box 44.1 outlines the primary care management of superficial and partial-thickness burns.

Patient and Parent Education

The following points are important components of patient and parent education:

- Emphasize injury prevention strategies (Chapter 24).
- Inform parents of serious or long-term consequences of burns: frequent and significant sunburns during early childhood can predispose to skin cancers in later life; electric burns cause thermal injury to skin (contact burn); if an arc is created and there is passage of electrical current through the body, there is a potential for cardiac dysrhythmias and neurologic impairment following the burn.
- Inform parents that the extent of scarring is difficult to predict with certainty; that scarring depends on depth of the burn, length of time needed for healing, whether grafting was done, and the child's age and skin color; and that scars remain immature for the first 12 to 18 months. Their color and texture changes as the child grows. Most minor scald injuries from hot liquids heal quickly with little or no scarring.

Contusions and Hematomas

A contusion, or bruise, is an injury in which the skin is not broken but trauma causes effusion into muscle and subcutaneous tissue with injury to the vessels and possibly the nerves. In children, contusions can occur anywhere on the body but are most often seen on the extremities.

Contusions are common in children and are caused by blunt trauma, most often as a result of falling or bumping into objects during play. Participation in contact sports puts children at increased risk for contusions. Bruises to the trunk, face, or head are red flags for possible child abuse. A careful history must be taken to determine whether the explanation of the injury is consistent with the child's condition and independent report of what happened.

Hematomas are localized collections of extravasated blood that are relatively or completely confined within a space or potential space. In essence, a hematoma is a raised, palpable ecchymosis or bruise. Hematomas can be associated with most types of minor and major wounds; they must be observed closely for signs of infection and, in some instances, drained.

Clinical Findings

History and Physical Examination. Inquire about a history of easy bleeding or bruising, or slow healing. The following should be determined:

- Circulatory status and discoloration, involvement of underlying structures

• BOX 44.1 **Management of Superficial and Partial-Thickness Burns in the Primary Care Setting**

1. Maintain proper nutrition and hydration to enhance healing.
2. Management of superficial burns (Wiktor and Richards, 2018):
   - Cleanse the burn and surrounding skin with lukewarm water and soap.
   - Burns with an intact epidermis, such as superficial or superficial partial-thickness wounds, do not require a topical antimicrobial agent.
   - A nonadherent dressing, such as Adaptic or Xeroform, followed by a gauze dressing may be applied for larger, more severe, superficial burns. Change twice a day or when soiled if risk of infection is present, such as on a hand. Otherwise leave the superficial burn open to air.
   - Aloe vera has antibacterial properties and may be used to help with skin healing and soothing. Lanolin may cause itching and is not recommended.
   - Administer analgesics, such as acetaminophen or ibuprofen, as indicated.
3. Management of superficial partial-thickness burns (Wiktor and Richards, 2018):
   - Administer adequate analgesic medication. Narcotics may be needed before performing wound care and for breakthrough pain. Switch to over-the-counter acetaminophen or ibuprofen as the pain subsides.
   - Cleanse the wound with mild soap and tap water.
   - Assess the burn the day after injury and then weekly (or more frequently if needed) to ensure proper healing and absence of infection. Dressing changes, debridement, and wound cleansing should be performed twice a day or as needed for soaked or soiled dressings until the burn has healed.
   - Leave small blisters intact as they provide a biological dressing and will rupture spontaneously and heal. Consider rupturing and unroofing the blister if large blisters are noted; the blister is on a

joint, hands, or feet; it limits range of motion; or it makes burn depth assessment difficult. (Tennehaus and Rennekampff, 2017).
   - Gently débride open blisters to remove devitalized tissue and residue from prior dressing changes.
   - Superficial partial thickness burns with an intact epidermis do not require a topical antimicrobial agent.
   - To prevent infection in any nonsuperficial burn, apply bacitracin or 1% silver sulfadiazine cream to the clean débrided area followed by the application of bismuth-impregnated petrolatum-based gauze such as Xeroform. Next apply a dry elastic gauze outer dressing such as kerlix.
   - One percent silver sulfadiazine cream (1% SSD) is an antimicrobial and soothing agent but should not be used if the patient has a sulfa allergy or the patient is younger than 2 months of age. Also, 1% SSD is oculotoxic and should not be used near the eyes.
   - Biologic and or synthetic dressings may be more beneficial depending on the burn. Consult with a burn specialist if considering use.
   - Itching occurs commonly during the healing process, often triggered by activity, heat, and stress. Use mittens for young children to prevent scratching if itching occurs. If needed, administer an antihistamine, such as diphenhydramine.
   - Individuals with circumferential extremity burns may need to be admitted to the hospital for observation to monitor for compartment syndrome.
   - Another option for partial-thickness burn management is the use of Aquacel Ag dressing (ConvaTec). This dressing is impregnated with silver ion, which helps prevent infection. Apply it after complete burn cleansing and débridement. Cover the burned area with sterile gauze and leave in place for 7 days, with close wound monitoring (Tenenhaus and Rennekampff, 2017).

- Motor and sensory function: sensation, mobility, and range of motion
- Referral is needed if there is any evidence of circulatory compromise, such as lack of pulse.

Differential Diagnosis

Hemophilia, von Willebrand disease, and conditions that cause purpura should be considered. Myositis ossificans, a complication of contusions rarely seen in children, can be confused with osteogenic sarcoma.

Management and Complications

For contusions involving extremities:
- Acute treatment (Murphy and Karlin, 2016):
  Prescribe protection, rest, ice, compression, and elevation (PRICE). Protect and rest the affected joint or limb during the acute phase. Consider use of slings, Ace wrap, or knee immobilizer depending on severity and location of the contusion. Apply ice to the injury for 20 minutes three to four times a day until the swelling improves or resolves. Apply a pressure bandage, such as an Ace wrap, to help prevent further edema or bleeding. Check the bandage to ensure it isn't too tight and affecting circulation. Elevate the affected body part (ideally, above the level of the heart) to help with venous blood return and decrease edema. Acetaminophen or a nonsteroidal antiinflammatory drug (NSAID), such as ibuprofen, are good analgesia choices.

- Post acute-phase treatment:
  Start range-of-motion and strengthening exercises as soon as possible to help the recovery process and not delay a return to normal activity. When the limb is pain free, gradually remove supportive/protective devices and return to normal activity.
- Reserve radiographs for suspected foreign objects or bone fracture. Refer severe injuries for orthopedic management.
  Most contusions heal quickly without sequelae. However, severe trauma to the quadriceps muscle can lead to myositis ossificans or, with large hemorrhage, to compartment syndrome.

Patient and Parent Education

Explain to parents the expected color changes of ecchymosis from purple to green, and that the ecchymosis may migrate to other surrounding tissues. Arrange for follow-up if discomfort continues or increases. Encourage injury prevention. The degree of injury and resolution of subjective symptoms determines return to activities. Physical therapy or an athletic trainer (for athletes) may be needed to help the patient return to activities of daily living and/or sports.

Bites and Stings

Animal and Child Bites

Pets, stray animals, or humans, especially other children, cause pediatric bite injuries. Most infants' and young children's animal bites involve the head and neck, while older children commonly have upper extremity bites. In contrast, most bites caused by young children occur on the upper extremities.

Each year, an estimated 1% of ED visits in the United States are due to animal or human bite wounds (Harper, 2017). About 80% to 90% of bites are dog bites (both provoked and unprovoked) (Ginsburg, 2016). Boys are attacked more often than girls. Dog and cat bites are often caused by animals known to the child. The risk of infection from a dog bite or human bite is between 15% and 20% (AAP, 2015a). The risk of infection from a cat bite (despite early medical attention) is at least 50%. Cat bites cause puncture wounds that tend to be deeper than dog bites. Dog bites cause abrasions, puncture wounds, and lacerations, with or without associated tissue avulsion. Limited data define the incidence of human bite injuries, but it is suspected that they are the leading cause of child care injury. All human bite wounds, regardless of mechanism of injury, are at high risk for infection. Other animal bites, such as rat bites, are not reportable, so their prevalence is unknown (Ginsburg, 2016). Clenched-fist bites (when the closed fist hits the another's teeth resulting in a laceration) are the most serious of human bites and are typically the result of fighting. Human bite injuries have high risk of infection and joint compromise.

Clinical Findings

History and Physical Examination. Ask about the circumstances surrounding the bite including the type of animal, domesticated or feral animal, provoked or unprovoked attack, and location of the attack. History of drug allergies and immunization status of the child also should be ascertained.

The wound should be assessed for the type, size, and depth of injury. Explore for the presence of foreign material and the status of underlying structures. If the bite is on an extremity, assess its range of motion and sensory intactness. Assess functioning of the facial nerve with deep facial bite injuries. A diagram of the injury should be recorded in the child's chart. It is best to photograph the injury.

Diagnostic Studies. Obtain aerobic and anaerobic cultures and Gram stain prior to starting antibiotics if wound infection is suspected (Harper, 2017). A radiograph of the affected part should be obtained if it is likely that a bone or joint could have been penetrated or fractured or if retained foreign material may be present.

Differential Diagnosis and Management. The differential diagnosis includes lacerations or puncture wounds from other causes.

Management involves both physical and psychological care of the child and includes the following (Carney and Roswell, 2016):

- Administer tetanus booster and rabies prophylaxis if indicated (consult with local animal control or public health department).
- Provide/administer appropriate analgesia or anesthesia.
- Debride avulsed or devitalized tissue and remove foreign matter.
- Using normal saline, irrigate the wounds using high pressure (>5 pounds per square inch) and high volume (>1 L).
- Isolated puncture wounds should not be irrigated; instead, soak the wound in a diluted solution of tap water and povidone-iodine for 15 minutes.
- Prescribe a 3- to 5-day course of prophylactic antibiotics for all human and cat bites, and for the following bite types or wound characteristics: hand, puncture, overlying bone fracture, substantial crushing tissue injuries, those that require debridement, or those involving tendons, muscles, or joint spaces. Immunosuppressed children require antibiotics.

Prescribe a broad-spectrum antibiotic, such as amoxicillin clavulanate (first choice). Treat penicillin-allergic individuals with an extended spectrum cephalosporin or trimethoprim-sulfamethoxazole plus clindamycin (Seeyave and Brown, 2016).

- Consider rabies exposure prophylaxis if there is any question about exposure. The CDC provides guidelines on rabies prophylaxis (see "Additional Resources"). The local health department is also a good resource for guidance on post-exposure rabies prophylaxis.
- Some controversy exists about whether bite wounds should be closed primarily with delayed closure (3 to 5 days after injury) or allowed to heal by secondary intention (leaving the wound open). Factors to consider are the type, size, and depth of the wound; the anatomic location; presence of infection; the time interval since the injury; and the potential for cosmetic disfigurement. Surgical consultation should be obtained for all deep or extensive wounds and those involving the bones, joints, or hands. Because of the excellent blood supply to the face, facial lacerations are at less risk for infection. Many plastic surgeons advocate primary closure of thoroughly irrigated and debrided facial bite wounds within 5 to 6 hours of injury. PCPs may refer patients with concerns about scarring or facial wounds for plastic surgery repair.
- Bites involving the hand or foot should not be sutured but allowed to drain. Hand and foot bites less than 1.5 cm are best healed by secondary intention; bites greater than 1.5 cm should have delayed primary closure.
- Bite wounds more than 8 to 12 hours old should not be sutured; facial wounds may be sutured up to 24 hours.
- A single layer of nonabsorbable sutures is best (avoid multiple closure layers).
- Refer children with severe bites. Obtain a surgical consult if there is evidence of or concern about nerve, tendon, and/or ligament injury or if a joint space was involved. Hospitalization, reconstructive surgery, and long-term follow-up may be indicated.
- Discuss the child's fears and management of any behavioral problems that may result (see Chapter 15).
- Report dog and wild animal bites to animal control.

Complications. Secondary infection is the most common complication of mammalian bites and can lead to cellulitis and lymphangitis, thus requiring hospitalization. *Streptococcus* and *Staphylococcus* are common organisms associated with infected animal and human bites; anaerobic infection is also possible. Species of gram-negative bacteria (e.g., *P. multocida* and *P. canis* from dog and cat bites and *Eikenella corrodens* from human bites) can also cause infections (Seeyave and Brown, 2016). The potential for rabies, human immunodeficiency virus (HIV), and hepatitis B and C exposure must also be considered.

Patient and Parent Education. Preventive education and actions should include the following (AAP, 2015b):

- Teach children to avoid stray animals, be cautious around domesticated animals, and not tease or provoke any animal.
- Emphasize the importance of parental supervision of children as they play with pets.
- Families with young children should not keep typically wild animals as pets.
- Never leave infants or young children alone with dogs or cats; animals with histories of aggression are inappropriate in households with children.
- Report stray animals promptly to animal control officials.

Hymenoptera (Bees, Wasps, and Ants)

Bees, hornets, yellow jackets, fire and harvester ants, and wasps belong to the Hymenoptera order of insects and have common venom antigens. Among the Hymenoptera order, the Vespidae (hornets, wasps, and yellow jackets), Apidae (honeybees and bumblebees), and Formicidae (fire ants) families cause allergic reactions from their sting. Cross-reactivity of the allergens present within family venoms occurs for all except the Apidae family (Casale and Burks, 2014). Immunoglobulin E–dependent hypersensitivity is the underlying cause of reactions. Histamines, leukotrienes, prostaglandins, and other inflammatory factors are released, causing local or systemic symptoms.

Bees and wasps ordinarily do not sting unless frightened, bothered, or hurt. Yellow jackets are aggressive. Fire ants may cause multiple, painful stings. Reactions to stings by these insects can vary from mild, local responses to life-threatening anaphylaxis with wheezing and urticaria. Most children experience only a local reaction, but some children suffer severe systemic reactions, which can progress to medical emergencies unless prompt intervention is initiated.

Clinical Findings

History and Physical Examination. The child usually reports being bitten or stung. There may be a past history of a local or systemic reaction following an insect bite.

Physical examination findings include the following:
- Mild reaction consists of local redness, pruritus, pain, edema, and possibly generalized urticaria.
- Severe reactions, including anaphylaxis, include local signs and urticaria, plus any of the following:
  - Watery eyes
  - Difficulty breathing, swallowing, or wheezing
  - Hoarseness, thickened speech
  - Gastrointestinal disturbances, abdominal pain
  - Dizziness, weakness, confusion
  - Collapse, unconsciousness, even death
  - Fire ant bites cause vesicles that develop into sterile pustules

Diagnostic Studies. Diagnosis of a Hymenoptera insect sting is usually based on history and physical examination alone. For systemic reactions, refer to an allergist for venom-specific immunoglobulin E testing and identification after resolution of the reaction.

Differential Diagnosis and Management

The differential diagnosis includes other insect bites, folliculitis, or urticaria.

The following management steps are taken:
- For *mild local* reactions:
  - Remove visible stingers with the edge of a sharp object (e.g., knife blade or credit card), taking care to not squeeze the attached venom sac.
  - Apply cool compresses or use cool baths.
  - Administer an antihistamine, such as diphenhydramine dosed every 4 to 6 hours at 6.25 mg (maximum 37.5 mg/day) for children 2-5 years old; 12.5-25 mg (maximum 150 mg/day) for 6 to 11 years old, and 25-50 mg (maximum 300 mg/day) for 12 years and older or hydroxyzine 2 mg/kg/day, in divided doses every 6 to 8 hours daily (50 mg/day maximum under 6 years old; 50 to 100 mg/day maximum over 6 years old), for pruritus.

- Topical glucocorticoid creams or ointments may help reduce itching.
- ⬤ For *moderate* to *severe* reactions:
- Moderate reactions may need to be treated with oral antihistamines, corticosteroids, and inhaled bronchodilators (if wheezing).
- Institute emergency measures for treatment of anaphylactic reactions and transport to the ED via emergency medical services (EMS) as quickly as possible.
- Hospitalize for anaphylactic shock.
- Epinephrine: 0.01 mg/kg (0.01 mL/kg/dose of 1 mg/mL solution) intramuscularly, not to exceed 0.3 mg to 0.5 mg, every 5 to 15 minutes. Usually the patient will respond after one or two doses.
- Give antihistamines immediately following epinephrine (and repeated every 6 hours for up to 3 days) but not as a substitute for epinephrine. Give both histamine type 1 (H_1) and type 2 (H_2) blockers to reduce hives, it is more effective than giving an H_1 blocker alone. Glucocorticoids are not helpful in treating acute reactions but may help to prevent a potential late-phase reaction also known as *biphasic anaphylaxis* (Campbell and Kelso, 2017).
- Consider giving oral prednisolone (1 mg/kg; 60 mg maximum).
- Nebulized albuterol (2.5 mg for <30 kg and 5 mg for >30 mg per dose repeated every 15 minutes as needed for children with bronchospasm or wheezing).
- Administer high-flow oxygen (warm humidified) by nonrebreather mask.

Referral to an allergist is indicated for any child who has life-threatening respiratory symptoms (e.g., stridor or wheezing) or hypotension. Venom immunotherapy desensitization is highly effective in preventing further systemic reactions. Children younger than 16 years old who have only urticaria or angioedema do not require venom immunotherapy, because few will have systemic reactions with subsequent stings.

Patient and Parent Education

Key issues to discuss with moderate to severe reactions include the following:
- Importance of wearing a medical alert tag or bracelet
- Proper use of an insect sting kit that includes two self-injectable epinephrine pens and the need to have a kit always readily available for emergency use
- Prevention of stings by avoiding areas likely to be infested with these insects, not wearing bright-colored clothing, and not using perfumed products

Mosquitoes, Fleas, and Chiggers (Red Bug or Harvest Mites)

Mosquito bites are the most common insect bites for infants and children. Mosquitoes are vectors of many important human diseases and their bites cause irritating local skin reactions. Flea and chigger (also known as *red bug* or *harvest mite*) bites produce local skin eruptions. The larvae of harvest mites secrete an irritating substance that cases the skin eruption characteristic of chigger bites. Chigger mites live on grain stems, shrubs, grass, and vines and attach to human or animals that pass by. Fleas that commonly attack humans in the United States include the human flea, cat flea, and dog flea. There is a seasonal pattern to mosquito, flea, and chigger bites.

Clinical Findings

History. The following may be reported:

- Mosquito or flea bites: known bite or seasonal time; presence of cat, dog, or furry animal in child's environment; complaints of a brief stinging sensation followed by itching
- Chigger bites: complaints of itching followed by dermatitis; history of playing or walking in grassy areas, parks, or other mite habitat near woods and water

Physical Examination and Diagnostic Studies. Mosquito bites are characterized by the following:

- Local irritation in unsensitized children
- In sensitized children urticarial wheals that itch and last several hours to days or firm papules or nodules that last a long time
- Central punctum (sometimes noted)
- Secondary impetigo from scratching of skin lesions
- Skeeter syndrome is a significant allergic reaction to the mosquito saliva that is difficult to distinguish from secondary infection, except that it occurs within hours of the bite. It is characterized by large, local areas of edema, erythema, and warmth.

Flea bites are characterized by the following:

- Urticarial wheal or papule surrounded by redness in a sensitized person that may progress into bullae, especially in young children.
- Central hemorrhagic puncta (often noted)
- Grouping of multiple lesions, commonly found on arms, ankles, legs, feet, thighs, waist, buttocks, and lower abdomen
- There is a classic linear configuration, which is referred to as the "breakfast, lunch, and dinner" sign
- Chigger bites are characterized by the following:
  - Discrete, bright-red papules 1 to 2 mm in diameter that often have hemorrhagic puncta
  - Lesions mainly seen on legs (sock area) and belt line but can be widespread
  - Wheals, papules, or papulovesicles in sensitized individuals
  - Bullae or purpuric lesions with secondary hypersensitivity reaction
  - Intense pruritus reaching a peak on the second day and decreasing over the next 5 to 6 days, but can persist for months
  - Possible secondary impetigo from scratching lesions
  - May see the embedded chiggers

The presence of fleas or harvest mites is diagnostic; otherwise, no studies are done.

Differential Diagnosis and Management

The diagnosis is often obvious, but the differential diagnosis can include insect bites that produce similar papular, vesicular lesions, or other skin conditions.

Management consists of controlling pruritus, including measures such as the following:

- Cool compresses
- Topical corticosteroids (e.g., 1% hydrocortisone cream)
- Topical antipruritic agents, such as calamine lotion; avoid topical diphenhydramine
- Oral antihistamines (e.g., diphenhydramine) if topical corticosteroids do not provide relief
- Removal of embedded chiggers (can be withdrawn by covering the insect with alcohol, mineral oil, nail polish, or ointment)
- Colloidal oatmeal baths (clean tub thoroughly after bath to avoid fall risk from oil residue left behind)

- Treatment of secondary skin lesions as indicated
- Elimination of fleas by treating animals and cleaning carpets, bedding, upholstered furniture; avoid areas that are potentially infested with mosquitoes, fleas, or chiggers
- Insecticides should be used with caution

Patient and Parent Education

Prevention of insect bites is a key educational component. Prevention includes eliminating mosquitoes, fleas, and chiggers from the environment, or by preventing their contact with the skin.

- Use insect repellents (generally effective against mosquitoes and harvest mites).
- Wear protective clothing to cover the body and tuck pants into shoes or socks.
- Wear neutral-colored clothes (white, green, tan, and khaki do not attract mosquitoes).
- Avoid scented hair sprays, powders, soaps, lotions, creams, and perfumes because they can attract all forms of stinging insects.
- Mosquitoes are attracted to bright clothing and sweaty skin and are drawn to humans by scent.
- Treat suspected animal carrier for fleas, and spray carpets and other infested areas; spray yards and grassy places for fleas in those environments that the child frequents.
- Vacuum carpets daily if fleas are seen on household pets.
- Avoid playing in areas of harvest mite habitat.
- Remove areas of standing water to decrease mosquito breeding

Spiders and Scorpions

Most spider bites are innocuous and do not cause reactions. If reactions occur, they are generally a minor, localized response that can be mistaken for a flea, bedbug, or some other insect bite. Most spiders cannot bite humans because of their short and fragile fangs, and almost all spiders avoid humans unless provoked. There are two main spiders common in the North American continent that can cause serious complications: the black widow (*Latrodectus mactans*) and the brown recluse (*Loxosceles reclusa*).

The black widow spider has a globular body about 1 cm across that is shiny black with a red or orange hourglass marking on its underside. It is found throughout the United States. The black widow spider prefers to live in cool, dark, dry places in buildings and little-used structures, such as wood piles, garages, basements, and tool sheds or less frequented outbuildings. This particular type of spider often spins its web on outdoor furniture, which explains why many black widow spider bites occur around the genitals and buttocks. The black widow has neurotoxic venom.

The brown recluse, one of the most dangerous spiders in the United States, has an oval light fawn to dark chocolate-brown body; it is approximately 1 cm long (adults range from 1 to 5 cm in total length) with a dark brown violin-shaped band extending from its eyes partially down its back. The brown recluse is endemic in the southern Midwest and southeastern states but have been reported in larger cities outside their typical geographic pattern (Otten, 2018). The brown recluse spider typically lives in dark, dry places (attics, basements, boxes) and storage closets among clothes. When living outdoors it resides in grasses, rocky bluffs, and barns. The brown recluse spiders are not aggressive and typically bite only in self-defense. The venom of the brown recluse can be hemolytic and necrotizing with extension caused by a spreading factor.

At least 30 of the 1400 reported scorpion species in the world produce fatal stings (LoVecchio, 2017). Scorpions have a stinging apparatus in their tail. They are nocturnal and found in the southwestern and southern United States. Scorpions commonly live in cool, dark places during the day and are known to crawl into sleeping bags, shoes, and discarded clothing. Scorpions prefer to avoid stinging unless they are provoked or attacked (Mayo Clinic Staff, 2016). Human stings by scorpions are usually accidental and most commonly occur when a person unintentionally steps on a scorpion or reaches under wood or rocks (LoVecchio, 2017).

Clinical Findings

History and Physical Examination. Assess the known history of a spider or scorpion bite or exposure to an environment where they live. The spider's characteristics help in identification. Children are more vulnerable to spider and scorpion bites than adults.

The characteristic physical features are identified for each type of spider bite:

- Black widow spider bites (Swanson et al., 2018):
  - Initially most bites are asymptomatic or include mild site pain.
  - The bite wound most often has a center punctum with a blanched circular patch and a surrounding erythema.
  - Symptoms start 30 to 120 minutes after the bite and may include tremors, weakness, shaking of the affected extremity, local paresthesias, diaphoresis, headaches, nausea, and/or vomiting.
  - Muscle pain is the most common symptom and usually occurs in the back, extremity muscles, or abdomen. Severe abdominal pain is characteristic with abdominal wall rigidity that can be confused with acute surgical conditions, such as appendicitis or cholecystitis. Muscle pain is self-limited and resolves within 24 to 72 hours without treatment.
  - Muscle rigidity and tenderness may also be noted adjacent to the bite site and/or include myoclonus of the affected limb.
  - Facial swelling and generalized erythema are common pediatric occurrences. Young infants and children are often distressed, inconsolable, and refuse to eat. There may be a history of using a crib that was just taken from storage.
  - Vital signs are normal in 70% of patients, but tachycardia, tachypnea, and hypertension have been noted secondary to anxiety, venom effects, or pain.
  - Rare findings include pulmonary edema, cardiovascular collapse, cardiomyopathy, priapism, rhabdomyolysis, hematuria, Horner syndrome, compartment syndrome, toxic epidermal necrolysis, and death.
- Brown recluse spider bites (Vetter and Swanson, 2019):
  - Brown recluse bites typically occur on the inner thigh, upper arm, or thorax and look like two small punctum marks with surrounding erythema. Central pallor eventually is noted around the punctum marks but is not usually seen immediately after the bite.
  - Usually the initial bite is painless, but some may report a burning sensation or pain.
  - Pain may develop 2 to 8 hours following the initial bite and increase in severity with resolution within 1 week of onset.
  - The wound may develop a dark, depressed center over 24 to 48 hours, resulting in a dry, ulcerative eschar. The ulcerative wound may evolve into a necrotic region several days following the bite. The necrotic and ulcerative regions are more common with bites over fatty areas like the buttocks and thighs. Necrotic lesions may expand for up to 10 days before healing, usually over several weeks, without needing surgical repair and without scarring.
  - Some patients develop itching or a morbilliform rash.
  - Systemically, malaise, nausea, vomiting, fever, or myalgias may occur.
  - Rarely, complications of acute hemolytic anemia, disseminated intravascular coagulopathy, coma, renal failure, myonecrosis, rhabdomyolysis, and/or death occur.
- Scorpion bites (LoVecchio, 2017):
  - In the United States and Mexico, most scorpion bites cause local symptoms or are painless with minimal swelling. Most puncture sites are difficult to see.
- Bites (Envenomations) from *Centruroides exilicauda*, *C. noxius*, and *C. suffusus* are the most dangerous and can cause:
  - Paresthesias, remote pain, and unexplained agitation with uncontrollable crying
  - Systemic reactions including abnormal eye movements, blurred vision, restlessness, fasciculations, shaking, limb and body jerking movements, stridor, wheezing, respiratory failure, hyperthermia, hypersalivation, rhabdomyolysis, multiple organ failure, pancreatitis, sterile cerebrospinal fluid pleocytosis, metabolic acidosis, and death
  - Children have a higher risk than adults of severe symptoms and death secondary to a scorpion bite.

Differential Diagnosis and Management

Differential diagnoses include other spider bites and conditions that result in similar cutaneous manifestations, systemic findings, or both.

When venomous spider bites are suspected or confirmed, refer to the appropriate medical specialist or toxicologist. Treatment for black widow spider bites includes cleansing the wound with soap and water, and administering pain medication, antiemetics, tetanus prophylaxis, and muscle relaxants (such as benzodiazepines) as needed (Vetter et al, 2017). For severe symptoms, consult with a medical toxicologist or a provider with experience in black widow bites. Most brown recluse bites tend to heal without incident. Bites with necrotic centers generally require tetanus prophylaxis, pain medication, cold compress application, extremity elevation, and surgical excision and skin grafts if extensive necrosis occurs. Scorpion stings may be managed immediately with cold compress application, elevation of the affected area, staying calm, and administering acetaminophen or ibuprofen for pain control. In the hospital setting, antivenin is administered, when available. Intensive care is needed for sedation and management of cardiorespiratory and neurologic complications.

Patient and Parent Education

The focus of patient and parent education is prevention. Careful monitoring of environments where spiders live and prompt treatment, if bitten, are important. Use caution when near woodpiles and attics, and always shake out shoes and sleeping bags before using them.

Snakebites

Worldwide, there are 600 different species of venomous snakes causing an average of at least 100,000 to 125,000 deaths per year (White, 2017). Approximately 5000 snake bites are reported to the American Association of Poison Control Centers annually, and most of the snakebite victims are males (Seifert, 2017). Venomous snakes include indigenous pit vipers (Crotalinae) (such as rattlesnakes, cottonmouths, water moccasins, and copperheads) and the Elapidae (coral snake).

Southern and western states including Texas, Florida, California, Arizona, Louisiana, Georgia, and North Carolina account for the highest venomous snakebite rates due to the warmer climate (Seifert, 2017). The snake injects venom that contains a variety of toxins into the soft tissue that may be carried throughout the body via the blood and lymph systems. Snake venom can be cytotoxic, hemotoxic, and/or neurotoxic. Cytotoxic envenomation presents with localized pain, swelling, and ecchymosis; compartment syndrome may develop in severe cases. Hematologic effects include hemolysis, fibrinogen activation, and thrombocytopenia. Neurologic toxicity includes taste abnormalities, local paresthesias, seizures, altered mental status, and fasciculations. Venomous snake bites may cause rhabdomyolysis, vomiting, nausea, diaphoresis, increased salivation, respiratory distress, and shock. Children bitten by snakes suffer more severe effects than adults. Rattlesnake bites typically produce more severe signs and symptoms than cottonmouths. Copperheads cause local cutaneous symptoms such as soft tissue swelling and pain, not systemic symptoms (Seifert, 2017).

Clinical Findings

History. Ask about the type of snake and history of present illness. Pit vipers have a large triangular head and vertically oriented elliptical pupils, unlike the round pupils of nonvenomous snakes. Copperheads and rattlesnakes have diamond-shaped patterns of varying colors. Coral snakes have blackheads, followed by yellow and red bands that are followed by black bands.

Physical Examination. Characteristic features of envenomation include the following:

- Severe local reaction soon after the bite with intense pain, burning, discoloration, edema, and hemorrhagic effects
- Proximal extension of ecchymosis and swelling during the first few hours after the bite with later fluid-filled or hemorrhagic bullae and necrosis
- Peripheral and central neurologic symptoms, including worsening weakness, numbness or tingling of the face and/or extremities, diplopia, and lethargy
- Increased salivation, metallic taste in the mouth, sweating, nausea, and vomiting
- Evidence of hematologic coagulopathy, such as hematemesis, melena, and hemoptysis
- Respiratory distress and shock that can lead to death

Diagnostic Studies. Coagulation studies and other laboratory tests may be indicated by the child's condition.

Management

For nonvenomous bites, clean the wound, give tetanus prophylaxis if necessary, and administer appropriate pain medication. Give oral antibiotic therapy for 5 days with amoxicillin/clavulanic acid if there is presence of a secondary infection or if the wound was heavily contaminated. If there is uncertainty about the identity of the snake, contact poison control and observe for venomous symptoms for at least 3 to 4 hours.

If a venomous snakebite is suspected, the effects (including possible death) depend on the size of the child, site of the bite, type of snake, and degree of envenomation, and the treatment effectiveness. Snakebite treatment for individuals with more than local symptoms or those with suspected envenomation includes rapid transportation to a medical center, referral to appropriate medical specialists, antivenin therapy, and treatment for shock and

respiratory difficulties. Up to a quarter of venomous snake bites are asymptomatic "dry" bites. Anti-venom (polyvalent Crotalidae-Fab) is indicated for pit viper bites that cause systemic symptoms or progressing local injury, ideally within 6 hours of envenomation (Dart, Rumac, Wang, 2016). For rattlesnake bites, there is a period of 6 to 8 hours between the bite and death during which effective treatment can be instituted to reverse the venom effects.

Patient and Parent Education

Prevention of snakebite is important. Families who live or vacation in areas where pit vipers are found should be familiar with emergency snakebite first-aid which includes (Seifert, 2017):

- Remove the patient from the area where the snakebite occurred.
- Splint the affected extremity and minimize the patient's movements.
- Remove jewelry, watches, or constrictive clothing from the affected extremity.
- Do not elevate the affected extremity; have them lay or sit down with the bite at the level of the heart.
- Do not give the person caffeinated beverages.
- Do not give drugs, such as narcotics, that could impair clinical evaluation.
- Cleanse the wound with soap and water.
- Do not use a tourniquet, compression dressing, or ice packs.
- Do not cut the bite area and attempt to suction out the venom.
- Transport immediately for medical evaluation.

Heat and Cold Injuries

Frostbite

Frostbite occurs when ice crystals form within the soft tissues due to cold exposure. The frozen tissue impairs circulation to the affected area and results in vasoconstriction and vaso-occlusion. This causes microvascular changes, cellular destruction, and the release of damaging inflammatory mediators. Frostbite most commonly involves distal, relatively poorly perfused regions of the body, such as fingertips, toes, earlobes, and the nose. In children, areas with poor heat-generating ability and insulation, including the cheeks and chin, are at high risk for frostbite. Any skin areas exposed to prolonged cold can be affected.

Exposure to temperatures ranging from 28.4°F to 14°F (–2°C to –10°C) can cause frostbite. The effects of cold are potentiated by factors such as exposure duration, increased wind velocity, dependency of the extremity (limb in a dependent, not elevated position), emollient application, fatigue, injury, high altitude, immobility, and general health. Exposure to very cold chemicals (e.g., liquid nitrogen or oxygen) produces instant frostbite.

Clinical Findings

History. The provider should assess the following:
- Exposure to cold temperatures
- Sensory changes (initial pain, then numbness if deeply frostbitten)
- Complaints of throbbing pain after thawing

Physical Examination. Typical initial findings include the following:
- Affected area is cold.
- Skin is red at first, then appears pale or waxy white or slightly yellow or may have a bluish tint if deeply frostbitten.
- In early stages, tissue blanches; in later stages, it feels doughy or rock hard.

TABLE 44.4 **Frostbite Categories**

Category by Degree	Description	Complication
First (frostnip)	Redness, central pallor, edema, transient discomfort; reversible within a few hours	Normal skin appearance within a few hours; may have mild desquamation
Second	Notable redness and swelling; numbness becomes burning pain in 12-24 h; bullae and vesicles form	Sensory neuropathy and cold sensitivity are residuals after healing, some soft tissue loss
Third	Hemorrhagic bullae or waxy mummified skin	Extensive tissue loss, unlikely amputation
Fourth	Involvement of full-thickness skin, muscle, tendon, bone	Amputation is likely

The extent of tissue damage becomes apparent after rewarming. Deep frostbite occurs when tissues are icy hard and without deep tissue resilience. Deep frostbite causes the following signs and symptoms with rewarming:

- Cyanosis or mottling
- Erythema and swelling
- Numbness that evolves into complaints of burning pain
- Vesicles and bullae that appear within 24 to 48 hours
- Gangrene in severe frostbite

Table 44.4 describes the four levels of frostbite.

Differential Diagnosis and Management

The differential diagnosis includes other conditions that produce similar cutaneous manifestations and injury; a history of exposure to extreme temperatures is the key to the diagnosis.

Initial treatment of mild frostbite includes the following:

- Cover affected area with other body surfaces and warm clothing.
- Avoid pressure or any rubbing of the affected area.
- Pain control as needed.
- Topical aloe and oral ibuprofen limit inflammation by inhibiting prostaglandins and thromboxane (Zafren and Crawford Mechem, 2018).
- *Do not apply topical dry heat*; this practice is dangerous and can cause tissue damage.

Severe frostbite requires specialist management. Treatment includes rapid rewarming procedures, pain management, medical and surgical management of tissue necrosis, infection prevention, and possible amputation.

Patient and Parent Education

Child and parent education about frostbite prevention and initial management is important. Essential points include the following:

- Use of appropriate clothing when exposed to extreme cold temperatures
- Survival skills for travelers, hikers, or winter sports participants who are exposed to cold temperatures or who become lost

- Immediate rewarming of whitened skin by covering with warm clothing or another body surface
- Danger of rubbing affected area with snow or ice or massaging; these practices are contraindicated because they lead to mechanical trauma

Hypothermia

Hypothermia occurs when body core temperature falls below 95°F (35°C), a point where the human body loses its ability to generate sufficient heat to maintain bodily functions. Body heat is lost by heat radiation to nearby objects, moisture evaporation from the skin and respiratory system, heat convection from the skin's surface into cooler air, or heat conduction to objects with direct body contact. Wind, moisture, and lack of appropriate clothing or shelter exacerbate cool ambient temperatures. Predisposing factors include malnutrition, anorexia nervosa, illness, adrenal insufficiency, sepsis, central nervous system (CNS) injury or anomalies, hypoglycemia, major trauma, burns, hypothyroidism, drug overdose, or child abuse/maltreatment that results in prolonged exposure to the elements. (Corneli, 2017). Although most cases are seen in winter, hypothermia can occur in other seasons during wet, windy weather. It occurs quickly with cold-water immersion.

Children are at increased risk of hypothermia because of their relatively larger BSA, proportionately larger head, smaller body fluid volume, less developed temperature-regulating mechanisms, and decreased body fat. Children are less able to independently leave a cold environment and are more likely to wander off from adult supervision. Those at high risk include newborns, particularly low-birth weight or premature infants, very young children, and children who are ill, fatigued, poorly nourished, or have experienced trauma.

Hypothermia results in cutaneous vasoconstriction and increased heat production by shivering and thyroxine releases. Hypothermia not associated with environmental exposure may be a sign of other life-threatening illnesses or injuries. Secondary hypothermia is not discussed here.

Clinical Findings

History, Physical Examination, and Diagnostic Studies. Assess the following history:

- Exposure to low ambient temperatures
- Risk factors (e.g., age, physical condition)

Signs of early to late stage hypothermia include:

- Decreasing body temperature
- Shivering stops in moderate hypothermia
- Pallor or blue lips and skin
- Disorientation, listlessness, sleepiness
- Decreased pulse and respiration
- Decreasing neurologic status and eventually coma and death

No diagnostic studies are needed if hypothermia is mild and responds to basic treatment measures.

Differential Diagnosis and Management. Shock is the differential diagnosis. For mild hypothermia (core body temperature 89.6°F [32°C]) remove the child from the cold environment, replace wet clothing, and provide warm liquids. Warm water baths can be effective. When the body cools and can no longer generate adequate heat, external heat sources must be provided. Use warm blankets, heat lamps, hot-water bottles, or, if none of these are available, place the child skin-to-skin in a sleeping bag or under a blanket with a person of normal body temperature. Heated humidified oxygen should be provided for all hypothermic children. Administration of warmed IV normal saline should be considered for treatment of mild hypothermia and is a necessity for treatment of moderate to severe hypothermia. ●Immediately refer hypothermic patients to emergency care for stabilization and treatment due to risk of cardiovascular instability and shock.

Patient and Parent Education

Instruct parents about the risks of hypothermia. Emphasize the need to monitor children's activities in cold weather and to provide adequate supervision and protection from exposure. The higher metabolic rate of normal, healthy children keeps them warm, and they may not feel the effects of short-term cold exposure. Thus, they may not want a jacket, sweater, hat, or mittens when their parents believe they need them. Families or teens on camping trips or traveling in uninhabited areas should have a survival kit.

Hyperthermia: Common Heat-Related Illness

Hyperthermia is a life-threatening increase in body core temperature. Heat cramps, heat exhaustion, and heatstroke are types of hyperthermia which are discussed in Chapter 19.

Acute Pediatric Poisoning

Poisoning occurs when a substance that interferes with normal body function is taken in by ingestion, inhalation, absorption, or injection. Poisoning generally refers to exposure and symptoms that are acute in nature. Toxic environmental exposures are more often chronic or insidious in nature (see also Chapter 4) and will be discussed later in this chapter.

Clinical Findings

History

The history may provide clues to an acute poisoning exposure. This could be as straightforward as a reported exposure, a witnessed exposure, or a caregiver suspecting an exposure. However, sometimes caregivers may be unwilling/unable to provide details, or the exposure went unrecognized. The history should include:

- The circumstances surrounding the possible exposure (e.g., location, activity just before onset of symptoms, timing).
- Cosmetics, personal care products, cleaning products, analgesics, cough and cold preparations, other medications (obtain a list), topical agents, plants, herbs, pesticides, and vitamins that the child has access to.
- Ask about illicit or recreational drug use in the home or used by anyone who lives in the home.
- Unknown pills or chemicals may be identifiable by consultation with a regional poison control center.

Physical examination

Common clinical manifestations seen on physical examination of a poisoning (Box 44.2) includes symptoms associated with an acute exposure. Physical examination should be tailored to the child's exposure and condition and include neurologic examination and assessing for signs of hypoxemia.

Management and Patient/Family Education

If the history or physical examination is suspicious of either an acute or suspected chronic exposure, the PCP should call the regional poison control center (1-800-222-1222) for advice while simultaneously attending to basic life support and consideration

---

• BOX 44.2 Clinical Manifestations of Poisoning in Children

Heart Rate: Bradycardia, tachycardia
Respirations: Bradypnea, tachypnea
Blood pressure: Hypotension, hypertension
Temperature: Hypothermia, hyperpyrexia (differing from hyperthermia)
Neurological:
- Central nervous system depression, including coma
- Agitation
- Delirium/psychosis
- Seizures
- Ataxia
- Weakness/paralysis
- Tremors/myoclonus
- Choreoathetosis
- Rigidity
Ophthalmologic:
- Miosis
- Mydriasis
- Nystagmus
Dermatologic:
- Jaundice
- Cyanosis
- Pink or red
Odors from patient:
- Acetone (fruity)
- Bitter almond
- Garlic
- Mothballs
- Oil of wintergreen
- Gasoline, turpentine, kerosene
- Rotten eggs

---

for transfer. ●If the patient demonstrates organ instability or failure, rapidly transfer them to an acute healthcare provider trained to provide ongoing care to the unstable child.

Basic life support focuses on airway, breathing, and circulation. For the poisoned (or suspected poisoned) child, additional considerations include neurologic examination, the need for empiric treatment (if poison identified), and emergent decontamination. Oxygen administration is warranted if the patient exhibits respiratory impairment or altered mental status (and is, thus, at risk for respiratory impairment), and/or requires antidote therapy (e.g., naloxone for opioid poisoning). Patients with depressed mental status, diminished respirations, miotic pupils, or other concerning evidence of opioid intoxication should receive naloxone intravenously, intramuscularly, subcutaneously, or intranasally—not orally. Decontamination strategies vary depending on the poison and are guided by poison control centers or a toxicology team. Inducing vomiting should not occur unless under the direction of poison control. General decontamination includes the following options:

- Ocular: copious saline lavage
- Skin: copious water rinse or gentle soap and water
- Gastrointestinal: dilution; gastric emptying; activated charcoal administration; catharsis; whole bowel irrigation (after consulting poison control)

Excretion of absorbed toxins can be enhanced by multi-dose activated charcoal, diuresis/urinary alkalization, dialysis, and hemoperfusion (similar to hemodialysis). Many of the antidote and decontamination therapies require hospitalization. Referral to a mental health specialist is needed for the child or adolescent with an intentional self-poisoning. ●Any child with concern for intentional poisoning by proxy (i.e., medical child abuse, formerly known as Munchausen's by proxy) should be promptly reported to child protective services.

All families should have the phone number of their local poison control center posted in a prominent location (e.g., refrigerator) in their homes. Stickers with this number should be given out by PCPs as part of routine well-child care.

Common Environmental Toxins: Heavy Metals and Pesticides

See Chapter 4 for a review of the general epidemiology and effects of exposure to lead, mercury, arsenic, and pesticides. The clinical findings and management, if toxic exposure is suspected to any of these substances, are discussed in this chapter.

Lead

Clinical Findings

History. Every infant and child seen by a PCP should have a history taken to determine risk for lead exposure. Boxes 4.1 and 4.2 contain information regarding environmental history content. Noteworthy risk factors include:

- The child exhibits pica
- The child lives near a lead smelter, battery recycling plant, or other industry likely to release lead
- A family member or caregiver works with lead-based materials
- Household members engage in hobbies that might include ceramics, stained glass, making own fishing tackle
- Painted or unusual materials are burned in wood stoves or fireplaces
- The family uses complementary, herbal, or folk remedies
- Food is prepared or stored in imported pottery or metal containers or water obtained from contaminated pipes

Physical Examination. Clinical signs of lead toxicity may not be noted during the physical examination because most lead retained by the body is stored in the bones and is not measured by blood lead levels (BLLs). A child can have high BLLs (e.g., 45 mcg/dL) with no obvious clinical signs on physical exam. Another child may complain of severe GI problems with a lower lead level (e.g., 15 to 20 mcg/dL). Many children have subclinical effects or have symptoms that are easily confused with other conditions such as anemia, constipation, abdominal pain, impaired hearing, learning disabilities, delayed growth, and/or hyperactivity. At higher levels, lead affects vitamin D metabolism, nerve conduction velocities, and hemoglobin synthesis that can lead to myocardial excitability, increased intracranial pressure, seizures, coma, and death. Many children do not demonstrate signs of acute toxicity until they have high lead levels.

Diagnostic Studies. All children at risk should be screened at 1 and 2 years of age for lead. Immigrant children or other children from 3 to 6 years of age who have not been previously tested should be screened. Also, children who have any sign of lead toxicity should be screened. If an elevated lead level is present, an assessment of free erythrocyte protoporphyrin (FEP) and zinc protoporphyrin (ZPP), and iron deficiency screening, including serum ferritin, are helpful in determining diagnosis and management.

Differential Diagnosis

GI infections, other causes of anemia, growth retardation, behavior disorders, attention deficit hyperactivity disorder (ADHD), and CNS infections are included in the differential diagnosis.

Management

Management involves preventing the child's exposure to lead in the environment, monitoring BLLs, correcting dietary deficiencies (if any), investigating and removing lead (i.e., lead abatement) from the child's daily environment, and treating the child for toxicity (see Table 44.5). Other children in the same household or environment where exposure could have occurred should be tested and treated as indicated. In all cases of lead toxicity (≥5 mcg/dL):

- Inform caregiver of level of toxicity.
- Provide caregiver dietary and environmental education.
- Remove child from source of lead if known.
- Report to public health department.
- Initiate environmental investigation. Some health department may do this.
- Initiate lead hazard control/abatement.
- Follow up BLL every 3 months until BLL declines.
- Refer to social services as appropriate.

Chelation therapy is recommended for levels higher than 45 mcg/dL (CDC, 2017) to treat acute, severe, and life-threatening poisoning. It is also critical that providers do follow-up testing for children with positive lead screens until levels return to normal. Further guidance on treatment is available at https://www.cdc.gov/nceh/lead/acclpp/actions_blls.html.

Patient and Family Education

Prevention of lead poisoning is a public health responsibility, and public health officials use geographic information systems (GIS) to identify high-risk areas. Population-based screening programs in Head Start classrooms can also identify prevalence of lead toxicity in children and promote early intervention programs. PCPs play a critical role in the process of preventing lead toxicity in children. Pediatric providers should take a lead exposure history on all children and families and identify all children who need to be screened, retested, and require appropriate intervention and treatment.

Parents need to be informed that it is critical to have professional assessment of the level of home contamination and professional abatement may be necessary. Public health officials can work with parents to identify ways to control lead dust and paint chips in older homes and can work with landlords on lead abatement of properties. Other strategies parents can use include:

- Cover smaller peeling paint areas with sticky-backed paper.
- Damp-mop and damp-dust with household cleaners or lead-specific cleaning products (e.g., Ledizolv) twice weekly to decrease lead dust in the air; do not dry mop or sweep.
- Pick up and dispose of paint chips with a disposable rag or paper towel soaked in phosphate cleaner.
- Run water until temperature changes to flush pipes of lead sediment.
- Do not store or cook food in lead crystal or pottery that contains lead.
- Remove work clothes and wash hands before returning home if job is lead-related.

TABLE 44.5 Management Recommendations for Lead Poisoning

Child has risk factors from screening criteria and/or there are no local or state guidelines on when to screen for lead levels

Screening Sample: Blood Lead Levels	Action to Be Taken	Follow-Up Blood Lead Levels Monitoring
<5 mcg/dL	Not considered lead poisoning: • Provide caregiver/parent dietary and environmental education • Refer to social services as appropriate • Conduct environmental assessment to determine if child is exposed to a lead source (e.g., pre-1978 housing)	• If high risk, retest in 6 months • If low risk, no further testing necessary; ongoing monitoring for changes in environment
≥5-9 mcg/dL	• Reference value requiring intervention: • Confirmatory venous blood test within 1-3 months	• Early follow-up (two to four tests) by 3 months • Later follow-up (after BLLs decline) at 6-9 months
10-44 mcg/dL	Confirmatory venous blood test within 1 week to 1 month[a]	
• 10-19 mcg/dL		• Early follow-up 1-3 months[b] • Later follow-up at 3-6 months
• 20-24 mcg/dL		• Early follow-up 1-3 months[b] • Later follow-up at 1-3 months
• 25-44 mcg/dL		• Early follow-up 2 weeks to 1 month • Later follow-up at 1 month • Retest every month until results <15 mcg/dL for at least 6 months, then retest every 3 months until child is 36 months old
45-59 mcg/dL	Confirmatory venous blood test within 48 h: • Complete history and physical examination • Complete neurologic examination • Lab work: Hgb or Hct and iron status (FEP or ZPP) • Abdominal x-ray with bowel decontamination if indicated • Chelation therapy, may be oral in ambulatory setting	• Early follow-up as soon as possible • Retest every month until results <15 mcg/dL for at least 6 months, then retest every 3 months until child is 36 months old
60-69 mcg/dL	Confirmatory venous blood test within 24 h: • Complete history and physical examination • Complete neurologic examination • Lab work: Hgb or Hct and iron status (TIBC or SF) • Abdominal x-ray with bowel decontamination if indicated • Chelation therapy, may be oral in ambulatory setting	• Early follow-up as soon as possible • Retest every month until results <15 mcg/dL for at least 6 months, then retest every 3 months until child is 36 months old
≥70 mcg/dL	Medical emergency: • Retest immediately as an emergency lab test with venous blood sample • Hospitalize for IV chelation • Proceed according to action for 45-69 mcg/dL	• Early follow-up as soon as possible • Retest every month until results <15 mcg/dL for at least 6 months, then retest every 3 months until child is 36 months old

[a]The higher the BLL, the sooner confirmatory testing should be done.

[b]May do at 1 month to ensure BLL are not rising rapidly.

BLL, Blood lead level; *FEP,* free erythrocyte protoporphyrin; *Hct,* hematocrit; *Hgb,* hemoglobin; *SF,* serum ferritin; *TIBC,* total iron-binding capacity; *ZPP,* zinc protoporphyrin.

Data adapted from Centers for Disease Control and Prevention (CDC). *Summary of Recommendations for Follow-up and Case Management of Children Based on Confirmed Blood Levels.* Atlanta: CDC; 2017; and Advisory Committee on Childhood Lead Poisoning Prevention of the Centers for Disease Control and Prevention (CDC). *Low Level Lead Exposure Harms Children: A Renewed Call for Primary Prevention.* Atlanta: CDC; 2012.

Inform parents that chelation therapy leads to a rapid fall in BLL, but most children have a rebound increase within days or weeks of treatment; repeated treatment may be necessary.

Mercury

Clinical Findings

History. The signs and symptoms of mercury poisoning may be easily attributed to other processes. A careful history is essential to identify any possible exposures. Questions should focus on potential exposure (e.g., industrial exposure, mercury spills, consumer goods, and diet) and whether others in the household are experiencing similar symptoms (see Chapter 4, Boxes 4.1 and 4.2).

Physical Examination. In the case of known or suspected mercury exposure, complete a full examination with special attention to the following systems:
• Respiratory system: Elemental mercury vapor produces chemical pneumonitis or necrotizing bronchitis, potentially

progressing to acute respiratory distress syndrome (qualifying as respiratory failure).

- Neurologic system: Subacute exposures may include insomnia, forgetfulness, loss of appetite, tremor, peripheral neuropathy, visual impairments, and behavioral changes (e.g., emotional lability).
- Skin/musculoskeletal: Acrodynia ("pink disease") is the constellation of findings in children with mercury poisoning. This hypersensitivity reaction prominently affects the extremities, causing swelling, pain, weakness (particularly of pelvic area), an erythematous maculopapular rash, and other organ disease.
- GI system: Gingivostomatitis may result from chronic exposure. Acute exposure such as the ingestion of button batteries may cause corrosive gastroenteritis, hematemesis, and pain with cardiovascular collapse or renal failure.
- Nephrology system: Renal tubular dysfunction and hypertension may develop.

Diagnostic Studies. Blood mercury levels can determine acute mercury exposure; however, due to mercury's half-life, the result may not accurately reflect the toxicity level. A blood level of less than 2 mcg/L is considered normal, but a normal level may not exclude mercury poisoning. A 24-hour urine sample can also be collected (<10 mcg/L is considered "normal"). Hair analysis done in a specialized controlled laboratory provides a more comprehensive look at mercury exposure. The specific type of suspected or known exposure (elemental, inorganic, or organic mercury; acute or chronic) will determine the best test, and its timing, in a specific circumstance. Poison control center personnel can assist with these determinations.

Differential Diagnosis

The differential diagnosis includes other poisonings, CNS, and/or psychiatric conditions. A high level of suspicion about environmental exposures is important when evaluating any rash. A patient with neurologic symptoms, along with rash, should always be evaluated for mercury and other poisonings.

Management

The initial management is mercury source removal from the child's environment. Public health officials should investigate and determine any sources of mercury and require a hazardous materials team or EPA-certified contractor for abatement. Other children in the environment should be evaluated for possible mercury poisoning. Consult with a pediatric toxicologist and the regional poison control center or pediatric environmental health specialty unit (PEHSU) regarding patient management.

Patient and Family Education

Education should focus on increasing awareness of sources of mercury and ways to prevent or limit exposure. Review common household items that contain mercury—old thermometers, healthcare supplies, antiques, and/or fluorescent light bulbs (including compact fluorescents lights [CFLs]). These should be recycled in accordance with local recommendations for hazardous materials. The Environmental Protection Agency (EPA) has specific instructions on how to clean up small mercury spills available at https://www.epa.gov/mercury/what-do-if-mercury-thermometer-breaks.

As with all environmental toxicants, PCPs and community activists should maintain awareness of local environmental issues (e.g., mercury emissions from industrial plants) and actively participate

---

> **• BOX 44.3** **Recommendations for Fish Consumption by Women of Childbearing Age and Children**
>
> - Eat 8-12 ounces of fish per week for women
> - Eat two to three servings of appropriate proportions per week for children
> - Choose fish lower in mercury (avoid predatory fish: shark, swordfish, king mackerel, tilefish)
> - Eat no more than 6 ounces of albacore tuna per week
> - When eating fish that have been caught from local streams, rivers, and lakes, pay attention to fish advisories on those bodies of water
>
> *From FDA and EPA updated advice for fish consumption lower in mercury for pregnant women and breastfeeding mothers to eat more fish accessed on 6/20/18 and available at https://www.fda.gov/downloads/Food/FoodborneIllnessContaminants/Metals/UCM537120.pdf*

---

in legislation and regulatory efforts to decrease pollution and, thus, improve the health of children. The EPA and Federal Drug Administration (FDA) have advice on fish consumption in children and women of childbearing age by promoting varieties of fish low in mercury (Box 44.3). Further information on regional varieties of fish lower in mercury can be accessed at https://www.fda.gov/media/102331/download.

Arsenic

Clinical Findings

History and Physical Examination. An exposure history is essential to determine the arsenic poisoning source and to form the differential diagnoses. Physical signs and symptoms depend on the exposure dose, route, and duration (see Box 4.1). The following symptoms and conditions can occur with arsenic poisoning:

- Cardiovascular: Hypotension, shock, arrhythmias, edema
- Respiratory: Respiratory tract irritation, pulmonary edema, bronchitis, pneumonia
- Neurologic: Sensorimotor peripheral axonal neuropathy, neuritis, muscle cramps, headache, weakness, lethargy, delirium, encephalopathy, hyperpyrexia, tremor, seizure, coma
- GI and hepatic: Garlic odor of breath, abdominal pain, nausea, vomiting, thirst, anorexia, gastroesophageal reflux, diarrhea, dysphagia, transaminitis, liver necrosis, cholangitis
- Renal: Hematuria, oliguria, proteinuria, uremia, tubular necrosis
- Hematologic: Hemolysis, anemia, leukopenia, thrombocytopenia, disseminated intravascular coagulation (DIC)
- Dermal: Mees' lines (transverse white lines in nail beds developing weeks to months after exposure), dermatitis, melanosis or pigment changes, hyperkeratosis
- Other: Rhabdomyolysis, conjunctivitis

Diagnostic Studies. A 24-hour urine sample is the most accurate measurement of arsenic levels and laboratory reference value of less than 35 mcg/L in a 24-hour urine is considered within normal limits for all age groups. Concentrations higher than 100 mcg/L indicate acute arsenic intoxication (ATSDR, 2016); however, intervention may be needed for lower levels. Serum levels can also be measured but are less accurate because the half-life is very short. Consult with a pediatric toxicologist to determine if exposure warrants laboratory evaluation and treatment.

Management

Minimizing exposure by identifying and removing the arsenic source is of utmost importance. For severe exposures, acute stabilization with gut decontamination (e.g., activated charcoal, gastric lavage) and/or chelation may be necessary. Monitor renal and hematologic function acutely and on follow-up. Treatment should be in consultation with a pediatric toxicologist.

Patient and Family Education

Parents and providers can work with schools and communities to assess for and manage arsenic contamination of play structures. Test water supplies that are suspected to be contaminated. Bottled water, distilled water, or home treatment units that remove arsenic should be used if drinking water is contaminated. Healthcare providers should support regulatory standards for the production and use of arsenic-containing products to ensure protection of children's health.

Pesticides

Clinical Findings

Adverse effects of pesticide exposure can be acute or chronic, and affect all body systems, depending on the nature of the toxin and the extent of exposure. In acute exposure, assessment is the same as with general poisoning. Acute poisoning with organophosphates or carbamates results in clinical signs of cholinergic excess (i.e., tearing, salivation, bronchospasm, urination/incontinence, emesis, diarrhea, and diaphoresis). Neurologic disorders may become apparent 24 to 96 hours after exposure and delayed neurotoxicity may occur weeks after exposure. Nephrotoxicity has also been reported.

Management

Pesticide exposure should be prevented. Specifics of exposure management depend on the type of pesticide, the amount, patient symptoms, and route of exposure. Foremost, information on ingredients and immediate treatment is available on product labels. When treating an individual who may have been exposed to pesticides, PCPs, by law, are entitled to access information about the implicated pesticides from the National Pesticide Information Center (http://npic.orst.edu/). The EPA's Worker Protection Standard (WPS) also mandates that providers be able to access information on general- and restricted-use pesticides. Under the WPS, this information can be obtained from employers or manufacturers. Patients/caregivers may be able to provide the clinician with the pesticide label. Treatment focuses on basic life support (as necessary) and the following:

- Antidote therapy (depends on the specific pesticide)
- Decontamination (e.g., remove patient's clothes; wash skin; gastric decontamination as indicated). Note that pesticides may penetrate standard healthcare personnel gloves; special protective gear may be required.
- Consultation with a poison control center (acute) and/or PEHSU (acute or chronic).
- Seizure control.
- Report pesticide exposure to the local and state health department.

Patient and Family Education

The risks pesticides present to children are significant to short- and long-term health outcomes, and acute or chronic exposure to pesticides may occur in unanticipated ways. Because exposures are additive, patterns of multiple contaminations must be recognized and a plan to regulate overall exposure developed. Families can choose foods that are local, in season, and organically grown as much as possible (see Chapter 4, Box 4.3). Not all foods labeled as organic are the same; check U.S. Department of Agriculture (USDA) labels, which include "100% organic," "organic" (i.e., at least 95% organic content), "made with organic" (i.e., 70% organic content for up to three ingredients), and "organic components" (i.e., products with <70% organic content). Organic foods are often more expensive than conventional foods, thus income disparities and environmental justice issues are important considerations. Regulation of pesticide use on foods should be considered in order to provide all children with safe foods, not just those families that "can afford it." Families should be advised to avoid conventionally grown foods in the "dirty dozen" category and buy those foods organic whenever possible, until improved agricultural regulations are in place to decrease pesticide content

Education and awareness are key to preventing pesticide poisoning in children. Steps can be taken to reduce or eliminate pesticide use, which in turn reduces exposure. *Integrated pest management* (IPM) combines physical, cultural, biologic, and other means of pest control with no, or minimal, use of pesticides. IPM is a coordinated use of pest and environmental information to prevent unacceptable levels of pest damage by the most economical means with the least possible hazard to people, property, and the environment (EPA, 2017). This involves pest prevention and nonchemical management methods as first-line measures. Some examples of IPM include: using cats by farmers to catch mice rather than using rodenticides, using bait traps for cockroaches rather than chemical sprays (in schools and homes), using boiling water to kill weeds, and caulking cracks in walls to prevent pest entry.

Additional Resources

American Association of Poison Control Centers (Poison Control Center). www.aapcc.org
1-800-222-1222 (24-7 Hotline)
American Burn Association.
www.ameriburn.org
Centers for Disease Control and Prevention, Tickborne Diseases of the United States.
https://www.cdc.gov/lyme/resources/tickbornediseases.pdf
Kid's Don't-Leave-Home-Without-It Equipment.
www.equipped.com/kidequip.htm
Sage II Burn Diagramming (Free calculator to estimate BSA and fluid resuscitation requirements). www.SageDiagram.com

References

American Academy of Pediatrics (AAP). *Treatment for Animal Bites*; 2015a (website). https://www.healthychildren.org/English/health-issues/conditions/from-insects-animals/Pages/Treatment-for-Animal-Bites.aspx. Accessed July 4, 2019.

American Academy of Pediatrics (AAP). *Prevent Bite Wounds*; 2015b (website). https://www.healthychildren.org/English/health-issues/conditions/prevention/Pages/Prevent-Bite-Wounds.aspx. Accessed July 4, 2019.

Antoon AY, Donovan MK. Burn injuries. In: Kliegman RM, Stanton BF, St. Geme JW, et al., eds. *Nelson's Textbook of Pediatrics*. 20th ed. Philadelphia: Saunders/Elsevier; 2016:568–576.

Attia M, Durani Y, Weihmiller SN. Minor trauma. In: Shaw KN, Bachur RG, et al., eds. *Fleisher and Ludwig's Textbook of Pediatric Emergency Medicine.* 7th ed. Philadelphia: Lippincott, Williams and Wilkins; 2016:1178–1179.

Baddour LM, Brown AM. *Infectious Complications of Puncture Wounds*; 2017 (website). https://www.uptodate.com/contents/infectious-complications-of-puncture-wounds?search=infectious%20complications%20of%20puncture%20wounds&source=search_result&selectedTitle=1~88&usage_type=default&display_rank=1. Accessed July 4, 2019.

Campbell RL, Kelso JM. *Anaphylaxis: emergency treatment* (website). https://www.uptodate.com/contents/anaphylaxis-emergency-treatment?search=anaphylaxis:%20emergency%20treatment&source=search_result&selectedTitle=1~150&usage_type=default&display_rank=1, accessed July 14, 2019.

Carney KP, Roswell K. Emergencies and injuries. In: Hay JR, Levin MJ, Deterding RR, et al., eds. *Current Diagnosis and Treatment: Pediatrics.* 23rd ed. New York: McGraw-Hill; 2016:308–330.

Casale TB, Burks AW. Hymenoptera-sting hypersensitivity. *New Eng J Med.* 2014;370(15):1432–1439.

Centers for Disease Control and Prevention (CDC). *Childhood Injury Report.* CDC; 2016 (website). https://www.cdc.gov/safechild/child_injury_data.html, accessed July 4, 2019.

Centers for Disease Control and Prevention (CDC). *Recommended actions based on blood lead level*; 2017 (website). https://www.cdc.gov/nceh/lead/acclpp/actions_blls.html. Accessed October 6, 2018.

Chiesa A, Sirotnak AP. Child abuse and neglect. In: Hay WW, Levin MJ, Deterding RR, et al., eds. *Current Diagnosis & Treatment: Pediatrics.* 23rd ed. New York: McGraw-Hill; 2016:216–224.

Chorley J. *Forefoot and midfoot pain in the active child or skeletally immature adolescent: overview of causes* (website). https://www.uptodate.com/contents/forefoot-and-midfoot-pain-in-the-active-child-or-skeletally-immature-adolescent-overview-of-causes?search=forefoot%20and%20midfoot%20pain%20in%20the%20active&source=search_result&selectedTitle=1~150&usage_type=default&display_rank=1, accessed July 4, 2019.

Corneli HM. *Hypothermia in children: clinical manifestations and diagnosis* (website). https://www.uptodate.com/contents/hypothermia-in-children-clinical-manifestations-and-diagnosis?search=hypothermia%20in%20chidlren:%20clinical%20manifestations%20and%20diagnosis&source=search_result&selectedTitle=1~150&usage_type=default&display_rank=1, accessed July 4, 2019.

Dart RC, Rumack BH, Wang GS. Poisoning. In: Hay WW, Levin MJ, Deterding RR, et al., eds. *Current Diagnosis & Treatment: Pediatrics.* 23rd ed. New York: McGraw-Hill; 2016:331–359.

Environmental Protection Agency (EPA). *About Pesticide Registration.* https://www.epa.gov/pesticide-registration/about-pesticide-registration, accessed July 4, 2019.

Erickson MA, Rhodes J, Niswander C. Orthopedics. In: Hay WW, Levin MJ, Deterding RR, et al., eds. *Current Diagnosis & Treatment: Pediatrics.* 23rd ed. New York: McGraw-Hill; 2016:815–839.

Ginsburg CM, Hunstad DA. Animal and human bites. In: Kliegman RM, Stanton BF, St. Geme JW, et al., eds. *Nelson's Textbook of Pediatrics.* 20th ed. Philadelphia: Saunders/Elsevier; 2016:3447–3459.

Harper M. *Clinical manifestations and initial management of animal and human bites* (website). https://www.uptodate.com/contents/clinical-manifestations-and-initial-management-of-animal-and-human-bites?search=clinical%20manifestations%20and%20initial%20management%20of%20human%20bites&source=search_result&selectedTitle=1~150&usage_type=default&display_rank=1, accessed July 4, 2019.

Lavoie M, Nance ML. Approach to the injured child. In: Shaw KN, Bachur RG, et al., eds. *Fleisher and Ludwig's Textbook of Pediatric Emergency Medicine.* 7th ed. Philadelphia: Lippincott Williams & Wilkins; 2016:9–19.

LoVecchio F. *Scorpion envenomation causing neuromuscular toxicity (United States, Mexico, Central America, and Southern Africa)* (website). https://www.uptodate.com/contents/scorpion-envenomation-causing-neuromuscular-toxicity-united-states-mexico-central-america-and-southern-africa?search=scorpion%20envenomation&source=search_result&selectedTitle=1~9&usage_type=default&display_rank=1, accessed July 4, 2019.

Mayo Clinic Staff. *Scorpion stings* (website). www.mayoclinic.org/diseases-conditions/scorpion-stings/basics/causes/con-20033894?p=1, accessed July 4, 2019.

Micak RP. *Inhalation injury from heat, smoke or chemical irritants* (website). https://www.uptodate.com/contents/inhalation-injury-from-heat-smoke-or-chemical-irritants?search=inhalation%20injury%20from%20heat&source=search_result&selectedTitle=1~150&usage_type=default&display_rank=1, accessed July 4, 2019.

Murphy KP, Karlin AM. Management of Musculoskeletal Injury. In: Kliegman RM, Stanton BF, St. Geme JW, et al., eds. *Nelson's Textbook of Pediatrics.* 20th ed. Philadelphia: Saunders/Elsevier; 2016:3336–3349.

Occupational Safety and Health Administration (OSHA). *Asbestos: OSHA standards, U.S. Department of Labor* (website). https://www.osha.gov/SLTC/asbestos/standards.html, accessed July 4, 2019.

O'Halloran A. Trauma, burns, and common critical care emergencies. In: Hughes HK, Kahl LK, eds. *The Harriet Lane Handbook.* 21st ed. Philadelphia: Elsevier; 2018.

Otten EJ. Venomous animal injuries. In: Walls RM, Hockberger RS, Gausche-Hill M, eds. *Rosen's Emergency Medicine Concepts and Clinical Practice.* 9th ed. Philadelphia: Elsevier; 2018:698–714.

Rice PL, Orgill DP. *Classification of burn injury* (Website). https://www.uptodate.com/contents/classification-of-burn-injury?search=classification%20of%20burns&source=search_result&selectedTitle=1~24&usage_type=default&display_rank=1, accessed July 4, 2019.

Seeyave DM, Brown KM. Environmental emergencies, radiological emergencies, bites and stings. In: Shaw KN, Bachur RG, et al., eds. *Fleisher and Ludwig's Textbook of Pediatric Emergency Medicine.* 7th ed. Philadelphia: Lippincott Williams & Wilkins; 2016:718–760.

Seifert SA. *Evaluation and management of Crotalinae (rattlesnake, water moccasin [cottonmouth], or copperhead) bites in the United States* (website). https://www.uptodate.com/contents/evaluation-and-management-of-crotalinae-rattlesnake-water-moccasin-cottonmouth-or-copperhead-bites-in-the-united-states?search=evaluation%20and%20management%20of%20crotalinae&source=search_result&selectedTitle=1~3&usage_type=default&display_rank=1, accessed July 4, 2019.

Swanson DL, Vetter RS, White J. *Clinical manifestations and diagnosis of widow spider bites* (website). https://www.uptodate.com/contents/clinical-manifestations-and-diagnosis-of-widow-spider-bites?search=clinical%20manifestations%20and%20diagnosis%20of%20widow%20spider%20bites&source=search_result&selectedTitle=1~150&usage_type=default&display_rank=1. Accessed July 4, 2019.

Tenenhaus M, Rennekampff HO. *Topical agents and dressings for local burn wound care* (website). https://www.uptodate.com/contents/topical-agents-and-dressings-for-local-burn-wound-care?search=topical%20agents%20and%20dressings%20for%20local%20burn%20wound%20care&source=search_result&selectedTitle=1~150&usage_type=default&display_rank=1Accessed, accessed July 4, 2019.

Vetter RS, Swanson DL. *Bites of recluse spiders* (website). https://www.uptodate.com/contents/bites-of-recluse-spiders?search=bites%20of%20recluse%20spiders&source=search_result&selectedTitle=1~150&usage_type=default&display_rank=1, accessed July 4, 2019.

Vetter RS, Swanson DL, White J. *Management of widow spider bites* (website). https://www.uptodate.com/contents/management-of-widow-spider-bites?search=management%20of%20widow%20spider%20bites&source=search_result&selectedTitle=1~150&usage_type=default&display_rank=1, accessed July 4, 2019.

White J. *Snakebites worldwide. Clinical manifestations and diagnosis* (website). https://www.uptodate.com/contents/snakebites-worldwide-clinical-manifestations-and-diagnosis?search=snakebites%20worldwide:%20clinical%20manife&source=search_result&selectedTitle=1~150&usage_type=default&display_rank=1, accessed July 4, 2019.

Wiktor A, Richards D. *Treatment of minor thermal burns* (website). https://www.uptodate.com/contents/treatment-of-minor-thermal-burns?search=treatment%20of%20minor%20thermal%20burns&source=search_result&selectedTitle=1~150&usage_type=default&display_rank=1, accessed July 4, 2019.

Zafren K, Crawford Mechem C. *Frostbite* (website). https://www.uptodate.com/contents/frostbite?search=frostbite&source=search_result&selectedTitle=1~26&usage_type=default&display_rank=1, accessed July 4, 2019.

45

Endocrine and Metabolic Disorders

ARLENE SMALDONE, BECKY J. WHITTEMORE, AND ALAN T. SCHULTZ

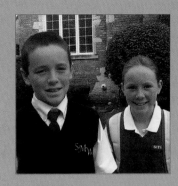

Endocrine and metabolic disorders affect a large number of children and may be rare (e.g., nephropathic cystinosis) or relatively common (e.g., type 1 and type 2 diabetes mellitus). Many children with endocrine and/or metabolic disorders are comanaged by primary care providers (PCPs) in collaboration with specialists. Although a great degree of overlap happens in these disorders, distinctive processes occur in each, and as such, specific conditions may involve different approaches to assessment and management. This chapter begins with an overview of anatomy, physiology, and pathophysiology of the endocrine and metabolic system and general issues related to assessment and management of the disorders.

Anatomy and Physiology

The endocrine system regulates growth, pubertal development and reproduction, homeostasis of the individual, and the production, storage, and utilization of energy. Classically, the endocrine system was understood to function via hormones produced in glands with action at a distant site. Currently, the understanding is that hormones may also act in a *para*crine fashion affecting cells adjacent to the hormone-secreting cell or in an *auto*crine fashion in which the hormone affects the secreting cell by diffusion. Many endocrine glands are controlled by the hypothalamic-pituitary axis. Many of the hormones of the hypothalamic-pituitary axis (or molecules that are structurally similar to such hormones) are also made in the gut and other tissues.

Hormones are often activated by a feedback loop; for example, thyrotropin-releasing hormone (TRH) from the hypothalamus stimulates pituitary thyrotropin (thyroid-stimulating hormone [TSH]) secretion, which in turn stimulates thyroid hormone production (triiodothyronine [T_3] and thyroxine [T_4]). Thyroid hormone levels provide feedback to the hypothalamus and pituitary, thereby suppressing TRH and TSH secretion so that a balance is reached. In similar fashion, the adrenal glands secrete corticosteroids and the gonads produce progesterone, androgens, and estradiol, all of which influence hypothalamic and pituitary hormone production. For some systems, the set point changes as individuals develop. Hormone secretion can be regulated by nerve cells and by factors important in the immune system (e.g., cytokines interact with hormones that influence weight homeostasis).

Metabolic function in the body involves complex biochemical processes to transform essential amino acids, carbohydrates, and lipids to substances or energy that can be used at the cellular level to produce molecules and to perform cell functions. These biochemical processes or metabolic pathways are driven by enzyme activity.

Pathophysiology

Endocrine abnormalities occur when an alteration in regulation of the normal feedback system results in hyposecretion or hypersecretion of one or more hormones. Multiple factors cause alterations in hormone production. These factors include tumors, trauma, infection, systemic disease, genetic disorders, congenital malformation or agenesis of an endocrine gland, idiopathic causes, and iatrogenic causes (e.g., medications). The defect or problem can originate at the pituitary-hypothalamic level, in organ abnormalities, or for unknown reasons that lead to unresponsiveness to endogenous hormone. Hypothyroidism and hyperthyroidism are examples of disease entities in which the interrelationships of the hypothalamic-pituitary-thyroid axis may be altered at any one of these sites.

Metabolic diseases are generally considered inborn errors of metabolism (IEMs). An alteration in genetic constitution results in disrupted biochemical functioning. For example, in children with phenylketonuria (PKU), a deficiency of the enzyme phenylalanine hydroxylase, the essential amino acid phenylalanine accumulates, which results in intellectual disability if not treated within the first weeks of life.

Assessment

Endocrine and metabolic disorders disrupt organs throughout the body and can alter various body functions. Assessment requires a thorough family history, physical examination, and specific diagnostic testing for the suspected disorder.

History

- What is the child's growth pattern since birth?
- Has there been a recent alteration in growth pattern?
- Is the child taking any medications, including herbs and supplements, that could affect endocrine or metabolic function?
- Any signs or symptoms of endocrine or metabolic dysfunction?

- Any maternal exposure to radioiodine, goitrogens, or iodine medication during pregnancy?
- When did the child first show signs of sexual development?
- What is the child's diet and exercise history?
- What are the parents' heights and at what age was the mother's menarche and father's growth spurt?
- Is there any family history of endocrine, autoimmune, or metabolic disorders (e.g., diabetes mellitus, thyroid disease)?
- Does the child have unusual odors, recurrent vomiting, or unexplained lethargy?

Physical Examination

A detailed examination should include the following:

Measure stature (length/height): Supine *length* is preferred for children younger than 2 years old or until walking well. *Height* is measured using a stadiometer for children older than 2 years and walking well. Plot height, weight, and head circumference on a standardized growth chart appropriate to the child's age and sex (see Appendix). The Centers for Disease Control and Prevention (CDC) recommends that the World Health Organization (WHO) growth charts be used to monitor growth in children younger than 2 years old and that the CDC growth charts be used for children from 2 to 20 years old (Rogol and Hayden, 2014). Serial measurements are critical to assess growth patterns over time. In addition, growth charts are available for children with certain genetic conditions, such as trisomy 21 (Down syndrome) and Turner (45, X0) syndrome, and should be used to assess growth patterns of children with these conditions. Growth charts for children with Down syndrome were updated based on serial measurements of 637 youth who participated in the Down Syndrome Growing Up Study (Zemel et al., 2015).

- Check for proportionate appearance: Measure sitting and standing heights for upper to lower segment (US:LS) ratio and arm span. See Appendix for how to measure.
- Assess *height age* (the age corresponding to the child's height when plotted at the 50th percentile on a growth chart) and *growth velocity* (linear growth in centimeters or inches over the past year).
- Inspect the child's genitalia for signs of normal, abnormal, or ambiguous genitalia.
- Identify the stage of sexual development using sexual maturity rating (Tanner staging).
- Note facial, axillary, and pubic hair for presence, distribution, and texture.
- Examine the skin for presence of striae and acanthosis nigricans of the neck, axilla, breast, knuckles, and skin folds.
- Palpate the thyroid gland for symmetry and size, noting enlargement or presence of nodules and/or Delphian node.
- Examine for presence of dysmorphic features.
- Examine the abdomen noting any organomegaly.
- Complete general neurologic examination.

Acquired endocrine disorders are often due to either hyposecretion or hypersecretion of a specific hormone or combination of hormones, and the child may or may not appear ill. Signs of dehydration, exophthalmos, and tachycardia are physical findings associated with endocrine pathology. Newborns with metabolic disorders may initially appear well, but physical signs develop with metabolic activity. Characteristic physical findings associated with specific disease entities are presented later in this chapter.

Diagnostic Studies

Measurement of hormone levels is a key tool in the diagnosis of endocrine disorders. Specific blood and urine studies that identify end products of abnormal metabolism, as well as elevated or diminished levels of various substances, such as ammonia, glucose, galactose, or amino acids, are important in the diagnosis of metabolic disorders. Accurate interpretation of data requires strict adherence to laboratory protocol for collecting and managing specimens. In addition, not all laboratories have the ability to conduct tests that are sensitive to the hormone or substance being measured (e.g., measurement of hormones in precocious puberty requires high sensitivity; measurement of ammonia levels requires strict procedures when obtaining the sample).

Radiographic and imaging studies (e.g., bone age, ultrasonography, computed tomography [CT], and magnetic resonance imaging [MRI]) are important diagnostic tools in evaluating certain endocrine and metabolic disorders. Many of these studies are expensive and can put additional emotional stress on a family that is already uncertain about their child's condition.

Management Strategies

General Measures

Clinical consequences for the child affected by an endocrine or metabolic disorder vary from mild to severe. If undiagnosed and untreated, some disorders may lead to irreversible intellectual disability, physical disability, neurologic damage, and/or death. Early detection, accurate diagnosis, and timely intervention are necessary to achieve favorable outcomes. Chronic disease issues and the effects of these diseases on lifestyle must also be addressed and include family, school, peer, and emotional adjustment; body image, self-esteem, and social competence; disease understanding, acceptance, and self-care; and regimen adherence. A successful outcome depends on the patient and family receiving support and encouragement in self-care, learning about the disease, and understanding the patient-parent role in managing a long-term illness or chronic condition.

Genetic Counseling

Genetic counseling is often necessary. Implications are significant for the family of a child with endocrine or metabolic disorders that are genetically linked (see Chapters 3 and 32).

Medications

Pharmacologic therapy, including hormone replacement, whether temporary or lifelong, is often essential. Short, clear instructions about medications are important; how much to give, when and how to administer, possible side effects, and when to make adjustments in medication are key messages to convey. Long-term adherence to medications can become problematic with chronic illnesses and requires constant vigilance on the part of providers who interact with the child.

Dietary Considerations

Metabolic diseases often require strict adherence to dietary plans and restrictions. Parents, patients, caregivers, and school personnel must be aware of the dietary needs and restrictions and the effect of diet on the disease process. Families must also be given support to adjust to the economic, social, and psychological demands created by such restrictions.

Patient and Family Education

Close supervision and frequent follow-up are necessary for children with metabolic and endocrine disorders. These children are best evaluated both initially and over time by an interprofessional team with expertise in pediatric endocrinology and metabolism or clinical genetics. Parent and patient education should include:
- Nature of the disorder, treatment plan, and possible complications
- Plan for long-term follow-up, including the timing and process of transition to adult care services
- Family self-management and appropriate level of responsibility for the child based on age and developmental stage

The interprofessional team can provide the education and support needed. The PCP, as a part of this team, is in an ideal position to reinforce the plan of care. In addition, essential primary healthcare needs and anticipatory guidance cannot be overlooked.

Disorders of Endocrine Function

The most common endocrine pathologies of childhood may be grouped into the following seven areas:
- Disturbance of growth
- Abnormalities of pubertal development
- Adrenal conditions
- Disorders of sexual maturation
- Thyroid conditions
- Diabetes mellitus, types 1 and 2
- Posterior pituitary gland dysfunction

Growth Disorders

Children grow in a predictable way, and deviation from a normal growth pattern can be the first sign of an endocrine disorder. Accurate and reliable serial growth measurements must be collected to assess a pattern of growth and current growth velocity. A child's predicted growth potential is based in large part on genetic potential and may change with altered nutritional status and illness patterns. An estimate of the child's expected stature (±2 standard deviations where 1 standard deviation equals 2 inches [4.5 cm] for a particular child) can be made by calculating a midparental target height:
- Target height for boys: (mother's height + 5 inches [13 cm]) + (father's height)/2
- Target height for girls: (father's height – 5 inches [13 cm]) + (mother's height)/2

Growth disorders may be classified as primary or secondary. *Primary* growth disorders include skeletal dysplasias, chromosomal abnormalities (e.g., Turner syndrome), and genetic short stature. *Secondary* growth disorders may result from undernutrition, chronic disease, endocrine disorder, and idiopathic constitutional growth delay (CGD) (Box 45.1).

The following discussion focuses on growth hormone deficiency (GHD) and CGD (Table 45.1).

Growth Hormone Deficiency

Growth hormone (GH) is an anterior pituitary hormone released in response to sleep, exercise, and hypoglycemia. Secretion of

• BOX 45.1 **Growth Abnormalities, Variants of Normal Growth, and U.S. Food and Drug Administration–Approved Indications for Growth Hormone Therapy**

Primary Growth Failure
- Genetic syndromes
  - Achondroplasia
  - Chondrodystrophy
  - Down syndrome
  - Noonan syndrome
  - Prader-Willi syndrome
  - Turner syndrome
  - Short stature homeobox-gene (SHOX) deficiency
- Small for gestational age (SGA) with failure of catch-up growth by 2 years

Secondary Growth Failure
- Endocrine disorders
  - Growth hormone deficiency (GHD), congenital or acquired
  - Hypothyroidism
  - Cushing syndrome
  - Disorders of the GH-insulin like growth factor 1 (IGF-1) axis
  - IGF-1 deficiency or resistance
  - Acid-labile subunit (ALS) deficiency
  - Consequence of precocious puberty
- Idiopathic short stature
  - Height greater than 2.25 standard deviations below the mean for age and gender
  - Unexplained short stature with poor height prognosis
- Malnutrition
- Chronic illness (see Box 45.2)
  - Chronic renal failure
- Systemic glucocorticoid therapy
- Treatment of childhood malignancy

Variants of Normal Growth
- Constitutional delay of growth and puberty
- SGA with catch up growth
- Early puberty with accelerated growth and bone maturation

Note: U.S. Food and Drug Administration–approved indications for growth hormone therapy are italicized

GH occurs in a series of irregular and pulsatile bursts throughout the day and night with most GH activity occurring during sleep. GHD may be either congenital or acquired. Individuals may also be resistant to GH, and GHD increases with age and immunodeficiency.

Clinical Findings

History. A history obtained to evaluate the short or slowly growing child should include:
- Details of pregnancy, delivery, and newborn period
  - Mother's health during pregnancy
  - Birthing process, type, and presence of complications
  - Birth length, weight, and head circumference
  - Neonatal course, including history of prolonged jaundice, hypoglycemia, and/or microphallus (often diagnostic of congenital GHD)
  - Dysmorphia, especially midline facial defects or eye abnormalities
- Parents' and siblings' height, weight, and growth pattern
- Age at which growth first noted to decelerate

TABLE 45.1 Short Stature: Characteristics of Growth Hormone Deficiency and Constitutional Growth Delay in Children

Condition	Etiology	Onset	Presentation	Endocrine/Metabolic Disturbance
Growth hormone deficiency (GHD)	Idiopathic (most common) Pituitary or hypothalamic disease Trauma Minor organic hypothalamic lesion Infection Radiation	Congenital or acquired	Slow growth rate with normal birth weight Signs and symptoms of increased intracranial pressure Microphallus Proportional short stature Delayed bone age	Deficiency or impairment in secretion of growth hormone-releasing hormone
Constitutional growth delay (CGD)	Variation of normal growth Not a disease	First years of life with impaired growth	Growth velocity is normal after 3 years of age Delayed puberty with pubertal growth spurt Delayed bone age Positive family history	None—final height is appropriate for parents' height

- Presence of chronic illness(es)
- Symptoms of hypothyroidism or other known pituitary hormone deficiency
- Trauma or insult to the central nervous system (CNS)
- Treatment with cranial radiation

Physical Examination. Physical examination of the short child or child who is not growing well should include:

- Identification of clinical clues to chronic illness or dysmorphic syndrome (e.g., childlike face with large, prominent forehead)
- Presence of midline defect
- Evaluation of the fundi for signs of increased intracranial pressure
- Palpation of the thyroid gland for the presence of a goiter
- Evaluation of the stage of sexual development
- Measurement of body proportions including arm span, height, and upper-to-lower (U/L) body segment ratio to exclude a skeletal dysplasia (dwarfing condition): Interpretation of the U/L body segment ratio is dependent on the age of the child. Body proportion varies during childhood. At birth, the U/L ratio is approximately 1.7; 1.3 at 3 years old; and 0.89 to 0.95 in postpubertal age children.
- Signs of an intracranial lesion

Diagnostic Studies. If growth velocity is subnormal (including when prior heights are not available), initial evaluation should include:

- Serum glucose (hypoglycemia or hyper glycemia)
- Complete blood count (CBC) and sedimentation rate (erythrocyte sedimentation rate [ESR])
- Urinalysis and chemistry panel
- Screening for gastrointestinal illness when appropriate (e.g., celiac disease screening [serum immunoglobulin A and transglutaminase], irritable bowel disease [ESR], stool for ova and parasites)
- Growth factors (insulin-like growth factor 1 [IGF-1] and insulin-like growth factor–binding protein 3 [IGFBP-3])
- Thyroid function tests: Free T_4 and TSH should be obtained to exclude both pituitary TSH deficiency and primary hypothyroidism
- Bone age x-ray of left wrist and hand

- Karyotype to rule out Turner syndrome in girls: Girls with Turner mosaicism may not manifest the typical clinical findings of Turner syndrome (e.g., cubitus valgus, webbing of the neck), thus highlighting the importance of karyotyping all females presenting with short stature (Rogol and Hayden, 2014) (see Chapter 32).
- Measurement of GH production may be necessary: Because secretion of GH is pulsatile, random serum measurement of the hormone is inadequate; stimulation testing using agents (such as, arginine, levodopa, clonidine, and/or glucagon) is needed to accurately assess GH production.

Differential Diagnosis. Individual children with short stature may not fit nicely into a single category but may have multiple factors contributing to their stature. Many chronic illnesses can slow linear growth, likely through a variety of mechanisms including malnutrition, acidosis, anorexia, and deficiencies of minerals (e.g., zinc, iron) and vitamins necessary for growth (Box 45.2). Typically, children with poor growth as a result of chronic illness are underweight for their height; their weight gain slows prior to growth deceleration. Deficiency of thyroid and/or sex hormones is characterized by subnormal growth velocity, normal to increased weight for height, and delay in bone age.

Management. Children should be referred to a pediatric endocrinologist for further assessment and testing if hypothyroidism, low IGF-1 and IGFBP-3, or other hormone deficiency is confirmed or for unexplained persistent slow growth without evidence of chronic illness. Updated clinical practice guidelines for GH IGF-1 treatment in children and adolescents (Grimberg et al., 2016) suggest that provocative GH stimulation testing may not be required in all cases to confirm a diagnosis of GHD. The U.S. Food and Drug Administration (FDA) has approved eight indications for GH therapy (see Box 45.1). Initial dose of GH (Genotropine) is based on a child's body weight, with doses ranging from 0.16 to 0.24 mg/kg/week (Grimberg et al., 2016).

During the first year of therapy, growth velocity may exceed normal growth rates as much as fourfold. Reported side effects of GH include glucose intolerance, pseudotumor cerebri, edema, growth of nevi, slipped capital femoral epiphyses, and

Gastrointestinal disease
   Celiac disease
   Inflammatory bowel disease
   Cystic fibrosis
Cardiovascular disease
   Cyanotic heart disease
   Congestive heart failure
Renal disease
   Uremia
   Renal tubular acidosis
Hematologic disorders
   Chronic anemia
Inborn errors of metabolism
Pulmonary disease
Chronic infection
Anorexia nervosa

scoliosis (Grimberg et al., 2016). The cost of GH therapy may present an economic burden to the family (Rose, Cook, and Fine, 2014), and referral to a social worker to assist in finding financial support may be appropriate. Timely initiation of GH therapy is instrumental in allowing children to achieve their genetic height potential. Findings from a large cohort study of 4297 youth treated with GH for a 5-year period (Ross, Lee, Gut, and Germak, 2015) demonstrate that, on average, treatment with GH was associated with increases in mean height standard deviation scores consistent with growth velocity approaching the child's genetic height potential. Height velocity over the first 4 months of treatment was the primary factor associated with long-term response to GH therapy. Other predictive factors were: younger age at GH initiation, male gender, taller parents, higher levels of IGF-1, and greater body mass index (BMI).

Constitutional Growth Delay

Constitutional delay of growth and puberty is a variant of normal growth and should not be considered a disease entity. When the child has no evidence of chronic illness, has a delay in bone age, and is growing at a normal rate for bone age, the likely diagnosis is CGD. These children generally reach normal adult height, although they may be slightly shorter compared with other family members.

Clinical Findings

History. The history may include the following:

- Normal length and weight at birth
- Slowed linear growth between 1 and 3 years old and then normal growth velocity; normal height velocity is the most critical factor in diagnosing CGD
- Height at or slightly below the third percentile on standardized growth charts
- Delayed pubertal development
- History of similar growth patterns in other family members: Often there is a family history of at least one family member with a delayed onset of puberty and/or growth than what would be expected.

Physical Examination. Findings on physical examination include:

- Delayed bone age with growth velocity normal for bone age

- Final height prediction based on bone age within range of calculated target height
- Neurologic examination within normal limits

Diagnostic Studies. The same screening tests used to evaluate GHD are performed to rule out pathologic conditions. A bone age x-ray can often be helpful in distinguishing between CGD and idiopathic short stature. The child with CGD will have a bone age consistent with his or her height age, whereas the child with idiopathic short stature will have a bone age consistent with his or her chronologic age (Rogol and Hayden, 2014).

Management. Reassurance and support should be provided to the child and family regarding ultimate height and development. An endocrine referral may be necessary to differentiate CGD from GHD and for possible hormone replacement therapy. For boys older than 11 years and girls older than 10 years where CGD is suspected, priming with sex steroids prior to provocative GH testing is recommended to prevent unnecessary GH treatment of children with CGD. Priming can be accomplished with either oral β-estradiol (boys and girls) or intramuscular testosterone (boys only) (Grimberg et al., 2016).

Growth Excess

In contrast to those with CGD, some children are tall for their family as young children and enter puberty early, yet ultimately reach a height within the normal range for their family. Rarely will this accelerated growth require referral to a pediatric endocrinologist. Tall stature in comparison with parents' height or rapid growth velocity in childhood may represent an underlying abnormality. These include:

- Primary skeletal abnormalities, such as Marfan syndrome, Klinefelter syndrome (47,XXY), and other overgrowth syndromes
- Overnutrition that advances the bone age and the timing of puberty: In these children, weight gain occurs first, and weight percentile is further above the growth curve than height percentile.
- Excess adrenal androgens or gonadal steroids: These children have physical examination findings of early puberty.

Pubertal Disorders

The physical changes of puberty occur in response to production of sex steroids by the ovaries or testes. Hypothalamic gonadotropin-releasing hormone (GnRH) regulates the release of luteinizing hormone (LH) and follicle-stimulating hormone (FSH) from the pituitary gland, which in turn stimulates gonadal hormone secretion.

By midgestation the fetal hypothalamic-pituitary-gonad (HPG) axis is intact; at term, GnRH, LH, and FSH are produced at low levels. When placental and maternal hormones are removed at delivery, unrestrained production of these hormones may occur in the newborn, with the infant experiencing a "mini puberty" between 2 weeks and 3 months of postnatal life. After infancy, the hypothalamic GnRH pulse generator is more sensitive to feedback inhibition from the brain, and by 1 year of age, LH and FSH decrease to the prepubertal range, and the child enters a "latency" period, which will continue until the time of puberty. Puberty occurs when the feedback inhibition is released and GnRH is again produced. The timing of the release correlates better with bone age than chronologic age.

Earlier data from the National Health and Nutrition Examination Survey as well as the more recently reported findings from the United Kingdom Millennium Cohort (Kelly, Zilanawala, Sacker, Hiatt, and Viner, 2017) demonstrate that the initiation of puberty in girls currently occurs earlier compared with past decades and varies by race, ethnicity, and social disadvantage. Sexual maturity rating (Tanner staging) stage 2 breast development occurs between the ages of 8 and 13 years in non-Hispanic white girls with normal BMI; however, thelarche (breast bud development) is a normal finding in non-Hispanic black and Mexican American girls before 8 years of age (Wolf and Long, 2016). Although girls are starting puberty at a younger age than in past generations, the timing of menarche and reaching sexual maturity rating stage 5 has not changed dramatically. Menarche typically occurs within 3 years from the start of breast development. Ninety-five percent of girls have signs of puberty by 12 years old and achieve menarche by 14 years old. Boys normally begin puberty anywhere from 9 years old to 14 years old. The first sign of puberty is increased testicular volume in 85% of boys. Clinicians should be concerned when puberty presents early or is delayed as well as if it occurs out of sequence.

Early Puberty/Precocious Puberty

Early puberty is divided into four categories: premature thelarche, premature adrenarche, isolated menarche, and true precocious puberty.

Premature thelarche, isolated breast development without any other features of puberty, occurs in infant and toddler girls and is sometimes present at birth. This breast development, likely due to increased sensitivity of breast primordia to estradiol, transient estradiol secretion from ovarian cysts, dietary estrogen intake, or transient activation of the HPG axis, has been proposed as a possible mechanism, resolves over time, and rarely progresses to true precocious puberty. It is important to note that for infants and toddlers with suspected premature thelarche, growth acceleration is not present, bone age is consistent with chronologic age, and there are no other signs of puberty.

Premature adrenarche is the early onset of pubic or axillary hair in either boys (prior to 10 years old) or girls (prior to 8 years old) not associated with other features of true puberty. Bone and height age may be slightly advanced in relation to chronologic age in children with premature adrenarche, and plasma dehydroepiandrosterone (DHEA) values may be slightly elevated but correlate with the sexual maturity rating of pubic hair development (Wolf and Long, 2016). Premature adrenarche may be caused by a mild form of congenital adrenal hyperplasia (CAH), exposure to topical testosterone, or rarely, adrenal tumor. Most often, the condition is idiopathic. Children with idiopathic premature adrenarche are at increased risk for polycystic ovary syndrome and metabolic syndrome (Long, 2015).

Isolated menarche is an uncommon condition in which girls have one to a few episodes of vaginal bleeding without breast development. In this condition, sexual abuse, vaginal tumor, a functional estrogen-producing ovarian cyst, and primary hypothyroidism all need to be excluded.

True precocious puberty refers to the onset of multiple features of puberty earlier than the normal range. It is defined as thelarche or pubarche (appearance of pubic hair) before 8 years old in girls and before 9 years old in boys, except in the case of non-Hispanic African-American and Mexican-American girls, for whom thelarche is considered within the normal range after 7 years

---

• BOX 45.3 Disorders of Puberty

Central Precocious Puberty
- Idiopathic (most frequent cause; more common in girls)
- Central nervous system (CNS) tumors
  - Hamartoma
  - Craniopharyngioma
- Post-CNS radiation
- CNS infection
- CNS trauma
- Congenital adrenal hyperplasia

Peripheral Precocious Puberty
- Girls
  - Ovarian cyst or tumor
  - Estrogen secreting ovarian or adrenal tumor
  - McCune-Albright syndrome
- Boys
  - Testicular tumor
  - Testotoxicosis (activating mutation of the luteinizing hormone receptor)
- Both genders
  - Human chorionic gonadotropin (HCG)-secreting tumor (rare; more common in boys)
  - Hypothyroidism

Normal Variants of Puberty
- Premature adrenarche
- Premature thelarche

---

old (Wolf and Long, 2016). Features of precocious puberty may include accelerated linear growth, breast development, testicular or penile enlargement, and pubic hair development. Depending on the duration of symptoms, the bone age may be advanced. Precocious puberty can be divided into two broad categories: (1) central, gonadotropin dependent; or (2) peripheral, gonadotropin independent (Box 45.3). Prolonged exposure to exogenous sex hormones (mother's birth control pills or father's topical testosterone) and exposure to chemicals that disrupt endocrine function can cause peripheral precocious puberty (Long, 2015).

In the United States, the incidence of precocious puberty is 1:5000 to 1:10,000 children. Precocious puberty is more common in females compared with males and in African-American children compared with Caucasian children. Any lesion that disrupts the normal connections between the brain and the hypothalamus can cause central precocious puberty. Although in 90% of girls central precocious puberty is idiopathic, in boys central precocious puberty is more likely to be associated with CNS pathology (Long, 2015).

Clinical Findings. Many children who present with features of early puberty do not require treatment. However, all children who exhibit signs of puberty at a younger age than normal should have an evaluation as to the etiology. Those children who start to develop signs of puberty at the early end of the normal range should be evaluated if they have either rapid progression of pubertal signs resulting in a bone age more than 2 years ahead of chronologic age or new CNS-related findings (e.g., headaches, seizures, and/or focal neurologic defects).

History. Evaluation includes the following:
- Age of onset and pattern of growth
- Type, duration, and progression of pubertal symptoms (i.e., breast tissue, pubic hair, phallic/testicular enlargement, acne, body odor, oily scalp)

- Any symptom suggestive of a CNS lesion
- Family pattern of pubertal changes
- Exposure to topical estrogens or testosterone, oral estrogens, or environmental hormone disruptors

Physical Examination. Physical examination should include:
- Assessment of stature and growth velocity
- Description of the child's sexual maturity rating (Tanner stage):
  - Presence of pubic and/or axillary hair and breast development: Breast development should be evaluated by palpation rather than inspection to differentiate between the presence of true breast tissue versus fat deposition
  - Presence of pubic and/or axillary hair and increase in penile length and/or testicular volume (boys)

Diagnostic Studies. Diagnostic studies should include:
- Premature thelarche: No laboratory studies are necessary in the infant or toddler girl unless other pubertal features are present or continued increase in breast size.
- Premature adrenarche: Serum 17-hydroxyprogesterone (17-OHP) to exclude CAH and a 24-hour urine collection for 17-ketosteroids or imaging of the adrenal glands to exclude an adrenal tumor.
- Isolated menarche: Thyroid function tests to exclude primary hypothyroidism, and pelvic ultrasound to rule out the presence of an ovarian cyst or pelvic tumor.
- True precocious puberty:
  - Bone age x-ray of left wrist and hand
  - LH, FSH, and estradiol or testosterone: Use a laboratory with a sensitive assay that will detect early pubertal values at the lower end of the range.
    - If LH and FSH are high (in pubertal range: indication of central etiology), an MRI is indicated to exclude CNS tumor.
    - If LH and FSH are low (in prepubertal range: indication of peripheral puberty), complete a GnRH stimulation test to distinguish central from peripheral puberty.
  - If etiology is peripheral puberty:
    - Pelvic ultrasonography of girls
    - Testicular ultrasonography of boys
    - Serum 17-OHP to rule out a severe form of CAH

Management. Treatment of early puberty depends on the etiology and should always be done with the guidance of a pediatric endocrinologist. Management depends on the underlying disorder, age of the child, degree of advancement of the bone age, and the child's and family's emotional response to the condition. Radiation, surgery, or chemotherapy is indicated in the case of CNS tumors. A long-acting GnRH agonist may be used to bring serum sex steroids to prepubertal levels. Treatment of precocious puberty is important to increase final adult height.

Delayed Puberty

Puberty is considered delayed when a boy 14 years old or older or a girl 13 years old or older has no clinical features of puberty on physical examination or if puberty has not progressed within a timely basis. Girls should progress to menarche within 5 years of breast budding; boys should attain sexual maturity rating stage 5 pubertal development within 4.5 years of initiation of puberty. If puberty is either delayed or has failed to progress, the child should be referred to an endocrinologist for evaluation of hypogonadism. Laboratory testing should begin with assessment of LH, FSH and estradiol in girls and LH, FSH and testosterone in boys. Children with delayed puberty and elevated FSH and/or LH levels should

• BOX 45.4   Etiology of Delayed Puberty

Chronic Illness
Gastrointestinal with poor weight gain
Chronic renal failure
Anorexia nervosa or bulimia
Chronic anemia
Respiratory or cardiac disease
Medication-induced poor weight gain

Constitutional Growth Delay
Endocrine diseases associated with delayed bone age
Hypothyroidism

Growth Hormone Deficiency
Failure of the hypothalamic-pituitary-gonadal axis

• BOX 45.5   Failure of the Hypothalamic-Pituitary-Gonadal Axis

Hypothalamic Pituitary Dysfunction (LH/FSH Deficiency)
Multiple pituitary hormone deficiency
Isolated gonadotropin deficiency
Kallmann syndrome (anosmia and gonadotropin deficiency)
Hyperprolactinemia
Functional deficiency associated with lack of calories or extreme exercise

Gonadal Failure
Girls
Turner syndrome
Oophoritis
Galactosemia
Chemotherapy induced

Boys
Vanishing testes syndrome (in utero testicular torsion)
Chemotherapy or radiation

FSH, Follicle-stimulating hormone; LH, luteinizing hormone.

be karyotyped to evaluate for Turner syndrome in girls and Klinefelter syndrome in boys (Wolf and Long, 2016).

Any chronic condition that delays the bone age may cause delayed puberty, because the timing of puberty correlates better with bone age than chronologic age (Box 45.4). In addition, failure of any part of the HPG axis may also delay puberty (Box 45.5). The most common cause of delayed puberty is CGD.

Clinical Findings

History and Physical Examination. History and physical examination should focus on clinical clues indicating a chronic illness, symptoms or signs of hypothyroidism (discussed later in this chapter), prior history of CNS insult, or new CNS symptoms suggesting hypopituitarism. Review of systems should include questions about pattern of growth, especially growth velocity, sense of smell (anosmia, absence of sense of smell, is suggestive of Kallman syndrome), and galactorrhea (suggestive of pituitary tumor).

Diagnostic Studies. Laboratory investigation should include:
- Focused screening for acute or chronic illness (CBC, sedimentation rate, C-reactive protein, urinalysis, liver enzymes, electrolytes [renal function])

- Bone age x-ray
- Free T$_4$ and TSH
- IGF-1 and IGFBP-3, if GHD is suspect
- Serum prolactin
- LH and FSH (when gonadal failure is present, LH and FSH are abnormally elevated)

Management. A referral to a pediatric endocrinologist is necessary to determine the etiology and necessary treatment. Hormonal replacement with recombinant GH is the treatment of choice for children with hypogonadism, whereas youth with CGD require reassurance that puberty will occur spontaneously albeit later compared with some peers (Shahid, McClellan, and Kapadia, 2016).

Gender-Affirming Hormonal Transition in Transgender and Gender Nonconforming Youth. Gender identity is a multifactorial construct representing the interaction of biologic, environmental, and cultural factors (Rosenthal, 2016). Transgender is a term used to describe a person whose gender identity does not match their natal gender. One's sexual orientation, the attraction to one or both genders, is not synonymous with one's gender identity. Any individual may have any sexual orientation.

Although the prevalence of transgender youth is not known (Rosenthal, 2016), data suggest that 1.4 million adults (Flores, Herman, Gates, and Brown, 2016) and 150,000 teens (Herman, Flores, Brown, Wilson, and Conron, 2017) identify as transgender. Therefore it is likely that PCPs will not only encounter but also assist in the planning and coordination of the interprofessional (mental health, endocrine, primary care) care needed by these youth. While recognizing the need for a multidisciplinary approach to care for these youth, this discussion is limited to hormonal interventions for transgender adolescents, specifically pubertal suppression at onset of puberty for youth experiencing a significant increase in gender dysphoria and prescription of cross-sex hormones to assist with transition to their affirmed gender (Rosenthal, 2016; Vance, Ehrensaft, and Rosenthal, 2014). Although evidence remains limited, this stepwise approach to treatment is supported by findings from a longitudinal study of 55 young transgender adults followed from the time of pubertal suppression to 1 year following gender reassignment surgery. In this cohort, well-being in young adulthood was similar to or better compared with similar age nontransgender peers (de Vries et al., 2014).

Pubertal Suppression. Gender nonconforming youth often experience heightened gender dysphoria (distress caused by the difference between one's assigned and affirmed gender) at onset of puberty. Gender dysphoric youth are eligible for pubertal suppression if they meet Diagnostic and Statistical Manual of Mental Disorders (DSM–5) criteria for gender dysphoria, are at least sexual maturity (Tanner) rating 2 or greater, have mental health and social support during treatment, psychiatric conditions that could impair treatment have been addressed, and have realistic expectations of pubertal suppression therapy. The input of a mental health professional regarding the youth's eligibility and readiness for suppression of puberty is essential in making the decision (*Guidelines for the primary and gender-affirming care of transgender and gender nonbinary people*, 2016). Use of GnRH analogues, leuprolide acetate or histrelin, more commonly used to delay pubertal progression in children with central precocious puberty, is a reversible intervention that interrupts puberty and development of undesired secondary sexual characteristics such as breast development and voice

changes. This temporary treatment allows time for readiness for the long-term decision regarding cross-sex hormonal therapy. Monitoring for adequate suppression of the HPG axis for pubertal suppression includes LH, FSH, and total testosterone for youth with testes and LH, FSH, and estradiol in those with ovaries with adjustment in dose of leuprolide acetate or histrelin as needed (*Guidelines for the primary and gender-affirming care of transgender and gender nonbinary people*, 2016). During this time, youth should be assessed regarding their desire to continue to the next phase of treatment, initiation of gender affirming hormones, typically initiated at age 16 or, in some cases, earlier. If gender identification changes, pubertal suppression regimens are reversible. Upon cessation of therapy, the normal pubertal process will resume (Vance et al., 2014).

Cross-Sex Hormonal Therapy. This stage of treatment induces secondary sexual characteristics consistent with the affirmed gender. For affirmed males, the goal of cross-sex hormone treatment with testosterone is masculinization and levels of testosterone consistent with adult males. At implementation of testosterone therapy, the GnRH analogue used to suppress puberty will often be continued to maintain suppression of the hypothalamic-pituitary axis and suppression of menses. Although some physical signs of masculinization induced by testosterone therapy, such as increased lean muscle mass and male pattern hair growth are partially reversible, other signs such as clitoromegaly and deepening of the voice are not. For affirmed females, cross-sex hormone therapy with both estrogen and a second agent, either a GnRH analogue or an antiandrogen such as spironolactone (*Guidelines for the primary and gender-affirming care of transgender and gender nonbinary people*, 2016), will be used. It is important for youth to have realistic expectations regarding goals and outcomes of cross-sex hormone therapy. For example, estrogen cannot reverse masculine features such as facial hair or lowered voice already present at estrogen initiation (Vance et al., 2014). Details regarding ongoing monitoring of transgender youth during pubertal suppression and cross-sex hormone treatment is fully described by Rosenthal (2016).

Polycystic Ovarian Syndrome. Hyperandrogenism, anovulation, and polycystic ovaries are characteristic features of polycystic ovarian syndrome (PCOS). The incidence ranges from 3% to 15% based on genetic background, race, and diagnostic criteria. PCOS is typically found in females of reproductive age who are overweight or obese; however, 5% with this syndrome are lean. Impaired glucose tolerance, increased insulin resistance, and obesity are associated with PCOS; insulin resistance is thought to be the major pathologic factor linked to this syndrome (Dashti et al., 2017).

Clinical Findings
- Irregular menstrual cycle—missed or fewer periods (<8 in a year), periods every 21 days or more often, or absent menses
- Hirsutism (70% have hair on face, chin, or on body where males typically have hair)
- Acne
- Thinning hair or hair loss on scalp; male-pattern baldness
- Obesity (central) or unexpected weight gain or difficulty losing weight
- Darkening of skin (neck creases, groin, underneath breasts)
- Skin tags

Diagnostic Testing. A pelvic exam should be performed. Cholesterol and glucose testing (see section on Type 2 Diabetes) as well as androgen and testosterone levels are basic studies. Diagnostic features include hyperandrogenemia, progressive hirsutism, menses cycle length of 45 days or more, and polycystic ovaries greater

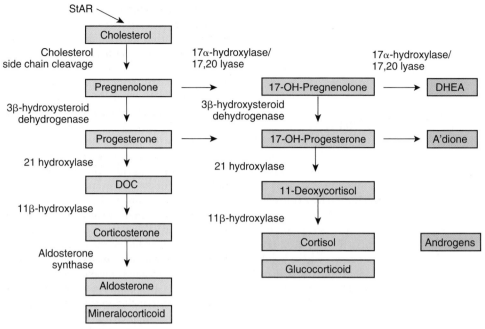

• **Fig 45.1** Adrenal Steroidogenesis. After the steroidogenic acute regulatory *(StAR)* protein–mediated uptake of cholesterol into mitochondria within adrenocortical cells, aldosterone, cortisol, and adrenal androgens are synthesized through the coordinated action of a series of steroidogenic enzymes in a zone-specific fashion. *A'dione,* Androstenedione; *DHEA,* dehydroepiandrosterone; *DOC,* deoxycorticosterone. (From Stewart PM. The adrenal cortex. In: Larsen PR, Kronenberg HM, Melmed S, et al., eds. *Williams Textbook of Endocrinology.* 10th ed. Philadelphia: WB Saunders; 2003:495.)

than 10 cm on sonogram (Francis and Menon, 2018). Recent guidelines note that ultrasound of the ovaries is not necessary for diagnosis (Teede et al., 2018); provider discretion is appropriate.

Differential Diagnosis. Late-onset CAH, androgen-secreting tumors, and Cushing disease should be included in the differential diagnosis.

Management. Referral to an endocrinologist is needed for optimal management. See section in this chapter on treatment of obesity and type 2 diabetes. Nonpharmacologic treatment of overweight and obese women involves lifestyle modification in diet, exercise, or both. Pharmacologic treatment may include one or a combination of the following agents: metformin, the thiazolidinediones, combination oral contraceptives (lower-dose preparation preferred), and orlistat. Metformin alone or in addition is recommended to treat metabolic features. It is the only agent that reduces fat distribution, BMI, and fasting blood sugar while increasing insulin sensitivity. It also reduces the risk of type 2 diabetes when given at higher doses (Dashti et al., 2017).

Refer to dermatology for hair removal products (antiandrogen agents) and procedures. See Chapter 34 for treatment of acne. Metformin typically has little effect on reducing acne and facial hair. Antidepressants may be needed for depression and anxiety, which is four times higher than in females without PCOS (Zhuang et al., 2013).

Complications

PCOS is associated with increased risk of type II diabetes, hypertension and cardiovascular disease, obstructive sleep apnea, depression and anxiety (mood disorders), endometrial hyperplasia, and endometrial cancer.

Adrenal Disorders

Anatomy and Physiology

Adrenal gland steroid production is under the control of the hypothalamic-pituitary axis. The hypothalamus secretes corticotropin-releasing hormone (CRH) in a pulsatile fashion, which stimulates production and secretion of adrenocorticotropic hormone (ACTH) by the pituitary gland. ACTH regulates adrenal glucocorticoid (cortisol) and androgen production. Cortisol is produced in a series of enzymatic steps (Fig 45.1) and is highest in the morning, low in the afternoon and evening, and lowest at midnight. Secreted in response to hypoglycemia, hypotension, pain, or other stressful events, cortisol has negative feedback on the synthesis and secretion of CRH, vasopressin, and ACTH.

The adrenal gland also produces mineralocorticoid hormones (aldosterone), regulated by renal production of renin interacting with angiotensinogen, to create angiotensin. The renin-angiotensin system is involved in regulation of salts, especially sodium, blood pressure; and renal blood flow. Aldosterone production also occurs in enzymatic steps, many of which are common to the cortisol production pathway.

Adrenal Insufficiency

Adrenal insufficiency is characterized by a deficiency of hormones produced by the adrenal cortex; deficits of cortisol and aldosterone are perhaps the most detrimental to body function. In *primary* adrenal insufficiency (hypofunctioning adrenal gland), glucocorticoid (cortisol), *and* mineralocorticoid (aldosterone) hormones are deficient, whereas in *secondary* adrenal insufficiency (hypothalamic or pituitary defect), only a glucocorticoid deficit is found. Thus children with both forms of adrenal insufficiency have hypoglycemia and hypotension caused by cortisol deficiency. Only those

• BOX 45.6 Adrenal Insufficiency

Deficiency of Corticotropin-Releasing Hormone or Adrenocorticotropin

Isolated deficiency
    Congenital
    Acquired as a result of hypophysitis
Multiple pituitary hormone deficiencies
    Congenital (e.g., septo-optic dysplasia, midline defects)
    Acquired (e.g., CNS trauma, infection, tumor, radiation)

Primary Adrenal

Congenital
    CAH (most common 21-OH deficiency)
    Adrenal hypoplasia (X-linked, autosomal recessive, ACTH receptor
        defect)
Acquired
    X-linked, adrenoleukodystrophy
    Autoimmune (Addison)
    Infection

21-OH, 21-Hydroxylase; ACTH, adrenocorticotropin; CAH, congenital adrenal hyperplasia; CNS, central nervous system.

---

with a primary adrenal insufficiency are at risk for salt-wasting crisis (hyponatremia, hyperkalemia, acidosis, and dehydration) caused by aldosterone deficiency.

Primary adrenal insufficiency may be due to an inability to produce cortisol secondary to an enzyme defect in the adrenal steroid pathway (e.g., CAH), hypoplasia of the adrenal gland, or an acquired defect (Box 45.6). Lesions of the hypothalamus or pituitary lead to secondary adrenal insufficiency. Suppression of the hypothalamic-pituitary-adrenal axis secondary to exogenous steroid use can also lead to adrenal insufficiency. Infants born extremely prematurely (24 to 28 weeks' gestation) sometimes demonstrate symptoms of adrenal insufficiency because of immaturity of the hypothalamic-pituitary-adrenal axis.

Secondary adrenal insufficiency can occur as a result of ACTH deficiency, as one of multiple hypothalamic-pituitary deficiencies, or rarely as an isolated problem. Most often the infant or child has a syndrome known to be associated with hypopituitarism (e.g., septo-optic dysplasia), has also been discovered to have GHD, or has a destructive lesion (e.g., tumor) or a history of prior radiation to the brain or CNS trauma.

CAH is caused by a deficiency of any of the enzymes in the cortisol pathway. In addition to interrupting normal cortisol production, the most common enzymatic abnormality, 21-hydroxylase (21-OH) deficiency, causes shunting of cortisol precursors to the androgen pathway, resulting in production of elevated levels of adrenal androgens in utero. Female infants born with classic CAH typically have ambiguous genitalia (e.g., enlarged clitoris and/or posterior fusion of the labia) from this excessive androgen exposure in utero. However, male infants have no signs of CAH at birth with the exception of subtle hyperpigmentation and possible mild enlargement of the penis (Fleming, Van Riper, and Knafl, 2017). Approximately 75% of children with CAH caused by 21-OH deficiency will also have aldosterone deficiency. Newborn screening programs currently routinely test for the presence of CAH caused by 21-OH deficiency to detect CAH early to avoid a potentially life-threatening salt-wasting crisis in affected infants.

Clinical Findings

History

- Symptoms of cortisol deficiency include a history of poor appetite, failure to thrive, or weight loss; weakness and vomiting
- Symptoms of aldosterone deficiency include vomiting, poor feeding, lethargy and dehydration

Physical Examination. The following signs are often seen:
- Dehydration and hypotension
- Excessive pigmentation of the skin and mucous membranes (present only with primary adrenal insufficiency)

Diagnostic Studies. The following diagnostic studies are indicated:
- Serum glucose (hypoglycemia)
- Blood gases and bicarbonate (metabolic acidosis)
- Electrolytes (low sodium, elevated potassium with aldosterone deficiency)
- Serum cortisol: A cortisol value greater than 20 µg/dL indicates adrenal sufficiency; a value less than that must be interpreted in the clinical context in which the sample was drawn. Often an ACTH stimulation test, performed in collaboration with a pediatric endocrinologist, is needed to conclusively diagnose both primary and secondary adrenal insufficiency.
- Serum ACTH (elevated in primary adrenal insufficiency)
- Serum 17-OHP (diagnostic in children with suspected CAH caused by 21-OH deficiency)
- Serum renin level (elevated in aldosterone deficiency)
- Aldosterone level (low in aldosterone deficiency)
- Plasma renin and aldosterone levels are interpreted best if they are drawn when serum sodium levels are low.

Management. Treatment of adrenal insufficiency includes hormone replacement and is best managed by a pediatric endocrinologist. Clinical practice guidelines of the Endocrine Society for diagnosis and treatment of primary adrenal insufficiency include specific recommendations for treatment and monitoring of primary adrenal insufficiency during childhood including management and prevention of adrenal crisis (Bornstein et al., 2016). Adrenal crisis is a medical emergency requiring immediate and vigorous administration of intravenous (IV) dextrose, normal saline, and stress doses of hydrocortisone succinate. IV stress doses of hydrocortisone succinate vary with age: 25 mg in children younger than 3 years old; 50 mg in children 3 to 12 years old; and 100 mg in children older than 12 years old, administered every 6 hours. Parents should be instructed regarding the need for stress doses of hydrocortisone succinate when their child has a febrile illness, surgery, or trauma; they should also be taught how to administer hydrocortisone succinate via intramuscular injection in case the child is vomiting or otherwise unable to swallow or retain oral medication. This injection allows parents extended time to seek further medical advice or intervention. Parent/caregiver education should include indications for when and how to administer hydrocortisone succinate, practice regarding drawing up medication, and review of injection technique and injection sites. This information should be reviewed with parents and/or caregivers on an annual basis.

Long-term therapy of CAH includes oral hydrocortisone in replacement doses of 8 to 10 mg/m^2 (8 to 10 mg per square meter of body surface per day, divided every 8 hours) in children with ACTH deficiency or primary adrenal insufficiency. Children with CAH tend to have higher hydrocortisone needs. If present, aldosterone deficiency must be treated with daily oral fludrocortisone acetate. Treatment of CAH requires a fine balancing act to replace steroids, thereby preventing androgen overproduction. Excess steroid intake can lead to delayed growth, whereas not enough steroids contribute to bone age advancement and ultimate short stature. Individual treatment plans are essential to meet the specific needs of individual children. The PCP should be familiar with the medical endocrinology treatment plan and reinforce it at routine well- and sick-child visits.

Hyperadrenal States

Cortisol excess is most commonly caused by exogenous glucocorticoid treatment of an illness (e.g., serious asthma, to prevent rejection after a transplant, or as part of chemotherapy protocols). Endogenous cortisol excess may be due to a pituitary tumor producing ACTH, adrenal tumor, or to ectopic production of ACTH from a nonpituitary tumor (rare in children).

Clinical Findings

History and Physical Examination. Features of cortisol excess include weight gain, growth failure, osteopenia, hypertension, plethora (hypervolemia), and delayed puberty. In addition, acne, purple striae, and hirsutism are common skin findings. Compulsive behaviors may be reported.

Diagnostic Studies. In situations where growth is slow or growth data are missing and cortisol excess needs to be excluded by laboratory evaluation, a 24-hour urine collection for free cortisol or a late evening serum or salivary cortisol are the best screening tests.

Differential Diagnosis. Obesity is in the differential diagnosis, but almost all children with simple obesity are tall for their age and cortisol excess can be excluded on physical examination alone.

Management. When children receive glucocorticoids for underlying illness for longer than 7 to 10 days, the steroid dose should be weaned rather than abruptly discontinued to allow the hypothalamic-pituitary-adrenal axis to recover normal function and sometimes to prevent a flare up of the underlying disease. Procedures for tapering the dose are empiric, but in general, the longer the child has been on glucocorticoids, the longer the taper. Withdrawal plans are based on the goal of treating the child with the least amount of glucocorticoids to avoid long-term adverse effects while avoiding potential adrenal insufficiency during withdrawal. Decreasing the dose to a physiologic dose while monitoring the cortisol level is one method to wean. A morning cortisol value of 20 μg/dL indicates that the hypothalamic-pituitary axis is intact and it is safe to wean further or, if the child is already on half maintenance dose, discontinue the medication (Liu et al., 2013). Even after the steroid has been safely discontinued, the patient may not be able to respond adequately to severe stress for as long as 6 to 12 months.

Disorders of Sex Development

Abnormalities of sexual differentiation usually present in infancy with ambiguous genitalia. The spectrum of physical examination findings ranges from the appearance of a normal male penis and normal scrotum but without palpable gonads, to an infant who looks mostly female with mild enlargement of the clitoris. True hermaphroditism, in which the infant has both male and female gonadal structures, is rare.

Infants with 46,XY chromosomes who have complete androgen insensitivity (androgen receptor defect) have genitalia that appear female; these children are not detected in the newborn period unless a karyotype is performed for some other reason. Children with complete androgen insensitivity may not be identified until the time of an inguinal hernia repair when a testis is discovered or during the teen years when they fail to develop pubic hair or menstruate.

Disorders of sex development occur when the XX fetus is exposed to excess androgen in utero, the XY fetus is unable to produce or respond to androgens, or, rarely, true hermaphroditism. The most common cause of disordered sex development is CAH that exposes an XX fetus to excess androgens during fetal life (see Fig 45.1). Less common virilizing conditions include aromatase deficiency or virilizing tumor in the mother. In an XY fetus, disordered sex development can result from inadequate androgen production or partial androgen insensitivity.

Clinical Findings

All infants should receive a complete genital examination before discharge from the nursery. The initial laboratory evaluation of an infant with ambiguous genitalia should be directed by a pediatric endocrinologist and includes:

- A karyotype test that can be done quickly (within 48 to 72 hours) if the cytogenetics laboratory is alerted to the urgency. Subsequent laboratory evaluation is based on karyotype results.
- In XY infants, measurement of the precursors of testosterone, testosterone, and dihydrotestosterone.
- In XX infants, serum 17-OHP to establish a diagnosis of 21-OH deficiency.
- Serum müllerian inhibitory substance can also be measured or can be assessed indirectly by obtaining an ultrasound or genitogram.

Management

The family needs to be counseled immediately. The PCP has a responsibility to document the abnormality and refer to a specialist team that includes a pediatric endocrinologist, medical geneticist, and pediatric urologist. The initial studies should be sent with the referral. The specialist team should meet with families and educate them about the normal process of genital development, the cause of their child's abnormality, the evaluation process, and the determination of gender for childrearing. Female is the appropriate sex of rearing for XX infants with CAH and for infants with complete androgen insensitivity. Determining the sex assignment for childrearing in incompletely masculinized XY infants is complicated, and waiting to assign the sex of rearing until the evaluation is complete is imperative. Initiation of treatment of the underlying cause, if known (e.g., CAH), is essential. More research is needed regarding how families manage the long-term challenges of raising youth with disorders of sexual development (Fleming, Van Riper, and Knafl, 2017).

Thyroid Disorders

Anatomy and Physiology

The hypothalamic-pituitary-thyroid axis begins functioning during fetal development (Fig 45.2). The hypothalamus produces TRH, which in turn stimulates pituitary production of TSH. TSH stimulates the thyroid gland to secrete primarily T_4. T_4 is converted in peripheral tissues to T_3. Both T_3 and T_4 bind to thyroid-binding proteins, primarily thyroid-binding globulin (TBG). The free, unbound form of T_3 and T_4 is biologically active. T_4 inhibits hypothalamic TRH and pituitary TSH secretion. Thyroid hormone has an important role in growth and development, basal metabolic activity, oxygen consumption, brain development, and metabolism of lipids, carbohydrates, and proteins.

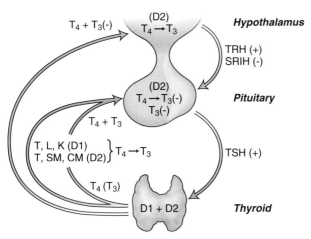

• **Fig 45.2** Interrelationships of the Hypothalamic-Pituitary-Thyroid Axis. *CM,* Cardiac muscle; *D1,* type 12 iodothyronine deiodinase; *D2,* type 2 iodothyronine deiodinase; *K,* kidney; *L,* liver; *SM,* skeletal muscle; *SRIH,* somatotropin release-inhibiting factor; *T₃,* triiodothyronine; *T₄,* thyroxine; *TRH,* thyrotropin-releasing hormone; *TSH,* thyroid-stimulating hormone. (From Wilson JD, Foster DW, eds. Williams Textbook of Endocrinology. 8th ed. Philadelphia: WB Saunders; 1992:169.)

Hypothyroidism

Primary hypothyroidism (hypothyroidism caused by a problem in the thyroid gland itself) may be either congenital or acquired. The incidence of congenital hypothyroidism (CH) is increasing globally. In North America, CH occurs in approximately 1 in 2500 infants and varies by geographic location and race/ethnicity (Diaz and Lipman Diaz, 2014). Female infants are more commonly affected. CH results from an abnormality in development of the thyroid gland during fetal life (dysgenesis or agenesis) or a problem with the ability of the thyroid to make thyroid hormone. Thyroid dysgenesis accounts for approximately 85% of cases of CH. Less frequently, CH may result from an abnormality at the level of the pituitary or hypothalamus (affecting 1 in 25,000 to 1 in 50,000 live births) (Diaz and Lipman Diaz, 2014). CH is the most common cause of preventable mental retardation. Untreated CH leads to irreversible brain damage and variable degrees of growth failure, deafness, and neurologic abnormalities. Earlier detection of CH through improvements in newborn screening combined with more aggressive thyroid hormone replacement regimens (10 to 15 µg/kg/day) at diagnosis have led to improved developmental outcomes for newborns with CH.

Newborn screening also identifies infants with TBG deficiency. Although this is not a condition that requires treatment, newborn screening tests appear abnormal with a low level of thyroid hormone (T_4) with low, normal, or slightly elevated thyrotropin (TSH) levels. The level of thyroid hormone is dependent on availability of binding proteins. For newborns with TBG deficiency, the level of thyroid binding globulin is low. However, the physical exam is within normal limits and there is no history (e.g., midline defect) to suggest central hypothyroidism. Laboratory testing for infants with suspected TBG deficiency includes assessment of free T_4 and TBG level. The free T_4 will be within normal limits because its level does not depend on binding proteins; the TBG level will be low which confirms TBG deficiency (Diaz and Lipman Diaz, 2014; Hanley, Lord, and Bauer, 2016).

The most common cause of acquired hypothyroidism in children in the Western world is Hashimoto thyroiditis, an autoimmune condition leading to destruction of the thyroid gland).

• **BOX 45.7** Acquired Primary Hypothyroidism

Etiology

Chronic lymphocytic thyroiditis (Hashimoto thyroiditis)
Drug induced (iodine, lithium, thioamides, resorcinol)
Thyroidectomy
I^{131} ablation
Infiltrative and storage disorders (histiocytosis X, cystinosis)
Subacute thyroiditis
Cranial/spinal radiation

Worldwide, iodine deficiency is the main cause of acquired primary hypothyroidism and has led to salt iodination as a public health measure in many countries. Hypothyroidism can also be due to a TSH deficiency that is secondary to pituitary disease or dysfunction of the hypothalamus (central hypothyroidism). Other causes of acquired hypothyroidism are listed in Box 45.7. Children with type 1 diabetes and/or other autoimmune conditions are at increased risk for Hashimoto thyroiditis.

Clinical Findings

History. Growth failure, goiter, delayed or arrested puberty, delayed dentition, weight gain, fatigue, dry skin, hyperlipidemia, decline in school performance, and menorrhagia can be present in the child with hypothyroidism. A family history of thyroid disease or other autoimmune conditions is frequently present. A past history of risk factors for hypopituitarism (e.g., CNS insult, frequent headaches, midline defects) is useful information when assessing the risk for TSH deficiency.

Physical Examination. The clinical manifestations of primary hypothyroidism vary with the age of the child.

• At birth, the newborn may appear completely normal, thus the importance of newborn screening programs for early identification of hypothyroidism. The most common neonatal signs are prolonged jaundice, constipation, and umbilical hernia. Infants with CH may also have large anterior and posterior fontanelles, macroglossia, decreased muscle tone, and be poor feeders. They may have respiratory distress and poor peripheral circulation with cool, cyanotic skin in the extremities.

• Older children who present with acquired hypothyroidism may exhibit delayed growth or subnormal growth velocity, goiter, weight gain, and delayed return of the deep tendon reflexes. Children with central hypothyroidism (thyroid deficiency secondary to pituitary or hypothalamus dysfunction) may show poor growth, increased weight for height, and features suggestive of hypopituitarism, such as midline facial or eye abnormalities.

Diagnostic Studies. For primary hypothyroidism:

• The diagnosis of CH is usually made during the first week of life, detected by newborn screening tests. Newborn screening programs test filter paper blood spots using one of two screening strategies: (1) a primary TSH/backup T_4 method or (2) a primary T_4/backup TSH method to identify newborns with either primary or central hypothyroidism. When a result is abnormal, the PCP or hospital of record is contacted to obtain a confirmatory free T_4 and TSH serum sample. A serum sample is also indicated if clinical features of CH are detected. Infants born with Down syndrome are at higher risk for CH, with males and females equally affected.

• In older children, TSH is abnormally elevated, whereas the free T_4 is either within the normal range or low.

TABLE 45.2 Thyroid Hormone Dosing

Age	Levothyroxine Sodium (L-thyroxine) mcg/kg/day (once daily)	Comments
Neonatal And 1-3 months	10-15	Targeted serum T_4 concentration (>10 mcg/dL); if risk for cardiac failure consult additional references
3-6 months	8-10	
6-12 months	6-8	
1-5 years	5-6	
6-12 years	4-5	
>12 years	2-3	Dose if incomplete growth and puberty
	1.7	Dose if growth and puberty complete

Data from Taketomo CK, Hodding JH, Kraus, DM. *Pediatric & Neonatal Dosage Handbook.* 24th ed. Hudson, Ohio: Wolters Kluwer, Lexicomp; 2018. T_4, Thyroxine.

- For central hypothyroidism:
- Free serum T_4 is low with a normal TSH.
- For children with TBG deficiency:
- Total T_4 will be low, but free T_4 and TSH will be normal. TBG level should then be measured to confirm TBG deficiency.

Management. Hypothyroidism is treated with replacement doses of levothyroxine sodium. Liquid suspensions of levothyroxine are not available in the United States; therefore parents need to be instructed regarding crushing the tablet and administering the medication via a spoon with a few drops of water, breast milk, or formula (Hanley et al., 2016). Brand name tablets are recommended over generic preparations because of increased reliability of dose (Leger et al., 2014). The dose (mg/kg) varies by age and weight (Table 45.2). Because of the long half-life of levothyroxine, if a dose is missed, the dose can be doubled the next day (Diaz and Lipman Diaz, 2014).

Ongoing laboratory monitoring and follow-up are also age dependent. Because normal thyroid function in the first 3 years of life is critical for normal cognitive development, more frequent monitoring is necessary for young infants and young children. Thyroid function testing is recommended 2 to 4 weeks after initiating therapy. The goal of treatment is to normalize TSH levels. Once this is accomplished, during the first year of life, thyroid function tests should be monitored every 1 to 3 months. From age 1 to 3 years, monitoring should be performed every 2 to 4 months (Hanley et al., 2016). Children older than the age of 3 years should be monitored every 6 to 12 months until growth is complete (Diaz and Lipman Diaz, 2014). In general, an elevated TSH (in primary hypothyroidism) or low free T_4 (in central hypothyroidism) indicates the need to increase the dose of medication. Following an adjustment in thyroid hormone replacement, thyroid function testing should be repeated in 4 weeks to be sure that the new dose is adequate.

Hyperthyroidism

Hyperthyroidism occurs in childhood when the thyroid gland overproduces thyroid hormone or when a child is given too large a dose of thyroid hormone replacement. Graves disease, an autoimmune condition, is the most common cause of hyperthyroidism (Srinivasan and Misra, 2015). In this condition, thyroid-stimulating immunoglobulin binds to the TSH receptor, resulting in excessive thyroid hormone production. Infants born to women with a current or past history of Graves disease sometimes present with neonatal Graves disease, secondary to passage of antibody from mother to fetus. Although neonatal Graves disease is self-limiting with dissipation of maternal antibodies by approximately 3 months old, early identification and management are critical because these infants are at risk for significant morbidity and mortality (van der Kaay, Wasserman, and Palmert, 2016). Some children with Hashimoto' thyroiditis will have a short (6 to 18 months) phase of hyperthyroidism (Hashimoto' thyrotoxicosis) at the onset of disease. Other causes of hyperthyroidism (e.g., autonomous thyroid nodules) are less common (Srinivasan and Misra, 2015).

Clinical Findings

History. The history of a child with hyperthyroidism may include:
- Palpitations, tremor, emotional lability
- Increased appetite often accompanied by weight loss
- Fatigue, muscle weakness, hyperdefecation
- Poor sleep and poor concentration with decreased school performance

Physical Examination. Often observed findings in hyperthyroidism include:
- Goiter (almost 100%)
- An audible thyroid bruit may be present
- Tachycardia, wide pulse pressure
- Underweight for height, warm moist skin, tremor, or hyperreflexia
- Eyelid lag or exophthalmos (approximately 50% of children with Graves disease have exophthalmos)
- A hyperfunctioning nodule in the thyroid may be present

Diagnostic Studies. The free T_4 and total T_4 levels are elevated and the TSH suppressed below the sensitivity of the assay. Measuring a T_3 level is helpful in hyperthyroidism because it may be more dramatically elevated than the T_4 and be a better marker to monitor.

Management. Children with hyperthyroidism should be referred to a pediatric endocrinologist for discussion of treatment options (i.e., medical therapy using antithyroid drugs, subtotal thyroidectomy or radioiodine) and ongoing management. Medical management with methimazole is considered first line therapy for children with Graves disease. Because of the risk of hepatotoxicity, use of propylthiouracil (PTU), another antithyroid drug option, is reserved for youth who are allergic to methimazole, have developed an adverse effect that warrants its discontinuation, or are pregnant (methimazole is contraindicated during pregnancy). Major adverse events for both methimazole and PTU occur in fewer than 2% of patients and include agranulocytosis, vasculitis, hepatitis, and liver failure (Srinivasan and Misra, 2015).

Diabetes Mellitus

Diabetes is one of the most common chronic diseases in childhood. Diabetes mellitus is a group of conditions characterized by inadequate insulin secretion, insulin resistance, or both. These

TABLE 45.3 Comparison of Type 1 and Type 2 Diabetes in Youth

	Type 1 Diabetes	Type 2 Diabetes
Age at onset	All ages	≥10 years old
Gender	Equal distribution by gender	More frequent in females
Race/ethnicity	Most frequent in non-Hispanic whites May occur in all racial and ethnic groups	More frequent in African Americans, Asians, Native Americans, Hispanics
Obesity	Similar to the general population; not related to type 1 diabetes	>90%
Family history of diabetes	5%-10% have first-degree relative affected	Approximately 80% have first-degree relative affected
Insulin secretion	Very low	Low, normal, or high
Insulin sensitivity	Normal	Decreased
Onset	Acute, severe	Subtle to severe
Ketosis, DKA	Approximately one-third of new cases	Uncommon
Hypertension	Uncommon	Common
Acanthosis nigricans	Rare	Common
Polycystic ovary syndrome	Rare	Common
Islet autoimmunity	Present	Uncommon

DKA, Diabetic ketoacidosis.

dynamics lead to defective metabolism of carbohydrate, protein, and fat and subsequent hyperglycemia. Diabetes (type 1 or 2) affects approximately 193,000 individuals younger than 20 years old in the United States, which is approximately 0.24% of American youth younger than 20 years of age (CDC, 2017).

Among youth, the majority (87%) have type 1 diabetes, 10.5% have type 2 diabetes, and 2.5% have other types (Pettitt et al., 2014). These include maturity-onset diabetes of youth (MODY), as well as diabetes related to chronic conditions (e.g. cystic fibrosis), induced by chronic medication use (e.g. steroids), or correlated with genetic disorders (e.g. Down syndrome). New cases of type 1 diabetes are more frequently diagnosed during the autumn and winter months. The incidence of both type 1 and type 2 diabetes is increasing dramatically in children in the United States and other countries throughout the world (Patterson et al., 2014; Pulgaron and Delamater, 2014). Table 45.3 shows the distinguishing features of type 1 and type 2 diabetes.

Type 1 Diabetes

Type 1 diabetes is caused by autoimmune destruction of pancreatic beta cells in the islets of Langerhans thought to be triggered by a preceding environmental event in genetically susceptible individuals. This destruction of beta cells results in an absolute deficiency in insulin secretion, reduced biologic effectiveness, or both. Normal metabolic function depends upon sufficient amounts of circulating insulin. Insulin deficiency results in uninhibited gluconeogenesis and a blockage in the use and storage of circulating glucose. Therefore high blood glucose levels are a result of the defective metabolism of carbohydrate, protein, and fats.

Based on 2009 data from the SEARCH for Diabetes in Youth study, 6666 of 3.4 million youth were diagnosed with type 1 diabetes and 558 of 1.7 million youth were diagnosed with type 2 diabetes in the United States (Dabelea, Mayer-Davis, et al., 2014).

Females and males were affected in equal numbers. The prevalence of type 1 diabetes varied by race and ethnicity and was highest among non-Hispanic white youth (2.55/1000 children). Native American children had a much lower prevalence of type 1 diabetes (0.35/1000 children), and only 32% of diabetes among Native American children was type 1.

The incidence of type 1 diabetes in the United States has increased. During the period 2002 to 2012, the incidence of type 1 diabetes increased from approximately 15,900 cases/year to approximately 17,900 cases/year, an increase of 1.8% annually after adjusting for age, sex, race, and ethnicity. The greatest increase in annual incidence was 4.2% in the Hispanic population (Mayer-Davis et al., 2017). Although children were most often diagnosed during the time of puberty and onset of symptoms can present at any age, increasing incidence occurred in all age groups of children older than 4 years (Mayer-Davis et al., 2017).

Clinical Findings. Although the onset of type 1 diabetes is gradual with destruction of pancreatic islet cells over time, children may become ill quite suddenly once symptoms manifest. As diabetes develops, the symptomatology reflects the decreasing degree of beta cell mass, increasing insulinopenia and hyperglycemia, and increasing ketoacids.

History. With type 1 diabetes, the child may have had a viral infection, cold, or flu; parents may notice increased urination and thirst during the recovery period, with additional signs and symptoms appearing over a period of days or weeks. The following early symptoms are often reported:

- Polydipsia, polyphagia, polyuria
- Nocturia, blurred vision
- Weight loss or poor weight gain
- Fatigue and lethargy
- Vaginal moniliasis

As ketoacids accumulate, the following history is reported:
- Abdominal pain, nausea and/or vomiting
- Fruity-smelling breath
- Weakness (caused by dehydration)
- Mental confusion
- Coma

Approximately 30% of children with new-onset type 1 diabetes present in diabetic ketoacidosis (DKA). Younger age, ethnic/race minority status, lower socioeconomic status, and lack of private health insurance are risk factors for presenting in DKA at diabetes onset (Dabelea, Rewers, et al., 2014).

Physical Examination. Although children typically have polyuria, polydipsia, and weight loss, the physical examination of children with new-onset type 1 diabetes may be remarkably benign. Findings can range from benign to severe and can include:
- Dehydration (child may not look clinically dehydrated unless actively vomiting)
- Weight loss or slow weight gain
- Muscle wasting
- Tachycardia
- Vaginal yeast, thrush, or other infection
  If ketosis develops:
- Slow, labored breathing (Kussmaul breathing)
- Flushed cheeks and face
- Fruity-smelling breath

Diagnostic Studies. Urine testing and blood glucose measurements are generally sufficient to make the diagnosis:
- Urine for glucose and ketones
- Metabolic screen for acid-base status to exclude DKA
- Hemoglobin A_{1c} (HbA_{1c})
- Blood glucose
- Screen for the presence of pancreatic autoantibodies: This should be considered to confirm the diagnosis of type 1 diabetes, particularly in those cases where there may be uncertainty regarding type (Chiang, Kirkman, Laffel, and Peters, 2014).

Capillary blood samples, reagent sticks, and glucose meters should be used only for monitoring diabetes control and not for diagnosing diabetes mellitus.

Diagnostic Criteria for Diabetes. The presence of one or more of the following criteria indicates a diagnosis of diabetes:
- $HbA_{1c} \geq 6.5\%$
- Fasting plasma glucose 126 mg/dL (7 mmol/L) or greater
- Random plasma glucose 200 mg/dL or greater plus presence of classic symptoms (polyuria, polydipsia, polyphagia)
- Postprandial (2 hours after eating) plasma glucose 200 mg/dL (11.1 mmol/L) or greater

Screening for Type 1 Diabetes in Family Members. When someone in the family develops type 1 diabetes, other family members may be at risk. Families concerned about risk to other family members should be directed to the Type 1 Diabetes TrialNet website (www.diabetestrialnet.org), where screening can be obtained from 18 clinical centers or more than 200 TrialNet network medical offices/physicians as part of an international clinical study. Children younger than 18 years old who test negative for the presence of antibodies associated with type 1 diabetes can be retested each year to determine if risk has changed. If antibodies are present, information will be provided regarding eligibility for participation in a diabetes prevention study.

Differential Diagnosis. Type 1 diabetes must be distinguished from stress-induced hyperglycemia, which in some studies occurs in up to 4% of normal children during a serious illness. Maturity-onset diabetes of the young (described later) may be misdiagnosed

as type 1 diabetes. Thyroiditis and/or celiac disease may be present at initial diagnosis of type 1 diabetes.

Management. The treatment goals for children with type 1 diabetes are to achieve normal growth and development, optimal glycemic control, and positive psychosocial adjustment to diabetes while minimizing acute or chronic complications. In 2014 the American Diabetes Association published a comprehensive position paper regarding the treatment goals of type 1 diabetes across the life span. Rather than base the glycemic goal on age, the new standard is to maintain a uniform glycemic level of HbA_{1c} less than 7.5% for all youth (American Diabetes Association, 2017). HbA_{1c} closely correlates with average blood glucose concentrations over the previous 3 months.

Diabetes treatment and education approaches for children and adolescents with type 1 diabetes are well defined and supported by strong evidence from the Diabetes Control and Complications Trial, a multicenter randomized controlled trial that demonstrated glycemic control through use of intensive insulin management prevents and/or delays development of microvascular complications of diabetes (The Diabetes Control Complications Trial Research Group, 1993, 1994). Each year, the American Diabetes Association publishes and makes available on their website standards of care for the management of diabetes in children (see Additional Resources).

Management of new-onset type 1 diabetes involves determining the insulin regimen and dose best suited to the individual child, target range for blood glucose levels, and best methods to manage the child's diet. Children and families must learn how to inject insulin, monitor blood glucose levels, quantify the amount of carbohydrates in food, prevent hypoglycemia, manage diabetes during illness, and adjust insulin dose or carbohydrate intake for strenuous activities. Diabetes education should be structured based on the child's age and developmental tasks, family management priorities, and family health literacy status. Beginning on or around 6 years old, the child should be incorporated into the educational experience (Chiang et al., 2014). These children and families need ongoing access to certified pediatric diabetes educators, pediatric registered dietician nutritionists, and psychologists or social workers when necessary. Each component of the treatment regimen is discussed in the following sections.

Initial Management. All children with type 1 diabetes should be started on insulin at diagnosis. Children with ketoacidosis should be admitted to the hospital for IV insulin treatment, fluid replacement, and careful monitoring to prevent cerebral edema that, although rare, can cause significant morbidity or mortality.

Whenever possible, children should be referred for ongoing care provided at a children's diabetes center for initiation of insulin therapy and diabetes education. Traditionally, most children with new-onset type 1 diabetes were hospitalized to initiate insulin therapy. Current practice in many diabetes centers is to routinely manage children with new-onset diabetes as an outpatient unless DKA is present. Outpatient management at initial diagnosis of type 1 diabetes has no disadvantages regarding glycemic control, complications, psychosocial factors, or total costs.

Initial management of new-onset diabetes also includes screening for concomitant associated autoimmune conditions:
- Screening for hypothyroidism by thyroid peroxidase and thyroglobulin antibody testing with annual screening thereafter. Approximately 25% of children with type 1 diabetes have thyroid autoantibodies present at the time of diagnosis, which is predictive of thyroid dysfunction, typically hypothyroidism. Screening for celiac disease by measuring tissue transglutaminase

TABLE 45.4	Insulin Dosages (units/kg/day)
Age	Total Daily Insulin (units/kg/day)
Partial Remission (Honeymoon) any age	<0.5
Prepubertal	0.7-1.0
Pubertal	1.0-2.0

Data from ISPAD Clinical Practice Consensus Guidelines 2018: Insulin treatment in children and adolescents with diabetes. Thomas Danne, Moshe Phillip, Bruce A. Buckingham, Przemyslawa Jarosz-Chobot, Banshi Saboo, Tatsuhiko Urakami, Tadej Battelino, Ragnar Hanas, Ethel Codner. Insulin treatment in children and adolescents with diabetes. *Pediatr Diabetes*. 2014;15(suppl 20):115–134. doi:10.1111/pedi.12184.

• BOX 45.8 Types of Insulin Analogues

Rapid acting
Duration: 3-5 h
- Aspart (NovoLog)
- Lispro (Humalog)
- Glulisine (Apidra)

Short acting
Duration: 5-8 h
- Regular insulin

Intermediate acting
Duration: 12-24 h
- NPH

Long acting
Duration: Up to 24 h
- Detemir (Levemir)
- Glargine (Lantus)
- Degludec (Tresiba) (duration up to 42 h per manufacturer)

Data from ISPAD 2018 Insulin guidelines
NPH, Neutral protamine hagedorn insulin.

or antiendomysial antibodies; screening thereafter if growth failure, abdominal symptoms, or failure to gain weight/weight loss are present. Celiac disease occurs more frequently in children with diabetes (1% to 16%) compared with children without diabetes (0.3% to 1%) (American Diabetes Association, 2017).

Insulin. In general, the goal of insulin therapy is to achieve optimal glycemic control typically defined as HbA_{1c} less than 7.5% and/or a fasting blood glucose level between 90 and 130mg/dL. For guidelines regarding insulin dosing by age and weight, see Table 45.4. There are several insulins available to treat diabetes, as well as several regimens. The most frequently used insulin preparations are listed in Box 45.8. The selection of an insulin regimen depends on the age of the child, family preferences and lifestyle, the family's social and educational resources, and the clinician's comfort level. All children require medical nutrition therapy (MNT) that must match the insulin schedule.

To achieve glycemic targets, exogenous insulin replacement that mimics physiologic insulin behavior is preferred for most children. In children without diabetes, the pancreas secretes a small amount of background or basal insulin throughout the day and a larger amount or bolus insulin when a meal is consumed. Intensive basal bolus insulin therapy attempts to match this. In general, basal insulin doses should be less than bolus insulin doses (Schulten, Piet, Bruijning, and de Waal, 2017; Strich, Balagour, Shenker, and Gillis, 2017).

Intensive basal bolus insulin therapy can be delivered using either multiple daily injections (MDIs), or continuous subcutaneous insulin infusion (CSII) using an insulin pump based on patient and family preferences. MDI regimens can be implemented using a long-acting insulin analogue administered typically once a day to provide a steady basal insulin replacement with boluses of rapid-acting insulin at meal and snack times. This regimen requires a minimum of four injections per day.

In CSII therapy, the pump infuses rapid-acting insulin into the subcutaneous tissue through a small, flexible, soft cannula. The cannula is replaced in a new site by the wearer or the family every 2 or 3 days. Basal insulin replacement is achieved by the delivery of small doses of rapid-acting insulin continuously throughout the day. These doses can be tailored to the child's physiologic requirements over the 24-hour period. Bolus insulin is delivered at meals and snacks. Bolus doses can be calculated by the pump if the user enters the amount of carbohydrate to be eaten and/or his/her blood glucose.

CSII via an insulin pump is particularly useful for delivering small bolus doses of insulin and varying the dose of basal insulin delivered over the 24-hour period. Insulin pumps are not "automatic," require

more work and deeper understanding of diabetes than subcutaneous injections, and put the child at risk for ketosis if the infusion catheter kinks or becomes obstructed or if the pump malfunctions. Use of insulin pumps is considered safe and efficacious even when used with young children and has become a popular way to deliver insulin in children with type 1 diabetes; approximately 60% of children in the national type 1 diabetes (T1D) Exchange registry report using an insulin pump (Miller et al., 2015).

Both MDI and CSII allow unreliable eaters to match their carbohydrate intake with insulin; children may be flexible with the timing of meals and snacks. Families learn to use a carbohydrate-to-insulin ratio (to cover the carbohydrate content of the meal/snack) and a blood sugar correction formula (if the blood glucose is above the target range) to determine each quick-acting insulin dose. If families either find MDI and/or CSII too demanding or needed support to maintain the regimen during the school day is inadequate, other insulin regimens may be considered including sliding scales although their use is waning.

The usual sites for insulin injection or infusion are the legs, arms, abdomen, hips, and buttocks. Young children with minimal subcutaneous abdominal fat may have difficulty with the abdominal site. Rotation of injection and infusion sites is necessary to prevent lipohypertrophy and poor absorption of insulin. Many of the insulin analogues are available in pen delivery systems.

After insulin treatment has been started, children may enter a "honeymoon period" during which insulin doses decrease. Close follow-up—often daily phone calls—after beginning insulin therapy is necessary to prevent hypoglycemic episodes. In general, insulin dose adjustments are based on the blood glucose patterns over several days. In general, the insulin dose would be decreased if any unexplained severe hypoglycemic events occur.

Monitoring Blood Glucose Levels. Frequent monitoring of blood glucose levels is required to dose insulin and prevent hypoglycemia/hyperglycemia. Children and families are taught to self-monitor blood glucose (SMBG) before meals, at bedtime, and sometimes in the middle of the night and during symptoms of hypoglycemia/hyperglycemia. Blood glucose meters have benefited from continued advances in technology; many blood glucose meters provide results within 5 seconds and automatically store and categorize blood glucose values by time of day or relation to meals.

The continuous glucose monitor (CGM) is different from a traditional glucose meter in that it measures interstitial glucose rather than blood glucose. Typically, there is a 5-minute lag between interstitial glucose reading and blood glucose readings. CGMs have three components: a sensor (small wire) that is placed in subcutaneous tissue, a transmitter that rests on the skin, and a receiver that displays the data. More recent systems have replaced the need for standalone receivers and instead display real-time interstitial glucose levels and trend graphs on mobile phones. Glucose data can be shared through the cloud in real time so that family members can be aware of their child's glucose level. Alarms warn of low and high blood glucose levels, using individually determined preset blood glucose ranges.

Due to recent advances in the accuracy of CGMs, the FDA has approved the use of the Dexcom G5 CGM for insulin dose calculations instead of the need for a fingerstick blood glucose measurement (FDA, March 29, 2017). However, currently CGMs in the United States still require at least two blood glucose calibrations a day.

Recent research indicates that use of CGMs can be effective in lowering HbA$_{1c}$ (Giani, Snelgrove, Volkening, and Laffel, 2017) but that children and adolescents are less likely than adults to continue its use (Wong et al., 2014). Data on CGM use and the reduction of hypoglycemia are unclear (Benkhadra et al., 2017). Although those who use CGMs report satisfaction, many barriers exist including fatigue from frequent alarms, cost, and variability of accuracy (Pickup, Ford Holloway, and Samsi, 2015; Rodbard, 2016).

Some CGMs are also integrated into insulin pumps. Known as "sensor-augmented pump therapy," these systems can adjust insulin doses based on CGM readings. Systems have features to pause basal insulin when the child's blood glucose is low. In 2017 the first hybrid–closed loop system became available on the U.S. market. This system can lower or increase basal rates to reduce hyperglycemia or hypoglycemia (Garg et al., 2017). However, it is important to note that these systems still require an attentive user to frequently monitor blood glucoses, count carbohydrates, bolus for meals, and/or elevated blood glucoses, and troubleshoot system errors.

Adjusting Insulin Dosages. Parents and teens can be educated to make insulin adjustments based on blood glucose patterns. They analyze what time of day the blood glucose is consistently outside of the target range (either too low or too high) and adjust the insulin dose that most directly is related to the problematic blood glucose pattern. Usually, parents can safely make up to a 10% adjustment to the basal or bolus insulin dose. With practice and guidance, many families eventually feel comfortable adjusting the insulin dose independently; others may feel more comfortable conferring with their diabetes care provider.

Medical Nutrition Therapy. Nutrition is an essential component of diabetes management. Diets should be healthy and daily calories spread over three meals and snacks. Caloric requirements are based on the child's age, body weight, and activity level. Calories are distributed between protein (15%), carbohydrates (55%), and fat (less than 30% of caloric intake with less than 7% in the form of saturated fats) and account for food preferences, including those pertinent to culture. The meal plan for a child with diabetes should include the same healthy foods recommended for all pediatric patients. The goal is to balance food intake with insulin dose and activity to maintain blood glucose levels within the target range and to prevent both hyperglycemic and hypoglycemic episodes.

A pediatric dietician nutritionist is essential to provide ongoing guidance to the child and family. Carbohydrate counting is an approach that allows greater flexibility for children using basal bolus insulin regimens. Children with diabetes can safely eat sugary treats on occasion by including those treats within their prescribed carbohydrate allotment. Low-calorie (e.g., saccharin, aspartame, sucralose, and acesulfame potassium) sweeteners are safe in moderation. Monitoring intake when eating out can be a challenge. Dieticians may help families to identify effective mobile phone applications that can be used to determine appropriate intake.

Exercise. Exercise is encouraged in all children, including those with diabetes, to promote cardiovascular fitness, control weight, and enhance social interaction and self-esteem. Children and adolescents with type 1 diabetes should not be excluded from participation in sports activities, including competitive sports. Any restrictions placed on an individual would be necessary only when optimal glycemic control cannot be maintained or if complications or comorbidities are not compatible with the activity. Youth with diabetes should follow the same physical activity guidelines as all children—striving for 60 minutes of physical activity daily (American Diabetes Association, 2017).

Control of the child's blood glucose level during exercise, especially rigorous exercise such as athletic competition, is a challenge. It requires ongoing blood glucose monitoring (before, during, and after exercise), careful planning of meals and carbohydrates, snacks around the time of exercise, and adjustment of insulin dosing to counterbalance the effect of exercise on blood glucose levels.

During physical exercise, the body's oxygen and energy demands increase greatly. To meet these energy needs, there is increased uptake of glucose into the tissues, and blood glucose levels fall. Skeletal muscle also relies on stores of glycogen, triglycerides, free fatty acids, and glucose production, largely from the liver. For athletes without diabetes, hormonal mediators maintain normal blood glucose levels even under high athletic conditions. In these individuals, exercise leads to decreased plasma insulin levels and increased glucagon that trigger hepatic glucose production. However, in youth with type 1 diabetes, this hormonal pathway is interrupted. Thus, if the level of insulin is too low, exercise can trigger release of high levels of glucose and ketone bodies, leading to hyperglycemia and eventually, if unchecked, to DKA. Conversely, if too much exogenous insulin is administered, the feedback loop for increased glucose mobilization is interrupted and hypoglycemia results.

Glucose levels can vary by the type, duration, and intensity of exercise performed. Typically, aerobic exercise, such as long distance running or cycling, results in a decrease in blood glucose levels, whereas anaerobic exercise, such as weight training, sprinting (running or cycling), or jumping, may temporarily increase glucose (Riddell et al., 2017). Therefore, to compensate for the effect of exercise on blood glucose levels, children and families are taught to either decrease the insulin dose or take extra carbohydrates prior to exercise. Anaerobic exercise requires conservative blood glucose correction for higher glucose post exercise as hypoglycemia can still occur later on in the day (Riddell et al., 2017). Because exercise may affect blood glucose levels for as long as 24 hours after exercise has occurred, parents need to be aware of the risk of nocturnal hypoglycemia on active days and monitor blood glucose levels more frequently including overnight.

It is generally recommended that athletes with type 1 diabetes have a medical team participating in their health care. This team ideally includes an endocrinologist and nutritionist who specialize in diabetes and are familiar with the energy requirements of the individual's sport. Depending on the level of athletic endeavor, an exercise physiologist may also be part of the team. It is essential that coaches, trainers, or other athletic staff be aware of the young athlete's diabetes care plan and be trained in aspects of care.

Ongoing Management. Children with type 1 diabetes should be seen every 3 to 4 months, with the visit tailored by age and developmental stage and careful attention paid to diabetes management including:

- Self-monitoring blood glucose results
- Frequency of hypoglycemia
- HbA_{1c}
- Physical activities
- Emotional adjustment to the disease
- Social issues, such as peer pressure
- Eating issues: Young women and men with diabetes have an increased incidence of eating disorders, such as "diabulemia" in which insulin dosage is decreased to lose weight (Doyle et al., 2017). Providers should have a high index of suspicion for disordered eating in youth with elevated BMIs and HbA_{1c} level
- A physical examination that focuses on:
  - Growth and weight gain
  - Blood pressure
  - Stage of puberty
  - Injection site assessment for lipodystrophy
  - Clues for other autoimmune disease (thyroiditis and celiac disease)

Ongoing management of type 1 diabetes also includes the following referrals:

- Referrals for nutritional review
- Collaboration with school nurses, teachers, and administrators to ensure treatment regimens are followed in the school or day care setting
- Continued well-child health supervision and appropriate immunizations (e.g., annual influenza vaccination)
- When the individual is ready, providers should discuss the process of transitioning to adult care. Many diabetes centers have structured programs in place to ameliorate the process (Schultz and Smaldone, 2017).

Complications. Morbidity and mortality in type 1 diabetes come from metabolic derangements and from long-term complications that affect the small and large blood vessels. Chronic high blood glucose levels have been shown to cause the long-term complications of microvascular disease (retinopathy, nephropathy, neuropathy, depression, and cognitive defects) and macrovascular disease (arterial obstruction with gangrene of extremities and ischemic heart disease). These complications can be prevented or their rate of progression slowed by improving glycemic control through use of intensive insulin regimens consisting of MDI or CSII.

Diabetes, types 1 or 2, is a known risk factor for atherosclerosis and early cardiovascular disease. Guidelines for lipid screening and treatment of dyslipidemia are consistent with those of the Expert Panel on Integrated Guidelines for Cardiovascular Health and Risk Reduction in Children, and Adolescents (2011) and the American Diabetes Association (2017) and apply to youth with diabetes regardless of type. For children 2 years and older with a family history of hypercholesterolemia or early cardiovascular event, a fasting lipid profile should be obtained shortly after diabetes diagnosis when glycemic control has been established. For those children with negative family history, the first lipid screening should begin at 10 years old. If lipid levels are abnormal, Expert Panel guidelines (2011) should be implemented with annual or more frequent monitoring as indicated. If low-density lipoprotein (LDL) cholesterol values are less than 100 mg/dL, lipid profiles may be repeated every 3 to 5 years (American Diabetes Association, 2017). If therapy is indicated, the treatment goal is an LDL cholesterol value less than 100 mg/dL.

Depression and anxiety rates are high in youth with type 1 diabetes (Buchberger et al., 2016). Appropriate screenings and referrals for psychological counseling, ideally by providers knowledgeable of the tasks required for diabetes management, are recommended.

Screening guidelines for complications and comorbidities are listed in Table 45.5.

Patient and Family Education. Providing families and children with information that helps them to gain control of a very difficult disease is crucial. The National Diabetes Education Program offers education materials specifically targeted to both type 1 and type 2 diabetes (see Additional Resources). Education of the child, family, and caregivers should include insulin therapy, self-monitoring of glucose, nutrition and meal planning (including carbohydrate counting), exercise, managing sick days, school issues, coping skills, and prevention of complications. Those with diabetes should always wear a form of medical identification. School personnel must be informed of the plan of care and must implement an individualized care plan for the child.

Type 2 Diabetes

The prevalence of type 2 diabetes in youth 10 to 19 years old is 0.46/1000 youth. Notably, the prevalence of type 2 diabetes has increased by approximately 30% over the period from 2001 to 2009. These estimates suggest that the number of youth diagnosed with type 2 diabetes will nearly quadruple by 2050. Type 2 diabetes in youth accounts for up to 11% of all new total diabetes cases among children in the United States (Dabelea, Mayer-Davis, et al., 2014). The incidence of type 2 diabetes is also on the rise with an increase of 4.8% from 2002 to 2012 after adjusting for age, sex, race, and ethnicity. It is highest among Native American youth, an average of 46.5 cases per 100,000 youths a year compared with 3.9 cases per year among non-Hispanic whites (Mayer-Davis et al., 2017). The overall prevalence rates may be underreported, especially because children may have no symptoms or mild symptoms for a long period of time. Children usually are diagnosed during the teenage years, between 10 and 19 years old.

Clearly, type 2 diabetes in youth is a serious and growing public health problem. Type 2 diabetes begins with increased tissue resistance to insulin, resulting in hyperinsulinemia and hyperglycemia. Although pancreatic beta cells initially produce insulin, hyperglycemia creates an increased insulin demand; with increasing demand for insulin over time, the pancreas loses its ability to effectively secrete insulin. Autoimmune destruction of pancreatic beta cells does not typically occur. During puberty, GH secretion as part of the pubertal growth spurt further increases resistance to insulin action for those predisposed to type 2 diabetes. Adolescents with normally functioning pancreatic beta cells secrete additional insulin to compensate for this puberty-related effect. However, when beta cells do not function properly, metabolic decompensation begins and leads to a state of prediabetes (impaired fasting

TABLE 45.5	Recommended Screening Parameters for Youth With Diabetes		
		FREQUENCY	
	Measure	**Type 1**	**Type 2**
Glycemic control	HbA$_{1c}$	• Every 3 months	• Every 3 months (every 6 months if stable)
Thyroid disease	Antithyroid peroxidase and antithyroglobulin antibodies	At diagnosis	• Not required
	TSH	• Every 1-2 years	• Not required
Celiac disease	tTG-IgA, IgA	• At diagnosis • 2 and 5 years later, and as clinically indicated	• Not required
Dyslipidemia	Fasting lipids	• If positive family history, shortly after diagnosis. • Otherwise start screening if ≥10 years of age. • If lipids are normal, repeat every 3-5 years. • If lipids are elevated, screen yearly	• At diagnosis, if ≥10 years of age, repeat every 3-5 years
Nephropathy	Random spot urine albumin to creatinine ratio	• 5 years after diagnosis • Repeat yearly	• At diagnosis, repeat yearly
Hypertension	Blood pressure	• At each visit	
Retinopathy	Dilated eye exam	• Yearly once ≥10 years old OR reached puberty AND diabetes duration of 3-5 years	• At diagnosis, repeat yearly
Neuropathy	Foot exam	• Yearly once ≥10 years old OR reached puberty AND diabetes duration of 5 years	• Yearly
Psychosocial		Screen for emotional well-being at each visit	

HbA$_{1c}$, Hemoglobin A$_{1c}$; *IgA*, immunoglobulin A; *TSH*, thyroid-stimulating hormone, *tTG-IgA*, tissue transglutaminase antibody-IgA.

glucose and/or impaired glucose tolerance) with eventual progression to type 2 diabetes (Halban et al., 2014).

Type 2 diabetes is strongly associated with environmental factors such as obesity, sedentary lifestyles, and high-caloric lipid-rich foods. Children born to a mother with gestational diabetes, who are small for gestational age at birth (sign of intrauterine undernutrition) (Zhang, Kris-Etherton, and Hartman, 2014), and those who are overweight and/or obese or have a family history of type 2 diabetes are at increased risk for type 2 diabetes (Pippitt, Li and Gurgle, 2016). Children who are breastfed are at lower risk of developing type 2 diabetes (Horta, Loret de Mola, and Victora, 2015).

Clinical Findings

Screening Guidelines. The symptoms of type 2 diabetes may be absent or subtle, so children at risk should be screened. The American Diabetes Association (2017) provides guidelines for screening children at risk:

- Screen if overweight (BMI is greater than 85th percentile for age and gender, or weight is greater than 120% of ideal weight), plus any two of following risk factors:
  - Family history of type 2 diabetes in first- or second-degree relative
  - Race/ethnicity (Native American, African American, Latino, Asian American, Pacific Islander)
  - Signs of insulin resistance or conditions associated with insulin resistance (e.g., acanthosis nigricans, polycystic ovary syndrome, hypertension, dyslipidemia)
  - Maternal history of diabetes or gestational diabetes during pregnancy with this child
- Screen every 3 years.

- Use fasting plasma glucose test following diagnostic criteria for diabetes discussed earlier.
- Use clinical judgment to screen for type 2 diabetes in high-risk patients who do not meet these guidelines.

History. The history of patients with type 2 diabetes may include:

- Polydipsia, polyphagia, polyuria
- Nocturia or bedwetting
- Blurred vision
- Obesity, especially central
- Report of a hyperpigmented, velvetlike rash in skin folds
- Frequent or slow-healing infections
- Fatigue, symptoms of sleep apnea
- History of premature adrenarche
- Family history of type 2 diabetes

Physical Examination. The physical examination should include assessment of height, weight, stage of pubertal development, and blood pressure. The following findings may be present:

- Dehydration
- Overweight (BMI greater than 85th percentile for age and gender) or obesity
- Weight loss (less common)
- Acanthosis nigricans noted in the axilla, base of the neck, groin, knuckles, and other skin folds
- Vaginal yeast, thrush, other infection
- Polycystic ovary syndrome symptoms (e.g., acne, hirsutism)
- Hypertension

Diagnostic Studies. Screening should be conducted in high-risk children without symptoms (see earlier "Screening Guidelines") and should include (American Diabetes Association, 2017):

- Urine for glucose and albumin (can be performed in the office)
- Children can have ketoacidosis if they have gone undiagnosed for a long time
- Fasting blood sample for blood glucose, HbA_{1c}, lipid panel, TSH and free T_4, and insulin level

Diagnostic Criteria for Diabetes. Diagnostic criteria are the same as type 1 diabetes.

Differential Diagnosis. Some obese children have type 1 diabetes and may be misdiagnosed as type 2. The presentation of type 1 diabetes can be of slower onset in older children and adults. A diagnosis of maturity-onset diabetes of the young (described later) should also be considered.

Management. Treatment of type 2 diabetes in youth remains in its infancy and currently lacks the strong evidence base of type 1 diabetes. The primary treatment for children and adolescents with type 2 diabetes is education and lifestyle modification, particularly improvement of nutritional practices and physical activity behaviors leading to weight loss. However, in the United States, fewer than 10% of children with type 2 diabetes are successful in achieving glycemic control with diet and exercise alone. If lifestyle changes are not successful in normalizing blood glucose levels, pharmacologic agents should be added to the treatment regimen. Two pharmacologic agents are approved for the use of type 2 diabetes in the pediatric population: metformin and insulin.

As with type 1 diabetes, the treatment plan for children with type 2 diabetes must be individualized. The treatment goal of both type 1 and type 2 diabetes is the same—the normalization of blood glucose values through the achievement of optimal glycemic control ($HbA_{1c} \leq 7.5\%$). This typically requires:

- Daily self-monitoring by the child: If the child is treated with multiple insulin injections or continuous pump therapy, check blood glucose levels three or more times each day; for those on less-frequent insulin injections, oral medication, or MNT alone, a daily check may be adequate.
- HbA_{1c} and plasma glucose levels monitored every 3 to 4 months for those whose therapy has changed or who are not meeting glycemic goals. Children who are meeting goals and have stable glycemic control can be monitored every 6 months.
- Follow-up every 3 to 4 months on lifestyle, nutrition, and other complications of obesity, discussed in more detail later.
- Screening and successful control of the associated complications, such as hypertension and hyperlipidemia, are important. See Table 45.5 for screening recommendations.

Lifestyle Changes: Nutrition and Exercise. When discovered early, type 2 diabetes may respond to lifestyle changes, such as alterations in diet and exercise. These changes must be comprehensive and family based. MNT is an important part of the treatment plan. Referral to a registered pediatric dietician nutritionist is essential, with the goals of weight loss and regulating nutritional intake. A low-fat diet, self-monitoring of weight, and being physically active are important components of MNT. Successful weight management may consist of weight maintenance rather than weight loss depending on the child's age and BMI. Changes in family eating patterns can contribute to weight maintenance or loss that may normalize insulin levels. Nutrition counseling should be provided both at the time of diagnosis of type 2 diabetes and as part of ongoing clinical management and should be consistent with guidelines of the Academy of Nutrition and Dietetics.

Inactivity and the increasing obesity epidemic are directly related to the escalating incidence of type 2 diabetes in young people. Physical activity is not only one of the major type 2 diabetes prevention messages, but it is also a critical component in treatment. Youth with type 2 diabetes should be strongly encouraged to be physically active by participating in sports and regular exercise. Daily vigorous exercise (30 to 60 minutes a day) helps to control weight, and even modest weight loss has been shown to reduce insulin resistance (American Diabetes Association, 2017).

Overweight or obese youth may initially be in poor physical condition with regard to sports endurance. Therefore activity and exercise plans should allow for a gradual and safe buildup in intensity and length. A nutritionist can be helpful in ensuring adequate calories for performance needs, as well as for safe weight loss. Overweight or obese adolescents may lack self-esteem or motivation to participate in school sports activities but may be willing to walk as a form of exercise. Use of mobile applications are feasible for youth; however, their effectiveness remains unclear (Chaplais, Naughton, Thivel, Courteix, and Greene, 2015). Wireless applications to monitor activity, caloric expenditure, heart rate, and fitness are gaining popularity.

The benefits of regular physical exercise for youth with type 2 diabetes include increased insulin effectiveness due to improving insulin-receptor sensitivity, weight control, reduced risk of cardiovascular disease, reduced dyslipidemia risk, and improved self-confidence and self-esteem. Glycemic control during exercise is generally not difficult to maintain. In addition to weight loss, regular physical activity of moderate to strenuous level improves body composition; furthermore, regular physical activity has been shown to improve HbA_{1c} levels, BMI, and high-density lipoprotein (HDL) levels (Herbst et al., 2015). For adolescents who are taking oral hypoglycemic medication or insulin for type 2 diabetes, the benefits of improved insulin sensitivity through regular exercise participation may enable them to reduce medication.

Pharmacotherapy. Little research has been done on the use of hypoglycemic agents in children. The Treatment Options for Type 2 Diabetes in Adolescents and Youth (TODAY) study compared the effectiveness of three treatment options for type 2 diabetes in youth 10 to 17 years old: (1) metformin, (2) metformin plus rosiglitazone, and (3) metformin plus an intensive behavioral intervention. The study found that treatment failure (defined as HbA_{1c} greater than or equal to 8% for 6 months or persistent metabolic decompensation) occurred in almost half of the study's subjects with any of the three treatments. Of the three treatment arms, rosiglitazone plus metformin was the most successful, yet 39% of subjects assigned to that group had treatment failure (TODAY Study Group, 2012). The implications for long-term health complications related to type 2 diabetes in youth are significant (Narasimhan and Weinstock, 2014).

Metformin is the only oral agent approved by the FDA for use in children with type 2 diabetes, and, although rosiglitazone is used in combination with metformin in adults, the FDA has found insufficient evidence to approve it for pediatric use. Many other medications prescribed for adults with type 2 diabetes are used off label in pediatrics. Metformin decreases the amount of glucose produced by the liver and increases insulin sensitivity of the liver and muscles.

Most children are started on metformin in doses up to 1000 mg twice a day. Metformin rarely causes hypoglycemia, so blood glucose needs to be checked only before breakfast and 2 hours after dinner. Mild gastrointestinal side effects may occur with metformin use but are usually self-limiting. Metformin users can experience vitamin B_{12} deficiency probably secondary to malabsorption, especially with higher doses and longer use. Providers should counsel youth taking metformin to increase foods high in vitamin B_{12}; they should also have a high suspicion of vitamin

B$_{12}$ deficiency if clinical signs appear (see Chapter 39). Although there is no consensus on requiring laboratory testing, youth taking metformin, especially long-term users, should probably be assessed regularly for vitamin B$_{12}$ deficits and high homocysteine levels (Thomas and Gregg, 2017). Liver function tests should also be monitored. Should the youth fail to respond to metformin, a combination of two oral agents may be used.

When a child or adolescent with type 2 diabetes has ketonuria or is in DKA, insulin therapy is needed initially. In addition, if the diagnosis is unclear regarding type 1 verses type 2 diabetes or if the patient's blood glucose is 250 mg/dL or greater or HbA$_{1c}$ is greater than 9%, insulin therapy should be initiated (American Diabetes Association, 2017). These children need to be started on the same insulin regimen with home glucose monitoring and a precise food plan as those with type 1 diabetes. Typically, the insulin needs are higher than in children with type 1 diabetes because of insulin resistance. Following stabilization of blood glucose levels, it may be possible to gradually wean the insulin and begin metformin. Over time, the natural course of type 2 diabetes can result in the body's inability to produce sufficient endogenous insulin, making treatment with oral agents ineffective. If this occurs, insulin replacement using long- and/or rapid-acting insulin will be necessary.

Medication may also be needed to control hypertension (see Chapter 38) and dyslipidemia (discussed later in this chapter), which are two frequent comorbidities of type 2 diabetes in youth.

Complications. Complications of type 2 diabetes are similar to those of type 1 diabetes (microvascular and macrovascular diseases). Nephropathy is a more common complication in those with type 2 than type 1 diabetes. Nonalcoholic fatty liver disease and eventual dependence upon insulin for control can occur.

Patient and Family Education. The same education needs apply to children with type 1 and type 2 diabetes: information about the nature of the disease; strategies and techniques to manage the physical disease (e.g., medication, insulin, nutrition, exercise); networks, support, and skills to cope with emotional and psychological issues; collaboration with school personnel; and wearing a form of medical identification. The National Diabetes Education Program is an invaluable resource for both providers and children and their families (see Additional Resources).

Maturity-Onset Diabetes of the Young. MODY is a group of autosomal dominant, single gene disorders that may clinically resemble type 1 or type 2 diabetes. MODY is characterized by impaired insulin secretion without significant defects in the action of insulin. To date, at least 13 genetic loci on different chromosomes have been identified as being related with MODY (American Diabetes Association, 2017). In comparison with type 1 diabetes, patients with MODY typically do not have pancreatic autoimmunity and have less insulin requirements. They have a positive family history of diabetes (Amed and Oram, 2016). On average, children with MODY are younger, less likely to be overweight or obese, and less likely to be from an ethnic minority group compared with children presenting with new-onset type 2 diabetes (Amed and Oram, 2016). Treatment for patients with MODY varies by type and includes insulin, sulfonylureas, or no treatment at all.

Obesity

The prevalence of obesity has dramatically increased in children and adults worldwide. Obesity in childhood is defined as a BMI greater than or equal to the 95th percentile for age and gender.

Approximately 17% of American youth meet this definition. Extreme obesity in childhood is defined as a BMI at or greater than 120% of the 95th percentile for age and gender. Approximately 5.8% of American youth meet this definition. For both obesity and extreme obesity, prevalence is highest among youth 12 to 19 years of age compared with younger children (Ogden et al., 2016). A more detailed discussion of obesity is found in Chapter 17.

In most children, overweight and obesity are thought to be due to an imbalance between calories consumed and calories burned. From an endocrine perspective, the mechanisms of weight homeostasis are complex and involve hypothalamic hormones, hormones produced by adipocytes (e.g., leptin), and the gut (e.g., ghrelin). In most children, hormone deficiency or excess does not explain obesity. Although several "classic" hormonal imbalances (such as, hypothyroidism, cortisol excess, and GHD) may be associated with overweight or obesity, the child with these endocrine conditions is likely to be either of short stature or growing at a subnormal growth velocity. Several rare genetic conditions predispose children to being overweight (e.g., Prader-Willi syndrome). Developmental delay and associated dysmorphic features are key to identifying these conditions.

Diagnostic Studies

Consistent with clinical practice guidelines developed jointly by the European Society of Endocrinology and the Pediatric Endocrine Society, children and adolescents with a BMI greater than 85th percentile for age and gender should be screened for a number of comorbidities (Styne et al., 2017):

- Prediabetes and type 2 diabetes (see diagnostic criteria for diabetes)
- Dyslipidemia with fasting lipid panel
- Nonalcoholic steatohepatitis with liver enzyme alanine aminotransferase (ALT)
- Obstructive sleep apnea by history of snoring, daytime somnolence. If history positive, refer to a pediatric pulmonologist for nocturnal polysomnography
- PCOS with a free and total testosterone level (if symptomatic with irregular menses, acne, or hirsutism)
- Prehypertension and hypertension with a blood pressure measurement
- Psychological issues by history of low self-esteem, behavior problems, or depression. If history positive, refer to mental health specialist

Management

Children with type 2 diabetes, PCOS, or other metabolic or endocrine disorders associated with obesity should be followed in concert with a pediatric endocrinologist. Recently published Endocrine Society guidelines recommend against routine evaluation for endocrine conditions in children with obesity unless the child's stature is inconsistent with his/her genetic potential or growth velocity is inconsistent with what is expected at the child's pubertal stage (Styne et al., 2017). All overweight and/or obese youth should be evaluated for potential comorbidities. Screening should be offered in the primary care setting and a treatment plan established with the family for nutritional counseling and ongoing support to achieve a more active lifestyle. In general, the goal is weight maintenance, not loss, in the overweight child without any of the aforementioned complications; it is expected that these children will eventually grow into their weight and achieve a BMI less than the 85th percentile. For children with an overweight-related complication, weight loss of 1 pound per month would be an appropriate goal; more rapid weight loss in children who have not yet reached their growth potential may be associated with slowing in linear growth.

Consensus is lacking as to the most effective way to manage childhood obesity. A recent systematic review and meta-analysis (O'Connor et al., 2017; Peirson et al., 2015) synthesized data from 42 lifestyle interventions to reduce BMI and/or BMI *z* score in overweight and obese youth age 2 to 18 years. Interventions with 26 or more hours of contact were successful in modest weight reduction and blood pressure reduction. Findings were mixed regarding the effect of these interventions on blood glucose and insulin measures, and there were no effects on serum lipid levels. Goals for reducing calories consumed and increasing daily exercise must be made within the context of each family; success is more likely to be achieved if the entire family participates in lifestyle changes. Providers must work closely with families to ensure consistent follow-up, to assess the effectiveness of interventions, and to modify the treatment strategy if necessary.

Posterior Pituitary Gland Disorders

Abnormal posterior pituitary function is uncommon in pediatrics. Children with inappropriately dilute urine for the clinical situation may be identified only when they develop hypernatremic dehydration, secondary enuresis, or polyuria. They may also be discovered in an evaluation of a child at risk for hypopituitarism. If a screening of first morning urine shows low specific gravity in the absence of urinary glucose, a pediatric endocrinologist should be consulted.

Introduction to Inborn Errors of Metabolism

IEMs encompass a wide range of inherited disorders with alterations of specific biochemical reactions. The term "inborn error of metabolism" was coined by Garrod in 1908 to describe the hereditary alteration in enzyme reactions that he observed in the first identified "inborn error," alkaptonuria, and use of the term has persisted (Garrod, 1908).

Although individually rare, IEMs have a collective incidence of approximately 1 in 800 live births and vary significantly by population and racial and ethnic groups (Mak, Lee, Chan, Lam, 2013; Weiner, 2017), and all healthcare providers will likely encounter a child with an IEM at some point in their career. Clinical consequences for the affected individual vary from mild to severe. Early detection, accurate diagnosis, rapid intervention, and patient/family education in managing the child's disorder are necessary to achieve favorable outcomes; prevent irreversible intellectual disability, physical disability, neurologic damage, or death; and reduce long-term financial burden and human suffering. This section discusses the classification and pathophysiology of IEMs; overviews newborn screening, including common clinical presentations and emergency management of conditions found in the newborn period; and presents a brief overview of the diagnosis and treatment of a few more common disorders.

Classification of Inborn Errors of Metabolism

Classification of IEMs presents a challenge because of the number and diversity of disorders. Proposed classification systems have suggested categorizing based on affected organ (e.g., neurologic or hepatic diseases), cellular organelle (e.g., mitochondrial or lysosomal disorders), age of presentation (e.g., neonatal or adult onset), large or small molecule diseases, or affected metabolic pathway (e.g., urea cycle defects [UCDs] or defects of amino acid metabolism) (see Box 45.9).

> ### • BOX 45.9 Classification of Inborn Errors of Metabolism With Partial List of Disorders
>
> **Amino Acid Disorders**
> MSUD
> PKU
> Tyrosinemia
> Homocystinuria
>
> **Organic Acidemias**
> Propionic acidemia
> Methylmalonic acidemia
>
> **Urea Cycle Disorders**
> Ornithine transcarbamylase deficiency
> Citrullinemia
>
> **Carbohydrate Disorders**
> Galactosemia
> Glycogen storage disease
> Hereditary fructose intolerance
>
> **Fatty Acid Oxidation Disorders**
> MCAD deficiency
> VLCAD deficiency
> LCHAD deficiency
>
> **Mitochondrial Disorders**
> Leigh disease
> MNGIE syndrome
> Pearson syndrome
>
> **Peroxisomal Disorders**
> Zellweger syndrome
> Adrenoleukodystrophy
> Infantile Refsum disease
>
> **Lysosomal Storage Disorders**
> Hurler syndrome
> Fabry disease
> Gaucher disease
> Niemann-Pick disease
>
> **Purine and Pyrimidine Disorders**
> Lesch-Nyhan disease
> Hereditary orotic aciduria
>
> **Metal Metabolism Disorder**
> Wilson disease
>
> *LCHAD, Long-chain 3-hydroxyacyl-coenzyme A dehydrogenase; MCAD, medium-chain acyl-coenzyme A dehydrogenase; MNGIE, mitochondrial neurogastrointestinal encephalopathy; MSUD, maple syrup urine disease; PKU, phenylketonuria; VLCAD, very-long-chain acyl-coenzyme A dehydrogenase.*

Pathophysiology

Most metabolic disorders are caused by an inherited defect, generally of a single enzyme or its cofactor, resulting in altered function of a metabolic pathway. Autosomal recessive inheritance patterns are most common. Fig 45.3 provides an overview of the major metabolic pathways. The majority of defects are caused by a single gene mutation encoding a specific enzyme whose function is to facilitate the conversion of various substances (substrates, [e.g., foodstuffs]) into others (metabolic products, [e.g., urea]). The block in the pathway variably leads to accumulation of substrate

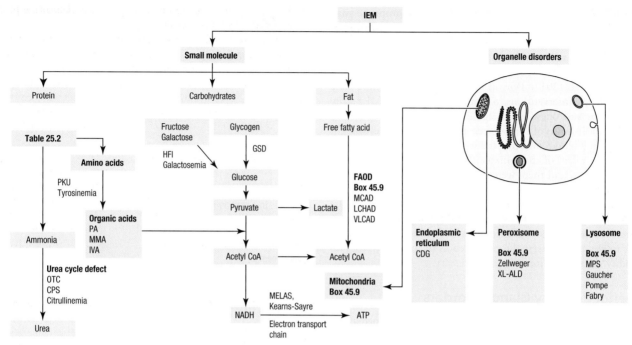

• **Fig 45.3** Overview of Major Metabolic Pathways. *Acetyl CoA*, Acetyl coenzyme A; *ATP*, adenosine triphosphate; *CDG*, congenital disorders of glycosylation; *CPS*, Carbamoyl Phosphate Synthetase I Deficiency; *FAOD*, Long-chain fatty acid oxidation disorders; *GSD*, glycogen storage disease; *HFI*, hereditary fructose intolerance; *IEM*, inborn errors of metabolism; *IVA*, Isovaleric Acidemia; *LCHAD*, long-chain 3-hydroxyacyl-coenzyme A dehydrogenase deficiency; *MCAD*, medium-chain acyl-coenzyme A dehydrogenase deficiency; *MMA*, Methylmalonic acidemia; *MPS*, Mucopolysaccharidosis; *NADH*, nicotinamide adenine dinucleotide; *OTC*, Ornithine transcarbamylase deficiency; *PA*, Phosphatidic acid; *PA*, Propionic Acidemia; *PKU*, phenylketonuria; *VLCAD*, very long-chain acyl-coenzyme A dehydrogenase deficiency; *XL-ALD*, X-linked adrenoleukodystrophy. (From Logan A. Metabolic disease. In: Cheng A, Williams BA, Sivarajan VB, eds. *The Hospital for Sick Children Handbook of Pediatrics*. 10th ed. Toronto: Saunders Canada; 2004:474.)

proximal to the block (e.g., lysosomal storage disorders); accumulation of toxic metabolites (e.g., galactose byproducts in galactosemia); deficiency of a product distal to the block (e.g., tyrosine in PKU); feedback inhibition or activation by the metabolite; or some combination thereof. Loss of enzyme function varies by degree, altering the clinical phenotype, the clinical course, and the response to treatment among individuals with the same diagnosis.

Assessment of Inborn Errors of Metabolism

IEMs are rare but should be included in the differential diagnosis of any critically ill neonate, as well as infants, children, adolescents, and adults, presenting with symptoms that are progressive or otherwise unexplained. The timing of symptom onset in relation to initiation of feedings can be an important clue. Infants with IEM commonly appear normal at birth with effects of the disease becoming apparent over the course of days to months. As substrates or toxic metabolites accumulate, such as in organic acidemias, nonspecific symptoms that may be indistinguishable from sepsis typically appear. However, finding a cause of symptoms does not necessarily rule out the possibility of an IEM (e.g., electrolyte abnormalities diagnosed as renal Fanconi syndrome may be caused by underlying cystinosis).

Clinical Findings

History. A thorough family and individual history is important to identify possibilities of IEMs. Details in a family and patient history that should raise suspicion include:

• Consanguinity, family history of IEM, siblings with unexplained infant or neonatal death

• Decompensation when ill greater than anticipated for the nature of the illness (commonly seen in acidosis)
• Developmental delay, psychomotor retardation, or loss of previously acquired milestones
• Failure to thrive
• Symptoms concurrent with a change in diet
• Unusual odor (sweat, urine, or cerumen)

Physical Examination. A complete examination is essential, with attention to dysmorphia, muscle tone, ocular symptoms, organomegaly, and respiratory function. Box 45.10 provides an overview of signs and symptoms suspicious for an inborn error at various ages.

Diagnostic Studies. Effective intervention for IEMs depends on the ability to identify the disorder before the onset of symptoms. Screening for the presence of IEMs allows the provider to identify the condition and, if possible, begin treatment before damage has occurred. However, not all IEMs are amenable to treatment, and in some cases supportive or palliative care may be the only option. The capability to screen for IEMs dates to the early 1960s, when an inexpensive test for PKU using a small blood sample collected on a filter paper was developed; 400,000 newborns in 29 states were part of a pilot study that confirmed the effectiveness of this test to detect PKU. As a result, states instituted screening programs for newborn infants, and currently, virtually all of the millions of infants born each year in the United States are screened.

Technologic advances have allowed for screening a wide array of disorders, and the newborn screening currently encompasses much more than screening for PKU. Further laboratory studies are generally necessary in the diagnosis of IEM; however, determining what studies to perform may not always be straightforward. Testing

Signs/Symptoms Suggesting an Inborn Error of Metabolism in Children by Age

Neonates and Infants
Abnormal neurologic examination
Acidosis
Cardiomyopathy
Coagulopathy
Coarse facial features
Dysmorphic features
Hyperammonemia
Hypotonia or hypertonia
Jaundice
Metabolic acidosis
Neutropenia and/or thrombocytopenia
Ocular findings (retinitis pigmentosa, cherry red spots, cataracts, or corneal clouding)
Organomegaly
Respiratory distress (apnea or tachypnea)
Seizures
Unexplained hypoglycemia
Vomiting
Xanthomas

Older Children and Adolescents (in Addition to Those of Neonates and Infants)
Ataxia
Dementia
Dystonia or chorea
Intellectual disability
Muscular weakness
Ophthalmoplegia
Progressive deterioration
Skeletal changes

for common (i.e., nonmetabolic) causes of presenting symptoms should not be sacrificed for metabolic testing, but it is not always prudent to wait for all routine tests to be performed and the results known before submitting samples for metabolic disease testing. This additional step facilitates work-up should the patient be referred to a metabolic specialist. When the ill child has signs and symptoms of what could be an IEM, the PCP should consult immediately with a metabolic specialist, rather than wait for results of tests. For chronic presentations, after common etiologies are ruled out, refer to a metabolic specialist for testing beyond routine analysis.

Initial laboratory studies for the neonate with a suspected IEM include:
- Newborn screening on any significantly ill neonate, unless proof of prior collection is obtained
- A second newborn screening at 10 to 14 days of age if the ill neonate was discharged early (before 24 hours of age)
- CBC with differential and urinalysis
- Blood glucose
- Blood urea nitrogen (BUN) and creatinine
- ALT, aspartate aminotransferase (AST), bilirubin
- Coagulation studies
- Blood gases
- Serum electrolytes with special attention to anion gap
- Plasma ammonia: Collected free flowing (no tourniquet, no heel stick) immediately placed on ice and analyzed within 45 to 60 minutes
- Plasma lactate: Collected free flowing
- Creatine kinase

- Plasma quantitative amino acids, plasma acylcarnitine profile, and plasma carnitine levels
- Ketones (if acidotic and hypoglycemic), organic acids, and mucopolysaccharides and oligosaccharides if storage disease is suspected

Some labs offer a metabolic screening panel, typically on urine; however, some labs prefer urine and blood. Metabolic panels vary between laboratories. Diagnostic testing may also consist of biochemical or molecular (DNA) analysis obtained from blood. Other more invasive tests may be needed, including cerebral spinal fluid (lactate, amino acids, glucose) or biopsy from skin, liver, or muscle (enzyme assays). In addition, for the child with chronic encephalopathy, consider an MRI and magnetic resonance spectroscopy (MRS) for brain imaging. Familiarity with the appropriate methods of specimen collection and handling (before and during shipment of the samples to the laboratory) is important because inappropriate practices alter the quality of the sample, potentially leading to unreliable results and thus either missed or erroneous cases.

Management

Management of metabolic disorders varies depending on the specific condition, its severity, and whether it is an acute or chronic presentation. Caregivers of children with a known diagnosis of inborn errors become very astute at early recognition of symptoms in their child and should be viewed as crucial partners in the healthcare team. Most families should have emergency protocol letters, sick day protocols, and 24-hour on-call contact information (Nyhan, Kolker, and Hoffmann, 2017).

Metabolic Emergencies

Emergency management of many metabolic disorders requires hospital admission and specialist care. The goal of emergency management is twofold: (1) prevent catabolism and (2) remove toxic substrates or metabolites. Aggressive management is necessary to avert or reduce neurologic sequelae. This acute care management may require IV medications (including glucose to halt catabolism), diet restriction (e.g., no protein for 24 to 48 hours or until mental status is back to baseline), hemodialysis, or life support (Aldubayan et al., 2017).

Stable Metabolic Disorders

The variability of IEMs requires individual management tailored to the patient's specific diagnosis and phenotype. However, the following strategies provide several broad categories from which treatments are drawn:
- Control substrate accumulation:
  - Restrict dietary intake (e.g., restricting phenylalanine intake in PKU) (Singh et al., 2016).
  - Control endogenous production of the substrate (e.g., give high-calorie, no-protein feeds during illness to prevent catabolism, which would release amino acids) (Aldubayan et al., 2017).
  - Accelerate removal of the substrate (e.g., administer sodium benzoate/phenylacetate in urea cycle disorders urea cycle disorders (UCDs) to increase elimination of waste nitrogen through an alternate pathway) (Litcher-Konecki, 2016).
- Dietary supplementation:
  - Replace or supplement the diet with products that become deficient distal to the metabolic block or if the diet is medically restricted (e.g., arginine or citrulline in UCD) (Tanaka et al., 2017).

- Vitamin and cofactor replacement:
  - Increase the supply of certain vitamins or medications (e.g., sapropterin dihydrochloride) that act as cofactors to metabolic reactions to improve function of the residual enzyme activity. Vitamin replacement is also important with severely restricted diets (Blau and Longo, 2015).
- Enzyme replacement therapy (ERT):
  - ERT (an IV infusion of enzyme replacement given every 1 to 2 weeks) is becoming widely available in the clinical setting for lysosomal storage diseases (Mistry et al., 2017).
- Bone marrow or organ transplant:
  - Stem cell transplantation using exogenous bone marrow or cord blood as a donor site is clinically available for some disorders, but it is in the early stage of widespread clinical use (Chiesa, Wynn, Veys, 2016).
  - Organ transplant can essentially "cure" some metabolic diseases by transplanting an organ in which the mutant genes are expressed. Liver transplantation has shown success in some IEMs (Pham, Enns, Esquivel, 2016).

Complications

Multiple complications such as renal failure, hypertension, spinal cord compression, and carpal tunnel syndrome may be seen with IEMs, often necessitating an interprofessional management team.

Specific Metabolic Disorders of Children

Disorders of Carbohydrate Metabolism

This group of disorders is caused by the inability to metabolize the monosaccharides (glucose, galactose, and fructose) and the polysaccharide glycogen. Aberrant glycogen synthesis or disorders of gluconeogenesis also contribute to faulty carbohydrate metabolism.

Glycogen Storage Diseases

Glycogen is a glucose polymer stored in muscle and the liver, and deficiency of any enzyme involved in the metabolic pathway of glycogen can affect biosynthesis or degradation of glycogen in the organ in which the enzyme is expressed. This deficiency results in a variety of presentations of disease. Glucose-6-phosphatase enzyme or translocase deficiency (type I), debrancher enzyme deficiency (type III), and liver phosphorylase kinase deficiency (type IX) are the most common early childhood presentations. Overall frequency of all forms is approximately 1:100,000 live births (National Institutes of Health [NIH] National Library of Medicine, 2018a).

Clinical Findings

Signs and symptoms may include cardiomegaly, hepatosplenomegaly, hypoglycemic seizures, lactic acidosis, ketosis, hyperlipidemia, elevated transaminases, easy fatigability, hypotonia, and muscle weakness.

Diagnostic Studies. Enzyme assays and mutation analysis are available for essentially all identified forms of glycogen storage disease.

Management

Treatment varies depending on the specific defect. Types I, III, and IX all affect enzyme activity in the liver, which is responsible for homeostasis of plasma glucose. Treatment is aimed at maintaining normal blood glucose levels and may require continuous feedings through a gastrostomy tube, frequent feedings, and/or ingestion of uncooked cornstarch or Glycosade (long-acting cornstarch) slurry at regular intervals throughout the day. Parents and children must be aware of symptoms of low blood sugar, and home glucose monitoring is recommended (Chou et al., 2015; Kishnani et al., 2014).

Galactosemia

Galactosemia results from a disorder of galactose metabolism. The classic form of galactosemia is caused by deficient galactose-1-phosphate uridyltransferase (GALT) activity. Dietary galactose is most commonly ingested as lactose, the principle carbohydrate in human milk and commercial nonsoy formulas. The metabolism of galactose undergoes many enzymatic reactions. A block at the level of the GALT enzyme results in accumulation of galactose-1-phosphate (gal-1-P) and other galactose derivatives, leading to clinical symptoms (Wellington et al., 2017). Incidence of the classic autosomal recessive form is estimated at 1 in 47,000 live births (Viggiano et al., 2017).

Clinical Findings

Infants with classic galactosemia appear normal at birth but demonstrate clinical manifestations after milk feeding. Although galactosemia is typically discovered on newborn screening, neonates may show clinical signs before results of the screening are known. Therefore galactosemia should remain in the differential diagnosis of any ill neonate. Clinical manifestations of severe, untreated galactosemia include poor weight gain, lethargy, jaundice, tubular kidney dysfunction, vomiting, coagulopathies, and *Escherichia coli* sepsis (Viggiano et al., 2017).

Diagnostic Studies. Measurement of GALT activity in red cells will be deficient, and liver enzymes and gal-1-P levels will be elevated (Viggino et al., 2017; Wellington et al., 2017).

Management

Treatment in classic galactosemia consists of eliminating dietary galactose. Ensure that the child is receiving appropriate calcium supplementation. Controversy surrounding appropriate treatment of variants (e.g., Duarte galactosemia) continues with some centers recommending dietary restriction, some recommending no therapy, and others using soy formula during the first year (Wellington et al., 2017).

Complications

Long-term complications of untreated galactosemia include cirrhosis, cataracts, and irreversible brain damage. Despite treatment, many children with classic galactosemia develop speech/language impairment, and some develop impaired motor and cognitive function (Wellington et al., 2017). Premature ovarian failure is also common (Thakur et al., 2017).

Urea Cycle Disorders

A defect in any enzyme of the urea cycle results in hyperammonemia secondary to the body's inability to detoxify waste nitrogen through its normal conversion to urea. Ammonia is an end product of amino acid catabolism and is highly toxic to the CNS. Five enzymes are required for the conversion of ammonia to urea, and deficiency in any of these enzymes results in disease. Incidence of the disorder is approximately 1:35,000 births (Litcher-Konecki, 2016).

Clinical Findings and Diagnostic Studies. In infants, symptoms related to the effects of hyperammonemia start after protein ingestion and include vomiting, lethargy, irritability, malaise, and potential seizures and coma. Older children may exhibit ataxia, confusion, agitation, irritability, and combativeness (Lichter-Konecki, 2016). No specific findings are typically found with initial laboratory testing, however:

- BUN may be low.
- Ammonia level greater than 100 mmol/L (or lower in older children) evokes concern (normal values are typically less than 35 mmol/L).
- Genetic mutation analysis may confirm the diagnosis of some IEM disorders.

Management and Complications. Treatment of acute hyperammonemia is completed by acute care staff with the goal being to establish a source of glucose and rapidly decreasing ammonia levels. Principles of treatment of chronic UCD are very similar, but they also include limiting endogenous protein catabolism and dietary protein consumption under the supervision of a metabolic dietician (Lichter-Konecki, 2016). Despite appropriate treatment, children with UCD are vulnerable to metabolic decompensation, mild to moderate mental retardation, and premature death.

Amino Acid Metabolism Disorders: Aminoacidopathies and Organic Acidurias and Acidemias

More than 30 defects of amino acid metabolism are attributed to enzyme or cofactor defects. Although all of these disorders result from defects in amino acid metabolism, they are generally classified as aminoacidopathies or organic acidurias or acidemias, depending on whether amino acids or organic acids are detected in urine or plasma. The more common aminoacidopathies include PKU, maple syrup urine disease (MSUD), tyrosinemias, and homocystinuria.

Phenylketonuria. Classic PKU is the most common form of PKU and results from deficiency of the enzyme phenylalanine hydroxylase, which converts phenylalanine to tyrosine. Untreated PKU leads to elevated phenylalanine concentrations in the blood and brain and results in CNS damage with profound mental retardation (Blau, 2016). The resulting lower level of tyrosine leads to impaired synthesis of other amines, including dopamine, norepinephrine, and melanin. More prevalent in Caucasians, PKU is an autosomal recessive disorder with an incidence of approximately 1:10,000 to 15,000 newborns in the United States (NIH National Library of Medicine Genetics Home Reference, 2018b).

Clinical Findings. No clinical manifestations are noted at birth, and the effects of high phenylalanine levels may not be apparent in the first few months, by which time, if untreated, irreversible brain damage has occurred. Children with more advanced, untreated disease tend to have lighter skin and hair than typical for their race and develop an eczematous rash and a musty or mousy odor related to build up of phenylacetate. (Blau, 2016). PKU should be detected on newborn screening. Infants with classic PKU ingesting a normal diet have serum phenylalanine levels greater than 1200 mmol/L on confirmatory plasma amino acid panel, whereas others with milder hyperphenylalaninemia have intermediate levels.

Differential Diagnosis. Biopterin is a cofactor for phenylalanine, tyrosine, and tryptophan hydroxylases. Children with biopterin defects may be detected on newborn screening but will continue to deteriorate despite usual dietary intervention for PKU (Nardecchia et al., 2017). Testing blood and urine pterins and biopterin enzymes is recommended in any child with high phenylalanine levels. Treatment for biopterin defects is different than routine PKU treatment.

Management

Treatment for PKU involves limiting the dietary intake of phenylalanine, with a goal of serum phenylalanine levels between 60 and 360 mmol/L in all patients (Vockley et al., 2014). Phenylalanine is an essential amino acid that cannot be eliminated entirely because patients need to receive enough to meet growth needs. To obtain the essential amino acids and to meet energy and other nutritional needs, the diet is supplemented with a medically modified formula, free of phenylalanine. Over the child's first few years of life, parents are educated on the phenylalanine content of foods; the child's phenylalanine level is frequently monitored; and a phenylalanine "allowance" is established based on the child's dietary tolerance. The current recommendation is "diet for life" to prevent long-term cognitive and neurologic sequelae. Medically modified low-phenylalanine food products are available online and in some stores, with insurance reimbursement in some states. Pregnant females with PKU must maintain very strict dietary restrictions to protect the fetus (Vockley et al., 2014; Waisbren et al., 2014) Consultation with or referral to a metabolic dietician is essential.

Classic Homocystinuria

Homocystinuria due to cystathionine synthase deficiency is the most common form of these disorders, with a prevalence of approximately 1:200,000 to 335,000 worldwide (NIH National Library of Medicine Genetics Home Reference, 2018c). Discussion of homocystinuria caused by defects in vitamin metabolism and deficiency of methylenetetrahydrofolate reductase (MTHFR) is beyond the scope of this chapter.

Clinical Findings and Diagnostic Studies. Clinical manifestations are nonspecific and include failure to thrive and developmental delay. Plasma and urine amino acid testing is completed to evaluate concentrations of:

- Methionine: Elevated levels may be found on the newborn screening, but values rise slowly, and high methionine levels may not be detected on specimens obtained from affected infants in the first few days after birth; a second newborn screening is necessary.
- Homocystine and total homocysteine

Management and Complications. Some children respond to vitamin B_6 therapy with greater than 30% reduction of either plasma total homocysteine and/or plasma methionine concentrations. If the child responds, treatment with vitamin B_6 is continued. Children who do not respond to vitamin B_6 are placed on a protein-restricted diet with frequent monitoring of plasma amino acids and total plasma homocysteine. Betaine is administered. Folate and vitamin B_{12} optimize conversion of homocystine to methionine (Sacharow et al., 2017; Kumar et al., 2016).

Treatment outcomes are variable, and these children are at high risk for metabolic stroke, although prognosis is good for those with the classical form of homocystinuria identified on newborn screening. Untreated patients develop ocular lens dislocation, progressive mental retardation, thromboembolic events, convulsions, and skeletal abnormalities resembling Marfan syndrome.

Disorders of Fatty Acid Oxidation

Medium-Chain Acyl-Coenzyme A Dehydrogenase Deficiency. Fatty acids are an important energy resource for the body, used during times of fasting and stress when glycogen stores become depleted. Defects can occur at any point in fatty acid transport or the mitochondrial beta-oxidation pathway, yielding more than 20 disorders in which individuals are unable to metabolize fatty acids. The more common fatty acid oxidation disorders are medium-chain acyl-coenzyme A dehydrogenase (MCAD) deficiency, very-long-chain acyl-coenzyme A dehydrogenase (VLCAD) deficiency, and long-chain 3-hydroxyacyl-coenzyme A dehydrogenase (LCHAD) deficiency. The incidence of all disorders ranges from 1:17,000 to 1:360,000. MCAD deficiency is quickly becoming one of the most common IEMs identified in infants by newborn screening, with an estimated incidence of 1:17, 0000 live births (NIH National Library of Medicine Genetics Home Reference, 2018d).

Clinical Findings and Diagnostic Studies. Individuals with MCAD deficiency may be asymptomatic for a lifetime or have premature death. Fasting, stress, or illness may lead to hypoketotic hypoglycemia, hypotonia, muscle weakness, lethargy, and vomiting progressing to seizures, coma, encephalopathy, and death. Any increase in energy demand may tip the balance and result in a metabolic crisis as vital organs are deprived of fuel. Historically, fatty acid oxidation disorders (all types) have been implicated as the cause of death in 5% of sudden unexpected deaths in infancy, but with comprehensive newborn screening the number of unexpected fatalities in infants should be close to none (Rosenthal et al., 2015). Expanded newborn screening will identify the majority of fatty acid oxidation defects.

Confirmatory tests for MCAD deficiency include:
- Plasma acylcarnitine profile
- Mutation analysis

Hypoglycemia or normoglycemia may be present during times of illness, and blood glucose monitoring is not a reliable measure of metabolic status in these children (Gartner et al., 2015).

Management. Treatment varies and may include fasting avoidance and carnitine supplementation to correct secondary carnitine deficiency. For individuals with MCAD deficiency, avoidance of fasting is the mainstay of treatment. Infants should not fast for longer than 3 hours for the first 3 months. For each month of age, 1 hour of fasting can be added up to a maximum of 12 hours of fasting. These guidelines do not apply during times of higher energy demand (Walter, 2009). Providers should maintain a low threshold for recommending IV glucose infusions during times of illness and fever when energy requirements increase. Monitor carnitine level, and supplement with oral carnitine 50 to 100 mg/kg/day in divided doses if the free carnitine level is less than the reference range (Ribas et al., 2014).

Complications

The most serious consequence of this group of disorders is the inability to use fatty acids for energy production and lack of ketone production (burned for energy) during times of fasting, which may result in death.

Lysosomal Storage Disorders

Lysosomal storage disorders are caused by an accumulation (storage) of glycoproteins, glycolipids, or glycosaminoglycans (e.g., mucopolysaccharide storage [MPS] diseases) within lysosomes and various tissues, which leads to the various clinical presentations and symptoms. Incidence for all lysosomal storage disorders is 1:7700 live births. Symptoms vary depending on the site of storage and the specific disorder and may include hepatosplenomegaly, coarse facies, corneal clouding, developmental regression, intellectual disability, thrombocytopenia, bone pain, abnormal liver function studies, respiratory problems, hydrocephalus, and cardiomyopathy. Enzymatic assay and mutation analysis are available for most disorders. Initial diagnostic testing for mucopolysaccharidosis consists of screening urinary glycosaminoglycans (urine MPS screen), both quantitative and qualitative (Zampini et al., 2017), but a normal screen does not rule out the diagnosis. Treatment varies from symptom management to ERT with varying degrees of success (Beck, 2018).

Dyslipidemia: Hypercholesterolemia and Hyperlipidemia

Dyslipidemias are disorders of lipoprotein metabolism, some of which lead to increased levels of total cholesterol and LDL cholesterol, a varied presentation of triglycerides, and/or decreased levels of HDL cholesterol. Dyslipidemias can be acquired (secondary) or genetic (primary). Secondary hyperlipidemias result from exogenous factors, such as obesity, drugs (e.g., isotretinoin, oral contraceptives, antipsychotics), and alcohol; endocrine or metabolic disorders (e.g., hypothyroidism, diabetes); storage disease (e.g., glycogen storage disease); obstructive liver disease (e.g., biliary atresia); and other causes, such as anorexia nervosa. Among primary dyslipidemia, familial hypercholesterolemia is most common; it is also the most commonly occurring congenital metabolic disorder (Martin et al., 2017). Familial hypercholesterolemia results from pathogenic mutation in the LDL receptor (LDLR [19p13.2]; most common), apolipoprotein B (ApoB) (2p24.1), or protein convertase subtilisin/kexin type 9 (PCSK9) (1p32.3) genes. These mutations compromise the receptor cells' ability to facilitate clearance of LDL cholesterol through the liver; as a result, LDL accumulates in the body. Triglycerides are usually normal. The two types of familial hypercholesterolemia are heterozygous, which is common (1:200 to 1:500) (de Ferranti et al., 2016), and homozygous, which is exceedingly rare (1:300,000) (Santos et al., 2016). Homozygous hypercholesterolemia is characterized by extremely high LDL levels (e.g., 600 mg/dL or more) and a poor outcome if the patient does not have extremely aggressive early treatment; treatment may include LDL apheresis, new specific medications that have been developed, and possible liver transplant. Even with treatment, atherosclerotic vascular disease is common by 30 years old (Santos et al., 2016).

Clinical Findings. Hyperlipidemia does not typically present as a clinical illness in children. Although not all children with dyslipidemia will have cardiovascular problems as adults, screening of children at risk is important to identify those with hyperlipidemia and hypercholesterolemia via cascade screening and intervene in an effort to prevent problems from occurring later in life (Knowles, Rader, Khoury, 2017).

History. Risk factors for hypercholesterolemia and hyperlipidemia found in the history include (Santos et al., 2016):
- Family history of premature heart disease (men ≤55 years old; women ≤65 years old)
- Increased age (men >30 years old; women >40 years old)
- Male sex; hypertension, smoking
- Type 2 diabetes
- Reduced HDL cholesterol concentration

Physical Examination. The child may have no clinical signs or symptoms or may have (Santos et al., 2016)
- Tendon xanthomas at any age (most common in finger extensor tendons and Achilles tendon)
- Arcus corneae (partial or complete) younger than 4 or 5 years old
- Tuberous xanthomas or xanthelasma

Diagnostic Studies. The clinical conditions of dyslipidemia can be determined by lipoprotein analysis. Universal screening for elevated serum cholesterol is recommended at 9 to 11 years old with a fasting lipid profile or nonfasting non-HDL cholesterol measurement. When the family history is positive for hypercholesterolemia or premature congenital heart disease (CHD), screening should be considered by 2 years old (Knowles, Rader, and Khoury, 2017).

Precise genetic etiology is not needed for therapeutic decisions, although conditions with overlapping signs and laboratory derangements and with different treatment (e.g., cerebrotendinous xanthomatosis, sitosterolemia, and cholesterol ester storage disease) should be considered and ruled out if appropriate.

Management

Lifestyle Changes. Prevention and/or control of hypercholesterolemia through lifestyle changes is a primary intervention. Dietary change has been the first step in treatment of children older than 2 years with hypercholesterolemia (LDL >110 mg/dL with total cholesterol of at least 200 mg/dL) and, combined with other lifestyle changes, remains a mainstay of treatment—even if medications are added to the regimen. The National Lipid Association (NLA) encourages individuals to change lifestyle patterns, as well as alter diet; educational materials related to this approach are available on the NLA website (see Additional Resources). Many issues arise with dietary changes in children (e.g., increasing dietary fiber may "fill up" the child and increase the risk of poor nutrient intake), so consultation with a pediatric dietitian nutritionist is essential to ensure that children receive adequate nutrition. Detailed guidelines are proposed by the Cardiovascular Health Integrated Lifestyle Diet (CHILD) 1 and 2, which is specific for age groups based on total cholesterol and LDL levels (Rohrs and Berger, 2015).

Pharmacotherapy. Drug therapy should be considered in children 8 years old or older who, after 6 to 12 months of therapy focused on diet and lifestyle changes, continue to have the following (Rohrs and Burger, 2015):
- LDL concentration greater than 190 mg/dL *or*
- LDL concentration between 160 and 190 mg/dL *and* positive family history of premature CHD or two risk factors
  - Risk factors:
    - Smoking
    - Hypertension
    - HDL level of less than 35 mg/dL
    - Obesity (greater than 30% more than ideal body weight)
    - Diabetes mellitus
    - Physical inactivity
    - Male sex
    - Renal disease, lupus, rheumatoid arthritis, human immunodeficiency virus infection, nephrotic syndrome, Kawasaki disease (without current aneurysms)

If the child is taking antipsychotic medication, a consult with the behavioral health provider is necessary before beginning treatment, because some antipsychotic medications increase the risk of hyperlipidemia. Use of HMG-CoA reductase inhibitors (statins) can be considered if the child has severe hypercholesterolemia. The statins function by inhibiting the rate-limiting enzyme in the synthesis of cholesterol. Because of the side effects of drugs and the uncertainty about their long-term use in the pediatric population, children who need drug therapy should be referred to a specialized pediatric lipid center for treatment.

Additional Resources

Academy of Nutrition and Dietetics (formerly American Dietetic Association). www.eatright.org
American Association of Diabetes Educators (AADE). www.diabeteseducator.org
American College of Medical Genetics and Genomics. www.acmg.net

American Diabetes Association. www.diabetes.org
American Heart Association. www.heart.org/HEARTORG/
American Thyroid Association. www.thyroid.org
Barbara Davis Center for Diabetes: University of Colorado Anschutz Medical Campus. www.barbaradaviscenter.org
Child Growth Foundation. www.childgrowthfoundation.org
Children with Diabetes. www.childrenwithdiabetes.com
Children's Diabetes Foundation. http://www.childrensdiabetesfoundation.org
Dwarfism/Short Stature Resources. www.kumc.edu/gec/support/dwarfism.html
Endocrine Society. www.endocrine.org
Gene Tests. https://genetests.org
Genetics Home Reference. https://ghr.nlm.nih.gov/
Human Growth Foundation. www.hgfound.org
Joslin Diabetes Center, Boston, MA. www.joslindiabetescenter.org/info/childhood-diabetes.html
Juvenile Diabetes Research Foundation (JDRF). www.jdrf.org
Little People of America. www.lpaonline.org
Magic Foundation. www.magicfoundation.org
March of Dimes. https://www.marchofdimes.org/
MedicAlert Foundation. www.medicalert.org
National Diabetes Education Program. www.ndep.nih.gov
National Heart, Lung, and Blood Institute. www.nhlbi.nih.gov
National Institutes of Health. www.nih.gov
National Lipid Association (NLA). www.lipid.org
Learn Your Lipids: Patient Information from the Foundation of the National Lipid Association. www.learnyourlipids.com
National Newborn Screening and Global Resource Center (NNSGRC). www.genes-r-us.uthscsa.edu
Online Mendelian Inheritance in Man (OMIM). www.omim.org
Pediatric Endocrinology Nursing Society (PENS). www.pens.org
Pituitary Network Association. www.pituitary.org
Screening, Technology, and Research in Genetics (STAR-G). www.newbornscreening.info
Society for Inherited Metabolic Disorders. www.simd.org
Treatment Options for Diabetes in Adolescents and Youth (TODAY) Study. https://portal.bsc.gwu.edu/web/today/home/

References

Aldubayan S, Rodan L, Berry G, Levy H. Acute illness protocol for organic acidemias. *Pediatic Emergency Care*. 2017;33(2):142–146.

Amed S, Oram R. Maturity-Onset Diabetes of the Young (MODY): making the right diagnosis to optimize treatment. *Can J Diabetes*. 2016;40(5):449–454. https://doi.org/10.1016/j.jcjd.2016.03.002.

American Diabetes Association. Standards of Medical Care in Diabetes. *Diabetes Care*. 2017;40(suppl 1). https://doi.org/10.2337/dc17-S015.

Beck M. Treatment strategies for lysosomal storage disorders. *Dev Med Child Neurol*. 2018;60(1):13–18. https://doi.org/10.1111/dmcn.13600. Epub 2017 Nov 1.

Benkhadra K, Alahdab F, Tamhane S, et al. Real-time continuous glucose monitoring in type 1 diabetes: a systematic review and individual patient data meta-analysis. *Clin Endocrinol (Oxf)*. 2017;86(3):354–360. https://doi.org/10.1111/cen.13290.

Blau N. Genetics of phenylketonuria: then and now. *Human Mutation*. 2016;37(6):508–515.

Blau N, Longo N. Alternative therapies to address the unmet medical needs of patients with phenylketonuria. *Expert Opinion on Pharmacotherapy*. 2015;16(6):791–800. https://doi.org/10.1517/14656566.2015.1013030.

Bornstein SR, Allolio B, Arlt W, et al. Diagnosis and treatment of primary adrenal insufficiency: an Endocrine Society clinical practice guideline. *J Clin Endocrinol Metab*. 2016;101(2):364–389. https://doi.org/10.1210/jc.2015-1710.

Buchberger B, Huppertz H, Krabbe L, Lux B, Mattivi JT, Siafarikas A. Symptoms of depression and anxiety in youth with type 1 diabetes: a systematic review and meta-analysis. *Psychoneuroendocrinology*. 2016;70:70–84. https://doi.org/10.1016/j.psyneuen.2016.04.01.

Centers for Disease Control and Prevention. *National Diabetes Statistics Report*; 2017. Retrieved from: https://www.cdc.gov/diabetes/pdfs/data/statistics/national-diabetes-statistics-report.pdf.

Chaplais E, Naughton G, Thivel D, Courteix D, Greene D. Smartphone interventions for weight treatment and behavioral change in pediatric obesity: a systematic review. *Telemed J E Health*. 2015;21(10):822–830. https://doi.org/10.1089/tmj.2014.0197.

Chiang JL, Kirkman MS, Laffel LMB, Peters AL. Type 1 Diabetes through the life span: a position statement of the American Diabetes Association. *Diabetes Care*. 2014;37(7):2034–2054. https://doi.org/10.2337/dc14-1140.

Chiesa R, Wynn RF, Veys R. Haematopoietic stem cell transplantation in inborn errors of metabolism. *Curr Opin Hematol*. 2016;23(6):530–535.

Chou J, Jun H, Mansfield B. Type I glycogen storage diseases: disorders of the glucose-6-phosphatase/glucose-6-phosphate transporter complexes. *J Inherit Metab Dis*. 2015;38(3):511–519.

Dabelea D, Mayer-Davis EJ, Saydah S, et al. Prevalence of type 1 and type 2 diabetes among children and adolescents from 2001 to 2009. *JAMA*. 2014;311(17):1778–1786. https://doi.org/10.1001/jama.2014.3201.

Dabelea D, Rewers A, Stafford JM, et al. Trends in the prevalence of ketoacidosis at diabetes diagnosis: the SEARCH for diabetes in youth study. *Pediatrics*. 2014;133(4):e938–945. https://doi.org/10.1542/peds.2013-2795.

Dashti S, Latiff LA, Zulkefli NA, et al. A review on the assessment of the efficacy of common treatments in polycystic ovarian syndrome on prevention of diabetes mellitus. *J Family Reprod Health*. 2017;11(2):56–66.

de Ferranti SD, Rodday AM, Mendelson MM, et al. Prevalence of familial hypercholesterolemia in the 1999 to 2012 United States National Health and Nutrition Examination Surveys (NHANES). *Circulation*. 2016;133(11):1067–1072.

de Vries AL, McGuire JK, Steensma TD, et al. Young adult psychological outcome after puberty suppression and gender reassignment. *Pediatrics*. 2014;134(4):696–704. https://doi.org/10.1542/peds.2013-2958.

Diaz A, Lipman Diaz EG. Hypothyroidism. *Pediatr Rev*. 2014;35(8):336–347; quiz 348-339. https://doi.org/10.1542/pir.35-8-336.

Doyle EA, Quinn SM, Ambrosino JM, Weyman K, Tamborlane WV, Jastreboff AM. Disordered eating behaviors in emerging adults with type 1 diabetes: a common problem for both men and women. *J Pediatr Health Care*. 2017;31(3):327–333. https://doi.org/10.1016/j.pedhc.2016.10.004.

Expert panel on integrated guidelines for cardiovascular health and risk reduction in children and adolescents: summary report. *Pediatrics*. 2011;128(suppl 5):S213–S256. https://doi.org/10.1542/peds.2009-2107C.

Fertil Steril. 2018 Aug;110(3):364-379. https://10.1016/j.fertnstert.2018.05.004. Epub 2018 Jul 19.

Fleming L, Van Riper M, Knafl K. Management of childhood congenital adrenal hyperplasia-an integrative review of the literature. *J Pediatr Health Care*. 2017;31(5):560–577. https://doi.org/10.1016/j.pedhc.2017.02.004.

Flores AR, Herman JL, Gates GJ, Brown TNT. *How Many Adults Identify as Transgender in the United States?* 2016. Retrieved from Los Angeles, CA: https://williamsinstitute.law.ucla.edu/wp-content/uploads/How-Many-Adults-Identify-as-Transgender-in-the-United-States.pdf.

Garrod A. The Croonian Lectures on inborn errors of metabolism. *Lancet*. 1908;172(1–7):73–79. 142–148, 214–220.

Gartner V, McGuire P, Lee P. Child neurology: medium chain acyl-coenzyme A dehydrogenase deficiency. *Neurology*. 2015;85:e37–e40. https://doi.org/10.1212/WNL.0000000000001786.

Garg SK, Weinzimer SA, Tamborlane WV, et al. Glucose outcomes with the in-home use of a hybrid closed-loop insulin delivery system in adolescents and adults with type 1 diabetes. *Diabetes Technol Ther*. 2017;19(3):155–163. https://doi.org/10.1089/dia.2016.0421.

Giani E, Snelgrove R, Volkening LK, Laffel LM. Continuous glucose monitoring (CGM) adherence in youth with type 1 diabetes: associations with biomedical and psychosocial variables. *J Diabetes Sci Technol*. 2017;11(3):476–483.

Grimberg A, DiVall SA, Polychronakos C, et al. Guidelines for growth hormone and insulin-like growth factor-I Treatment in children and adolescents: growth hormone deficiency, idiopathic short stature, and primary insulin-like growth factor-I deficiency. *Horm Res Paediatr*. 2016;86(6):361–397. https://doi.org/10.1159/000452150.

Guidelines for the Primary and Gender-Affirming Care of Transgender and Gender Nonbinary People; 2016. Retrieved from San Francisco: http://transhealth.ucsf.edu/trans?page=guidelines-youth.

Halban PA, Polonsky KS, Bowden DW, et al. beta-cell failure in type 2 diabetes: postulated mechanisms and prospects for prevention and treatment. *Diabetes Care*. 2014;37(6):1751–1758. https://doi.org/10.2337/dc14-0396.

Hanley P, Lord K, Bauer A. J. Thyroid disorders in children and adolescents: a review. *JAMA Pediatr*. 2016;170(10):1008–1019. https://doi.org/10.1001/jamapediatrics.2016.0486.

Herbst A, Kapellen T, Schober E, et al. Impact of regular physical activity on blood glucose control and cardiovascular risk factors in adolescents with type 2 diabetes mellitus–a multicenter study of 578 patients from 225 centres. *Pediatr Diabetes*. 2015;16(3):204–210. https://doi.org/10.1111/pedi.12144.

Herman JL, Flores AR, Brown TNT, Wilson EDM, Conron KJ. *Age of Individuals who Identify as Transgender in the United States*; 2017. Retrieved from: http://williamsinstitute.law.ucla.edu/wp-content/uploads/TransAgeReport.pdf.

Horta BL, Loret de Mola C, Victora CG. Long-term consequences of breastfeeding on cholesterol, obesity, systolic blood pressure and type 2 diabetes: a systematic review and meta-analysis. *Acta Paediatr*. 2015;104(467):30–37. https://doi.org/10.1111/apa.13133.

Jonklaas J, Bianco AC, Bauer AJ, et al. Guidelines for the treatment of hypothyroidism: prepared by the American Thyroid Association task force on thyroid hormone replacement. *Thyroid*. 2014;24(12):1670–1751. https://doi.org/10.1089/thy.2014.0028.

Kelly Y, Zilanawala A, Sacker A, Hiatt R, Viner R. Early puberty in 11-year-old girls: Millennium Cohort Study findings. *Arch Dis Child*. 2017;102(3):232–237. https://doi.org/10.1136/archdischild-2016-310475.

Kishnani PS, Austin S, Abdenur J, Arn P, Bali D, Boney A. Diagnosis and management of glycogen storage disease type 1: A practice guideline of the American College of Medical Genetics and Genomics. *Genet Med*. 2014;16(e1). https://doi.org/10.1038/gim.2014.128.

Knowles J, Radar D, Khoury M. Cascade screening for familial hypercholesterolemia and the use of genetic testing. *JAMA*. 2017;318(4):381–382. https://doi.org/10.1001/jama.2017.8543.

Kumar T, Sharma G, Singh L. Homcystinuria: therapeutic approach. *Clinica Acta*. 2016;458:55–62. https://doi.org/10.106/j.cca.2016.04.002.

Leger J, Olivieri A, Donaldson M, et al. European Society for Paediatric Endocrinology consensus guidelines on screening, diagnosis, and management of congenital hypothyroidism. *J Clin Endocrinol Metab*. 2014;99(2):363–384. https://doi.org/10.1210/jc.2013-1891.

Lichter-Konecki U. Defects of the urea cycle. *Transl Sci Rare Dis*. 2016;1:23–43.

Liu D, Ahmet A, Ward L, et al. A practical guide to the monitoring and management of the complications of systemic corticosteroid therapy. *Allergy Asthma Clin Immunol*. 2013;9(30).

Long D. Precocious puberty. *Pediatr Rev*. 2015;36(7):319–321. https://doi.org/10.1542/pir.36-7-319.

MakC M, Lee HC, Chan AY, Lam CW. Inborn errors of metabolism and expanded newborn screening: review and update. *Crit Rev Clin Lab Sci*. 2013;50(6):142–162. https://doi.org/10.3109/10408363.2013.847896.

Mayer-Davis EJ, Lawrence JM, Dabelea D, et al. Incidence trends of type 1 and type 2 diabetes among youths, 2002–2012. *N Engl J Med*. 2017;376(15):1419–1429. https://doi.org/10.1056/NEJMoa1610187.

Miller KM, Foster NC, Beck RW, et al. Current state of type 1 diabetes treatment in the U.S.: updated data from the T1D Exchange Clinic Registry. *Diabetes Care*. 2015;38(6):971–978. https://doi.org/10.2337/dc15-0078.

Mistry PK, Lopes G, Schiffmann R, Barton N, Weinreb N, Sidransky E. Gaucher disease: progress and ongoing challenges. *Mol Genet Metab Rep.* 2017;120(1):8–21.

Narasimhan S, Weinstock RS. Youth-onset type 2 diabetes mellitus: lessons learned from the TODAY study. *Mayo Clin Proc.* 2014;89(6):806–816. https://doi.org/10.1016/j.mayocp.2014.01.009.

Nardecchia F, Chiarotti F, Carducci C, et al. Altered tetrahydrobiopterin metabolism in patients with phenylalanine hydroxylase deficiency. *Eur J Pediatr.* 2017;176:917–924.

NIH National Library of Medicine. *Glycogen Storage Disease*; 2018a. https://ghr.nlm.nih.gov/condition/glycogen-storage-disease-type-ix#statistics.

NIH National Library of Medicine. *Phenylketonuria.* 2018b. https://ghr.nlm.nih.gov/search?query=PKU.

NIH National Library of Medicine. *Homocystinuria.* 2018c. https://ghr.nlm.nih.gov/condition/homocystinuria#statistics.

NIH National Library of Medicine. *Medium-Chain Acyl-Coenzyme A Dehydrogenase Deficiency*; 2018d. https://ghr.nlm.nih.gov/condition/medium-chain-acyl-coa-dehydrogenase-deficiency#statistics.

Nyhan WL, Kölker S, Hoffmann GF. Emergency Treatment of Inherited Metabolic Diseases. In: Hoffmann G, Zschocke J, Nyhan W, eds. *J Inherit Metab Dis.* Berlin, Heidelberg: Springer; 2017.

O'Connor EA, Evans CV, Burda BU, Walsh ES, Eder M, Lozano P. Screening for obesity and intervention for weight management in children and adolescents: evidence report and systematic review for the US Preventive Services Task Force. *JAMA.* 2017;317(23):2427–2444. https://doi.org/10.1001/jama.2017.0332.

Ogden CL, Carroll MD, Lawman HG, et al. Trends in obesity prevalence among children and adolescents in the United States, 1988-1994 through 2013-2014. *JAMA.* 2016;315(21):2292–2299. https://doi.org/10.1001/jama.2016.6361.

Patterson C, Guariguata L, Dahlquist G, Soltesz G, Ogle G, Silink M. Diabetes in the young – a global view and worldwide estimates of numbers of children with type 1 diabetes. *Diabetes Res Clin Pract.* 2014;103(2):161–175. https://doi.org/10.1016/j.diabres.2013.11.005.

Peirson L, Fitzpatrick-Lewis D, Morrison K, Warren R, Usman Ali M, Raina P. Treatment of overweight and obesity in children and youth: a systematic review and meta-analysis. *CMAJ Open.* 2015;3(1):E35–E46. https://doi.org/10.9778/cmajo.20140047.

Pettitt DJ, Talton J, Dabelea D, et al. Prevalence of diabetes in U.S. youth in 2009: the SEARCH for diabetes in youth study. *Diabetes Care.* 2014;37(2):402–408. https://doi.org/10.2337/dc13-1838.

Pham TA, Enns GM, Esquivel CO. Living donor liver transplantation for inborn errors of metabolism – An underutilized resource in the United States. *Pediatr Transplant.* 2016;20(6):770–773. https://doi.org/10.1111/petr.12746. Epub 2016 Jul 8.

Pickup JC, Ford Holloway M, Samsi K. Real-time continuous glucose monitoring in type 1 diabetes: a qualitative framework analysis of patient narratives. *Diabetes Care.* 2015;38(4):544–550. https://doi.org/10.2337/dc14-1855.

Pippitt K, Li M, Gurgle HE. Diabetes mellitus: screening and diagnosis. *Am Fam Physician.* 2016;93(2):103–109.

Pulgaron ER, Delamater AM. Obesity and type 2 diabetes in children: epidemiology and treatment. *Curr Diab Rep.* 2014;14(8):508. https://doi.org/10.1007/s11892-014-0508-y.

Ribas G, Vargas C, Wajner M. L-carnitine supplementation as a potential antioxidant therapy for inherited neurometabolic disorders. *Gene.* 2014;533(2):469–476. https://doi.org/10.1016/j.gene.2013.10.017.

Riddell MC, Gallen IW, Smart CE, et al. Exercise management in type 1 diabetes: a consensus statement. *Lancet Diabetes Endocrinol.* 2017;5(5):377–390. https://doi.org/10.1016/S2213-8587(17)30014-1.

Rodbard D. Continuous glucose monitoring: a review of successes, challenges, and opportunities. *Diabetes technology & therapeutics.* 2016;18(S2):S23–S213.

Rogol AD, Hayden GF. Etiologies and early diagnosis of short stature and growth failure in children and adolescents. *J Pediatr.* 2014;164(suppl 5):S1–S14 e16. https://doi.org/10.1016/j.jpeds.2014.02.027.

Rohr F. Nutrition management of urea cycle disorders. In: Bernstein L, Rohr F, Helms J, eds. *Nutrition Management of Inherited Metabolic Diseases.* Springer Cham; 2015. https://doi.org/10.1007/978-3-319-14621-8_15.

Rohrs H, Berger S. *Pediatric Lipid Disorders in Clinical Practice Treatment and Management*; 2015. http://emedicine.medscape.com/article/1825087-overview.

Rose SR, Cook DM, Fine MJ. Growth hormone therapy guidelines: clinical and managed care perspectives. *Am J Pharm Benefits.* 2014;6(5):e134–e146.

Rosenfield RL. The Diagnosis of polycystic ovary syndrome in adolescents. *Pediatrics.* 2015;36(6):1154–1165.

Rosenthal N, Currier R, Baer R, Feuchtbaum L, Jelliffe-Pawlowski L. Undiagnosed metabolic dysfunction and sudden infant death syndrome-a case control study. *Paediatr Perinat Epidemiol.* 2015;29:151–155.

Rosenthal SM. Transgender youth: current concepts. *Ann Pediatr Endocrinol Metab.* 2016;21(4):185–192. https://doi.org/10.6065/apem.2016.21.4.185.

Ross JL, Lee PA, Gut R, Germak J. Attaining genetic height potential: analysis of height outcomes from the ANSWER Program in children treated with growth hormone over 5 years. *Growth Horm IGF Res.* 2015;25(6):286–293. https://doi.org/10.1016/j.ghir.2015.08.006.

Sacharow S, Picker J, Levey H. Homocystinuria caused by cystathionine beta-synthase deficiency. In: Adam M, Ardinger H, Pagon R, et al., eds. *GeneReviews.* Seattle: University of Washington; 2017.

Santos R, Gidding S, Hegele R, et al. Defining severe familial hypercholesterolaemia and the implications for clinical management: A consensus statement from the International Atherosclerosis Society Severe Familial Hypercholesterolemia Panel. *Lancet.* 2016;4(10):850–861.

Schulten RJ, Piet J, Bruijning PC, de Waal WJ. Lower dose basal insulin infusion has positive effect on glycaemic control for children with type I diabetes on continuous subcutaneous insulin infusion therapy. *Pediatric Diabetes.* 2017;18(1):45–50. https://doi.org/10.1111/pedi.12352.

Schultz AT, Smaldone A. Components of interventions that improve transitions to adult care for adolescents with type 1 diabetes. *J Adolesc Health.* 2017;60(2):133–146. https://doi.org/10.1016/j.jadohealth.2016.10.002.

Shahid M, McClellan D, Kapadia C. Case 1: absent pubertal development in a 17.5-year-old girl. *Pediatr Rev.* 2016;37(7):301–303. https://doi.org/10.1542/pir.2015-0004.

Singh RH, Cunningham AC, Mofidi S, et al. Updated web-based nutrition management guidelines for PKU: An evidence and consensus based approach. *Genet Metab.* 2016;118(2):72–83.

Srinivasan S, Misra M. Hyperthyroidism in children. *Pediatr Rev.* 2015;36(6):239–248. https://doi.org/10.1542/pir.36-6-239.

Strich D, Balagour L, Shenker J, Gillis D. Lower basal insulin dose is associated with better control in type 1 diabetes. *J Pediatr.* 2017;182:133–136. https://doi.org/10.1016/j.jpeds.2016.11.029.

Styne DM, Arslanian SA, Connor EL, et al. Pediatric obesity-assessment, treatment, and prevention: An Endocrine Society Clinical Practice Guideline. *J Clin Endocrinol Metab.* 2017;102(3):709–757. https://doi.org/10.1210/jc.2016-2573.

Tanaka K, Nakamura K, Matsumoto S, et al. Citrulline for urea cycle disorders in Japan. *Pediatr Int.* 2017;59(4):422–445. https://doi.org/10.1111/ped.13163. Epub 2016 Dec 22.

Teede HJ, Misso ML, Costello MF, Dokras A, Laven J, Moran L, Piltonen T, Norman RJ; International PCOS Network.

Thakur M, Feldman G, Puscheck E. Primary ovarian insufficiency in classic galactosemia: current understanding and future research opportunities. *J Assist Reporod Genet.* 2017. https://do.org/10.1007/s10815-017-1039-7.

The Diabetes Control and Complications Trial Research Group. The effect of intensive treatment of diabetes on the development and progression of long-term complications in insulin-dependent diabetes mellitus. *N Engl J Med.* 1993;329(14):977–986. https://doi.org/10.1056/nejm199309303291401.

The Diabetes Control and Complications Trial Research Group. Effect of intensive diabetes treatment on the development and progression of long-term complications in adolescents with insulin-dependent diabetes mellitus: Diabetes Control and Complications Trial. *J Pediatr.* 1994;125(2):177–188.

Thomas I, Gregg B. Metformin; a review of its history and future: from lilac to longevity. *Pediatr Diabetes.* 2017;18(1):10–16. https://doi.org/10.1111/pedi.12473.

TODAY Study Group. A clinical trial to maintain glycemic control in youth with type 2 diabetes. *N Engl J Med.* 2012;366(24):2247–2256. https://doi.org/10.1056/NEJMoa1109333.

U.S. Food and Drug Administration. *FDA Expands Indication for Continuous Glucose Monitoring System, First to Replace Fingerstick Testing for Diabetes Treatment Decisions*; 2017. Retrieved from: http://www.fda.gov/NewsEvents/Newsroom/PressAnnouncements/ucm534056.htm.

van der Kaay DC, Wasserman JD, Palmert MR. Management of neonates born to mothers with Graves' disease. *Pediatrics.* 2016;137(4). https://doi.org/10.1542/peds.2015-1878.

Vance SR, Ehrensaft D, Rosenthal SM. Psychological and medical care of gender nonconforming youth. *Pediatrics.* 2014;134(6):1184–1192. https://doi.org/10.1542/peds.2014-0772.

Viggiano E, Marabotti A, Politano L, Burlina A. *Clinical Genetics.* 2017:1–10. https://doi.org/10.1111/cge.13030.

Vockley J, Andersson H, Antshel K, et al. Phenylalanine hydroxylase deficiency: diagnosis and management guideline. *Genet Med.* 2014;16(2):188–200.

Waisbren S, Rohr F, Anastasoaie V, et al. Maternal phenylketonurias: long term outcomes in offspring and post-pregnancy maternal characteristics. *JIMD Reports.* 2014;21:23–32.

Walter J. Tolerance to fast: rational and practical evaluation with children with hypoketonaemia. 2009;2:214–217.

Wellington L, Bernstein L, Berry G, et al. International clinical guidelines for the management of classical galactosemia: diagnosis, treatment and follow-up. *J Inherit Metab Dis.* 2017;40:171–176.

Weiner DL. Inborn errors of metabolism. *Medscape.* 2017. https://emedicine.medscape.com/article/804757-overview.

Wolf RM. Long D. Pubertal development. *Pediatr Rev.* 2016;37(7):292–300. https://doi.org/10.1542/pir.2015-0065.

Wong JC, Foster NC, Maahs DM, et al. Real-time continuous glucose monitoring among participants in the T1D Exchange Clinic Registry. *Diabetes Care.* 2014;37(10):2702–2709.

Yu L, Rayhill S, Hsu E, Landis C. Liver transplantation for urea cycle disorders: analysis of the United Network for Organ Sharing database. *Transplant Proc.* 2015;47:2413–2418.

Zemel BS, Pipan M, Stallings VA, et al. Growth charts for children with Down syndrome in the United States. *Pediatrics.* 2015;136(5):e1204–1211. https://doi.org/10.1542/peds.2015-1652.

Zhang Z, Kris-Etherton PM, Hartman TJ. Birth weight and risk factors for cardiovascular disease and type 2 diabetes in US children and adolescents: 10 year results from NHANES. *Maternal Child Health J.* 2014;18(6):1423–1432. https://doi.org/10.1007/s10995-013-1382.

Zampini L, Padell L, Marchesiello R, et al. Importance of combine urinary procedure for the diagnosis of mucopolysaccharidoses. *Clinica Chimica Acta.* 2017;464:165–169.

46

Neurologic Disorders

RUTH K. ROSENBLUM AND DANIEL J. CRAWFORD

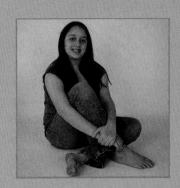

Central nervous system (CNS) problems can affect many systems and present in a variety of ways and degrees. No other body system has as much influence on a child's overall development. The challenge for healthcare providers is to be able to screen and identify neurologic problems, know when to appropriately refer to specialists, be able to monitor the general health of the patient and provide routine preventive care, serve as a case manager based on school and healthcare issues, help coordinate resources, and support families with children who have neurologic deficits as they deal with the challenges of grief and long-term care.

Anatomy and Physiology

Anatomy

Briefly, the nervous system is divided into two parts: the CNS and the peripheral nervous system (PNS). The CNS consists of the brain and spinal cord. The anatomic units of the brain and their functions are listed in Table 46.1 and shown in Figs 46.1 and 46.2. The PNS can be subdivided into three groups based on function: the somatic nervous system, the autonomic nervous system (ANS), and the enteric nervous system. The somatic nervous system mediates voluntary control of skeletal muscles and is made up of a network of nerves that send information to the brain (afferent nerves) and out to the body (efferent nerves) for responses. Descending tracts from the brain to the gray matter of the spinal cord include the extrapyramidal tract, which conveys information from the cerebellum to the motor cells of the anterior column, and the pyramidal tract, which is the main motor pathway from the cerebral cortex to the spinal nerves, and carries messages for voluntary movement. Most pyramidal tract fibers cross in the medulla, so the left half of the brain controls the right side of the body and vice versa. The ANS mediates control of the smooth muscles and glands. The enteric nervous system is a component of the ANS, but it does not play a role specifically in neurology. This system consists of a meshwork of nerve fibers that innervate the digestive system.

Autonomic Nervous System

The visceral activities of the body (i.e., blood vessels, glandular secretions, gastrointestinal tract, and cardiac muscle) are controlled by the ANS. The ANS is composed of the sympathetic system and the parasympathetic system, which are principally under the control of the hypothalamus. When the hypothalamus receives information from the cortical centers (e.g., visual, auditory, and olfactory) and sensory stimuli from the various parts of the body (e.g., organs and glands), it functions as a "switchboard" between the two systems. In general, both systems supply the same organs, glands, and smooth muscles. The sympathetic system begins in the thoracolumbar area of the spinal cord and extends distally; its function is often referred to as the "fight-or-flight" reaction. It is most active when an individual is physically or mentally stressed. The parasympathetic system begins in the medulla and midbrain with relays to the thalamus and higher centers. Stimulation of this system results in slowed activity, a decreased metabolic rate, and the conservation of energy; this system is active when an individual is mentally or physically relaxed. The principal sympathetic system neurotransmitters are epinephrine and norepinephrine. The parasympathetic fibers produce acetylcholine. The two systems function in balance—one excites and the other inhibits (Box 46.1).

Physiology

Nerve impulses are transmitted along a nerve fiber through changes in polarization of the membrane, during which electrical activity is produced. Certain chemicals diffuse across the synapses between nerves and end organs. There are approximately 50 substances that act as neurotransmitters in the brain. The main categories of neurotransmitters are acetylcholine (a primary transmitter released by neurons projecting through the cerebral cortex and limbic system), amino acids (e.g., glutamate, aspartate, glycine, γ-aminobutyric acid [GABA]), biogenic amines (e.g., norepinephrine, dopamine, serotonin, histamine), and the largest family, neuropeptides (e.g., endorphins, angiotensin II, melatonin, oxytocin, and many others). All of the neurotransmitters play an important role in either excitation or inhibition of neurons.

Pathophysiology and Defense Mechanisms

The nervous system is intimately related to the functioning of the entire body; problems in any part of the system can have neurologic implications. Examples include uncontrolled firing of cerebral neurons (seizures), the inability of cerebral neurons to fire or the inability of the CNS to process stimuli and respond accordingly (coma), or the inability of peripheral nerves to respond to or receive signals through the pyramidal system of afferent and efferent nerves (paralysis). Other problems occur when special areas of the nervous system or individual nerves are damaged. Additional causative factors for CNS disorders include:

| TABLE 46.1 | **Anatomic Units of the Nervous System and Functions** |

Anatomic Unit	Functions
I. Central nervous system	
A. Brain	
1. Forebrain—cerebrum	
a. Cortex (gray matter)	Posterior—motor skills
(1) Frontal area	Anterior—decision-making, emotions, memory, judgment, ethics, abstract thinking
	Broca area—speech
(2) Parietal area	Sensory integration, language, reading, writing, pattern recognition
(3) Temporal area	Memory storage, auditory processing, olfaction, limbic system in deep temporal lobe—arousal
(4) Occipital area	Visual processing
b. Diencephalon	
(1) Thalamus	Receives and sorts sensory input, modulates motor impulses from cortex
(2) Hypothalamus	Integrates autonomic functions
2. Midbrain	Connects brain with cerebellum, pons, medulla
3. Hindbrain	
a. Pons	Bridges cerebellum, medulla, midbrain; cranial nerves (CN V, CN VI, CN VIII) arise here
b. Medulla	Proximal end of spinal cord; contains reticular system—arousal; CN IX to CN XII arise here
c. Cerebellum	Coordination and movement; balance; smooth movements
B. Cranial nerves	Sensory and motor components; olfaction; vision; hearing; facial, tongue, pharyngeal, eye, shoulder movements
II. Spinal cord	
A. Dorsal roots	Afferent sensory fibers
B. Ventral roots	Efferent motor fibers
III. Protective layers	
A. Meninges	Protection of delicate nervous tissues
B. Ventricles	
C. Cerebrospinal fluid	

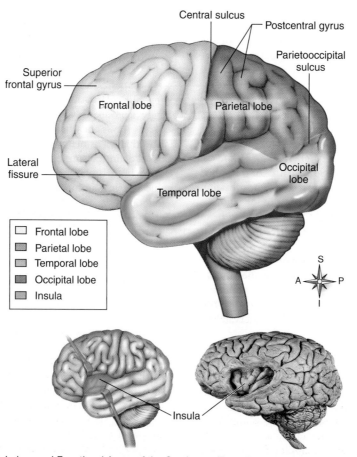

• **Fig 46.1** Lobes and Functional Areas of the Cerebrum. (From Patton K. *Anatomy and Physiology.* 9th ed. St Louis: Mosby/Elsevier; 2015.)

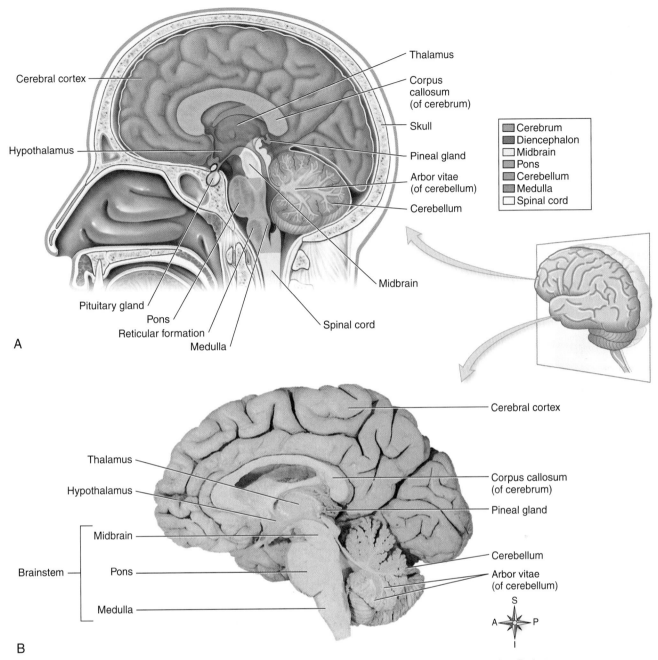

• **Fig 46.2** Midsagittal Section of the Brain Showing the Major Portions of the Diencephalon, Brainstem, and Cerebellum. (From Patton K. *Anatomy and Physiology.* 9th ed. St. Louis: Mosby/Elsevier; 2015.)

• Systemic problems: The brain is extremely sensitive to changes in physiology anywhere in the body. Thus any metabolic change, whether from external or internal factors (autoimmune, inflammatory, and/or infectious causes), may affect the CNS. Examples include delirium from toxins, diabetic coma, meningitis, ataxias, and chorea.

• Neurodegenerative disorders: Neurodegenerative disorders result from a loss of structure or function of neurons in the brain or spine, including death of neurons. Many neurodegenerative diseases are caused by genetic mutations (e.g., multiple sclerosis [MS] and Rett syndrome).

• Genetic problems: Many medical disorders have a genetic component that directly affects the nervous system. Some of the single-gene defects may have direct neurologic effects (such

as neurofibromatosis), whereas others, typically inborn errors of metabolism, can have indirect effects via the abnormal metabolites released (e.g., phenylketonuria). Other examples of disorders with a genetic component include Down and Rett syndromes.

• Structural defects: Because the CNS is structurally complex, there are many opportunities for defects to occur in utero. Examples of such defects include cortical migration defects, hydrocephaly, anencephaly, and spina bifida.

• Trauma: Head and spinal cord injuries occur frequently and can have long-term, serious consequences for the child. Recovery from head trauma can be lengthy and require a long rehabilitation time. Even then, return to baseline does not always occur. Peripheral nerves can regenerate somewhat if conditions

Parasympathetic System

Pupil constriction
Increased watery saliva
Lacrimal gland vasodilation
Coronary vessel vasoconstriction
Bronchial muscle constriction
Stomach and colon peristalsis
Genitalia vasodilation
Urinary bladder constriction
Skin vessel dilation

Sympathetic System

Pupil dilation
Increased viscous/thick saliva
Coronary vessel vasodilation
Bronchial muscle relaxation
Stomach and colon constriction
Adrenaline secretion
Sphincter relaxation or constriction
Genitalia vasoconstriction
Urinary bladder relaxation
Skin vessel constriction

are optimal. In the spinal cord, the axons of injured neurons cannot regrow within the cord, but they can grow in peripheral nerves outside the cord. In this case, if the cut ends are reconnected with special attention to the myelin sheath, regeneration of the injured nerve begins at the proximal end of the neuron soon after injury.

- Tumors and cancer: Benign or malignant tumors evolve when there is a problem with cellular division, which can cause unrestricted growth. Problems with the body's immune system can also lead to such tumors.
- Neurotransmitter abnormalities: When neurotransmitters do not work properly, problems may ensue. Examples include depression (serotonin) and attention-deficit/hyperactivity disorder (ADHD) and movement disorders in children.

Assessment of the Nervous System

Assessment of the nervous system requires a careful history from the child and family and a detailed physical examination. The examiner needs to determine if a neurologic disorder exists and, if so, the disorder's location and the patterns of impairment. For children with complex or severe neurologic problems, social, environmental, developmental, and family issues need thorough exploration. Historical information from children older than 3 years and from one or more family members provides the most accurate picture. Imaging or laboratory studies may be required. See Chapter 30 for guidelines on neurodevelopmental assessments of children.

History

History of Present Illness

- Onset: When did the first symptoms appear? Was the onset insidious or sudden? Was it associated with an injury or other event, such as an illness, surgery, poisoning, ingestion, or recent

exacerbating event? If yes, describe the event. Was the onset accompanied by any constitutional symptoms? How has the disorder evolved?
- Duration: How long have the symptoms been present? If intermittent, how long do symptoms last when they are present?
- Pain and/or headache: Location and character, path of radiation, severity, extent of disability produced, effect of various activities or stimuli (including light and sound sensitivity), aggravating or alleviating factors (e.g., changes in position or worse in the morning versus the evening or from day to nighttime), effects of previous treatment, and/or presence of pain or discomfort in other parts of the body. Morning awakening with headaches, vomiting, double vision, and/or balance problems require immediate referral.
- Sensory deficits: Changes in hearing, vision, taste, or smell; loss of pain sensation; vertigo; dizziness; numbness; and/or tingling.
- Injury: How, when (time and date), why, where? Mechanism or manner in which the injury was produced: accidental or nonaccidental? Immediate treatment provided? If past injury, at what age did the injury occur?
- Reflexive responses: Vomiting, coughing, primitive reflexes, tics, and/or clonus.
- Behavioral changes: Irritability, stupor, changes in appetite, lack of attention, random activity such as lip smacking, emotional lability, and/or changes in school performance.
- Motor and balance changes: Ataxia, spasticity, and/or increased or decreased tone.
- Review all systems plus:
  - Allergies, immunizations, hearing, vision, dental, skin integrity, behavior, nutritional status, and eating disorders
  - Medications (over-the-counter and prescription drugs) and recreational drug use
  - Other health conditions, treatments, providers, or resources involved with patient

Medical History

- Prenatal history: Maternal and paternal ages, alcohol, drug ingestion (including environmental toxins, such as fish contaminated with mercury and workplace exposures), radiation exposure, nutrition, prenatal care, injuries, hyperthermia, smoking, human immunodeficiency virus (HIV) or other infectious disease exposure, maternal illness, bleeding, preeclampsia, diabetes, previous abortions and stillbirths
- Birth history and neonatal course: Unusual circumstances around the birth, vaginal or C-section, complications, labor and delivery, birth weight/length/head circumference, resuscitation, trauma, congenital anomalies, feeding history (reflux, colic, frequent formula changes), jaundice, convulsions, infection, gestational age, sleep disturbances, multiple birth (premature, low birth weight, and infants who are small for gestational age face particular challenges regarding future development)
- Injuries or infections: Meningitis, encephalitis, head injuries, frequent musculoskeletal injuries that can suggest coordination disturbance or impulsive behavior
- Cardiovascular or respiratory disorders
- Environmental exposure to toxins (e.g., lead exposure)
- Metabolic disorders: Diabetes mellitus, thyroid disease
- Past neurologic disease and tests: TIcs, hydrocephalus, history of seizuers—type, description, frequency, onset, medications; genetic screening, or imaging studies done.

- Psychiatric disorders: Hallucinations, delusions, illusions
- Drug or other ingestions: Lead poisoning, dietary/herbal supplements, pharmaceuticals, maternal drug use while pregnant
- Urinary tract disease: Uremic syndrome manifests with confusion, convulsions, coma
- Physical growth

Family Disease History
- Family members with similar symptoms and features or genetic disorders; obtain a pedigree
- Consanguinity
- Neurologic disorders (i.e., migraine, epilepsy, neurodegenerative disorder, etc.)
- Intellectual functioning of family members

Developmental, Functional Health, and Social Context
- Review achievement plateau or loss of skills in all developmental milestone categories—language, gross motor skills, fine motor skills, social skills, and cognitive skills—and school performance. A variety of standardized assessment tools exist and should be used for this purpose. If concerns are identified, further evaluation with a neuropsychologist or healthcare provider with special expertise in child neurology or developmental pediatrics can be considered.
- Inquire about the effects of symptoms on all areas of health promotion and safety, nutrition, elimination, activity, communication, role relationships, values and beliefs, sexuality, sleep, family coping and resilience (management style), and stress tolerance, temperament, and self-concept. Masten (2014) describes resilience as the capacity of a dynamic system to adapt successfully to disturbances that threaten system function, viability, or development. Neurobiology, epigenetics, and developmental timing may play a role in resilience (or the ability to rebound) in children. Resilience in children ranges from the micro (how they function in their day-to-day lives) to the macro (their response to global threats and surprises).
- Inquire about the family composition including critical family events, such as additions or losses of family members, military deployment; home, neighborhood, and school environment; culture and ethnicity; exposure to violence or other stressors; strengths; resources; child care; financial issues (socioeconomic status, poverty); identified social supports (e.g., family, friends, health professionals); and community agencies involved with the family and child.

Physical Examination

The following should be noted:
- Growth pattern, including height, weight, body mass index (BMI), and head circumference
- Abnormalities of the skin (café au lait macules, angiomas, neurofibromas, ash leaf spots, or other pigmentation changes)
- Anomalies (e.g., unusual facies, shape and number of digits, low-set ears, symmetry of body)
- Cardiovascular system (including blood pressure)
- Musculoskeletal system: Gowers sign, calf muscle hypertrophy, muscle atrophy, and muscular function (strength and range of motion)
- Hearing

- Vision: Eye problems, including cataract, corneal clouding, cherry-red spot, change of visual function
- Tanner stage
- Hepatomegaly/splenomegaly

Specifics of the Neurologic Examination

The neurologic examination moves from the highest level of functioning to the lowest. Cerebral function is tested first; then cranial nerves (CNs), motor function, sensory function, coordination; and finally reflexes. The neonate's neurologic functioning is largely subcortical. Therefore, the examination is more limited than in an older infant or child. In infants and children, watching them carefully while collecting the history and actively playing with them in an age-appropriate manner provide a great deal of neurologic information. A tennis ball, some small toys (e.g., a small car), a bell, and something that attracts attention (e.g., a pinwheel) are useful throughout the examination.

Behavior and Mental Status
Test the following cortical functions:
- Responsiveness
- Judgment
- Language and speech (receptive, expressive, written); speech flow, voice quality, organization of thoughts
- Memory
- General knowledge
- Ability to relate to others: parents versus strangers
- Mood and affect

Cranial Nerve Function
The majority of the neurologic examination to test for CN function assesses CN II through CN XII because CN I (the olfactory) is difficult to assess in children and is not functional until the infant is 5 to 7 months old. Details for age-specific CN assessment techniques can be found in Table 46.2.

Motor Examination
Gait, posture, fine motor coordination, strength, muscle symmetry, quality of movement, and tone are aspects of the motor examination. Information can be gained from questioning the parent, because it is often difficult to elicit the needed information about these skills in the time and environment given for the examination.
- Muscle strength and size: Look at muscle size, contour, and symmetry. Have the child stand from a lying position. Look for Gower sign (i.e., a child using the arms to push off from bent knees and gradually climbing the body and straightening up, which is common in children with muscular dystrophy). Ask the child to move extremities against resistance and to grip your fingers hard. The presence of muscular hypertrophy or hypotrophy should be noted.
- Muscle tone: Muscle tone might be considered the resting strength of the muscle. Is the trunk control and/or extremities floppy, rigid, or somewhat stiff when the child is resting or active? How difficult is it to move body parts passively? Tone may be increased or decreased all over or differ between the legs and the trunk and arms. In addition, symmetry of muscle tone, bulk, and power should be noted.

TABLE 46.2	Cranial Nerve Assessment in the Young Child Versus the Older Child	
	Young Child	**Older Child**
CN I	Difficult to assess, typically not present prior to 5-7 months of age; grossly assess by observing grimace/response to strong odors	Differentiation of smells
CN II	Recognition of objects introduced into visual fields; funduscopic exam if tolerated	Visual acuity, visual fields, funduscopic exam
CN III, IV, VI	Pupillary response to light, extraocular movements with tracking object of interest, ptosis	Pupillary response to light, extraocular movements, ptosis
CN V	Grossly assess by noting response to light facial touch	Sensation to light facial touch, temporalis and masseter strength
CN VII	Note symmetry of facial expressions	Symmetry of smile and rise of eyebrows, orbicularis oculi strength, strength with cheeks puffed out
CN VIII	Response to soft sounds made outside of visual fields, observe for lateralization of sounds	Weber and Rinne; can use whisper test
CN IX, X	Symmetrical rise of soft palate, gag reflex	Symmetrical rise of soft palate, gag reflex
CN XI	Difficult to assess if unable to follow directions but can evaluate symmetry of sternocleidomastoid (SCM) movements	Turns head against resistance, shoulder shrug
CN XII	Tongue lies and/or protrudes midline	Tongue protrudes midline

- Fine motor coordination: Fine motor coordination is tested by having the child pick up small pieces, write, stack blocks, copy pictures, turn book pages, put puzzles together, or do other hand activities. In older children, assessment of their handwriting appropriateness for their age should be observed.
- Involuntary movements: Tremors are fine involuntary movements. *Chorea* or *choreiform movements* are large, irregular jerking and writhing movements. *Athetoid movements* are slow writhing movements, especially of the hands and feet. *Dystonia* is an uncontrolled change in tone with movement and a tendency to hyperextend the joints.
- Posture: *In an infant, assessing posture and muscle tone is fundamental.* Motor testing should include observation for symmetry of movements, consistent fisting of the hands, opisthotonos, scissoring, abnormal tone, and tremors. The infant's cry can be an indicator of several diseases (e.g., it is high pitched with increased intracranial pressure, it resembles mewing in cri du chat syndrome, and it is hoarse with hypothyroidism).

Sensory Examination

Evaluate functioning of the spinothalamic tract and dorsal column. The spinothalamic tract can be assessed by evaluating sharp/dull sensation and/or temperature sensation. The dorsal column can be assessed by evaluating joint position sense and/or vibratory sensation. If abnormality is identified, the examiner should attempt to localize the abnormality. The accuracy of interpretation of this part of the examination is always limited in infants and young children.

Reflexes

- Deep tendon reflexes include the biceps, brachioradialis, triceps, patellar, and Achilles jerk reflex.
- Superficial reflexes include the upper abdominal, lower abdominal, cremasteric, gluteal, and plantar.

- Primitive reflexes include sucking, rooting, asymmetric tonic neck, grasp, trunk incurvation, stepping (may be absent or decreased in a satiated or sleepy infant). In older children and adults, a positive Babinski is an important sign of upper motor neuron disease.

Coordination

Gait, balance, and coordination of movements are important parts of the neurologic evaluation. Gait should be assessed with the patient walking, and, if indicated based on history or exam findings, running. Patients should be asked to walk on their toes and then on their heels. For children school-aged and older, tandem gait should also be assessed. For younger children, balancing on each foot independently, hopping on each foot or jumping can be considered for assessment based on developmentally appropriateness. The Romberg test should be performed as a part of the balance assessment. Coordination of movements should be assessed using a developmentally appropriate combination of finger to nose movements, rapid alternating movements, and heel to shin movements. Abnormalities with the coordination examination such as ataxia, poor coordination and/or balance, dysmetria or dysdiadochokinesia should be noted and likely require further evaluation.

Cranium Examination

The neurologic examination should always include measurement of head circumference until the child is 2 years old (The American Academy of Pediatrics *Bright Futures*) or until 36 months old, per the Centers for Disease Control and Prevention (CDC), and if it appears abnormally large or small in an older child. Inspect the skull for symmetry and shape. Auscultation over the skull or above the eyes may reveal a cranial bruit. Percussion of the skull can give a sound resembling a cracked pot when the sutures are separated, as with increased intracranial pressure. The anterior fontanelle should normally be slightly depressed with very faintly perceived pulsations until its closure between 18 and 24 months.

Autonomic Nervous System

Alterations in blood pressure, sweating, or body temperature can be indicators of ANS problems.

Meningeal Signs

Evidence of meningeal irritation, such as with meningitis, includes positive Kernig and Brudzinski signs. A Kernig sign is positive if resistance and head or neck pain are elicited when the patient bends over from the waist and touches fingers to toes. In an infant, the Kernig sign can be tested by extending the leg at the knee with the infant lying supine. A positive sign can be as subtle as facial grimacing. A positive Brudzinski sign is evidenced by the patient spontaneously flexing the hip and knees after the examiner passively flexes the neck.

Diagnostic Studies

- Radiographs have relatively little diagnostic value for the neurologic system since the advent of computed tomography (CT) and magnetic resonance imaging (MRI). CT scans display differences in density of the intracranial tissues and structures. CT scans have a limited spectrum of use as routine study given the large amount of radiation exposure and evidence suggesting risk for neoplasia as a result of repeated exposure. MRI provides a higher quality image without radiation exposure and can provide additional information related to structure of the neurologic system (e.g., tumors, CNS, spinal cord, and malformations). There may be a medical need to order more specific tests, such as a magnetic resonance angiogram/venogram (used to detect blood vessel stenosis and aneurysms), magnetic resonance spectroscopy (used to detect metabolic changes in an isolated location of the brain), functional magnetic resonance imaging (fMRI; used to detect subtle metabolic changes in the brain that indicate how certain parts of the brain are working), or a positron emission tomography (PET) scan to assess blood flow, oxygen use, and sugar (glucose) metabolism. A neurologic consultant can advise when these would be necessary.
- Laboratory studies provide indicators of systemic disease, infection, or inflammation. They are especially important for children receiving medication for seizures. Drug levels, liver function, and blood studies may need to be monitored routinely.
- Genetic studies can be a valuable diagnostic tool for evaluation of etiology of various neurologic disorders.
- Lumbar puncture (LP) provides information about metabolism, neurotransmitters, infections, and trauma.
- EEG provide information about the electrical activity of the CNS, which is important in assessing function rather than structure.
- Ultrasonography can be useful in infants to evaluate brain tissue.
- Other studies can include polysomnography (helps assess narcolepsy, apnea of infancy, certain movement disorders, nocturnal seizures, and obstructive or central sleep apnea); electromyography (EMG; tests muscle activity); nerve conduction studies; evoked responses (brainstem—auditory, somatosensory, and visual); electronystagmography (measures eye movements to assess vertigo and post-concussion syndrome); and cerebral arteriography (visualizes cerebral blood vessels to

evaluate vascular anomalies and tumors). Children needing such studies would typically need to be referred to a neurology provider.

Management Strategies

Neurologic Development

Families are sometimes concerned about problems that providers believe are within normal limits. No neurology referral is necessary in these situations. The family needs to understand the anticipated pattern of neurologic development, including timelines and markers that they can use to monitor their child's development. Misperceptions about the implications of minor variations should be dealt with in the primary care setting, and the family should always be given the opportunity to return for further assessment or discussion if concerns remain. The temperament of the child and the child's learned social behavior versus pathologic symptoms may need to be addressed (e.g., breath holding versus seizures).

Educational Needs

Many neurologic problems in children affect learning, although neurologic problems are not synonymous with intellectual disability. Sensory problems may affect the child's ability to receive the input necessary for learning. Motor problems may affect both the child's ability to interact with the environment and the ability to communicate or indicate understanding. Management strategies should always include the educational needs of the child. Special infant or preschool early intervention educational programs can assist the child to learn by using the most appropriate learning modalities. Teachers often need assistance in understanding the limitations and strengths of the child. Parents need to be encouraged to develop close communication with the educational staff because this relationship is mutually beneficial for optimizing the learning experience of the child.

Referrals for Other Key Assessments

Many neurologic conditions are genetic in origin. Genetic implications are best communicated through formal genetics counseling; feelings of parental guilt need to be addressed. Physical therapy can be useful to help restore or maintain function or to teach new motor skills. The physical therapist should be accustomed to dealing with children. Physical therapy services are often combined with occupational and speech therapy to promote maximal development. Early intervention programs offer such assistance in many states and are generally free to qualifying patients. Should any services be denied, families should be advised to inquire about the appeal process in their state. Federal funding is available in most states for therapy programs for children from birth through 2 years old. For children where concerns about possible cognitive problems exist, referral to neuropsychology for formal cognitive functioning evaluation should be considered. Referral for social services is another key intervention. Children and families with children who experience multiple handicapping conditions frequently have ongoing issues of coping, monitoring, and management of medical and financial resources. Medical social workers, public health nurses, and case managers can provide invaluable assistance for these families for continuity and coordination of care.

Medications

A variety of medications are used to control the effects of neurologic problems. The majority of the time, these medications are used off-label in children when treating neurologic disorders. These may include antiepileptic drugs (AEDs), mood stabilizers, and antidepressants. Most require time for the effects to become apparent, need dosage adjustments, and are affected by the metabolism of the individual child. Periodic measurement of blood levels for some medications is needed either for dosing decisions or to monitor for potential side effects. Side effects of medications need to be weighed against their beneficial effects. Many medications require tapering of dosages when treatment is to be discontinued.

Specific Neurologic Problems of Children: Headaches and Head Injury

Headaches

Headaches of all types are one of the most common reasons for referral to a pediatric neurology practice (Kacperski, Kabbouche, O'Brien, and Weberding, 2016). They are common during childhood, increasing in frequency and incidence during adolescence. Headaches fall into two classifications—acute and chronic. Box 46.2 lists the more common types found in these classifications. A person may experience different types of headaches. Migraines may be particularly difficult to diagnose because manifestations in addition to description of symptoms are generally expressed differently and with less clarity during childhood.

The exact physiologic mechanism and etiology for many headaches have not been conclusively determined. Headache pain occurs when pain-sensitive intracranial structures are activated. Such structures include the arteries of the circle of Willis and some of their branches, meningeal arteries, large veins and dural venous sinuses, and part of the dura near blood vessels. Muscles around the head, neck, scalp, eyes, jaw, teeth, sinuses, and the external carotid artery and its branches are pain-sensitive structures external to the skull. Stimulation of these structures results in more localized pain that is carried by CN V, CN VII, CN IX, and CN X. In contrast, intracranial stimulation refers pain imprecisely (e.g., occipital lobe tumor). Regardless of the pathophysiologic basis for the headache, identifying treatment modalities that provide optimal management and relief is a key consideration for providers.

Prevalence rates for migraine headaches are reported to be: age 3 (3% to 8%), age 5 (19.5%), age 7 (37% to 51%), and 7 to 15 years old (57% to 82%; Antonaci et al., 2014). Children as young as 2 years have been described as having migraine-like symptoms. Before 10 years old, the incidence is higher in males than females. During teenage years, females have a higher headache incidence, with hormonal influences likely playing a role.

The provider must discern between symptoms that suggest that a headache is primary (e.g., tension-type, cluster, migraine type) or due to a secondary cause (e.g., tumor, hydrocephalus, infection, intoxication [lead, carbon monoxide], idiopathic intracranial hypertension, increased intracranial pressure). Key historical questions and a thorough workup are mandatory in order to exclude secondary headache etiology. In the absence of findings suggestive of a secondary headache, a more certain diagnosis of a primary headache disorder can be made. For nonorganic headaches, there may be no known etiology (e.g., no tumor, aneurysm, or

---

• BOX 46.2 **Most Common Types of Primary Headaches Seen in Primary Care Settings**

Diagnostic Criteria Based on History

Pediatric Migraine Headache
A. More than five attacks fulfilling features of B through D
B. Duration: 2-72 h
C. At least two of the following features:
 1. Bilateral or unilateral (commonly bilateral in young children; unilateral pain usually emerges in late adolescence or early adult life)
  a. Usually frontal/temporal
  b. Occipital location is unusual and should be carefully evaluated (occipital headache in children whether unilateral or bilateral is rare and calls for diagnostic caution; many cases are attributable to structural lesions)
 2. Pulsating quality
 3. Moderate to severe intensity aggravated by routine physical activity
 4. At least one of the following:
  a. Nausea and/or vomiting
  b. Photophobia and phonophobia (can infer from behavior)
 5. Not attributed to another disorder

Infrequent Episodic Tension Type Headache
A. At least 10 episodes occurring on <1 day per month on average (<12 days/year) and fulfilling criteria B through D
B. Headache lasting from 30 min to 7 days
C. Headache has at least two of the following characteristics:
 1. Bilateral location
 2. Pressing/tightening (non-pulsating) quality
 3. Mild or moderate intensity
 4. Not aggravated by routine physical activity, such as walking or climbing stairs
D. Both of the following:
 1. No nausea or vomiting (anorexia may occur)
 2. No more than one of photophobia or phonophobia
E. Not attributed to another ICHD-3 diagnosis

Chronic Tension Headache
A. Headache occurring on 15 days per month on average for >3 months (180 days/year) and fulfilling criteria B through D
B. Headache lasts hours to days or may be continuous
C. Headache has at least two of the following characteristics:
 1. Bilateral location
 2. Pressing/tightening (nonpulsating) quality
 3. Mild or moderate intensity
 4. Not aggravated by routine physical activity such as walking or climbing stairs
D. Both of the following:
 1. No more than one of photophobia, phonophobia, or mild nausea
 2. Neither moderate or severe nausea nor vomiting
E. Not attributed to another ICHD-3 diagnosis

ICHD-3, International Classification of Headache Disorders, 3rd edition.

Adapted from Headache Classification Committee of the International Headache Society (IHS). The international classification of headache disorders, 3rd edition (beta version). Cephalalgia. 2013;33(9):644–645, 660–661.

---

metabolic or structural cause). The International Headache Society (IHS) provides succinct clinical criteria (available at www.ihs-classification.org/en/) to help the provider evaluate, delineate between, and classify primary headaches (e.g., including migraines with or without aura and migraine subtypes) and secondary headaches. The International Classification of Headache Disorders 3 (ICHD) and IHS recommendations are the "gold standard" for current migraine and associated headache management. The ICDH-3 uses pediatric modifiers to further delineate pediatric migraine definition.

Clinical Findings

History. It is important to ask the child, not the parent (when possible), open-ended questioning and use drawings or other methods of eliciting information. Headache diaries may be used to gather history and track symptoms over time. Sample diaries can be downloaded at www.achenet.org/resources/headache_diaries/. There are also readily available online "apps" at no charge that can be used for monitoring headache frequency and severity. Children and teens can also use the calendar or other method on their personal device. Important questions to ask the child and parent(s) include:

- Duration: Recent severe onset is considered a worrisome history and warrants further investigation.
- Frequency and triggers: Children with recurrent, low-intensity headaches, with no neurologic changes, and who recover completely between episodes are unlikely to have serious intracranial etiology. Triggers can include ovulation or menstruation, exercise, food or odors, and stress. Other triggers can include chocolate, processed meats, aged cheeses, nuts, altered amounts of caffeine intake, dairy products, shellfish, and some dried fruits. Consistent findings such as perimenstrual exacerbation, food triggers, and a stable pattern to the headache with intervals of wellness over a long time period are reassuring symptoms that suggest a primary headache. In most cases, a specific trigger or etiology is not ever identified.
- Location: Occipital or consistently localized headaches can indicate underlying pathology. Facial pain might be sinusitis. Oculomotor imbalance can produce a dull periorbital discomfort, whereas temporomandibular joint pain tends to localize around the periauricular or temporal areas. The child should be asked if the pain is unilateral or bifrontal.
- Quality and severity of pain: Sharp, throbbing, or pounding pain may indicate vascular migraine. Dull and constant pain may be tension or organic. Severity can be assessed by asking about limitations to activities and missed school days, although there are other factors that contribute to missed school and limited activities. How many "different kinds of headaches" are experienced?
- Age of onset: Progression of the headaches over time and longest period of time without symptoms.
- Home management and medication dosages.
- Associated symptoms can include nausea, vomiting, visual changes, dizziness, paresthesia, neck/shoulder pain, back pain, otalgia, abdominal pain, hypersomnia, food cravings, confusion, ataxia, pallor, photophobia, and phonophobia. Changes in gait, personality, vision, mentation, or behavior that do not occur at the same time as the headache are worrisome and merit further evaluation with referral. There are some precursor symptoms and conditions that can indicate a predisposition to migraines. These include cyclic vomiting and abdominal migraine (see Chapter 40) and benign paroxysmal vertigo (BPV; discussed later in the chapter). Alone, they do not warrant extensive or expensive workups unless the diagnosis is unclear.
- Head trauma: If associated with headache, a subdural hematoma or post-concussive syndrome must be considered.
- Psychologic symptoms: Evaluate for the presence of depression, school stressors, or concerns about family functioning. Additional factors to consider include bullying or peer issues at

TABLE 46.3	Pediatric and Adolescent Migraine: With or Without Aura	
Classic Migraine With Aura	**Common Migraine Without Aura**
	No aura
Represent about one-third of children with migraines	Represent about two-thirds of children with migraines
Prodrome may precede headache up to 24 h characterized by irritability, elation/sadness, talkativeness/social withdrawal, food craving/anorexia, water retention, sleep disturbance	Also has similar prodrome features but more pronounced
Severe, unilateral often throbbing headache follows aura >30 min later; lasts 5-20 min; may generalize About 5% of children with classic migraine do not have headache with their auras	Headache in young children: Commonly bilateral, orbital, or frontotemporal; pain may radiate to face, occiput, neck Headache throbbing or pulsating; typically lasts <4 h but can last up to 72 h; moderate or severe intensity Activity aggravates, and sleeps relives headache Nausea or vomiting or both Sensitivity to light, sound, and movement

Information from Robertson WC. Migraine in children, Medscape (website) updated 2016. http://emedicine.medscape.com/article/1179268-overview#aw2aab6b3. Accessed January 8, 2018.

school, "over programming" and family expectations, and meal, hydration, and sleep status.
- Family history: Some children with headache, especially migraine, have a family history of headaches.

Distinguishing Features of Headache Types

- Migraine and migraine with aura: These can be differentiated by the presence or absence of aura symptoms (Table 46.3). Characteristics of migraines include nausea, abdominal pain, vomiting, unilateral pain, pulsating pain, relief with sleep, an aura, visual changes such as dark or blind spots, and a history of a family member (usually on the maternal side) with migraine without aura. Dizziness and motion sickness may be described. Infants and toddlers may present with irritability, sleepiness, and pallor. In preadolescents, common migraine symptoms are more likely. Nausea and vomiting might not occur, and the pain can be more frontal. Lethargy and sleep can follow. Visual changes are rare, and the pain quality is variable. Times between headaches are pain free. Pediatric migraine modifiers (variations in characteristics specific to pediatrics) include a duration of 1 to 72 hours and some evidence of pulsating (self-reported with heartbeat).
- Muscle contraction or tension headaches: The pain is dull and bifrontal or occipital, with nausea and vomiting occurring only rarely; there is no prodrome. Characteristic tension headaches feel like a band is squeezing the head. Tension headaches can last for days or weeks but generally do not interfere with activities. In children, it can be difficult to differentiate migraine and tension-type headaches. Psychosocial stress seems to be a

major factor in tension and chronic daily headaches in both children and adolescents.

- Medication overuse headaches: Resulting from the overuse of agents such as acetaminophen, NSAIDs, and "migraine medications" (e.g., Excedrin migraine), these headaches are comorbid with primary headache disorders and are increasing in frequency in children. Medication overuse is generally defined as the use of medications more than 15 days per month, manifested by a gradual increase in headache frequency even in the face of increasing analgesic treatment.
- Abdominal migraine: Discussed in Chapter 40, symptoms include midline pain, nausea, and vomiting with minimal or no headache. This rare and somewhat controversial diagnosis can be suggestive of complex partial seizures and may merit further evaluation.
- Secondary headaches (or those headaches that have a pathologic process): Key historical markers are sudden onset of hyper acute or increasing pain severity or accompanying neurologic signs. Box 46.3 describes red flags indicative of a pathologic process requiring immediate referral.

Physical Examination. A complete physical and neurologic examination is needed:

- Blood pressure, height and weight, and head circumference (all ages)
- Vision screen
- Eyes: Palpate for tenderness; check for papilledema, movements
- Ears: Patency of canals, normal tympanic membranes
- Neck: Palpate muscles; check range of motion for nuchal rigidity
- Sinuses (frontal and maxillary)
- Teeth and temporomandibular joints (mouth and jaw): Palpate and check range of motion
- Thyroid gland
- Bones and muscles of skull: Palpate for tenderness; listen for cranial bruits; check range of motion of cervical spine

- Extremities: Tandem gait
- Nerves: Palpate supraorbital, trochlear, occipital nerves; assess CN IX to CN XII
- Reflexes: Pronator drift test (Romberg)

Diagnostic Studies. Imaging studies are rarely indicated unless the history suggests intracranial pressure (see Box 46.3); there is a sudden onset, increased severity, or change in headache pattern (Box 46.4); the neurologic examination is abnormal; or when a complaint of "dizziness" is accompanied by double vision, a sensation of whirling, or confusion. CTs are generally out of favor due to radiation exposure. MRI is the first-line treatment unless imaging is extremely urgent and cannot be obtained immediately. Neuroimaging must be considered in children whose headaches do not meet specific criteria for a primary headaches syndrome, or who have an abnormal physical examination (Kacperski, Kabbouche, O'Broen, and Weberding, 2016). Neuroimaging should be obtained within a reasonable time period (2 to 4 weeks) to avoid progression of symptoms or a delay in treatment if an abnormality is found. An EEG should be obtained if the history and physical examination suggest a seizure process. If there is a history of external trauma, such as from a motor vehicle accident, cervical and spinal x-rays should be ordered.

Hemoglobin/iron studies and vitamin D levels may be helpful with persistent headaches.

Differential Diagnosis. Determining the correct headache classification or entity is part of the differential diagnosis. The need for corrective lenses is often considered a possible cause of headaches; however, the literature does not support this assumption. Brain tumors, abscesses, hematomas, and arteriovenous malformations are termed *space occupying lesions* because they crowd out other intracranial structures, precipitating edema and interfering with the normal actions of cerebrospinal fluid (CSF) and vessels. In children they are generally associated with ataxia, papilledema, intellectual changes, or behavioral changes. Infants may initially accommodate well to the increase in intracranial pressure because of the ability of their cranial sutures to expand.

Differential diagnosis is broad, including sinusitis, trigeminal neuralgia, pseudotumor cerebri, sleep disorder, hyperthyroidism,

---

• BOX 46.3 Red Flags Suggestive of Secondary or Pathologic Headaches

- Headache upon awakening from sleep that then fades; increases in frequency and severity over a period of only a few weeks; is persistent and unilateral
- First or worst headache
- Pain that awakens the child from sleep
- Vomiting but not nauseated that may relieve the headache, or intractable vomiting
- Visual disturbances, diplopia, edema of the optic disc (papilledema)
- Increased pain with straining, sneezing, coughing, defecation, or changes in position
- Occipital region and neck pain
- Educational, mental, personality, or behavioral alterations; irritability
- New onset seizures or facial or extremity numbness
- Unsteadiness or dramatic changes in balance, gait abnormalities
- Fever with or without nuchal rigidity
- Family history of neurologic disorders (e.g., brain tumors, neurofibromatosis, vascular malformations)
- Child has a history of a ventriculoperitoneal shunt, meningitis, hydrocephalus, tumor, or prior history of a malignancy.

From Kacperski, J, Kabbouche MA, O'Brien HL, Weberding JL. The optimal management of headaches in children and adolescents. Ther Adv Neurol Disord. 2016;9(1):53–68.

• BOX 46.4 Red Flags Suggestive of Intracranial Structural Pathology

Infants

Full anterior fontanelle
Open metopic and coronal sutures
Poor growth
Impaired upward gaze
Abnormal head growth
Shrill cry
Lethargy
Vomiting

Children

Headache described as severe, excruciating of recent onset, unlike any previously experienced headache, no period of normal functioning between episodes, *or* persistent and unilateral
Papilledema or abnormal eye movements (or one or both eyes suddenly turn in)
Ataxia, hemiparesis, or abnormal deep tendon reflexes
Cranial bruits
Personality changes

hypertension, cyclic vomiting, abdominal migraine, BPV, and temporomandibular joint dysfunction (see Table 46.4).

Management. Parents seek medical attention for pain relief for their child, in addition to reassurance that there are no intracranial processes occurring (brain tumors). Each child with headaches requires an individually tailored strategy that may include pharmacologic and nonpharmacologic modalities. The goals of treating acute-onset migraines include reducing frequency, severity, duration, and disability; improving overall quality of life and optimizing self-care abilities of the patient and family; reducing headache-related distress and associated psychologic symptoms; using beneficial and cost-effective treatment when needed and minimizing medication side effects; avoiding escalation of medications and reliance on those that are poorly tolerated or ineffective.

Medication. Nonsteroidal anti-inflammatory drugs are the first-line pharmaceutical for acute treatment. These include acetaminophen, ibuprofen, and naproxen sodium. Zofran can be used for vomiting associated with headaches. Many of the newer medications for migraines (e.g., triptans) have not been adequately tested for safety and efficacy in children and adolescents, with the

exception of sumatriptan and zolmitriptan (Table 46.5). Abortive medications should be taken at the onset of the headache and in the prescribed dosage, and should be available at home, school, or work. Importantly, the overuse of analgesics is to be avoided (more than three doses per week), as this can lead to medication overuse headaches (see "Complications").

Prophylactic therapy is considered when migraines cause a child to miss school regularly and/or when the child suffers severe migraine headaches two to four times a month or tension or migraine three to four times per week with a clear sense of functional disability. Medication classifications to consider include specific β-blockers, antidepressants, anticonvulsants, or calcium channel blockers (Table 46.6). The recent CHAMP (Childhood and Adolescent Migraine Prevention) study (2017) by Powers, Coffey, and Chamberlin found no significant difference in headache frequency between the use of placebo versus preventive headache medications (amitriptyline, topiramate, and placebo). The study postulated that pharmacotherapy may need to be reconsidered in this population.

Other treatments that are increasing in use include nutraceuticals. These are not regulated by the FDA and are used mainly for

TABLE 46.4 Differential Diagnosis for Headaches in Children

Cause	Characteristics
Drugs	
Cocaine	Migraine-like pain in patient with no history of migraine headaches
Marijuana	Frontal, mild
Analgesics, methylphenidate, oral contraceptives, steroids, and cardiovascular agents	Pain follows administration (of drug) or withdrawal (typical of analgesics)
Food additives (nitrites and/or monosodium glutamate are common)	Pain occurs only in individual genetically sensitive; pain is diffuse, throbbing after ingestion
Physiologic	
Vasculitis	Uncommon in children; can occur as part of a collagen-vascular disease, such as systemic lupus erythematosus
Chronic hypertension	Low-grade occipital pain on awakening or frontal during day
Eyestrain	Dull, aching pain behind eyes relieved when eyes are closed; caused by muscular fatigue during prolonged ocular convergence; not a refractive error
Temporomandibular joint (TMJ) syndrome	>8 years old; pain on one side of face and vertex of TMJ; may be a history of jaw injury
Whiplash and neck injury	Pain dull, aching in neck, shoulders, upper arms with poor neck rotation; no nausea or vomiting; caused by muscles contracted to "splint" area of dysfunction in cervical joint areas or soft tissue
Following partial or generalized seizure	Diffuse pain
Infectious illness (viral or bacterial): meningitis, sinusitis, pharyngitis, upper respiratory infection; fever	Pain may be nonspecific
Dental disease	Uncommon
Malfunctioning shunt or hydrocephalus	History of ventriculoperitoneal, ventriculopleural, or ventriculoatrial shunt
Toxins—carbon monoxide, lead	Dull, aching pain
Tumor, brain abscess, subarachnoid or intracranial hemorrhage	Progressive worsening; can be severe; worst in early morning and with lying down (brain tumors); occipital location
Exertional	Sharp and occurs after exercise
Posttraumatic head injury	Pain can be severe when associated with epidural hematoma; if not associated with epidural hematoma, can start within hours up to weeks following injury

TABLE 46.5 Therapies for Acute Pediatric Migraine

Drug	Dosage	Side Effects and Comments
Medications (These Should Be Tried First in Acute Management)		
Acetaminophen (gel capsule)	10-15 mg/kg PO every 4 h up to 500 mg every 4 h	For mild to moderate pain, acetaminophen has faster onset of action than ibuprofen.
Ibuprofen	7.5-10 mg/kg/dose PO every 6-8 h; maximum daily dose of 2400 mg	Use at onset of attack. Greater headache resolution than acetaminophen (rebound headache can occur). Take with food.
Naproxen sodium	Children >2 years old: 5-7 mg/kg PO every 8-12 h; Adolescents: 400 mg as initial dose; 200 mg PO every 8-12 h (maximum 1000 mg/24 h)	Safe and effective.
Ondansetron (Zofran)	Ages 4-11 years old, one 4-mg tablet *or* ODT tablet *or* 5 mL	For vomiting associated with headaches.
Migraine-Specific Abortive Acute Medications		
Sumatriptan: Children >12 years old when no response to analgesics	Nasal spray: 5 mg/spray; 5-20 mg each nostril once (may repeat every 2 h if headache unresolved; maximum dosage 40 mg/24 h) Subcutaneous (self-administered): 3-6 mg single dose Oral: 25-100 mg once (may be repeated every 2 h; maximum 200 mg/24 h); available in tablets: 25, 50, or 100 mg	Triptans are FDA approved for ≥18 years old; regarded as safe and well tolerated ≥12 years old. Used off-label in children <12 years old who have not responded to typical analgesic regimens. If the first dose is given in the outpatient setting, the patient should be monitored for 1 hour. Do not use in basilar-type and hemiplegic migraine or in those with cardiovascular disease, uncontrolled hypertension, or who have used MAOI in prior 2 weeks. Use with caution in patients who have migraine with aura.

FDA, U.S. Food and Drug Administration; *MAOI,* monoamine oxidase inhibitor; *ODT,* orally disintegrating tablet.

TABLE 46.6 Prophylaxis Therapies for Pediatric Migraine

Drug	Dosage	Side Effects and Comments
Antidepressants		
Amitriptyline	0.25 mg/kg/day PO at bedtime; may increase dose by 0.25 mg/kg/day every 2 weeks; maximum dosage 1 mg/kg/day	One of the most widely used agents, but off-label. Use with caution in children <12 years old. Order ECG if dosage exceeds 25 mg/day. Adverse effects: Somnolence, dry mouth, dysrhythmia.
Anticonvulsants		
Divalproex sodium	Dosage depends on preparation and age—consult pharmacology text.	Not for use in children younger than 2 years old. Adverse effects: Weight gain, heartburn, hair loss, dizziness.
Topiramate	Adolescent/adult immediate release oral preparation: Initially 25 mg once daily (in evening); may increase weekly by 25 mg daily up to 100 mg daily divided in two equal doses.	Gaining wide acceptance for efficacy. Indicated in epilepsy for children as young as 2 years old. Adverse effects: Weight loss, episodes of paresthesia, cognitive slowing, loss of appetite, dizziness, irritability; monitor any change in school/cognitive performance.
Anti-Serotonergic Agents		
Cyproheptadine	Not recommended <2 years old. ≥3 years and adolescents: 0.2-0.4 mg/kg/day divided in two equal doses; maximum daily dose 0.5 mg/day	Effective in migraine prophylaxis in ages 3-12 years. Adverse effects: Weight gain (due to appetite stimulation) and somnolence; sedation more problematic at doses higher than 4-8 mg/24 h.
Antihypertensives		
Propranol	35 kg: 10-20 mg three times a day >35 kg: 20-40 mg three times a day Adults: 80 mg/day divided every 6-8 h with a maximum of 160-240 mg/day in divided doses every 6-8 h	May take several weeks to a month to be effective. Do not use in children with history of asthma; use with caution in children with depression. Adverse effects: lowers blood pressure, depressive effects or exercise-induced asthma.

Maintain use for at least 4 to 6 months and then wean slowly.

5-HT, 5-hydroxtryptamine; *ECG,* electrocardiogram; *PO, per os* (by mouth, orally); *prn, pro re nata* (when necessary).

Data from Chawla J. Migraine headache medication, Medscape (website); 2017. http://emedicine.medscape.com/article/1142556-medication#2. Accessed January 8, 2018. Hershey AD. Migraine. In: Kliegman RM, Stanton BF, St. Geme JW, et al., eds. *Nelson Textbook of Pediatrics.* 19th ed. Philadelphia: Saunders/Elsevier; 2011:2040–2045; and Taketomo CK, Hodding JH, Kraus DM: *Pediatric & Neonatal Dosage Handbook.* 21st ed. Hudson, OH: Lexi-Comp; 2014.

headache prevention, not acute treatment. Some nutraceuticals currently under study are magnesium (400 mg qd in adolescent, 200 mg in younger children), Coenzyme Q10, Riboflavin, butterbur, omega-3 fish oil, and Migraleif (riboflavin, puracol, magnesium). Melatonin is sometimes used to help establish good sleep patterns (Meehan and O'Brien, 2018).

Common wisdom now recommends treating migraines throughout the school year and then gradually curtailing daily agents during the summer months. However, this is patient and provider dependent and requires discussion. An alternative for younger children is to use shorter courses of preventive medications (6 to 8 weeks) followed by gradual weaning.

Complementary Therapies. Biofeedback and cognitive-behavioral therapies, acupressure and acupuncture, nerve blocks or needling, osteopathic manipulation, yoga (downward facing dog and half warrior), physical therapy, and massage therapy can all contribute significantly to the management of chronic headaches. Essential oils and aromatherapy may also have a role. See Chapter 27 for further information.

Referral. Refer all patients with suspected organic (structural) headaches. Any patient with persisting chronic headaches may also benefit from referral to a headache subspecialist.

Complications. School absence, anxiety, and depression are known complications.

Patient and Parent Education. Family and patient education is key to migraine and chronic headache management. A self-administered rescue plan and headache hygiene or lifestyle modifications are essential to maximizing care.

1. Headache plan: Develop step-by-step plan for rescue, complementary, and headache hygiene. This plan should include a piece for school management. Include ice, rest, and a dark environment.
2. Headache diary: These are extremely helpful in figuring out triggers and monitoring patient progress.
3. Trigger factors: Every person's triggers are different, so identify and avoid them as possible. Consider dietary, physiologic, and environmental possibilities. Common food triggers contain tyramine, nitrates, or MSG, such as aged cheese, artificial sweeteners, caffeine, chocolate, citrus fruit, cured meats, nuts, onions, and salty foods. Physiologic triggers include hormonal changes, emotional anxiety, irregular eating or sleep, and stress. Environmental triggers include such things as weather changes, altitude, lighting, sun and odors, motion or activity (too little or too much).
4. Nutrition: Stress the importance of eating something for breakfast even if just a healthy smoothie or power bar, three meals a day at regular hours, and not skipping meals. Every meal should contain a protein and be high fiber and low fat to keep sugar and sodium levels normal. Avoid foods that trigger headaches (multiple lists are available online).
5. Fluid intake: Adequate hydration (4 to 8 glasses of water) to prevent dehydration-related headaches. Caffeine should be avoided. Sports drinks without caffeine may help during a headache.
6. Sleep: Get plenty of regular sleep (8 to 12 hours at night) and do not oversleep. Try to go to bed and wake up every day at close to the same time. Turn off all electronic devices 1 to 2 hours before bedtime. Do not keep phone in bedroom.
7. Exercise: Aerobic activity 30 to 45″ with increased heart rate and 5 to 10″ of stretching most days. Weight lifting does not count.
8. School: Headaches can result in significant loss of school attendance, but attendance should be mandatory. Develop a home/school headache plan. A quiet rest period may be allowed at school if needed, and school nurses can be helpful in developing a plan for this. If the child remains home, activities should be restricted to bed and all homework completed. The child should be returned to school if the pain improves during the school day. Minimize attention to the headache. Consider posture and lighting.
9. Electronic use: Limit total use of devices requiring screen time (TV, movies, videogames, computer, phones). Use nightlight/lowlight setting on devices in the later hours of the day.
10. Stress: Plan activities sensibly to avoid overcrowded schedules and stressful situations. The child and parents should be taught pain and stress management techniques, as well as relaxation exercises, including progressive muscle relaxation. If there are issues with posture and neck muscle tension, warm compresses before stretching can decrease tightness, and rolling the neck area with a tennis or racquetball also helps loosen tight muscles. If parent and child do not achieve relief, referral to a physical therapist is often helpful. Biofeedback training is also used.

Head Injury or Concussion

Traumatic brain injury (TBI) involves tissue damage to the brain and its surrounding structures, and injury can range from mild to severe. This discussion of head injury is limited to minor traumatic brain injuries, and indications of impending CNS compromise are presented. Most TBIs occur secondary to acceleration-deceleration or rotational forces, and long-term sequelae are much more likely in children with developing brains. Head injuries can be either open or closed. Open head trauma produces more focal injuries. Closed head trauma causes more multifocal or diffuse damage. Primary effects are from the initial injury and are related to mechanical forces that tear connections within the brain and cause contusions where the brain hits the skull surfaces (e.g., shaken baby syndrome). Axons to distant areas, fibers in the corpus callosum connecting the two hemispheres, or both can be torn. Contusions and hemorrhage can occur. Secondary effects of the trauma, such as hypoxia, ischemia, hypotension, brain swelling, hemorrhage, contusion, and seizures, can affect recovery.

TBI is a common cause of trauma in pediatrics, resulting in almost 3000 deaths, 29,000 hospitalizations, and 473,947 ED visits annually in the United States for children 0 to 14 years old (Faul, 2016). In the United States, approximately 2 to 5 million infants, children, and adolescents sustain head traumas of varying intensities each year when all ages during childhood and adolescence are considered. Common causes of TBI that are treated in the emergency department (ED) include falls, sports-related injuries, motor vehicle accidents, violence and assaults, and being struck by or against objects. Boys experience head injury twice as frequently as girls. Children with impulse control issues may experience more head trauma. Children who survive their injuries may have significant long-term disability.

TABLE 46.7	Glasgow Coma Scale	
Category	Best Response	Score[a]
Eye opening (E)	Spontaneous	4
	To speech (command)	3
	To pain	2
	None	1
Motor (M)	Obeys (command)	6
	Localizes	5
	Withdraws	4
	Abnormal flexion	3
	Extensor response	2
	None	1
Verbal (V)	Oriented	5
	Confused conversation	4
	Inappropriate words	3
	Incomprehensible sounds	2
	None	1

[a]Total score (E + M + V): maximum 15; minimum 3.

From Coulter DL. Head trauma. In Finberg LL, ed. *Saunders Manual of Pediatric Practice.* Philadelphia: Saunders; 1998:883–885.

The most common causes of head trauma differ according to age. Infants and toddlers are more likely to sustain head trauma from falls and nonaccidental trauma. Children 0 to 4 years old and 15 to 24 years old have the highest risk of TBI. Young children suffer head injuries from falls and pedestrian and bicycle accidents, whereas adolescents TBI most often occur from motor vehicle accidents, sports-related injuries, and assaults (CDC, 2017).

Young children are particularly vulnerable to mild traumatic brain injury (MTBI), also known as *concussion*. The CDC defines MTBI as a complex pathologic brain process that results from primary or secondary forces on the head that disrupt brain processes and functioning. MTBI results in physical, cognitive, emotional, and sleep symptoms (Table 46.7 or https://www.aan.com/go/ practice/concussion). Various types of head injuries can result in pathologic conditions: skull fracture, concussion, posttraumatic seizure, cerebral contusion, epidural hematoma, subdural hematoma, cerebral edema, and penetrating injury. Children can also experience subtle symptoms of TBI that may not appear until days or weeks after the injury.

Clinical Findings

History. Symptoms of TBI can mimic those of other medical conditions, thus making the diagnosis challenging. It is recommended that providers use an evidence-based assessment tool like the CDC's Acute Concussion Evaluation (ACE) tool (available at www.cdc.gov/headsup/pdfs/providers/ace-a.pdf).

The following information should be obtained:
- History of how injury occurred; if injury involved a fall, the height from which the child fell. Specifically, providers should ascertain injury cause, body part affected, forces, and circumstances.

- Loss of or alteration in consciousness or memory, confusion, irritability, inappropriate behavior, repetitive questioning
- Presence of vomiting and frequency
- Presence of headache, description of the headache pain
- Presence of blurred vision, diplopia, or other vision problem
- Numbness or loss of sensation, loss of balance, or difficulty walking
- Specific symptoms occurring at the time of injury and interval changes

Nonaccidental trauma should be strongly suspected when a head injury is present in a child without a history of a fall or with a history of a fall from a relatively low height of less than 4 feet. It is also recommended that a skeletal survey be obtained in children younger than 3 years old when head injuries are suspected, because younger children are at higher risk for skeletal trauma as well. With concerns about radiation exposure, there are data suggesting that skeletal surveys may be modified to limit radiation exposure (Bregstein et al., 2014).

Physical Examination
- Check vital signs (temperature, blood pressure, pulse, and respiration) and compare findings with normal parameters expected for children of varying ages. Changes in vital signs can indicate shock or intracranial hypertension.
- Perform a thorough physical examination (including a careful oral examination) and a careful neurologic examination including level of consciousness, mental status, motor function (both gross and fine motor), sensory function, CN functioning, and reflexes.
- Be alert to any signs of CNS involvement. The Glasgow Coma Scale (GCS; Table 46.7) and/or the Pediatric GCS (Table 46.8) has traditionally been used to measure the severity of head injury.
- Evaluation of concussion symptoms includes physical, cognitive, emotional and sleep (see Table 46.9) can be accomplished by questionnaire or "apps" such as the CDC Heads Up. (https://www.cdc.gov/headsup/resources/app.html) and ImPACT (https://www.impacttest.com/products/?ImPACT-Immediate-Post-Concussion-Assessment-and-Cognitive-Test-2).
- Examine the entire child for other signs of trauma, such as neck injury, internal abdominal injuries, or bone fractures. Periorbital hemorrhage ("raccoon-eyes"), ecchymosis behind the ear (Battle sign), blood behind the eardrum, and bleeding from the ears or nose indicate a basilar skull fracture and warrant immediate attention in an ED.
- Table 46.10 has a classification of head injuries based on key characteristics.

Diagnostic Studies. The severity of the head trauma dictates the need for investigative studies. All children with moderate (GCS 9 to 12) and severe (GCS 3 to 8) acute trauma should have a cranial CT scan. In addition, the need for skull radiographs and other views is determined by the severity of the head trauma. Indications for obtaining a CT scan include any of the following:
- Penetrating trauma or depressed skull fracture or signs of basilar injury
- Altered level of consciousness (excessive irritability or lethargy)
- Loss of consciousness (exceeding 1 minute)
- Amnesia about the injury
- Focal neurologic signs or deficit
- Persistent vomiting or seizures
- History of coagulopathy

CT is the preferred imaging technique for emergency situations, because it can be obtained rapidly, and the child can be

TABLE 46.8	Pediatric Glasgow Coma Scale		
	>1 Year	**<1 Year**	**Score**
Eye opening	Spontaneously	Spontaneously	4
	To verbal command	To shout	3
	To pain	To pain	2
	No response	No response	1
Motor response	Obeys	Spontaneous	6
	Localizes pain	Localizes pain	5
	Flexion-withdrawal	Flexion-withdrawal	4
	Flexion-abnormal (decorticate rigidity)	Flexion-abnormal (decorticate rigidity)	3
	Extension (decerebrate rigidity)	Extension (decerebrate rigidity)	2
	No response	No response	1

	>5 Years	**2-5 Years**	**0-23 months**	
Verbal response	Oriented	Appropriate words/phrases	Smiles/coos appropriately	5
	Disoriented/confused	Inappropriate words	Cries and is consolable	4
	Inappropriate words	Persistent cries and screams	Persistent inappropriate crying and/or screaming	3
	Incomprehensible sounds	Grunts	Grunts, agitated, and restless	2
	No response	No response	No response	1

TABLE 46.9	Mild Traumatic Brain Injury (Concussion) Symptoms		
Physical	**Cognitive**	**Emotional**	**Sleep**
Headache	Confusion	Abnormal irritability	Drowsiness
Nausea/vomiting	Altered concentration	Feelings of sadness or being "emotional"	Insomnia or hypersomnia
Difficulty with balance	Mental torpor	Abnormal feelings of being nervous	Difficulty falling asleep
Changes in vision	Altered memory		
Dizziness	Forgetfulness (especially conversations or recent events)		
Light or sound sensitivity	Needs to repeat or slowly answer questions		
Paresthesias			
Feelings of being dazed or stunned			

Adapted from Centers for Disease Control and Prevention (CDC). Heads up: facts for physicians about mild traumatic brain injury (MTBI). https://www.cdc.gov/headsup/partners/index.html. Accessed January 12, 2018.

monitored easily during the study. Skull fractures are better visualized on skull radiographs. Acute hemorrhage is detected more easily by CT (without contrast) than by MRI. If CT is ordered after several days (3 or more days past injury), it should be done both with and without contrast (to pick up extravasated blood). CT can demonstrate brain edema, midline displacements, hydrocephalus, loss of brain tissue, and most skull fractures. Although CT itself is a safe procedure, some healthy children require sedation or anesthesia (with some risk), so the benefits gained from CT should be carefully weighed against the possible harm of sedating or anesthetizing a child. In addition, CT scans obtained for asymptomatic children may show incidental findings

TABLE 46.10	Classification of Head Injuries Based on Key Characteristics			
Classification	Glasgow Coma Scale[a]	Neurologic Focal Deficit[b]	Loss of Consciousness	Other Neurologic Findings
Mild	13-15	No	No or brief loss (<30 min)	May have linear skull fractures
Moderate	9-12	Focal signs	Variable loss	May have depressed skull fracture or intracranial hematoma
Severe	≤8	Focal signs	Prolonged loss	Often have depressed skull fractures and intracranial hematoma

[a]Either initial or subsequent scores.
[b]Neurologic focal deficit (e.g., hemiparesis, reflex asymmetry, Babinski sign, abnormal cranial nerve findings).

that lead to subsequent unnecessary medical or surgical interventions. There also are current concerns regarding the amount of radiation in a CT; however, it remains the imaging of choice for closed head injuries. Schonfeld et al. (2014), working with the Pediatric Emergency Care Applied Research Network (PCARN), found that age-based TBI prediction rules identify children at low risk who can safely avoid CT. Further, they identify observation as an important strategy and note that parent and patient preference should also play a role.

In 2018, the FDA approved the Brain Trauma Indicator (BTI), a blood test to evaluate mild TBI in adults. Results, which are available in 3 to 4 hours, measure two brain specific biomarkers that appear within 12 hours of injury and predict which patients may have detectable intracranial lesions and require CT. Reliability for the presence of lesions was 97.5%, and for no visible lesion, it was 99.6% (FDA, 2018).

Differential Diagnosis. The history of a head injury is the key to diagnosis. Differentiating minor head trauma that will resolve on its own from more extensive brain injury is problematic at times. Head trauma may cause injuries of the scalp, skull, dentition, and intracranial contents. Children with intracranial lesions after minor closed head injury are not easily distinguishable clinically from the large majority with no intracranial injury. Children with mild nonspecific signs such as headache, vomiting, or lethargy after minor closed head injury may be more likely to have intracranial lesions than children without such signs. However, these clinical signs are of limited predictive value, and most children with headache, lethargy, or vomiting after minor closed head injury do not have demonstrable intracranial injury. Some children with intracranial injury do not have any of these symptoms and have a normal neurologic assessment. Because of these findings, some experts recommend a liberal policy on the ordering of cranial CT scans following any head trauma.

Management. Management issues related to only mild and moderate head injuries are discussed in this chapter. The level of consciousness is a key determinant of the child's prognosis. Prompt identification of a deteriorating level of consciousness and quick medical and/or surgical intervention are essential components of the management plan.

Management of the Child With Minor Closed Head Injury and No Loss of Consciousness. Observation in the clinic, office, ED, or home, under the care of a competent caregiver, who understands what signs and symptoms to watch for, is able to closely and reliably monitor, and can quickly bring the child back for treatment or access emergency medical services if necessary, is

recommended for children with minor closed head injury and no loss of consciousness. Observation implies regular monitoring by a competent adult who would be able to recognize abnormalities and seek appropriate assistance.

Management of the Child With Minor Closed Head Injury and Brief Loss of Consciousness. For children with minor closed head injury and brief loss of consciousness (several minutes) and no other neurologic or physical deficits reported or detected on examination, observation in the office, clinic, ED, hospital, or home, when under the care of a competent caregiver may be used. However, CT scanning along with observation is also accepted. If the provider is not assured that the child will be closely and reliably monitored at home, hospitalization is indicated.

Management of the Child With Moderate Head Injury or Worrisome Symptoms. A child with a skull fracture or transient neurologic findings whose level of consciousness is normal may be admitted for overnight observation. Children with moderate head injuries (GCS 9 to 12) may require admission or prolonged observation in the ED until their mental status stabilizes. Children with severe head injuries (GCS less than 8 or coma and physical findings) need immediate hospital admission and consultation with a neurologist and critical care team. Children with any of the following should be hospitalized:
- Changing vital signs
- Seizures, altered mental status or slurred speech
- Prolonged unconsciousness (>30 seconds)
- Persisting memory deficit or focal neurologic signs
- Depressed or basilar skull fractures
- Persistent headache (particularly with stiff neck)
- Recurrent vomiting or unexplained fever
- Unexplained injury (suspected child abuse)
- CT scan or MRI findings that are worrisome

Complications. Initial complications of head injury can include concussion, posttraumatic seizures, cerebral contusion, epidural hematoma, subdural hematoma, intracerebral hematoma, subarachnoid hemorrhage, acute brain swelling, and penetrating injuries. Second impact syndrome (SIS) occurs when the brain swells catastrophically, after a person suffers a second concussion prior to resolution of symptoms from an earlier injury. This second impact can occur any time after an initial concussion, and even a mild concussion can lead to catastrophic results. SIS is a concern. Intracranial lesions, particularly epidural hematomas, are life threatening and have significant complications. Features indicative of serious injury include loss of consciousness (longer than 1 minute), persistent vomiting, depressed level of consciousness, seizures, unequal pupil size, severe headache, and GCS less than 15.

Posttrauma Sequelae and Post-Concussion Syndrome. Minor head injury without neurologic changes generally has no resulting physical deficit. However, subtle cognitive deficits may be present for weeks to months. TBI severity is correlated with a risk for psychiatric conditions and long-term neurologic deficits (CDC, 2017). After a more severe injury, cognitive function changes generally will not improve after 12 months, but speech and motor difficulties may continue to improve for up to several years. A neuropsychological evaluation may be helpful to plan appropriate educational and behavioral management for selective cases of concussion. Such testing can provide an objective measure of brain-behavior relationships. Ransom (2015) found that children with post injury academic issues such as failure to complete schoolwork or memory issues without any supports in place may lead to depression and anxiety. Conclusions call for a key partnership between provider and school in guiding a successful return to school.

Children (2 to 6 years old) may be more impaired than adolescents secondary to immature brain development and general vulnerability. However, children and adolescents are more likely to show improvement in cognitive and social skills evolving slowly over several years than adults who suffered the same degree of head trauma.

Typical postconcussive syndrome in adolescents is manifested by headache, dizziness, irritability, and impaired ability to concentrate. In younger children, it is manifested as aggression, disobedience, behavioral regression, inattention, and anxiety. Sleep-related issues also occur. Cognitive and physical brain rest are the essential components of the management plan. The treatment plan must be communicated to school personnel—teachers and coaches—and should identify a gradual/step-wise return to school with modifications outlined related to academics. Once academics are stabilized, return-to-play guidelines can be initiated. Chapter 19 discusses this aspect. Because sports-related head injuries are common in children and teens, prescreening using standardized neuropsychological testing is often encouraged for student athletes as a baseline measure. Assessments are then completed at various intervals after an injury has occurred to assess for cognitive deficits.

Patient and Parent Education. Give caregivers written patient education materials and make every effort to ensure that they not only understand the instructions about observing the child and indications for immediate follow-up but will also comply with them (Box 46.5).

In addition, parents should also be informed that sometimes symptoms from head trauma occur days, weeks, or months after the initial trauma. Eisenberg and colleagues (2014) found the following sequence of events: headache is prevalent immediately after a head injury, emotional symptoms may develop later during the recovery, and cognitive symptoms span the entire injury spectrum. Long-term complications may include cognitive difficulties, concentration problems, sleep issues, and irritability.

Neurologic sequelae following mild head injury in children often improve or resolve within 9 to 12 months. These sequelae include:

- Headache, vertigo or dizziness
- Difficulty concentrating or loss of memory
- Poor school performance and neurobehavioral problems
- Depression, fatigue

• BOX 46.5 Head Injury Education Key Points for Parents

Parents or caregivers should be given specific instructions regarding:
- Waking the child every 2-4 h for the first 24 h after injury, ensuring the child wakes easily and is able to stay awake for a few minutes.
- Making sure child is moving his or her arms and legs normally.
- Giving only acetaminophen, if needed, for headache or relief of soft tissue pain.

Contact the health care provider or take the child to an ED if the following symptoms are observed:
- Increased drowsiness, sleepiness, inability to wake up, unconsciousness
- Vomiting more than twice
- Neck pain
- Watery or bloody drainage from ear or nose
- Seizures or fainting
- Unusual irritability, personality change, confusion, or any unusual behavior
- Headache that gets worse or lasts more than a day
- Unequal pupils, blurred vision, abnormal or changing hearing, or speech
- Gait abnormality (e.g., clumsiness or stumbling), weakness of any muscle of arms, legs, or face

Prevention

- Use appropriate seat restraints when riding in motor vehicles.
- Protect children from falls in the home or from playground equipment. Discourage the purchase of residential trampolines.
- Wear helmets when using bicycles, skateboards, scooters, motorcycles, inline skates, snowboarding, ski racing, and when appropriate for sports participation. The proper fitting of helmets is important.
- Ensure that sports teams and trainers use state of the art helmets and training equipment and follow state laws with regard to concussion prevention.

Disturbances of Head Growth

Macrocephaly

Macrocephaly is defined as a head circumference more than two standard deviations above the mean for age and gender or one that increases too rapidly. "Large" heads may be genetic and not clinically significant; the provider's initial evaluation should include measuring both parents' head circumferences. Macrocephaly can also be attributed to hydrocephalus, megalencephaly (enlarged brain), subdural hematoma, tumor, thickening of the skull, or other problems. Benign familial macrocephaly may occur as a part of, or be related to, a genetic syndrome (anatomic or metabolic), such as Soto syndrome (cerebral gigantism) or neurofibromatosis type 1 (NF1). Infants with anatomic megalencephaly have macrocephaly at birth, but those with a metabolic etiology are normocephalic at birth. In cases of excessive volumes of CSF, the fluid may be located within the brain (in the ventricular cavities) or outside the brain, in the subarachnoid spaces.

A CT scan can be diagnostic with consultation or referral if abnormal. A CT interpretation of benign enlargement of the subarachnoid spaces (BESS) generally requires no further treatment. The subarachnoid enlargement resolves by school age, although the macrocephaly remains. The use of CT scans remains controversial due to the radiation exposure, especially if serial CTs are done, increasing cumulative exposure over time.

Hydrocephalus

See Chapter 29 for the discussion on congenital hydrocephalus.

Acquired hydrocephalus has a variety of different etiologies, pathologies, and diagnostic criteria. In general, hydrocephalus is acquired from several means, including transitional (diagnosed as a child); longstanding ventriculomegaly or chronic congenital hydrocephalus; an identifiable etiology, which may include hemorrhage, cerebral trauma, infection, or mass; and those with idiopathic normal pressure hydrocephalus (Hamilton, Gruen, and Luciano, 2016).

Clinical recognition of the signs and symptoms of hydrocephalus is imperative because acute presentation, if untreated, can lead to catastrophic results. Investigation and intervention is paramount to avoid morbidity and mortality. A cardinal feature of acute hydrocephalus is increased intracranial pressure, which itself is associated with a well-recognized pattern of symptoms that may include altered level of consciousness, headaches, nausea, and vomiting, which is worse in the morning. Box 46.4 presents red flags for increasing intracranial pressure in infants and children. Other signs and symptoms may include a new onset of esotropia or horizontal diplopia, which is caused by an abducens nerve palsy occurring from increased intracranial pressure and possible herniation of the brainstem. New onset of a gait disturbance may also be present. These findings are urgent and indicate an immediate need for further evaluation by a neurologist or neurosurgeon.

Hydrocephalus may be associated with a Type 1 Chiari Malformation, which may cause recognizable symptoms including motor deficits, ataxia, nystagmus, and others, but also may be asymptomatic until early adulthood (Witiw, Hachem, and Bernstein, 2017). Often these malformations are not diagnosed until early adulthood and may be associated with occipital-suboccipital headaches.

Microcephaly

Microcephaly is defined as head circumference two standard deviations below the mean for age and gender, or a head in which the growth decelerates from the normal pattern. On examination the skull appears to be normally shaped; palpation may reveal some overlapping bones along the suture lines. This disorder can result from conditions in which the brain never formed correctly because of genetic or chromosomal abnormalities. Disease processes that interfere with normal brain growth can also be causative (these infants have normal head circumferences at birth). Brain damage that occurs prenatally may or may not always be evident initially in the newborn; a decreasing or plateauing head circumference curve may start to occur after the infant reaches 3 to 6 months of age. Infants with microcephaly due to a perinatal event such as hypoxic-ischemic encephalopathy frequently also have developmental delay, disorders of tone, and sometimes seizures.

Management of microcephaly is supportive, may involve an interdisciplinary team, and is directed toward optimizing functionality from resulting deficits. Referral to a neurology provider should be made for diagnostic purposes and a brain MRI should be done as a baseline at some point.

Craniosynostosis

Skull malformations may be due to primary or secondary causes. Congenital (or "true" or "primary") craniosynostosis involves premature fusion of one or more cranial sutures. Syndromic craniosynostosis accounts for about 8% of craniosynostosis cases and is associated with many familial syndromes including Apert and Crouzon in addition to several other less familiar syndromes

(Governale, 2015). Craniosynostosis syndromes usually have an autosomal dominant inheritance pattern, however penetrance and expression are quite variable (Governale, 2015). In addition, spontaneous mutations can occur. In this disorder, premature closure of a major suture, such as sagittal, results in cranial deformity as the skull flattens over the closed suture(s). Increased intracranial pressure may result as the brain tries to grow within the confined space, but this does not always occur. Primary craniosynostosis occurs in 1 per 2,000 to 2,500 births (Governale, 2015), is ethnically neutral, and can vary in type and prominence between genders. The sagittal suture is most commonly fused (referred to as *scaphocephaly* or *dolichocephaly*), is found in 1 in 5000 births, and accounts for about half of all cases. Fig 46.3 illustrates the different descriptions for skull deformities seen.

Secondary synostosis results when outside forces put pressure on the growing cranium, causing the skull to become misshapen, referred to as *deformational plagiocephaly*. This is most commonly seen with premature infants (termed *deformational scaphocephaly*), after shunting an infant with hydrocephalus, in children who have microcephaly and aberrant positioning in utero, during birth, or perinatally because of torticollis or positioning traditions. Many infants who were not premature have positional plagiocephaly, partially due to the success of the "Back to Sleep campaign" and lack of enough time prone ("tummy time") to avoid this. This occipital deformity is not accompanied by compensatory suture line growth that would be seen with a primary lambdoidal synostosis.

Clinical Findings

Physical Examination. Monitor cranial symmetry for the first year. This is best done by looking down at the top of the head, noting the position of the ears and cheekbones. Typically, a deformational plagiocephaly will form a parallelogram characterized by unilateral occipital flattening and contralateral occipital bossing, ipsilateral ear displacement anteriorly, and associated parietal bossing and cheekbone prominence on the side of the occipital flattening. In contrast, the deformity of lambdoidal craniosynostosis does not assume a parallelogram shape, may be present at birth, and has less frontal asymmetry than positional plagiocephaly. The ear ipsilateral to the occipital flattening is posterior and displaced inferiorly to the contralateral ear, and this deformity may become more severe over time. Fig 46.4 compares these deformities.

Symmetry of neck rotation should also be included in the examination to rule out torticollis. Infants with torticollis typically have some limitation of neck rotation away from the side of their occipital flattening and may require physical therapy for symptom management and parental education.

Diagnostic Studies. A CT scan is standard for a skull shape deformity; 3D CT scans are also becoming more available and aid in this diagnosis. Deformational plagiocephaly does not require imaging studies in most situations when the history and physical examination are diagnostic. Consider further neuroimaging with MRI if the neurologic examination is abnormal.

Differential Diagnosis. In about 5% of young infants, the frontal metopic suture may normally be prominent and identified as "frontal bossing." This prominence is not clinically significant, does not signify craniosynostosis, and does not require intervention.

Management. If craniosynostosis is suspected, refer the child to an experienced pediatric neurosurgeon or craniofacial plastic surgeon. Treatment is often surgical, but in some cases reassurance and education, repositioning, exercises for any associated

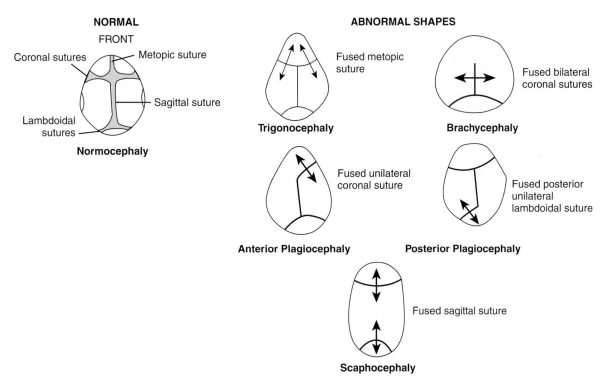

• **Fig 46.3** Characteristics of Skull Deformities Seen With Craniosynostosis. (Adapted from Cohen MM Jr. Craniosynostosis update 1987. *Am J Med Genet Suppl.* 1988;4:99–148.)

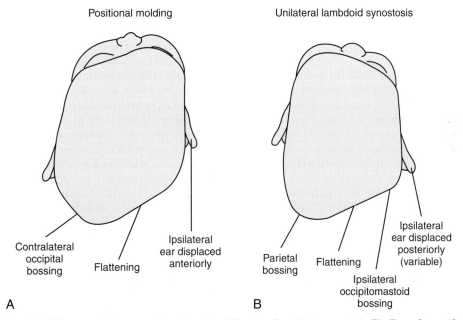

• **Fig 46.4** Differences between positional molding (A) and unilambdoid synostosis (B). (From Gruss JS, Ellenbogen RG, Whelan MF. Lambdoid synostosis and posterior plagiocephaly. In: Lin KY, Ogle RC, Jane JA, eds. *Craniofacial Surgery: Science and Surgical Technique.* Philadelphia: Saunders; 2002.)

torticollis, and clinical follow-up are sufficient. If the condition is noted to be genetic, management needs to be planned according to the problems associated with the syndrome, including genetic counseling and long-term follow-up.

PCPs can anticipate concern about deformational plagio-cephaly by counseling parents at the newborn visit to (1) lay infant down in the Back to Sleep position for sleep, alternating positions (i.e., left and right occiputs); (2) when awake and

observed, place infants prone for "tummy time" or in a side posi-tion to reduce the flattening; (3) during feedings, have parents avoid holding an infant in a manner that puts pressure on the flattened part of the skull; and (4) have infants spend minimal time in car seats or other upright devices that maintain supine positioning. Improvement should occur over a 2- to 3-month period if interventions are instituted early. Throughout the first year, emphasize tummy time. Monitor head shape during all

ILAE 2017 Classification of Seizure Types Expanded Version

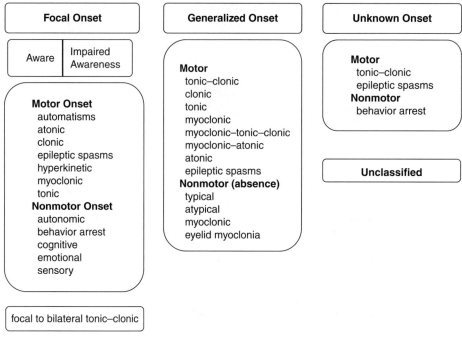

• **Fig 46.5** ILEA 2017 Classification of Seizure Types. (From Fisher RS. An overview of the 2017 ILAE operational classification of seizure types. *Epilepsy Behav.* 2017;70:271–273. https://doi.org/10.1016/j. yebeh.2017.03.022.)

well-child visits. The majority of positional plagiocephalies are self-limited; sometimes physical therapy is indicated in recalcitrant cases (e.g., with torticollis).

For positional plagiocephaly, orthotic cranial molding helmet therapy may be prescribed when repositioning and exercises are not successful. The helmet is individually engineered to allow growth where needed and restrict it where the head is prominent; it needs to be worn for 23 hours a day for 4 to 6 months, can lead to odor and skin breakdown, is costly, and may not be covered by health insurance. However, Ditthakasem and Kolar (2017) identify a lack of evidence supporting the use of helmets including controversies around cost and long-term outcomes. In addition, they postulate that prevention of positional plagiocephaly is paramount, via parent and caregiver education about the importance of proper head positioning. Of concern, Martiniuk, Vujoivich-Dunn, et al. (2017) reviewed 19 articles in a systematic review about deformational plagiocephaly. Their review suggested that plagiocephaly is a marker of elevated risk of developmental delays meriting close monitoring of infants and prompt referral for intervention services, though there may be confounding factors in this conclusion such as parenting, socioeconomic status, and so forth.

Epilepsy, Febrile Seizures and Benign Paroxysmal Vertigo

Epilepsy

Epilepsy is a neurologic disorder characterized by recurrent unprovoked seizures. A seizure is an event caused by an abnormal electrical signal arising from within the cerebral cortex. Seizures can present in many different ways. The two primary types of seizures are generalized (arising across the cortex) and focal (arising from one specific area of the cortex). The International League Against Epilepsy (ILAE) has created a system for classification of seizure types and presentation (Fig 46.5). The primary care provider (PCP) should be familiar with the presentation for various types of seizures. The diagnostic criteria for epilepsy is a single unprovoked seizure with a known increased risk for future provoked seizures OR two unprovoked seizures that occur greater than 24 hours apart OR diagnosis of an epilepsy syndrome (Fisher et al., 2014). Within epilepsy, there are several types of epilepsies. The ILAE has also published a classification of the types of epilepsies which factors etiology along with seizure type (see Fig 46.6). It is important for providers to remember that epilepsy is a clinical diagnosis based on the aforementioned criteria. Although diagnostic studies can be of great value, the diagnosis itself is often based on historical and physical findings.

Clinical Findings

History. Historical questioning should include the following:
- Description of the seizure: Focal or generalized (if known), semiology (presentation characteristics of the seizure), loss of consciousness, aura, length of postictal sleep or confusion, duration of the episode, history of prior seizures and associated illness or injury
- Any underlying medical diagnosis (e.g., diabetes, renal disease, cardiovascular disorder)
- Previous CNS infection or birth trauma
- Intrauterine infection, trauma, bleeding
- Toxic exposure or drug use
- AED noncompliance (stopped abruptly or doses missed) or changes in drug manufacturer or change to generic from name brand
- Family history of seizures
- Any history of developmental or learning delay or regression

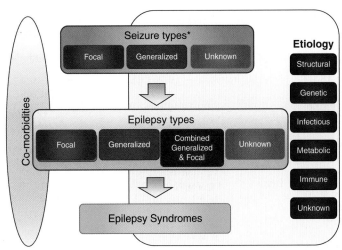

• **Fig 46.6** Framework for the Classification of Seizures. *Denotes onset of seizures. (From Scheffer IE, Berkovic S, Capovilla G, et al. ILAE classification of the epilepsies: position paper of the ILAE Commission for Classification and Terminology. *Epilepsia*. 2017;58:512–521. https://doi.org/10.1111/epi.13709.) http://onlinelibrary.wiley.com/doi/10.1111/epi.13709/full

Physical Examination. The following should be determined on physical examination:
- Weakness or focal abnormalities on the neurologic exam
- Presence of seizure activity during the examination
- Hypertension (for renal disease)
- Signs of systemic disease or cardiovascular disorder
- Skin findings suggestive of neurocutaneous syndromes (i.e., café au lait spots, ash leaf spots, hypopigmented macules, or facial hemangiomas)
- Signs of head trauma
- Transillumination of the skull in infants

For children presenting with staring spells that are questionable for childhood absence epilepsy (CAE), the provider can perform 2 to 3 minutes of hyperventilation using a pinwheel or similar object. Often times, this will provoke a seizure, which is diagnostic for CAE. Appropriate safety precautions should be taken prior to performing this, and the child and family should also be informed of the intent prior to proceeding.

Diagnostic Studies. These are the typical diagnostic test recommendations:
- Complete blood count (CBC), including platelets and liver function tests (LFTs)—useful for diagnostic purposes or as a baseline before AED therapy is started.
- Metabolic screen may be considered later in the workup, not initially.
- Blood glucose—standard in all patients.
- Urine and serum toxicology—only if illicit drug exposure is suspected.
- Genetic testing—expanding use in epilepsy assessment but not routinely ordered. Need typically determined by specialist.
- LP—only if child is younger than 6 months; child of any age with persistent changes in mental status or failure to return to baseline functioning; patients with meningeal signs.
- EEG—standard in all children after first unprovoked seizure. An abnormal EEG supports the diagnosis and can be useful in differentiating the type of epilepsy. However, a normal EEG when the child is not seizing does not rule out epilepsy. Video electroencephalogram (VEEG) over 1 to 6 days is another option to help characterize events concerning for seizures.

- MRI—imaging studies are not routinely indicated for generalized seizures provided the seizure is followed by a normal neurologic examination and return to baseline mental status. Imaging is recommended: (1) following a focal seizure or if the EEG reveals focal electrographic abnormality; (2) if the patient demonstrates cognitive changes after several hours and postictal focal dysfunction (signs of increased intracranial pressure, such as found with tumors, abscesses, strokes, or vascular malformations); (3) if the seizure lasted more than 15 minutes; (4) in infants younger than 6 months old; and (5) if any new onset of focal neurologic deficit has occurred.
- CT scan—used only in emergent cases of marked cognitive, motor, or neurologic dysfunction of unknown etiology
- Polysomnography (simultaneous EEG, electromyogram, electrocardiogram [ECG], and electrooculogram) can be useful to assess symptoms occurring during sleep.

Differential Diagnosis

Consider breath-holding, inattentive staring, benign movements (sleep myoclonus, infant jitteriness, etc.), self-stimulation, tantrums, cyclic vomiting, BPV, syncope, migraine headaches, gastroesophageal reflux, night terrors, conversion disorder, nonepileptic seizures, metabolic problems, tumors or other CNS problems, or a cardiovascular problem. Tics (involuntary, spasmodic, nonrhythmic, repetitive movements) are stereotypic but not associated with impaired consciousness and at times can be suppressed by the patient.

Management

Referral. If epilepsy is suspected, refer to a provider with expertise in child neurology for diagnosis and initiation of treatment. The PCP can monitor stable children with epilepsy, including continuing the prescription for their AED, monitoring laboratory studies, and performing case management. However, most neurology providers will perform these tasks at routine follow up visits.

Initial Management of Epilepsy. Medication is generally the first-line treatment for epilepsy. The goal for treating epilepsy should always be two-fold: no seizures and no side effects. AED

TABLE 46.11 Common Antiepileptic Medications Used in Children

Medication	Seizure Type	Metabolism	Drug Level	Common (Severe) Adverse Effects
Levetiracetam	Focal, Generalized	Enzymatic hydrolysis	6-20 mg/L	Mood changes, headache, **significant aggression or depression**
Lamotrigine	Focal, Generalized	Liver	1-15 mg/L	Somnolence, headache, dizziness, **Stevens-Johnson syndrome (SJS)**
Oxcarbazepine	Focal	Liver	13-28 mg/L	Hyponatremia, dizziness, ataxia, drowsiness, **SJS, blood cell count changes**
Topiramate	Focal, Generalized	Liver	2-25 mg/L	Paresthesia, weight loss, cognitive change, renal stones, **glaucoma, metabolic acidosis**
Lacosamide	Focal, Generalized	Liver	5-10 mcg/mL	Dizziness, headache, vision change, ataxia, **syncope, arrhythmia, suicide**
Valproic acid	Focal, Generalized	Liver	50-100 mcg/mL	Weight gain, tremor, hair loss, liver toxicity, pancreatitis, bone marrow suppression
Ethosuximide	Childhood Absence Epilepsy	Liver	40-100 mcg/mL	Upset stomach, headache, weight gain, **blood cell count changes, SJS**
Carbamazepine	Focal	Liver	4-12 mcg/mL	Tiredness, dizziness, photosensitivity reaction, **SJS, hypersensitivity**
Phenobarbital	Neonatal seizures, Status Epilepticus	Liver	15-40 mcg/mL	Sleep change, sedation, gastrointestinal symptoms, **irreversible cognitive change, blood cell count changes, SJS**

selection should be individualized based on type of epilepsy but should also account for other factors, such as potential side effects, medical history, gender, and age. Providers should be aware that much of AED use in children is done off-label, but there is a large body of evidence supporting this practice. Medication information including potential side effects should be reviewed with the patient and family prior to initiating therapy. Table 46.11 provides a vital overview of common AEDs used in children. For children who fail treatment with two AEDs (achieving maximum therapeutic dose with continued seizures), their epilepsy is considered to be intractable. Nonpharmacologic treatment options should be considered for intractable epilepsy.

Therapeutic Considerations. Therapeutic considerations include medication compliance, the presence of side effects, and (when appropriate) the therapeutic drug level. Laboratory testing for potential side effects is dictated by the risks associated with each specific AED. Key points include:

- Some children with epilepsy can be controlled with subtherapeutic blood levels.
- Some children can be free of side effects at levels beyond the therapeutic range.
- Half-lives and steady state concentrations can vary when new AEDs are introduced or when other non-AEDs are being taken (e.g., antibiotics, antipyretics). Half-lives can be longer with the introduction to a new drug; steady concentrations (and elimination) of the drug are achieved at five half-lives.
- If gastrointestinal side effects occur, decreasing the dosage and increasing the frequency of administration may help; try changing to an enteric-coated pill or taking the medication after eating.
- Administration of AEDs no more frequently than twice daily can achieve better compliance.

- The first signs of toxicity usually include sedation, changes in behavior, and changes in cognition and balance; other drug toxicities may cause decreases in memory and attention span or interpersonal relationship difficulties. It is important to note that some children may exhibit these changes and have drug levels within the normal range.
- Metabolites of the drugs can cause hypersensitivity side effects.
- Monitor routine drug levels based on the clinical picture with trough levels for some AEDs.
- Some herbal products interfere with seizure control.

Antiepileptic Drug Withdrawal. For many children with epilepsy, it may be possible to taper medication if the child is able to go 2 years without a seizure. Historically, child neurology providers obtain an EEG prior to medication withdrawal, but more recent literature suggests that this test is not necessary (Tolaymat et al., 2015). Some children are not considered candidates for AED withdrawal based on type of epilepsy, etiology, or exam/diagnostic findings, but the decision remains individualized. Most AEDs can be tapered for withdrawal over a period of 6 to 8 weeks, but the provider should always review this prior to beginning taper (Tolaymat et al., 2015). Only one AED should be withdrawn at a time. If seizures do recur, most likely within the first 6 months off medication, the child should be placed back on AED therapy, typically the same medication and dose prior to withdrawal. Epilepsy can be considered resolved when a child is able to go for 10 years without a seizure, with 5 of those years being off medication (Fisher et al., 2014).

Ketogenic Diet. The ketogenic diet is a valuable nonpharmacologic treatment option that should be considered for children with intractable epilepsy (particularly nonsurgical candidates) or as a first-line treatment for specific types of epilepsy (such as GLUT1 transporter deficiency). The ketogenic diet is a very rigid diet that allows for high ratios of fats to protein plus carbohydrates in order to transform the body's primary source of energy from glucose to ketones (ketosis). The traditional ketogenic diet ratio is 4:1, but more recently, lesser ratios have been implemented successfully. Strict adherence to the prescribed ratio is necessary as deviation from this ratio can often result in breakthrough seizures. The ketogenic diet is typically co-managed by a healthcare provider with expertise in child neurology and a dietician with special knowledge related to the ketogenic diet. Prior to initiating the ketogenic diet, specific metabolic conditions must be ruled out. Many centers also screen children and/or families to determine if they are capable to follow the diet and also to assess emotional functioning and problem solving. Children must be screened for growth and nutritional status prior to starting the ketogenic diet. The ketogenic diet is typically initiated in the hospital setting to allow for more extensive education and monitoring. However, outpatient initiation can be completed successfully under the right conditions. Side effects of the ketogenic diet include vitamin and mineral deficiency, abdominal pain, constipation or diarrhea, fatigue, slowed growth, and renal stones.

Surgical Interventions. Surgical intervention for intractable epilepsy can be another effective nonpharmacologic treatment option. Surgery is now considered earlier in the treatment process than it was in the past. All children with intractable focal epilepsy should be evaluated at a comprehensive epilepsy center to determine if they may be a candidate for surgical intervention. There are a variety of surgical options that can be considered and are individualized based on the patient. These can range from resection of a seizure focus or hemisphere (sometimes curative) to procedures that disrupt pathways in the brain (generally palliative), such as with a corpus callosotomy or multiple subpial transection. Postoperatively, some children will be able to reduce the number of AEDs they are taking, but this is not always the case.

An additional surgical option is implantation of a vagus nerve stimulator (VNS). This is an option that can be considered for intractable epilepsies, particularly those that may not be candidates for resective surgical intervention. The VNS is an implanted device where the generator is typically placed in the left anterior chest wall inferior to the clavicle. A wire lead is then run from the device and coiled around the ipsilateral vagus nerve. While the mechanism is not entirely well understood, electrical impulses are sent regularly from the generator up the vagus nerve to the brain. Many patients with a VNS see improvement in seizure control, and some are able to decrease AED use. The VNS also has a magnet that can be swiped across the generator in case of a prolonged seizure to function as a rescue option to stop the seizure. Device programming can be done in the office setting, and standard dosing increments are available from the device manufacturer.

Counseling. It is important that children and their parents understand the diagnosis, treatment, plan for follow up and prognosis. For children, this should be presented in an age appropriate manner. Children often experience psychosocial stress surrounding their diagnosis, and providers should address psychosocial stress and the child's coping skills. Parents are encouraged to treat the child as they normally would. Support groups or similar resources can be helpful to both children and their families. Many AEDs are teratogenic; therefore, contraception and thorough patient and family education is essential for females of child-bearing age.

Safety. Uncontrolled seizures can present safety hazards for an unsupervised child. The child and family need to consider situations that the child will be in and be sure that someone knows what to do if a seizure occurs, including school personnel. Seizure first aid should be taught to family members. Swimming alone is never recommended, but swimming, contact sports, and climbing are to be allowed if the child is well controlled and there is constant supervision during these activities. Children should be counseled to wear a helmet any time they are riding a toy with wheels (bike, skateboard, scooter, etc.). Safety helmets worn at all times are sometimes warranted if falls and head injury occur frequently. Driving is often a concern for adolescents with epilepsy. While driving laws vary by state, it is generally recommended that adolescents be restricted from driving until they have been seizure-free for 6 months.

Immunizations. The decision to give the diphtheria-tetanus-acellular pertussis (DTaP) vaccine to children with epilepsy or other neurologic conditions needs to be made on an individual basis. Oftentimes, consultation with the child's neurology provider may be warranted. The CDC recommends deferring DTaP until a child's neurologic status is clarified and stabilized from a known progressive neurologic disorder, such as infantile spasms, uncontrolled epilepsy, or progressive encephalopathy. This vaccine is contraindicated in children who have experienced encephalopathy (e.g., coma, decreased level of consciousness, or prolonged seizures), not attributable to another identifiable cause within 7 days of administration of a previous dose of DTP or DTaP (Kroger, Duchin, and Vazquez, n.d.).

Complications. Status epilepticus (SE) are seizures that may be continuous, or frequent, without recovery between episodes. SE can either be classified as Convulsive SE or Nonconvulsive SE based on clinical presentation. In general, SE refers to a seizure that lasts for greater than 30 minutes or multiple seizures without recovery between events. A child who has Convulsive SE may be at increased risk for morbidity and mortality due to lack of oxygenation, decreased cerebral perfusion, metabolic acidosis, hypoglycemia, hyperkalemia, lactic acidosis, increased temperature, and increased intracranial pressure. Such an occurrence needs to be handled as a medical emergency. SE can be triggered by an acute brain infection, progressive neurologic disease, medication failure or noncompliance, electrolyte imbalance, or rarely, a febrile seizure in an otherwise healthy child without other risk factors. Adverse outcomes can include behavioral problems, acquired intellectual disability, and focal deficits. Administration of a rescue medication in the prehospital setting by parents or caregivers (including school personnel) is recommended. Medications that are commonly used for this purpose include rectal diazepam, intranasal midazolam, or buccal clonazepam. The need for a rescue medication prescription and medication selection is typically determined by the neurology provider. Not all children with epilepsy require a prescription for a rescue medication. Patients who are given a rescue medication should be evaluated by a healthcare provider following administration.

Febrile Seizures

Febrile seizures are the most common type of seizures in childhood and occur in up to 5% of children. A febrile seizure is a seizure that occurs in conjunction with a fever. The fever is typically defined as 38°C and can occur before or after the seizure. Febrile seizures typically occur between the ages of 6 to 60 months. Seizures occurring with fever outside of those age parameters warrants further evaluation. Febrile seizures can be classified as either simple febrile seizures or complex febrile seizures. Simple febrile seizures present as generalized seizures and last for less than 15 minutes. Complex febrile seizures can present with generalized or focal seizures, duration greater than 15 minutes, and/or with clustering of seizures (multiple seizures without recovery between). In rare cases, children may experience febrile SE (seizure lasting >30 minutes), which rarely stops spontaneously and requires prompt intervention. Most children in febrile SE require one or more medications to end the seizure.

The etiology of febrile seizures is unclear and by definition excludes seizures that are caused by intracranial illness or are related to an underlying CNS problem. The risk is higher in children with a family medical history for febrile seizures or in those with predisposing factors (e.g., neonatal intensive care unit [NICU] stay more than 30 days, developmental delay, day care attendance). Nearly two-thirds of children will experience only an isolated febrile seizure without recurrence. Risk factors for recurrence include (1) first febrile seizure prior to 18 months of age, (2) low degree of temperature at time of the seizure, (3) fever not present until after the seizure, or (4) family history of febrile seizures.

Clinical Findings

History. Include the following:
- Description of seizure duration, type (generalized or focal), frequency in 24 hours
- Relationship of the seizure to a febrile episode and level of temperature
- Any abnormal neurologic findings noted before the seizure (is not consistent with a febrile seizure)
- Family history of afebrile or febrile seizures
- Maternal smoking in the perinatal period
- Prematurity or neonatal hospitalizations for more than 28 days
- Parents' perception of development of child

Physical Examination. The physical examination is the same as that described earlier for epilepsy.

Diagnostic Studies. Diagnostic studies include the following:
- An LP should be considered if history or physical suggest acute bacterial meningitis or other CNS infection (Kimia et al., 2015).
- Blood glucose, CBC, calcium, electrolytes, and urinalysis are not routinely recommended solely for febrile seizure. However, age, gender, and findings from the H&P should direct decision-making for these laboratory studies.
- EEG should be performed for all complex febrile seizures. EEG is not typically indicated for simple febrile seizures.
- MRI for complex febrile seizure or for focal exam findings.

Differential Diagnosis

Consider sepsis, meningitis, metabolic or toxic encephalopathies, hypoglycemia, anoxia, trauma, tumor, and hemorrhage. Febrile delirium and febrile shivering can be confused with seizures. Breath-holding spells can mimic febrile seizures; however, breath-holding is always related to crying or tantrums. Epileptic seizures are unprovoked but may occur during an illness.

Management

Routine seizure first aid should be initiated as follows:
- Protect the airway, breathing, and circulation if the seizure is still occurring. Place the child in a side-lying position to prevent aspiration or airway obstruction.
- Do not put anything into the child's mouth during the seizure.
- Time the duration of the seizure. For seizures lasting greater than 5 minutes, call 911.
  Fever management:
- Reduce the fever with acetaminophen or ibuprofen (oral or suppository) after the seizure has stopped, although the use of antipyretics will not necessarily prevent another febrile seizure.

Prophylaxis for Recurrent Febrile Seizures. Prophylactic pharmacologic management is not indicated. Providers can prescribe a rescue medication (rectal diazepam, intranasal midazolam or buccal clonazepam) to be used for prolonged febrile seizures or clusters of febrile seizures in the prehospital setting. Antipyretics can reduce the discomfort associated with a fever but do not alter the risk of having another febrile seizure.

Patient and Parent Education

The family should receive information about febrile seizures, risks, first aid, and management. Education should include risk factors for recurrence, reassurance that nothing can be done to prevent the seizures, and that no long-term consequences are associated with simple febrile seizures and most complex febrile seizures. The PCP can reassure parents that simple febrile seizures are adequately managed in the primary care setting. However, with complex febrile seizures, further evaluation and/or referral may be warranted. Families should be advised to report any future febrile seizures to the PCP.

Complications

Death or persisting motor deficits do not occur in patients with febrile seizures outside of febrile SE. No indication has been found that intellect or learning is impaired. Children with complex febrile seizures may have a slightly increased risk to develop epilepsy later in life.

Psychogenic Nonepileptic Seizures. A psychogenic nonepileptic seizure (PNES) may be difficult to distinguish from epileptic seizures, even after direct observation. It is a common manifestation of a conversion disorder in children. Many children with PNES have an existing diagnosis of epilepsy, making the diagnostic evaluation process much more complicated. In such cases, the PNES serve as attention-seeking behaviors for the child who misses the attention gained before seizure control was achieved with their epilepsy diagnosis. PNES are most commonly seen in adolescent females (Takasaki, Stransky, and Miller, 2016). Psychosocial stressors (family, peers, school) and/or traumatic events are often revealed during the history if the provider inquires.

Distinguishing characteristics of PNES include the following:
- Unilaterally or bilaterally coordinated motor activity, more like thrashing and jerking (scissor-like movements), rather than characteristic tonic-clonic movements; no aura or complaints of malaise; heart palpitations; feeling like choking before seizure onset
- Occur only before a witness; occur at home; do not interrupt play, may occur at school
- Normally reactive pupils to light
- Are situation specific and have a gradual onset
- No associated tongue biting or injury
- Have an abrupt recovery—no postictal state
- Discomfort, distress expressed; sometimes ataxia, fumbling; consciousness may be impaired, but the patient is not unconscious
- No incontinence
- No EEG changes, even during episodes

Treatment for PNES is generally directed by psychology/psychiatry and often centers around cognitive behavioral therapy (Takasaki, Stransky, and Miller, 2016). Most instances of PNES improve or cease after the diagnosis is made and interventions are in place. Previous somatic complaints, stress factors, peers, family, and illness modeled in the home should be assessed. If suspected, but the history is unclear, a VEEG or admission to an Epilepsy

Monitoring Unit (EMU) may be helpful. No AEDs are used in the case of children who do not have an underlying epilepsy diagnosis.

Benign Paroxysmal Vertigo

BPV is a syndrome characterized by episodic vertigo. BPV is one of the most common causes of episodic vertigo in children (Gioacchini et al., 2014). Symptoms generally present before the child is 4 years of age. BPV is commonly associated with a family history of migraine headaches and the development of migraine headaches later in childhood. If the child also presents with a history suggestive of migraine headaches, consider vestibular migraine as a possible differential diagnosis.

The history may include rapid onset of an attack (vertigo, disequilibrium, and nausea) that lasts seconds to minutes, daily attacks that occur in clusters over several days and then may not recur for weeks or months, and a possible history of motion sickness. Symptoms are likely to have resolved by the time the child is examined. BPV is not associated with hearing loss, tinnitus, or loss of consciousness. The physical examination findings consist of

- Acute unsteadiness: The child may fall or refuse to walk or sit; the child may grab on to a parent or object for steadiness.
- Nystagmus may be present within but not between attacks (Robertson, 2015).
- Vomiting and nausea may be present and be quite prominent.
- Child appears frightened and/or pale.
- Child may be lethargic or drowsy; some children may sleep and return to normal activities on awakening.
- Neurologic examination is essentially negative except for abnormal vestibular function.

Because the symptoms of BPV can appear to mimic cranial neuropathies, MRI of the brain will often be ordered to assess for tumor or other structural abnormality. An MRI of the brain would be essential if abnormalities were identified during the neurologic examination between episodes. One possible diagnostic study involves ice water caloric testing to detect abnormal vestibular function. However, this test is rarely done due to the intense discomfort that it produces. Other diagnostic studies are available if questions about the diagnosis persist. Referral to a vestibular specialist should be considered to pursue additional diagnostic testing.

Typically pharmacologic intervention is not indicated, given the short duration of the attacks (Jahn, 2016). Once a diagnosis is made, parental reassurance is key. Spontaneous resolution of symptoms associated with BPV should be expected by 8 to 10 years of age (Jahn et al., 2015).

Cerebral Palsy and Hypotonia

Cerebral Palsy

Cerebral palsy (CP) is a chronic nonprogressive motor disorder that is the result of damage to the areas in the brain that control motor function. Symptoms appear within the first few years of life. Early detection of CP is very important because this allows for early diagnosis and treatment, which can have a significant impact on long-term outcomes. Depending on the area affected and the extent of damage, children with CP can also have disturbances in sensation, perception, cognition, communication, and behavior. In addition, epilepsy and musculoskeletal problems secondary to the motor impairment are often present (Ketelaar et al., 2014). The degree of brain injury is individual, and the degree of impairment may not be directly associated with the degree of injury. There are three major types of CP: (1) spastic, (2) athetoid (or dyskinetic), and (3) ataxic. See Table 46.12 for more details related to each type of CP, as well as descriptors for presenting symptoms.

The prevalence of CP is 1.5 to more than 4 per 1000 live births (or 1 in 323) across many studies (CDC, 2019). CP was once believed to be caused only by birth complications (neonatal or perinatal asphyxia or trauma); however, it is now believed that there are a wide range of factors that may contribute to the development of CP. One more recent development was the discovery that some cases of CP are of genetic etiology (Novak et al., 2017). The etiology remains unknown in a large percentage of cases. The current diagnostic critieria for CP is motor dysfunction and either abnormal neuroimaging or risk factors for CP (Novak et al., 2017).

Clinical Findings

History. The history should include prenatal and birth histories and assessment for the presence of associated comorbid, developmental, and functional health problems. Risk factors are listed in Box 46.6. Inquire about the following in history taking:

- Prenatal/birth history risk factors
- Hearing and vision or ocular problems, such as strabismus, nystagmus, and optic atrophy
- Change in growth parameters, especially decreased head circumference
- Early head injury, meningitis, or seizures
- Muscle tone: hypotonic/hypertonic; tone can be hypotonic before 6 months old, then become hypertonic in the affected extremities
- Developmental milestones: They may be delayed but should still be attained depending on the extent of CP; persistent primitive reflexes are common (e.g., Moro and tonic neck). Hand preference before 1 year old is highly suspect.
- Feeding history of regurgitating through the nose, inability to coordinate suck and swallow, inability to advance the diet to textured foods—oral-motor coordination problems
- Irritability or depressed affect (including unusual sleepiness) as a neonate
- Difficulty with movement, grasp and release, self-feeding, and head control to look around; inability to change position per developmental level
- Communication problems, either in language or speech proficiency

Physical Examination

- Skin: Dermatologic signs of other syndromes should be evaluated. Skin lesions suggestive of a neurocutaneous syndrome should be examined.
- Orthopedic examination: Scoliosis, contractures, and dislocated hip(s) may be present after they have had months or years to develop.
- Neurologic examination: The following may be seen:
  - Asymmetric or abnormal deep tendon reflexes and movement
  - Ankle clonus, no fasciculations
  - Tone increased although tone is occasionally decreased; hypotonia before 6 months of age is common; tone may also be mixed
  - Minimal muscle atrophy

TABLE 46.12　Terms Used to Describe Abnormal Motor Exam

Term	Description	Associated Impairments
Movement Type		
Spastic	Inability of a muscle to relax	Often evident after 4-6 months; retarded speech; convergent strabismus; toe-walking; flexed elbows; delayed walking until 18-24 months; one third have seizures
Athetoid	Inability to control muscle movement (continuous, writhing movements)	Infant has difficulty feeding as a result of tongue thrust, is initially hypotonic with head lag; increasing tone with rigidity over time; speech delay
Ataxic	Problems with balance and coordination	Tremors
Body Part Involved		
Diplegic	Affects both legs more than both arms	Most have limited use of legs; can walk often with aids; walk typically "scissor-like" with knees bent in and crisscross over each other
Hemiplegic	Affects one side of the body (upper extremity more than the lower extremity)	Often not detected at birth; right side often more affected than left; 50% develop seizures; growth arrest of affected limb(s); individuals usually able to walk
Tetraplegic/ quadriplegic	Affects all four extremities, trunk and head	Affects upper extremities more than lower; 50% with grand mal seizures; IQ impairment can be severe; most unable to walk or stand
Specific Problems With Movement or Function		
Dystonia	Involuntary, slow, sustained muscle contraction	Abnormal posture, writhing motion of arms, legs, trunk
Choreic	Disorganized tone	Uncontrollable jerky movements fingers/toes
Tremor	Involuntary, rhythmic movements of opposing muscles; can affect extremities, head, face, vocal cords, trunk	
Ballismus	Violent, jerky movements; may affect only one side of body	
Rigidity	Stiffness	

IQ, Intelligence quotient.

• BOX 46.6　Risk Factors for Cerebral Palsy

Congenital
Maternal vaginal bleeding between the 6th and 9th month of pregnancy
Severe proteinuria late in pregnancy; preeclampsia
Antepartal hemorrhage, maternal stroke, seizure
Maternal hyperthyroidism and/or maternal intellectual disability
Maternal/intrauterine infection exposure (evidenced by chorioamnionitis)
Labor and delivery complications; breech presentation; traumatic delivery
Fetal distress; APGAR score of less than 3 at 10 min
Small for gestation age; low birth weight (<1000 g); prematurity, post maturity
Multiple births; microcephaly; intrauterine drug exposure
Intracranial hemorrhage; neonatal seizure; coagulopathy in fetus or newborn

Acquired
Meningitis, encephalitis
Head trauma, nonaccidental trauma, motor vehicle accident, falls, near drowning

- Persistent primitive reflexes (e.g., tonic neck and Moro after 6 months of age)
- Delayed reflexes (e.g., parachute reflex remains absent after 9 to 10 months of age; side-protective reflexes remain absent after 5 months of age)
- Preferred handedness before 1 to 2 years of age
- Abnormalities of head size such as macrocephaly or microcephaly
- Vision and hearing: Visual refractive errors occur in half of children; strabismus is found in a third. Hearing problems may have resulted from the initial brain insult.
- Development: Assess gross motor, fine motor, language, and personal social skills. Motor milestones are commonly delayed. Note quality of movements (e.g., smoothness of gait, grasping, and clarity of speech). Standardized tools to assess motor dysfunction should be used within the appropriate age groups including the Hammersmith Infant Neurological Examination (ages 2 to 24 months) and the Gross Motor Function Classification System Extended and Revised (GMFCS). It should be noted that the GMFCS score is more reliable in children over the age of 2 years (Novak et al., 2017).
- Feeding: Note a reversed swallow wave; uncoordinated suck and swallow, which may cause reflux and respiratory problems; decreased tone of the lips, tongue, and cheeks; increased gag reflex; involuntary tongue and lip movements; increased sensitivity to food stimuli; poor occlusion; and delayed inhibition of the suck reflex.
- Evaluate the diet, height, weight, and BMI for adequate nutrition.

Diagnostic Studies

- Imaging studies: An MRI of the brain aids in visualizing potential structural abnormalities of the brain.
- Chromosomal and metabolic studies: These studies can be done to identify genetic causes of CP or other genetic disorders that could explain the presenting symptoms. It has been suggested that genetic testing may become a routine part of the diagnostic evaluation for CP in the future (Novak et al., 2017).
- LP if sepsis is suspected.

Differential Diagnosis

The first and main requirement is to differentiate central from peripheral disorders. CP is always a central disorder. Exam findings in patients with CP will support this distinction. Many other conditions can have CP-like motor involvement. These conditions include organic causes, such as sepsis from intrauterine infections, fetal alcohol syndrome, hydrocephalus, tumors, agenesis of the corpus callosum or other brain malformations, Tay-Sachs disease, phenylketonuria, Lesch-Nyhan syndrome, spinal cord injury, hypothyroidism, muscle diseases, seizures, and many genetic and metabolic disorders (e.g., cerebral folate deficiency), or acquired causes, such as a severe TBI.

Management

The management of a child with CP requires dealing with multiple associated problems (see Box 46.7). The care described here can serve as a model for the management of children with a variety of neurologic problems.

- *Referral of suspected cases:* Children with CP should be evaluated and cared for at centers that have an established interdisciplinary team of healthcare professionals, including providers with expertise in developmental pediatrics, gastroenterology, orthopedics, neurology, nursing and/or advanced practice nursing, speech pathology, physical and occupational therapy, education and psychology, and social work. Care may also involve an ophthalmologist, feeding clinic and nutritionist services, and genetic counseling.
- *Family education about the diagnosis:* It is imperative that families understand that CP is nonprogressive, but without intervention, motor dysfunction may progressively worsen. They need to understand that the extent of brain damage is not always related to the level of disability; no one can predict what the future for a given child will be. Children who receive special services—physical therapy, occupational therapy, speech therapy, and other interventions—have better outcomes than children who do not, and early intervention typically leads to better outcomes. United CP has educational materials and a variety of services available.
- *Family support:* In general, families grieve when given the diagnosis of CP and need support during this time. Support groups or opportunities to meet other families with affected children are often helpful. The emotional needs of siblings must not be overlooked. A social worker can be helpful to families trying to cope with complex health problems.
- *Financial resources:* CP services are long term and expensive and adaptive equipment, such as leg braces and wheelchairs, need periodic maintenance and replacement. Many children will be eligible for Supplemental Security Income or state program benefits for the severely handicapped. Respite care may be available. The Individuals with Disabilities Education Act of 1997 (IDEA) requires children with disabilities to be assessed for and instructed in the use of assistive devices along with

appropriate referrals to regional centers. Medical social workers and public health nurses can help in connecting families to appropriate services.

- *Nutrition:* Children with CP may be at risk for inadequate nutrition if they have oral-motor coordination problems. In addition, children with athetosis may need as much as 50% to 100% more calories to support their constant writhing movements. Children with spasticity, on the other hand, may need fewer calories because of their decreased movements (for more about nutrition, see Chapter 17). Occasionally, oral-motor coordination problems are so severe that a gastrostomy is needed, sometimes with fundoplication to prevent reflux and aspiration. Feeding clinics are often helpful as feeding therapy, modified positioning during feedings, and special feeding devices can help.
- *Elimination:* For children with significant motor impairment, constipation is common because of lack of exercise, inadequate fluid and fiber intake, medications, poor positioning, low abdominal muscle tone, or other factors. Stool softeners, such as docusate sodium, may help. Laxatives, such as senna concentrate or milk of magnesia, may be useful but should not be used long term. Osmotic agents may also be used (e.g., polyethylene glycol). Bladder control and urinary retention are also problems in CP; these children are at risk for urinary tract infections (UTIs). Most children achieve bladder control between 3 and 10 years old. For some, toilet training may be difficult, especially for those with intellectual disability.
- *Dentistry:* Orofacial muscle tone can contribute to malocclusion. Problems with oral mobility make daily dental hygiene difficult, leading to gum disease. For children with CP and epilepsy, the side effects of some seizure medications can include swollen gums and tooth decay. A diligent dental care program is necessary.
- *Drooling:* Inability to manage oral secretions results in drooling. Drooling can lead to social isolation, wet clothing, skin

---

• BOX 46.7　Problems Associated With Cerebral Palsy

Cognitive: learning disabilities, intellectual disability

Seizure Disorders: various types

Language and Speech Disorders: articulation, vocal strength and quality, language processing

Vision: refractive errors, strabismus, amblyopia, cataracts, retinopathy of prematurity, cortical blindness, homonymous hemianopsia (hemiplegia)

Hearing: conductive and/or sensorineural disorders

Other Sensory: tactile hypersensitivity or hyposensitivity, dyspraxia, balance and movement problems, proprioceptive difficulties, stereognosis

Motor: prolonged primitive reflexes, absence of protective reflexes, delayed motor milestones, hip subluxation and dislocation, scoliosis, contractures

Feeding and Eating Problems: chewing, sucking, and swallowing deficits, drooling, hypoxemia, fatigue, underweight and overweight, gastroesophageal reflux, aspiration

Bowel: constipation, encopresis

Urinary: bladder control, urinary retention, urinary tract infections

Dental: malocclusions, enamel deficits and caries, gum hyperplasia (with phenytoin)

Pulmonary: respiratory infections, pneumonia

Skin: pressure ulcers, latex allergy

Behavioral and Emotional: behavioral disorders, attention-deficit disorder, with and without hyperactivity, self-injurious behaviors, depression, autism, growth failure excoriation, malodorous breath, and discomfort. Furthermore, poor oral secretion management can lead to choking, gagging, and aspiration. The anticholinergic glycopyrrolate is approved for use in those 3 to 16 years old with chronic excessive drooling from neurologic conditions. Oral dosage is 20 mcg/kg/dose three times a day initially, with increases of 20 mcg/kg dose every 5 to 7 days if needed; maximum dosage is 100 mcg/kg/dose three times daily, not exceeding 1500 to 3000 mcg/dose. Oral solutions should be given 1 hour before or 2 hours after meals. Side effects may be problematic (e.g., dry mouth, vomiting, constipation, flushing, urinary retention, and nasal congestion). Clinical improvement resulting in a reduction in drooling has been demonstrated with this treatment. Surgical intervention is a last resort and commonly involves removing the submandibular gland or nerves or cutting or rerouting the salivary duct.

- *Respiratory:* Positioning problems, an increase in gastroesophageal reflux disorder, and difficulty in clearing secretions place children with CP at higher risk for respiratory problems, notably pneumonias (especially from aspiration). The duration of respiratory symptoms with upper respiratory infections (URIs) may be increased in these children because they may have sleep-related obstruction or other positioning difficulties, which slow respiratory return to baseline. A tracheotomy may be necessary in severe cases of upper airway obstruction or difficulty. Suctioning equipment may be required.

- *Skin:* The skin in sedentary children is more likely to break down and cause a pressure ulcer(s). Furthermore, significant spasticity may lead to the development of skin lesions over bony prominences. Of note, there is an increased incidence of skin latex allergies with CP.

- *Movement and mobility:* Functional mobility including positioning and seating, standing, transportation, bathing, dressing, play, and mobility in the school setting is important to assess and manage. Involvement of occupational and physical therapist is key as families need their help incorporating various strategies into their homes and lifestyles. The goals of therapy are to improve physical conditioning and gain maximal independence in mobility, fine motor activities, self-care, and communication by promoting efficient movement patterns, inhibiting primitive reflexes, and achieving isolated extremity movements. Bracing, postural support and seating systems, adaptive devices, and early intervention programs beginning in infancy are important. Open-front walkers, quadrupedal canes, gait poles, wheelchairs, and motorized wheelchairs are beneficial in helping children explore their environment more efficiently. Although the condition is not progressive in terms of the brain lesion, contractures, scoliosis, dislocated hips, and other deformities can develop if the child is allowed to maintain in abnormal positions for long periods; range-of-motion exercises are a long-term need. Orthopedic care may be necessary.

- *Medications:* Antispasmodic medications (baclofen, tizanidine, diazepam, and dantrolene) may be used to minimize contractures and spasticity. They are appropriate for children needing only a mild decrease in their muscle tone or in those with widespread spasticity. For optimal results, dosages often need to be high, and side effects can result (drowsiness, upset stomach, high blood pressure, and possible liver damage with chronic use).
  - Botulinum toxin A injections are used as treatment for spasticity, which can be helpful with improving function, decreasing pain, or reducing contractures. Although

botulinum toxin A has become standard treatment for spasticity in children, it is used off-label (NINDS, 2015b). Its use is dependent on the evaluation recommendations made by a healthcare provider with expertise in pediatric physiatry, pediatric neurology, or pediatric orthopedic surgery. Input from the child's therapy team and family should also be factored into this decision. Botulinum toxin A is injected directly into muscles (sometimes guided by an electromyogram or electrical stimulation). The child may experience mild flulike symptoms and transient worsening of spasticity. Injections are most effective when used in conjunction with an appropriate therapy regimen that helps strengthen the antagonist and agonist muscles (NINDS, 2015b). The dosage administered depends on which muscles are being selected and muscle size. Results are generally seen within 5 to 7 days and last 3 to 4 months. Botulinum toxin A has been safely used in infants older than 1 month. Resistance can occur because neutralizing antibodies can develop. Therefore, only the smallest possible effective dose must be used, and at least 3 months must lapse between injections. Injection of botulinum toxin A into salivary glands is also being used to reduce severity of drooling. Providers must be aware of the several contraindications and adverse effects that may be associated with this treatment option prior to prescribing. https://link.springer.com/article/10.1007/s40272-019-00344-8.

- *Communication:* With the combined problems of lack of oral-motor control and the high incidence of intellectual disability, communication can be a problem. Speech therapy may be of assistance. Augmentative devices, such as computers with voices, can allow for language development and communication of needs for children with severe speech impairment. Hearing deficits need to be identified and managed by an audiologist.

- *Vision:* Visual acuity, eye tracking, and binocularity are key factors to be assessed by a provider with expertise in pediatric ophthalmology/optometry.

- *Osteopenia:* Individuals with CP are at risk of bone density loss secondary to their inability to ambulate and place weight on their bones. Some medical providers prescribe bisphosphonates off-label to children (NINDS, 2015b). Monitoring of calcium and vitamin D should be strongly considered and supplemental vitamin D prescribed if levels are low.

- *Pain:* Spastic muscles, strain on compensatory muscles, and frequent or irregularly occurring muscle spasms can cause chronic and acute pain. Diazepam, gabapentin, and complementary therapies (distraction, biofeedback, relaxation, and therapeutic massage) can help (NINDS, 2015b).

- *Special education:* Early intervention programs and specialized educational programs through school systems are often beneficial.

- *Surgery:* At times surgery is used to release contractures or to sever over activated nerves (called a *selective dorsal root rhizotomy*). Selective dorsal root rhizotomy (of spinal nerves) plus intrathecal baclofen decrease spasticity and increase range of motion of affected limbs. An implantable pump is used to deliver intrathecal baclofen, a muscle relaxant. The pump is programmable with an electronic telemetry wand. Pumps have been successfully implanted in children as young as 3 years of age; this treatment has few but significant risks of complications. It is most efficacious in children who have some motor movement control and who have few muscles to treat that are not fixed or rigid (NINDS, 2015b). As an added benefit, it overcomes the problem of CNS adverse effects associated with the administration of large oral doses of baclofen. Intense physical therapy is an instrumental adjunct treatment.

- *Strength training* can help with balance and weakness. Functional electrical stimulation (involves insertion of a microscopic wireless device into specific muscles or nerves) has been used to activate and strengthen muscles in the hand, shoulder, and ankle. It should be regarded as experimental in CP and is used only as an alternative treatment if other treatments fail to relax muscles or relieve pain (NINDS, 2015b).

Complications. An Autism and Developmental Disabilities Monitoring (ADDM) Network study noted approximately 41% of children with CP had epilepsy and 7% had co-occurring autism spectrum disorder, with nonspastic CP having an 18% association with ASD (Christensen et al., 2014). Children who receive no intervention have poorer functional abilities; they make less progress developmentally and are at risk for unnecessary contractures and deformities. Box 46.7 lists additional problems that may be seen in children with CP.

The Hypotonic Infant

When supported with a hand under the chest, the normal infant will hold the back straight or nearly so, the arms flexed and slightly abducted at the elbows, and the head slightly up at less than 45 degrees. The "floppy" or hypotonic infant will droop over the hand. A hypotonic infant is alert but may have depressed spontaneous movements, which should arouse suspicion. By history, movement may have been abnormal in utero. Hypotonia may also be seen in the child with seizures, abnormal reaction to painful stimuli, muscle wasting, abnormal reflexes, tongue fasciculation, and asymmetric movement of extremities. Etiologies usually focus on a metabolic or CNS dysfunction or a systemic illness. Hypotonia can result from ischemic or hemorrhagic brain insults, congenital brain malformations, genetic syndromes, metabolic disease, prematurity, or for idiopathic reasons. Many conditions involving hypotonia are long term and require physical therapy for the infant/child to attain optimal function; others may be transitory, such as brachial plexus nerve palsy after birth or congenital myasthenia gravis.

Hypotonic infants can increase their tone over the first year of life and then demonstrate spastic CP. A baby can have low tone but still not lack strength when actively moving. The infant may also be weak, which means that its maximal effort lacks strength. Floppy infants with brisk reflexes almost certainly have a CNS disorder. All hypotonic babies need to be referred to a multidisciplinary team, which may include a neurology practitioner, physical and/or occupational therapy, and genetics. The diagnostic tool of choice is the MRI; sometimes muscle biopsies or various neurophysiologic studies are used.

Injuries and Congenital Conditions

Brachial Palsy

A stretch injury of the brachial plexus in neonates can occur during a difficult vaginal delivery; such injury has also been reported following cesarean births. Injury involves the upper cervical nerve roots C5 and C6 (Erb-Duchenne palsy) and the lower cervical nerve roots C7, C8, and T1 (Klumpke palsy). The injuries are attributed to traction of the involved nerves (with mild effect) to more serious complete nerve root avulsion from the spinal cord. Partial diaphragmatic paralysis can result because innervation comes from C3, C4, and C5.

Neonatal risk factors for plexus injuries include high birth weight, macrosomia, prolonged labor, breech delivery, maternal gestational diabetes, and instrumented delivery. The risk of brachial plexus palsy at birth is increased by 100 times when shoulder dystocia is present. (Buterbaugh, Kristin, and Shah, 2016). The incidence is approximately 3 per 1000 live births for Erb palsy. Klumpke palsy is rare (about 0.5% of plexus palsies) and is believed to be caused by delivering the head before the upper arm in a breech baby whose arms are extended. The incidence of brachial palsy at birth is cited as 0.4 to 4 per 100 live births. Some hypothesize that multiparity, increased labor induction, and increased Caesarean sections may contribute to a decreasing incidence. (Buterbaugh and Shah, 2016). Brachial plexus injuries can also occur in children restrained with a seatbelt during an automobile accident.

Clinical Findings

Physical Examination. Soon after birth, the infant is found to have asymmetric active range of motion of the arms, specifically lack of spontaneous upper extremity movement. Most frequently, Erb palsy is noted, consisting of positioning of the arm with shoulder adduction and internal rotation with wrist flexion (waiter's tip), with possibly some sensory impairment. Brachial plexus injuries are classified into preganglionic and postganglionic lesions, with postganglionic lesions having a better prognosis and more amenable to repair by direct surgery (Buterbaugh and Shah, 2016). Total plexus avulsion is defined as a completely flaccid upper extremity and portends a poorer prognosis.

The neonatal physical examination should include a careful evaluation of the Moro reflex (for symmetry), respiratory effort, evidence of Horner syndrome (ptosis, myosis [pupillary contraction], anhidrosis [absence of sweat]), and the neuromuscular function of the involved extremity. After the neonatal period, examine for posterior shoulder dislocation (would present as markedly limited external rotation) or bony deformity of the glenoid. Ability to fist is a favorable sign for a good outcome. Serial examinations and the use of available examination scoring scales allow the clinician to track recovery and function and evaluate ongoing recovery or plateau of recovery. Buterbaugh and Shah (2016) support that the key prognostic sign is recovery of antigravity elbow flexion.

Diagnostic Studies. Current expert opinion is that brachial palsy remains a diagnosis based on clinical examination. Radiographs can be considered to the evaluate humerus and clavicular fractures, if suspected. CT or MRI can be used to help characterize injury patterns; MRI is currently preferred because it eliminates radiation exposure. There is controversy regarding the role of EMG for determining prognosis.

Differential Diagnosis

Consider ipsilateral clavicle fracture with resultant pain that can explain the immobility of the extremity and Horner syndrome, which presents with ptosis, myosis, and anhidrosis in addition to avulsion of the T1 nerve root.

Management

Gentle range-of-motion exercises by parents and scheduled follow-up appointments to assess progress by the PCP are the current clinical standard. A referral to physical therapy may be indicated.

Surgical exploration and repair of neurolysis and nerve grafting may be undertaken in those with nerve root avulsion. Outcomes and comparisons between treatment modalities have been inconclusive. Older children with permanent functional limitations may be candidates for corrective shoulder surgery. Tang et al. (2016) studied infants with brachial plexus palsy and found that 64% (*n* = 28) had positional plagiocephaly. They postulate that an increased prevalence of positional plagiocephaly is present in the neonatal brachial plexus population and encourage parents and providers to use upper extremities to change position to reduce the occurrence of cranial asymmetry.

Prognosis

The majority of brachial plexus palsies spontaneously resolve over several weeks to several months. By the 3rd month, recovery of biceps function (active motion against gravity) is evidenced. Should wrist, thumb, and finger extension occur by this time, a complete recovery can be expected. In those with nerve root avulsions, early intervention is crucial to achieve some functional recovery. A quarter to a third of infants with brachial palsy will have residual neurologic deficits, so immediate intervention and assessment is vital. Newer treatment modalities such as botulinum toxin, microsurgery, and secondary shoulder and elbow procedures are controversial and unstudied, but promising.

Bell Palsy

Bell palsy is an acute unilateral paralysis or weakening of the facial nerve that may include individual or all branches of the facial nerve. Symptoms are attributed to edema of CN VII and venous congestion in areas of the nerve canal. A viral etiology is suspected, but the exact mechanism or etiology of Bell palsy remains unknown (Holland and Bernstein, 2014). It can occur across the life-span but is most common in individuals 15 to 40 years of age (Holland and Bernstein, 2014). Onset is rapid and can progress to maximal intensity within hours. Symptoms generally spontaneously resolve without intervention but may last for up to 5 months (Holland and Bernstein, 2014). A small percentage of children will experience recurrence of Bell palsy during childhood.

Clinical Findings

History. The child may initially experience localized pain or tingling in one ear and then experience sagging of the facial features corresponding to the affected branches of the facial nerve on the affected side. If there is a history of severe preceding pain, this should prompt the provider to consider other differential diagnoses. The history often reveals a viral illness or symptomatology within the two weeks preceding onset.

Physical Examination. A neurologic assessment of all facial nerve functions may be difficult in children and is not critical to make an accurate diagnosis. However, the provider should make their best effort to assess facial nerve functioning in an age appropriate manner and as completely as possible. In addition to facial nerve assessment, all other CNs should be assessed for dysfunction in an age appropriate manner. The clinician should observe for the following on examination:

- Unilateral motor changes in the forehead, cheek, and perioral area; face muscles pull to the normal side when the child makes facial expressions
- Normal blood pressure

- Dribbling liquids from the weak side; eating and drinking are more difficult
- Hypersensitivity to loud noises
- Eyelid fails to close on the affected side, and complete blinking may be absent; exposure keratitis may be present
- Lacrimation, taste (half of patients); anterior two-thirds of tongue and salivation may be impaired
- No limb weakness
- Any skin lesions to suggest herpes on the affected side of the face (would indicate active viral infection of the nerve or its motor neurons)
- Otoscopic examination to evaluate for symptoms of infection

Diagnostic Studies. It is widely accepted that diagnostic testing is not indicated unless other cranial neuropathies or focal abnormalities are present on neurologic examination, the patient fails to improve over a 6-week period, or other neurologic symptoms occur.

Differential Diagnosis

Included in the differential diagnosis are Ramsay Hunt syndrome (includes unilateral rash near or over ear with ipsilateral facial weakness), Guillain-Barré syndrome (GBS; usually includes an additional symptom of absent tendon reflexes of limbs), hypertension, congenital absence of the depressor angularis oris muscle, infection, trauma (forcep use during during delivery can cause a facial nerve compression neuropathy that spontaneously resolves within a few days to weeks), Melkersson-Rosenthal syndrome (involves recurrent facial palsies with swollen lips, tongue, cheeks, or eyelids), Möbius syndrome, acute otitis media, poliomyelitis, histiocytosis X, varicella, facial nerve tumors, neurofibroma, infiltration of facial nerves with leukemic cells, rhabdomyosarcoma of the middle ear, and brainstem infarcts.

Management

If eyelid closure is incomplete, prescribe methylcellulose eye drops or ocular lubricant to the affected eye several times daily and patch the eye if the child plays outdoors, during active play, and when sleeping. The American Academy of Neurology and the American Academy of Otolaryngology agree that steroids should be used in newly diagnosed patients (oral prednisone is dosed at 1 mg/kg/day for 1 week, then tapered for 1 week; starting within the first 3 to 5 days) (Schwartz et al., 2014). Holland and Bernstein (2014) acknowledge lack of strong evidence for the efficacy of combined steroid and antiretroviral therapy. For children who do not experience full recovery of symptoms, facial retraining has been explored as a possible treatment, but evidence on this intervention is limited (Holland and Bernstein, 2014).

Complications

Approximately 85% of children recover spontaneously within 3 weeks while the remaining children may take up to 5 months to see recovery of symptoms (Holland and Bernstein, 2014). If recovery is incomplete, lack of salivation in response to food, lack of lacrimation, facial contractures, and tics may occur.

Tethered Cord

The spinal cord is attached to the base of the brain and free at the caudal end, allowing for freedom of movement during growth, activities, and skeletal changes (including such abnormalities as scoliotic curves). With a tethered cord, however, the caudal end is fixed by a ropelike filum terminale at or below the L2 level. This can cause abnormal stretching and damage to nerve cells, fibers, and blood vessels. Eventually, symptoms of neurologic deterioration may occur. Tethered cord often associated with a congenital spinal anomaly, such as spina bifida (90%), but tethering can also result from bony protrusions, tough membranous bands, lipomas, tumors, cysts, scarring, and trauma in the area of the cauda equina.

Not all tethering leads to clinical symptoms. If symptoms do occur, they manifest as functional deficits to nerves that emanate from the area of the cauda equina. In children, symptoms may include lesions, hairy patches, dimples, or fatty tumors on the lower back; foot and spinal deformities; weakness in the legs; low back pain; scoliosis; and incontinence. This type of tethered spinal cord syndrome appears to be the result of improper growth of the neural tube during fetal development and is closely linked to spina bifida. Tethered spinal cord syndrome may go undiagnosed until adulthood, when pain, sensory and motor problems, and loss of bowel and bladder control emerge (NINDS, 2017). Symptoms are not necessarily evident in infancy but can be manifested in early childhood to adulthood. Skin changes are often seen in individuals later diagnosed with tethered cord or other spinal abnormalities; these may include dimples above the gluteal cleft or within the cleft (dimples at the coccyx are generally benign), spinal hair tufts, a deviated gluteal fold, spinal fatty deposits, midline birthmarks, and sacral sinuses or tracts (Fig 46.7).

If a provider is suspicious of a tethered cord, an MRI of the spine is the gold standard for viewing the parenchymal anatomy. A referral to a pediatric neurosurgeon is also indicated for further evaluation of surgical suitability. Surgery is usually the treatment of choice and can halt and prevent further neurologic dysfunction. If a child has reached full skeletal height with minimal symptoms, monitoring is all that is often done. Be watchful for retethering in children who have had surgery for tethered cord; this can occur as the child gets older and will be made apparent with symptom progression. A child with a history of repaired spina bifida must be closely monitored for early symptoms of tethered cord. Children with tethered cord syndrome in the 3-6 years age range have lower surgical morbidity compared with older or younger patients (Kashlan, Wilkinson, Morgenstern, and Maher, 2016).

Arnold-Chiari Malformation

Arnold-Chiari malformations consist of two types of uncommon congenital spinal cord anomalies whose sequelae are usually not evident until late childhood or into adulthood. Type I malformation involves the downward elongation (herniation) of the caudal end of the cerebellar vermis through the foramen magnum with frequency of about 0.61% and a female to male ratio of 3:1 (Poretti, Ashmawy, et al., 2016). Type II malformation is present in 0.5 to 1 per 1000 of children with spina bifida myelomeningocele. The herniation can lead to brainstem and upper cervical cord compression that may ultimately cause necrosis of both structures. The etiology is believed to be a structural anomaly at the base of the skull due to mesodermal insufficiency (Poretti, Ashmawy, et al., 2016). Historically, this disorder was attributed to disruption of the process of neural tube closure but the modern view postulates that no closure disorder is associated with this malformation. Other causes such as a segmental defect or underdevelopment of the occipital bone are considered to play a role in pathogenesis. The symptoms of a malformation may not be readily apparent. Type I malformation can cause headache, neck pain, atrophy and decreased reflexes in the lower extremities, sensory losses, and scoliosis. Any child with

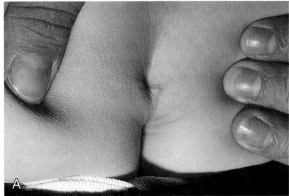

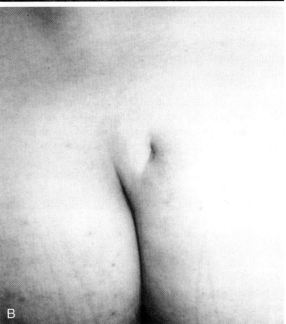

• **Fig 46.7** (A) Deep sacral dimple above the gluteal crease. Most sacral dimples that fall within the gluteal crease are normal. Dimples that are deep, large (>0.5 cm), located in the superior portion or above the gluteal crease (>2.5 cm from the anal verge), or that are associated with a deviated gluteal crease or other cutaneous markers should be radiologically imaged. (B) Buttocks of teenage boy with tethered cord secondary to lipomeningocele. Note sacral dimple and deviation of gluteal fold to the left.

myelomeningocele should be suspected of having type II malformation. Type II malformation involves the same herniation as type I plus an alteration in the shape and development of the medulla. Further symptoms of type II may include hydrocephaly, respiratory distress, syncope, poor feeding, vomiting, dysphagia, tongue paralysis, and cardiopulmonary failure. Epilepsy is not related. Diagnosis is made by MRI and the condition may inadvertently be found at the time of an MRI for a possibly unrelated reason (e.g., headache).

Management strategies are not always successful; surgery to relieve the compression or a ventriculoperitoneal shunt may be tried in symptomatic cases. Langridge, Phillips, and Choi (2017) conclude that the natural history of this disorder is generally benign and nonspecific; surgical decompression and its risk must be weighed against symptom severity at presentation. **Due to the risk of brainstem herniation, an LP should never be attempted in a child with an Arnold-Chiari malformation.** Always consult with neurosurgery prior to LP when this is present.

Myelomeningocele

Failure during embryogenesis of the vertebrae, skull, meninges, brain, or spinal cord to be encapsulated by the lamina of the vertebrae along the dorsal midline of the body is referred to as a *dysraphic defect*. Therefore, the posterior neural tube and the vertebral column are not closed. *Myelomeningocele* refers to the protrusion of both the spinal cord nerve roots *(myelo)* and the three layers of membranes *(meninges)* that cover the spinal cord and brain through this spinal defect. At times, the protruding dural sac may contain only the meninges or both meninges and nerve roots (the remaining cases). The term *spina bifida cystica* is often used interchangeably with myelomeningocele. When the vertebral arches fail to close but there is no subsequent herniation of cord or meninges, the term *spina bifida occulta* is used. Most cases of spina bifida cystica occur in the thoracolumbar area. Meningoceles may also protrude through the skull and may or may not be covered with skin. Such a cranial meningocele consists only of a CSF-filled meningeal sac; no nerve roots are involved, and therefore no neurologic deficits exist. However, there may be brain malformation under the mass that does have neurologic consequences. Encephaloceles or cephaloceles refer to cranial lesions that contain a meningocele sac plus cerebral cortex, cerebellum, or portions of brainstem that protrude from fissures in the occipital (most common), frontal, or nasal cavity areas of the skull.

Closure of the neural tube usually occurs during the 3rd and 4th weeks of gestation. Genetic and environmental factors are believed to play a causative role in the failure of the closure to occur. CDC estimates show that neural tube defects account for 3.5 in 10,000 births in the United States (Antiel et al., 2016), with Hispanic women having the highest rate of having a child affected by spina bifida, when compared with non-Hispanic white and non-Hispanic black women. The rate of affected pregnancies with neural tube defects dramatically dropped after the mandatory fortification of cereal grains with folic acid. Since 2004, the incidence has leveled off to about 3000 affected pregnancies in the United States, rather than continuing to decline. One study using data from 19 state-based birth defects tracking programs estimated the change in prevalence of NTDs before and after the introduction of folic acid fortification. Overall, a 28% reduction in prevalence was observed for anencephaly (a birth defect of the brain) and spina bifida. A greater reduction (35% reduction) was observed among programs that actively looked for a neural tube defect during a women's pregnancy (prenatal ascertainment) than for programs that did not (21% reduction; Williams, Mai, et al., 2015). A woman wishing to conceive, or who has had a prior pregnancy that resulted in a neural tube defect, should take 4 mg/day for 4 weeks before conception and through the first trimester. Intake of certain drugs and toxins is associated with neural tube defects: folic acid antagonists (trimethoprim, carbamazepine, phenytoin, phenobarbital, and primidone), retinoic acid derivatives (e.g., vitamin A, a paradox given that insufficient levels also cause the defect), valproic acid, and alcohol.

There is speculation that this leveling may be due to overall decreases in serum folate, red blood cell (RBC) folate concentrations in nonpregnant women, and some nonfolate risk factors yet to be identified (CDC, 2015). Proposed explanations for the decline in serum folate include increasing obesity rates (obese individuals metabolize folate differently), low-carbohydrate diet trends (which requires the elimination of breads, cereals, and other products that contain the mandatory fortified folic acid-enriched flour), the popularity of whole-grain breads (which have lower natural folate levels), the reduction in the mean folate content of certain enriched breads, and maternal diabetes.

A maternal serum test showing an increase in the concentration of alpha-fetoprotein is diagnostic; if elevated, an ultrasound and amniocentesis are performed (α-fetoprotein is the primary plasma protein found within the fetus and in the amniotic fluid and is elevated if there is a defect in the skin of the fetus). Cranial ultrasounds should be done to look for hydrocephalus and cephaloceles (and in turn the Arnold-Chiari type II malformation). It is preferable that these infants be delivered by cesarean section. Some pregnancies are terminated when a diagnosis of a neural tube defect is made.

The *MTHFR* gene is critical in providing instructions for making an enzyme called *methylenetetrahydrofolate reductase*. This enzyme is critical in B-vitamin folate (also called *folic acid* or *vitamin B₉*) chemical reactions. *MTHFR* mutations are associated with neural tube defects. It is also a possible risk factor for preeclampsia and cancer among others. Genetic testing for this gene mutation is widely available and used with women with certain risk factors.

Clinical Findings

- Poor intake of folic acid, exposure to known toxins, or no known risk factors
- Saclike cyst containing meninges and spinal fluid covered by a thin layer of partially epithelialized skin; 75% found in the lumbosacral area
- Flaccid paralysis of lower extremities
- Absence of deep tendon reflexes
- Lack of response to touch and pain in lower extremities
- Incontinence issues including constant urinary dribbling, encopresis

Other physical anomalies can accompany myelomeningocele including cleft lip and palate, omphalocele, diaphragmatic hernia, tracheoesophageal fistula, congenital heart disease, bladder exstrophy, and imperforate anus.

Management and Complications

In the neonatal period, serial cranial ultrasounds are conducted to watch for the development of hydrocephalus if this condition has not shown up prenatally. Surgical resection and closure of the involved neural tube structures are done within a week after birth; often shunting for hydrocephalus is also required. Intrauterine surgery has also been successful in closing the defect and preventing exposure of the neural tube to amniotic fluid and possible postnatal infection. If the defect occurs in a high spinal region or there is clinical hydrocephalus at birth, survival is also compromised. Multidisciplinary supportive management is indicated. The overall impact on families caring for a child with myelomeningocele having prenatal surgery compared with the postnatal surgery group was significantly lower (Antiel, Adzick, et al., 2016).

The PCP's role includes delivering well-child care, assessing and treating acute illnesses (especially UTIs and constipation), monitoring shunt function, checking for skin breakdown, and communicating with and often coordinating services between the myriad of specialists who will be involved (e.g., orthopedists, ophthalmologists [strabismus is common], neurologists, nephrologists, physical therapists, social workers, and geneticists).

Genitourinary management entails teaching parents (and eventually the child) how to regularly catheterize a neurogenic bladder. Periodic urine cultures, assessing renal function (with serum electrolytes, creatinine), and, depending on the child's course, ordering appropriate imaging studies (renal scans, intravenous pyelograms [IVPs], ultrasounds) fit within the PCP's role. In addition, the PCP needs to be alert to the onset of symptoms indicative of Arnold-Chiari type II malformation and tethered cord, and watch for seizures, learning difficulties, and ADHD. Bowel training can help control stool incontinence.

Prognosis

With aggressive early treatment, survival rates can be quite high, and children can be maintained with current interventions; deaths more commonly occur before 4 years of age. Normal intelligence is seen in 70% of survivors, but they experience more learning and seizure problems. Continence can sometimes be achieved with an artificial urinary sphincter or bladder augmentation when the child is older. Functional mobility depends on the level and degree of the defect and on the intact function of the iliopsoas muscle. A child with a defect in the sacral and lumbosacral area almost certainly will be able to achieve functional ambulation; those with a higher defect may have variable function with mobility aids.

Prevention

Folic acid supplementation (400 mcg/day) with a daily multivitamin is helpful in preventing neural tube defects and should be taken by all females of childbearing age. Prenatal vitamins have at least 400 mcg/vitamin; however, additional folic acid supplementation (4000 mcg) is recommended for those women who have had a child with a neural tube defect (CDC, 2015).

Infection and Immune Disorders

Central Nervous System Infections

Infections of the CNS have similar symptoms. These infections can be manifested acutely (over 1 to 24 hours) or chronically (over 1 to 7 days or more). Bacteria, viruses, fungi, spirochetes, protozoa, and parasites can all cause CNS infection. The meninges, superficial cortical structures, blood vessels, and brain parenchyma can be involved. The most common microbes are:

- Infants: *Escherichia coli* (42%), followed by group B *Streptococcus* (23%). Streptococcus pneumoniae is more likely in older infants (Ouchenir et al., 2017).
- Children: Bacterial infections—*Haemophilus influenzae* type B, *Neisseria meningitidis*, and *Streptococcus pneumoniae* are the most common. In those with immune deficiencies, *Pseudomonas aeruginosa*, *Staphylococcus aureus*, coagulase-negative staphylococci, *Salmonella* spp., and *Listeria monocytogenes* can be implicated.

Pathology generally includes colonization of the nasopharynx by adhesion to the mucosa via various mechanisms. Invasion of the mucosa and penetration into the bloodstream between or through epithelial cells then occurs. Eventually, the bacteria invade the blood-brain barrier (BBB), multiply in the CSF, and trigger an inflammatory response, resulting in increased permeability of the BBB.

The poorest end results lead to cerebral edema, derangements of cerebral metabolism, neuronal damage, strokes, and severe impairment or death.

Clinical Findings

History. The following may be reported:
- Upper respiratory tract or gastrointestinal symptoms accompanied by fever

- Increasing lethargy and irritability or behavioral change
- Recent head injury or neurosurgical procedure
- Immunocompromised host
- History of travel, sick contact, insect bites, animal contacts

Physical Examination. Findings on physical examination include the following:
- Systemic signs, including fever, malaise, and/or impaired heart, lung, or kidney function, "ill-appearing" infant or child
- CNS signs, including headache; stiff neck and spine; nausea and vomiting; fever or hypothermia; changes in mental status, ranging from irritability to lethargy or coma; seizures; and focal or sensory deficits in CNs, notably CN III, CN IV, and CN VI
- Presence of Kernig or Brudzinski signs of meningeal irritation (may be absent in a young infant)
- Bulging fontanelle and increasing head circumference in a young infant
- Papilledema—a late finding in older children or adolescents
- CN dysfunction

By age, the most common findings are as follows:
- From 0 to 3 months old: Fever, hypothermia, lethargy, irritability, poor feeding, apnea, focal seizures, enteric or respiratory symptoms, nuchal rigidity, and a bulging fontanelle
- From 3 months to 5 years old: Petechial rash, localized CNS signs as described earlier
- From 6 to 18 years old: Petechial rash, CN VII palsy (Lyme disease), sinusitis symptoms, localized CNS signs

Diagnostic Studies. Blood cultures, CBC with differential, urinalysis, chemistry panel, and LP for CSF studies are done. Enterovirus meningitis and herpes simplex virus rapid tests are available. EEG and/or brain biopsy may be needed. Imaging may include head CT without contrast to rule out space-occupying lesions, hemorrhage, or trauma; a MRI of brain and spine should be done if there is a concern for myelitis/encephalitis. In addition, abscess or inflammation may be identified. Cerebral edema is often not demonstrated on scans. CSF culture remains the gold standard for diagnosis of CNS infection.

Management and Complications

The PCP needs to refer all children with potential CNS infection as rapidly as possible. Hypovolemia, hypoglycemia, hyponatremia, acidosis, septic shock, increased intracranial pressure, and other complications can occur quickly and need aggressive management. Hearing loss can occur in all forms of meningitis, and all children with meningitis merit post infection auditory evaluation. Blindness, hydrocephalus, CP, seizures, and global developmental delays can also occur depending on the type of organism involved. Outcomes are typically based on the type of infectious agent and severity of initial infection, age of the child (the younger, the worse the outcome), length of symptoms before the diagnosis and initiation of treatment, and antibiotic and dosage.

Zika Virus

Zika virus came to the world's attention in 2015 when there was a cluster of cases in Brazil. Zika is an emerging mosquito-borne flavivirus and is transmitted via mosquito to humans. Zika infection is manifested by fever, headache, arthralgia, myalgia, and maculopapular rash (Mlakar et al., 2016). The disease itself is self-limiting; however, there is an association between Zika infection in pregnancy and fetal malformations. These malformations may include microcephaly, gross intrauterine growth retardation, subcortical white matter brain calcifications, and pachygyria or

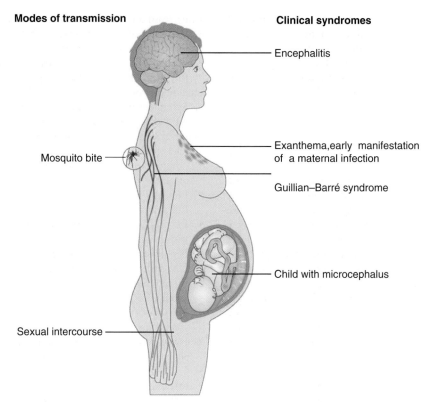

Modes of transmission

Clinical syndromes

- Encephalitis

- Exanthema, early manifestation of a maternal infection

- Guillian–Barré syndrome

Mosquito bite —

- Child with microcephalus

Sexual intercourse —

• **Fig 46.8** Modes of transmission and clinical syndromes related to Zika virus.

polymicrogyria in the frontal lobes. There is no treatment for infants exposed to Zika during pregnancy; multidisciplinary supportive care is recommended. Of note, an increase in Guillain Barre syndrome is associated with Zika virus (Fig 46.8).

Zika virus is commonly transmitted by the Aedes aegypti mosquito, but sexual transmission has also been reported. Zika virus infection presents with exanthema and might lead to abrogation of neurogenesis during fetal brain development, resulting in microcephaly. During or after Zika virus infection, acute demyelinating inflammatory polyneuropathy can develop. In rare cases, Zika virus causes encephalitis.

Reye Syndrome

Reye syndrome is an encephalopathy process often associated with a viral infection primarily affecting those under 18 years of age. Infrequently, cases are seen with varicella or nonspecific respiratory infections, notably *H. influenzae* type B. A decline in incidence has been associated with the decreased use of salicylates in children and also possibly related to improvements in the diagnosis of underlying inborn errors of metabolism. Fatty changes of the liver and sudden, acute cerebral edema are hallmarks of Reye syndrome, along with elevated liver enzymes and hyperammonemia. For the past 3 decades, since Reye syndrome was at a peak, due to the association between salicylates and the development of Reye syndrome, it is recommended that children under age 18 avoid salicylates.

The clinical course in Reye syndrome proceeds in predictable stages after the initial prodromal symptoms of the illness: severe vomiting progresses to irrational behavior; stupor and coma; apnea, fixed pupils, and decorticate posturing with increasing brain edema; and finally, death. Management involves immediate referral with admission to a hospital

equipped for tertiary supportive care. Treatment includes respiratory support and methods to control cerebral edema and reduce ammonia levels. Survivors of Reyes syndrome may have severe neurologic sequelae. Infants are more severely affected than older children.

Myasthenia Gravis

MG is an autoimmune disorder that produces an immune-mediated neuromuscular blockade or neuromuscular junction disorder. It originates when circulating receptor-binding antibodies decrease the number of available acetylcholine receptors (AChRs) on the postsynaptic muscle membrane or motor endplate, leaving the motor endplate less responsive than normal.

MG is nonhereditary in most cases; however, three rare presynaptic congenital forms exist. Symptoms of congenital MG start at or close after birth and persist. Mothers with MG may have infants with a transient neonatal myasthenic syndrome as a result of the transfer of placental anti-AChR antibodies. Once the infant's own receptors regenerate and reinsert into synaptic membranes, the symptoms resolve. Children with MG can also experience other autoimmune diseases (e.g., systemic lupus erythematosus, thyroiditis, rheumatoid arthritis, and/or diabetes mellitus).

MG affects approximately 40 per 1 million population; about one-fifth of these develop symptoms before 20 years of age. It is estimated that between 10% and 15% of cases occur in the pediatric population (Peragallo, 2017). Juvenile myasthenia gravis patients are classified into two subgroups—the very early onset group (<8 years) and the puberty onset group (8 to 18 years) (Hong, Skeie, Zismopoulou, et al 2017). There is also a neonatal form of this disorder. Twelve percent of infants born to mothers with MG develop symptoms within 72 hours of birth—respiratory insufficiency, dysphagia, hypotonia, weakness, poor spontaneous motor activity, weak cry, poor sucking, choking, expressionless face, and absent Moro reflex. Symptoms generally resolve within 12 weeks. With congenital MG, symptoms are permanent, there is no remission, and these children do not experience myasthenic crises. There is no racial or geographic predilection.

Clinical Findings

Physical Examination. The key findings of this disorder include:

- Ptosis and some degree of extraocular muscle weakness (usually the first symptom): Older children may complain of double vision; younger children may endeavor to hold their eyelids open with their fingers. The ocular signs may be asymmetric.
- Dysphagia: Infants commonly have feeding problems; older children fatigue when chewing. There may be slurred speech and a snarling appearance when trying to smile.
- Muscular weakness of neck flexor muscles (infants), limb-girdle, and distal muscles of hands: Limb weakness is not a common symptom of onset, and symptoms do not include muscle fasciculations, myalgias, or sensory symptoms. Other times, the weakness may be so mild as to only occur after exercise.
- Rapid muscular fatigue as evidenced by inability to:
  - Hold an upward gaze for 30 to 90 seconds
  - Sustain a chin to chest position while supine
  - Maintain arm abduction for more than 1 to 2 minutes
  - Sustain rapid hand-fisting movements for long periods of time

Diagnostic Studies

- A short-acting cholinesterase inhibitor (edrophonium chloride) is given as a clinical test; it should cause spontaneous improvement in the ptosis and ophthalmoplegia within seconds; other muscles should fatigue less rapidly.
- An EMG is more diagnostic than a muscle biopsy.
- AchR antibody testing is commercially available and should be performed. However, this test is often inconclusive; only one-third of adolescents and an occasional prepubertal child exhibit these antibodies.
- Other tests can include serologic antinuclear antibodies and immune complexes; thyroid profile; CK level (normal with MG); chest x-ray (any enlarged thymus needs to be followed up with a tomography or CT scan of the anterior mediastinum); ECG (should be normal); muscle biopsy may be considered.

Differential Diagnosis

Hypothyroidism (caused by Hashimoto thyroiditis), polymyalgia rheumatica, MS, progressive external ophthalmoplegia, GBS, Möbius syndrome, congenital ptosis, congenital myopathies, myotonic dystrophy, and glycogen-storage disease are in the differential.

Management

MG (including neonatal MG) is treated with anticholinesterase therapy (pyridostigmine), because it is longer acting and produces less severe side effects than neostigmine. Pyridostigmine should be part of the initial treatment in most patients with MG. Pyridostigmine dose should be adjusted as needed based on symptoms. The ability to discontinue pyridostigmine can be an indicator that the patient has met treatment goals and may guide the tapering of

other therapies. Corticosteroids or immunosuppressant therapy should be used in all patients with MG who have not met treatment goals after an adequate trial of pyridostigmine (Sanders, Wolfe, Benatar, et al., 2016). The initial dosage is age and weight dependent and is then titrated upward until the patient responds, side effects are controlled, or until increases are no longer effective. Corticosteroids, cytotoxic agents (azathioprine and cyclosporine), or thymectomy may also be considered, especially if symptoms are severely debilitating (bulbar or respiratory involvement). Corticosteroids should be administered on an alternate-day regimen. Plasmapheresis and IVIG are alternative treatments with limited use.

Complications

Complications include growth retardation from steroids and possible immunodeficiency in adulthood after thymectomy. Long-term therapy with anticholinergics may lead to cholinergic crises that present similarly to myasthenic crises.

Neurofibromatosis

NF1 is a disorder that is dominantly inherited and stems from a genetic mutation in the NF1 tumor suppressor gene. NF1 affects about 1:2500 to 3000 people worldwide with no differentiation of gender or ethnic origin (Hirbe and Gutmann, 2014). About 50% of those affected are de novo or spontaneous mutations, meaning that there is no family history of the disease. As phenotype and genotype testing becomes more and more accurate, correlations of severity are emerging indicating that some have more severe genotypes depending on the genetic microdeletion and the amount of the gene that is affected (Hirbe and Gutmann, 2014). NF1, called von Recklinghausen disease in the past, was first described in 1882, and diagnostic criteria were published by the National Institutes of Health in 1987 (Hirbe and Gutmann, 2014).

NF1 should be suspected in individuals when two of these findings are present:

- Six or more café au lait macules greater than 5 mm in greatest diameter in prepubertal individuals and greater than 15 mm in greatest diameter in post pubertal individuals
- Two or more neurofibromas of any type or one plexiform neurofibroma
- Freckling in the axillary or inguinal regions
- Optic glioma
- Two or more Lisch nodules (iris hamartomas)
- A distinctive osseous lesion such as sphenoid dysplasia or tibial pseudarthrosis
- A first-degree relative (parent, sib, or offspring) with NF1 as defined by the above criteria

NF1 carries with it the potential for a number of comorbid diagnoses, including nonmalignant clinical features such as pigmentary abnormalities, neurofibromas, plexiform neurofibromas (different from cutaneous or pigment neurofibromas in that they are internal and grow along the length of a nerve), skeletal deformities such as osteopenia or scoliosis, cardiovascular abnormalities (which may include congenital heart disease or vasculopathies and hypertension), and neurocognitive deficits. These are examples only, and manifestations may be different or more severe than described here.

Malignant features of NF1 include optic pathway or brainstem gliomas which occur in about 15% to 20% of the NF1 population, glioblastomas, and malignant peripheral nerve sheath tumors. Recent evidence (Anastaki, Morris, et al., 2017) indicates that some NF1 children who harbor a specific mutation in a specific gene location are more likely to develop gliomas; this is similar to findings in other research. Noncentral nervous system malignancies may include breast cancers, leukemia and lymphoma, pheochromocytoma, rhabdomyosarcoma, and GI tumors.

The following evaluations are recommended when monitoring NF1 patients to determine the extent of their disease and individual needs:

- Personal medical history with particular attention to features of NF1
- Physical examination with particular attention to the skin, skeleton, cardiovascular system, and neurologic systems, measurement, and assessment of changes in neurocutaneous features, serial blood pressure measurements, baseline cardiology examination
- Ophthalmologic evaluation, including slit lamp examination of the irides and infrared reflectance imaging or optical coherence tomography of the fundus
- Developmental assessment in children
- Routine head MRI scanning in individuals is controversial due to the requirement for sedation in small children in the absence of related symptoms, but is done at the time of diagnosis in most centers to obtain a baseline.
- Other studies as indicated on the basis of clinically apparent signs or symptoms
- Consultation with a clinical geneticist and/or genetic counselor to obtain a thorough family history with particular attention to NF1 features

Management of NF1 in children consists of referral to specialists for assessment of various body systems that may become involved including the eye, central or PNS, cardiovascular system, endocrine system, spine, or long bones; future interventions may include surgical removal of disfiguring or uncomfortable discrete cutaneous or subcutaneous neurofibromas. Treatment of optic gliomas is generally unnecessary, as they are usually asymptomatic and clinically stable.

The PCP must be familiar with diagnostic criteria and monitoring and be able to coordinate needed services with specialists or a neurofibromatosis center. Frequently, however, the PCP will be the initial contact when and if the child begins to exhibit neurodevelopmental disorders. Vogel, Gutmann, and Morris (2017) describe the spectrum of neuropsychiatric symptoms including IQ variations affecting school performance (but not intellectual disability), ADHD, ASD, and intellectual disability. Estimates are that 4% to 8% of the NF1 population have an intellectual disability (Vogel, Gutmann, Morris, 2017). Children with NF1 are at high risk for learning disabilities involving math, writing, and reading skills, and also may have social deficits. The combination of these issues may make school particularly challenging for these children. Early recognition and intervention is critical for optimal school performance (see Chapter 30).

Nutakki, Varni, et al. (2017) used the Health-related Quality of Life (HRQOL) Peds QL NF1 Module with 23 children, adolescents, and young adults who also participated in semistructured interviews. Ultimately, they identified 15 domains reflecting specific concerns in this population: skin, pain, pain impact and management, cognitive functioning, worry, balance and fine motor skills, school activities, and interactions with peers. The authors found that NF1 symptoms have a significant effect on day to day function of the patients and their parents.

Guillain-Barré Syndrome

GBS is an acute polyradiculoneuropathy that primarily affects peripheral nerves and is characterized by progressive weakness and diminished or absent reflexes (Verboon, van Doorn, and Jacobs, 2016). The paralysis frequently follows a respiratory (notably *Mycoplasma pneumoniae*) or gastrointestinal (notably *Campylobacter jejuni* or *Helicobacter pylori*) infection by approximately 10 days. Infection with Epstein-Barr virus has also been implicated, linked to a milder form of GBS. Notably, there may have been an association of GBS with the H1N1 vaccination campaign in 2009, but this was mainly in the elderly not children. This association remains controversial; however, it continues to be investigated by the World Health Organization (Roodbol, deWit, van den Berg, et al., 2017). Most children diagnosed with GBS have muscle weakness of varying severity and decreased reflexes in weak limbs. Additional studies may include CSF examination and nerve conduction studies. Most diagnoses include acute demyelinating neuropathy. Known variants include acute motor axonal degeneration (as evidenced by ophthalmoparesis, ataxia, and areflexia) and acute sensory neuropathy.

Clinical Findings

History. The following are reported:
- Fever
- Nonspecific viral infection (gastrointestinal or respiratory) occurring within recent past
- Weakness or neurologic changes in sensory, motor, or visual systems: Onset is gradual, progressing in an ascending order (known as *Landry ascending paralysis*), starting in the lower extremities and progressing to the bulbar muscles over days or weeks; maximum weakness reached within 2 to 3 weeks.

Physical Examination
- Tenderness and pain in muscles with palpation
- Irritability
- Inability or refusal to walk due to flaccid tetraplegia or quadriplegia
- Paresthesia may or may not be present
- Respiratory insufficiency (may occur later as progression of the disease)
- Dysphagia, facial weakness
- Extraocular muscle involvement rare; papilledema and visual acuity changes may be seen
- Miller-Fisher syndrome may be seen (acute external ophthalmoplegia, ataxia, areflexia)
- Signs of viral meningitis or meningoencephalitis
- Urinary retention or incontinence (20% of cases and is usually transient in nature)
- Blood pressure and cardiac rate changes, including bradycardia, postural hypotension, asystole

Diagnostic Studies
- CSF studies: Elevated CSF protein (usually greater than twice upper limit of normal); normal glucose, no pleocytosis (fewer than 10 white blood cells [WBCs]/mm^3)
- Negative blood cultures; viral cultures rarely conclusive
- Normal or mildly elevated creatine kinase (CK) level; antiganglioside antibodies (against GM1, GD1) may be elevated in axonal neuropathy form of the disease.
- Decreased motor nerve conduction velocities; slowed sensory nerve conduction
- EMG: Shows acute denervation of muscle

Differential Diagnosis

Bickerstaff brainstem encephalitis, meningitis, meningoencephalitis, spinal muscle atrophy, HIV, metabolic diseases, and West Nile virus are included in the differential diagnoses.

Management

Hospitalization is paramount for observation and for handling complications of respiratory muscle paralysis. IVIG for 5 days is standard protocol. In some cases, a second course of IVIG may be used due to the severity of neurologic deterioration. However, 97% of children have a monophasic disease course. Plasmapheresis and/or immunosuppressive drugs may be used in cases unresponsive to IVIG; however, use of these is empiric and not well studied via randomized trials in children (Verboon, van Doorn, and Jacobs, 2016). Care is supportive and includes respiratory support, prevention of decubitus, and treatment of secondary bacterial infections. Rehabilitative therapy should begin early. Children with GBS may have neuropathic and nociceptive pain, which may be severe. Nonsteroidal anti-inflammatory drugs may not provide adequate relief, and opioids may exacerbate autonomic symptoms. Chronic pain must be addressed during treatment and rehabilitation therapy.

Complications

Chronic varieties of Guillain-Barré can occur, as evidenced by recurrence or lack of improvement of symptoms over months or years. Unresolved weakness, flaccid tetraplegia or quadriplegia, and bulbar and respiratory muscle compromise may linger or remain and last longer than 2 months. This is then considered chronic inflammatory demyelinating radiculopathy. GBS with occurrences shortly after, and then greater than 20 years after the first episode are reported (Roodbol, deWit, van den Berg, et al., 2017).

Neurodegenerative Disorders

Neurodegenerative disorders occur when the gray or white matter of the brain is affected. These are believed to be the result of biochemical or metabolic dysfunctions (in turn caused by genetic, immune-mediated demyelination or by unknown etiologies) that lead to anatomic or functional insults to major portions of the brain. These insults can affect the basal ganglia, cerebellum, brainstem, spinal cord, peripheral and CNs, or cerebrum. Such insults can also follow infections or an altered immune state.

Gray matter diseases involve neurons, and their onset is heralded by seizures, a decrease in cognitive functioning, and visual changes. Gray matter disorders that are exceedingly rare include Menkes syndrome (also called *kinky hair syndrome*), progressive infantile poliodystrophy, neuronal ceroid-lipofuscinoses, and Rett syndrome. White matter diseases are characterized by demyelination and are evidenced by decreasing motor skills, ataxia, and spasticity. Such disorders include Schilder disease, acute disseminating encephalomyelitis, acute hemorrhagic leukoencephalitis, leukodystrophies, and MS. The diagnosis is based on age of onset, clinical features (signs and symptoms), family history (genetic pedigree), and diagnostic studies that may include neuroimaging as well as chemical and genetic studies. It also must be determined if the episodes of disability are single (monophasic) or polyphasic (relapses close to initial onset of symptoms with similar areas of involvement as in MS).

In the case of inflammatory demyelination, separate events are determined by whether or not they occur more than 30 days apart and involve separate white matter pathways. In an initial acute demyelinating event, it may be difficult to determine a diagnosis; the extent of motor, visual, and neurologic involvement needs to be determined in all events. If a demyelinating event is suspected, the child should be referred to a neurology provider (preferably pediatric) for a comprehensive evaluation and diagnosis.

Rett Syndrome

Rett syndrome is a genetic neurodevelopmental disorder characterized by developmental arrest and regression and multisystem comorbidities. The gene mutation most commonly associated with Rett syndrome is a mutation in the X-linked, methyl-CpG-binding protein 2 (MECP2) gene. Other genes that have been identified and are associated with this disorder include CDKL5 and FOXG1. Despite this being a genetic disorder, inheritance of the gene mutation is uncommon with most cases representing de novo mutations. These mutations alone are not sufficient to make a Rett diagnosis; therefore, clinical criteria for diagnosis remains key. Standardized diagnostic criteria for Rett syndrome exist (Neul et al., 2010).

Rather than cause brain degeneration, Rett syndrome arrests maturation of certain areas of the brain. This syndrome most commonly affects females, although males can also be affected. The typical age where the onset of symptoms occurs is between 5 and 18 months old. Children with Rett syndrome typically experience developmental regression, including partial or complete loss of purposeful hand skills and partial or complete loss of acquired spoken language, followed by a plateau of developmental milestones. They often develop bruxism, apraxia, gait abnormalities, and stereotypic hand movements (e.g., wringing/squeezing, clapping/tapping, hand-mouthing or biting and handwashing/rubbing automatisms). Head growth deceleration is an early red flag for the diagnosis. Rett syndrome can affect many body systems potentially including respiratory dysregulation, gastrointestinal dysfunction, scoliosis, sleep disturbance, and less commonly prolonged QTc interval. Neurologic comorbidities may include seizures and spasticity, which are often late developments in the syndrome. Due to the risk for seizures associated with Rett Syndrome, arrangement of a screening EEG is advised for children with this diagnosis.

Physical, occupational, and speech therapies and seizure management are important to preserve functional abilities. As with all neurodevelopmental problems, families need significant support and social services. Life expectancy varies depending on complicating factors. Differential diagnoses include CP, autism, psychosis, other neurodevelopmental disorders, genetic disorders, or other neurodegenerative diseases.

Multiple Sclerosis

MS is a chronic, relapsing disorder of the CNS that involves demyelination of the brain, spinal cord, and optic nerves. MS is rare in children, and it is uncommon to see symptoms before a child is 10 years old. The median age of disease onset of pediatric cases is 14 years old, with the median age at diagnosis age 15 (range of 11 to 19 years old; Boesen et al., 2014). Two to three times as many females as males are affected. It is widely believed that MS is an autoimmune inflammatory neurodegenerative disorder of the CNS. Macrophages, activated T-lymphocytes, and other destructive molecules

• BOX 46.8   **Symptoms of Multiple Sclerosis**

Unilateral weakness, ataxia or other cerebellar symptoms (frequent presenting symptom)

Symptoms that last for more than 24 h

Headache (may be severe, prolonged, generalized)

Motor symptoms (vague paresthesias of lower extremities, distal portions of hands, feet and face)

Visual disturbance (diplopia, blurred vision, or sudden loss of vision as a result of optic neuritis)

Vertigo, dysarthria, and sphincter disturbances uncommon; neurogenic bladder may present in acute transverse myelitis

Repeated episodes frequently preceded by fever, nausea, vomiting, and lethargy; may occur within months or years of each other

From Boesen MS, Sellebjerg F, Blinkenberg M. Onset symptoms in paediatric multiple sclerosis. Dan Med J. 2014;61(4):A4800.

are stimulated by yet not fully understood events. These inflammatory cells cause both CNS demyelination and axon damage within the white brain matter, including the optic nerve. No specific virus has been isolated, although the most likely agent seems to be the Epstein-Barr virus. Some scientists propose that it is multifactorial (National Multiple Sclerosis Society, n.d.a).

Overall, the clinical course is variable. The disease is typified by two phases: (1) initial relapse and remittance and (2) secondary progression. The episodes of focal neurologic dysfunction can last weeks or months, followed by partial or complete recovery. Children are noted to have acute exacerbations three times as frequently as adults. Frequent relapses early in the disease process may lead to a more rapid progression to irreversible disability. However, once irreversible disability begins, the rate of progression is independent of the frequency of relapses.

Most symptoms seen in children are the same as for all other ages (Box 46.8). However, seizures and mental status changes (lethargy) are seen in children but are not typically seen in adults with MS. A diagnosis of pediatric MS can be given after two episodes of demyelinating events, lasting longer than 24 hours, separated by more than 30 days, involving a distinct CNS region(s) and with no other plausible diagnosis (Karussis, 2016).

Diagnostic studies are typically ordered by the neurology provider and include:

- Neuroimaging: An MRI (gadolinium enhanced) early in the course of the disease can be important in predicting the clinical future. In children, demyelination of white matter presents as well defined and perpendicular to the corpus callosum. Evidence of disturbance of the BBB is thought to be a better predictor than the number of T2 white matter lesions for developing inflammatory MS lesions and atrophy. Gray matter lesions are believed to play a role but are undetectable using current imaging.
- Other studies may include an LP (may show oligoclonal bands) and visual-evoked responses.

Because of the frequency of other childhood conditions and disorders that have similar presentations and symptoms, determining a diagnosis of MS in a child may be challenging. Differential diagnoses may include acute disseminated encephalomyelitis (ADEM), other demyelinating disorders, brain tumor, focal encephalitis, nonviral infections with focal cerebritis or abscess formation, cerebrovascular diseases, leukodystrophies, systemic vasculitis, mitochondrial disorder, vitamin B_{12} deficiency (with macrocytic anemia), and spinal cord disorders. If MS is suspected, prompt referral for evaluation to a child neurology provider should be initiated.

Additional Resources

Brain Injury Association of America.
www.biausa.org
Centers for Disease Control and Prevention (CDC): HEADS UP.
www.cdc.gov/headsup/index.html
National Headache Foundation.
www.headaches.org
National Institute of Neurological Disorders and Stroke.
www.ninds.nih.gov
Rettsyndrome.org
www.rettsyndrome.org
Spina Bifida Association.
spinabifidaassociation.org
Tourette Association of America.
www.tsa-usa.org
United Cerebral Palsy.
www.ucp.org
United Spinal Association: Spinal Cord Resource Center.
www.spinalcord.org
https://www.aan.com/tools-and-resources/practicing-neurologists-administrators/patient-resources/sports-concussion-resources/

References

Antiel RM, Adzick NS, Thom EA, et al. Management of myelomeningocele study investigators. impact on family and parental stress of prenatal vs postnatal repair of myelomeningocele. *Am J Obstet Gynecol.* 2016;215(4). 522–e1.

Antonaci F, Voiticovschi-Iosob C, Di Stefano AL, et al. The evolution of headache from childhood to adulthood: a review of the literature. *J Headache Pain.* 2016;15(1):15.

Boesen MS, Sellebjerg F, Blinkenberg M. Onset symptoms in paediatric multiple sclerosis. *Dan Med J.* 2014;61(4):A4800.

Bregstein JS, Lubell TR, Ruscica AM, et al. Nuking the radiation: minimizing radiation exposure in the evaluation of pediatric blunt trauma. *Curr Opin Pediatr.* 2014;26(3):272–278.

Buterbaugh KL, Shah AS. The natural history and management of brachial plexus birth palsy. *Curr Rev Musculoskelet Med.* 2016;9(4):418–426.

Centers for Disease Control and Prevention (CDC). Cerebral Palsy: Data & Statistics. Available at: https://www.cdc.gov/ncbddd/cp/data.html. Accessed August 10, 2019.

Centers for Disease Control and Prevention (CDC). Folic acid: recommendations, CDC (website). Available at: www.cdc.gov/ncbddd/folic acid/recommendations.html.

Centers for Disease Control and Prevention (CDC). Injury prevention & control: traumatic brain injury. Available at: www.cdc.gov/traumaticbraininjury/basics.html; 2015.

Christensen D, Van Naarden BK, Doernberg NS, et al. Prevalence of cerebral palsy, co-occurring autism spectrum disorders, and motor functioning—autism and developmental disabilities monitoring network, USA, 2008. *Dev Med Child Neurol.* 2014;56(1):59–65.

Ditthakasem K, Kolar JC. Deformational plagiocephaly: a review. *Pediatr Nurs.* 2017;43(2):59.

Eisenberg MA, Meehan WP, Mannix R. Duration and Course of Post-Concussive Symptoms Pediatrics. Jun 2014;133(6):999–1006. https://doi.org/10.1542/peds.2014-0158.

Faul M, Xu L, Wald MM, et al. *Traumatic Brain Injury in the United States: Emergency Department Visits, Hospitalizations and Deaths 2002–2006.* Atlanta: Centers for Disease Control and Prevention, National Center for Injury Prevention and Control; 2010.

Fisher RS, Cross JH, D'Souza C, et al. Instruction manual for the ILAE 2017 operational classification of seizure types. *Epilepsia.* 2017;58(4):531–542. https://doi.org/10.1111/epi.1367, 2017.

Gioacchini FM, Alicandri-Ciufelli M, Kaleci S, et al. Prevalence and diagnosis of vestibular disorders in children: A review. *Int J Pediatr Otorhinolaryngol.* 2014;78(5):718–724. https://doi.org/10.1016/j.ijporl.2014.02.009.

Governale LS. Craniosynostosis. *Pediatr Nurs.* 2015;53(5):394–401.

Hamilton M, Gruen JP, Luciano MG. Adult hydrocephalus. *Neurosurg Focus.* 2016;41(3). https://doi.org/10.3171/2016.6.FOCUS16272. [E1].

Headache Classification Committee of the International Headache Society (IHS). The international classification of headache disorders, 3rd edition (beta version). *Cephalalgia.* 2013;33(9):629–808.

Hirbe AC, Gutmann DH. Neurofibromatosis type 1: a multidisciplinary approach to care. *Lancet Neurol.* 2014;13(8):834–843.

Holland NJ, Bernstein JM. Bell's palsy. *BMJ Clinical Evidence.* 2014;04(1204):1–19. Available at http://clinicalevidence.bmj.com/x/systematic-review/1204/overview.html.

Hong Y, Skeie GO, Zisimopoulou P, et al. Juvenile-onset myasthenia gravis: autoantibody status, clinical characteristics and genetic polymorphisms. *J neurol.* 2017;264(5):955–962.

Jahn K, Langhagen T, Heinen F. Vertigo and dizziness in children. *Curr Opinions Neurol.* 2015;28(1):78–82. https://doi.org/10.1097/WCO.0000000000000157.

Jahn K. Vertigo and dizziness in children. In: 3rd ed. Furman JM, Lempert T, eds. *Handbook of Clinical Neurology Neuro-Otology.* 137. 2016;353–363. https://doi.org/10.1016/b978-0-444-63437-5.00025-x.

Kacperski J, Kabbouche MA, O'Brien HL, et al. The optimal management of headaches in children and adolescents. *Ther Adv Neurol Disord.* 2016;9(1):53–68.

Karussis D. The diagnosis of multiple sclerosis and the various related demyelinating syndromes: a critical review. *J Autoimmunity.* 2014;48–49. https://doi.org/10.1016/j.jaut.2014.01.022. 134–142.

Kashlan O, et al. 202 Predictors of surgical treatment and postoperative complications in the pediatric patient with isolated tethered cord syndrome. *Neurosurgery.* 2016;63:179.

Ketelaar M, Gorter JW, Westers P, et al. Developmental trajectories of mobility and self-care capabilities in young children with cerebral palsy. *J Pediatr.* 2014;164(4):769–774.

Kimia AA, Bachur RG, Torres A, et al. Febrile seizures: emergency medicine perspective. *Curr Opinions Pediatrics.* 2015;27(3):292–297. https://doi.org/10.1097/MOP.0000000000000220.

Kroger AT, Duchin J, Vazquez M. *General best practice guidelines for immunization: best practices guidance of the Advisory Committee on Immunization Practices* (ACIP). Available at https://www.cdc.gov/vaccines/hcp/acip-recs/general-recs/downloads/general-recs.pdf. Accessed August 19, 2019.

Langridge B, Phillips E, Choi D. Chiari Malformation Type 1: a systematic review of natural history and conservative management. *World Neurosurgery.* 2017;104:213–219.

Martiniuk ALC, Vujovich-Dunn C, Park M, et al. Plagiocephaly and developmental delay: a systematic review. *J Dev Behav Pediatr.* 2017;38(1):67–78.

Masten AS. Global perspectives on resilience in children and youth. *Child Dev.* 2014;85(1):6–20.

Meehan WP, O'Brien MJ. Concussion in children and adolescents: Management. Up to Date Topic 91282 Version 32.0. Available at https://www.uptodate.com/contents/concussion-in-children-and-adolescents-management?search=melatonin%20in%20pediatrics%20for%20sleep%20in%20headache&source=search_result&selectedTitle=3~150&usage_type=default&display_rank=3#H2832495. Accessed August 19, 2019.

National Institute of Neurological Disorders and Stroke (NINDS). Cerebral palsy: hope through research, NIH (website). Available at: https://www.ninds.nih.gov/Disorders/Patient-Caregiver-Education/Hope-Through-Research/Cerebral-Palsy-Hope-Through-Research Accessed August 15, 2019.

National Multiple Sclerosis Society: Epidemiology of MS, National Multiple Sclerosis Society (website). n.d. Available at: www.nationalmssociety.org/about-multiple-sclerosis/what-we-know-about-ms/who-gets-ms/epidemiology-of-ms/index.aspx. Accessed August 19, 2019.

Neul JL, Kaufmann WE, Glaze DG, et al. Rett syndrome: Revised diagnostic criteria and nomenclature. *Annals of Neurology.* 2010;68(6):944–950. https://doi.org/10.1002/ana.22124.

Novak I, Morgan C, Adde L, et al. Early, accurate diagnosis and early intervention in cerebral palsy: advances in diagnosis and treatment. *JAMA Pediatrics.* 2017:E1–E11. https://doi.org/10.1001/jamapediatrics.2017.1689.

Nutakki K, Varni JW, Steinbrenner S, et al. Development of the pediatric quality of life inventory neurofibromatosis type 1 module items for children, adolescents and young adults: qualitative methods. *J Neurooncol.* 2017;132(1):135–143.

Ouchenir L, Renaud C, Khan S, et al. The epidemiology, management, and outcomes of bacterial meningitis in infants. *Pediatrics.* 2017:e20170476.

Peragallo JH. *Pediatric Myasthenia Gravis. Seminars in Pediatric Neurology.* WB Saunders; 2017.

Poretti A, Ashmawy R, Garzon-Muvdi T, et al. Chiari type 1 deformity in children: pathogenetic, clinical, neuroimaging, and management aspects. *Neuropediatrics.* 2016;47(5):293–307.

Powers SW, Coffey CS, Chamberlin LA, et al. Trial of amitriptyline, topiramate, and placebo for pediatric migraine. *N Engl J Med.* 2017;376(2):115–124.

Ransom DM, Vaughn CG, Pratson L, et al. Academic effects of concussion in children and adolescents. *Pediatrics.* 2015. peds-2014.

Robertson WC. Migraine in children, Medscape (website), update. Available at: http://emedicine.medscape.com/article/1179268-overview#aw2aab6b3; 2015.

Roodbol J, de Wit MY, van den Berg B, et al. Diagnosis of Guillain–Barré syndrome in children and validation of the Brighton criteria. *J Neurol.* 2017;264(5):856–861.

Sanders D, Wolfe GI, Benatar M, et al. International consensus guidance for management of myasthenia gravis executive summary. *Neurology.* 2016;87(4):419–425.

Scheffer IE, Berkovic S, Capovilla G, et al. Neurodevelopmental disorders in children with neurofibromatosis type 1. *Dev Med Child Neurol.* 2017;59(11):1112–1116.

Schonfeld D, Bressan S, Da Dalt L, et al. *Pediatric Emergency Care Applied Research Network Head Injury Clinical Prediction Rules are Reliable in Practice.* Archives of Disease in Childhood Archdischild-2013; 2014.

Schwartz SR, Jones SL, Getchius TS, et al. Reconciling the clinical practice guidelines on Bell's palsy from the AAO-HNSF and the AAN. *Otolaryngol Head Neck Surg.* 2014;150(5):709–711.

Stumpf DA, Alksne JF, Annegers F, et al. NIH consensus development conference: neurofibromatosis conference statement. *Arch Neurol.* 1988;45:575–578.

Takasaki K, Stransky AD, Miller G. Psychogenic nonepileptic seizures: diagnosis, management, and bioethics. *Pediatr Neurol.* 2016;62:3–8. https://doi.org/10.1016/j.pediatrneurol.2016.04.011.

Tang M, Gorbutt KA, Peethambaran A, et al. High prevalence of cranial asymmetry exists in infants with neonatal brachial plexus palsy. *J Pediatr Rehabil Med.* 2016;9(4):271–277.

Tolaymat A, Nayak A, Geyer JD, et al. Diagnosis and management of childhood epilepsy. *Curr Probl Pediatr Adolesc Health Care.* 2015;45:3–17. https://doi.org/10.1016/j.cppeds.2014.12.002.

US Food and Drug Administration *FDA authorizes marketing of first blood test to aid in the evaluation of concussion in adults.* Available at https://www.fda.gov/NewsEvents/Newsroom/PressAnnouncements/ucm596531.htm. Accessed August 17, 2019.

Verboon C, van Doorn P, Jacobs BC. Treatment dilemmas in Guillain-Barré syndrome. *J Neurol Neurosurg Psychiatry.* 2016;88(4):346–352.

Vogel AC, Gutmann DH, Morris SM. Neurodevelopmental disorders in children with neurofibromatosis type 1. *Dev Med Child Neurol.* 2017;59(11):1112–1116.

Williams J, Mai CT, Mulinare J, et al. Updated estimates of neural tube defects prevented by mandatory folic acid fortification—United States, 1995–2011. *Centers Dis Control Prev.* 2015;64(1):1–5.

Witiw C, Hachem L, Bernstein M. Clinical presentation of hydrocephalus in adults. In: Ammar A, ed. *Hydrocephalus.* Cham: Springer; 2017.

Appendix A

Growth Charts

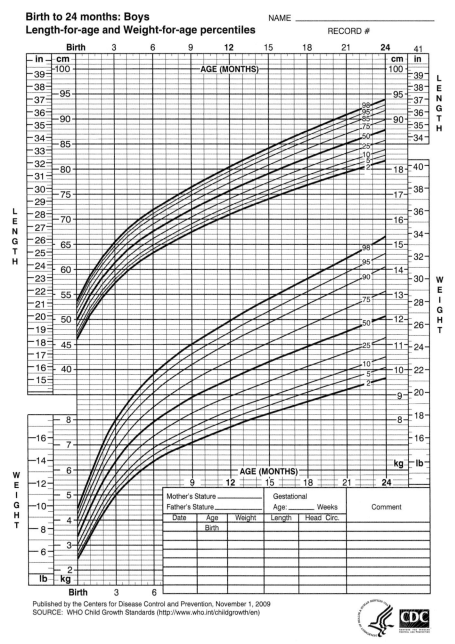

Birth to 24 months: Boys
Length-for-age and Weight-for-age percentiles

NAME _____

RECORD # _____

Published by the Centers for Disease Control and Prevention, November 1, 2009
SOURCE: WHO Child Growth Standards (http://www.who.int/childgrowth/en)

● **Fig A.1** (1) Birth to 24 months: boys' length-for-age and weight-for-age percentiles. (2) Birth to 24 months: boys' head circumference-for-age and weight-for-length percentiles. (Published by the Centers for Disease Control and Prevention, November 1, 2009. From WHO Child Growth Standards. Available at www.cdc. gov/growthcharts.) (3) Two to 20 years old: boys' stature-for-age and weight-for-age percentiles. (4) Two to 20 years old: boys' body mass index-for-age percentiles. (From the National Center for Health Statistics in collaboration with the National Center for Chronic Disease Prevention and Health Promotion, 2000.) Note: When plotting length, weight, and head circumference, use corrected age for most premature infants until age 2 years. Corrected age may need to be used until age 3 years for some premature infants whose birth weights is less than 1000 g. For those who "catch up" before 24 to 36 months of age, chronologic age is then used for plotting measurements. (http://depts.washington.edu/growth/cshcn/text/page4a.htm).

Birth to 24 months: Boys
Head circumference-for-age and
Weight-for-length percentiles

NAME _____

RECORD # _____

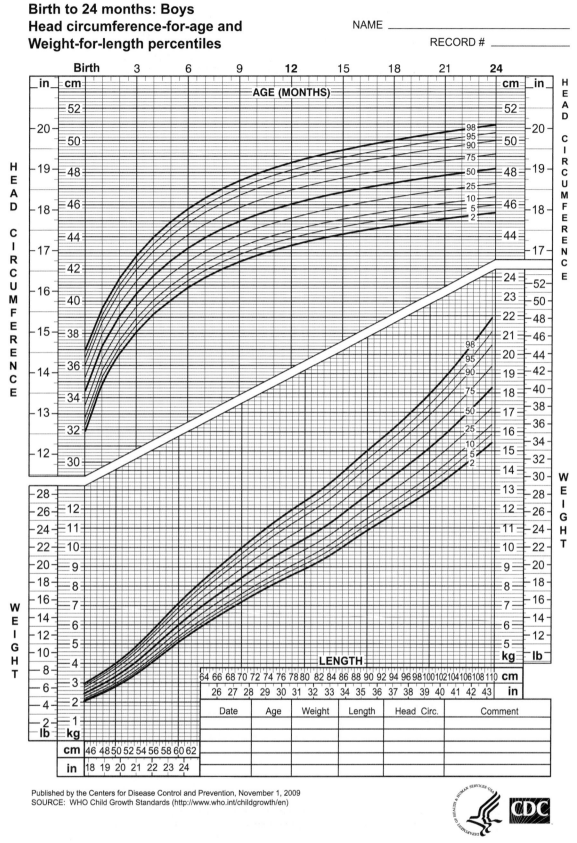

Published by the Centers for Disease Control and Prevention, November 1, 2009
SOURCE: WHO Child Growth Standards (http://www.who.int/childgrowth/en)

• **Fig A.1, cont'd**

2 – 20 years: Boys
Stature-for-age and Weight-for-age percentiles

NAME _____

RECORD# _____

Mother's Stature _____		Father's Stature _____		
Date	Age	Weight	Stature	BMI*

*To Calculate BMI: Weight (kg) ÷ Stature (cm) ÷ Stature (cm) x 10,000
or Weight (lb) ÷ Stature (in) ÷ Stature (in) x 703

AGE (YEARS)

Published May 30, 2000 (modified 11/21/00)..

SOURCE: Developed by the National Center for Health Statistics in collaboration with
the National Center for Chronic Disease Prevention and Health Promotion (2000).
http://www.cdc.gov/growthcharts

SAFER · HEALTHIER · PEOPLE™

• **Fig A.1, cont'd**

2 – 20 years: Boys
Body mass index-for-age percentiles

NAME _____

RECORD# _____

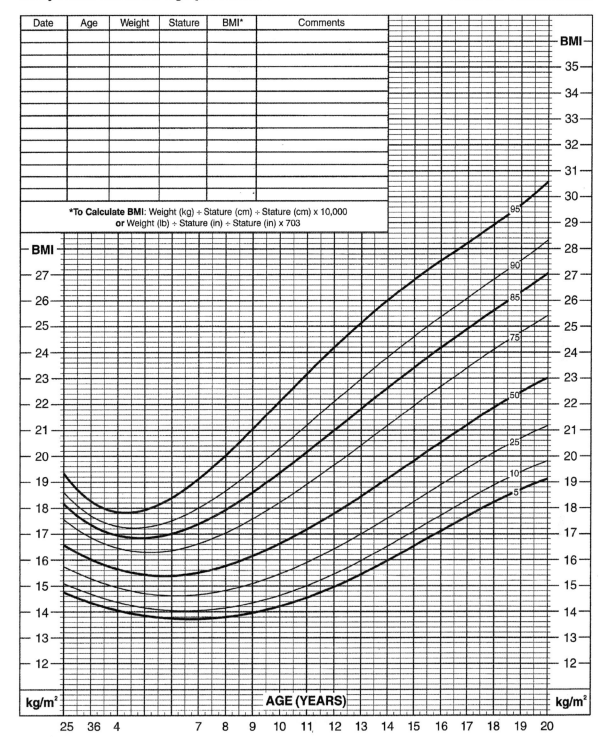

Date	Age	Weight	Stature	BMI*	Comments

*To Calculate BMI: Weight (kg) ÷ Stature (cm) ÷ Stature (cm) x 10,000
or Weight (lb) ÷ Stature (in) ÷ Stature (in) x 703

AGE (YEARS)

Published May 30, 2000 (modified 10/16/00).
SOURCE: Developed by the National Center for Health Statistics in collaboration with
the National Center for Chronic Disease Prevention and Health Promotion (2000).
http://www.cdc.gov/growthcharts

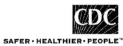

SAFER · HEALTHIER · PEOPLE™

● **Fig A.1, cont'd**

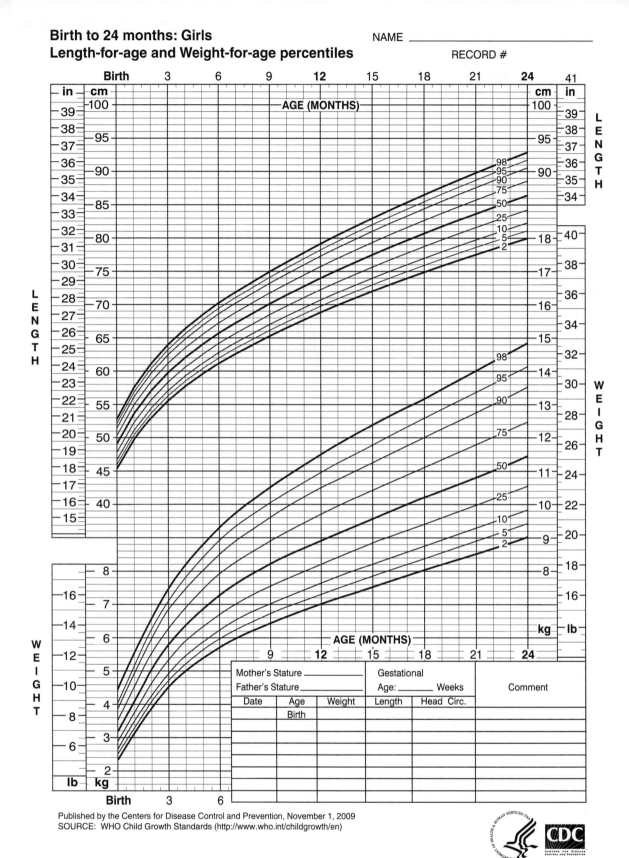

Birth to 24 months: Girls
Length-for-age and Weight-for-age percentiles

NAME _____

RECORD # _____

Published by the Centers for Disease Control and Prevention, November 1, 2009
SOURCE: WHO Child Growth Standards (http://www.who.int/childgrowth/en)

• **Fig A.2** (1) Birth to 24 months: girls' length-for-age and weight-for-age percentiles. (2) Birth to 24 months: girls' head circumference-for-age and weight-for-length percentiles. (Published by the Centers for Disease Control and Prevention, November 1, 2009. From WHO Child Growth Standards. Available at www.cdc. gov/growthcharts.) (3) Two to 20 years old: girls' stature-for-age and weight-for-age percentiles. (4) Two to 20 years old: girls' body mass index-for-age percentiles. (From the National Center for Health Statistics in collaboration with the National Center for Chronic Disease Prevention and Health Promotion, 2000.) Note: When plotting length, weight and head circumference, use corrected age for most premature infants until age 2 years. Corrected age may need to be used until age 3 years for some premature infants whose birth weights is less than 1000 g. For those who "catch up" before 24 to 36 months of age, chronologic age is then used for plotting measurements. (http://depts.washington.edu/growth/cshcn/text/page4a.htm).

Birth to 24 months: Girls
Head circumference-for-age and
Weight-for-length percentiles

NAME _____

RECORD # _____

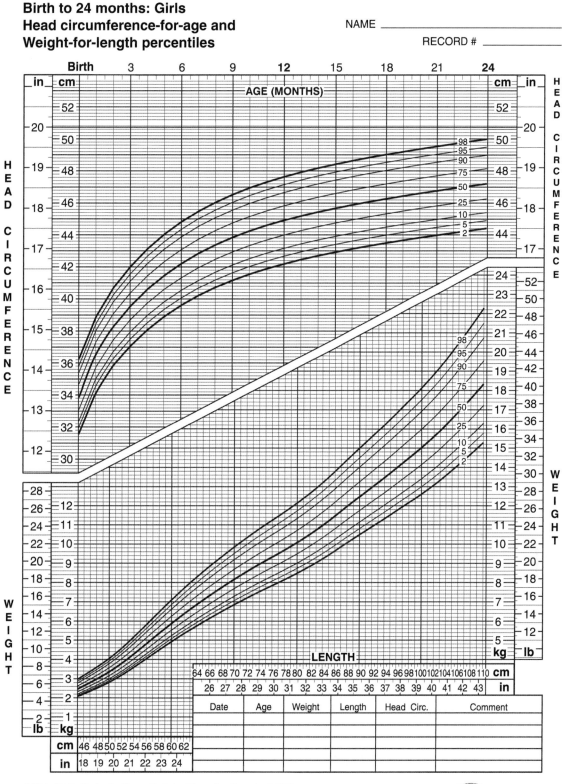

Published by the Centers for Disease Control and Prevention, November 1, 2009
SOURCE: WHO Child Growth Standards (http://www.who.int/childgrowth/en)

• **Fig A.2, cont'd**

2 to 20 years: Girls
Stature-for-age and Weight-for-age percentiles

NAME _____

RECORD # _____

Mother's Stature _____		Father's Stature _____		
Date	Age	Weight	Stature	BMI*

***To Calculate BMI:** Weight (kg) ÷ Stature (cm) ÷ Stature (cm) x 10,000
or Weight (lb) ÷ Stature (in) ÷ Stature (in) x 703*

AGE (YEARS)

STATURE

WEIGHT

Published May 30, 2000 (modified 11/21/00).
SOURCE: Developed by the National Center for Health Statistics in collaboration with
the National Center for Chronic Disease Prevention and Health Promotion (2000).
http://www.cdc.gov/growthcharts

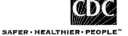

● **Fig A.2, cont'd**

2 to 20 years: Girls
Body mass index-for-age percentiles

NAME _____

RECORD# _____

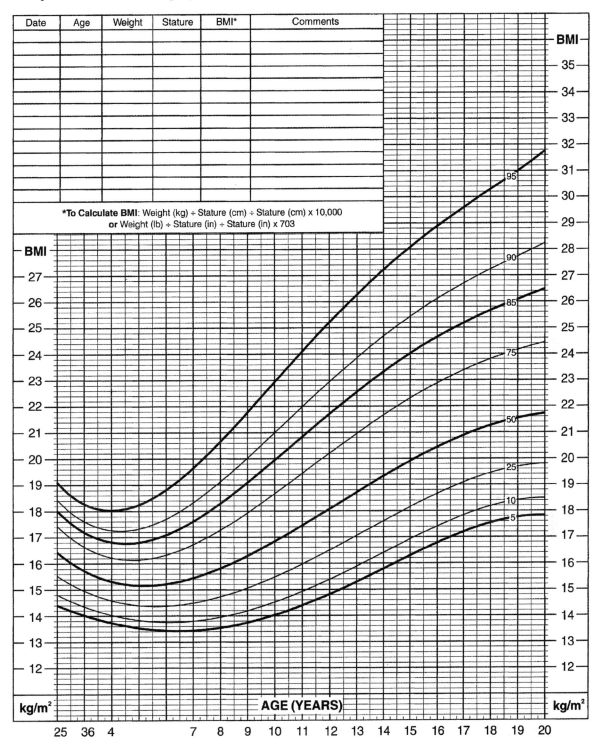

Date	Age	Weight	Stature	BMI*	Comments

*To Calculate BMI: Weight (kg) ÷ Stature (cm) ÷ Stature (cm) x 10,000
or Weight (lb) ÷ Stature (in) ÷ Stature (in) x 703

AGE (YEARS)

Published May 30, 2000 (modified 10/16/00).
SOURCE: Developed by the National Center for Health Statistics in collaboration with
the National Center for Chronic Disease Prevention and Health Promotion (2000).
http://www.cdc.gov/growthcharts

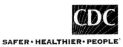

SAFER · HEALTHIER · PEOPLE

• Fig A.2, cont'd

BOYS

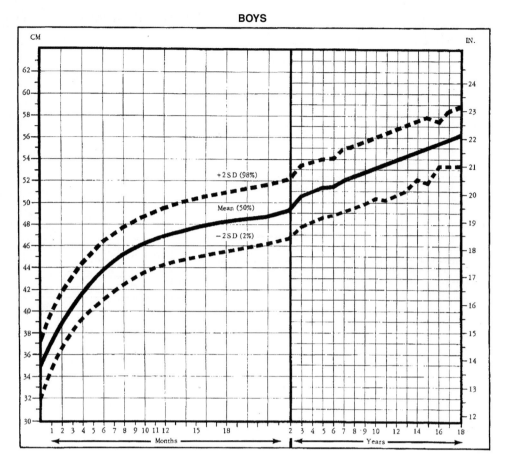

GIRLS

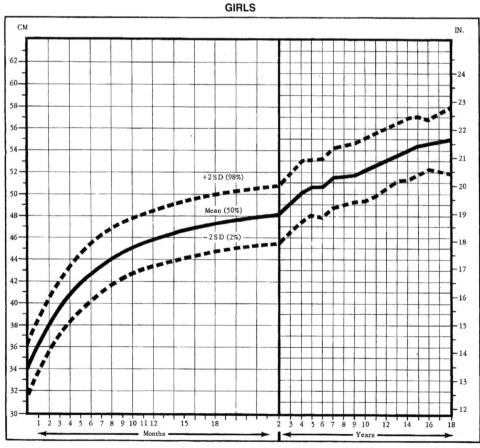

• **Fig A.3** (1) Birth to 18 years old: boys' head circumference percentiles. (2) Birth to 18 years old: girls' head circumference percentiles. (From Nellhaus G. Head circumference from birth to eighteen years. Practical composite international and interracial graphs. *Pediatrics.* 1968;41:106–114.)

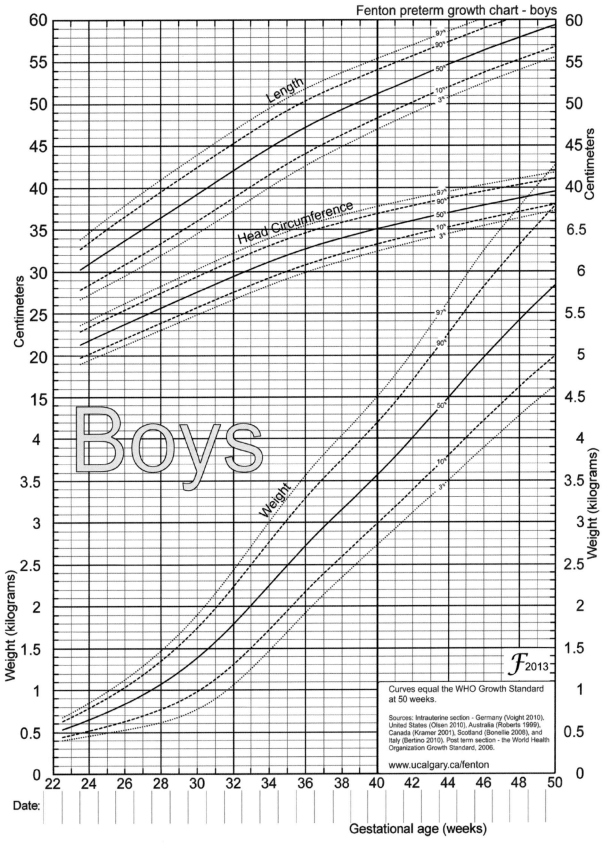

● **Fig A.4** (1) Boys preterm infant. (2) Girls' preterm infant. (From Fenton TR, Kim JH. A systematic review and meta-analysis to revise the Fenton growth chart for preterm infants. *BMC Pediatr.* 2013;13:59.)

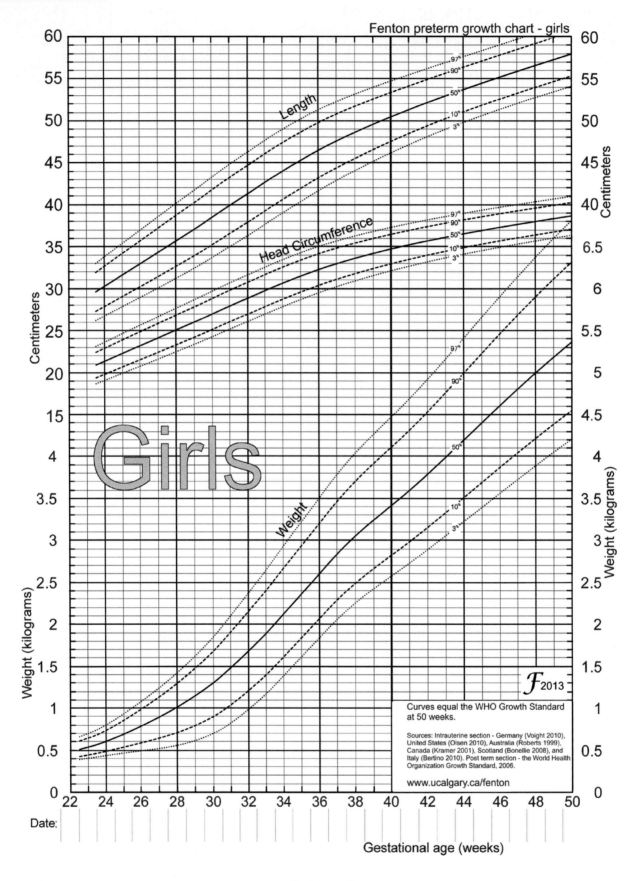

Fenton preterm growth chart - girls

Curves equal the WHO Growth Standard at 50 weeks.

Sources: Intrauterine section - Germany (Voight 2010), United States (Olsen 2010), Australia (Roberts 1999), Canada (Kramer 2001), Scotland (Bonellie 2008), and Italy (Bertino 2010). Post term section - the World Health Organization Growth Standard, 2006.

www.ucalgary.ca/fenton

$\mathcal{F}$2013

Date:

Gestational age (weeks)

• **Fig A.4, cont'd**

Appendix B

Body Measurements

Crown-Rump Length and Sitting Height

Sitting height and crown-rump length can be used as a proxy measure for stature and length when a child cannot stand but can sit erect.

Crown-rump length is measured using a recumbent length board (Fig A.5).

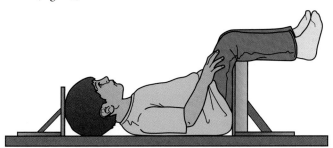

● **Fig A.5** Crown to Rump Measurement.

Measurement Technique, Plotting, and Interpretation

Position head as done with a length measurement. Raise legs so that thighs are at a 90-degree angle to the board and held in that position during the measurement. To take the measurement, bring sliding footboard up against the buttocks with firm pressure. Plot the measurement on the Centers for Disease Control and Prevention charts for stature for age or length for age. Measurements can fall to less than the 5th percentile but are used to establish a growth pattern over time.

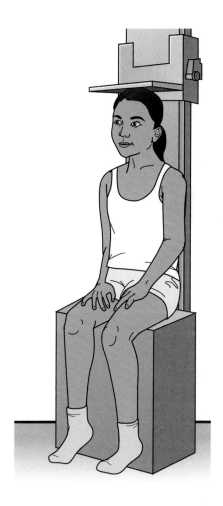

● **Fig A.6** Sitting Height Measurement.

Measurement Technique, Plotting, and Interpretation

Place the child on a sitting base of a known height backed up against a wall-mounted stadiometer. Place the child as erect as possible with buttocks, shoulders, and head in contact with stadiometer backboard. Total height is measured. Subtract the height of the sitting surface from the total height. Plot the measurement on the Centers for Disease Control and Prevention charts for stature for age. Measurements can fall to less than the 5th percentile but are used to establish a growth pattern over time (Fig A.6).

Segmental Lengths: Upper Arm Length and Lower Leg Length and Upper Arm Length

Segmented lower leg and upper arm lengths can serve as a proxy measurement when a child's stature cannot be measured accurately because of neuromuscular conditions.

Measurement Technique, Plotting, and Interpretation

Leg lengths in children ages 6 to 18 years who have contractures and or cannot stand can be measured using a steel or plastic tape or an anthropometer. Accuracy in leg length measurement is difficult because of the potential for error in selecting correct measurement points (Fig A.7).

Upper Arm Length

To measure the upper arm length, have the child extend arms perpendicular to his body with the anthropometer touching the extended middle fingers of both hands (Fig A.8).

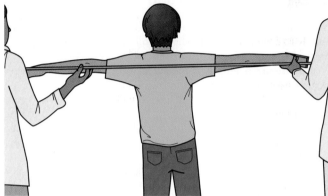

• **Fig A.8** Upper Arm Length Measurement.

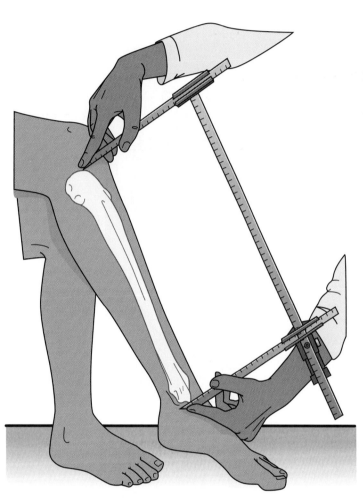

• **Fig A.7** Lower-Leg Length Measurement.

Appendix C

Nutrition

TABLE A.1   Estimated Caloric Needs of Infants and Children Through Age 18 Years

Estimated Energy Requirement (EER) Equations (Calculate Calories/Day)

Infants and Young Children

0-3 months: EER = [89 × weight (kg) − 100] + 175
4-6 months: EER = [89 × weight (kg) − 100] + 56
7-12 months: EER = [89 × weight (kg) − 100] + 22
13-35 months: EER = [89 × weight (kg) − 100] + 20

Boys Aged 3-18 Years

3-8 years: EER = 88.5 − [61.9 × age (year)] + [PA × 26.7 × weight (kg)] + [903 × height (m)] + 20
9-18 years: EER = 88.5 − [61.9 × age (year)] + [PA × 26.7 × weight (kg)] + [903 × height (m)] + 25

Girls Aged 3-18 Years

3-8 years: EER = 135.3 − [30.8 × age (year)] + [PA × 10 × weight (kg)] + [934 × height (m)] + 20
9-18 years: EER = 135.3 − [30.8 × age (year)] + [PA × 10 × weight (kg)] + [934 × height (m)] + 25

Pregnancy (14-18 Years)

EER = adolescent EER + pregnancy energy deposition:
   First trimester = adolescent EER + 0 kcal
   Second trimester = adolescent EER + 340 kcal
   Third trimester = adolescent EER + 452 kcal

Lactation (14-18 Years)

EER = adolescent EER + milk energy output − weight loss:
   First 6 months = adolescent EER + 500 − 170
   Second 6 months = adolescent EER + 400 − 0

PA, Physical activity coefficient.

TABLE A.2   Physical Activity Coefficients: By Gender and Level of Activity

	Sedentary Activity (Physical Activity Levels Required for Independent Living)	Low Active (30 to 45 min Sustained Daily Activity)	Active (60 min Sustained Daily Activity)	Very Active (≥90 min Sustained Daily Activity)
PAL	≥1.0 but <1.4	≥1.4 but <1.6	≥1.6 but <1.9	≥1.9 but <2.5
PA (boys ages 3-18)	1.00	1.13	1.26	1.42
PA (girls ages 3-18)	1.00	1.16	1.31	1.56

PA, Physical activity coefficient; *PAL*, physical activity level.

From Johns Hopkins Hospital, Hughes JK, Kahl LK. *The Harriet Lane Handbook.* 21st ed. Philadelphia: Elsevier; 2018.

Appendix D

Gesell Figures

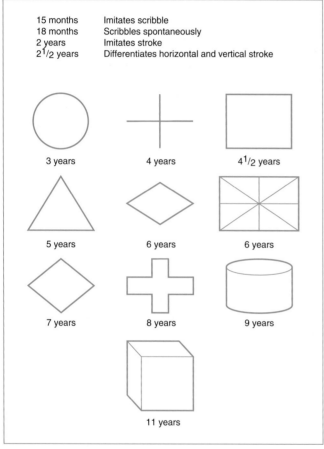

15 months   Imitates scribble
18 months   Scribbles spontaneously
2 years   Imitates stroke
2$^{1}/_{2}$ years   Differentiates horizontal and vertical stroke

3 years

4 years

4$^{1}/_{2}$ years

5 years

6 years

6 years

7 years

8 years

9 years

11 years

• **Fig A.9** Gesell Figures. (From Illingsworth RS. *The Development of the Infant and Young Child, Normal and Abnormal.* 5th ed. Baltimore: Williams & Wilkins; 1972:229–232; and Cattel P. *The Measurement of Intelligence of Infants and Young Children.* New York: Psychological Corporation; 1960:97–261.)

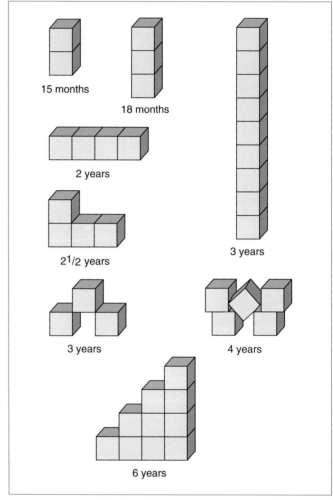

15 months

18 months

2 years

2$^{1}/_{2}$ years

3 years

3 years

4 years

6 years

• **Fig A.10** Block Skills. (From Capute AJ, Accardo PJ. *The Pediatrician and the Developmentally Disabled Child: A Clinical Textbook on Mental Retardation.* Baltimore: University Park Press; 1979:122.)

Index

Note: Page numbers followed by *"f"* indicate figures, *"t"* indicate tables, and *"b"* indicate boxes.